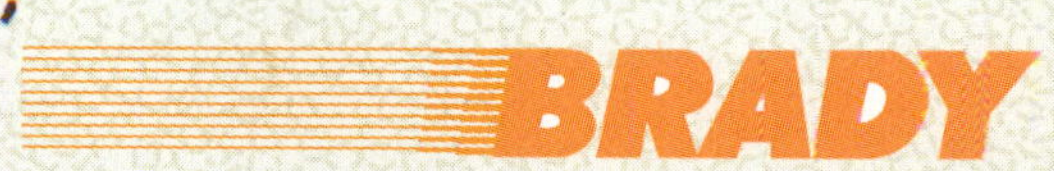

Essentials of Paramedic Care

SECOND EDITION

UPDATE

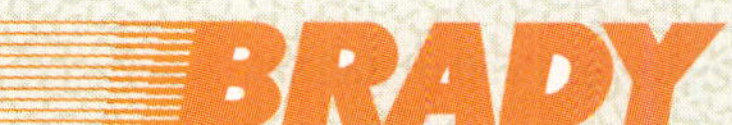

Essentials of Paramedic Care

SECOND EDITION

UPDATE

BRYAN E. BLEDSOE, DO, FACEP, FAAEM, EMT-P

Clinical Professor of Emergency Medicine
Director, EMS Fellowship
University of Nevada School of Medicine
and
Attending Emergency Physician
University Medical Center of Southern Nevada
Las Vegas, Nevada

ROBERT S. PORTER, MA, NREMT-P

Senior Advanced Life Support Educator
Madison County Emergency Medical Services
Canastota, New York
and
Flight Paramedic (retired)
AirOne, Onondaga County Sheriff's Department
Syracuse, New York

RICHARD A. CHERRY, MS, NREMT-P

Director of Training
Northern Onondaga Volunteer Ambulance
Liverpool, New York

Brady
is an imprint of

Pearson

Boston Columbus Indianapolis New York San Francisco Upper Saddle River
Amsterdam Cape Town Dubai London Madrid Milan Munich Paris Montreal Toronto
Delhi Mexico City Sao Paulo Sydney Hong Kong Seoul Singapore Taipei Tokyo

Library of Congress Cataloging-in-Publication Data

Bledsoe, Bryan E.

Essentials of paramedic care: principles & practice/Bryan E. Bledsoe, Robert S. Porter, Richard A. Cherry.—2nd ed. update. p. ; cm.

Includes bibliographical references and index.

ISBN-13: 978-0-13-215689-9

ISBN-10: 0-13-215689-X

1. Emergency medicine. 2. Emergency medical technicians. I. Porter, Robert S. II. Cherry, Richard A. III. Title.

[DNLM: 1. Emergency Treatment—methods. 2. Emergencies. 3. Emergency Medical Services—methods. 4. Physical Examination—methods. WB 105 B646ea 2011]

RC86.7.B594 2011

616.02'5—dc22

2010005192

Publisher: Julie Levin Alexander
Publisher's Assistant: Regina Bruno
Editor-in-Chief: Marlene McHugh Pratt
Senior Managing Editor for Development: Lois Berlowitz
Editorial Assistant: Jonathan Cheung
Project Manager for Second Edition: Sandra Breuer
Project Manager for Second Edition Update: Deborah Wenger
Managing Photography Editor: Michal Heron
Director of Marketing: David Gesell
Executive Marketing Manager: Katrin Beacom
Marketing Manager: Harper Coles
Marketing Specialist: Michael Sirinides
Marketing Assistant: Judy Noh
Managing Editor for Production: Patrick Walsh
Production Liaison: Faye Gemmellaro
Production Editor: Heather Willison, S4Carlisle Publishing Services
Manufacturing Manager: Ilene Sanford
Manufacturing Buyer: Pat Brown
Art Director: Christopher Weigand
Cover Design: Blair Brown
Cover Image: Eddie Sperling
Interior Photographers: Michael Gallitelli, Michal Heron, Richard Logan
Interior Illustrations: Rolin Graphics
Interior Design: Jill Little
Media Project Manager: Lorena Cerisano
Composition: S4Carlisle Publishing Services
Printing and Binding: Courier/Kendallville
Cover Printer: Lehigh-Phoenix Color/Hagerstown

Brady
is an imprint of

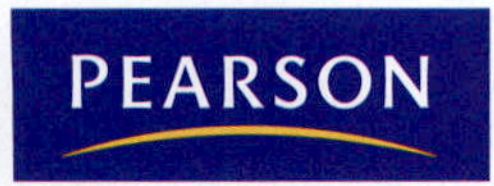

www.bradybooks.com

Notices

It is the intent of the authors and publishers that this textbook be used as part of a formal paramedic education program taught by a qualified instructor and supervised by a licensed physician. The care procedures presented here represent accepted practices in the United States. They are not offered as a standard of care. Paramedic-level emergency care is to be performed only under the authority and guidance of a licensed physician. It is the reader's responsibility to know and follow local care protocols as provided by medical advisors directing the system to which he or she belongs. Also, it is the reader's responsibility to stay informed of emergency care procedure changes.

Notice on Drugs and Drug Dosages

Every effort has been made to ensure that the drug dosages presented in this textbook are in accordance with nationally accepted standards. When applicable, the dosages and routes are taken from the American Heart Association's *Advanced Cardiac Life Support Guidelines.* The American Medical Association's publication *Drug Evaluations,* the *Physicians' Desk Reference,* and the *Prentice Hall Health Professional's Drug Guide* are followed with regard to drug dosages not covered by the American Heart Association's guidelines. It is the responsibility of the reader to be familiar with the drugs used in his or her system, as well as the dosages specified by the medical director. The drugs presented in this book should only be administered by direct order, whether verbally or through accepted standing orders, of a licensed physician.

Notice on Gender Usage

The English language has historically given preference to the male gender. Among many words, the pronouns "he" and "his" are commonly used to describe both genders. Society evolves faster than language, and the male pronouns still predominate in our speech. The authors have made great effort to treat the two genders equally, recognizing that a significant percentage of paramedics and patients are female. However, in some instances, male pronouns may be used to describe both male and female paramedics and patients solely for the purpose of brevity. This is not intended to offend any readers of the female gender.

Notice on Photographs

Please note that many of the photographs contained in this book are taken of actual emergency situations. As such, it is possible that they may not accurately depict current, appropriate, or advisable practices of emergency medical care. They have been included for the sole purpose of giving general insight into real-life emergency settings.

10 9 8 7 6 5 4 3 2 1
ISBN 13: 978-0-13-215689-9
ISBN 10: 0-13-215689-X

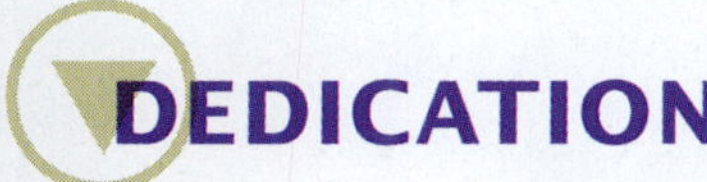

DEDICATION

This text is respectfully dedicated to all EMS personnel who have made the ultimate sacrifice. Their memory and good deeds will forever be in our thoughts and prayers.

BEB, RSP, RAC

Contents

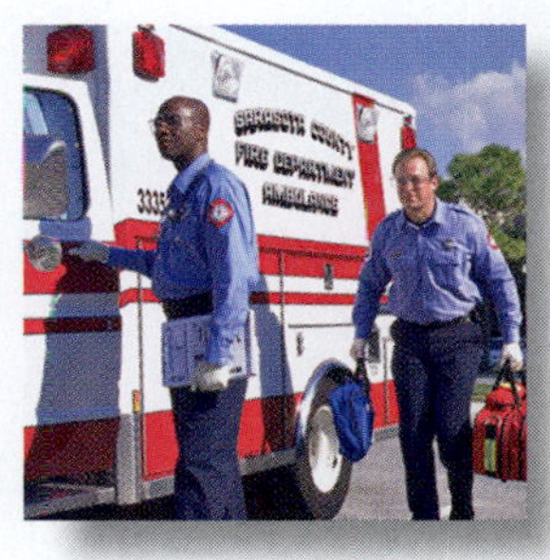

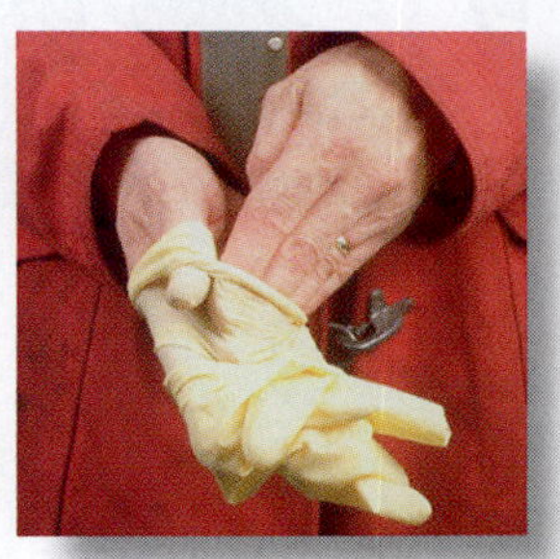

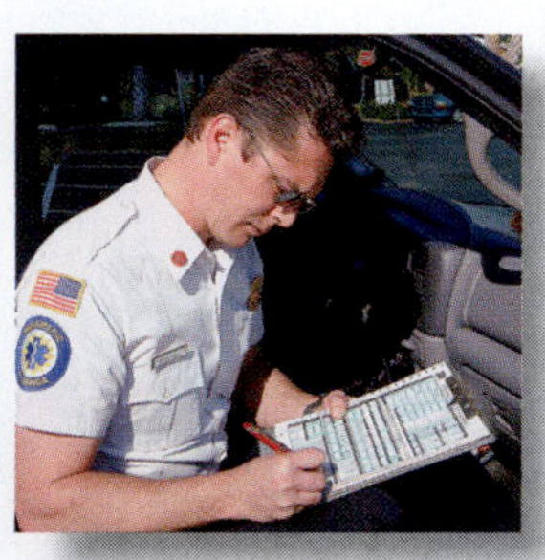

Chapter 3 Anatomy and Physiology 84

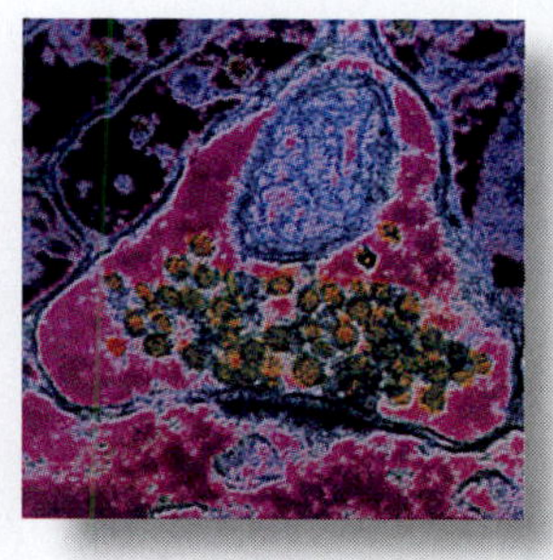

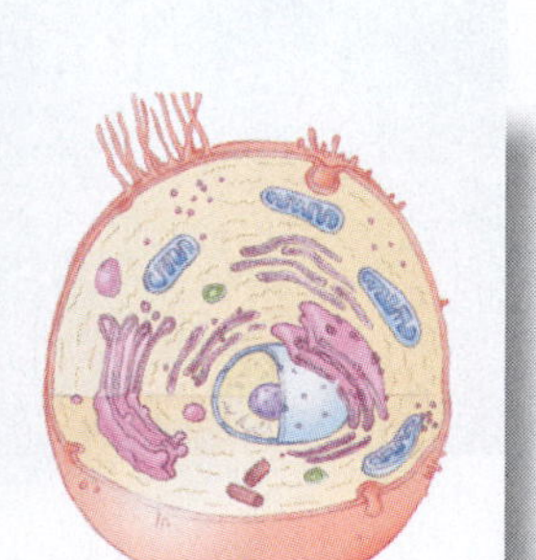

Chapter 4 General Principles of Pathophysiology 239

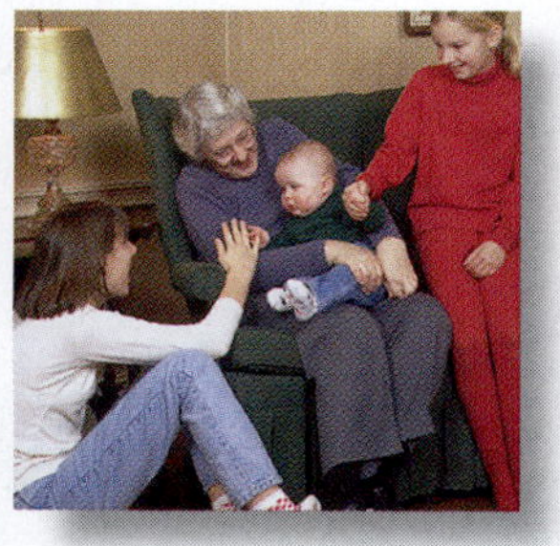

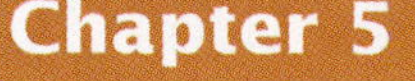

Chapter 5 Life-Span Development 291

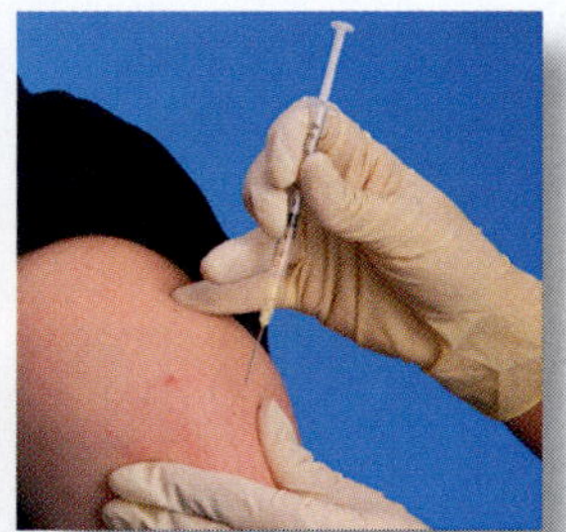

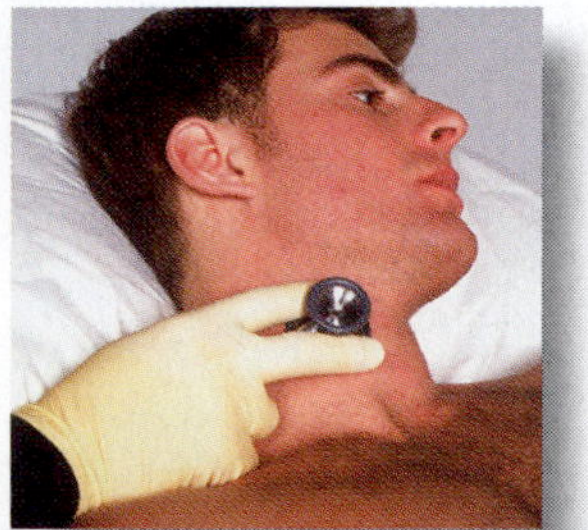

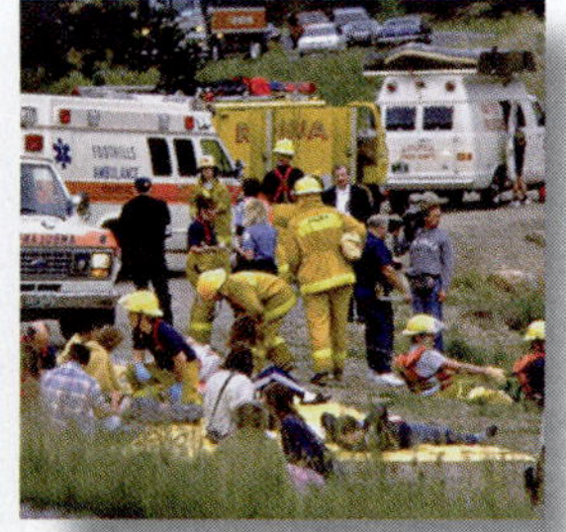

DIVISION 3 TRAUMA EMERGENCIES 759

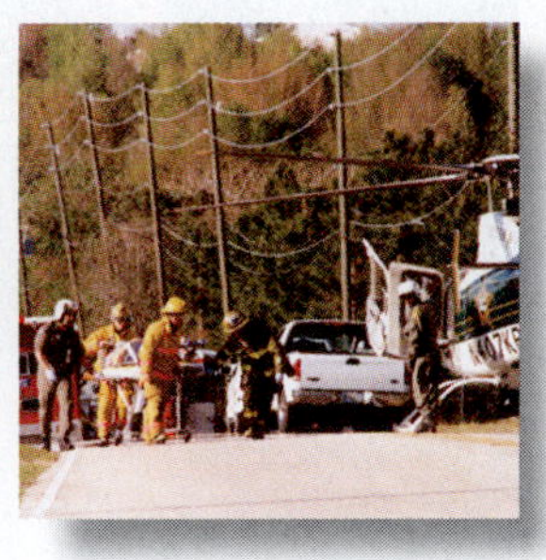

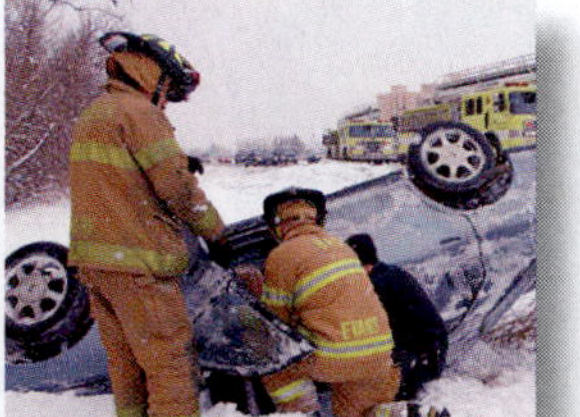

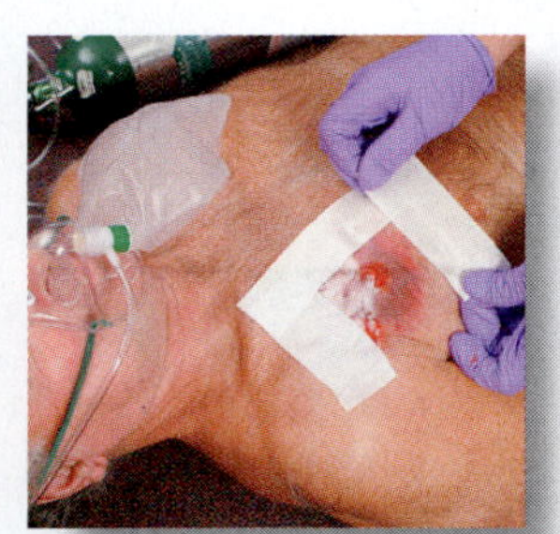

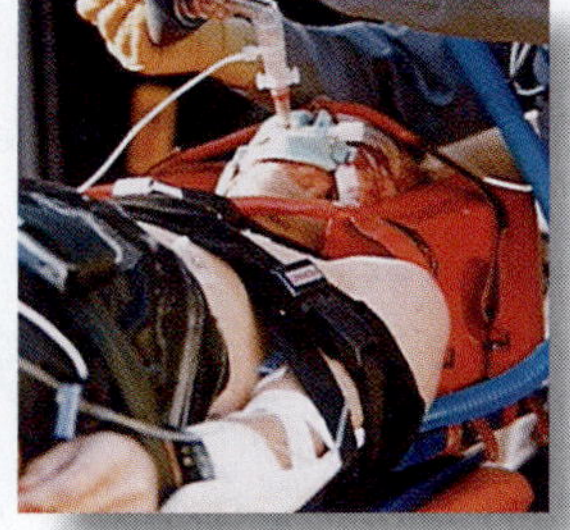

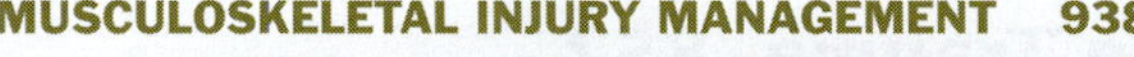

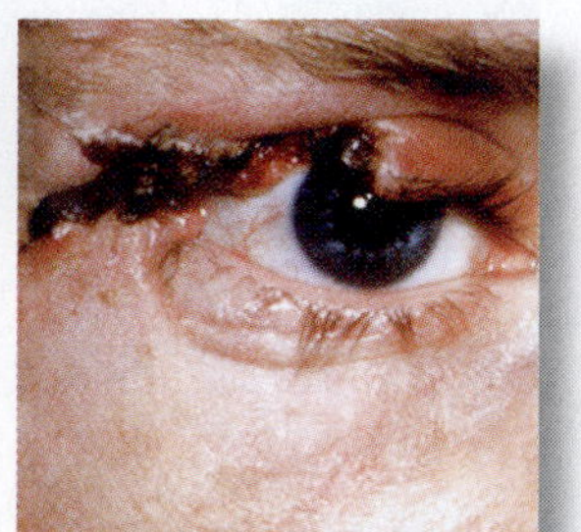

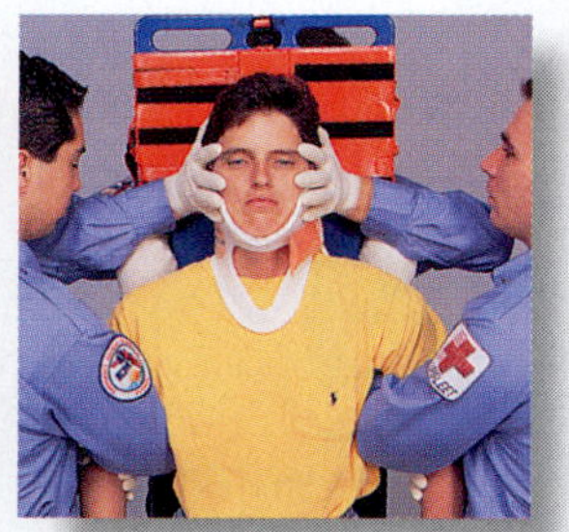

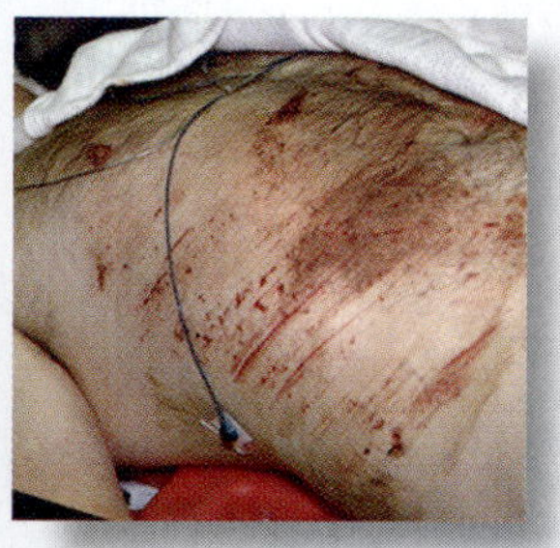

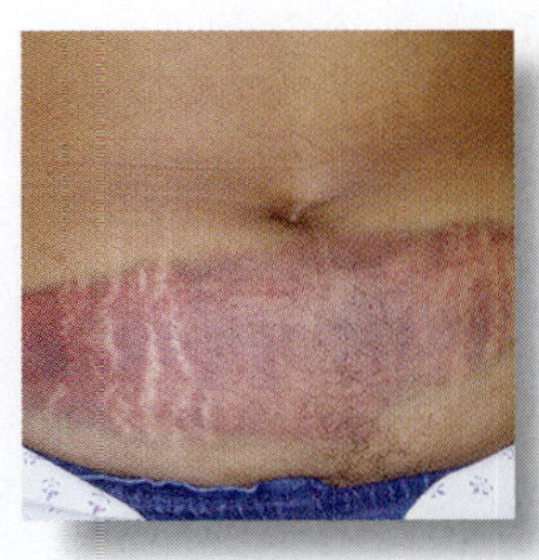

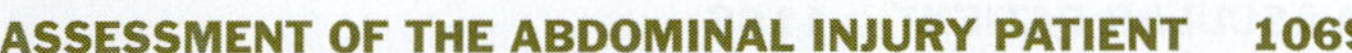

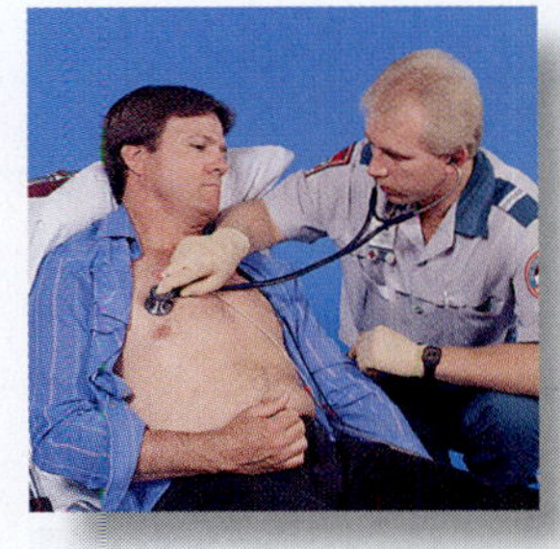

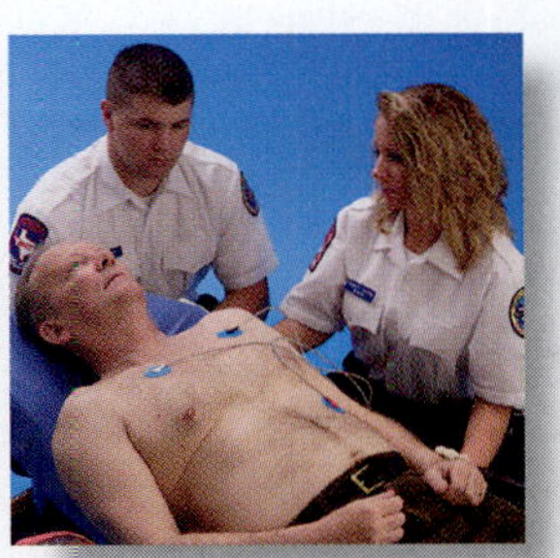

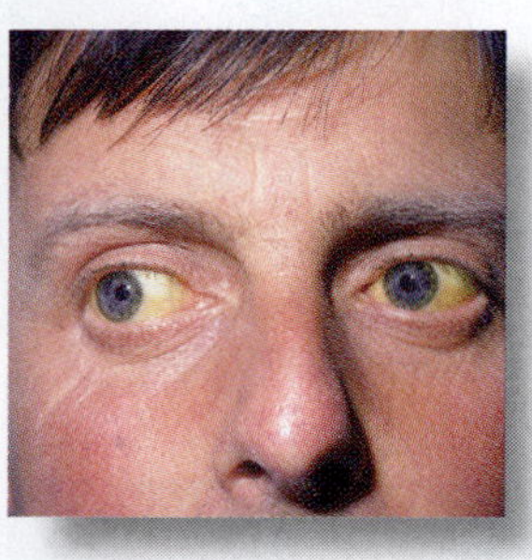

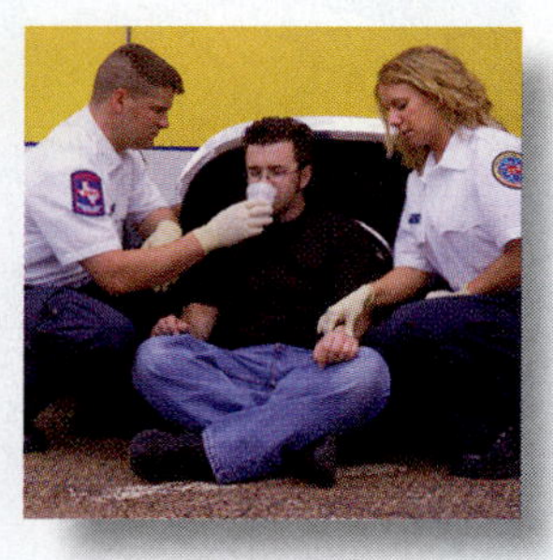

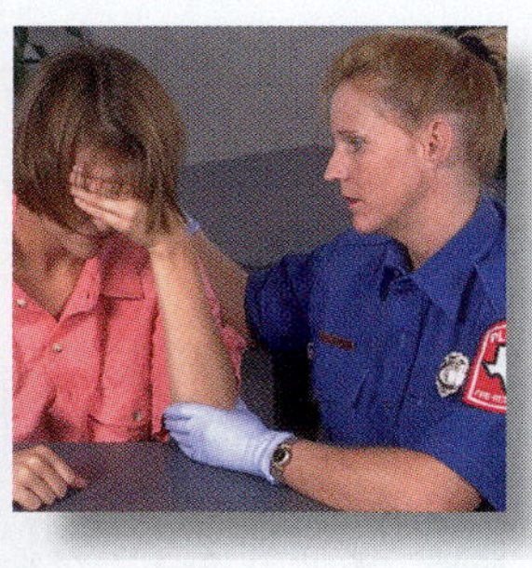

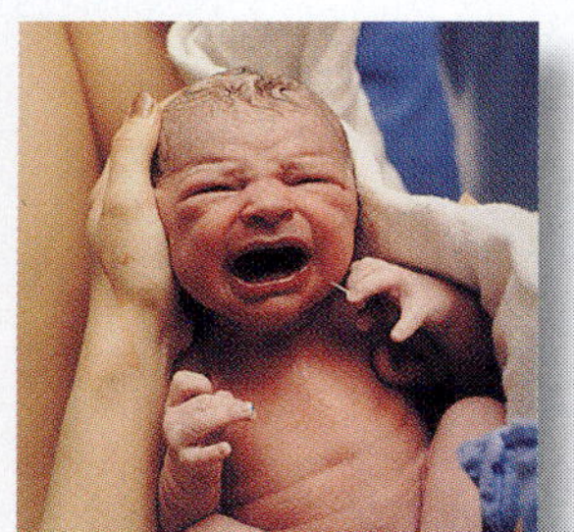

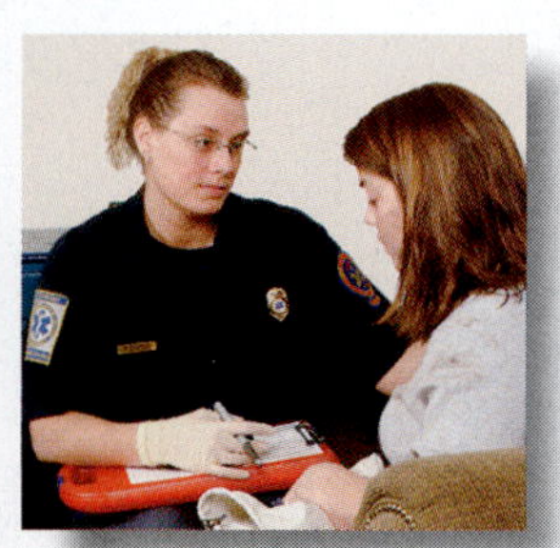

Chapter 44 Abuse and Assault 1715

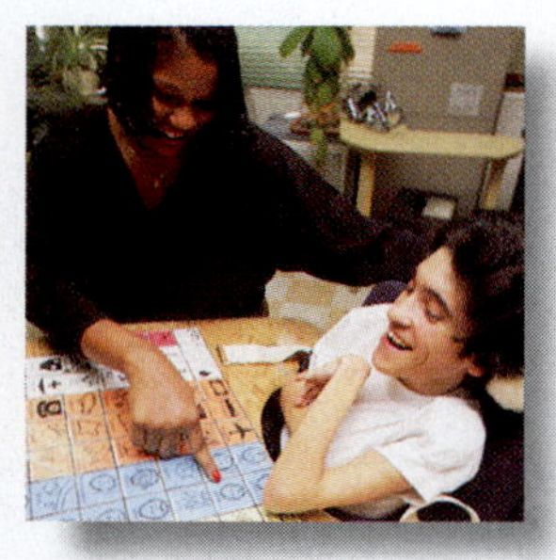

Chapter 45 The Challenged Patient 1729

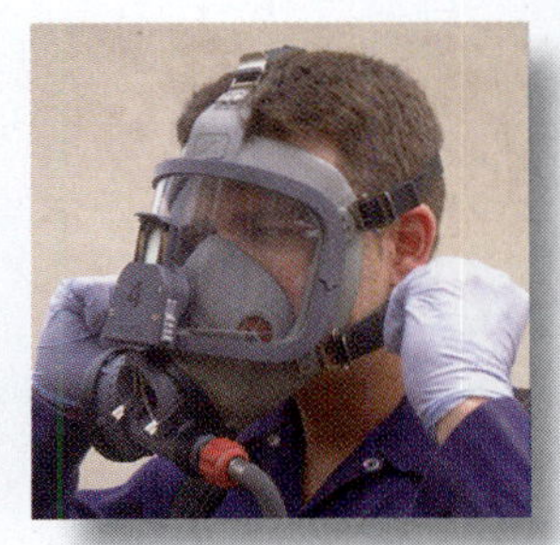

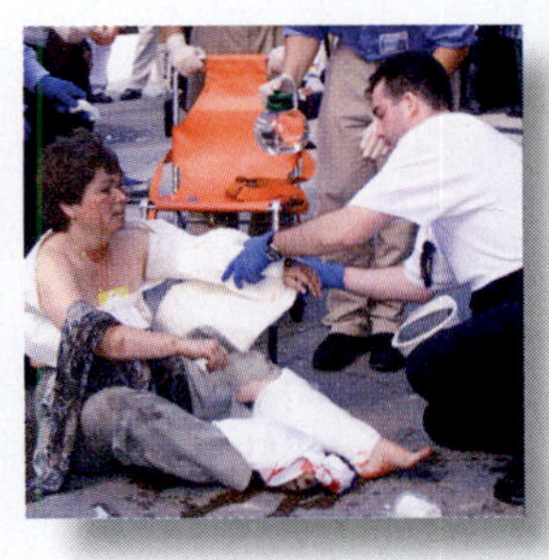

Photo Scans/Procedures

BRADY

It's Your Profession

Dear Student:

Thank you for using Brady's ***Essentials of Paramedic Care,*** 2nd edition Update. This text, based on the widely used *Paramedic Emergency Care* text we developed more than 20 years ago, will provide the core foundation for your paramedic education. Coupled with quality classroom instruction and clinical rotations, you are assured of receiving the knowledge and skills required of a quality paramedic. We know you want to pass your certification exam, and you also want to be prepared for the challenges you'll encounter on the street. ***Essentials of Paramedic Care*** is the textbook that will help you accomplish both goals.

We are proud to tell you that Brady has made a top-down commitment to quality, a commitment that is evident in the book you now hold. William A. Foster once wrote, "Quality is never an accident; it is always the result of high intention, sincere effort, intelligent direction, and skilled execution; it represents the wise choice of many alternatives." Every person at Brady involved in the preparation of this text has made a sincere commitment to quality, beginning with our efforts as authors. We know you have made a significant investment in your program, and we have gone to great effort to ensure that our paramedic program is accurate, current, and complete. The second edition has been extensively reviewed and revised to reflect changes in EMS as well as new AHA guidelines that have occurred since the first edition was published. The three of us, as well as contributors to this work, have made a tremendous effort to ensure that the material accurately reflects the current state of and best practices in EMS.

Brady makes a considerable investment in "development editing," and its development team is among the most dedicated and skilled in the publishing industry. Development editing ensures that content is reviewed appropriately for accuracy and currency, explanations are consistent, and the material remains at the appropriate level for the paramedic student. Brady's editors have worked hard toward these goals. Another of Brady's strongest assets is its production team. These publishing experts have many years of experience in the business and an undeniable commitment to producing books with distinctive designs and clear formatting. Working together, Brady's development and production teams help to ensure that our books are the best on the market. Brady's commitment to a standard of excellence continues with the customer service and feedback system provided by the sales team, a highly dedicated, skilled, and enthusiastic group.

In summary, EMS is about quality. Welcome. Be safe. Have fun. We wish you all the best in your education and in the practice of EMS.

Sincerely,

Bryan E. Bledsoe   Robert S. Porter   Richard A. Cherry

The Twenty-First Century EMS System: All That Glitters Is Not Gold

Although EMS has made some significant improvement, considerably more work needs to be done. Certainly, EMS in the twenty-first century is changing rapidly. The terrorist attacks on the World Trade Center in New York City and the Pentagon on September 11, 2001 forever changed EMS and the world. In addition to the carnage, these attacks pointed out the problems and inefficiencies with the United States emergency response system. Governmental oversight of various emergency response agencies was uneven and uncoordinated. Many of these agencies were subsequently combined into the Department of Homeland Security (DHS). However, in 2005, the southern United States was struck by Hurricanes Katrina and Rita. Hurricane Katrina virtually destroyed the city of New Orleans and similar communities along the Gulf coast. The emergency response to these disasters was far from adequate, and additional adjustments to DHS and other entities were made.

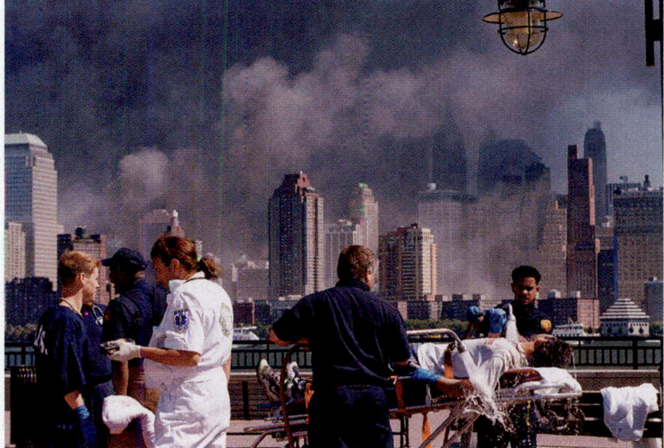

(© Reuters/CORBIS)

In 2006, the National Academies of Science, Institute of Science published an evaluation of the status of emergency services in the United States. This document, titled *Emergency Medical Services: At the Crossroads,* was critical of many EMS practices. The study found that there were significant problems at the federal level. Despite the advances made in EMS, sizable challenges remain. At the federal policy level, government leadership in emergency care is fragmented and inconsistent. As it is currently organized, responsibility for prehospital and hospital-based emergency and trauma care is scattered across multiple agencies and departments. Similar divisions are evident at the state and local levels. In addition, the current delivery system suffers in a number of key areas:

- ★ *Insufficient coordination.* EMS care is often uncoordinated among providers. Multiple EMS agencies are often serving within a single population center and do not operate cohesively. Agencies in adjacent jurisdictions frequently are unable to communicate with one another. In many cases, EMS and other public safety agencies cannot talk to one another because they operate with incompatible communications equipment or on different frequencies.
- ★ *Coordination of transport within regions is limited.* The management of the regional flow of patients is poor, and patients may not be transported to facilities that are optimal and ready to receive them. Communications and handoffs between EMS and hospital personnel are frequently ineffective and often omit important clinical information.
- ★ *Disparities in response times.* The speed with which ambulances respond to emergency calls is highly variable. In some cases this variability is related to geography. In dense population centers, for example, the distances ambulances must travel are small, but traffic and other problems can cause delays; rural areas, on the other hand, involve longer travel times and sometimes difficult terrain. This

is further worsened by problems in the organization and management of EMS services, the communications and coordination between 911 dispatch and EMS responders, and the priority placed on response time given the resources available.

- ★ *Uncertain quality of care.* There is very little known about the quality of care delivered by EMS services in the United States because there are no standardized measures of EMS quality, no nationwide standards for the training and certification of EMS personnel, no accreditation of institutions that educate EMS personnel, and virtually no accountability for the performance of EMS systems. Even though most Americans assume that their communities are served by competent EMS services, the public has no idea whether this is true, and no way to know.
- ★ *Lack of readiness for disasters.* Although EMS personnel are among the first to respond in the event of a disaster, they are the least prepared component of community response teams. Most EMS personnel have received little or no disaster response training for terrorist attacks, natural disasters, or other public health emergencies. Despite the massive amounts of federal funding directed to homeland security, only a tiny proportion of those funds has been directed to medical response. Furthermore, EMS representation in disaster planning at the federal level has been highly limited.
- ★ *Divided professional identity.* EMS is a unique profession, one that straddles both medical care and public safety. Among public safety agencies, however, EMS is often regarded as a secondary service, with police and fire taking more prominent roles; within medicine, EMS personnel often lack the respect afforded to other professionals, such as physicians and nurses. Despite significant investments in education and training, salaries for EMS personnel are often well below those for comparable positions, such as police officers, firefighters, and nurses. In addition, there is a cultural divide among EMS, public safety, and medical care workers that contributes to the fragmentation of these services.
- ★ *Limited evidence base.* The evidence base for many practices routinely used in EMS is limited. Strategies for EMS have often been adapted from settings that differ substantially from the prehospital environment and, consequently, their value in the field is questionable, and some may even be harmful. For example, field intubation of children, which is still widely practiced, has been found to do more harm than good in many situations. Although some recent research has added to the EMS evidence base, a host of critical clinical questions remain unanswered because of limited federal research support, as well as inherent difficulties associated with prehospital research due to its sporadic nature and the difficulty of obtaining informed consent for the research.

A similar study was published in 2006 by the American College of Emergency Physicians. The paper, titled *The National Report Card on the State of Emergency Medicine: Evaluating the Environment of Emergency Care Systems State by State,* pointed out the significant problems in all aspects of emergency care. This paper primarily addressed problems in hospital emergency departments but also examined EMS issues. Overall, the report detailed that emergency services in the United States are so overstressed that the quality of care has been compromised. Multiple causes were identified and included such factors as inadequate funding, patient overcrowding, lack of alternate care facilities, problems with medical liability, the effect of illegal immigration, and many others. Each state was given a letter grade that reflected the reported standard of emergency care in that state.

Despite these deficiencies and ongoing problems, EMS is still a rewarding and noble profession. Together, we must work together to make the system better. Strategies to achieve this include improved education, improved public image, a unified identity, adequate system funding, and more. Regardless, as a paramedic you can improve the system by ensuring that you treat each patient competently and professionally. This will go a long way toward improving the EMS system. The image of the modern EMS hinges on every call, and each paramedic can make a difference.

—B.E.B.

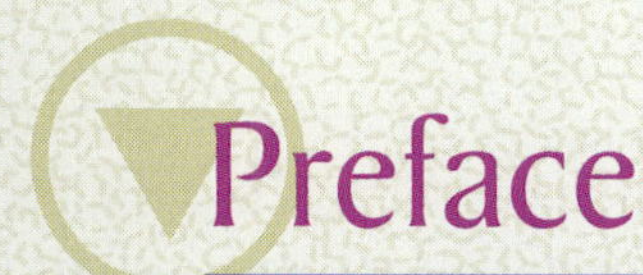

Preface

Congratulations on your decision to further your EMS career by undertaking the course of education required for certification as a Paramedic! The world of paramedic emergency care is one that you will find both challenging and rewarding. Whether you will be working as a volunteer or a paid paramedic, you will find the field of advanced prehospital care very interesting.

This textbook, ***Essentials of Paramedic Care,*** 2nd edition Update, will serve as your guide and reference to advanced prehospital care. It is based on the 1998 U.S. Department of Transportation's *Emergency Medical Technician–Paramedic National Standard Curriculum* and is divided into five divisions:

Division 1 *Introduction to Advanced Prehospital Care*

Division 2 *Patient Assessment*

Division 3 *Trauma Emergencies*

Division 4 *Medical Emergencies*

Division 5 *Special Considerations/Operations*

Division 1, *Introduction to Advanced Prehospital Care,* presents the foundations of paramedic practice as well as an introduction to pathophysiology, pharmacology, medication administration, and airway management and ventilation. **Division 2, *Patient Assessment,*** adds the cognitive and psychomotor skills of patient assessment, communications, and documentation. This knowledge base expands as the series applies it to the trauma patient in **Division 3, *Trauma Emergencies,*** and to the medical patient in **Division 4, *Medical Emergencies.* Division 5, *Special Considerations/Operations,*** enriches these general patient care concepts and principles with applications to special patients and circumstances we commonly see as paramedics. The product of this complete and integrated series is a set of principles of care you will be required to practice as a twenty-first-century paramedic.

Your paramedic education program should include ample classroom, practical laboratory, in-hospital clinical, and prehospital field experience. These educational experiences must be guided by instructors and preceptors with special training and experience in their areas of participation in your program.

DEVELOPING ADVANCED SKILLS

The psychomotor skills of fluid and medication administration, advanced airway care, ECG monitoring and defibrillation, and advanced medical and trauma patient care are best learned first in the classroom and the skills laboratory and then in the clinical and field settings. Commonly required advanced prehospital skills are discussed in the text as well as outlined in the accompanying procedure sheets. Review these before and while practicing each skill.

It is important to underscore that neither this nor any other text can teach skills. Care skills are learned only under the watchful eye of a paramedic instructor and perfected during your clinical and field internship.

CONTENT OF THE FIVE DIVISIONS

It is intended that your program coordinator will assign reading from ***Essentials of Paramedic Care*** in preparation for each classroom lecture and discussion section. The knowledge gained from reading this text will form the foundation of the information you will need in order to function effectively as a paramedic in your EMS system. Your instructors will build on this information to strengthen your knowledge and understanding of advanced prehospital care so that you may apply it in your practice.

The content of each division of ***Essentials of Paramedic Care*** is summarized below, with an emphasis on "what's new" in this second edition update.

DIVISION 1: INTRODUCTION TO ADVANCED PREHOSPITAL CARE

Division 1 addresses the fundamentals of paramedic practice, including paramedic roles and responsibilities, pathophysiology, pharmacology, medication administration, and advanced airway management.

What's New in Division 1?

- ★ In Chapter 1, "Introduction to Advanced Prehospital Care," the "EMS Systems" section has added a discussion of **The EMS Agenda for the Future** and a section on **Evidence-Based Medicine.** In the "Well-Being of the Paramedic" section, former discussions of critical incident stress management (a technique that is no longer recommended) have been replaced with new sections on specific **EMS stresses** and on **general mental health services** and **disaster mental health services** available to EMS personnel. UPDATE: The definitions of the certification levels have been revised.
- ★ Chapter 2, "Medical/Legal Aspects of Advanced Prehospital Care," contains a new section on the **Health Insurance Portability and Accountability Act (HIPAA) privacy rules.**
- ★ Chapter 4, "General Principles of Pathophysiology," and Chapter 7, "Intravenous Access and Medication Administration," include new sections on **HBOCs (hemoglobin-based oxygen-carrying substances),** which are considered to have significant advantages over standard crystalloids and colloids for fluid resuscitation. UPDATE: Referrals to flowcharts in mybradykit have been added.
- ★ Chapter 6, "General Principles of Pharmacology," includes updated information on **insulin preparations,** an updated **immunization schedule,** and discussion of **new drugs for erectile dysfunction.**
- ★ Chapter 8, "Airway Management and Ventilation," includes a new section on **capnography,** particularly its uses in monitoring tube placement during endotracheal intubation. New sections are also included on the **Intubating LMA (laryngeal mask airway),** the **Cobra Perilaryngeal Airway,** and the **Ambu Laryngeal Mask.** For assistance in intubation, the **bougie** device is newly discussed and illustrated as are techniques for **nasotracheal intubation.** UPDATE: Sections have been added on new equipment and documentation.

DIVISION 2: PATIENT ASSESSMENT

Division 2 builds on the assessment skills taught in the basic EMT course, emphasizing advanced-level patient assessment and clinical decision making at the scene. UPDATE: Terminology for assessment stages has been revised.

What's New in Division 2?

- ★ Chapter 11, "Physical Exam Techniques," includes much-expanded information and photos to illustrate the **ophthalmic (eye) exam** and the **otoscopic (ear) exam.**
- ★ Chapter 11, "Physical Exam Techniques," and Chapter 12, "Patient Assessment in the Field," feature new sections on **capnography** as an assessment tool.
- ★ Chapter 14, "Communications," includes new information on **wireless phones and 911 calls** (new technology for identifying locations and call-back numbers). There is a section on the promising new technology of **automatic collision notification** (ACN) and also a discusison of the importance of **speaking to medical direction on a recorded line** (which will help in the event of a lawsuit).

DIVISION 3: TRAUMA EMERGENCIES

Division 3 discusses advanced prehospital care of the trauma patient, from mechanism-of-injury analysis to care of specific types of trauma.

What's New in Division 3?

- ★ Chapter 17, "Blunt Trauma," includes new information on **side air bags** and on **deactivation of undeployed air bags.** Notes are included regarding **terrorist use of explosives** that contain nails, screws, and other materials intended to cause maximum injury and destruction.
- ★ Chapter 19, "Hemorrhage and Shock," includes a new section on the use of **capnography** as a guide to ventilation rates and volumes as well as for ensuring proper tube placement. A new section has been added on the use of two techniques to improve ventilatory efficiency: **positive end-expiratory pressure (PEEP)** and **continuous positive airway pressure (CPAP).**
- ★ In Chapter 20, "Soft-Tissue Trauma," **fentanyl** is introduced as a drug for pain control.
- ★ Chapter 21, "Burns," includes new information on **keratitis,** an eye injury welders may suffer; on the unreliability of **pulse oximetry** to measure oxygen saturation in the patient who has inhaled carbon monoxide; and on **fentanyl** as a pain management drug. Illustrations and text on factors affecting **radiation injury** have been revised and expanded.
- ★ In Chapter 22, "Musculoskeletal Trauma," discussions and illustrations of the **vacuum splint** and the **pelvic sling** have been added. The Hare splint has been deleted from the section on traction splinting and the **Fernotrac splint** has been added. Under pain control medications, **fentanyl** has been added and nalbuphine has been deemphasized. **UPDATE:** The section on **compartment syndrome** has been replaced.
- ★ Chapter 23, "Head, Facial, and Neck Trauma," has an added discussion of **capnography** as an assessment tool with the head injury patient and as a tool for confirmation of tube placement. A section on **recognition of herniation** is newly included. Both **adult and pediatric Glasgow Coma Scales** are now included. The importance of obtaining **blood glucose readings** in the head injury patient is newly emphasized. In the directed intubation section, the **bougie** device is introduced. Recommended **ventilation rates and volumes for the head injury patient** have been updated, as has information on **maintenance of blood pressure in the head injury patient.** Caveats regarding the use of **rapid-sequence intubation** in the prehospital setting have been included. In the discussion of medications, mannitol has been deleted as a diuretic, **atracurium** has been added as a paralytic, and **etomidate** and **fentanyl** have been added as sedatives. **UPDATE:** A new section has been added on the **Sellick maneuver.**
- ★ In Chapter 24, "Spinal Trauma," extensive discussions of **spinal clearance** and a spinal clearance protocol have been added. A term that is gaining acceptance, **spinal motion restriction,** is discussed. Use of the **full-body vacuum mattress** is discussed. **Capnography** is now included, along with pulse oximetry, as an aid in ensuring adequate oxygenation. An explanation is included as to why routine use of **steroids in spine injury is no longer recommended.**

DIVISION 4: MEDICAL EMERGENCIES

Division 4 addresses the paramedic level of care in medical emergencies. Particular emphasis is placed on respiratory and cardiovascular emergencies, which are the most common EMS medical calls.

What's New in Division 4?

- ★ Chapter 27, "Pulmonology," features new information on **capnography** as a prehospital diagnostic tool and means of monitoring the patient's respiratory status, specifically in upper airway obstruction and asthma emergencies. New material on **severe acute respiratory syndrome** (SARS) is included.
- ★ Chapter 28, "Cardiology," introduces the use of the **15-lead and 18-lead ECGs in right ventricular and left ventricular posterior wall infarctions. The 2005 AHA algorithms** for cardiac rhythms, arrest, and acute coronary syndrome are included. UPDATE: The sections on management of **congestive heart failure** and **CPAP** have been revised.
- ★ Chapter 29, "Neurology," has added information on the **pediatric Glasgow Coma Scale The 2005 AHA stroke algorithm** is included. UPDATE: A section on CO oximetry has been added.
- ★ Chapter 33, "Urology and Nephrology," has a new section on **priapism.**
- ★ UPDATE: Chapter 34, "Toxicology and Substance Abuse," has a new section on Africanized honeybees.
- ★ Chapter 37, "Infectious Disease"—like Chapter 1—includes new information on **SARS.** UPDATE: A section on hepatitis G has been added.
- ★ Chapter 38, "Psychiatric and Behavior Disorders," features completely revised text and photos regarding **restraint of violent patients** to emphasize supine placement and monitoring the airway and breathing of the restrained patient.

DIVISION 5: SPECIAL CONSIDERATIONS/OPERATIONS

Division 5 addresses such topics as neonatal, pediatric, and geriatric care; home health care and challenged patients; and incident command, ambulance service, rescue, hazardous material, crime scene operations, and responding to terrorist acts.

What's New in Division 5?

- ★ Chapter 41, "Neonatology," includes expanded text regarding congenital anomalies and, in particular, more information on **congenital heart problems. The 2005 AHA Neonatal Flow algorithm** is included.
- ★ Chapter 42, "Pediatrics," has a new section on **verification of tube placement in the pediatric patient. The 2005 AHA algorithms for pediatric tachycardia, bradycardia, and arrest** are included. UPDATE: A section on multiple casualty incidents involving children has been added.
- ★ Chapter 44, "Abuse and Assault," features a new section on **date rape drugs.**
- ★ In Chapter 48, "Operations," the section on "Ambulance Operations" includes **updated criteria for air medical dispatch.** The "Medical Incident Management" section makes reference to the new **U.S. Department of Homeland Security National Incident Management System (NIMS).** The former emphasis on critical incident stress debriefings has been deleted and replaced by new sections on **mental health support** and **disaster mental health services.**
- ★ Chapter 49, **"Responding to Terrorist Acts," is an entirely new chapter** that did not appear in the first (pre-September 11, 2001) edition of *Paramedic Care.* It includes information on **explosive, nuclear, chemical, and biological agents** as well as **scene safety, recognizing a terrorist attack,** and **responding to a terrorist attack.**

Acknowledgments

CHAPTER CONTRIBUTORS

We wish to acknowledge the remarkable talents and efforts of the following people who contributed to ***Essentials of Paramedic Care.*** Individually, they worked with extraordinary commitment on this new program. Together, they form a team of highly dedicated professionals who have upheld the highest standard of EMS instruction.

B.E.B., R.S.P., R.A.C.

Beth Lothrop Adams, MA, RN, NREMT-P, ALS Coordinator, EHS Programs, Adjunct Assistant Professor, Emergency Medicine, The George Washington University. Chapters 30, 39, 40

J. Nile Barnes, BS, NREMT-P, Associate Professor of EMS Professions, Austin Community College, Austin, Texas and Paramedic, Williamson County (Texas) EMS Department. Chapter 1

Brenda Beasley, RN, BS, EMT-P, EMS Program Director, Calhoun College, Decatur, Alabama. Chapter 42

Sandra Bradley, Pleasant Hill, California. Chapter 45

Lawrence C. Brilliant, MD, FACEP, Clinical Assistant Professor, Department of Primary Care Education and Community Services, Hahnemann University; Emergency Physician, Doylestown Hospital, Doylestown, Pennsylvania. Chapters 23, 28

Eric C. Chaney, MS, NREMT-P, Administrator, Office of the State EMS Medical Director, Maryland Institute for Emergency Medical Services Systems, Baltimore, Maryland. Chapter 1

Elizabeth Coolidge-Stolz, MD, Medical Writer, Health Educator, North Reading, Massachusetts. Chapters 30, 32, 33

Robert A. De Lorenzo, MD, FACEP Lieut. Colonel, Medical Corps, U.S. Army; Associate Clinical Professor of Military and Emergency Medicine, Uniformed Services University of the Health Sciences, Bethesda, Maryland. Chapters 20, 21, 49

Kate Dernocoeur, BS, EMT-P, Lowell, Michigan. Chapters 1, 9

Clyde Deschamp, MEd, NREMT-P, Chairman and Assistant Professor, Department of Emergency Medical Technology, Director, Helicopter Transport, University of Mississippi Medical Center. Chapter 37

James W. Drake, MS, NREMT-P, EMS Coordinator, Jameson Memorial Hospital, New Castle, Pennsylvania. Chapter 7

Bob Elling, MPA, REMT-P, Faculty Member, Institute of Prehospital Emergency Medicine, Hudson Valley Community College, Troy, New York. Chapter 48

Robert Feinberg, EMT-P, PA-C, Emergency Medicine, Wayne, Pennsylvania. Chapter 24

Joseph P. Funk, MD, FACEP, Peachtree Emergency Associates, Piedmont Hospital, Atlanta, Georgia. Chapter 8

Kathleen G. Funk, MD, FACEP, Emergency Medicine Physician, Atlanta, Georgia. Chapter 8

Eric W. Heckerson, RN, MA, NREMT-P, EMS Coordinator, Mesa Fire Department, Mesa, Arizona. Chapters 1, 22, 29, 37, 38

Chris Hendricks, NREMT-P, Field Instructor, Paramedic, Pridemark Paramedics, Boulder, Colorado. Chapter 46

Sandra Hultz, BS, NREMT-P, EMS Instructor, University of Mississippi Medical Center, Jackson, Mississippi. Chapter 1

Jeffrey L. Jarvis, MS, LP, Medical Student, University of Texas Medical Branch, Galveston, Texas. Chapter 6

Deborah Kufs, RN, BS, CCRN, CEN, NREMT-P, Clinical Instructor, Hudson Valley Community College, Institute for Prehospital Emergency Medicine, Troy, New York. Chapters 35, 43

Daniel Limmer, EMT-P, Kennebunk Fire Rescue, Kennebunk, Maine; Adjunct Faculty, Southern Maine Community College, Portland, Maine. Chapters 38, 48

William Marx, DO, Associate Professor of Surgery and Critical Care; Director, Surgical Critical Care SUNY Upstate Medical University, Syracuse, New York. Chapter 26

Michael O'Keefe, MS, NREMT-P, EMS Training Coordinator, Vermont Department of Health. Chapter 1

John M. Saad, MD, Medical Director of Emergency Services, Navarro Regional Hospital, Corsicana, Texas; Medical Director of Emergency Services, Medical Center at Terrell, Terrell, Texas. Chapters 34, 36

John S. Saito, MPH, EMT-P, Director, EMS/Paramedic Education, Assistant Professor, Oregon Health Sciences University, School of Medicine, Department of Emergency Medicine, Portland, Oregon. Chapters 4, 37

Jo Anne Schultz, BA, NREMT-P, Paramedic, Lifestar Ambulance Inc., Salisbury, Maryland; Level II Emergency Medical Services Instructor, Maryland Fire and Rescue Institute, University of Maryland; Paramedic Instructor, Maryland Institute of Emergency Medical Services Systems, University of Maryland; ACLS, BTLS, and PALS instructor. Chapters 5, 36, 41, 47

Craig A. Soltis, MD, FACEP, Assistant Professor of Clinical Emergency Medicine, Northeastern Ohio Universities College of Medicine; Chairman, Department of Emergency Medicine, Forum Health, Youngstown, Ohio. Chapters 25, 35

Marian D. Streger, RN, BSN, CEN, Lawrenceville, New Jersey. Chapters 45, 47

Matthew R. Streger, MPA, NREMT-P, Distinguished Lecturer, Emergency Medicine Special Operations Institute, University of Cincinnati, College of Medicine, Cincinnati, Ohio. Chapters 44, 46, 48

Emily Vacher, Esq., MPA, EMT-CC, Associate Director of Judicial Affairs, Syracuse University, Syracuse, New York. Chapter 2

Kevin Waddington, MedStar, Fort Worth, Texas. Chapter 28

Gail Weinstein, MA, EMT-P, Director of Paramedic Training, State University of New York Upstate Medical University, Syracuse, New York. Chapter 43

Howard A. Werman, MD, FACEP, Associate Professor of Clinical Emergency Medicine, The Ohio State University College of Medicine and Public Health, Columbus, Ohio; Medical Director, MedFlight of Ohio. Chapter 27

Matthew S. Zavarella, BSAS, NREMT-P, CCTEMT-P, Instructor, Department of Emergency Medical Technology, School of Health Related Professions, University of Mississippi Medical Center, Jackson, Mississippi. Chapters 4, 32

MEDICAL REVIEW BOARD

Our special thanks to the following physicians for their review of material in our paramedic program. Their reviews were carefully prepared, and we appreciate the thoughtful advice and keen insight each shared with us.

Dr. Robert De Lorenzo, Lieutenant Colonel, Medical Corps, U.S. Army; Associate Clinical Professor of Military and Emergency Medicine, Uniformed Services University of Health Sciences.

Dr. Edward T. Dickinson, Assistant Professor and Director of EMS Field Operations in the Department of Emergency Medicine, University of Pennsylvania School of Medicine in Philadephia.

Dr. Christopher W. Lentz, Associate Professor of Surgery and Pediatrics and Medical Director, Strong Regional Burn Center, University of Rochester Department of Surgery, Rochester, New York.

Dr. Howard A. Werman, Associate Professor, Department of Emergency Medicine, The Ohio State University College of Medicine and Public Health, Columbus, Ohio.

INSTRUCTOR REVIEWERS

The reviewers of ***Essentials of Paramedic Care,*** 2nd edition, have provided many excellent suggestions and ideas for improving the text. The quality of the reviews has been outstanding, and the reviews have been a major aid in the revision of the text. The assistance provided by these EMS experts is deeply appreciated.

Trisha Appelhans, NREMT-P
Division of EMS Education
Medical University of Ohio
Toledo, OH

Deborah Atwood, RN, BSN, CCRN, CEN, NREMT-P
Mechanicville, NY

John L. Beckman, AA, FF/PM Instructor
EMS Instructor
Technical Center of DuPage County
Addison, IL

Christopher L. Carver, BA, EMT-P (LP)
Associate Professor
EMS Professions
Austin Community College
Austin, TX

Harvey Conner, AS, NREMT-P
EMS Programs
Oklahoma City Community College
Oklahoma City, OK

Steven V. Day, NREMT-P
Instructor/Training Coordinator
EMS Education Department
Baxter Regional Medical Center
Mountain Home, AK

Joseph J. Gadoury, BA, MICP
JeffSTAT EMS Training Center
Thomas Jefferson University Hospital
Philadelphia, PA

Captain Rudy Garrett
Training Coordinator
Somerset Fire/EMS
Somerset, KY

Attila Hertelendy, MS, MHSM, NREMT-P, CCEMT-P, ACP
Department of Health Sciences
School of Health Related Professions
University of Mississippi Medical Center
Jackson, MS

Raymond Klein, AAS, NREMT-P
EMS Training Director, Pima Community College
Captain, Tucson Fire Department
Tucson, AZ

Bill Locke, EMS, I/C
Emergency Medical Training Instructor-Coordinator
Moraine Park Technical College
Fond du Lac, WI

Earl D. Morgan, MD, FACFE
Regional EMS Medical Director
EMMCO East
Kersey, PA

Nikhil Natarajan, NREMT-P, CCEMT-P, I/C
Paramedic Program Coordinator
SUNY Ulster
Stone Ridge, NY

Warren J. Porter, MS, BA, NREMT-P
EMS Programs Manager
Garland Texas Fire Department
Garland, TX

Fredrick H. (Ted) Rogers, BA, NREMT-P
EMS Faculty
St. Petersburg College EMS Program
St. Petersburg, FL

We also wish to express appreciation to the following EMS professionals who reviewed ***Essentials of Paramedic Care,*** 1st edition. Their suggestions and perspectives helped to make this program a successful teaching tool.

Division 1

Brenda Beasley, RN, BS, EMT-P
EMS Program Director
Calhoun College
Decatur, AL

Tom Blake, MS, EMT-P
Director, Paramedic Associates Degree Program
Southern Maine Technical College
South Portland, ME

Alan Brower, RN, NREMT-P
Ricks College Paramedic Program
Rexbury, ID

Kerry Campbell, NREMT-P
Lakeshore Technical College
Cleveland, WI

Albert Dimmitt, Jr.
Penn Valley Community College
Kansas City, MO

Robert Dotterer, BSEd, MEd, NREMT-P
Phoenix Fire Department
Phoenix College
Phoenix, AZ

Bill Gentry, MICP
Paramedic Program Coordinator
Northern California Training Institute
Sacramento, CA

Blaine Griffiths, BS, NREMT-P
Youngstown State University
Youngstown, OH

Jeffrey Grunow, MSN, NREMT-P
Director, Prehospital Education
Carolinas Medical Center
Charlotte, NC

Linda Honeycutt, EMT-P, I/C
HealthStream, Inc.
Nashville, TN

Samuel D. Marciano, MS, EMT-I
Assistant Professor
Erie Community College
Lancaster, NY

Larry W. Masterman, MICP, CEM
Northern California EMS Agency
Redding, CA

Vicki L. May
Houston Community College
Houston, TX

Michael E. Murphy, RN, EMT-P
Deputy Chief
Rockland Paramedic Services
Orangeburg, NY

Gerard Oncale, RN, BSN, CEN, REMT-P
EMS Faculty
University of South Alabama
Mobile, AL

Judith Ruple, PhD, RN
Associate Professor
The University of Toledo
Toledo, OH

Larry Ryland
Director of Emergency Medical Services
L.B. Wallace College
Andalusia Rescue Squad
Andalusia, AL

John Saito, EMT-P, MPH
EMS/Paramedic Education
Oregon Health Sciences University
Portland, OR

Christopher D. Scott, MEd, NREMT-P
Paramedic Program Director
Assistant Professor
Springfield College EMSM
Springfield, MA

Brad L. Sparks
Paramedic Program Coordinator
St. Francis Hospital and Health Centers
Indianapolis, IN

Andrew W. Stern, NREMT-P, MPA, MA
Senior Paramedic/Flightmedic
Town of Colonie Emergency Medical Services
Colonie, NY

Regina M. Twisdale, AS, MICP
Director, School of Paramedic Sciences
Virtua Health/Camden County College
Camden County, NJ

Michael D. Zemany
Director of Education
Mt. Lakes Regional EMS Program
Saranac Lake, NY

Division 2

Linda M. Abrahamson, RN, EMT-P
EMS Education Coordinator
Will Grundy EMS
Silver Cross Hospital
Joliet, IL

Brenda Beasley, RN, BS, EMT-P
EMS Program Director
Calhoun College
Decatur, AL

Jeffery L. Beinke, BS, REMT-P, CCEMT-P
Division Chair, Allied Health Sciences
Montgomery Community College
Troy, NC

Ed Carlson, Med, REMT-P
Department of EMS Education
University of South Alabama
Mobile, AL

Chuck Carter, RN, NREMT-P, CEN
Mississippi State Department of Health
Division of EMS
Jackson, MS

Claudette Dirzanowski, EMT-P
Certified Instructor/Examiner for the State of Texas, AHA, ARC, PHTLS
Sweeney Community Hospital and Brazosport College
Sweeney, TX

Bob Elling, MPA, REMT-P
Faculty Member, Institute of Prehospital Emergency Medicine
Hudson Valley Community College
Troy, NY

Joseph J. Mistovich
Chairperson and Associate Professor
Department of Health Professions
Youngstown State University
Youngstown, Ohio

Catherine Pattison, RN, MSN, EMT-B
EMS Program Coordinator
Bishop State Community College
Mobile, AL

Steven A. Weinman, RN, BSN, CEN
Instructor, Emergency Department
New York Presbyterian Hospital
New York Cornell Campus
New York, NY

Division 3

Philip Adams, EMT-P, RN, BSN
Paramedic Course Coordinator
Paducah Community College
Paducah, KY

Kim Dickerson, EMT-P, RN
EMS Coordinator
Edison Community College
Fort Myers, FL 33906

Rudy Garrett
Paramedic Training Coordinator
Somerset-Pulaski County EMS
Somerset, KY

Ted S. Goldman, EMT-P
City of Philadelphia Fire Department
Director of EMS Programs
Star Technical Institute
Philadelphia, PA

Linda Groarke, MPH/MS, NREMT-P
Paramedic Program Director
Assistant Professor
Natural and Applied Sciences
LaGuardia Community College/CUNY
New York, NY

Theresa Jordan, RN, TNS, EMT
Arkansas Emergency Transport
Jacksonville, AR

Scott Kar, MEd, NREMT-P
Bevill State Paramedic Program
Sumiton, AZ

David LaCombe, NREMT-P
Center for Research in Medical Education
University of Miami School of Medicine
Miami, FL

Shelby Louden, BS, EMT-P
Safety and Compliance Coordinator
Butler County Joint Vocational Schools
Hamilton, OH

Joseph J. Mistovich
Chairperson and Associate Professor
Department of Health Professions
Youngstown State University
Youngstown, Ohio

Becky A. Morris, BS, NREMT-P, IC
EMS Department Head
Trenholm State College
Montgomery, AL

John Eric Powell, MS, NREMT-P
Flight Paramedic
UT-Lifestar Aeromedical Service
University of Tennessee Medical Center
Level 1 Trauma Facility
Knoxville, TN

Larry Richmond
Mountain Plains Health Consortium
Fort Meade, SD

Captain Michael W. Robinson
EMS Training Coordinator
Baltimore County Fire Department
Baltimore, MD

Tom Rothrock, RN, BSN, CEN, PHRN
Flight Nurse, University Medevac
Paramedic Coordinator, Lehigh Valley Hospital
Allentown, PA

Andrew W. Stern, NREMT-P, MPA, MA
Senior Paramedic/Flightmedic
Town of Colonie Emergency Medical Services
Colonie, NY

Michael Tretola, BS, EMT-P
Administrative Coordinator
EMS Institute/Department of Emergency Medicine
Catholic Medical Center of Brooklyn and Queens, NY

Peter H. Viele, MS, NREMT-P
Operations Manager
Action Ambulance Service, Inc.
Stoneham, MA

Division 4

John L. Beckman
Fire Fighter/Paramedic Instructor
Lincolnwood Fire Department
Lincolnwood, IL

Mike Coakley
EMS Director
Alabama Fire College
Program in Emergency Medicine
Tuscaloosa, AL

Janice Dorsey, RN, BS
EMS Coordinator, Education
Christ Hospital and Medical Center
Oaklawn, IL

Darren K. Ellenburg, BS, EMT-P
Assistant Professor, Paramedic Education
Northeast State Technical Community College
Blountville, TN

Joseph P. Funk, MD, FACEP
Emory University
Department of Emergency Medicine
Atlanta, GA

Mary Gillespie, RN, EMT-P, I/C
Allied Health Division Chair
Davenport College
Grand Rapids, MI

Blaine Griffiths, BSAS, RN, NREMT-P
Youngstown State University
Paramedic Program
Youngstown, OH

J. Scott Hartley, NREMT-P, EMS-I
A.L.S. Affiliates
Omaha, NE

Arthur Hsieh, MA, NREMT-P
Assistant Professor, Emergency Health Services Program
Department of Emergency Medicine
George Washington University
Washington, DC

Larry Impson, AS, NREMT-P
Dean of Prehospital Education
METS Inc.
Lodi, CA

Kevin McCoy, CCEMT-P
EMS Administrator/Paramedic Instructor
Cherokee Nation EMS
Tahlequah, OK

Robert G. Nixon, BA, EMT-P
Lifecare Medical Training
Walnut Creek, CA

Robert C. Rajsky, MSEd, NREMT-P
Manager of the Department of EMS Education
Chair-Southern Tier Regional EMS Council
Education Supervisor Erway Ambulance
President-Southern Tier ALS

Andria Savary, RN, MSN, ANP, EMT-P
Assistant Director
Institute for Emergency Medical Services
Northeastern University
Boston, MA

Andrew Stern, NREMT-P, MPA, MA
Senior Medic/Flightmedic
Town of Colonie Emergency Medical Services
Colonie, NY

Eric Strokley, AAS, NREMT-P
Program Director
Global Education Services
Lilburn, GA

Dave Tauber, NREMT-P, I/C
Executive Director Advanced Life Support Institute
Paramedic/Firefighter
Conway, NH

Timothy Walsh, RN, ANP, NREMT-P
Assistant Professor
Community College of Rhode Island
Lincoln, RI

Steve Weinman, RN, BSN, CEN
Emergency Department Instructor
New York Hospital–Cornell Medical Center
New York, NY

Gail Weinstein
Paramedic Instructor
SUNY Health Science Center
Department of Emergency Medicine
Syracuse, NY

Paul A. Werfel, NREMT-P
Director Paramedic Program SUNY
Stony Brook, NY

Division 5

Stanley A. Bell, Jr.
MICP Lead Instructor
Trinitas Hospital Mobile ICU
Elizabeth, NJ

Michael D. Berg, NREMT-P
Medical Liaison Officer
Austin/Travis County EMS
Austin, TX

Robert Carter
Clinical Associate Pediatric Intensive Care Unit
Johns Hopkins Children's Center
Paramedic, Baltimore City Fire Department
Baltimore, MD

Edna Deacon, EMT
EMT Coordinator Sussex County Community College
Mine Hill First Aid Squad President
Newton, NJ

Robert De Lorenzo, MD, FACEP
Lieutenant Colonel, Medical Corps
United States Army
Associate Clinical Professor of Military and Emergency Medicine
Uniformed Services University of Health Sciences
Bethesda, MD

Robert Dotterer, BSEd, MEd NREMT-P
Phoenix Fire Department
Phoenix College
Phoenix, AZ

Julie M. Falcone, BS, BM
Fire Fighter/Paramedic
Walla Walla Fire Department
Walla Walla, WA

Jonathan Hockman, Paramedic, ACLS, EMSIC
Goldrush Consulting
Detroit, MI

Darin Hoggatt, MS, FF/NREMT-P
Clarian Health and Greenwood Fire Department
Indianapolis, IN

Tony Hyre, BA, REMT-P
C.E. Officer
West Virginia EMS

James L. Jenkins, Jr., BA, NREMT-P
Confidential Assistant to the Governor
Office of the Secretary of Public Safety
Virginia Department of Fire Programs
Richmond, VA

Anthony T. Kramer, RN, BSN, NREMT-P
Field Service Assistant Professor
Clinical Coordinator, Center for Prehospital Education
University of Cincinnati
Cincinnati, OH

Nick Meacher, NREMT-P
Instructor, Public Safety Center
Harrisburg Area Community College
York Springs, PA

Steven L. Poffenberger, BS, EMT-P
Paramedic Program Clinical Coordinator
Harrisburg Area Community College
Harrisburg, PA

Jackie L. Richey, RN, NREMT-P
Rural/Metro Ambulance
Indianapolis, IN

Captain Michael W. Robinson
EMS Training Coordinator
Baltimore County Fire Department
Baltimore, MD

Michael G. Rubin, BS, NREMT-P
State University of New York at Stony Brook
Stony Brook, NY

Daniel L. Sponsler, BS, NREMT-P
Division Chair, Emergency Services
Northwest Technical College
East Grand Forks, MN

Andrew W. Stern, NREMPT-P, MPA, MA
Senior Paramedic/Flightmedic
Town of Colonie Emergency Medical Services
Colonie, NY

Matthew R. Streger, MPA, NREMT-P
Distinguished Lecturer
Emergency Medicine Special Operations Institute
University of Cincinnati, College of Medicine
Cincinnati, OH

Anthony Tucci, EMT-P
Western Berks Ambulance Association
West Lawn, PA

Charles N. Zarrelli
Coordinator, EMT Training
Camden County College
Blackwood, NJ

PHOTO ACKNOWLEDGMENTS

All photographs not credited to the photographer or in the photo credit section below are photographed on assignment for Brady/Prentice Hall Health.

Organizations

We wish to thank the following people and organizations for their valuable assistance in creating the photo program.

Marshall Eiss, REMT
Special Events Coordinator
Indian Rocks Volunteer Firemen's Association
Indian Rocks Beach, FL

Steve Fravel, NREMT-P
Pinellas County EMS & Fire Administration
Largo, FL

C.T. "Chuck" Kearns, MBA, EMT-P
Director, Pinellas County EMS/Sunstar
Largo, FL

Chief John R. Leahy, Jr.
Pinellas Suncoast Fire & Rescue
Indian Rocks Beach, FL

Darryl Quigley
TLC Ambulance Service
Dallas, TX

Rural-Metro Medical Services, Syracuse, NY
North Area Volunteer Ambulance Corps (NAVAC)
North Syracuse, NY

Chief David Schrodt
Midlothian Fire Department
Midlothian, Texas

Rev. Robert A. Wagenseil, Jr.
Chaplain—Pinellas Suncoast Fire & Rescue
Rector—Cavalry Episcopal Church
Indian Rocks Beach, FL

Robert A. Walley, REMT
District Chief
Pinellas Suncoast Fire & Rescue
Indian Rocks Beach, FL

Special thanks to Jeff Goethe of Phillips Medical Systems for provision of electronic monitors.

Technical Advisors

Thanks to the following people for providing valuable technical support during the photo shoots:

Richard A. Cherry, MS, EMT-P
Director of Training
Northern Onondaga Volunteer Ambulance
Liverpool, NY

Michael Cox, Instructor
Division of State Fire Marshal
Florida Bureau of Fire Standards and Training
Florida State Fire College
Ocala, FL

Richard T. Walker, EMT-P
District Chief
Pinellas Suncoast Fire & Rescue
Indian Rocks Beach, FL

Digital Postproduction: Richard Carter, Tampa, FL

About the Authors

BRYAN E. BLEDSOE, DO, FACEP, FAAEM, EMT-P

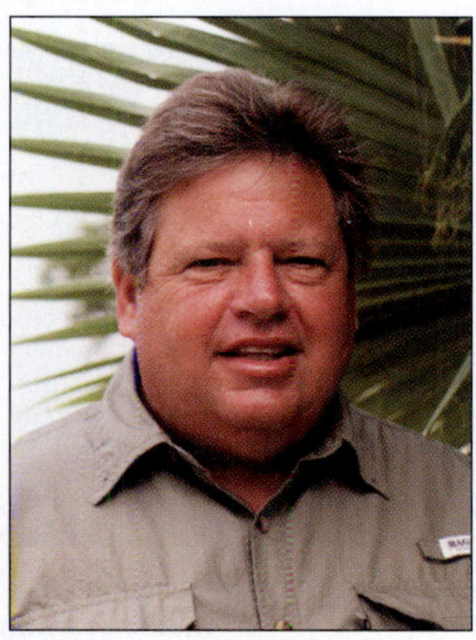

Dr. Bryan Bledsoe is an emergency physician, researcher, and EMS author. He is currently Clinical Professor of Emergency Medicine and Director of the EMS Fellowship program at the University of Nevada School of Medicine and an Attending Emergency Physician at the University Medical Center of Southern Nevada in Las Vegas. He is board certified in emergency medicine.

Prior to attending medical school, Dr. Bledsoe worked as an EMT, a paramedic, and a paramedic instructor. He completed EMT training in 1974 and paramedic training in 1976 and worked for 6 years as a field paramedic in Fort Worth, Texas. In 1979, he joined the faculty of the University of North Texas Health Sciences Center and served as coordinator of EMT and paramedic education programs at the university. Dr. Bledsoe is active in emergency medicine and EMS research. He is a popular speaker at state, national, and international seminars and writes regularly for numerous EMS journals. He is active in educational endeavors with the United States Special Operations Command (USSOCOM) and the University of Nevada at Las Vegas.

Dr. Bledsoe is the author of numerous EMS textbooks and has almost 1 million books in print. Dr. Bledsoe was named a "Hero of Emergency Medicine" in 2008 by the American College of Emergency Physicians as a part of its 40th anniversary celebration and was named a "Hero of Health and Fitness" by *Men's Health* magazine in its 20th anniversary edition in November 2008. He is frequently interviewed in the national media. Dr. Bledsoe is married and divides his time between his two residences in Midlothian, Texas and Las Vegas, Nevada.

ROBERT S. PORTER, MA, NREMT-P

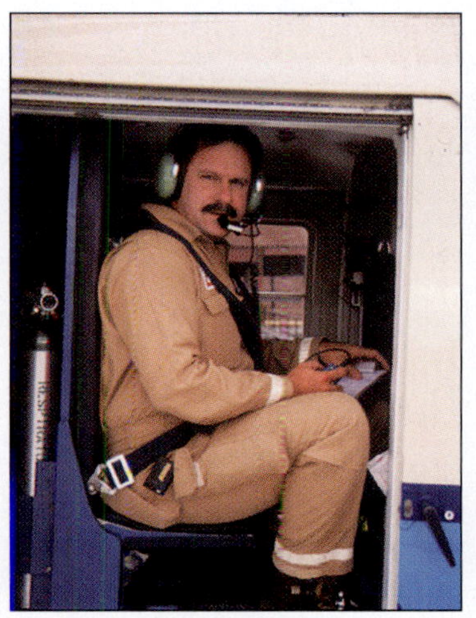

Robert Porter has been teaching in emergency medical services for 30 years and currently serves as the Senior Advanced Life Support Educator for Madison County, New York. For 15 years, he was a Flight Paramedic with the Onondaga, New York, County Sheriff's Department helicopter service, AirOne. Mr. Porter is a Wisconsin native and received his bachelor's degree in education from the University of Wisconsin. He completed his paramedic training at Northeast Wisconsin Technical Institute in 1978 and earned a master's degree in health education at Central Michigan University in 1990.

Mr. Porter has been an EMT and EMS educator and administrator since 1973 and obtained his national registration as an EMT-Paramedic in 1978. He has taught both basic and advanced EMS courses in the states of Wisconsin, Michigan, Louisiana, Pennsylvania, and New York. Mr. Porter served for more than 10 years as a paramedic program accreditation-site evaluator for the American Medical Association and is a past chair of the National Society of EMT Instructor/Coordinators. He has authored Brady's *Paramedic Care: Principles & Practice, Essentials of Paramedic Care, Intermediate Emergency Care: Principles & Practice, Tactical Emergency Care,* and *Weapons of Mass Destruction: Emergency Care,* as well as the workbooks accompanying this text, *Paramedic Emergency Care,* and *Intermediate Emergency Care.* When not writing or teaching, Mr. Porter enjoys offshore sailboat racing and historic home restoration.

RICHARD A. CHERRY, MS, EMT-P

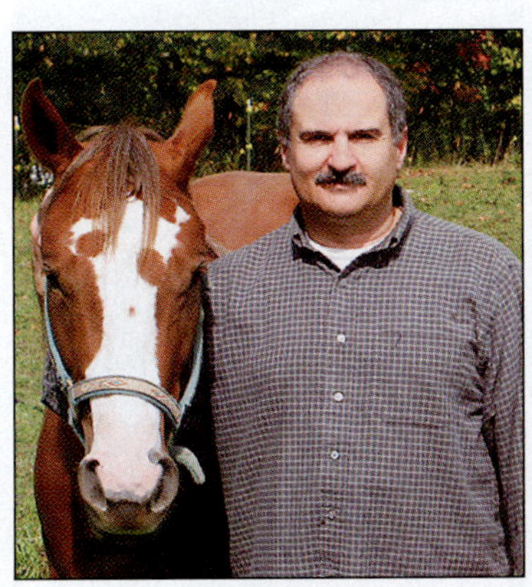

Richard Cherry is the Director of Training for the Northern Onondaga Volunteer Ambulance in Liverpool, New York. His experience includes years of classroom teaching and emergency fieldwork. A native of Buffalo, Mr. Cherry earned his bachelor's degree at nearby St. Bonaventure University in 1972. He taught high school for the next 10 years while he earned his master's degree in education from Oswego State University in 1977. He holds a permanent teaching license in New York State.

Mr. Cherry entered the emergency medical services field in 1974 with the DeWitt Volunteer Fire Department, where he served his community as a firefighter and EMS provider for more than 15 years. He took his first EMT course in 1977 and became an ALS provider 2 years later. He earned his paramedic certificate in 1985 as a member of the area's first paramedic class. He then became Clinical Assistant Professor of Emergency Medicine and the Director of Paramedic Training at Upstate Medical University, a position he held for more than 20 years until his retirement last year.

Mr. Cherry has authored several books for Brady. Most notable are *Paramedic Care: Principles & Practice, Essentials of Paramedic Care, Intermediate Emergency Care: Principles & Practice,* and *EMT Teaching: A Common Sense Approach.* He has made presentations at many state, national, and international EMS conferences on a variety of teaching topics. He and his wife, Sue, run a horse-riding camp for children with special needs on their property in West Monroe, New York. He also plays guitar in a Christian band.

Welcome to Paramedic Care

BRADY

Brady
Prentice Hall Health
Upper Saddle River, NJ 07458

Dear Instructor:

Brady, your partner in education, is pleased to present the 2nd edition Update of our best-selling ***Essentials of Paramedic Care.*** Expanding on the many innovations made in the third edition of ***Paramedic Care: Principles & Practice***, we continued to stay on top of science, practice, and trends and updated our ***Essentials*** to be the most current product on the market.

We know that Paramedic programs are varied in length, depth, focus, and even curricula, so we created ***Essentials*** to give you a choice. Part of our responsibility as the #1 publisher in the EMS market is to continue to provide you with top-quality, innovative, and effective products in a world of change. We rely on our experience, commitment, and your trust to create solutions that will benefit any program, any time. The following walkthrough outlines the features found in each chapter of ***Essentials.*** We've retained the tried-and-true and added some new ones based on what we've discovered works in educational publishing and in EMS.

The walkthrough also provides information for each of our student and instructor supplements, which have been updated and reviewed extensively. Our ***mybradykit*** site houses all student and instructor resources in a single place for easy and complete access. A new addition is the Clinical & Internship Tracking Program, a tool you can use to keep your students' activities and performance in check. Also, we introduce several related products that can be used to make your program the best it can be. We are truly proud to be able to offer you a complete set of resources for education.

We know you have choices for educational products, and we appreciate the vote of confidence you've given Brady year in and year out. Your confidence and trust enables us to continue to bring you up-to-date, accurate, and innovative solutions for all areas of EMS education. We're committed to helping teachers and students become the best professionals possible. After all, it's you who may help us in an emergency some day. This update is an extension of our promise to both of you.

Sincerely,

Julie Levin Alexander
VP/Publisher

Katrin Beacom
Executive Marketing Manager

Marlene McHugh Pratt
Executive Editor

Thomas Kennally
National Sales Manager

Lois Berlowitz
Senior Managing Editor

Emphasizing Principles

Objectives

Part 1: Cardiovascular Anatomy and Physiology, ECG Monitoring, and Dysrhythmia Analysis (begins on p. 1127)

After reading Part 1 of this chapter, you should be able to:

1. Describe the incidence, morbidity, and mortality of cardiovascular disease. (p. 1126)
2. Discuss prevention strategies that may reduce the morbidity and mortality of cardiovascular disease. (p. 1126)
3. Identify the risk factors most predisposing to coronary artery disease. (p. 1126)
4. Describe the anatomy of the heart, including the position in the thoracic cavity, layers of the heart, chambers of the heart, and location and function of cardiac valves. (pp. 1127–1128; also see Chapter 3)

◀ **Chapter Objectives with Page References.** List the objectives that form the basis of each chapter, in addition to the page on which each objective is covered.

Key Terms

aberrant conduction, p. 1184
absolute refractory period, p. 1140
acute arterial occlusion, p. 1235
acute pulmonary embolism, p. 1234
aneurysm, p. 1233
angina pectoris, p. 1211
arrhythmia, p. 1143
compensatory pause, p. 1166
congestive heart failure (CHF), p. 1221
coronary heart disease (CHD), p. 1126
coupling interval, p. 1173
cystic medial necrosis, p. 1234
deep venous thrombosis,
interpolated beat, p. 1172
myocardial infarction (MI), p. 1214
noncompensatory pause, p. 1152
non-ST-elevation myocardial infarction (non-STEMI), p. 1214
normal sinus rhythm, p. 1142
paroxysmal nocturnal

◀ **Key Terms with Page References.** Present important terminology at the beginning of each chapter, along with the page on which each term is introduced.

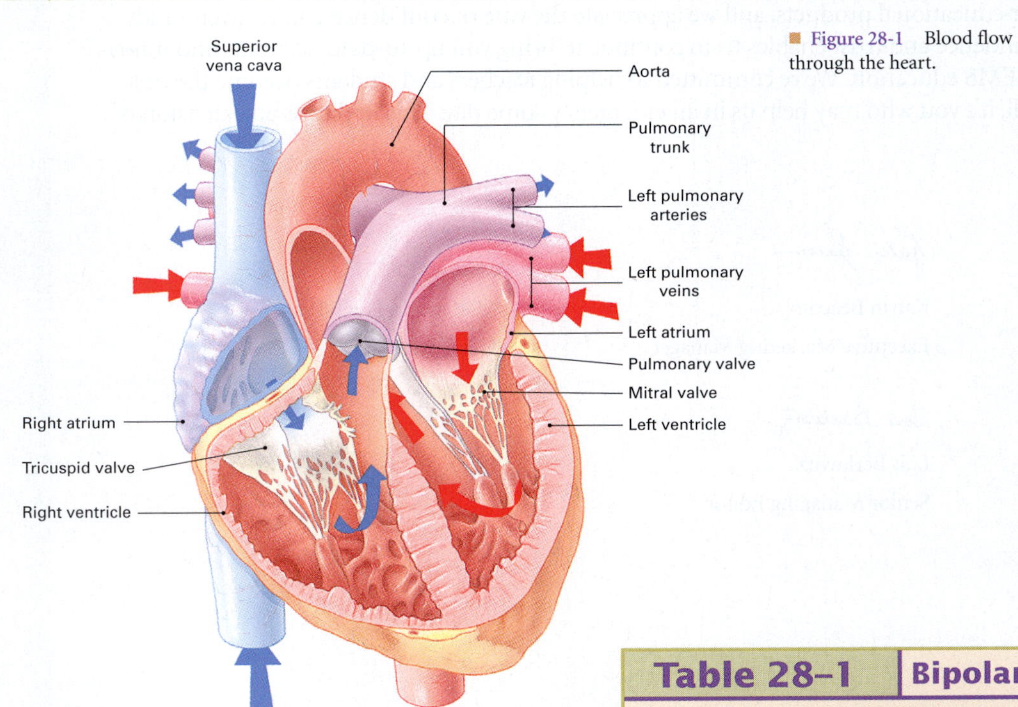

■ Figure 28-1 Blood flow through the heart.

◀▼ **Illustrations and Tables.** Provide visual support to enhance understanding.

Table 28–1 Bipolar Lead Placement Sites

Lead	Positive Electrode	Negative Electrode
I	Left arm	Right arm
II	Left leg	Right arm
III	Left leg	Left arm

Emphasizing Principles

One of your most important skills as a paramedic will be obtaining and interpreting ECG rhythm strips.

▲ **Key Points.** Help students identify and learn fundamental points.

cardiovascular disease (CVD) *disease affecting the heart, peripheral blood vessels, or both.*

▲ **Margin Definitions.** Located in margins near the paragraphs in which they first appear, these help students master new terminology.

Content Review

ECG Leads

- Bipolar (limb)
- Augmented (unipolar)
- Precordial (chest)

▲ **Content Review.** Summarizes important content, giving students a format for quick review.

► **Summary.** Provides students with a concise review of important chapter information.

Summary

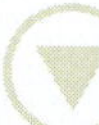

Cardiovascular disease is the number-one cause of death in the United States and Canada. Many deaths from heart attack occur within the first 24 hours—frequently within the first hour. With the advent of fibrinolytic therapy, time is of the essence when managing the patient with suspected ischemic heart disease. EMS plays an ever-increasing role in the early recognition of patients suffering coronary ischemia. In certain areas, EMS provides definitive care by initiating fibrinolytic therapy in the field. This is especially important in cases where transport times can be long. With cardiovascular disease, EMS can truly mean the difference between life and death.

Review Questions

1. ___________ refers to the strength of a cardiac muscular contraction.
   a. Atropy
   b. Inotropy
   c. Dromotropy
   d. Chronotropy
2. Due to the property of ___________, the individual cells of the conductive system can depolarize without any impulse from an outside source.
   a. Excitability
   b. Conductivity
   c. Automaticity
   d. Contractility
3. ___________ results from an increased rate of SA node discharge.
   a. Sinus bradycardia
   b. Sinus tachycardia
   c. Sinus dysrhythmia
   d. Atrial tachycardia

◄ **NEW Review Questions.** Ask students to recall information and to apply the principles they've just learned.

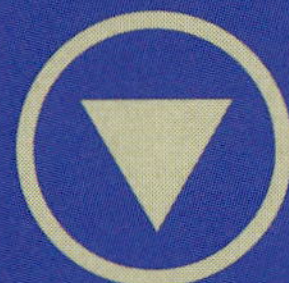

Emphasizing Practice

Procedure 28–2 Defibrillation

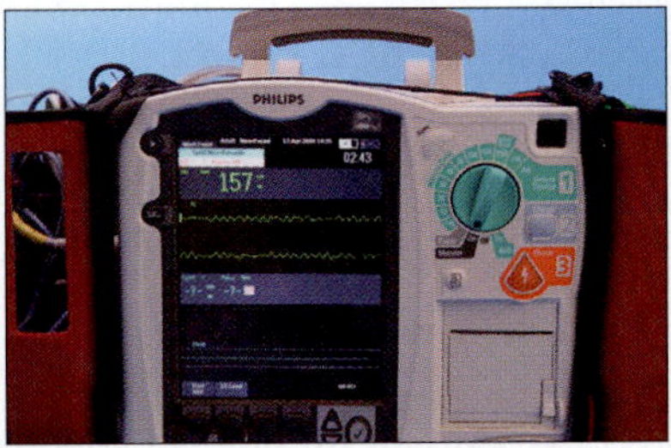

28-2a Identify rhythm on the cardiac monitor.

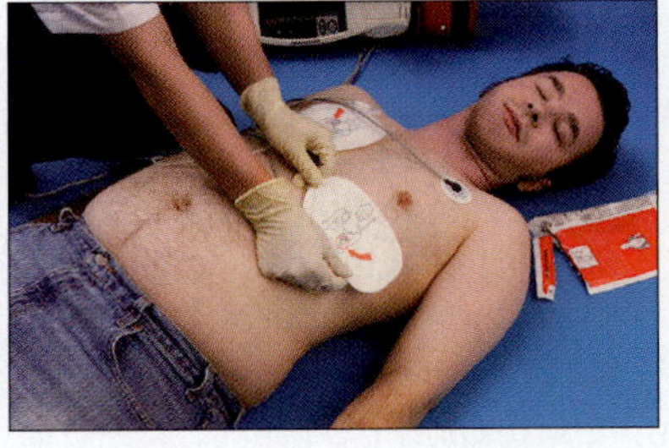

28-2b Place commercial defibrillation pads on the patient's exposed thorax.

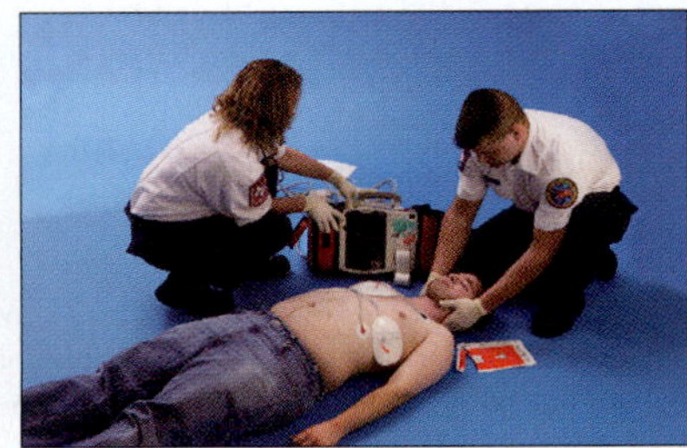

28-2c Charge the defibrillator.

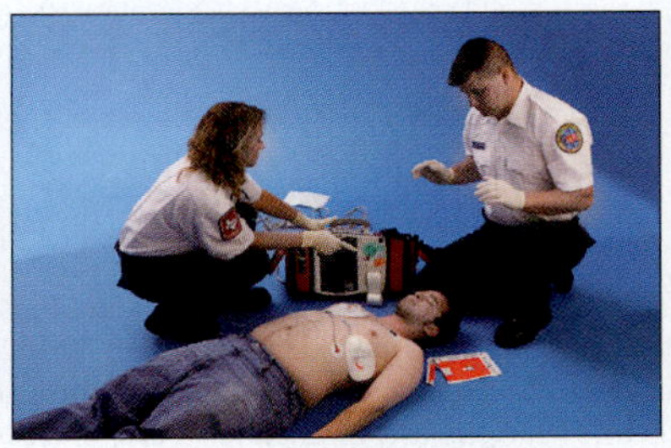

28-2d Reconfirm the rhythm on the cardiac monitor.

Procedure Scans. Provide step-by-step visual support on how to perform skills.

Procedure 28–2 Defibrillation *(continued)*

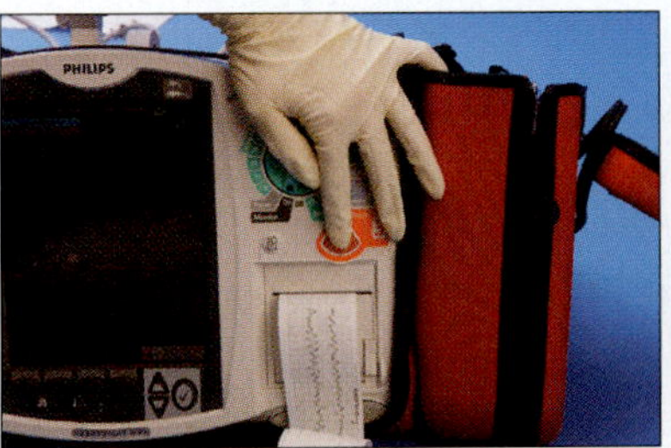

28-2e Verbally and visually clear everybody, including yourself, from the cardiac patient.

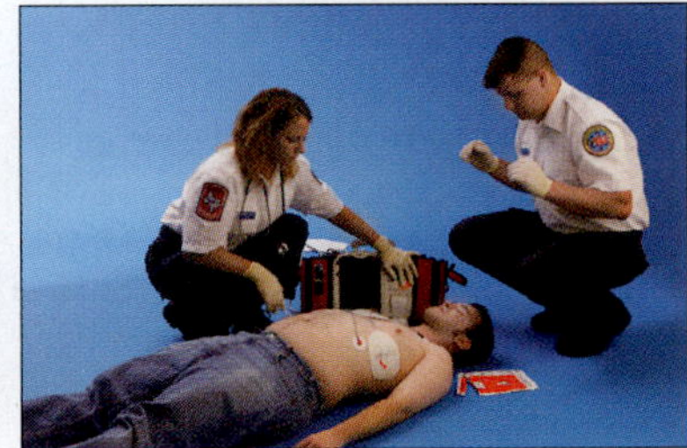

28-2f Deliver a shock by pressing the button.

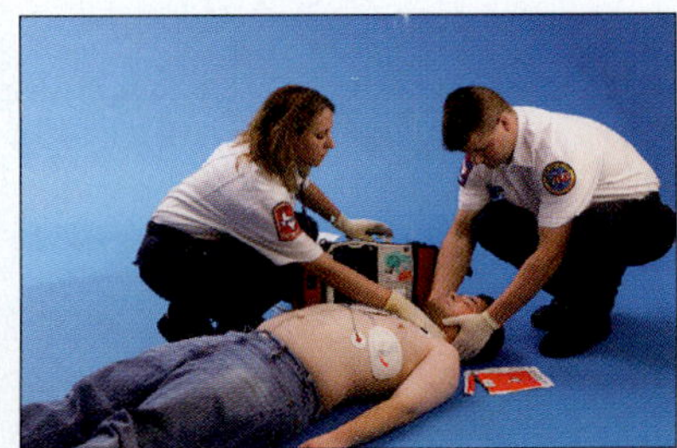

28-2g Reconfirm the rhythm on the cardiac monitor.

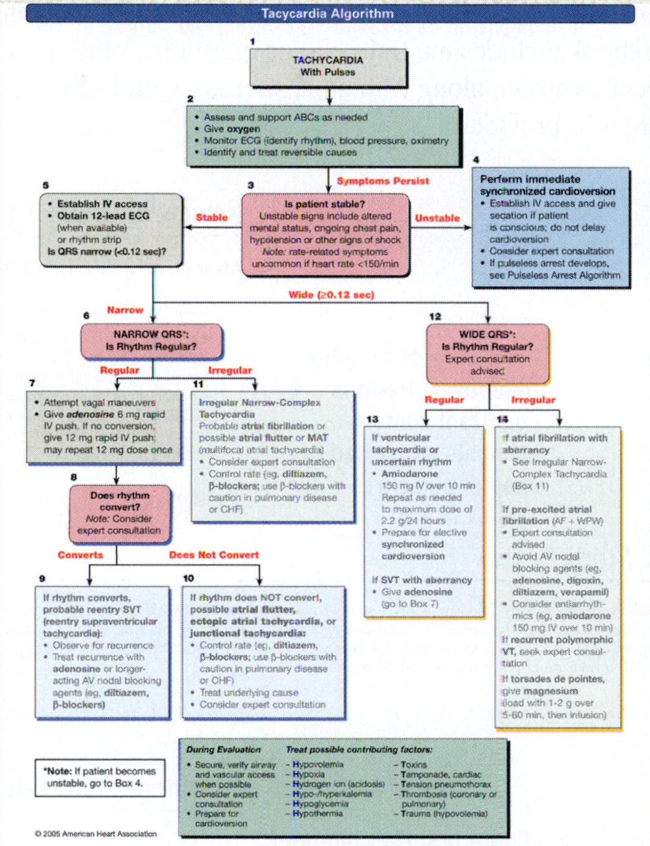

Patient Care Algorithms. Provide graphic "pathways" that integrate assessment and care procedures.

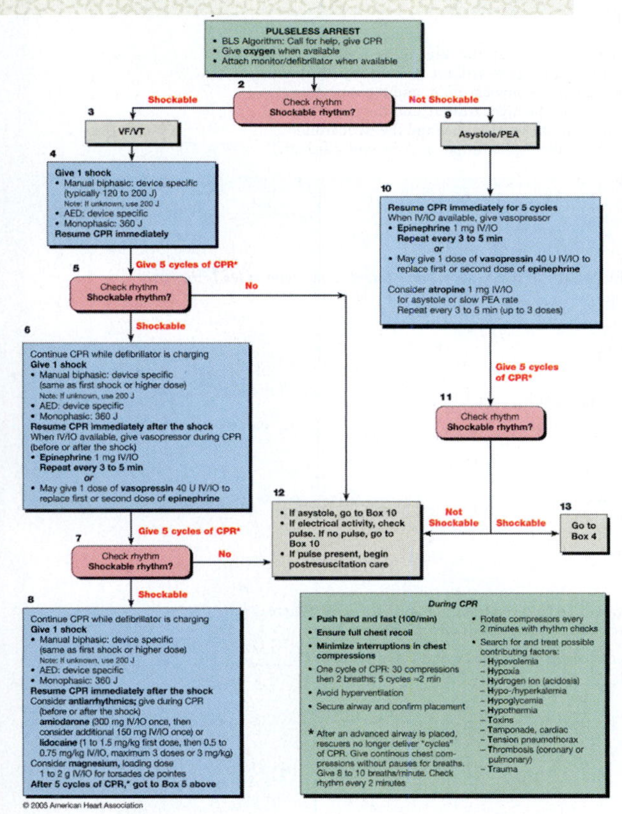

Student Workbook

A student workbook with review and practice activities accompanies this text. The workbook includes multiple-choice questions, other exercises, case studies, and special projects, along with an answer key with text page references. Flash Cards are also provided.

Review of Chapter Objectives. Reviews important content elements addressed by chapter objectives.

Review of Chapter Objectives

After reading this part of the chapter, you should be able to:

1. Describe the incidence, morbidity, and mortality of cardiovascular disease.

   Cardiovascular disease (CVD) is serious and extremely common, with more than 60 million Americans affected. Morbidity is considerable: An American has a nonfatal heart attack (myocardial infarction, MI) roughly every 29 seconds. Coronary heart disease (CHD), one type of CVD, is the single largest killer of Americans and Canadians. Roughly 466,000 Americans die annually from CHD, half of them before reaching a hospital. Many deaths from CHD are sudden and involve lethal cardiac dysrhythmias. Many deaths from MI occur within the first 24 hours, frequently within the first hour.

Case Study Review

Paramedic supervisor John Bigelow is presented with an "elderly man with abdominal pain." He begins his investigation of the history by introducing himself, identifying his role at the scene, and expressing his desire to help Mr. O'Donnell. He also asks for and uses Mr. O'Donnell's name to place the conversation on a more comfortable and personal level.

Case Study Review. Reviews and points out essential information and applied principles.

Content Self-Evaluation. Multiple-choice, matching, and short-answer questions to test reading comprehension.

Content Self-Evaluation

Multiple Choice

_____ 1. From innermost to outermost, the three tissue layers of the heart are:
- A. the endocardium, the pericardium, and the myocardium.
- B. the endocardium, the myocardium, and the syncytium.
- C. the endocardium, the myocardium, and the pericardium.
- D. the myocardium, the epicardium, and the pericardium.
- E. the epicardium, the myocardium, and the endocardium.

Matching

Write the letter of the ECG leads in the space provided next to the type of leads they are.

A. I, II, III

B. V_1, V_2, V_3, V_4, V_5, V_6

C. aVR, aVL, aVF

_____ 9. unipolar (augmented)

_____ 10. bipolar

_____ 11. precordial

Fill-in-the-Blanks

56. The ___________ valves lie between the atria and ventricles, whereas the ___________ valves lie between the ventricles and the arteries into which they open.

57. The four properties of cells in the cardiac conductive system are ___________ , ___________ , ___________ , and ___________ .

Student Workbook

Special Project

Assessing Respiratory Emergencies

Read the assessment written for each of three patients evaluated in a prehospital setting and identify the probable cause for each emergency. Check the Assessment section of the textbook for each disorder to refamiliarize yourself with characteristic findings on history and physical examination.

Scenario 1: You are called to an elementary school where a student has become "suddenly ill" during a class birthday party. You find a distressed seven-year-old child who is breathing rapidly and shallowly and whose skin tone is becoming dusky. The use of accessory muscles to breathe is evident. The school nurse offers you a box containing an inhaler that she says the child uses on an "as needed" basis and states she isn't sure what ingredients were in the cupcakes brought for the party. She adds that the boy has several severe food allergies.

Probable cause: ____________________

Scenario 2: You are called to a home where an elderly man is "short of breath." On arrival, you find a thin, elderly man with a broad chest whose breathing is labored despite use of a home supplemental oxygen setup. His daughter tells you that he has had a cold recently, and he suddenly became "shorter of breath" this morning. On exam, the man has a fever of

◀ **Special Projects.** Experiences designed to help students remember information and principles.

EMT-Paramedic Form

National Registry of Emergency Medical Technicians
Advanced Level Practical Examination

PATIENT ASSESSMENT - TRAUMA

Candidate: ____________________ Examiner: ____________________

Date: ____________________ Signature: ____________________

Scenario # ________

Time Start: ________ NOTE: Areas denoted by "**" may be integrated within sequence of Initial Assessment

	Possible Points	Points Awarded
Takes or verbalizes body substance isolation precautions	1	
SCENE SIZE-UP		
Determines the scene/situation is safe	1	
Determines the mechanism of injury/nature of illness	1	
Determines the number of patients	1	
Requests additional help if necessary	1	
Considers stabilization of spine	1	

▶ **National Registry Practical Evaluation Forms.** Give a clearer picture of what is expected during the practical exam.

Name/Class: ADENOSINE (Adenocard)/Antidysrhythmic

Description: Adenosine is a naturally occurring agent that can "chemically cardiovert" PSVT to a normal sinus rhythm. It has a half-life of 10 seconds and does not cause hypotension.

Indications: Narrow, complex paroxysmal supraventricular tachycardia refractory to vagal maneuvers.

Contraindications: Hypersensitivity, 2nd- and 3rd-degree heart block, sinus node disease, or asthma.

Precautions: It may cause transient dysrhythmias. COPD.

Dosage/Route: 6 mg rapidly (over 1 to 2 sec) IV, then flush the line rapidly with saline. If ineffective, 12 mg in 1 to 2 min, may be repeated. Ped: 0.1 mg/kg (over 1 to 2 sec) IV followed by rapid saline flush, then 0.2 mg/kg in 1 to 2 min to max 12 mg.

◀ **Emergency Drug Cards.** Alphabetized perforated flash cards can be detached. They allow you to test your knowledge of correct route, dosage, and other important information on each drug.

Teaching and Learning Package

FOR THE INSTRUCTOR

PEARSON mybradykit™

This *new* robust companion website has all your instructor resources in one location! It provides a one-stop shop for online chapter support materials and all your teaching resources. Available for download are:

Curriculum Management Resources. These include

- Classroom Management material
- Lesson Plans with teaching suggestions and discussion questions
- Media Resources with exercises
- Objectives Checklists
- Reinforcement and Assessment Handouts

TestGen. Program containing more than 2,000 questions that support and reinforce text content and including text page references to where answers can be found. TestGen software can be used to customize your tests chapter by chapter and provide the questions electronically or on paper. You can also add your own questions to the database.

PowerPoint Slides. With a complete library of all images in the text.

The above resources are also available on the Instructor's Resource Center at ***www.pearsonhighered.com.***

To access ***mykit*** for this text, please visit ***www.bradybooks.com.*** Click on ***mybradykit***, followed by ***myemskit*** and then the cover for ***Essentials of Paramedic Care, 2nd Edition Update.***

CourseCompass. Provides a dynamic, interactive online learning environment. You can easily create a course and customize it with your own materials. All instructor resources for this edition are already loaded to enable you to run your online course. You'll find a link to CourseCompass in the ***mybradykit*** for this text.

FOR THE STUDENT

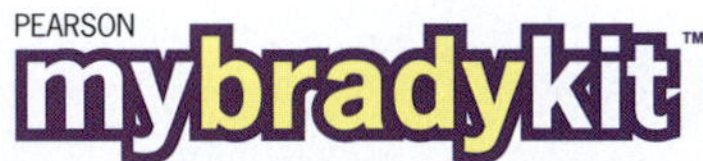

Mybradykit. Provides a one-stop shop for online chapter support materials and resources. You can prepare for class and exams with

- Multiple Choice Quizzes
- Anatomy Labeling Exercises
- Case Study Activities
- Video Vignettes
- Media Resources with Exercises
- 3D Animations
- Narrated Virtual Tours
- Breath Sounds
- Interactive Drag-and-Drop Exercises
- Resource Weblinks
- Medical Terminology
- Drug Guide
- Trauma Gallery
- Audio Glossary
- Resume Builder

To access ***mykit*** for this text, please visit ***www.bradybooks.com.*** Click on ***mybradykit***, followed by ***myemskit*** and then the cover for ***Essentials of Paramedic Care, 2nd Edition Update.***

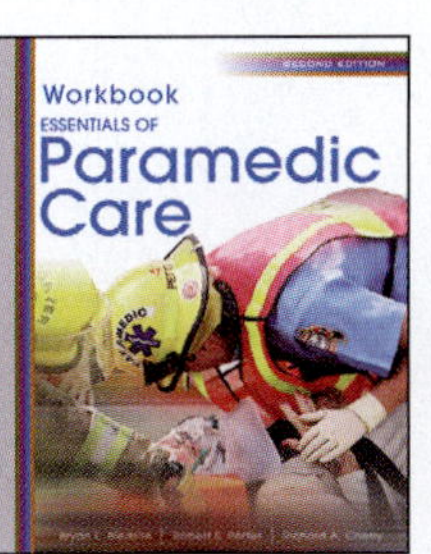

Workbook. Contains a review of objectives with summary information for each chapter; case study review; multiple-choice, matching, and short-answer questions; emergency drug flashcards.

Other Titles of Interest

SKILLS

Brady Skills Series: Advanced Life Support (0-13-119307-4—video; 0-13-119326-0—CD)
26 skills presented in step-by-step format with introduction, equipment, overview, and close-up, including assessment.

Advanced Life Support Skills (0-13-093874-2)
26 skills presented in full color, with step-by-step photos and rationales.

REVIEW & REFERENCE

Beasley, Mistovich, *EMT Achieve: Paramedic Test Preparation* (0-13-119269-8)
Online test preparation, with full-length exams and quizzes, with rationales and supporting text, artwork, and video.

Cherry, SUCCESS! for the Paramedic, 4th edition (0-13-238550-3)
Best-selling review, containing test questions with DOT and text page references and rationales.

Miller, *Paramedic National Standards Self-Test*, 5th edition (0-13-199987-7)
Based on the 1998 DOT curriculum, uses self-test format to target areas students need to study further. Includes multiple-choice and scenario-based questions.

Bledsoe, Clayden, *Pocket Reference for ALS Providers*, 3rd edition (0-13-170728-0)
Drugs, dosages, algorithms, tables and charts, pediatric emergencies, advanced skills, and home medications provided in an easy-to-use field guide.

Cherry, Bledsoe, *Drug Guide for Paramedics*, 2nd edition (0-13-193645-X)
Handy field resource for accurate, easily accessed information about patient medication.

ANATOMY & PHYSIOLOGY

Martini, Bartholemew, Bledsoe, *Anatomy & Physiology for Emergency Care*, 2nd edition (0-13-234298-7)
EMS-specific applications at the end of every chapter provide an emergency care focus to A&P discussions.

CARDIAC/EKG

Walraven, *Basic Arrhythmias*, 7th edition (0-13-500238-9)
Classic best-seller covers all the basics of EKG. Also contains appendices on clinical implications, cardiac anatomy & physiology, 12-lead EKG, basic 12-lead interpretation, and pacemakers.

Beasley, *Understanding EKGs: A Practical Approach*, 3rd edition (0-13-506906-8)
A direct approach to EKG interpretation that presents all the essential concepts for mastering the basics of this challenging field, while assuming no prior knowledge of EKGs.

Page, *12-Lead ECG for Acute and Critical Care Providers* (0-13-022460-X)
This full-color text presents ECG interpretation in a practical, easy-to-understand, and user-friendly manner.

Beasley, *Understanding 12-Lead EKGs: A Practical Approach*, 2nd edition (0-13-170789-2)
This comprehensive, reader-friendly text teaches beginning students basic 12-lead EKG interpretation.

MEDICAL

Dalton, et al., *Advanced Medical Life Support*, 3rd edition (0-13-172340-5)
This groundbreaking text offers a practical approach to adult medical emergencies. Each chapter discusses realistic methods that a seasoned EMS practitioner would use.

Other Titles of Interest

MEDICAL TERMINOLOGY

Fremgen, *Medical Terminology*, 4th edition (0-13-158998-9)
A consistent and logical system helps students build vocabulary. Also provides a tour of medical terminology as it applies to the human body and health professions.

PHARMACOLOGY

Bledsoe, Clayden, *Prehospital Emergency Pharmacology*, 6th edition (0-13-150711-7)
This text and handy reference is a complete guide to the most common medications used in prehospital care.

TRAUMA

Campbell, *International Trauma Life Support for Paramedics and Advanced Providers*, 6th edition (0-13-237982-1)
Best-selling BTLS text provides a complete course that covers all the skills necessary for rapid assessment, resuscitation, stabilization, and transportation of the trauma patient.

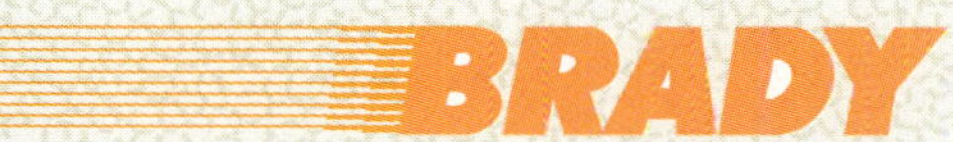

Essentials of Paramedic Care

SECOND EDITION

UPDATE

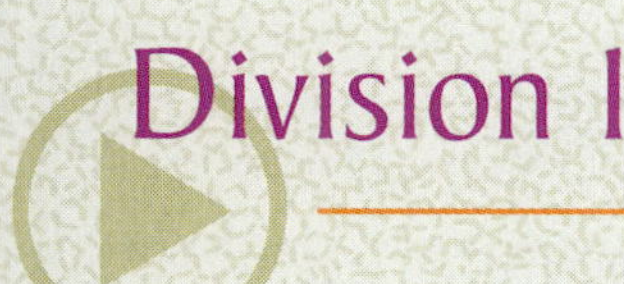

Division 1

Introduction to Advanced Prehospital Care

Chapter

1

Introduction to Advanced Prehospital Care

Objectives

Part 1: Introduction to Advanced Prehospital Care (begins on p. 6)

After reading Part 1 of this chapter, you should be able to:

1. Describe the relationship between the paramedic and other members of the allied health professions. (pp. 6–7)
2. Identify the attributes and characteristics of the paramedic. (p. 7)
3. Explain the elements of paramedic education and practice that support its stature as a profession. (p. 7)
4. Define and give examples of the expanded scope of practice for the paramedic. (p. 8)

Part 2: EMS Systems (begins on p. 8)

After reading Part 2 of this chapter, you should be able to:

1. Describe key historical events that influenced the national development of Emergency Medical Services (EMS) systems. (pp. 9–12)
2. Define the following terms:

   certification (p. 16), EMS systems (p. 8), ethics (p. 53), health care professional (p. 17), licensure (p. 16), medical direction (pp. 13–14), peer review (p. 21), profession (p. 16), professionalism (p. 21), protocols (p. 14), and registration (p. 16).
3. Identify national groups important to the development, education, and implementation of EMS as well as the role of national associations, the National Registry of EMTs, and the roles of various EMS standard-setting agencies. (pp. 17–18)
4. Identify the standards (components) of an EMS system as defined by the National Highway Traffic Safety Administration. (p. 11)

5. Differentiate among EMS provider levels: First Responder, Emergency Medical Technician-Basic, Emergency Medical Technician-Intermediate, and Emergency Medical Technician-Paramedic. (p. 17)
6. Describe what is meant by "citizen involvement in the EMS system." (p. 14)
7. Discuss the role of the EMS physician in providing medical direction, prehospital and out-of-hospital care as an extension of the physician, the benefits of on-line and off-line medical direction, and the process for the development of local policies and protocols. (pp. 13–14)
8. Describe the relationship between a physician on the scene, the paramedic on the scene, and the EMS physician providing on-line medical direction. (p. 13)
9. Describe the components of continuous quality improvement and analyze its contribution to system improvement, continuing medical education, and research. (pp. 20–21)
10. Describe the importance, basic principles, process of evaluating and interpreting, and benefits of research. (pp. 21–23)

Part 3: Roles and Responsibilities of the Paramedic (begins on p. 23)

After reading Part 3 of this chapter, you should be able to:

1. Describe the attributes of a paramedic as a health care professional. (pp. 27–30)
2. Describe the benefits of paramedic continuing education and the importance of maintaining one's paramedic license/certification. (pp. 30–31)
3. List the primary and additional responsibilities of paramedics. (pp. 23–27)
4. Define the role of the paramedic relative to the safety of the crew, the patient, and bystanders. (p. 25)
5. Describe the role of the paramedic in health education activities related to illness and injury prevention. (p. 26)
6. Describe examples of professional behaviors in the following areas: integrity, empathy, self-motivation, appearance and personal hygiene, self-confidence, communications, time management, teamwork and diplomacy, respect, patient advocacy, and careful delivery of service. (pp. 28–30)
7. Identify the benefits of paramedics teaching in their community. (p. 26)
8. Analyze how the paramedic can benefit the health care system by supporting primary care for patients in the prehospital setting. (p. 25)
9. Describe how professionalism applies to the paramedic while on and off duty. (p. 28)

Part 4: The Well-Being of the Paramedic (begins on p. 31)

After reading Part 4 of this chapter, you should be able to:

1. Discuss the concept of wellness and its benefits, components of wellness, and role of the paramedic in promoting wellness. (p. 31)
2. Discuss how cardiovascular endurance, weight control, muscle strength, and flexibility contribute to physical fitness. (pp. 31–34)
3. Describe the impact of shift work on circadian rhythms. (pp. 42–43)
4. Discuss the contributions that periodic risk assessments and warning sign recognition make to cancer and cardiovascular disease prevention. (pp. 32–33)

5. Differentiate proper from improper body mechanics for lifting and moving patients in emergency and nonemergency situations. (pp. 33–34)
6. Describe the problems that a paramedic might encounter in a hostile situation and the techniques used to manage the situation. (pp. 45–50)
7. Describe the considerations that should be given to using escorts, dealing with adverse environmental conditions, using lights and siren, proceeding through intersections, and parking at an emergency scene. (pp. 46–47)
8. Discuss the concept of "due regard for the safety of all others" while operating an emergency vehicle. (p. 47)
9. Describe the equipment available in a variety of adverse situations for self-protection, including body substance isolation steps for protection from airborne and bloodborne pathogens. (pp. 35–38, 45, 46–47)
10. Given a scenario where equipment and supplies have been exposed to body substances, plan for the proper cleaning, disinfection, and disposal of the items. (p. 37)
11. Describe the benefits and methods of smoking cessation. (p. 33)
12. Identify and describe the three phases of the stress response, factors that trigger the stress response, and causes of stress in EMS. (pp. 41–43)
13. Differentiate between normal/healthy and detrimental physiological and psychological reactions to anxiety and stress. (pp. 43–44)
14. Describe behavior that is a manifestation of stress in patients and those close to them, and describe how that behavior relates to paramedic stress. (pp. 44–45)
15. Identify and describe the defense mechanisms and management techniques commonly used to deal with stress, discuss research about possible problems in the use of critical incident stress management (CISM), and identify the appropriate mental health services that should be available to EMS personnel. (pp. 44–45)
16. Given a scenario involving a stressful situation, formulate a strategy to help adapt to the stress. (pp. 44–45)
17. Describe the stages of the grieving process (Kübler-Ross) and the unique challenges for paramedics in dealing with themselves, adults, children, and other special populations related to their understanding or experience of death and dying. (pp. 38–41)
18. Given photos of various motor-vehicle collisions, assess scene safety and propose ways to make the scene safer. (pp. 46–47)

Part 5: Illness and Injury Prevention (begins on p. 47)

After reading Part 5 of this chapter, you should be able to:

1. Describe the incidence; morbidity; and mortality; and the human, environmental, and socioeconomic impact of unintentional and alleged unintentional injuries. (pp. 47–48)
2. Identify health hazards and potential crime areas within the community. (pp. 50–51)
3. Identify local municipal and community resources available for physical, socioeconomic crises. (pp. 48–49, 52–53)
4. List the general and specific environmental parameters that should be inspected to assess a patient's need for preventive information and direction. (pp. 50–53)

5. Identify the role of EMS in local municipal and community prevention programs. (pp. 47, 48–53)
6. Identify the injury and illness prevention programs that promote safety for all age populations. (pp. 50–53)
7. Identify patient situations where the paramedic can intervene in a preventive manner. (pp. 50–53)
8. Document primary and secondary injury prevention data. (pp. 50–53)

Part 6: Ethics in Advanced Prehospital Care (begins on p. 53)

After reading Part 6 of this chapter, you should be able to:

1. Define ethics and morals and distinguish between ethical and moral decisions in emergency medical service. (pp. 53–54)
2. Identify the premise that should underlie the paramedic's ethical decisions in prehospital care. (pp. 54–55)
3. Analyze the relationship between the law and ethics in EMS. (p. 53)
4. Compare and contrast the criteria used in allocating scarce EMS resources. (pp. 59–60)
5. Identify issues surrounding advance directives in making a prehospital resuscitation decision and describe the criteria necessary to honor an advance directive in your state. (pp. 56–58)

Key Terms

advanced life support (ALS), p. 9
allied health professions, p. 6
anchor time, p. 43
autonomy, p. 55
basic life support (BLS), p. 9
beneficence, p. 54
bioethics, p. 54
burnout, p. 43
certification, p. 16
circadian rhythms, p. 42
cleaning, p. 37
continuous quality improvement (CQI), p. 20
disinfecting, p. 37
Emergency Medical Dispatcher (EMD), p. 15
Emergency Medical Services (EMS) system, p. 8
epidemiology, p. 47
ethics, p. 53
exposure, p. 37
health care professionals, p. 17
incubation period, p. 35
infectious disease, p. 35
injury, p. 47
injury risk, p. 47
injury-surveillance program, p. 48
intervener physician, p. 13
isometric exercise, p. 31
isotonic exercise, p. 31
justice, p. 55
licensure, p. 16
medical direction, p. 10
medical director, p. 13
morals, p. 53
nonmaleficence, p. 54
off-line medical direction, p. 14
on-line medical direction, p. 13
pathogens, p. 35
pathophysiology, p. 23
peer review, p. 21
personal protective equipment (PPE), p. 35
primary care, p. 25
primary prevention, p. 48
profession, p. 16
professionalism, p. 21
protocols, p. 14
quality assurance (QA), p. 20
quality improvement (QI), p. 11
reciprocity, p. 16
registration, p. 16
rules of evidence, p. 21
secondary prevention, p. 48
Standard Precautions, p. 35
standing orders, p. 14
sterilizing, p. 37
stress, p. 41
stressor, p. 41
teachable moment, p. 48
tertiary prevention, p. 48
trauma, p. 10
trauma center, p. 11
triage, p. 9
years of productive life, p. 47

INTRODUCTION

Congratulations on your decision to become an EMT-Paramedic. Before you begin this rewarding endeavor, it is important to understand what the job of a twenty-first century EMT-Paramedic entails.

Emergency Medical Services (EMS) has made significant advances. Roles and responsibilities of the paramedic have advanced accordingly.

Emergency Medical Services (EMS) has made significant advances over the last 30 years. Not that long ago, the ambulance was simply a vehicle that provided rapid, horizontal transportation to the hospital. Today, equipped with the latest in equipment and technology, the ambulance is truly a mobile emergency department. The twenty-first century paramedic is a highly trained health care professional.

Part 1: Introduction to Advanced Prehospital Care

DESCRIPTION OF THE PROFESSION

The paramedic is the highest level of prehospital care provider and the leader of the prehospital care team.

allied health professions *ancillary health care professions, apart from physicians and nurses.*

The paramedic is the highest level of prehospital care provider and the leader of the prehospital care team. As a member of the **allied health professions** (ancillary health care professions, apart from physicians and nurses), the paramedic is highly regarded by society.

The roles and responsibilities of the paramedic are diverse and encompass the disciplines of health care, public health, and public safety. Any of these might come into play on a given day. As EMS research evolves, it is becoming clear that illness and injury prevention are just as important as acute health care and public safety responsibilities (Figure 1-1 ■).

There are many types of EMS system designs and operations. As a paramedic, you may work for a fire department, private ambulance service, third city service, hospital, police department, or other operation. Regardless of the type of service you work for, you are an essential component in the continuum of care. Furthermore, paramedics often serve as a link between various health resources. While twenty-first century paramedics will continue to fill the traditional role of 911 response, they will also find themselves taking on a variety of additional responsibilities. Emerging roles and responsibilities include public education, health promotion, and participation in injury and illness prevention programs. As a consequence of the need to cut costs, you may be charged

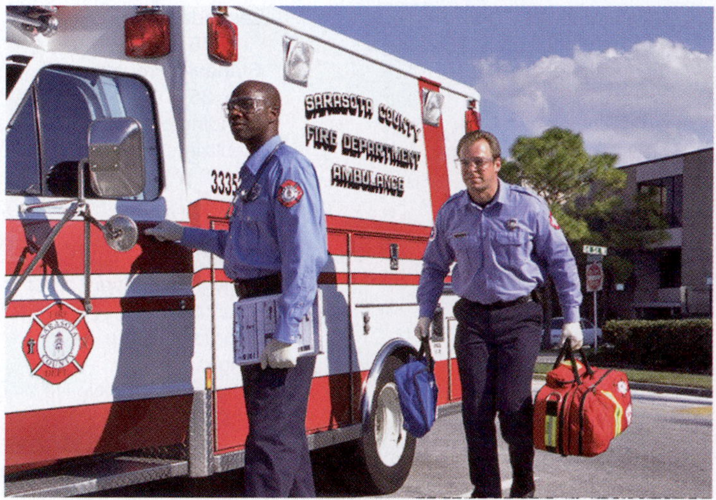

■ **Figure 1-1** The paramedic is the highest level of prehospital care provider and the leader of the prehospital care team.

with assuring that your patient gets to the appropriate health care facility, which may be a facility other than the hospital emergency department. Thus, the paramedic may begin to function as a facilitator of access to care as well a treatment provider.

Paramedics must always strive toward maintaining high-quality health care at a reasonable cost. Nevertheless, you must always be an advocate for your patient and assure that the patient receives the best possible care—without regard to the patient's ability to pay or insurance status.

Paramedics are responsible and accountable to the system medical director, their employer, the public, and their peers. Although this may seem like a difficult standard to meet, if you always act in the patient's best interest, you will seldom run into problems.

You must always be an advocate for your patient and assure that the patient receives the best possible care—without regard to the patient's ability to pay.

Paramedics are accountable to their medical director, their employer, the public, and peers. However, if you always act in the best interest of the patient, you will seldom have problems.

PARAMEDIC CHARACTERISTICS

As a paramedic, you must be a confident leader who can accept the challenge and responsibility of the position. You must have excellent judgment and be able to prioritize decisions so as to act quickly in the patient's best interest. You must be able to develop rapport with a wide variety of patients so that, for example, you can safely interview hostile patients and communicate with members of diverse cultural groups and the various ages within those groups. Overall, you must be able to function independently at an optimum level in a nonstructured, constantly changing environment. The job is never easy and always challenging.

You must be a confident leader—able to function independently at an optimum level in a nonstructured, constantly changing environment. The job is never easy and always challenging.

THE PARAMEDIC: A TRUE HEALTH PROFESSIONAL

Despite its relative youth as a profession, the field of Emergency Medical Services is now recognized as an important part of the health care system. As a paramedic, you must never take this status for granted. Instead, you must always strive to earn your acceptance as a health care professional. Consider the completion of your initial paramedic course to be the start of your professional education, not the end. Participate in continuing education programs. Frequently review and practice skills, especially those less frequently used. Participate in routine peer-evaluation and assume an active role in professional and community organizations.

You must always strive to earn your status as a health care professional.

The current *EMT-Paramedic: National Standard Curriculum* provides for a much improved understanding of the pathophysiology of the various illness and injury processes.

A major step toward the development of EMS as a true health care profession has been to raise the standards of education for prehospital personnel. A significant advance was the 1998 publication by the U.S. Department of Transportation of the revised *EMT-Paramedic: National Standard Curriculum,* which has taken paramedic education to a much higher level. The paramedic course now requires a far more extensive foundation of medical knowledge to underlie the required skills. The 1998 DOT paramedic curriculum is the guideline for this textbook. In 2005, the federal government published the *National EMS Scope of Practice Model* as a part of an integrated plan to strengthen the infrastructure of EMS education as proposed in the *EMS Education Agenda for the Future: A Systems Approach.* This document calls for four levels of EMS providers and details the essential knowledge base and psychomotor skills for each.

As a paramedic, you must actively participate in the design, development, evaluation, and publication of research on topics relevant to your profession. For years, paramedic practice was based on anecdotal data and tradition. Only during the 1990s did we truly begin applying the scientific method to various aspects of prehospital practice. Surprisingly, we found that there were little or no scientific data to support many of our prehospital practices. As a result of research, many traditional EMS treatments have been abandoned or refined. There are still many unanswered questions about paramedic practice, and these can only be answered by sound, ongoing scientific research.

Participation in research projects relevant to EMS is an important part of your profession as a paramedic.

Another essential aspect of a health professional is acceptance and adherence to a code of professional ethics and etiquette. The public must feel confident that, for the paramedic, the patient's and public's interests are always placed above personal, corporate, or financial interests. You must never forget that the patient is your primary concern.

An essential aspect of a health professional is acceptance and adherence to a code of professional ethics and etiquette. The patient is always your primary concern.

EXPANDED SCOPE OF PRACTICE

Paramedics have a very bright future. New technologies and therapies can literally bring the emergency department to the patient. Paramedics must be willing to step up to these expanding roles, or persons from other health care disciplines will fill them. There are many aspects of prehospital care that can provide you with the opportunity to work in an environment other than the typical 911 response vehicle. These include:

- ★ *Critical care transport.* Paramedics manage complicated interhospital transports—typically from one intensive care unit to another—in specially equipped ambulances or aircraft designed to provide a higher level of care.
- ★ *Primary care.* In the era of managed care, one goal is to keep patients with non-emergency problems out of the hospital emergency department. As a result, the EMS system has been involved in triaging and directing patients to the proper nonhospital facilities. In many cases, cost-effective, convenient medical care can be provided in the field by paramedics with additional skills.
- ★ *Tactical EMS.* Paramedics accompany specially trained law enforcement officers on tactical operations such as hostage rescue, drug raids, and similar high-risk emergencies. The tactical paramedic is a member of the operations team but is also trained to provide sophisticated, prolonged, definitive patient care.
- ★ *Industrial medicine.* Paramedics specially trained in occupational health are used to staff construction sites, oil rigs, and other facilities where unique skills are required. These personnel may also serve as safety officers and inspectors.
- ★ *Sports medicine.* Many sports teams hire paramedics to complement their trainers. In this role, paramedics participate in pregame preparation and assume responsibility for injury prevention. They are also trained to deal with injuries specific to the sport, such as orthopedic injuries, with the goal of returning players to action as quickly and safely as possible.

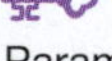

Paramedics are now stepping into new, nontraditional roles because of their unique education and ability to think and work independently.

Paramedics are now stepping into nontraditional roles such as these because of their unique education and ability to think and work independently.

Part 2: EMS Systems

Emergency Medical Services (EMS) system *a comprehensive network of personnel, equipment, and resources established for the purpose of delivering aid and emergency medical care to the community.*

An **Emergency Medical Services (EMS) system** is a comprehensive network of personnel, equipment, and resources established to deliver aid and emergency medical care to the community. An EMS system is comprised of both out-of-hospital and in-hospital components. The out-of-hospital component includes:

- ★ Members of the community who are trained in first aid and CPR
- ★ A communications system that allows public access to emergency services dispatch and allows EMS providers to communicate with each other
- ★ EMS providers, including paramedics
- ★ Fire/rescue and hazardous-materials services
- ★ Public utilities, such as power and gas companies
- ★ Resource centers, such as regional poison control centers

The in-hospital component includes:

- ★ Emergency nurses
- ★ Emergency physicians and specialty physicians
- ★ Ancillary services, such as radiology and respiratory therapy
- ★ Specialty physicians, such as trauma surgeons and cardiologists
- ★ Rehabilitation services

A typical EMS operation begins with citizen activation when someone contacts a 911 dispatch center. EMS dispatch collects essential information and sends out the closest appropriately staffed and equipped unit. In many EMS systems, the dispatcher also provides prearrival instructions to the caller.

The first EMS provider at the scene may be a police officer, firefighter, lifeguard, teacher, or other community member who has been trained as a First Responder. The first responder's role is to stabilize the patient until more advanced personnel arrive. The next EMS provider likely to arrive depends on the type of EMS system. In most areas, the dispatcher will send either a **basic life support** (BLS) or an **advanced life support** (ALS) ambulance. Other EMS systems use a "tiered response," sending multiple levels of emergency care personnel to the same incident. In still other areas, ALS personnel respond to every incident regardless of the level of care needed.

basic life support (BLS) *refers to basic life-saving procedures such as artificial ventilation and cardiopulmonary resuscitation (CPR).*

Once care has been initiated, EMS providers must quickly decide on the medical facility to which the patient should be transported—based on the type of care needed, transport time, and local protocols. Where specialty centers have been designated (such as pediatric, trauma, and burn centers), it may be necessary to transport the patient to a facility other than the closest hospital. At the receiving medical facility, an emergency nurse or physician assumes responsibility, and the patient is assigned a priority of care. If needed, a surgeon or other specialist will be summoned.

advanced life support (ALS) *refers to advanced life-saving procedures such as intravenous therapy, drug therapy, intubation, and defibrillation.*

HISTORY OF EMS

There is evidence that emergency medicine has a very long history.

ANCIENT TIMES

Emergency medicine may be traced back to biblical times when it was recorded that a "good Samaritan" provided care to a wounded traveler by the side of a road. In fact, about 4,000 to 5,000 years ago, Sumerians inscribed clay tablets with some of the earliest medical records. Similar to EMS protocols today, the tablets provided step-by-step instructions for care based on the patient's description of symptoms as well as instructions on how to create and administer medications. The most striking difference between these first "protocols" and EMS today is the absence of a physical exam.

In 1862, the Egyptologist Edwin Smith purchased a papyrus scroll dating to about 1500 B.C.E. It contained 48 medical case histories with data arranged in head-to-toe order and in order of severity, an arrangement very similar to today's patient assessment. One section, the "Book of Wounds," explains the treatment of injuries such as fractures and dislocations.

At about the same time, King Hammurabi of Babylon created a code of laws known today as the "Code of Hammurabi." A section of the code regulated medical fees and penalties based on the social class of the patient. For example, if a surgeon operated successfully on a commoner, he would be paid only half of what his fee would be if he had operated on a rich man. If a surgeon caused the death of a rich man, the surgeon's hand would be cut off, but if a slave died under his care, he only had to replace the slave.

EIGHTEENTH AND NINETEENTH CENTURIES

During the Napoleonic Wars of the early nineteenth century, one of Napoleon's chief surgeons, Jean Larrey, formed the *ambulance volante,* or "flying ambulance," which focused efforts on providing emergency surgery as close to the battlefield as possible. Though the *ambulance volante* was little more than a covered horse-drawn cart, Larrey is credited with the development of the first prehospital system that used **triage** and transport.

triage *a method of sorting patients by the severity of their injuries.*

Between 1861 and 1865, during the U.S. Civil War, a nurse named Clara Barton coordinated care for the sick and injured. Defying army leaders, she persisted in going to the front where wounded men suffered and often died from lack of the simplest medical attention. She organized the triage and transport of injured soldiers to improvised hospitals in nearby houses, barns, and churches away from the battlefield.

The first civilian ambulance service was formed about the same time (1865) in Cincinnati, Ohio. Four years later, in 1869, the New York City Health Department Ambulance Service began operating out of Bellevue Hospital. The ambulances of both services were specially designed horse-drawn carts, which were staffed with physician interns from the various hospital wards.

TWENTIETH CENTURY

During World War I, a high mortality rate of soldiers was associated with an average evacuation time of 18 hours. As a result, in World War II a system was created in which battlefield ambulance corps transported wounded soldiers from the front lines to the echelons (levels) of care. However, many of the echelons were so far from the battlefield and each other that there were huge delays in patient care. In many cases, it was often days from the injury itself to definitive surgery.

During the Korean and Vietnam conflicts, there were great advances in the patient care delivery system. The wounded soldier was treated on the battlefield when the injury occurred and evacuated by helicopter to a field hospital to receive definitive surgery. In Vietnam, in many cases, this occurred within 10 to 20 minutes. Once stabilized and able to be moved (generally within 24 to 48 hours), the patient would be flown by jet to Clark Air Force Base in the Philippines for further treatment. The decrease in the amount of time to definitive care plus the advances in medical procedures significantly reduced mortality rates.

trauma *a physical injury or wound caused by external force or violence.*

Throughout history, significant advances in **trauma** care occurred during wartime. However, until the late 1960s, few areas of the United States provided adequate civilian prehospital emergency care. Medical care began in the hospital emergency department. Rescue techniques were crude, ambulance attendants poorly educated, and equipment minimal. Police, fire, and EMS personnel had no radio communication. Proper medical direction was not available, and the only interaction between physicians and EMS personnel was at the receiving facility.

Eventually, as costs and demand for additional services forced many rural mortician-operated ambulances to withdraw, local police and fire departments found that they had to provide the ambulance service. In many areas, volunteer ambulance services made up of local, independent EMS provider agencies proliferated. In the urban setting, the increased demand on hospital-based EMS systems resulted in the development of municipal services operated on city, county, or regional levels. However, because they could not communicate with each other, it was impossible to coordinate a response to any but the simplest local calls.

Content Review

1973 EMSS Act: 15 Components of EMS Systems

- Manpower
- Training
- Communications
- Transportation
- Emergency facilities
- Critical care units
- Public safety agencies
- Consumer participation
- Access to care
- Patient transfer
- Standardized record keeping
- Public information and education
- System review and evaluation
- Disaster management plans
- Mutual aid

In 1966 the publication of *Accidental Death and Disability: The Neglected Disease of Modern Society* by the National Academy of Sciences, National Resource Council, focused attention on the problem. "The White Paper," as the report was called, spelled out the deficiencies in prehospital emergency care. It suggested guidelines for the development of EMS systems, the training of prehospital emergency medical providers, and the upgrading of ambulances and their equipment. This landmark publication set off a series of federal and private initiatives, including these:

★ *1966.* Congress passed the National Highway Safety Act, which established the U.S. Department of Transportation (DOT), a cabinet-level department. It provided matching grants to states for emergency medical services and forced them to develop effective EMS systems or risk losing federal highway construction funds. In 1969 the Emergency Medical Technician–Ambulance program was made public. The first paramedic curriculum followed in 1977.

★ *1971.* The White House gave nearly $9 million to EMS model demonstration projects.

★ *1972.* The Department of Health, Education, and Welfare funded a $16 million five-state initiative for the development of regional EMS systems. The next year, the Robert Wood Johnson Foundation provided approximately $15 million in grants for establishing regional EMS projects and communication systems.

Then, in 1973 Congress passed the Emergency Medical Services Systems Act, which provided additional funding for a series of projects related to the delivery of trauma care. As a result, the development of regional EMS systems continued from 1974 through 1981. A total of $300 million was allocated to study the feasibility of EMS planning, operations, expansion, and research.

medical direction *medical policies, procedures, and practices that are available to providers either on-line or off-line.*

In order to be eligible for this funding, an EMS system had to include the following 15 components: manpower, training, communications, transportation, emergency facilities, critical care units, public safety agencies, consumer participation, access to care, patient transfer, standardized record keeping, public information and education, system review and evaluation, disaster management plans, and mutual aid. Unfortunately, the designers of this legislation omitted two major components: system financing and **medical direction.** The Emergency Medical Services Systems Act was amended in 1976 and again in 1979, and a total of $215 million was appropriated over a 7-year period toward the establishment of regional EMS systems.

In 1981, the passage of the Consolidated Omnibus Budget Reconciliation Act (COBRA) essentially wiped out federal funding for EMS. The small amount of funding that remained was placed into state preventive-health and health-services block grants. The National Highway Traffic Safety Administration (NHTSA) attempted to sustain the efforts of the Department of Health and Human Services, but with its other EMS responsibilities and no additional funding, the momentum for continued development was lost.

In 1988, the Statewide EMS Technical Assessment Program was established by the NHTSA. It defines elements necessary to all EMS systems. Briefly, they are:

- ★ *Regulation and policy.* Each state must have laws, regulations, policies, and procedures that govern its EMS system. It also is required to provide leadership to local jurisdictions.
- ★ *Resources management.* Each state must have central control of EMS resources so all patients have equal access to acceptable emergency care.
- ★ *Human resources and training.* A standardized EMS curriculum should be taught by qualified instructors, and all personnel who transport patients in the prehospital setting should be adequately trained.
- ★ *Transportation.* Patients must be safely and reliably transported by ground or air ambulance.
- ★ *Facilities.* Every seriously ill or injured patient must be delivered in a timely manner to an appropriate medical facility.
- ★ *Communications.* A system for public access to the EMS system must be in place. Communication among dispatchers, the ambulance crew, and hospital personnel must also be possible.
- ★ *Trauma systems.* Each state should develop a system of specialized care for trauma patients, including one or more **trauma centers** and rehabilitation programs. It also must develop systems for assigning and transporting patients to those facilities.
- ★ *Public information and education.* EMS personnel should participate in programs designed to educate the public. The programs are to focus on the prevention of injuries and how to properly access the EMS system.
- ★ *Medical direction.* Each EMS system must have a physician as its medical director. This physician delegates medical practice to nonphysician caregivers and oversees all aspects of patient care.
- ★ *Evaluation.* Each state must have a **quality improvement** (QI) system in place for continuing evaluation and upgrading of its EMS system.

Many EMS providers today fail to realize that each component of the EMS system has gone through many stages of development. Nevertheless, in this technologically advanced country, there are still startling regional differences in the quality of prehospital care.

Review

Content

1988 NHTSA: "10 System Elements"

- Regulation and policy
- Resources management
- Human resources and training
- Transportation
- Facilities
- Communications
- Trauma systems
- Public information and education
- Medical direction
- Evaluation

trauma center *medical facility that has the capability of caring for the acutely injured patient. Trauma centers must meet strict criteria to use this designation.*

quality improvement (QI) *an evaluation program that emphasizes service and uses customer satisfaction as the ultimate indicator of system performance.*

THE EMS AGENDA FOR THE FUTURE

The EMS Agenda for the Future was published in 1996 as an opportunity to examine what has been learned during the prior three decades and to create a vision for the future for EMS in the United States. This opportunity came at an important time, when those agencies, organizations, and individuals that affect EMS were evaluating its role in the context of a rapidly evolving health care system—an ongoing process of evaluation.

The EMS Agenda for the Future project was supported by the National Highway Traffic Safety Administration and the Health Resources and Services Administration, Maternal and Child Health Bureau. This document focuses on aspects of EMS related to emergency care outside of traditional health care facilities. It recognizes the changes occurring in the health care system of which EMS is a part. EMS of the future will be a community-based health management system that is fully integrated with the overall health care system. EMS of the future will have the ability to identify and modify illness and injury risks, provide acute illness and injury care and follow-up, and contribute to the treatment of chronic conditions and to community health monitoring. EMS will be integrated with other health care providers and public health and public safety agencies in the effort to improve community health, which will result in more appropriate use of acute health care resources. EMS will remain the public's emergency medical safety net.

To realize this vision, *The EMS Agenda for the Future* proposes continued development of 14 EMS attributes. They are:

- ★ Integration of health services
- ★ EMS research
- ★ Legislation and regulation
- ★ System finance
- ★ Human resources
- ★ Medical direction
- ★ Education systems
- ★ Public education
- ★ Prevention
- ★ Public access
- ★ Communication systems
- ★ Clinical care
- ★ Information systems
- ★ Evaluation

This document serves as guidance for EMS providers, health care organizations and institutions, governmental agencies, and policy makers who must be committed to improving the health of their communities and to ensuring that EMS efficiently contributes to that goal. They must invest the resources necessary to provide the nation's population with emergency health care that is reliably accessible, effective, subject to continuous evaluation, and integrated with the remainder of the health system.

The EMS Agenda for the Future provides a vision for out-of-facility EMS. Achieving such a vision requires deliberate action and application of the knowledge gained during the past decades of EMS experience. If pursued conscientiously, it will be an achievement that greatly benefits all of society.

TODAY'S EMS SYSTEMS

Though EMS systems across the country and the world will vary, certain elements are essential to ensure the best possible patient care.

LOCAL AND STATE-LEVEL AGENCIES

At the municipal and regional levels, an administrative agency manages the local EMS system's resources, develops operational protocols, and establishes standards and guidelines. The agency's planning board should include emergency physicians, the emergency nurse association, the firefighter association, state and local police, and "consumers." It develops a budget and selects a qualified administrative staff. The agency designates who may function within the system, develops policies consistent with existing state requirements, and creates a quality assurance or quality improvement program.

State EMS agencies are typically responsible for allocating funds to local systems; sponsoring legislation concerning the prehospital practice of medicine, licensing, and certification; enforcing state EMS regulations; and appointing regional advisory councils.

In essence, EMS is made up of a series of systems within a system. The integration of these systems and the cooperation of all participants help to result in the best quality of emergency care.

MEDICAL DIRECTION

An EMS system must retain a **medical director**—a physician who is legally responsible for all clinical and patient-care aspects of the system. Prehospital medical care provided by nonphysicians is considered an extension of the medical director's license; that is, prehospital care providers are the medical director's designated agents, regardless of who their employers may be.

medical director *a physician who is legally responsible for all of the clinical and patient-care aspects of an EMS system. Also referred to as medical direction.*

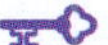

All prehospital care providers are the medical director's designated agents, regardless of who their employer may be.

The medical director's role in an EMS system is to:

★ Educate and train personnel
★ Participate in personnel and equipment selection
★ Develop clinical protocols in cooperation with expert EMS personnel
★ Participate in quality improvement and problem resolution
★ Provide direct input into patient care
★ Interface between the EMS system and other health care agencies
★ Advocate within the medical community
★ Serve as the "medical conscience" of the EMS system, including advocating for quality patient care

In addition to the responsibilities listed previously, the medical director is the ultimate authority for all on-line (direct) and off-line (indirect) medical direction.

On-Line Medical Direction

On-line medical direction occurs when a qualified physician gives direct orders to a prehospital care provider by either radio or telephone (Figure 1-2 ■). Medical direction may be delegated to a mobile intensive care nurse (MICN), a physician assistant (PA), or a paramedic. In all circumstances, ultimate on-line responsibility remains with the medical director.

on-line medical direction *occurs when a qualified physician gives direct orders to a prehospital care provider by either radio or telephone.*

On-line medical direction offers several benefits to the patient, including immediate medical consultation and use of telemetry to provide instant diagnostic information to the medical director. In most systems, on-line consultations can be recorded for review and quality improvement.

At the emergency scene, the provider with the most knowledge and experience in the delivery of prehospital emergency care should be in charge. When a nonaffiliated physician, or **intervener physician,** is on scene and on-line medical direction does not exist, the paramedic should relinquish responsibility to the physician. However, the intervener physician must first identify himself, demonstrate a willingness to accept responsibility, and document the intervention as required by the local EMS system. If his treatment differs from established protocol, the intervener physician must accompany the patient in the ambulance to the hospital. If an intervener physician is on scene and on-line medical direction does exist, the on-line physician is ultimately responsible. In case of a disagreement, the paramedic must take orders from the on-line physician.

intervener physician *a licensed physician, professionally unrelated to patients on scene, who attempts to assist EMS providers with patient care.*

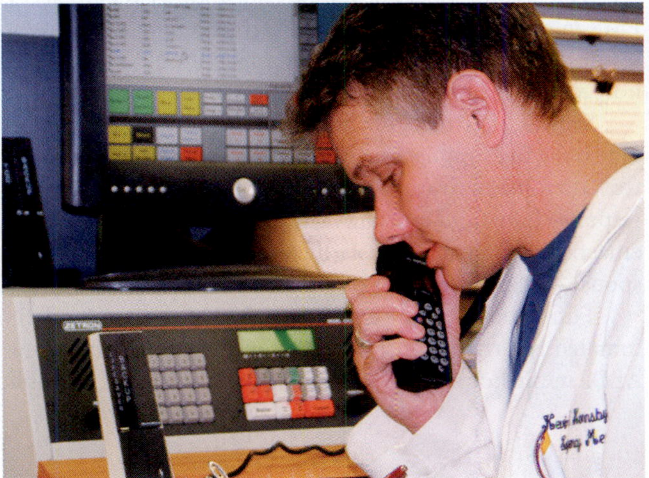

■ **Figure 1-2** The medical director can provide on-line guidance to EMS personnel in the field. *(© Ken Kerr)*

Off-Line Medical Direction

off-line medical direction *refers to medical policies, procedures, and practices that medical direction has set up in advance of a call.*

protocols *the policies and procedures for all components of an EMS system.*

Off-line medical direction refers to medical policies, procedures, and practices that a system physician has set up in advance of a call. It includes "prospective medical direction," such as guidelines on the selection of personnel and supplies, training and education, and protocol development. It also includes "retrospective medical direction," such as auditing, peer review, and other quality assurance processes.

Protocols are the policies and procedures of an EMS system. They provide a standardized approach to common patient problems, a consistent level of medical care, and a standard for accountability. Based on such protocols, the on-line physician can assist prehospital personnel in interpreting the patient's complaint, understanding assessment findings, and providing the appropriate treatment. Protocols are designed around the four "Ts" of emergency care:

Content Review

Four "Ts" of Emergency Care

- Triage
- Treatment
- Transport
- Transfer

★ *Triage.* Guidelines that address patient flow through an EMS system, including how system resources are allocated to meet the needs of patients.

★ *Treatment.* Guidelines that identify procedures to be performed upon direct order from medical direction and procedures that are preauthorized protocols called **standing orders.**

★ *Transport.* Guidelines that address the mode of travel (air vs. ground) based on the nature of the patient's injury or illness, the condition of the patient, the level of care required, and estimated transport time.

★ *Transfer.* Guidelines that address receiving facilities to ensure that the patient is admitted to the one most appropriate for definitive care.

standing orders *preauthorized treatment procedures; a type of treatment protocol.*

Protocols also are established for special circumstances, such as "Do Not Resuscitate" orders, patients who refuse treatment, sexual abuse, abuse of children or elderly people, termination of CPR, and intervener physicians. Although protocols standardize field procedures, they should allow the paramedic the flexibility to improvise and adapt to special circumstances.

PUBLIC INFORMATION AND EDUCATION

The public is an essential, yet often overlooked, component of an EMS system. EMS should have a plan to educate the public on recognizing an emergency, accessing the system, and initiating basic life support procedures.

Recognizing an emergency can save lives. For example, the American Heart Association (AHA) estimates that over 300,000 cardiac arrests per year occur before the patient reaches the hospital. Such arrests are called "sudden death" because most happen within 2 hours of the onset of cardiac symptoms. Many patients delay calling for help when symptoms occur. If the patient and bystanders are taught to recognize the emergency and call for help in time, many cases of sudden death could be prevented.

The second aspect of public education is system access. Citizens must know how to activate EMS in an emergency to avoid life-threatening delays. Whether access is by way of 911 or a local seven-digit phone number, the number should be well publicized, and citizens should be taught how to give the necessary information to the emergency medical dispatcher.

Finally, after recognizing an emergency and activating EMS, citizens must know how to provide basic life support assistance, such as cardiopulmonary resuscitation (CPR) and bleeding control after major trauma. Abundant research indicates that a relationship exists between EMS response times and mortality (death) rates of patients. Communities have proven that when many citizens are trained in basic life support—and there is a rapid advanced life support (ALS) response—a larger number of patients can be successfully resuscitated.

Future public involvement may include bystander defibrillation. With the development of automated external defibrillator (AED) technology, it is now possible to place affordable, portable AEDs in the homes of cardiac patients as well as in all public places.

COMMUNICATIONS

The communications network is the heart of a regional EMS system. A communications plan should include:

- ★ *Citizen access.* A well-publicized universal number, such as 911, provides direct citizen access to emergency services. Multiple community numbers add life-threatening minutes to emergency response times. Enhanced 911, or E-911, gives automatic locations of the caller, instant routing of the call to the appropriate emergency service (fire, police, or EMS), and instant callback capability.
- ★ *Single control center* (Figure 1-3 ■). One control center that can communicate with and direct all emergency vehicles within a large geographical area is best. Ideally, all public service agencies should be dispatched from the same communications center.
- ★ *Operational communications capabilities.* With these, EMS dispatch can manage all aspects of system response and assess the system's readiness for the next response. Emergency units can communicate with each other and with other agencies during mutual aid and disaster operations. Hospitals also can communicate with other hospitals in the region to assess specialty capabilities.
- ★ *Medical communications capabilities.* EMS providers can communicate with the receiving facility and, in many areas, transmit ECG telemetry signals to the on-line physician. Hospitals also can communicate with each other to facilitate patient transfer.
- ★ *Communications hardware.* Radios, consoles, pagers, cell phone transmission towers, repeaters, telephone landlines, and other telecommunications equipment are required.
- ★ *Communications software.* This includes radio frequencies and, in many systems, satellite and high-tech computer programs that track ambulances. Procedures, policies consistent with FCC standards and local protocols, and backup communications plans for disaster operations are essential.

Emergency Medical Dispatcher (EMD)

The **Emergency Medical Dispatcher** (EMD) is crucial to the operation of EMS. EMDs not only send ambulances to the scene, but they also make sure that system resources are in constant readiness to respond. EMDs must be both medically and technically trained. The course should be standardized and include certification by a government agency.

Emergency Medical Dispatcher (EMD) *EMS person medically and technically trained to assign emergency medical resources to a medical emergency.*

EMS Dispatch

Emergency medical dispatching is the nerve center of an EMS system. It should be under the full control of the medical director and the EMS agency. In general, EMS system status management relies on projected call volumes and locations to make strategic placement of ambulances and crews. This method helps to reduce response times. Another management method, "priority dispatching," was first used by the Salt Lake City Fire Department. Using a set of medically approved

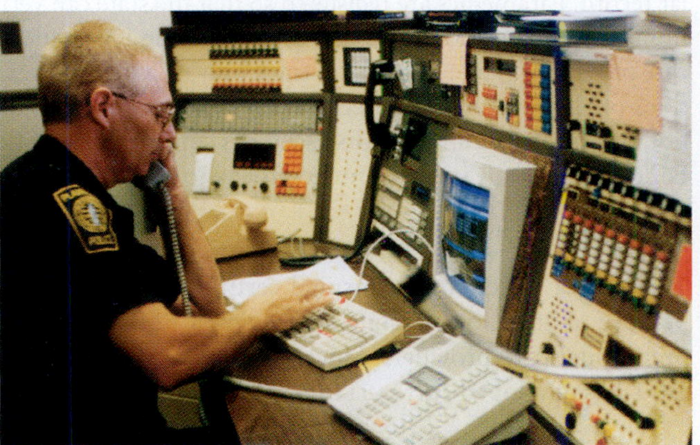

■ Figure 1-3 The ideal communications center can communicate with and control the movement of all emergency units within an EMS system.

protocols, EMDs are trained to medically interrogate a distressed caller, prioritize symptoms, select an appropriate response, and give lifesaving prearrival instructions.

In 1974, the Phoenix Fire Department introduced a prearrival instruction program developed by medically trained dispatchers. In that program, callers initiate lifesaving first aid with the dispatcher's help while they wait for emergency units to arrive on scene. In 1985, the Seattle EMS system initiated a successful program of instructing callers in CPR. Prearrival instruction may result in increased liability, but the liability risk of *not* providing it may far outweigh the risk of providing it.

An effective EMS dispatching system places BLS care on scene within 4 minutes of onset and ALS care in less than 8 minutes.

An effective EMS dispatching system places the first responding units on scene within 4 minutes of the onset of the emergency. The American Heart Association (AHA) reports that brain resuscitation will not be successful unless there is proper BLS intervention (CPR) within 4 minutes. Studies also suggest that defibrillation within 8 minutes can reverse sudden-death mortality. So, the goal of emergency response is: BLS care in less than 4 minutes and ALS care in less than 8 minutes after the event. High-performance systems meet this standard more than 90 percent of the time.

EDUCATION AND CERTIFICATION

EMS education includes both initial and continuing programs. *Initial education* programs are the original training courses for prehospital providers. *Continuing education* programs include refresher courses for recertification and periodic in-service training.

Initial Education

A paramedic's initial education is completion of a course that follows the new National EMS Standards and Instructional Guidelines published by the U.S. DOT, which establishes the minimum content and sets a nationwide standard for paramedic programs. The educational guidelines are divided into three specific learning domains:

- ★ *Cognitive,* which consists of facts, or information knowledge
- ★ *Affective,* which requires students to assign emotions, values, and attitudes to that information
- ★ *Psychomotor,* which consists of hands-on skills students learn while in laboratory and clinical settings

certification *the process by which an agency or association grants recognition to an individual who has met its qualifications.*

licensure *the process by which a governmental agency grants permission to engage in a given occupation to an applicant who has attained the degree of competency required to ensure the public's protection.*

profession *refers to the existence of a specialized body of knowledge or skills.*

registration *the process of entering your name and essential information within a particular record. In EMS this is done in order for the state to verify the provider's initial certification and to monitor recertification.*

reciprocity *the process by which an agency grants automatic certification or licensure to an individual who has comparable certification or licensure from another agency.*

Once initial education is completed, the paramedic will become either certified or licensed, depending on the state. **Certification** is the process by which an agency or association grants recognition to an individual who has met its qualifications. Many states certify paramedics.

Licensure is a process of occupational regulation. Through licensure, a governmental agency (usually a state agency) grants permission to engage in a given trade or **profession** to an applicant who has attained the degree of competency required to ensure the public's protection. Some states choose to license paramedics instead of certifying them. (Note that there is an unfounded general belief that a licensed professional has greater status than one who is certified or registered. However, a certification granted by a state, conferring a right to engage in a trade or profession, is in fact a license.)

Registration is accomplished by entering your name and essential information within a particular record. Paramedics are registered so that the state can verify the provider's initial certification and monitor recertification. Almost every state has an EMS office that tracks the registration of emergency care providers. While some states track only ALS providers, others maintain registers on the certifications of all provider levels. **Reciprocity** is the process by which an agency grants automatic certification or licensure to an individual who has comparable certification or licensure from another agency. For example, some states grant reciprocity to paramedics who are certified in another state.

Certification Levels

There are a variety of prehospital certification levels for communities to choose from. In 1983, because of variations in state and regional EMS terminology, there were as many as 30 levels of prehospital care providers. Since then, the National Registry of EMTs has recognized—and the DOT has developed curricula for—four different levels of providers. They are:

- ★ *First Responder.* Usually the first EMS-trained provider to arrive on scene, the First Responder's role is to stabilize the patient until more advanced EMS personnel arrive.

He is trained to perform a general patient assessment and to provide emergency care such as bleeding control, spinal stabilization, and CPR. He also may assist in emergency childbirth. In some areas, he is trained in the administration of oxygen and in the use of an automated external defibrillator (AED). The first responder level will be called Emergency Medical Responder (EMR) when the new curriculum is developed and ratified.

★ *Emergency Medical Technician-Basic (EMT-B).* This EMS provider is trained to do all that a First Responder can do, plus perform complex immobilization procedures, restrain patients, and drive and staff ambulances. The EMT-Basic also may assist in the administration of certain medications and, in some areas, perform an endotracheal intubation. The EMT-B will be simply referred to as an EMT when the new curriculum is developed and ratified.

★ *Emergency Medical Technician-Intermediate (EMT-I).* The EMT-Intermediate should possess all EMT-Basic skills and be competent in advanced airway management, intravenous fluid therapy, and certain other advanced skills. In some states, the EMT-Intermediate may be trained as a cardiac technician and authorized to administer additional medications. The EMT-I will be referred to as an Advanced EMT (AEMT) when the new curriculum is developed and ratified.

★ *Emergency Medical Technician-Paramedic (EMT-P).* As the most advanced EMS provider, the paramedic is trained in all EMT-I skills, plus advanced patient assessment, trauma management, pharmacology, cardiology, and other medical skills. He should successfully complete advanced cardiac life support (ACLS) and pediatric advanced life support (PALS) courses offered by the American Heart Association. Basic trauma life support (BTLS) or prehospital trauma life support (PHTLS) course completion is also desirable. The EMT-Paramedic will be simply referred to as a Paramedic when the new curriculum is developed and ratified.

Content Review

EMS Certification Levels

- First Responder
- EMT-Basic
- EMT-Intermediate
- EMT-Paramedic

The training of prehospital personnel is a critical phase of EMS system design. In addition to gaining the knowledge and skills necessary to perform their jobs well, paramedics should graduate with the high regard for human dignity and passion for excellence expected of all **health care professionals.**

health care professionals *properly trained and licensed or certified providers of health care.*

National Registry of EMTs

The National Registry of Emergency Medical Technicians (NREMT) prepares and administers standardized tests for the First Responder, EMT-Basic, EMT-Intermediate, and EMT-Paramedic. It establishes the qualifications for registration and serves as a major tool for reciprocity by providing a process for EMTs to become certified when moving from one state to another. The National Registry also develops and evaluates EMT training programs. Currently, the majority of states use National Registry examinations. Several states instead offer locally developed examinations.

Professional Organizations

Belonging to a professional organization is a good way to keep informed and share ideas. National EMS organizations include:

★ National Association of Emergency Medical Technicians (NAEMT)
★ National Association of Search and Rescue (NASAR)
★ National Association of State EMS Directors (NASEMSD)
★ National Association of EMS Physicians (NAEMSP)
★ International Flight Paramedics Association (IFPA)
★ National Council of State EMS Training Coordinators (NCSEMSTC)
★ National EMS Management Association (NEMSMA)

These are just some examples of organizations through which EMS providers can enrich themselves and pursue their particular interests. Such organizations assist in the development of educational programs, operational policies and procedures, and the implementation of EMS. The Joint Review Committee on Educational Programs for the EMT-Paramedic is an example of a standard-setting organization. With input from national professional groups such as the NAEMT, it establishes national standardization within the didactic and clinical portion of paramedic education programs.

Professional Journals

The following is just a partial list of the many journals that are available to keep the paramedic aware of the latest changes in this ever-changing industry. They also offer an opportunity for EMS professionals to write and publish articles:

- ★ *Annals of Emergency Medicine*
- ★ *Emergency Medical Services*
- ★ *Journal of Emergency Medical Services*
- ★ *Journal of Emergency Medicine*
- ★ *Journal of Pediatric Emergency Medicine*
- ★ *Journal of Trauma*
- ★ *Prehospital Emergency Care*

PATIENT TRANSPORTATION

Patients who are transported under the direction of an EMS system should be taken to the nearest appropriate medical facility whenever possible. Medical direction should designate that facility, based on the needs of the patient and the availability of services. In some cases, the patient's need for special services (such as care for burns) means designating a facility that is not nearby. At other times, the closest facility will be designated for stabilization of the patient while transfer is arranged. The ultimate authority for this decision remains with on-line medical direction.

Patients may be transported by ground or air. Today, trauma care systems use law enforcement, municipal, hospital-based, private, and military helicopter transport services to transfer patients. Fixed-wing aircraft also are used when patients must be transported long distances, usually more than 200 miles.

All transport vehicles must be licensed and meet local and state EMS requirements. In 1983, the American College of Surgeons Committee on Trauma recommended a standard set of equipment to be carried by providers of BLS services. In 1988, the American College of Emergency Physicians (ACEP) recommended a list of ALS supplies and equipment. These recommendations serve as guidelines for all prehospital EMS systems. Regional standardization of equipment and supplies is most effective in facilitating interagency efforts during disaster operations.

In 1974, in response to a request from the DOT, the General Services Administration developed the "KKK-A-1822 Federal Specifications for Ambulances." This was the first attempt at standardizing ambulance design. The act defined the following basic types of ambulances:

- ★ *Type I.* A conventional cab and chassis on which a module ambulance body is mounted, with no passageway between the driver's and patient's compartments.
- ★ *Type II.* A standard van, body, and cab form an integral unit. Most have a raised roof.
- ★ *Type III.* A specialty van with forward cab, integral body, and a passageway from the driver's compartment to the patient's compartment.

Only these certified ambulances may display the registered "Star of Life" symbol as defined by the National Highway Traffic Safety Administration (NHTSA). The word *ambulance* should appear in mirror image on the front so that other drivers can identify the ambulance in their rear-view mirrors.

Many services now place a variety of specialized equipment on board ambulances, including specialty rescue, HAZMAT, and additional advanced life support equipment. This has often meant exceeding the gross vehicle weight and has resulted in introduction of a medium-duty truck chassis built for rugged durability and large storage and work areas. Another newer type of ambulance, developed for fuel economy, is the diesel hybrid ambulance. Ambulance standards will continue to evolve.

In 1980, the revision "KKK-A-1822A" aimed at improving ambulance electrical systems by designing a low-amp lighting system to replace antiquated light bars and beacons. In 1985, another revision "KKK-A-1822B" specified changes based on the National Institute for Occupational Safety and Health (NIOSH) standards. These include reduced internal siren noise, high engine temperatures, and exhaust emissions; safer cot-retention systems; wider axles; handheld spotlights; battery conditioners for longer life; and venting systems for oxygen compartments. In 2002, revision "KKK-A-1822E" provided guidelines to improve occupant protection in the patient compartment including additional occupant restraints, more rounded interior corners, and more secure locations of the sharps container for needles and other potentially dangerous items.

All ambulances purchased with federal funds must comply with the KKK criteria. However, some states have adopted their own stricter criteria.

RECEIVING FACILITIES

Not all hospitals are equal in emergency and support service capabilities. So how do you get the right patient to the right facility in an appropriate amount of time? EMS systems categorize hospitals according to their ability to receive and treat emergency patients. EMS coordinators use these categories to quickly identify the most appropriate facility for definitive treatment or life-saving stabilization. Regionalizing available services also helps give all patients reasonable access to the appropriate facility. Burn, trauma, pediatric, psychiatric, perinatal, cardiac, spinal, and poison centers are examples of specialty service facilities that offer high-level care for specific groups of patients in a wide region. Large EMS systems should designate a resource hospital that will coordinate specialty resources and ensure appropriate patient distribution.

To select the appropriate receiving facility for your patient, it is important to know which facilities in your area offer the following services:

- ★ Fully staffed and equipped emergency department
- ★ Trauma care capabilities
- ★ Operating suites available 24 hours a day and 7 days a week
- ★ Critical care units, such as post-anesthesia recovery rooms and surgical intensive care units
- ★ Cardiac facilities with on-staff cardiologists
- ★ Neurology department that provides a "stroke team"
- ★ Acute hemodialysis capability
- ★ Pediatric capabilities, including pediatric and neonatal intensive care units
- ★ Obstetric capabilities, including facilities for high-risk delivery
- ★ Radiological specialty capabilities, such as computerized tomography (CT) and magnetic resonance imaging (MRI)
- ★ Burn specialization for infants, children, and adults
- ★ Acute spinal-cord and head-injury management capability
- ★ Rehabilitation staff and facilities
- ★ Clinical laboratory services
- ★ Toxicology, including hazmat decontamination facilities
- ★ Hyperbaric oxygen therapy capability
- ★ Microvascular surgical capabilities for replants
- ★ Psychiatric facilities

Receiving facilities are categorized by the level of care they can provide. For example, the American College of Surgeons categorizes trauma centers by levels:

- ★ *Level I*—provides the highest level of trauma care
- ★ *Level II*—may not have specialty pediatrics or a neurosurgeon on site
- ★ *Level III*—generally does not have immediate surgical facilities available

A fourth designation may be given to specialty referral centers, which offer unique services. They include burn, pediatric, psychiatric, perinatal, cardiac, spinal, and poison centers.

Ideally, all receiving facilities should have the following capabilities: an emergency department with an emergency physician on duty at all times, surgical facilities, a lab and blood bank, X-ray capabilities available around the clock, and critical and intensive care units. They should have a documented commitment to participate in the EMS system, a willingness to receive all emergency patients in transport regardless of their ability to pay, and medical audit procedures to ensure quality care and medical accountability. Finally, receiving facilities should exhibit a desire to participate in multiple-casualty preparedness plans.

MUTUAL AID AND MASS-CASUALTY PREPARATION

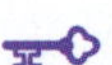

Each EMS system should have a disaster plan that is practiced frequently.

The only acceptable quality of an EMS system is excellence.

The resources of any one EMS system can be overwhelmed. A mutual-aid agreement ensures that help is available when needed. Such agreements may be between neighboring departments, municipalities, systems, or states. Cooperation must transcend geographical, political, and historical boundaries.

Each EMS system should have a disaster plan for catastrophes that can overwhelm available resources. There should be a coordinated central management agency, integration of all EMS system components, and a flexible communications system. Frequent drills should test the plan's effectiveness and practicality.

Content Review

Guidelines for Quality Improvement

- Leadership
- Information and analysis
- Strategic quality planning
- Human resources development and management
- EMS process management
- EMS system results
- Satisfaction of patients and other stakeholders

QUALITY ASSURANCE AND IMPROVEMENT

The only acceptable quality of an EMS system is excellence. In 1997, the National Highway Traffic Safety Administration (NHTSA) released a manual called *A Leadership Guide to Quality Improvement for Emergency Medical Services Systems.* Its guidelines are based on the following components:

★ Leadership
★ Information and analysis
★ Strategic quality planning
★ Human resources development and management
★ EMS process management
★ EMS system results
★ Satisfaction of patients and other stakeholders

quality assurance (QA) *a program designed to maintain continuous monitoring and measurement of the quality of clinical care delivered to patients.*

continuous quality improvement (CQI) *a program designed to refine and improve an EMS system, emphasizing customer satisfaction.*

A **quality assurance (QA)** program monitors and measures the quality of clinical care delivered to patients through evaluation of objective data such as response times, adherence to protocols, patient survival, and other key indicators. QA programs document the effectiveness of the care provided. They also help to identify problems and selected areas that need improvement. A common complaint about QA programs is that they tend to identify only the problems and therefore focus only on punitive corrective action. Thus, prehospital personnel often view QA programs negatively.

As a result, many EMS systems have taken QA a step further with a **continuous quality improvement (CQI)** program. A CQI program emphasizes customer satisfaction and includes evaluations of such aspects as billing and maintenance. In contrast to QA programs, CQI focuses on recognizing, rewarding, and reinforcing good performance. The dynamic process of CQI includes six basic steps: researching and identifying systemwide problems; elaborating on the probable causes; listing possible solutions; outlining a plan of corrective action; providing the resources and support needed to ensure the plan's success; and reevaluating results continuously.

In general, EMS quality can be divided into two categories: "take-it-for-granted" quality and service quality.

"Take-It-for-Granted" Quality

People must be able to take it for granted that EMS will respond quickly to a 911 call and act at the highest level of **professionalism,** providing care that is safe, appropriate, and the best that is available.

professionalism *the conduct or qualities that characterize a practitioner in a particular field or occupation.*

When considering a new medication, process, or procedure, we must follow set rules before permitting its use in EMS. These rules, often called **rules of evidence,** were developed by Joseph P. Ornato, MD, PhD. They include the following guidelines:

rules of evidence *guidelines for permitting a new medication, process, or procedure to be used in EMS on the basis of proven efficacy.*

- ★ *There must be a theoretical basis for the change.* That is, the change must make sense based on relevant medical science.
- ★ *There must be ample research.* Any device or medication for patient care must be justified by adequate scientific human research.
- ★ *It must be clinically important.* The device, medication, or procedure must make a significant clinical difference to the patient. For example, a defibrillator may mean the difference between living and dying for some patients, while color-coordinated stretcher linen has little clinical significance.
- ★ *It must be practical, affordable, and teachable.* Some medical devices remain too expensive and too impractical for use in routine prehospital emergency care.

Another way to accomplish "take-it-for-granted" quality improvement is through the ongoing education of personnel. Paramedics can improve their skills by reading, taking classes, soliciting feedback on clinical performance from receiving hospitals, and following up on patients. **Peer review**—the process of EMS personnel reviewing each other's patient reports, emergency care, and interactions with patients and families—is another way for paramedics to improve their knowledge and skills.

peer review *an evaluation of the quality of emergency care administered by an individual, which is conducted by that individual's peers (others of equal rank). Also, an evaluation of articles submitted for publication.*

Ethics are the standards that govern the conduct of a group or profession. Prehospital providers at all levels have an ethical responsibility to their patients and to the public. The public expects excellence from the EMS system, and we should accept no less than excellence from ourselves.

Service Quality

In the business world, service quality is called "customer satisfaction." This is the kind of quality that individual customers get excited about, feel good about, and tell stories about. These are the little extras that exceed a customer's expectations and elicit thank-you letters. Prime examples of customer satisfaction include patient statements such as: "You fed my cat before we left." "You remembered my name and introduced me to the nurse." "You held my hand." "You seemed like a friend when I needed one."

Customer satisfaction can be created or destroyed with a simple word or deed. A significant part of the way we communicate with one another is through body language and tone of voice. Paramedics who genuinely care about their patients communicate it in many subtle ways. From the patient's perspective this is much more important than IVs, backboards, and ECGs.

Customer satisfaction can be created or destroyed with a simple word or deed.

RESEARCH

The future enhancement of EMS is strongly dependent on the availability of quality research. The current trend of introducing "new and improved" ideas or new "high tech" equipment to existing procedures must be evaluated scientifically. Unfortunately, many EMS protocols and procedures in use today have evolved without clinical evidence of usefulness, safety, or benefit to the patient. One area that will rely heavily on research is funding. As managed care increases its influence, EMS systems will be forced to validate their effectiveness. Restrictions on reimbursement will drive the push for quality EMS research. Outcome studies will also be required to justify funding and assure the future of EMS.

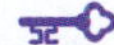

The future enhancement of EMS is strongly dependent on the availability of quality research.

Future EMS research must address the following issues: Which prehospital interventions actually reduce morbidity and mortality? Are the benefits of certain field procedures worth the potential risks? What is the cost-benefit ratio of sophisticated prehospital equipment and procedures? Is field stabilization possible, or should paramedics begin immediate transport in every case?

Paramedics can play a valuable role in data collection, evaluation, and interpretation of research. The components of a research project include the following:

- ★ Identify a problem, explain the reason for the proposed study, and state the hypothesis or a precise question.
- ★ Identify the body of published knowledge on the subject.
- ★ Select the best design for the study, clearly outline all logistics, examine all patient-consent issues, and get them approved through the appropriate investigational review process.
- ★ Begin the study, and collect raw data.
- ★ Analyze and correlate your data in a statistical application.
- ★ Assess and evaluate the results against the original hypothesis or question.
- ★ Write a concise, comprehensive description of the study for publication in a medical journal.

Current EMS practice must be justified by hard clinical data derived from an objective, valid program of ongoing research. EMS providers at all levels share the responsibility for identifying research opportunities, conducting peer review programs, and publishing the results of their projects. As leaders in the prehospital care environment, paramedics should set an example in the development of and participation in research projects.

Evidence-Based Medicine

For many years, EMS practice has been based on anecdotes and unproven theories. Today, EMS personnel must base their practice on sound scientific evidence. Because of this, all paramedics must fundamentally understand EMS research.

A movement has been building in the house of medicine called *evidence-based medicine (EBM)*. This movement has been widely embraced by those in emergency medicine. It is only logical that the principles of EBM be applied to EMS. After all, EMS is an extension of the practice of emergency medicine. There is really nothing all that new about EBM. Its roots can be traced back to the mid-nineteenth century and earlier. The current resurgence of EBM began in Great Britain and has spread throughout the medical world.

EBM is the conscientious, explicit, and judicious use of the current best evidence in making decisions about the care of individual patients. It requires combining clinical expertise with the best available clinical evidence from systematic research. Thus, to practice effective EBM, EMS personnel must first be proficient in prehospital care and exercise sound clinical judgment. These traits can only be developed following a comprehensive initial education program, followed by clinical experience and practice.

To move to the next level, prehospital personnel must be familiar with the current and past research pertinent to prehospital care and be able to integrate that knowledge into the care of individual patients. An essential skill is knowing how to read and interpret the scientific literature and to determine whether the information is sound. (Again, refer to the Appendix, Research in EMS, which discusses how to read and evaluate research.)

External clinical evidence can invalidate previously accepted treatments and procedures and replace them with new ones that are more powerful, more effective, and safer. Good paramedics can become excellent paramedics by using both their clinical expertise and the best available external evidence. In today's medical setting, neither clinical experience nor external evidence alone is enough; there must always be a balance between the two.

Some might say that EBM is simply "cookbook" medicine. This is simply not true. As previously noted, EBM requires paramedics to be, first, clinically proficient. Anybody can follow simple "cookbook" directions and provide some level of patient care. But to achieve excellent patient care, external evidence can inform but never replace the individual paramedic's clinical expertise. Clinical expertise is required to form the best determination of the optimum treatment for each individual patient.

There has been a trend in EMS over the last decade or so to study the various practices and procedures of prehospital care. When studied, some treatments, such as pneumatic anti-shock garments (PASG), did not stand up to the test. Likewise, some treatments, such as early defibrillation, were found to have significant positive impact on survival following out-of-hospital cardiac arrest.

Looking at this from a different perspective, by using the best research data available, we were able to abandon a practice (PASG) that helped few if any patients. Later, we were able to embrace a practice (early defibrillation) that has saved countless lives through diverse programs that include bystander defibrillation.

Practicing EBM helps to assure that we are providing our patients the best possible care at the lowest possible price.

SYSTEM FINANCING

At present in the United States, a wide variety of EMS system designs exist. EMS can be hospital-based, fire- or police-department-based, a municipal service, a private commercial business, a volunteer service, or some combination. Major differences exist in methods of EMS system finance, too. They range from fully tax-subsidized municipal systems to all-volunteer squads supported solely by contributions.

EMS funding can come from many sources. The most common is fee-for-service revenue, which may be generated from Medicare, Medicaid, private insurance companies, specialty service contracts, or private paying patients. Most of these sources of revenue are referred to as "third-party payers," because payment comes from someone other than the patient. To date, almost all third-party payers require the patient to be transported or the EMS service will not be compensated for a response. Reimbursement may also be based on the level of care the patient receives during transport.

Because of the high costs of health care and complex billing and reimbursement systems, the "Public Utility Model" and the "Failsafe Franchise" are becoming increasingly popular. In these systems, a municipality establishes the design and standards for the contract bid, then periodically—usually every 3 or 4 years—holds a wholesale competition open to the market. The provider firm that wins the contract must manage services properly and efficiently throughout the contract term or face severe penalties, usually in the form of fines. The use of models such as these shifts the financial burden of operating an EMS system from the local community to the service franchise.

Part 3: Roles and Responsibilities of the Paramedic

The roles and responsibilities of the paramedic are dramatically different than they were 10 years ago. Today, paramedic emergency care is an enormous responsibility for which you must be mentally, physically, and emotionally prepared. You will be required to have a strong knowledge of **pathophysiology** and of the most current medical technology. You will have to be capable of maintaining a professional attitude while making medical and ethical decisions about severely injured and critically ill patients (Figure 1-4 ■). You will be required to provide not only competent emergency care but also emotional support to your patients and their families.

pathophysiology *the study of how disease affects normal body processes.*

PRIMARY RESPONSIBILITIES

A paramedic's responsibilities include emergency medical care for the patient and a variety of other responsibilities before, during, and after a call.

Content Review

Primary Responsibilities

- Preparation
- Response
- Scene size-up
- Patient assessment
- Patient management
- Disposition and transfer
- Documentation
- Cleanup, maintenance, and review

PREPARATION

Preparation includes making sure that inspection and routine maintenance have been completed on your emergency vehicle and on all equipment. It means restocking medications and intravenous solutions and checking their expiration dates. In addition, you must be very familiar with:

- ★ All local EMS protocols, policies, and procedures
- ★ Communications system hardware (radios) and software (frequency utilization and communication protocols)

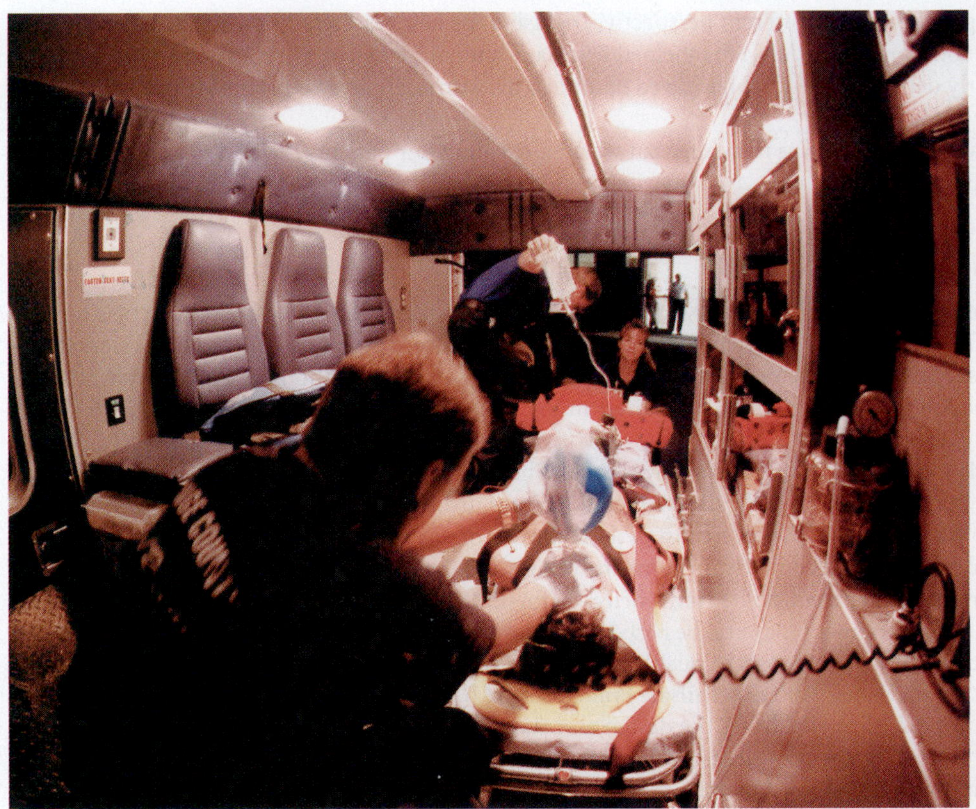

■ **Figure 1-4** A paramedic provides emergency medical care to ill and injured patients. *(© Craig Jackson/In the Dark Photography)*

- ★ Local geography, including populations during peak utilization times, and alternative routes during rush hours
- ★ Support agencies, including services available from neighboring EMS systems and the methods by which efforts and resources are coordinated

RESPONSE

During an emergency response, remember that personal safety is your number one priority. If your ambulance crashes en route to an incident because of speeding or running red traffic lights, you will be of no benefit to the patient. Always follow basic safety precautions en route to an incident. Wear a seat belt, obey posted speed limits, and monitor the road for potential hazards.

You must also get to the scene in a timely manner. Make certain you know the correct location of the incident and, en route, request any additional personnel or services that you think may be needed. Don't wait to ask for such assistance until you get to a chaotic scene. Learn to anticipate potential high-risk situations based on dispatch information and experience. For example, if any of the following is reported to be on scene, you may need to call for assistance:

- ★ Multiple patients
- ★ Motor-vehicle collisions
- ★ Hazardous materials
- ★ Rescue situations
- ★ Violent individuals (patients or bystanders)
- ★ Use of a weapon
- ★ Knowledge of previous violence

PATIENT ASSESSMENT AND MANAGEMENT

Your primary responsibilities as a paramedic involve scene size-up and assessment and management of the patient (Figure 1-5 ■). These topics will be discussed fully in subsequent chapters. Keep in mind that your primary concern is the safety of yourself, your crew, the patient, and bystanders.

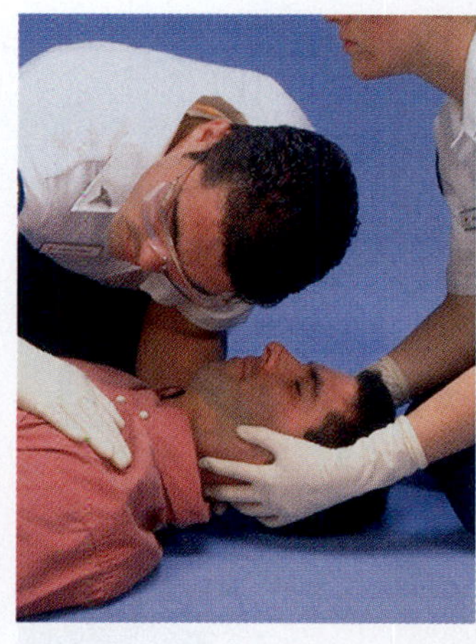

■ Figure 1-5 During the initial assessment of your patient, you will look for and immediately treat any life-threatening conditions.

APPROPRIATE DISPOSITION

As noted earlier, the mode of transport and the selection of receiving facility are critical decisions to be made for your patient. For example, you might opt for ground or air transport. You might choose the nearest medical facility or a facility with special treatment capabilities like burn care or hyperbaric oxygen therapy.

Most patients request transportation to the nearest medical facility. However, patients enrolled in managed care programs, such as health maintenance organizations (HMOs) or designated provider groups, may request transport to a facility approved by their group, which may be a facility other than the nearest hospital. Other patients may ask you to transport them to a facility outside of your run area. Even though the requested facility may be appropriate for the patient, there may be an equally appropriate hospital that is closer. Remember, you are responsible for patient care and, therefore, also ultimately responsible for selecting the transport destination. When in doubt, contact on-line medical direction for advice and support.

In some areas, paramedics provide **primary care.** They have well-defined protocols that allow them to treat patients at the scene and transfer them to facilities other than a hospital. For example, a child cuts his arm on a shard of glass. There is a simple 2-inch laceration. Instead of transporting the patient to the hospital, using resources that are not needed for this patient, and incurring a costly emergency department fee for the family, the paramedics contact medical direction and request permission to transport the child to a local outpatient center.

primary care *basic health care provided at the patient's first contact with the health care system.*

Another type of disposition is "treat and release" in which paramedics assess the patient and provide emergency care. If they determine there is no need for further medical attention, they contact medical direction and request orders not to transport. In some systems, paramedics may then contact a specialized dispatch center where an office appointment is made with a local physician.

While disposition systems such as these are not widely accepted, the increasing numbers of people in managed care programs (which generally attempt to achieve optimum care while controlling costs) may change that. Innovative programs such as these are setting standards for the future of EMS.

PATIENT TRANSFER

The managed-care environment has caused many people—both laypersons and health care providers—to occasionally question whether certain actions that are intended to reduce the cost of medical care are actually in the patient's best interest. For example, to avoid the cost of duplicating equipment and services in a number of facilities that serve the same geographic area, managed care systems have encouraged facilities to specialize and, often, to transfer patients to a facility that can provide the specific care needed.

Occasionally, there may be a question as to whether the transfer of a patient from one facility to another has been approved for cost reasons but may not actually be in the patient's best interest. When you are assigned to transport a patient, you share responsibility—with the receiving and accepting physician—for the treatment and care of the patient. When you are in doubt about the patient's stability for the duration of transport, or about the capabilities of the receiving facility, contact medical direction.

Prior to removing the patient from a hospital, request a verbal report from the primary-care provider (usually a registered nurse or a physician). Also request a copy of essential parts of the patient's chart, including a summary of the patient's past and present medical history. However, if the

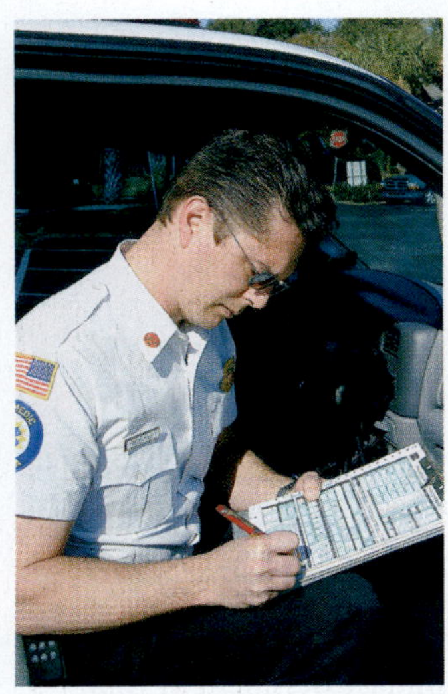

■ Figure 1-6 A paramedic's responsibility does not end with delivering the patient to the emergency department. Documentation, restocking, and a run critique are as important as the call itself.

results of diagnostic tests taken at the facility are not ready when you are prepared to leave, do not delay patient transport. The data can be sent by fax, e-mailed, or telephoned to the receiving facility.

Your first priority during transport is the patient. While en route, contact the receiving facility and provide them with an estimated time of arrival (ETA) and an update on the patient's condition. Upon arrival at your destination, seek out the contact person (usually a registered nurse or physician). Provide that person with an updated patient report, including any treatment or changes in status while en route. All documents provided by the sending facility should be turned over to the receiving care provider along with a copy of your run report. If required by your service, obtain appropriate billing/insurance information at this time.

DOCUMENTATION

Maintaining a complete and accurate written patient care report is essential to the flow of patient information, to research efforts, and to the quality improvement of your EMS system. Documentation will be discussed in detail in Chapter 15.

RETURNING TO SERVICE

Once you have completed patient care, turned the patient over to the hospital staff, and completed all documentation, immediately prepare to return to service (Figure 1-6 ■). Clean and decontaminate the unit, properly discard disposable materials, restock supplies, and replace and stow away equipment. If necessary, refuel the unit on the way back to your station or post. Review the call with crew members, including any problems that may have occurred. Such a dialogue can lead to solutions that enhance the delivery of quality patient care. Finally, the paramedic team leader should check crewmembers for signs of critical incident stress and assist anyone who needs help.

Content Review

Additional Responsibilities

- Community involvement
- Support for primary care
- Citizen involvement
- Personal and professional development

ADDITIONAL RESPONSIBILITIES

The role of the paramedic involves duties in addition to those associated with emergency response. They may include training civilians in CPR, EMS demonstrations and seminars, teaching first aid classes, organizing prevention programs, and engaging in professional development activities. All involve taking an active role in promoting positive health practices in your community.

COMMUNITY INVOLVEMENT

Prehospital providers should take the lead in helping the public learn how to recognize an emergency, how to provide basic life support (BLS), and how to properly access the EMS system. A successful effort can save lives. Providing educational programs can also encourage positive health practices in the community, such as the American Heart Association's "prudent heart living" campaign. EMS injury prevention projects, such as seat belt awareness and the proper use of child safety seats, are essential to the reduction of long-term disability and accidental death.

In order to decide what injury prevention projects need to be developed in a community, EMS systems often conduct illness and injury risk surveys. For example, an EMS service reviews run reports for a 6-month period and finds they responded to 10 vehicle collisions at railroad crossings. A public safety campaign directed at the safe crossing of railroad tracks may be appropriate. Once an EMS service has identified a problem and target audience, they should seek community agencies—including the local political structure—to assist in the development, promotion, and delivery of the campaign.

Additional benefits of community involvement are the following: It enhances the visibility of EMS, promotes a positive image, and puts forth EMS personnel as positive role models. It also creates opportunities to improve the integration of EMS with other health care and public safety agencies through cooperative programs.

COST CONTAINMENT

Promoting wellness and preventing illness and injury will be important components of EMS in the future. Some systems have already begun to direct resources toward the development of prevention and wellness programs that decrease the need for emergency services. The theory is to reduce the cost of the services provided to the community by decreasing the burden on the system.

One strategy is to establish protocols that specify the mode of transportation for nonemergency patients. Some systems already operate vans rather than ambulances to transport such patients to and from nursing facilities or from their residences to a doctor's office. Though an additional expense to the system, this service reduces emergency equipment costs and the demand for emergency personnel. The result is a decrease in the overall operating expense, which results in an increase in revenue.

Another strategy being used in many areas of the country is having EMS and hospitals team up to provide an alternative to the emergency department. They transport patients to freestanding outpatient centers or clinics, which ultimately reduces the cost of care to the patient and the system. The development of such alliances will undoubtedly continue. However, caution should be taken to ensure that the patient always receives the appropriate emergency care based on need, not cost.

CITIZEN INVOLVEMENT IN EMS

Citizen involvement in EMS helps to give "insiders" an outside, objective view of quality improvement and problem resolution. Whenever possible, members of the community should be used in the development, evaluation, and regulation of the EMS system. When considering the addition of a new service or the enhancement of an existing one, community members should help to establish what is needed. After all, they are your "customers," and their needs are your priority.

PROFESSIONALISM

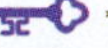

The paramedic is a health care professional.

A paramedic is a member of the health care profession. The word *profession* refers to a specialized body of knowledge or skills. Generally self-regulating, a profession will have recognized standards, including requirements for initial and ongoing education. When you have satisfied the initial education requirements as a paramedic, you may then be either certified or licensed. The EMS profession has regulations that ensure that members maintain standards. For the paramedic, these regulations come in the form of periodic recertification with a specified amount of continuing education time.

The term *professionalism* refers to the conduct or qualities that characterize a practitioner in a particular field. Health care professionals promote quality patient care and pride in their profession, setting and striving for the highest standards and earning the respect of team members and the public. Attaining professionalism requires an understanding of what distinguishes the professional from the nonprofessional.

PROFESSIONAL ATTITUDES

A commitment to excellence is a daily activity. While on duty, health care professionals place their patients first; nonprofessionals place their egos first. True professionals establish excellence as their goal and never allow themselves to become complacent about their performance. They practice their skills to the point of mastery and then keep practicing them to stay sharp and improve. They also take refresher courses seriously, because they know they have forgotten a lot and because they are eager for new information. Nonprofessionals believe their skills will never fade.

Professionals set high standards for themselves, their crew, their agency, and their system. Nonprofessionals aim for the minimum standard and can be counted on to take the path of least resistance. Professionals critically review their performance, always seeking ways to improve. Nonprofessionals look to protect themselves, hide their inadequacies, and place blame on others. Professionals check out all equipment prior to the emergency response. Nonprofessionals hope that everything will work, supplies will be in place, batteries will be charged, and oxygen levels will be adequate.

A professional paramedic is responsible for acting in a professional manner both on and off duty. Remember, the community you serve will judge other EMS providers, the service you work for, and the EMS profession as a whole by your actions.

Professionalism is an attitude, not a matter of pay. It cannot be bought, rented, or faked. Although it is a young industry, EMS has achieved recognition as a bona fide allied health profession. Gaining professional stature is the result of many hard-working, caring individuals who refused to compromise their standards. Always strive to maintain that level of performance and commitment.

Content Review

Professional Attributes

- Leadership
- Integrity
- Empathy
- Self-motivation
- Professional appearance and hygiene
- Self-confidence
- Communication skills
- Time management skills
- Diplomacy in teamwork
- Respect
- Patient advocacy
- Careful delivery of service

PROFESSIONAL ATTRIBUTES

Leadership

Leadership is an important but often forgotten aspect of paramedic training. Paramedics are the prehospital team leaders (Figure 1-7 ■). They must develop a leadership style that suits their personalities and gets the job done. Although there are many successful styles of leadership, certain characteristics are common to all great leaders. They include:

- Self-confidence
- Established credibility
- Inner strength
- Ability to remain in control
- Ability to communicate
- Willingness to make a decision
- Willingness to accept responsibility for the consequences of the team's actions

The successful team leader knows the members of the crew, including each one's capabilities and limitations. Ask crew members to do something beyond their capabilities and they will question your ability to lead, not their ability to perform.

Integrity

The patient and other members of the health care team assume that you, as a paramedic, have integrity. The single most important behavior that you will be judged by is honesty. Your work will often put you in the patient's home or in charge of the patient's wallet and other personal possessions, such as jewelry and items left in a vehicle. You must be trustworthy. The easiest way to lose respect is to be dishonest. Additionally, in acting as an agent of the medical director, you are entrusted with carefully following protocols, providing the best possible care, and accurately documenting it.

Empathy

One of the most important components to successful interaction with a patient and family is empathy. To have empathy is to identify with and understand the circumstances, feelings, and motives of

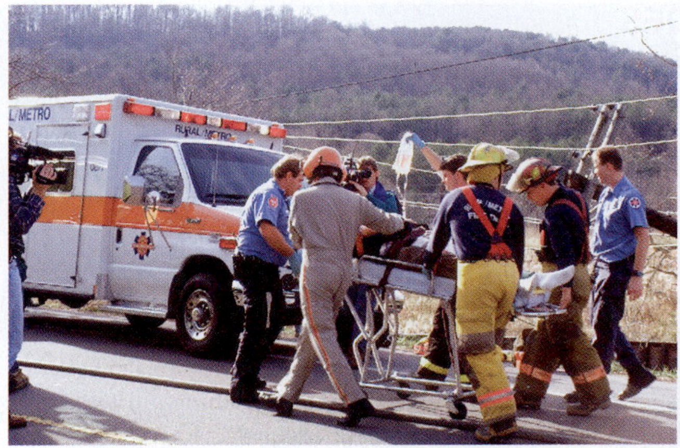

■ Figure 1-7 As leader of the EMS team, the paramedic must interact with patients, bystanders, and other rescue personnel in a professional and efficient manner. *(© Glenn Jackson)*

others. As a professional, you will often have to place your own feelings aside to deal with others, even when you are having a bad day. Paramedics who act in a professional manner can show empathy by:

- ★ Being supportive and reassuring
- ★ Demonstrating an understanding of the patient's feelings and the feelings of the family
- ★ Demonstrating respect for others
- ★ Having a calm, compassionate, and helpful demeanor

Self-Motivation

You will often work without direct supervision, so it is up to you to be able to motivate yourself and establish a positive work ethic. Examples of a positive work ethic are:

- ★ Completing assigned duties without being asked or told to do so
- ★ Completing all duties and assignments without the need for direct supervision
- ★ Correctly completing all paperwork in a timely manner
- ★ Demonstrating a commitment to continuous quality improvement
- ★ Accepting constructive feedback in a positive manner
- ★ Taking advantage of learning opportunities

Appearance and Personal Hygiene

From the moment you arrive at the scene of an emergency, you are judged by the way you present yourself. Good appearance and personal hygiene are critical. If you have a sloppy appearance, your patient may suspect that your medical care will be sloppy, too. Slang, foul, abusive, or off-color language is not acceptable and will alienate you from your patients. Your appearance, as well as your behavior, are vital to establishing credibility and instilling confidence.

Always wear a clean, pressed uniform. Multiple pagers and holsters with tape hanging from them, or rubber gloves pulled through a belt loop, simply do not give you a professional appearance. Also, avoid wearing an abundance of patches and pins on your uniform. Remember that it is the care you provide, not the patches and pins you wear, that will impress the patient. Keep hair off the collar. If facial hair is allowed, keep it neat and trimmed. A light-colored tee shirt may be worn under your uniform shirt, which should be buttoned up, with only the top collar button open. Jewelry, other than a wedding ring, a watch, or small plain earrings for a female, is unprofessional. Long fingernails that have the potential to puncture protective gloves also should be avoided.

Self-Confidence

The patient and family will not trust you if they sense you do not trust yourself. A lack of self-confidence shows and is the basis of many lawsuits. The easiest way to gain self-confidence is to accurately assess your strengths and limitations, then seek every opportunity to improve any weaknesses. Also, keep in mind that self-confidence does not equal cockiness. When a self-confident paramedic is presented with a complex situation, he will ask for assistance.

Communication

Communication is a skill often underestimated in EMS services. Providing emergency care in the prehospital environment requires constant communication with the patient, family, and bystanders, as well as with other EMS providers and rescuers from other public agencies. Communication skills are discussed in detail in later chapters.

Time Management

The experienced paramedic who plans ahead, prioritizes tasks, and organizes them to make maximum use of time will generally be more effective in the field. A paramedic with good time-management skills is punctual for shifts and meetings and completes tasks such as paperwork and maintenance duties on or ahead of schedule.

Some simple time-management techniques that you can use are making lists, prioritizing tasks, arriving at meetings or appointments early, and keeping a personal calendar. By implementing just one or two of these techniques, you may find your schedule to be more manageable and less stressful.

Teamwork and Diplomacy

The paramedic is a leader. Leadership implies the ability to work with other people—to foster teamwork. Teamwork requires diplomacy, or tact and skill in dealing with people, even when you are under siege from the patient or family. Diplomacy requires the paramedic to place the interests of the patient or team ahead of his own interests. It means listening to others, respecting their opinions, and being open-minded and flexible when it comes to change. A strong leader of any team realizes that he will be successful only if he has the support of all team members. A confident leader will:

- Place the success of the team ahead of personal self-interests
- Never undermine the role or opinion of another team member
- Provide support for members of the team, both on and off duty
- Remain open to suggestions from team members and be willing to change for the benefit of the patient
- Openly communicate with everyone
- Above all, respect the patient, other care providers, and the community you serve

Respect

To respect others is to show—and feel—deferential regard, consideration, and appreciation for them. A paramedic respects all patients, and provides the best possible care to each and every one of them, no matter what their race, religion, sex, age, or economic condition. Showing that you care for a patient's or family member's feelings, being polite, and avoiding the use of demeaning or derogatory language toward even the most difficult patients are simple ways to demonstrate respect.

Patient Advocacy

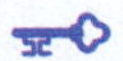

The paramedic should always be an advocate for the patient.

A paramedic is an advocate for patients, defending them, protecting them, and acting in their best interests. Except when your safety is threatened, you should always place the needs of your patient above your own.

Careful Delivery of Service

Professionalism requires the paramedic to deliver the highest quality of patient care with very close attention to detail. Examples of behaviors that demonstrate a careful delivery of service include:

- Mastering and refreshing skills
- Performing complete equipment checks
- Careful and safe ambulance operations
- Following policies, procedures, and protocols

CONTINUING EDUCATION AND PROFESSIONAL DEVELOPMENT

Only through continuing education and recertification can the public be assured that quality patient care is being delivered consistently. So after you are certified and/or licensed, you have an important responsibility to continue your personal and professional development. Remember, everyone is subject to the decay of knowledge and skills over time. Use this as a rule of thumb: As the volume of calls decreases, training should correspondingly increase. Refresher requirements and courses vary from state to state, but the goal is the same: to review previously learned materials and to receive new information.

Since EMS is a relatively young industry, new technology and data emerge rapidly. Make a conscious effort to keep up. A variety of journals, seminars, computer news groups, and learning experiences are available to help. So are professional EMS organizations at the local, state, and national levels. Additionally, by participating in activities designed to address work-related issues—such as case reviews and other quality improvement activities, mentoring programs, research projects, multiple-casualty incident drills, in-hospital rotations, equipment in-services, refresher courses, and self-study exercises—you can expect substantial career growth.

The paramedic must continually strive to stay abreast of changes in EMS.

Part 4: The Well-Being of the Paramedic

Well-being, or wellness, is a fundamental aspect of top-notch performance in EMS. It includes your physical well-being as well as your mental and emotional well-being.

This section discusses the many elements of well-being. If you listen now and enhance your knowledge later, you stand a good chance of enjoying a long and rewarding career of helping others—all because you helped yourself.

Well-being is a fundamental aspect of top-notch performance.

BASIC PHYSICAL FITNESS

The benefits of achieving acceptable physical fitness are well known. They include a decreased resting heart rate and blood pressure, increased oxygen-carrying capacity, increased muscle mass and metabolism, and increased resistance to illness and injury. Quality of life is enhanced, as is self-image. Other benefits are improved mental outlook, reduced anxiety levels, and enhanced ability to maintain sound motor skills throughout life.

CORE ELEMENTS

Core elements of physical fitness are cardiovascular endurance (aerobic capacity), muscular strength, and flexibility. Like a three-legged stool, if any one of the three is deficient, the whole becomes unstable. Each is equally important.

Be careful about plunging into a well-intended effort to get in shape. For example, before starting an exercise or stretching regimen, it can be helpful to measure your current state of fitness. There are various methods of assessing the three core elements of fitness. Many EMS agencies have access to facilities where precise assessment methods—with trained personnel—are available. Take advantage of any information available to you.

Content Review

Basics of Physical Fitness

- Cardiovascular endurance
- Strength and flexibility
- Nutrition and weight control
- Disease prevention
- Freedom from harmful habits and addictions
- Back safety

Muscular strength is achieved with regular exercise that may be isometric or isotonic. **Isometric exercise** is active exercise performed against stable resistance, where muscles are exercised in a motionless manner. **Isotonic exercise** is active exercise during which muscles are worked through their range of motion. Weight lifting is an obvious way to achieve muscular strength, and it is excellent all-around training for the body. Rotate between training the muscles of your upper body and shoulders, chest and back, and lower body. Do abdominal exercises daily. Take time to get in-depth information about the best approach from a trainer or other knowledgeable person.

isometric exercise *active exercise performed against stable resistance, where muscles are exercised in a motionless manner.*

isotonic exercise *active exercise during which muscles are worked through their range of motion.*

Cardiovascular endurance results from exercising at least 3 days a week vigorously enough to raise your pulse to its target heart rate (Table 1–1). There is no need to become a marathon runner to gain aerobic capacity. Try a brisk walk, or ride a stationary bike while watching TV. Make it a daily habit. Even modest exercise helps. Walking briskly from the outer reaches of the employee parking lot, using stairs whenever possible, and playing actively with your children can all "count" toward physical fitness.

Flexibility seems to be the forgotten element of fitness. Without an adequate range of motion, your joints and muscles cannot be used efficiently or safely. A body builder with tight hamstrings may be as much at risk for back injury as anyone else. To achieve (or regain) flexibility, stretch the main muscle groups regularly. Try to stretch daily. Never bounce when stretching; this causes microtears in muscle and connective tissues. Hold a stretch for at least 60 seconds. A side benefit of good flexibility is prevention or reduction of back pain. Stretching is an excellent TV-time activity. If you are interested, consider studying yoga.

Table 1-1 Finding Your Target Heart Rate

1. Measure your resting heart rate. (You will use this total later.)
2. Subtract your age from 220. This total is your estimated maximum heart rate.
3. Subtract your resting heart rate from your maximum heart rate, and multiply that figure by 0.7.
4. Add the figure you just calculated to your resting heart rate.

EXAMPLE: In a 44-year-old woman whose resting heart rate is 52, maximum heart rate would be 176 (220 – 44). Maximum heart rate minus resting heart rate is 124 (176 – 52). Multiply 124 by 0.7 for a value of 86.8. Resting heart rate plus the calculated figure is 138.8 (52 + 86.8). Rounded up, this person's target heart rate is 140 beats per minute.

Content Review

Major Food Groups

- Whole grains
- Fruits and vegetables
- Fats and oils
- Milk and dairy products
- Meat, fish, and beans

NUTRITION

Exercise and good nutrition are fundamental to your well-being. The following are exercise and diet guidelines published as "My Pyramid" by the U.S. Department of Agriculture.

- ★ *Physical activity.* Be physically active at least 30 minutes most days.
- ★ *Whole grains.* Eat at least 3 ounces of whole grain bread, cereal, crackers, rice, or pasta per day.
- ★ *Fruits and vegetables.* Eat 2 cups of fruit and 2½ cups of vegetables each day. Eat more dark green and orange vegetables. Eat a variety of fresh, frozen, canned, or dried fruit (go easy on fruit juices).
- ★ *Fats.* Get most of your fats from fish, nuts, and vegetable oils. Limit solid fats like butter, stick margarine, shortening, and lard.
- ★ *Milk.* Drink 3 cups per day of fat free or low fat milk.
- ★ *Meat and beans.* Choose broiled, baked, or grilled lean meats and poultry. Vary it with fish, beans, peas, nuts, and seeds.

In short, exercise and eat (in moderation) a balanced variety of wholesome foods. (The USDA website MyPyramid.gov provides details about how you can tailor the guidelines to meet your own needs.)

Food labels (Figure 1-8 ■) contain abundant information about nutritional content. Learn to read them. Standardization of food labels has reduced much of the confusion. Be sure to check the serving size to avoid misinterpreting the food's overall nutritional value.

Eating on the run, as EMS providers must often do, can be less detrimental if you plan ahead and carry a small cooler filled with whole-grain sandwiches, cut vegetables, fruit, and other wholesome foods. If you must, stop at a local market instead of the fast-food place next door. Buy fresh fruit, yogurt, and sensible deli selections. They are more nutritious and much cheaper than "fast foods." Monitor your fluid intake. Your body needs plenty of fluids to flush food through your system and eliminate toxins. Fill a "go-cup" with fresh ice water when you stop by the emergency department instead of spending your money on soft drinks.

Nutrition Facts
Serving Size 8 fl oz (240 mL)
Servings Per Container 8

Amount Per Serving	
Calories 110 Calories from Fat 0	
	% Daily Value*
Total Fat 0g	0%
Sodium 0mg	0%
Potassium 450mg	13%
Total Carbohydrate 26g	9%
Sugars 22g	
Protein 2g	
Vitamin C 120% • Calcium 2%	
Thiamin 10% • Niacin 4%	
Vitamin B6 6% • Folate 15%	

Not a significant source of saturated fat, cholesterol, dietary fiber, vitamin A and iron.

* Percent Daily Values are based on a 2,000 calorie diet.

■ Figure 1-8 Example of a standardized food label.

PREVENTING CANCER AND CARDIOVASCULAR DISEASE

Exercising and eating well can help you prevent both cancer and cardiovascular disease. Although for the typically youthful EMS provider, the likelihood of being hit by either of these diseases seems remote, it happens. You can do a lot to prevent it. Minimizing stress through healthy stress management practices, for example, can work wonders. In addition, assess yourself and your family history.

Exercise will improve cardiovascular endurance, help lower blood pressure, and tip the balance of your body composition favorably—all good measures against cardiovascular disease. Know your cholesterol and triglyceride levels, and keep them in check. For women who are menopausal, be informed about the risks and benefits of using hormone replacement therapy (particularly estrogen).

Diet can also do much to minimize the chances of getting certain cancers. Certain foods, such as broccoli and high-fiber foods, can help reduce the incidence of cancer; others, such as charcoal-cooked foods, can increase it. The connection between sun exposure and skin cancer is well known. So, take the precaution of using sunblocks and wear sunglasses and a hat when you can. Watch out for the warning signs of cancer, such as blood in the stools (even in young people, especially men), a changing mole, unexplained weight loss, unexplained chronic fatigue, and lumps.

Be sure to include appropriate periodic risk-assessment screening and self-examination habits in your personal well-being program. That includes tests like mammograms and prostate exams as you gain in years.

HABITS AND ADDICTIONS

Many people who work high-stress jobs overuse and abuse substances such as caffeine and nicotine. These bad habits are rampant in EMS. Each can contribute to long-term diseases such as cancer and cardiovascular disease. Choose a healthier life, and avoid overindulging in these and other harmful substances such as alcohol. For example, smoking cessation programs are usually easily accessed in local areas or on the Internet. Whatever it takes, the message is clear: get free of addictions, particularly those that threaten your well-being. Substance abuse programs, nicotine patches, 12-step groups—all exist to help you help yourself. But the first step has to be yours.

BACK SAFETY

EMS is a physically demanding endeavor. Of the host of movements needed (scrambling down embankments, climbing ladders or trees, squeezing into narrow spaces, and so on), none will be more frequent than lifting and carrying equipment and patients. To avoid back injury, you must keep your back fit for the work you do. You also must use proper lifting techniques each time you pick up a load, whether the load is heavy or light.

Pay particular attention to keeping your back fit for the work you do. Always use the proper techniques for lifting and moving patients and equipment.

Back fitness begins with conditioning the muscles that support the spinal column. These are the "guy wires" that stabilize the spine, much the way cables help keep telephone poles upright. Note that the muscles of the abdomen are also crucial to overall spinal-column strength and safe lifting. Never perform old-fashioned sit-ups. They can seriously strain your lumbar spine. Instead, use abdominal crunches, which target only the stomach muscles. Consult an exercise coach or trainer for specifics.

Correct posture will minimize the risk of back injury (Figure 1-9 ■). Good nutrition helps to maintain healthy connective tissue and intervertebral discs. Excess weight contributes to disc deterioration. So does smoking. Thus, proper weight management and smoking cessation are relevant to back health. Finally, adequate rest gives the spine non-weight-bearing time to nourish discs and repair itself.

Proper lifting techniques should ideally be taught by and practiced with a trainer who understands the variety of challenges faced by EMS providers. Important principles of lifting are as follows:

- ★ Move a load only if you can safely handle it.
- ★ Ask for help when you need it—for *any* reason.
- ★ Position the load as close to your body and center of gravity as possible.
- ★ Keep your palms up whenever possible.
- ★ Do not hurry. Take the time you need to establish good footing and balance. Keep a wide base of support with one foot ahead of the other.
- ★ Bend your knees, lower your buttocks, and keep your chin up. If your knees are bad, do not bend them more than 90 degrees.
- ★ "Lock in" the spine with a slight extension curve, and tighten the abdominal muscles to support spinal positioning.
- ★ Always avoid twisting and turning.
- ★ Let the large leg muscles do the work of lifting, not your back.

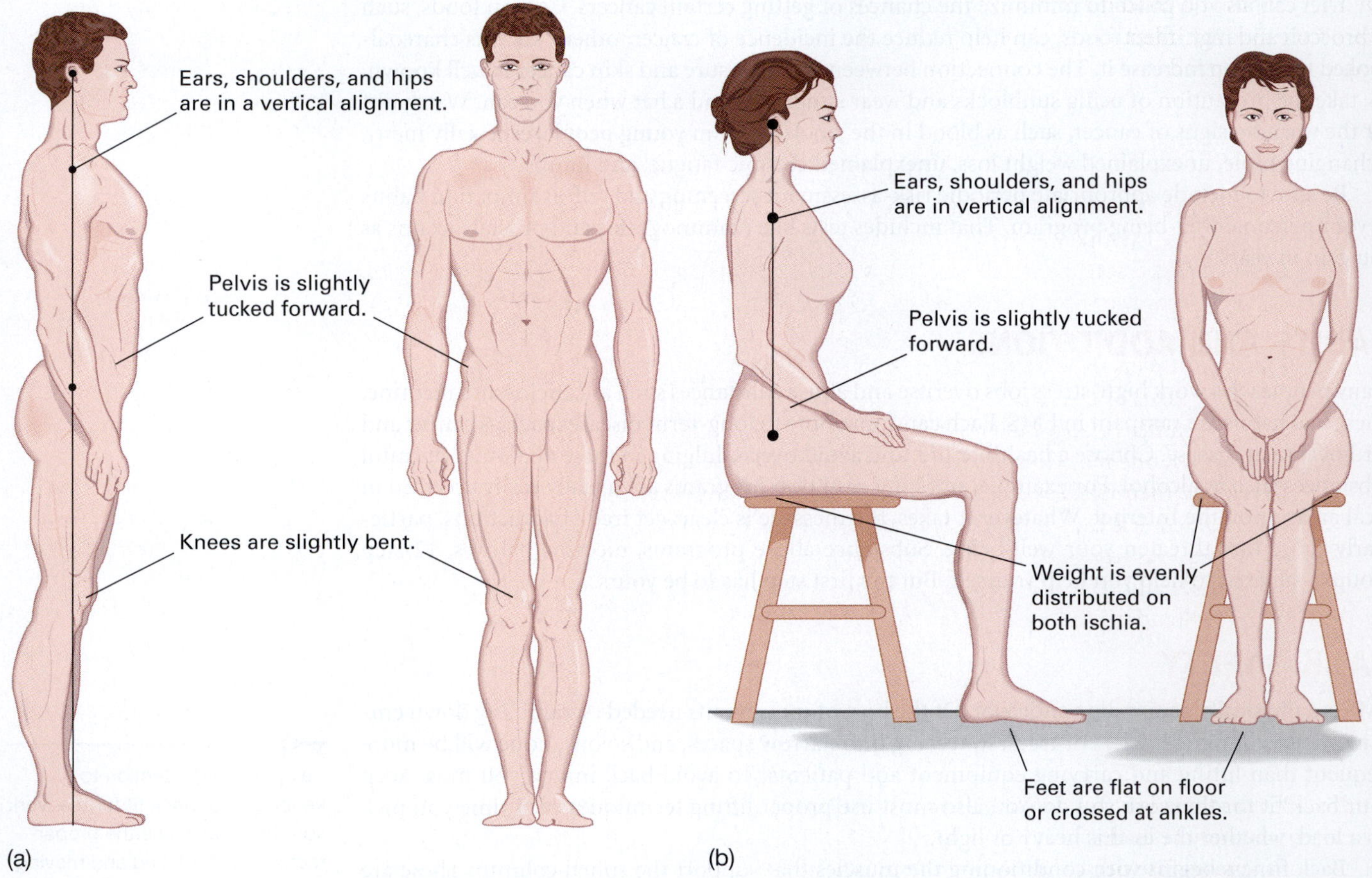

■ **Figure 1-9** (a) Correct standing posture. (b) Correct sitting posture. Note the straight line from the ear through the shoulder and hip and from the knee to arch of the foot.

★ Exhale during the lift. Do not hold your breath.

★ Given a choice, push. Do not pull.

★ Look where you are walking or crawling. Take only short steps, if you are walking. Move forward rather than backward whenever possible.

★ When rescuers are working together as a team to lift a load, only one person should be in charge of verbal commands.

Heed your own body's signals. You are stronger some days than others. Know when you are physically depleted due to exhaustion, lack of food, or minor illness. Use volunteers wisely, and be sure to ask if their backs are strong enough for the job.

Never reach for an item, or attempt to lift it, and twist at the same time. Most back injuries occur because of the cumulative effect of such low-level everyday stresses. Everything you do on behalf of back safety adds up to choices that can mean the difference between a long and rewarding career in EMS, or one shortened by an injury. Be careful!

PERSONAL PROTECTION FROM DISEASE

In recent years the emphasis on infection control has focused on the most devastating diseases, such as HIV/AIDS, hepatitis B, and tuberculosis—and rightly so. Fortunately, there is a lot you can do to minimize your risk of infection. A good first step is to develop a habit of doing the things promoted in this chapter. Eating well, getting adequate rest, and managing stress are among the building blocks of a good defense against infection. In addition, it is a good idea to periodically assess your risk for infection, such as noticing when you are run down or when your hands are dangerously chapped.

infectious disease *any disease caused by the growth of pathogenic microorganisms, which may be spread from person to person.*

INFECTIOUS DISEASES

Infectious diseases are caused by **pathogens** such as bacteria and viruses, which may be spread from person to person. For example, infection by way of bloodborne pathogens can occur when the blood of an infected person comes in contact with another person's broken skin (cuts, sores, chapped hands) or by way of parenteral contact (stick by a needle or other sharp object). Infection by airborne pathogens can occur when an infected person sneezes or coughs, causing body fluids in the form of tiny droplets to be inhaled or to come in contact with the mucous membranes of another person's eyes, nose, or mouth.

pathogens *microorganisms capable of producing disease, such as bacteria and viruses.*

HIV/AIDS, hepatitis B, and tuberculosis are diseases of great concern because they are life threatening. However, one may be exposed to many different infectious diseases. See Table 1–2 for some common ones, their modes of transmission, and **incubation periods.**

incubation period *the time between contact with a disease organism and the appearance of the first symptoms.*

Even when someone is carrying pathogens for disease, signs of an illness may not be apparent. For this reason, *you must consider the blood and body fluids of every patient you treat as infectious.* Safeguards against infection are mandatory for all medical personnel. They involve a form of infection control called Standard Precautions.

Treat all blood and other body fluids as if they are infectious, and take appropriate body substance isolation (BSI) precautions whenever you treat a patient.

INFECTION CONTROL PRACTICES

Standard Precautions

Standard Precautions is a strategy that is based on the assumption that all blood and body fluids are infectious. It dictates that all EMS personnel use Standard Precautions with every patient. To achieve this, appropriate **personal protective equipment (PPE)** should be available in every emergency vehicle. The minimum recommended PPE includes the following:

Standard Precautions *a strict form of infection control that is based on the assumption that all blood and other body fluids are infectious.*

personal protective equipment (PPE) *equipment used by EMS personnel to protect against injury and the spread of infectious disease.*

- ★ *Protective gloves.* Wear disposable protective gloves before initiating any emergency care. When an emergency involves more than one patient, change gloves between

Table 1–2 Common Infectious Diseases

Disease	Mode of Transmission	Incubation Period
AIDS (Acquired Immune Deficiency Syndrome)	AIDS- or HIV-infected blood via intravenous drug use, semen and vaginal fluids, blood transfusions, or (rarely) needle sticks. Mothers also may pass HIV to their unborn children.	Several months or years
Hepatitis B, C	Blood, stool, or other body fluids, or contaminated objects.	Weeks or months
Tuberculosis	Respiratory secretions, airborne or on contaminated objects.	2 to 6 weeks
Meningitis, bacterial	Oral and nasal secretions.	2 to 10 days
Pneumonia, bacterial and viral	Oral and nasal droplets and secretions.	Several days
Influenza	Airborne droplets, or direct contact with body fluids.	1 to 3 days
Staphylococcal skin infections	Contact with open wounds or sores or contaminated objects.	Several days
Chickenpox (varicella)	Airborne droplets, or contact with open sores.	11 to 21 days
German measles (rubella)	Airborne droplets. Mothers may pass it to unborn children.	10 to 12 days
Whooping cough (pertussis)	Respiratory secretions or airborne droplets.	6 to 20 days
SARS (severe acute respiratory syndrome)	Airborne droplets and personal contact.	4 to 6 days

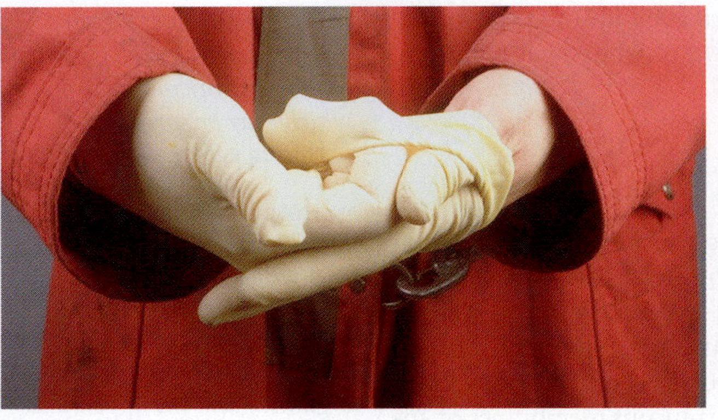
(a)

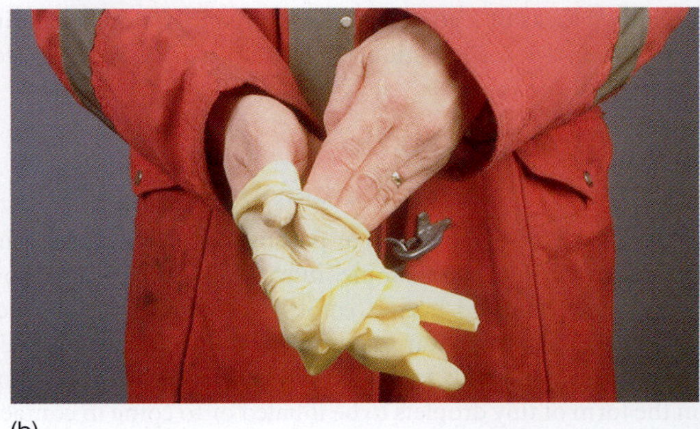
(b)

■ **Figure 1-10** (a) To remove gloves, first hook the gloved fingers of one hand under the cuff of the other glove. Then pull that glove off without letting your gloved fingers come in contact with bare skin. (b) Then slide the fingers of the ungloved hand under the remaining glove's cuff. Push that glove off, being careful not to touch the glove's exterior with your bare hand.

patients. When gloves have been contaminated, remove and dispose of them properly as soon as possible (Figure 1-10 ■).

★ *Masks and protective eyewear.* These should be worn together whenever blood spatter is likely to occur, such as with arterial bleeding, childbirth, endotracheal intubation and other invasive procedures, oral suctioning, and cleanup of equipment that requires heavy scrubbing or brushing. Both you and your patient should wear masks whenever the potential for airborne transmission of disease exists.

★ *HEPA and N-95 respirators.* Due to the resurgence of tuberculosis (TB), you must protect yourself from infection through the use of a high-efficiency particulate air (HEPA) or N-95 respirator. Wear one whenever you care for a patient with confirmed or suspected TB, especially during procedures that involve the airway, such as the administration of nebulized medications, endotracheal intubation, or suctioning.

★ *Gowns.* Disposable gowns protect your clothing from splashes. If large splashes of blood are expected, such as with childbirth, wear an impervious gown.

★ *Resuscitation equipment.* Use disposable resuscitation equipment as your primary means of artificial ventilation in emergency care.

Perhaps the most important infection-control practice is hand washing.

These garments and equipment will assist you in achieving, to the extent possible, the Standard Precautions recommended by the Centers for Disease Control. Infectious diseases also are minimized through the use of appropriate work practices and equipment especially engineered to minimize risk. For example, use disposable invasive equipment once, then dispose of it properly. Launder reusable clothing with infection control in mind.

Content Review

Hand Washing

- Lather with soap and water.
- Scrub for at least 15 seconds.
- Rinse under running water.
- Dry on a clean towel.

Probably the most important infection-control practice is hand washing as soon as possible after every patient contact and decontamination procedure. First remove any rings or jewelry from your hands and arms. Lather your hands vigorously front and back, for at least 15 seconds up to 2 or 3 inches above the wrist. Lather and rub between your fingers and in the creases and cracks of your knuckles. Scrub under and around the fingernails with a brush. Rinse well under running water, holding your hands downward so that the water drains off your fingertips. Dry your hands on a clean towel. Plain soap works perfectly well for hand washing. When soap is not available, use an antimicrobial hand washing solution or an alcohol-based foam or towelette.

Vaccinations and Screening Tests

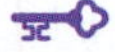

Monitor your personal medical history accurately, and be sure to get all appropriate vaccinations, boosters, and screenings on a regular basis.

Immunizations against many illnesses are available. Get them. Even "nuisance" illnesses can be avoided if you get vaccinated. Immunizations are available for rubella (German measles), measles, mumps, chickenpox, and other childhood diseases, as well as for tetanus/diphtheria, polio, influenza, hepatitis B, and Lyme disease. Some, such as tetanus, may require booster shots periodically, so monitor your personal medical history well. Also arrange for routine tuberculosis (TB) screenings.

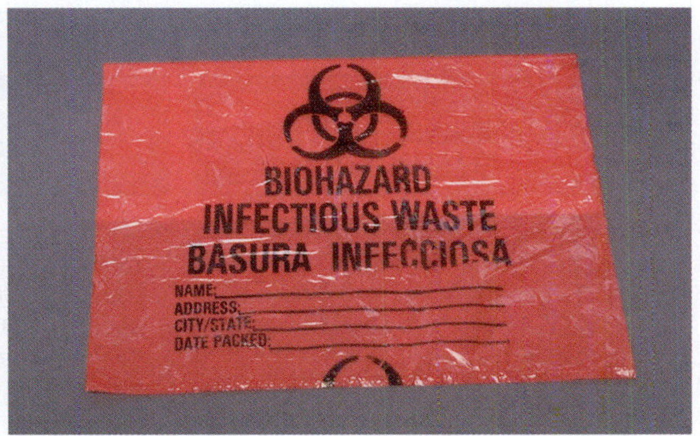

■ **Figure 1-11** Dispose of biohazardous wastes in a properly marked bag.

Decontamination of Equipment

Infection control includes properly cleaning, disinfecting, sterilizing, or properly discarding all equipment after contact with a patient.

Any personal protective equipment (PPE) designed for a single use should be properly disposed of after use. The same is true of medical devices designed for a single use. Such materials should be discarded in a red bag marked with a biohazard seal (Figure 1-11 ■). Needles and other sharp objects should be discarded in properly labeled, puncture-proof containers. Containers should be disposed of according to local guidelines.

Nondisposable equipment that has been contaminated must be cleaned, disinfected, or sterilized:

- **Cleaning** refers to washing an object with soap and water. After caring for a patient, wash your work areas down with approved soaps. Throw away single-use cleaning supplies in a proper biohazard container.
- **Disinfecting** includes cleaning with a disinfecting agent, which should kill many microorganisms on the surface of an object. Disinfect equipment that had direct contact with the intact skin of a patient, such as backboards and splints. Use a commercial disinfectant or bleach diluted in water (one part bleach to 10 parts water, or follow local guidelines).
- **Sterilizing** is the use of a chemical, or a physical method such as pressurized steam, to kill all microorganisms on an object. Items that were inserted into the patient's body (a laryngoscope blade, for example) should be sterilized by heat, steam, or radiation. There are also EPA-approved solutions for sterilization.

cleaning *washing an object with cleaners such as soap and water.*

disinfecting *cleaning with an agent that can kill some microorganisms on the surface of an object.*

sterilizing *use of a chemical or physical method such as pressurized steam to kill all microorganisms on an object.*

If your equipment needs more extensive cleaning, bag it and remove it to an area designated for this purpose. Disposable work gloves worn during cleaning and decontamination should be properly discarded. If your clothing has become contaminated, bag the items and wash them in accordance with local guidelines. After removing contaminated clothing, take a shower before dressing again.

Postexposure Procedures

By definition, an **exposure** is any occurrence of blood or body fluids coming in contact with nonintact skin, the eyes or other mucous membranes, or parenteral contact (needle stick). In most areas, an EMS provider who has had an exposure should (Figure 1-12 ■):

- Immediately wash the affected area with soap and water.
- Get a medical evaluation.
- Take the proper immunization boosters.
- Notify the agency's infection control liaison.
- Document the circumstances surrounding the exposure, including the actions taken to reduce chances of infection.

exposure *any occurrence of blood or body fluids coming in contact with nonintact skin, mucous membranes, or parenteral contact (needle stick).*

Follow your EMS system guidelines on all management and documentation of any exposure to a patient's blood or body fluids.

In general, the EMS provider should cooperate with the incident investigation and comply with all required reporting responsibilities and time frames.

■ Figure 1-12 A federal regulation called the Ryan White Comprehensive AIDS Resources Emergency (CARE) Act outlines procedures to follow after an occupational exposure to HIV, hepatitis B, diphtheria, meningitis, plague, hemorrhagic fever, rabies, or tuberculosis.

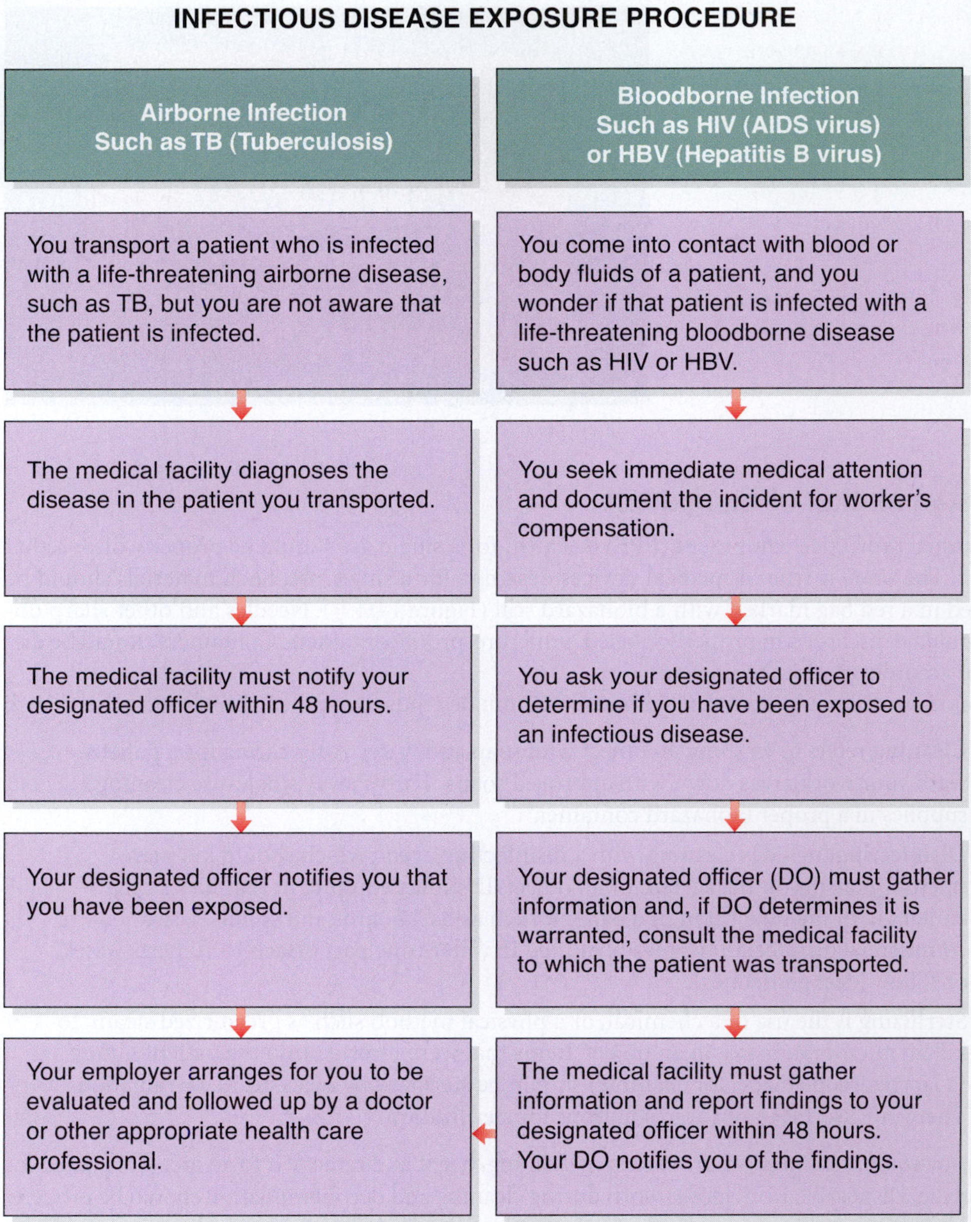

INFECTIOUS DISEASE EXPOSURE PROCEDURE

Airborne Infection Such as TB (Tuberculosis)	Bloodborne Infection Such as HIV (AIDS virus) or HBV (Hepatitis B virus)
You transport a patient who is infected with a life-threatening airborne disease, such as TB, but you are not aware that the patient is infected.	You come into contact with blood or body fluids of a patient, and you wonder if that patient is infected with a life-threatening bloodborne disease such as HIV or HBV.
↓ The medical facility diagnoses the disease in the patient you transported.	↓ You seek immediate medical attention and document the incident for worker's compensation.
↓ The medical facility must notify your designated officer within 48 hours.	↓ You ask your designated officer to determine if you have been exposed to an infectious disease.
↓ Your designated officer notifies you that you have been exposed.	↓ Your designated officer (DO) must gather information and, if DO determines it is warranted, consult the medical facility to which the patient was transported.
↓ Your employer arranges for you to be evaluated and followed up by a doctor or other appropriate health care professional.	↓ The medical facility must gather information and report findings to your designated officer within 48 hours. Your DO notifies you of the findings. ←

DEATH AND DYING

Paramedics encounter death much more frequently than other people do. They often see it as it happens. This can lead to a sense of cumulative overload, which the paramedic needs to recognize and deal with in a healthy manner.

Review Content

Stages of Loss

- Denial
- Anger
- Bargaining
- Depression
- Acceptance

LOSS, GRIEF, AND MOURNING

A long-standing taboo against discussing death and dying changed when pioneer Elisabeth Kübler-Ross braved the backlash to meet with terminally ill hospital patients to discuss their feelings about death and dying. Before then, it was assumed dying people did not want to talk about the experience. What Kübler-Ross learned is that there are five predictable stages of loss:

★ *Denial, or "not me."* This is the inability or refusal to believe the reality of the event. It is a defense mechanism, during which the patient puts off dealing with the inevitable end of life.

- ★ *Anger, or "why me?"* The patient's anger is really frustration related to his inability to control the situation. That anger could focus on anyone or anything.
- ★ *Bargaining, or "okay, but first let me. . . ."* In the patient's mind, he tries to make a deal to "buy additional time" to put off or change the expected outcome.
- ★ *Depression, or "okay, but I haven't. . . ."* The patient is sad and despairing, often mourning things not accomplished and dreams that will not come true. The patient withdraws, or retreats, into a private world, unwilling to communicate with others.
- ★ *Acceptance, or "okay, I'm not afraid."* The patient may come to realize his fate and achieve a reasonable level of comfort with the anticipated outcome. At this stage, the family may need more support than the patient.

Given enough time, a person experiencing a significant loss usually works through the five predictable stages: denial, anger, bargaining, depression, and acceptance.

A person experiencing any significant loss usually works through these stages, given enough time. Although there is a tendency to progress from one stage to the next in order, both dying patients and their loved ones experience the stages in their own unique ways. They may jump around among the stages, they may go back and forth, or they may never finish them. It is important for you to remain flexible in your expectations, so you can decide how best to help, if asked.

Because paramedics encounter death and dying often, there is a mistaken belief that they handle it better. However, paramedics are human, too. Let yourself deal with death and dying when it occurs. Do not shirk the support of friends and family. Do not try to "tough it out." Use every opportunity to process a specific incident in a healthy manner, through appropriately grieving losses that have an impact on you.

Grief is a feeling. Mourning is a process. A grieving person feels mostly sadness or distress. A person in mourning is immersed in the process of displaying and ultimately dissipating the feelings of grief. The sense of loss is predictably most intense immediately after the news is received. Although numerous models for the mourning process exist, a good rule of thumb is that after the loss of a close friend or relative, a period of 1 year of mourning is normal.

Upon initially hearing the news of a death, a person experiences a "paralyzing, totally incapacitating surge of grief that is exactly comparable to the incapacitating pain of an acute blow to an eye or a testicle in that the whole world shrinks down to that acute pain." Typically, the feeling lasts for 5 to 15 minutes. When you deliver the news of a death, remember that a survivor cannot function during this grief spike. After delivering the news, wait until it is past and the survivor is ready and able to receive information and make decisions.

A period of intense feelings that continues for around 4 to 6 weeks follows the grief spike. Feelings may include loss, anger, resentment, sadness, and even guilt, depending on the relationship and the circumstances surrounding the death. Gradually, the intensity and immediacy of the loss fades into a phase dominated by a sense of loneliness, which lasts about 6 months. Finally, a period of recovery ensues. The survivor begins to view the loss more objectively and rediscovers an interest in living. Key to the process of mourning is the passage of significant dates and anniversaries, such as birthdays, holidays, and the monthly (then annual) date when the loss occurred (anniversary phenomenon).

How different people cope with difficult moments, such as death, varies. If you are dealing with a child, understand that children's perceptions are different from an adult's. (See Table 1–3 for a summary.) This is true of all the special populations you will encounter, such as the elderly and people with mental disabilities. The elderly, for example, may be particularly concerned about the effects of the loss on other family members, about further loss of their own independence, and about the costs of a funeral and burial. There is a wide variety of responses to death among different peoples and cultures as well. Be flexible, and be ready for anything.

WHAT TO SAY

As "Do Not Resuscitate" orders and other out-of-hospital death situations increase, EMS personnel are more often placed in the position of telling people that someone has died. It would be nice to have a script for those difficult moments, but the reality is that you have to assess the scene and the people in each situation to determine the safest and most compassionate way to deliver the sad news.

In terms of safety, you never know how people will respond, even if you know them. Most people accept the news quietly. However, some allow their grief to flood out of them in very physical ways, such as throwing things, kicking walls, or screaming and running in circles. Before speaking,

Table 1–3	Needs and Expectations of Children Regarding Death	
Age Range	**Characteristics**	**Suggestions**
Newborn to age 3	Senses that something has happened in family, and notices that there is much activity in the household. Realizes that people are crying and sad. Watch for irritability and changes in eating, sleeping, or other behavioral patterns.	Be sensitive to the child's needs. Try to maintain consistency in routines. Maintain consistency with significant people in child's life.
Ages 3 to 6	Believes death is a temporary state, and may ask continually when the person will return. Believes in magical thinking, and may feel responsible for the death or it is punishment for own behavior. May be fearful of catching the same illness and die, or may believe that everyone else he loves will die also. Watch for changes in behavior patterns with friends and at school, difficulty sleeping, and changes in eating habits.	Emphasize that the child was not responsible for the death. Reinforce that when people are sad, they cry, and that crying is normal and natural. Encourage the child to talk about and/or draw pictures of his feelings, or to cry.
Ages 6 to 9	May prefer to hide or disguise feelings to avoid looking babyish. Is afraid significant others will die. Seeks out detailed explanations for death, and differences between fatal illness and "just being sick." Has an understanding that death is real, but may believe that those who die are too slow, weak, or stupid. Fantasizes in an effort to make everything the way it was. Denial is most helpful coping skill.	Talk about the normal feelings of anger, sadness, and guilt. Share your own feelings about death. Do not be afraid to cry in front of the child. This and other expressions of loss help to give the child permission to express his feelings.
Ages 9 to 12	Begins to understand the irreversibility of death. May seek details and specifics of the situation, and may need repeated, explicit explanations. Hard-won sense of independence becomes fragile, and may show concern about the practical matters of his lifestyle. May try to act "adult," but then regress to earlier stage of emotional response. When threatened, expresses anger toward the ill/deceased, himself, or other survivors.	Set aside time to talk about feelings. Encourage sharing of memories to facilitate grief response.
Ages 12 to 18	Demanding developmental processes are an awkward fit with need to take on different family roles. Retreats to safety of childhood. Feels pressure to act as an adult, while still coping with skills of a child. Suppresses feelings in order to "fit in," leaving teen isolated and vulnerable.	Encourage talking, but respect need for privacy. See if a trusted, reliable friend or adult can provide appropriate support. Locate support group for teens.

consciously position yourself between them and the door or another escape route. Remember, initially the grief spike has its grip on the survivors. There is little you can do but give them a safe, private place to get through it. Also, for safety, do not deliver the news to a large group. Ask the primary people (no more than four or five) to step aside with you to a private place. Let them tell the others in their own way.

Find out who is who among the survivors. Do not make assumptions. Then address the closest survivor, preferably in a way that shows compassion. That is, avoid standing above the survivor. Instead, sit or squat so that your eyes are at the same level. If the survivor is alone, call for a friend, neighbor, clergy member, or relative. Wait to tell the survivor the news until that person has arrived.

Introduce yourself by name and function ("My name is Kate. I'm a paramedic with West End Ambulance."). A careful choice of words is helpful. Although it may seem blunt, use the words *dead* and *died,* rather than euphemisms that may be misinterpreted or misunderstood. Use gentle eye contact and, if appropriate, the power of touching an arm or holding a hand. Basic elements of your message should include:

- ★ A loved one has died.
- ★ There is nothing more anyone could have done.
- ★ Your EMS service is available to assist the survivors if needed. (Sometimes, medical emergencies occur in survivors in the wake of such stressful news.)
- ★ Information about local procedures for out-of-hospital death, such as the inspection of the scene by the medical examiner or coroner, and so on.

Do not include statements about God's will or relief from pain or any subjective assumption. You do not know the people well enough to know the details about their relationship or their religious preferences.

WHEN IT IS SOMEONE YOU KNOW

Many paramedics are called to serve in small communities, where calls often involve people you know. Elements of this are both rewarding and heart-wrenching. People may be greatly relieved to see a familiar, trusted face among the EMS team. There also is a lot of support for paramedics in small communities because you are there to help others during their most fearful moments. However, being involved when the life of someone you know is threatened—or lost—can have a powerful impact upon your own emotions. If it is too much, you must find a way to manage the stress. Oftentimes, you must grieve as well. Your well-being demands it.

STRESS AND STRESS MANAGEMENT

Many aspects of EMS are stressful. Stress, according to researcher Hans Selye, is "the nonspecific response of the body to any demand." The word **stress** also refers to a hardship or strain, or a physical or emotional response to a stimulus. A person's reactions to stress are individual. They are affected by previous exposure to the stressor, perception of the event, general life experience, and personal coping skills.

stress *a hardship or strain; a physical or emotional response to a stimulus.*

A stimulus that causes stress is known as a **stressor.** Stress is usually understood to generate a negative effect, or *distress,* in an individual. There is also "good" stress, which is called *eustress* (for example, seeing a lost loved one for the first time in years). However, even eustress generates physiological and psychological signs and symptoms.

stressor *a stimulus that causes stress.*

Adapting to stress is a dynamic, evolving process. As a person adapts, he develops:

- ★ *Defensive strategies.* While sometimes helpful for the short term, these strategies deny and distort the reality of a stressful situation.
- ★ *Coping.* This is an active process during which a person confronts the stressful situation and changes or adjusts as necessary. Coping may not serve as the best strategy for the long term.
- ★ *Problem-solving skills.* These skills are regarded as the healthiest approach to everyday concerns. Reflected in the ability to analyze a problem and recognize multiple options and potential solutions, mastery generally comes only as a result of extensive experience with similar situations.

EMS has abundant stressors, which provide ample opportunities for the development of problem-solving skills. There are administrative stressors, such as waiting for calls, shift work, loud pagers, and inadequate pay. There are scene-related stressors, such as violent and abusive people, flying debris, vomit, loud noises, and chaos. There are emotional and physical stressors, such as fear, demanding bystanders, abusive patients, frustration, exhaustion, hunger or thirst, and lifting heavy objects.

Environmental stress may be in the form of siren noise, inclement weather, confined work spaces, and the frequent urgency of rapid scene responses and life-or-death decisions. In addition, the often difficult world of EMS can strain a paramedic's family relationships and possibly lead to conflicts with supervisors and coworkers. Add this to the common personality traits of paramedics, which include a strong need to be liked and often unrealistically high self-expectations, and the combination can lead to disturbing feelings of guilt or anxiety. All these stressors take a toll on the paramedic.

Your job in managing stress is to learn these things:

To manage stress, identify your own personal stressors, the amount of stress you can take before it becomes a problem, and what specific stress-management techniques work for you.

- ★ *Your personal stressors.* Each person has an individual list. What is stressful to you may be enjoyable to someone else. What was stressful to you last year may be replaced by new stressors this year.
- ★ *Amount of stress you can take before it becomes a problem.* Stress occurs in a tornado-like continuum. It starts with a few breezes, but it can increase in force until it is whirling out of control. Stopping the "storm" early is key to your well-being. You need to know which stress responses are early indicators for you, so you can deal with them at that point.
- ★ *Stress management strategies that work for you.* Again, this is totally individual. Those who seek personal well-being must become well-versed about personally appropriate options.

Content Review

Phases of a Stress Response

- Alarm
- Resistance
- Exhaustion

If a person piles on stressor after stressor without regard for the consequences, the results are likely to be bad. Stress-related disease is avoidable if you make a habit of doing what is necessary to preserve your personal well-being.

There are three phases of a stress response: alarm, resistance, and exhaustion. At the end comes a period of rest and recovery.

- ★ *Stage I: Alarm.* The alarm phase is the "fight-or-flight" phenomenon. It occurs when the body physically and rapidly prepares to defend itself against a perceived threat. The pituitary gland begins by releasing adrenocorticotropic (stress) hormones. Hormones continue to flood the body via the autonomic nervous system, coordinated by the hypothalamus. Epinephrine and norepinephrine from the adrenal glands increase heart rate and blood pressure, dilate pupils, increase blood sugar and slow digestion, and relax the bronchial tree. This reaction ends when the event is recognized as not dangerous.
- ★ *Stage II: Resistance.* This stage starts when the individual begins to cope with the stress. Over time, an individual may become desensitized or adapted to stressors. Physiological parameters, such as pulse and blood pressure, may return to normal.
- ★ *Stage III: Exhaustion.* Prolonged exposure to the same stressors leads to exhaustion of an individual's ability to resist and adapt. Resistance to all stressors declines. Susceptibility to physical and psychological ailments increase. A period of rest and recovery is necessary for a healthy outcome.

It would be great if we could manage each stressor to the point of recovery before the next one hits, but that is not how it works. Typically, people are still dealing with one stress (or the same ongoing one, such as the chronic stress of shift work) when additional stressors pile on, resulting in cumulative stress. If stress accumulates without intervention, the consequences can be serious.

SHIFT WORK

There will always be shift work in EMS. Because EMS is a 24-hour, 7-days-a-week endeavor, someone has to be functional at all times. This is inherently stressful because of disruptions in the biorhythms of the body, known as **circadian rhythms,** and sleep deprivation.

circadian rhythms *physiological phenomena that occur at approximately 24-hour intervals.*

Circadian rhythms are biological cycles that occur at approximately 24-hour intervals. These include hormonal and body temperature fluctuations, appetite and sleepiness cycles, and other bodily processes. When life patterns disrupt the circadian rhythms, biological effects can be stressful. For example, sleep deprivation is common among people who work at night. The inherent dangers to paramedics are clear. If you have to sleep in the daytime, there are some tips to minimize the stress:

- ★ Sleep in a cool, dark place that mimics the nighttime environment.
- ★ Stick to sleeping at your **anchor time** (times you can rest without interruption), even on days off. Do not try to revert to a daytime lifestyle on days off. For example, if you work 9 p.m. to 5 a.m. and your anchor time is 8 a.m. to 12 noon, then go to bed "early" on days off and on workdays sleep from 8 a.m. to 3 p.m.
- ★ Unwind appropriately after a shift in order to rest well. Do not eat a heavy meal or exercise right before bedtime.
- ★ Post a "day sleeper" sign on your front door, turn off the phone's ringer, and lower the volume of the answering machine.

anchor time *set of hours when a night-shift worker can reliably expect to rest without interruption.*

SIGNS OF STRESS

A variety of factors can trigger a stress response. They include the loss of something valuable, injury or the threat of injury, poor health or nutrition, general frustration, and ineffective coping mechanisms. Remember, each individual is susceptible to different stressors and therefore has a different constellation of signs and symptoms.

These signs and symptoms (Table 1–4) are a blessing in a way, because they are the body's way of warning that corrective stress management is needed. The warnings typically are mild at first, but left uncorrected they will build in intensity until you are forced to rest. If it means having a heart attack or collapsing, that is what the body will do. So, pay attention. If you catch a warning sign of excessive stress early and manage it, there is no need to reach the extreme endpoint commonly referred to as **burnout.**

burnout *a condition that occurs when coping mechanisms no longer buffer stressors, which can compromise personal health and well-being.*

Table 1–4 Warning Signs of Excessive Stress

Physical	Cognitive	Emotional	Behavioral
Nausea/vomiting	Confusion	Anticipatory anxiety	Change in activity
Upset stomach	Lowered attention span	Denial	Hyperactivity, hypoactivity
Tremors (lips, hands)	Calculation difficulties	Fearfulness	Withdrawal
Feeling uncoordinated	Memory problems	Panic	Suspiciousness
Diaphoresis (profuse sweating), flushed skin	Poor concentration	Survivor guilt	Change in communications
Chills	Difficulty making decisions	Uncertainty of feelings	Change in interactions with others
Diarrhea	Disruption in logical thinking	Depression	Change in eating habits
Aching muscles and joints	Disorientation, decreased level of awareness	Grief	Increased or decreased food intake
Sleep disturbances	Seeing an event over and over	Hopelessness	Increased smoking
Fatigue	Distressing dreams	Feeling overwhelmed	Increased alcohol intake
Dry mouth	Blaming someone	Feeling lost	Increased intake of other drugs
Shakes		Feeling abandoned	Being overly vigilant to environment
Headache		Feeling worried	Excessive humor
Vision problems		Wishing to hide	Excessive silence
Difficult, rapid breathing		Wishing to die	Unusual behavior
Chest tightness or pain, heart palpitations, cardiac rhythm disturbances		Anger	Crying spells
		Feeling numb	
		Identifying with victim	

COMMON TECHNIQUES FOR MANAGING STRESS

There are two main groups of defense mechanisms and techniques for managing stress: beneficial and detrimental. Detrimental techniques may provide a temporary sense of relief, but they will not cure the problem. They only make things worse. They include substance abuse (alcohol, nicotine, illegal and prescription drugs), overeating or other compulsive behaviors, chronic complaining, freezing out or cutting off others and the support they could give you, avoidance behaviors, and dishonesty about your actual state of well-being ("I'm just fine!").

It is far better for you to spend your energy on beneficial, or healthy, techniques that serve to dissipate the accumulation of stress and promote actual recovery. In situations where your stress response threatens your ability to handle the moment, you can:

- ★ *Use controlled breathing.* Focus attention on your breathing. Take in a deep breath through your nose. Then exhale forcefully but steadily through your mouth, so that you can hear the air rush out. Press all the air out of your lungs with your abdomen. Do this two or more times, until you feel steadier. This technique helps to reduce your adrenaline levels and slow your heart rate, so you can do your job appropriately.
- ★ *Reframe.* Mentally reframe interfering thoughts, such as "I can't do this" or "I'm scared." Be sure to deal with the thoughts later, or they will continue to interfere with the performance of your duties.
- ★ *Attend to the medical needs of the patient.* Even if you know the people involved, do not let those relationships interfere with your responsibilities as an EMS provider. Later, when it is appropriate to do so, address your stress about the call.

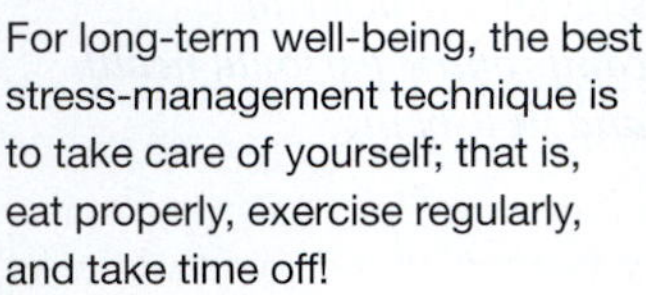

For long-term well-being, the best stress-management technique is to take care of yourself; that is, eat properly, exercise regularly, and take time off!

For long-term well-being, one of the best stress management techniques is to take care of yourself—physically, emotionally, and mentally. Remember that regular exercise does not have to be extreme. Do something that you enjoy and find relaxing. At stressful times, pay especially close attention to your diet. If you smoke, make it a goal to quit.

Create a non-EMS circle of friends, and renew old friendships or activities. Take a vacation or a few days off. Say "no!" to the next offer of an overtime shift. Listen to music, meditate, and learn positive thinking. Try the soothing techniques of guided imagery and progressive relaxation. Some paramedics have even quit EMS for a while. In general, you can make many choices. The key principle is to generate positive options for yourself, and keep choosing them until you have recovered.

SPECIFIC EMS STRESSES

There are three types of clearly defined EMS stresses:

- ★ *Daily stress.* Most EMS stress is unrelated to critical incidents and disasters. Instead, it is related to such things as pay, working conditions, dealing with the public, administrative matters, and other hassles of day-to-day living. To help deal with daily stress, all emergency personnel should develop personal stress management strategies such as a personal support system made up of coworkers, family, clergy, and others.
- ★ *Small incidents.* Incidents involving only one or two patients, including incidents that result in injuries or deaths of emergency workers, are best handled by competent mental health personnel in individual or small group settings. Mental health professionals should be familiar with EMS and be ready to respond when needed. They should then continue to screen affected emergency workers for signs and symptoms of abnormal response to stress and, if these are detected, refer these workers, as appropriate, to other competent mental health professionals who use accepted treatment methods.
- ★ *Large incidents and disasters.* Most EMS personnel will never encounter a disaster situation. However, all must be ready in case such a catastrophe occurs. The stress of large-scale disasters can be mitigated by a well-coordinated and organized response. Use of the Incident Management System (IMS) or Incident Command System (ICS) in large incidents and disasters serves to appropriately direct responding personnel. It also provides for rotating personnel through rehabilitation and surveillance stations.

Those who are showing signs of stress or fatigue are removed from duty, at least temporarily. Here, too, there is a role for competent mental health professionals, who should be readily available to provide psychological first aid.

MENTAL HEALTH SERVICES

Mental health professionals can provide the information and education needed for rescuers to understand trauma, what to expect, and where to get help if needed. In addition, competent mental health personnel should be available at all major incidents to provide psychological first aid to rescuers and victims. Psychological first aid includes:

- ★ Listening
- ★ Conveying compassion
- ★ Assessing needs
- ★ Ensuring that basic physical needs are met
- ★ Not forcing personnel to talk
- ★ Providing or mobilizing family or significant others
- ★ Encouraging, but not forcing, social support
- ★ Protecting rescuers and victims from additional harm

Psychological first aid is not a treatment or packaged proprietary intervention technique. It is an attempt to provide practical palliative care and contact while respecting the wishes of those who may not be ready to deal with the possible onslaught of emotional responses in the early days following an incident. It entails providing comfort and information and meeting people's immediate practical and emotional needs.

DISASTER MENTAL HEALTH SERVICES

The emotional well-being of both rescuers and victims is an important concern in any multiple-casualty incident. In the past, Critical Incident Stress Management (CISM) was recommended for use in emergency services. However, recent evidence has clearly shown that CISM and Critical Incident Stress Debriefing (CISD) do not appear to mitigate the effects of traumatic stress and, in fact, may interfere with the normal grieving and healing process and should not be used.

However, there remains an important role for competent mental health professionals in any multiple-casualty incident. Mental health personnel should be available on scene to provide psychological first aid to all those affected by an incident—including EMS personnel. At the same time, they can survey rescuers and victims for the development of abnormal stress-related symptoms. In addition, mental health professionals should be available during the 2 months following a critical incident to screen and assist anyone who may be developing stress-related symptoms. Persons so affected may be referred for additional counseling or mental health care.

The current recommendation of major organizations (such as the World Health Organization) for the management of critical stress is the resiliency-based model and psychological first aid. This model advocates the development of good coping and stress management strategies early in your career. In the event of a critical incident, psychological first aid simply assures that physical needs are met and information provided.

GENERAL SAFETY CONSIDERATIONS

The topic of scene safety is vast and requires career-long attention. Considering the many problems that can occur, it is impressive how few injuries there are. Your risks include violent people, environmental hazards, structural collapse, motor vehicles, and infectious disease. Many of these hazards can be minimized with protective equipment, such as helmets, body armor, reflective tape for night visibility, footwear with ankle support, and Standard Precautions against infectious disease. Whatever protective equipment you have should be used.

INTERPERSONAL RELATIONS

Safety issues that arise in prehospital care often stem from poor interpersonal relations. Paramedics are public ambassadors of health care. Interpersonal safety begins with effective communication. If you can build a rapport with the strangers you have been sent to serve, you will gain their trust. Suspicious, angry, and upset people are far more likely to be defensive and inflict harm than those who see a reason to trust what you are doing.

Treat every person you meet with dignity and respect, no matter what his or her race, sex, age, religion, economic background, or present condition.

Building rapport depends on the ability to put your personal prejudices aside. Everyone has prejudices. But as a representative of an institution far greater than yourself, you must never allow them to interfere with appropriate patient and bystander management. In fact, go beyond curbing prejudice, and challenge yourself to treat every person you meet with dignity and respect.

You can begin by taking time to pay attention to the rich array of cultural diversity and learning to see those differences as valuable and positive. In particular, learn about the different cultural backgrounds of people in your area and how to work with them effectively. For example, although you may like a lot of eye contact, understand that it is regarded as more polite in several cultures to avoid eye contact. Therefore, someone showing you esteem might avoid eye contact with you. This is not wrong. It is just different. Listen well to the stories of other people and see what you can learn. When a person can accept differences easily, it becomes easier to work toward win-win situations on the streets.

ROADWAY SAFETY

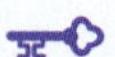

One of the greatest hazards in EMS is the motor vehicle. Be sure to obey roadway laws and follow all driving safety guidelines.

Roadways are unsafe places. There are good books, classes, and mentors to help you become aware of the various roadway hazards. Learn the principles of:

★ Safely following an emergency escort vehicle
★ Intersection management, when traffic is moving in several directions
★ Noting hazardous conditions, such as spilled hazardous materials (gasoline, industrial chemicals, and so on), downed power lines, and proximity to moving traffic; also noting adverse environmental conditions
★ Evaluating the safest parking place when arriving at a roadway incident
★ Safely approaching a vehicle in which someone is slumped over the wheel
★ Patient compartment safety—in particular, bracing yourself against sudden deceleration or swerving to avoid roadway hazards; and making a habit of hanging on consistently, especially when changing positions
★ Safely using emergency lights and siren

An ambulance escort can create additional hazards. Inexperienced ambulance operators often follow the escort vehicle too closely and are unable to stop when the escort does. Inexperienced operators also may assume that other drivers know the ambulance is following an escort. In fact, other drivers do not know another emergency vehicle is coming and often pull out in front of the ambulance just after the escort vehicle passes.

Multiple-vehicle responses can be just as dangerous, especially when responding vehicles travel in the same direction close together. When two vehicles approach the same intersection at the same time, not only may they fail to yield to each other, but other drivers may yield for the first vehicle only, not the second one. Extreme caution must be taken when approaching intersections.

Certain equipment is intended to promote your safety on roadways. For example, to be visible to oncoming drivers, who may have dirty, smeared, pitted windshields and may not be sober, wear reflective tape and orange or lime-green safety vests. In fact, you also may be issued other protective gear, especially if you are in the fire service. Using respiratory protection, gloves, boots, turnout coat and pants (or coveralls), and other specialty safety equipment is the mark of an aware, professional paramedic. Ask nonmedical personnel to set out flares or cones, if needed. Leave some emergency lights flashing, although you should be careful not to blind oncoming drivers.

To park safely at a roadway incident, make it a habit to scan each individual setting. Notice curves, hilltops, volume, and the speed of surrounding traffic. Ideally, park in the front of a crash site on the same side of the street. This facilitates access to the patient compartment and equipment, and it protects you from traffic coming from behind. However, when responding to an incident such as "person slumped behind wheel," maintain the defensive advantage by staying behind the vehicle, and use spotlights to "blind" the person until you know there are no hostile intentions. Walk to the vehicle with cautious alertness until you are sure it is not a trap.

The use of seat belts in the front of an ambulance should be an obvious habit, both for safety and for role modeling. Less obvious is the use of safety restraints in the patient compartment. An improper assumption is that the paramedic is too busy attending the patient and passengers to wear a seat belt. However, buckling into a seat belt for a safer ride is, in fact, possible during much or most of ambulance transport times. Death and major disability is common when someone is in the patient compartment during a crash. For your well-being, wear a seat belt whenever possible, even "in back."

Because ambulances represent help and hope, it is doubly tragic when a paramedic crew is involved in a motor-vehicle crash caused by the misuse of lights and siren. Lights and siren are tools, not toys. They are the paramedic's means for gaining quick access to people in dire need. Those who misuse the mandate to operate them chip away at the public's trust in EMS. Whether using lights and siren or not, in most states, the paramedic has a legal responsibility to drive with "due regard for the safety of all others." As a professional, you are obligated to study and use safe driving practices at all times.

Part 5: Illness and Injury Prevention

How often do EMS crews respond to incidents that could easily have been prevented? How often have you thought to yourself "I wish there was something I could have done" in the wake of senseless circumstances surrounding an accidental injury or illness? But what if EMS personnel asked these questions *before* an incident occurred? How many injuries could be prevented? How many lives could be saved? This section focuses on these questions and discusses illness and injury prevention as a paramedic's crucial duty and responsibility.

EPIDEMIOLOGY

Injury is one of our nation's most important health problems. Consider the following facts offered by the U.S. Department of Transportation:

- ★ Injury has surpassed stroke as the third leading cause of death in the United States, and it is the leading cause of death in people ages 1 to 44.
- ★ Injuries that are unintentional result in nearly 70,000 deaths and millions of nonfatal injuries each year. The leading causes of death from unintentional injuries are motor-vehicle collisions, fires, burns, falls, drownings, and poisonings.
- ★ The estimated lifetime cost of injuries will exceed $114 billion.
- ★ For every one death caused by injury, there are an estimated 19 hospitalizations and 254 emergency department visits.

Injury is one of our nation's most important health problems.

Injuries result from interaction with potential hazards in the environment, which means that they may be predictable and preventable.

Though many people believe that injuries "just happen," evidence shows that injuries result from interaction with potential hazards in the environment. Thus, it has been suggested that "MVAs" (motor-vehicle accidents) should be called "MVCs" (motor-vehicle collisions), since driving drunk or at 80 mph and crashing is no accident. In other words, many injuries may be predictable and preventable. The study of the factors that influence the frequency, distribution, and causes of injury, disease, and other health-related events in a population is called **epidemiology.**

Concepts related to epidemiology that you should know include **years of productive life,** a calculation made by subtracting the age at death from 65. (For example, in a liability suit concerning the death of a 45-year-old, a jury might assess damages based on the deceased's loss of 20 years as a wage-earner.) Another concept is **injury,** which refers to the intentional or unintentional damage to a person resulting from acute exposure to thermal, mechanical, electrical, or chemical energy or from the absence of such essentials as heat and oxygen. An accident is an *unintentional injury,* but an injury that is purposefully inflicted either on oneself (e.g., suicide) or on another person (e.g., homicide) is an *intentional injury.* Intentional injuries make up about a third of all injury deaths. Other categories of intentional injury include rape, assault, and domestic, elder, and child abuse.

Other concepts related to epidemiology include **injury risk,** which is a real or potentially hazardous situation that puts people in danger of sustaining injury. As medical professionals, EMS

epidemiology *the study of factors that influence the frequency, distribution, and causes of injury, disease, and other health-related events in a population.*

years of productive life *age at death subtracted from 65.*

injury *intentional or unintentional damage to a person resulting from exposure to mechanical or any other form of energy or from absence of essentials such as heat or oxygen.*

injury risk *a situation that puts people in danger of injury.*

injury-surveillance program *ongoing systematic collection, analysis, and interpretation of injury data important to public health practice.*

teachable moment *the time shortly after an injury when patients and observers may be more receptive to teaching about how similar injuries may be prevented in the future.*

primary prevention *keeping an injury or illness from ever occurring.*

secondary prevention *medical care after an injury or illness that helps to prevent further problems from occurring.*

tertiary prevention *rehabilitation after an injury or illness that helps to prevent further problems from occurring.*

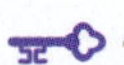

The more than 600,000 EMS providers in the United States comprise a great arsenal in the war to prevent injury and disease.

EMS organizational commitment is vital to the development of prevention activities.

Content Review

Organizational Commitment

- Protect EMS providers
- Provide initial and continuing education
- Collect and distribute illness and injury data
- Empower EMS personnel

providers should assess every scene and situation for injury risk and maintain statistics as part of an **injury-surveillance program,** or the ongoing systematic collection, analysis, and interpretation of injury data essential to the planning, implementation, and evaluation of public health practice.

An injury-surveillance program must also include a component for the timely dissemination of data to those who need to know. The final link in the injury-surveillance chain is the application of these data to prevention and control. **Teachable moments** occur shortly after an injury when the patient and observers remain acutely aware of what has happened and may be more receptive to learning about how similar injury or illness could be prevented in the future.

By becoming involved in injury prevention, EMS providers can focus on **primary prevention,** or keeping an injury from ever occurring. Medical care and rehabilitation activities that help to prevent further problems from occurring are referred to, respectively, as **secondary prevention** and **tertiary prevention.**

PREVENTION WITHIN EMS

Even armed with the best equipment and technology, EMS providers cannot save every life. However, by working as partners in public health and safety, members of the EMS community can go beyond their normal daily routine and work with the public to prevent avoidable illness and injury.

EMS providers are widely distributed in the population, often reflecting the composition of their communities. They are often considered to be champions of the health care consumer and are welcome in schools and other community institutions. Medical personnel are high-profile role models and, as such, can have a significant impact on the reduction of injury rates. In rural areas, EMS providers are sometimes the most medically educated individuals and are often looked to for advice and direction. Essentially, the more than 600,000 EMS providers in the United States comprise a great arsenal in the war to prevent injury and disease.

ORGANIZATIONAL COMMITMENT

EMS organizational commitment is vital to the development of prevention activities in the following areas:

- ★ *Protection of EMS providers.* The leadership of EMS agencies must assure that policies are in place to promote response, scene, and transport safety. The appropriate body substance isolation (BSI) and personal protective equipment should be issued to protect against exposure to bloodborne and airborne pathogens as well as environmental hazards. An overall commitment to safety and wellness should be emphasized and supported.
- ★ *Education of EMS providers.* A "buy-in" from employees at every level is key to the success of any prevention program. EMS managers have the responsibility of instructing employees in the fundamentals of primary prevention. Public and private sector specialty groups may be called upon for specific training (Figure 1-13 ■). EMS providers should also have the skills and training necessary to defend against violent patients or other hostile attackers. Classes in on-scene survival techniques should be commonplace in every EMS agency.
- ★ *Data collection.* Monitoring and maintaining records of patient illnesses and injuries is essential in determining trends and in developing and measuring the success of prevention programs. Each agency should contribute data to local, regional, state, and national systems that track such information.
- ★ *Financial support.* An agency's internal budget should reflect support for prevention strategies as a priority. If necessary, support must be sought from outside the organization. Large corporations are often willing to donate funds in exchange for standby coverage at an event or company function. State highway safety offices can offer funding for traffic-related projects, such as those involving child safety seats, seat belts, and drunk driving. Advertising agencies may contribute billboards for safety messages and public service announcements. Partnerships with local hospitals can

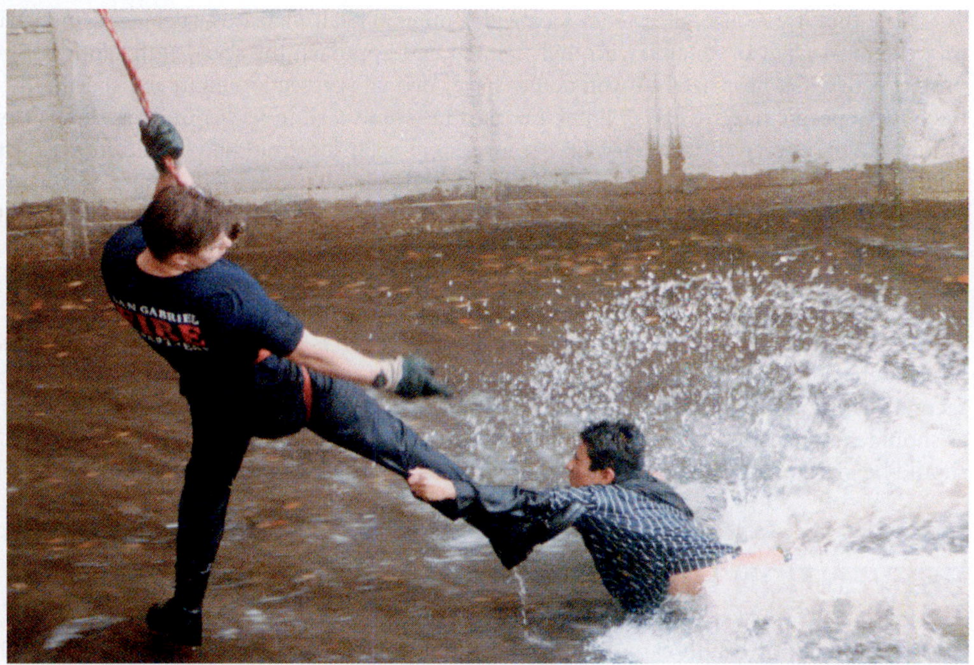

■ **Figure 1-13** Training in specialized safety procedures should be available to you. *(© Jonathan Alcorn/ZUMA/Corbis)*

result in advertising safety messages in newsletters and flyers. Community groups such as Mothers Against Drunk Driving (MADD) and junior auxiliaries also are great resources for initiating community and school programs.

★ *Empowerment of EMS providers.* Frontline personnel are the ultimate factor in achieving success in a prevention program. Managers should identify, encourage, foster, and reward employee interest, support, and involvement. In addition, managers should rotate assignment to prevention programs and provide salary for off-duty injury prevention activities.

EMS PROVIDER COMMITMENT

Illness and injury prevention should begin at home and be carried over into the workplace. The priority for EMS providers is to protect themselves from harm. Employers have an obligation to provide a safe environment. Written guidelines and policies should promote wellness and safety among employees, emphasizing the following areas (Part 4 of this chapter provided more information on the points listed):

★ Standard Precautions
★ Physical fitness
★ Stress management
★ Professional care and counseling
★ Safe driving

Content Review

EMS Illness and Injury Prevention

- Use Standard Precautions
- Maintain physical fitness and use proper lifting and moving techniques
- Manage stress
- Seek professional care when needed
- Drive safely

SCENE SAFETY

Safety is always your first priority. Once your unit is dispatched to a call, evaluate the dispatch information prior to arrival. Focus your attention on response and equipment needed. Upon arrival, park the unit in the safest and most convenient place to load the patient as well as to leave the scene. Consider traffic, road conditions, and all other possible hazards. Directing traffic is primarily the responsibility of local law enforcement agencies. The safest method for traffic control at serious vehicle collisions is to stop all traffic and reroute it to different roads. This is for the safety of patients, bystanders, and rescue personnel.

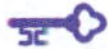

Safety is always your first priority.

Note that if you are called to an area with potential health hazards, such as an industrial park or a chemical plant or an area with high crime rates, approach the scene with caution. Be sure to protect yourself appropriately. If you do not have adequate protection or are not specifically trained to control specific hazards, never enter a hazardous scene. Call in specialized teams, such as a hazardous materials crew, if necessary. Law enforcement agencies should be contacted for any violent, potentially violent, or dangerous scene, including those involving domestic abuse or other crimes.

If the scene is safe to enter, be sure to wear reflective clothing to provide added protection on the scene. With Standard Precautions in place, approach patients with your safety in mind. Determine the mechanisms of injury (forces that caused injury) or the nature of illness. Treat the patient according to protocol.

After patient care is addressed and a transport decision is made, make sure your unit is secure before departure. Have your partner check the outside of the unit to make certain that all doors are secured. The patient should be secured on an ambulance stretcher with at least three straps as well as shoulder straps if available. If a family member is allowed to accompany the patient, that person should be placed in the passenger seat in the front compartment with vehicle restraints in place.

PREVENTION IN THE COMMUNITY

EMS has a responsibility to prevent injury and illness not only among EMS workers but also among members of the public.

As a component of health care, EMS has a responsibility to not only prevent injury and illness among EMS workers, but also to promote prevention among the members of the public.

Content Review

Areas in Need of Prevention Activities

- Low birth weight
- Unrestrained children in motor vehicles
- Bicycle-related injuries
- Household fire and burn injuries
- Unintentional firearm-related deaths
- Alcohol-related motor-vehicle collisions
- Fall injuries in the elderly
- Workplace injuries
- Sports and recreation injuries
- Misuse or mishandling of medications
- Early discharge of patients

AREAS OF NEED

Infants and Children

Each year, nearly 290,000 infants are born weighing less than 5.5 pounds (2,500 grams), often as a result of inadequate prenatal care. Low birth weight is a key indicator of poor health at the time of birth. Babies born too small or too soon are far more likely to die in the first year of life. Annually, over 4,000 die of low birth weight and prematurity. Among those who survive, an estimated 2 to 5 percent have a disability, and one quarter of the smallest survivors (born weighing less than 1,500 grams) have serious disabilities such as mental retardation, cerebral palsy, seizure disorders, or blindness.

One of every three deaths among children in the United States results from an injury. The number of injuries, of course, far exceeds the number of deaths. The most common causes of fatal injuries in children include motor-vehicle collisions, pedestrian or bicycle injuries, burns, falls, and firearms. Injuries generally can be classified into intentional events (such as shootings and assaults), unintentional events (such as motor-vehicle collisions), and alleged unintentional events (such as suspicious injury patterns that suggest possible abuse).

In motor-vehicle collisions, young children are easily thrown on impact. Because a young child's head is large in proportion to the body, unrestrained children tend to fly head first into the windshield or out of the car when a collision occurs. The back seat is the best seat for children 12 years old or younger. In this location, the properly restrained child is least likely to sustain injuries in a crash. Car safety seats and seat belts can prevent most severe injuries to passengers of all ages if they are used correctly. Air bags are designed to save people's lives when used with seat belts, and they can protect drivers and passengers who are correctly buckled.

Infants and toddlers are commonly injured by cars backing up in driveways or parking lots. Children between the ages of 5 and 9 who are struck by cars typically dart out in front of traffic. Children riding bicycles can be injured when they collide with cars or other fixed objects or when they are thrown from the bicycle. The most serious bicycle-related injuries are head injuries, which can cause death or permanent brain damage.

Falls are the most frequent cause of injury to children younger than 6 years old. About 200 children die from falls each year. Fire and burn injuries occur in the highest numbers in the very young. Most are caused by scalding from a hot liquid such as when children grab pot handles and spill the contents.

In this modern age of media and the Internet, children and young adults are bombarded with an incredible amount of information and are often faced with some of the same stressors as adults. Sometimes those stressors become overwhelming. One of the most troubling recent trends is the number of violent acts among young people, occurring in the form of self-destructive behavior, gang violence, and assaults. In addition, firearm injury is becoming more common as a result of the accessibility of hand guns to children. Injuries and deaths occur when children and adolescents take guns to school. The number of firearm deaths has doubled since 1953. About 15 percent of all firearm-related deaths are unintentional, often resulting from improper handling and lack of safety mechanisms.

Geriatric Patients

Falls account for the largest number of preventable injuries for persons over 75 years of age. As a result of slower reflexes, failing eyesight and hearing, and arthritis, the elderly are at increased risk of injury from falls. Falls frequently result in fractures since the bones become weaker and more brittle with age.

The aging process also places the elderly at greater risk for serious head injury as well as other injuries. Although many geriatric patients are completely coherent, many others suffer from some degree of dementia. Alzheimer's disease is merely one of the mental conditions that can affect the elderly. The associated confusion can contribute to dangerous behaviors such as wandering away from home or into a roadway.

Motor-Vehicle Collisions

As noted earlier, EMS and law enforcement have long referred to vehicular collisions as motor-vehicle accidents (MVAs). However, the term motor-vehicle collision (MVC) more accurately reflects the fact that no collision is an accident: something caused the crash to occur. Such crashes are responsible for over half of all deaths from unintentional injuries. Alcohol use is a factor in about half of all motor-vehicle fatalities.

Work and Recreation Hazards

In the workplace, back injuries account for 22 percent of all disabling injuries. Injuries to the eyes, hands, and fingers are responsible for another 22 percent. Even the quietest office setting can be hazardous. Never underestimate the potential dangers in an area that appears to be safe. Copy machines, electrical cords, faulty wiring, and shoddy building construction can be hazardous.

Sports injuries are commonly seen in persons of all ages due to the increased popularity and participation in outdoor recreational activities. Football, soccer, and baseball, as well as running, hiking, and biking, are among popular sports that can result in fractures, dislocations, sprains, and strains.

Medications

When an illness or injury occurs and treatment is sought, medications are often part of the treatment regimen. These medications are occasionally taken improperly (too much or not enough), or they are taken by others, sometimes causing serious medical problems. Medications of any kind should be taken only by those for whom they are prescribed. They should be stored according to label directions. They should also be continued until the prescription is completed. Following the physician's, the pharmacist's, and the label directions is imperative.

Early Discharge

Managed-care organizations such as HMOs and insurance companies often mandate shorter hospital stays and early discharges from the hospital, urgent care centers, and other outpatient facilities. Such policies often result in more patients being at home sooner with illnesses that are less completely treated. These patients may call upon 911 for supportive care and intervention.

IMPLEMENTATION OF PREVENTION STRATEGIES

The following is a list of prevention strategies that you should be able to implement:

★ *Preserve the safety of the response team.* Always remember that your first priority is your safety and the safety of your fellow crew members. The next priorities are the patient and, finally, bystanders. Do what you can and what is within your training to

Content Review

Prevention Strategies

- Preserve the safety of the response team
- Recognize scene hazards
- Document findings
- Engage in on-scene education
- Know community resources
- Conduct a community needs assessment

maintain a safe and secure working area. Do not hesitate to contact backup units and law enforcement personnel if necessary.

- ★ *Recognize scene hazards.* Size up the scene for potential risks or dangers before entering. Be aware of your surroundings. Is there anyone or anything that could cause harm to you, your crew, or the patient? Does the mechanism that injured the patient still pose a threat to the rescuers? Are there any hazardous materials in the area? Has any crime been committed? Are there structural risks? Are there temperature extremes for which you are unprepared? Call for the appropriate assistance.
- ★ *Document findings.* Document your patient-care findings at the end of every call. Note that EMS patient forms often can be designed to include specific data on injury prevention in order to benefit researchers and implement future prevention programs. Such a form should include space to describe scene conditions at the time of EMS arrival, the mechanism of injury, and any risks that were overcome. If protective devices were used (or not used) during the emergency, these should be documented, too. (See Figure 1-14 ■ for an example.)
- ★ *Engage in on-scene education.* Take advantage of a teachable moment to decrease future emergency responses. Remain objective, nonjudgmental, and nonthreatening. Inform your listeners of how they can prevent the recurrence of a similar emergency and, if needed, instruct them on the use of protective devices.
- ★ *Know your community resources.* Determine what your patient's needs are and how you may assist him. Your patient may require a referral to an outside agency such as a prenatal clinic; a social service organization that offers food, shelter, clothing, mental health resources, or counseling; or other services. Your system may also allow for referral or transportation to a clinic, urgent care, or alternative form of health care. Be aware of the presence of both licensed and unlicensed child care centers in your area.

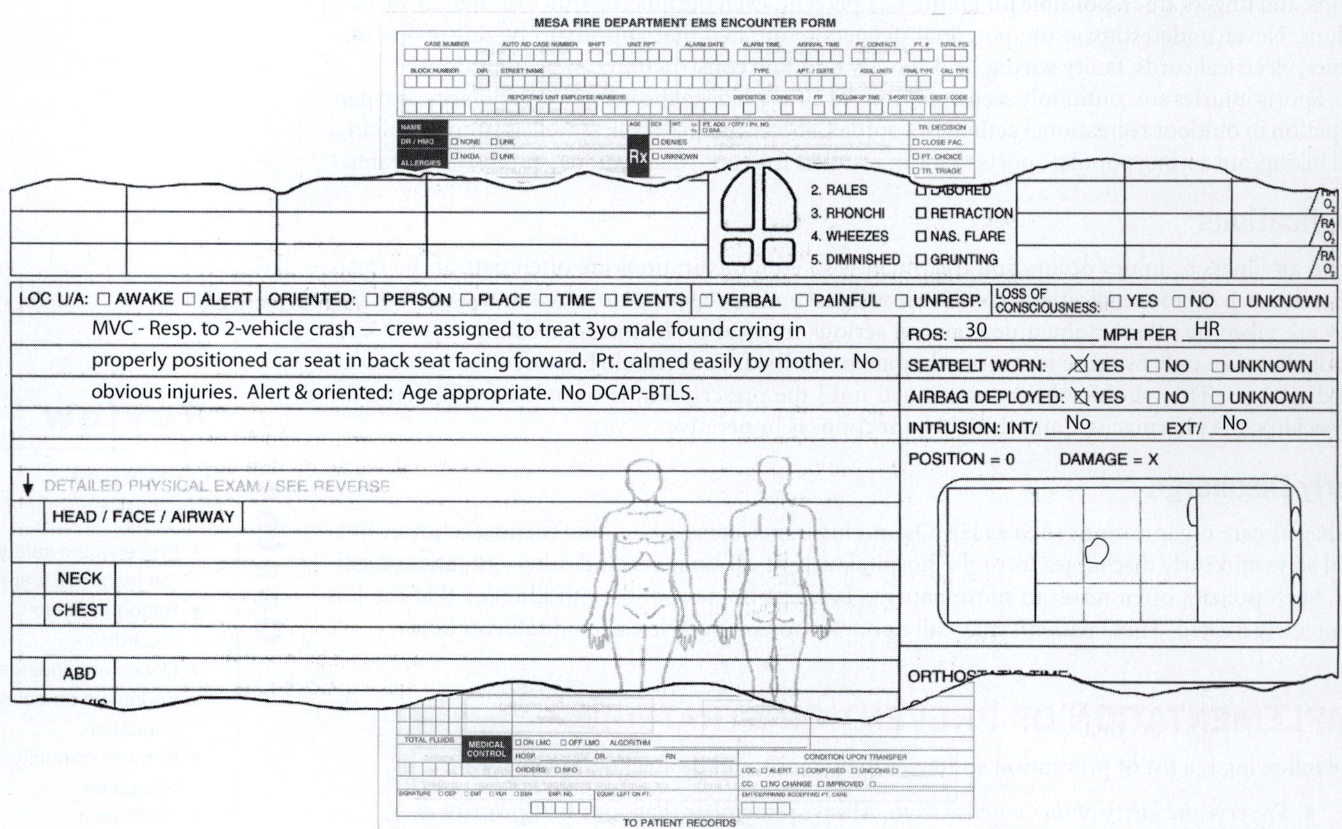
MESA FIRE DEPARTMENT EMS ENCOUNTER FORM

2. RALES ☐ LABORED
3. RHONCHI ☐ RETRACTION
4. WHEEZES ☐ NAS. FLARE
5. DIMINISHED ☐ GRUNTING

LOC U/A: ☐ AWAKE ☐ ALERT | ORIENTED: ☐ PERSON ☐ PLACE ☐ TIME ☐ EVENTS | ☐ VERBAL ☐ PAINFUL ☐ UNRESP. | LOSS OF CONSCIOUSNESS: ☐ YES ☐ NO ☐ UNKNOWN

MVC - Resp. to 2-vehicle crash — crew assigned to treat 3yo male found crying in properly positioned car seat in back seat facing forward. Pt. calmed easily by mother. No obvious injuries. Alert & oriented: Age appropriate. No DCAP-BTLS.

ROS: 30 MPH PER HR
SEATBELT WORN: ☒ YES ☐ NO ☐ UNKNOWN
AIRBAG DEPLOYED: ☒ YES ☐ NO ☐ UNKNOWN
INTRUSION: INT/ No EXT/ No
POSITION = 0 DAMAGE = X

DETAILED PHYSICAL EXAM / SEE REVERSE
HEAD / FACE / AIRWAY
NECK
CHEST
ABD

TO PATIENT RECORDS

■ **Figure 1-14** Documentation of primary and secondary injury prevention data is available.

Encourage parents to provide preexisting consent for treatment and transport in case of illness or injury at a child care facility. Follow local protocols to report suspected abuse situations. Consider developing a social service resource guide for your organization to provide solutions and ideas for these and other situations.

★ *Conduct a community needs assessment.* Conducting a needs assessment will assist in identifying community priorities. Consider the following:

– Childhood and flu immunizations
– Prenatal and well-baby clinics
– Elder-care clinics
– Defensive driving classes
– Workplace safety courses
– Health clinics (cosponsored by local hospitals or health care organizations)
– Prevention information on your agency's Internet website

The population served and its ethnic, cultural, and religious makeup may affect the needs and approaches that are most appropriate. Also consider community members who are learning disabled or physically challenged. These are just a few of the ideas that may be appropriate for your organization.

Part 6: Ethics in Advanced Prehospital Care

When asked what the most difficult part of the job is, most paramedics do not say "ethics." Nonetheless, a significant percentage of advanced life support calls do pose possible ethical conflicts, for example regarding refusal of care, choice of hospital destination, and advance directives. So, whether or not you are consciously thinking about ethics, you are almost certain to be called upon to decide what is the ethical thing to do from time to time in the course of your work.

OVERVIEW OF ETHICS

Ethics and morals are closely related concepts. **Morals** are generally considered to be social, religious, or personal standards of right and wrong. **Ethics** more often refers to the rules or standards that govern the conduct of members of a particular group or profession. Both ethics and morals address a question Socrates asked: "How should one live?"

morals *social, religious, or personal standards of right and wrong.*

ethics *the rules or standards that govern the conduct of members of a particular group or profession.*

RELATIONSHIP OF ETHICS TO LAW AND RELIGION

Ethics and the law have a great deal in common, but they are distinct. In general, laws have a much narrower focus. Laws frequently describe what is wrong in the eyes of society. Ethics goes beyond what is wrong and examines what is right, or good. As a result, the law frequently has little or nothing to say about ethical problems. In fact, laws themselves can be unethical; for example, laws that once perpetuated racial segregation. Even though ethics and the law are different, ethical discussions can sometimes benefit from techniques developed in the law. In particular, the law emphasizes impartiality, consistency, and methods to identify and balance conflicting interests.

Just as ethics differs from the law, it also differs from religion. In a pluralistic society such as ours, ethics must be understood by and applied to people who hold a broad range of religious beliefs or no religious beliefs at all. Thus, ethics cannot derive from a single religion. It is true, however, that religion can enhance and enrich one's ethical principles and values.

MAKING ETHICAL DECISIONS

There are many approaches to determining how a medical professional should behave. One is to say that each person must decide how to behave and whatever decision that person makes is okay. This is known as *ethical relativism.* However, people typically do not find ethical relativism satisfactory. For example, no reasonable person would say that it was acceptable for the Nazis to behave as they did. A similar approach is to say, "Just do what is right." This sounds fine, but different people have different beliefs about what is "right." Even the Golden Rule—"Do unto others as you would have them do unto you"—is not a sufficient guideline. What happens when the care provider's desires and values differ from the patient's? It becomes clear that reason and logic must be used and emotion must be excluded as much as possible from the decision-making process.

Reason must be used and emotion must be excluded as much as possible from the decision-making process.

CODES OF ETHICS

Over the years, a number of organizations have drafted codes of ethics for the members of their organizations. The American Medical Association has a code of ethics for physicians. The American College of Emergency Physicians has a code of ethics specifically for emergency physicians. The American Nurses Association and Emergency Nurses Association both have codes for practitioners in their fields. In 1948, the World Medical Association adopted the "Oath of Geneva." The National Association of EMTs adopted a code of ethics for EMTs in 1978.

Most codes of ethics address broad humanitarian concerns and professional etiquette. Few provide solid guidance on the kind of ethical problems commonly faced by practitioners. For example, a paramedic is expected to work in an uncontrolled environment that is sometimes dangerous. A person who is unwilling to enter a scene until every risk has been totally eliminated is not acting in accordance with the expectations of the profession. Conversely, a paramedic is expected to refrain from entering a hazardous area until the risks have been made manageable. Common sense should help in resolving conflicts such as these.

THE FUNDAMENTAL QUESTIONS

The single most important question a paramedic has to answer when faced with an ethical challenge is "What is in the patient's best interest?"

The single most important question a paramedic has to answer when faced with an ethical challenge is "What is in the patient's best interest?" Usually the answer is obvious, but not always. For example, what is in the best interest of a terminally ill patient who goes into cardiac arrest—to resuscitate, or not to start resuscitation in order to prevent further suffering?

A paramedic must be very cautious in accepting a family's description of what a patient desires. The family is often under a great deal of stress when the paramedic encounters them. The paramedic must also realize that the family may not agree with the patient's desires. They may be led to substitute their own desires for the patient's.

Under ideal circumstances, a written statement describing the patient's desires will be available. In many states, such a statement (which meets other specified state and local requirements) is required by law before a paramedic may elect not to start resuscitation efforts. In less extreme circumstances, the patient may state verbally what he wishes you to do and not do. It may sometimes be difficult for a paramedic to agree or to comply with a patient's wishes, but as long as the patient is competent and the desires are consistent with good practice, the paramedic is obligated to respect the patient's wishes.

FUNDAMENTAL PRINCIPLES

bioethics *ethics as applied to the human body.*

beneficence *the principle of doing good for the patient.*

nonmaleficence *the obligation not to harm the patient.*

A common approach to resolving problems in **bioethics** today is to employ four fundamental principles or values. These principles are beneficence, nonmaleficence, autonomy, and justice.

- ★ **Beneficence** is related to a more familiar term, *benevolence.* Both come from Latin and concern doing good. However, *benevolence* means the desire to do good (usually the main reason people become paramedics), whereas *beneficence* means actually doing good (the paramedic's obligation to the patient).
- ★ **Nonmaleficence** means *not* doing harm. (*Maleficence* means doing harm, the opposite of *beneficence.*) Few medical interventions are without risk of harm. Under the principle of nonmaleficence, however, the paramedic is obligated to minimize that risk as much as possible. This includes, for example, making the scene safe and protecting the patient from impaired or unqualified health care providers. The Latin phrase, *primum non nocere,* which means "first, do no harm," sums up nonmaleficence very well.

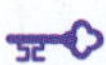

First, do no harm (primum non nocere).

- ★ **Autonomy** refers to a competent adult patient's right to determine what happens to his own body, including treatment for medical illnesses and injuries. Under ordinary conditions, a patient must give consent before the paramedic can begin treatment. There are, of course, exceptions to this (see the discussion of consent later in this chapter and in Chapter 2), but the implication is that the paramedic must be truthful in describing to the patient his condition and the risks and benefits of treatment. It also implies respect for the patient's privacy.
- ★ **Justice** refers to the paramedic's obligation to treat all patients fairly, without regard to sex, race, ability to pay, or cultural background, among other conditions.

autonomy *a competent adult patient's right to determine what happens to his own body.*

justice *the obligation to treat all patients fairly.*

RESOLVING ETHICAL CONFLICTS

The paramedic needs to have a system for resolving ethical conflicts. One such method of resolving ethical issues is illustrated in the following scenario:

> *You represent your service at the regional EMS coordinating agency. The head nurse for the emergency department of a large hospital mentions how recent cutbacks in support staff have led to difficulty retrieving patients' medical records in a timely manner. This has led to a number of difficulties in treating patients. As a result, the ED was considering asking incoming ambulances to give patients' names and dates of birth on the radio. This would give the ED staff additional time to search for the patient's medical records.*
>
> *You consider the issue's ethical aspects. First, you identify the problem: Is it justifiable to breach patient confidentiality in order to expedite the retrieval of medical records? Second, you list the possible actions that might be taken in this situation:*
>
> - *Provide all patients' names and dates of birth on the radio.*
> - *Continue, as now, to identify patients only by age and sex.*
> - *Provide selected patients' names and dates of birth on the radio.*

To reason out an ethical problem, first state the action in a universal form. Then list the implications or consequences of the action. Finally, compare them to relevant values, as follows:

Content Review

Solving an Ethical Problem

1. State the action in a universal form.
2. List the implications or consequences of the action.
3. Compare them to relevant values.

1. *State the action in a universal form. Describe what should be done, who should do it, and under what conditions.* For example, EMS (who) will volunteer names and dates of birth for all patients (what) on the radio (condition).
2. *List the implications, or consequences, of the action.* Positive consequences: The ED will be able to get records sooner for patients who have records at that hospital. There will be no change for most patients because hospital records are often irrelevant to emergency care. The ED admitting staff may be able to admit patients more quickly. Negative consequences: Patients' names and dates of birth will be broadcast to thousands of people listening with scanners. Long term, people with scanners will learn more about patients who go to the hospital via EMS. Because private information may be broadcast, patients may become reluctant to call EMS. Conceivably, there may be more burglaries at homes of patients who use EMS.
3. *Compare the consequences to relevant values.* A list of values that pertain to this case might include: beneficence, nonmaleficence, autonomy, and confidentiality. That is, if EMS provided names and dates of birth for all patients on the radio, what would be the benefit to the patient (beneficence)? A few patients might be cared for sooner because their records arrived sooner. Most patients will see no benefit because they have no records at that hospital or time is not a significant issue (such as for a laceration that requires sutures). Autonomy suffers under this arrangement because the patient is not given the opportunity to consent (or decline). The patient's name and date of birth go out over the air without his permission. And, in this case, nonmaleficence and confidentiality are intertwined. There is potential for harm to the patient and to future patients who lose faith in the EMS system's ability to maintain privacy.

Since the possible consequences of providing all patients' names and dates of birth on the radio are not compatible with the values we consider important and relevant, you must go back and test another action using this same method.

What about the second option, simply to continue the current policy of identifying all patients over the radio only by age and sex? The consequences might be that people listening to scanners can learn about patients EMS is transporting but not their identities, and a few patients may get delayed care because their records do not arrive quickly enough. A comparison with relevant values reveals that patient confidentiality and patient confidence in EMS are unchanged, but the patients who might benefit from earlier arrival of their records may be suffering.

What about the third option, to provide names and dates of birth of selected patients, for example, those in serious condition whose treatment must not be delayed? A comparison with relevant values shows that there is potential benefit for selected patients, a breach of confidentiality for those patients, but no breach of confidentiality for any other patients. So, the scenario may conclude as follows:

> *The third option sounds closer to being acceptable, but you wonder if there is a way to further limit loss of confidentiality. You suggest revising the rule to read, "EMS broadcasts the names and dates of birth of selected patients who (1) meet predetermined criteria, (2) when there is no other private means of communication available." This strictly limits the loss of confidentiality to patients who may benefit from it and encourages both EMS and the ED to find other less public means of identifying patients. For example, having someone at the scene telephone the ED to relay the patient's name and date of birth privately.*

Content Review

Quick Ways to Test Ethics

- Impartiality test
- Universalizability test
- Interpersonal justifiability test

The previously described method is useful when you come upon a new ethical problem and time is not an issue. In situations where time is limited, an abbreviated method can sometimes be used. First, ask yourself whether the current problem is similar to other problems for which you have already formulated a rule. If the answer is yes, follow that rule. If the answer is no, analyze the potential action against three tests suggested by Iserson: the impartiality test, the universalizability test, and the interpersonal justifiability test:

- ★ *Impartiality test*—asks whether you would be willing to undergo this procedure or action if you were in the patient's place. This is really a version of the Golden Rule (Do unto others as you would have them do unto you), which helps to reduce the possibility of bias.
- ★ *Universalizability test*—asks whether you would want this action performed in all relevantly similar circumstances, which helps the paramedic to avoid shortsightedness.
- ★ *Interpersonal justifiability test*—asks whether you can defend or justify your actions to others. It helps to ensure that an action is appropriate by asking the paramedic to consider whether other people would think the action reasonable.

When there is little time to consider a new ethical problem, these three questions can help a paramedic navigate murky waters, allowing him to find an acceptable solution in a short time.

ETHICAL ISSUES IN CONTEMPORARY PARAMEDIC PRACTICE

The preceding discussion described principles and methods for dealing with ethical issues. The following discussion is meant to help you apply those principles to several commonly encountered situations as well as some less common situations you may face.

RESUSCITATION ATTEMPTS

Consider the following scenario:

> *You are leaving the emergency department in your ambulance when a woman jumps out of a window of the hospital and lands on the road in front of you. Your partner stops the vehi-*

cle, and you grab your kit. As you reach the patient, a breathless aide runs out the door and says, "Don't do anything! She's got a DNR order!" How does this affect the care you administer? Your instincts say, treat her now and let the hospital sort things out later if she survives.

In this case, your instincts are probably steering you in the right direction for a number of reasons. First, state law requires that you see the order and verify its legitimacy in some manner. In this case, the order is not available for you to see so you are under no legal obligation to withhold care.

Second, if the patient is alive (as she appears to be), even a valid DNR order would not prevent you from assessing the patient and administering basic care, including comfort care.

Third, the principle of nonmaleficence says do no harm. Refraining from helping her might cause irreversible harm, perhaps death. The principle of beneficence also urges you to help the patient. The potential conflict arises when you consider autonomy. The competent patient of legal age has a right to determine what happens to her body, but you are unable to verify her wishes regarding resuscitation.

The conclusion of the scenario is as follows:

You and your partner go ahead and assess the patient. She responds to verbal stimuli by moaning, her airway is open, ventilations are adequate, and she has several lacerations and apparent fractures. Since you are literally in front of the hospital, you limit your interventions to quick immobilization on a spine board with bleeding control and oxygen by mask. You rapidly move her to the ED and turn her over to the team there.

Later you discover that she had originally been admitted for evaluation of new-onset seizures. When the doctors told her she might have a brain tumor, she signed a DNR form. Fortunately, no tumor was found and her prognosis is actually quite good. The trauma team finds no life-threatening injuries from her fall and expects her to be able to begin psychiatric treatment before she leaves the hospital. This additional information makes you very glad you decided to go ahead with treatment.

More and more states are passing laws or regulations allowing prehospital personnel to withhold certain treatment when the patient has a DNR order. A valid order consists of a written statement describing interventions a particular patient does not wish to have that is recognized by the authorities of that state. (See Chapter 2 for legal aspects of DNR orders.)

Paramedics spend a great deal of time and energy learning how to assess and treat patients with life-threatening problems. It becomes difficult, then, for a paramedic to watch someone die without doing something to try to stop it. You must nonetheless respect the patient's wishes when a competent patient has clearly communicated what he really wants. DNR orders make this easier because they typically must be signed or approved by a physician, increasing the likelihood that the decision was thoroughly thought through.

When there is no such order, however, it becomes more difficult for the paramedic to determine what the patient's wishes truly are. Family members may be able to describe the patient's desires, but they can have conflicts of interest that make their statements less credible. For example, the patient may have accepted his impending death before his family has. They may want you to attempt resuscitation when that was clearly against the patient's expressed wishes. A less common situation is one in which the patient wishes all resuscitation efforts, but the family does not because they do not wish to prolong their own suffering or they have other less noble motivations.

The general principle for paramedics to follow in cases such as these is: "When in doubt, resuscitate." This usually satisfies the principles of beneficence and nonmaleficence, admittedly perhaps at the expense of autonomy, but one of the biggest advantages to this approach is that, unlike the alternative, it is not irreversible. If you refrain from attempting resuscitation, it is certain that the patient will die. If you attempt resuscitation, there is no guarantee the patient will survive, but the patient can be removed from life-sustaining equipment later if that is deemed appropriate. Another advantage is that there will be more time later to sort out competing interests.

The general principle for paramedics to follow is "When in doubt, resuscitate."

What about not attempting resuscitation when the situation appears futile? This option may appear attractive at first glance. After a little investigation, though, the issue becomes much more complex. How would a reasonable person or society define "futile"? Except at the extreme ends of the spectrum, there is no consensus on what constitutes a futile attempt at resuscitation. In addition, there is the issue of who would actually make the decision that a resuscitation attempt is futile in a particular case. Is it the experienced paramedic who has seen very few lives saved under similar circumstances or the new paramedic who is still excited about the prospect of saving lives every day? How can it be fair to have such wide disparities in such an important decision? Clearly, the concept of futility does not provide a useful guide for whether or not to attempt resuscitation.

Another related topic is what to do when an advance directive is presented to you after you have begun resuscitation. Once you have verified the validity of the order and the identity of the patient, you are obligated ethically (and perhaps legally, depending on your state) to cease resuscitation efforts. This can be a very difficult situation for you emotionally, but you have an obligation to respect the patient's autonomy and stop doing something to him that he did not want. Follow your local protocols regarding procedures for cessation of resuscitation efforts.

CONFIDENTIALITY

Consider this scenario:

> *You are called at one o'clock in the morning to a local hotel for a man reported to be unresponsive (but breathing) at the front desk. When you arrive, one of the guests at the hotel meets you and tells you he found the clerk slumped over in his chair, apparently unconscious, with what smelled like alcohol on his breath.*
>
> *You approach the patient. His skin appears normal, and he is moving air well. He does not respond when you call him by the name on his name plate, Howard. He has a strong, regular radial pulse that is within normal limits. You do not smell anything except for a faint minty odor. When you shake his shoulder and call his name again, he opens his eyes, looks around, and asks, "Who are you?"*
>
> *You explain to Howard that you were called by a concerned guest who could not wake him up. Howard says he is fine now and does not want to go to a hospital. He is alert and oriented to person, place, and time. He denies any complaints, takes no medications, and has no past medical history. His vital signs are within normal limits. He denies any alcohol intake or use of any other drugs. The physical exam is unremarkable.*
>
> *By your protocols and standard operating procedures, you have no reason to attempt to force the patient to go to a hospital. You complete the appropriate documentation for a refusal of transport and are leaving the lobby when the guest who called 911 stops you. "Aren't you going to take him to the hospital?" he asks. No, you reply, he does not want to go. "But what if there's a fire in the hotel and he's passed out and unable to help guests evacuate?"*
>
> *This makes you stop and think, and you begin to weigh the rights of the hotel guests against the rights of your patient.*

Your obligation to the patient is to maintain as confidential the information you obtained as a result of your participation in this medical situation. If you reported his condition to hotel management, what would you report? You have found no objective evidence that he is under the influence of alcohol or drugs. Depending on the state you are in, you may actually have a legal obligation to maintain confidentiality under circumstances such as these. However, what if there is an emergency in which the desk clerk's assistance is needed and he is unable to provide it? That is a conceivable but unlikely possibility. There is no clear and present danger that would require you to report.

There are a number of reasons to respect confidentiality in general. In an emergency, a patient assumes that he can be honest with these strangers who have come to help him because they will protect his privacy. If that trust was violated without sufficient cause, patients might very well be embarrassed or humiliated. This would undermine the public's trust in EMS. If word got around that private information was being made public, patients might not be forthcoming in giving their medical histories, potentially leading to disastrous consequences. For example, a man who had recently taken sildenafil (Viagra) for erectile dysfunction might deny taking it before you give him nitroglycerin. That drug interaction is potentially serious, possibly even fatal.

There are nonetheless times when it is appropriate and necessary to breach confidentiality. Every state has laws requiring the reporting of certain health facts such as births, deaths, particular infectious diseases, child neglect and abuse, and elder neglect and abuse. These last requirements have the most applicability to EMS. They are considered justifiable reasons to breach confidentiality because, in the eyes of society, the benefit to someone who is defenseless (protection from harm and perhaps even death) and to the public (a safer environment for children and the elderly) outweighs the right to privacy of a particular person. A valid court order is also considered a reasonable justification for breaching confidentiality. So is a clear threat by a patient to a specific person, as well as informing other health care professionals who will care for the patient.

Clearly, patient confidentiality is an important principle, but not an inviolable one. When determining whether it is appropriate to breach confidentiality, take into account the probability of harm, the magnitude of the expected harm, and alternative methods of avoiding harm that do not require encroaching on confidentiality.

In the previous scenario, factors do not justify breaching confidentiality. The person who called 911 for emergency assistance, however, is under no such obligation. The scenario comes to an end as follows:

You inform the hotel guest that you are unable to discuss the case with anyone because of confidentiality. However, you point out, the guest is not under the same obligation. He replies, "OK, you may not be able to do anything about it, but I'm calling the manager!"

CONSENT

Consider this scenario:

Bob, a 58-year-old male, has been having crushing substernal pain radiating to his left arm for several hours. He also is pale, sweaty, and nauseated. He denies shortness of breath. His condition remains unchanged after you give him oxygen and nitroglycerin. When you ask Bob which hospital he wants to go to, he tells you, "I'm not going to any hospital." Surprised, you find it difficult to understand why someone in this much pain would not want to go to a hospital. You try to enlist the help of relatives over the telephone (Bob lives alone), but they are unable to persuade the patient. He has no regular physician, so that option is not available to you. Finally, you decide to try on-line medical direction. While you are waiting for the physician to come to the phone, you wonder: If the patient continues to refuse, can you force him to go? How can you act in the best interest of a patient who refuses to accept what you feel certain is best for him?

A competent patient of legal age has the fundamental right to decide what health care he will receive and will not receive. This is at the core of patient autonomy. To exercise this right, a patient must have the information necessary to make an informed decision, the mental faculties to weigh the risks and benefits of various treatment options, and the freedom from restraints that might hamper his ability to exercise his options (such as threats).

It is sometimes appropriate to use the doctrine of implied consent to force the patient to go to the hospital. For the paramedic to use this approach, the patient must be unable to give consent. Typically, the doctrine is invoked when the patient is unable to communicate, but it also can be employed when the patient is incapacitated because of drugs, illness, or injury. In this scenario, however, the patient shows no signs of being incapacitated. He is alert and oriented, making judgments and answering questions in a manner completely compatible with competence. The fact that the patient refuses something you recommend does not, in itself, indicate that he is incompetent.

Before you leave the patient, you must not only do the things you need to do to protect yourself legally, but you must also assure yourself that the patient truly understands the issues at hand and is able to make an informed decision. As difficult as it may be for you, if the patient is able to do these things, you may have to accept the patient's desires and leave him.

ALLOCATION OF RESOURCES

Paramedics do not usually think of themselves as guardians of finite resources, but occasionally they are. The most obvious example of this is when there are more patients present than the paramedic is able to manage, such as in a multiple-casualty incident (MCI). While learning how to provide emergency medical care for multiple patients at the same scene, you might ask: What are the ethics of triage?

There are several possible approaches to consider in parceling out scarce resources. Patients could all receive the same amount of attention and resources (true parity). They could receive resources based on need. Or they could receive what someone has determined they've earned.

The civilian method of triage, where the most seriously injured patients receive the most care, is based on need. This is intended to produce the most good for the most people. However, other methods of triage are in use. Military triage, for example, has traditionally concentrated on helping the least seriously injured because this approach produces the greatest number of soldiers who can return to duty. When the president or vice president visits a town or city, there is typically an ambulance dedicated for the dignitary's use if needed. The ambulance is not to be used for anyone else. Because these officials are so important and because so many others need them, the typical order of care is changed.

A controversy exists in emergency medicine as to whether or not celebrities should be treated ahead of others. The argument for doing so typically emphasizes the disorder brought to the ED by the presence of a celebrity and the need to get the person out of the ED as quickly as possible to restore normal operation. The argument against takes the position that giving preferential treatment to a celebrity is an affront to justice and fairness.

All of these methods have their proponents for different situations. The key to resolving the issue of allocation of scarce resources is to examine the competing theories in light of the circumstances at hand.

OBLIGATION TO PROVIDE CARE

Those who provide emergency care have a special obligation to help all those in need. Many other health care professionals are free to pick and choose their patients, accepting only those who have health insurance or who can themselves pay for the services delivered by the health care professional. This is not the case in emergency medicine. Paramedics, like other emergency professionals, are obligated to provide medical care for those in need without regard to ability to pay. They also have an ethical obligation to prevent and report instances of patient "dumping," where those without insurance are transferred against their will to public or charity hospitals.

A particular issue arises regarding the patient who is a member of a managed care organization such as a health maintenance organization (HMO). The HMO may insist that the patient be treated at a particular facility with which it has a contract. This must not be allowed to interfere with the patient's emergency care. The paramedic, like every other member of the EMS system, has an obligation to act in the patient's best interest, even when that goes against the HMO's economic interests.

Another situation is offering assistance when off duty. Although only two states require paramedics, among others, to stop and render help when they come upon someone in need of emergency care, there is still a strong ethical obligation to do so. This does not extend to situations where the paramedic would put himself in danger (such as getting into a car teetering on the edge of a cliff), if assisting would interfere with important duties owed to others (such as leaving young children unattended in a car), or when someone else is already providing assistance. In return, society offers limited liability in the form of Good Samaritan statutes in every state in the United States (as discussed in Chapter 2).

TEACHING

When patients call for EMS, they generally expect to receive care from qualified, credentialed individuals. EMS systems with students working in them should make sure students are clearly identified by the uniform they wear. The paramedic acting as preceptor should also, when appropriate, inform patients of the presence of a student and request the patient's consent before the student performs a procedure. This sounds more cumbersome than it actually is. Patients who are unable to consent obviously do not fall into this category. Implied consent is invoked in this case. Patients who are able to consent are frequently very understanding of the student's need for experience. As long as the preceptor stresses that he is overseeing the student, the vast majority of patients usually consent.

Another issue related to students is how many attempts they should be allowed in order to perform procedures such as intravenous placement and endotracheal intubation before the preceptor steps in. Factors to consider include the student's skill level, the anticipated difficulty of the procedure, and the relative importance of the procedure. It is important to have a limit, at least initially, for the number of times a student will be allowed to attempt a procedure. Such a number will need to be decided by each system in consultation with the medical director.

PROFESSIONAL RELATIONS

As a health care professional, the paramedic answers to the patient. As a physician extender, the paramedic answers to a physician medical director. As an employee (or volunteer), the paramedic answers to the EMS system. These competing interests can sometimes make life difficult. Each can lead to ethical challenges.

In general, there are three potential sources of conflict between paramedics and physicians. One possibility is a case in which a physician orders something the paramedic believes is contraindicated. For example, suppose a physician ordered a paramedic to transport a critical blunt-trauma patient without attempting any intravenous access, either at the scene or en route during the anticipated 45-minute transport. This order would run counter to standard medical practice.

A different situation arises when the physician orders something the paramedic believes is medically acceptable but not in the patient's best interests. For example, imagine you are transporting a patient with stable vital signs who is complaining of abdominal pain. In accordance with your protocols, you and your partner have each tried twice to start an IV line without success. The patient's veins are some of the worst you have ever seen, and you have no expectation that you will be successful on further attempts. The patient experienced considerable pain with each attempt and is now crying, asking you not to try any more. The physician, however, insists you continue attempts to gain access.

A third potential source of conflict is the situation in which the physician orders something the paramedic believes is medically acceptable but morally wrong. For example, say you are ordered to stop CPR on a young male found in cardiac arrest after blunt trauma. His initial rhythm of asystole has remained unchanged, and you know it is almost always associated with death. Nonetheless, although there is a very slim chance of recovery for the patient if you continue your resuscitation efforts, you would not be able to live with yourself if you did not at least try.

In each of the three cases, it is certainly appropriate for the paramedic to start by confirming the order and asking the physician to repeat it. If the order is confirmed, the medic would be prudent to ask the physician for an explanation, given the controversial nature of the orders. The next steps will depend on the physician's explanation, the patient's condition, the need for the intervention in the judgment of the paramedic, the feasibility of performing the intervention (like gaining IV access), and the amount of time available to discuss the issue.

Ultimately, the paramedic must determine for himself how the patient's interests are best served. This typically does not lead to conflict, but on occasion the paramedic may run into situations like the ones previously described. In these cases, the medic must consider the competing interests of beneficence, nonmaleficence, autonomy, and justice; the roles of the physician and the paramedic; the relative confidence (or lack thereof) the paramedic has in his own medical and ethical judgment; how far the paramedic is willing to go as an advocate for his patient; and the degree of risk acceptable to the paramedic in contravening physician orders.

It is important for the paramedic to understand that no matter what decision he makes, he will have to defend it. The explanation that he was just following the doctor's orders (or, conversely, just doing what he felt was right) will not be sufficient in and of itself. A paramedic is expected to be more than a robot. He is expected to simultaneously be a physician extender, working under a physician's license, and a clinician with the ability and independence to recognize and question inappropriate orders. The paramedic should also understand that he is not expected to act in ways he feels are immoral. However, if the individual's morals are significantly out of step with the expectations of the profession, he needs to reconsider his profession.

Disagreements with physician orders happen rarely. Usually they are the result of poor communication (such as, saying one thing while meaning another or static interfering with the radio transmission) or lack of sufficient information. Conflicts with physicians that reach the level in the previous examples are fortunately rare. When they happen, the paramedic must be willing to be an advocate for the patient and act in the patient's best interests.

RESEARCH

EMS research is only in its infancy, but it will clearly become more important and more common as the field establishes the foundation necessary to introduce, modify, and justify field interventions. As this occurs, paramedics will become instrumental in implementing research protocols and gathering data. It is essential that a paramedic participating in a research project understand the importance of gaining expressed patient consent or following federal, state, and local regulations regarding implied consent.

The goal of patient care is to improve the patient's condition. The goal of research, however, is to help future patients. The two goals are not the same, so patients must be protected from untoward outcomes as much as possible.

One very important way of protecting the patient is by gaining the patient's expressed consent. There are several difficulties with this. One is the concern that a patient experiencing an emergency may not be able to truly consent because of the emotional pressures he is feeling. This pressure may occur in spite of the paramedic's best efforts to explain matters calmly and impartially.

Another concern is with the patient who is unable to consent. An excellent example of this occurs in cardiac arrest research. By the very nature of the problem being studied, the investigators will be unable to gather consent from the patient. In this case, the federal government has strict rules, for example, about community notification before the study begins and gaining consent from the patient or an appropriate family member as soon as possible after a patient is entered into the study. A paramedic participating in such a study needs to be familiar with these rules and their implications.

Although many interventions have been tested and found to be life saving, there are unfortunately documented instances of patients denied treatment for life-threatening conditions in the name of research in the United States (e.g., the Tuskegee syphilis research project in which treatment for the disease was withheld). The paramedic has an obligation to prevent such things from happening in EMS research.

Summary

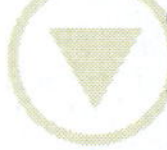

This is an exciting time for EMS and prehospital medicine. The paramedic of the twenty-first century is a true health care professional who can provide a significant impact on health care.

EMS has evolved over many years. Today, a comprehensive EMS system provides a continuum of care from First Responder to hospital and rehabilitative staff, from the mechanic who maintains the ambulance fleet to the emergency physician. It is a total team effort. The paramedic is the leader of the prehospital emergency medical team. You must undertake the responsibility of preparing yourself to do the job and of continually updating your knowledge and skills. The best paramedics are those who make a commitment to excellence.

The best paramedics are those who make a commitment to excellence.

As a paramedic, you must attend first to your own well-being in order to maintain the health and fitness to help others and to be a positive role model. Additionally, each member of EMS shares the responsibility of promoting wellness and preventing illness and injury among coworkers and in the community.

As a paramedic, you also have the responsibility to behave ethically by acquiring a foundation in ethical values and having a system for making ethical decisions.

Review Questions

1. Paramedics may only function under the direction and license of the EMS system's:
   a. town council.
   b. company owner.
   c. medical director.
   d. board of directors.
2. Verbal orders about patient management given by a physician to a paramedic by radio or telephone are examples of:
   a. direct medical direction.
   b. indirect medical direction.
   c. intermittent medical direction.
   d. reciprocal medical direction.
3. Medical direction can best be described as:
   a. paramedic development of patient care protocols.

b. on-scene physician's direction of all patient care.
c. delegated practice involving physicians on scene in the field.
d. physician direction of the actions of his designated agents.

4. The process by which an agency or association grants recognition to an individual who has met its qualifications is called:
a. profession.
b. licensure.
c. registration.
d. certification.

5. During an emergency response, remember that __________ is your number one priority.
a. patient care
b. personal safety
c. documentation
d. medical direction

6. A __________ trauma center provides the highest level of trauma care.
a. level I
b. level II
c. level III
d. specialty referral

7. Correct techniques are necessary to avoid on-the-job injury. Of all the movements you will make as a paramedic, the most common—and commonly associated with back injury—is:
a. crouching.
b. climbing.
c. lifting.
d. pushing.

8. A strict form of infection control that is based on the assumption that all blood and other body fluids are infectious is termed:
a. personal protective equipment.
b. mode of transmission.
c. incubation period.
d. Standard Precautions.

9. For safety at a roadway incident it is appropriate to do all of the following except:
a. ask nonmedical personnel to set out flares or cones.
b. wear reflective tape and an orange or lime-green vest.
c. blind a slumped-over passenger with a spotlight as you approach.
d. park on the opposite side of the street from the crashed vehicle.

10. The study of the factors that influence the frequency, distribution, and causes of injury, disease, and other health-related events in a population is called:
a. logistics.
b. census gathering.
c. epidemiology.
d. pathophysiology.

11. __________ means not doing harm.
a. Nonfeasance
b. Misfeasance
c. Nonmaleficence
d. Beneficence

12. Every state has laws requiring the reporting of certain health facts such as:
a. births.
b. deaths.
c. child neglect or abuse.
d. all of the above

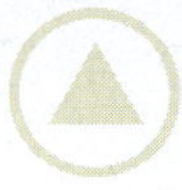

See Answers to Review Questions at the back of this book.

Chapter 2

Medical/Legal Aspects of Advanced Prehospital Care

Objectives

After reading this chapter, you should be able to:

1. Differentiate among legal, ethical, and moral responsibilities. (p. 66)
2. Describe the basic structure of the legal system and differentiate civil and criminal law. (pp. 66–67)
3. Differentiate licensure and certification. (p. 68)
4. List reportable problems or conditions and to whom the reports are to be made. (p. 69)
5. Define: Abandonment (p. 78); Advance directives (p. 80); Assault (p. 78); Battery (p. 78); Breach of duty (p. 70); Confidentiality (p. 73); Consent (expressed, implied, informed, involuntary) (p. 75); Do Not Resuscitate orders (p. 80); Duty to act (p. 70); Emancipated minor (p. 76); False imprisonment (p. 78); Immunity (p. 69); Liability (p. 66); Libel (p. 74); Minor (p. 76); Negligence (p. 70); Proximate cause (p. 71); Scope of practice (p. 68); Slander (p. 74); Standard of care (p. 70); Tort (p. 67).
6. Discuss the legal implications of medical direction. (pp. 68, 72)
7. Describe the four elements necessary to prove negligence. (pp. 70–71)
8. Explain liability as it applies to emergency medical services. (pp. 66, 70–73)
9. Discuss immunity, including Good Samaritan statutes, as it applies to the paramedic. (pp. 69, 72)
10. Explain necessity and the standards for maintaining patient confidentiality that apply to the paramedic. (pp. 73–74)
11. Differentiate expressed, informed, implied, and involuntary consent and describe the process used to obtain informed or implied consent. (pp. 75–76)

12. Discuss appropriate patient interaction and documentation techniques regarding refusal of care. (pp. 76–77)
13. Identify legal issues involved in the decision not to transport a patient, or to reduce the level of care. (pp. 77, 79)
14. Describe the criteria and the role of the paramedic in selecting hospitals to receive patients. (p. 79)
15. Differentiate assault and battery. (p. 78)
16. Describe the conditions under which the use of force, including restraint, is acceptable. (pp. 78–79)
17. Explain advance directives and how they impact patient care. (pp. 80–81)
18. Discuss the paramedic's responsibilities relative to resuscitation efforts for patients who are potential organ donors. (pp. 80–81)
19. Describe how a paramedic may preserve evidence at a crime or accident scene. (p. 81)
20. Describe the importance of providing accurate documentation of an EMS response. (pp. 81–82)
21. Describe what is required to make a patient care report an effective legal document. (pp. 81–82)

Key Terms

abandonment, p. 78
actual damages, p. 71
administrative law, p. 66
advance directive, p. 80
assault, p. 78
battery, p. 78
breach of duty, p. 70
civil law, p. 67
common law, p. 66
competent, p. 75
confidentiality, p. 73
consent, p. 75
constitutional law, p. 66
criminal law, p. 66
defamation, p. 74
Do Not Resuscitate (DNR) order, p. 80
duty to act, p. 70
emancipated minor, p. 76
expressed consent, p. 75
false imprisonment, p. 78
Good Samaritan laws, p. 69
immunity, p. 69
implied consent, p. 75
informed consent, p. 75
involuntary consent, p. 75
legislative law, p. 66
liability, p. 66
libel, p. 74
living will, p. 80
malfeasance, p. 70
minor, p. 76
misfeasance, p. 70
negligence, p. 70
nonfeasance, p. 70
proximate cause, p. 71
reasonable force, p. 78
res ipsa loquitur, p. 71
scope of practice, p. 68
slander, p. 74
standard of care, p. 70
tort, p. 67

INTRODUCTION

To practice competent prehospital care today, paramedics must become familiar with the legal issues they are likely to encounter in the field. As a paramedic, you must be prepared to make the best medical decisions and the most appropriate legal decisions. This chapter addresses general legal principles in addition to specific laws and legal concepts that affect the paramedic's daily practice.

Note that since laws vary from state to state, and protocols can vary from county to county, the information contained in this chapter cannot be used as a substitute for competent legal advice. Just like the practice of medicine, the practice of law involves some art, some science, and is always heavily dependent on the unique facts present in each situation. If you are faced with a specific legal question, you must rely on the advice of your attorney.

LEGAL DUTIES AND ETHICAL RESPONSIBILITIES

liability *legal responsibility.*

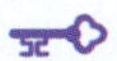

Your best protection from liability is to perform systematic assessments, provide appropriate medical care, and maintain accurate and complete documentation.

As a paramedic, you have specific legal duties. Failure to perform your job appropriately can result in civil or criminal liability. Your best protection from **liability** (legal responsibility) is to perform a systematic patient assessment, provide the appropriate medical care, and maintain accurate and complete documentation of all incidents.

A paramedic also is responsible for meeting ethical standards. Ethical standards are not laws. They are principles that identify desirable conduct by members of a particular group. Your ethical responsibilities include:

- ★ Promptly respond to the needs of every patient.
- ★ Treat all patients and their families with courtesy and respect.
- ★ Maintain mastery of your skills and medical knowledge.
- ★ Participate in continuing education and refresher training.
- ★ Critically review your performance, and seek improvement.
- ★ Report honestly and with respect for patient confidentiality.
- ★ Work cooperatively with and respect other emergency professionals.

In addition, you will encounter moral issues. Morality concerns right and wrong as governed by individual conscience. Always strive to meet the highest legal, ethical, and moral standards when providing patient care.

THE LEGAL SYSTEM

Sources of Law

In the United States, there are four primary sources of law: constitutional law, common law, legislative (or statutory) law, and administrative (or regulatory) law.

constitutional law *law based on the U.S. Constitution.*

common law *law that is derived from society's acceptance of customs and norms over time. Also called* case law *or* judge-made law.

Constitutional law is based on the Constitution of the United States, which sets forth our basic governmental structures and protects people against governmental abuse. For example, the Fourth Amendment protects people from unreasonable searches and seizures.

Common law, also referred to as "case law" or "judge-made" law, originated with the English legal system and is derived from society's acceptance of customs and norms over time. Common law changes and grows over the years. As a part of common law, precedents set by the courts are generally followed by other courts. In 2000, the Supreme Court upheld the rules set forth in *Miranda,* affirming that a confession will not be admissible at trial if it is found that the defendant was not advised of his rights before making his statement.

legislative law *law created by law-making bodies such as Congress and state assemblies. Also called* statutory law.

administrative law *law that is enacted by governmental agencies at either the federal or state level. Also called* regulatory law.

Legislative law (or statutory law) does not come from court decisions. It is created by law-making or legislative bodies. Statutes are enacted at the federal, state, and local levels by the legislative branches of government. Examples of legislative bodies include the U.S. Congress, state assemblies, city councils, and district boards. Legislative law takes precedence over common-law decisions.

Administrative law (or regulatory law) is enacted by an administrative or governmental agency at either the federal or state level. Administrative agencies, such as the Occupational Safety and Health Administration (OSHA), will take a statute enacted by a legislative body and will produce rules and regulations necessary to implement it. The agency is given the authority to make regulations based on that statute; enforce rules, regulations, and statutes under its authority; and hold administrative hearings to carry out penalties for any violations of its rules.

Categories of Law

criminal law *division of the legal system that deals with wrongs committed against society or its members.*

The United States has two general categories of law: civil law and criminal law. **Criminal law** deals with crime and punishment. It is an area of law in which the federal, state, or local government will prosecute an individual on behalf of society for violating laws meant to protect society. Homicide, rape, and burglary are examples of criminal wrongs. Violations of criminal laws are punished by imprisonment, fines, or a combination of the two.

Civil law deals with noncriminal issues, such as personal injury, contract disputes, and matrimonial issues. In civil litigation, which involves conflicts between two or more parties, the *plaintiff* (person initiating the litigation) will seek to recover damages from the *defendant* (person against whom the complaint is made). **Tort** law, which is a branch of civil law, deals with civil wrongs committed by one individual against another (rather than against society). Tort law claims include negligence, medical malpractice, assault, battery, and slander.

Note that the United States has a *federal court system* and a *state court system.* The federal court system was created by the U.S. Constitution. Generally, only cases that involve a question of federal law or cases in which the parties are citizens of different states will be heard in a federal court. The state court system is the location for most of the cases in which a paramedic may become involved. In *trial courts,* a judge or jury determines the outcome of individual cases. *Appellate courts* hear appeals of decisions by trial courts or other appeals courts. The decisions of appellate courts may set precedents for later cases.

civil law *the division of the legal system that deals with noncriminal issues and conflicts between two or more parties.*

tort *a civil wrong committed by one individual against another.*

ANATOMY OF A CIVIL LAWSUIT

If you have ever been served with legal papers, you know that being sued or even being called to testify at a trial can be very unsettling. A basic understanding of the legal system can help. The following is a brief description of the components of a civil lawsuit:

★ *Incident.* For example, a person is driving on a road and fails to see a stop sign. When he passes through the intersection, he hits another car and that driver sustains several injuries.

★ *Investigation.* The injured driver's attorney makes a preliminary inquiry into the facts and circumstances surrounding the incident to determine if the case has merit.

★ *Filing of the complaint.* The injured driver (now called the "plaintiff") commences the lawsuit by filing a complaint with the court. The complaint contains information such as the names of the parties, the legal basis for the claim, and the damages sought by the plaintiff. A copy of the complaint is served on the defendant.

★ *Answering the complaint.* The defendant's attorney then prepares an answer, which addresses each allegation made in the complaint. The answer is then filed with the court, and a copy is given to the plaintiff's attorney.

★ *Discovery.* Before any lawsuit appears in front of a judge or jury, both parties to an action participate in pretrial discovery. This is the stage of the lawsuit when all relevant information about the incident is shared so that parties can prepare trial strategies. Discovery may include the following:
  - *An examination before trial,* which is also called a "deposition," allows a witness to answer questions under oath with a court stenographer present.
  - *An interrogatory,* used by either side, is a set of written questions that requires written responses.
  - *Requests for document production* entitle each side to request relevant documents, including the patient care report, records of the receiving hospital, any subsequent medical records, police records, and other records necessary to help prove or defend the lawsuit.

★ *Trial.* A trial will be commenced at the lowest level of court in the state. In many states, they are called "superior" courts. At the trial, each side will be given the opportunity to present all relevant evidence and testimony from witnesses.

★ *Decision.* After deliberations, the judge or jury determines the guilt or liability of the defendant and then decides the amount of damages to award the plaintiff, if any.

★ *Appeal.* After the jury's decision is entered by the court, either party may be entitled to an appeal. Generally, grounds for an appeal are limited to errors of law made by the court. Appeals will not be heard at the lower-level court, but by the higher-level appellate court.

Content Review

Components of a Civil Lawsuit
- Incident
- Investigation
- Filing of complaint
- Answering of complaint
- Discovery
- Trial
- Decision
- Appeal
- Settlement

★ *Settlement.* This can occur at any stage of the lawsuit. Generally, the defendant will offer the plaintiff an amount of money that is less than the amount for which he is being sued. The plaintiff may then agree to accept the reduced amount on the condition, for example, that he will no longer pursue the case.

LAWS AFFECTING EMS AND THE PARAMEDIC

Most of the laws that affect EMS and paramedics are state laws. Although these laws vary from state to state, they share common principles.

Scope of Practice

scope of practice *range of duties and skills paramedics are allowed and expected to perform.*

The range of duties and skills paramedics are allowed and expected to perform is called the **scope of practice.** Usually, the scope of practice is set by state law or regulation and by local medical direction. Often, a state will have a general "medical practice act" that governs the practice of medicine and all health care professionals. These acts prescribe how and to what extent a physician may delegate authority to a paramedic. As you learned in Chapter 1, paramedics may function only under the direct supervision of a licensed physician through a delegation of authority. Generally, paramedics should follow orders given by on-line and off-line medical direction. However, you should not blindly follow orders that you know are medically inappropriate.

You may function as a paramedic only under the direct supervision of a licensed physician through a delegation of authority.

Circumstances in which an order from medical direction may be legitimately refused include when you are ordered to provide a treatment that is beyond the scope of your training and inconsistent with established protocols or procedures and when you are ordered to administer a treatment that you reasonably believe would be harmful to the patient. For example, imagine that a paramedic is en route to the hospital with a 200-pound (100-kg) patient who is having 15 multifocal premature ventricular contractions (PVCs) per minute. The treatment protocol for such a condition is to administer 1.0 to 1.5 mg/kg of lidocaine, or 100 to 150 mg to a 200-pound patient. The on-line physician orders the paramedic to administer 1 g (1,000 mg) of lidocaine. The paramedic knows this amount of medication would seriously harm the patient. What should he do? He should first raise the concern with the physician. If the physician still insists, the paramedic should refuse to follow the order and document the incident thoroughly on the patient care report.

In addition, every EMS system should have a policy in place to guide paramedics in dealing with intervener physicians (on-scene licensed physicians who are professionally unrelated to the patient and who are attempting to assist with patient care). Generally, such a policy requires that certain conditions be met before the paramedic allows the intervener physician to assume control of patient care. That is, the physician must be properly identified to the paramedic, licensed to practice medicine in the state, willing to accept the responsibility of continuing medical care until the patient reaches the hospital, and willing to document the intervention as required by the local EMS system.

Licensure and Certification

Other laws that directly affect the paramedic's ability to practice relate to certification and licensure requirements. *Certification* refers to the recognition granted to an individual who has met predetermined qualifications to participate in a certain activity. It is usually given by a certifying agency (not necessarily a government agency) or professional association. For example, after completing an approved paramedic program in New York State, a student who passes an approved written and practical examination will become a certified New York State paramedic.

Licensure is a process used to regulate occupations. Generally, a governmental agency, such as a state medical board, grants permission to an individual who meets established qualifications to engage in a particular profession or occupation. Certification or licensure, or perhaps both, may be required by your state or local authorities for you to practice as a paramedic.

Most states have laws that govern paramedic practice and set forth the requirements for certification, licensure, recertification, and relicensure. It is your responsibility to understand fully the EMS laws and regulations in your state.

Motor-Vehicle Laws

As with other EMS-related laws, motor-vehicle laws vary from state to state. Generally, there are special motor-vehicle laws that govern the operation of emergency vehicles and the equipment they carry. These laws apply to areas such as vehicle maintenance and use of the siren and emergency lights. It is important that you become familiar with the laws of your state. Keep up-to-date with local regulations, too.

Mandatory Reporting Requirements

Each state enacts different laws designed to protect the public. For example, most states have laws that require a health care worker to report to local authorities any suspected spousal abuse, child abuse or neglect, or abuse of the elderly. In many states, violent crimes, such as sexual assault, gunshot wounds, and stab wounds, must be reported to law enforcement. Emergencies that threaten public health, such as animal bites and communicable diseases, also must be reported to the proper authorities. The content of such reports and to whom they must be made are set by law, regulation, or policy. Become familiar with the circumstances under which you are required to make a report. If you fail to make a required report, you may be criminally and civilly liable for your inaction.

Content Review

Commonly Mandated Reports

- Spouse abuse
- Child abuse and neglect
- Elder abuse
- Sexual assault
- Gunshot and stab wounds
- Animal bites
- Communicable diseases

Legal Protection for the Paramedic

In addition to the laws that protect patients, legislative bodies have enacted laws to protect paramedics. For example, some jurisdictions have enacted laws that criminally punish a person who commits assault or battery against a paramedic while he is providing medical care. Others have laws prohibiting the obstruction of paramedic activity.

Immunity, or exemption from legal liability, is another form of protection. Governmental immunity is a judicial doctrine that prohibits a person from bringing a lawsuit against a government without its consent. However, most states today have waived their immunity rights, and courts are becoming increasingly likely to strike down the ones that still exist. This type of liability protection, even if allowed under law, generally serves to protect only the government agency, not the individual paramedic. Therefore, you should not rely on governmental immunity to protect you from claims of negligence.

immunity *exemption from legal liability.*

Virtually every state has **Good Samaritan laws,** which provide immunity to people who assist at the scene of a medical emergency. Though these laws vary from state to state, generally they protect a person from liability if that person acts in good faith, is not negligent (most states will cover acts of simple negligence but not ones of gross negligence), acts within his scope of practice, and does not accept payment for services. The Good Samaritan laws of many states have been expanded to protect both paid and volunteer prehospital personnel.

Good Samaritan laws *laws that provide immunity to certain people who assist at the scene of a medical emergency.*

Good Samaritan laws vary from state to state. Some provide protection for paid EMS personnel, while others exclude paid personnel. Learn the Good Samaritan laws in effect in the area where you work.

As a paramedic, you should also become familiar with local laws and regulations governing the use of physical restraints for dangerous or violent patients. There also may be regulations governing entry into restricted areas such as military installations, nuclear power plants, and sites with hazardous materials. Since the laws affecting paramedic practice vary from state to state, your agency should obtain the advice of an attorney in order to minimize potential exposure to liability.

Other laws are designed to protect the paramedic in the event of exposure to bloodborne or airborne pathogens. For example, the Ryan White Comprehensive AIDS Resources Emergency Act (Ryan White CARE Act) requires hospitals and EMS agencies to create a notification system to provide information and assist the paramedic when an exposure occurs. This law allows the paramedic who has been exposed to certain diseases (such as hepatitis B, AIDS, and tuberculosis) access to medical records to determine if the patient has tested positive for, or is exhibiting signs and symptoms of, an infectious disease. The Ryan White CARE Act is a federal law, but many states have enacted similar or even more comprehensive laws to protect paramedics who may have been exposed to infectious diseases. The Ryan White CARE Act was set to expire in 2009 but new legislation, the Ryan White HIV/AIDS Treatment Extension Act of 2009, replaced the original law. It is important for each agency to appoint an infection control officer and for this individual to implement protocols and an appropriate infection control plan.

LEGAL ACCOUNTABILITY OF THE PARAMEDIC

As a paramedic, you are required to provide a level of care to your patients that is consistent with your education and training and equal to that of any other competent paramedic with equivalent training. You also are expected to perform your duties in a reasonable and prudent manner, as any other paramedic would in a similar situation. Any deviation from this standard might open you to allegations of negligence and liability for any resulting damages.

negligence *deviation from accepted standards of care recognized by law for the protection of others against the unreasonable risk of harm.*

Content Review

The Four Elements of Negligence

- Duty to act
- Breach of that duty
- Actual damages
- Proximate cause

NEGLIGENCE AND MEDICAL LIABILITY

Negligence is defined as a deviation from accepted standards of care recognized by law for the protection of others against the unreasonable risk of harm. It can result in legal accountability and liability. In the health care professions, negligence is synonymous with malpractice.

Components of a Negligence Claim

In a negligence claim against a paramedic, the plaintiff must establish and prove four particular elements in order to prevail: a duty to act, a breach of that duty, actual damages to the patient or other individual, and proximate cause (causation of damages).

duty to act *a formal contractual or informal legal obligation to provide care.*

breach of duty *an action or inaction that violates the standard of care expected from a paramedic.*

standard of care *the degree of care, skill, and judgment that would be expected under like or similar circumstances by a similarly trained, reasonable paramedic in the same community.*

First, the plaintiff must establish that the paramedic had a **duty to act.** That is, he must prove that the paramedic had a formal contractual or informal legal obligation to provide care. Note that the act of voluntarily assuming care of a patient may imply that there was a duty to act, which creates a continuing duty to act. For example, in some states if an off-duty paramedic witnesses a person choking, he may be under no legal duty to act. However, if that paramedic initiates care, then he has a duty to continue care. The rationale behind this rule is if bystanders see that a victim is being helped, they may walk away. If the paramedic rendering assistance walks away after initiating treatment, but not completing it, the patient may actually be left in a worse condition than if the paramedic never tried to help.

Duties that are expected of the paramedic include:

- ★ Duty to respond to the scene and render care to ill or injured patients
- ★ Duty to obey federal, state, and local laws and regulations
- ★ Duty to operate the emergency vehicle reasonably and prudently
- ★ Duty to provide care and transportation to the expected standard of care
- ★ Duty to provide care and transportation consistent with the paramedic's scope of practice and local medical protocols
- ★ Duty to continue care and transportation through to appropriate conclusions

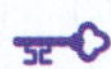

Always exercise the degree of care, skill, and judgment expected under like circumstances by a similarly trained, reasonable paramedic in the same community.

Second, the plaintiff must prove there was a **breach of duty** by the paramedic. A paramedic always must exercise the degree of care, skill, and judgment that would be expected under like circumstances by a similarly trained, reasonable paramedic in the same community. The **standard of care** specific to the paramedic's practice is generally established by court testimony and referenced to published codes, standards, criteria, and guidelines applicable to the situation. A breach of duty may occur by **malfeasance, misfeasance,** or **nonfeasance:**

malfeasance *a breach of duty by performance of a wrongful or unlawful act.*

misfeasance *a breach of duty by performance of a legal act in a manner that is harmful or injurious.*

nonfeasance *a breach of duty by failure to perform a required act or duty.*

- ★ *Malfeasance* is the performance of a wrongful or unlawful act by the paramedic. For example, a paramedic commits malfeasance if he assaults a patient.
- ★ *Misfeasance* is the performance of a legal act in a manner that is harmful or injurious. For example, a paramedic commits misfeasance when he inadvertently intubates a patient's esophagus, fails to confirm tube placement, and leaves the tube in place.
- ★ *Nonfeasance* is the failure to perform a required act or duty. For example, it would be an act of nonfeasance to fail to fully immobilize a collision patient who is complaining of neck and back pain.

In some cases, negligence may be so obvious that it does not require extensive proof. Unlike criminal cases, which require proof "beyond a reasonable doubt," civil cases require only a proof of guilt by a "preponderance of evidence." In most cases, the burden of proving negligence rests on the plaintiff. As a result, when it is difficult to do so, a plaintiff may sometimes invoke the doctrine of ***res ipsa loquitur,*** which is Latin for "the thing speaks for itself."

res ipsa loquitur *a legal doctrine invoked by plaintiffs to support a claim of negligence, it is a Latin term that means "the thing speaks for itself."*

To support a claim of *res ipsa loquitur,* the complainant must prove that the damages would not have occurred in the absence of somebody's negligence, the instruments causing the damages were under the defendant's control at all times, and the patient did nothing to contribute to his own injury. After the doctrine of *res ipsa loquitur* is invoked in court, the burden of proof shifts from the plaintiff to the defendant.

For example, a classic situation in which *res ipsa loquitur* might be used occurs when a patient has an appendectomy and wakes to find that a surgical instrument has been left inside his abdomen. To prove negligence in this case, the plaintiff's attorney would show that the damage would not have occurred without the physician's negligence, that the surgical instrument was under the physician's control at all relevant times, and that the patient did not contribute to the injury. Many cases in which *res ipsa loquitur* would be successful are settled out of court.

Another situation in which little proof is required occurs when the paramedic violates a statute and injury to a plaintiff results. Some laws state that if a statute is violated and an injury results, a person will be guilty of *negligence per se,* or automatic negligence. For example, if a paramedic who is driving in nonemergency mode fails to stop at a red light and hits a pedestrian, the paramedic's negligence is obvious. He violated vehicle and traffic statutes that prohibit a vehicle from running a red light, and he is therefore guilty of *negligence per se.*

After a duty to act and a breach of that duty have been proven, **actual damages** is the third required element of proof in a negligence claim. That is, the plaintiff must prove that he was actually harmed in a way that can be compensated by the award of damages. This is an essential component. A lawsuit cannot be won if the paramedic's action caused no ill effects. The plaintiff must prove that he suffered compensable physical, psychological, or financial damage such as medical expenses, lost wages, lost future earnings, conscious pain and suffering, or wrongful death.

actual damages *refers to compensable physical, psychological, or financial harm.*

In addition, the plaintiff may seek punitive (punishing) damages. These are awarded only when a defendant commits an act of gross negligence or willful and wanton misconduct. An act of ordinary negligence, such as accidentally allowing an IV to infiltrate, will not support an award of punitive damages. If punitive damages are awarded to the plaintiff, most insurance policies will not cover them. Therefore, the paramedic may become personally liable for any punitive damages awarded to the plaintiff.

Finally, to prove negligence, the plaintiff must show that the paramedic's action or inaction was the **proximate cause** of the damages; that is, the action or inaction of the paramedic immediately caused or worsened the damage suffered by the plaintiff. For example, a cardiac patient who breaks his arm during an ambulance collision while en route to the hospital will likely be able to prove that his injuries resulted from the incident; that is, the collision was the proximate cause of his injuries. However, a patient with a sprained wrist who happens to suffer a stroke while in the ambulance would have difficulty proving the ambulance ride was the proximate cause of the stroke.

proximate cause *action or inaction of the paramedic that immediately caused or worsened the damage suffered by the patient.*

Proximate cause may also be thought of in terms of "foreseeability." To show the existence of proximate cause, the plaintiff needs to prove that the damage to the patient was reasonably foreseeable by the paramedic. This is usually established by expert testimony. For example, imagine that a paramedic negligently crashes into a telephone pole with the ambulance. As a result, two people are injured—the patient who was in the back of the ambulance and, two blocks away, a baby who was dropped by his mother when the loud crash startled her. It should be easy for the patient to prove proximate cause, because it was reasonably foreseeable that an ambulance crash could hurt passengers. However, if the woman who dropped her baby sued the paramedic, she probably would not be able to establish proximate cause. Although the crash was the reason her baby was injured, it was not a foreseeable injury resulting from the ambulance crash.

Defenses to Charges of Negligence

If you are accused of negligence, you may be able to avoid liability if you can establish a defense to the plaintiff's claim. The following is a list of potential defenses to negligence:

- ★ *Good Samaritan laws.* If the paramedic can establish that his actions were protected by a Good Samaritan law, liability may be avoided. Note that such laws generally do not protect providers from acts of gross negligence, reckless disregard, or willful or wanton conduct, and they do not prohibit the filing of lawsuits.
- ★ *Governmental immunity.* These laws do not offer much protection for the individual paramedic accused of negligence. Though governmental immunity laws vary from state to state, the current legal trend is toward limiting this type of protection.
- ★ *Statute of limitations.* This is a law that sets the maximum time period during which certain actions can be brought in court. After the time limit is reached, no legal action can be brought regardless of whether or not a negligent act occurred. Statutes of limitations vary from state to state, so carefully review the laws in your state. Note that they may vary for different negligent acts and for cases involving children.
- ★ *Contributory or comparative negligence.* Some state laws will reduce or eliminate a plaintiff's award of damages if the plaintiff is found to have caused or worsened his own injury. For example, imagine that a patient involved in a car crash complained of neck pain but refused to let the paramedics properly immobilize his spine. The paramedics explained the risks of refusing treatment, but the patient signed a "release-from-liability" form anyway. Later, the patient learns that he has permanent spinal-cord damage and sues the paramedics for negligence. Many courts will find that the paramedics were not negligent because, by refusing necessary treatment, the patient contributed to the exacerbation of his own injury.

It is essential for all paramedics to be covered by liability insurance.

To protect yourself against claims of negligence, you should receive appropriate education, training, and continuing education; receive appropriate medical direction, both on-line and off-line; always prepare accurate, thorough documentation; have a professional attitude and demeanor at all times; always act in good faith, and use your own common sense. In addition, it is essential for all paramedics to be covered by liability insurance. Although many employers and agencies carry coverage, it is a good idea to obtain your own because your agency's coverage may be inadequate.

SPECIAL LIABILITY CONCERNS

Medical Direction

If a paramedic makes a mistake in the field and is sued by the injured patient, it is possible that the patient will also sue the paramedic's medical director and the on-line physician. The on-line physician may be liable to a patient for giving the paramedic medically incorrect orders or advice, for the refusal to authorize the administration of a medically necessary medication, or for directing an ambulance to take a patient to an inappropriate medical facility.

A paramedic's medical director may be liable to the patient for the negligent supervision of the paramedic. In order for the patient to be successful in this type of claim, he would have to prove that the physician breached a duty to supervise the paramedic and that breach was the proximate cause of the patient's injuries. Examples include: the medical director failed to establish medication protocols or standing orders consistent with the current standards of medical practice for the paramedic to use in the field; the medical director observed and then failed to correct a paramedic's poor intubation technique; or the medical director received complaints of inappropriate care by a paramedic and then failed to effectively investigate and resolve the problem.

Borrowed Servant Doctrine

As a paramedic, you may find yourself in the position of supervising other emergency care providers, such as EMT-Basics or EMT-Intermediates. When doing so, it will be your responsibility to make sure they perform their duties in a professional and medically appropriate manner. Depending on the degree of supervision and the amount of control you have, you may be liable for any negligent act they commit. This is called the "borrowed servant" doctrine. For it to apply, the paramedic accused of negligence must have taken the employees of another employer under his control and exercised supervisory powers over them.

Civil Rights

In addition to suing you for negligence, a patient may be able to sue you under certain circumstances for violating his civil rights if you fail to render care for a discriminatory reason. As a paramedic, you may not withhold medical care for reasons such as race, creed, color, gender, national origin, or (in some cases) ability to pay. Also, all patients should be provided with appropriate care regardless of their status, condition, or disease (including AIDS/HIV, tuberculosis, and other communicable diseases).

Off-Duty Paramedics

Liability also may arise in a situation in which an off-duty paramedic renders assistance at the scene of an illness or injury. Generally, any person who provides basic emergency first aid to another person would be protected from liability under a Good Samaritan law. However, when the off-duty paramedic provides advanced life support, a problem may arise. In most states, paramedics cannot practice advanced skills unless they are practicing within an EMS system. Performing paramedic skills and procedures that require delegation from a physician while off-duty may constitute the crime of practicing medicine without a license. Learn the law in your jurisdiction.

PARAMEDIC-PATIENT RELATIONSHIPS

The relationship you establish with your patient is a very important one. Not only must you provide the best medical care, but you also have legal and ethical duties to protect the patient's privacy and treat him with honesty, respect, and compassion.

CONFIDENTIALITY

All records related to the emergency care rendered to a patient must be kept strictly confidential. Keeping patient **confidentiality** means that any medical or personal information about a patient—including medical history, assessment findings, and treatment—will not be released to a third party without the express permission of the patient or legal guardian. However, there are specific circumstances under which a patient's confidential information may be released:

confidentiality *the principle of law that prohibits the release of medical or other personal information about a patient without the patient's consent.*

★ *Patient consents to the release of his records.* A patient may request a copy of his medical records for any reason. If the patient is a child, consent for release of medical records must be obtained from the child's parent or other legal guardian. The request should be accepted only if it is in writing, specifically authorizes the agency to release the records, and contains the patient's signature (or other authorized signature). If the request so directs, it is permissible to forward the records to the patient's physician, insurance company, attorney, or any other party the patient specifies. Be sure your agency retains a copy of the consent document.

★ *Other medical care providers have a need to know.* For example, it is not a breach of patient confidentiality to discuss the patient's condition with on-line medical direction or to give a patient report to an emergency nurse upon arrival at the hospital. This is permitted because it allows medical care appropriate for the patient to be continued. It is not acceptable, however, to discuss confidential patient information with medical providers who have no responsibility for the patient's care.

★ *EMS is required by law to release a patient's medical records.* Records may be requested by a court order that is signed by a judge, or they may be requested by *subpoena* (a command to appear at a certain time and place to give testimony). When an agency receives a court order or subpoena, it is good practice to consult with an attorney to make sure the order is valid and for assistance with compliance. Failure to comply with a court order or subpoena may result in severe penalties.

★ *There are third-party billing requirements.* For EMS agencies that bill patients for services, it is generally necessary to release certain confidential information to receive reimbursement from private insurance companies, Medicaid, or Medicare. If possible, the agency should obtain patient authorization for this purpose.

The law provides penalties for the breach of confidentiality. The improper release of information may result in a lawsuit against the paramedic for defamation (libel or slander), breach of confidentiality, or invasion of privacy. If found guilty, the paramedic may be responsible for paying money damages to the patient.

Health Insurance Portability and Accountability Act (HIPAA)

The Health Insurance Portability and Accountability Act of 1996 (HIPAA) changed the methods EMS providers use to file for insurance and Medicare payments. It also adds important new layers of privacy protection for EMS patients. The privacy protections provide, among other things, that all EMS employees be trained in HIPAA compliance. Furthermore, EMS providers must develop administrative, electronic, and physical barriers to unauthorized disclosure of patients' protected health information. Disclosures of information—except for purposes of treatment, obtaining payment for services, health care operations, and disclosures mandated or permitted by law—must be preauthorized in writing. HIPAA requires providers to post notices in prominent places advising patients of their privacy rights and provides both civil and serious criminal penalties for violations of privacy.

Patients are given the right to inspect and copy their health records, restrict use and disclosure of their individually identifiable health information, amend their health records, require a provider to communicate with them confidentially, and account for disclosures of their protected health information except for treatment, payment, health care operations, and legally required reporting purposes. The requirements of HIPAA are detailed and every EMS provider must become familiar with them.

Defamation

defamation *an intentional false communication that injures another person's reputation or good name.*

libel *the act of injuring a person's character, name, or reputation by false statements made in writing or through the mass media with malicious intent or reckless disregard for the falsity of those statements.*

slander *act of injuring a person's character, name, or reputation by false or malicious statements spoken with malicious intent or reckless disregard for the falsity of those statements.*

Defamation occurs when a person makes an intentional false communication that injures another person's reputation or good name. A patient may sue a paramedic for defamation if the paramedic communicates an untrue statement about a patient's character or reputation without legal privilege or consent. Defamation can occur in written form or through verbal statements.

Libel is the act of injuring a person's character, name, or reputation by false statements made in writing or through the mass media with malicious intent or reckless disregard for the falsity of those statements. Allegations of libel can be avoided by completing an accurate, professional, and confidential patient care report. Do not use slang and value-loaded words or phrases in your report (for example, do not refer to a patient as "stupid" or use any derogatory race-based terms). Since many states consider the patient care report part of the public record, never write anything on it that could be considered libelous.

Slander is the act of injuring a person's character, name, or reputation by false or malicious statements spoken with malicious intent or reckless disregard for the falsity of those statements. An allegation of slander can be avoided by limiting oral reporting of a patient's condition to appropriate personnel only. Note that many EMS systems record ambulance-hospital radio transmissions. In addition, scanners, which give the public access to EMS transmissions, are common in the United States. Therefore, information transmitted over the radio should be limited to essential matters of patient care. In most cases, the patient's name and insurance status should not be transmitted over the radio.

Invasion of Privacy

A paramedic may be accused of invasion of privacy for the release of confidential information, without legal justification, regarding a patient's private life, which might reasonably expose the patient to ridicule, notoriety, or embarrassment. That includes, for example, the release of information regarding HIV status or other sensitive medical information. The fact that released information is true is not a defense to an action for invasion of privacy.

CONSENT

By law, you must get a patient's consent before you can provide medical care or transport. **Consent** is the granting of permission to treat. More accurately, it is the granting of permission to touch. It is based on the concept that every adult human being of sound mind has the right to determine what should be done with his own body. Touching a patient without appropriate consent may subject you to charges of assault and battery.

consent *the patient's granting of permission for treatment.*

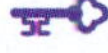

By law, you must get a patient's consent before you can provide medical care or transportation.

A patient must be **competent** in order to give or withhold consent. A competent adult is one who is lucid and able to make an informed decision about medical care. He understands your questions and recommendations, and he understands the implications of his decisions made about medical care. Although there is no absolute test for determining competency, keep the following factors in mind when making a determination: the patient's mental status, the patient's ability to respond to questions, statements regarding the patient's competency from family or friends, evidence of impairment from drugs or alcohol, or indications of shock.

competent *able to make an informed decision about medical care.*

Informed Consent

Conscious, competent patients have the right to decide what medical care to accept. However, for consent to be legally valid, it must be **informed consent,** or consent given based on full disclosure of information. That is, a patient must understand the nature, risks, and benefits of any procedures to be performed. Therefore, before providing medical care, you must explain the following to the patient in a manner he can understand:

informed consent *consent for treatment that is given based on full disclosure of information.*

- ★ Nature of the illness or injury
- ★ Nature of the recommended treatments
- ★ Risks, dangers, and benefits of those treatments
- ★ Alternative treatment possibilities, if any, and the related risks, dangers, and benefits of accepting each one
- ★ Dangers of refusing treatment and/or transport

Informed consent must be obtained from every competent adult before treatment may be initiated. Conscious, competent patients may revoke consent at any time during care and transport. In most states, a patient must be 18 years of age or older in order to give or withhold consent. Generally, a child's parent or legal guardian must give informed consent before treatment of the child can begin.

Expressed, Implied, and Involuntary Consent

There are three more types of consent: expressed, implied, and involuntary. **Expressed consent** is the most common. It occurs when a person directly grants permission to treat—verbally, nonverbally, or in writing. Often, the act of a patient requesting an ambulance is considered an expression of a desire to be treated. However, just because the patient consents to a ride to the hospital does not mean he has consented to all types of treatment (such as the initiation of an IV and/or the administration of medications). You must obtain consent for each treatment you plan to provide. Consent from the patient does not always need to be granted verbally. It may be expressed by allowing care to be rendered.

expressed consent *verbal, nonverbal, or written communication by a patient that he wishes to receive medical care.*

Unconscious patients cannot grant consent. When treating them or any patient who requires emergency intervention but is mentally, physically, or emotionally unable to grant consent, treatment depends on **implied consent** (sometimes called "emergency doctrine"). That is, it is assumed that the patient would want lifesaving treatment if he were able to give informed consent. Implied consent is effective only until the patient no longer requires emergency care or until the patient regains competence.

implied consent *consent for treatment that is presumed for a patient who is mentally, physically, or emotionally unable to grant consent. Also called emergency doctrine.*

Occasionally, a court will order patients to undergo treatment, even though they may not want it. This is called **involuntary consent.** It is most commonly encountered with patients who must be held for mental-health evaluation or as directed by law enforcement personnel who have the patient under arrest. It also is used on occasion to force patients to undergo treatment for a disease that threatens the community at large (tuberculosis, for example). Law-enforcement personnel often will accompany patients who are undergoing court-ordered treatment.

involuntary consent *consent to treatment granted by the authority of a court order.*

Consent issues also can arise when a paramedic is called by law-enforcement officials to treat a sick or injured prisoner or arrestee. The officers may tell you that they have the legal authority to give consent to treatment for the patient simply because the patient is in police custody. However, a competent adult in police custody does not necessarily lose the right to make medical decisions for himself. In fact, many prisoners have successfully sued health care providers for rendering treatment without consent. Generally, forced treatment is limited to emergency treatment necessary to save life or limb or treatment ordered by the court. Be sure that you are familiar with your local protocols and laws on this issue.

Special Consent Situations

minor *depending on state law, this is usually a person under the age of 18.*

In the case of a **minor** (depending on state law, this is usually a person under the age of 18), consent should be obtained from a parent, legal guardian, or court-appointed custodian. The same is true of a mentally incompetent adult. If a responsible person cannot be located, and if the child or mentally incompetent adult is suffering from an apparent life-threatening injury or illness, treatment may be rendered under the doctrine of implied consent.

emancipated minor *a person under 18 years of age who is married, pregnant, a parent, a member of the armed forces, or financially independent and living away from home.*

Generally, an **emancipated minor** is considered an adult. This is a person under 18 years of age who is married, pregnant, a parent, a member of the armed forces, or financially independent and living away from home. As an adult, an emancipated minor may legally give informed consent. Anyone else under the age of 18 may not grant informed consent.

Withdrawal of Consent

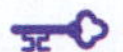

Refusal of care by a patient must be informed and properly documented.

A competent adult may withdraw consent for any treatment at any time. However, refusal must be informed. That is, the patient must understand the risks of not continuing treatment or transport to the hospital in terms he can fully understand. A common example of a patient withdrawing consent occurs after a hypoglycemic patient regains full consciousness with the administration of dextrose. The patient should be encouraged—*but may not be forced*—to go to the emergency department. If he is competent, the patient may refuse transport. In such cases, advanced life support measures, such as IV fluids, which were initiated when the patient was unconscious, should be discontinued. The patient also should complete a release-from-liability form (Figure 2-1 ■).

Sometimes patients choose to accept one recommended treatment but refuse others. For example, a patient involved in a motor-vehicle crash may refuse to be fully immobilized but ask to be transported to the hospital. It is very important for you to do everything in your power to be sure he understands why spinal precautions are necessary and what may happen if they are not taken. If a competent adult continues to refuse care, be sure to thoroughly document his reason for refusal and your attempts to convince him to change his mind. Have the patient and a witness sign a release-from-liability form.

REFUSAL OF TREATMENT AND TRANSPORTATION

I, THE UNDERSIGNED, HAVE BEEN ADVISED THAT MEDICAL ASSISTANCE ON MY BEHALF IS NECESSARY AND THAT REFUSAL OF SAID ASSISTANCE AND TRANSPORTATION MAY RESULT IN DEATH, OR IMPERIL MY HEALTH. NEVERTHELESS, I REFUSE TO ACCEPT TREATMENT OR TRANSPORT AND ASSUME ALL RISKS AND CONSEQUENCES OF MY DECISION AND RELEASE GOLD CROSS AMBULANCE COMPANY AND ITS EMPLOYEES FROM ANY LIABILITY ARISING FROM MY REFUSAL.

SIGNATURE OF PATIENT

WITNESSED BY

DATE SIGNED

■ **Figure 2-1** Example of a "release-from-liability" form.

Refusal of Service

Not every EMS run results in the transportation of a patient to a hospital. Emergency care should always be offered to a patient, no matter how minor the injury or illness may be. However, often, the patient will refuse. If this occurs, you must:

- ★ Be sure that the patient is legally permitted to refuse care; that is, the patient must be a competent adult.
- ★ Make multiple and sincere attempts to convince the patient to accept care.
- ★ Enlist the help of others, such as the patient's family or friends, to convince the patient to accept care.
- ★ Make certain that the patient is fully informed about the implications of his decision and the potential risks of refusing care.
- ★ Consult with on-line medical direction.
- ★ Have the patient and a disinterested witness, such as a police officer, sign a release-from-liability form.
- ★ Advise the patient that he may call you again for help if necessary.
- ★ Attempt to get the patient's family or friends to stay with the patient.
- ★ Document the entire situation thoroughly and accurately on your patient care report.

Remember, the refusal of care must be informed. That is, the patient must be told of and understand all possible risks of refusal. Decisions not to transport should involve medical direction. It is a good idea to put the patient directly on the phone with the on-line physician. If all efforts fail, be sure to thoroughly document the reasons for refusal and your efforts to change the patient's mind. If an on-line physician was involved, it is a good idea to obtain his signature on your patient care report.

Problem Patients

As a paramedic, you will occasionally encounter a "problem patient": one who is violent, a victim of a drug overdose, an intoxicated adult or minor, or an ill or injured minor with no adult available to provide consent for medical treatment. Such a patient can present you with a medical-legal dilemma. For example, consider the patient who has allegedly taken an overdose of medication. Concerned family members may panic and activate the EMS system. However, upon your arrival at the scene, you find the patient alert, oriented, denying that he has taken any medication, and refusing to give consent for treatment or transport.

In a case such as this, attempt to develop trust and some rapport with the patient. If he continues to refuse and remains alert and oriented, a refusal form should be completed and witnessed by a police officer. If the patient will not sign the form, have a police officer or family member sign it, indicating that the patient verbally refused care. If, however, the situation becomes dangerous, or you have reason to suspect the patient has tried to injure himself, police officers or family members should consider legal measures to force the patient to receive treatment.

The intoxicated person who refuses treatment and transport also poses a problem for the paramedic. Every effort should be made to encourage the patient to accept care and transport to the hospital. If the patient refuses, explain to him in a calm and detailed manner the implications of refusal. However, if you determine that the patient cannot understand the nature of his illness or the consequences of his refusal, then he may not refuse treatment because he is not competent to do so. Involve law enforcement at this point. If the patient is competent to make such a decision, then have him sign a refusal form. Your conversation with the patient and his refusal should be witnessed by a disinterested third party such as a police officer.

Regardless of the type of problem patient, always document the encounter in detail. Your records should include a description of the patient, the results of any physical examination (or reasons for the lack of one), important statements made by the patient and other persons at the scene, and the names and addresses of any witnesses. If you are going to include an important statement from the patient or witnesses in your patient care report, put the exact statement in quotation marks.

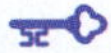

Involve the police and document in detail any encounter with a "problem patient."

Ideally, a police officer should respond to the scene of all problem patients and should either sign the patient care report as a witness or, if the paramedic's safety is at risk, accompany the patient and paramedic to the emergency department.

LEGAL COMPLICATIONS RELATED TO CONSENT

There are many legal complications related to consent to treatment. If the paramedic does not obtain the proper consent to treat or fails to continue appropriate treatment, he may be liable for damages based on a tort cause of action, such as abandonment, assault, battery, or false imprisonment.

Abandonment

abandonment *termination of the paramedic-patient relationship without assurance that an equal or greater level of care will continue.*

Abandonment is the termination of the paramedic-patient relationship without providing for the appropriate continuation of care while it is still needed and desired by the patient. You cannot initiate patient care and then discontinue it without sufficient reason. You cannot turn the care of a patient over to personnel who have less training than you without creating potential liability for an abandonment action. For example, a paramedic who has initiated advanced life support should not turn the patient over to an EMT-Basic or an EMT-Intermediate for transport.

Abandonment can occur at any point during patient contact, including in the field or in the hospital emergency department. Physically leaving a patient unattended, even for a short time, may also be grounds for a charge of abandonment. If, for example, you leave a patient at a hospital without properly turning over his care to a physician or nurse, you may be liable for abandonment. It is always a good idea to have the nurse or physician to whom you have passed responsibility for patient care sign your patient care report.

Assault and Battery

assault *an act that unlawfully places a person in apprehension of immediate bodily harm without his consent.*

battery *the unlawful touching of another individual without his consent.*

Failure to obtain appropriate consent before treatment could leave the paramedic open to allegations of assault and battery. **Assault** is defined as unlawfully placing a person in apprehension of immediate bodily harm without his consent. For example, your patient states that he is scared of needles and refuses to let you start an IV. If you then show him an IV catheter and bring it toward his arm as if to start an IV, you may be liable for assault.

Battery is the unlawful touching of another individual without his consent. It would be battery to actually start an IV on a patient who does not consent to such treatment. A paramedic can be sued for assault and battery in both criminal and civil contexts.

False Imprisonment

false imprisonment *intentional and unjustifiable detention of a person without his consent or other legal authority.*

False imprisonment may be charged by a patient who is transported without consent or who is restrained without proper justification or authority. It is defined as intentional and unjustifiable detention of a person without his consent or other legal authority, and may result in civil or criminal liability. Like assault and battery, a charge of false imprisonment can be avoided by obtaining appropriate consent.

This is a particular problem with psychiatric patients. In most cases, you can avoid allegations of false imprisonment by having a law enforcement officer apprehend the patient and accompany you to the hospital. If no officer is available, you should attempt to consult with medical direction and carefully judge the risks of false imprisonment against the benefits of detaining and treating the patient. You should determine whether medical treatment is immediately necessary and whether the patient poses a threat to himself or to the public when you are making your decision to treat or transport.

REASONABLE FORCE

reasonable force *the minimal amount of force necessary to ensure that an unruly or violent person does not cause injury to himself or others.*

If it is safe to do so, you may use a reasonable amount of force to control an unruly or violent patient. The definition of **reasonable force** depends on the amount of force necessary to ensure that the patient does not cause injury to himself, you, or others. Excessive force can result in liability for the paramedic. Force used as punishment will be considered assault and battery for which the patient may be able to recover damages and the paramedic may face criminal charges. When you believe it is necessary to use force, involve law enforcement if possible.

The use of restraints may be indicated for a combative patient. Restraints must conform to your local protocols. Restraining devices typically used by EMS providers include straps, jackets, and restraining blankets. In this circumstance, an EMS team's goal is to use the least amount of force necessary to safely control the patient while causing him the least amount of discomfort. If the use of restraints is indicated, involve law enforcement officials.

Patient restraint has become a particularly thorny legal issue for EMS personnel. Because physical restraint has been associated with significant problems, all EMS systems must have detailed protocols and standing orders that specifically deal with restraint.

PATIENT TRANSPORTATION

The transportation of patients to a health care facility is an integral part of the patient-care continuum. During transportation to a health care facility, be sure to maintain the same level of care as was initiated at the scene. This means that if you, as a paramedic, initiate advanced emergency care procedures, you must either ride with the patient to the hospital or ensure that another paramedic will accompany the patient. If you fail to do so, and the patient is harmed as a result, you may be liable for abandonment.

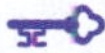

During transport of a patient to a health care facility, be sure to maintain the same level of care as was initiated at the scene.

One of the greatest areas of potential liability for paramedics is emergency vehicle operations. It is essential that you become familiar with your state and local laws. The laws that provide exceptions from driving rules and regulations may allow you, for example, to drive at a rate of speed in excess of a posted speed limit, but if you are negligent at any time during the operation of your vehicle, you will not be protected from liability.

Another issue that will arise is patient choice of destination. If you work in a small area with only one hospital, you are not likely to encounter difficulties. However, many paramedics work in areas that have many hospitals and medical centers to choose from. Over the past few years, increasing numbers of lawsuits involving facility selection have been brought by patients. Some have sued paramedics themselves, claiming negligence based on the failure to transport to the nearest or most appropriate hospital.

An additional issue you may need to address involves the patient's insurance company protocols. In some situations, it may be appropriate to respect a patient's choice of facility based on his insurance company's facility-choice protocols. Local restrictions by insurance companies and health care maintenance organizations may determine under what conditions and to what facilities patient transport may be authorized and paid for. While most areas are not yet being confronted with restrictions on service provision, it may be only a matter of time. However, never put patient care in jeopardy by transporting to a less appropriate facility because of insurance concerns.

In general, facility selection should be based on patient request, patient need, and facility capability. Local written protocols, the paramedic, on-line medical direction, and the patient should all play a role in facility selection. The patient's preference, however, should be honored unless the situation or the patient's condition dictates otherwise.

RESUSCITATION ISSUES

Advances in medical technology have saved and prolonged thousands of lives. However, in some instances, the use of sophisticated medical technology may only prolong pain, suffering, and death. When a person is seriously injured or gravely ill, family members must make difficult decisions regarding the medical care to be provided, including the use or withdrawal of life-support systems.

Generally, you are under obligation to begin resuscitative efforts when summoned to the scene of a patient who is unresponsive, pulseless, and apneic (not breathing). There are times, however, when you will determine that resuscitation is not indicated. This occurs with patients who have a valid Do Not Resuscitate (DNR) order, with patients who are obviously dead (decapitated, for example), with patients with obvious tissue decomposition or extreme dependent lividity (gravitational pooling of blood in dependent areas of the body), or with a patient who is at a scene that is too hazardous to enter.

Always follow your state laws, local protocols, and medical direction. The role of medical direction should be clearly delineated and included in your agency's protocols. If you are authorized to determine that resuscitative efforts are not indicated, be sure to thoroughly document your decision and the criteria upon which it was based.

ADVANCE DIRECTIVES

To improve communication between patients, their family members, and physicians regarding such matters, the federal government enacted the Patient Self-Determination Act of 1990. This act requires hospitals and physicians to provide patients and their families with sufficient information to make informed decisions about medical treatment and the use of life-support measures, including cardiopulmonary resuscitation (CPR), artificial ventilation, nutrition, hydration, and blood transfusions.

Patients and their families are therefore more likely than ever to have prepared a written statement of the patient's own preference for future medical care, or an **advance directive.** An advance directive is a document created to ensure that certain treatment choices are honored when a patient is unconscious or otherwise unable to express his choice of treatments. They come in a variety of forms. The most common encountered in the field are: living wills, durable powers of attorney for health care, Do Not Resuscitate orders, and organ donor cards.

advance directive *a document created to ensure that certain treatment choices are honored when a patient is unconscious or otherwise unable to express his choice of treatment.*

The types of advance directives recognized in each state are governed by state law and local protocols. Medical direction must establish and implement policies for dealing with advance directives in the field. Those policies should clearly define the obligations of a paramedic who is caring for a patient with an advance directive. They should also provide for reasonable measures of comfort to the patient and emotional support to the patient's family and loved ones. Some states do not allow paramedics to honor living wills in the field, but do allow them to honor valid Do Not Resuscitate orders. Be sure you are familiar with your state law and local policies.

Review Content

Advance Directives

- Living wills
- Durable powers of attorney for health care
- DNR orders
- Organ donor cards (such as found on a driver's license)

Living Will

A **living will** is a legal document that allows a person to specify the kinds of medical treatment he wishes to receive should the need arise. For example, many states allow patients to include in living wills their wishes concerning dying in a hospital or at home, receiving CPR, and donation of their organs and other body parts. In addition, patients with prolonged illnesses sometimes invoke the right to choose a person who may make health care decisions for them in the event that their mental functions become impaired. They might formalize this decision by way of a special notation in a living will. (They may also do this through execution of a document called a "Durable Power of Attorney for Health Care" or "Health Care Proxy.") Living wills, once signed and witnessed, are effective until they are revoked by the patient.

living will *a legal document that allows a person to specify the kinds of medical treatment he wishes to receive should the need arise.*

Be sure you know your local protocols concerning living wills. If any question arises on scene, contact medical direction for instructions.

Do Not Resuscitate Orders

A **Do Not Resuscitate (DNR) order** is a common type of advance directive. Usually signed by the patient and his physician, the DNR order is a legal document that indicates to medical personnel which, if any, life-sustaining measures should be taken when the patient's heart and respiratory functions have ceased. DNR orders generally direct EMS personnel to withhold CPR in the event of a cardiac arrest. When you honor a DNR order, do not simply pack up your equipment and leave the scene. You still may have the patient's family and loved ones to attend to. Provide emotional support as appropriate.

Do Not Resuscitate (DNR) order *legal document, usually signed by the patient and his physician, that indicates to medical personnel which, if any, life-sustaining measures should be taken when the patient's heart and respiratory functions have ceased.*

DNR orders pose a particular problem in the field. Paramedics are often called to nursing homes or residences where they find a patient in cardiac arrest and in need of resuscitation. As a rule, you are legally obligated to attempt resuscitation. If a physician has written a specific order to avoid it, the paramedics should not have been summoned. Even so, people tend to panic and will call for help. Valid DNR orders should be honored as your protocols allow. Note, however, that if there is any doubt as to the patient's wishes, resuscitation should be initiated.

Occasionally, you may be requested to treat a patient as a "slow code" or "chemical code only." This is not legally permitted. Cardiac resuscitation is an all-or-nothing proposition. Treating a cardiac arrest with only medications would mean abandoning airway management and defibrillation. To do so, even at the request of the family, amounts to negligence and must be avoided.

Potential Organ Donation

Over the past few years, advances in medicines have led to an increased number of organ transplants. As organs and tissues are in very high demand and short supply, many EMS systems are now becoming a vital link in the organ procurement and transplant process. Some have developed protocols that specifically address organ viability after a patient's death. These include providing circulatory support through IV fluids and CPR and ventilatory support via endotracheal tube. Whether or not your EMS has protocols in place for potential organ donation, it is important for you to consult with on-line medical direction when you have identified a patient as a potential donor.

Some states require that relatives of a recently deceased person be asked about the possibility of organ donation.

DEATH IN THE FIELD

Whether you arrive at the scene of a patient who has died prior to your arrival or you make an authorized decision to terminate resuscitative efforts, a death in the field must be appropriately dealt with and thoroughly documented. Follow state and local protocols and contact medical direction for guidance.

CRIME AND ACCIDENT SCENES

Preserve evidence at a crime scene whenever possible.

You may be called to treat a patient at a crime scene. You must not sacrifice patient care to preserve evidence or to become involved in detective work. You can best assist investigating officers by properly treating the patient and by doing your best to avoid destroying any potential evidence. As a paramedic, your responsibilities at a crime scene include the following:

- ★ If you believe a crime may have been committed on scene, immediately contact law enforcement if they are not already involved.
- ★ Protect yourself and the safety of other EMS personnel. This should always be your primary consideration. You will not be held liable for failing to act if a scene is not safe to enter.
- ★ Once a crime scene has been deemed safe, initiate patient contact and medical care.
- ★ Do not move or touch anything at a crime scene unless it is necessary to do so for patient care. Observe and document the original placement of any items moved by your crew. If the patient's clothing has holes made by a gunshot or a stabbing, leave them intact if possible. If the patient has an obvious mortal wound, such as decapitation, try not to touch the body at all. Do your best to protect any potential evidence.
- ★ If you need to remove items from the scene, such as an impaled weapon or bottle of medication, be sure to document your actions and notify investigating officers.

Treat the scene of an accident in the same way. Ensure your own safety and the safety of your crew and treat your patients as medically indicated.

DOCUMENTATION

The treatment of your patient does not end until you have properly documented the entire incident. A complete patient care report is your best protection in a malpractice action. In fact, a well-written report may actually discourage a plaintiff from filing a malpractice case in the first place. In general, a plaintiff's attorney will request copies of all medical records, including the paramedic's report, before filing a lawsuit. If the paramedic's report is sloppy, incomplete, or otherwise not well written, this may encourage the plaintiff to sue.

A well-documented patient care report has the following characteristics:

- ★ *It is completed promptly after patient contact.* It should be made in the course of business, not long after the event. Any delay could cause you to forget important observations or treatments. If possible, a copy of the completed report should be left with the emergency department staff before you leave the hospital. This copy will become part of the patient's permanent medical records. *Note:* Never delay patient care to attend to a patient care report.
- ★ *It is thorough.* The main purpose is not simply to record patient data, but also to support the diagnosis and treatment that you provided to the patient. All actions, procedures, and administered medications should be documented. Remember: "If you didn't write it down, you didn't do it."

★ *It is objective.* Avoid the use of emotional and value-loaded words. They are irrelevant and also may be the cause of a libel suit.

★ *It is accurate.* Be precise, avoiding abbreviations and jargon that are not commonly understood. Try to limit your report to information that you have personally seen or heard. If you document something that you do not have personal knowledge of, indicate the source of your information. Document your observations, not your assumptions, and do not draw a medical conclusion that you are not competent to make. For example, you cannot conclusively diagnose a patient as having pneumonia. You can, however, report your suspicion of pneumonia and document consistent findings.

★ *It maintains patient confidentiality.* Follow your agency's policies regarding the release of patient information. Whenever possible, patient consent should be obtained prior to the release of information.

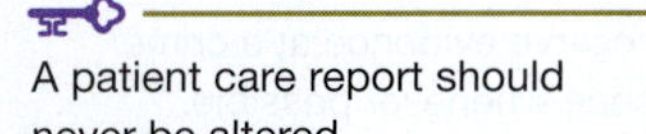

A patient care report should never be altered.

Intentional alteration of a medical record amounts to an admission of guilt by the paramedic. If a patient care report is found to be incomplete or inaccurate, a written amendment should be attached with the date and time the amendment was written, not the date of the original report. Send a copy of the addendum to the receiving hospital to become a part of the patient's medical records. Medical records need to be maintained for a period prescribed by state law. Become familiar with the record retention requirements in your state.

Summary

It is in your best interest to learn and follow all state laws and local protocols related to your practice as a paramedic. Also be sure to receive good training and keep current by pursuing continuing education, reading industry journals, and obtaining recertification or relicensure as required by state law. Always act in good faith and use your common sense. High-quality patient care and high-quality documentation are always your best protection from liability.

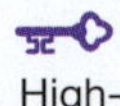

High-quality patient care and high-quality documentation are always your best protection from liability.

Review Questions

1. ___________ ___________ originated with the English legal system and is also called "case law" or "judge-made law."
   a. Common law
   b. Civil law
   c. Criminal law
   d. Constitutional law
2. ___________ ___________ is enacted by an administrative or governmental agency at either the federal or state level.
   a. Civil law
   b. Criminal law
   c. Legislative law
   d. Administrative law
3. The ___________ ___________ ___________ is the location of most of the cases in which a paramedic may become involved.
   a. appellate court system
   b. state court system
   c. federal court system
   d. supreme court system

4. On-scene licensed physicians who are professionally unrelated to the patient and who are attempting to assist with patient care are called:
   a. intervener physicians.
   b. direct control physicians.
   c. on-line medical control.
   d. indirect control physicians.
5. Legislative statutes that generally protect the person who provides care at no charge at the scene of a medical emergency are called:
   a. medical practice laws.
   b. scope of practice laws.
   c. Good Samaritan laws.
   d. standard of care laws.
6. In a negligence claim against a paramedic, the plaintiff must establish and prove four particular elements in order to prevail. Which of the following is *not* one of those elements?
   a. proximate cause
   b. duty to act
   c. level of compensation
   d. breach of the duty to act
7. The law provides penalties for the breach of confidentiality. The improper release of information may result in a lawsuit against the paramedic for:
   a. defamation.
   b. invasion of privacy.
   c. breach of confidentiality.
   d. all of the above
8. This court-ordered type of consent is most commonly encountered with patients who must be held for mental-health evaluation or as directed by law enforcement personnel who have the patient under arrest.
   a. implied
   b. expressed
   c. involuntary
   d. guardianship
9. ___________ is the termination of the paramedic-patient relationship without providing for the appropriate continuation of care while it is still needed and desired by the patient.
   a. libel
   b. slander
   c. neglect
   d. abandonment
10. A well-documented patient care report is:
   a. accurate.
   b. objective.
   c. thorough.
   d. all of the above

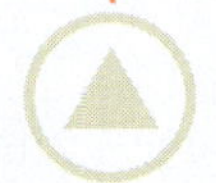

See Answers to Review Questions at the back of this book.

Chapter

3

Anatomy and Physiology

Objectives

Part 1: The Cell and the Cellular Environment (begins on p. 88)

After reading Part 1 of this chapter, you should be able to:

1. Describe the structure and function of the normal cell. (pp. 88–90)
2. List types of tissue. (pp. 90–91)
3. Define organs, organ systems, the organism, and system integration. (pp. 91–94)
4. Discuss the cellular environment (fluids and electrolytes), including osmosis and diffusion. (pp. 94–101)
5. Discuss acid–base balance and pH. (pp. 101–104)

Part 2: Body Systems (begins on p. 105)

After reading Part 2 of this chapter, you should be able to:

1. Describe the anatomy and physiology of the integumentary system, including the skin, hair, and nails. (pp. 105–107)
2. Describe the anatomy and physiology of the hematopoietic system, including the components of the blood, and discuss hemostasis, the hematocrit, and hemoglobin. (pp. 107–116)
3. Describe the anatomy and physiology of the musculoskeletal system, including bones, joints, skeletal organization, and muscular tissue and structure. (pp. 117–138)
4. Describe the anatomy and physiology of the head, face, and neck and their relation to the physiology of the central nervous system. (pp. 138–151)
5. Describe the anatomy and physiology of the spine, including the cervical, thoracic, lumbar, and sacral spine and the coccyx. (pp. 151–155)
6. Describe the anatomy and physiology of the thorax, including its skeletal and muscular structure and the organs and vessels contained within it. (pp. 155–160)
7. Describe the anatomy and physiology of the nervous system, including the neuron, the central nervous system (brain and spine), and the peripheral nervous system (somatic, autonomic, sympathetic, and parasympathetic divisions). (pp. 160–178)

8. Describe the anatomy and physiology of the endocrine system, including the glands and other organs with endocrine activity. (pp. 177–188)
9. Describe the anatomy and physiology of the cardiovascular system, including the heart and the circulatory system. (pp. 188–200)
10. Describe the physiology of perfusion. (pp. 200–205)
11. Describe the anatomy of the respiratory system (upper and lower airway and pediatric airway) and the physiology of the respiratory system (respiration and ventilation and measures of respiratory function). (pp. 205–217)
12. Describe the anatomy and physiology of the abdomen, including its divisions and the organs and vessels contained within it. (pp. 217–220)
13. Describe the anatomy and physiology of the digestive system, including the digestive tract and the accessory organs of digestion, and also the spleen. (pp. 220–223)
14. Describe the anatomy and physiology of the urinary system, including the kidneys, ureters, urinary bladder, and urethra. (pp. 223–228)
15. Describe the anatomy and physiology of the female reproductive system, the menstrual cycle, and the pregnant uterus. (pp. 228–234)
16. Describe the anatomy and physiology of the male reproductive system. (pp. 234–235)

Key Terms

2,3-diphosphoglycerate (2,3-DPG), p. 109
abduction, p. 119
acidosis, p. 102
action potential, p. 197
active transport, p. 100
adduction, p. 119
adenosine triphosphate (ATP), p. 89
afterload, p. 202
alkalosis, p. 102
alveoli, p. 209
amphiarthrosis, p. 119
anastomosis, p. 192
anatomy, p. 92
anion, p. 98
anterior medial fissure, p. 167
antidiuresis, p. 227
apnea, p. 216
appendicular skeleton, p. 122
aqueous humor, p. 146
arachnoid membrane, p. 140
articular surface, p. 118
ascending loop of Henle, p. 224
ascending tracts, p. 167
aspiration, p. 208
atelactasis, p. 209
autoimmune disease, p. 113
automaticity, p. 197
autonomic ganglia, p. 171
autonomic nervous system, p. 160
autoregulation, p. 143
axial skeleton, p. 122
blood pressure, p. 203
Bohr effect, p. 109
Bowman's capsule, p. 224
brainstem, p. 142
bronchi, p. 208
buffer, p. 98
bursae, p. 120
cancellous, p. 118
cardiac contractile force, p. 202
cardiac cycle, p. 193
cardiac depolarization, p. 196
cardiac output, p. 202
cartilage, p. 119
cation, p. 98
cell, p. 88
cell membrane, p. 88
central nervous system, p. 160
cerebellum, p. 142
cerebral perfusion pressure (CPP), p. 143
cerebrospinal fluid, p. 141
cerebrum, p. 141
chemotaxis, p. 111
chronotropy, p. 194
chyme, p. 222
circumduction, p. 120
clitoris, p. 230
collecting duct, p. 224
conductivity, p. 197
conjunctiva, p. 146
connective tissue, p. 91
contractility, p. 197
cornea, p. 146
cortex, p. 224
cranial nerves, p. 171
cranium, p. 139
creatinine, p. 227
cricothyroid membrane, p. 208
cytoplasm, p. 89
dehydration, p. 96
dermatome, p. 169
dermis, p. 106
descending loop of Henle, p. 224
descending tracts, p. 167
devascularization, p. 117
diaphysis, p. 117
diarthrosis, p. 119
diastole, p. 193
diffusion, p. 99
digestive tract, p. 220
dissociate, p. 98
distal tubule, p. 224
diuresis, p. 226
dromotropy, p. 194
dura mater, p. 140
ejection fraction, p. 201
electrolyte, p. 98
endometrium, p. 231
endotracheal intubation, p. 207
epidermis, p. 105

INTRODUCTION

An understanding of basic human anatomy and physiology is fundamental to paramedic practice. Part 1 of this chapter presents an organizational overview of human body systems, including:

- ★ The cell
- ★ Tissues
- ★ Organs
- ★ Organ systems
- ★ The organism
- ★ System integration
- ★ Fluids and electrolytes
- ★ Acid–base balance

Part 2 describes the major body systems:

- ★ The integumentary system
- ★ The blood
- ★ The musculoskeletal system
- ★ The head, face, and neck
- ★ The spine and thorax
- ★ The nervous system
- ★ The endocrine system
- ★ The cardiovascular system
- ★ The respiratory system
- ★ The abdomen
- ★ The digestive system and spleen
- ★ The urinary system
- ★ The reproductive system

Part 1: The Cell and the Cellular Environment

THE NORMAL CELL

cell *the basic structural unit of all plants and animals. A membrane enclosing a thick fluid and a nucleus. Cells are specialized to carry out all of the body's basic functions.*

The fundamental unit of the human body is the **cell** (Figure 3-1 ■). It contains all necessary components to turn essential nutrients into energy, remove waste products, reproduce, and carry on other essential life functions.

There are two kingdoms of cells: *prokaryotes* and *eukaryotes.* Prokaryotes are the cells of lower plants and animals such as blue-green algae and bacteria. Their structure is very simple, with an indistinct nucleus that is not encased in a membrane, and containing no other internal structures. Eukaryotes are the cells of higher plants and animals such as most algae, fungi, protozoa—and humans. Eukaryotes are, of course, more complex than prokaryotes. The cell structure discussed on the following pages relates to the eukaryotes.

Review

Content

Main Elements of the Cell

- Cell membrane
- Cytoplasm
- Organelles

CELL STRUCTURE

A cell is something like a small, self-sustaining city. Within the cell, specialized structures perform specific functions. In a normal cell, all the structures and functions work together to maintain a normal, balanced environment. Each cell has three main elements: the cell membrane, the cytoplasm, and the organelles.

The Cell Membrane

cell membrane *the outer covering of a cell; also called plasma membrane.*

semipermeable *able to allow some, but not all, substances to pass through. Cell membranes are semipermeable.*

The **cell membrane** (sometimes called the *plasma membrane*) is the outer covering that encircles and protects the cell.

The membrane is selectively permeable, or **semipermeable,** which means that it allows certain substances to pass from one side to another but does not allow others to pass. Vital functions of the cell membrane, made possible by its selective permeability, include electrolyte and fluid balance and the transfer of enzymes, hormones, and nutrients into and out of the cell. These functions will be discussed in greater detail later.

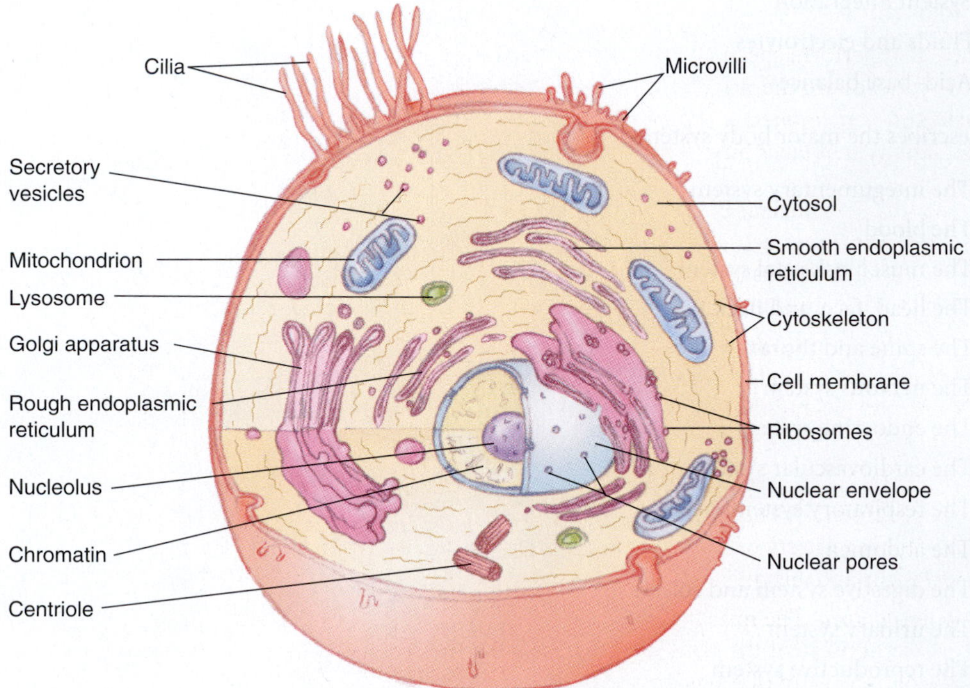

■ **Figure 3-1** The cell.

Without the cell membrane, the interior contents of a cell would become exposed to the extracellular environment and quickly die. That is why the cellular membrane of bacteria is the site targeted by many antibiotic drugs—because destroying the cell membrane kills the cell.

The Root CYT

To understand the discussion of cells, take note of the root cyt—which means "cell." Words with this root include:

cytokine	*protein produced by a white blood cell that instructs neighboring cells to respond in a genetically preprogrammed fashion.*
cytoplasm	*thick fluid that fills a cell.*
cytoskeleton	*structure of protein filaments that supports a cell's internal structure.*
cytosol	*clear liquid portion of the cytoplasm in a cell.*
cytotoxic	*poisonous (toxic) to cells.*
cytotoxin	*substance that is poisonous to cells.*
erythrocyte	*red blood cell.*
granulocyte	*white cell with multiple nuclei that has the appearance of a bag of granules.*
leukocyte	*white blood cell.*
lymphocyte	*a type of leukocyte, or white blood cell, that attacks foreign substances as part of the body's immune response.*
monocyte	*white blood cell with a single nucleus; the largest normal blood cell.*
phagocyte	*a cell that has the ability to ingest other cells and substances such as bacteria and cell debris.*
phagocytosis	*ingestion and digestion of bacteria and other substances by phagocytes.*
thrombocyte	*blood cell responsible for clotting; also called a* platelet.

The Cytoplasm

Cytoplasm is the thick, viscous fluid that fills and gives shape to the cell, also called *protoplasm.* The clear liquid portion of the cytoplasm is called *cytosol.* Substances dissolved in the cytosol are mainly electrolytes, proteins, glucose (sugar), and lipids (fatty substances). Structures of various sizes and functions are dispersed throughout the cytosol.

cytoplasm *the thick fluid that fills a cell; also called* protoplasm.

The Organelles

Structures that perform specific functions within the cell are called **organelles.** Six of the most important organelles are the *nucleus,* the *endoplasmic reticulum,* the *Golgi apparatus, mitochondria, lysosomes,* and *peroxisomes.* A brief discussion of a few of their functions provides an idea of the complex activity that takes place within a cell.

organelles *structures that perform specific functions within a cell.*

- ★ *Nucleus.* The **nucleus** contains the genetic material, deoxyribonucleic acid (DNA), and the enzymes necessary for replication of DNA. DNA determines our inherited traits and also plays a critical ongoing role within our bodies. DNA must be constantly copied and transferred to the cells.
- ★ *Endoplasmic reticulum.* The endoplasmic reticulum is a network of small channels that has both rough and smooth portions. Rough endoplasmic reticulum functions in the synthesis (building) of proteins. Smooth endoplasmic reticulum functions in the synthesis of lipids, some of which are used in the formation of cell membranes, and carbohydrates.
- ★ *Golgi apparatus.* The Golgi apparatus is located near the nucleus of most cells. It performs a variety of functions including synthesis and packaging of secretions such as mucus and enzymes.
- ★ *Mitochondria.* The mitochondria are the energy factories, sometimes called the "powerhouses," of the cells. They convert essential nutrients into energy sources, often in the form of **adenosine triphosphate** (ATP).

nucleus *the organelle within a cell that contains the DNA, or genetic material; in the cells of higher organisms, the nucleus is surrounded by a membrane.*

adenosine triphosphate (ATP) *a high-energy compound present in all cells, especially muscle cells; when split by enzyme action it yields energy. Energy is stored in ATP.*

★ *Lysosomes.* Lysosomes contain digestive enzymes. Their functions include protection against disease and production of nutrients, breaking down bacteria and organic debris that has been taken into the cells and releasing usable substances such as sugars and amino acids.

★ *Peroxisomes.* Peroxisomes are similar to lysosomes. Especially abundant in the liver, they absorb and neutralize toxins such as alcohol.

A wide variety of other structures and functions exist within the cell. Within the nucleus, for example, there are one or more smaller organelles called *nucleoli* (plural of *nucleolus*). Another component of the nucleus is *chromatin* (tangles of chromosome filaments containing DNA). Additional organelles exist in the cytoplasm (cytosol) outside the nucleus, including the *cytoskeleton* (a structure of protein filaments that supports the internal structure of the cell), *ribosomes* (granular structures that manufacture proteins—some float free, others attach to the surface of the endoplasmic reticulum, which creates the "rough" endoplasmic reticulum), *vesicles* (which play a role in transferring and storing secretions from the rough endoplasmic reticulum and Golgi complex), and *centrioles* (which play a role in cell division). On the surface of some cells are *microvilli* (folds on the cell surface), and, on some cells, whiplike *cilia* and *flagella* (which move fluids across cell surfaces and move cells through the surrounding extracellular fluid).

Review

Content

Structural Hierarchy of the Body

Cells
↓
Tissues
↓
Organs
↓
Organ systems
↓
Organism

CELL FUNCTION

All the cells of the human body have the same general structure and contain the same genetic material but, through a process called *differentiation,* or *maturation,* cells become specialized. Eventually, cells perform specific functions that are different from the functions performed by other cells. There are seven major functions of cells:

★ *Movement* is performed by muscle cells. Skeletal muscles move arms and legs. The smooth muscle around blood vessels causes them to dilate or constrict as necessary. Other smooth muscle moves food and wastes through the digestive tract. Cardiac muscle causes the chambers of the heart to contract. (See Muscle Tissue in the next section.)

★ *Conductivity* is the function of nerve cells that creates and transmits an electrical impulse in response to a stimulus.

★ *Metabolic absorption* is a function of cells of the intestines and kidneys, which take in nutrients that pass through the body.

★ *Secretion* is performed by glands that produce substances such as hormones, mucus, sweat, and saliva.

★ *Excretion* is a function all cells perform as they break down nutrients and expel wastes.

★ *Respiration* is the function by which cells take in oxygen, which is used to transform nutrients into energy.

★ *Reproduction* is the process by which cells enlarge, divide, and reproduce themselves, replacing dead cells and enabling new tissue growth and healing of wounds. Some cells, such as nerve cells, cannot reproduce—for instance, a severed spinal cord cannot repair itself.

tissue *a group of cells that perform a similar function.*

epithelial tissue *the protective tissue that lines internal and external body tissues. Examples: skin, mucous membranes, the lining of the intestinal tract.*

TISSUES

Tissue refers to a group of cells that perform a similar function. The following are the four basic types of tissue:

★ **Epithelial tissue** lines internal and external body surfaces and protects the body. In addition, certain types of epithelial tissue perform specialized functions such as secretion, absorption, diffusion, and filtration. Examples of epithelial tissue are skin, mucous membranes, and the lining of the intestinal tract.

★ **Muscle tissue** has the capability of contraction when stimulated. There are three types of muscle tissue (see Figure 3-42 in the Musculoskeletal System section later in this chapter).

—*Cardiac muscle* is tissue that is found only within the heart. It has the unique capability of spontaneous contraction without external stimulation.

—*Smooth muscle* is the muscle found within the intestines and encircling blood vessels. Smooth muscle is generally under the control of the involuntary, or autonomic, component of the nervous system.

—*Skeletal muscle* is the most abundant muscle type. It allows movement and is mostly under voluntary control.

★ **Connective tissue** is the most abundant tissue in the body. It provides support, connection, and insulation. Examples of connective tissue include bones, cartilage, and fat. Blood is also sometimes classified as connective tissue.

★ **Nerve tissue** is tissue specialized to transmit electrical impulses throughout the body. Examples of nerve tissue include the brain, the spinal cord, and peripheral nerves.

muscle tissue *tissue that is capable of contraction when stimulated. There are three types of muscle tissue:* cardiac *(myocardium, or heart muscle),* smooth *(within intestines, surrounding blood vessels), and* skeletal, *or* striated *(allows skeletal movement). Skeletal muscle is mostly under voluntary, or conscious, control; smooth muscle is under involuntary, or unconscious, control; cardiac muscle is capable of spontaneous, or self-excited, contraction.*

connective tissue *the most abundant body tissue; it provides support, connection, and insulation. Examples: bone, cartilage, fat, blood.*

nerve tissue *tissue that transmits electrical impulses throughout the body.*

ORGANS, ORGAN SYSTEMS, AND THE ORGANISM

A group of tissues functioning together is an **organ.** For example, the pancreas consists of epithelial tissue, connective tissue, and nervous tissue. Together, these tissues perform the essential functions of the pancreas. These functions include production of certain digestive enzymes and regulation of glucose metabolism.

A group of organs that work together is referred to as an **organ system.** The following are important organ systems:

★ *Cardiovascular system.* The cardiovascular system consists of the heart, blood vessels, and blood. It transports nutrients and other essential elements to all parts of the body.

★ *Respiratory system.* The respiratory system consists of the lungs and associated structures. It provides oxygen to the body, while removing carbon dioxide and other waste products.

★ *Gastrointestinal system.* The gastrointestinal system consists of the mouth, salivary glands, esophagus, stomach, intestines, liver, pancreas, gallbladder, rectum, and anus. It takes in complex nutrients and breaks them down into a form that can be readily used by the body. It also aids in the elimination of excess wastes.

★ *Genitourinary system.* The genitourinary system consists of the kidneys, ureters, bladder, and urethra. It is important in the elimination of various waste products. It also plays a major role in the regulation of water, electrolytes, blood pressure, and other essential body functions.

★ *Reproductive system.* The reproductive system provides for reproduction of the organism. In the female, it consists of the ovaries, fallopian tubes, uterus, and vagina. In the male, it consists of the testes, prostate, seminal vesicles, vas deferens, and penis.

★ *Nervous system.* The nervous system consists of the brain, spinal cord, and all of the peripheral nerves. It controls virtually all bodily functions and is the seat of intellect, awareness, and personality.

★ *Endocrine system.* The endocrine system is a control system closely associated with the nervous system. It consists of the pituitary gland, pineal gland, pancreas, testes (male), ovaries (female), adrenal glands, thyroid gland, and parathyroid glands. There is evidence that other organs—such as the heart, kidney, and intestines—have endocrine functions. As noted earlier, the endocrine system exerts its effects through the release of chemical messengers called hormones.

★ *Lymphatic system.* The lymphatic system is often considered a part of the cardiovascular system. It consists of the spleen, lymph nodes, lymphatic channels,

organ *a group of tissues functioning together. Examples: heart, liver, brain, ovary, eye.*

organ system *a group of organs that work together. Examples: the cardiovascular system, formed of the heart, blood vessels, and blood; the gastrointestinal system, comprising the mouth, salivary glands, esophagus, stomach, intestines, liver, pancreas, gallbladder, rectum, and anus.*

Content Review

Organ Systems

- Cardiovascular
- Respiratory
- Gastrointestinal
- Genitourinary
- Reproductive
- Nervous
- Endocrine
- Lymphatic
- Muscular
- Skeletal

organism *the sum of all the cells, tissues, organs, and organ systems of a living being. Examples: the human organism, a bacterial organism.*

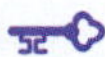

The failure of any component of an organism—from the cellular level to the organ system level—can result in a serious medical emergency.

thoracic duct, and the lymph fluid itself. It is important in fighting disease, in filtration, and in removing waste products of cellular metabolism.

★ *Muscular system.* The muscular system is responsible for movement, posture, and heat production. It consists, primarily, of the skeletal muscles.

★ *Skeletal system.* The skeletal system consists of the bones, cartilage, and associated connective tissue. It provides for support, protection, and movement. The bone marrow is the site for production of various blood cells, including the red blood cells and certain types of white blood cells.

The sum of all cells, tissues, organs, and organ systems is the **organism.** The failure of any component, from the cellular level to the organ-system level, can result in the development of a serious medical emergency.

SYSTEM INTEGRATION

homeostasis *the natural tendency of the body to maintain a steady and normal internal environment.*

anatomy *the structure of an organism; body structure.*

physiology *the functions of an organism; the physical and chemical processes of a living thing.*

metabolism *the total changes that take place during physiological processes.*

The human body is not just a static structure of bones, cavities, and tubes. It is a dynamic organization in which cells, tissues, organs, and organ systems perform functions essential to the organism's preservation. **Homeostasis** is the term for the body's natural tendency to keep the internal environment and metabolism steady and normal. At the cellular level, the body will strive to maintain a very constant environment, because cells do not tolerate extreme environmental fluctuations.

A significant amount of energy is needed to maintain the order that is evident in the structures (**anatomy**) and functions (**physiology**) of the organism. Potential energy is stored in the biochemical bonds of cells and tissues in plants and animals, and the kinetic energy necessary to maintain homeostasis is obtained by the breaking of those bonds. Food provides energy substrates such as sugar, fats, and proteins which, when broken down, produce the energy for the maintenance of homeostasis. **Metabolism** refers to the building up (*anabolism*) and breaking down (*catabolism*) of biochemical substances to produce energy.

The body's cells interact and intercommunicate, rather like a multicellular "social" organism. Communication between the cells consists of electrochemical messages. When something interferes with the normal sending or receiving of these messages, a disease process can begin or advance.

When something interferes with the electrochemical messages cells send to each other, a disease process can begin or advance.

Many intercellular messages are conveyed by substances secreted by various body glands. *Endocrine glands,* sometimes called ductless glands (including the pituitary, thyroid, parathyroid, and adrenal glands, the islets of Langerhans in the pancreas, the testes, and the ovaries), secrete hormones directly into the circulatory system, where they travel to the target organ or tissue. *Exocrine glands* secrete substances such as sweat, saliva, mucus, and digestive enzymes onto the body's epithelial surfaces (the skin or linings of body cavities and organs) via ducts.

Several types of signaling take place among cells. *Endocrine signaling* (via hormones distributed throughout the body) is one mode of intercellular communication. *Paracrine signaling* (nonendocrine, nonhormonal) involves secretion of chemical mediators by certain cells that act only on nearby cells. In *autocrine signaling,* cells secrete substances that may act on themselves. In *synaptic signaling,* cells secrete specialized chemicals called neurotransmitters, such as norepinephrine, acetylcholine, serotonin, and dopamine, that transmit signals across synapses, the junctions between neurons.

These chemical signals—in the form of hormones and neurotransmitters—are received by various kinds of receptors. Receptors can be nerve endings, sensory organs, or proteins that interact with, and then respond to, the chemical signals and other stimuli. Many of the medications administered by paramedics act on these receptors. *Chemoreceptors* respond to chemical stimuli. Chemoreceptors within the brain respond to increasing levels of CO_2 in the cerebrospinal fluid, stimulating respiratory centers in the brainstem to increase the rate and depth of respirations. *Baroreceptors* respond to pressure changes. Baroreceptors in the arch of the aorta and in the carotid sinuses along the carotid artery sense changes in blood pressure, which then cause the cardiac centers in the medulla to alter the heart rate. *Alpha and beta adrenergic receptors* on the surfaces of cells in the bronchi, heart, and blood vessels respond to neurotransmitters and medications, resulting in a variety of cardiovascular and respiratory responses.

When normal metabolism is disturbed the body attempts to restore normal metabolism, (i.e., homeostasis).

As the previous examples demonstrate, when normal intercellular communication is interrupted and normal metabolism is disturbed, the body will respond in various ways to compensate and attempt to restore the normal metabolism (i.e., homeostasis).

Each organ system plays a role in maintaining homeostasis. An example is the body's response to the accumulation of cellular carbon dioxide that occurs during exercise. The respiratory system immediately attempts to return the internal environment to its normal state by increasing the respiratory rate and depth to eliminate excess carbon dioxide—which is why runners pant.

The organization of the human body is very complex, with constant interactions occurring within and among the systems to maintain homeostasis. When disease interrupts these interactions, it can cause both local effects (at the specific site of the illness or injury) and systemic effects (throughout the body). When this happens, body cells and systems will respond to restore normal conditions.

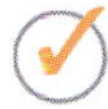

Content Review

Effects of Disease

- Local (at the site of the illness or injury)
- Systemic (throughout the body)

To understand how human systems interact, physiologists sometimes view them from an engineering perspective. Various body systems respond to *inputs,* or stressors, that may be sensed by other systems. The system receiving the input responds in some fashion, creating an *output.* The portion of the system creating the output, be it a cell or an organ, is known as the *effector.* For example, consider a large laceration to an extremity with severe blood loss. The drop in blood pressure resulting from the blood loss is sensed by the baroreceptors, which in turn cause messages to be sent from the cardiac center in the medulla to the heart, resulting in an increase in the rate and strength of contractions in an attempt to restore normal blood pressure. By definition, the input would be the drop in pressure sensed by the baroreceptors; the effector would be the heart, which increased its rate in response to signals from the medulla; and the output would be the resultant increase in blood pressure.

This kind of feedback is essential for maintaining stability within a system and homeostasis for the organism. When the output of a system corrects the situation that created the input, it is said to loop, or feedback on the input, and a **negative feedback loop** exists—"negative" because the feedback negates the input caused by the original stressor. To elaborate on the example of the baroreceptors, the output or increase in blood pressure resulting from the increased heart rate feeds back on, or cancels out, the original input (low blood pressure), and the heart (effector) no longer has to maintain an elevated rate. This particular feedback loop is known as the baroreceptor reflex mechanism.

negative feedback loop *body mechanisms that work to reverse, or compensate for, a pathophysiological process (or to reverse any physiological process, whether pathological or nonpathological).*

Unfortunately, the grim reality of this model is that blood loss often overwhelms the heart's ability to respond with an increased rate. At that point, the system has lost the ability to compensate, and, as a paramedic, you must intervene by administering fluids and taking other necessary therapeutic measures. When the outputs of effector organs are ineffective in correcting the input condition, *decompensation* is said to have occurred.

In the case of decompensation, the feedback system doesn't or can't restore homeostasis. The opposite problem can occur when the feedback system goes too far and overcompensates for the original problem. To prevent this, it is important for the body to have some way to stop the output—to restore the heart rate to normal, because the inability to control the pulse rate would cause instability in the cardiovascular system and danger to the organism. In fact, the body does have numerous means of controlling or halting output.

Biological systems generally employ negative feedback loops to maintain stability. Positive feedback systems do exist in human physiology. (Positive feedback enhances, rather than negates, the effects of input.) An example would be some short-lived positive feedback loops involved in follicular (egg) development in females. However, these loops work in conjunction with negative feedback loops to maintain stability.

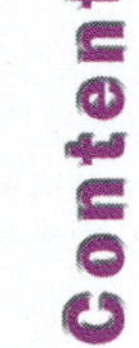

Content Review

Control Systems

- Nervous system
- Endocrine system

Feedback activity must be orchestrated and synchronized to maintain homeostasis. Two systems work together to maintain homeostasis and to integrate the responses of different systems: the nervous system and the endocrine system. They are functionally and anatomically coupled to allow for this integration. For example, the pituitary gland of the endocrine system is joined with the hypothalamus of the nervous system by a stalklike structure called the infundibulum. This allows for rapid communication between these two body control systems.

There are important temporal (time-related) differences in the responses of these two systems. Nervous system response is generally rapid in onset but short-lived. An example is the baroreceptor reflex mechanism, mentioned earlier, which is primarily mediated by the nervous system. Conversely, endocrine responses generally take longer—that is, they have a slower onset of action but a longer duration. For example, the pituitary gland secretes antidiuretic hormone (ADH) in response to low blood pressure. ADH acts on the renal (kidney) tubules, causing water to be reabsorbed into the blood instead of being eliminated from the body. This causes an increase in intravascular fluid volume that compensates for the decrease in intravascular volume caused by the blood loss. All these responses are stimulated by pathological alterations or events.

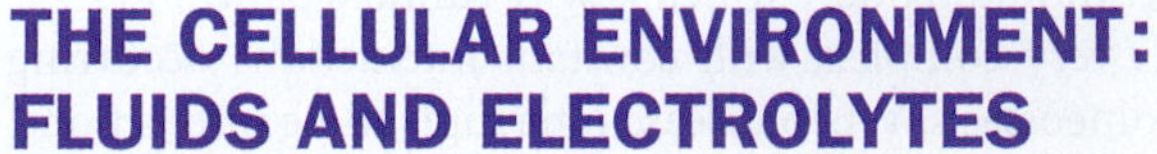

THE CELLULAR ENVIRONMENT: FLUIDS AND ELECTROLYTES

Some fluid and electrolyte derangements can result in death.

Many pathological conditions, both medical and traumatic, adversely affect the fluid and electrolyte balance of the body. Certain disease processes, such as diabetic ketoacidosis and heat emergencies, are associated with certain electrolyte abnormalities. Severe derangements in fluid and electrolyte status can result in death. For this reason, as a paramedic, you need to have a good understanding of the fluids and electrolytes present in the human body.

total body water (TBW) *the total amount of water in the body at a given time.*

intracellular fluid (ICF) *the fluid inside the body cells.*

extracellular fluid (ECF) *the fluid outside the body cells. Extracellular fluid is comprised of intravascular fluid and interstitial fluid.*

intravascular fluid *the fluid within the circulatory system; blood plasma.*

WATER

Water is the most abundant substance in the human body. In fact, water accounts for approximately 60 percent of the total body weight (the average for all ages). The total amount of water in the body at any given time is referred to as the **total body water** (TBW). In an adult weighing 70 kilograms (154 pounds), the amount of total body water would be approximately 42 liters (11 gallons) (Figure 3-2 ■).

Water is distributed into various compartments of the body (Table 3–1). These compartments are separated by cell membranes. The largest compartment, the *intracellular compartment*, contains the **intracellular fluid** (ICF), which is all of the fluid found inside body cells. Approximately 75 percent of all body water is found within this compartment. The *extracellular compartment* contains the remaining 25 percent of all body water. It contains the **extracellular fluid** (ECF), all of the fluid found outside the body cells.

There are two divisions within the extracellular compartment. The first contains the **intravascular fluid**—the fluid found outside of cells and within the circulatory system. It is essentially the

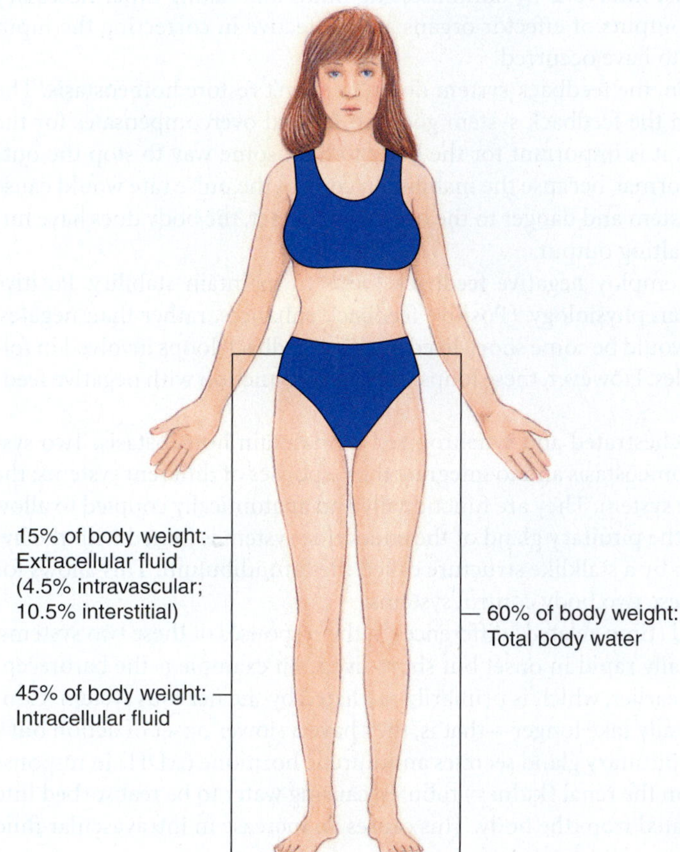

■ **Figure 3-2** Percentage of total body weight due to water as distributed into various fluid compartments.

Table 3–1 Body Fluid Compartments

Compartment	Percentage of Total Body Water	Volume in 70 kg Adult
Intracellular fluid	75.0%	31.50 L
Extracellular fluid	25.0%	10.50 L
Interstitial fluid	17.5%	7.35 L
Intravascular fluid	7.5%	3.15 L

same as the blood plasma. The remaining compartment contains the **interstitial fluid**—all the fluid found outside of the cell membranes, yet not within the circulatory system. For example, minute amounts of fluid are found in the synovial fluid that lubricates the joints; the aqueous humor of the eye; secretions including saliva, gastric juices, and bile; and so on.

interstitial fluid *the fluid in body tissues that is outside the cells and outside the vascular system.*

Total body water and its distribution vary with age and physiological condition. At birth, an infant's TBW is about 75 to 80 percent of its body weight, compared to the 65 percent TBW of the average adult. Infants have a higher TBW for two reasons. First, infants have less fat than adults. (Fat does not absorb water, so the less fat in the body, the more water.) Second, water is essential for the high rates of metabolism that are necessary to promote growth in the infant. The TBW slowly decreases to approximately 70 to 75 percent by age 1. Diarrhea is especially worrisome in the infant, because it can mean the loss of a significant percentage of TBW. In addition, body systems that compensate for fluid loss are still immature; therefore, infants can rapidly become dangerously dehydrated and subject to electrolyte imbalances. By late childhood the TBW decreases to 65 to 70 percent.

By early adulthood, the TBW of males and females begins to differ. In adult males, TBW constitutes approximately 65 to 70 percent of the body weight, while in adult females the average TBW is 60 to 65 percent. The gender difference is the result of hormonal differences that result in the male's greater muscle mass and the female's greater percentage of body fat.

As the human body ages, the loss of muscle mass, increased percentage of fat, and the body's decreasing ability to regulate fluid levels lowers the TBW to around 45 to 55 percent. Due to a decreasing ability to regulate electrolytes and fluid levels, the elderly, like the very young, are at high risk for dehydration and disorders related to electrolyte imbalances.

Hydration

Water is the universal **solvent.** That is, most substances dissolve in water. When they do, various chemical changes take place. For this reason, the water content of the body is crucial to virtually all of the body's biochemical processes. Normally, the total volume of water in the body, as well as the distribution of fluid in the three body compartments, remains relatively constant. This occurs despite wide fluctuations in the amount of water that enters and is excreted from the body on a daily basis. The water coming into the body is referred to as intake. The water excreted from the body is referred to as output. To maintain relative homeostasis, the intake must equal the output, as shown in the following text.

solvent *a substance that dissolves other substances, forming a solution.*

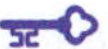

Water is the universal solvent. Water is crucial to virtually all of the body's biochemical processes.

Intake

digestive system:	
liquids:	1,000 mL
food (solids):	1,200 mL
metabolic sources:	300 mL
TOTAL:	2,500 mL

Output

lungs (water vapor):	400 mL
kidneys (urine):	1,500 mL
skin (perspiration):	400 mL
intestines (feces):	200 mL
TOTAL:	2,500 mL

Several mechanisms work to maintain a relative balance between input and output. For example, as explained earlier, when the fluid volume drops, the pituitary gland secretes antidiuretic hormone (ADH), which causes the kidney tubules to reabsorb more water into the blood and to excrete less urine. This process helps to restore the fluid volume to normal values.

Thirst also regulates fluid intake. The sensation of thirst normally occurs when body fluids decrease, stimulating the person to take in more fluids orally. Conversely, when too many fluids enter the body, the kidneys are activated and more urine is excreted, thus eliminating excess fluid. The body also maintains fluid balance by shifting water from one body space to another.

dehydration *excessive loss of body fluid.*

Review

Content

Some Causes of Dehydration

- Vomiting
- Diarrhea
- Perspiration
- Peritonitis
- Malnutrition
- Burns
- Open wounds

Dehydration **Dehydration** is an abnormal decrease in the total body water and can result from several factors:

- ★ *Gastrointestinal losses* result from prolonged vomiting, diarrhea, or malabsorption disorders.
- ★ *Increased insensible loss* is loss of water through normal mechanisms that is difficult to detect or measure (e.g., perspiration, water vapor from the lungs, saliva). These can be increased in fever states, during hyperventilation, or with high environmental temperatures.
- ★ *Increased sweating* (also called perspiration or diaphoresis) can result in significant fluid loss. This can occur with many medical conditions or high environmental temperatures.
- ★ *Internal losses* are commonly called "third space" losses because fluid is lost from intravascular or intracellular spaces into the interstitial space. With dehydration, fluid is typically lost from the intravascular compartment into the interstitial compartment, which effectively takes it out of the circulating volume. This can occur with peritonitis, pancreatitis, or bowel obstruction. It can also occur in poor nutritional states where there is not enough protein in the vascular system to retain water.
- ★ *Plasma losses* occur from burns, surgical drains and fistulas, and open wounds.

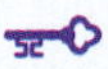

Dehydration usually involves loss of both water and electrolytes.

Dehydration rarely involves only the loss of water. More commonly, there is also a loss of electrolytes. At the hospital, fluid replacement will be based on both fluid and electrolyte deficits, once the patient's electrolyte abnormalities are determined through laboratory testing.

turgor *normal tension in a cell; the resistance of the skin to deformation. (In a normally hydrated person, the skin, when pinched, will quickly return to its normal formation. In a dehydrated person, the return to normal formation will be slower.)*

overhydration *the presence of retention of an abnormally high amount of body fluid.*

Clinically, the dehydrated patient will exhibit dry mucous membranes and poor skin **turgor.** There often is excessive thirst. As it becomes more severe, dehydration will be accompanied by an increased pulse rate, decreased blood pressure, and orthostatic hypotension (increased pulse and decreased blood pressure on rising from a supine position). In infants, the anterior fontanelle may be sunken and the diaper may be dry or reveal the presence of highly concentrated (dark yellow, strong-smelling) urine. The absence of tears in a crying infant, a capillary refill time greater than 2 seconds, dry mucosa, and a decrease in urinary output are signs that indicate severe dehydration. The treatment for dehydration is replacement of fluid.

Overhydration **Overhydration** can occur as well. The major sign of overhydration is edema. Patients with heart disease may manifest overhydration much earlier than patients without heart disease. In severe cases of overhydration, overt heart failure may be present. Treatment is directed at removing the excessive fluid.

How to Read Chemical Notation

To describe chemical substances and reactions, scientists use chemical notation, a kind of "shorthand."

Every chemical element has a one- or two-letter abbreviation. Just four elements— hydrogen, oxygen, carbon, and nitrogen—make up over 99 percent of the body's atoms. These are called the "major elements." Nine "trace elements" account for the remaining less-than-1 percent.

Major Element	Symbol	Percent	Trace Element	Symbol
Hydrogen	H	62.0%	Calcium	Ca
Oxygen	O	26.0%	Chlorine	Cl
Carbon	C	10.0%	Iodine	I
Nitrogen	N	1.5%	Iron	Fe
			Magnesium	Mg
			Phosphorus	Ph
			Potassium	K
			Sodium	Na
			Sulfur	S

An *atom* is the smallest particle of an element. A *molecule* is a combination of atoms. The notation for a molecule combines the notations of the included elements. A subscript number after an element indicates the number of atoms of that element. If there is just one atom, there is no number. For example:

NaCl (Sodium chloride, or table salt. A sodium chloride molecule has 1 sodium atom and 1 chlorine atom.)

H_2O (Water. A water molecule has 2 hydrogen atoms and 1 oxygen atom.)

H_2CO_3 (Carbonic acid. A carbonic acid molecule has 2 hydrogen, 1 carbon, and 3 oxygen atoms.)

Ions

Each atom is made up of even smaller particles: electrons (that have a negative electrical charge), protons (that have a positive electrical charge), and neutrons (that are uncharged). Protons and neutrons are in the inner core, or nucleus, of the atom while electrons occupy outer orbits around the nucleus. Sometimes an atom of an element can lose one or more of its outer electrons or can capture one or more extra electrons from another element.

An *ion* is an atom that has lost one or more negatively charged electrons and now has a positive charge, or an atom that has gained one or more electrons and now has a negative charge. A superscript plus ($^+$) indicates a positively charged cation. A superscript minus ($^-$) indicates a negatively charged anion. For example:

Na^+ (A sodium ion has lost an electron and has a positive charge.)

Ca^{++} (A calcium ion has lost two electrons and has a double positive charge.)

Cl^- (A chloride ion has gained an electron and has a negative charge.)

Electrolytes are substances that form ions when they break down, or dissociate, in water. Remember that the body and its blood are mostly water. The ions formed by dissociation of electrolytes in the body's fluids is a major factor in body metabolism.

Chemical Reactions

Notations for chemical reactions use a plus sign (+) to indicate substances that are combined and an arrow (→) to show the direction of the reaction. The reactants are usually on the left, with the product of the reaction on the right.

$$2H + O \rightarrow H_2O$$

(2 hydrogen atoms + 1 oxygen atom → 1 water molecule)

In some circumstances, a reaction may be reversible. That is, separate elements may synthesize (combine), or the synthesized substance may dissociate (break down) into separate components. A two-directional arrow (⟷) shows that a reaction is reversible and can be read in either direction.

$$CO_2 + H_2O \leftrightarrow H_2CO_3$$

Read as: (carbon dioxide + water → carbonic acid) or (carbonic acid → water + carbon dioxide).

Notice that no atoms are gained or lost in a chemical reaction. In the previous example, the two oxygen atoms in CO_2 and the single oxygen atom in H_2O combine to equal the three oxygen atoms in H_2CO_3. The hydrogen and carbon atoms are also equal on both sides of the reaction.

Up and down arrows (↑ ↓) are used to indicate an increase or decrease in the substance that follows the arrows. For example:

↑ **H^+** (an increase in hydrogen ions)
↓ **CO_2** (a decrease in carbon dioxide)

ELECTROLYTES

electrolyte *a substance that, in water, separates into electrically charged particles.*

dissociate *separate; break down. For example, sodium bicarbonate, when placed in water, dissociates into a sodium cation and a bicarbonate anion.*

ion *a charged particle; an atom or group of atoms whose electrical charge has changed from neutral to positive or negative by losing or gaining one or more electrons. (In an atom's normal, nonionized state, its positively charged protons and negatively charged electrons balance each other so that the atom's charge is neutral.)*

cation *ion with a positive charge—so called because it will be attracted to a cathode, or negative pole.*

anion *ion with a negative charge—so called because it will be attracted to an anode, or positive pole.*

buffer *a substance that tends to preserve or restore a normal acid–base balance by increasing or decreasing the concentration of hydrogen ions.*

The various chemical substances present throughout the body can be classified either as electrolytes or nonelectrolytes. **Electrolytes** are substances that **dissociate** into electrically charged particles when placed into water. The charged particles are referred to as **ions**. Ions with a positive charge are called **cations**, while ions with a negative charge are called **anions**.

An example of this would be the dissociation of the drug sodium bicarbonate when placed into water. Sodium bicarbonate is a neutral salt. When placed into water, it dissociates into two charged particles, as shown below.

$$NaHCO_3 \rightarrow Na^+ + HCO_3^-$$

sodium bicarbonate → sodium cation + bicarbonate anion
neutral salt → cation + anion

Sodium bicarbonate is an example of an electrolyte that is taken into the body as a medication. However, there are many naturally occurring electrolytes present in the body.

The most frequently occurring cations include:

- ★ *Sodium (Na^+).* Sodium is the most prevalent cation in the extracellular fluid. It plays a major role in regulating the distribution of water because water is attracted to and moves with sodium. In fact, it is often said that "water follows sodium." Sodium is also important in the transmission of nervous impulses. An abnormal increase in the relative amount of sodium in the body is called *hypernatremia,* while an abnormal decrease is referred to as *hyponatremia.*
- ★ *Potassium (K^+).* Potassium is the most prevalent cation in the intracellular fluid. It is also important in the transmission of electrical impulses. An abnormally high potassium level is called *hyperkalemia,* while an abnormally low potassium level is referred to as *hypokalemia.*
- ★ *Calcium (Ca^{++}).* Calcium has many physiological functions. It plays a major role in muscle contraction as well as nervous impulse transmission. An abnormally increased calcium level is called *hypercalcemia,* while an abnormally decreased calcium level is called *hypocalcemia.*
- ★ *Magnesium (Mg^{++}).* Magnesium is necessary for several biochemical processes that occur in the body and is closely associated with phosphate in many processes. An abnormally increased magnesium level is called *hypermagnesemia*; an abnormally decreased magnesium level is called *hypomagnesemia.*

The most frequently occurring anions include:

- ★ *Chloride (Cl^-).* Chloride is an important anion. Its negative charge balances the positive charge associated with the cations. It also plays a major role in fluid balance and renal function. Chloride has a close association with sodium.
- ★ *Bicarbonate (HCO_3^-).* Bicarbonate is the principal **buffer** of the body. This means that it neutralizes the highly acidic hydrogen ion (H^+) and other organic acids. (Buffering will be discussed in more detail later in this chapter.)
- ★ *Phosphate (HPO_4^-).* Phosphate is important in body energy stores. It is closely associated with magnesium in renal function. It also acts as a buffer, primarily in the intracellular space, in much the same manner as bicarbonate.

Many other compounds carry negative charges. Among these are some of the proteins, certain organic acids, and other compounds. Electrolytes are usually measured in *milliequivalents* per liter (mEq/L).

Nonelectrolytes are molecules that do not dissociate into electrically charged particles. These include glucose, urea, proteins, and similar substances.

OSMOSIS AND DIFFUSION

As discussed earlier, the various fluid compartments are separated by cell membranes. These membranes are semipermeable, allowing the passage of certain materials while restricting the passage of others. Compounds with small molecules, such as water (H_2O), pass readily through the membrane; larger compounds, such as proteins, are restricted. This selective movement of fluids results from the presence of pores (openings) in the membrane. Electrolytes do not pass as readily as water through the membrane. This is due not so much to their size as to their electrical charge.

When solutions on opposite sides of a semipermeable membrane are equal in concentration, the relationship is said to be **isotonic.** When the concentration of a given solute (dissolved substance) is greater on one side of the membrane than on the other, it is said to be **hypertonic.** When the concentration is less on one side of the cell membrane, as compared to the other, it is referred to as **hypotonic.** This difference in concentration is known as the **osmotic gradient.**

The natural tendency of the body is to keep the balance of electrolytes and water equal on both sides of the cell membrane. This is an example of homeostasis. If one side of a cell membrane has an increased quantity of a given electrolyte (is hypertonic), there will be a shift of the electrolyte from that side and a shift of water from the other side to restore balance in concentration—the balanced state.

The tendency of molecules to move from an area of higher concentration to an area of lower concentration is referred to as **diffusion** and does not require energy (Figure 3-3 ■). The diffusion of a solute (usually an electrolyte) across a cell membrane from the area of higher concentration to the area of lower concentration continues until the natural balance is again attained. This movement from an area of higher concentration to an area of lower concentration is termed a movement *with the osmotic gradient.*

Water also moves across the cell membrane so as to dilute the area of increased electrolyte concentration. The movement of water is more rapid than the movement of electrolytes. This form of

isotonic *equal in concentration of solute molecules; solutions may be isotonic to each other.*

hypertonic *having a greater concentration of solute molecules; one solution may be hypertonic to another.*

hypotonic *having a lesser concentration of solute molecules; one solution may be hypotonic to another.*

osmotic gradient *the difference in concentration between solutions on opposite sides of a semipermeable membrane.*

diffusion *the movement of molecules through a membrane from an area of greater concentration to an area of lesser concentration.*

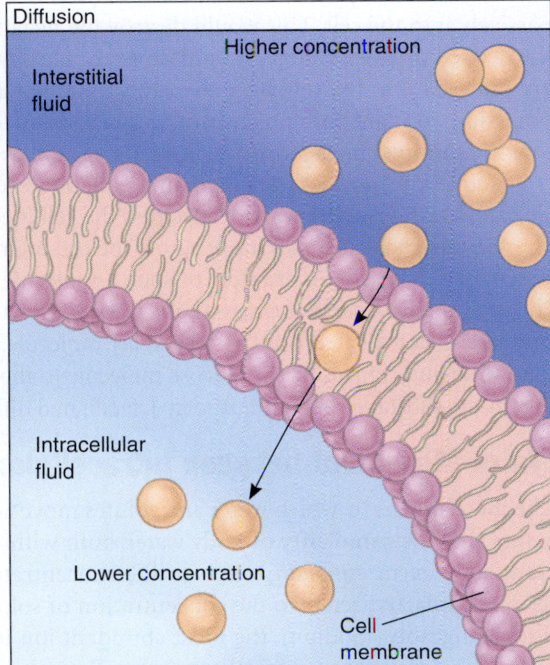

■ **Figure 3-3** Diffusion is the movement of a substance from an area of greater concentration to an area of lesser concentration.

Figure 3-4 Osmosis is the movement of water from an area of higher WATER concentration to an area of lesser WATER concentration. Because water is a solvent, it moves from an area of lower SOLUTE concentration to an area of higher SOLUTE concentration.

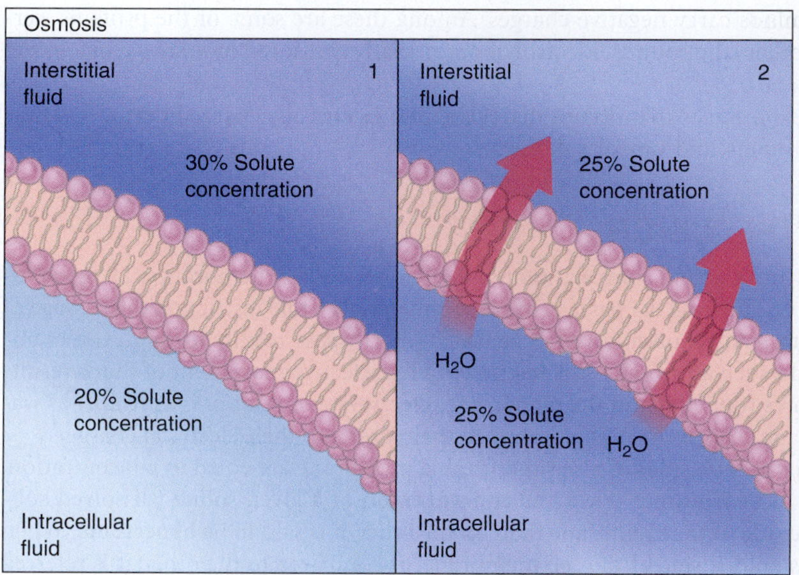

osmosis *the passage of a solvent such as water through a membrane.*

active transport *movement of a substance through a cell membrane against the osmotic gradient; that is, from an area of lesser concentration to an area of greater concentration, opposite to the normal direction of diffusion.*

facilitated diffusion *diffusion of a substance such as glucose through a cell membrane that requires the assistance of a "helper," or carrier protein; also called* carrier mediated diffusion.

osmolality *the concentration of solute per kilogram of water. See also* osmolarity.

osmolarity *the concentration of solute per liter of water (often used synonymously with* osmolality*).*

diffusion (the passage of any solvent, usually water, through a membrane) is referred to as **osmosis** (Figure 3-4 ■). It occurs in the direction opposite to the direction of solute movement. For example, if a semipermeable membrane separates solutions of water and sodium, and if the concentration of sodium is two times higher on one side of the membrane than on the other, then two things will occur. Sodium will diffuse from the area of higher concentration (the hypertonic side) to the area of lesser concentration (the hypotonic side). Concurrently, water will diffuse in the opposite direction. That is, water will leave the hypotonic side and diffuse across the membrane to the hypertonic side. These actions will continue until the concentration of water and sodium on both sides has equalized.

In addition to diffusion, two other mechanisms—active transport and facilitated diffusion—can transport substances across cell membranes. **Active transport** is the movement of a substance across the cell membrane *against the osmotic gradient* (that is, toward the side that already has more of the substance).

For example, the body requires cells of the myocardium to be negatively charged on the inside of the cells as compared to the outside. However sodium, with its positive charge, tends to diffuse passively into the cell. This would destroy the negative charge inside the cell. In order to maintain the desired negative charge, sodium ions are actively pumped out of the cell, while potassium ions are pumped into the cell, by a mechanism known as the sodium-potassium pump. (Sodium and potassium ions are both positive, but more sodium ions are pumped out of the cell than potassium ions are pumped in, creating the desired negative charge inside the cell.)

Active transport is faster than diffusion, but it requires the expenditure of energy, which diffusion does not. Proteins are moved across the cell membrane in a similar fashion.

Certain molecules can move across the cell membrane by another process known as **facilitated diffusion.** Glucose is an example of such a molecule. Facilitated diffusion requires the assistance of "helper proteins," parts of a membrane transport system, on the surface of the cell membrane. These proteins, once activated, bind to the glucose molecule. Following binding, the protein changes its configuration and transports the glucose molecule to the inside of the cell, where it is released. Depending on the substance being transported, facilitated diffusion may or may not require energy.

Water Movement between Intracellular and Extracellular Compartments

The mechanisms by which water and solutes move across cell membranes, as previously described, assure that the **osmolality** of body water, both within and outside the cells, is normally in equilibrium. (The term *osmolality* refers to the concentration of solute per kilogram of water; a related term, **osmolarity,** refers to the concentration of solute per liter of water. The terms are often used interchangeably.) Sodium, the most abundant ion in the extracellular fluid, is responsible for the osmotic balance of the extracellular space. Potassium plays the same role in the intracellular space.

Generally, the osmolality of intracellular fluid does not change very rapidly. However, when there is a change in the osmolality of extracellular fluid, water will move from the intracellular to the extracellular compartment, or vice versa, until osmotic equilibrium is regained.

Water Movement between Intravascular and Interstitial Compartments

Within the extracellular compartment, movement of water between the plasma in the intravascular space and the interstitial space is primarily a function of forces at play in the capillary beds.

In general, the movement of water and solutes across a cell membrane is governed by **osmotic pressure.** Osmotic pressure is the pressure exerted by the concentration of solutes on one side of a semipermeable membrane, such as a cell membrane or the thin wall of a capillary. Osmotic pressure can be thought of as a "pull" rather than a "push," because a hypertonic concentration of solutes tends to pull water from the other side of the membrane.

Generally, this is a two-way street as solutes move out of a space while water moves into the space to balance the concentration of solutes on both sides of the membrane. However, there is a somewhat different osmotic mechanism that operates between the plasma inside a capillary and the interstitial space outside the capillary. Blood plasma generates **oncotic force,** which is sometimes called *colloid osmotic pressure.* Plasma proteins are colloids, large particles that do not readily move across the capillary membrane. They tend to remain within the capillary. At the same time, there is very little water in the interstitial space. The small amount of water that does get into the interstitial space is usually taken up by the lymphatic system. Therefore, since there is little water outside the capillary, and because plasma proteins do not readily move outside the capillary, the forces governing movement of water between the capillary and the interstitial space are almost all on one side, governed by the plasma on the inside of the capillary.

Another force inside the capillaries is **hydrostatic pressure,** which is the blood pressure, or force against the vessel walls, created by contractions of the heart. Hydrostatic pressure does tend to force some water out of the plasma and across the capillary wall into the interstitial space, a process that is called **filtration.** Hydrostatic pressure (a force that favors filtration, pushing water out of the capillary) and oncotic force (a force opposing filtration, pulling water into the capillary) together are responsible for **net filtration,** which is described in *Starling's hypothesis:*

$$\text{Net filtration} = (\text{Forces favoring filtration}) - (\text{Forces opposing filtration})$$

Net filtration in a capillary is normally zero. It works this way: As plasma enters the capillary at the arterial end, hydrostatic pressure forces water to cross the capillary membrane into the interstitial space. This loss of water increases the relative concentration of plasma proteins. By the time the plasma reaches the venous end of the capillary, the oncotic force exerted by the increased concentration of plasma proteins is great enough to pull the water from the interstitial space back into the capillary. The outcome is that water is retained in the intravascular space and does not remain in the interstitial space.

osmotic pressure *the pressure exerted by the concentration of solutes on one side of a membrane that, if hypertonic, tends to "pull" water (cause osmosis) from the other side of the membrane.*

oncotic force *a form of osmotic pressure exerted by the large protein particles, or colloids, present in blood plasma. In the capillaries, the plasma colloids tend to pull water from the interstitial space across the capillary membrane into the capillary. Oncotic force is also called* colloid osmotic pressure.

hydrostatic pressure *blood pressure or force against vessel walls created by the heartbeat. Hydrostatic pressure tends to force water out of the capillaries into the interstitial space.*

filtration *movement of water out of the plasma across the capillary membrane into the interstitial space.*

net filtration *the total loss of water from blood plasma across the capillary membrane into the interstitial space. Normally, hydrostatic pressure forcing water out of the capillary is balanced by an oncotic force pulling water into the capillary for a net filtration of zero.*

ACID–BASE BALANCE

Acid–base balance is a dynamic relationship that reflects the relative concentration of hydrogen ions (H^+) in the body. Hydrogen ions are acidic and the concentration of these within the body must be maintained within fairly strict limits. Any deviation in the hydrogen ion concentration adversely affects all of the biochemical events that occur in the body. The hydrogen ion concentration is dynamic, changing from second to second.

THE pH SCALE

The total number of hydrogen ions present in the body at any given time is very high. Because of this, the **pH** system of measurement is used. The pH scale is inversely related to hydrogen ion concentration. That is, the greater the hydrogen ion concentration, the lower the pH. The lower the hydrogen ion concentration, the higher the pH.

pH *abbreviation for* potential of hydrogen. *A measure of relative acidity or alkalinity. Since the pH scale is inverse to the concentration of acidic hydrogen ions, the lower the pH the greater the acidity and the higher the pH the greater the alkalinity. A normal pH range is 7.35 to 7.45.*

Table 3–2 The pH Scale and Hydrogen Ion Concentrations

pH		Example	H^+ Concentration*	
Acidic	0	Hydrochloric acid	10^{-0}	(1.0)
	1	Stomach secretions	10^{-1}	(0.1)
	2	Lemon juice	10^{-2}	(0.01)
	3	Cola drinks	10^{-3}	(0.001)
	4	White wine	10^{-4}	(0.0001)
	5	Tomato juice	10^{-5}	(0.00001)
	6	Coffee, urine, saliva	10^{-6}	(0.000001)
Neutral	7	Distilled water	10^{-7}	(0.0000001)
Basic	8	Blood, semen	10^{-8}	(0.00000001)
	9	Bile	10^{-9}	(0.000000001)
	10	Bleach	10^{-10}	(0.0000000001)
	11	Milk of magnesia	10^{-11}	(0.00000000001)
	12	Ammonia water	10^{-12}	(0.000000000001)
	13	Drain opener	10^{-13}	(0.0000000000001)
	14	Lye	10^{-14}	(0.00000000000001)

*Hydrogen ion concentrations are expressed in moles per liter, a quantity based on molecular weight.

The pH scale is logarithmic, with each number representing a value 10 times that of its neighboring number, so that pH 6 represents a hydrogen ion concentration 10 times as great as that represented by pH 7. The following formula represents pH:

$$pH = \log\frac{1}{[H^+]}$$

The pH scale ranges from 1 to 14. A pH of 1 means that only hydrogen ions are present. A pH of 14 means that there are virtually no hydrogen ions present. The pH of water is 7.0, which is a neutral pH. The pH of the body is normally 7.35 to 7.45 (Table 3–2).

acidosis *a high concentration of hydrogen ions; a pH below 7.35.*

alkalosis *a low concentration of hydrogen ions; a pH above 7.45.*

Because hydrogen ions are acidic, a pH below 7.35 is referred to as **acidosis.** A substance that produces negatively charged ions that can neutralize the positively charged hydrogen ions (or other acids) is called an alkali or a base. An excess of alkaline (base) substances or a deficit of acids will produce a pH above 7.45, which is referred to as **alkalosis.** In humans, a variation of only 0.4 of a pH unit in either direction from normal (6.9 or 7.8) can be fatal.

BODILY REGULATION OF ACID–BASE BALANCE

Content Review

Three Mechanisms of Hydrogen Ion Removal

- Bicarbonate buffer system
- Respiration
- Kidney function

The body is constantly producing hydrogen ions (acids) through metabolism and other biochemical processes. To maintain the acid–base balance, these hydrogen ions must be constantly eliminated from the body. There are three major mechanisms to remove hydrogen ions from the body. The fastest mechanism is often referred to as the *buffer system* or the *bicarbonate buffer system.*

The two components of the bicarbonate buffer system are bicarbonate ion (HCO_3^-) and carbonic acid (H_2CO_3). These two compounds are in equilibrium with hydrogen ion (H^+), as follows: In some circumstances hydrogen ion will combine with bicarbonate ion to produce carbonic acid. In other circumstances, carbonic acid will dissociate into bicarbonate ion and hydrogen ion:

$$H^+ + HCO_3^- \leftrightarrow H_2CO_3$$

hydrogen ion + bicarbonate ion ↔ carbonic acid

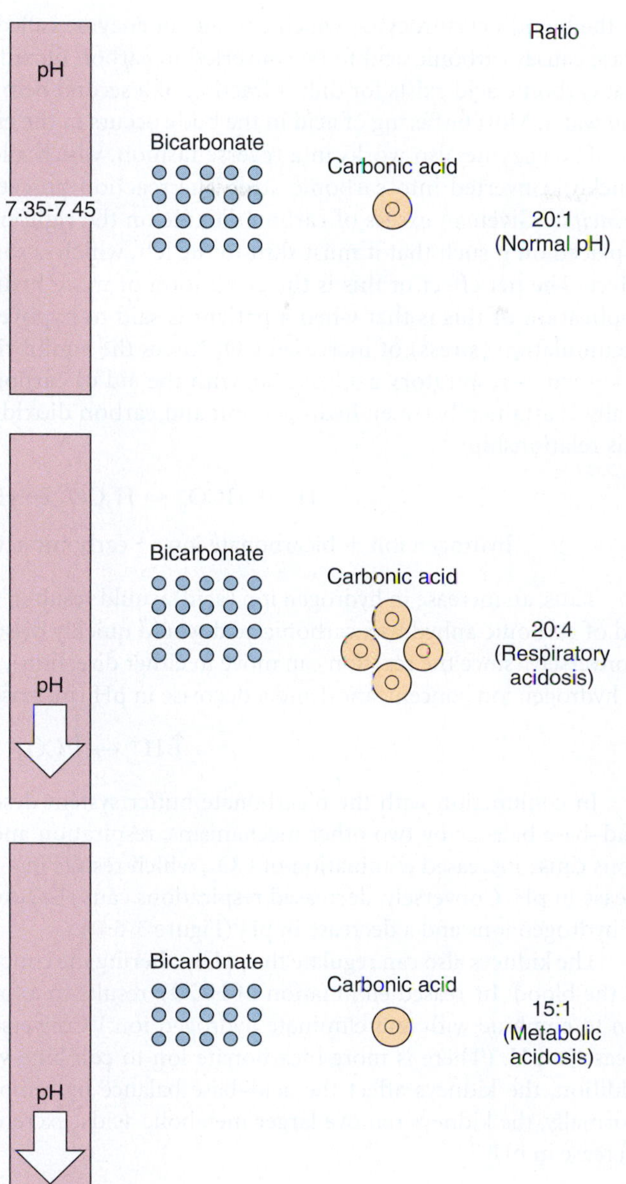

■ **Figure 3-5** Acid–base ratios relevant to pH.

In a healthy individual, for every molecule of carbonic acid, there are 20 molecules of bicarbonate ion. Any change in this 20:1 ratio is immediately corrected without significant change in the total body pH. This occurs in the following manner: An increase in hydrogen ions (acidosis) is corrected as the excess hydrogen ions combine with bicarbonate ions to form carbonic acid. (Thus, an increase in hydrogen ions leads to an increase in carbonic acid—driving the previous equation to the right.) Conversely, when there is a deficit in hydrogen ions (alkalosis), carbonic acid will dissociate into bicarbonate ions and hydrogen ions. (Thus, a decrease in hydrogen ions leads to a decrease in carbonic acid—driving the previous equation to the left.) (Figure 3-5 ■):

$$\text{Increased Acid: } \uparrow H^+ + HCO_3^- \rightarrow \uparrow H_2CO_3$$
$$\text{Decreased Acid: } \downarrow H^+ + HCO_3^- \rightarrow \downarrow H_2CO_3$$

Carbonic acid is a weak acid that is better tolerated by the body than pure hydrogen ion. However, the body carries this reaction further. Any increase in carbonic acid must also be eliminated.

The elimination of excess carbonic acid takes place as follows: Carbonic acid is unstable and will eventually dissociate into carbon dioxide and water. This normally slow process is made faster by the blood's erythrocytes, which contain an enzyme called *carbonic anhydrase.* Carbonic anhydrase causes carbonic acid to be converted to carbon dioxide and water very rapidly—so rapidly that carbonic acid exists for only a fraction of a second before it is converted into carbon dioxide and water. Most buffering of acid in the body occurs in the erythrocytes.

The enzyme also works in a reverse fashion, which allows carbon dioxide and water to be quickly converted into carbonic acid. The reaction proceeds in accordance with *LeChetalier's Principle.* Given an excess of carbon dioxide on the right hand side of the equilibrium, a stress is placed on it such that it must shift to the left, which is sometimes referred to as a mass action effect. The net effect of this is the generation of more hydrogen ion, and acidosis. The clinical application of this is that when a patient is said to hypoventilate, that is, retain CO_2, then the accumulation (stress) of increased CO_2 forces the equilibrium to shift to the left, causing what is known as respiratory acidosis. So, with the aid of carbonic anhydrase, an equilibrium eventually is attained between hydrogen ion and carbon dioxide. The following equation illustrates this relationship:

$$H^+ + HCO_3^- \leftrightarrow H_2CO_3 \leftrightarrow H_2O + CO_2$$

hydrogen ion + bicarbonate ion ↔ carbonic acid ↔ water + carbon dioxide

Thus, an increase in hydrogen ion (acid) would result in an increase in carbonic acid. With the aid of carbonic anhydrase, carbonic acid would quickly dissociate into water and carbon dioxide. Conversely (since the reaction can move in either direction), an increase in CO_2 causes an increase in hydrogen ion concentration and a decrease in pH (increase in acidity), such as:

$$\uparrow H^+ \leftrightarrow \uparrow CO_2$$

In conjunction with the bicarbonate buffer system described previously, the body regulates acid–base balance by two other mechanisms, respiration and kidney function. Increased respirations cause increased elimination of CO_2, which results in a decrease in hydrogen ions and an increase in pH. Conversely, decreased respirations cause CO_2 to be retained. This causes an increase in hydrogen ions and a decrease in pH (Figure 3-6 ■).

The kidneys also can regulate the pH by altering the concentration of bicarbonate ion (HCO_3^-) in the blood. Increased elimination of HCO_3^- results in a lowered pH. (There is less bicarbonate ion to combine with and eliminate hydrogen ion.) Conversely retention of HCO_3^- causes an increase in pH. (There is more bicarbonate ion to combine with and eliminate hydrogen ion.) In addition, the kidneys affect the acid–base balance by removing or retaining various chemicals. Normally, the kidneys remove larger metabolic acids, excreting them in the urine, resulting in an increase in pH.

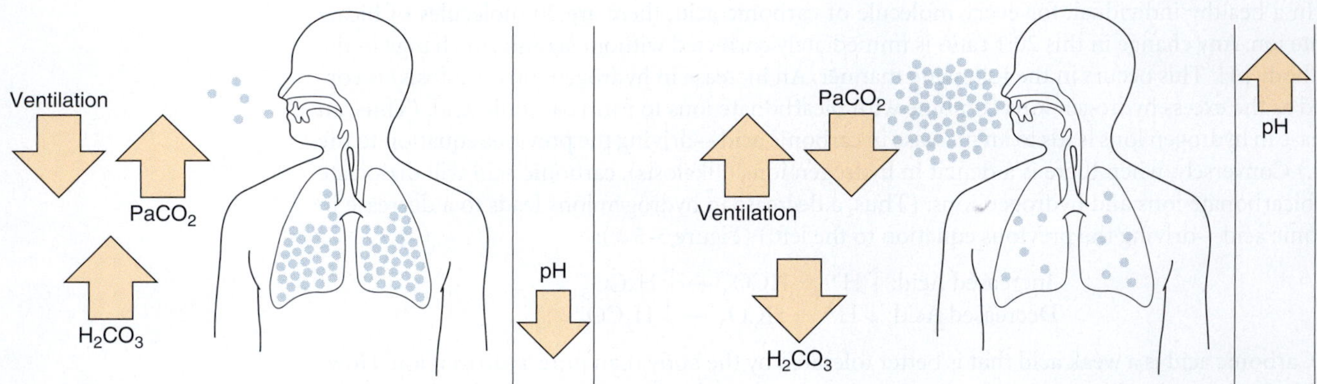

■ **Figure 3-6** The respiratory component of acid–base balance.

Part 2: Body Systems

THE INTEGUMENTARY SYSTEM

The protective envelope we call the skin is a complex structure. Understanding how it is put together and how it functions will help you appreciate the importance of injuries to it and the value of its proper care.

Content Review

Layers of the Skin

- Epidermis
- Dermis
- Subcutaneous tissue

THE SKIN

The epidermis, dermis, and subcutaneous tissue layers comprise what is commonly known as the skin (Figure 3-7 ■). Each of these layers performs functions essential to helping the body maintain homeostasis and each plays an important role in the wound repair process.

Epidermis

The outermost skin layer is the **epidermis.** It is generated by a layer of cells just above the dermis (stratum germinativum). These cells divide rapidly, generating a movement of cells upward toward the epidermal surface. As the epidermis contains no vasculature, the further these cells are pushed away from the dermis, the less circulation they receive, and they eventually die. As they die, they flatten and interlock, providing a firm and secure barrier around the body (stratum corneum). The outermost cells are eventually abraded or washed away and then replaced, allowing the epidermis to maintain its thickness. It normally takes 2 weeks for a cell to move from the dermal border to the surface of the epidermis and another 2 to 4 weeks until it is abraded away. This outward movement of cells helps the body resist invasion by bacteria.

epidermis *outermost layer of the skin comprised of dead or dying cells.*

A waxy substance called **sebum** lubricates the surface of the epidermis. This lubrication acts much like oil on leather. It keeps the outer layers of the skin flexible, strong, and resistant to penetration by

sebum *fatty secretion of the sebaceous gland that helps keep the skin pliable and waterproof.*

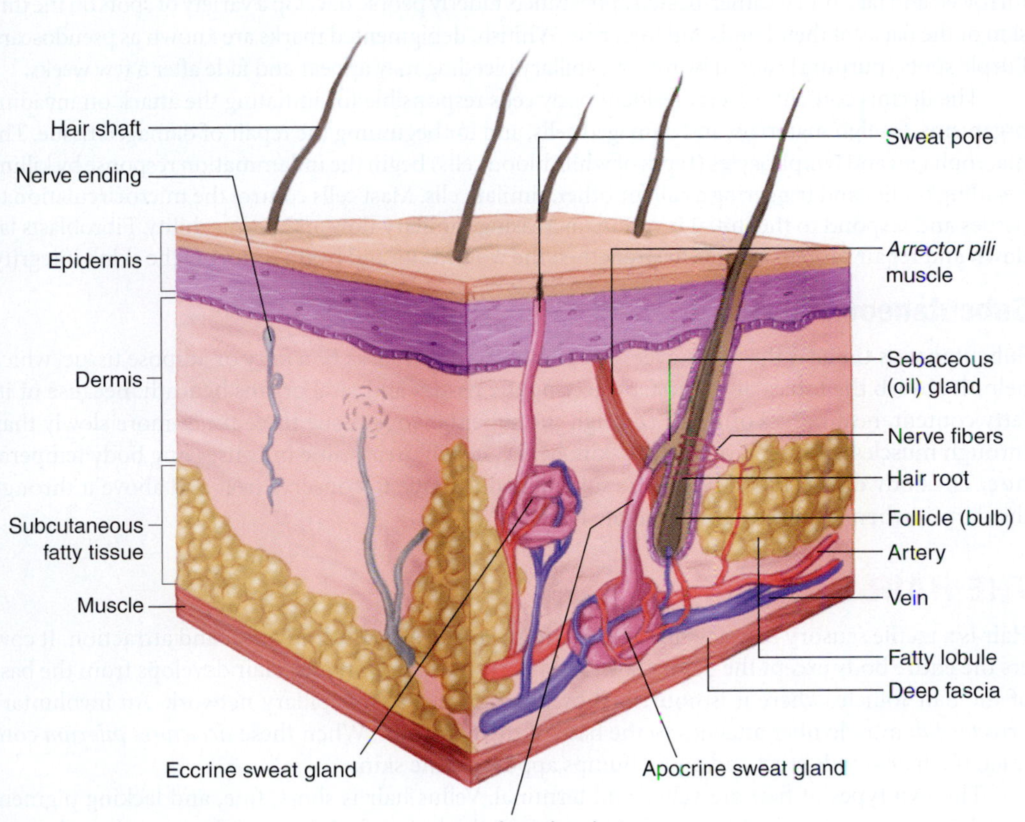

■ Figure 3-7 Layers and major structures of the skin.

water. The epidermis is also responsible for the pigmentation that protects the skin from the harmful effects of ultraviolet radiation. The thickness of the epidermis varies greatly, depending on the amount of abrasion and pressure it receives. On the soles of the feet, it is very thick and strong, while over the eye it is microscopic in thickness and very delicate.

Dermis

dermis *true skin, also called the corium; it is the layer of tissue producing the epidermis and housing the structures, blood vessels, and nerves normally associated with the skin.*

sebaceous glands *glands within the dermis secreting sebum.*

sudoriferous glands *glands within the dermis that secrete sweat.*

Directly beneath the epidermis is the **dermis,** a connective tissue that helps contain the body and supports the functions of the epidermis. The upper layer of the dermis is the papillary layer, consisting of loose connective tissue, capillaries, and nerves supplying the epidermis. The reticular layer is the deeper dermis made up of strong connective tissue that integrates the dermis firmly with the subcutaneous layer below. This tissue also holds the skin firmly around the body and permits the stretching and flexibility necessary for articulation.

The dermis contains blood vessels, nerve endings, glands, and other structures. It is here that **sebaceous glands** produce sebum and secrete it directly onto the surface of the skin or into hair follicles. **Sudoriferous glands** secrete sweat to help move heat out of and away from the body through evaporation. Hair follicles produce hair that helps to reduce surface abrasion and conserve heat.

The two types of sweat glands are *eccrine glands* and *apocrine glands.* Eccrine glands, also known as merocrine glands, open onto the skin surface and help control body temperature through water excretion. They are widely distributed but are most heavily concentrated in the axilla and genital areas. Apocrine glands are found exclusively in the armpits and genital region, and they open into hair follicles. These glands respond to emotional stress. During adolescence, the apocrine glands enlarge and actively increase the axillary sweating that causes adult body odor. Also during this period, the sebaceous glands increase their activity, giving the skin an oily appearance. This predisposes the teenager to acne problems.

As we age, sebaceous and sweat gland activity decreases. As a result, the skin becomes drier and produces less perspiration. The epidermis thins and flattens, and the dermis loses some of its vascularity. The skin wrinkles as it loses turgor. In warmer climates, the skin can become thickened, yellowed, and furrowed and take on a weather-beaten appearance. Elderly people develop a variety of spots on the thin skin of the backs of their hands and forearms. Whitish, depigmented marks are known as pseudoscars. Purple spots (purpura) caused by minor capillary bleeding may appear and fade after a few weeks.

The dermis contains several resident body cells responsible for initiating the attack on invading organisms, foreign materials, and damaged cells, and for beginning the repair of damaged tissue. The macrophages and lymphocytes (types of white blood cells) begin the inflammation response by killing invading bodies and triggering a call for other, similar cells. Mast cells control the microcirculation to tissues and respond to the initial invasion, increasing capillary flow and permeability. Fibroblasts lay down and repair protein strands to strengthen the wound site and begin restoring the skin's integrity.

Subcutaneous Tissue

subcutaneous tissue *body layer beneath the dermis.*

Subcutaneous tissue is the body layer beneath the dermis. It is rich in fatty or adipose tissue, which helps it absorb the forces of trauma, protecting the tissues and vital organs beneath. Because of its fatty content, heat moves outward through the subcutaneous tissue three times more slowly than through muscles or other layers of the skin; hence, it is of great value in conserving body temperature. The body directs blood below the subcutaneous tissue to conserve heat and above it through the dermis when it is necessary to radiate heat.

THE HAIR

Hair is a tactile sensory organ, while also playing a role in sexual stimulation and attraction. It covers the entire body except the palms, soles, and parts of the sex organs. Hair develops from the base of the hair follicle, where it is nourished by the papilla, a vast capillary network. An involuntary *arrector pili* muscle fiber attaches to the base of the hair shaft. When these *arrectores pilorum* contract, the hair stands erect and goose bumps appear on the skin.

The two types of hair are vellus and terminal. Vellus hair is short, fine, and lacking pigment (similar to "peach fuzz"). Terminal hair is coarser, thicker, and pigmented. It appears on the eyebrows and scalp, in the armpits and groin of both sexes, and on the faces and bodies of males.

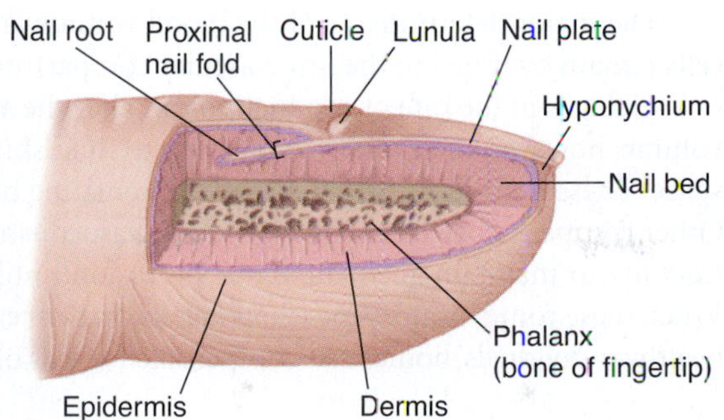

■ **Figure 3-8** The nail.

With aging the hair turns gray from a decrease in pigmentation and its growth declines. A transition from terminal to vellus hair on the scalp causes baldness in both men and women. The opposite occurs in the nares and ears of men, where terminal hair replaces vellus hair. Both genders generally experience a decrease in body hair as they age. Loss of the lateral third of the eyebrow is also normal in the elderly.

THE NAILS

Nails are found at the most distal ends of fingers and toes and are primarily for protection. Nails are strong yet flexible and provide a sharp edge for scratching, scraping, and clawing. They are made up of the nail plate, the nail bed, the proximal nail fold, and the nail root (Figure 3-8 ■). The angle between the proximal nail fold and the nail plate should be less than 180 degrees. Fingernails grow approximately 0.1 mm daily, slightly faster in the summertime. The nail plate lies on a highly vascular nail bed that gives the nail a pink appearance. Nail edges should be smooth and rounded. The nail plates should be smooth, flat, or slightly curved and should feel hard and uniformly thick. As we age, nail growth diminishes because of decreased peripheral circulation. The nails, especially the toenails, become hard, thick, brittle, and yellowish.

THE BLOOD

The **hematopoietic system** consists of blood (both cells and plasma), bone marrow, the liver, the spleen, and the kidneys. The cellular components of blood are formed by the differentiation of a **pluripotent stem cell** in a process termed **hematopoiesis.** In the fetus, hematopoiesis occurs first outside of the bone marrow (*extramedullary hematopoiesis*) in the liver, spleen, lymph nodes, and thymus. By the fourth month, the developing bone marrow begins to produce blood cells (*intramedullary hematopoiesis*). After birth, the bone marrow is the primary site of blood cell production and extramedullary hematopoiesis greatly diminishes, occurring mostly in the liver and spleen. By adulthood, hematopoiesis occurs exclusively in the bone marrow unless a pathological state exists.

In hematopoiesis, the stem cell reproduces to maintain a constant population of cells. Some stem cells then further differentiate into myeloid multipotent stem cells that, in turn, differentiate into unipotent progenitors. These unipotent progenitors ultimately mature into basophils, eosinophils, neutrophils, monocytes (types of white blood cells), erythrocytes (red blood cells), and thrombocytes (platelets). Pluripotent stem cells may also differentiate into common lymphoid stem cells that ultimately mature into lymphocytes (another type of white cell). The kidney, and to a lesser extent the liver, produce **erythropoietin,** the hormone responsible for red blood cell production. The liver also removes toxins from the blood and produces many of the clotting factors and proteins in plasma. The spleen, an important part of the immune system, has cells that scavenge abnormal blood cells and bacteria.

Blood volume normally remains relatively constant at about 6 percent of total body weight. With an average of 80–85 mL of blood per kilogram of body weight, a person who weighs 75 kg has approximately 6 L of blood. The body can easily handle up to about 0.5 L of lost blood or fluid. An example is routine blood donations where healthy donors tolerate the blood loss without complication.

hematopoietic system *body system having to do with the production and development of blood cells, consisting of the bone marrow, liver, spleen, kidneys, and the blood itself.*

Review Content

Hematopoietic System Components

- Bone marrow
- Liver
- Spleen
- Kidneys
- Blood

pluripotent stem cell *a cell from which the various types of blood cells can form.*

hematopoiesis *the process through which pluripotent stem cells differentiate into various types of blood cells.*

erythropoietin *the hormone responsible for red blood cell production.*

The major determinants of the blood volume are red cell mass and plasma volume. Red blood cells remain confined to the intravascular compartment. If their destruction remains constant, then only changes in the rate of production can alter the size of the circulating red cell mass. The plasma volume, however, can rapidly change due to fluid shifts between the intravascular and extravascular space. These fluid shifts help to preserve circulating blood volume in the event of acute hemorrhage. Other compensatory mechanisms include vasoconstriction, tachycardia, and increased cardiac contractility to maintain adequate tissue perfusion until significant losses overwhelm these measures. When these compensatory measures fail, the patient enters decompensated shock. Fortunately, young healthy individuals' bodies can compensate for loss of as much as 25–30 percent of blood volume.

Content Review

Components of Blood

- Plasma
- Formed elements
- Red blood cells
- White blood cells
- Platelets

COMPONENTS OF BLOOD

Blood consists of liquid, or plasma, and formed elements—red blood cells, white blood cells, and platelets.

Plasma

plasma *thick, pale yellow fluid that makes up the liquid part of the blood.*

Plasma is a thick, pale yellow fluid that is 90–92 percent water and 6–7 percent proteins. Fats, carbohydrates, electrolytes, gases, and certain chemical messengers comprise the remaining 2–3 percent. Plasma transports the cellular components of blood and dissolved nutrients throughout the body and, at the same time, transports waste products from cellular metabolism to the liver, kidneys, and lungs, where they can be removed from the body.

Most plasma components can move back and forth across the capillary membranes to the interstitial fluid. However, plasma proteins, such as albumin, are large molecules and have great difficulty diffusing across the membranes. This is fortunate, since they remain in the plasma to help retain water in the capillaries. As noted earlier, this is known as *oncotic force,* or *colloid osmotic pressure.* Plasma proteins perform many other functions, including clotting of blood, dismantling of clots, buffering of the blood's acid–base balance, transporting hormones and regulating their effects, and providing a source of energy.

Electrolytes are also found in the plasma. (As noted earlier, these are chemical substances that dissociate into charged particles in water.) They are essential for nerve conduction, muscle contraction, and water balance. They can easily diffuse across capillary membranes based on their concentration gradients. Carbohydrates in plasma are generally in the form of glucose, the primary energy source for all body tissues. Glucose is especially important to brain cells as they cannot obtain energy from fat metabolism. (Glucose cannot diffuse across most cell membranes without assistance from the hormone insulin.) Plasma also performs a role in gas transport. In addition to being carried by red blood cells, carbon dioxide and oxygen are dissolved and transported in plasma.

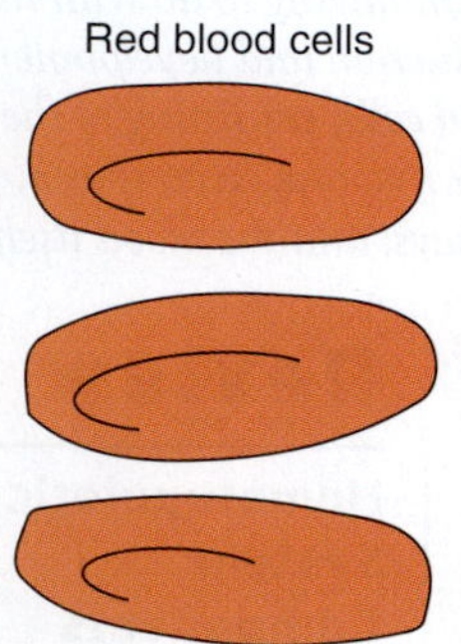

■ Figure 3-9 Red blood cells.

Red Blood Cells

erythrocyte *red blood cell.*

hemoglobin *oxygen-bearing molecule in the red blood cells. It is made up of iron-rich red pigment called* heme *and a protein called* globin.

The primary function of blood is to transport oxygen from the lungs to the tissues. At rest, the body consumes about 4 mL of oxygen per kilogram of body weight every minute. Because it stores little oxygen, the body would quickly succumb to anoxia without the continued transport provided by the blood.

The red blood cell (RBC), or **erythrocyte,** is a biconcave disc that does not have a nucleus when mature (Figure 3-9 ■). It contains **hemoglobin** molecules that transport oxygen. Hemoglobin comprises four subunits of *globin,* each bonded to a *heme* (iron-containing) molecule. Each globin subunit can bind with one oxygen molecule; thus, each complete hemoglobin molecule can carry up to four oxygen molecules. When all four subunits are carrying an oxygen molecule, the hemoglobin is 100 percent saturated. When fully saturated, each gram of hemoglobin can transport 1.34 mL of oxygen.

PO_2 *partial pressure of oxygen;* (partial pressure *is the pressure exerted by a given component of a gas containing several components).*

Oxygen Transport The effectiveness of oxygen transport depends on many factors. Red blood cell mass (the number of red blood cells present) is obviously a factor in oxygen transport. The greater the number of red blood cells, the greater will be the potential oxygen carrying capacity. The percentage of oxygen bound to hemoglobin increases as the **PO_2** increases. This is illustrated in the oxygen-hemoglobin dissociation curve (Figure 3-10 ■). Normal PO_2 is approximately 95 mmHg. Based on this, the oxygen-hemoglobin dissociation curve indicates that normal oxygen saturation

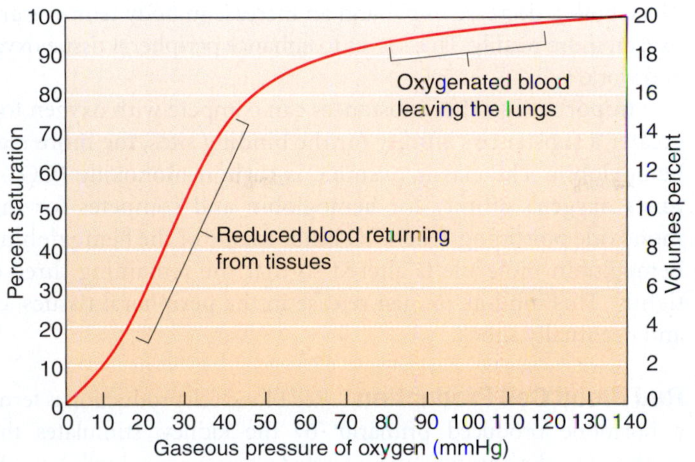

■ **Figure 3-10** The oxygen-hemoglobin dissociation curve.

is about 97 percent. Hemoglobin's affinity for oxygen is also a factor in oxygen transport. Several factors affect oxygen affinity, including pH, PCO_2, concentration of 2,3-DPG, and temperature.

The lower the pH (that is, the more acidic the blood), the more readily hemoglobin will release oxygen. This shifts the oxygen-hemoglobin dissociation curve to the right. In contrast, alkalosis makes hemoglobin bind to oxygen more tightly. This shifts the oxygen-hemoglobin dissociation curve to the left (Figure 3-11 ■). The PCO_2 is directly related to the pH. Thus, in the lungs, as PCO_2 decreases with diffusion of CO_2 into the alveoli, the quantity of oxygen that binds with the hemoglobin increases. The opposite effect occurs when the blood reaches the tissues. There, waste CO_2 from the tissues diffuses into the blood, causing the hemoglobin to give up more oxygen to the tissues. This is called the **Bohr effect.**

Except for hemoglobin, the most abundant chemical in red blood cells is **2,3-diphosphoglycerate (2,3-DPG).** During prolonged periods of hypoxia, the level of 2,3-DPG increases. This shifts the oxygen-hemoglobin dissociation curve to the right and can increase the PO_2 in the plasma as much as 10 percent more than it otherwise would have been. However, the increased 2,3-DPG makes it more difficult for oxygen to combine with hemoglobin in the lungs. This effect casts doubt on whether 2,3-DPG's effect in hypoxia is as beneficial as was once thought.

An elevation in the body temperature causes a shift to the right of the oxygen-hemoglobin dissociation curve and a decrease in hemoglobin's affinity for oxygen. Conversely, a fall in body temperature causes hemoglobin to bind oxygen more tightly. During periods of hyperthermia and pyrexia (fever), hemoglobin's decreased affinity for oxygen enhances oxygenation of the peripheral tissues and end organs.

Exercise has several effects on oxygen affinity. First, exercise causes the production and release of carbon dioxide and other acids, especially from the large muscles. It also increases body temperature.

PCO_2 *partial pressure of carbon dioxide;* (partial pressure *defined—see PO_2).*

Bohr effect *phenomenon in which a decrease in PCO_2/acidity causes an increase in the quantity of oxygen that binds with the hemoglobin; conversely, an increase in PCO_2/acidity causes the hemoglobin to give up a greater quantity of oxygen.*

2,3-diphosphoglycerate (2,3-DPG) *chemical in the red blood cells that affects hemoglobin's affinity for oxygen.*

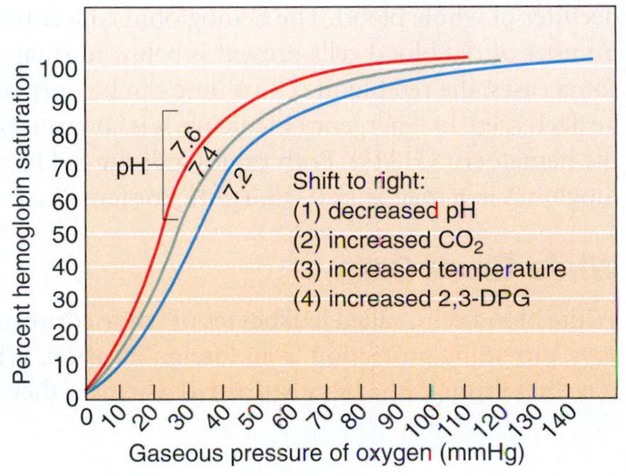

■ **Figure 3-11** Effects of pH, increased carbon dioxide, temperature, and 2,3-DPG on the oxygen-hemoglobin dissociation curve.

Thus, both a decrease in pH and an increase in body temperature will cause hemoglobin to release oxygen more readily. This serves to enhance peripheral tissue oxygenation during strenuous exercise and work.

Importantly, other substances can compete with oxygen for hemoglobin's binding sites. The greater a substance's affinity for the binding sites, the more readily the substance will bind with hemoglobin. The classic example is carbon monoxide (CO). Carbon monoxide has 210–250 times oxygen's affinity for hemoglobin and competes for the same binding sites. In carbon monoxide poisoning, when CO binds to one of the hemoglobin molecule's four binding sites, the hemoglobin molecule is altered so that the remaining three oxygen molecules are held more tightly. This inhibits oxygen release in the peripheral tissues, contributing to hypoxia, acidosis, and eventually shock.

erythropoiesis *the process of producing red blood cells.*

Red Blood Cell Production Red blood cell production is termed **erythropoiesis.** Erythropoietin, a hormone produced primarily by the kidney, stimulates the bone marrow's production of erythrocytes. Erythropoietin is secreted when the renal cells sense hypoxia. This in turn stimulates the bone marrow to increase RBC production, resulting in increased red cell mass. Although a relatively slow process, this effectively increases the oxygen-carrying capacity of blood, thereby increasing oxygen delivery to the tissues.

hemolysis *destruction of red blood cells.*

sequestration *the trapping of red blood cells by an organ such as the spleen.*

The red blood cell lives approximately 120 days. Hemorrhage, **hemolysis** (destruction of the RBC), or **sequestration** of the RBCs by the liver or spleen may significantly reduce its life span. Hemorrhage may occur outside the body or be hidden within a body cavity such as the peritoneum, retroperitoneum, or GI tract. Hemolysis may occur within the circulatory system in sickle cell disease and in rare autoimmune anemias. The spleen and liver contain specialized scavenger cells called macrophages (a type of white blood cell) that can remove damaged or abnormal red blood cells from the circulation.

Laboratory Evaluation of Red Blood Cells and Hemoglobin Red blood cells (RBCs) are quantified or measured and reported in two ways: red blood cell count and hematocrit. The red blood cell count is the total number of RBCs reported in millions per cubic millimeter (mm^3) of blood. Normal values vary with age and sex but in general run between 4.2 and 6.0 million/mm^3.

hematocrit *the packed cell volume of red blood cells per unit of blood.*

The **hematocrit** is the packed cell volume of red blood cells per unit of blood (Figure 3-12 ■). This measurement is obtained by placing a sample of blood in a centrifuge and spinning it at high speed so that the cellular elements separate from the plasma. The red blood cells are the heaviest blood component since they carry the iron-containing pigment hemoglobin. They are forced to the bottom of the tube. Above the red blood cells are the white blood cells. On the top of the specimen is the plasma, which consists primarily of water. The RBCs' column height is divided by the blood's total column height (cellular component plus plasma) and reported as a percentage. Normal values range between 40 and 52 percent, with females generally running a few percentage points below males.

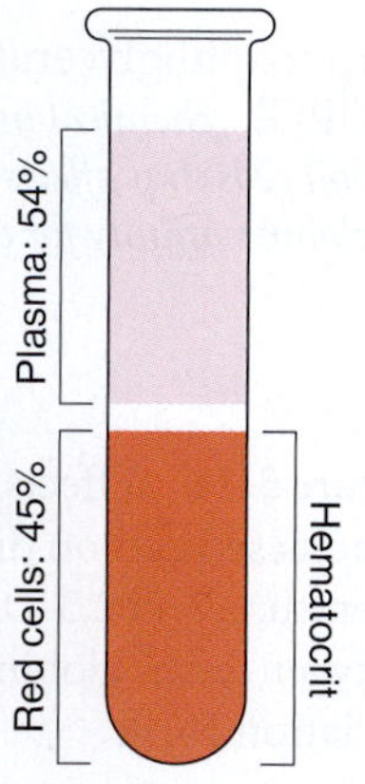

■ Figure 3-12 Hematocrit, including plasma.

Another way to determine the status of the red blood cell is to measure the concentration of hemoglobin present. This is typically expressed as the number of grams of hemoglobin present per deciliter of whole blood. The hemoglobin concentration will decrease in two ways. First, when the number of red blood cells present is below normal, the hemoglobin will also be below normal. In some cases, the red blood cell volume can be normal, but the amount of hemoglobin present may be decreased. In emergency medicine, it is commonplace to measure the hemoglobin in addition to the hematocrit (H&H). Both values indicate red blood cell volume and capability. The normal hemoglobin in a man is 12.0–15.0 g/dL; for females, it is 10.5–14.0 g/dL.

leukocyte *white blood cell.*

White Blood Cells

White blood cells, called **leukocytes** or white corpuscles, circulate through the bloodstream and tissues, providing protection from foreign invasion. White blood cells (WBCs) are extremely mobile, traveling through the bloodstream to wherever they are needed in order to fight infection.

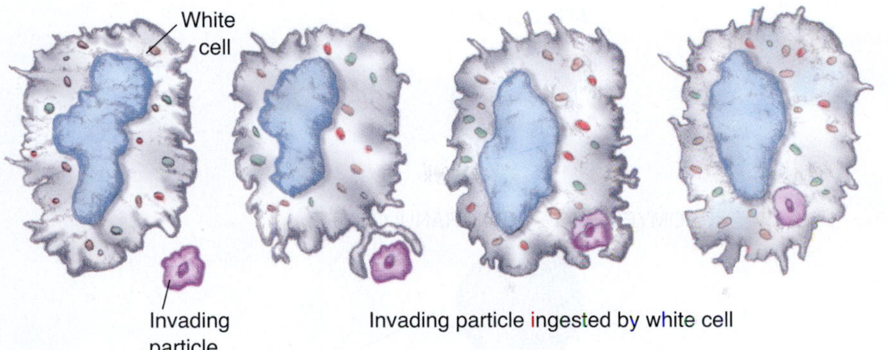

■ **Figure 3-13** White blood cells engulfing and destroying an invader in the process called phagocytosis.

A large population of leukocytes does not move freely within the bloodstream but instead is attached to the blood vessels' walls. These *marginated* leukocytes may quickly return to the circulating pool in response to stress, corticosteroids, seizures, epinephrine, and exercise. This process is called *demargination.* Marginated leukocytes that attach more firmly to the vascular lining through *adhesion* may then leave the blood vessels by *diapedesis.* This enables the leukocytes to squeeze between the cells lining the blood vessels and to follow chemical signals (**chemotaxis**) to the infection site. There, they may engulf and destroy an invader by **phagocytosis** (Figure 3-13 ■). Others stimulate either chemical or immune responses to fight infection.

chemotaxis *the movement of white blood cells in response to chemical signals.*

phagocytosis *process in which white blood cells engulf and destroy an invader.*

leukopoiesis *the process through which stem cells differentiate into the white blood cells' immature forms.*

Healthy people have from 5,000 to 9,000 white blood cells per microliter of blood. An infection can increase that number to more than 16,000 white blood cells. An increase in the white blood cell number is a classic sign of bacterial infection. White blood cells originate in the bone marrow from undifferentiated stem cells. Through a process termed **leukopoiesis,** these stem cells respond to specific growth factors that allow them to differentiate into three main blasts (immature forms): myeloblasts, monoblasts, and lymphoblasts.

White blood cells are categorized as *granulocytes, monocytes,* or *lymphocytes* (Figure 3-14 ■).

Content Review

White Blood Cell Blasts

- Myeloblasts
- Monoblasts
- Lymphoblasts

Granulocytes Granulocytic white blood cells, so named for the granules they contain, form from stem cells that differentiate in the bone marrow in response to hormonal stimulation. These cells mature through several stages from myeloblast to promyelocyte, myelocyte, metamyelocyte, band form, and mature form (Figure 3-15 ■). Their mature forms are classified by the type of stain

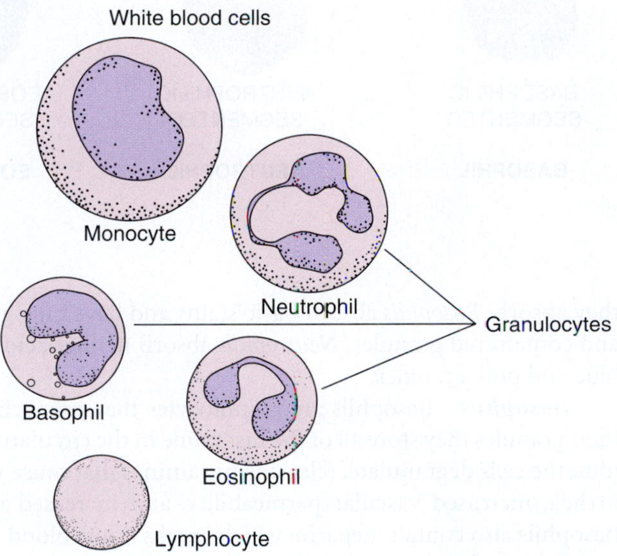

■ **Figure 3-14** Types of white blood cells.

■ Figure 3-15 Granulocyte maturation.

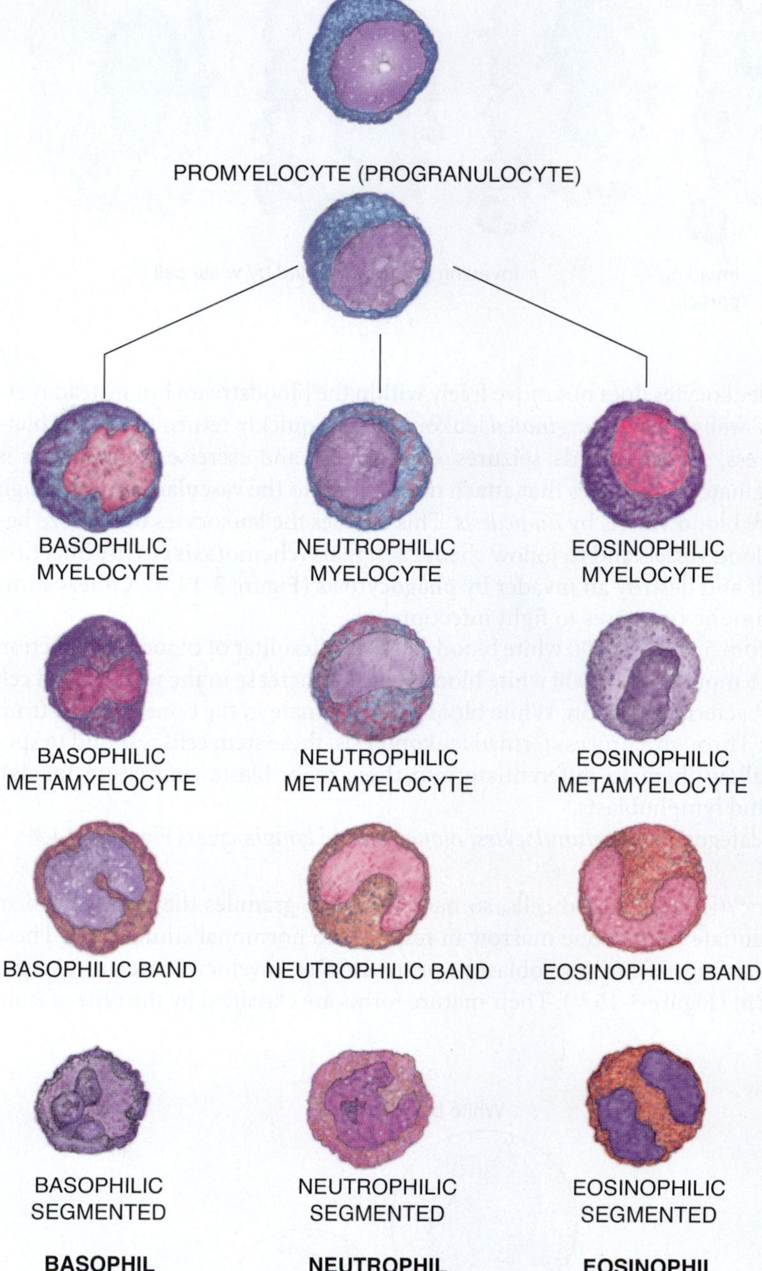

Content Review

White Blood Cell Categories

- Granulocytes
- Monocytes
- Lymphocytes

they absorb. *Basophils* absorb basic stains and have blue granules. *Eosinophils* absorb acidic stains and contain red granules. *Neutrophils* absorb neither acidic nor basic stains well and contain pale blue and pink granules.

Basophils Basophils are granulocytes that primarily function in allergic reactions. Within their granules they store all of the histamine in the circulating blood. In response to an allergic stimulus, the cells degranulate, releasing histamines that cause vasodilation, bronchoconstriction, rhinorrhea, increased vascular permeability, and increased neutrophil and eosinophil chemotaxis. Basophils also contain heparin, which breaks down blood clots.

Eosinophils Eosinophils are highly specialized members of the granulocytic series. They can inactivate the chemical mediators of acute allergic reactions, thereby modulating the anaphylactic response. They also contain **major basic protein (MBP),** which they release in conjunction with an antibody response shown to fight parasitic infections.

Neutrophils The neutrophils' primary function is to fight infection. They leave the bloodstream by diapedesis and engulf and kill microorganisms that have invaded the body. Once they have phagocytized the microorganism, primary and secondary granules within the neutrophil fuse with the phagosome, and the organism is killed and digested. In severe infections the total neutrophil count may rise rapidly, with immature (band) forms apparent on the peripheral blood smear under microscopic examination. If the neutrophil count is low (**neutropenia**), the body cannot mount an appropriate response to infection, and the infection may overwhelm the body's defenses and kill the individual. Neutropenia may result from primary bone marrow disorders that decrease production; from overwhelming infection, viral syndrome, autoimmune disease, or drugs; and from nutritional deficiencies.

Review

Content

Granulocyte Classifications

- Basophils
- Eosinophils
- Neutrophils

major basic protein (MBP) *a larvacidal peptide.*

neutropenia *a low neutrophil count.*

Monocytes Monocytes are unique in that after their initial phase of maturation they are released into the circulation and can remain there as circulating monocytes or migrate to distant sites to further mature into free or fixed tissue macrophages. Macrophages, the "garbage collectors" of the immune system, engulf both foreign invaders and dead neutrophils. They also can attack tumor cells and participate in tissue repair. Monocytes and macrophages also secrete growth factors to stimulate production of granulocytes and red blood cells. Some macrophages are fixed within tissues, residing in the liver, spleen, lungs, and lymphatic system. These cells are part of the reticuloendothelial system. They remove foreign matter, cellular debris, and proteins from the blood. After engulfing foreign proteins or infectious agents, these fixed macrophages of the reticuloendothelial system can stimulate lymphocyte production in an immune response against these agents.

Lymphocytes Lymphocytes are the primary cells involved in the body's immune response. They are located throughout the body in the circulating blood as well as in other tissues such as lymph nodes, circulating in lymph fluid, bone marrow, spleen, liver, lungs, intestine, and skin. Lymphocytes are characteristically small, round, white blood cells containing no granules on staining. However similar they may appear, these cells are highly specialized. They contain surface receptor sites specific to a single antigen (foreign protein) and stand ready to initiate the immune response to rid the body of that particular substance or infectious agent.

Immunity The two basic subpopulations of lymphocytes are T cells and B cells. T cells mature in the thymus gland, located in the mediastinum, and then migrate throughout the body. They are responsible for developing *cell-mediated immunity,* also called *cellular immunity.* Once an antigen activates them, they generate other cells called effector cells that are responsible for delayed-type hypersensitivity reactions, tumor suppression, graft rejection (organ transplant rejections), and defense against intracellular organisms. B cells produce antibodies to combat infection, which is termed *humoral immunity.* They originate in the bone marrow and then migrate to peripheral lymphatic tissues. There they can be exposed to antigens from invading organisms and respond by producing the specific antibodies necessary to defend against them. Some of these B cells' lines are maintained and give the body a "memory" of the previous infection. When the body is subsequently exposed to the same antigen or infection, it generates a rapid response to quickly overwhelm the infection.

Autoimmune Disease **Autoimmune disease** occurs when the body makes antibodies against its own tissues. These antibodies may be limited to specific organs, such as the thyroid, as occurs in *Hashimoto's thyroiditis.* Or, they may involve virtually every tissue type as in the antinuclear antibodies of *systemic lupus erythematosis (SLE)* that attack the body's cell nuclei. Several anemias result from autoimmunity. Mechanisms for the development of autoimmune disease include genetic factors and viral infections.

autoimmune disease *condition in which the body makes antibodies against its own tissues.*

Alterations in Immune Response Several factors can alter the body's immune response. For example, patients who receive an organ transplant must take drugs that inhibit cellular immunity and prevent graft rejection. If they do not, the T cells will recognize the new organ as "not self" and begin the process of attacking it. This is called *rejection.* Unfortunately, organ recipient

immunosuppressed patients are at risk for infections from many different organisms including bacteria, viruses, fungi, and protozoa. Human immunodeficiency virus (HIV) effectively destroys cell-mediated immunity by selectively attacking and ultimately killing T cells. This also leaves the patient at risk for opportunistic infections against which the body cannot defend itself, ultimately causing death. Patients who have cancer are often immunocompromised by the disease itself or by chemotherapy agents that also attack the bone marrow. These agents decrease leukocyte production to extremely low levels, leaving the body defenseless against infection. As a paramedic, you must protect your immunosuppressed patients from undue exposure to infection by good hand washing technique, correct IV technique, and proper wound care. If you have an infection, you must take precautions not to transmit it to your patients. If the infection is highly contagious, as in influenza or chickenpox, you may have to work in a non-patient-care setting.

Protect your immunosuppressed patients from undue exposure to infection by good hand washing technique, correct IV technique, and proper wound care.

inflammatory process *a nonspecific defense mechanism that wards off damage from microorganisms or trauma.*

Inflammatory Process The **inflammatory process** is a nonspecific defense mechanism that wards off damage from microorganisms or trauma. It attempts to localize the damage while destroying the source, at the same time facilitating repair of the tissues. Causes of the inflammatory process may be an infectious agent, trauma, chemical, or immunologic. After local tissue injury occurs, the damaged tissues release chemical messengers that attract white blood cells (chemotaxis), increase capillary permeability, and cause vasodilation. If bacteria are present, responding neutrophils or macrophages will phagocytize them and tissue repair begins. The greater capillary permeability and vasodilation allows increased blood flow to the area and enables fluid to leak out of the capillaries. The process of local inflammation results in redness, warmth, swelling, and usually pain. The pain serves as a reminder against overuse, allowing time for rest and repair. Systemic inflammation is an inflammatory reaction, often in response to a bacterial infection. Fever is a common symptom and likely occurs in response to chemical mediators that macrophages release in response to the infectious agent. These chemical mediators act on the brain and lead to stimulation of the sympathetic nervous system, which causes vasoconstriction, heat conservation, and fever. The macrophages also release factors that stimulate the release of leukocytes from the bone marrow, leading to an elevated white blood cell count.

Platelets

thrombocyte *blood platelet.*

Platelets, or **thrombocytes,** are small fragments of large cells called *megakaryocytes.* Like the other blood cells described so far, megakaryocytes come from an undifferentiated stem cell in the bone marrow. The hormone *thrombopoietin* stimulates these stem cells to differentiate through several stages into megakaryocytes, which then mature and break up into platelets—small fragments without nuclei. The normal number of platelets ranges from 150,000 to 450,000 per microliter of blood. As they function to form a plug at an initial bleeding site and also secrete factors important in clot formation, too few platelets, a condition called *thrombocytopenia,* can lead to bleeding problems and blood loss. Too many platelets, *thrombocytosis,* may cause abnormal clotting, plugs in vessels, and emboli that may travel to the extremities, heart, lungs, or brain. Platelets survive from 7 to 10 days and are removed from circulation by the spleen.

Platelets are activated when they contact injured tissue. This contact stimulates an enzyme within the platelet, causing the surface to become "sticky," which in turn leads the platelets to aggregate and form a plug. Platelets also adhere to the damaged tissue to keep the plug in place. As the platelets aggregate, they release chemical messengers that also activate the blood clotting system.

HEMOSTASIS

hemostasis *the combined mechanisms that work to prevent or control blood loss.*

Hemostasis—from *hemo* (blood) and *stasis* (standing still)—is the term used to describe the combined three mechanisms that work to prevent or control blood loss. These mechanisms include:

- Vascular spasms
- Platelet plugs
- Stable fibrin blood clots (coagulation)

When a blood vessel tears, the smooth muscle fibers (*tunica media*) in the vessel walls contract. This causes vasoconstriction and reduces the size of the tear. Less blood flows through the constricted

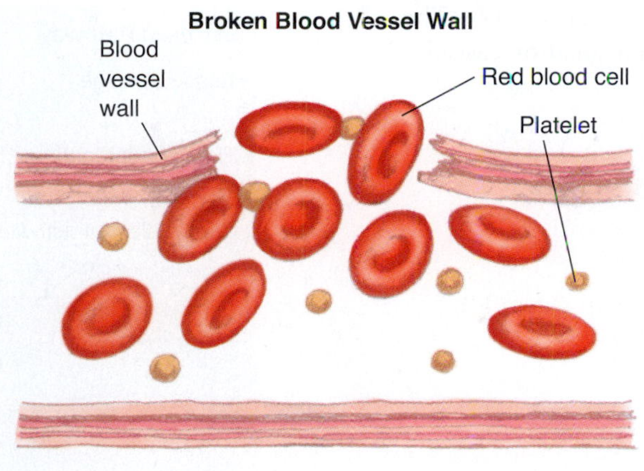

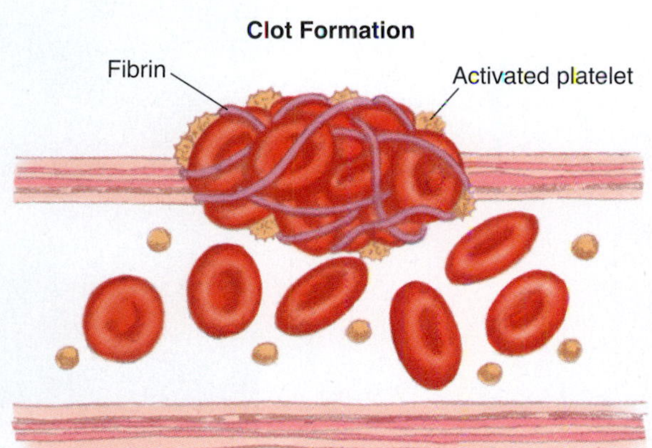

■ **Figure 3-16** Clot formation.

area, effectively limiting blood loss, and the smaller tear makes it easier for a platelet plug to develop and stop blood loss. At any tear in a blood vessel, platelets aggregate and adhere to collagen, a connective tissue that supports the blood vessels. This forms a platelet plug, which acts much like bubble gum stuck into a hole. The plug is unstable, however, and would permit the vessel to bleed again if not for the formation of a stable fibrin clot. This process, blood coagulation, is initiated in part by the platelet plug (Figure 3-16 ■).

Due to the smoothness of the *tunica intima,* the blood vessels' innermost lining, blood normally flows through the vessels without frictional damage to cells or platelets. Damage to cells or to the vessel lining, however, starts the coagulation cascade. This cascade, or sequence of events, can be activated either by damage to vessels (extrinsic pathway) or by trauma to blood from turbulence (intrinsic pathway). Either results in the cascade's progression to a clot. Most clotting proteins are produced in the liver and circulate in an inactive state. The best known of these are *prothrombin* and *fibrinogen.* The damaged cells send out a chemical message that activates a specific clotting factor. This activates each protein in turn, until a stable fibrin clot forms. To completely stop the bleeding, the coagulation cascade relies on the platelet plug and the clotting factors to interact. Once the bleeding stops, the inflammatory and healing processes can begin. The coagulation cascade can be summarized thus (Figure 3-17 ■):

1. **a.** *Intrinsic pathway.* Platelets release substances that lead to the formation of prothrombin activator

   or

   b. *Extrinsic pathway.* Tissue damage causes platelet aggregation and the formation of prothrombin activator.
2. *Common pathway.* The prothrombin activator, in the presence of calcium, converts prothrombin to thrombin.
3. *Thrombin.* In the presence of calcium, thrombin converts fibrinogen to stable fibrin, which then traps blood cells and more platelets to form a clot.

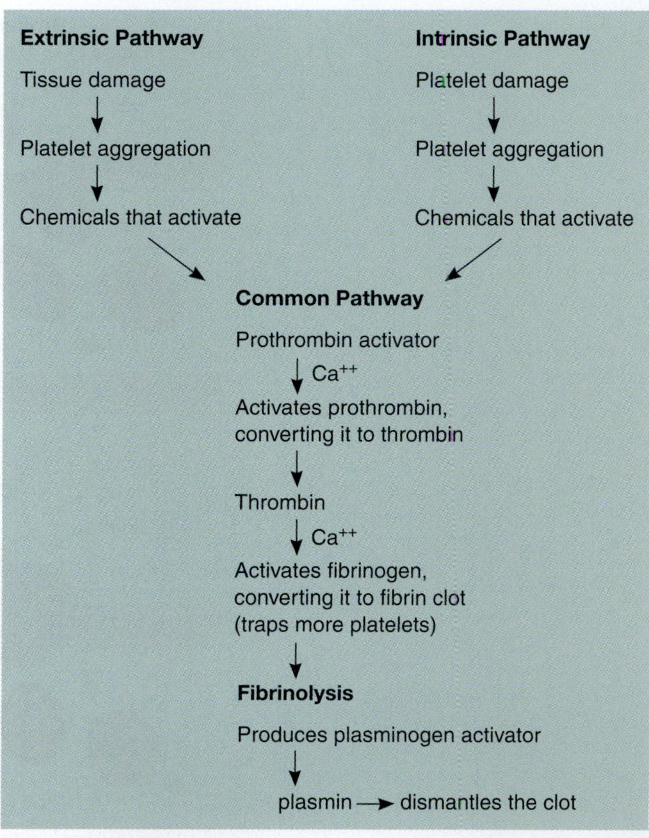

■ **Figure 3-17** The coagulation cascade.

The development of a clot does not end the coagulation cascade. What the body can do it usually can undo, given sufficient time. Once a fibrin clot is formed, it releases a chemical called *plasminogen.* Plasminogen is converted to *plasmin* and is then capable of dismantling, or lysing, a clot through the process of **fibrinolysis.** A clot's dismantling generally takes from hours to days. By that time, scarring has begun.

fibrinolysis *the process through which plasmin dismantles a blood clot.*

thrombosis *clot formation, which is extremely dangerous when it occurs in coronary arteries or cerebral vasculature.*

Thrombosis (clot formation), when it occurs in coronary arteries or cerebral vasculature, may lead to heart attack and stroke. To stimulate or speed fibrinolysis and thus break down clots, medical researchers have developed several fibrinolytic agents. These agents may help reestablish blood flow to these vital organs, limiting or preventing tissue death, and thus helping to prevent the patient's disability or death. Fibrinolytics are effective only against blockages whose components include a fibrin clot.

Patients who lack certain clotting factors can have bleeding disorders that may complicate their assessment and treatment. Other patients take medications that decrease the effectiveness of platelets or the coagulation cascade. Recall that an enzyme on a platelet membrane makes the membrane sticky. Certain medications such as aspirin, dipyridamole (Persantine), and ticlopidine (Ticlid) irreversibly alter the enzyme, thus decreasing the platelets' ability to aggregate and initiate the coagulation cascade. Other medications such as heparin and warfarin (Coumadin) cause changes within the clotting cascade that prevent clot formation. Heparin, in conjunction with antithrombin III (a naturally occurring thrombin inactivator), rapidly inactivates thrombin, which then prevents formation of the fibrin clot. Warfarin (Coumadin) blocks vitamin K activity necessary to generate the activated forms of clotting factors II, VII, IX, and X, effectively interrupting the clotting cascade.

Vitamin K (AquaMEPHYTON) enhances clotting. Certain by-products of tobacco smoking (especially in females on birth control pills) also enhance clotting. Relative or complete immobility, trauma, polycythemia (high red blood cell count), and cancer may also lead to increased clotting as blood becomes relatively stagnant. This allows platelet activation to begin, which leads to clotting. To counteract the effects of decreased activity, many patients take aspirin or other antiplatelet inhibitors and wear compressive stockings to facilitate venous drainage from the lower extremities.

THE MUSCULOSKELETAL SYSTEM

The musculoskeletal system is a complex arrangement of levers and fulcrums, powered by biochemical motors, that provides motion and support for the body. It consists of two distinct subsystems, the skeleton and the muscles. The skeleton is the human body's superstructure, while the muscles supply the power of motion to this superstructure, the organs, and the other body components. These subsystems also produce body heat, store essential salts and energy sources, and create the majority of blood cells for transporting oxygen and combating disease.

The musculoskeletal system is covered by the skin and subcutaneous tissue. These elements protect the skeleton and muscles, as well as other body systems, from trauma, fluid loss, infection, and fluctuations in body temperature. The skin also provides some cushioning for the skeletal components, as on the soles of the feet during walking.

Review Content

Functions of the Skeleton

- Gives the body structural form
- Protects vital organs
- Allows for efficient movement
- Stores salts and other materials for metabolism
- Produces red blood cells

SKELETAL TISSUE AND STRUCTURE

As the body's living framework, the skeleton has a structure and design that permits it to perform a variety of functions and to repair itself as needed within limits. The skeleton is a complex, living system of cells, salt deposits, protein fibers, and other specialized elements. It serves five important purposes:

- ★ It gives the body its structural form.
- ★ It protects the vital organs.
- ★ It allows for efficient movement despite the forces of gravity.
- ★ It stores many salts and other materials needed for metabolism.
- ★ It produces the red blood cells used to transport oxygen.

Although the skeleton is not often thought of as alive, it is exactly that. Its cells live within a matrix of protein fibers and salt deposits. These living cells constantly change the structure and dynamics of the human frame. In fact, 20 percent of the total bone mass (salts, protein fiber, and bone cells) is replaced each year by the remodeling process.

Some 20 percent of the total bone mass is replaced each year by the remodeling process.

Bone Structure

The structure of a typical bone consists of numerous aligned cylinders of bone. Minute blood vessels travel lengthwise along the bone through small tubes, called **haversian canals.** These blood vessels are surrounded by layers of salts deposited in collagen fibers. Bone cells called **osteocytes** are trapped within the matrix and maintain the collagen and the calcium, phosphate, carbonate, and other salt crystals. Other bone cells, osteoblasts and osteoclasts, build or dissolve these salt deposits as necessary. **Osteoblasts** lay down new bone in areas of stress during growth and during the bone repair cycle. **Osteoclasts** dissolve bone structures that are not carrying the pressures of articulation and support or when the body requires more salts for electrolyte balance. These three types of bone cells maintain a dynamic and efficient structure for supporting and moving the body.

A continuous blood supply brings oxygen and nutrients to the bones and removes carbon dioxide and waste products from them. The blood vessels enter and exit the bone shaft through **perforating canals** and distribute blood to both the bone tissue and the structures located within the medullary canal of the shaft and bone ends. As with any other body tissue, bone tissue becomes ischemic and will eventually die if the blood supply is reduced or cut off. The bone does not show evidence of such degeneration for quite some time, and certainly not during prehospital emergency care. However, the long-term effects of **devascularization** may result in loss of bony integrity and failure of the bone to support weight or forces.

The long bones, such as those of the forearm (humerus) and thigh (femur), best demonstrate the organization of bone tissue into structural body elements (Figure 3-18 ■). The major areas and tissues of the long bones include the diaphysis, the epiphysis, the metaphysis, the medullary canal, the periosteum, and the articular cartilage.

The Diaphysis The **diaphysis** is the central portion or shaft of the long bone. It consists of a very dense and relatively thin layer of compact bone. Because of its tubular structure, the diaphysis

haversian canals *small perforations of the long bones through which the blood vessels and nerves travel into the bone itself.*

osteocyte *bone-forming cell found in the bone matrix that helps maintain the bone.*

osteoblast *cell that helps in the creation of new bone during growth and bone repair.*

osteoclast *bone cell that absorbs and removes excess bone.*

perforating canals *structures through which blood vessels enter and exit the bone shaft.*

devascularization *loss of blood vessels from a body part.*

diaphysis *hollow shaft found in long bones.*

■ **Figure 3-18** The internal anatomy of a long bone.

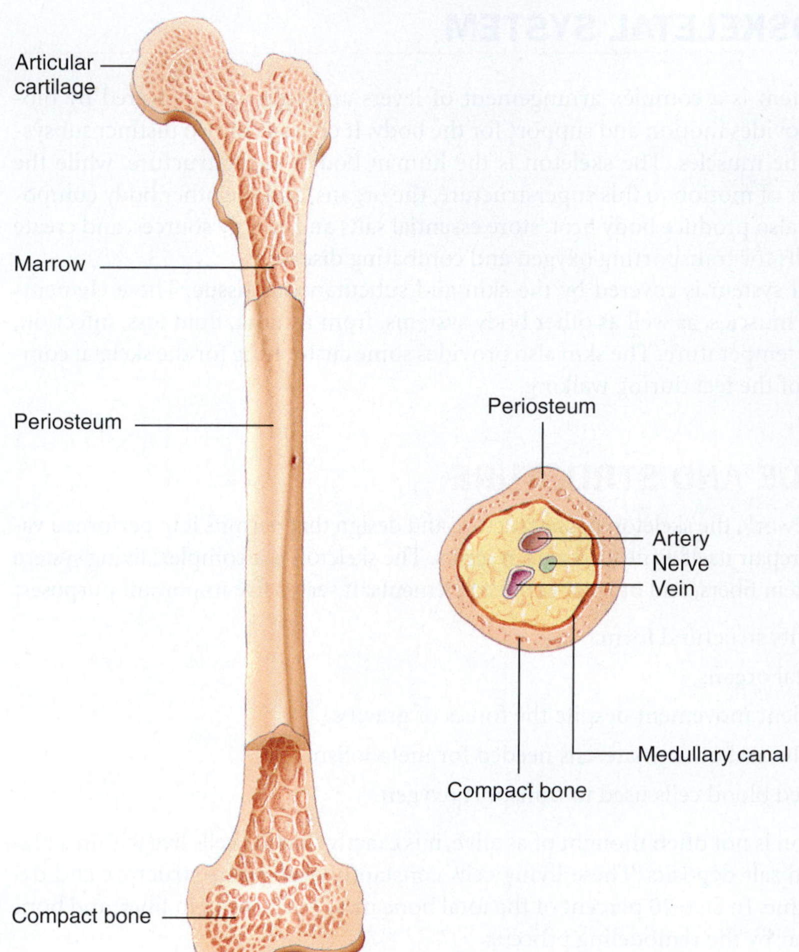

epiphysis *end of a long bone, including the epiphyseal, or growth plate, and supporting structures underlying the joint.*

cancellous *having a latticework structure, as in the spongy tissue of a bone.*

articular surface *surface of a bone that moves against another bone.*

metaphysis *growth zone of a bone, active during the development stages of youth. It is located between the epiphysis and the diaphysis.*

epiphyseal plate *area of the metaphysis where cartilage is generated during bone growth in childhood; growth plate.*

medullary canal *cavity within a bone that contains the marrow.*

yellow bone marrow *tissue that stores fat in semiliquid form within the internal cavities of a bone.*

efficiently supports weight yet is relatively light. While the design of the bone shaft enables it to carry weight well, lateral forces may cause the shaft to break rather easily.

The Epiphysis Toward the ends of the long bone, its structure changes. The bone's diameter increases dramatically, and the underlying thin, hard, compact bone of the shaft changes to a network of skeletal fibers and strands. This network spreads the stresses and pressures of weight bearing over a larger surface. This widened articular end of the bone is called the **epiphysis.** The tissue within the epiphysis in cross section resembles a rigid bony sponge and is called spongy or **cancellous** bone. Covering this network of fibers is a very thin layer of compact bone supporting the surface that meets and moves against another bone, the **articular surface.**

The Metaphysis The **metaphysis** is an intermediate region between the epiphysis and diaphysis. It is where the diaphysis's hollow tube of compact bone makes the transition to the bone-fiber honeycomb of the epiphysis's cancellous bone. In this region is the **epiphyseal plate,** or *growth plate.* During childhood, cartilage is generated here and the plate widens. Osteoblasts from the end of the diaphysis deposit salts within the cartilage's collagen matrix to create new bone tissue. This results in the lengthening of the infant's and then the child's bone. During the growth period, the epiphyseal plate is also weaker than the rest of the bone and associated joints and is thus a frequent site of fractures in pediatric patients.

The Medullary Canal The chamber formed within the hollow diaphysis and the cancellous bone of the epiphysis is called the **medullary canal.** The central medullary canal is filled with **yellow bone marrow** that stores fat in a semiliquid form. The fat is a readily available energy source the body can use quickly and easily. **Red bone marrow** fills the cancellous bone chambers of the larger long bones, the pelvis, and the sternum. It is responsible for the manufacture of erythrocytes and other blood cells.

The Periosteum A tough fibrous membrane called the **periosteum** covers the exterior of the diaphysis. With extensive vasculature and innervation, it transmits sensations of pain when the bone fractures and then initiates the bone repair cycle. Blood vessels and nerves penetrate both the periosteum and compact bone by traveling through the small perforating canals. Tendons intermingle with the collagen fibers of the periosteum and with the collagen fibers of the bony matrix to form strong attachments.

Cartilage A layer of connective tissue called **cartilage** is a continuous collagen extension of the underlying bone and covers a portion of the epiphyseal surface. It is a smooth, strong, and flexible material that functions as the actual surface of articulation between bones. Cartilage is very slippery and somewhat compressible. It permits relatively friction-free joint movement and absorbs some of the shock associated with activity, such as walking.

Bones are classified according to their general shape. Those previously described are considered long bones and include the humerus, radius, ulna, tibia, fibula, metacarpals (hand), metatarsals (foot), and phalanges (fingers and toes). The bones of the wrists and ankles, the carpals and tarsals, are short bones. The bones of the cranium, sternum, ribs, shoulder, and pelvis are classified as flat. Irregularly shaped bones include the bones of the vertebral column and the facial bones. Another special type of bone is the **sesamoid bone,** a bone that grows within tendinous tissue; one example is the kneecap, also called the patella.

Joint Structure

Bones move at, and are held together by, a relatively sophisticated structure called a **joint.**

Types of Joints There are three basic types of joints, which are classified by the amount of movement they permit.

Synarthroses are immovable joints, such as the sutures of the skull or the juncture between the jaw and the teeth (which is called a gomphosis). **Amphiarthroses** are joints that allow some very limited movement. Examples include the joints between the vertebrae and between the sacrum and the ilium of the pelvis. **Diarthroses,** or **synovial joints,** permit relatively free movement. Such joints include the elbow, knee, shoulder, and hip.

Diarthroses are divided into three categories of joints based on the movements they allow (Figure 3-19 ■). These include:

★ *Monaxial joints*

Hinge joints permit bending in a single plane. Examples include the knees, elbows, and fingers.

Pivot joints are characterized by the articulation between the atlas (the first cervical vertebrae) and the axis of the spine. They allow the head to rotate through about 180 degrees of motion.

★ *Biaxial joints*

Condyloid, or gliding, joints provide movement in two directions. They are located at the joints of carpal bones in the wrist and between the clavicle and sternum.

Ellipsoidal joints provide a sliding motion in two planes, as between the wrist and the metacarpals.

Saddle joints allow for movement in two planes at right angles to each other. Examples are the joints at the bases of the thumbs.

★ *Triaxial joints*

Ball-and-socket joints permit full motion in a cone of about 180 degrees and allow a limb to rotate. Examples include the hip and shoulder.

These joints permit various types of motion. **Flexion/extension** is the bending motion that reduces/increases the angle between articulating elements. **Adduction/abduction** is the movement of

red bone marrow *tissue within the internal cavity of a bone responsible for manufacture of erythrocytes and other blood cells.*

periosteum *the tough exterior covering of a bone.*

cartilage *connective tissue providing the articular surfaces of the skeletal system.*

sesamoid bone *bone that forms in a tendon.*

Bones are classified according to their general shape.

joint *area where adjacent bones articulate.*

Content Review

Types of Joints

- Synarthroses—immovable
- Amphiarthroses—very limited movement
- Diarthroses (synovial joints)—relatively free movement:
  - Monaxial
  - Biaxial
  - Triaxial

synarthrosis *joint that does not permit movement.*

amphiarthrosis *joint that permits a limited amount of independent motion.*

diarthrosis *a synovial joint.*

synovial joint *joint that permits the greatest degree of independent motion.*

flexion *bending motion that reduces the angle between articulating elements.*

extension *bending motion that increases the angle between articulating elements.*

adduction *movement of a body part toward the midline.*

abduction *movement of a body part away from the midline.*

■ Figure 3-19 Types of joints.

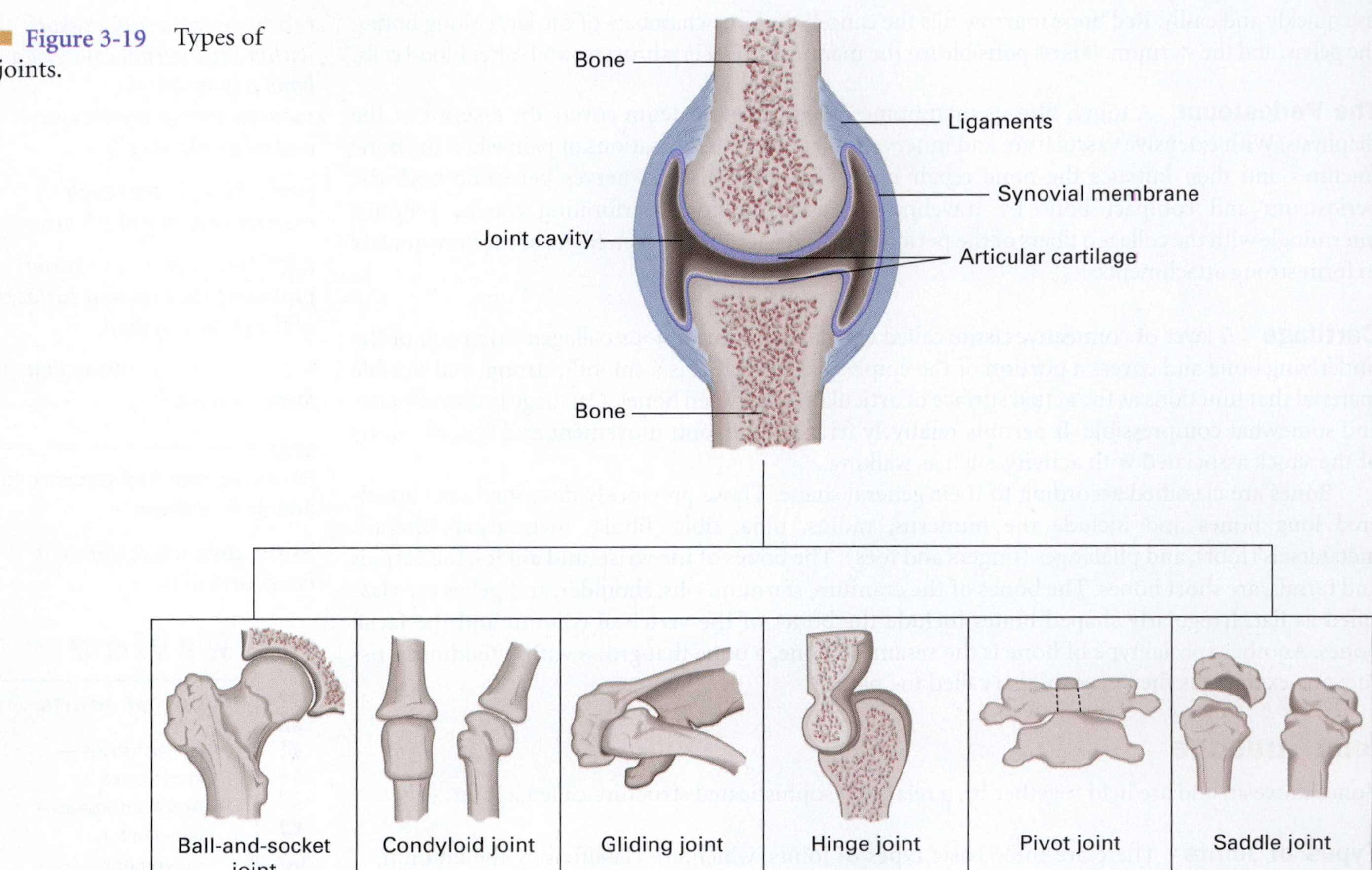

a body part toward/away from the midline. **Rotation** refers to a turning along the axis of a bone or joint. **Circumduction** refers to movement through an arc of a circle.

rotation *a turning along the axis of a bone or joint.*

circumduction *movement at a synovial joint where the distal end of a bone describes a circle but the shaft does not rotate; movement through an arc of a circle.*

ligaments *connective tissue that connects bone to bone and holds joints together.*

joint capsule *the ligaments surround a joint;* synovial capsule.

synovial fluid *substance that lubricates synovial joints.*

bursae *sacs containing synovial fluid that cushion adjacent structures; singular* bursa.

Ligaments

Ligaments Ligaments are bands of connective tissue that hold bones together at joints. They stretch and permit motion at the joint while holding the bone ends firmly in position. The ends of the ligaments attach to the joint ends of each of the associated bones. Ligaments surround the articular region and cross it at many oblique angles. This arrangement ensures that the joint is held together firmly but flexibly enough to permit movement through a designed range of motion.

Joint Capsule

Joint Capsule The ligaments surrounding a joint form what is known as the **joint capsule** or *synovial capsule* (Figure 3-20 ■). This chamber holds a small amount of fluid to lubricate the articular surfaces. This oily, viscous substance, known as **synovial fluid,** assists joint motion by reducing friction. Its lubrication reduces friction to about one fifth that of two pieces of ice sliding together. Small sacs filled with synovial fluid, known as **bursae,** are also located between tendons and ligaments or cartilage in the elbows, knees, and other joints to reduce friction and absorb shock. Synovial fluid flows into and out of the articular cartilage as the joint undergoes pressure and movement. The cartilage acts like a sponge, pushing out fluid as it is compressed and drawing in fluid when it is relaxed. This movement of synovial fluid circulates oxygen, nutrients, and waste products to and from the joint cartilage.

SKELETAL ORGANIZATION

The human skeleton is made up of approximately 206 bones (Figure 3-21 ■). These bones form two major divisions, the axial and the appendicular skeletons.

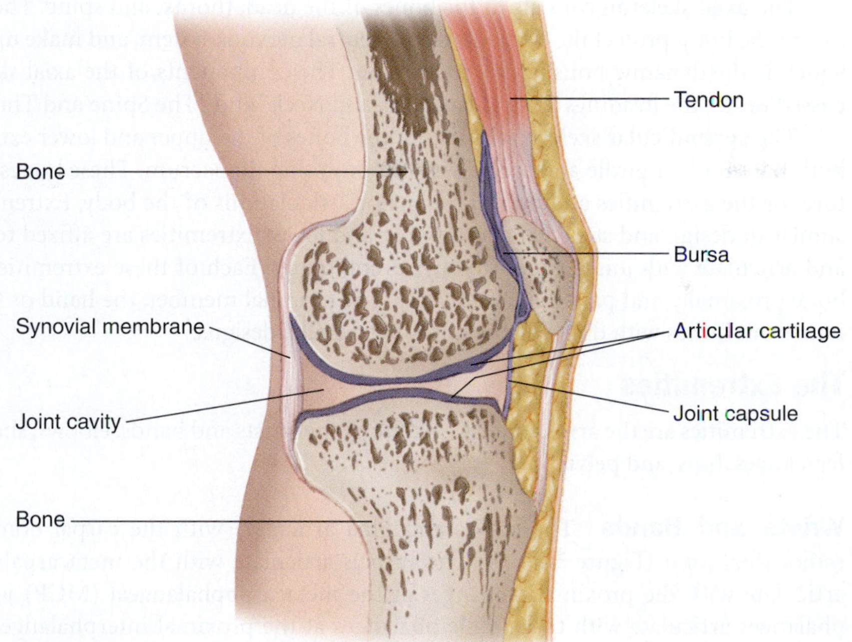

Figure 3-20 Structure of a joint.

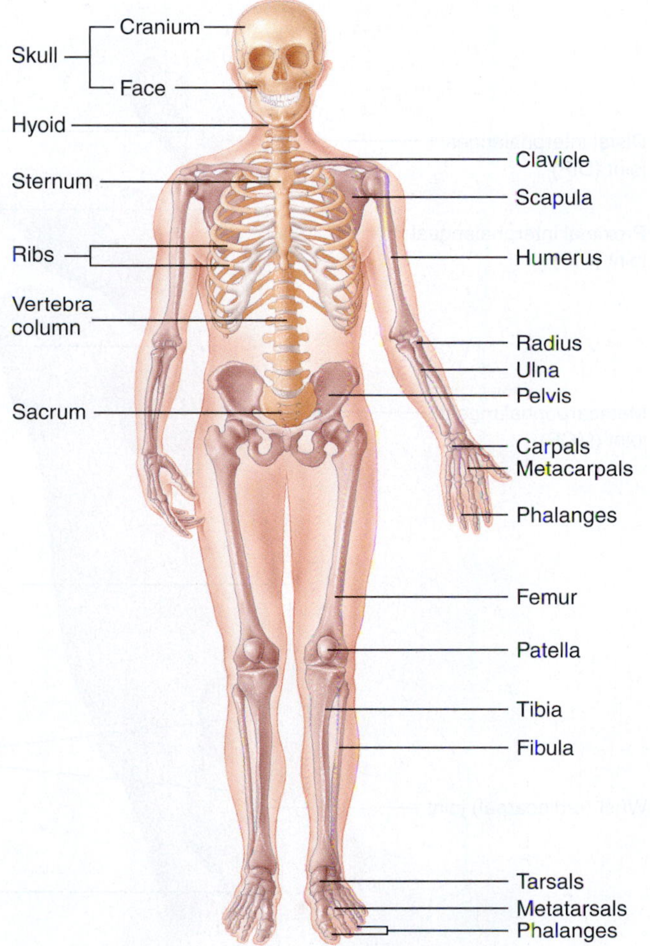

Figure 3-21 The human skeleton.

axial skeleton *bones of the head, thorax, and spine.*

appendicular skeleton *bones of the extremities, shoulder girdle, and pelvis (excepting the sacrum).*

The **axial skeleton** consists of the bones of the head, thorax, and spine. These bones form the axis of the body, protect the elements of the central nervous system, and make up the thoracic cage, which is the dynamic housing for respiration. The components of the axial skeleton will be discussed under the headings "The Head, Face, and Neck" and "The Spine and Thorax."

The **appendicular skeleton** consists of the bones of the upper and lower extremities, including both the shoulder girdle and the pelvis, and excepting the sacrum. These bones provide the structure for the extremities and permit the major articulations of the body. Extremity long bones are similar in design and structure. Both upper and lower extremities are affixed to the axial skeleton and articulate with joints supported by several bones. Each of these extremities has a single long bone proximally and paired bones distally. The terminal member, the hand or foot, is made up of numerous bones with differing purposes, yet parallel designs.

The Extremities

The extremities are the arms and legs, including the wrists and hands, elbows, shoulders, ankles and feet, knees, hips, and pelvis.

Wrists and Hands The radius and ulna articulate with the carpal bones at the wrist, or radiocarpal joint (Figure 3-22 ■). The carpals articulate with the metacarpals. The metacarpals articulate with the proximal phalanges at the metacarpophalangeal (MCP) joint. The proximal phalanges articulate with the middle phalanges at the proximal interphalangeal (PIP) joint. The middle phalanges articulate with the distal phalanges at the distal interphalangeal (DIP) joint. Movement at the wrist includes flexion, extension, radial deviation, and ulnar deviation. Movement at the MCP, PIP, and DIP joints includes flexion and extension. The MCP joints also allow abduction (spreading the fingers out) and adduction (bringing them back together). The major

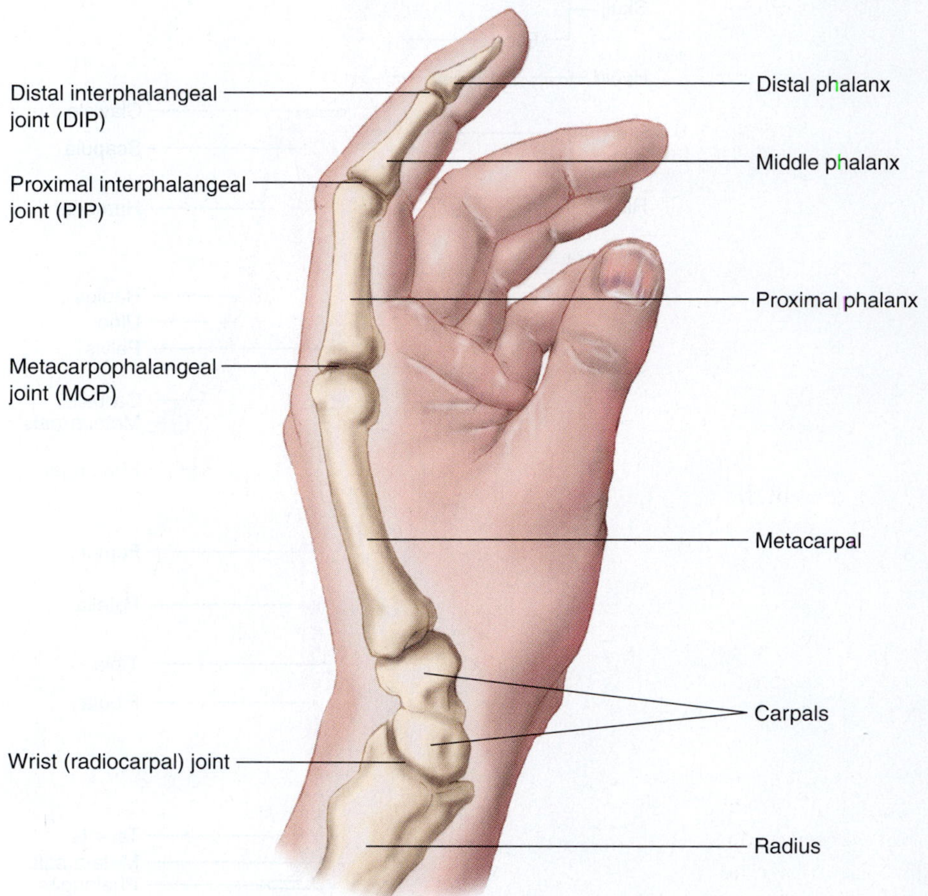

■ Figure 3-22 Bones and joints of the hand and wrist.

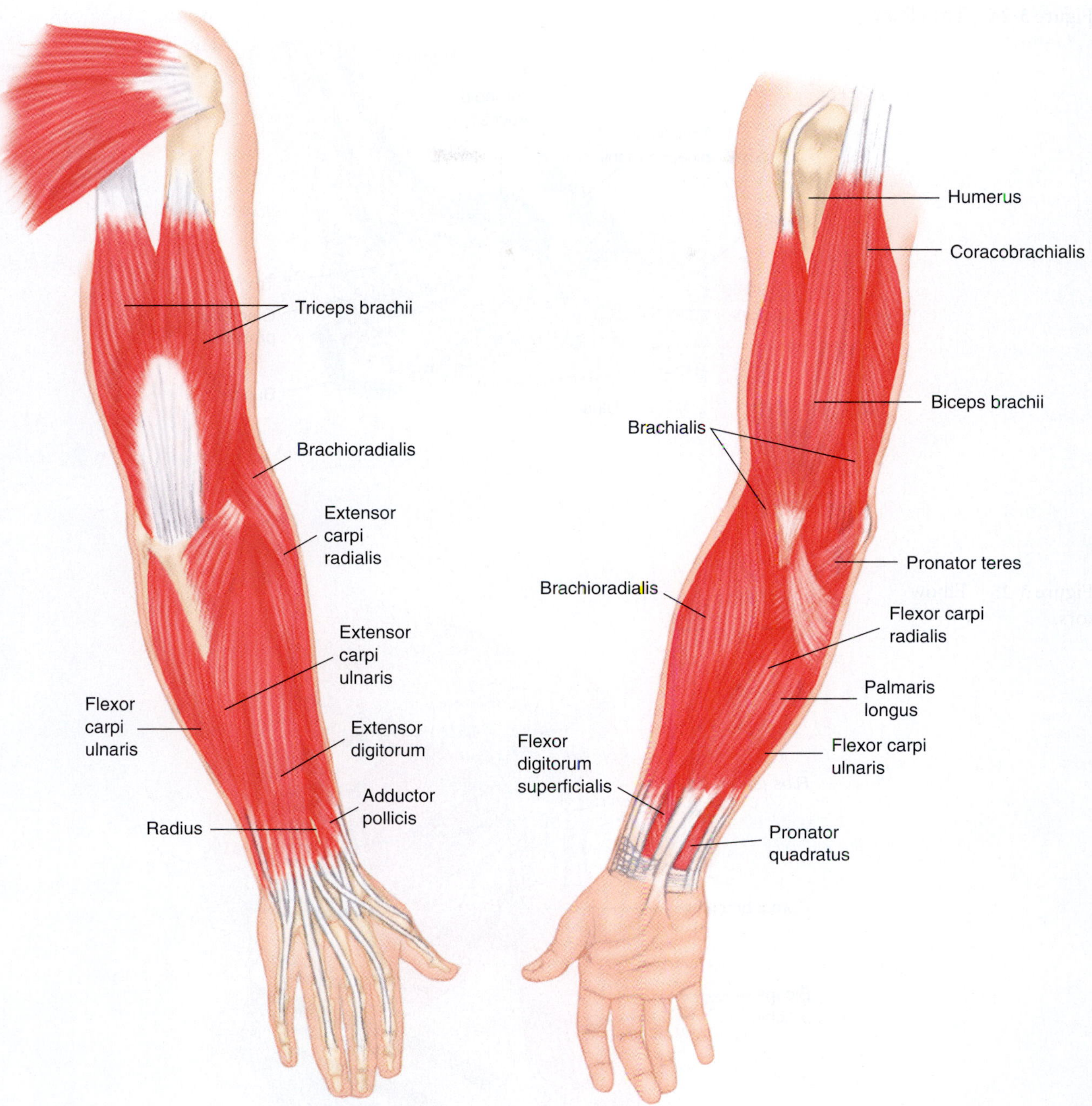

■ Figure 3-23 Muscles of the arm.

flexor muscles are the flexor carpi radialis and flexor carpi ulnaris (Figure 3-23 ■). The major extensor muscles are the extensor carpi radialis longus, extensor carpi radialis brevis, and extensor carpi ulnaris.

Elbows The lateral and medial epicondyles (large rounded edges) of the distal humerus, the olecranon process of the proximal ulna, and the proximal radius comprise the elbow joint (Figure 3-24 ■). Between the olecranon process and skin lies a bursa. The ulnar nerve (funny bone) extends through the groove between the olecranon process and the medial epicondyle. The elbow is a hinge joint, allowing flexion and extension. The major flexor muscles are the biceps (Figure 3-25 ■). The

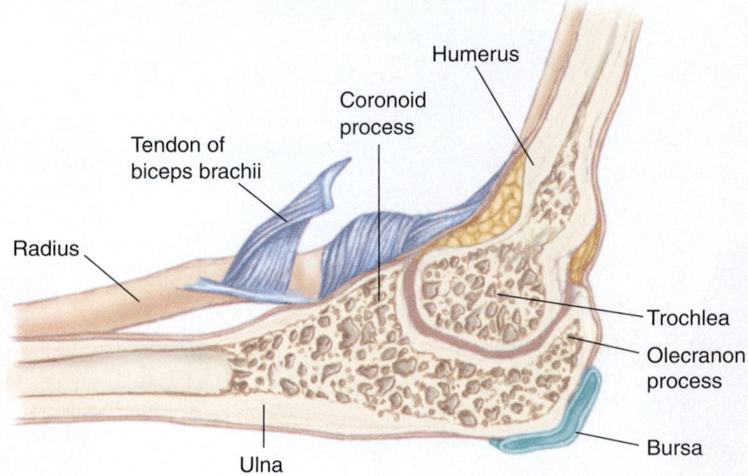

■ **Figure 3-24** The elbow.

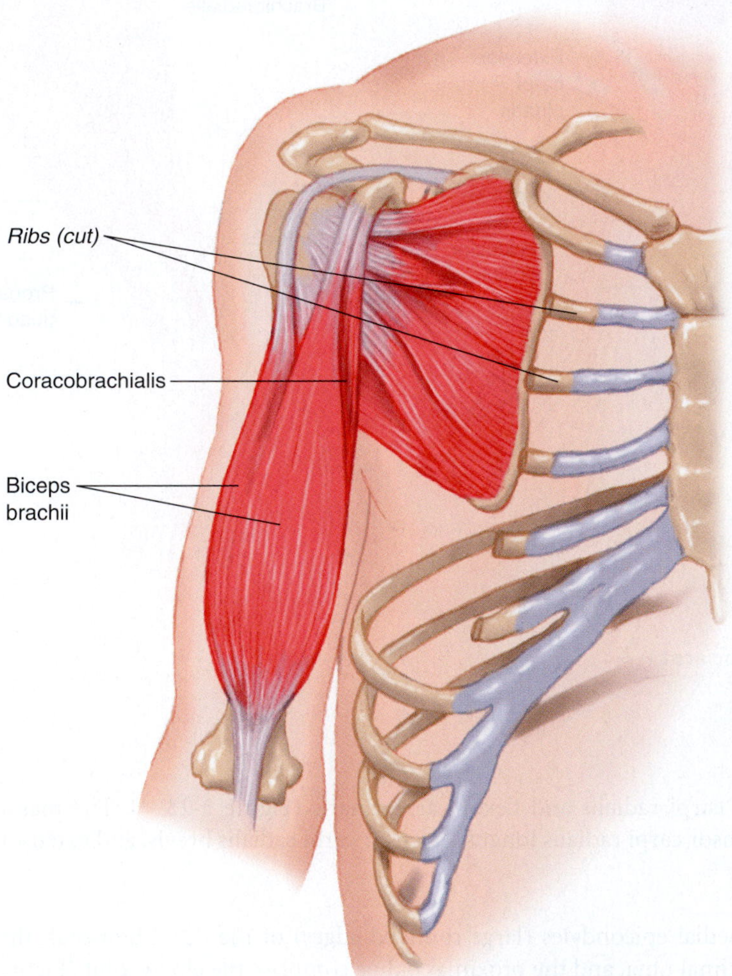

■ **Figure 3-25** Elbow flexors.

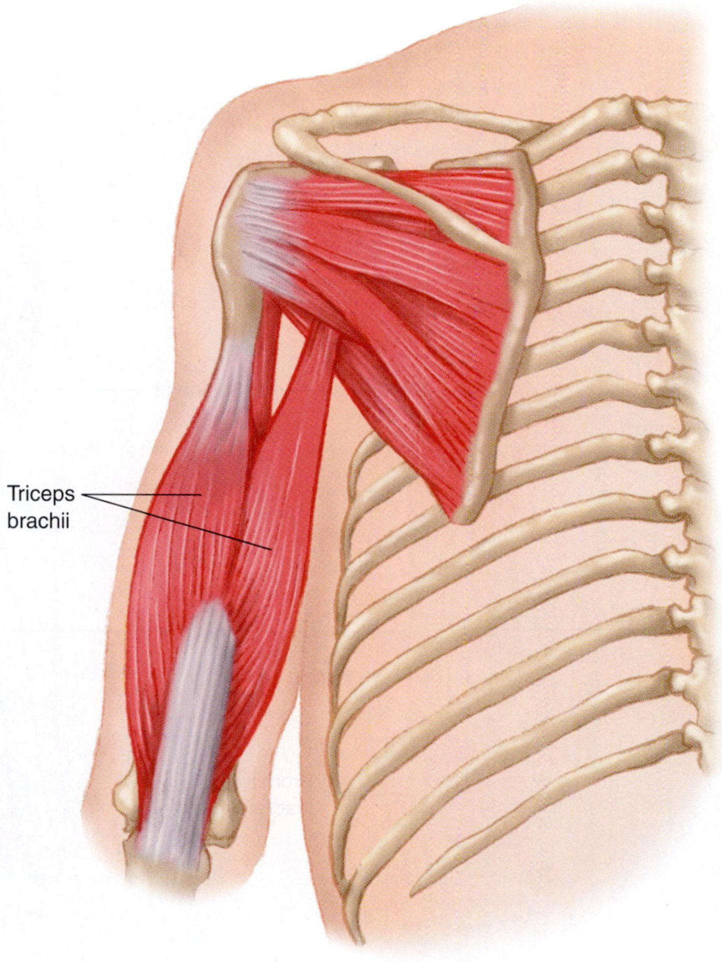

■ Figure 3-26 Elbow extensors.

major extensor muscles are the triceps (Figure 3-26 ■). Just below the elbow, the relationship of the radius and ulna to the pronator and supinator muscles allows the forearm to supinate (turn palm up) and pronate (turn palm down) (Figure 3-27 ■).

Shoulders The shoulder girdle consists of articulations between the clavicle and the scapula and between the scapula and the head of the humerus (Figure 3-28 ■). The sternoclavicular joint, which joins the clavicle and the manubrium, is the only bony link between the upper extremity and the axial skeleton. Movement at this joint is largely passive and occurs as a result of active movements of the scapula. The distal clavicle articulates with the acromion, or acromion process, of the scapula at the acromioclavicular (AC) joint. The clavicle acts as a strut, keeping the upper limb away from the thorax and permitting a greater range of motion. The AC joint also helps provide stability to the upper limb, reducing the need for muscle energy to keep the shoulder in its proper alignment.

The glenohumeral joint is a ball-and-socket joint that allows flexion, extension, internal and external rotation, abduction, and adduction. It has the greatest range of motion of any joint in the body and as a result is the most frequent site for dislocation. The head of the humerus (ball)

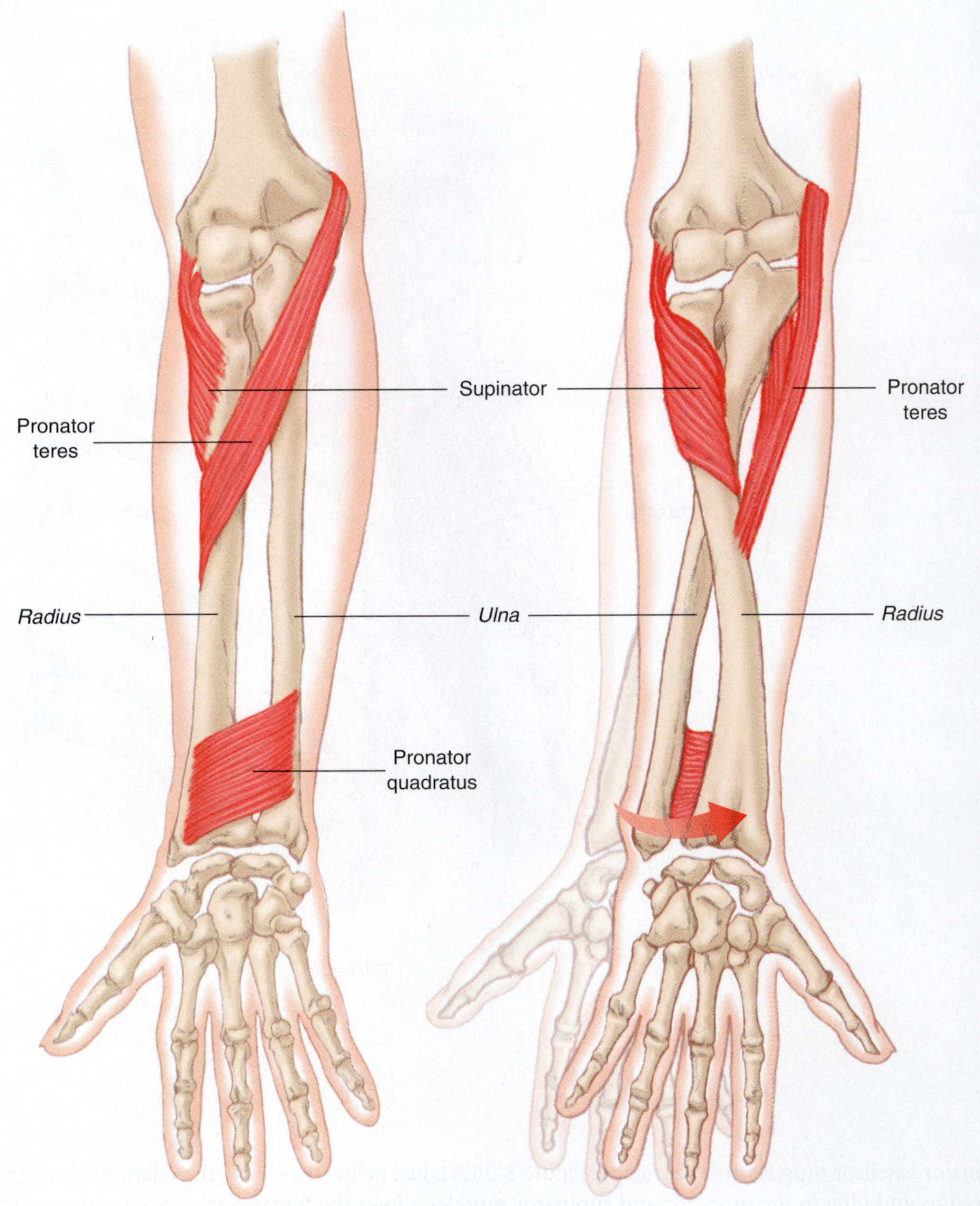

■ **Figure 3-27** Pronator-supinator muscles.

fits into the glenoid cavity (socket) of the scapula. The proximal humerus has two rounded protrusions called the greater and lesser tubercles. The biceps tendon runs through the bicipital groove between the greater and lesser tubercles and is easily palpable on the lateral surface of the shoulder. The glenohumeral joint is encapsulated and reinforced by the tendons and four muscles that make up the rotator cuff and by the large deltoid muscle (Figures 3-29 ■ and 3-30 ■). The muscles of the rotator cuff include the supraspinatus, the infraspinatus, the teres minor, and the subscapularis muscles.

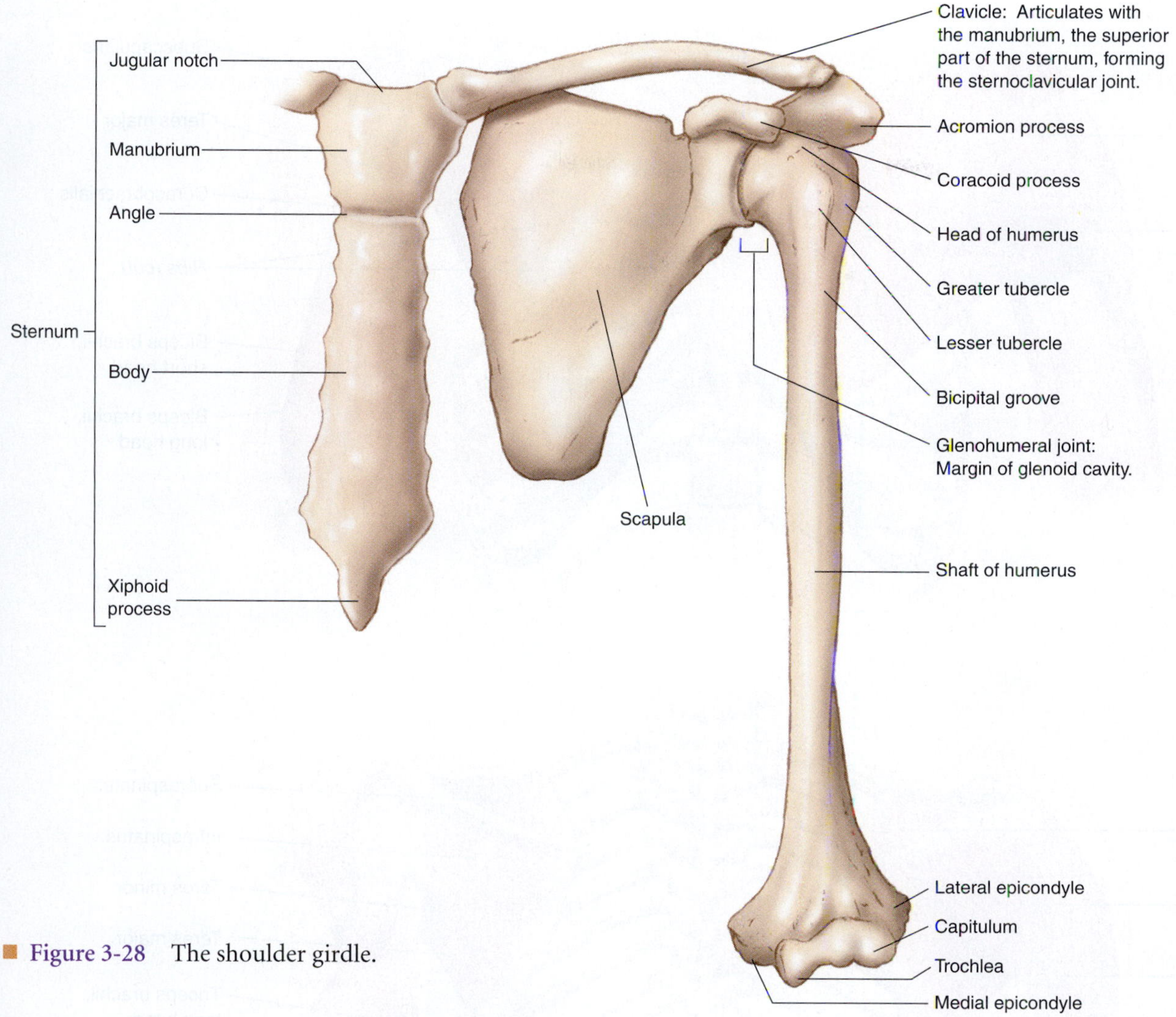

Jugular notch
Manubrium
Angle
Sternum
Body
Xiphoid process
Scapula
Clavicle: Articulates with the manubrium, the superior part of the sternum, forming the sternoclavicular joint.
Acromion process
Coracoid process
Head of humerus
Greater tubercle
Lesser tubercle
Bicipital groove
Glenohumeral joint: Margin of glenoid cavity.
Shaft of humerus
Lateral epicondyle
Capitulum
Trochlea
Medial epicondyle

■ **Figure 3-28** The shoulder girdle.

Coracoacromial ligament
Acromioclavicular ligament
Acromion
Subacromial bursa
Tendon of *infraspinatus muscle*
Glenohumeral ligaments
Glenoid fossa
Glenoid labrum
Articular capsule
Teres minor muscle
Clavicle
Coracoclavicular ligament
Coracoid process
Subcoracoid bursa
Coracohumeral ligament (cut)
Tendon of *biceps brachii muscle*
Subscapular bursa
Subscapularis muscle

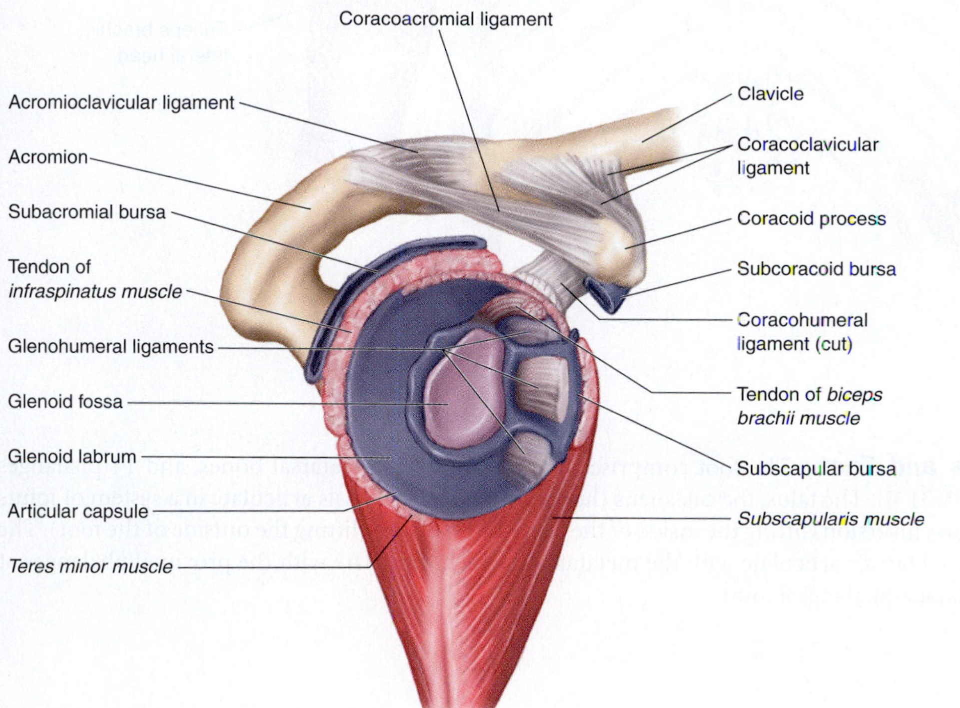

■ **Figure 3-29** Shoulder girdle ligaments.

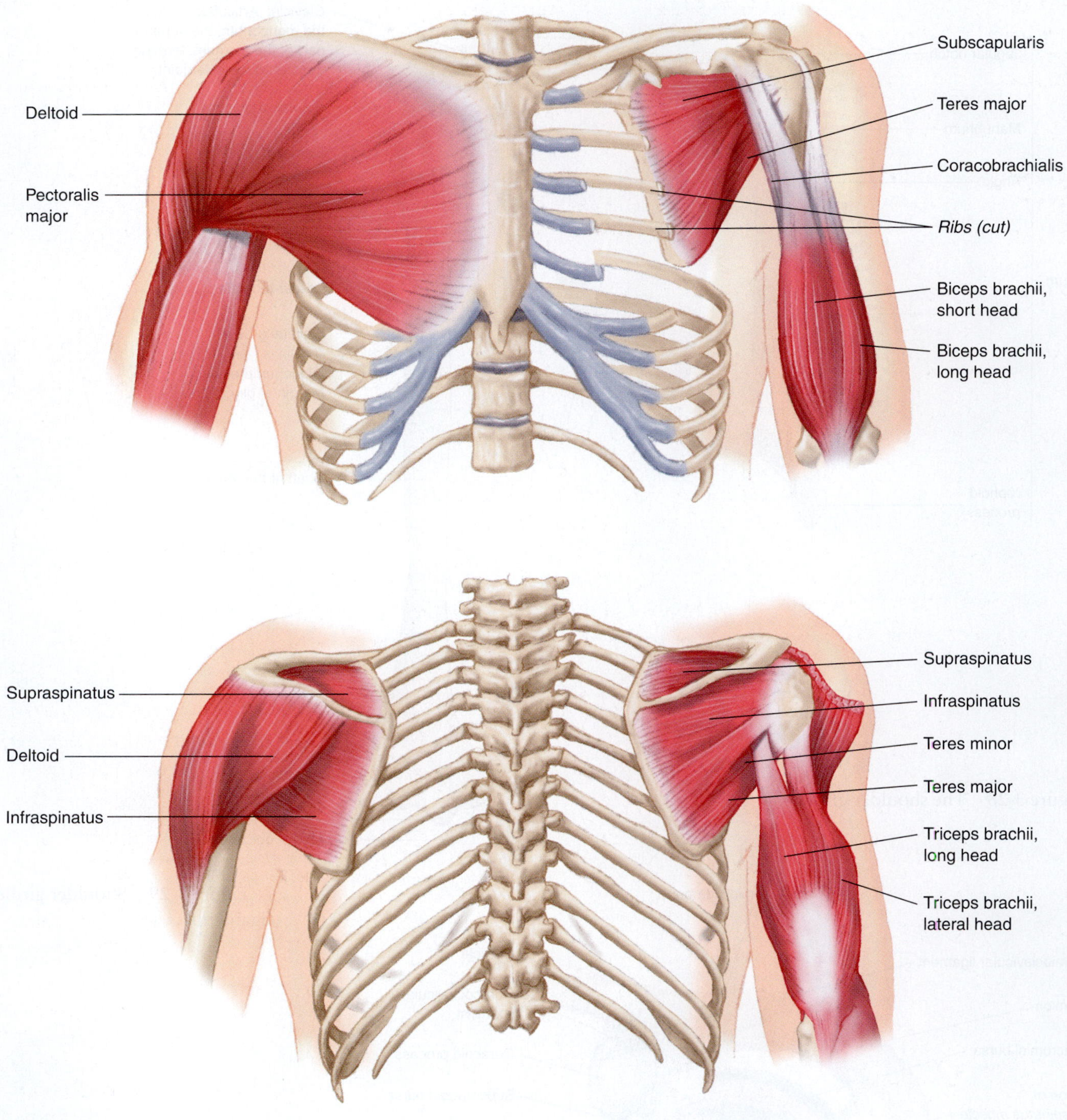

■ **Figure 3-30** Shoulder muscles.

Ankles and Feet The foot comprises 7 tarsal bones, 5 metatarsal bones, and 14 phalanges (Figure 3-31 ■). The talus, the calcaneus (heel), and the other tarsals articulate in a system of joints that allows inversion (lifting the inside of the foot) and eversion (lifting the outside of the foot). The most distal tarsals articulate with the metatarsals, which articulate with the proximal phalanges at the metatarsophalangeal joints.

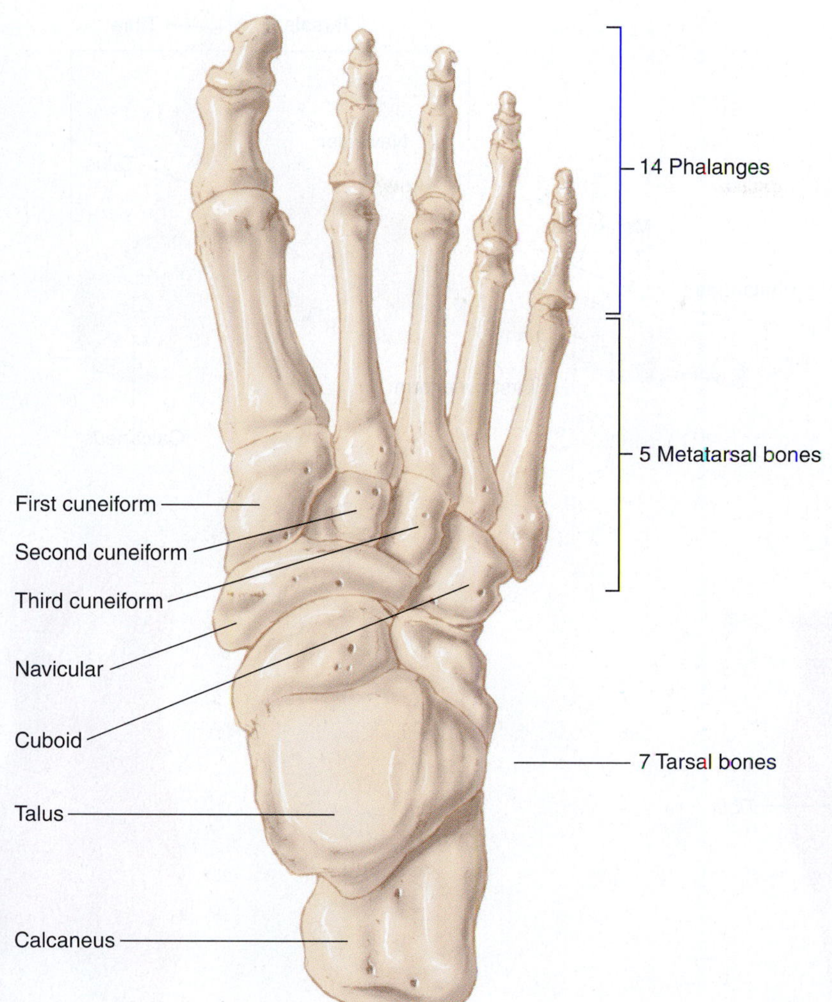

■ **Figure 3-31** Bones of the foot.

At the ankle joint, the distal tibia (medial malleolus) and the distal fibula (lateral malleolus) articulate with the talus (Figure 3-32 ■). Ligaments stretching from each malleolus to the foot itself hold the ankle joint together. The strong Achilles tendon, which inserts on the calcaneus (heel), also helps maintain the ankle's integrity. Movement in the ankle is limited to dorsiflexion (raising the foot) and plantar flexion (lowering the foot). The major dorsiflexor muscle is the tibialis anterior (Figure 3-33 ■). The major plantar flexor is the gastrocnemius (calf muscle) (Figure 3-34 ■).

Knees The knee joint involves the distal femur, the proximal tibia, and the patella (Figure 3-35 ■). The distal femur and the proximal tibia meet at this joint and are cushioned by the lateral meniscus and the medial meniscus, which form a cartilaginous surface for pain-free movement. The joint capsule contains synovial fluid. Several ligaments surround the knee joint and help maintain its integrity. The medial and lateral collateral ligaments provide side-to-side stability and are easily palpable. The anterior and posterior cruciate ligaments, which give the knee front-to-back stability, lie deep within the joint capsule and are not palpable.

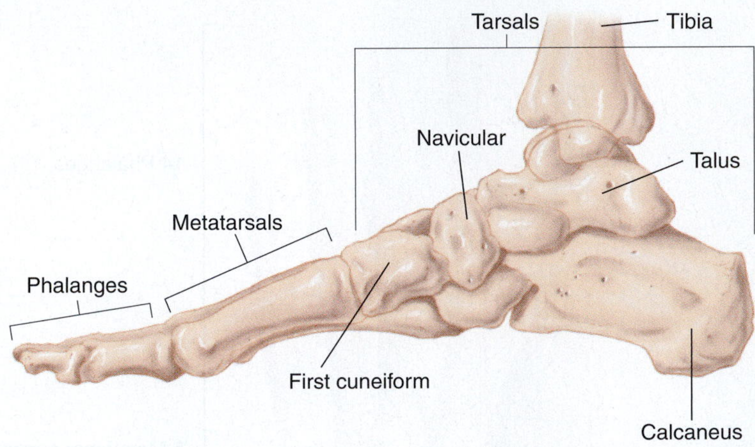

■ **Figure 3-32** The foot and ankle.

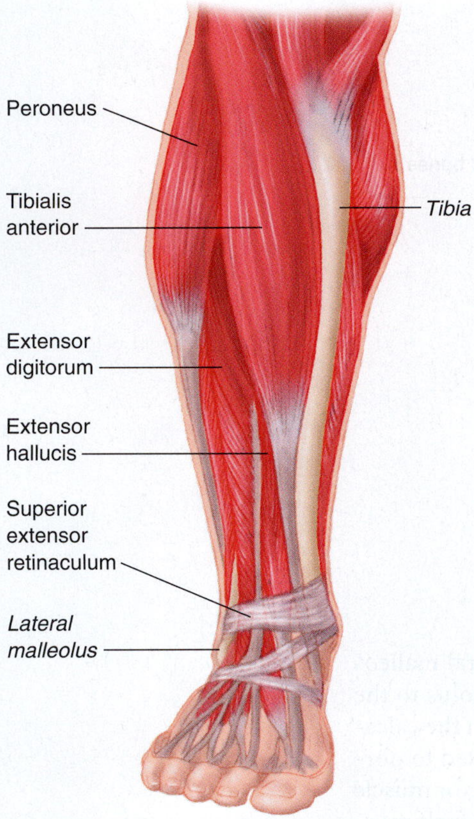

■ **Figure 3-33** The dorsiflexors.

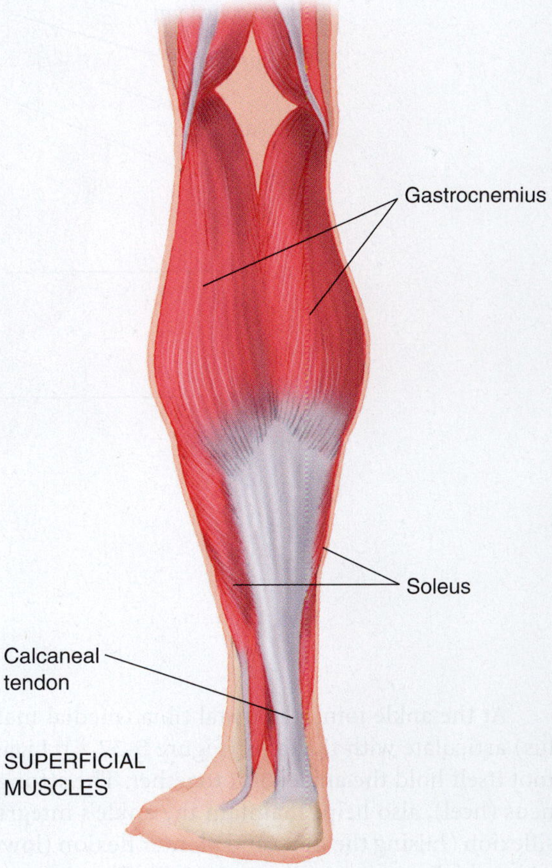

■ **Figure 3-34** The plantar flexors.

The knee is a modified hinge joint, allowing flexion and extension, with some rotation during flexion. The major flexors are a group of three muscles (biceps femoris, semimembranosus, and semitendinosus) known as the hamstrings (Figure 3-36 ■). The major extensors are a group of four muscles (vastus lateralis, vastus intermedius, vastus medialis, and rectus femoris) known as the quadriceps (Figure 3-37 ■). The femur can rotate on the tibia slightly. The patella lies deep in the middle of the quadriceps tendon, which inserts on the tibial tuberosity below the knee. Concave areas at each side of the patella and below it contain synovial fluid.

Lateral condyle
Anterior cruciate ligament
Fibular (lateral) collateral ligament
Lateral meniscus
Cut tendon
Tibia
Tibial (medial) collateral ligament
Fibula
Patellar surface
Posterior cruciate ligament
Medial condyle
Medial meniscus
Synovial membrane
Joint capsule
Gastrocnemius muscle
Soleus muscle
Tibialis posterior muscle
Knee extensor muscles
Femur
Extensor tendon
Suprapatellar bursa
Patella
Prepatellar bursa
Fat pad
Lateral meniscus
Patellar ligament
Tibia

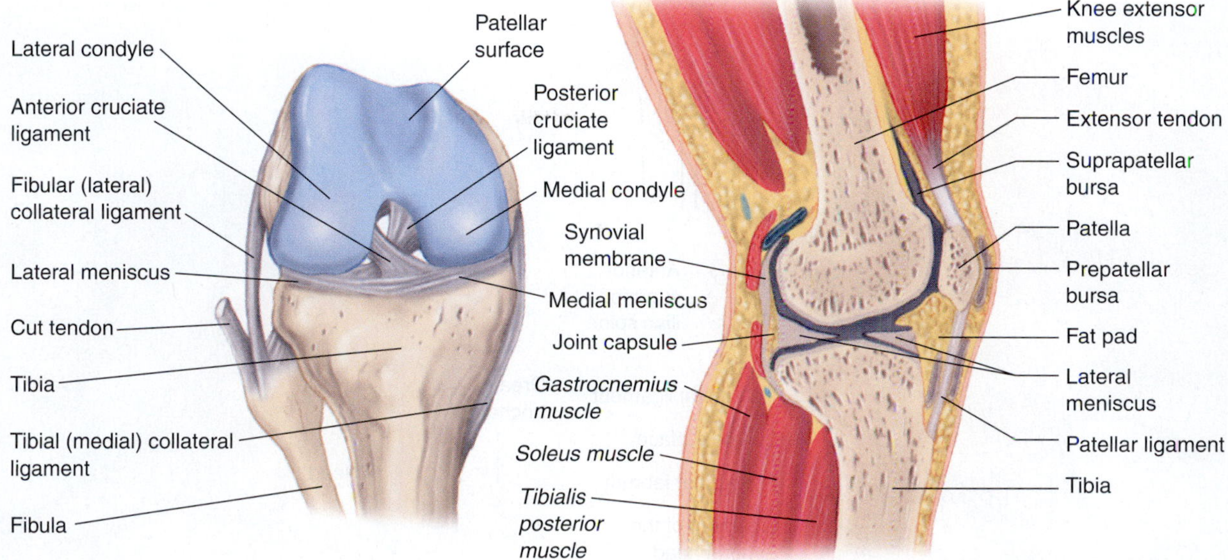

Figure 3-35 The knee.

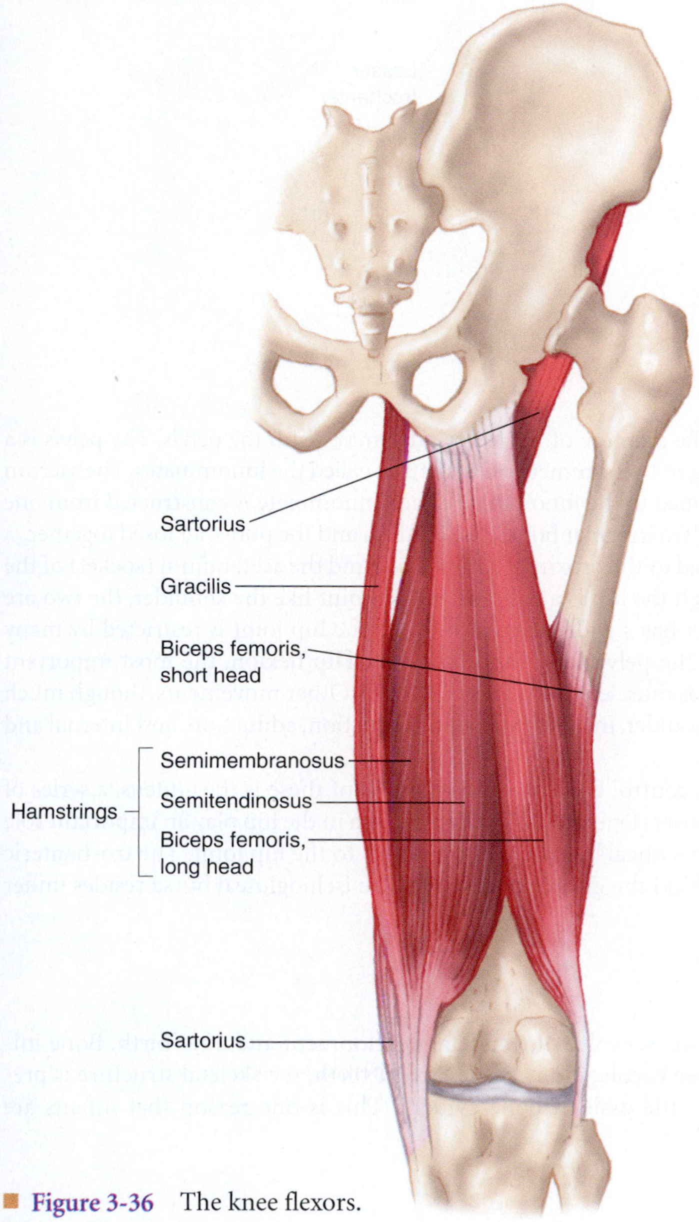

Sartorius
Gracilis
Biceps femoris, short head
Hamstrings
Semimembranosus
Semitendinosus
Biceps femoris, long head
Sartorius

Figure 3-36 The knee flexors.

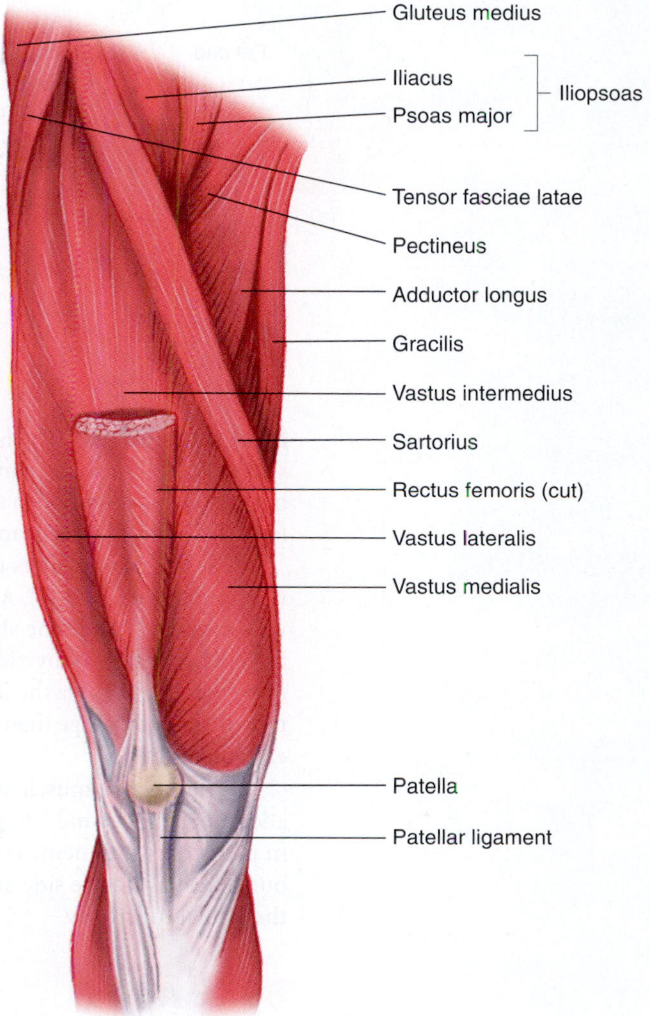

Gluteus medius
Iliacus
Psoas major
Iliopsoas
Tensor fasciae latae
Pectineus
Adductor longus
Gracilis
Vastus intermedius
Sartorius
Rectus femoris (cut)
Vastus lateralis
Vastus medialis
Patella
Patellar ligament

Figure 3-37 The knee extensors. (The vastus intermedius is behind the rectus femoris.)

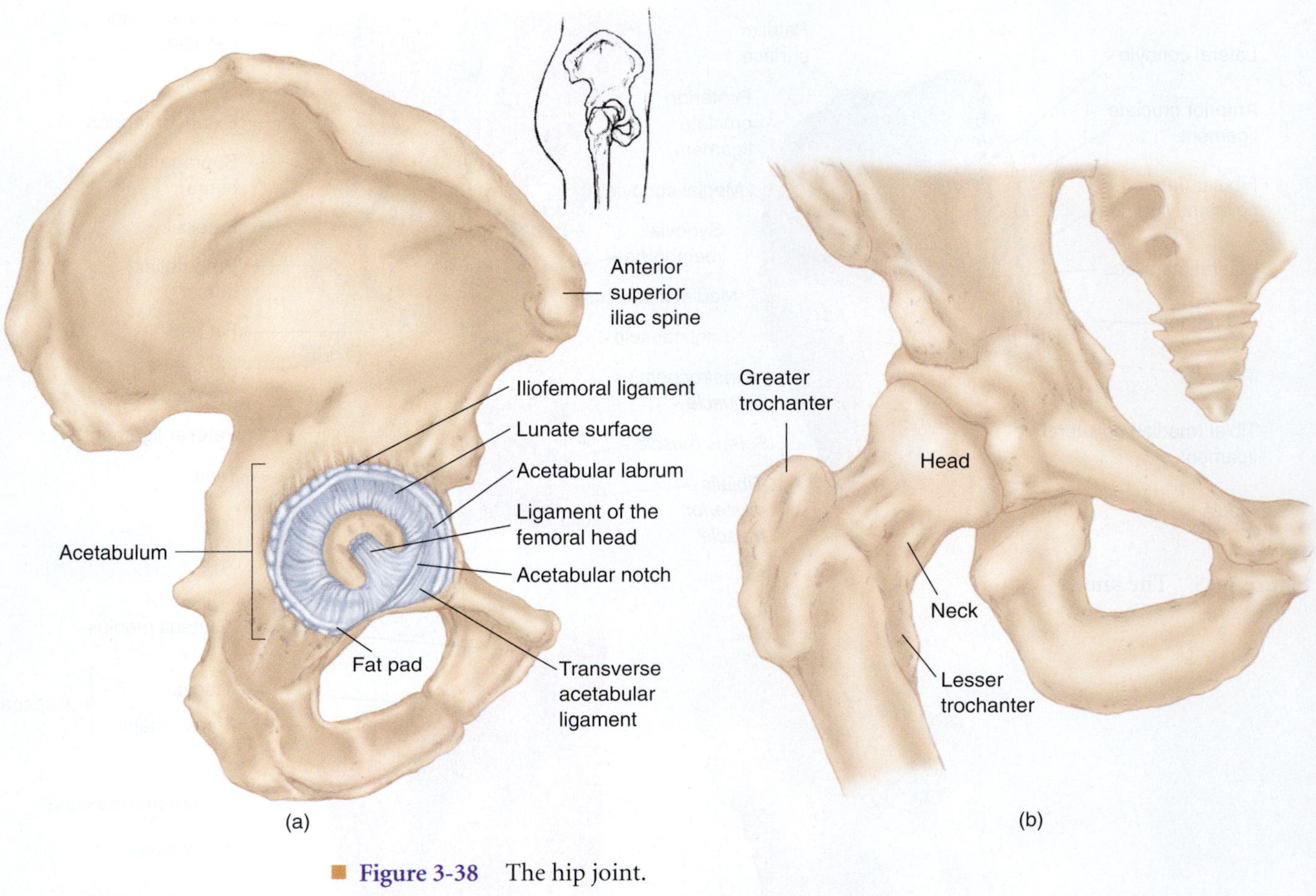

■ **Figure 3-38** The hip joint.

Hips and Pelvis The hip is the juncture of the lower extremities with the pelvis. The pelvis is a strong skeletal structure consisting of two symmetrical structures called the innominates. The sacrum of the spine is posterior to and joined to the innominates. Each innominate is constructed from one large flat bone, the ilium, and the two irregular bones, the ischium and the pubis, all fused together.

The hip joint involves the head of the proximal femur (ball) and the acetabulum (socket) of the ischium (Figure 3-38 ■). Although the hip is a ball-and-socket joint like the shoulder, the two are very different. While the shoulder has a wide range of motion, the hip joint is restricted by many large ligaments, a bony ridge in the pelvis, and capsular fibers. Hip flexion, the most important movement, occurs via the iliopsoas muscle group (Figure 3-39 ■). Other movements, though much more limited in range than the shoulder, include extension, abduction, adduction, and internal and external rotation.

A number of muscle groups control these movements. One of these is the gluteus, a series of adductor muscles and lateral rotators (Figure 3-40 ■). Three bursa in the hip play an important role in pain-free movement. The iliopectineal bursa sits just anterior to the hip joint. The trochanteric bursa lies just to the side and behind the greater trochanter. The ischiogluteal bursa resides under the ischial tuberosity.

BONE AGING

The bones, like all other body tissues, evolve during fetal development and after birth. Bone initially forms in the embryo as loose cartilaginous tissue. Before birth, the skeletal structure is predominantly cartilage, with very little ossified bone evident. This is one reason that infants are

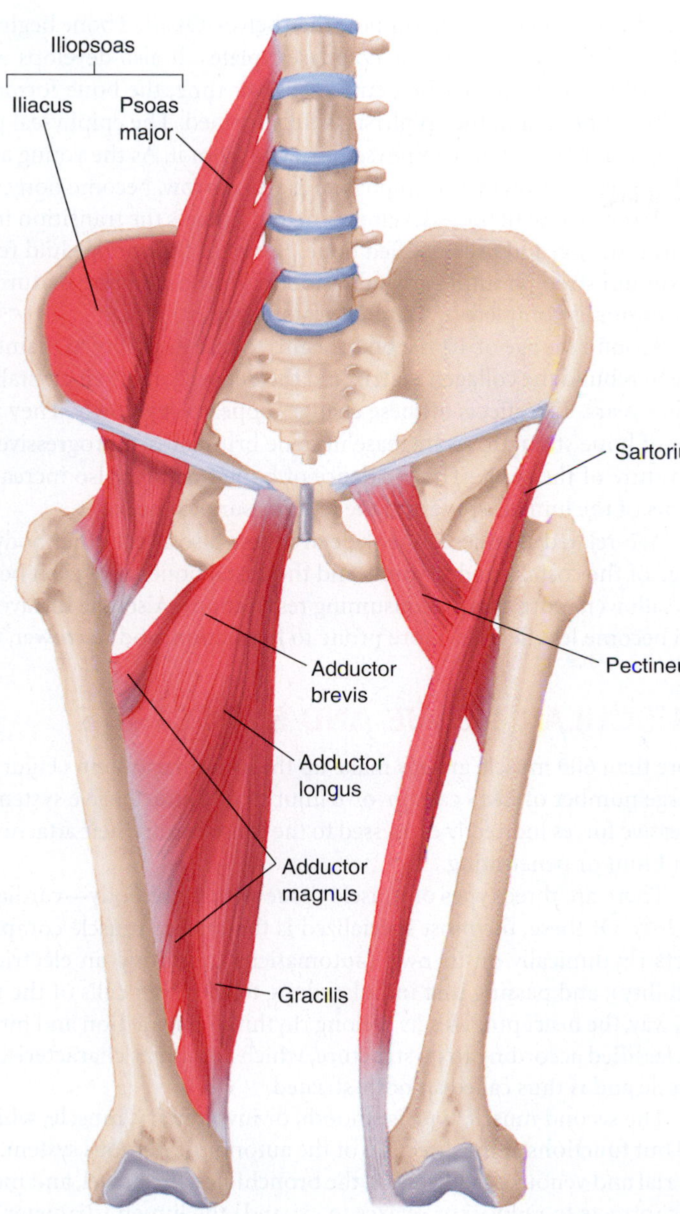

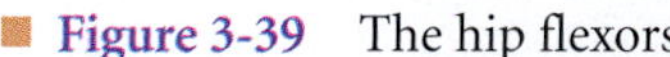

■ **Figure 3-39** The hip flexors.

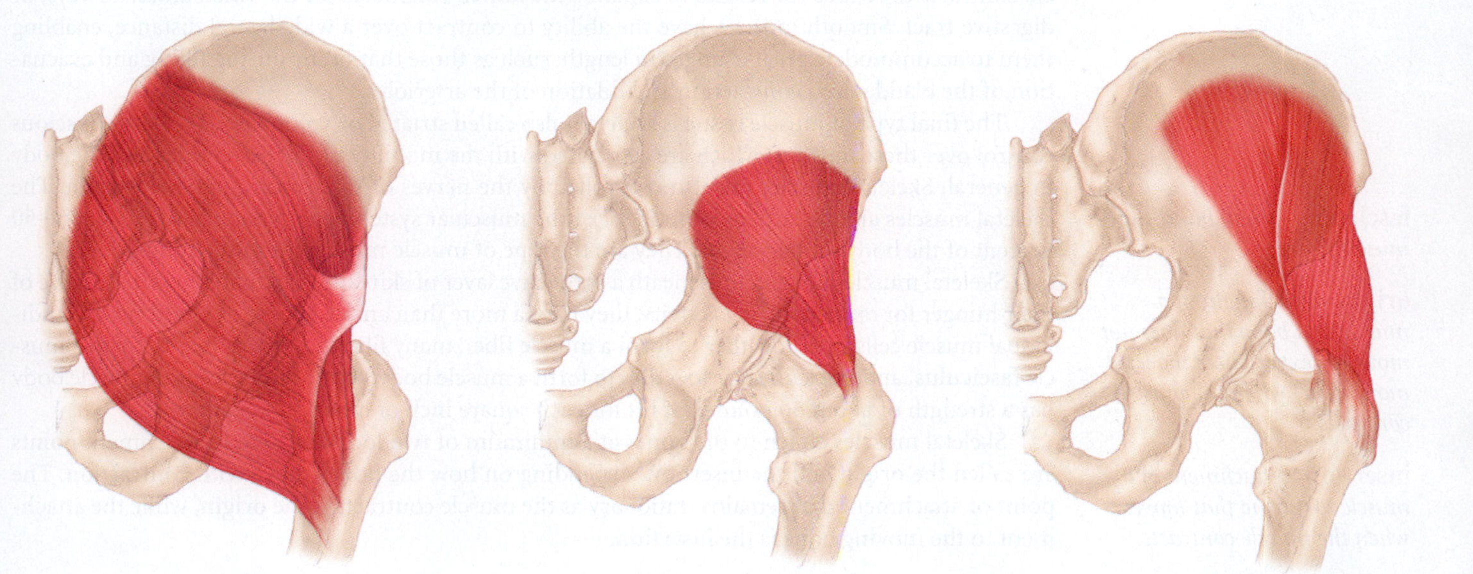

■ **Figure 3-40** The gluteus muscles.

highly flexible yet unable to support themselves. Ossified bone begins to appear along the long bone shafts and then extends to the epiphyseal plates. It also develops within the epiphyses and grows outward to form the articular surfaces. Over time, the bone formation becomes complete to the epiphyseal plate, and the epiphysis is fully formed. The epiphyseal plate continues to generate cartilage, with the shaft and epiphyses growing from it. As the young adult reaches full height and the end of skeletal growth, the epiphyseal plates narrow, become bony, and cease to produce cartilage.

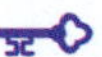

Bones of the young child remain flexible and do not reach maximum strength until maturation, which is usually completed by 18 to 20 years of age.

Associated with bone development and aging is the transition from flexible, cartilaginous bone to firm, strong, and fully ossified bone. Bones of the young child remain flexible and do not reach maximum strength until early adulthood. While each bone matures at a different time, almost all maturation is complete by 18 to 20 years of age.

After approximately the age of 40, the body begins to lose the ability to maintain bone structure.

Around the age of 40, the body begins to lose its ability to maintain the bone structure. It is unable to rebuild the collagen matrix and the deposition of salt crystals is reduced from what it was in earlier years. The effects of these changes appear very slowly. They include a very gradual diminution of bone strength, an increase in bone brittleness, a progressive loss of body height, and some curvature of the spine. The incidence of bone fractures also increases, especially at the high stress points of the lumbar spine and the femur's surgical neck.

Age-related changes in the skeletal system also affect other body systems. For example, the cartilage of the costal-condral joints and the costal bones (the ribs) becomes less flexible, which leads to shallower, more energy-consuming respirations. Also, the intravertebral disks lose water content and become less flexible, more prone to herniation, and narrower, thus shortening the trunk.

MUSCULAR TISSUE AND STRUCTURE

More than 600 muscle groups make up the muscular system (Figure 3-41 ■). As you might expect, a large number of EMS calls involve injuries to this extensive system. Injuries to it may result from excessive forces indirectly expressed to the muscles and their attachments or from direct trauma, either blunt or penetrating.

Content Review

Types of Muscle

- Cardiac muscle
- Smooth muscle
- Skeletal muscle

There are three types of muscle tissue within the body—cardiac, smooth, and skeletal (Figure 3-42 ■). Of these, the most specialized is the cardiac muscle comprising the myocardium. It contracts rhythmically on its own (automaticity), emitting an electrical impulse in the process (excitability), and passing that impulse along to the other cells of the myocardium (conductivity). In this way, the heart provides its lifelong rhythmic contraction and pumping. Cardiac muscle can also be classified according to its structure, which combines characteristics of both skeletal and smooth muscle and is thus called smooth-striated.

The second muscle type is smooth, or involuntary, muscle, which is not under conscious control but functions at the direction of the autonomic nervous system. These muscles are found in the arterial and venous blood vessels, the bronchioles, the bowel, and many other organs. Smooth muscle contracts to reduce (or relaxes to expand) the lumen (diameter) of the vasculature, airways, or digestive tract. Smooth muscles have the ability to contract over a wide lateral distance, enabling them to accommodate great changes in length, such as those that occur during filling and evacuation of the bladder and contraction and dilation of the arterioles.

The final type of muscle tissue is skeletal (also called striated or voluntary). We have conscious control over these muscles, which are associated with the mobility of the extremities and the body in general. Skeletal muscles are also controlled by the nerves of the somatic nervous system. The skeletal muscles are the largest component of the muscular system, comprising between 40 and 50 percent of the body's total weight. They are the type of muscle most commonly traumatized.

fasciculus *small bundle of muscle fibers.*

origin *attachment of a muscle to a bone that does not move (or experiences the least movement) when the muscle contracts.*

insertion *attachment of a muscle to a bone that moves when the muscle contracts.*

Skeletal muscles lie directly beneath a protective layer of skin and subcutaneous fat. Because of their hunger for oxygen during activity, they have a more than ample supply of blood vessels. Individual muscle cells layer together to form a muscle fiber, many fibers layer together to form a muscle **fasciculus,** and fasciculi layer together to form a muscle body, such as the triceps. A muscle body has a strength of about 50 pounds of lift for each square inch of cross-sectional area.

Skeletal muscles attach to the bones at a minimum of two locations. These attachment points are called the origin and the insertion, depending on how the bones move with contraction. The point of attachment that remains stationary as the muscle contracts is the **origin,** while the attachment to the moving bone is the **insertion.**

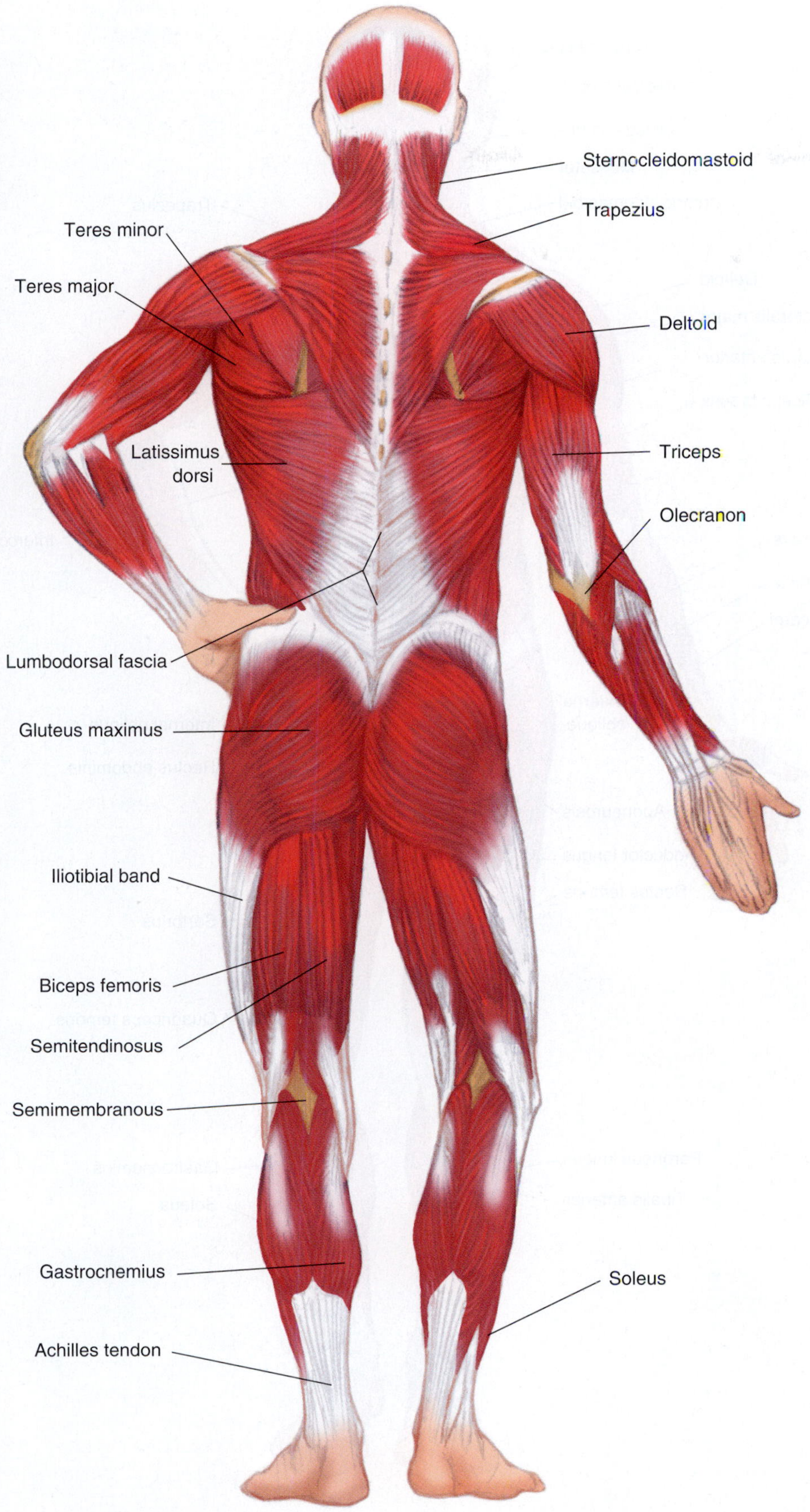

■ **Figure 3-41** (a) The muscular system (posterior view).

Sternocleidomastoid
Trapezius
Teres minor
Teres major
Deltoid
Latissimus dorsi
Triceps
Olecranon
Lumbodorsal fascia
Gluteus maximus
Iliotibial band
Biceps femoris
Semitendinosus
Semimembranous
Gastrocnemius
Soleus
Achilles tendon

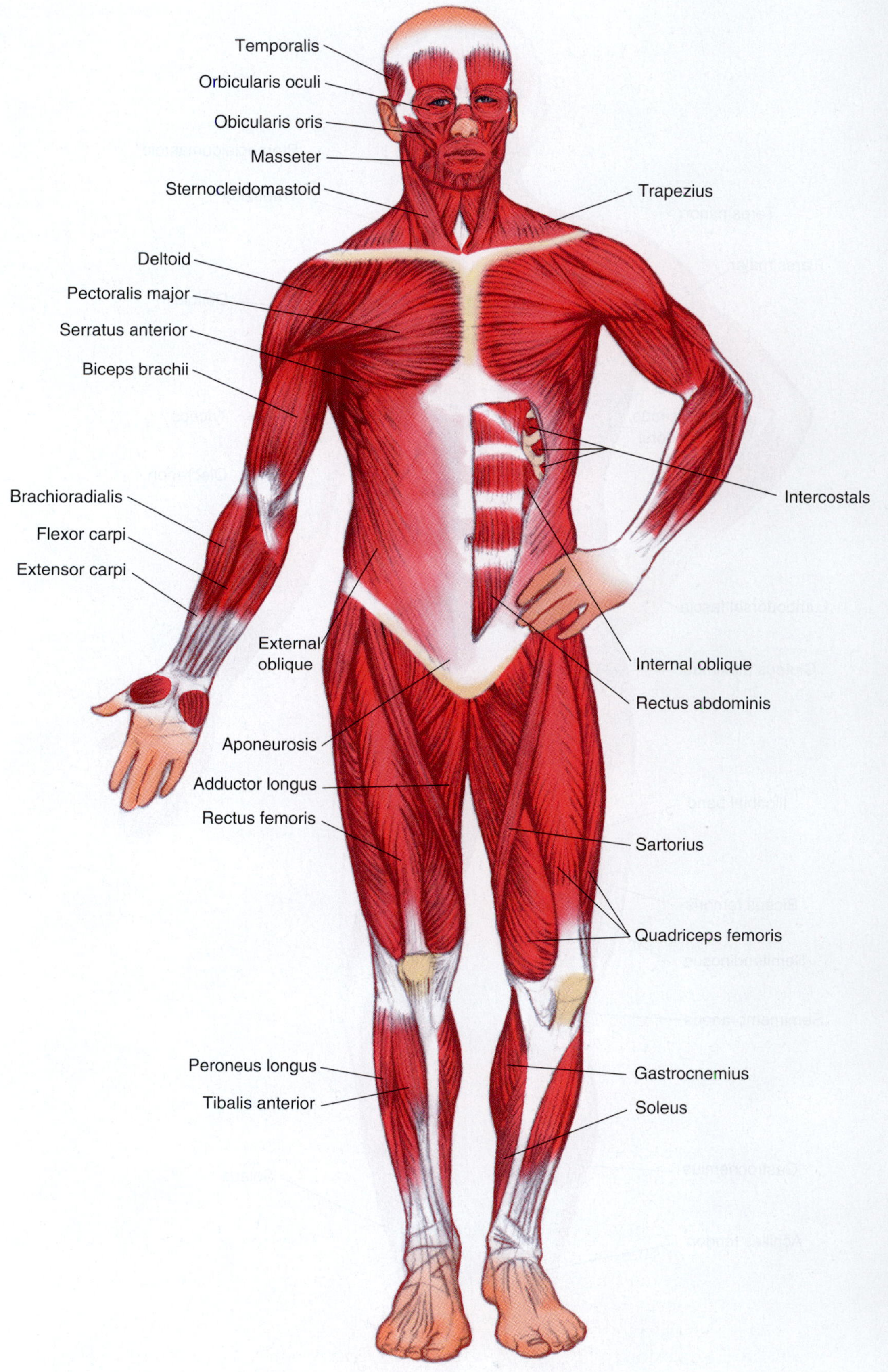

■ **Figure 3-41** ***Continued***
(b) The muscular system (anterior view).

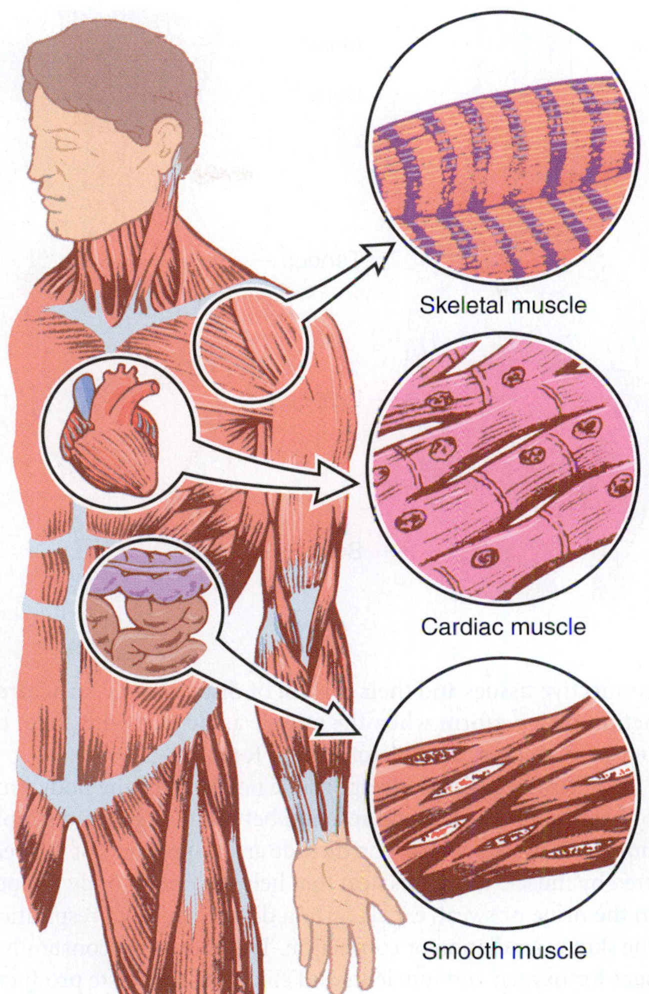

■ **Figure 3-42** Three types of muscle.

Muscles usually pair, one on each side of a joint. This configuration is essential because muscles can actively contract, not lengthen. One muscle moves the extremity in one direction by contraction, while the opposing (and relaxed) muscle stretches. The opposing muscle can then in turn contract, stretching the first muscle and moving the extremity in the opposite direction. This arrangement, called **opposition,** permits the straightening (extension) and then bending (flexion) of the limbs.

opposition *pairing of muscles that permits extension and flexion of limbs.*

With several muscles attached to a joint with different origins and insertions, the body enjoys a wide variety of motions. In the shoulder, for example, the humerus can travel through several types and ranges of motion. These include moving the extremity away from the body (abduction) and toward the body (adduction), turning the humerus (rotation) through about 60 degrees, and circling the entire extremity (circumduction) through a 180-degree arc.

Tendons are specialized bands of connective tissue that accomplish the attachment of muscle to bone at the insertion and, in some cases, at the origin (Figure 3-43 ■). These very fibrous ribbons, actually parts of the muscles, are extremely strong and do not stretch. They are so strong that in some instances they will break an area of bone loose rather than tear. The Achilles tendon demonstrates the strength of this particular tissue. It can be felt as the band posterior to the malleoli of the ankle. This tendon is the muscle-controlled cord that allows a person to lift the entire body weight when standing on the toes.

The forearm demonstrates the sophistication of the muscle-tendon relationship. As the muscles controlling finger flexion contract, you can feel them tensing in the dorsal forearm. You can also visualize and palpate tendon movement in the distal forearm and wrist as the fingers flex and extend. It is easy to appreciate the damage a deep transverse laceration can cause to the underlying

■ Figure 3-43 How muscle attaches to bone.

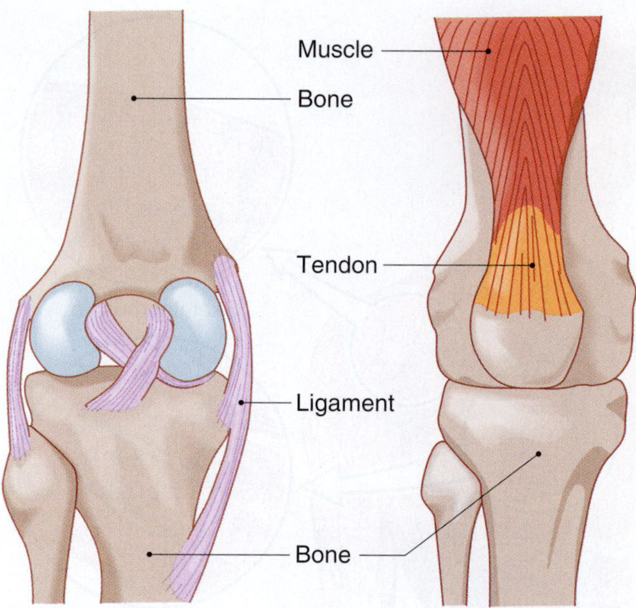

connective tissues and their control of distal skeletal structures. Tendons are often classified by the action they perform when the muscle associated with them contracts—for example, flexor or extensor, abductor or adductor, and so forth.

The muscle tissue is responsible not only for the body's movement but also for the production of heat energy. A chemical reaction between oxygen and simple sugars produces the energy of motion. Heat, water, and carbon dioxide are by-products of this reaction. More than half the energy created by muscle motion is heat that helps maintain body temperature. The body then excretes water in the urine or sweat, expels carbon dioxide through respiration, and dissipates excess heat through the skin via radiation or convection. The body must constantly meet the requirements of muscle tissues for oxygen and nutrients and eliminate the waste products of those tissues, including heat.

tone *state of slight contraction of muscles that gives them firmness and keeps them ready to contract.*

Muscles are found in a condition of slight contraction called **tone.** Even while the body is at rest, the central nervous system sends some limited impulses to the muscle fibers, causing a few to contract. These impulses give the muscles firmness and assure that they are ready to contract when the need arises. Muscle tone may be very significant in a well-conditioned athlete or absent (flaccid muscle tone) in someone with peripheral motor nerve disruption.

THE HEAD, FACE, AND NECK

THE HEAD

The head is made up of three structures that cover the brain: the scalp, the cranium, and the meninges. Each of these structures provides essential protection from the environment and from trauma.

The Scalp

The scalp is a strong and flexible mass of skin, fascia (bands of connective tissue), and muscular tissue that is able to withstand and absorb tremendous kinetic energy. The scalp is also extremely vascular in order to help maintain the brain at the body's core temperature. Scalp hair further insulates the brain from environmental temperatures and, to a lesser degree, from trauma.

galea aponeurotica *connective tissue sheet covering the superior aspect of the cranium.*

The scalp is only loosely attached to the skull and is made up of the overlying skin and a number of thin layers of muscle and connective tissue underneath. Directly beneath the skin and covering the most superior surface of the head is a fibrous connective tissue sheet called the **galea aponeurotica.** Connected anteriorly to it and covering the forehead is a flat sheet of muscle, the frontal muscle. Connected posteriorly and covering the posterior skull surface is the occipitalis muscle. Laterally, the auricularis muscles cover the areas above the ears and between the lateral brow ridge and the occiput. A layer of loose connective tissue beneath these muscles and the galea and just above the periosteum is called the areolar tissue. It contains emissary veins that permit venous blood to flow from the dural sinuses into the venous vessels of the scalp. These emissary veins also exist in the upper reaches of the nasal cavity. These veins become potential routes for infection in scalp wounds or nasal injuries. A helpful way to remember the layers of skin protecting the scalp is the mnemonic SCALP: S—skin; C—connective tissue; A—aponeurotica; L—layer of subaponeurotica (areolar) tissue; P—the periosteum of the skull (the pericranium).

The Cranium

The bony structure supporting the head and face is the skull. It can be subdivided into two components, the vault for the brain, called the **cranium,** and the facial bones that form the skeletal base for the face (Figure 3-44 ■). The cranium actually consists of several bones fused together at pseudojoints called **sutures.** These bony plates are constructed of two narrow layers of hard compact bone, separated by a layer of spongy cancellous bone. The plates form a strong, light, rigid, and spherical container for the brain. The cranium is, therefore, quite effective in protecting its contents from the direct effects of trauma. This cranial vault, however, provides very little space for internal swelling or hemorrhage. Any expanding lesion within the cranium results in an increase in **intracranial pressure (ICP).** This reduces cerebral perfusion and can severely damage the delicate brain tissue.

cranium *vaultlike portion of the skull encasing the brain.*

sutures *pseudojoints that join the various bones of the skull to form the cranium.*

intracranial pressure (ICP) *pressure exerted on the brain by the blood and cerebrospinal fluid.*

The cranial bones form regions that are helpful in describing the cerebral structures beneath. The anterior or frontal bone begins at the brow ridge and covers the upper and anterior surface of the

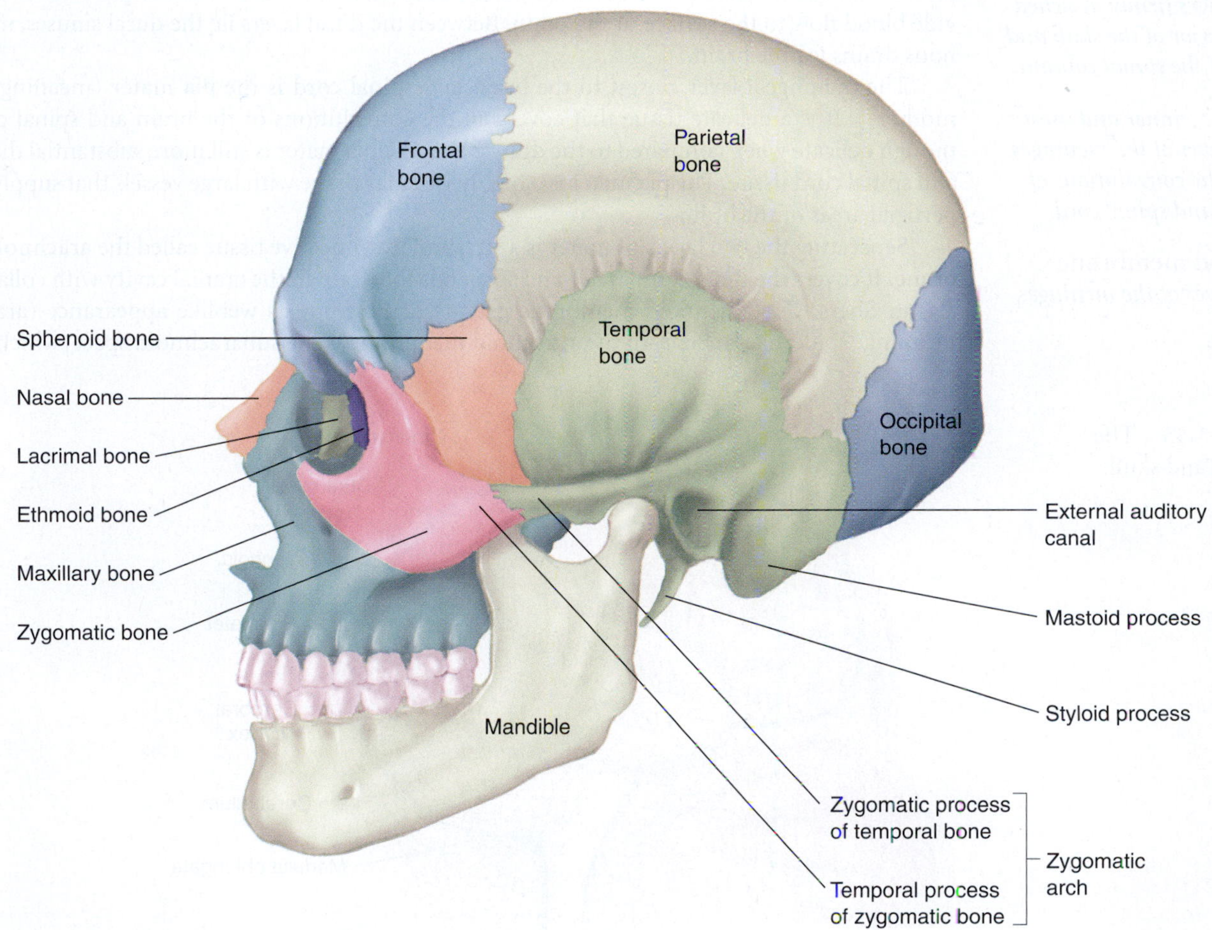

■ **Figure 3-44** Bones of the human skull.

brain. The parietal bones, one on either side, begin just behind the lateral brow ridge and form the skull above the external portions (pinnae) of the ears. The occipital bone forms the posterior and inferior aspect of the cranium, extending to and forming the foramen magnum. The temporal bones form the lateral cranial surfaces anterior to the ears, while the ethmoid and sphenoid bones, which are very irregular in shape, form the portion of the cranium concealed and protected by the facial bones.

The base of the skull consists of portions of the occipital, temporal, sphenoid, and ethmoid bones. This area is important in cases of trauma because the openings, or foramina, for blood vessels, the spinal cord, the auditory canal, and the cranial nerves pass through it. These openings weaken the area, leaving it prone to fracture with serious trauma.

Other anatomical points of interest within the cranium are the cribriform plate and the foramen magnum. The cribriform plate is an irregular portion of the ethmoid bone and a portion of the base of the cranium. It and the remainder of the base of the cranium have rough surfaces against which the brain may abrade, lacerate, or contuse during severe deceleration. The foramen magnum is the largest opening in the skull. It is located at the base of the skull where it meets the spinal column and is where the spinal cord exits the cranium.

The Meninges

meninges *three membranes that surround and protect the brain and spinal cord. They are the dura mater, pia mater, and arachnoid membrane.*

dura mater *tough layer of the meninges firmly attached to the interior of the skull and interior of the spinal column.*

pia mater *inner and most delicate layer of the meninges. It covers the convolutions of the brain and spinal cord.*

arachnoid membrane *middle layer of the meninges.*

The final protective mechanisms for the brain and the spinal cord are the **meninges** (Figure 3-45 ■). They are three layers of tissue that lie between the cranium and the brain and also between the spinal column and the spinal cord. The outermost layer is the **dura mater** (meaning, literally, "tough mother"), which consists of a tough connective tissue. The dura mater is actually two layers. The outer layer is the cranium's inner periosteum. The dural layer is made up of tough, continuous connective tissue that extends into the cranial cavity where it forms partial structural divisions (the falx cerebri and the tentorium cerebelli). Above the dura mater lie some of the larger arteries that provide blood flow to the surface of the brain. Between the dural layers lie the dural sinuses, major venous drains for the brain.

The meningeal layer closest to the brain and spinal cord is the **pia mater** (meaning "tender mother"). It is a delicate tissue that covers all the convolutions of the brain and spinal cord. Although delicate when compared to the dura mater, the pia mater is still more substantial than brain and spinal cord tissue. The pia mater is a highly vascular tissue with large vessels that supply the superficial areas of the brain.

Separating the two layers of mater is a stratum of connective tissue called the **arachnoid membrane.** It covers the inner dura mater and suspends the brain in the cranial cavity with collagen and elastin fibers. The arachnoid membrane gets its name from its weblike appearance (arachnoid, meaning "spiderlike"). Beneath the arachnoid membrane is the subarachnoid space, which is filled

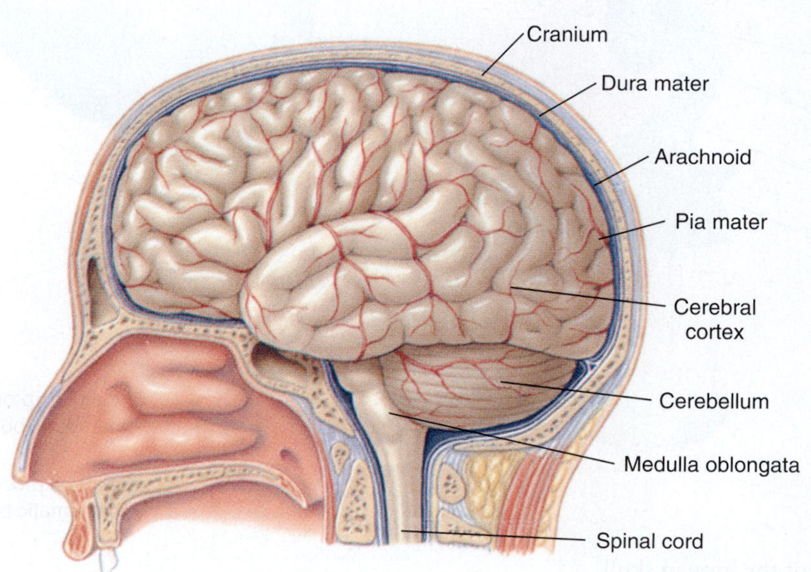

■ Figure 3-45 The meninges and skull.

with cerebrospinal fluid. This region provides cushioning for the brain when the head is subjected to strong forces of acceleration or deceleration.

Cerebrospinal Fluid

Cerebrospinal fluid is a clear, colorless solution of water, proteins, and salts that surrounds the central nervous system and absorbs the shock of minor acceleration and deceleration. The brain constantly generates cerebrospinal fluid in the largest two of four spaces (or ventricles) within the substance of the brain. The fluid circulates through the ventricles, then through the subarachnoid space, where it is returned to the venous circulation through the dural sinuses. The cerebrospinal fluid provides buoyancy for the brain and actually floats it in a near-weightless environment within the cranial cavity. This fluid also is a medium through which nutrients and waste products such as oxygen, proteins, salts, and carbon dioxide are diffused into and out of the brain tissue.

cerebrospinal fluid *fluid surrounding and bathing the brain and spinal cord (the elements of the central nervous system).*

The Brain

The brain occupies about 80 percent of the interior of the cranium. It is made up of three major structures essential to human function—the cerebrum, the cerebellum, and the brainstem.

The **cerebrum** is the largest element of the nervous system and occupies most of the cranial cavity. It consists of an exterior cortex of gray matter (cell bodies) and is the highest functional portion of the brain. The central portion of the cerebrum is predominantly white matter, mostly communication pathways (axons). The cerebrum is the center of conscious thought, personality, speech, motor control, and of visual, auditory, and tactile (touch) perception. The cerebrum is regionalized into lobes roughly lying beneath the bones of the cranium (and given the same names). The frontal region is anterior and determines personality. The parietal region, which is superior and posterior, directs motor and sensory activities as well as memory and emotions. The occipital region, which is posterior and inferior, is responsible for sight. Laterally, the temporal regions are the centers for long-term memory, hearing, speech, taste, and smell.

cerebrum *largest part of the brain. It consists of two hemispheres separated by a deep longitudinal fissure. It is the seat of consciousness and the center of the higher mental functions such as memory, learning, reasoning, judgment, intelligence, and emotions.*

A structure called the falx cerebri divides the cerebrum into right and left hemispheres. A dural partition, the falx cerebri extends into the cranial cavity from the interior and superior surface of the cranium (Figure 3-46 ■). Corresponding to the falx cerebri is a fissure in the cerebrum called the central sulcus. This fissure physically splits the cerebrum into the left and right hemispheres, each of which controls (for the most part) the activities of the opposite side of the body. The crossing of nerve impulses from one side to the other takes place just below the medulla oblongata. The

The crossing of nerve impulses from one side of the body to the other takes place just below the medulla oblongata.

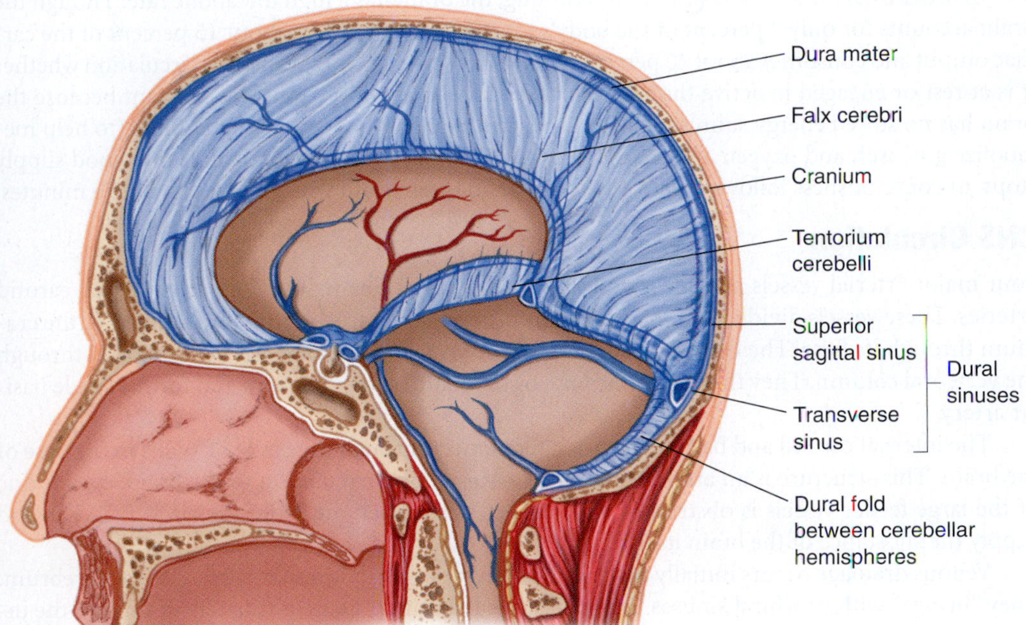

■ **Figure 3-46** The partitions extending into the skull, the falx cerebri and tentorium cerebellum.

tentorium cerebelli is a similar fibrous sheet within the occipital region, running at right angles to the falx cerebri. It separates the cerebrum from the cerebellum. The brainstem perforates the tentorium through an opening called the tentorium incisura.

The oculomotor nerve (CN-III), which controls pupil size, travels along the tentorium. It is likely to be compressed as intracranial pressure rises or the brain is displaced due to edema, a growing mass, or hemorrhage. This compression causes pupillary disturbances that manifest most commonly on the same side as the problem. If the pressure is great enough, it may affect both sides and both pupils may dilate and fix.

cerebellum *portion of the brain located dorsally to the pons and medulla oblongata. It plays an important role in the fine control of voluntary muscular movements.*

brainstem *the part of the brain connecting the cerebral hemispheres with the spinal cord. It is comprised of the medulla oblongata, the pons, and the midbrain.*

midbrain *portion of the brain connecting the pons and cerebellum with the cerebral hemispheres.*

hypothalamus *portion of the brain important for controlling certain metabolic activities, including the regulation of body temperature.*

thalamus *switching station between the pons and the cerebrum in the brain.*

reticular activating system (RAS) *a series of nervous tissues keeping the human system in a state of consciousness.*

pons *process of tissue responsible for the communication interchange between the cerebellum, the cerebrum, midbrain, and the spinal cord.*

medulla oblongata *lower portion of the brainstem containing the respiratory, cardiac, and vasomotor centers.*

Though the brain accounts for only 2 percent of the body's total weight, it consumes about 20 percent of the body's oxygen.

The left cerebral hemisphere is identified as the dominant hemisphere in most of the population, excepting a few left-handed individuals. It is responsible for mathematical computations (occipital region) and writing (parietal region) and is the center for language interpretation (occipital region) and speech (frontal region). The right, nondominant cerebral hemisphere processes nonverbal imagery (occipital region).

The **cerebellum** is located directly under the tentorium. It lies posterior and inferior to the cerebrum. The cerebellum "fine tunes" motor control and allows the body to move smoothly from one position to another. Additionally, it is responsible for balance and maintenance of muscle tone.

The **brainstem** is an important central processing center and the communication junction among the cerebrum, spinal cord, cranial nerves, and cerebellum. It includes the midbrain, the pons, and the medulla oblongata. The **midbrain** makes up the upper portion of the brainstem and consists of the hypothalamus, thalamus, and associated structures. The **hypothalamus** controls much of the endocrine function, the vomiting reflex, hunger, thirst, kidney function, body temperature, and emotions. The **thalamus** is the switching center between the pons and the cerebrum and is a critical element in the **reticular activating system (RAS),** the system that establishes consciousness. This region also provides the major tracts, or pathways, for the optic and olfactory nerves.

The **pons** acts as the communication interchange between the various components of the central nervous system—the cerebellum, the cerebrum, the midbrain, and the spinal cord. It is a bulb-shaped structure directly above the medulla oblongata and appears to be responsible for the sleep component of the reticular activating system.

The last nervous system structure still within the cranial vault is the **medulla oblongata.** It is recognizable as a bulge in the very top of the spinal cord. The medulla contains three important centers—the respiratory center, the cardiac center, and the vasomotor center. The cardiac center regulates the rate and strength of cardiac contractions. The vasomotor center controls the distribution of blood and maintains blood pressure. The respiratory center controls respiratory depth, rate, and rhythm.

In order to maintain its advanced functioning, the brain has a high metabolic rate. Though the brain accounts for only 2 percent of the body's total weight, it receives about 15 percent of the cardiac output and consumes about 20 percent of the body's oxygen. It requires this circulation whether it is at rest or engaged in active thought. Further, this blood supply must be constant because the brain has no stored energy sources. It needs constant availability of glucose, thiamine (to help metabolize glucose), and oxygen and relies almost solely on aerobic metabolism. If the blood supply stops, unconsciousness follows within 10 seconds, and brain death will ensue within 4 to 6 minutes.

CNS Circulation

Four major arterial vessels provide blood flow to the brain. The first two are the internal carotid arteries. These vessels divide from the common carotid at the carotid sinus and then enter the cranium through its base. The two posterior vessels, the vertebral arteries, ascend along and through the vertebral column. They then enter the base of the skull, where they join and form a single basilar artery.

The internal carotid and basilar arteries interconnect through the circle of Willis in the base of the brain. This structure is an arterial circle that assures good circulation to the brain, even if one of the large feeder vessels is obstructed. Various arteries branch out from the circle of Willis and supply the substance of the brain itself.

Venous drainage occurs initially through bridging veins that drain the surface of the cerebrum. They "bridge" with the dural sinuses (large, thin-walled veins). These ultimately drain into the internal jugular veins and then into the superior vena cava.

Blood–Brain Barrier

The capillaries of the brain are special in that their walls are thicker and not as permeable as those found elsewhere in the body. They do not permit the interstitial flow of proteins and other materials as freely as do other body capillaries. This assures that many substances found in the circulatory system, such as some hormones, do not affect the central nervous system cells. Lymphatic circulation is also lacking in the brain and is replaced by the cerebrospinal fluid flow system. This results in a very special and protected environment for central nervous system cells. If frank blood seeps into the central nervous system tissue, it acts as an irritant, initiating an inflammatory response, resulting in edema.

Cerebral Perfusion Pressure

Cerebral perfusion is exceptionally critical and depends on many factors. Primarily, the pressure within the cranium (intracranial pressure or ICP) resists blood flow and limits perfusion to the central nervous system tissue. Usually the pressure is less than 10 mmHg and does not significantly impede blood flow as long as the mean arterial blood pressure (MAP is the diastolic blood pressure plus one third the pulse pressure) is at least 50 mmHg. The pressure moving blood through the cranium is the **cerebral perfusion pressure (CPP).** This is calculated as the mean arterial pressure (MAP) minus the intracranial pressure (ICP). Changes in ICP are met with compensatory changes in blood pressure to assure adequate cerebral perfusion pressure and cerebral blood flow. This compensating reflex is called **autoregulation.**

cerebral perfusion pressure (CPP) *the pressure moving blood through the brain.*

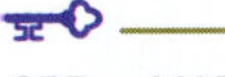

CPP = MAP − ICP

autoregulation *process that controls blood flow to the brain tissue by causing alterations in the blood pressure.*

Since the cranium is a fixed vault for the structures of the brain, its volume and the pressure within are shared by the occupants. Any expanding mass (tumor), hemorrhage, or edema within the cranium will displace some other occupant, particularly the cerebrospinal fluid or blood, since they are the only readily movable media. This displacement maintains the intracranial pressure very effectively, up to a point. When the volumes of cerebrospinal fluid and venous blood are reduced to their limits, however, the intracranial pressure begins to rise. Autoregulation then raises the blood pressure to assure there is enough differential (CPP) to provide good cerebral perfusion. However, this increase in blood pressure causes the intracranial pressure to rise still higher and cerebral blood perfusion to diminish even more. As this cycle of increasing intracranial pressure and increasing blood pressure continues, brain injury and death are close at hand.

Cranial Nerves

The cranial nerves are nerve roots originating within the cranium and along the brainstem. They comprise 12 distinct pathways that account for some of the more important senses, innervate the facial area, and control significant body functions (see Figure 3-72 in the Nervous System section later in this chapter).

Ascending Reticular Activating System

The ascending reticular activating system is a tract of neurons within the upper brainstem, the pons, and the midbrain that is responsible for the sleep-wake cycle. It is a complex control system that monitors the amount of stimulation the body receives and regulates important bodily functions such as respiration, heart rate, and peripheral vascular resistance. Injury to the midbrain may result in unconsciousness or coma, while injury to the pons may result in a protracted waking state.

THE FACE

Facial bones make up the anterior and inferior structures of the head and include the zygoma, maxilla, mandible, and nasal bones (Figure 3-47 ■). The **zygoma** is the prominent bone of the cheek. It protects the eyes and the muscles controlling eye and jaw movement. The **maxilla** comprises the upper jaw, supports the nasal bone, and provides the lower border of the orbit. The nasal bone is the attachment for the nasal cartilage as it forms the shape of the nose. The last of the facial bones is the **mandible,** or jawbone. It resembles two horizontal "L's," which join anteriorly and hinge underneath the posterior zygomatic arch. Besides forming the beginning of the airway and the alimentary canal, the facial bones form supporting and protective structures for several sense organs, including the tongue (taste), eye (sight), and olfactory nerve (smell).

zygoma *the cheekbone.*

maxilla *bone of the upper jaw.*

mandible *the jawbone.*

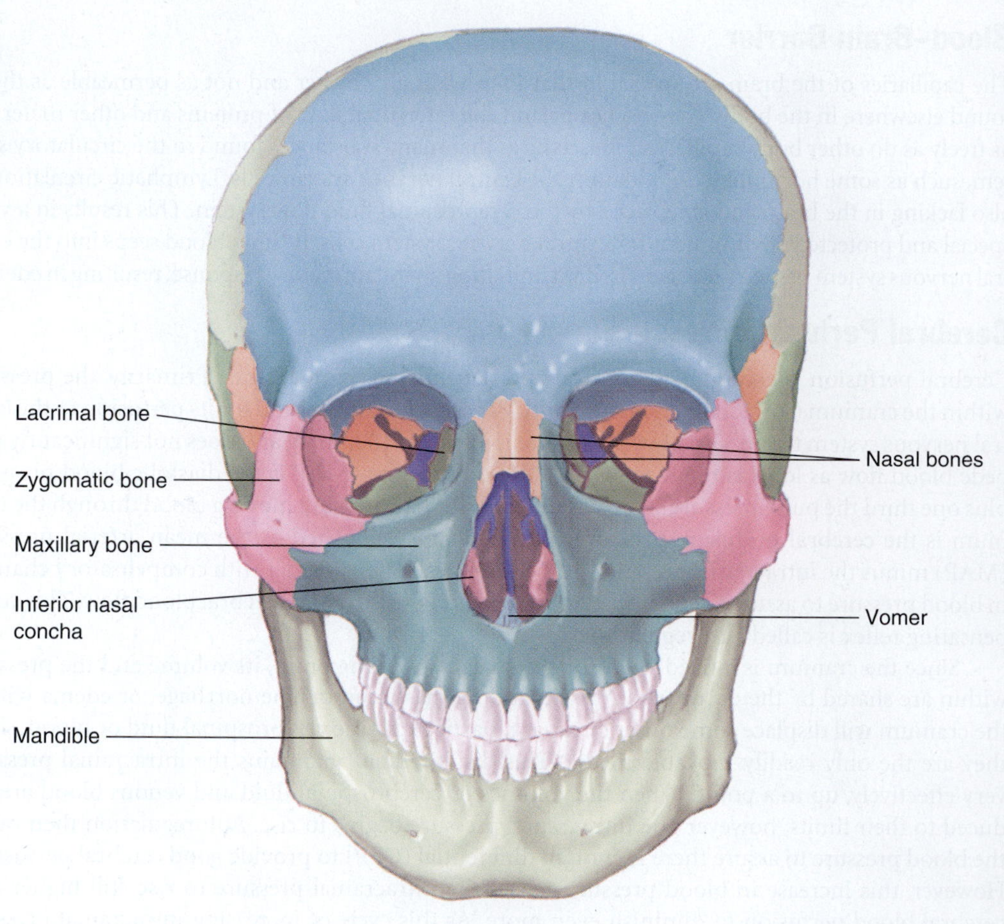

■ **Figure 3-47** The facial bones.

The facial region, like most other areas of the body, is covered with skin that serves to protect the tissue underneath from trauma and against adverse environmental effects. In the facial region, the skin is very flexible and relatively thin. It also has a very good vascular supply and hemorrhages freely when injured. Beneath the skin is a minimal layer of subcutaneous tissue and, beneath that, there are many small muscles that control facial expression and the movements of the mouth, eyes, and eyelids.

Circulation for the facial area is provided by the external carotid artery as it branches into the facial, temporal, and maxillary arteries. The facial artery crosses the mandible, then travels up and along the nasal bone. The maxillary artery runs under the mandible and zygoma, then provides circulation to the cheek area. The temporal artery runs anterior to the ear just posterior to the zygoma. Each major artery has an associated vein paralleling its path.

The most important cranial nerves traversing this area are the trigeminal (CN-V) and the facial (CN-VII). The trigeminal nerve provides sensation for the face and some motor control over eye movement as well as enabling the chewing process. The facial nerve provides motor control to the facial muscles and contributes to the sensation of taste.

The nasal cavity is formed by the juncture of the ethmoid, nasal, and maxillary bones. It is a channel running posteriorly with a bony septum dividing it into left and right chambers and plates protruding medially from the lateral sides. These plates, called turbinates, form support for the vascular mucous membranes that serve to warm, humidify, and collect particulate matter from the incoming air. The lower border of the nasal cavity is formed by the bony hard palate and then, posteriorly, by the more flexible cartilaginous soft palate. The soft palate moves upward to close off the opening of the posterior nasal cavity during swallowing. The nasal bone lies anterior and inferior to the eyes and provides a base for the nasal cartilage. The nasal cartilage defines the shape of the nose and divides the nostrils and their openings, which are called the **nares**.

nares *the openings of the nostrils.*

The oral cavity is formed by the concave shape of the maxillary bone, the palate, and the upper teeth meeting the mandible and the lower teeth. The floor of the chamber consists of musculature and connective tissue that span the mandible and support the tongue. The tongue is a large muscle that occupies much of the oral cavity, provides the taste sensation, moves food between the teeth during chewing (mastication), and propels the chewed food posteriorly, then inferiorly during swallowing. The tongue connects with the hyoid bone, a free-floating U-shaped bone located inferiorly and posteriorly to the mandible. The mandible articulates with the temporal bone at the temporomandibular joint, under the posterior zygoma, and is moved by the masseter muscles. The lip muscles (obicularis oris) are responsible for sealing the mouth during chewing and swallowing.

Special structures are found in and around the oral cavity. Salivary glands provide saliva, the first of the digestive juices. These glands are located just anterior and inferior to the ear, under the tongue, and just inside the inferior mandible. Specialized lymphoid nodules, the tonsils, are located in the posterior wall of the pharynx.

Prominent cranial nerves serving the oral area include the hypoglossal, the glossopharyngeal, the trigeminal, and the facial nerves. The hypoglossal nerve (CN-XII) directs swallowing and tongue movement. The glossopharyngeal nerve (CN-IX) controls saliva production and taste. The trigeminal nerve (CN-V) carries sensations from the facial region and assists in chewing control. The facial nerve (CN-VII) controls the muscles of facial expression and taste.

Posterior and inferior to the oral cavity is a collection of soft tissue called the pharynx. The process of swallowing begins in the pharynx once the bolus of food has been propelled back and down by the tongue. The epiglottis moves downward while the larynx moves up, sealing the lower airway opening. The food or liquid moves into the esophagus where a peristaltic wave begins its trip to the stomach. This area is of great importance because it maintains the critical segregation of materials between the digestive tract and the airway.

Sinuses are hollow spaces within the bones of the cranium and face that lighten the head, protect the eyes and nasal cavity, and help produce the resonant tones of the voice. They also strengthen this region against the forces of trauma.

The Ear

The outer, visible portion of the ear is termed the **pinna.** It is composed of cartilage and has a poor blood supply. It connects to the external auditory canal, which leads to the eardrum. The external auditory canal contains glands that secrete wax (cerumen) for protection. The ear's important structures are interior and exceptionally well protected from nearly all trauma (Figure 3-48 ■). Only trauma involving great pressure differentials (e.g., blast and diving injuries) or basilar skull fractures are likely to damage this area.

pinna *outer, visible portion of the ear.*

The ear provides the body with two very useful functions, hearing and positional sense. The middle and inner ear contain the structures needed for hearing. Hearing occurs when sound waves cause the tympanic membrane (eardrum) to vibrate. The eardrum transmits the vibrations through three very small bones (the ossicles) to the cochlea, the organ of hearing. These vibrations stimulate the auditory nerve, which in turn transmits the signal to the brain.

The **semicircular canals** are responsible for sensing position and motion. They are three hollow, fluid-filled rings set at different angles. When the head moves, fluid in these rings shifts. Small cells with hairlike projections sense the motion and signal the brain to help maintain balance. This positional sense is present even when the eyes are closed. If injury or illness disturbs this area, it transmits excess signals to the brain. Patients then experience a continuous moving sensation known as vertigo.

semicircular canals *the three rings of the inner ear. They sense the motion of the head and provide positional sense for the body.*

The Eye

The eyes provide much of the input we use to interact with our environment. Although they are placed prominently on the face, the eyes are well protected from trauma by a series of facial bones. The frontal bones project above the globe of the eye, while the nasal bones and cartilage protect medially. The bone of the cheek, or zygoma, completes the physical protection both laterally and inferiorly. These bones collectively form the eye socket or **orbit.** The soft tissue of the eyelid and the eyelashes give additional protection to the critical ocular surface.

orbit *the eye socket.*

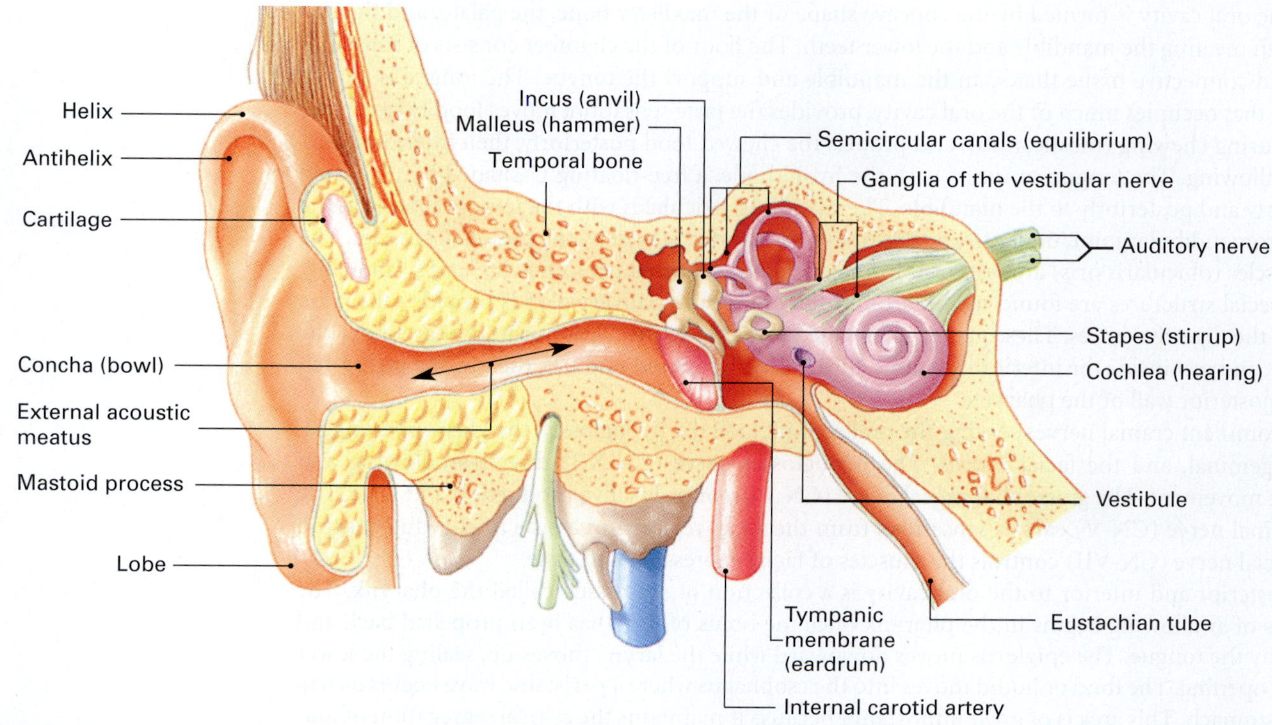

Figure 3-48 The anatomy of the ear.

vitreous humor *clear watery fluid filling the posterior chamber of the eye. It is responsible for giving the eye its spherical shape.*

retina *light- and color-sensing tissue lining the posterior chamber of the eye.*

aqueous humor *clear fluid filling the anterior chamber of the eye.*

iris *pigmented portion of the eye. It is the muscular area that constricts or dilates to change the size of the pupil.*

pupil *dark opening in the center of the iris through which light enters the eye.*

sclera *the "white" of the eye.*

cornea *thin, delicate layer covering the pupil and the iris.*

conjunctiva *mucous membrane that lines the eyelids.*

lacrimal fluid *liquid that lubricates the eye.*

The eye is a spherical globe, filled with liquid (Figure 3-49 ■). Its major compartment (the posterior chamber) contains a crystal-clear gelatinous fluid called **vitreous humor.** Lining the posterior of the compartment is a light- and color-sensing tissue known as the **retina.** Images focused on the retina are transmitted to the brain via the optic nerve. The lens separates the posterior and anterior chambers. The lens is responsible for focusing light and images on the retina by the action of small muscles that change its thickness. A fluid called **aqueous humor,** which is similar to vitreous humor, fills the anterior chamber. The anterior chamber also contains the **iris,** the muscular and colored portion of the eye that regulates the amount of light reaching the retina. Light enters the eye through the dark opening in the center of the iris called the **pupil.**

By examining the eye, you can easily identify several of its components such as the colored iris and the central black pupil. Bordering the iris is the **sclera,** the white and vascular area that forms the remaining, underlying surface of the exposed eye. The **cornea,** a very thin, clear, and delicate layer, covers both the pupil and iris. Contiguous with the cornea and extending out to the eyelid's interior surface is the **conjunctiva,** another delicate, smooth layer that slides over itself and the cornea when the eye closes or blinks.

The eye is bathed in **lacrimal fluid,** which is produced by almond-shaped lacrimal glands located along the brow ridge just lateral and superior to the eyeball. Lacrimal fluid flows through lacrimal ducts and then over the cornea. Because the cornea does not have blood vessels, the fluid provides crucial lubrication, oxygen, and nutrients. If injury or some other mechanism—for example, a contact lens left in an unconscious patient's eye—prevents this fluid from reaching the cornea, the surface of the eye may be damaged. The lacrimal fluid is drained from the eye into the lacrimal sac, located along the medial orbit, and empties then into the nose.

The last major functional elements of the eye are the muscles that move them and their controlling cranial nerves. These small muscles are attached to the eyeball in the region of the conjunctival fold and are hidden within the eye socket and under the zygomatic arch. The oculomotor (CN-III), trochlear (CN-IV), and abducens (CN-VI) nerves control these muscles, which in turn control the eye's motion. The oculomotor nerve controls pupil dilation, conjugate movement (movement of the eyes together), and most of the eye's travel through its normal range of motion. The trochlear nerve moves the eye downward and inward, while the abducens nerve is responsible for eye abduction (outward gaze).

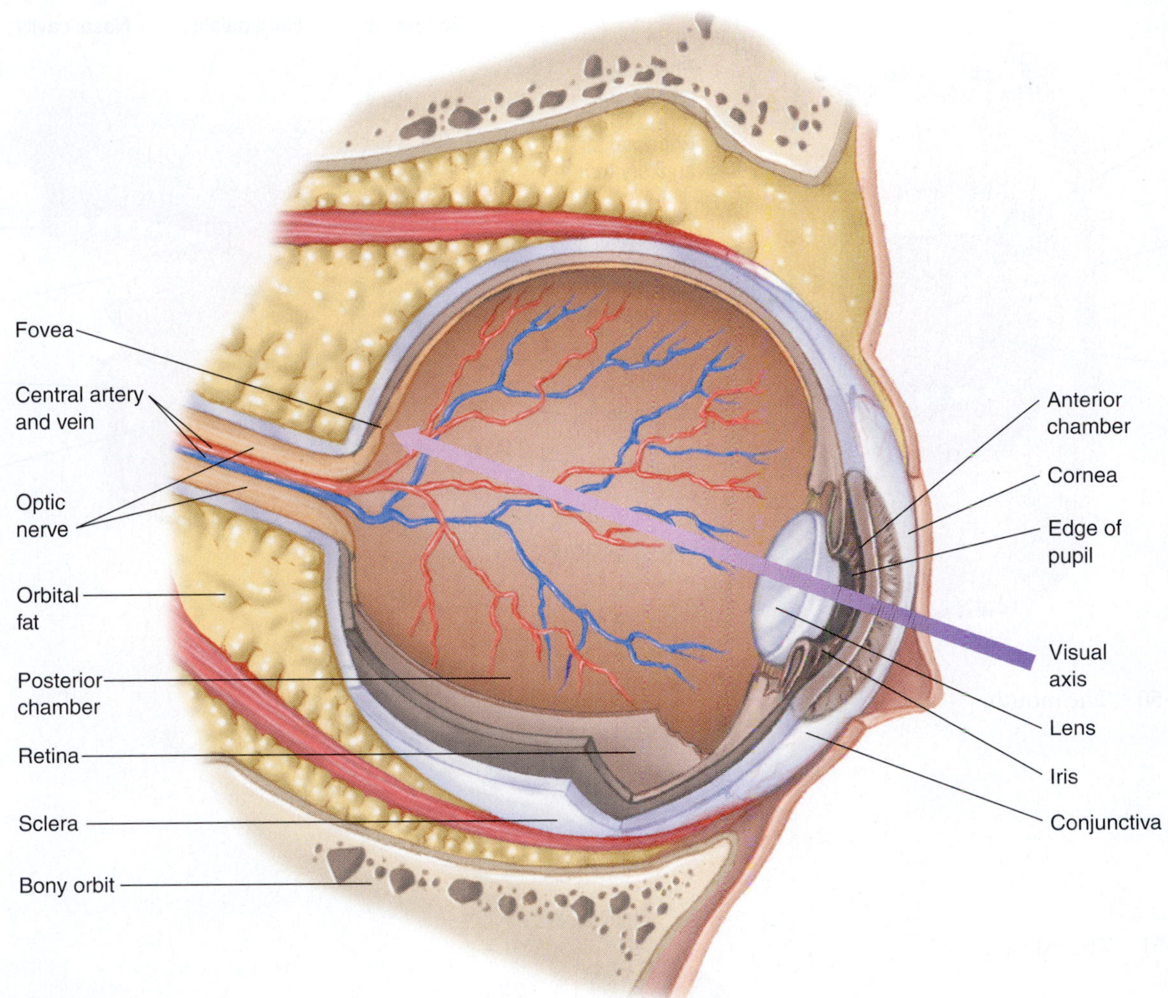

■ **Figure 3-49** The anatomy of the eye.

The Mouth

The lips mark the entrance to the mouth and play a role in the articulation of speech. The mouth houses the tongue, the gums (gingiva), and the teeth (Figure 3-50 ■). The roof of the mouth is formed by the hard palate and the soft palate. The uvula is the peninsular extension of the soft palate that hangs in the back of the mouth. The oral cavity, lined with buccal (cheek/mouth) mucosa, is rich in mucous membranes. The parotid glands, just in front of the ears, and the submandibular glands, just beneath the mandible, secrete digestive enzymes and saliva into the oral cavity (Figure 3-51 ■). The sublingual glands secrete enzymes just beneath the tongue. You can easily palpate these glands under the chin.

The tongue, a large, mobile muscle covered by mucous membranes, has many functions. It helps in chewing by keeping food on the teeth, and it assists in swallowing by moving the food into the oropharynx. It also contains the taste buds and is essential in forming words when we speak.

A highly vascular mucosa lines the gingiva, giving it a pink color. The teeth are anchored in bony sockets; only their white enamel-covered crowns are visible. An adult normally has 32 permanent teeth, including incisors, canines, premolars, and molars. The pharynx consists of three distinct areas: the nasopharynx (behind the nasal cavity), the oropharynx (back of the throat), and the laryngopharynx (just above the epiglottis). At the back of the throat on either side, the tonsils help separate the oropharynx (food processing) from the nasopharynx (air passage).

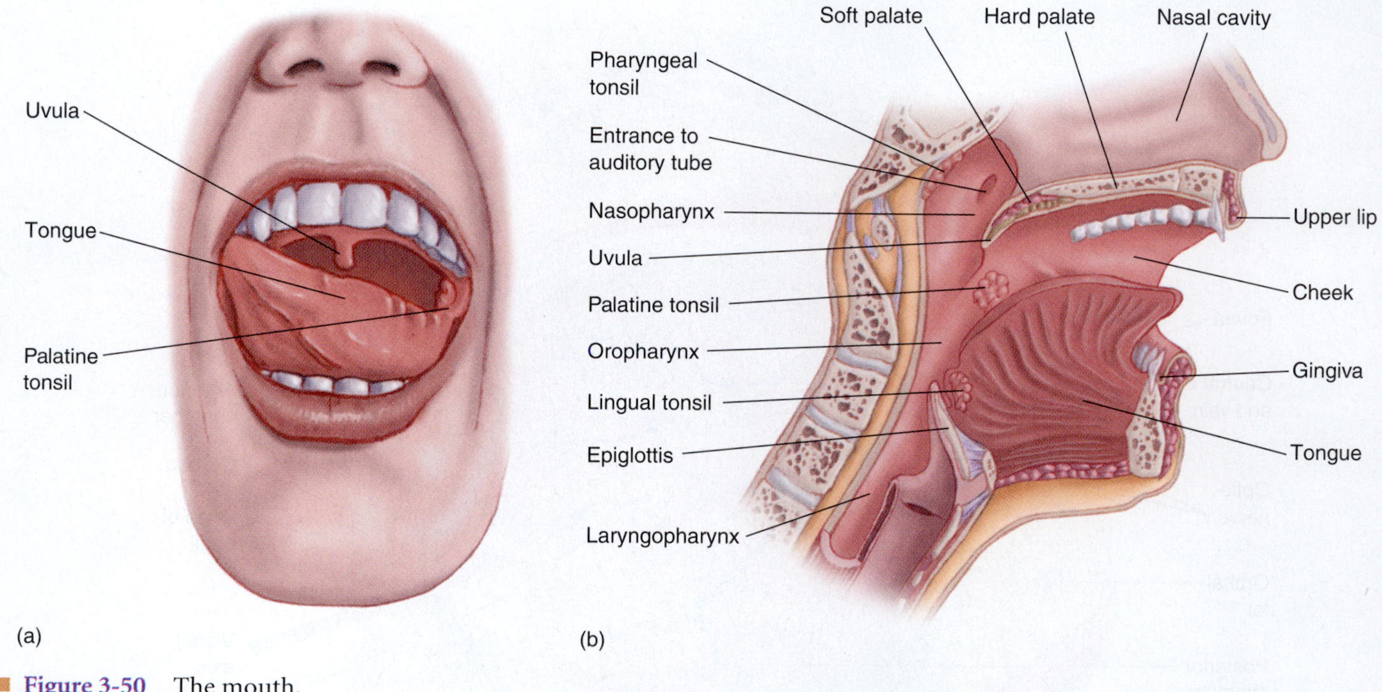

Figure 3-50 The mouth.

Figure 3-51 The salivary glands.

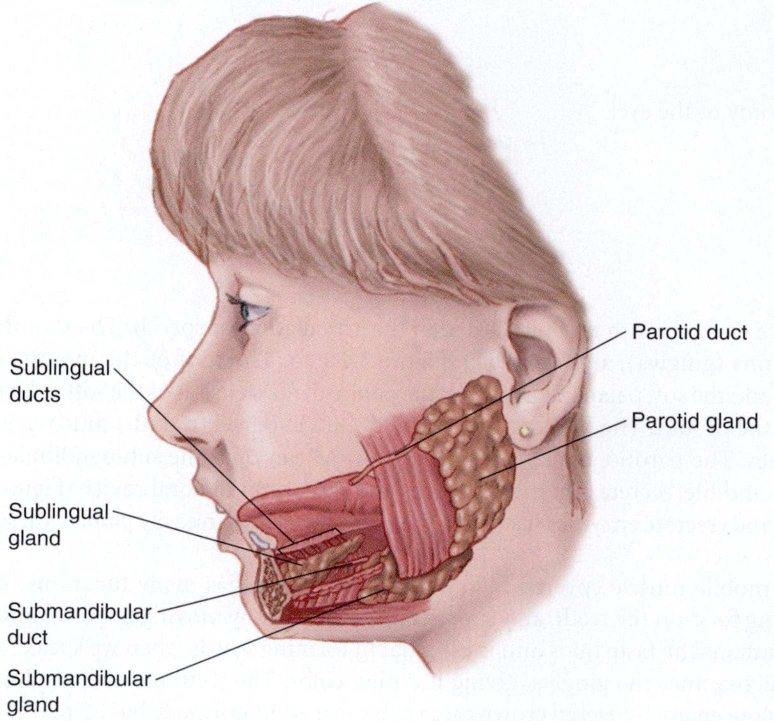

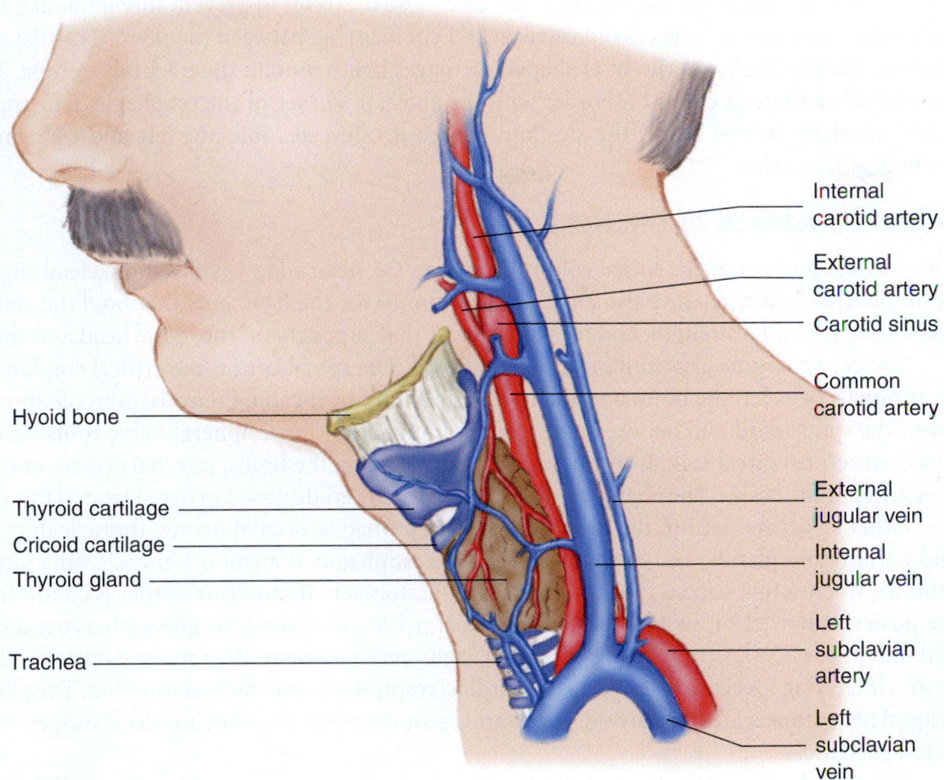

■ **Figure 3-52** The neck.

THE NECK

The neck (Figure 3-52 ■) is the region that links the head to the rest of the body. Traveling through this anatomical area are blood for the facial region and brain, air for respiration, food for digestion, and neural communications to sense the body and its environment and to control both the voluntary and involuntary muscles and glands of the body. The neck also contains some of the important muscles used to provide head and shoulder movement as well as the thyroid and parathyroid glands of the endocrine system.

Vasculature of the Neck

The major blood vessels traversing the neck are the carotid arteries and the jugular veins. The carotid arteries arise from the brachiocephalic artery on the right and the aorta on the left. They travel upward and medially along the trachea and split into internal and external carotid arteries at about the level of the larynx's upper border. At this split are the carotid bodies and carotid sinuses, which are responsible for monitoring carbon dioxide and oxygen levels in the blood and the blood pressure, respectively. The jugular veins are paired on each side of the neck. The internal jugular vein runs in a sheath with the carotid artery and vagus nerve, while the external jugular vein runs superficially just lateral to the trachea. The jugular veins join the brachiocephalic veins just beneath the clavicles.

Airway Structures

The airway structures of the neck begin with the larynx. It is a prominent hollow cylindrical column made up of the thyroid and cricoid cartilages, atop the trachea. The thyroid opening is covered during swallowing by a cartilaginous and soft-tissue flap, the epiglottis. The vocal cords, two folds of connective tissue sitting atop the opening of the larynx, further protect the airway. These cords vibrate with air passage and form sounds; they may also close in spasm to prevent foreign bodies from entering the lower airway. The cricoid cartilage is a circular ring between the thyroid cartilage and the trachea. The trachea is a series of C-shaped cartilages that maintain the tracheal opening. The posterior trachea shares a common border with the anterior surface of the esophagus. The trachea extends inferiorly to just below the sternum, where it bifurcates into the left and right mainstem bronchi at the carina.

Other Structures of the Neck

The cervical portion of the spinal column traverses the neck and provides the skeletal support for both the head and neck. It is also an attachment point for the ligaments that hold the column together and give it its strength, and for the tendons that support and move the head and shoulders.

The cervical spine also contains the spinal cord. The spinal cord is the critical conduit for nervous signals between the brain and the body, and injury to it can be serious, even life threatening. From the spinal cord and between each vertebral junction, the peripheral nerve roots branch out. These structures direct signals to, and receive signals from, the limbs, internal organs, and sensory structures of the body. (The anatomy of the cervical spine is addressed in detail later in this chapter.)

Other structures within the neck include the esophagus, cranial nerves, thoracic duct, thyroid and parathyroid glands, and brachial plexus. The esophagus is a smooth muscle tube located behind the trachea that carries food and liquid to the stomach. Its anterior border is continuous with the posterior border of the trachea. Some cranial nerves, including the glossopharyngeal (CN-IX) and the vagus (CN-X), traverse the neck. The vagus nerve is essential for many parasympathetic activities including speech, swallowing, and cardiac, respiratory, and visceral function. The glossopharyngeal nerve innervates the carotid bodies and carotid sinuses, monitoring blood oxygen levels and blood pressure.

lymphatic system *a network of vessels that drains fluid, called lymph, from the body tissues. Lymph nodes help filter impurities en route to the subclavian vein and then to the heart.*

The **lymphatic system** helps drain fluid from the head and face and assists in fighting infection. A long chain of lymph nodes runs along the side of the neck, behind the ears, and under the chin (Figure 3-53 ■). They are palpable when congested with infectious products. (The lymphatic

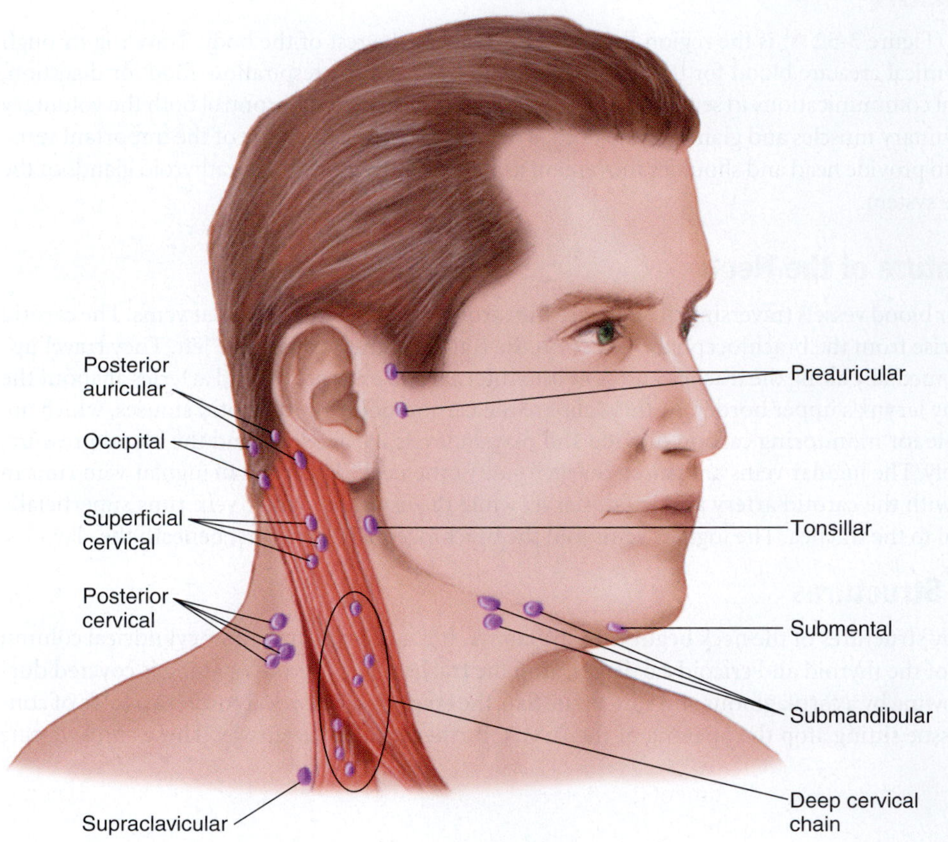

■ **Figure 3-53** The lymph nodes of the head and neck.

system is discussed further in the Cardiovascular System section, later in this chapter.) The right and left thoracic ducts deliver lymph to the venous system at the juncture of the jugular and subclavian veins.

The thyroid gland sits over the trachea just below the cricoid cartilage and controls the rate of cellular metabolism as well as the systemic levels of calcium. The brachial plexus is a network of nerves in the lower neck and shoulder responsible for lower arm and hand function. Lastly, numerous muscles (including the sternocleidomastoid, platysma, and upper trapezius), fascia, and soft tissues are found in the neck.

THE SPINE AND THORAX

THE SPINE

The spine consists of a supporting skeletal structure, the vertebral column, and a central nervous system pathway, the spinal cord. These are important functional elements both for body posture and movement and for communication among the body's many systems. The vertebral column provides skeletal support for and permits movement of the head, assists in maintaining the shape of the thoracic cage, supports the upper body, and forms the posterior aspect of the pelvis. The spinal cord, contained and protected within the vertebral column, is the main communication conduit of the central nervous system. It is responsible for transmitting messages from the brain to the body organs and tissues and from the sensory nerves in the organs, skin, and other tissues back to the brain.

The Vertebral Column

The vertebral column is a hollow skeletal tube made up of 33 irregular bones, called **vertebrae.** This column attaches to the head, to the bones of the rib cage, and to the pelvis. It provides the central skeletal support structure and a major portion of the axial skeleton. At the same time, the vertebrae provide a protective container for the spinal cord. Several components with differing functions may make up the structure of each individual vertebra.

vertebrae *the 33 bones making up the vertebral column; singular vertebra.*

The major weight-bearing component of a vertebra is the **vertebral body.** It is a cylinder of skeletal tissue made up of cancellous bone surrounded by a layer of hard, compact bone. It lies anterior to the other components of the vertebra.

vertebral body *short column of bone that forms the weight-bearing portion of a vertebra.*

The size of the vertebral body varies with its location along the spinal column (Figure 3-54 ■). The first two cervical vertebrae (C-1 and C-2) do not have vertebral bodies because of their specialized functions. Below C-1 and C-2, the size of the vertebral bodies increases progressively as you move down the spine because the vertebral column is supporting an increasing portion of the upper body's weight. The lumbar spine has the strongest and largest vertebral bodies due to the weight they bear. Because of the fused nature of the sacrum and coccyx, these regions have no discernable bodies.

A component of the vertebra posterior to the vertebral body is the **spinal canal,** which is the opening, or foramen, that accommodates the spinal cord. This opening is formed by small fused bony structures that are joined together to create a ring. The lateral structures of the ring are called **pedicles,** while the two posterior structures are called **laminae.** The inferior surface of the pedicle contains a notch, called the intervertebral foramen. This notch permits the exit of a peripheral nerve root and spinal vein and the entrance of a spinal artery on each side of the spinal canal and at each vertebral junction.

spinal canal *opening in the vertebrae that accommodates the spinal cord.*

pedicles *thick, bony struts that connect the vertebral bodies with the spinous and transverse processes and help make up the opening for the spinal canal.*

laminae *posterior bones of a vertebra that help make up the foramen, or opening, of the spinal canal.*

At the juncture of the pedicle and lamina on each side of a vertebra, there is a bony outgrowth called the **transverse process.** There is also a bony outgrowth where the laminae join, which is called the **spinous process.** The spinous process is the posteriorly and inferiorly oriented bony protrusion that you can feel along the spine.

transverse process *bony outgrowth of the vertebral pedicle that serves as a site for muscle attachment and articulation with the ribs.*

The spinous and transverse processes are points of attachment for ligaments and tendons. Ligaments hold the vertebrae firmly together and in place while they permit limited motion. The tendons attach muscles to the vertebral column and permit these muscles to move the spine, other bones, and the body. This attachment of muscles and capsule of ligaments protects and strengthens the vertebral column against the forces of trauma.

spinous process *prominence at the posterior part of a vertebra.*

■ **Figure 3-54** Changing dimensions of the vertebral column.

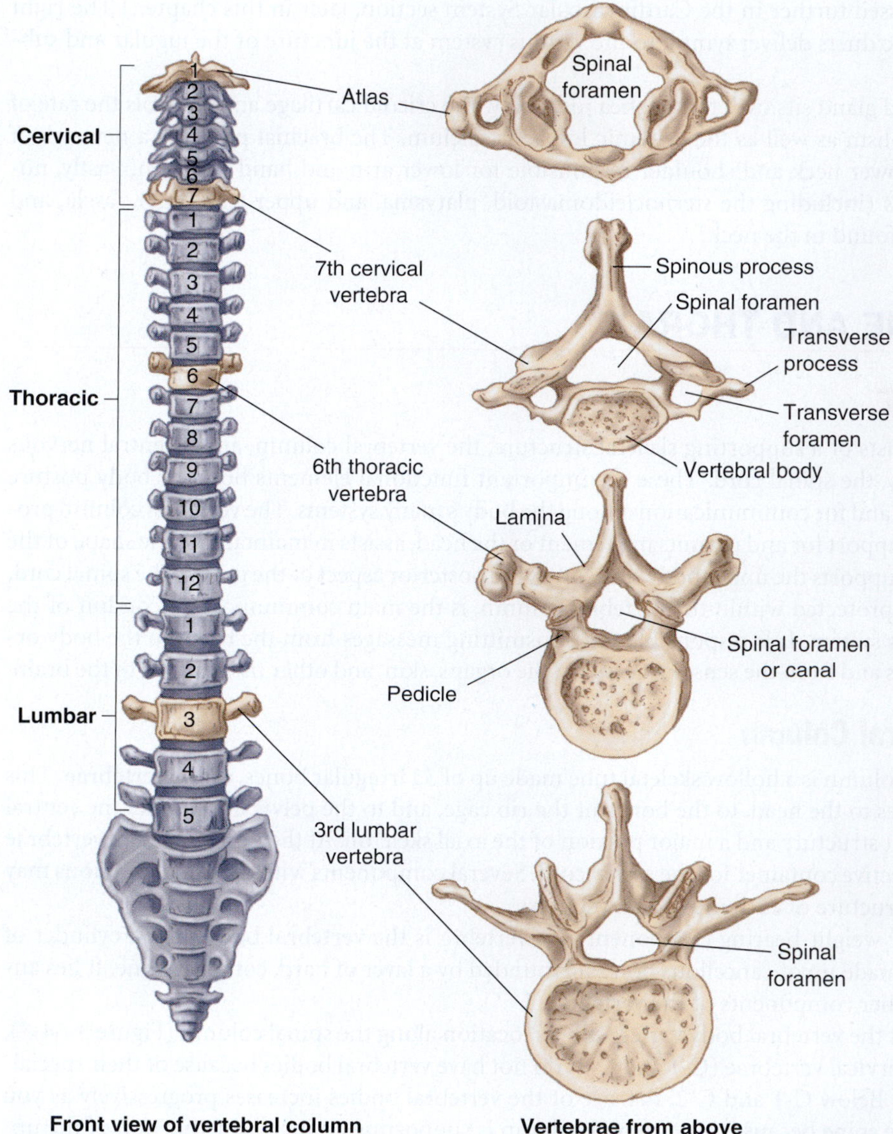

intervertebral disk
cartilaginous pad between vertebrae that serves as a shock absorber.

Between the vertebral bodies are cartilaginous **intervertebral disks.** These disks are formed of a strong yet somewhat flexible outer cover called the annulus fibrosus and a soft and gelatinous inner region called the nucleus pulposus. The intervertebral disks accommodate some motion of the adjacent vertebrae, limit bone wear, and absorb shock along the length of the spinal column. The intervertebral disks make up about 25 percent of the total length of the spinal column, and their degeneration accounts for much of the height loss associated with advancing age.

The elements of the spinal column also have numerous articular surfaces. These surfaces are found on the vertebral bodies, the pedicles, and on the transverse and spinous processes. The articular surfaces enable the spinal column to move around the spinal cord without compressing it, permit articulation with the skull and ribs, and make possible the formation of the rigid, immobile joint of the pelvis.

The vertebral bodies are held firmly together by strong ligaments to assure that the spinal foramen safely accommodates the spinal cord and that the body has a reasonable range of motion. The anterior longitudinal ligament travels along the anterior surfaces of the vertebral bodies. It provides the major stability of the spinal column and resists hyperextension. The posterior longitudinal ligament travels along the posterior surfaces of the vertebral bodies, within the spinal canal. This ligament helps to prevent hyperflexion; when it is disrupted, the result is, frequently, a spinal cord injury. Other ligaments encapsulate the spinous processes (interspinous ligaments) and the transverse processes. These ligaments strengthen and stabilize the column against excessive lateral bending, rotation, and flexion.

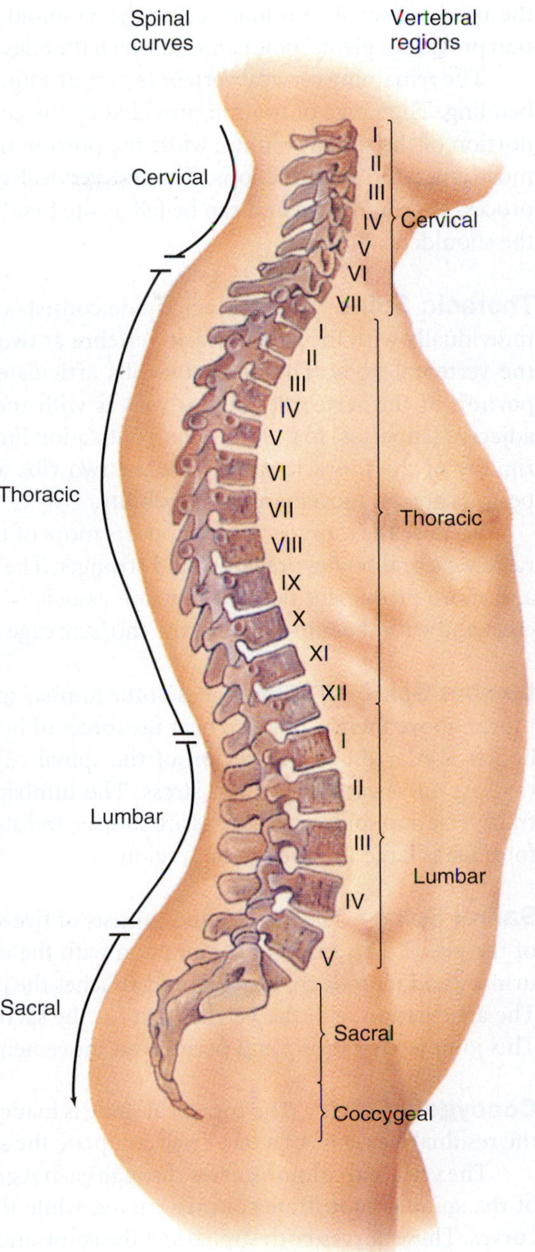

■ Figure 3-55 Divisions of the vertebral column.

Divisions of the Vertebral Column

The vertebral column is divided into five regions: the cervical, the thoracic, the lumbar, the sacral, and the coccygeal (Figure 3-55 ■). Each region is unique in its design and function and has a curve that reverses the curve of the spinal section(s) adjacent to it. The individual vertebrae of the column are identified by the first letter of their region and numbered from superior to inferior. For example, the most inferior of the seven cervical vertebrae is identified as C-7.

Content Review

Divisions of the Vertebral Column

- Cervical spine
- Thoracic spine
- Lumbar spine
- Sacral spine
- Coccygeal spine

Cervical Spine The cervical spine consists of seven cervical vertebrae located between the base of the skull and the shoulders. The cervical spine is the sole skeletal support for the head, which weighs about 16 to 22 pounds.

The first two cervical vertebrae have a unique relationship with the head and each other that permits rotation to the left and right and nodding of the head. The first cervical vertebra, C-1, is called the atlas (after the Greek god who held up the world) and supports the head. It is securely affixed to the occiput and permits nodding but does not accommodate any twisting or turning motion. It and the next vertebra, C-2, differ from most vertebrae in not having discernable vertebral bodies. Vertebra C-2, called the axis, has a small bony tooth, called the odontoid process or dens, that projects upward. This projection provides a pivotal point around which the atlas and head can rotate from side to side.

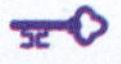

The range of motion provided by the cervical spine is the greatest allowed by any region, yet the cord in this region is critical to life functions.

The remaining cervical vertebrae permit some rotation as well as flexion, extension, and lateral bending. The range of motion provided by the cervical spine is greater than allowed by any other portion of the spinal column, while the portion of the spinal cord traveling through the region is most critical to life functions. The last cervical vertebra (C-7) is quite noticeable as its spinous process is pronounced and can be felt as the first bony prominence along the spine and just above the shoulders.

Thoracic Spine The thoracic spine consists of 12 thoracic vertebrae. The first rib articulates individually with the first thoracic vertebra at two locations, with the transverse process and with the vertebral body. The next nine ribs articulate with the transverse process and the superior portion of the vertebral body as well as with the inferior portion of the vertebral body that is adjacent (superior) to it. This system of fixation limits rib movement and increases the strength and rigidity of the thoracic spine. The last two ribs articulate only with the vertebral bodies, which permits greater movement and flexibility.

Because the thoracic spine supports more of the human body than the cervical spine, the thoracic vertebral bodies are larger and stronger. The spinous and transverse processes are also larger and more prominent because they are associated with the musculature holding the upper body erect and with the movement of the thoracic cage during respiration.

Lumbar Spine The five bones of the lumbar spine each carry the weight of the head, neck, and thorax above them. They also bear the forces of bending and lifting above the pelvis. The vertebral bodies are largest in this region of the spinal column, and the intervertebral disks are also the thickest and bear the greatest stress. The lumbar pedicles and lamina are also thick, while the transverse and spinous processes are shorter and stouter than those in the thoracic spine. The spinal foramen is largest in the lumbar region.

Sacral Spine The sacral spine consists of five sacral vertebrae that fuse into the posterior plate of the pelvis. This plate, in conjunction with the two innominate bones of the pelvis, protects the urinary and reproductive organs and attaches the pelvis and lower extremities to the axial skeleton. The articulation with the pelvis occurs at the sacroiliac joint on the lateral surface of the sacrum. This joint is very strong and permits no movement. The upper body balances on the sacrum.

Coccygeal Spine The coccygeal spine is made up of three to five fused vertebrae that represent the residual elements of a tail. They comprise the short skeletal end of the vertebral column.

The vertebral column curves through each region of the spine. The cervical and lumbar regions of the spine demonstrate concave curves, while the thoracic and sacral regions represent convex curves. These curves both strengthen the spine and permit a greater range of supported motion.

The Spinal Meninges

The spinal meninges are similar to those covering and protecting the structures within the cranium. They consist of the dura mater, the arachnoid, and the pia mater. The meninges cover the entire spinal cord and the peripheral nerve roots as they leave the spinal column. However, the spinal meninges are not as strongly secured to the spinal column as the meninges are to the cranium. The dura mater is firmly attached to the base of the skull and to a collagen fiber called the coccygeal ligament at the top of the sacrum. These attachments and the dura mater's attachments associated with each pair of peripheral nerve roots help position the cord centrally within the spinal canal yet permit the column to move around the cord (Figure 3-56 ■).

As it does in the brain, cerebrospinal fluid bathes the spinal cord by filling the subarachnoid space. The fluid provides a medium for the exchange of nutrients and waste products and absorbs the shocks of sudden movements. Cerebrospinal fluid is produced in the ventricles of the brain and then circulates through the ventricles and through the arachnoid space of the spinal meninges. The fluid is absorbed by specialized cells (the arachnoid villi) in the lower portion of the lumbar meninges, a region called the spinal cistern.

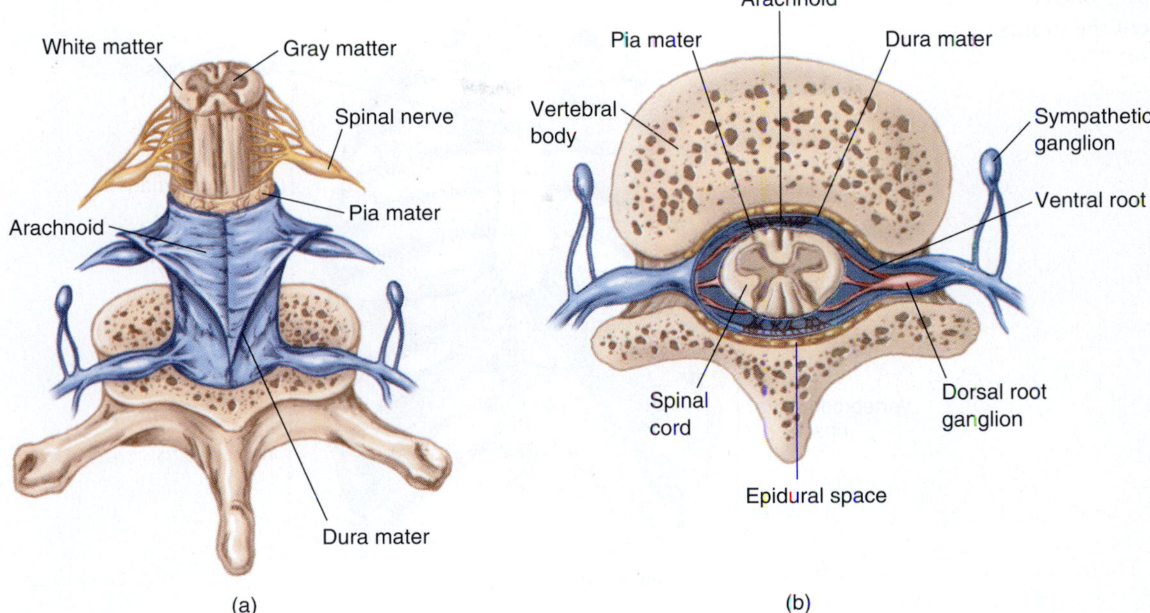

■ **Figure 3-56** Structural protection of the spinal cord.

The distance between the spinal cord and the interior of the vertebral foramen varies in the different spinal regions. The region with the closest tolerance between the cord and the interior surfaces of the spinal foramen is the thoracic spine, where movement of the spinal column is most limited. Although this region is injured only infrequently, just a slight displacement into the vertebral foramen is likely to cause spinal cord injury. The greatest spacing between the cord and the interior of the vertebral column is found in upper lumbar and upper cervical (C-1 and C-2) regions.

Injuries to the mid- or lower lumbar regions do not endanger the spinal cord because the cord ends at the L-1 or L-2 level in mature adults. Injury to the lumbar spine can, however, damage the peripheral nerve roots there. The vertebral foramen below L-1 or L-2 is filled with cerebrospinal fluid and is where the fluid may be most safely removed for diagnostic testing (spinal tap).

THE THORAX

The thoracic cage is the chamber that moves air in and out and where oxygen and carbon dioxide are exchanged to support the body's metabolism. It consists of the thoracic skeleton, diaphragm, and associated musculature. It is also the location of the heart, major blood vessels, and other important structures essential for body function. It contains the trachea, bronchi, lungs, and the mediastinum. Finally, the dynamics of the chest (ventilation) are controlled by a series of centers in the brain and blood vessels.

The Thoracic Skeleton

The thoracic skeleton is defined by 12 pairs of C-shaped ribs, which articulate posteriorly with the thoracic spine and then extend in an anterior and inferior direction (Figure 3-57 ■). The upper seven pairs join the sternum at their cartilaginous endpoints. The 8th through 10th ribs have cartilage at their distal anterior ends that join the cartilage of the 7th rib at the inferior margin of the sternum. The 11th and 12th ribs are often termed the floating ribs and have no anterior attachment.

The sternum completes the anterior bony structure of the thorax and is made up of three sections: the manubrium, the body of the sternum, and the xiphoid process. The manubrium is the superior portion of the sternum and is the medial endpoint of the clavicle and first rib. The sternal angle (also known as the angle of Louis) is the junction of the manubrium and the body of the sternum and is palpable through the skin as an elevation or prominence. This structure has clinical significance as it is the site of attachment of the second rib and quickly allows the paramedic to identify

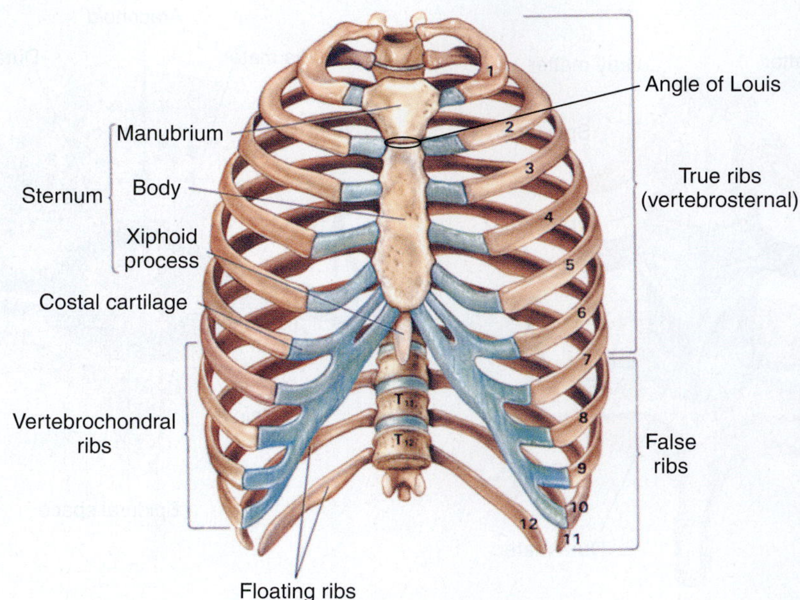

■ **Figure 3-57** Skeletal components of the thorax.

the second intercostal space. This location is important because it is where you may be required to perform a needle decompression of the chest in the event of a tension pneumothorax. The xiphoid process is the most inferior portion of the sternum and meets the body at the junction of the costal cartilages of the lower ribs.

The thorax is divided by imaginary vertical lines used to describe positions lateral to the sternum. These lines include the midclavicular line, the anterior axillary line, the midaxillary line, and the posterior axillary line. When combined with a rib level, these lines serve as good landmarks for describing wounds, locating underlying structures, and for identifying locations to perform procedures. The space just inferior to each rib is called an intercostal space and is given the number of the rib above it. For example, the anterior axillary line extends from the anterior margin of the axilla (armpit) inferiorly along the thoracic wall. Its intersection with the fifth intercostal space is generally used in the emergency department to place a thoracostomy tube in patients with pneumothorax or hemothorax. It is not frequently used for prehospital needle decompression because this site is often obscured by the patient's arms or by immobilization devices, strapping, and blankets.

The thoracic inlet is the superior opening in the thorax. It is narrow in comparison to the thoracic outlet, and is defined by the curvature of the first rib, with its posterior attachment at the first thoracic vertebra and ending anteriorly, at the manubrium. The thoracic outlet is formed posteriorly by the 12th vertebra, laterally by the curvature of the 12th rib, and extends anteriorly and superiorly along the costal margin to the **xiphisternal joint.**

xiphisternal joint *union between xiphoid process and body of the sternum.*

The Diaphragm

The diaphragm is a muscular, domelike structure that separates the abdominal cavity from the thoracic cavity. It is affixed to the lower border of the rib cage, while its central and superior margin may extend to the level of the fourth intercostal space anteriorly and the sixth intercostal space posteriorly during maximal expiration. This superior positioning may allow penetrating wounds of the lower half of the thorax to penetrate the diaphragm and enter the abdominal cavity. The aorta, esophagus, and inferior vena cava exit the thoracic cavity through separate openings in this structure. The diaphragm is a major muscle of respiration, contracting to displace the floor of the thoracic cavity downward during inspiration and relaxing and moving upward with expiration.

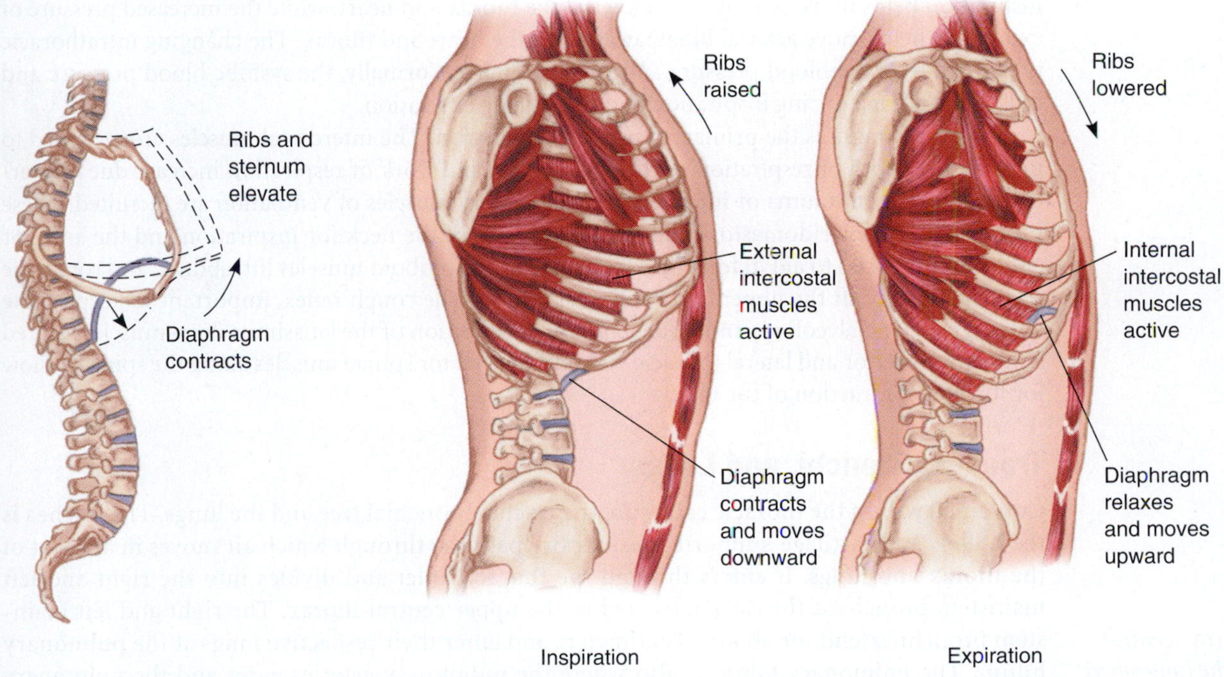

■ **Figure 3-58** The diaphragm and muscles of the chest change its volume to effect respirations.

Associated Musculature

The chest wall musculature along with the shoulder musculature, clavicles, scapula, and humerus provide additional protection to the vital structures within the upper thorax (Figure 3-58 ■). The clavicles articulate laterally with the acromion process of the scapula. The scapula covers the posterior and lateral aspects of the first six ribs and articulates with the humerus to complete the shoulder girdle.

Chest wall muscles between the ribs, called the intercostal muscles, along with the diaphragm and the sternocleidomastoid muscles are the major muscles of respiration. The sternocleidomastoid muscles raise the upper rib and sternum and, with the sternum, the anterior attachments of the next nine ribs. The intercostal muscles contract to further elevate the ribs and increase the anterior-posterior dimension of the thorax. Simultaneously, the diaphragm, which forms the floor of the thorax, contracts and flattens to further increase the volume of the thoracic cavity. As the thoracic volume increases, the pressure within it becomes less than atmospheric. Air rushes in through the tracheobronchial tree and into the alveoli to equalize this pressure gradient, filling the lungs.

As the musculature relaxes, the diaphragm again intrudes upward into the thoracic cavity, the ribs and sternum move inferiorly, and the ribs move closer together in an inferior and posterior direction. This decreases the thoracic volume and increases the intrathoracic pressure. When the pressure within the thorax exceeds that of the surrounding atmosphere, air rushes out. Therefore exhalation in the resting state is largely a passive activity aided by the elastic recoil of the lungs. Gravity helps facilitate this action with downward displacement of the ribs in either the upright or supine position. This changing of volume to move air in and out is called the bellows effect.

> Normal inspiration is an active process, while normal expiration is a passive process.

The changing volume and pressure within the thoracic cage also assist with the pumping of blood to and venous return from the systemic circulation. The decreased intrathoracic pressure of inspiration helps move venous blood toward the thorax and heart, while the increased pressure of expiration helps move arterial blood away from the heart and thorax. The changing intrathoracic pressure affects the blood pressure and pulse strength. Normally, the systolic blood pressure and pulse strength fall during inspiration and rise during expiration.

The diaphragm is the primary muscle of respiration. The intercostal muscles are recruited to increase the depth of respiration. As the rate, depth, and work of respiration increase due to exercise or stress from trauma or infection, more accessory muscles of ventilation are recruited. These include the sternocleidomastoid and scalene muscles of the neck for inspiration and the anterior abdominal muscles to aid in forceful exhalation. The rhomboid muscles lift, abduct, and rotate the scapulae to help lift the upper chest with inspiration. The cough reflex, important to keeping the airways clear and alveoli expanded, depends on the addition of the latissimus dorsi muscles located along the posterior and lateral thoracic wall and the erector spinae muscles along the spine to allow for forceful contraction of the thorax.

Trachea, Bronchi, and Lungs

Contained within the thoracic cavity are the tracheobronchial tree and the lungs. The trachea is the hollow and cartilage-supported respiratory pathway through which air moves in and out of the thorax and lungs. It enters through the thoracic inlet and divides into the right and left mainstem bronchi at the carina, located in the upper central thorax. The right and left mainstem bronchi extend for about 3 centimeters and enter their respective lungs at the **pulmonary hilum.** The pulmonary hilum is also where the pulmonary arteries enter and the pulmonary veins exit the lungs and is the sole point of fixation of the lung in the thoracic cage. The bronchi then further divide into bronchioles, which ultimately terminate in the alveoli. The lungs contain millions of these tiny "grape"-shaped alveoli, which are the basic unit of structure and function in the lungs.

pulmonary hilum *central medial region of the lung where the bronchi and pulmonary vasculature enter the lung.*

Each lung occupies one side of the thoracic cavity and is divided into lobes. The right lung has three lobes: the upper, middle, and lower. The left lung has two lobes, the upper and lower. The left upper lobe contains the cardiac notch against which the heart rests. The lower section of the left upper lobe (the lingula) projects around the lateral border of the heart and corresponds to the middle lobe of the right lung.

The lungs are covered by the visceral pleura, a smooth membrane that lines the exterior of the lungs. It folds over on itself at the pulmonary hilum and then lines the inside of the thoracic cavity, becoming the parietal pleura. This dual layer forms a potential space called the pleural space. It contains a small amount of serous (pleural) fluid for lubrication and permits the lungs to expand and contract easily. This dual layer also creates the seal that causes the lungs to expand and contract with the changing volume of the thoracic cavity.

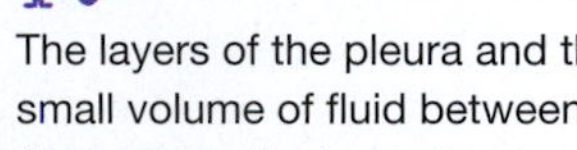

The layers of the pleura and the small volume of fluid between them cause the lungs to move with the thoracic cage.

The trachea, bronchi, and lungs are discussed further in the Respiratory System section later in this chapter.

Mediastinum and Heart

The mediastinum (Figure 3-59 ■) is the central space within the thoracic cavity bounded laterally by the lungs, inferiorly by the diaphragm, and superiorly by the thoracic inlet. The heart is located within and fills most of the mediastinum. (The heart is discussed in detail in the Cardiovascular System section, later in this chapter.) Through the mediastinum, the great vessels (see the next section) traverse to and from the heart, and the trachea and esophagus enter the thorax. The esophagus then courses anterior to the aorta before exiting through the diaphragm at the thoracic outlet (esophageal hiatus or foramen).

The vagus nerve, which provides parasympathetic innervation of thoracic and abdominal viscera, enters the thorax bilaterally through the thoracic inlet and traverses the mediastinum giving branches to the larynx, esophagus, trachea, bronchi, and heart. The vagus nerve then ex-

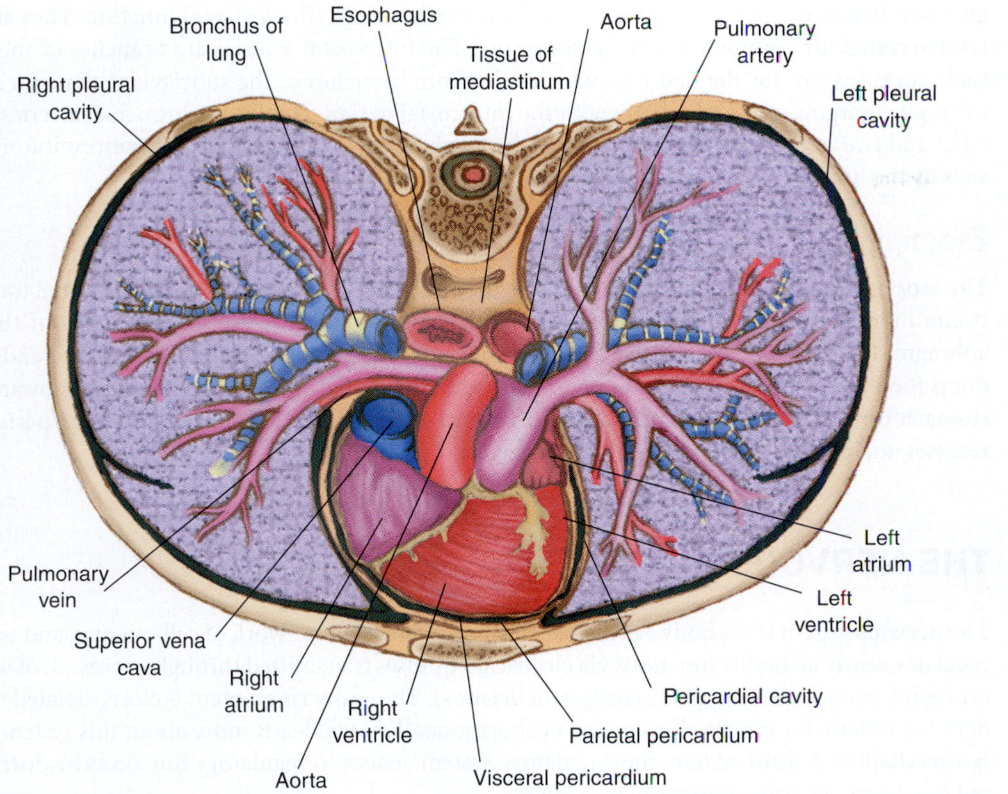

Figure 3-59 Structures of the mediastinum and thorax.

its the thorax through the esophageal opening in the diaphragm to innervate the abdominal viscera. The phrenic nerve (originating from the third, fourth, and fifth cervical nerve roots) also enters the thorax through the thoracic inlet and traverses the thorax to innervate the diaphragm.

The thoracic duct (part of the lymphatic system) also traverses the thorax from the thoracic outlet where it enters through the aortic opening in the diaphragm. It typically crosses the midline from the right side of the aorta in the posterior mediastinum at the level of the fifth thoracic vertebra and then ascends above the level of the left clavicle before arching back downward to empty into the left internal jugular vein. The thoracic duct carries most of the body's lymphatic drainage (all but the right side of the head, neck, thorax, and right upper extremity).

Great Vessels

The **great vessels** are those large arteries and veins that enter and leave the heart and are found in the mediastinum. They are the aorta, the superior and inferior vena cava, the pulmonary arteries, and the pulmonary veins. Injury to these large vascular structures can lead to significant blood loss and death if the condition is not quickly recognized and repaired. The aorta, which is fixed at three positions within the thorax, is not only susceptible to penetrating injury, but also to blunt injury by rapid deceleration or shear forces. It is fixed at the annulus where it attaches to the heart, at the **ligamentum arteriosum** near the bifurcation of the pulmonary artery, and at the aortic hiatus where it passes through the diaphragm and enters the abdomen.

great vessels *the large arteries and veins located in the mediastinum that enter and exit the heart; the aorta, superior and inferior vena cava, pulmonary arteries, and pulmonary veins.*

ligamentum arteriosum *cordlike remnant of a fetal vessel connecting the pulmonary artery to the aorta at the aortic isthmus.*

Other major vessels that branch from the great vessels in the upper thorax include the subclavian arteries and veins, the common carotid arteries, and the brachiocephalic artery (which is the first large branch off the aortic arch dividing into the right common carotid and right subclavian). The internal mammary vessels are inferior branches of the subclavians running along the anterior surface of the pleura, posterior to the costochondral (rib-cartilage) junction. They are often harvested for coronary artery bypass grafts. The intercostal arteries are branches of the thoracic aorta (except for the first two, which arise from branches of the subclavian) that run along the lower margins of the ribs along with the intercostal nerves. Finally, the bronchial arteries (one right and two left) are usually branches of the thoracic aorta that nourish the nonrespiratory tissues of the lung.

The nervous system is the body's principal control system.

central nervous system *the brain and the spinal cord.*

peripheral nervous system *part of the nervous system that extends throughout the body and is composed of the cranial nerves arising from the brain and the peripheral nerves arising from the spinal cord. Its subdivisions are the somatic and the autonomic nervous systems.*

somatic nervous system *part of the nervous system controlling voluntary bodily functions.*

autonomic nervous system *part of the nervous system controlling involuntary bodily functions. It is divided into the sympathetic and the parasympathetic systems.*

sympathetic nervous system *division of the autonomic nervous system that prepares the body for stressful situations. Sympathetic nervous system actions include increased heart rate and dilation of the bronchioles and pupils. Its actions are mediated by the neurotransmitters epinephrine and norepinephrine.*

parasympathetic nervous system *division of the autonomic nervous system that is responsible for controlling vegetative functions. Parasympathetic nervous system actions include decreased heart rate and constriction of the bronchioles and pupils. Its actions are mediated by the neurotransmitter acetylcholine.*

neuron *nerve cell; the fundamental component of the nervous system.*

Esophagus

The esophagus enters the thorax through the thoracic inlet with and just posterior to the trachea. It continues the length of the mediastinum and exits through the esophageal hiatus of the diaphragm. It is a muscular tube that is contiguous with the posterior wall of the trachea and conducts food and drink from the oral pharynx to the stomach. It moves food and liquid toward the stomach through a rhythmic muscular contraction called peristalsis. During vomiting, peristalsis reverses and propels the emesis up the esophagus.

THE NERVOUS SYSTEM

The nervous system is the body's principal control system. This network of cells, tissues, and organs regulates nearly all bodily functions via electrical impulses transmitted through nerves, all of which are highly susceptible to hypoxia (oxygen deficiency). The endocrine system is closely related to the nervous system. It exerts bodily control via hormones. You will learn more about this system later in this chapter. A third system, the circulatory system, assists in regulatory functions by distributing hormones and other chemical messengers.

The nervous system consists of two main divisions—the central nervous system and the peripheral nervous system. The **central nervous system** (CNS) consists of the brain and the spinal cord. The **peripheral nervous system** (PNS) is somewhat more complex. As you look at Figure 3-60 ■, note that the peripheral nervous system is divided into two major subdivisions—the **somatic nervous system,** which governs voluntary functions (those we control consciously), and the **autonomic nervous system,** which has two subdivisions—the **sympathetic nervous system** and the **parasympathetic nervous system.** These two subdivisions of the autonomic nervous system work together to carry out involuntary physiological processes such as regulation of blood pressure, heart rate, and digestion.

You will learn more about these divisions of the nervous system as you continue through the next pages. As you read, it will be helpful if you think of the nervous system as a "living computer." The central nervous system is the central processing unit and the various divisions of the peripheral nervous system carry on the input and output processes.

FUNDAMENTAL UNIT: THE NEURON

The fundamental unit of the nervous system is the nerve cell, or **neuron.** The neuron includes the *cell body* (soma), containing the nucleus; the *dendrites,* which transmit electrical impulses to the cell body; and the *axons,* which transmit electrical impulses away from the cell body (Figure 3-61 ■).

The transmission of impulses in the nervous system resembles the conduction of electrical impulses through the heart. In its resting state, the neuron is positively charged on the outside and negatively charged on the inside. When electrically stimulated, sodium rapidly surges into the cell and potassium rapidly leaves it to eliminate the difference in electrical charge between the inside and the outside. This "depolarization," or loss of the charge difference, is subsequently transmitted down the neuron at an extremely high rate of speed.

The neuron joins with other neurons at junctions called *synapses* (Figure 3-62 ■). The neurons never come into direct contact with each other at these synapses. Instead, on reaching the synapse,

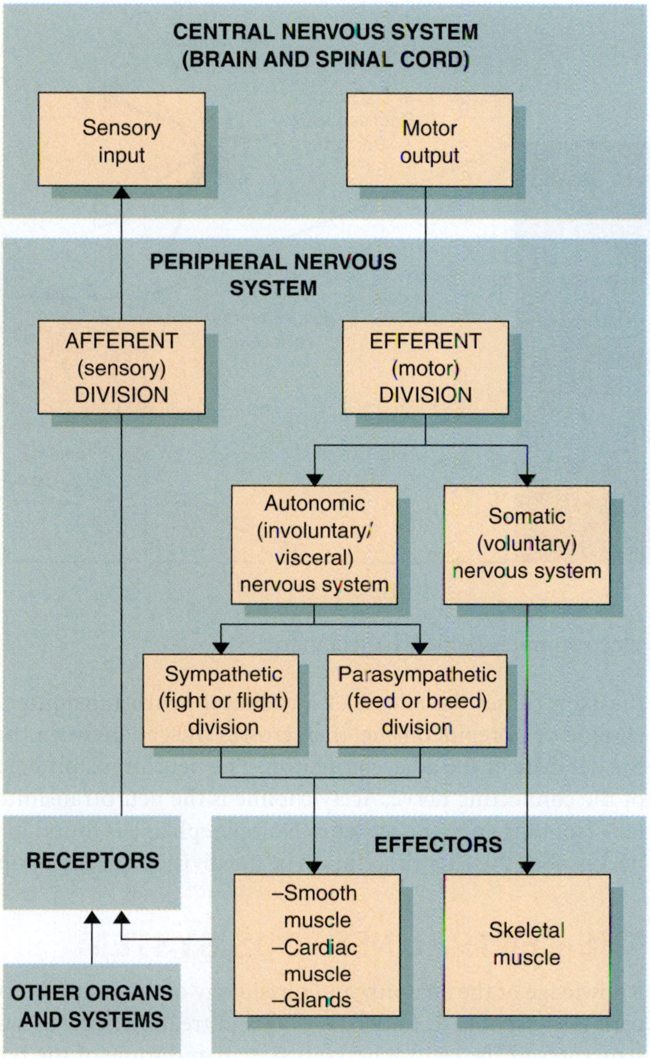

CENTRAL NERVOUS SYSTEM
(BRAIN AND SPINAL CORD)
Sensory input
Motor output
PERIPHERAL NERVOUS SYSTEM
AFFERENT (sensory) DIVISION
EFFERENT (motor) DIVISION
Autonomic (involuntary/ visceral) nervous system
Somatic (voluntary) nervous system
Sympathetic (fight or flight) division
Parasympathetic (feed or breed) division
RECEPTORS
EFFECTORS
–Smooth muscle
–Cardiac muscle
–Glands
Skeletal muscle
OTHER ORGANS AND SYSTEMS

■ **Figure 3-60** Overview of the nervous system.

Dendrites
Soma
Axon
Synaptic terminals
Stimulated by environmental changes or the activities of other cells
Contains the nucleus and most of the metabolic machinery (mitochondria, ribosomes, and so on)
Conducts nerve impulse (action potential) away from the soma
Affect another neuron or effector (muscle, gland, and so on)

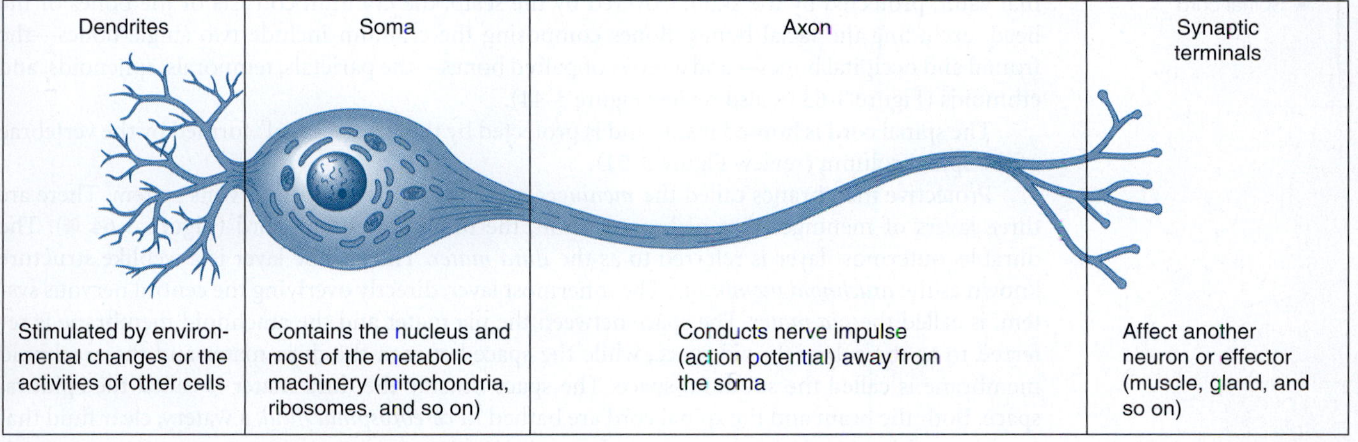

■ **Figure 3-61** Anatomy of a neuron.

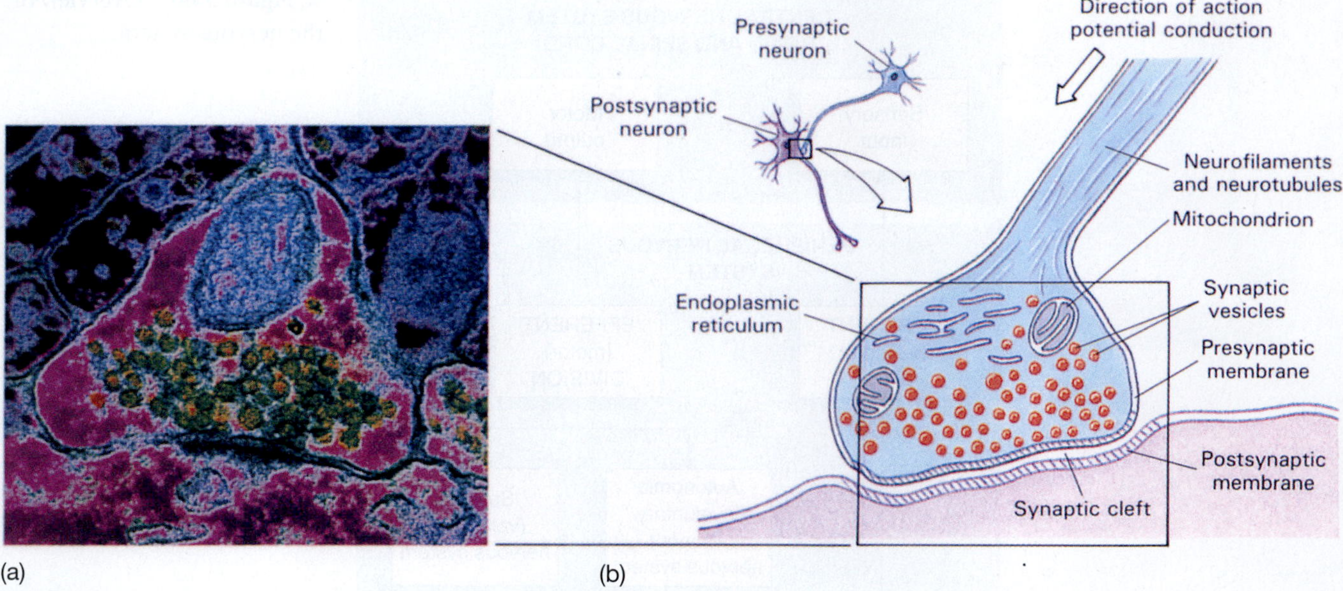

■ **Figure 3-62** The synapse: (a) electron micrograph, (b) schematic.

neurotransmitter *a substance that is released from the axon terminal of a presynaptic neuron on excitation and that travels across the synaptic cleft to either excite or inhibit the target cell. Examples include acetylcholine, norepinephrine, and dopamine.*

Content Review

Central Nervous System

- Brain
- Spinal cord

the axon causes the release of a chemical **neurotransmitter.** This neurotransmitter, either acetylcholine or norepinephrine, then crosses the gap between the axon of the depolarized neuron and the dendrite of the adjacent neuron. The neurotransmitter stimulates the postsynaptic membrane of the connecting nerve. Acetylcholine is the neurotransmitter of the parasympathetic and voluntary (somatic) nervous systems. Norepinephrine is found in the synaptic terminals of sympathetic nerves. (See the later description of the divisions of the peripheral nervous system.)

THE CENTRAL NERVOUS SYSTEM

Knowledge of the anatomy and physiology of the central nervous system—the brain and the spinal cord—is essential to understanding and treating nervous system emergencies. Note that the basic structures of the central nervous system and some of the related terminology were presented earlier in the chapter under the headings "The Head, Face, and Neck" and "The Spine and Thorax."

Protective Structures

Most of the central nervous system is protected by bony structures. The brain lies within the cranial vault, protected by the skull. Covered by the scalp, the cranium consists of the bones of the head, excluding the facial bones. Bones composing the cranium include two single bones—the frontal and occipital bones—and a series of paired bones—the parietals, temporals, sphenoids, and ethmoids (Figure 3-63 ■; also review Figure 3-44).

The spinal cord is housed inside and is protected by the "spinal canal" formed by the vertebrae of the spinal column (review Figure 3-54).

Protective membranes called the *meninges* cover the entire central nervous system. There are three layers of meninges that pad, or cushion, the brain and spinal cord (Figure 3-64 ■). The durable, outermost layer is referred to as the *dura mater.* The middle layer is a weblike structure known as the *arachnoid membrane.* The innermost layer, directly overlying the central nervous system, is called the *pia mater.* The space between the pia mater and the arachnoid membrane is referred to as the subarachnoid space, while the space between the dura mater and the arachnoid membrane is called the subdural space. The space outside the dura mater is called the epidural space. Both the brain and the spinal cord are bathed in *cerebrospinal fluid,* a watery, clear fluid that acts as a cushion to protect these organs from physical impact.

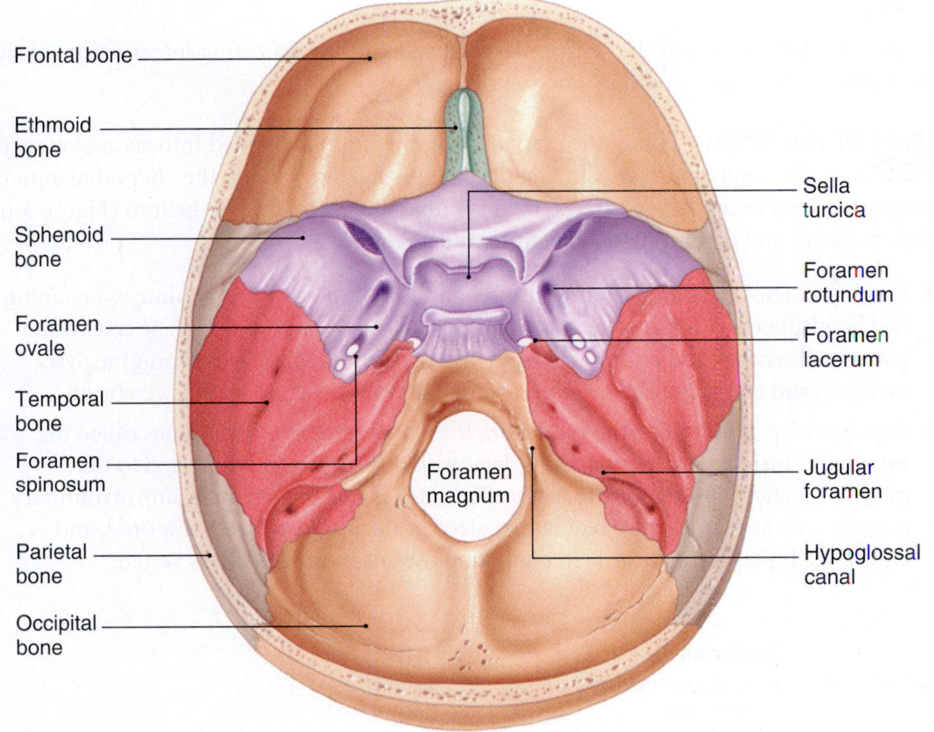

■ **Figure 3-63** The bones of the skull.

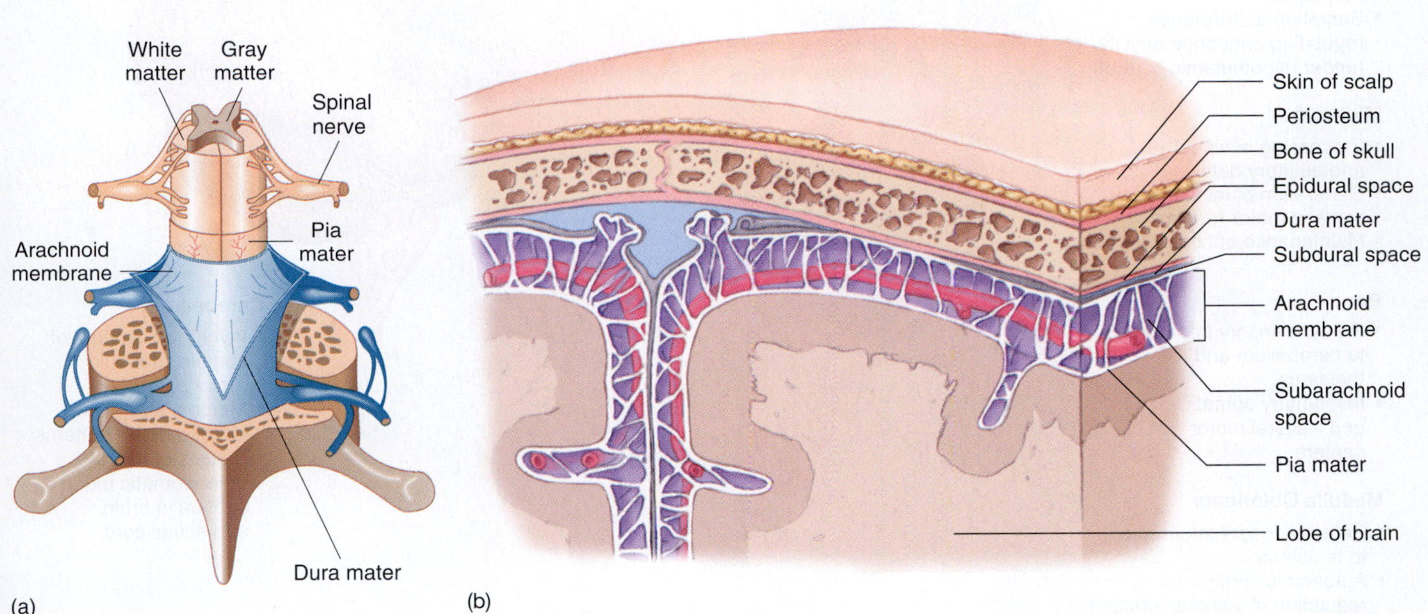

■ **Figure 3-64** The meninges: (a) posterior view of the spinal cord showing the meningeal layers; (b) the meninges of the brain.

The Brain

The brain is the largest part of the central nervous system. The following information provides a general profile of the brain's anatomy and physiology.

Divisions of the Brain Filling the cranial vault, the brain is divided into six major parts: the cerebrum, the diencephalon (which includes the thalamus and the hypothalamus), the mesencephalon (midbrain), the pons, the medulla oblongata, and the cerebellum (Figure 3-65 ■).

The cerebrum and diencephalon constitute the *forebrain.*

- ★ *Cerebrum.* The cerebrum is in the anterior and middle area of the cranium. Containing two hemispheres, it is joined by a structure called the *corpus callosum.* The cerebrum governs all sensory and motor actions. It is the seat of intelligence, learning, analysis, memory, and language. The *cerebral cortex* is the outermost layer of the cerebrum.
- ★ *Diencephalon.* Covered by the cerebrum, the diencephalon is sometimes called the *interbrain.* Inside it are the *thalamus, hypothalamus* (which is connected to the pituitary gland), and the *limbic system.* This area is responsible for many involuntary actions such as temperature regulation, sleep, water balance, stress response, and emotions. It plays a major role in regulating the autonomic nervous system.

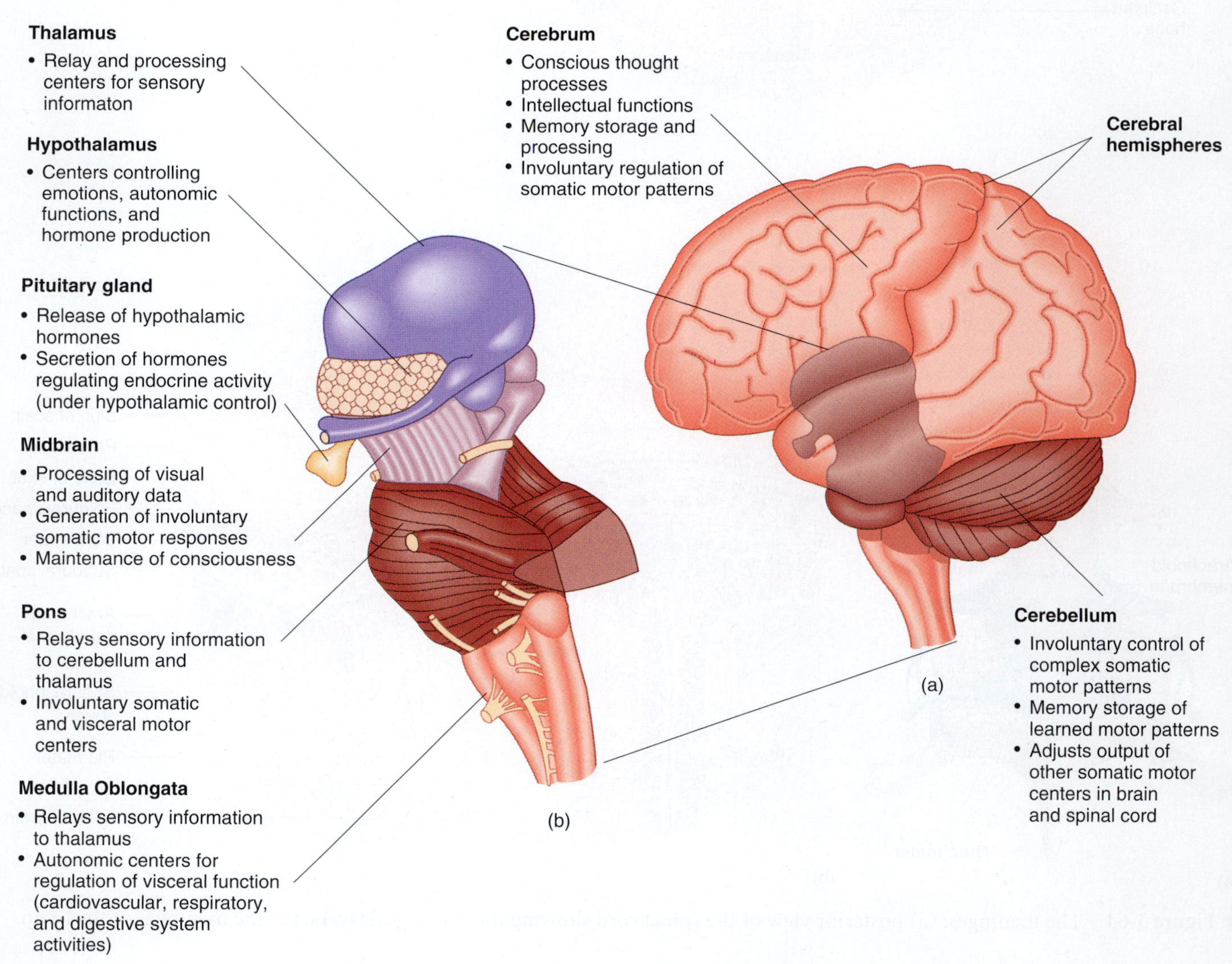

■ **Figure 3-65** The human brain: (a) superficial view of the brain; (b) components of the brainstem.

The mesencephalon (midbrain), pons, and the medulla oblongata collectively form the *brainstem.* The brainstem and the cerebellum together constitute the *hindbrain.*

- ★ *Mesencephalon,* or *midbrain.* The mesencephalon, located between the diencephalon and the pons, is responsible for certain aspects of motor coordination. The mesencephalon is the major region controlling eye movement.
- ★ *Pons.* Between the midbrain and the medulla oblongata, the pons contains connections between the brain and the spinal cord.
- ★ *Medulla oblongata.* The medulla oblongata is located between the pons and the spinal cord. It marks the division between the spinal cord and the brain. Located here are major centers for controlling respiration, cardiac activity, and vasomotor activity.
- ★ *Cerebellum.* The cerebellum is located in the posterior fossa of the cranial cavity. It consists of two hemispheres closely related to the brainstem and higher centers. The cerebellum coordinates fine motor movement, posture, equilibrium, and muscle tone.

Areas of Specialization Several areas of specialization are recognized within the brain and have clinical application (Figure 3-66 ■). These include:

- ★ *Speech.* Located in the temporal lobe of the cerebrum.
- ★ *Vision.* Located in the occipital cortex of the cerebrum.
- ★ *Personality.* Located in the frontal lobes of the cerebrum.
- ★ *Balance and coordination.* Located in the cerebellum.
- ★ *Sensory.* Located in the parietal lobes of the cerebrum.
- ★ *Motor.* Located in the frontal lobes of the cerebrum.
- ★ *Reticular activating system.* The reticular activating system (RAS) operates in the lateral portion of the medulla, pons, and especially the midbrain. The RAS sends impulses to and receives impulses from the cerebral cortex. It is a diffuse system of interlacing nerve cells responsible for maintaining consciousness and the ability to respond to stimuli (Figure 3-67 ■).

Vascular Supply The brain receives about 20 percent of the body's total blood flow per minute. Blood flow to the brain is provided by two systems. The *carotid system* is anterior, while the *vertebrobasilar system* is posterior. Both join at the *circle of Willis* before entering the structures of the brain (Figure 3-68 ■). The system is designed so that interruption of any part will not cause significant loss of blood flow to the tissues. Venous drainage of the brain is through the venous sinuses and the internal jugular veins.

Besides blood flow, cerebrospinal fluid bathes the brain and spinal cord. Several chambers within the brain, called ventricles, contain most of the intracranial volume of this fluid.

The Spinal Cord

The **spinal cord** is the central nervous system (CNS) pathway responsible for transmitting sensory input from the body to the brain and for conducting motor impulses from the brain to the body muscles and organs. Through this pathway, the brain monitors and controls most body functions. Additionally, the spinal cord acts as a reflex center, intercepting sensory signals and initiating short-circuited (reflex) signaling to muscle bodies as needed. If this pathway is compromised, control of the body below the injury is lost.

spinal cord *central nervous system pathway responsible for transmitting sensory input from the body to the brain and for conducting motor impulses from the brain to the body muscles and organs.*

In the fetus, the cord fills the entire length of the vertebral column. However, the growth of cord does not keep pace with the growth of the vertebral column. This discrepancy means that, as a person grows, the peripheral nerve roots are pulled into the spinal foramen. The sheath of the dura below L-2 is thus filled with numerous strands of peripheral nerves. The resulting structure resembles the tail of a horse and is called the cauda equina (Latin for horse's tail). In the adult, the spinal cord extends from the base of the brain (the medulla oblongata) to approximately the L-1 or L-2 level.

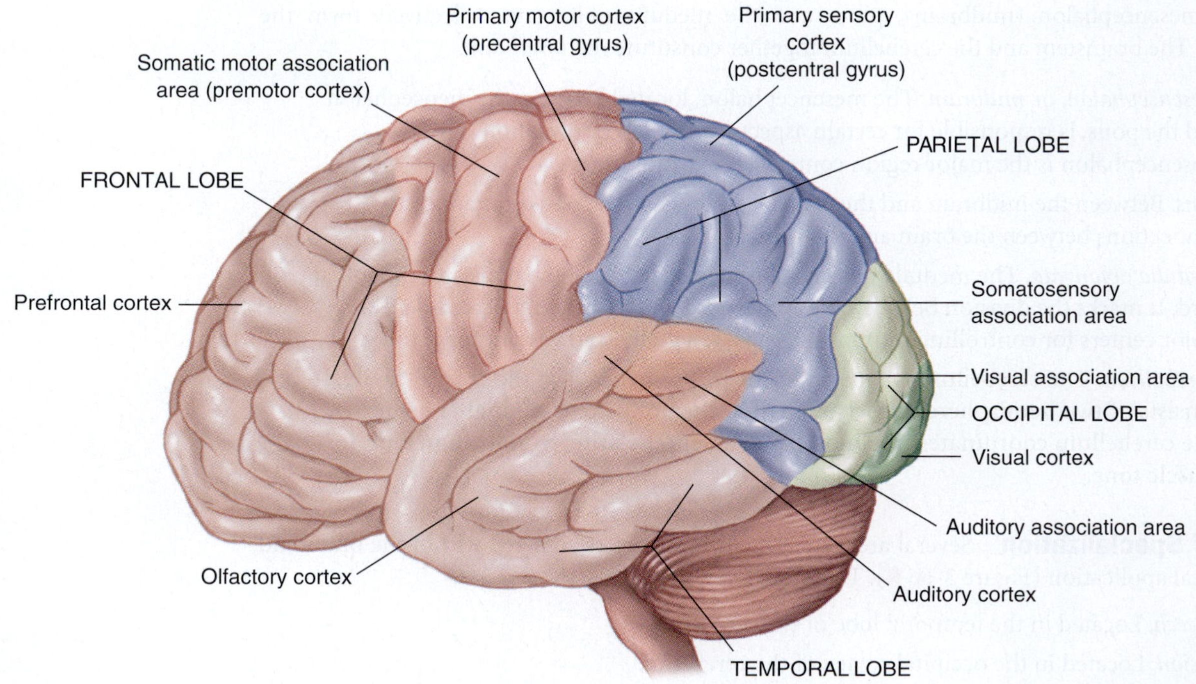

Figure 3-66 External anatomy of the brain.

Figure 3-67 The reticular activating system (RAS), which sends and receives messages from various parts of the brain.

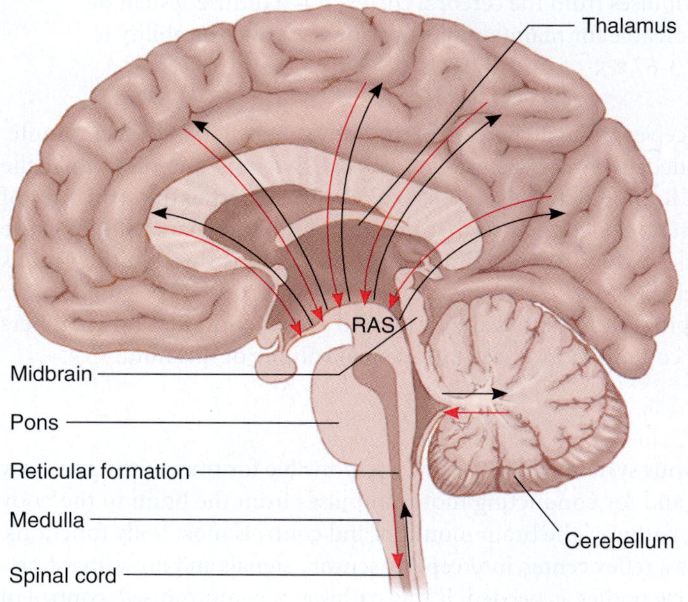

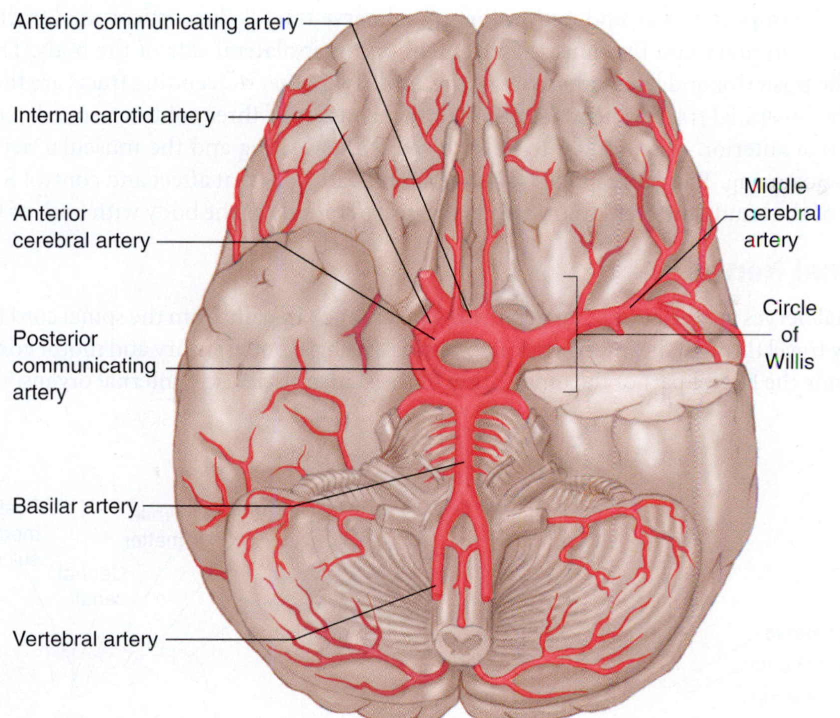

Figure 3-68 An interior view of the brain showing the circle of Willis, which is formed by the anterior and posterior communicating arteries.

Like all central nervous system tissue, the spinal cord constantly needs oxygenated blood. This blood is supplied through paired spinal arteries that branch off the vertebral, cervical, thoracic, and lumbar arteries. These spinal arteries travel through intervertebral foramina, then split into anterior and posterior arteries. On the surface of the spinal cord there are numerous interconnections (anastomoses) between the arteries to provide a better chance for adequate circulation in case of vascular blockage or injury.

Anatomically, the spinal cord is a long cylinder divided into left and right halves by the **anterior medial fissure** and by the **posterior medial sulcus.** In cross section, the central part of the cord has a butterfly or "H" shape and appears gray in color. This **gray matter** is made up largely of neural cell bodies and plays an important role in the reflex system.

The remaining areas, or **white matter,** then form three bundles or columns of myelinated (covered with a protein sheath) nerve fibers on each side of the cord around the gray matter: the anterior white column, the lateral white column, and the posterior white column. This white matter is composed of nerve cell pathways, called axons. It contains bundles of axons that transmit signals upward to the brain in what are called **ascending tracts** and bundles that transmit signals downward to the body in what are called **descending tracts.** These tracts are paired, one ascending and one descending on each side, and injury may affect either or both.

A thorough discussion of organization and functions of the ascending and descending spinal tracts is beyond the scope of this textbook. However, knowing the functions of some motor and sensory pathways can aid you in recognizing spinal cord injury.

The important ascending (sensory) tracts or fasciculi include the fasciculus gracilis, fasciculus cutaneous, and the spinothalamic tracts. The fasciculus gracilis and fasciculus cutaneous carry sensory impulses of light touch, vibration, and positional sense from the skin, muscles, tendons, and joints to the brain. They are located on the posterior portion of the cord (posterior columns). Their injury causes disruption on the ipsilateral (same side) of the body because the left to right switching occurs at the medulla. The spinothalamic tracts include both lateral and anterior tracts. The anterior pathway conducts pain and temperature, while the lateral pathway conducts touch and pressure sensation. These pathways cross as they enter the cord; hence, injury results in contralateral (opposite side) deficits.

anterior medial fissure *deep crease along the ventral surface of the spinal cord that divides the cord into right and left halves.*

posterior medial sulcus *shallow longitudinal groove along the dorsal surface of the spinal cord.*

gray matter *areas in the central nervous system dominated by nerve cell bodies; the central portion of the spinal cord.*

white matter *material that surrounds gray matter in the spinal cord; made up largely of axons.*

ascending tracts *bundles of axons along the spinal cord that transmit signals from the body to the brain.*

descending tracts *bundles of axons along the spinal cord that transmit signals from the brain to the body.*

The important descending (motor) spinal nerve tract is the corticospinal tract. It is responsible for voluntary and fine muscle movement on the ipsilateral side of the body. This pathway lies on the posterior and lateral portions of the cord. Two other descending tracts are the reticulospinal and rubrospinal tracts. The reticulospinal tract consists of three subtracts: one lateral, one medial, and one anterior. It is thought to be involved with sweating and the muscular activity associated with posturing. The rubrospinal tracts are lateral pathways that affect and control fine motor function of the hands and feet. Injury affects the ipsilateral side of the body with both of these pathways.

Spinal Nerves

spinal nerves *31 pairs of nerves that originate along the spinal cord from anterior and posterior nerve roots.*

Spinal nerves are the peripheral nerve roots that branch in pairs from the spinal cord (Figure 3-69 ■). They travel through the intervertebral foramina and have both sensory and motor components. They provide the largest part of the innervation of the skin, muscles, and internal organs.

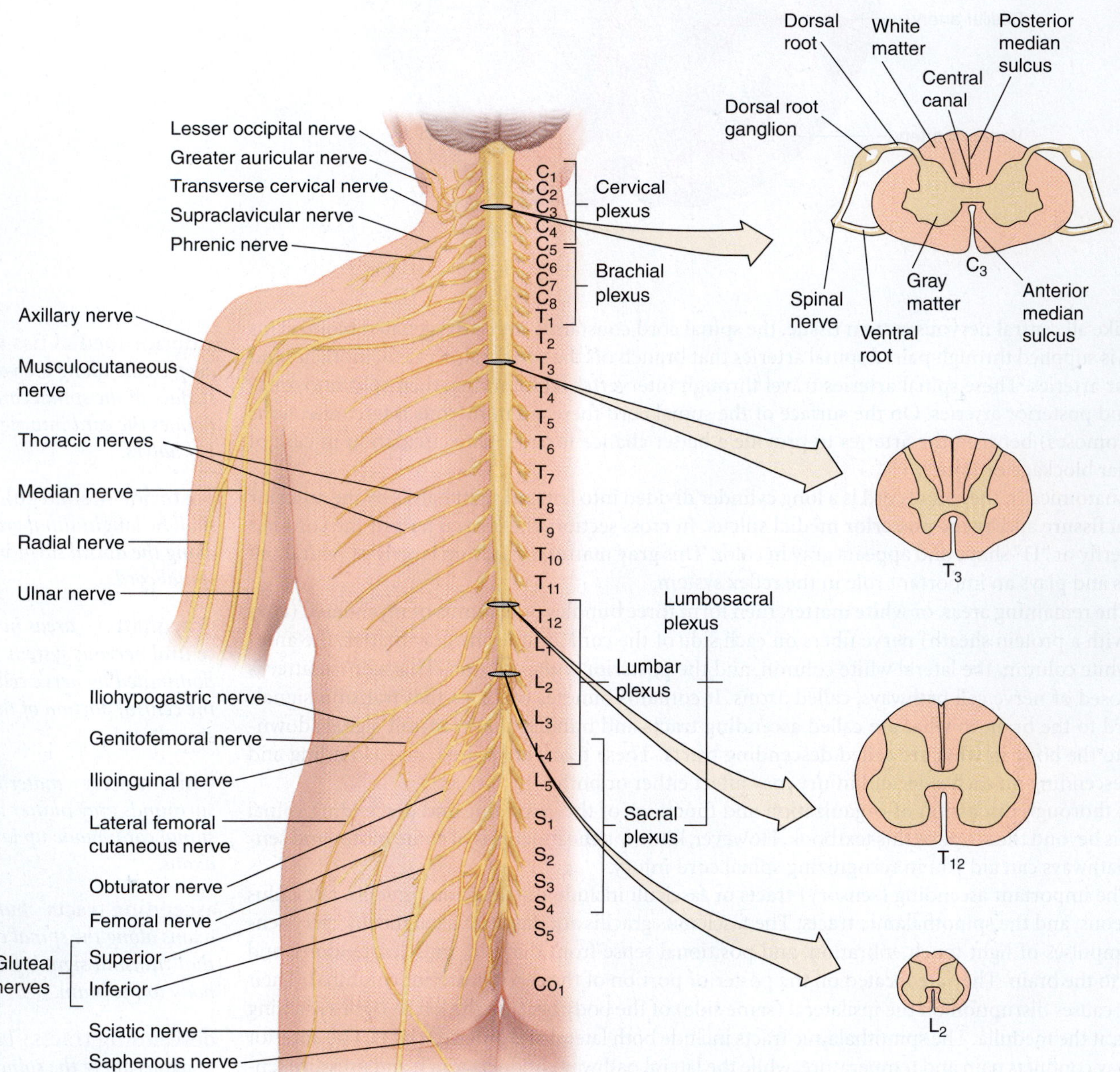

■ **Figure 3-69** The spinal cord and spinal nerves.

Table 3–3	Spinal Nerve Plexuses			
Plexus	**Origin**	**Nerve**	**Control**	**Result of Injury**
Cervical	C-1 to C-5	Phrenic	Diaphragm	Respiratory paralysis
Brachial	C-5 to C-8, T-1	Axillary	Deltoid/skin of shoulder	Deltoid muscle paralysis
		Radial	Triceps/forearm	Wristdrop
		Median	Flexor muscles, forearm, arm	Decreased usage
		Musculocutaneous	Flexor muscles of arm	Decreased usage
		Ulnar	Wrist/hand	Claw hand; inability to spread fingers
Lumbar	T-12 to L-4	Femoral	Lower abdomen, gluteus, thighs	Inability to extend leg, flex hip
		Obturator	Adductor muscles medial thigh	Decrease in usage
Sacral	L-4 to S-3	Sciatic	Lower extremity	Decreased usage

There are 31 pairs of spinal nerve roots. The first pair exits the spinal column between the skull and the first cervical vertebra. Each of the next seven pairs exits just below one of the cervical vertebrae and is identified as C-2 through C-8. (While there are only seven cervical vertebrae, there are eight cervical spinal nerves.) There are 12 pairs of thoracic nerves, 5 lumbar, 5 sacral, and 1 coccygeal. Each of these pairs originates just below the vertebra with whose name it is identified. Each spinal nerve pair has two dorsal and two ventral roots. The ventral roots carry motor impulses from the cord to the body, while the dorsal roots carry sensory impulses from the body to the cord. (C-1 and Co [coccygeal]-1 do not have dorsal [sensory] roots.)

The nerve roots often converge in a cluster of nerves called a plexus (Table 3–3). A plexus (or braiding) permits peripheral nerve roots to rejoin and function as a group. The cervical plexus, made up of the first five cervical nerve roots, innervates the neck and produces the phrenic nerve. The phrenic nerve (consisting of peripheral nerve roots C-3 through C-5) is responsible for diaphragm control. The brachial plexus joins the nerves controlling the upper extremity (C-5 through T-1). The lumbar and sacral plexuses control the innervation of the lower extremity.

The sensory components of the spinal nerves innervate specific and discrete areas of the body surface. These areas are called **dermatomes** and are distributed from the occiput of the head to the heel of the foot and buttocks (Figure 3-70 ■). Key locations to recognize for assessment include the collar region (C-3), the little finger (C-7), the nipple line (T-4), the umbilicus (T-10), and the small toe (S-1).

dermatome *topographical region of the body surface innervated by one nerve root.*

The motor components of the spinal nerve roots also innervate discrete tissues and muscles of the body in regions called **myotomes.** However, as the body grows and matures, some muscles merge and their control is not as specific as it is with the dermatomes. Key myotomes for neurologic evaluation include arm extension (C-5), elbow extension (C-7), small finger abduction (T-1), knee extension (L-3), and ankle flexion (S-1). Evaluation of areas controlled by both dermatomes and myotomes can help you identify the spinal cord region associated with an injury.

myotome *muscle and tissue of the body innervated by a spinal nerve root.*

The spinal cord also performs some primary processing functions, speeding body responses and helping the brain maintain balance and muscle tone. These responses, called reflexes, occur as special neurons in the cord, called interneurons, intercept sensory signals (Figure 3-71 ■). For example, if you touch a hot stove, the severe pain sends an intense signal to the brain. This strong signal simultaneously triggers an interneuron in the spinal cord to direct a signal to the flexor muscles telling them to contract. The limb withdraws without waiting for the signal sent to the brain to reach it, be processed, and trigger a command to be sent back to the limb. The speed of this reflex action reduces the seriousness of injury. Other reflexes help stabilize the body if it stands in one position for a length of time. As the stretch receptors report the body is moving, the interneurons signal muscles to counteract the movement to help maintain position. This again reduces the body's reaction time and allows the body to stand or maintain a steady position.

The spinal nerves can be further subdivided according to the division of the autonomic nervous system they serve and to their spinal origin. The parasympathetic nervous system controls rest and

Figure 3-70 The dermatomes. Each dermatome corresponds to a spinal nerve.

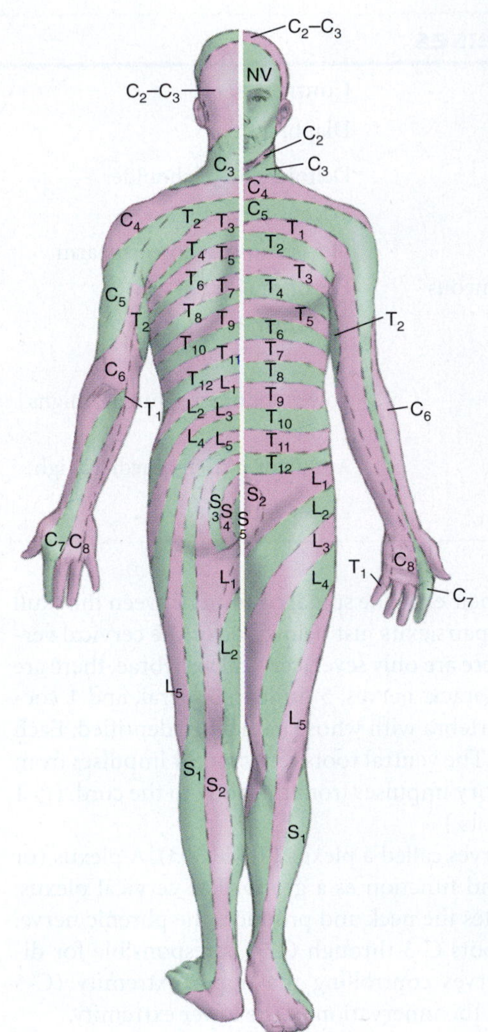

Figure 3-71 The reflex response.

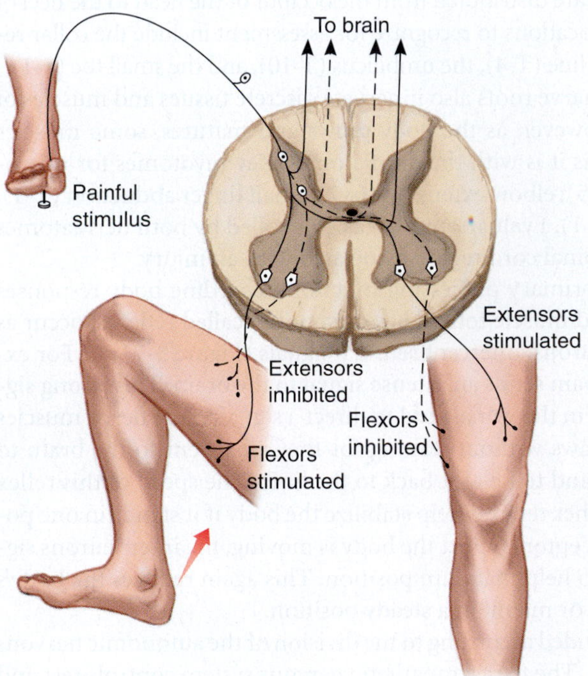

regenerative functions and consists of the peripheral nerve roots branching from the sacral region and the cranial nerves (predominantly the vagus nerve). The parasympathetic nervous system's major tasks are to slow the heart and increase digestive system activity; the system also plays a role in sexual stimulation. The sympathetic nervous system adjusts the body's metabolic rate to waking activity, provides "fight-or-flight" functions, and branches from nerves originating in the thoracic and lumbar regions. This system decreases organ and digestive activity through vasoconstriction, constricts the venous blood vessels, and affects the body's metabolic rate through the release of the adrenal hormones norepinephrine and epinephrine. In shock, the sympathetic nervous system causes systemic vasoconstriction to reduce the venous blood volume and increase peripheral vascular resistance. It also increases the heart rate to increase cardiac output in response to dropping preload and blood pressure.

THE PERIPHERAL NERVOUS SYSTEM

Consisting of the cranial and the peripheral nerves, the peripheral nervous system has both voluntary and involuntary components. The 12 pairs of **cranial nerves** originate in the brain and supply nervous control to the head, neck, and certain thoracic and abdominal organs (Figure 3-72 ■). The peripheral nerves, as described previously, originate in the spinal cord and supply nervous control to the periphery.

cranial nerves *twelve pairs of nerves that extend from the lower surface of the brain.*

The four categories of peripheral nerves are:

- ★ *Somatic sensory.* These afferent nerves transmit sensations involved in touch, pressure, pain, temperature, and position (proprioception).
- ★ *Somatic motor.* These efferent fibers carry impulses to the skeletal (voluntary) muscles.
- ★ *Visceral (autonomic) sensory.* These afferent tracts transmit sensations from the visceral organs. Sensations such as a full bladder or the need to defecate are mediated by visceral sensory fibers.
- ★ *Visceral (autonomic) motor.* These efferent fibers exit the central nervous system and branch to supply nerves to the involuntary cardiac muscle and smooth muscle of the viscera (organs) and to the glands.

Content Review

Peripheral Nervous System

- Voluntary (Somatic)
- Involuntary (Autonomic)
  - Sympathetic
  - Parasympathetic

The Somatic (Voluntary) Nervous System

The voluntary component of the peripheral nervous system, often called the somatic nervous system, is responsible for the conscious control of movement, primarily controlling the skeletal muscles.

The Autonomic (Involuntary) Nervous System

The involuntary component of the peripheral nervous system, commonly called the autonomic nervous system, is responsible for the unconscious control of many body functions, including those governed by the smooth muscle, cardiac muscle, and the glands. The two functional divisions of the autonomic nervous system are the sympathetic nervous system and the parasympathetic nervous system.

The autonomic nervous system arises from the central nervous system. The nerves of the autonomic nervous system exit the central nervous system and subsequently enter specialized structures called **autonomic ganglia.** In the autonomic ganglia, the nerve fibers from the central nervous system interact with nerve fibers that extend from the ganglia to the various target organs. Autonomic nerve fibers that exit the central nervous system and terminate in the autonomic ganglia are called **preganglionic nerves.** Autonomic nerve fibers that exit the ganglia and terminate in the various target tissues are called **postganglionic nerves.** The ganglia of the sympathetic nervous system are located close to the spinal cord, while the ganglia of the parasympathetic nervous system are located close to the target organs (Figure 3-73 ■).

autonomic ganglia *groups of autonomic nerve cells located outside the central nervous system.*

preganglionic nerves *nerve fibers that extend from the central nervous system to the autonomic ganglia.*

postganglionic nerves *nerve fibers that extend from the autonomic ganglia to the target tissues.*

The sympathetic and parasympathetic systems are antagonistic. In their normal state, they exist in balance with each other. During stress, the sympathetic system dominates. During rest, the parasympathetic system dominates.

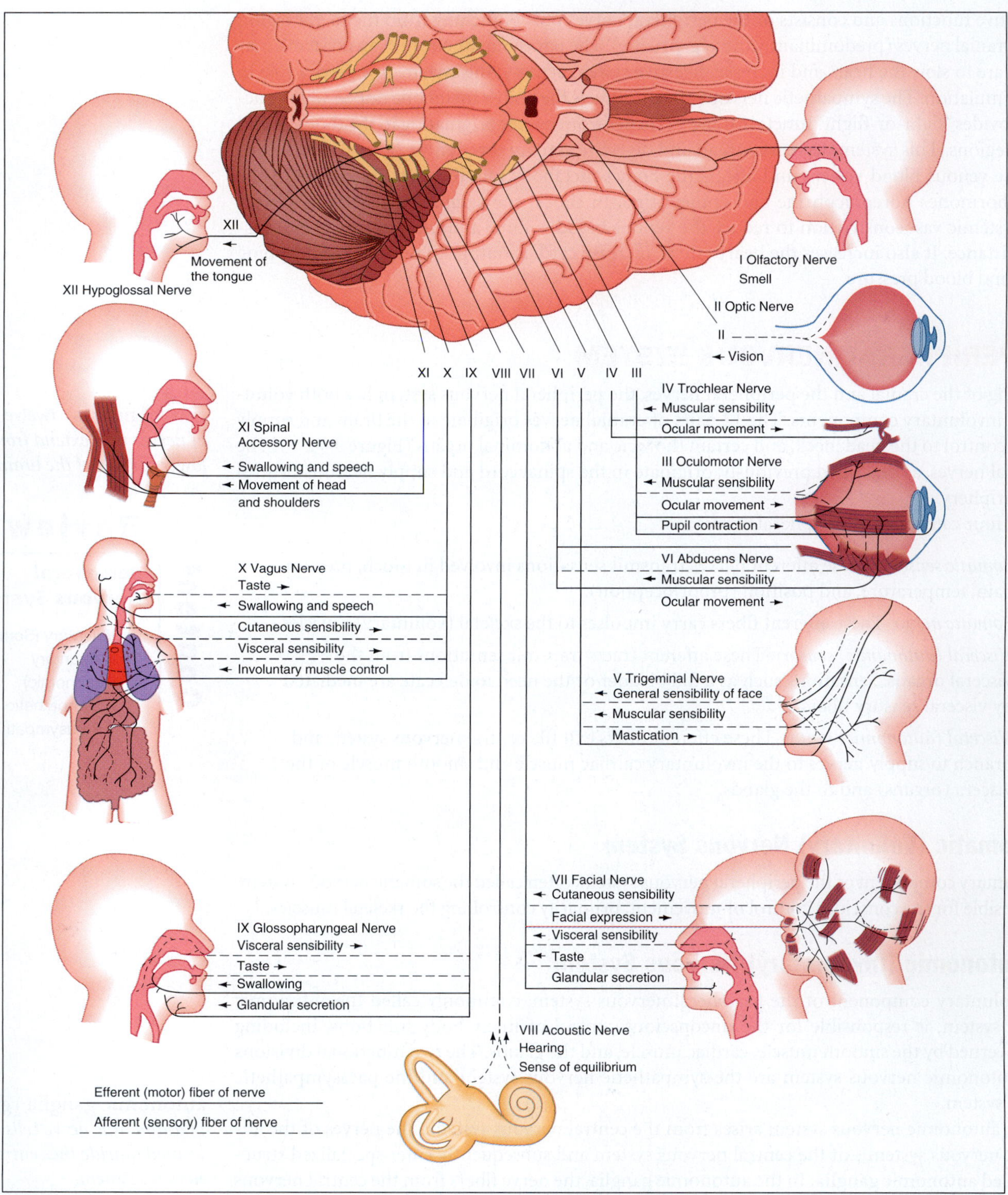

■ **Figure 3-72** The cranial nerves.

The Sympathetic Nervous System The sympathetic nervous system, often referred to as the "fight-or-flight" system, prepares the body for stressful situations. It is located near the thoracic and lumbar part of the spinal cord.

Preganglionic nerves leave the spinal cord through the spinal nerves and end in the sympathetic ganglia. There are two types of sympathetic ganglia: sympathetic chain ganglia and collateral ganglia (Figure 3-74 ■). In addition, special preganglionic sympathetic nerve fibers innervate the

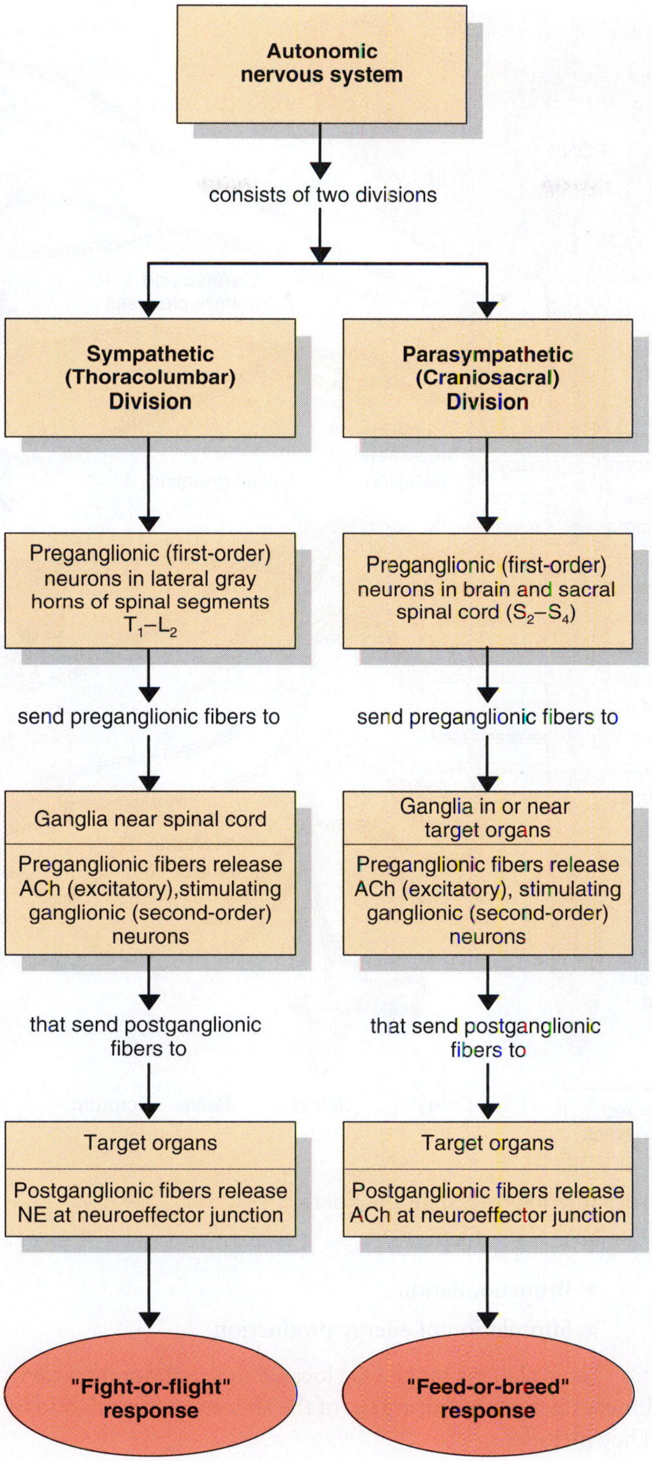

Autonomic nervous system

consists of two divisions

Sympathetic (Thoracolumbar) Division	Parasympathetic (Craniosacral) Division
Preganglionic (first-order) neurons in lateral gray horns of spinal segments T_1–L_2	Preganglionic (first-order) neurons in brain and sacral spinal cord (S_2–S_4)
send preganglionic fibers to	send preganglionic fibers to
Ganglia near spinal cord	Ganglia in or near target organs
Preganglionic fibers release ACh (excitatory),stimulating ganglionic (second-order) neurons	Preganglionic fibers release ACh (excitatory), stimulating ganglionic (second-order) neurons
that send postganglionic fibers to	that send postganglionic fibers to
Target organs	Target organs
Postganglionic fibers release NE at neuroeffector junction	Postganglionic fibers release ACh at neuroeffector junction
"Fight-or-flight" response	"Feed-or-breed" response

■ **Figure 3-73** Components of the autonomic nervous system.

adrenal medulla. Postganglionic nerves that exit the sympathetic chain ganglia extend to several peripheral target tissues of the sympathetic nervous system. When stimulated, these fibers have several effects. They include:

- ★ Stimulation of secretion by sweat glands
- ★ Constriction of blood vessels in the skin
- ★ Increase in blood flow to skeletal muscles
- ★ Increase in the heart rate and force of cardiac contractions

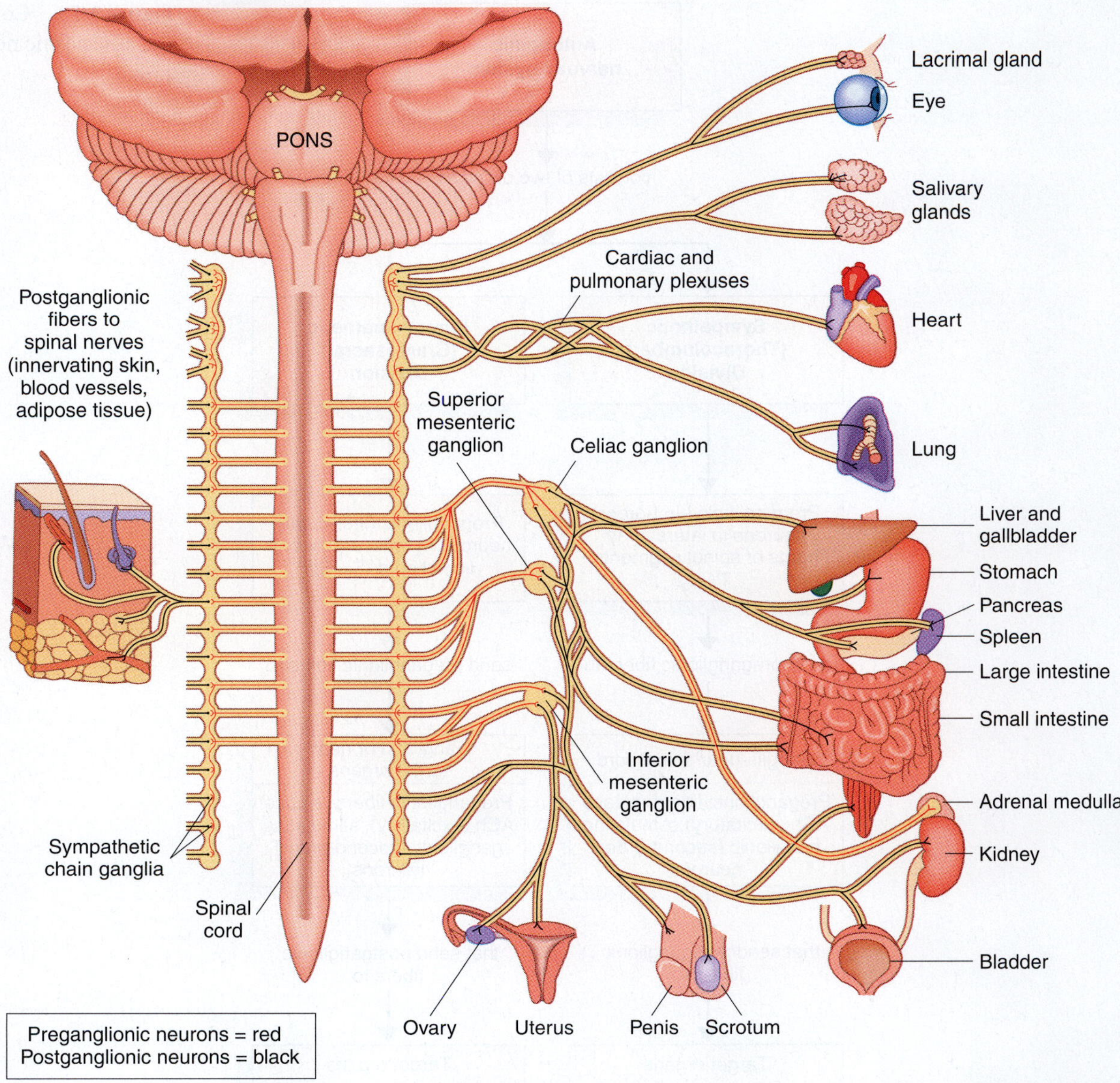

■ **Figure 3-74** Distribution of sympathetic postganglionic fibers.

- ★ Bronchodilation
- ★ Stimulation of energy production

The collateral ganglia are located in the abdominal cavity. Nerves leaving the collateral ganglia innervate many of the organs of the abdomen. Stimulation of these fibers causes several conditions. They include:

- ★ Reduction of blood flow to abdominal organs
- ★ Decreased digestive activity
- ★ Relaxation of smooth muscle in the wall of the urinary bladder
- ★ Release of glucose stores from the liver

Sympathetic nervous system stimulation also results in direct stimulation of the adrenal medulla, the inner portion of the adrenal gland (Figure 3-75 ■). The adrenal medulla in turn releases the hormones norepinephrine (noradrenalin) and epinephrine (adrenalin) into the circulatory system. Approximately 80 percent of the hormones released by the adrenal medulla are

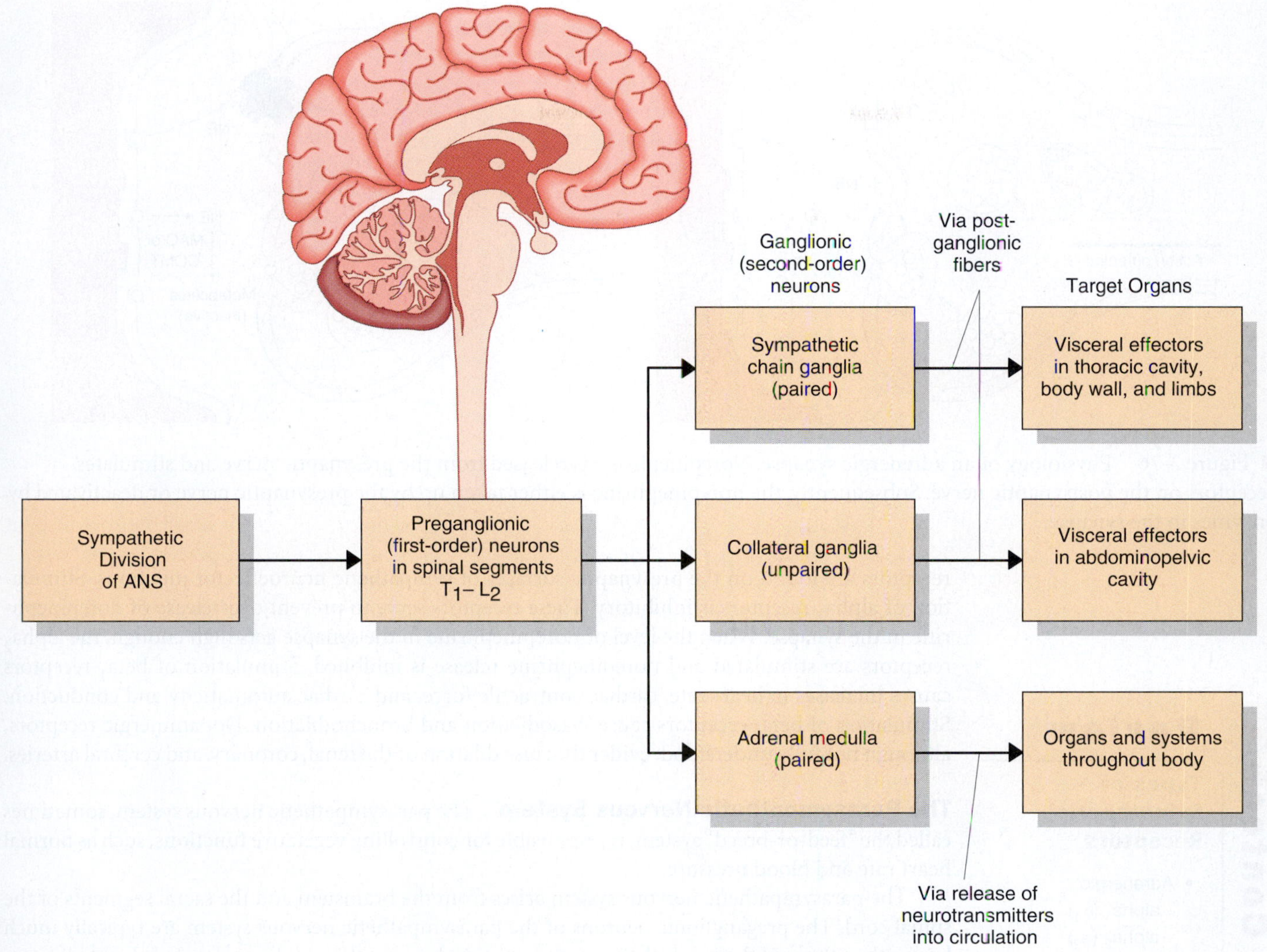

■ Figure 3-75 Organization of the sympathetic division of the autonomic nervous system.

epinephrine, while norepinephrine constitutes the remaining 20 percent. Once released, these hormones are carried throughout the body where they cause their intended effects by acting on hormone receptors. The release of norepinephrine and epinephrine by the adrenal medulla stimulates tissues that are not innervated by sympathetic nerves. In addition, it prolongs the effects of direct sympathetic stimulation. All of these effects serve to prepare the body to deal with stressful and potentially dangerous situations.

Sympathetic stimulation ultimately results in the release of the hormone norepinephrine from postganglionic, presynaptic nerves. The norepinephrine subsequently crosses the synaptic cleft and interacts with adrenergic receptors on the postsynaptic nerves. Shortly thereafter, the norepinephrine is either taken up by the presynaptic neuron for reuse or broken down by enzymes present within the synapse (Figure 3-76 ■). Sympathetic stimulation also results in the release of the hormones epinephrine and norepinephrine from the adrenal medulla. In addition, both epinephrine and norepinephrine interact with specialized adrenergic receptors on the membranes of the target organs. These receptors are located throughout the body. Once stimulated by the appropriate hormone, they cause a response in the organ or organs they control.

The two known types of sympathetic receptors are the *adrenergic receptors* and the *dopaminergic receptors.* The adrenergic receptors are generally divided into four types. These four receptors are designated alpha$_1$ (α_1), alpha$_2$ (α_2), beta$_1$ (β_1), and beta$_2$ (β_2). The α_1 receptors cause peripheral vasoconstriction, mild bronchoconstriction, and stimulation of metabolism. The alpha$_2$

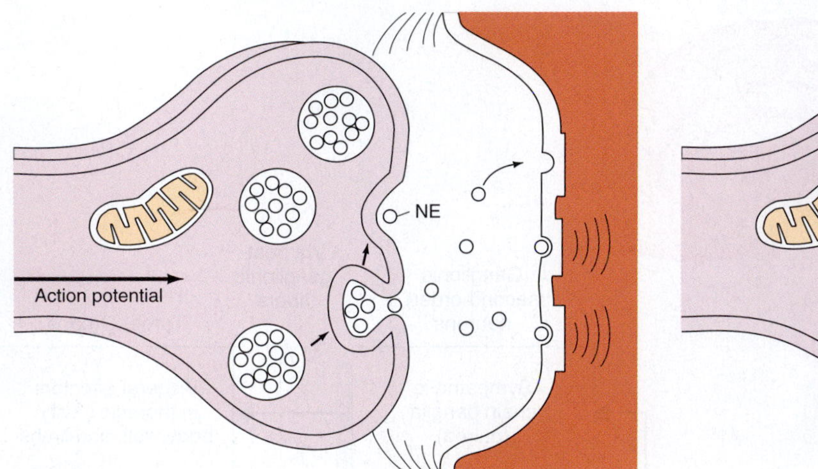

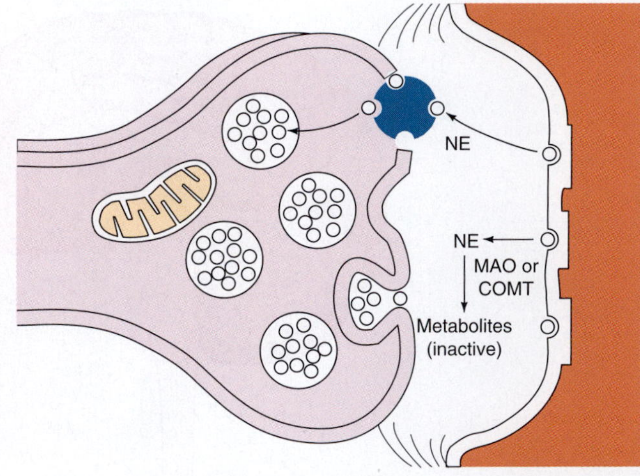

■ Figure 3-76 Physiology of an adrenergic synapse. Norepinephrine is released from the presynaptic nerve and stimulates receptors on the postsynaptic nerve. Subsequently, the norepinephrine is either taken up by the presynaptic nerve or deactivated by enzymes in the synapse.

receptors are found on the presynaptic surfaces of sympathetic neuroeffector junctions. Stimulation of $alpha_2$ receptors is inhibitory. These receptors serve to prevent overrelease of norepinephrine in the synapse. When the level of norepinephrine in the synapse gets high enough, the $alpha_2$ receptors are stimulated and norepinephrine release is inhibited. Stimulation of $beta_1$ receptors causes increases in heart rate, cardiac contractile force, and cardiac automaticity and conduction. Stimulation of $beta_2$ receptors causes vasodilation and bronchodilation. Dopaminergic receptors, although not fully understood, evidently cause dilation of the renal, coronary, and cerebral arteries.

Content Review

Types of Sympathetic Receptors

- Adrenergic
  - $alpha_1$ (α_1)
  - $alpha_2$ (α_2)
  - $beta_1$ (β_1)
  - $beta_2$ (β_2)
- Dopaminergic

The Parasympathetic Nervous System The parasympathetic nervous system, sometimes called the "feed-or-breed" system, is responsible for controlling vegetative functions, such as normal heart rate and blood pressure.

The parasympathetic nervous system arises from the brainstem and the sacral segments of the spinal cord. The preganglionic neurons of the parasympathetic nervous system are typically much longer than those of the sympathetic nervous system, because the ganglia are located close to the target tissues. Parasympathetic nerve fibers that leave the brainstem travel within four of the cranial nerves including the oculomotor nerve (III), the facial nerve (VII), the glossopharyngeal nerve (IX), and the vagus nerve (X). These fibers synapse in the parasympathetic ganglia with short postganglionic fibers that then continue to their target tissues. Postsynaptic fibers innervate much of the body, including the intrinsic eye muscles, the salivary glands, the heart, the lungs, and most of the organs of the abdominal cavity. The sacral segment of the parasympathetic nervous system forms distinct pelvic nerves that innervate ganglia in the kidneys, bladder, sex organs, and the terminal portions of the large intestine (Figure 3-77 ■). Stimulation of the parasympathetic nervous system results in the following conditions:

Content Review

Cranial Nerves Carrying Parasympathetic Fibers

- III
- VII
- IX
- X

★ Pupillary constriction

★ Secretion by digestive glands

★ Reduction in heart rate and cardiac contractile force

★ Bronchoconstriction

★ Increased smooth muscle activity along the digestive tract

These and other functions facilitate the processing of food, energy absorption, relaxation, and reproduction (Figure 3-78 ■).

All preganglionic and postganglionic parasympathetic nerve fibers use acetylcholine as a neurotransmitter. Acetylcholine, when released by presynaptic neurons, crosses the synaptic cleft and activates receptors on the postsynaptic neurons or on the neuroeffector junction. Acetylcholine is also the neurotransmitter for the somatic nervous system and is present in the neuromuscular junction. Acetylcholine is very short-lived. Within a fraction of a second after its release, it is deactivated

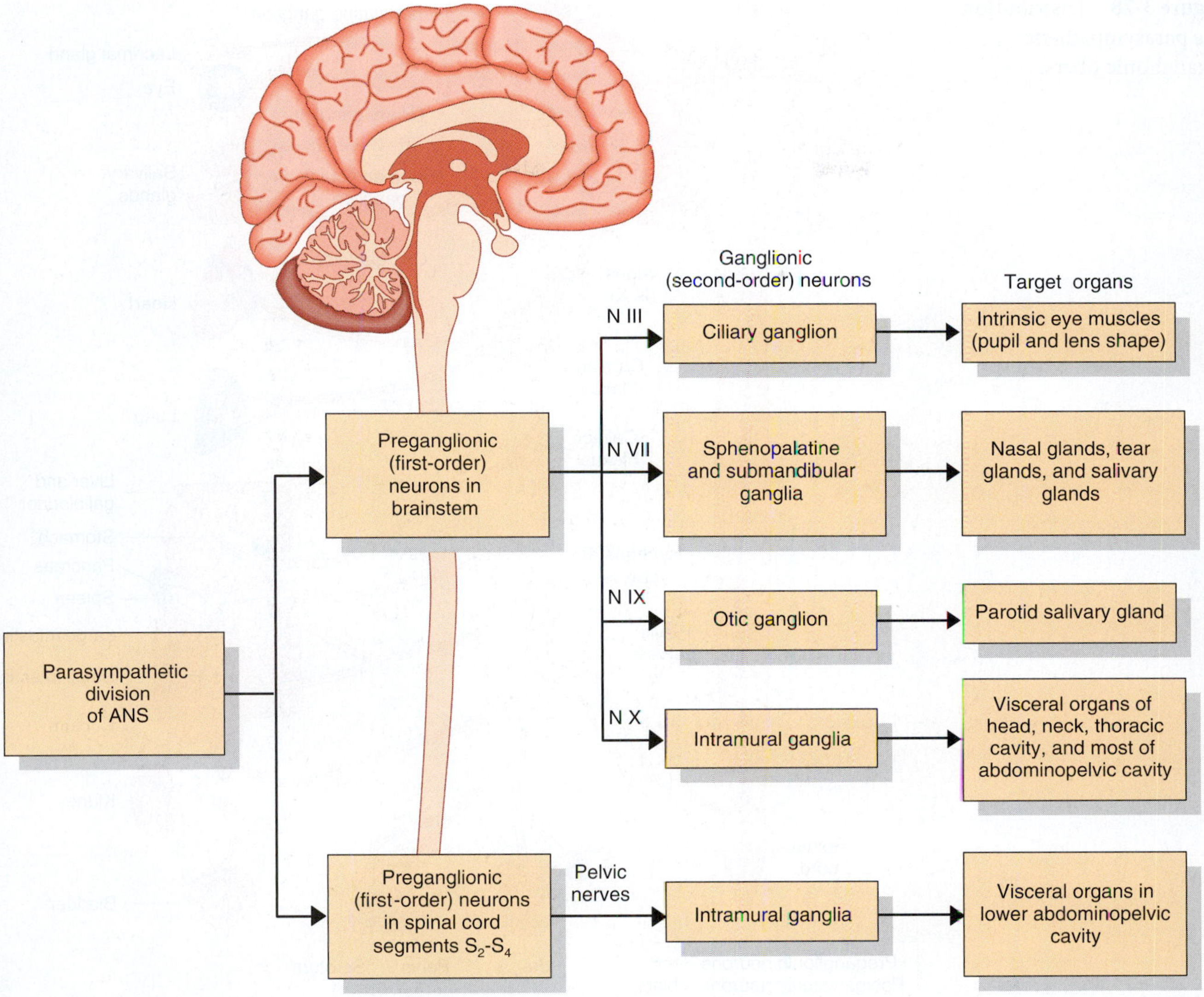

Ganglionic (second-order) neurons

Target organs

Parasympathetic division of ANS

Preganglionic (first-order) neurons in brainstem

N III → Ciliary ganglion → Intrinsic eye muscles (pupil and lens shape)

N VII → Sphenopalatine and submandibular ganglia → Nasal glands, tear glands, and salivary glands

N IX → Otic ganglion → Parotid salivary gland

N X → Intramural ganglia → Visceral organs of head, neck, thoracic cavity, and most of abdominopelvic cavity

Preganglionic (first-order) neurons in spinal cord segments S_2-S_4

Pelvic nerves → Intramural ganglia → Visceral organs in lower abdominopelvic cavity

■ **Figure 3-77** Organization of the parasympathetic division of the autonomic nervous system.

by another chemical called acetylcholinesterase. Acetic acid and choline, which are produced when acetylcholine is deactivated, are taken back up by the presynaptic neuron (Figure 3-79 ■).

The parasympathetic system has two main types of ACh receptors, nicotinic and muscarinic. Knowing these receptors' locations and functions will greatly simplify learning the functions of drugs in this class. Nicotinic$_N$ (neuron) receptors are found in all autonomic ganglia, where acetylcholine serves as the presynaptic neurotransmitter of both the parasympathetic and sympathetic nervous systems. Nicotinic$_M$ (muscle) receptors are found at the neuromuscular junction and initiate muscular contraction as part of the somatic nervous system. Muscarinic receptors are found in many organs throughout the body and are primarily responsible for promoting the parasympathetic response. Table 3–4 summarizes the locations and actions of the muscarinic receptors.

THE ENDOCRINE SYSTEM

There are eight major glands in the endocrine system: the hypothalamus, pituitary gland, thyroid gland, parathyroid glands, thymus, pancreas, adrenal glands, and gonads. The pineal gland is also an endocrine gland, but much of its function remains unclear. In addition to the endocrine glands, many body tissues have been found to have endocrine function. These include the kidneys, heart, placenta, and parts of the digestive tract.

Content Review

Endocrine Glands

- Hypothalamus
- Pituitary
- Thyroid
- Parathyroid
- Thymus
- Pancreas
- Adrenals
- Gonads
- Pineal

■ **Figure 3-78** Distribution of the parasympathetic postganglionic fibers.

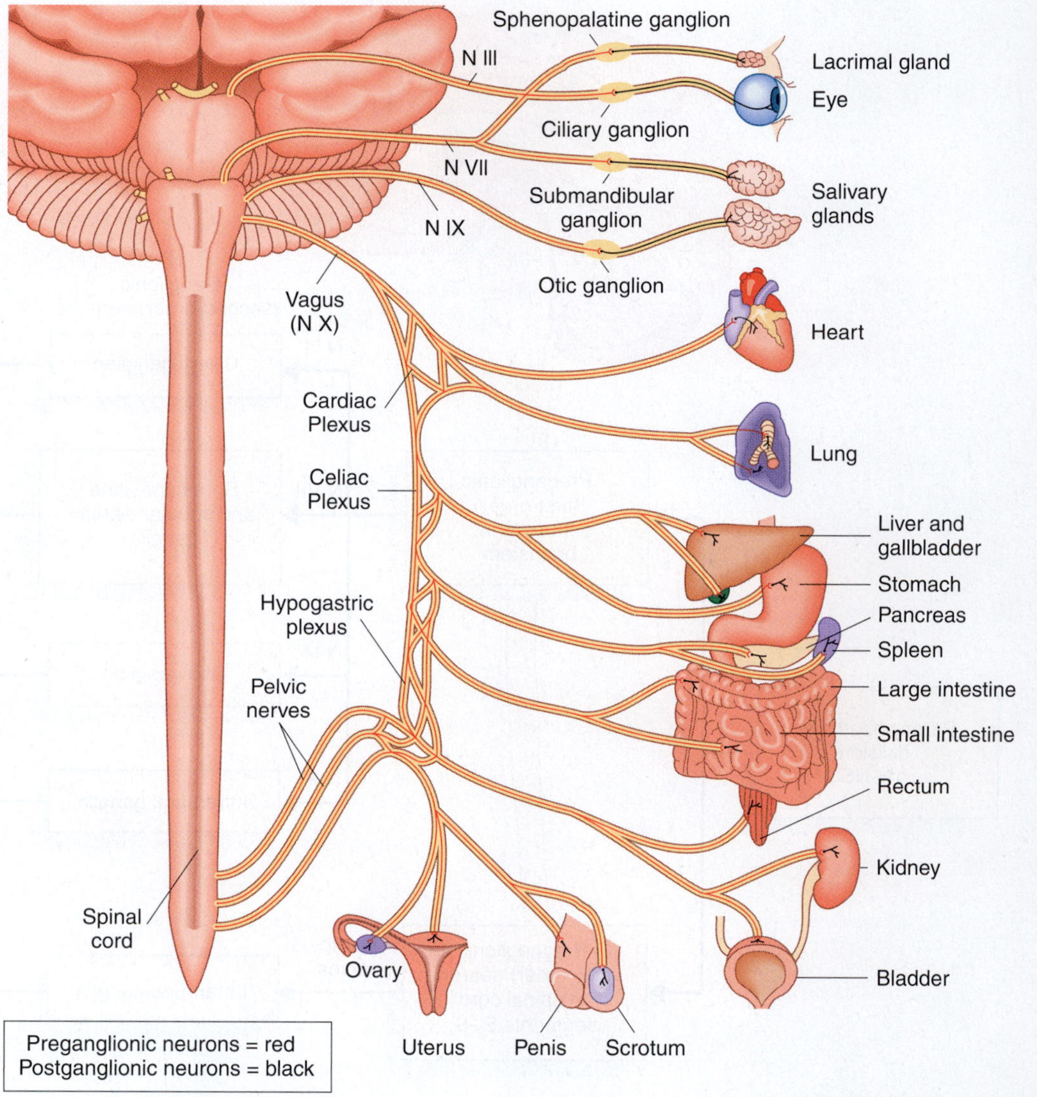

Preganglionic neurons = red
Postganglionic neurons = black

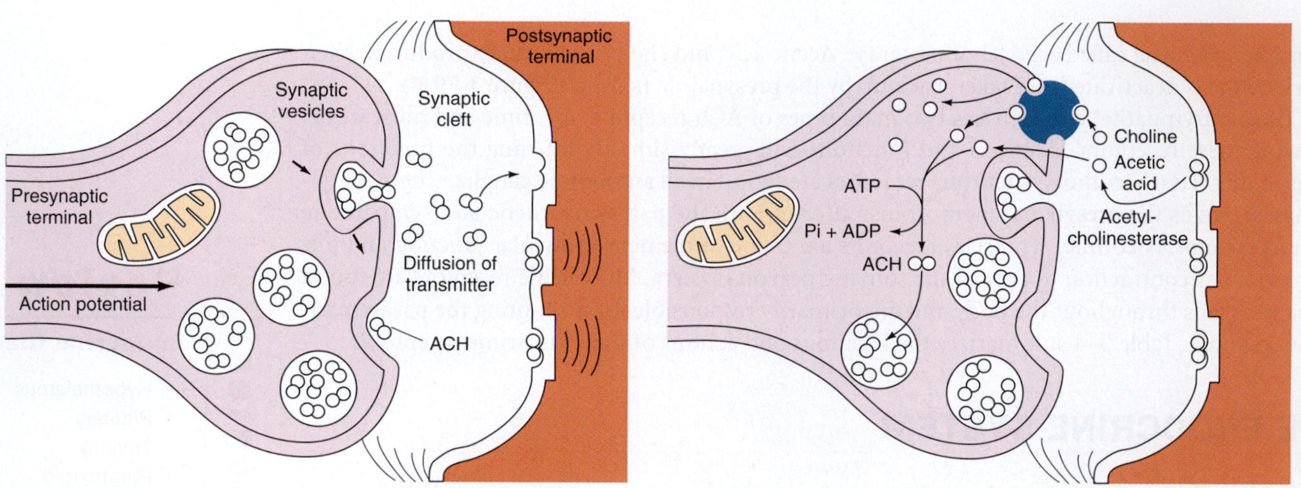

■ **Figure 3-79** Physiology of a cholinergic synapse. Acetylcholine is released from the presynaptic nerve and stimulates receptors on the postsynaptic nerve. Subsequently, acetylcholinesterase breaks down the acetylcholine and the presynaptic nerve fiber takes up the products.

Table 3–4	Location and Effect of Muscarinic Receptors	
Organ	**Functions**	**Location**
Heart	Decreased heart rate	Sinoatrial node
	Decreased conduction rate	Atrioventricular node
Arterioles	Dilation	Coronary
	Dilation	Skin and mucosa
	Dilation	Cerebral
GI tract	Relaxed	Sphincters
	Increased	Motility
	Increased salivation	Salivary glands
	Increased secretion	Exocrine glands
Lungs	Bronchoconstriction	Bronchiole smooth muscle
	Increased mucus production	Bronchial glands
Gallbladder	Contraction	
Urinary bladder	Relaxation	Urinary sphincter
	Contraction	Detrusor muscle
Liver	Glycogen synthesis	
Lacrimal glands	Secretion (increased tearing)	Eye
Eye	Contraction for near vision	Ciliary muscle
	Constriction	Pupil
Penis	Erection	

The endocrine glands are located throughout the body (Figure 3-80 ■). Although the figure shows an adult, remember that the thymus is primarily active during childhood, when it plays a role in maturation of the immune system. By adulthood, the thymus is so small that it is not visualized on chest X-rays. The hormones secreted by endocrine glands, their target tissues, and their effects are listed in Table 3–5.

HYPOTHALAMUS

The *hypothalamus* is located deep within the cerebrum of the brain. Hypothalamic cells act both as nerve cells, or neurons, and as gland cells. The hypothalamus is the junction, or connection, between the central nervous system and the endocrine system. As neurons, many hypothalamic cells receive messages from the autonomic nervous system—peripheral nerves that, among other functions, detect internal conditions such as blood pressure or blood glucose level and convey that information to the central nervous system through nerve impulses. Some hypothalamic cells respond by producing nerve impulses that travel to cells in the posterior pituitary gland. Other hypothalamic cells respond as gland cells by producing and releasing hormones into the stalk of tissue that connects the hypothalamus and the anterior pituitary gland.

In response to impulses from the autonomic nervous system, the hypothalamus—and other organs of the endocrine system—can release the hormones that promote homeostasis:

- ★ *Growth hormone releasing hormone (GHRH)*
- ★ *Growth hormone inhibiting hormone (GHIH)*
- ★ *Corticotropin releasing hormone (CRH)*
- ★ *Thyrotropin releasing hormone (TRH)*
- ★ *Gonadotropin releasing hormone (GnRH)*

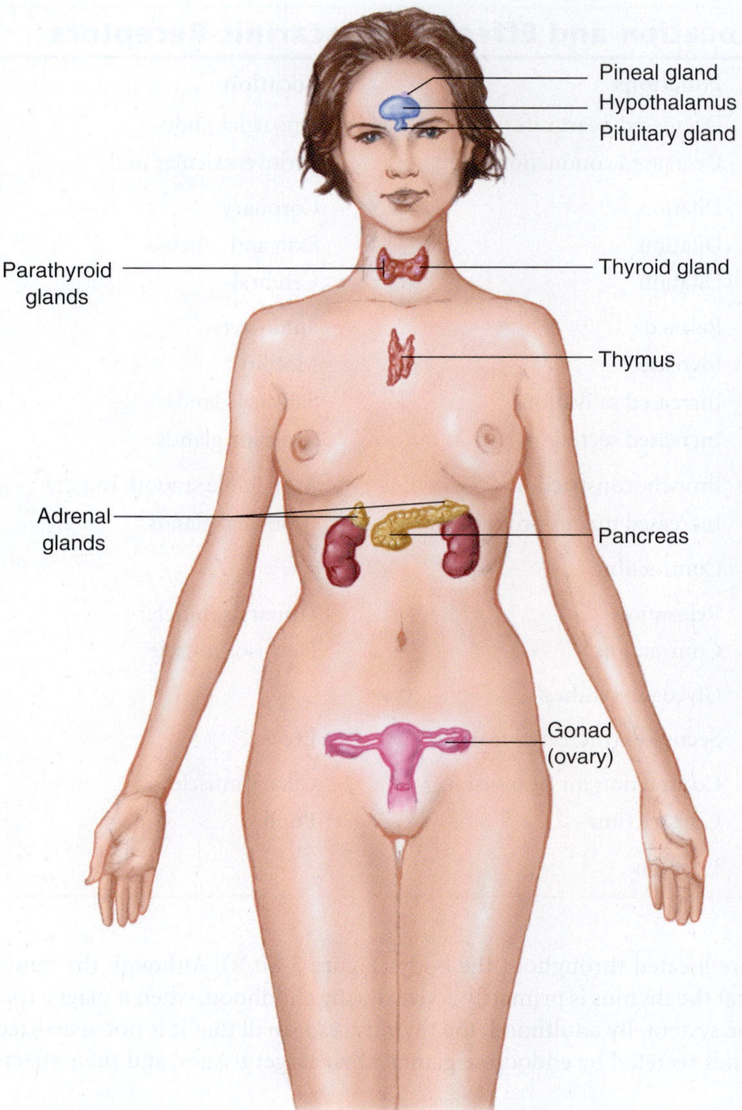

■ **Figure 3-80** The major glands of the endocrine system.

★ *Prolactin releasing hormone (PRH)*

★ *Prolactin inhibiting hormone (PIH)*

As shown in Table 3–5, most hypothalamic hormones, including thyrotropin releasing hormone (TRH) and growth hormone releasing hormone (GHRH), stimulate secretion of pituitary hormones that rouse yet another endocrine gland or body tissue to increased activity. For example, in response to TRH the anterior pituitary releases thyroid stimulating hormone, and thyroid stimulating hormone then acts on the thyroid gland to increase thyroid activity.

The pair of hypothalamic hormones—growth hormone releasing hormone (GHRH) and growth hormone inhibitory hormone (GHIH)—demonstrate a major trait of endocrine function: Many hormonal activities are driven not by one hormone, but by two hormones with opposing effects. GHRH stimulates secretion of growth hormone, and GHIH suppresses secretion of growth hormone. The actual amount of growth hormone secreted by the anterior pituitary depends on the net amount of stimulation (Figure 3-81 ■).

PITUITARY GLAND

The *pituitary gland* is only about the size of a pea. It is divided into posterior and anterior pituitary lobes. These tissues have different embryonic origins and different functional relationships with the hypothalamus. The *posterior pituitary gland* responds to nerve impulses from the hypothalamus,

Table 3–5 Endocrine System: Glands, Hormones, Target Tissues, Hormone Effects

Gland and Major Hormone(s)	Target Tissues	Major Hormone Effect(s)
Hypothalamus		
Growth hormone releasing hormone, GHRH	Anterior pituitary	Stimulates release of growth hormone
Growth hormone inhibiting hormone, GHIH (or somatostatin)	Anterior pituitary	Suppresses release of growth hormone
Corticotropin releasing hormone, CRH	Anterior pituitary	Stimulates release of adrenocorticotropin
Thyrotropin releasing hormone, TRH	Anterior pituitary	Stimulates release of thyroid-stimulating hormone
Gonadotropin releasing hormone, GnRH	Anterior pituitary	Stimulates release of luteinizing hormone and follicle stimulating hormone
Prolactin releasing hormone, PRH	Anterior pituitary	Stimulates release of prolactin
Prolactin inhibiting hormone, PIH	Anterior pituitary	Suppresses release of prolactin
Posterior Pituitary Gland		
Antidiuretic hormone, ADH	Kidneys	Stimulates increased reabsorption of water into blood volume
Oxytocin	Uterus and breasts of females, kidneys	Stimulates uterine contractions and milk release
Anterior Pituitary Gland		
Growth hormone, GH	All cells, especially growing cells	Stimulates body growth in childhood; causes switch to fats as energy source
Adrenocorticotropic hormone, ACTH	Adrenal cortexes	Stimulates release of corticosteroidal hormones cortisol and aldosterone
Thyroid-stimulating hormone, TSH	Thyroid	Stimulates release of thyroid hormones thyroxine and triiodothyronine
Follicle-stimulating hormone, FSH	Ovaries or testes	FSH stimulates development of sex cells (ovum or sperm)
Luteinizing hormone, LH	Ovaries or testes	LH stimulates release of hormones (estrogen, progesterone, or testosterone)
Prolactin, PRL	Mammary glands	Stimulates production and release of milk
Thyroid Gland		
Thyroxine, T_4	All cells	Stimulates cell metabolism
Triiodothyronine, T_3	All cells	Stimulates cell metabolism
Calcitonin	All cells	Stimulates calcium uptake by bones, decreasing blood calcium level
Parathyroid Glands		
Parathyroid hormone, PTH	Bone, intestine, kidneys	Stimulates calcium release from bone, calcium uptake from GI tract, calcium reabsorption in kidney, all increasing blood calcium level
Thymus		
Thymosin	White blood cells, primarily T lymphocytes	Stimulates reproduction and functional development of T lymphocytes

(Continued)

Table 3–5 Endocrine System: Glands, Hormones, Target Tissues, Hormone Effects *(Continued)*

Gland and Major Hormone(s)	Target Tissues	Major Hormone Effect(s)
Pancreas		
Glucagon	All cells, particularly in liver, muscle, and fat	Stimulates hepatic glycogenolysis and gluconeogenesis, increasing blood glucose level
Insulin	All cells, particularly in liver, muscle, and fat	Stimulates cellular uptake of glucose, increased rate of synthesis of glycogen, proteins, and fats, decreasing blood glucose level
Somatostatin	Alpha and Beta cells in the pancreas	Suppresses secretion of glucagon and insulin within islets of Langerhans
Adrenal Medulla		
Epinephrine (or adrenaline)	Muscle, liver, cardiovascular system	Stimulates features of "Fight-or-Flight" response to stress
Norepinephrine	Muscle, liver, cardiovascular system	Stimulates vasoconstriction
Adrenal Cortex		
Glucocorticoids		
Cortisol	Most cells, particularly white blood cells (cells responsible for inflammatory and immune responses)	Stimulates glucagonlike effects, acts as anti-inflammatory and immuno-suppressive agent
Mineralocorticoids		
Aldosterone	Kidneys, blood	Contributes to salt and fluid balance by stimulating kidneys to increase potassium excretion and decrease sodium excretion, increasing blood volume
Androgenic hormones		
Estrogen	Most cells	See effects under Gonads (Ovaries and Testes)
Progesterone	Uterus	
Testosterone	Most cells	
Ovaries		
Estrogen	Most cells, particularly those of female reproductive tract	Stimulates development of secondary sexual characteristics, plays role in maturation of egg prior to ovulation
Progesterone	Uterus	Stimulates uterine changes necessary for successful pregnancy
Testes		
Testosterone	Most cells, particularly those of male reproductive tract	Stimulates development of secondary sexual characteristics; plays role in development of sperm cells
Pineal Gland		
Melatonin	Exact action unknown	Releases melatonin in response to light; may help determine daily, lunar, and reproductive cycles; may affect mood

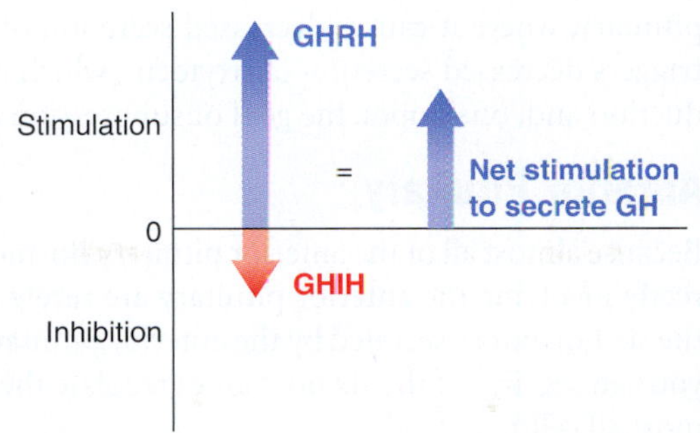

■ **Figure 3-81** Regulation by hormone pairs. The net level of stimulation created by the opposing actions of growth hormone releasing hormone (GHRH) and growth hormone inhibitory hormone (GHIH) determines the amount of growth hormone (GH) secreted by the anterior pituitary.

whereas the *anterior pituitary gland* responds to hypothalamic hormones that travel down the stalk that connects the anterior pituitary and hypothalamus. As you look at the target tissues of the anterior pituitary in Table 3–5, you will understand why physiologists once thought of the pituitary gland as the "master gland." Its hormones have a direct impact on endocrine glands throughout the body. The term is used little today, because the dependence of the pituitary on the hypothalamus has been made clear.

As noted, the pituitary gland has two lobes, the posterior and the anterior.

Posterior Pituitary

The posterior pituitary produces two hormones:

- ★ *Antidiuretic hormone (ADH)*—causes retention of body water
- ★ *Oxytocin*—causes uterine contraction and lactation

Antidiuretic hormone (ADH), also known as vasopressin, causes the kidneys to increase water reabsorption. This retention of water, or antidiuretic effect, results in increased circulating blood volume and decreased urine volume. Increased secretion of ADH is part of the homeostatic mechanism that can counteract losses of blood volume up to about 25 percent. Clinically, you will see increased ADH secretion in early shock states associated with dehydration or hemorrhage. Note that the opposite effect, decreased secretion of ADH, occurs after ingestion of alcohol and when there is a significant rise in circulating blood volume.

Although it is unlikely that a disorder in ADH secretion will present as a medical emergency, you should understand such endocrine dysfunction when patients discuss their medical histories. *Diabetes insipidus,* a disorder marked by large volumes of urine, is caused by inadequate ADH secretion relative to blood volume. The resultant reduction of blood volume, or diuretic effect, appears as excessive urine production. In a 24-hour period, the kidneys normally produce 1 to 1.5 liters of urine. In diabetes insipidus, it is not uncommon for urine output to increase to almost 20 liters per day. You can remember the characteristic urine presentation of diabetes insipidus by remembering that dilute urine has an insipid, or neutral, odor (and taste).

Oxytocin, the natural form of the drug Pitocin, stimulates uterine contraction and lactation in women who have just delivered a baby. Oxytocin actually causes the "letdown" of milk by stimulating contractile cells within the mammary glands. An infant suckling at the breast stimulates receptors in the nipples that causes the release of oxytocin from the posterior pituitary. This, in turn, causes discharge of milk so that the infant can feed. Following delivery, it is recommended that the infant be placed on the breast to suckle, thus stimulating the release of oxytocin. In addition to stimulating milk letdown, the oxytocin stimulates uterine contraction, which can help minimize postpartum bleeding.

In both sexes, oxytocin has a mild antidiuretic effect, which is similar to that of ADH due to their chemical similarity. The relationship between oxytocin and ADH has direct application to emergency medicine. Women in preterm labor are often given an IV fluid bolus in an attempt to suppress uterine contractions without the use of drugs. This works in the following way: The administration of an IV fluid bolus causes an increase in circulating blood volume, which is detected by autonomic nerves in the kidneys. An impulse is sent through the hypothalamus to the posterior pituitary, where it causes decreased secretion of ADH. This inhibition of ADH secretion in turn triggers decreased secretion of oxytocin, which contributes to the observed increase in urine production and, one hopes, the goal of suppression of preterm labor.

Anterior Pituitary

Because almost all of the anterior pituitary hormones regulate other endocrine glands, disorders directly involving the anterior pituitary are rarely a factor in endocrine emergencies. Table 3–5 lists the six hormones secreted by the anterior pituitary, as well as target tissues and hormone effects. As you can see, five of the six hormones regulate the activity of target glands, while the sixth affects almost all cells:

Five anterior pituitary hormones affect target glands.

- ★ *Adrenocorticotropic hormone (ACTH)*—targets the adrenal cortexes
- ★ *Thyroid-stimulating hormone (TSH)*—targets the thyroid
- ★ *Follicle-stimulating hormone (FSH)*—targets the gonads, or sex organs
- ★ *Luteinizing hormone (LH)*—also targets the gonads
- ★ *Prolactin (PRL)*—targets the mammary glands of women

The sixth anterior pituitary hormone has a broader effect.

- ★ *Growth hormone (GH)*—targets almost all body cells

GH has its most significant effects in children because it is the primary stimulant of skeletal growth. In adults, GH has several physiologic effects, but the most significant is metabolic. GH causes adipose cells to release their stored fats into the blood and causes body cells to switch from glucose to fats as the primary energy source. The net effect is that the body uses up fat stores and conserves its sugar stores.

THYROID GLAND

The two lobes of the *thyroid gland* are located in the neck anterior to and just below the cartilage of the larynx, with one lobe on either side of the midline. The two lobes are connected by a small isthmus, or band of tissue, that crosses the trachea at the level of the cricoid cartilage. The thyroid produces three hormones:

- ★ *Thyroxine (T_4)*—stimulates cell metabolism
- ★ *Triiodothyronine (T_3)*—stimulates cell metabolism
- ★ *Calcitonin*—lowers blood calcium levels

The thyroid is composed of tiny hollow sacs called follicles, which are filled with a thick fluid called *colloid*. The hormones *thyroxine (T_4)* and *triiodothyronine (T_3)* are produced within the colloid. When stimulated by the pituitary hormone TSH or by environmental conditions such as cold, the thyroid gland releases these hormones to increase the general rate of cell metabolism.

The thyroid gland also contains perifollicular cells called C cells which produce a different hormone, *calcitonin*. Calcitonin lowers blood calcium levels by increasing uptake of calcium by bones and inhibiting breakdown of bone tissue. Parathyroid hormone has the opposite, or antagonistic, effect on the blood calcium level, which is covered in the following discussion of the parathyroid glands.

Disorders of excessive or deficient production of thyroid hormones T_4 and T_3 are called hyperthyroidism and hypothyroidism, respectively.

PARATHYROID GLANDS

Each *parathyroid gland* is very small, with a maximum diameter of 5 mm and weight of only 35–40 mg. Normally, four parathyroid glands are located on the posterior lateral surfaces of the thyroid, one pair above the other. Sometimes there are more than four parathyroid glands, but only rarely are there fewer. The parathyroid glands secrete:

- ★ *Parathyroid hormone (PTH)*—increases blood calcium levels

PTH increases blood calcium levels through actions on three different target tissues. In bone, the primary target, PTH causes release of calcium into the blood. In the intestines, PTH converts vitamin D into its active form, causing increased absorption of calcium. In the kidneys, PTH causes increased reabsorption of calcium. PTH is the antagonist of calcitonin, and the balance of PTH and calcitonin determines the level of blood calcium. The parathyroid glands rarely cause clinical problems. However, they can be accidentally damaged or removed during surgery or they may be damaged if the thyroid gland is irradiated. In either case, the loss of parathyroid function may result in hypocalcemia, low blood calcium levels.

THYMUS GLAND

The *thymus* is in the mediastinum just behind the sternum. It is fairly large in children but shrinks into a small remnant of fat and fibrous tissue in adults. Although the thymus is usually considered a lymphatic organ on the basis of its anatomy, its most important function is as an endocrine gland: During childhood, it secretes:

★ *Thymosin*—promotes maturation of T lymphocytes

Thymosin is critical to maturation of T lymphocytes, the cells responsible for cell-mediated immunity. The T of T lymphocyte stands for thymus.

PANCREAS

The *pancreas,* located in the upper retroperitoneum behind the stomach and between the duodenum and spleen, is composed of both endocrine and exocrine tissues. The exocrine tissues, known as acini, secrete digestive enzymes essential to digestion of fats and proteins into a duct that empties into the small intestine.

The microscopic clusters of endocrine tissue found within the pancreas are known as *islets of Langerhans.* Although 1 to 2 million islets are interspersed throughout the pancreas, they comprise only about 2 percent of its total mass. The three most important types of endocrine cells in the islets of Langerhans are termed *alpha* (α), *beta* (β), and *delta* (δ) (Figure 3-82 ■). Each type produces and secretes a different hormone. In addition, the islets contain a much smaller number of cells called polypeptide cells. These cells produce pancreatic polypeptide (PP), the function of which is still unclear.

The alpha and beta cells produce two hormones essential for homeostasis of blood glucose:

★ *Glucagon*—increases blood glucose

★ *Insulin*—decreases blood glucose

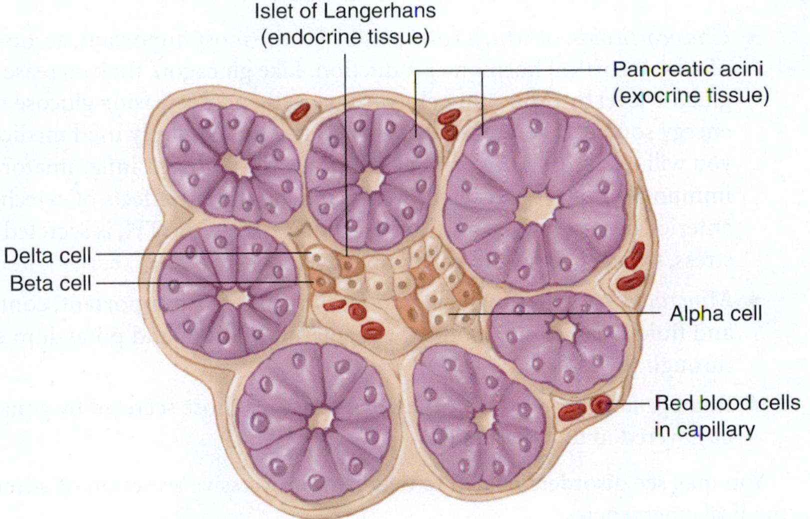

■ **Figure 3-82** The internal anatomy of the pancreas.

glycogenolysis *the breakdown of glycogen to glucose, primarily by liver cells.*

gluconeogenesis *conversion of protein and fat to form glucose.*

Approximately 25 percent of islet tissue is made up of alpha cells. Alpha cells produce the hormone *glucagon.* When blood glucose level falls, alpha cells increase secretion of glucagon. Glucagon stimulates breakdown of glycogen, the complex carbohydrate that is the storage form of glucose, into individual glucose molecules that are released into the blood. This process, called **glycogenolysis,** takes place in more than one tissue, but activity in the liver is by far the most important in raising blood glucose level.

The liver is the largest and heaviest of the internal organs and so it has many cells that can contain glycogen. In addition, liver cells have the greatest capacity to store glycogen—liver cells can store 5 to 8 percent of their weight as glycogen. Compare this with the capacity of skeletal muscle (1 to 3 percent), another important storage tissue in the body. In addition to stimulating glycogenolysis, the hormone glucagon also stimulates liver breakdown of body proteins and fats with subsequent chemical conversion to glucose. This second process, which produces glucose from nonsugar sources, is called **gluconeogenesis.** Both processes contribute to homeostasis by raising the blood glucose level.

Beta cells make up about 60 percent of islet tissue, and they produce the hormone *insulin.* Insulin is the antagonist of glucagon: Insulin lowers the blood glucose level by increasing the uptake of glucose by body cells. In addition, insulin promotes energy storage in the body by increasing the synthesis of glycogen, protein, and fat. Because the liver removes circulating insulin within 10 to 15 minutes from time of secretion, it must be secreted constantly to sustain an appropriate balance of glucagon and insulin—a balance that results in a steady supply of glucose for immediate use as an energy source and for appropriate energy storage. Loss of functional beta cells leads to increased blood glucose levels as seen in diabetes.

Delta cells, which comprise about 10 percent of islet tissue, produce *somatostatin.* This hormone acts within islets to inhibit secretion of glucagon and insulin. Somatostatin also retards nutrient absorption from the intestines, although its mechanisms of action in the gut are poorly understood. As you look at Table 3–5, note that somatostatin is the same substance as growth hormone inhibiting hormone (GHIH).

ADRENAL GLANDS

The paired *adrenal glands* are located on the superior surface of the kidneys. Each gland has two distinct anatomical divisions with different functions. The inner portion of the adrenal gland is called the *adrenal medulla,* and its cells behave both as nerve cells and as gland cells. The adrenal medulla is intimately related to the sympathetic component of the autonomic nervous system. When sympathetic nerves carry an impulse into the adrenal medulla, its cells respond by secreting the catecholamine hormones *epinephrine* (or adrenalin) and *norepinephrine* into the bloodstream. The outer portion of the adrenal gland is called the *adrenal cortex,* and it consists of endocrine tissue. The adrenal cortex secretes three classes of steroidal hormones that differ only slightly in chemical structure but have very distinct effects in the body:

- ★ *Glucocorticoids,* of which *cortisol* is by far the most important, account for 95 percent of adrenocortical hormone production. Like glucagon, they increase the blood glucose level by promoting gluconeogenesis and decreasing glucose utilization as an energy source. If you recall that cortisone is a commonly used medical glucocorticoid, you will realize that this class of hormones also inhibits inflammatory reactions and immune-system responses, as well as potentiates the effects of catecholamines. The anterior pituitary hormone that promotes release, ACTH, is secreted in response to stress, trauma, or serious infection.
- ★ *Mineralocorticoids,* of which *aldosterone* is the most important, contribute to salt and fluid balance in the body by regulating sodium and potassium excretion through the kidneys.
- ★ *Androgenic* hormones have the same effects as those secreted by gonads, and they will be covered in that discussion.

You may see disorders related to deficient or excessive secretion of adrenal hormones present as medical emergencies.

GONADS

Some differences in the *gonads* are obvious: Ovaries produce eggs, whereas testes produce sperm cells. However, the gonads of both sexes share one vital function: They are the endocrine glands chiefly responsible for the sexual maturation of puberty and any subsequent reproduction.

Ovaries

The *ovaries,* or female gonads, are paired organs about the size of an almond that are located in the pelvis on either side of the uterus. Under the regulation of the anterior pituitary hormones FSH and LH, the ovaries produce:

- ★ *Estrogen*
- ★ *Progesterone*

The hormone *estrogen* promotes the development and maintenance of secondary female sexual characteristics. Estrogen also plays a role in the egg development that precedes ovulation during each menstrual cycle. *Progesterone* is familiarly known as the "hormone of pregnancy" because it is necessary for implantation of the fertilized egg and maintenance of the uterine lining throughout pregnancy. Estrogen also serves to protect the female against heart disease. When estrogen levels fall at menopause, the female's risk of developing heart disease quickly increases to the level of the male's. In addition, the ovaries produce small amounts of *testosterone,* which influences some body changes associated with puberty.

Testes

The male gonads, or *testes,* are located outside of the abdominal cavity in the scrotum. Under the regulation of the anterior pituitary hormones FSH and LH, the testes produce:

- ★ *Testosterone*

The hormone *testosterone* promotes the development and maintenance of secondary male sexual characteristics and plays a role in the development of sperm.

PINEAL GLAND

The *pineal gland* is located in the roof of the thalamus in the brain. Its function has remained somewhat elusive. However, it has been shown that the pineal gland releases the hormone *melatonin* in response to changes in light. For example, melatonin production is lowest during daylight hours and highest in the dark of the night. Because of this, the pineal is felt to help determine day-length and lunar cycles and plays a role in controlling the reproductive "biological clock." Melatonin may affect a person's mood. The pineal gland has been implicated in "seasonal affective disorder (SAD)," which is characterized by severe depression during the winter months. Further research will help clarify the role of melatonin.

OTHER ORGANS WITH ENDOCRINE ACTIVITY

We have discussed the principal glands of the endocrine system. Many tissues not considered part of the endocrine system have important endocrine functions. Certain organs in other systems secrete hormones directly into the blood. The placenta can be considered an endocrine gland because of its secretion of *human chorionic gonadotropin (hCG)* throughout gestation. It is the early secretion of hCG that is detected by at-home pregnancy tests. In the digestive tract, gastric and intestinal mucosa produce the hormones *gastrin* and *secretin,* both of which regulate digestive function.

Additionally, there are hormone-producing cells in the atrial walls of the heart. *Atrial natriuretic hormone (ANH)* is secreted by certain atrial cells in response to increased stretching of the atrial walls due to abnormally high blood volume or blood pressure. The hormone ANH is an antagonist to ADH and inhibits secretion of aldosterone, thus contributing to a homeostatic reduction in blood volume by increasing urine production.

The kidneys also have some endocrine function. Certain kidney cells will react to a decrease in blood volume or blood pressure by releasing the enzyme *renin*. Renin acts on *angiotensinogen*, converting it to *angiotensin I*. In the lungs, angiotensin I is converted to *angiotensin II* by *angiotensin-converting enzyme (ACE)*. Angiotensin II stimulates the adrenal production of aldosterone, which causes water retention by the kidneys. This leads to increased blood volume and blood pressure. In addition to renin, the kidneys secrete the hormone erythropoietin that stimulates the production of red blood cells by the bone marrow.

THE CARDIOVASCULAR SYSTEM

The cardiovascular system's two major components are the heart and the peripheral blood vessels.

ANATOMY OF THE HEART

The *heart* is a muscular organ, approximately the size of a closed fist. It is in the center of the chest in the mediastinum, anterior to the spine and posterior to the sternum (Figure 3-83 ■). Approximately two thirds of the heart's mass is to the left of the midline, with the remainder to the right. The bottom of the heart, or *apex*, is just above the diaphragm, left of the midline. The top of the heart, or *base*, lies at approximately the level of the second rib. The great vessels connect to the heart through the base.

Tissue Layers

The heart consists of three tissue layers: endocardium, myocardium, and pericardium (Figure 3-84 ■). The *endocardium*, the innermost layer, lines the heart's chambers and is bathed in blood. The *myocardium* is the thick middle layer of the heart. Its cells are unique in that they physically resemble skeletal muscle but have electrical properties similar to smooth muscle. These cells also contain specialized structures that help to rapidly conduct electrical impulses from one muscle cell to another, enabling the heart to contract.

The *pericardium* is a protective sac surrounding the heart. It consists of two layers, visceral and parietal. The *visceral pericardium*, also called the *epicardium*, is the inner layer, in contact

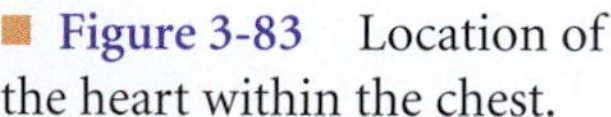

■ Figure 3-83 Location of the heart within the chest.

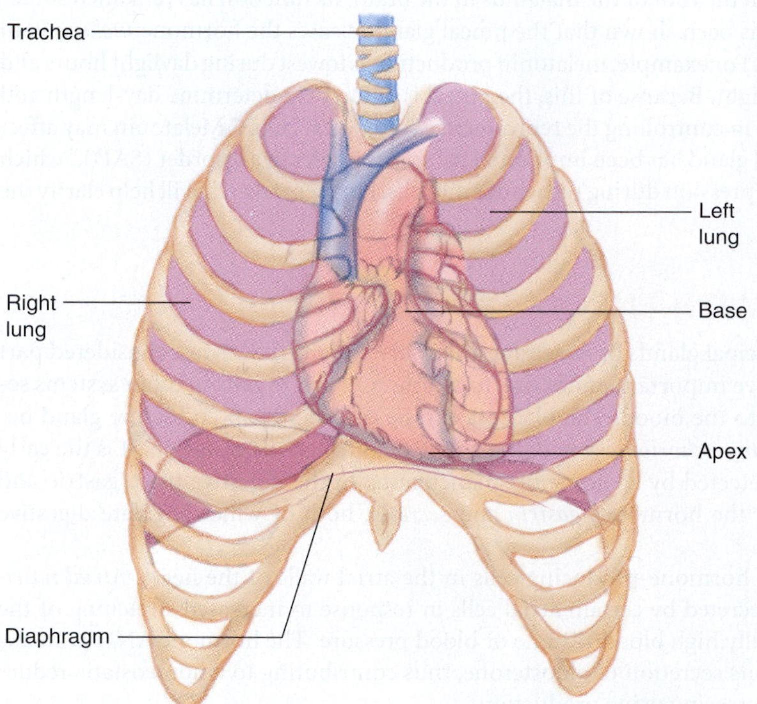

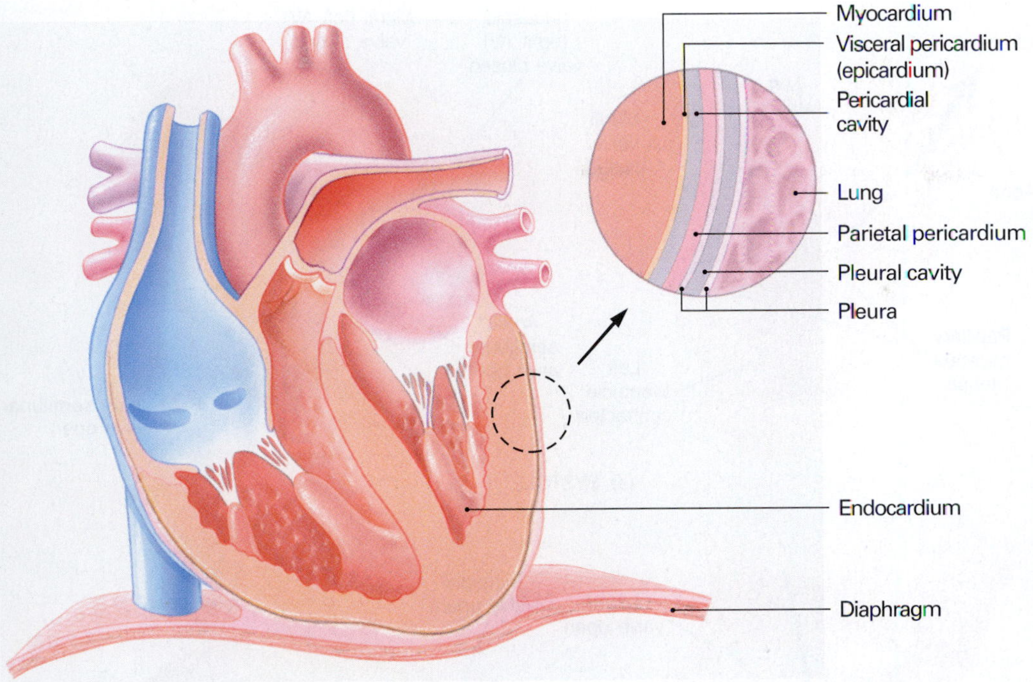

Myocardium
Visceral pericardium (epicardium)
Pericardial cavity
Lung
Parietal pericardium
Pleural cavity
Pleura
Endocardium
Diaphragm

■ **Figure 3-84** Layers of the heart.

with the heart muscle itself. The *parietal pericardium* is the outer, fibrous layer. In the pericardial cavity, between these two layers, is about 25 milliliters of pericardial fluid, a straw-colored lubricant that reduces friction as the heart beats and changes position. Certain disease processes and injuries can increase the amount of fluid in this sac, compressing the heart and decreasing cardiac output.

Chambers

The heart contains four chambers (Figure 3-85 ■). The *atria,* the two superior chambers, receive incoming blood. The *ventricles,* the two larger, inferior chambers, pump blood out of the heart. The

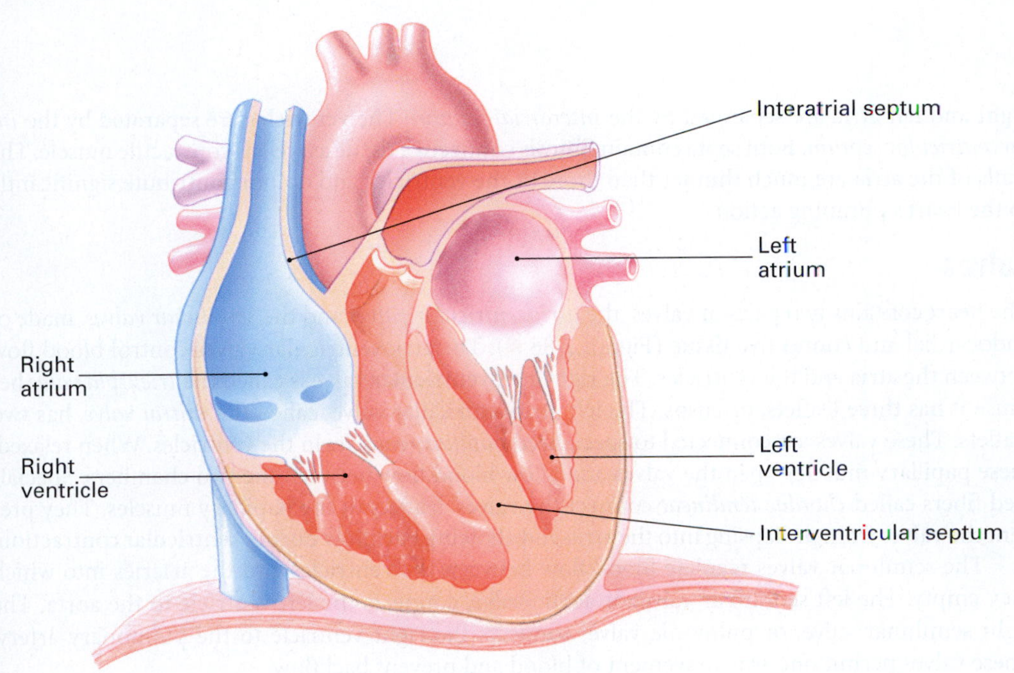

■ **Figure 3-85** The chambers of the heart.

■ **Figure 3-86** The valves of the heart.

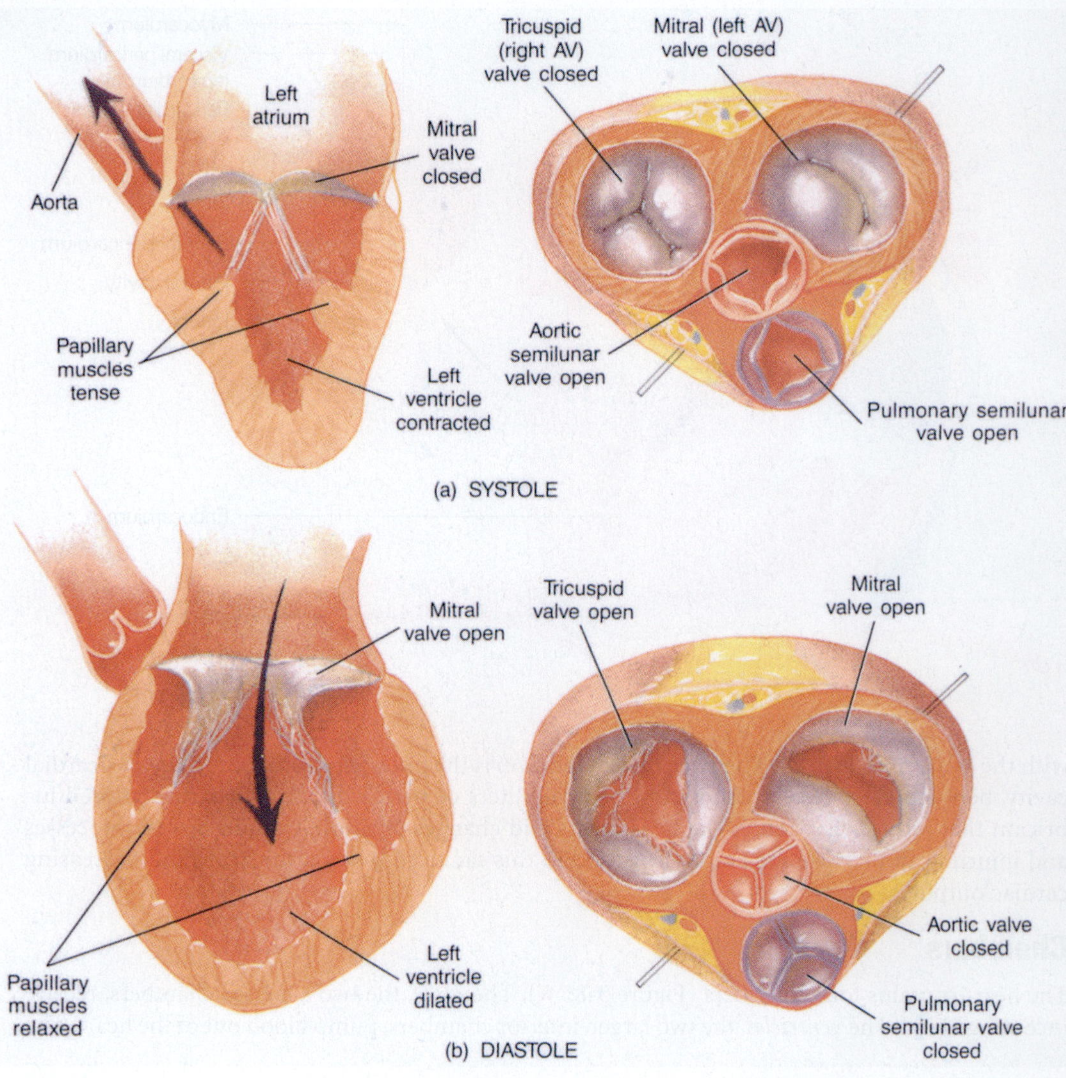

right and left atria are separated by the *interatrial septum.* The ventricles are separated by the *interventricular septum.* Both septa contain fibrous connective tissue as well as contractile muscle. The walls of the atria are much thinner than those of the ventricles and do not contribute significantly to the heart's pumping action.

Valves

The heart contains two pairs of valves, the *atrioventricular valves* and the *semilunar valves,* made of endocardial and connective tissue (Figure 3-86 ■). The atrioventricular valves control blood flow between the atria and the ventricles. The right atrioventricular valve is called the *tricuspid valve* because it has three leaflets, or cusps. The left atrioventricular valve, called the *mitral valve,* has two leaflets. These valves are connected to specialized *papillary muscles* in the ventricles. When relaxed, these papillary muscles open the valves and allow blood flow between the two chambers. Specialized fibers called *chordae tendineae* connect the valves' leaflets to the papillary muscles. They prevent the valves from prolapsing into the atria and allowing backflow during ventricular contraction.

The semilunar valves regulate blood flow between the ventricles and the arteries into which they empty. The left semilunar valve, or aortic valve, connects the left ventricle to the aorta. The right semilunar valve, or pulmonic valve, connects the right ventricle to the pulmonary artery. These valves permit one-way movement of blood and prevent backflow.

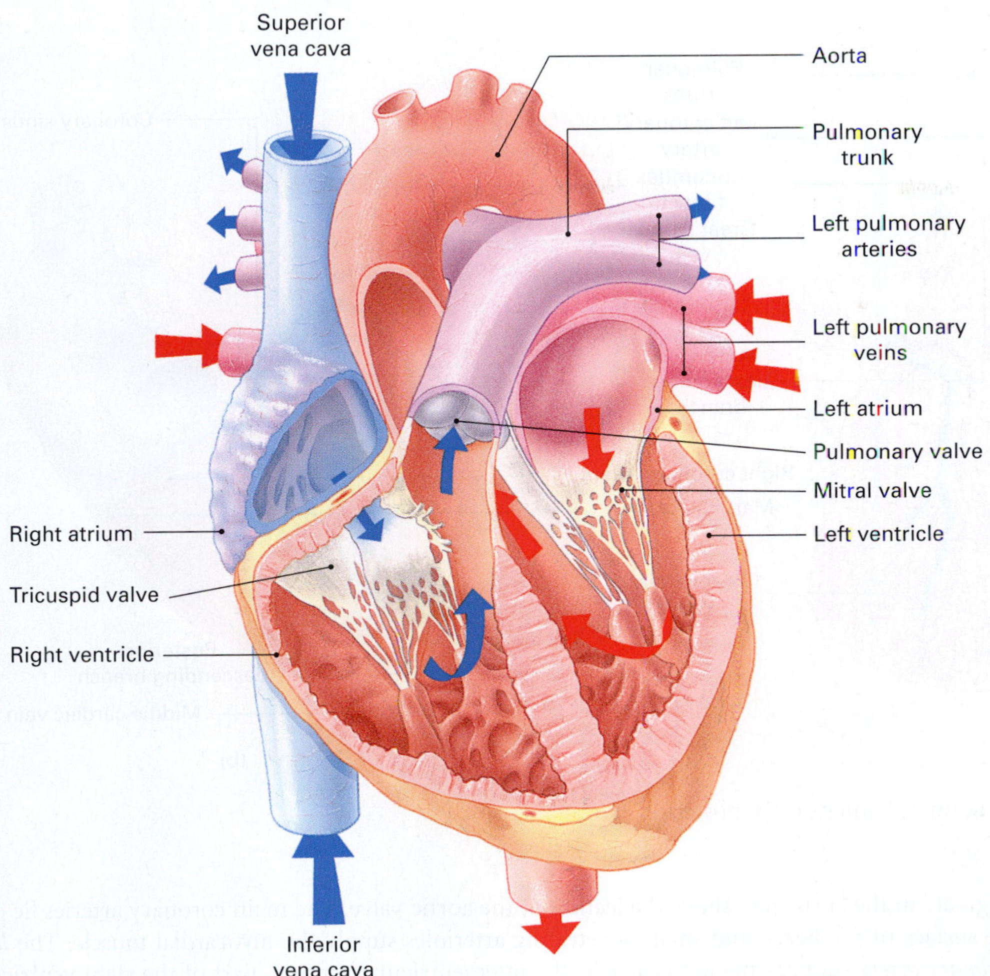

■ **Figure 3-87** Blood flow through the heart.

Blood Flow

The right atrium receives deoxygenated blood from the body via the superior and inferior venae cavae (Figure 3-87 ■). The *superior vena cava* receives deoxygenated blood from the head and upper extremities, the *inferior vena cava* from the areas below the heart. The right atrium pumps this blood through the tricuspid valve and into the right ventricle. The right ventricle then pumps the deoxygenated blood through the pulmonic valve to the *pulmonary artery* and on to the lungs. (The pulmonary artery is the only artery in the body that carries deoxygenated blood.)

After the blood circulates through the lungs and becomes oxygenated, it returns to the left atrium via the *pulmonary veins.* (The pulmonary veins are the only veins in the body that carry oxygenated blood.) The left atrium sends this oxygenated blood through the mitral valve and into the left ventricle. Finally the left ventricle pumps the blood through the aortic valve to the aorta, which feeds the oxygenated blood to the rest of the body. Intracardiac pressures are higher on the left than on the right because the lungs offer less resistance to blood flow than the systemic circulation. Thus, the left myocardium is thicker than the right.

The major vessels of the body all branch off of the aorta, which has three main parts. The *ascending aorta* comes directly from the heart. The *thoracic aorta* curves inferiorly and goes through the chest (or thorax). The *abdominal aorta* goes through the diaphragm and enters the abdomen.

Coronary Circulation

Although the endocardium is bathed in blood, the heart does not receive its nutrients from the blood within its chambers but from the *coronary arteries* (Figure 3-88 ■). The coronary arteries

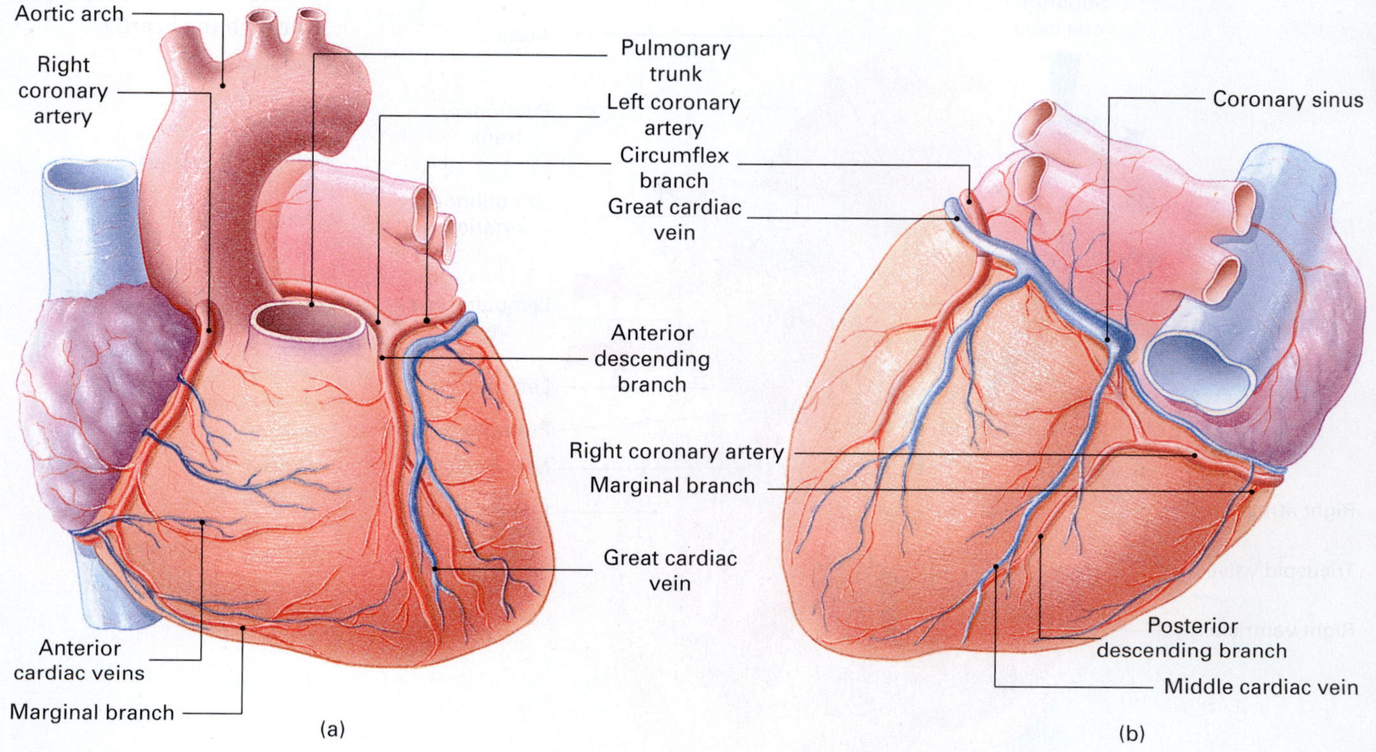

Figure 3-88 The coronary circulation: (a) anterior; (b) posterior.

originate in the aorta, just above the leaflets of the aortic valve. The main coronary arteries lie on the surface of the heart, and small penetrating arterioles supply the myocardial muscle. The *left coronary artery* supplies the left ventricle, the interventricular septum, part of the right ventricle, and the heart's conduction system. Its two major branches are the *anterior descending artery* and the *circumflex artery.*

The *right coronary artery* supplies a portion of the right atrium and right ventricle and part of the conduction system. Its two major branches are the *posterior descending artery* and the *marginal artery.* (Although the blood supply to most people's hearts follows this pattern, anatomical variants do exist.) The coronary vessels receive blood during diastole, when the heart relaxes, because the aortic valve leaflets cover the coronary artery openings (*ostia*) during systole, when the heart contracts.

Blood drains from the left coronary system via the *anterior great cardiac vein* and the *lateral marginal veins.* These empty into the *coronary sinus.* The right coronary vein empties directly into the right atrium via smaller cardiac veins.

anastomosis
communication between two or more vessels.

Many **anastomoses** (communications between two or more vessels) among the various branches of the coronary arteries allow *collateral circulation.* Collateral circulation is a protective mechanism that provides an alternative path for blood flow in case of a blockage somewhere in the system. This is analogous to a river's developing small tributaries to reach a larger body of water.

CARDIAC PHYSIOLOGY

The Cardiac Cycle

Although the heart's right and left sides perform different functions, they act as a unit. The right and left atria contract at the same time, filling both ventricles to their maximum capacities. Both ventricles then contract at the same time, ejecting blood into the pulmonary and systemic circulations. The pressure of the contraction closes the tricuspid and mitral valves and opens the aortic and pulmonic valves at the same time.

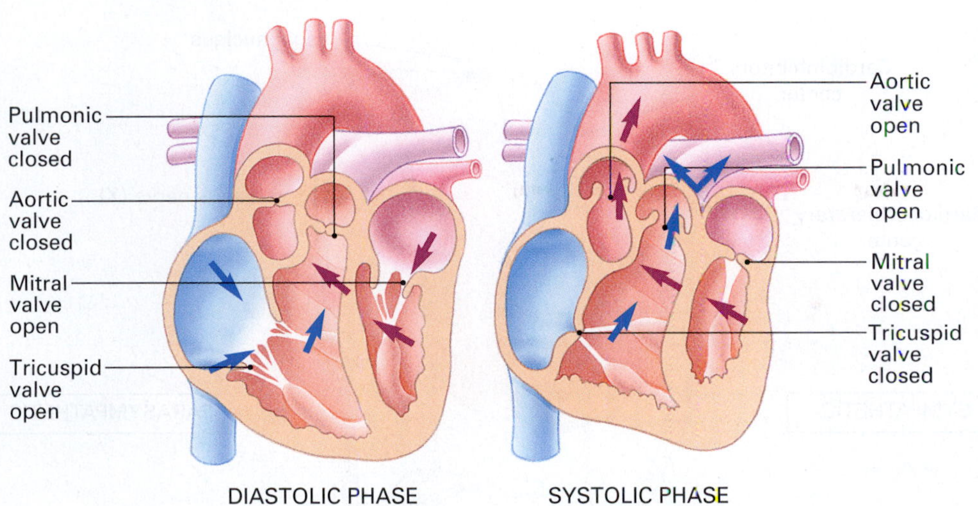

■ **Figure 3-89** Relation of blood flow to cardiac contractions.

The **cardiac cycle** is the sequence of events that occurs between the end of one heart contraction and the end of the next. To evaluate heart sounds and read electrocardiographs, you must thoroughly understand the pumping action of the cardiac cycle (Figure 3-89 ■). **Diastole,** the first phase of the cardiac cycle, is the relaxation phase. This is when ventricular filling begins. Blood enters the ventricles through the mitral and tricuspid valves. The pulmonic and aortic valves are closed.

cardiac cycle *the period of time from the end of one cardiac contraction to the end of the next.*

diastole *the period of time when the myocardium is relaxed and cardiac filling and coronary perfusion occur.*

systole *the period of the cardiac cycle when the myocardium is contracting.*

During the second phase, **systole,** the heart contracts. The atria contract first, to finish emptying their blood into the ventricles. Atrial systole is relatively quick and occurs just before ventricular contraction; in healthy hearts, this atrial "kick" boosts cardiac output. The pressure in the ventricles now increases until it exceeds the pressure in the aorta and pulmonary artery. At this point blood flows out of the ventricles through the pulmonic and aortic valves and into the arteries. The pressure also closes the mitral and tricuspid valves and, if working properly, prevents backflow of blood into the atria. When pressures in the artery exceed the pressures in the ventricles, the valves close and diastole begins again.

Nervous Control of the Heart

The sympathetic and parasympathetic components of the autonomic nervous system work in direct opposition to one another to regulate the heart. In the heart's normal state the two systems balance. In stressful situations, however, the sympathetic system becomes dominant, while during sleep the parasympathetic system dominates. The sympathetic nervous system innervates the heart through the *cardiac plexus,* a network of nerves at the base of the heart (Figure 3-90 ■).

The sympathetic nerves arise from the thoracic and lumbar regions of the spinal cord, then leave the spinal cord and form the sympathetic chain, which runs along the spinal column. The cardiac plexus arises in turn from ganglia in the sympathetic chain and innervates both the atria and ventricles. The chemical neurotransmitter for the sympathetic nervous system, and thus for the cardiac plexus, is norepinephrine. Its release increases heart rate and cardiac contractile force, primarily through its actions on beta receptors.

As noted earlier, the sympathetic nervous system has two principal types of receptors, alpha and beta. Alpha receptors are located in the peripheral blood vessels and are responsible for vasoconstriction. Beta$_1$ receptors, primarily located in the heart, increase the heart rate and contractility. Beta$_2$ receptors, principally located in the lungs and peripheral blood vessels, cause bronchodilation and peripheral vasodilation. Medications specific to these various receptors cause different physiological effects. For instance, beta-blockers slow the heart rate and lower blood pressure by blocking the beta$_1$ receptors, whose job is to increase heart rate and contractility.

Parasympathetic control of the heart occurs through the *vagus nerve* (the 10th cranial nerve). The vagus nerve descends from the brain to innervate the heart and other organs. Vagal nerve fibers primarily innervate the atria, although some innervate the upper ventricles. The neurotransmitter

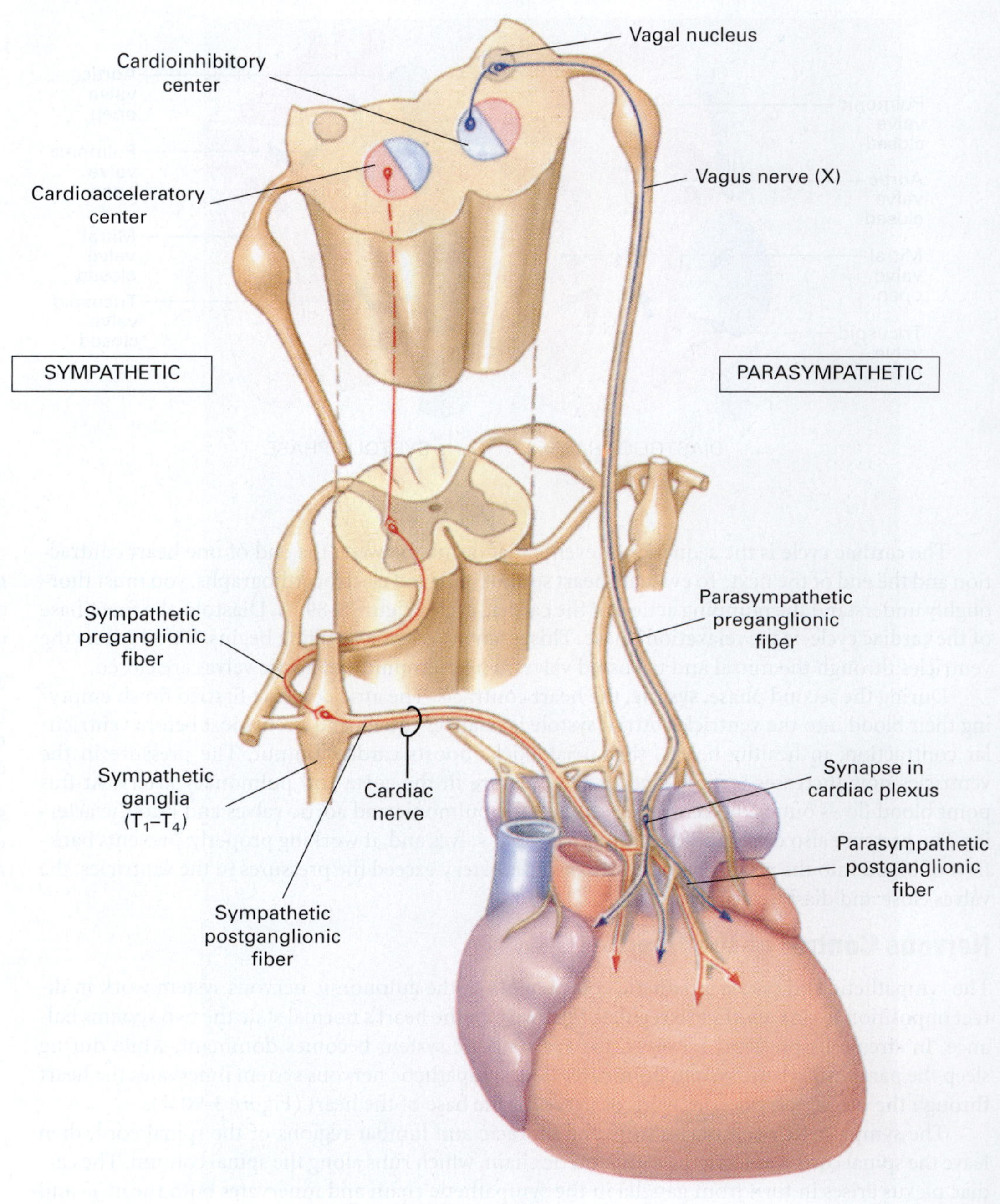

■ **Figure 3-90** Nervous control of the heart.

for the parasympathetic nervous system, and thus the vagus nerve, is acetylcholine. Its release slows both the heart rate and the atrioventricular conduction. Several maneuvers can stimulate the vagus nerve, including Valsalva maneuver (forced expiration against a closed glottis, which can occur when lifting heavy objects), pressure on the carotid sinus (carotid sinus massage), and distention of the urinary bladder.

chronotropy *pertaining to heart rate.*

inotropy *pertaining to cardiac contractile force.*

dromotropy *pertaining to the speed of impulse transmission.*

The terms *chronotropy, inotropy,* and *dromotropy* describe autonomic control of the heart. **Chronotropy** refers to heart rate. A positive chronotropic agent increases the heart rate. Conversely, a negative chronotropic agent decreases the heart rate. **Inotropy** refers to the strength of a cardiac muscular contraction. A positive inotropic agent strengthens the cardiac contraction, while a negative inotropic agent weakens it. **Dromotropy** refers to the rate of nervous impulse conduction. A positive dromotropic agent speeds impulse conduction, while a negative dromotropic agent slows conduction.

Role of Electrolytes Cardiac function, both electrical and mechanical, depends heavily on electrolyte balances. Electrolytes that affect cardiac function include sodium (Na^+), calcium (Ca^{++}), potassium (K^+), chloride (Cl^-), and magnesium (Mg^{++}). Sodium plays a major role in depolarizing the myocardium. Calcium takes part in myocardial depolarization and myocardial contraction. Hypercalcemia can result in increased contractility, whereas hypocalcemia is associated with decreased myocardial contractility and increased electrical irritability. Potassium influences repolarization. Hyperkalemia decreases automaticity and conduction, whereas hypokalemia increases irritability. New research is also investigating the roles of magnesium and chloride in the cardiac cycle.

Electrophysiology

The heart comprises three types of cardiac muscle: atrial, ventricular, and specialized excitatory and conductive fibers. The atrial and ventricular muscle fibers contract in much the same way as skeletal muscle, with one major difference. Within the cardiac muscle fibers are special structures called **intercalated discs** (Figure 3-91 ■). These discs connect cardiac muscle fibers and conduct electrical impulses quickly—400 times faster than the standard cell membrane—from one muscle fiber to the next. This speed allows cardiac muscle cells to function physiologically as a unit. That is, when one cell becomes excited, the action potential spreads rapidly across the entire group of cells, resulting in a coordinated contraction. This functional unit is a **syncytium.**

intercalated discs *specialized bands of tissue inserted between myocardial cells that increase the rate in which the action potential is spread from cell to cell.*

syncytium *group of cardiac muscle cells that physiologically function as a unit.*

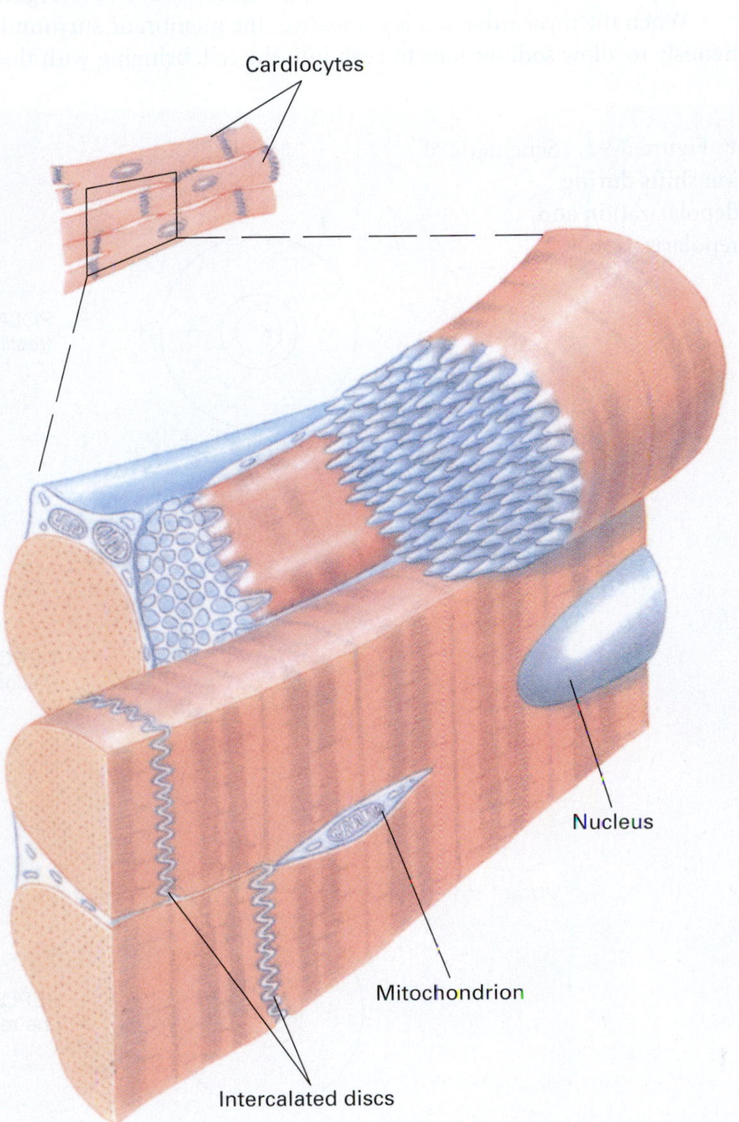

■ **Figure 3-91** Microscopic appearance of cardiac muscle. The intercalated discs speed transmission of the electrical potential quickly from one cell to the next.

The heart has two syncytia—the *atrial syncytium* and the *ventricular syncytium.* The atrial syncytium contracts from superior to inferior, so that the atria express blood to the ventricles. The ventricular syncytium, however, contracts from inferior to superior, expelling blood from the ventricles into the aorta and pulmonary arteries. The syncytia are separated from one another by the fibrous structure that supports the valves and physically separates the atria from the ventricles. The only way an impulse can be conducted from the atria to the ventricles is through the *atrioventricular (AV) bundle.* Cardiac muscle functions according to an "all-or-none" principle. That is, if a single muscle fiber becomes *depolarized,* the action potential will spread through the whole syncytium. Stimulating a single atrial fiber will thus completely depolarize the atria, and stimulating a single ventricular fiber will completely depolarize the ventricles.

cardiac depolarization *a reversal of charges at a cell membrane so that the inside of the cell becomes positive in relation to the outside; the opposite of the cell's resting state in which the inside of the cell is negative in relation to the outside.*

resting potential *the normal electrical state of cardiac cells.*

Cardiac Depolarization

Understanding **cardiac depolarization** is essential to interpreting electrocardiograms (ECGs). Normally, an ionic difference exists on the two sides of a cell membrane. The cell's sodium-potassium pump expels sodium (Na^+) from the cell. This leaves more negatively charged anions inside the cell than positively charged cations. Thus, the inside of the cell is more negatively charged than the outside. This difference, called the **resting potential,** can be measured experimentally by placing one probe inside the cell and another outside the cell and determining the difference in millivolts. The resting potential in a myocardial cell is approximately 290 mV (Figure 3-92 ■).

When the myocardial cell is stimulated, the membrane surrounding the cell changes instantaneously to allow sodium ions to rush into the cell, bringing with them their positive charge. This

■ **Figure 3-92** Schematic of ion shifts during depolarization and repolarization.

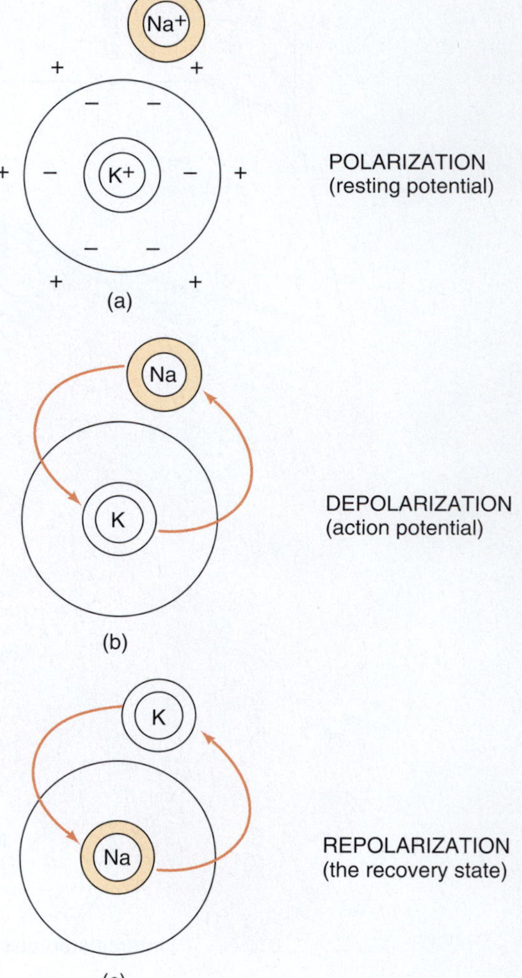

charge is so strong that it gives the inside of the cell a positive charge approximately +20 mV greater than the outside. This influx of sodium and change of membrane polarity is the **action potential.** After the influx of sodium, a slower influx of calcium ions (Ca^{++}) through the calcium channels increases the positive charge inside the cell. Once depolarization occurs in a muscle fiber, it is transmitted throughout the entire syncytium, via the intercalated discs, until the entire muscle mass is depolarized. Contraction of the muscle follows depolarization.

action potential *the stimulation of myocardial cells, as evidenced by a change in the membrane electrical charge, that subsequently spreads across the myocardium.*

The cell membrane remains permeable to sodium for only a fraction of a second. Thereafter, sodium influx stops and potassium escapes from inside the cell. This returns the charge inside the cell to normal (negative). In addition, sodium is actively pumped outside the cell, allowing the cell to **repolarize** and return to its normal resting state.

repolarization *return of a cell to its preexcitation resting state.*

Cardiac Conductive System

The cardiac conductive system stimulates the ventricles to depolarize in the proper direction. As mentioned earlier, the atria contract from superior to inferior, the ventricles from inferior to superior. If the depolarization impulse originated in the atria and spread passively to the ventricles, then the ventricles would depolarize from superior to inferior and would be ineffective. The cardiac conduction system, therefore, must initiate an impulse, spread it through the atria, transmit it quickly to the apex of the heart, and then stimulate the ventricles to depolarize from inferior to superior. To do this, the conduction system relies on specialized conductive fibers comprising muscle cells that transmit the depolarization potential through the heart much faster than can regular myocardial cells.

To accomplish their task, the cells of the cardiac conductive system have the important properties of excitability, conductivity, automaticity, and contractility.

- ★ **Excitability.** The cells can respond to an electrical stimulus, like all other myocardial cells.
- ★ **Conductivity.** The cells can propagate the electrical impulse from one cell to another.
- ★ **Automaticity.** The individual cells of the conductive system can depolarize without any impulse from an outside source. This property is also called self-excitation. Generally, the cell in the cardiac conductive system with the fastest rate of discharge, or automaticity, becomes the heart's pacemaker. As a rule, the highest cell in the conductive system has the fastest rate of automaticity. Normally, this cell is in the sinoatrial (SA) node, high in the right atrium; however, if one pacemaker cell fails to discharge and depolarize, then the cell with the next fastest rate becomes the pacemaker.
- ★ **Contractility.** Since the cells of the cardiac conductive system are specialized cardiac muscle cells, they retain the ability to contract.

excitability *ability of the cells to respond to an electrical stimulus.*

conductivity *ability of the cells to propagate the electrical impulse from one cell to another.*

automaticity *pacemaker cells' capability of self-depolarization.*

contractility *ability of muscle cells to contract, or shorten.*

Internodal atrial pathways connect the SA node to the AV node (Figure 3-93 ■). These internodal pathways conduct the depolarization impulse to the atrial muscle mass and through the atria to the AV junction. The AV junction (the "gatekeeper") slows the impulse and allows the ventricles time to fill. Then, the impulse passes through the AV junction into the AV node and on to the AV fibers, which conduct the impulse from the atria to the ventricles. In the ventricles the AV fibers form the *bundle of His.*

The bundle of His subsequently divides into the right and left bundle branches. The *right bundle branch* delivers the impulse to the apex of the right ventricle. From there the *Purkinje system* spreads it across the myocardium. The *left bundle branch* divides into *anterior and posterior fascicles* that also ultimately terminate in the Purkinje system. At the same time that the impulse is transmitted to the right ventricle, the Purkinje system spreads it across the mass of the myocardium. Repolarization predominantly occurs in the opposite direction.

Each component of the conductive system has its own intrinsic rate of self-excitation:

SA node = 60–100 beats per minute

AV node = 40–60 beats per minute

Purkinje system = 15–40 beats per minute

■ Figure 3-93 The cardiac conductive system.

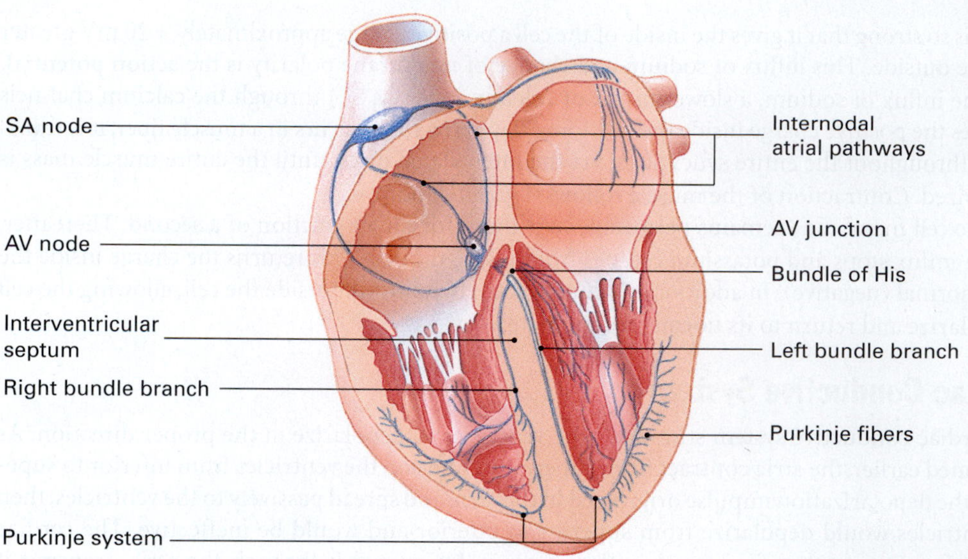

ANATOMY OF THE PERIPHERAL CIRCULATION

The peripheral circulation (Figure 3-94 ■) transports oxygenated blood from the heart to the tissues and subsequently transports deoxygenated blood back to the heart. Oxygenated blood leaves the heart via the arterial system, while deoxygenated blood returns via the venous system. (As noted earlier, the exceptions to this rule are the pulmonary artery and the pulmonary veins.)

A capillary wall consists of a single layer of cells. The walls of arteries and veins, however, comprise several layers (Figure 3-95 ■). The arteries' and veins' innermost lining, the *tunica intima,* is a single cell layer thick. The middle layer, the *tunica media,* consists of elastic fibers and muscle. It gives blood vessels their strength and recoil, which results from the difference in pressure inside and outside the vessel. The tunica media is much thicker in arteries than in veins. The outermost lining is the *tunica adventitia,* a fibrous tissue covering. It gives the vessel strength to withstand the pressures generated by the heart's contractions. The cavity inside a vessel is the *lumen.*

Poiseuille's law *a law of physiology stating that blood flow through a vessel is directly proportional to the radius of the vessel to the fourth power.*

The vessels' diameters vary significantly and are directly related to the amount of blood they can transport. The larger the diameter, the greater the blood flow. In fact, according to **Poiseuille's law** the blood flow through a vessel is directly proportional to the fourth power of the vessel's radius. For example, a vessel with a relative radius of 1 would transport 1 mL per minute of blood at a pressure difference of 100 mmHg. If the vessel's radius were increased to 4, keeping the pressure difference constant, the flow would increase to 256 mL (4^4) per minute.

The Arterial System

The *arterial system,* which carries oxygenated blood from the heart, functions under high pressure. The larger arterial vessels are the *arteries.* The arteries branch into smaller structures called *arterioles,* which control blood flow to various organs by their degree of resistance. The arterioles continue to divide until they become *capillaries,* which are the connection points between the arterial and venous systems. The vascular system and the tissues are able to exchange gases, fluids, and nutrients through the very thin capillary walls.

The Venous System

The *venous system* transports blood from the peripheral tissues back to the heart. It functions under low pressure with the aid of surrounding muscles and one-way valves within the veins. Blood enters the venous system through the capillaries, which drain into the *venules.* The venules, in turn, drain into the *veins,* the veins into the venae cavae, and the venae cavae into the atria.

The Lymphatic System

The *lymphatic system* is a network of vessels that drains fluid, called lymph, from the body tissues and delivers it to the subclavian vein (Figure 3-96 ■). Lymph nodes in the neck, the axilla, and the

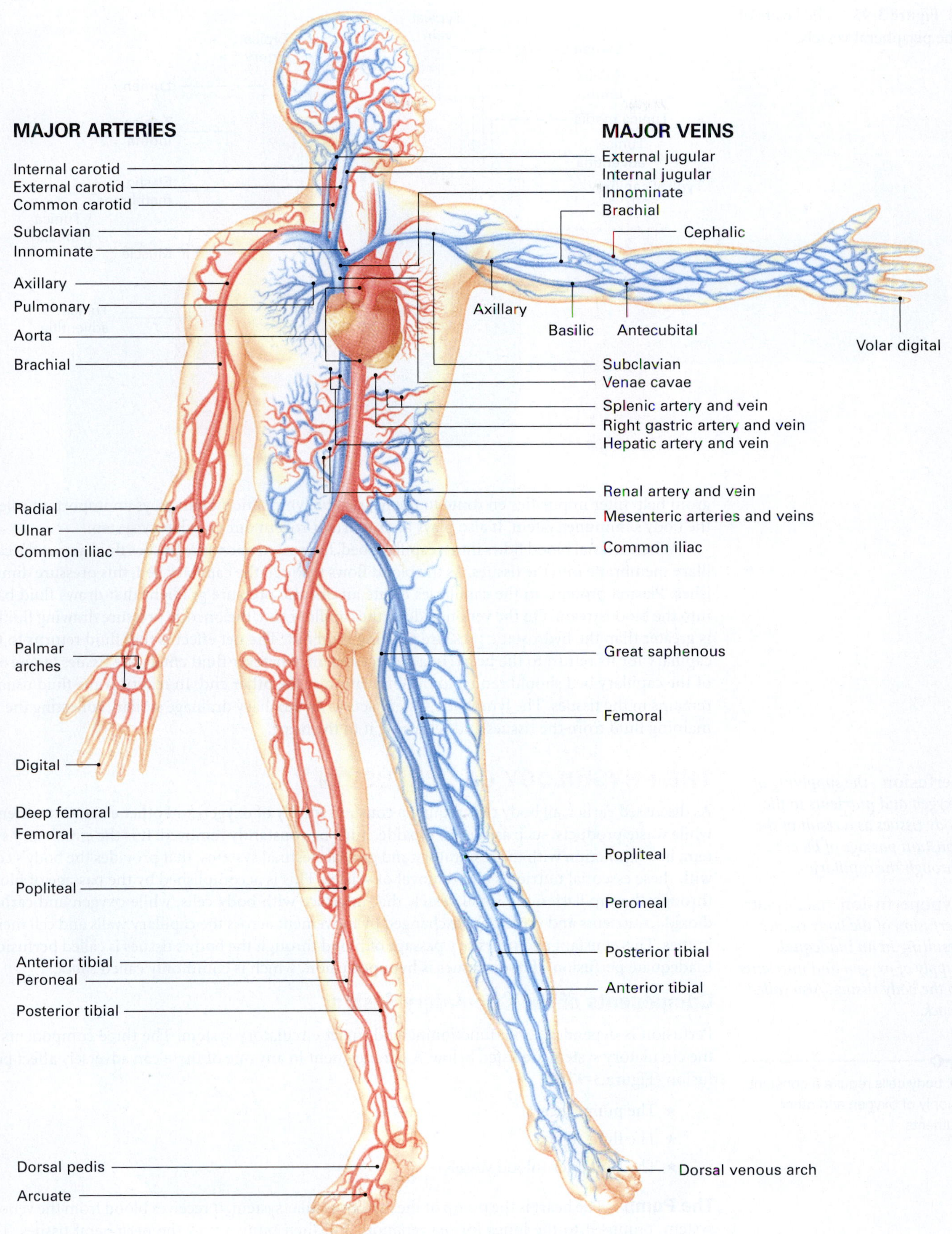

■ **Figure 3-94** The circulatory system.

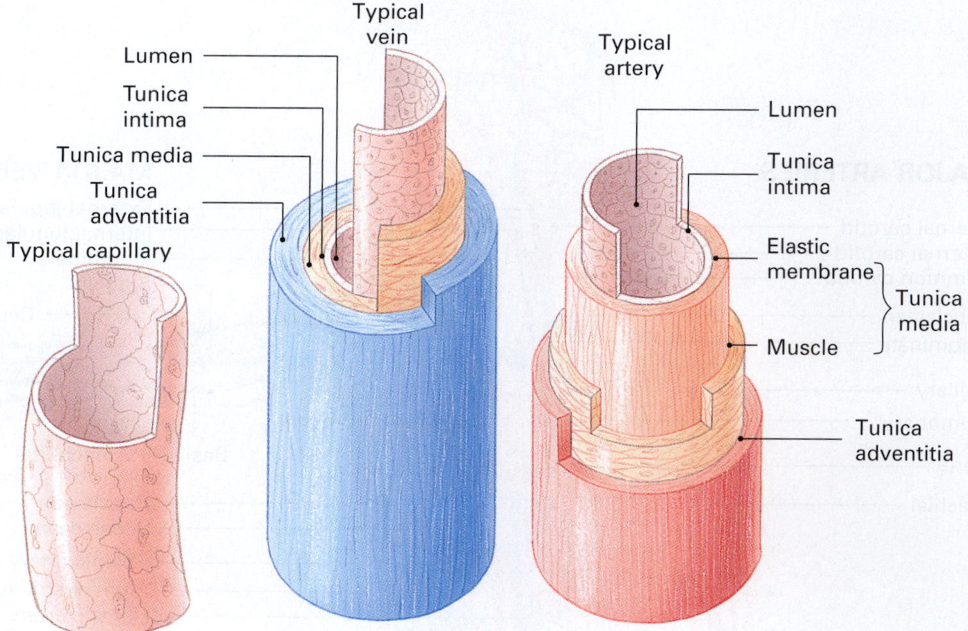

■ **Figure 3-95** The layers of the peripheral vessels.

groin help filter impurities en route to the heart. The lymphatic system plays an important role in the body's immune system. It also plays an important role in our circulatory system.

When arterial blood flows into a capillary bed, hydrostatic pressure pushes fluid across the capillary membrane into the tissues. As the blood flows through the capillary bed, this pressure diminishes. Plasma proteins in the capillaries create an oncotic pressure gradient that draws fluid back into the bloodstream. On the venous side of the capillary bed, the oncotic pressure drawing fluid in is greater than the hydrostatic pressure pushing fluid out. The net effect is that fluid returns to the capillary for its return to the heart. In a perfect system, whatever fluid enters the tissues at one end of the capillary bed should return to the circulation at the other end. In reality, some fluid usually remains in the tissues. The lymphatic system acts as an auxiliary drainage system, collecting the remaining fluid from the tissues and returning it to the heart.

THE PHYSIOLOGY OF PERFUSION

perfusion *the supplying of oxygen and nutrients to the body tissues as a result of the constant passage of blood through the capillaries.*

hypoperfusion *inadequate perfusion of the body tissues, resulting in an inadequate supply of oxygen and nutrients to the body tissues. Also called shock.*

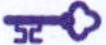

All body cells require a constant supply of oxygen and other nutrients.

As discussed earlier, all body cells require a constant supply of oxygen and other essential nutrients, while waste products, such as carbon dioxide, must be constantly removed. It is the circulatory system, in conjunction with the respiratory and gastrointestinal systems, that provides the body's cells with these essential nutrients and removal of wastes. This is accomplished by the passage of blood through the capillaries, the small vessels that interface with body cells, while oxygen and carbon dioxide, nutrients and wastes, are exchanged by movement across the capillary walls and cell membranes. This constant and necessary passage of blood through the body's tissues is called **perfusion.** Inadequate perfusion of body tissues is **hypoperfusion,** which is commonly called *shock*.

Components of the Circulatory System

Perfusion is dependent on a functioning and intact circulatory system. The three components of the circulatory system are listed below. A derangement in any one of these can adversely affect perfusion (Figure 3-97 ■).

- ★ The pump (heart)
- ★ The fluid (blood)
- ★ The container (blood vessels)

The Pump The heart is the pump of the cardiovascular system. It receives blood from the venous system, pumps it to the lungs for oxygenation, and then pumps it to the peripheral tissues. The

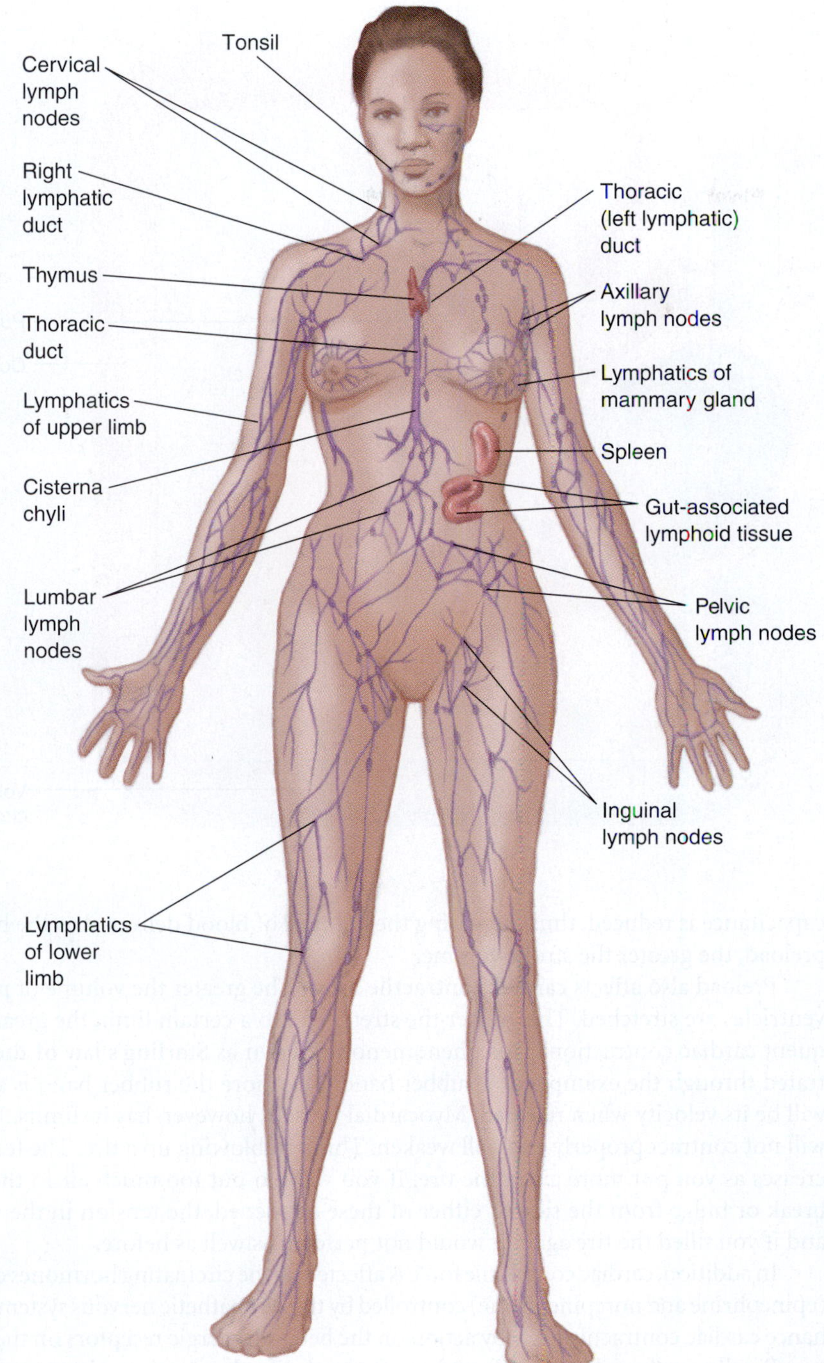

■ **Figure 3-96** The lymphatic system.

normal ventricle ejects about two-thirds of the blood it contains at the end of diastole. This ratio is the **ejection fraction.** The amount of blood ejected by the heart in one contraction is referred to as the **stroke volume.** Each time the ventricle pumps blood into the aorta, it generates a pressure wave along the major arteries, which we feel as a pulse. Stroke volume varies between 60 and 100 mL, with the average being 70 mL. Three factors affect stroke volume: preload, cardiac contractile force, and afterload.

Preload is the amount of blood delivered to the heart during diastole (when the heart fills with blood between contractions). Preload depends on venous return. The venous system is a capacitance, or storage system. That is, it can be contracted or expanded, to some extent, as needed to meet the physiological demands of the body. When additional oxygenated blood is required, the venous

ejection fraction *ratio of blood pumped from the ventricle to the amount remaining at the end of diastole.*

stroke volume *the amount of blood ejected by the heart in one cardiac contraction.*

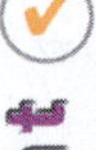

Review

Content

Factors Affecting Stroke Volume

- Preload
- Cardiac contractility
- Afterload

preload *the pressure within the ventricles at the end of diastole, commonly called the* end-diastolic volume.

■ Figure 3-97 Components of the circulatory system.

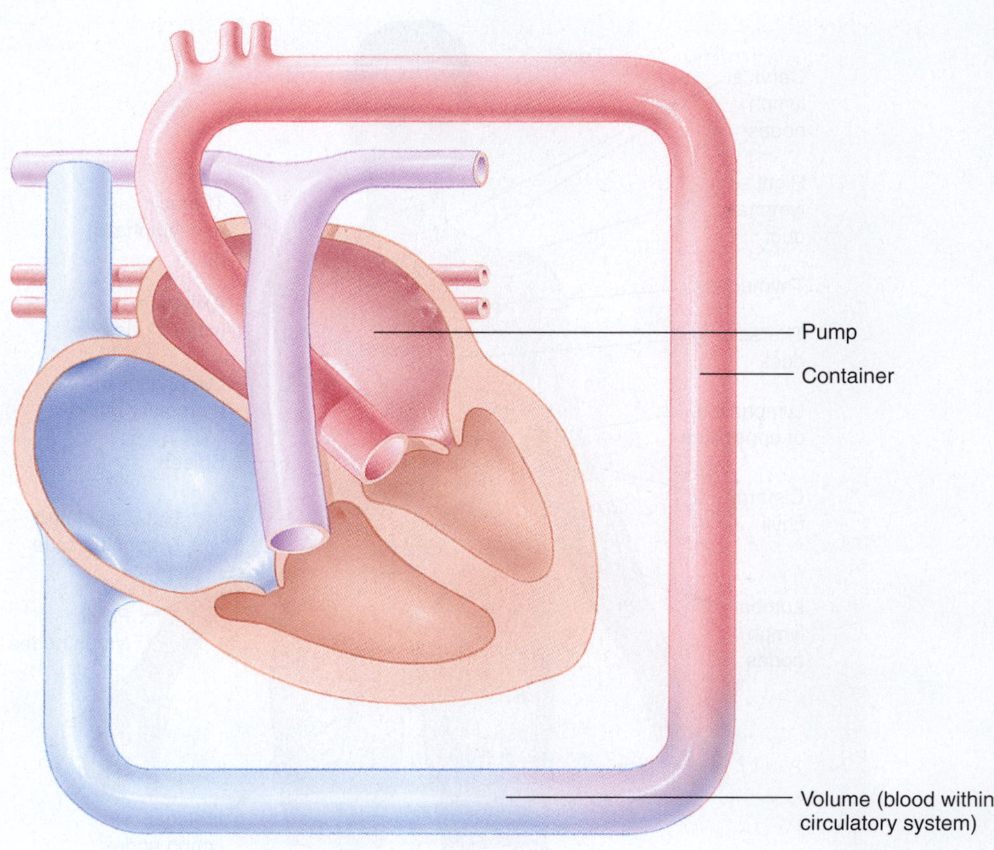

capacitance is reduced, thus increasing the amount of blood delivered to the heart. The greater the preload, the greater the stroke volume.

cardiac contractile force *force of the strength of a contraction of the heart.*

Starling's law of the heart *law of physiology stating that the more the myocardium is stretched, up to a certain limit, the more forceful the subsequent contraction will be.*

Preload also affects **cardiac contractile force.** The greater the volume of preload, the more the ventricles are stretched. The greater the stretch, up to a certain limit, the greater will be the subsequent cardiac contraction. This phenomenon (known as **Starling's law of the heart**) can be illustrated through the example of a rubber band. The more the rubber band is stretched, the greater will be its velocity when released. Myocardial muscle, however, has its limits. If stretched too far, it will not contract properly and will weaken. Think of blowing up a tire. The tension in the walls increases as you put more air in the tire. If you were to put too much air in the tire, the tire would break or bulge from the side. If either of these happened, the tension in the wall would decrease, and if you filled the tire again it would not perform as well as before.

In addition, cardiac contractile force is affected by the circulating hormones called catecholamines (epinephrine and norepinephrine) controlled by the sympathetic nervous system. Catecholamines enhance cardiac contractile force by action on the beta-adrenergic receptors on the surface of the cells.

afterload *the resistance against which the heart must pump.*

Finally, stroke volume is affected by afterload. **Afterload** is the resistance against which the ventricle must contract. This resistance must be overcome before ventricular contraction can result in ejection of blood. Afterload is determined by the degree of peripheral vascular resistance, which depends on the amount of vasoconstriction present. (The arterial system can be expanded and contracted to meet the metabolic demands of the body.) An increase in peripheral vascular resistance will decrease stroke volume, and conversely, a decrease in peripheral vascular resistance will allow stroke volume to increase.

cardiac output *the amount of blood pumped by the heart in 1 minute.*

The amount of blood pumped by the heart in 1 minute is referred to as the **cardiac output.** It is a function of stroke volume (milliliters per beat) and heart rate (beats per minute). Cardiac output is usually expressed in liters per minute. It can be defined by this equation:

$$\text{Stroke volume (mL/b)} \times \text{Heart rate (bpm)} = \text{Cardiac output (mL/min)}$$

Since the average stroke volume is 70 mL and the normal heart rate is about 70 beats per minute, the average cardiac output is 4,900 milliliters per minute (rounded to 5,000 mL/min or 5 liters per minute).

The foregoing equation illustrates the factors that can affect cardiac output. An increase in stroke volume or an increase in heart rate can increase cardiac output. Conversely, a decrease in stroke volume (in turn governed by preload, contractile force, and afterload) or a decrease in heart rate can decrease cardiac output.

Blood pressure, the tension exerted by blood against the arterial walls, is dependent on both cardiac output and peripheral vascular resistance:

blood pressure *the tension exerted by blood against the arterial walls.*

$$\text{Blood pressure} = \text{Cardiac output} \times \text{Peripheral vascular resistance}$$

Peripheral vascular resistance is the pressure against which the heart must pump. Since the circulatory system is a closed system, increasing either cardiac output or peripheral vascular resistance will increase blood pressure. Likewise, a decrease in cardiac output or a decrease in peripheral vascular resistance will decrease blood pressure.

peripheral vascular resistance *the resistance of the vessels to the flow of blood: increased when the vessels constrict, decreased when the vessels relax.*

The body strives to keep the blood pressure relatively constant by employing compensatory mechanisms and negative feedback loops to regulate the elements of the previous formula. As noted earlier, baroreceptors in the carotid sinuses and in the arch of the aorta closely monitor blood pressure. If blood pressure increases, the baroreceptors send signals to the brain that cause the blood pressure to return to its normal values. This is accomplished by decreasing the heart rate, decreasing the preload, or decreasing peripheral vascular resistance.

The baroreceptors are also stimulated if the blood pressure falls. The heart rate is increased, as is the strength of the cardiac contractions. There is also arteriolar constriction, venous constriction (which results in decreased container size), and overall increased peripheral vascular resistance. Also, the adrenal medulla (the inner portion of the adrenal gland) is stimulated. This results in the secretion of epinephrine and norepinephrine, which further enhance the response.

The Fluid Blood is the fluid of the cardiovascular system. It is a viscous fluid; that is, it is thicker and more adhesive than water. As a result, blood flows more slowly than water. Blood, which consists of the plasma and the formed elements (red cells, white cells, and platelets), transports oxygen, carbon dioxide, nutrients, hormones, metabolic waste products, and heat.

An adequate amount of blood is required for perfusion. Since the cardiovascular system (the heart and blood vessels) is a closed system, the volume of blood present must be adequate to fill the container, as described in the following section.

The Container Blood vessels (arteries, arterioles, capillaries, venules, and veins) serve as the container of the cardiovascular system. The blood vessels can be thought of as a continuous, closed, and pressurized pipeline by which blood moves throughout the body. While the heart functions as the pump of the circulatory system, the blood vessels—under the control of the autonomic nervous system—can regulate blood flow to different areas of the body by adjusting their size as well as by selectively rerouting blood through the microcirculation.

While the arteries and veins, like the heart, are subject to direct stimulation from sympathetic portions of the autonomic nervous system, the microcirculation (comprised of the small vessels: the arterioles, capillaries, and venules) is primarily responsive to local tissue needs. The capability of some vessels in the capillary network to adjust their diameter permits the microcirculation to selectively supply undernourished tissue, while temporarily bypassing tissues with no immediate need. Capillaries have a sphincter at the origin of the capillary (between arteriole and capillary), called the *precapillary sphincter,* and another at the end of the capillary (between capillary and venule), called the *postcapillary sphincter.* The precapillary sphincter responds to local tissue conditions, such as acidosis and hypoxia, and opens as more arterial blood is needed. The postcapillary sphincter opens when blood is to be emptied into the venous system.

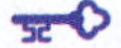

The precapillary sphincter responds to local tissue demands such as acidosis and hypoxia.

Blood flow through the vessels is regulated by two factors: peripheral vascular resistance and pressure within the system. Peripheral vascular resistance, as noted earlier, is the resistance to blood flow. Vessels with larger inside diameters offer less resistance, while vessels with smaller inside diameters offer greater resistance. Peripheral vascular resistance is governed by three factors—the length of the vessel, the diameter of the vessel, and blood viscosity.

There is very little resistance to blood flow through the aorta and arteries, but a significant change in peripheral resistance occurs at the arterioles and precapillary sphincters. This is because the inside diameter of the arteriole is much smaller, as compared to that of the aorta and arteries. Additionally, the arteriole has the ability to make a pronounced change in its diameter, as much as fivefold. It tends to do this in response to local tissue needs and autonomic nervous signals.

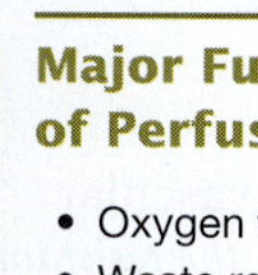

Content Review

Major Functions of Perfusion

- Oxygen transport
- Waste removal

Contraction of the venous side of the vascular system results in decreased capacitance and increased cardiac preload. The arterial system, however, provides systemic vascular resistance. An increase in arterial tone increases resistance, which increases blood pressure.

Oxygen Transport

Oxygen is brought into the body via the respiratory system. During inspiration, approximately 500 to 800 mL of atmospheric air is taken in through the upper and lower airways, coming to rest in the alveoli of the lungs.

Surrounding the alveoli are capillaries that are perfused by the pulmonary circulation. The blood that comes into the pulmonary capillaries is oxygen-depleted blood that was returned from the body to the right atrium of the heart, then pumped by the right ventricle of the heart into the pulmonary arteries and then into the pulmonary capillaries.

The air in the alveoli contains a concentration of about 13.6 percent oxygen. This is less than the 21 percent concentration of oxygen in atmospheric air because of various factors, including the fact that some air always remains in the alveoli from earlier respirations and oxygen is constantly being absorbed from this air. Nevertheless, alveolar air is far richer in oxygen than blood that enters the pulmonary capillaries.

Another way of stating this is that the *partial pressure of oxygen* present in air in the alveoli of the lungs is greater than the partial pressure of oxygen in the blood within the pulmonary circulation. (In a mix of gases, the portion of the total pressure exerted by each component of the mix is known as the partial pressure of that component.) For this reason, oxygen from the alveoli diffuses across the alveolar-capillary membrane and into the bloodstream—from the area of greater partial pressure to the area of lower partial pressure.

Content Review

Fick Principle

The movement and utilization of oxygen by the body is dependent on:

- Adequate concentration of inspired oxygen
- Appropriate movement of oxygen across the alveolar/capillary membrane into the arterial bloodstream
- Adequate number of red blood cells to carry the oxygen
- Proper tissue perfusion
- Efficient offloading of oxygen at the tissue level

The red blood cells "pick up" this oxygen while passing through the pulmonary capillary bed. Oxygen binds to the hemoglobin molecules of the red blood cells, which serve as the primary carriers of oxygen within the bloodstream. Normally, between 95 and 100 percent of the hemoglobin is saturated with oxygen. The oxygen-enriched blood then circulates back to the heart through the venous side of the pulmonary circulation. Passing through the left atrium and into the left ventricle, the oxygen-enriched blood is pumped throughout the body via the systemic circulation.

On reaching capillaries throughout the body, the oxygen-rich blood interfaces with the tissues. The tissues contain cells that are oxygen-deficient as a result of normal metabolic activity. Since the partial pressure of oxygen is greater in the bloodstream than in the cells, oxygen will diffuse from the red blood cells across the capillary wall-cell membrane barrier, into the cells and tissues.

Overall, the movement and utilization of oxygen in the body is dependent on the following conditions:

★ Adequate concentration of inspired oxygen
★ Appropriate movement of oxygen across the alveolar/capillary membrane into the arterial bloodstream
★ Adequate number of red blood cells to carry the oxygen
★ Proper tissue perfusion
★ Efficient off-loading of oxygen at the tissue level

The dependence on this set of conditions for oxygen movement and utilization is known as the Fick Principle.

Waste Removal

The waste products of cellular metabolism are expelled from the cells and carried away by the blood. Carbon dioxide leaves the bloodstream during the oxygen-carbon dioxide exchange, which occurs through the alveolar/capillary membranes. Carbon dioxide is ultimately eliminated by exhalation from the lungs. Some cellular waste products are expelled into the interstitial fluid and picked up by the lymphatic system. These ultimately flow through the lymph channels into the thoracic duct. The thoracic duct empties the waste products into the venous side of the circulatory system. Other wastes are cleansed from the blood by the kidneys and excreted as urine. Finally, some cellular waste products are emptied into the gastrointestinal system and expelled in the feces.

There is some local control of both tissue perfusion and waste removal. When the amounts of metabolic waste products (such as lactic acid) increase, the tissues subsequently become acidotic. This local acidosis causes nearby precapillary sphincters to relax, thus opening the capillaries and increasing perfusion of the affected tissues. This provides increased capacity for waste elimination and response to local metabolic demands.

THE RESPIRATORY SYSTEM

The respiratory system provides a passage for oxygen, a gas necessary for energy production, to enter the body and for carbon dioxide, a waste product of the body's metabolism, to exit. This gas exchange, called **respiration,** requires a patent, open airway as well as adequate respiratory function. Many pathological processes can inhibit respiration. To understand the interventions that you will use to maintain adequate airway and ventilatory function, you must thoroughly understand the anatomy of the upper and lower airway.

respiration *the exchange of gases between a living organism and its environment.*

UPPER AIRWAY ANATOMY

The upper airway extends from the mouth and nose to the larynx (Figure 3-98 ■). It includes the nasal cavity, oral cavity, and pharynx. The larynx joins the upper and lower airways.

Content Review

Upper Airway Components

- Nasal cavity
- Oral cavity
- Pharynx

The Nasal Cavity

The nasal cavity is the most superior part of the airway. The maxillary, frontal, nasal, ethmoid, and sphenoid bones comprise the lateral and superior walls of the nasal cavity. The hard palate forms the floor of the nasal cavity. The cartilaginous and highly vascular **nasal septum** separates the right and left nasal cavities.

Several different structures connect with the nasal cavity. These include the sinuses, the eustachian tubes, and the nasolacrimal ducts. The **sinuses** are air-filled cavities that are lined with a mucous membrane. There are four pairs of sinuses: the ethmoid sinuses, the frontal sinuses, the maxillary sinuses, and the sphenoid sinuses. The sinuses, named for the bone where they are contained, help reduce the overall weight of the head and are thought to assist in heating, purifying, and moistening the inhaled air. The sinuses help trap bacteria entering the nasal cavity. Because of this, they can become infected. Fractures of the upper sinuses (sphenoids) can occasionally cause cerebrospinal fluid (CSF) to leak from the cranial cavity into the nasal cavity. Clinically this presents with clear fluid draining from the nose (rhinorrhea) and can provide a direct route for the transmission of pathogens to the brain and associated structures.

The **eustachian tubes,** or auditory tubes, connect the ear with the nasal cavity and allow for equalization of pressure on each side of the tympanic membrane. Swallowing can assist in equalizing this pressure. The **nasolacrimal ducts** drain tears and debris from the eyes into the nasal cavity. This can cause the nose to run when someone cries.

Air enters the nasal cavity through the external nares (nostrils). Nasal hairs just inside the external nares initially filter the incoming air. The air then proceeds into the nasal cavity, where it strikes three bony projections, the superior, middle, and inferior turbinates, or conchae. These shelflike structures, which are parallel to the nasal floor, serve as conduits into the sinuses, increase the surface area of the nasal cavity, and cause turbulent airflow. This turbulence helps to filter the

nasal septum *cartilage that separates the right and left nasal cavities.*

sinus *air cavity that conducts fluids from the eustachian tubes and tear ducts to and from the nasopharynx.*

eustachian tube *a tube that connects the ear with the nasal cavity.*

nasolacrimal duct *narrow tube that carries into the nasal cavity tears and debris that have drained from the eye.*

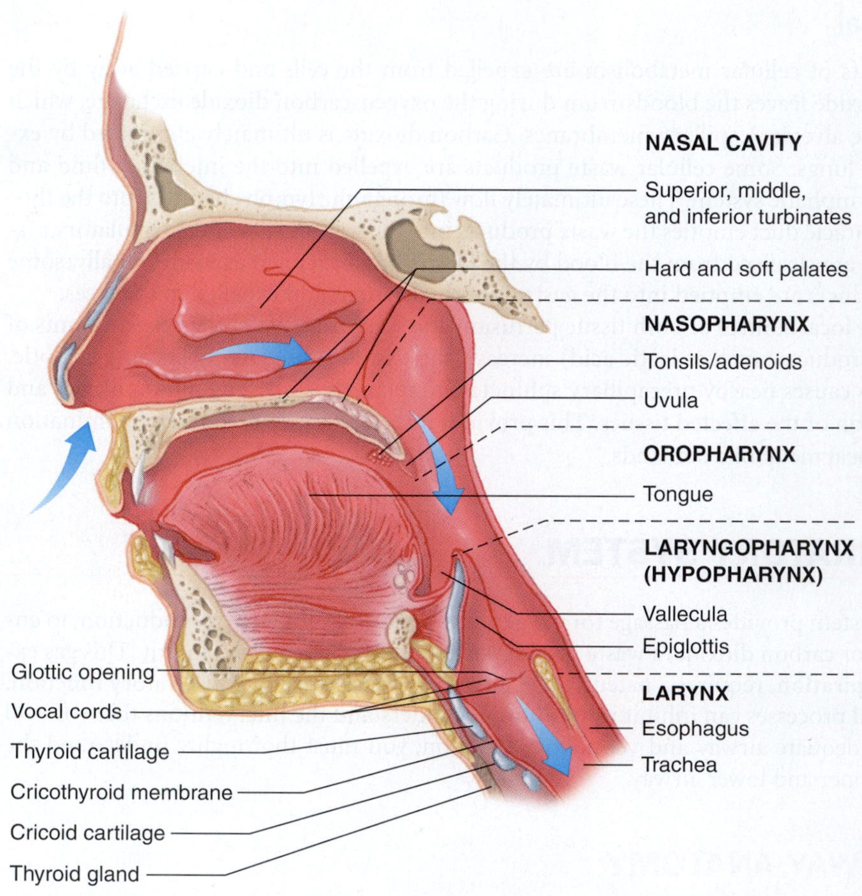

Figure 3-98 Anatomy of the upper airway.

air by depositing airborne particles on the **mucous membrane** lining the nasal cavity. Hairlike fibers called cilia propel those trapped particles to the back of the pharynx, where they are swallowed.

mucous membranes *tissues lining body cavities that communicate with the air; usually contain mucus-secreting cells.*

mucus *slippery secretion that lubricates and protects airway surfaces.*

Because the mucous membrane is covered with **mucus** and has a rich blood supply, it also immediately warms and humidifies the air entering the nose. By the time the air reaches the lower airway, it is at body temperature (37°C), 100 percent humidified, and virtually free of airborne particles. Air proceeds from the nasal cavity through internal nares into the nasopharynx. The tissue of the nasal cavity is extremely delicate and vascular. Because of this, it is susceptible to trauma.

The Oral Cavity

The cheeks, the hard and soft palates, and the tongue form the mouth, or oral cavity. The lips that surround the mouth's opening are fleshy folds of skin. Behind the lips lie the gums and teeth, normally numbering 32 in the adult. Significant force is required to avulse (dislodge) or fracture the teeth. Broken or dislodged teeth can potentially obstruct the airway. The hard palate anteriorly and the soft palate posteriorly form the top of the oral cavity and separate it from the nasal cavity.

The tongue, a large muscle on the bottom of the oral cavity, is the most common airway obstruction. It attaches to the mandible and the hyoid bone through a series of muscles and ligaments. The U-shaped hyoid bone is located just beneath the chin. The hyoid bone is unique. It is the only bone in the axial skeleton that does not articulate with any other bone. Instead, it is suspended by ligaments from the styloid process of the temporal bone and serves to anchor the tongue and larynx, as well as to support the trachea.

The Pharynx

pharynx *a muscular tube that extends vertically from the back of the soft palate to the superior aspect of the esophagus.*

The **pharynx** is a muscular tube that extends vertically from the back of the soft palate to the superior aspect of the esophagus. It allows the air to flow into and out of the respiratory tract and food and liquids to pass into the digestive system. It contains several openings, including the internal nares, the mouth, the larynx, and the esophagus.

The pharynx is divided into three regions: the nasopharynx, the oropharynx, and the laryngopharynx (hypopharynx). The nasopharynx is the uppermost region, extending from the back of the nasal opening to the plane of the soft palate. The oropharynx extends from the plane of the soft palate to the hyoid bone. The adenoids, lymphatic tissue in the mouth and nose, filter bacteria. Either hypertrophy or swelling of the adenoids from infection may make them large enough to obscure your view. The laryngopharynx extends posteriorly from the hyoid bone to the esophagus and anteriorly to the larynx. The laryngopharynx is especially important in airway management.

Because the mouth and pharynx serve dual purposes for respiration and digestion, a number of mechanisms help prevent accidental blockage. To prevent foreign material from entering the trachea and lungs, sensitive nerves activate the body's cough and swallowing mechanisms as well as the **gag reflex.**

Located anteriorly in the hypopharynx is the epiglottis, a leaf-shaped cartilage that prevents food from entering the respiratory tract during swallowing. Just anterior and superior to the epiglottis is the **vallecula,** a fold formed by the base of the tongue and the epiglottis. It is an important landmark for **endotracheal intubation.** A series of ligaments and muscles connect the epiglottis to the hyoid bone and mandible. Immediately behind the hypopharynx are the fourth and fifth cervical vertebral bodies.

The Larynx

The **larynx** is the complex structure that joins the pharynx with the trachea (Figure 3-99 ■). Lying midline in the neck, it is attached to and lies just inferior to the hyoid bone and anterior to the esophagus. It consists of the thyroid and cricoid cartilage (both considered tracheal cartilage), glottic opening, vocal cords, arytenoid cartilage, pyriform fossae, and cricothyroid membrane.

The main laryngeal cartilage is the shield-shaped thyroid cartilage. Larger in males than in females, the thyroid cartilage forms the anterior prominence called the Adam's apple. The arytenoid cartilage, which forms a pyramid-shaped attachment for the vocal cords posteriorly, is an important landmark for endotracheal intubation. Posteriorly, smooth muscle closes a gap in the thyroid cartilage. Directly behind the Adam's apple, the thyroid cartilage houses the glottic opening, the narrowest part of the adult trachea, which is bordered by the vocal cords. The patency of the glottic opening, or **glottis,** depends heavily on muscle tone. On either side of the glottic opening are the pyriform fossae, recesses that form the lateral borders of the larynx. The thyrohyoid membrane attaches the upper end of the thyroid cartilage to the hyoid bone.

Within the laryngeal cavity lie the true vocal cords, white bands of cartilage that regulate the passage of air through the larynx and produce voice by contraction of the laryngeal muscles. The

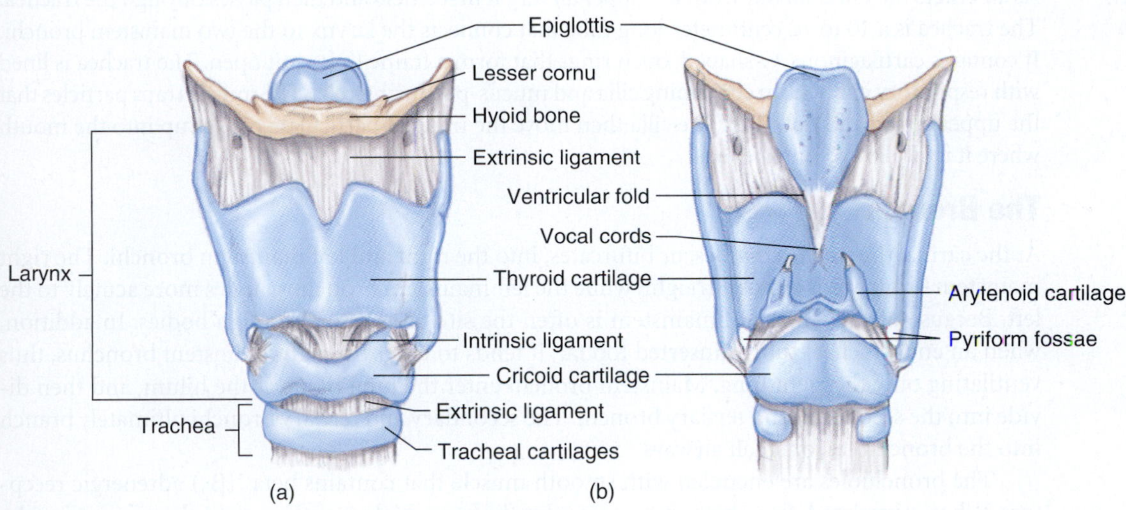

■ Figure 3-99 Internal anatomy of the upper airway.

Content Review

Regions of the Pharynx

- Nasopharynx
- Oropharynx
- Laryngopharynx

gag reflex *mechanism that stimulates retching, or striving to vomit, when the soft palate is touched.*

vallecula *depression between the epiglottis and the base of the tongue.*

endotracheal intubation *passing a tube into the trachea to protect and maintain the airway and to permit medication administration and deep suctioning.*

larynx *the complex structure that joins the pharynx with the trachea.*

glottis *liplike opening between the vocal cords.*

vocal cords can also close together to prevent foreign bodies from entering the airway. The passage of an endotracheal tube between the vocal cords interferes not only with the creation of sound, but also with the protective function of coughing.

Sellick maneuver *pressure applied in a posterior direction to the anterior cricoid cartilage to occlude the esophagus.*

aspiration *inhaling foreign material, such as vomitus, into the lungs.*

cricothyroid membrane *membrane between the cricoid and thyroid cartilages of the larynx.*

Beneath the thyroid cartilage is the cricoid cartilage, which forms the inferior border of the larynx. Often it is considered the first tracheal ring. Unlike the thyroid and other tracheal cartilages, whose posterior surfaces are open and not fused, the cricoid cartilage forms a complete ring. The esophagus lies behind the cricoid cartilage, so pressure applied in a posterior direction to the anterior cricoid cartilage occludes the esophagus (**Sellick maneuver**), thus inhibiting vomiting and subsequent **aspiration** during airway management. In children, the cricoid cartilage is the narrowest part of the laryngeal airway. The fibrous **cricothyroid membrane** connects the inferior border of the thyroid cartilage with the superior aspect of the cricoid cartilage. It is the site for surgical airway techniques.

A mucous membrane lines most of the larynx. Rich with nerve endings from the vagus nerve, it is so sensitive that any irritation sparks a cough, or forceful exhalation of a large volume of air. First, air is drawn into the respiratory passageways. Next, the glottic opening shuts tightly, trapping the air within the lungs. Then the abdominal and thoracic muscles contract, pushing against the diaphragm and increasing intrathoracic pressure. The vocal cords suddenly open, and a burst of air forces foreign particles out of the lungs. The laryngeal mucous membrane is so sensitive that its stimulation by a laryngoscope or endotracheal tube can cause bradycardia (slow pulse rate), hypotension (low blood pressure), and decreased respiratory rate.

Other structures proximate to the larynx and of particular interest when you perform surgical airways are the thyroid gland, carotid arteries, and jugular veins. The thyroid gland is a "bow-tie" shaped endocrine gland located in the neck. It is highly vascular and lies inferior to the cricoid cartilage. It contains two lobes, one on each side of the trachea. These lobes are joined in the middle by the isthmus that extends across the trachea. The carotid arteries run closely along the trachea. Several branches of the carotid arteries cross the trachea. Likewise, the jugular veins lie very close to the trachea. Several branches of the jugular veins, such as the superior thyroid vein, cross the trachea.

Content Review

Lower Airway Components

- Trachea
- Bronchi
- Alveoli
- Lung parenchyma
- Pleura

LOWER AIRWAY ANATOMY

The lower airway extends from below the larynx to the alveoli (Figure 3-100 ■). This is where the respiratory exchange of oxygen and carbon dioxide occurs. Helpful landmarks are the fourth cervical vertebra at the posterior superior border, and the xiphoid process anterior inferiorly, though the posterior lung extends beyond this inferiorly.

The Trachea

trachea *tube that connects the larynx to the mainstem bronchi.*

As air enters the lower airway from the upper airway, it first enters and then passes through the **trachea.** The trachea is a 10 to 12 centimeter-long tube that connects the larynx to the two mainstem bronchi. It contains cartilaginous, C-shaped, open rings that form a frame to keep it open. The trachea is lined with respiratory epithelium containing cilia and mucus-producing cells. The mucus traps particles that the upper airway did not filter. The cilia then move the trapped particulate matter up into the mouth where it is swallowed or expelled.

The Bronchi

bronchi *tubes from the trachea into the lungs.*

At the carina, the trachea divides, or bifurcates, into the right and left mainstem **bronchi.** The right mainstem bronchus is almost straight, while the left mainstem bronchus angles more acutely to the left. Because of this, the right mainstem is often the site of aspirated foreign bodies. In addition, when an endotracheal tube is inserted too far, it tends to enter the right mainstem bronchus, thus ventilating only the right lung. Mainstem bronchi enter the lung tissue at the hilum, and then divide into the secondary and tertiary bronchi. The secondary and tertiary bronchi ultimately branch into the bronchioles, or small airways.

The bronchioles are encircled with smooth muscle that contains beta$_2$ (β_2) adrenergic receptors. When stimulated, these beta$_2$ receptors relax the bronchial smooth muscle, thus increasing the airway's diameter. This bronchodilation can increase the amount of air transported through the bronchiole. Conversely, parasympathetic receptors, when stimulated, cause the bronchial smooth

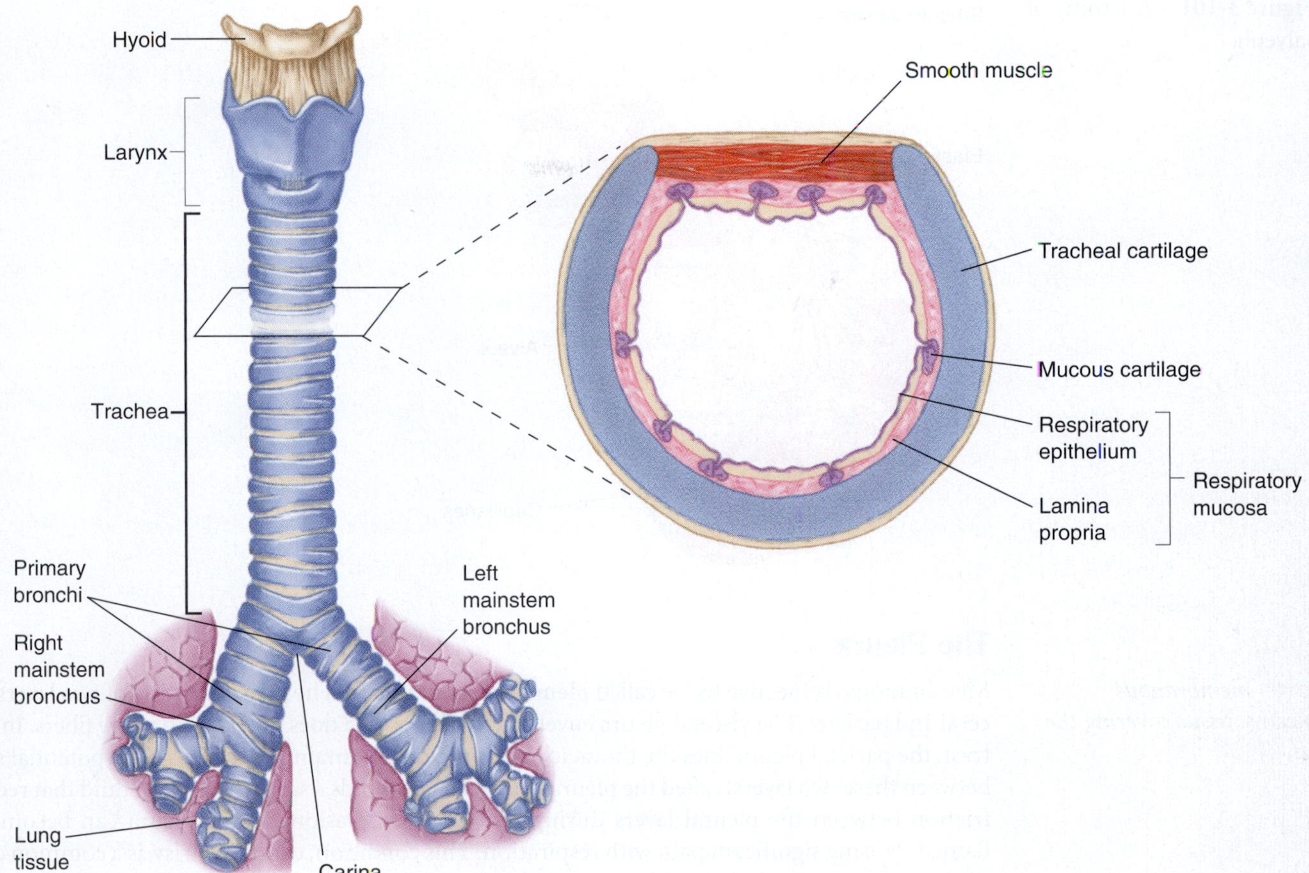

■ **Figure 3-100** Anatomy of the lower airway.

muscles to contract, thus reducing the diameter of the bronchiole. This bronchoconstriction can inhibit the movement of air through the bronchiole.

After approximately 22 divisions, the bronchioles turn into the respiratory bronchioles. These structures contain only muscular connective tissue and have a limited capacity for gas exchange. The respiratory bronchioles terminate at the alveoli.

The Alveoli

The respiratory bronchioles divide into the alveolar ducts, which terminate in balloonlike clusters of **alveoli** called alveolar sacs (Figure 3-101 ■). The alveoli contain an alveolar membrane that is only one or two cell layers thick. Because of this, the alveoli comprise the key functional unit of the respiratory system. Most oxygen and carbon dioxide gas exchanges take place here, although limited gas exchange may occur in the alveolar ducts and respiratory bronchioles. The alveoli become thinner as they expand. This facilitates diffusion of oxygen and carbon dioxide.

alveoli *microscopic air sacs where most oxygen and carbon dioxide gas exchanges take place.*

The alveoli's surface area is massive, totaling more than 40 square meters—enough to cover half of a tennis court. These hollow structures resist collapse largely because of the presence of surfactant, a chemical that decreases their surface tension and makes it easier for them to expand. Alveolar collapse (**atelectasis**) can occur if surfactant is insufficient or if the alveoli are not inflated. No gas exchange takes place in atelectatic alveoli.

atelactasis *alveolar collapse.*

The Lung Parenchyma

The alveoli are the terminal ends of the respiratory tree and the functional units of the lungs. As such, they are the core of the lung **parenchyma.** The lung parenchyma is arranged in two pulmonary lobules that form the anatomic division of the lungs. These lobules are further organized into lobes. The right lung has three lobes, the upper lobe, the middle lobe, and the lower lobe. The left lung, which shares thoracic space with the heart, has only two lobes, the upper lobe and the lower lobe.

parenchyma *principle or essential parts of an organ.*

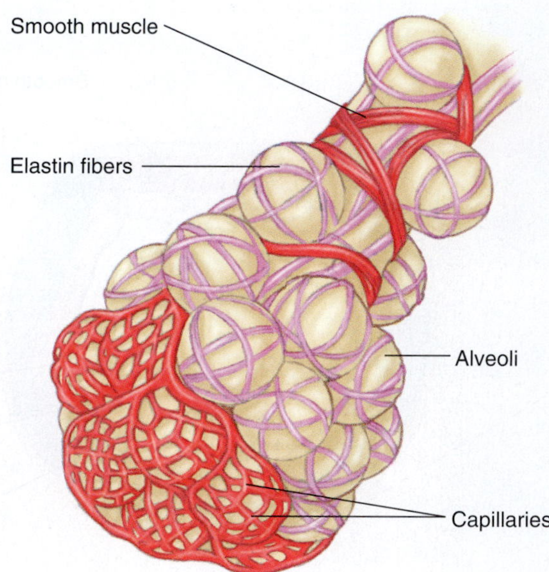

■ **Figure 3-101** Anatomy of the alveoli.

The Pleura

pleura *membranous connective tissue covering the lungs.*

Membranous connective tissue called **pleura** covers the lungs. The pleura consists of two layers, visceral and parietal. The visceral pleura envelopes the lungs and does not contain nerve fibers. In contrast, the parietal pleura lines the thoracic cavity and does contain nerve fibers. The potential space between these two layers, called the pleural space, usually holds a small amount of fluid that reduces friction between the pleural layers during respiration. Occasionally, the pleura can become inflamed, causing significant pain with respiration. This condition, called pleurisy, is a common cause of chest pain, particularly in cigarette smokers.

THE PEDIATRIC AIRWAY

The pediatric airway is fundamentally the same as an adult's, but you will need to know the differences in relative size and position of some components. The airway is smaller in all aspects, particularly the diameters of the openings and passageways.

In the pharynx, the jaw is smaller and the tongue relatively larger, resulting in greater potential airway encroachment (Figure 3-102 ■). The epiglottis is much floppier and rounder ("omega" shaped). The dental (alveolar) ridge and teeth are softer and more fragile than an adult's and potentially more subject to damage from airway maneuvers.

The larynx lies more superior and anterior in children and is funnel-shaped because the cricoid cartilage is undeveloped. Before the age of 10, the cricoid cartilage is the narrowest part of the airway. Most significantly, even a small foreign body or a limited degree of swelling in the pediatric airway can be life threatening. Because of this, young children tend to suffer more problems related to the trachea than do older children. A common example is croup (laryngotracheobronchitis), a viral infection that causes the soft tissues below the glottis to swell. This can reduce the diameter of the airway, potentially causing serious problems.

The ribs and the cartilage of the pediatric thoracic cage are softer and more pliable. This lack of rigidity lessens the thoracic wall's and accessory muscles' ability to assist lung expansion during inspiration. As a result, infants and children tend to rely more on their diaphragms for breathing. Always pay close attention to these differences when treating pediatric patients, especially those with respiratory complaints.

PHYSIOLOGY OF THE RESPIRATORY SYSTEM

Just as successful airway management requires a firm understanding of airway anatomy, a good outcome for these patients requires a working knowledge of the mechanics of oxygenation and ventilation. Your knowledge of normal respiratory physiology will lay the groundwork for your

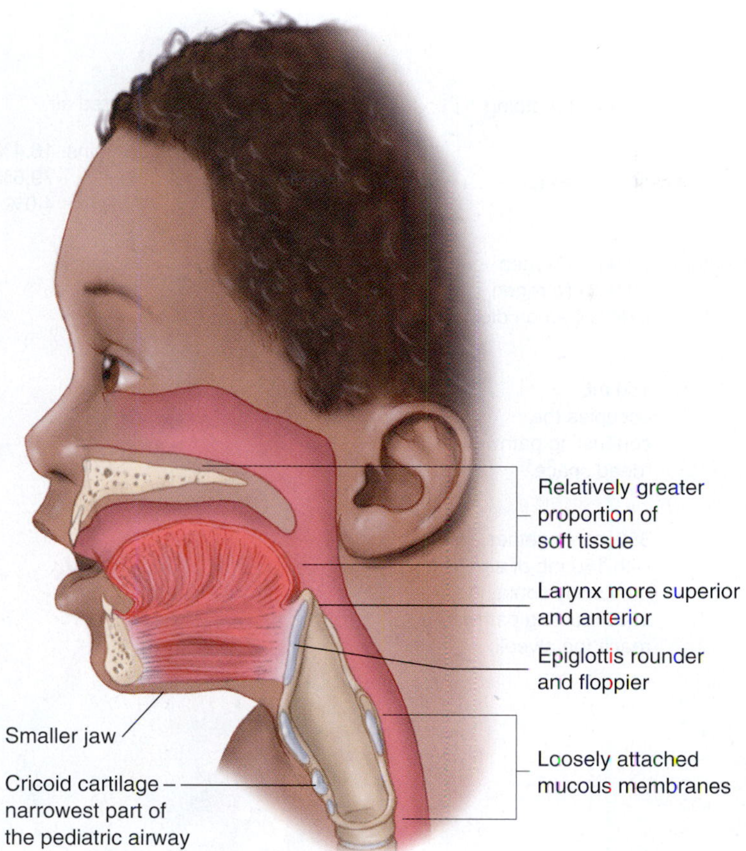

■ **Figure 3-102** Anatomy of the pediatric airway.

comprehension of important pathophysiology and will help you to determine which actions will assure optimal patient care.

Respiration and Ventilation

Respiration is the exchange of gases between a living organism and its environment. Pulmonary, or external, respiration occurs in the lungs when the respiratory gases are exchanged between the alveoli and the red blood cells in the pulmonary capillaries through the capillary membranes (Figure 3-103 ■). Cellular, or internal, respiration occurs in the peripheral capillaries. It is the exchange of the respiratory gases between the red blood cells and the various body tissues. Cellular respiration in the peripheral tissue produces carbon dioxide (CO_2). The blood picks up this waste product in the capillaries and transports it as bicarbonate ions through the venous system to the lungs. While respiration describes the process of gas exchange in the lungs and peripheral tissues, **ventilation** is the mechanical process that moves air into and out of the lungs. Ventilation is necessary for respiration to occur.

ventilation *the mechanical process that moves air into and out of the lungs.*

The Respiratory Cycle Nothing within the lung parenchyma makes it contract or expand. Pulmonary ventilation, therefore, depends on changes in pressure within the thoracic cavity. These changes occur in a respiratory cycle involving coordinated interaction among the respiratory system, the central nervous system, and the musculoskeletal system.

The thoracic cavity is a closed space, opening to the external environment only through the trachea. The diaphragm separates the thoracic cavity from the abdomen. When the diaphragm contracts, it draws downward, away from the thoracic cavity, thus enlarging it. Likewise, when the muscles between the ribs, or intercostal muscles, contract, they draw the rib cage upward and outward, away from the thoracic cavity, further increasing its volume.

The respiratory cycle begins when the lungs have achieved a normal expiration and the pressure inside the thoracic cavity equals the atmospheric pressure. At this point, respiratory centers in the brain communicate with the diaphragm by way of the phrenic nerve, signaling it to contract and

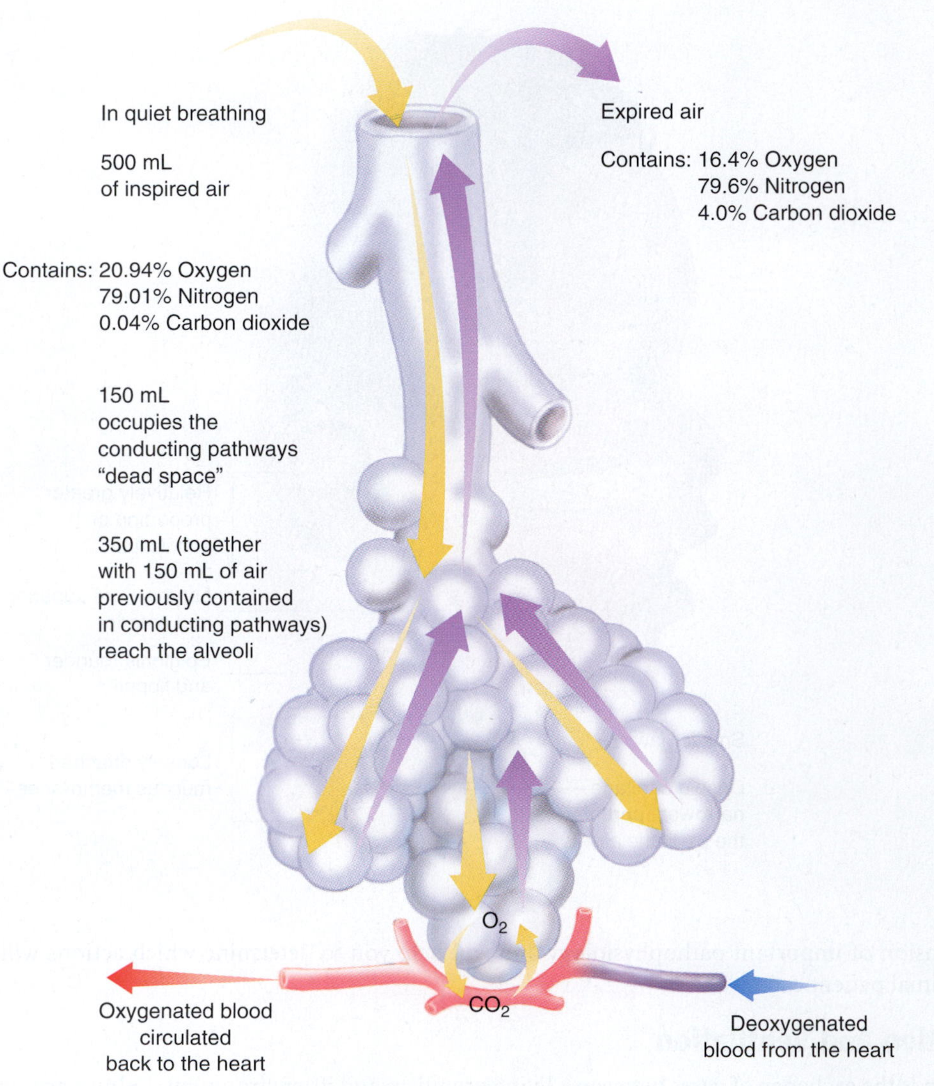

Figure 3-103 Diffusion of gases across an alveolar membrane.

thus initiate the respiratory cycle. As the size of the thorax increases in relation to the volume of air it holds, pressure within the thorax decreases, becoming lower than atmospheric pressure. This negative intrathoracic pressure invites air into the thorax through the airway. Because the visceral and parietal pleura remain in contact with each other under normal circumstances, the highly elastic lungs immediately assume the thoracic cavity's internal contour. These combined factors move air into the lungs (inspiration). At the same time, the alveoli inflate with the lungs. They become thinner as they expand, allowing oxygen and carbon dioxide to diffuse across their membranes.

When the pressure in the thoracic cavity again reaches that of the atmosphere, the alveoli are maximally inflated. Pulmonary expansion stimulates microscopic stretch receptors in the bronchi and bronchioles. These receptors signal the respiratory center by way of the vagus nerve to inhibit inspiration, and the air influx stops. This process is primarily protective, as it prevents overinflation of the lungs.

At the end of inspiration, the respiratory muscles now relax, thus decreasing the size of the chest cavity, and in turn increasing the intrathoracic pressure. The naturally elastic lungs recoil, forcing air out through the airway (expiration) until intrathoracic and atmospheric pressure are equal once again. Normal expiration is a passive process, while inspiration is an active process, using energy. In respiratory inadequacy, when this process fails to provide satisfactory gas exchange, the patient may use accessory respiratory muscles such as the strap muscles of his neck and his abdominal muscles to augment his efforts to expand the thoracic cavity.

Pulmonary Circulation Respiration also requires an intact circulatory system. In fact, during each cardiac cycle, the heart pumps as much blood to the lungs as it pumps to the peripheral tissues.

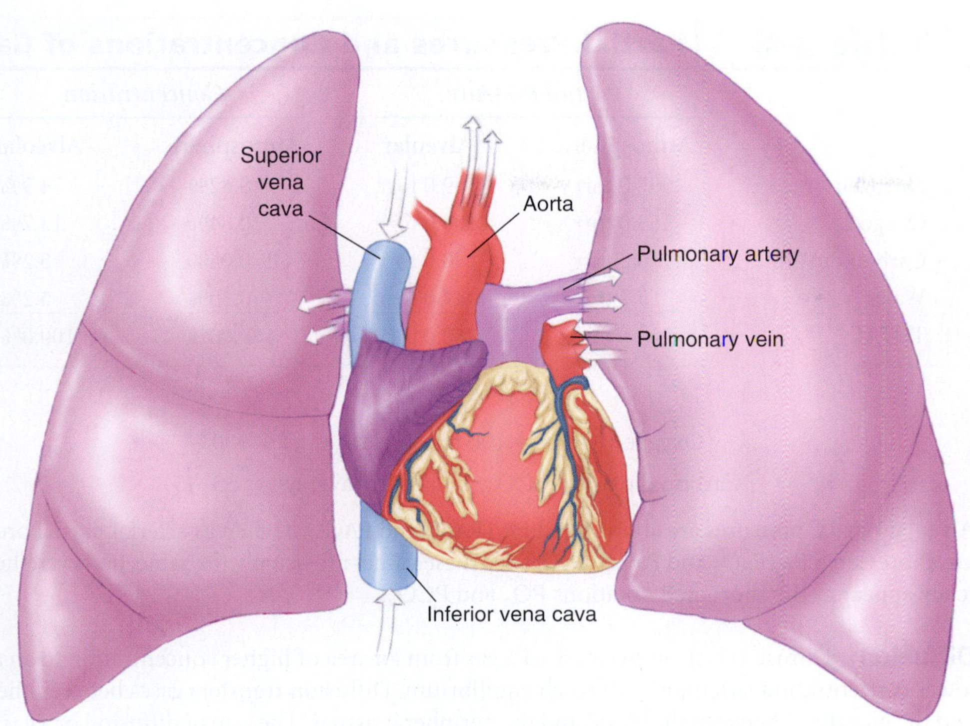

■ Figure 3-104 Pulmonary circulation.

In the capillaries, these cells take oxygen from red blood cells coming from the arterial system and give up carbon dioxide to blood returning to the venous system. The venous system carries this deoxygenated blood to the right side of the heart, and the right ventricle pumps it into the pulmonary artery (Figure 3-104 ■).

The pulmonary artery immediately branches into the right and the left pulmonary arteries, each supplying its respective lung. In turn, both branches quickly fan into smaller arteries that end in the pulmonary capillaries. These capillaries are spread over the surfaces of the alveoli, where the red blood cells exchange carbon dioxide for oxygen. The pulmonary capillaries recombine into larger veins, eventually terminating in the pulmonary vein. The pulmonary vein empties the oxygenated blood into the left atrium of the heart. Finally, the heart transports the oxygenated blood through the left ventricle and into the systemic arterial system via the aorta and its tributaries.

The lungs themselves receive little of their blood supply from the pulmonary arteries or veins. Instead, bronchial arteries that branch from the aorta supply most of their blood. Bronchial veins return this blood from the lungs to the superior vena cava.

Measuring Oxygen and Carbon Dioxide Levels

You can determine the amount of oxygen and carbon dioxide in the blood by measuring their partial pressures. **Partial pressure** is the pressure exerted by each component of a gas mixture. In other words, the partial pressure of a gas is its percentage of the mixture's total pressure. The partial pressure of oxygen at normal atmospheric pressure, for example, is the percentage of oxygen in atmospheric air (21 percent) multiplied by the atmospheric pressure at sea level (760 torr, or 14.7 pounds per square inch):

partial pressure *the pressure exerted by each component of a gas mixture.*

$$0.21 \times 760 \text{ torr} = 159.6 \text{ torr}$$

(Note that torr and mmHg are the same measures of pressure.) Earth's atmosphere consists of four major respiratory gases: nitrogen (N_2), oxygen (O_2), carbon dioxide (CO_2), and water (H_2O). Although nitrogen is metabolically inert, it is needed to inflate gas-filled body cavities such as the chest. Table 3–6 lists these four respiratory gases' partial pressures and concentrations in the environment and in the alveoli.

Since alveolar partial pressure and arterial partial pressure are essentially the same in the normal lung, normal arterial partial pressures for oxygen and carbon dioxide may be expressed:

Table 3–6 Partial Pressures and Concentrations of Gases

	Partial Pressure		*Concentration*	
	Atmospheric	**Alveolar**	**Atmospheric**	**Alveolar**
Nitrogen	597.0 torr	569.0 torr	78.62%	74.9%
Oxygen	159.0 torr	104.0 torr	20.84%	13.7%
Carbon dioxide	0.3 torr	40.0 torr	0.04%	5.2%
Water	3.7 torr	47.0 torr	0.50%	6.2%
TOTAL	760.0 torr	760.0 torr	100.00%	100.0%

$$\text{Oxygen } (PaO_2) = 100 \text{ torr (average} = 80\text{–}100)$$

$$\text{Carbon dioxide } (PaCO_2) = 40 \text{ torr (average} = 35\text{–}45)$$

PA *alveolar partial pressure.*

Pa *arterial partial pressure.*

Alveolar partial pressures are abbreviated **PA** (PAO_2 and $PACO_2$) whereas arterial partial pressures are abbreviated **Pa** (PaO_2 and $PaCO_2$). Because these values are usually the same, however, they typically appear as the shortened notations PO_2 and PCO_2.

Diffusion Diffusion is the movement of a gas from an area of higher concentration to an area of lower concentration, attempting to reach equilibrium. Diffusion transfers gases between the lungs and the blood and between the blood and the peripheral tissues. The rate of diffusion of a gas across the pulmonary membranes depends on the gas's solubility in water. For example, carbon dioxide is 21 times more soluble in water than oxygen and readily crosses the pulmonary capillary membranes. In the peripheral tissues, the gradient (direction of diffusion) for CO_2 is from the tissue, where its concentration is high, to the capillary blood, where its concentration is low.

In the lungs, oxygen dissolves in water at the alveolar membrane and leaves the area of higher concentration, the alveoli, and enters the area of lower concentration, the venous blood in the pulmonary capillaries. Concurrently, carbon dioxide leaves the area of higher concentration, the arterial blood, and enters the area of lower concentration, the alveoli. The blood returns from the pulmonary vein to the heart and then moves into the systemic circulation.

Oxygen Concentration in the Blood Oxygen diffuses into the blood plasma, where most of it combines with hemoglobin and is measured as oxygen saturation (SpO_2). The remainder is dissolved in the blood and is measured as the PaO_2. Hemoglobin approaches 100 percent saturation when the PaO_2 of dissolved oxygen reaches 90 to 100 torr. Each gram of saturated hemoglobin carries 1.34 milliliters of oxygen. Oxygen saturation is the ratio of the blood's actual oxygen content to its total oxygen-carrying capacity:

$$\text{Oxygen saturation} = O_2 \text{ content}/O_2 \text{ capacity} \times 100(\%)$$

The hemoglobin molecule carries the vast majority of oxygen in the blood (approximately 97 percent). Very little oxygen dissolves in the plasma. Since partial pressure measurements detect only the amount of oxygen dissolved in the plasma and do not always reflect the total oxygen saturation, they can be misleading. For example, a patient who has suffered carbon monoxide poisoning cannot transport enough oxygen to the peripheral tissues since carbon monoxide displaces oxygen from the hemoglobin molecule. But an arterial blood gas sample might reveal a normal or high PaO_2. This would indicate that adequate oxygen was reaching the blood. In fact, however, an inadequate amount of hemoglobin would be available to transport the oxygen to the peripheral tissues, thus resulting in peripheral hypoxia.

Several factors can affect oxygen concentrations in the blood:

★ *Decreased hemoglobin concentration* (anemia, hemorrhage)

★ *Inadequate alveolar ventilation* due to low inspired-oxygen concentration, respiratory muscle paralysis, and pulmonary conditions such as emphysema, asthma, or pneumothorax

- ★ *Decreased diffusion across the pulmonary membrane* when diffusion distance increases or the pulmonary membrane changes; for example, when fluid enters the space between the alveolar membrane and the pulmonary capillary membrane, as in pneumonia, chronic obstructive pulmonary disease (COPD), or pulmonary edema (swelling).
- ★ *Ventilation/perfusion mismatch* occurs when a portion of the alveoli collapses, as in atelectasis. Blood travels past these collapsed alveoli without oxygenation (shunting), without carbon dioxide, and without oxygen uptake. This can result from **hypoventilation,** which can occur secondary to pain or inability to inspire (traumatic asphyxia). When the lung collapses, as in **pneumothorax, hemothorax,** or a combination of the two, less surface area is available for gas exchange. Alternatively, a ventilation/perfusion mismatch can occur when blood is prevented from reaching the alveolar capillary membranes but alveolar ventilation remains adequate. This occurs when a blood clot travels to or is formed in the pulmonary arterial system, a condition known as pulmonary thromboembolism.

hypoventilation *reduction in breathing rate and depth.*

pneumothorax *accumulation of air or gas in the pleural cavity.*

hemothorax *accumulation in the pleural cavity of blood or fluid containing blood.*

You can correct oxygen derangements by increasing ventilation, administering supplemental oxygen, using intermittent positive-pressure ventilation (IPPV), or administering drugs to correct underlying problems such as pulmonary edema, asthma, or **pulmonary embolism.** The emergency being treated determines the desired fractional concentration of oxygen (FiO_2) to be delivered. It is crucial to remember not to withhold oxygen from any patient whose clinical condition indicates its need.

pulmonary embolism *blood clot that travels to the pulmonary circulation and hinders oxygenation of the blood.*

FiO_2 *concentration of oxygen in inspired air.*

Carbon Dioxide Concentration in the Blood

The blood transports carbon dioxide mainly in the form of bicarbonate ion (HCO_3^-). It carries approximately 70 percent as bicarbonate and approximately 20 percent combined with hemoglobin. Less than 7 percent is dissolved in the plasma. Several factors influence carbon dioxide's concentration in the blood, including increased CO_2 production and/or decreased CO_2 elimination:

- ★ *Hyperventilation lowers CO_2 levels* and can be the result of an increased respiratory rate or deeper respiration, both of which increase the minute volume. (We will discuss minute volume more completely later.)
- ★ *Increased CO_2 production* can be caused by:
  - Fever
  - Muscle exertion
  - Shivering
  - Metabolic processes resulting in the formation of metabolic acids
- ★ *Decreased CO_2 elimination* (increased CO_2 levels in the blood) resulting from decreased alveolar ventilation is commonly caused by hypoventilation due to:
  - Respiratory depression by drugs
  - Airway obstruction
  - Impairment of the respiratory muscles
  - Obstructive diseases such as asthma and emphysema

Increased CO_2 levels (**hypercarbia**) are usually treated by increasing the rate and/or volume of ventilation and by correcting the underlying cause.

hypercarbia *excessive pressure of carbon dioxide in the blood.*

Regulation of Respiration

Voluntary and Involuntary Respiratory Controls

The number of times a person breathes in 1 minute, the **respiratory rate,** is unique in that both voluntary and involuntary nervous system mechanisms control it. We do not ordinarily need to make a conscious effort to breathe; our brains automatically regulate this function. However, we can voluntarily override our involuntary respirations until physical and chemical mechanisms signal the nervous system's respiratory centers to involuntarily provide impulses and correct any breathing irregularities.

respiratory rate *the number of times a person breathes in 1 minute.*

Nervous Impulses from the Respiratory Center The main respiratory center lies in the *medulla oblongata* in the brainstem. Various neurons within the medulla initiate impulses that result in respiration. A rise in the frequency of these impulses increases the respiratory rate. Conversely, a decrease in their frequency decreases the respiratory rate. The medulla is connected to the respiratory muscles primarily via the vagus nerve. This is an involuntary pathway. If the medulla fails to initiate respiration, an additional control center in the pons, called the *apneustic center,* assumes respiratory control to ensure the continuation of respirations. A third center, the *pneumotaxic center,* also in the pons, controls expiration.

Stretch Receptors During inspiration, the lungs become distended, activating stretch receptors. As the degree of stretch increases, these receptors fire more frequently. The impulses they send to the brainstem inhibit the medullary cells, decreasing the inspiratory stimulus. Thus, the respiratory muscles relax, allowing the elastic lungs to recoil and expel air from the body. As the stretch decreases, the stretch receptors stop firing. This process, called the *Hering-Breuer reflex,* prevents overexpansion of the lungs.

Chemoreceptors Other involuntary respiration controls include central chemical receptors in the medulla and peripheral chemoreceptors in the carotid bodies and in the arch of the aorta. These chemoreceptors are stimulated by decreased PaO_2, increased $PaCO_2$, and decreased pH. (The pH scale expresses the degree of acidity or alkalinity. A lower pH indicates greater acidity; a higher pH indicates greater alkalinity. Chapter 4 discusses pH in greater detail.) Cerebrospinal fluid (CSF) pH is the primary control of respiratory center stimulation. The CSF pH responds very quickly to changes in arterial PCO_2. Any increase in PCO_2 will decrease CSF pH, which will in turn stimulate the central chemoreceptors to increase respiration. Conversely, low $PaCO_2$ levels will raise CSF pH, in turn decreasing chemoreceptor stimulation and slowing respiratory activity. Because $PaCO_2$ is inversely related to CSF pH, $PaCO_2$ is seen as the normal neuroregulatory control of respirations. Additionally, any increase in the arterial $PaCO_2$ stimulates the peripheral chemoreceptors to signal the brainstem to increase respiration, thus speeding CO_2 elimination from the body.

hypoxemia *decreased blood oxygen level.*

hypoxic drive *mechanism that increases respiratory stimulation when blood oxygen falls and inhibits respiratory stimulation when blood oxygen climbs.*

apnea *absence of breathing.*

Hypoxic Drive The body also constantly monitors the PaO_2 and the pH. In fact, **hypoxemia** (decreased partial pressure of oxygen in the blood) is a profound stimulus of respiration in a normal individual. People with chronic respiratory disease such as emphysema and chronic bronchitis tend to retain CO_2 and, therefore, have a chronically elevated $PaCO_2$. Chemoreceptors in the periphery eventually become accustomed to this chronic condition, and the central nervous system stops using $PaCO_2$ to regulate respiration. This activates a default mechanism called **hypoxic drive,** which increases respiratory stimulation when PaO_2 falls and inhibits respiratory stimulation when PaO_2 climbs. High-volume oxygen administration to people with this condition can cause respiratory arrest. Because high-flow, high-concentration oxygen can quickly double or even triple the PaO_2, peripheral chemoreceptors stop stimulating the respiratory centers, causing **apnea** (cessation of breathing). Although this is a potential threat, it is never appropriate to withhold oxygen from a patient for whom oxygen therapy is indicated; if the respiratory effort becomes inadequate, ventilatory assistance will be necessary.

Measures of Respiratory Function

The respiratory rate is the number of respiratory cycles per minute, normally 12 to 20 breaths per minute in adults, 18 to 24 in children, and 40 to 60 in infants. Several factors affect respiratory rate:

- ★ Fever—increases rate
- ★ Emotion—increases rate
- ★ Pain—increases rate
- ★ Hypoxia (inadequate tissue oxygenation)—increases rate
- ★ Acidosis—increases rate

★ Stimulant drugs—increase rate

★ Depressant drugs—decrease rate

★ Sleep—decreases rate

Paramedics must fully understand ventilatory mechanics and capacities for the average adult's respiratory system. This knowledge will enable you to adapt your mechanical ventilation techniques to your patient's size, lung compliance, need for hyperventilation, or other individual requirements. It is especially crucial in situations that call for advanced mechanical ventilator skills. Respiratory capacities and measurements with which you must be familiar include:

★ ***Total lung capacity*** (TLC). This is the maximum lung capacity—the total amount of air contained in the lung at the end of maximal inspiration. In the average adult male, this volume is approximately 6 liters.

total lung capacity *maximum lung capacity.*

★ ***Tidal volume*** (V_T). The tidal volume is the average volume of gas inhaled or exhaled in one respiratory cycle. In the adult male this is approximately 500 mL (5–7 mL/kg).

tidal volume *average volume of gas inhaled or exhaled in one respiratory cycle.*

★ *Dead space volume* (V_D). The dead space volume is the amount of gas in the tidal volume that remains in air passageways unavailable for gas exchange. It is approximately 150 mL in the adult male. Anatomic dead space includes the trachea and bronchi. Obstructions or diseases such as chronic obstructive pulmonary disease or atelectasis can cause physiologic dead space.

★ *Alveolar volume* (V_A). The alveolar volume is the amount of gas in the tidal volume that reaches the alveoli for gas exchange. It is the difference between tidal volume and dead-space volume (approximately 350 mL in the adult male):

$$V_A = V_T - V_D$$

★ ***Minute volume*** (V_{min}). The minute volume is the amount of gas moved in and out of the respiratory tract in 1 minute:

$$V_{min} = VT \times \text{Respiratory rate}$$

minute volume *amount of gas inhaled and exhaled in 1 minute.*

★ *Alveolar minute volume* ($V_{A\text{-}min}$). The alveolar minute volume is the amount of gas that reaches the alveoli for gas exchange in 1 minute:

$$V_{A\text{-}min} = (V_T - V_D) \times \text{Respiratory rate}$$

or

$$V_{A\text{-}min} = V_A \times \text{Respiratory rate}$$

★ *Inspiratory reserve volume* (IRV). The inspiratory reserve volume is the amount of air that can be maximally inhaled after a normal inspiration.

★ *Expiratory reserve volume* (ERV). The expiratory reserve volume is the amount of air that can be maximally exhaled after a normal expiration.

★ *Residual volume* (RV). The residual volume is the amount of air remaining in the lungs at the end of maximal expiration.

★ *Functional residual capacity* (FRC). The functional residual capacity is the volume of gas that remains in the lungs at the end of normal expiration:

$$FRC = ERV + RV$$

★ *Forced expiratory volume* (FEV). The forced expiratory volume is the amount of air that can be maximally expired after maximum inspiration.

THE ABDOMEN

The abdominal cavity is bound by the diaphragm, superiorly; the pelvis, inferiorly; the vertebral column, the posterior and inferior ribs, and the back muscles (psoas and paraspinal muscles), posteriorly; the muscles of the flank, laterally; and the abdominal muscles, anteriorly (Figure 3-105 ■). The cavity is divided into three spaces: the **peritoneal space** (containing those organs or portions of

peritoneal space *division of the abdominal cavity containing those organs or portions of organs covered by the peritoneum.*

■ Figure 3-105 Muscles protecting the organs of the abdominal cavity.

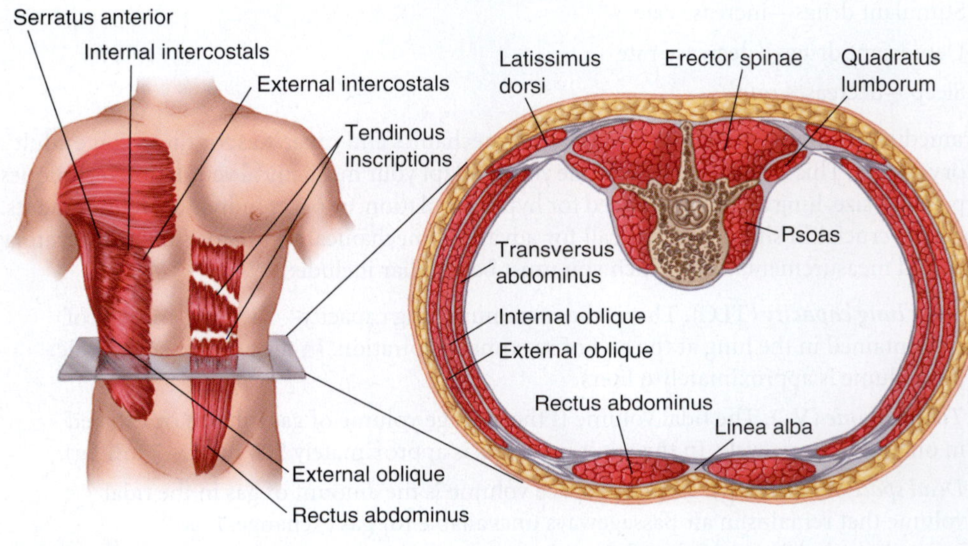

a. Anterior view of the trunk, showing superficial and deep members of the oblique and rectus groups.

b. Diagrammatic sectional view through the abdominal region.

retroperitoneal space *division of the abdominal cavity containing those organs posterior to the peritoneal lining.*

pelvic space *division of the abdominal cavity containing those organs located within the pelvis.*

organs covered by the abdominal (peritoneal) lining); the **retroperitoneal space** (containing those organs posterior to the peritoneal lining); and the **pelvic space** (containing the organs within the pelvis). Anatomical landmarks of this area include the centrally located umbilicus (the navel), the xiphoid process (tip of the sternum) at the upper and central abdominal border, the bony ridges of the pelvis (the iliac crests) inferiorly and laterally, and the pubic prominence inferiorly.

The abdomen is divided into four subregions by imaginary vertical and horizontal lines intersecting at the umbilicus (navel) and forming the right and left upper and lower quadrants. The right upper quadrant contains the gallbladder, right kidney, most of the liver, some small bowel, a portion of the ascending and transverse colon, and a small portion of the pancreas. The left upper quadrant contains the stomach, spleen, left kidney, most of the pancreas, and a portion of the liver, small bowel, and transverse and descending colon. The right lower quadrant contains the appendix, and portions of the urinary bladder, small bowel, ascending colon, rectum, and female genitalia. The left lower quadrant contains the sigmoid colon and portions of the urinary bladder, small bowel, descending colon, rectum, and female genitalia.

The major structures within the abdomen include the digestive tract, the accessory organs of digestion, the spleen, the structures and organs of the urinary system, and the female reproductive organs. (The male reproductive organs, or genitalia, are considered to be part of the urinary system. The female reproductive organs are separate from the urinary system, and include the reproductive organs within the abdomen as well as the external genitalia.)

ABDOMINAL VASCULATURE

The abdominal contents are supplied with blood via the abdominal aorta, which travels along and to the left of the spinal column. It sends forth many branches to discrete organs and the bowel (Figure 3-106 ■). The abdominal aorta bifurcates at the upper sacral level into two large iliac arteries. These eventually become the femoral arteries as they traverse and then exit the pelvis. The attachment of these arteries to the pelvic structure is quite firm and may result in their tearing if the pelvis is fractured and displaced. The inferior vena cava is located along the spinal column and collects venous blood from the lower extremities and the abdomen, relatively parallel to the arterial system, returning it to the heart. The abdomen also houses a special circulatory system, the portal system. This venous subsystem collects venous blood as well as the fluid and nutrients absorbed by the bowel and transports them to the liver. The liver detoxifies the fluid, stores excess nutrients, adds nutrients when they are deficient, and then sends the blood/nutrient/fluid mixture into the inferior

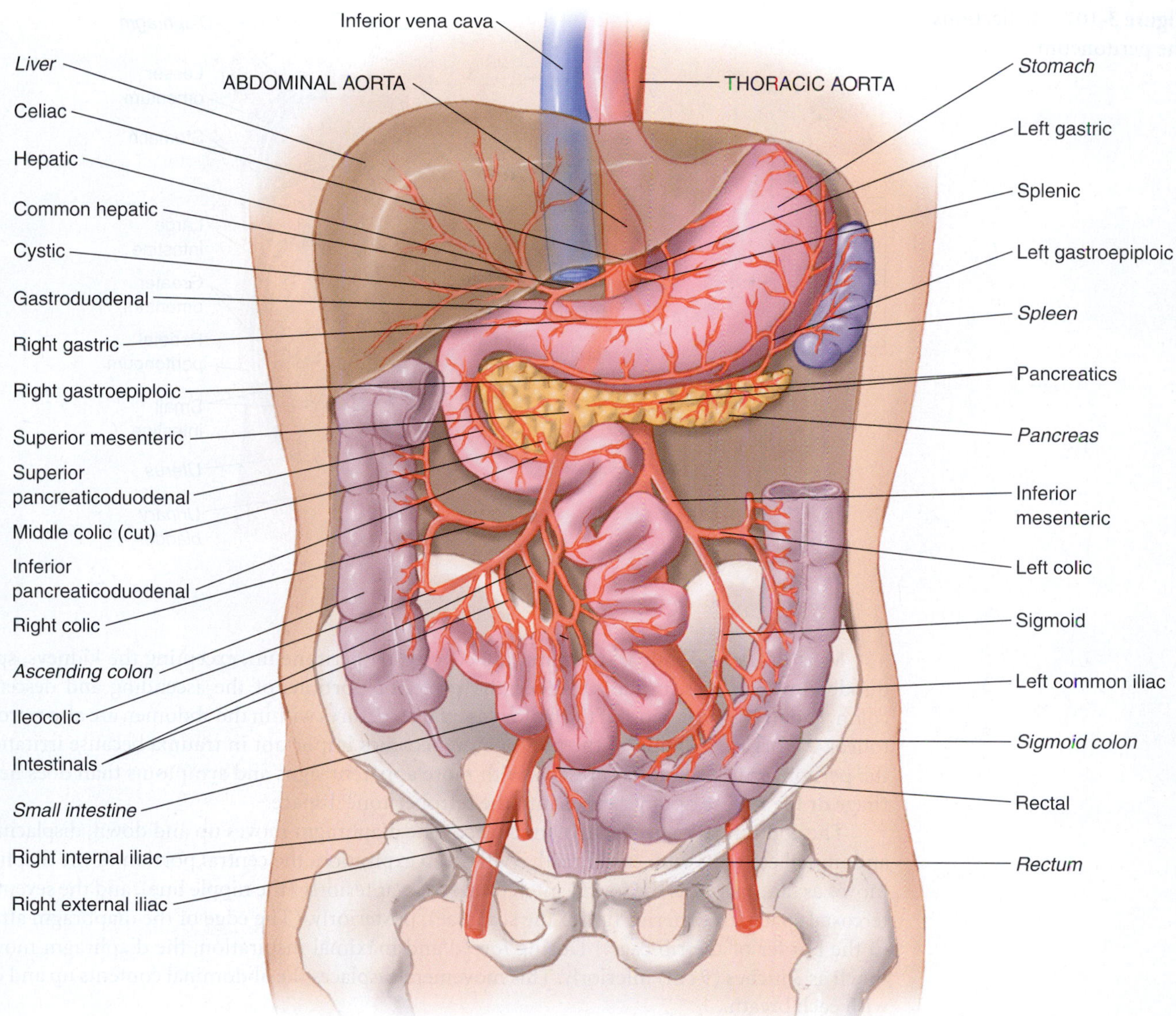

■ Figure 3-106 The abdominal arteries.

vena cava, just below the heart. There it mixes with venous blood and is circulated through the heart and then the rest of the body.

THE PERITONEUM

Many of the abdominal organs are covered by a serous membrane called the **peritoneum** (Figure 3-107 ■). This tissue resembles the pleura of the lungs and functions in a similar manner. The parietal peritoneum covers most of the interior surface of the anterior and lateral abdominal cavity, while the visceral peritoneum covers the individual organs. A small amount of fluid is found between the peritoneal layers and permits free movement of the bowel during digestion.

peritoneum *fine fibrous tissue surrounding the interior of most of the abdominal cavity and covering most of the small bowel and some of the abdominal organs.*

The digestive tract is restrained and prevented from tangling by a structure called the **mesentery.** The mesentery is a double fold of peritoneum containing blood vessels, lymphatic vessels, nerves, and fatty tissue. It suspends the bowel from the posterior abdominal wall. An additional fold of mesentery, called the omentum, also covers, insulates, and protects the anterior surface of the abdomen. The thickness of the omentum varies with the size and percentage of body fat of the patient. It may be several inches thick in the obese patient or very narrow in the thin and muscular patient.

mesentery *double fold of peritoneum that supports the major portion of the small bowel, suspending it from the posterior abdominal wall.*

■ **Figure 3-107** Reflections of the peritoneum.

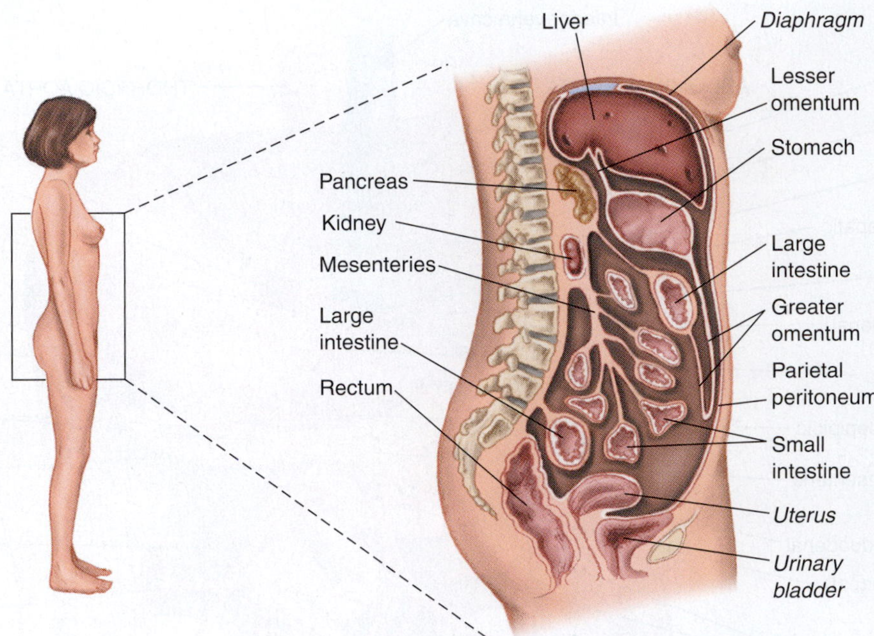

Most of the abdominal structures are covered by peritoneum, excepting the kidneys, spleen, duodenum, pancreas, urinary bladder, the posterior portions of the ascending and descending colon, and the rectum. Most of the major vascular structures within the abdomen are also retroperitoneal. An organ's relation to the peritoneum becomes important in trauma because irritation of the peritoneum (peritonitis) presents with more apparent signs and symptoms than does hemorrhage or the release of other fluids into the retroperitoneal space.

The abdominal cavity is a dynamic place. The diaphragm moves up and down, displacing the abdominal contents with each breath. With deep expiration, the central portion of the diaphragm moves as far upward as the fourth intercostal space, anteriorly (the nipple line), and the seventh intercostal space (the inferior tips of the scapulae), posteriorly. (The edge of the diaphragm attaches to the border of the rib cage.) During forced and maximal inspiration, the diaphragm moves as much as 3 inches (9 cm) inferiorly. This movement displaces the abdominal contents up and down with each breath.

Additionally, the volume of substance within the hollow organs varies—an empty (10 mL) versus a distended (500 mL) bladder or a full (1.5 L) versus an empty stomach. The digestive tract is also suspended from the back of the abdominal cavity and is permitted some movement as it digests food. This dynamic movement becomes an important consideration when anticipating abdominal injury due to blunt or penetrating trauma.

THE DIGESTIVE SYSTEM

The digestive system includes the digestive tract and the accessory organs of digestion (Figure 3-108 ■). The digestive tract (also called the *alimentary canal*) is the muscular tube that physically and chemically breaks down and absorbs the fluids and nutrients from the food we eat. The accessory organs of digestion include the liver, gallbladder, and pancreas. These organs prepare and store digestive enzymes and perform other important body functions.

THE DIGESTIVE TRACT

digestive tract *internal passageway that begins at the mouth and ends at the anus; also called the* alimentary canal.

The **digestive tract** is a thin, 25-foot-long hollow muscular tube responsible for churning the material to be digested, for excreting digestive juices to be mixed with it, and for absorbing nutrients and then water. Abdominal components of the digestive tract consist of the stomach, the small

The Digestive System

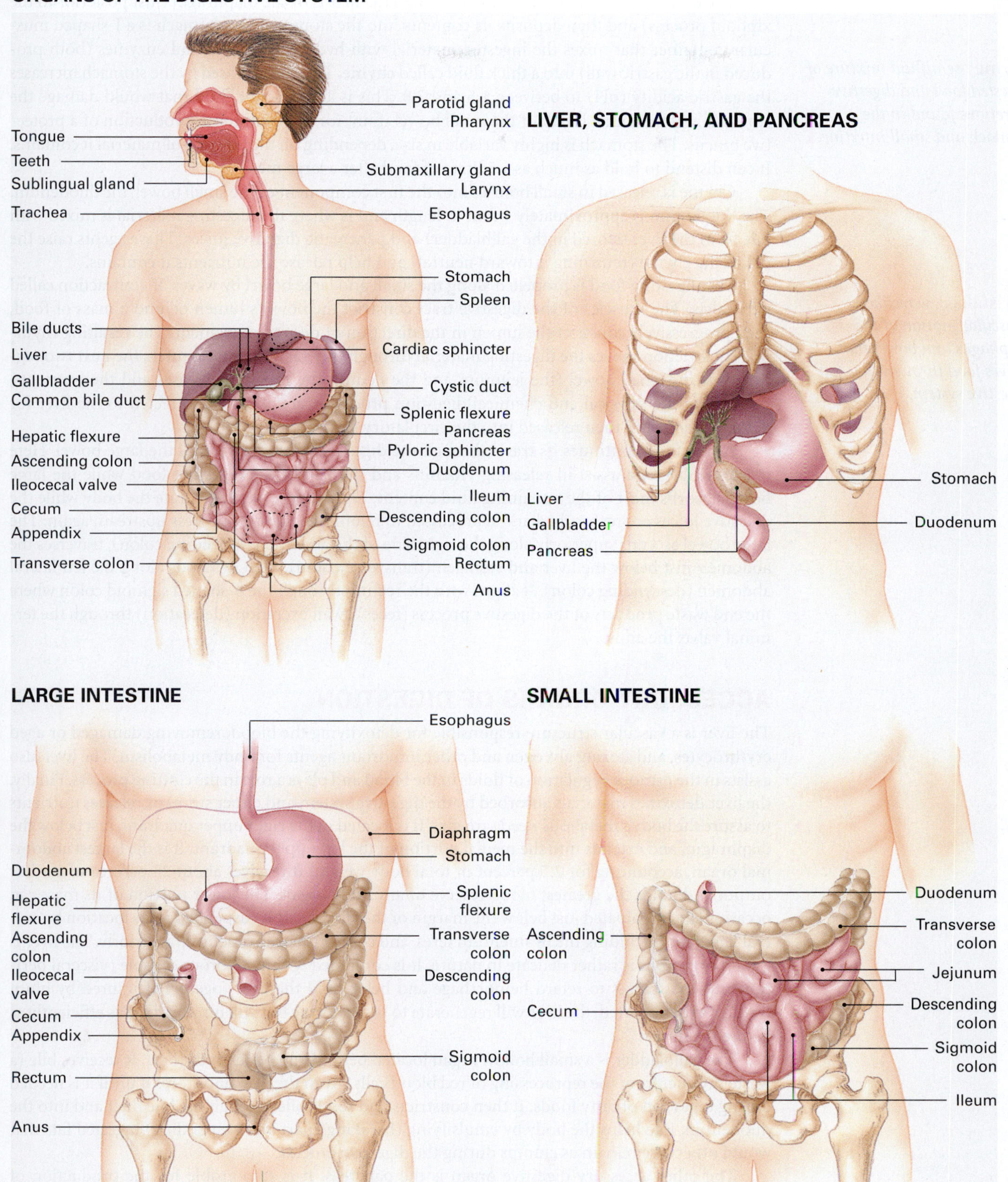

■ **Figure 3-108** The digestive tract and accessory organs.

bowel (duodenum, jejunum, and ileum), the large bowel (or colon), the rectum, and the anus. These structures fill the anterior and lateral aspects of the abdominal cavity, except for the area occupied by the liver.

The esophagus enters the abdomen through the hiatus of the diaphragm (just posterior to the xiphoid process) and then deposits its contents into the stomach. The stomach is a J-shaped muscular container that mixes the ingested material with hydrochloric acid and enzymes (both produced in the gastric wall) into a thick fluid called **chyme.** The acid released by the stomach increases the gastric acidity (pH) to between 1.5 and 2.0. This is a very acidic fluid that would damage the stomach and the initial lining of the small bowel if not for the continuous production of a protective mucus. The stomach is highly variable in size, depending on the amount of material it contains. It can distend to hold as much as 1.5 liters of food after a large meal.

chyme *semifluid mixture of ingested food and digestive secretions found in the stomach and small intestine.*

Chyme is released in small boluses into the first component of the small bowel, the duodenum. The duodenum is approximately 1 foot in length and is where the digesting material is mixed with bile from the liver (stored in the gallbladder) and pancreatic digestive juices. These agents raise the pH of the chyme (returning it toward neutral) and help release the nutrients it contains.

The digesting food is propelled along the small and large bowel by waves of contraction called **peristalsis.** The muscles of the digestive tract constrict the bowel's lumen behind a mass of food, then progressively constrict the lumen in the direction of desired movement. The resulting rhythmic constriction moves the digesting material through the tract. As chyme enters the next two segments of the small bowel (the jejunum and the ileum), the mixing decreases and the nutrients, released by the physical and chemical digestion processes, are absorbed, directed to the liver for detoxification, and then released into the circulatory system.

peristalsis *wavelike muscular motion of the esophagus and bowel that moves food through the digestive system.*

As the food continues its travel through the digestive tract, it arrives at the large bowel. Here masses of bacteria assist in releasing vitamins and fluid from the digesting food while the large bowel absorbs most of the remaining fluid content. The water serves to hydrate the body while the digestive juices are reabsorbed and reprocessed to rejoin the digestive process upstream again. The large bowel ascends superiorly along the right side of the abdomen (ascending colon), traverses the abdomen just below the liver and stomach (transverse colon), then descends along the left lateral abdomen (descending colon). It aligns with the rectum through the S-shaped sigmoid colon where the end waste products of the digestive process (feces) await excretion (defecation) through the terminal valve, the anus.

ACCESSORY ORGANS OF DIGESTION

The liver is a vascular structure responsible for detoxifying the blood, removing damaged or aged erythrocytes, and storing glycogen and other important agents for body metabolism. The liver also assists in the osmotic regulation of fluids in the blood and plays a role in the clotting process. Finally, the liver detoxifies materials absorbed by the digestive system and either stores or releases nutrients to assure the body's metabolic needs are met. It is located in the right upper quadrant, just below the diaphragm, and extends into the medial portion of the left upper quadrant. It is the largest abdominal organ, accounting for 2.5 percent of total body weight. It receives about 25 percent of cardiac output and holds the greatest blood reserve of any body organ. The lower portion of its mass can occasionally be palpated just below the margin of the rib cage. It is suspended in its location by several ligaments including the ligamentum teres, and connects to the omentum inferiorly. The liver is a solid organ but is rather delicate in nature. It is contained within a fibrous capsule (visceral peritoneum) that serves to retard hemorrhage and helps hold the liver together if injured by blunt trauma. When injured, the liver will regenerate to some degree but will not function as efficiently as before the injury.

The gallbladder is a small hollow organ located behind and beneath the liver. It receives bile (a waste product from the reprocessing of red blood cells) from the liver and stores it until it is needed during digestion of fatty foods. It then constricts and sends bile through the bile duct and into the duodenum. Bile helps the body by emulsifying (breaking apart and suspending) ingested fats that would otherwise remain as clumps during the digestive process.

The other accessory digestive organ is the pancreas. It is responsible for the production of glucagon and insulin, hormones responsible for the regulation of blood glucose levels and the transport of glucose across cell membranes. The pancreas also produces very powerful digestive enzymes that help return the pH of the chyme toward normal and break down proteins. These enzymes enter the duodenum through the common bile duct. Like the liver, the pancreas is a solid, though delicate, organ, encapsulated in a serous membrane. It is located in the medial and lower portion of the left upper quadrant and extends into the medial portion of the right upper quadrant. The duodenum wraps around the right pancreatic border. If the cells of the pancreas are damaged, the pancreatic enzymes may become active and begin to "self-digest" pancreatic tissue. If these enzymes are released into the retroperitoneal space, they will also damage surrounding tissue.

THE SPLEEN

The spleen is not an accessory organ of digestion but rather a part of the immune system. It is a very vascular organ about the size of the palm of the hand and is located behind the stomach and lateral to the kidney in the left upper quadrant. The spleen performs some immunological functions and also stores a large volume of blood. It is the most fragile abdominal organ, though well protected in its location by the rib cage, spine, and **flank** and back muscles. The spleen, however, can be injured during blunt trauma, especially with impacts affecting the left flank. When injured, the spleen bleeds heavily.

flanks *the part of the back below the ribs and above the hip bones.*

THE URINARY SYSTEM

The urinary system contains four major structures: the kidneys, ureters, urinary bladder, and urethra (Figure 3-109 ■). First we will discuss the structures and functions of the urinary system, focusing on the kidneys. Then we will cover the additional structures of the male genitourinary system.

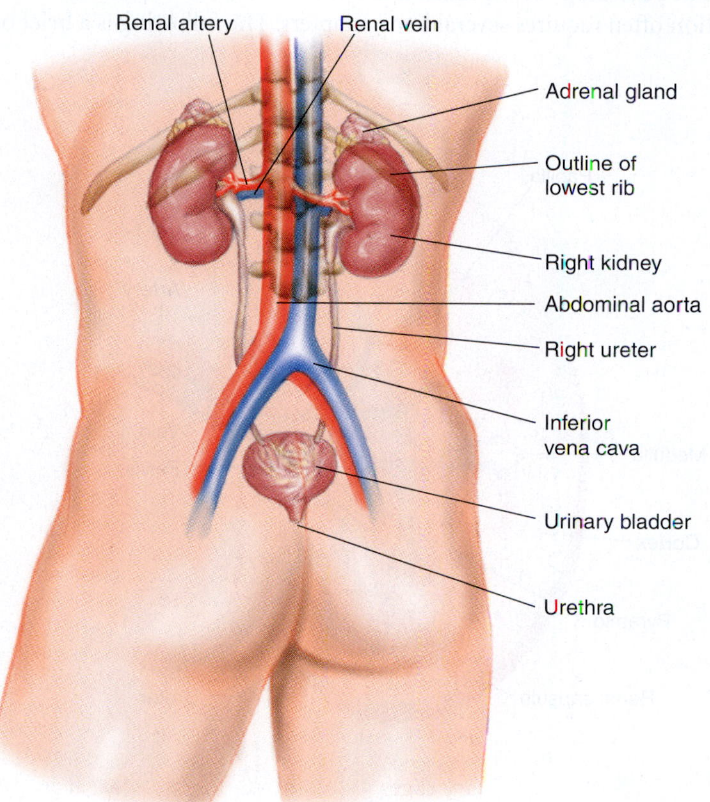

■ Figure 3-109 Anatomy of the urinary system, posterior view.

THE KIDNEYS

The left kidney lies in the upper abdomen behind the spleen, and the right kidney lies behind the liver. These locations correspond to the left and right areas of the small of the back, or the flanks. A healthy **kidney** in a young adult is about the size of a fist and contains about 1 million **nephrons,** the microscopic structures that produce urine. With aging comes a normal loss of nephrons—10 percent per decade of life after age 40—so you should always be alert to the possibility of compromised kidney function in elderly patients.

kidney *an organ that produces urine and performs other functions related to the urinary system.*

nephron *a microscopic structure within the kidney that produces urine.*

hilum *the notched part of the kidney where the ureter and other structures join kidney tissue.*

cortex *the outer tissue of an organ such as the kidney.*

medulla *the inner tissue of an organ such as the kidney.*

pyramids *the visible tissue structures within the medulla of the kidney.*

papilla *the tip of a pyramid; it juts into the hollow space of the kidney.*

renal pelvis *the hollow space of the kidney that junctions with a ureter.*

glomerulus *a tuft of capillaries from which blood is filtered into a nephron.*

Bowman's capsule *the hollow, cup-shaped first part of the nephron tubule.*

proximal tubule *the part of the tubule beyond Bowman's capsule.*

descending loop of Henle *the part of the tubule beyond the proximal tubule.*

ascending loop of Henle *the part of the tubule beyond the descending loop of Henle.*

distal tubule *the part of the tubule beyond the ascending loop of Henle.*

collecting duct *the larger structure beyond the distal tubule into which urine drips.*

Gross and Microscopic Anatomy of the Kidney

The renal artery and vein, as well as nerves, lymphatic vessels, and the ureter, pass into the kidney through the notched region called the **hilum.** The tissue of the kidney itself is visibly divided into an outer region, the **cortex,** and an inner region, the **medulla.** Medullary tissue is divided into fan-shaped regions, or **pyramids.** Each pyramid ends in a portion of tissue called the **papilla,** which projects into the hollow space of the **renal pelvis** (Figure 3-110 ■). The spaces of the pelvis come together at the origin of the ureter. Urine forms in the cortical and medullary tissue of the kidney and leaves the kidney through the renal pelvis and ureter.

The functional unit of the kidney, the nephron, forms urine (Figure 3-111 ■). Each nephron consists of a tubule divided into structurally different portions and capillaries that form a complex net of vessels covering the surface of the tubule. Blood that has entered the kidney through the renal artery flows through successively smaller vessels until it reaches a **glomerulus,** a cluster of capillaries surrounded by **Bowman's capsule,** the cup-shaped, hollow structure that is the first part of the nephron. Water and chemical substances enter the tubule through Bowman's capsule. After passage through successive parts of the tubule—the **proximal tubule, descending loop of Henle, ascending loop of Henle,** and **distal tubule**—urine drips into the **collecting duct** before entering the renal pelvis and ureter.

Kidney Physiology

The physiology of the kidneys is one of the most complex topics in human physiology. Its explanation often requires several book chapters. The following is a brief overview.

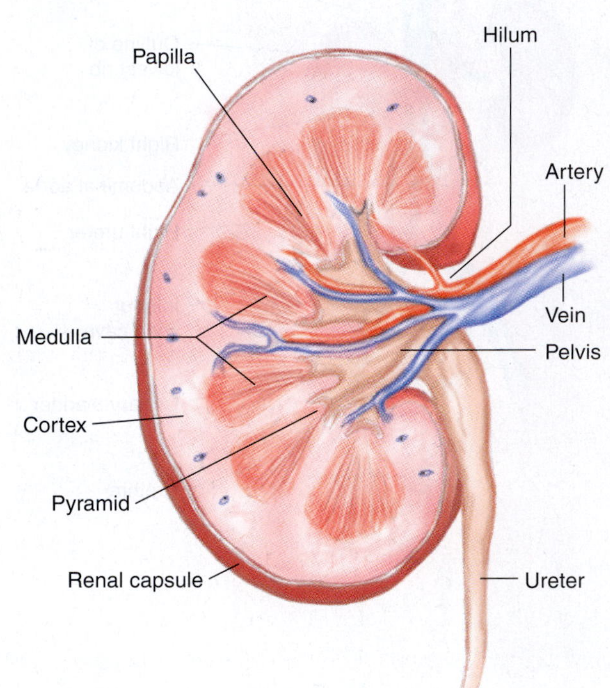

■ Figure 3-110 Cross-section of the kidney.

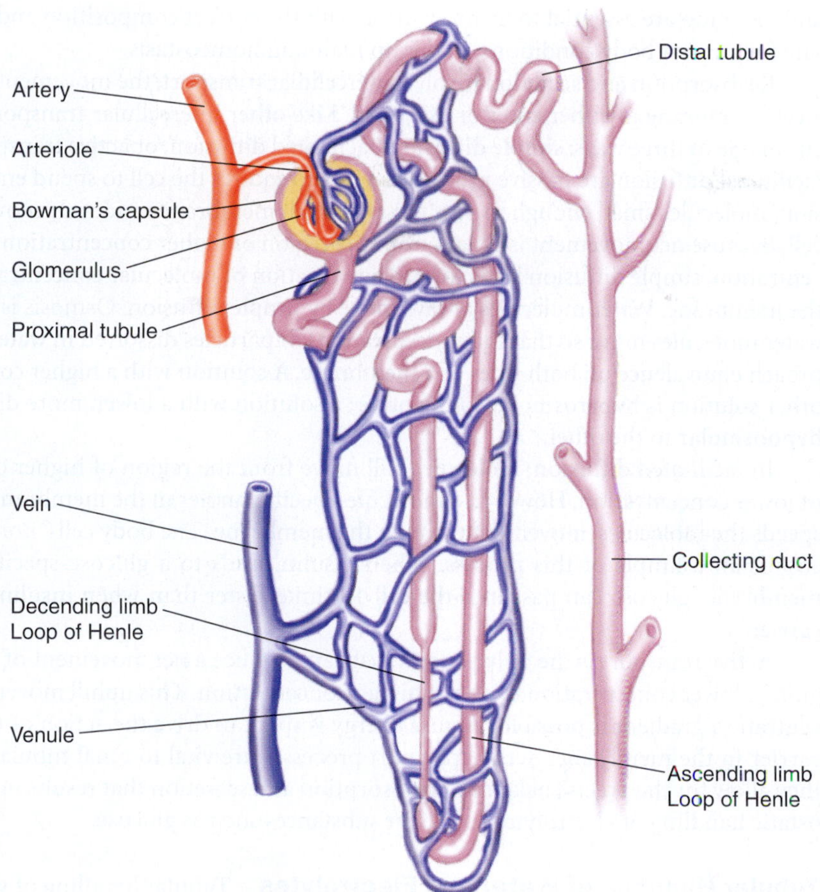

■ **Figure 3-111** Anatomy of the nephron.

Overview of Nephron Physiology Forming and eliminating urine are the basis for two of the kidneys' major functions: (1) maintaining blood volume with proper balance of water, electrolytes, and pH and (2) retaining key compounds such as glucose while excreting wastes such as urea. A third function, controlling arterial blood pressure, relies both on urine formation and on a second mechanism that does not involve urine production. Last, kidney cells regulate erythrocyte development, but this process does not involve urine formation in any way.

Urine is produced through the interactions among capillary blood flowing over the nephron tubule, the fluid flowing inside the tubule, and the capillary and tubular cells themselves. Three general processes are involved in formation of urine: **glomerular filtration, reabsorption** of substances from the renal tubule into blood, and **secretion** of substances from blood into the renal tubule.

The first step in urine formation is filtration of blood. As blood flows through the capillaries of the glomerulus, water and numerous chemical materials are filtered out of the blood and into Bowman's capsule. Normally, the only blood elements that are not freely filtered into the capsule are blood cells and the plasma proteins, all of which are too large to pass through the pores formed by cell junctions in the capillary walls. Consequently, the fluid formed in the capsule—the **filtrate**—roughly resembles blood plasma except for the absence of proteins.

The rate at which blood is filtered, the **glomerular filtration rate (GFR),** averages 180 L/day, the equivalent of 60 complete passages of blood plasma through the glomerular filters. This remarkable efficiency underlies the kidneys' ability to excrete toxic or foreign substances such as urea or drug metabolites so quickly that the substances do not accumulate in the blood.

Filtration is a nonselective process based primarily on molecular size (electrical charge is a secondary factor), and it is essential to urine formation. In contrast, reabsorption of substances into the blood and secretion of substances into the renal tubule are highly selective processes. Almost all elements of filtrate are handled independently of the other elements. The processes of reabsorption

glomerular filtration *the removal from blood of water and other elements, which enter the nephron tubule.*

reabsorption *the movement of a substance from a nephron tubule back into the blood.*

secretion *the movement of a substance from the blood into a nephron tubule.*

filtrate *the fluid produced in Bowman's capsule by filtration of blood.*

glomerular filtration rate (GFR) *the volume per day at which blood is filtered through capillaries of the glomerulus.*

and secretion are essential to forming urine with the correct composition and volume to compensate for current body conditions, that is, to maintain homeostasis.

Reabsorption and secretion involve intercellular transport, the movement of a molecule across a cell membrane to either enter or exit a cell. Like other intercellular transport processes, they occur in one of three ways: **simple diffusion,** facilitated diffusion, or active transport. Both simple and facilitated diffusion are passive processes: neither requires the cell to spend energy. In simple diffusion, molecules small enough to pass through a cell membrane randomly move into and out of the cell. Because net movement is always from the region of higher concentration to that of lower concentration, simple diffusion leads toward equalization of molecular concentration on both sides of the membrane. Water molecules always move by simple diffusion. Osmosis is the process in which water molecules move so that the concentrations of particles dissolved in water (or osmolarity) approach equivalence on both sides of a membrane. A solution with a higher concentration than another solution is **hyperosmolar** to the other; a solution with a lower, more dilute concentration is **hypoosmolar** to the other.

simple diffusion *the random motion of molecules from an area of high concentration to an area of lower concentration.*

hyperosmolar *a solution that has a concentration of the substance greater than that of a second solution.*

hypoosmolar *a solution that has a concentration of the substance lower than that of a second solution.*

In facilitated diffusion, molecules still move from the region of higher concentration to that of lower concentration. However, a molecule-specific carrier in the membrane acts as a tunnel and speeds the molecules' movement through the membrane. The body cells' normal handling of glucose is an example of this process. When insulin binds to a glucose-specific carrier in the cell membrane, glucose can pass into the cell 10 times faster than when insulin is not bound to the carrier.

Active transport is the only process that can produce a net movement of molecules from a region of lower concentration to one of higher concentration. This uphill movement against the concentration gradient is possible because energy is spent to drive the action of the molecule-specific carrier in the membrane. Active transport processes are vital to renal tubular physiology because they allow for the precise balance of reabsorption and secretion that results in independent, homeostatic handling of electrolytes and other substances such as glucose.

Tubular Handling of Water and Electrolytes Tubular handling of water and electrolytes including sodium (Na^+), potassium (K^+), hydrogen (H^+), and chloride (Cl^-) is the basis for control of blood volume and maintenance of electrolyte balance, including pH. As you recall, Na^+ is the dominant cation in the body's extracellular fluids, including blood, whereas K^+ is the dominant cation in intracellular fluid. Appropriate retention of Na^+ in the body, along with osmotic retention of water, is key to maintaining blood volume. Selective retention of K^+ and H^+, along with anions such as Cl^-, maintains the balance of blood electrolytes and blood pH.

Filtrate formed in Bowman's capsule enters the proximal tubule (review Figure 3-111). The cells of the proximal tubule have an extensive brush border that maximizes contact between the cell membrane and filtrate. They also have high concentrations of molecule-specific carriers in their membranes and maintain a high level of metabolic activity, producing energy that can support active transport. Under normal conditions, about 65 percent of filtered Na^+ and Cl^- is reabsorbed in the proximal tubule, along with osmotic reabsorption of about the same percentage of filtered water. Reabsorption takes place by both passive and active transport processes. Much of the active Na^+ reabsorption is coupled with secretion of H^+ into the tubule; H^+ secretion raises the pH of the arterial-derived blood flowing in capillaries surrounding the tubule. Further handling of H^+ as the filtrate moves through the tubule determines the pH both of the venous blood leaving the kidneys and of the urine excreted from the body.

As filtrate moves through the next part of the nephron, the loop of Henle, its volume and composition change further. Simple diffusion is the dominant process in the first part of the loop. By the time filtrate has moved through the descending limb of the loop, roughly another 20 percent of the filtrate's original water load has been reabsorbed. The cells of the second, ascending limb of the loop of Henle are normally virtually impermeable to water; however, passive and active reabsorption of significant amounts of electrolytes occurs in the same part of the tubule. This reabsorption of electrolytes without reabsorption of water produces a relatively dilute fluid that may exit the collecting duct as dilute urine. Healthy kidneys can produce urine with an osmolarity as low as one-sixth the osmolar concentration of blood plasma, an action termed **diuresis.** A number of hormones alter tubular handling of water and electrolytes (Table 3–7). Some increase the perme-

diuresis *formation and passage of a dilute urine, decreasing blood volume.*

Table 3–7	Hormones That Affect Tubular Handling of Water and Key Electrolytes	
Hormone	**Target Tissue**	**Effect(s)**
Aldosterone	Distal tubule, collecting duct	Increase in reabsorption of Na^+, Cl^-, and water Increase in secretion of K^+
Angiotensin II	Proximal tubule	Increase in reabsorption of Na^+, Cl^-, and water Increase in secretion of H^+
Antidiuretic Hormone (ADH)	Distal tubule, collecting duct	Increase in reabsorption of water
Atrial Natriuretic Hormone (ANH)	Distal tubule, collecting duct	Decrease in reabsorption of Na^+ and Cl^-

Note: Aldosterone, ADH, and ANH are discussed in detail in "Endocrinology," Chapter 30; angiotensin II is discussed in "Cardiology," Chapter 28.
Table derived from Guyton, Arthur C., and John E. Hall, *Textbook of Medical Physiology.* 9th ed. Philadelphia: W. B. Saunders Company, 1996.

ability of the distal tubule, collecting duct, or both, so that far more water is reabsorbed. **Antidiuresis,** the result of this hormonal activity, can form a very concentrated urine with an osmolarity as high as four times that of plasma.

antidiuresis *formation and passage of a concentrated urine, preserving blood volume.*

The ability of healthy kidneys to handle significant swings in water and electrolyte intake is remarkably large. Studies have shown that an individual can increase his sodium intake to 10 times the average amount or decrease it to roughly one-tenth the average, and the kidneys will still compensate properly. Blood volume and sodium content will change only modestly from their baseline, normal levels.

Tubular Handling of Glucose and Urea Glucose and urea represent substances that the kidneys handle in opposite fashion. Critical substances such as glucose are retained in the body, and wastes such as urea are excreted.

Glucose is freely filtered into Bowman's capsule as an element of filtrate. Normally, glucose is completely reabsorbed through an active transport process by the time filtrate leaves the proximal tubule. The body's absolute retention of glucose is usually maintained until the blood glucose level reaches about 180 mg/dL; above that level, glucose begins to be lost in urine. This pattern, in which glucose is completely reabsorbed until a ceiling, or threshold level of blood glucose, is reached is due to saturation of the active-transport process responsible for reabsorption of glucose. At excessively high blood glucose levels, so much glucose enters the filtrate that the proximal tubule's transport capacity to reabsorb it is insufficient. When this occurs, as in uncontrolled diabetes mellitus type I, the body loses not only glucose but also large amounts of water through **osmotic diuresis.**

osmotic diuresis *greatly increased urination and dehydration that results when high levels of glucose cannot be reabsorbed into the blood from the kidney tubules and the osmotic pressure of the glucose in the tubules also prevents water reabsorption.*

Urea, a waste product, is also freely filtered into Bowman's capsule. However, tubular handling of this small molecule is very different from that of glucose. Urea is passively reabsorbed throughout most of the tubule, and about half of the filtered load will remain in urine. Thus, the kidneys' ability to excrete urea efficiently depends on the glomerular filtration rate, or GFR. If blood passes through the glomerular capillaries at an adequate rate, the net result of filtration and passive reabsorption will keep the blood level from rising toward a toxic level. The blood urea nitrogen test, or BUN, directly measures blood concentration of urea and is an indirect indicator of GFR. **Creatinine,** another waste product of metabolism, has larger molecules than urea and is not reabsorbed. Because all of the filtered creatinine will be eliminated in urine, the blood concentration of creatinine is a direct indicator of GFR.

creatinine *a waste product caused by metabolism within muscle cells.*

BUN and creatinine are both important indications of renal function.

Control of Arterial Blood Pressure The kidneys regulate systemic arterial blood pressure in several ways. Over the long term, they control the body's balance of water and electrolytes, thus maintaining blood volume at a healthy level. In addition, juxtaglomerular cells, specialized cells adjacent to glomerular capillary cells, respond to low blood pressure by releasing an enzyme called **renin.** Within seconds of its release renin produces significant amounts of the active hormone angiotensin I. As angiotensin I flows through the lungs, angiotensin converting enzyme (ACE) produces angiotensin II, the powerful vasoconstrictor that immediately raises arterial blood pressure.

renin *an enzyme produced by kidney cells that plays a key role in controlling arterial blood pressure.*

Angiotensin II acts both on kidney tubular cells (Table 3–7) and on adrenal cells, causing the latter to secrete aldosterone. The renin-angiotensin system has an important role in the maintenance of blood pressure, as noted earlier.

Control of Erythrocyte Development The kidneys produce 90 percent of the body's erythropoietin, a hormone that regulates the rate at which erythrocytes mature in bone marrow. The exact mechanism that produces erythropoietin is unclear. The impact of renal tissue death, however, is clear and profound; the nonkidney sources of erythropoietin can produce only about one-third to one-half the red cell mass (measured as hematocrit) needed by the body.

THE URETERS

ureter *a duct that carries urine from kidney to urinary bladder.*

Urine drains from the renal pelvis into the **ureter,** the long duct that runs from the kidney to the urinary bladder (review Figure 3-109). Each ureter is about 25 cm long and, like the kidney, is located in the retroperitoneum of the abdomen. A thin muscular layer in the ureters' walls limits their ability to distend in response to internal pressure. The ureters' nerves derive from renal, gonadal, or hypogastric nerve trunks. The microscopic structure of the ureters and the nature of their nerve supply are important in understanding the symptoms caused by kidney stones caught in a ureter.

THE URINARY BLADDER

urinary bladder *the muscular organ that stores urine before its elimination from the body.*

The **urinary bladder,** the anterior-most organ in the pelvis of both men and women, stores urine. The muscular bladder usually contains at least a small amount of urine, which produces its roughly spherical shape. The bladder neck, through which urine passes during urination, is held in place by ligaments. In women, connective tissue loosely attaches the bladder's posterior wall to the anterior vaginal wall. In men, the bladder wall is structurally continuous with the prostate gland.

THE URETHRA

urethra *the duct that carries urine from the urinary bladder out of the body; in men, it also carries reproductive fluid (semen) to the outside of the body.*

The **urethra** is the duct that carries urine from the bladder to the exterior of the body. In women, the urethra is only about 3 to 4 cm long and opens to the external environment via a small orifice just anterior to that of the vagina. In men, the urethra is about 20 cm long and ends at the tip of the penis. The female urethra's shortness is probably one reason the female urinary system is more vulnerable to bacterial infection from environmental (largely skin) sources. Because the male urethra carries both urine and male reproductive fluid, it can be an entry way for sexually transmitted diseases.

THE REPRODUCTIVE SYSTEM

It is important to have an understanding of both the female and the male reproductive systems.

THE FEMALE REPRODUCTIVE SYSTEM

The most important female reproductive organs are internal and are located within the pelvic cavity. These include the ovaries, fallopian tubes, uterus, and vagina, which are essential to reproduction. The external genitalia have accessory functions, in that they protect body openings and play an important role in sexual functioning.

The External Genitalia

The female external genitalia are known collectively as the *vulva,* or *pudendum* (Figure 3-112 ■). These external genitalia consist of highly vascular tissues that protect the entrance to the birth canal. They include the perineum, mons pubis, labia, and clitoris.

The external genital organs begin to mature and take adult proportions during adolescence. Puberty also marks the appearance of breast buds, pubic hair, and the first period (menarche). The

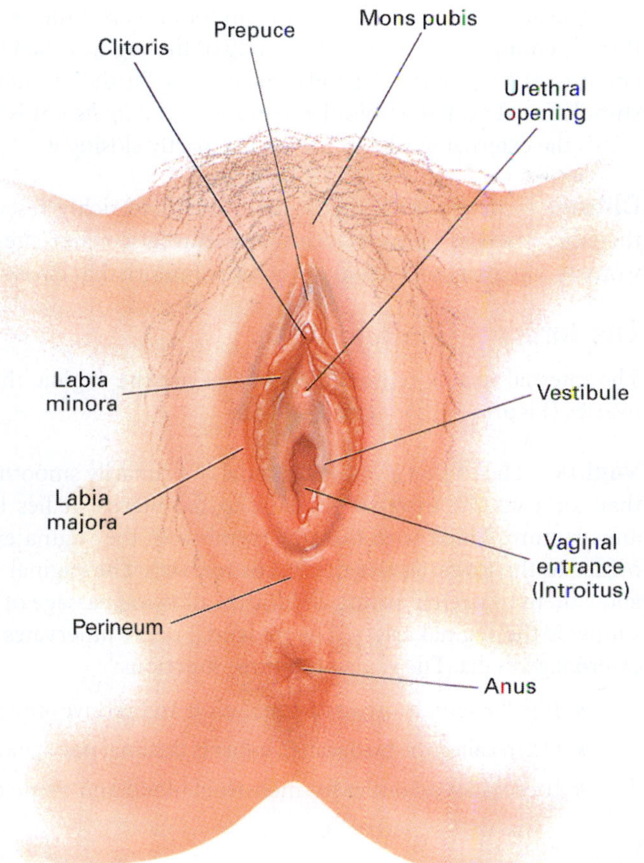

■ **Figure 3-112** The vulva.

age in which sexual development occurs varies among individuals. As women grow older, ovarian function diminishes, menstrual periods cease, and pubic hair becomes gray and sparse. The labia and clitoris become smaller; the vagina narrows and shortens and its lining (the mucosa) becomes thin, pale, and dry. The ovaries and uterus decrease in size.

Perineum The **perineum** is a roughly diamond-shaped, skin-covered muscular tissue that separates the vagina and the anus. These tissues form a slinglike structure supporting the internal pelvic organs and are able to stretch during childbirth. This area is sometimes torn as a result of sexual assault or during childbirth. An *episiotomy,* or incision of the perineum, may be done to facilitate delivery of the baby and to prevent spontaneous tearing, which may cause significant injury to the perineum and adjacent structures. Sometimes the term *perineum* is used to include the entire vulvar area.

perineum *muscular tissue that separates the vagina and the anus.*

Mons Pubis The **mons pubis** is a fatty layer of tissue over the pubic symphysis, the junction of pubic bones. During puberty, the hormone estrogen causes fat to be deposited under the skin, giving it a moundlike shape. This serves as a cushion that protects the pubic symphysis during intercourse. Also during puberty, the mons becomes covered with pubic hair and its sebaceous and sweat glands become more active.

mons pubis *fatty layer of tissue over the pubic symphysis.*

Labia The **labia** are the structures that protect the vagina and the urethra. There are two distinct sets of labia. The labia majora are located laterally, while the labia minora are more medial. Both sets of labia are subject to injury during trauma to the vulvar area, such as occurs with sexual assault.

The *labia majora* are two folds of fatty tissue that arise from the mons pubis and extend to the perineum, forming a cleft. During puberty, pubic hair grows on the lateral surface, and sebaceous glands on the hairless medial surface begin to secrete lubricants. The labia majora serve to protect the inner structures of the vulva. The *labia minora,* lying medially within the labia majora, are two smaller, thinner folds of highly vascular tissue, well supplied with nerves and sebaceous glands, which secrete lubricating fluid. During sexual arousal the labia minora become engorged with blood.

labia *structures that protect the vagina and urethra, including the* labia majora *and the* labia minora.

The area protected by the labia minora is called the *vestibule.* The vestibule contains the urethral opening and the external opening of the vagina called the vaginal orifice, or *introitus.* The secretions of two pairs of glands (Skene and Bartholin) lubricate these structures during sexual stimulation. Located within the vestibule is the *hymen.* It is a thin fold of mucous membrane that forms the external border of the vagina, partly closing it.

clitoris *highly innervated and vascular erectile tissue anterior to the labia minora.*

Clitoris The **clitoris** is highly innervated and richly vascular erectile tissue that lies anterior to the labia minora. This cylindrical structure is a major site of sexual stimulation and orgasm in women. The *prepuce* is a fold of the labia minora that covers the clitoris.

The Internal Genitalia

The internal female reproductive organs are the vagina, the uterus, the fallopian tubes, and the ovaries (Figures 3-113 ■ and 3-114 ■).

vagina *canal that connects the external female genitalia to the uterus.*

Vagina The **vagina** is an elastic canal of primarily smooth muscle, 9 to 10 centimeters in length, that connects the external genitalia to the uterus. It lies between the urethra/bladder and the anus/rectum. Lined with mucous membrane, the vagina extends up and back from the vaginal orifice to the lower end of the uterus (cervix). The vaginal walls are crisscrossed with ridges that allow them to stretch during childbirth, allowing passage of the fetus. The vagina's primary blood supply is the vaginal artery. The pudendal nerve innervates the lower third of the vagina and the external genitalia. The vagina has three functions:

- ★ It is the female organ of copulation and receives the penis during sexual intercourse.
- ★ Often called the birth canal, it forms the final passageway for the infant during childbirth.
- ★ It provides an outlet for menstrual blood and tissue to leave the body.

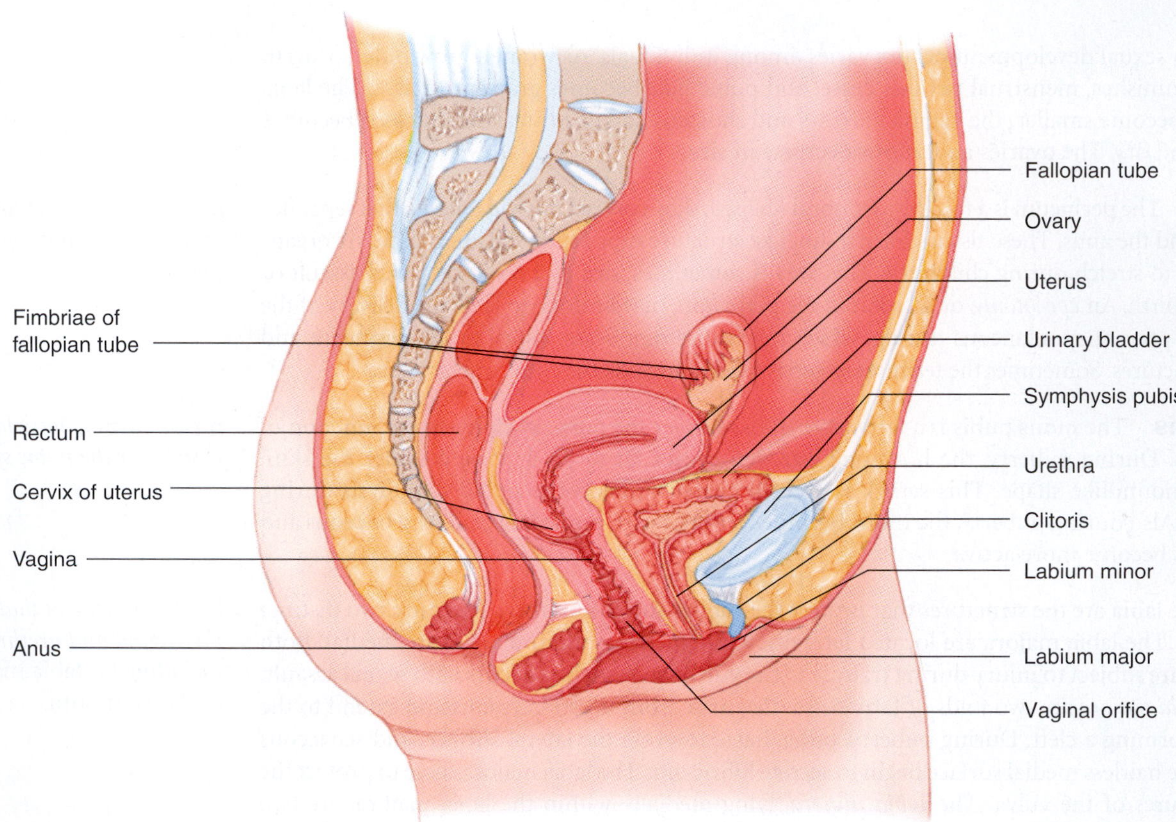

■ **Figure 3-113** Cross-sectional anatomy of the female reproductive system.

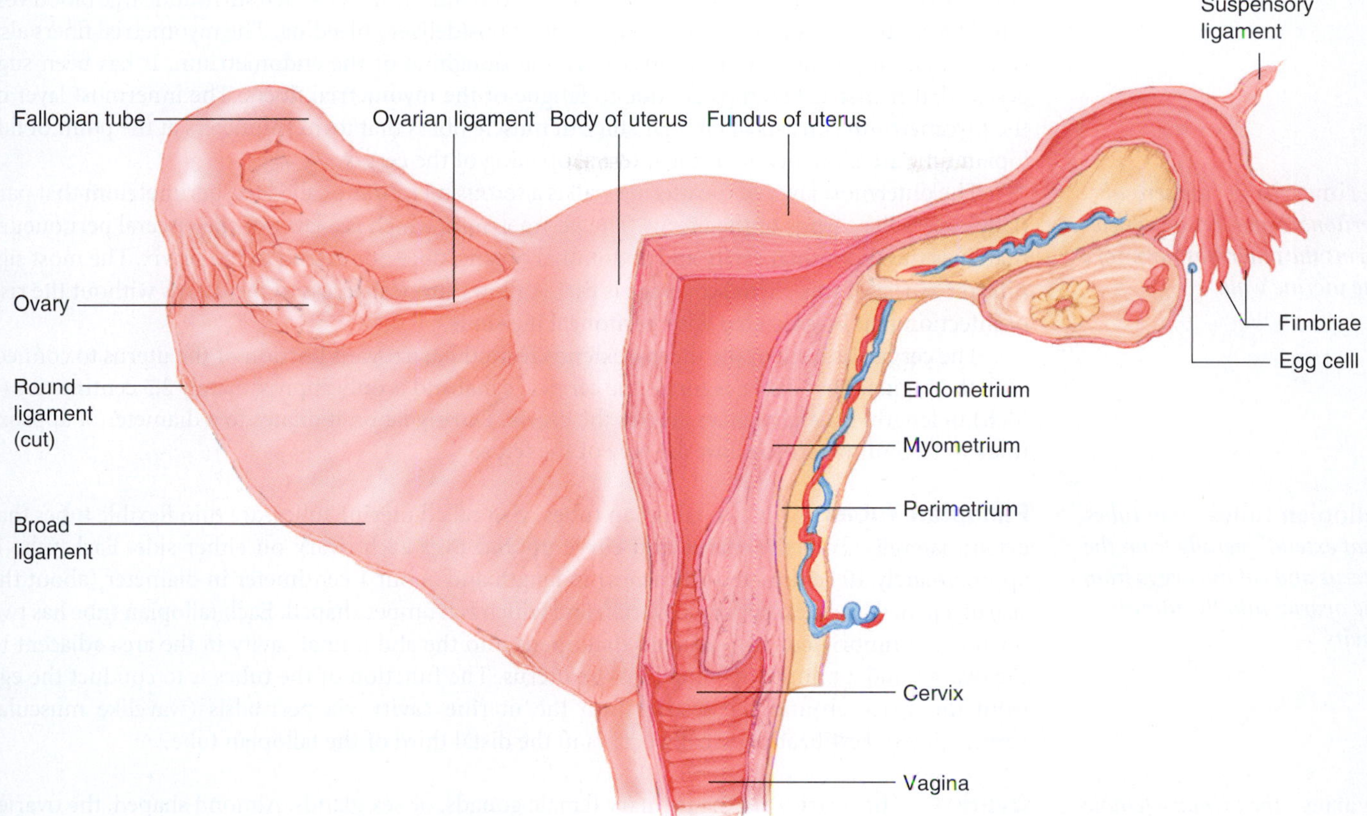

■ **Figure 3-114** The uterus, fallopian tubes, and ovaries.

Uterus The **uterus** is a hollow, thick-walled, muscular, inverted-pear-shaped organ that connects with the vagina. It lies in the center of the pelvis and is flexed forward between the bladder and rectum above the vagina. Approximately 7.5 centimeters (3 inches) long and 5 centimeters (2 inches) wide, the uterus is held loosely in position by ligaments, peritoneal folds, and the pressure of adjacent abdominal structures. The primary function of the uterus is to provide a site for fetal development. During pregnancy, the uterus stretches to a size capable of containing the fetus, placenta, and the associated membranes and amniotic fluid. At term, the gravid uterus measures approximately 40 centimeters (16 inches) in length. The uterus has an extensive blood supply, primarily from the uterine arteries which are branches of the internal iliac artery. The autonomic nervous system innervates the uterus. In a nonpregnant state, the uterine cavity is flat and triangular.

uterus *hollow organ in the center of the abdomen that provides the site for fetal development.*

The uterus has two major parts: the *body* (or corpus) and the *cervix*, or neck. The upper two-thirds of the uterus forms the body and is comprised of smooth muscle layers. The lower third is the cervix.

The rounded uppermost portion of the body of the uterus is the *fundus*, which lies above the point where the fallopian tubes attach. Measurement of fundal height (distance from the symphysis pubis to the fundus) may be used to estimate gestational age during pregnancy. The fundal height measured in centimeters is generally comparable to the weeks of gestation. For instance, if the fundal height is 30 centimeters, the gestational age is about 30 weeks. This method of assessing uterine size is most accurate from 22 to 34 weeks.

The body of the uterus has three layers of tissue that make up the uterine wall. The innermost layer or lining is called the **endometrium.** Each month, stimulated by estrogen and progesterone, the endometrium builds up in preparation for the implantation of a fertilized ovum. If fertilization does not occur, the lining degenerates and sloughs off. This sloughing of the uterine lining is referred to as the *menses*, or menstrual period.

endometrium *the inner layer of the uterine wall where the fertilized egg implants.*

The thick middle layer of the uterine wall, called the **myometrium,** consists of three distinct layers of smooth muscle fibers. In the outer layer, primarily over the fundus, the fibers run longitudinally, which allows expulsion of the fetus following cervical dilation. The middle (and thicker)

myometrium *the thick middle layer of the uterine wall made up of smooth muscle fibers.*

layer is made up of figure-eight patterns of interlaced muscle fibers which surround large blood vessels. The contraction of these fibers helps control postdelivery bleeding. The myometrial fibers also contract during menstruation to maximize the sloughing of the endometrium. It has been suggested that menstrual cramps are due to fatigue of the myometrial fibers. The innermost layer of the myometrium consists of circular smooth muscle fibers that form sphincters at the point of fallopian tube attachment and at the internal opening of the cervix.

perimetrium *the serosal peritoneal membrane which forms the outermost layer of the uterine wall.*

The outermost layer of the uterine wall is a serous membrane called the **perimetrium** that partially covers the corpus of the uterus. The perimetrium, which is a layer of the visceral peritoneum that lines the abdominal cavity and abdominal organs, does not extend to the cervix. The most significant aspect of this partial coverage is that it allows surgical access to the uterus without the risk of infection that is associated with peritoneal incisions.

The cervix, or neck of the uterus, extends from the narrowest portion of the uterus to connect with the vagina. That distance forms the cervical canal and is only approximately 2.5 centimeters (1 inch) in length. Elasticity characterizes the cervix. During labor, it dilates to a diameter of approximately 10 centimeters to allow delivery of the fetus.

fallopian tubes *thin tubes that extend laterally from the uterus and conduct eggs from the ovaries into the uterine cavity.*

Fallopian Tubes The two **fallopian tubes,** also called uterine tubes, are thin flexible tubes that extend laterally from the uterus and curve up and over each ovary on either side. Each tube is approximately 10 centimeters (4 inches) in length and about 1 centimeter in diameter (about the size of a pencil lead), except at its ovarian end which is trumpet shaped. Each fallopian tube has two openings, a fimbriated (fringed) end that opens into the abdominal cavity in the area adjacent to the ovaries and a minute opening into the uterus. The function of the tubes is to conduct the egg from the space around the ovaries into the uterine cavity via peristalsis (wavelike muscular contractions). Fertilization usually occurs in the distal third of the fallopian tube.

ovaries *the primary female sex glands that secrete estrogen and progesterone and produce eggs for reproduction.*

Ovaries The **ovaries** are the primary female gonads, or sex glands. Almond shaped, the ovaries are situated laterally on either side of the uterus in the upper portion of the pelvic cavity. They have two functions. One function is the secretion of the hormones estrogen and progesterone in response to stimulation from follicle stimulating hormone (FSH) and luteinizing hormone (LH) secreted from the anterior pituitary gland. The second function of the ovaries is the development and release of eggs (ova) for reproduction.

The Menstrual Cycle

menarche *the onset of menses, usually occurring between ages 10 and 14.*

The female undergoes a monthly hormonal cycle, generally every 28 days, that prepares the uterus to receive a fertilized egg. The onset of the menstrual cycle, that is, the onset of ovulation at puberty, establishes female sexual maturity. This onset, known as **menarche,** usually begins between the ages of 10 and 14. At first, the periods are irregular. Later they become more regular and predictable. The length of the menstrual cycle may vary from 21 to 32 days. A "normal" menstrual cycle is what is normal for the woman in question. Because of this, it is important to inquire as to the normal length of the patient's menstrual cycle. Regardless of the length of the menstrual cycle, the period of time from ovulation to menstruation is always 14 days. Any variance in cycle length occurs during the preovulatory phase.

From puberty to menopause, the female sex hormones (estrogen and progesterone) control the ovarian-menstrual cycle, pregnancy, and lactation. These hormones are not produced at a constant rate, but rather their production surges and diminishes in a cyclical fashion. The secretion of estrogen and progesterone by the ovaries is controlled by the secretion of FSH and LH.

ovulation *the release of an egg from the ovary.*

The Proliferative Phase The first 2 weeks of the menstrual cycle, known as the proliferative phase, are dominated by estrogen, which causes the uterine lining (endometrium) to thicken and become engorged with blood. In response to a surge of LH at approximately day 14, **ovulation** (release of an egg) takes place.

At birth, each female's ovary contains some 200,000 ova within immature ovarian follicles known as graafian follicles. This is the female's lifetime supply of ova, which are gradually "used up" through ovulation during her lifetime.

In response to FSH and increased estrogen levels, once during every menstrual cycle, a follicle reaches maturation and ruptures, discharging its egg through the ovary's outer covering into the abdominal cavity. The ruptured follicle, under the influence of LH, develops the corpus luteum, a small yellowish body of cells, which produces progesterone during the second half of the menstrual cycle. If the egg is not fertilized, the corpus luteum will atrophy about 3 days prior to the onset of the menstrual phase. If the egg is fertilized, the corpus luteum will produce progesterone until the placenta takes over that function.

The cilia (fine, hairlike structures) on the fimbriated ends of the fallopian tubes draw the egg into the tube and sweep it toward the uterus. If the woman has had sexual intercourse within approximately 24 hours of ovulation, fertilization may take place. If the egg is fertilized, it normally implants in the thickened lining of the uterus, where the fetus subsequently develops. If it is not fertilized, it passes into the uterine cavity and is expelled.

The Secretory Phase The stage of the menstrual cycle immediately surrounding ovulation is referred to as the secretory phase. If the egg is not fertilized, the woman's estrogen level drops sharply while the progesterone level dominates. Uterine vascularity increases during this phase in anticipation of implantation of a fertilized egg.

The Ischemic Phase If fertilization does not occur, estrogen and progesterone levels fall. Vascular changes cause the endometrium to become pale and small blood vessels to rupture.

The Menstrual Phase During the menstrual phase, the ischemic endometrium is shed, along with a discharge of blood, mucus, and cellular debris, a process known as **menstruation.** A "normal" menstrual cycle depends on the regular pattern in the individual woman. The first day of the menstrual cycle is the day on which bleeding begins and the menstrual flow usually lasts from 3 to 5 days, although this varies from woman to woman. An average blood loss of about 50 mL is common. The absence of a menstrual period in any woman in the childbearing years (generally ages 12 to 55) who is sexually active and whose periods are usually regular should raise the suspicion of pregnancy.

menstruation *sloughing of the uterine lining (endometrium) if a fertilized egg is not implanted. It is controlled by the cyclical release of hormones. Menstruation is also called a* period.

Some women regularly experience marked physical signs and symptoms immediately prior to the onset of their menstrual period. These are collectively known as **premenstrual syndrome (PMS).** Although you may hear crude jokes made about PMS, there is no denying the reality of the physical changes that accompany the changing hormonal levels. It is not uncommon for women to report breast tenderness or engorgement, transient weight gain or bloating as a result of fluid retention, excessive fatigue, and/or cravings for specific foods. Women who are prone to migraine headaches may see them increase during the premenstrual period. Other women may have only minimal physical symptoms, but are more affected by emotional responses such as irritability, anxiety, or depression. The severity of PMS varies with each individual and may require treatment focused on relief of symptoms.

premenstrual syndrome (PMS) *a variety of signs and symptoms, such as weight gain, irritability, or specific food cravings associated with the changing hormonal levels that precede menstruation.*

Menopause, the cessation of menses, marks the cessation of ovarian function and the cessation of estrogen secretion. Menstrual periods generally continue to occur until a woman is 45 to 55, at which time they begin to decline in frequency and length until they ultimately stop. The end of reproductive life is also known as the "climacteric," which is derived from Greek meaning "critical time of life." Occasionally, physicians use the term *surgical menopause,* which means that a woman's periods have stopped because of surgical removal of her uterus, ovaries, or both. The decrease in estrogen levels causes many women to experience hot flashes, night sweats, and mood swings during menopause. It is not uncommon for hormone replacement therapy (oral estrogen, or estrogen and progesterone) to be prescribed to help relieve these complaints and to provide other health benefits associated with continuing adequate levels of these hormones.

menopause *the cessation of menses and ovarian function resulting from decreased secretion of estrogen.*

The Pregnant Uterus

The dynamics of pregnancy greatly affect the anatomy of the female abdominal cavity (Figure 3-115 ■). The uterus and its contents grow rapidly from the time of conception until delivery and are well protected during the first trimester (3 months) of pregnancy. During the second trimester (12 to 24 weeks),

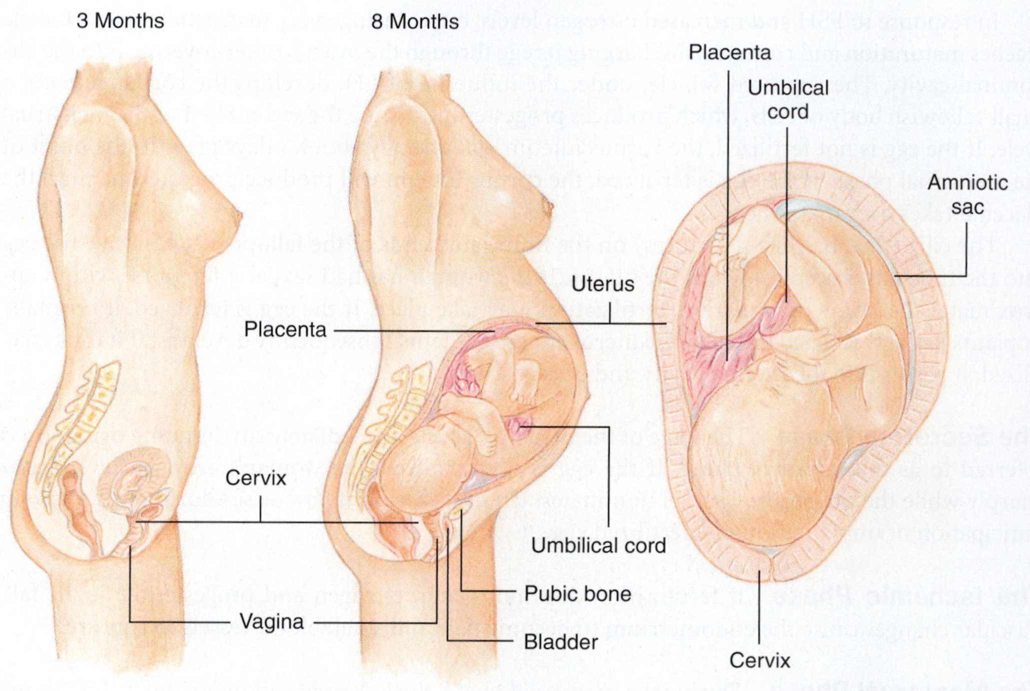

■ **Figure 3-115** The pregnant uterus.

the progressive enlargement of the uterus displaces most of the abdominal contents upward as the growing uterus rises out of the pelvis and its upper border extends above the umbilicus. By 32 weeks and until the end of the pregnancy, the uterus fills the abdominal cavity to the level of the lower rib margin. This enlarging mass in the abdomen also increases the intra-abdominal pressure and displaces the diaphragm upward. This displacement reduces lung capacity at the same time that the physiological changes of pregnancy increase the tidal volume.

Pregnancy also affects the maternal physiology by raising the circulatory volume by about 45 percent and, by the third trimester, raising the cardiac rate by about 15 beats per minute and the cardiac output by up to 40 percent. The increase in the vascular volume is accompanied by a less significant increase in the number of erythrocytes. The result is a relative anemia that becomes an important consideration with aggressive fluid resuscitation for the mother in shock. In the last trimester of pregnancy, the uterus is significant in both size and weight and may compress the vena cava, reducing venous return to the heart and inducing a temporary hypotension in the supine patient (supine hypotensive syndrome). Finally, the developing fetus means there are now two lives to protect when the mother suffers any trauma, especially involving the abdomen.

THE MALE REPRODUCTIVE SYSTEM

As noted earlier, the male reproductive organs are considered to be part of the urinary system (Figure 3-116 ■). Like the female reproductive system, the male reproductive system includes both external and internal genitalia.

testes *primary male reproductive organs that produce hormones responsible for sexual maturation and sperm; singular* testis.

epididymis *small sac in which sperm cells are stored.*

vas deferens *duct that carries sperm cells to the urethra for ejaculation.*

Testes

The **testes** are the primary male reproductive organs. They produce both the hormones responsible for sexual maturation and sperm cells, male sex cells. The testes lie outside of the abdomen in a muscular sac called the scrotum. Normal scrotal temperature is about 2–3°C lower than abdominal temperature, which is critical for development of sperm.

Epididymis and Vas Deferens

Sperm cells pass from the testis into the **epididymis,** a small sac where they are stored. Each testis with its paired epididymis is palpable inside the scrotum. Sperm are channeled from the epididymis into the **vas deferens,** a muscular duct that carries them into the pelvis and through the substance of the prostate gland to its opening into the urethra. Sperm cells mix with special fluid before passing into the urethra for ejaculation, elimination from the body.

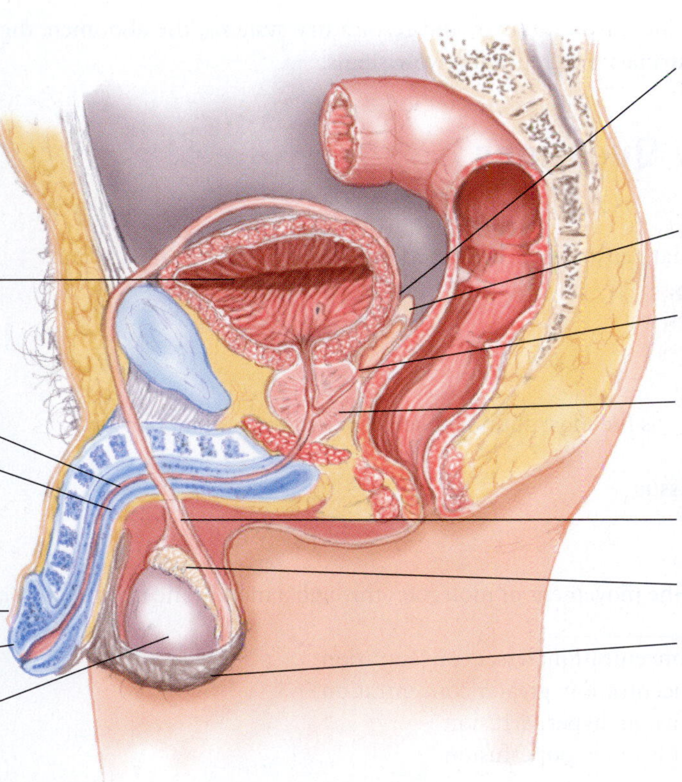

Figure 3-116 Anatomy of the male genitourinary system.

The vas deferens passes through an opening in the inguinal ligament known as the *inguinal canal.* The testicular blood supply also runs through this opening, an anatomical weak point that is the site of male hernias.

Prostate Gland The **prostate gland** surrounds the male urinary bladder neck, and the first part of the urethra runs through its tissue. The prostate gland is a major source of the fluid that combines with sperm to form semen, the ejaculated male reproductive fluid. In emergency care, the prostate is probably most important in its role as part of the urinary system. Because the first part of the urethra passes through the prostate, enlargement of the prostate can narrow or obstruct the urethra and block urine flow.

prostate gland *gland that surrounds the male urinary bladder neck and is a major source of the fluid that combines with sperm to form semen.*

Penis The **penis** is the male organ of copulation. Its spongy internal tissues fill with blood to produce penile erection. The skin covering the end of the penis, the *foreskin,* is often surgically removed in infancy through circumcision; the difference in appearance is noticeable.

penis *male organ of copulation.*

The male genital organs begin to mature and take adult proportions during adolescence. Puberty also marks a noticeable increase in the size of the testes. As in the female, the actual age in which sexual development occurs will vary widely. As men grow older, the penis decreases in size and the testes hang lower in the scrotum. The pubic hair becomes gray and sparse.

Summary

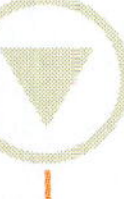

An understanding of human anatomy and physiology is basic to paramedic practice. This begins with an understanding of the basic organization of the human body, beginning with the cell and moving on to more complex structures: the tissues, organs, organ systems, and system integration within the organism itself.

Also critical is an understanding of the important body systems including the integumentary system; the blood; the musculoskeletal system; the head, face, and neck; the spine and thorax, the nervous, endocrine, cardiovascular, and respiratory systems; the abdomen, digestive system, and spleen, and the urinary and reproductive systems.

Review Questions

1. Structures that perform specific functions within a cell are called:
   a. cytokines.
   b. organelles.
   c. phagocytes.
   d. ganglia.
2. ___________ is the most abundant substance in the human body.
   a. Blood
   b. Muscle tissue
   c. Plasma
   d. Water
3. Diffusion is the movement of molecules through a membrane from an area of ___________ to an area of ___________.
   a. greater concentration; lesser concentration
   b. lesser concentration; greater concentration
   c. hypoperfusion; hyperperfusion
   d. hyperperfusion; hypoperfusion
4. The lower the pH, the higher the concentration of ___________ in the body.
   a. hydrogen ions
   b. hemoglobin
   c. bicarbonate
   d. water molecules
5. The outermost layer of the skin is the:
   a. epidermis.
   b. cutaneous layer.
   c. dermis.
   d. sebaceous layer.
6. Which of the following would not be considered a formed element of the blood?
   a. platelets
   b. red blood cells
   c. white blood cells
   d. plasma
7. During childhood, cartilage is generated at the:
   a. diaphysis.
   b. periosteum.
   c. epiphyseal plate.
   d. medullary canal.
8. Which of the following is not a part of the axial skeleton?
   a. head
   b. thorax
   c. spine
   d. pelvis
9. Which of the following is not one of the three types of muscle?
   a. cardiac
   b. autonomic
   c. smooth
   d. skeletal

10. Which of the following occupies the largest part of the brain and is the seat of consciousness?
   a. cerebellum
   b. cerebrum
   c. brainstem
   d. hypothalamus
11. The ___________ is the fluid that fills the major compartment of the eye.
   a. aqueous humor
   b. lacrimal fluid
   c. vitreous humor
   d. conjunctival fluid
12. The ___________ are the pads that serve as shock absorbers between the vertebrae of the spine.
   a. intervertebral disks
   b. transverse processes
   c. pedicles
   d. laminae
13. The mediastinum of the thorax is filled principally by the:
   a. aorta.
   b. trachea.
   c. lungs.
   d. heart.
14. The fundamental unit of the nervous system is the nerve cell, which is also known as a:
   a. dendrite.
   b. axon.
   c. synapse.
   d. neuron.
15. The subdivision of the nervous system that prepares the body to handle stressful situations is the ___________ nervous system.
   a. somatic
   b. afferent
   c. sympathetic
   d. parasympathetic
16. Which gland produces the hormone insulin?
   a. pituitary
   b. hypothalamus
   c. pancreas
   d. thyroid
17. Which of the following formulas represents cardiac output?
   a. stroke volume × heart rate
   b. preload × afterload
   c. blood pressure × peripheral vascular resistance
   d. heart rate × ejection fraction
18. The major functions of perfusion are:
   a. oxygen transport and waste removal.
   b. respiration and ventilation.
   c. inhalation and exhalation.
   d. depolarization and repolarization.
19. The average volume of gas inhaled or exhaled in one respiratory cycle is known as the:
   a. minute volume.
   b. tidal volume.
   c. dead space volume.
   d. residual volume.

20. Compared to the adult airway, which of the following is/are true about the pediatric airway?
    a. Within the pharynx, the pediatric tongue is relatively smaller.
    b. Before age 10, the cricoid cartilage is the widest part of the airway.
    c. The pediatric epiglottis is floppier and rounder than the adult's.
    d. all of the above
21. Which of the following structures is/are not covered by the peritoneum?
    a. kidneys
    b. pancreas
    c. urinary bladder
    d. all of the above
22. Which of the following structures is not a part of the digestive tract?
    a. esophagus
    b. duodenum
    c. transverse colon
    d. urinary bladder
23. The organ that filters blood and produces urine is the:
    a. liver.
    b. kidney.
    c. gallbladder.
    d. pancreas.
24. In the female, eggs are produced for reproduction in the:
    a. fallopian tube.
    b. ovaries.
    c. uterus.
    d. endometrium.
25. In the male, sperm cells are produced in the:
    a. epididymis.
    b. vas deferens.
    c. testes.
    d. prostate gland.

See Answers to Review Questions at the back of this book.

Chapter 4

General Principles of Pathophysiology

Objectives

Part 1: How Normal Body Processes Are Altered by Disease and Injury (begins on p. 241)

After reading Part 1 of this chapter, you should be able to:

1. Discuss cellular adaptation, injury, and death. (pp. 241–246)
2. Discuss factors that precipitate disease in the human body. (pp. 246–251)
3. Analyze disease risk. (pp. 252–257)
4. Describe environmental risk factors and combined effects and interaction among risk factors. (pp. 252–257)
5. Discuss familial diseases and associated risk factors. (pp. 254–257)
6. Discuss hypoperfusion. (pp. 257–261)
7. Define cardiogenic, hypovolemic, neurogenic, anaphylactic, and septic shock. (pp. 261–265)
8. Describe multiple organ dysfunction syndrome. (pp. 265–267)

Part 2: The Body's Defenses against Disease and Injury (begins on p. 268)

After reading Part 2 of this chapter, you should be able to:

1. Define the characteristics of the immune response. (pp. 271–273)
2. Discuss induction of the immune system. (pp. 272–273)
3. Describe the inflammation response and its systemic manifestations. (pp. 273–279)
4. Discuss the role of mast cells, the plasma protein system, and cellular components plus resolution and repair as part of the inflammation response. (pp. 274–279)
5. Discuss hypersensitivity. (pp. 279–280)
6. Describe deficiencies in immunity and inflammation. (pp. 280–282)
7. Describe homeostasis as a dynamic steady state. (p. 283)
8. Describe neuroendocrine regulation. (pp. 284–286)
9. Discuss the interrelationships between stress, coping, and illness. (pp. 286–288)

Key Terms

ABO blood groups, p. 273
acquired immunity, p. 272
aerobic metabolism, p. 258
AIDS, p. 281
albumin, p. 249
allergy, p. 279
anabolism, p. 245
anaerobic metabolism, p. 258
anaphylactic shock, p. 264
anaphylaxis, p. 264
antibiotics, p. 268
antibody, p. 271
antigen, p. 271
apoptosis, p. 246
atrophy, p. 242
autoimmunity, p. 279
B lymphocytes, p. 272
bacteria, p. 268
cardiogenic shock, p. 261
catabolism, p. 245
cell-mediated immunity, p. 272
cellular swelling, p. 245
chemotactic factors, p. 277
chemotaxis, p. 277
colloids, p. 249
compensated shock, p. 260
cortisol, p. 285
crystalloids, p. 249
decompensated shock, p. 260
degranulation, p. 275
delayed hypersensitivity reaction, p. 279
dilation, p. 242
diuretic, p. 251
dynamic steady state, p. 283
dysplasia, p. 242
edema, p. 247
endotoxins, p. 269
erythrocytes, p. 247
exotoxins, p. 269
fatty change, p. 245
fibroblasts, p. 278
general adaptation syndrome (GAS), p. 283
granuloma, p. 278
hematocrit, p. 248
hemoglobin, p. 248
hemoglobin-based oxygen-carrying solutions (HBOCs), p. 249
histamine, p. 277
HIV, p. 281
humoral immunity, p. 272
hyperplasia, p. 242
hypersensitivity, p. 279
hypertrophy, p. 242
hypoperfusion, p. 257
hypovolemic shock, p. 262
hypoxia, p. 243
immediate hypersensitivity reaction, p. 279
immune response, p. 271
immunity, p. 271
immunogens, p. 272
inflammation, p. 273
irreversible shock, p. 260
ischemia, p. 243
isoimmunity, p. 279
leukocytes, p. 247
leukotrienes, p. 277
lymphocyte, p. 272
mast cells, p. 274
metabolic acidosis, p. 251
metabolic alkalosis, p. 251
metaplasia, p. 242
mitosis, p. 242
multiple organ dysfunction syndrome (MODS), p. 265
natural immunity, p. 272
necrosis, p. 246
neurogenic shock, p. 263
osmotic diuresis, p. 262
pathogen, p. 244
pathology, p. 241
pathophysiology, p. 241
physiological stress, p. 283
plasma, p. 247
progressive shock, p. 260
prostaglandins, p. 277
psychoneuroimmunological regulation, p. 284
pus, p. 278
repair, p. 278
resolution, p. 278
respiratory acidosis, p. 251
respiratory alkalosis, p. 251
Rh blood group, p. 273
Rh factor, p. 273
septic shock, p. 265
septicemia, p. 269
serotonin, p. 277
stress, p. 282
stress response, p. 284
stressor, p. 283
T lymphocytes, p. 272
thrombocytes, p. 247
tonicity, p. 249
turnover, p. 283
virus, p. 269

INTRODUCTION

As a paramedic, you will assess your patient (noting the patient's complaints, signs, and symptoms) and plan a course of treatment. If you understand basic human physiology (how the body functions normally) and pathophysiology (how the body functions in the presence of disease or injury), you will be better able to understand the probable causes of common assessment findings and, consequently, better able to choose effective treatments.

General principles of pathophysiology are presented in this chapter. Before reading this chapter, be familiar with the fundamentals of anatomy and normal physiology as presented in Chapter 3—especially the sections on the cell and cellular environment.

This chapter is divided into two parts:

Part 1: How Normal Body Processes Are Altered by Disease and Injury

Part 2: The Body's Defenses against Disease and Injury

Part 1: How Normal Body Processes Are Altered by Disease and Injury

PATHOPHYSIOLOGY

Pathology, from the root *patho* meaning "disease," is the study of disease and its causes. **Pathophysiology** is the study of how diseases alter or result from an alteration in the normal physiological processes of the human body. The concept "disease" may include both medical illness and injury.

As a paramedic, you should realize that your understanding of pathophysiology, as a consequence of basic science and clinical outcome research, is constantly expanding. This has resulted in many changes and improvements in how we care for patients.

One example of this is the assessment and management of shock. From the origin of EMS until the mid-1980s, emergency department and EMS personnel depended on hypotension with tachycardia (low blood pressure with an accelerated pulse rate) as the primary indicators of shock in trauma and medical patients. Basic scientific research has revealed the pathophysiology of shock to be a cellular event, with many compensatory mechanisms occurring before a patient actually presents with hypotension and tachycardia. A patient with this combination of vital signs has already been in shock for an undeterminable amount of time without any intervention, and will probably not have a good outcome. Clinical research validated what had been deduced from basic scientific research, and the standard of care shifted from using the presence of hypotension and tachycardia to using the mechanism of injury and earlier, more subtle clinical signs and symptoms as the catalysts for responding to shock before it has advanced beyond the stage where it can be effectively reversed.

In this chapter, we will discuss the elements of physiology and pathophysiology: more about the cell (its function and environment), the role of genetics, the interplay and integration of systems to maintain homeostasis, and the impact of system disorders that result in stress, disease, and death. You will confirm, as you read, that an understanding of the cell is critical to an understanding of all these topics.

pathology *the study of disease and its causes.*

pathophysiology *the physiology of disordered function.*

Keep in mind that our understanding of pathophysiology, as a consequence of basic science and clinical outcomes research, is constantly expanding. This has resulted in changes and improvements in how we care for patients.

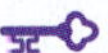

In shock, many physiological changes occur before the classic signs, hypotension and rapid pulse, become evident. Therefore, you must treat for shock promptly based on the mechanism of injury and early, subtle signs and symptoms, without waiting for the classic signs to appear.

HOW CELLS RESPOND TO CHANGE AND INJURY

Keep in mind the concept of homeostasis: the body's tendency to maintain a constantly balanced environment and to correct or compensate for any change that upsets the balance. In this section, we will look at a variety of mechanisms by which cells respond to change and potential or actual injury.

CELLULAR ADAPTATION

Cells, tissues, organs, and even entire organ systems can adapt to both normal and injurious (pathological) conditions. For example, the growth of the uterus during pregnancy is a response to a normal change in condition. Dilation of the left ventricle after a myocardial infarction is an example of response to a pathological condition.

Adaptation to external stressors results in alterations in structure and function at the cellular level. These alterations are classified as atrophy, hypertrophy, hyperplasia, metaplasia, and dysplasia.

Many of these cellular adaptations are successful, at least in the short run, but may also be part of the process of a disease. Therefore, it is sometimes hard to distinguish an adaptive change that is a successful response to a functional demand from one that is pathological in nature.

Review

Content

Cellular Adaptations

- Atrophy
- Hypertrophy
- Hyperplasia
- Metaplasia
- Dysplasia

Atrophy

The size of an individual cell is generally determined by its workload. The cell's size will be sufficient to meet the demands placed on it by the body without wasting energy or vital nutrients. If demands decrease, cell size will also decrease to meet the demands efficiently, using minimal energy and nutrients. The cell will use less oxygen and ATP, due to its decrease in size, and the number of

atrophy *a decrease in cell size resulting from a decreased workload.*

organelles within the cytoplasm will decrease. The process of decreasing size and increasing efficiency is known as **atrophy.**

In addition to a decrease in workload, a variety of other causes of atrophy have been identified. Atrophy may occur as a result of disuse, lack of stimulation, lack of nervous system impulses, decreased nutrient supply, ischemia (lack of oxygen), or a decreased vascular (blood) supply.

Atrophy generally affects the cells found in skeletal muscle, the heart, the brain, and sex organs.

Hypertrophy

hypertrophy *an increase in cell size resulting from an increased workload.*

dilation *enlargement. In reference to the heart, an abnormal enlargement resulting from pathology.*

When there is an increase in workload, a cell will often respond, in the opposite direction from atrophy, as **hypertrophy.** Hypertrophy is an increase in the size of the cell and its functional mass, including an increase in the number of organelles. The increased functional mass allows the cell to meet the increased demand. Hypertrophy of the myocardium (heart muscle) gradually occurs in response to aerobic exercise. When the heart enlarges as a consequence of a pathological event, such as after an AMI (acute myocardial infarction, or heart attack), the term applied is **dilation.** In a dilated state, the heart muscle cells have increased in size, but often result in a decrease in the force of contraction due to their expanded mass.

It is thought that cells that undergo hypertrophy are those that must enlarge in mass because they are unable to increase their numbers through division as in hyperplasia. Hypertrophy most commonly affects cells of the heart and kidneys (enlarged heart, enlarged kidney).

Hyperplasia

hyperplasia *an increase in the number of cells resulting from cell division caused by an increased workload.*

mitosis *cell division with division of the nucleus; each daughter cell contains the same number of chromosomes as the mother cell. Mitosis is the process by which the body grows.*

Another type of response to an increased workload is **hyperplasia.** Hyperplasia is an increase in the number of cells through cell division. Cell division and duplication also includes duplication of the genetic material (DNA) and the nucleus in a process called **mitosis.** Cells capable of undergoing hyperplasia include epithelial, glandular, and epidermal cells. Others, such as skeletal, cardiac, and nerve tissues, cannot divide by mitosis and therefore cannot undergo hyperplasia.

Hyperplasia is very commonly seen along with hypertrophy, because the demands placed on cells in a specific area often affect cells and tissues throughout the body, some of which respond through hypertrophy and others of which respond through hyperplasia.

Metaplasia

metaplasia *replacement of one type of cell by another type of cell that is not normal for that tissue.*

Sometimes, damaged or destroyed cells of one type are replaced by cells of another type in a process called **metaplasia.** Metaplasia often involves replacement of one type of epithelial cell with another type of epithelial cell.

This process can be seen in chronic inflammation or irritation of the respiratory tract from inhalation of irritants, commonly cigarette smoke. The irritants in the smoke will damage and destroy the ciliated columnar epithelial cells of the trachea and larger airways. The response by the body will be to replace these cells with stratified squamous epithelial cells. The squamous epithelium is less likely to be damaged by the carcinogens in the smoke. However, the squamous epithelial cells do not secrete mucus or have cilia, thus causing loss of a vital protective mechanism. The particles once removed by the ciliated columnar cells now accumulate. In addition, the stratified squamous epithelial cells have a higher tendency to become malignant (cancerous).

Metaplasia is reversible if the causative factor is removed in time. If the person stops smoking before a malignancy (cancer) develops, the body will replace the stratified squamous cells with normal ciliated columnar cells.

Dysplasia

dysplasia *a change in cell size, shape, or appearance caused by an external stressor.*

The last adaptive mechanism of cellular response is **dysplasia.** Dysplasia is an abnormal change in cell size, shape, and appearance due to some type of external stressor. (Dysplasia is related to hyperplasia and is often called abnormal or atypical hyperplasia.)

With dysplasia, the external stressor is usually chronic inflammation due to chronic irritation of the tissue. The changes seen result from the irritation and inflammation of the cells. As a result, there is cellular proliferation to protect underlying cells. If the irritant is removed early on, then the cellular changes are often reversible.

Dysplastic cells have a high tendency to cause malignant changes if they are present for an extended period of time. For example, dysplasia of the cervix potentially leads to cervical cancer.

CELLULAR INJURY

Review

Content

Forms of Cellular Injury

- Hypoxia
- Chemicals
- Infectious agents
- Inflammatory reactions
- Physical agents
- Nutritional factors
- Genetic factors

In addition to the cellular adaptations just described, there is an enormous variety of cellular responses to injury or insult. In this section, we will discuss the seven most common mechanisms of cellular injury—hypoxia, chemicals, infectious agents, immunologic/inflammatory reactions, physical agents, nutritional factors, and genetic factors—and provide examples of the ways cells respond to these types of injury in the effort to restore homeostasis.

Hypoxic Injury

The most common cause of cellular injury is **hypoxia,** or oxygen deficiency. Hypoxia can have various causes, such as a deficit in the respiratory or cardiovascular system. Such causes include an inadequate amount of oxygen being taken into the lungs (as from a lack of oxygen in the environment, an occluded airway, or inadequate respiration), a condition that prevents oxygen in the lungs from passing into the bloodstream (as with emphysema), inadequate pumping of blood throughout the body (as in congestive heart failure), or a blockage in the arterial system that prevents oxygenated blood from reaching the cells (as in myocardial infarction or stroke). A blockage or reduction of the delivery of oxygenated blood to the cells is known as **ischemia.**

hypoxia *oxygen deficiency.*

ischemia *a blockage in the delivery of oxygenated blood to the cells.*

Ischemia can also result if there is a deficiency of red blood cells to carry the oxygenated hemoglobin, a deficiency in hemoglobin in the blood, a chemical transformation of hemoglobin as occurs with exposure to nitrates and other chemicals, or a lack of available binding sites as occurs with carbon monoxide poisoning. As the cell becomes progressively more ischemic, the intracellular metabolism becomes *anaerobic* (without oxygen). With anaerobic metabolism, there is a marked decrease in cellular ATP production and an increase in the production of harmful acids (ketoacids), primarily lactic acid. The cell and some of its organelles then begin to swell due to increased levels of sodium that result from the breakdown of the sodium-potassium ATPase pump. In those cells that use fats as their primary sources of energy, fat may accumulate within the cells, worsening the swelling.

If oxygen is supplied to the cell in time, the injury is reversible. But if oxygen is not supplied, the cell begins to break down and the cell membrane ruptures, releasing lysosomes, digestive enzymes, and intracellular potassium into the extracellular environment. As a result, the cellular injury has progressed from reversible to irreversible. The result is the cellular and tissue death called *infarction.*

A patient suffering a heart attack should be thought of as having myocardial ischemia. Myocardial infarction is irreversible, and we hope to intervene before this occurs.

Chemical Injury

Cellular injury due to chemical products is very common. Deadly chemicals can be found under our sink, in our walls, in our work environment, and everywhere around us. Harmful chemical agents include heavy metals such as lead, carbon monoxide, ethanol (alcohol), drugs (misused medicinal drugs as well as street drugs), and insecticides, among others. Some, such as cyanide, cause cell damage and death within minutes. Others, such as common air pollutants, cause injury through prolonged exposure.

Children make up a large percentage of those affected by chemicals. From ingestion of poisons, such as cleaning products, to ingestion of lead-based-paint chips, to ingestion of ethanol products, children lead the way. However, persons of all ages can suffer injury from chemical agents.

Chemicals can damage the body in many ways. Injuries to the cells cause disruption of the cellular membrane resulting in enzymatic reactions, alteration of coagulation, and eventually death of the cell.

Infectious Injury

Infectious, or disease-causing, agents are a common cause of cellular injury. A healthy person harbors many microorganisms (living things so tiny they are invisible to the naked eye) in various body sites. These include bacteria, viruses, fungi, and parasites. The vast majority are harmless, and

pathogen *a microorganism capable of producing infection or disease.*

Review

Content

Pathogens vs. the Body: Three Possible Outcomes

- Pathogen wins.
- Pathogen and body battle to a draw.
- Body defeats pathogen.

some are even useful to their human hosts. Only a few cause infection or disease. Those that do are known as **pathogens.**

The body has a variety of entry-blocking barriers and mechanisms that ward off most pathogens. The chief barrier is the skin. Mucous secretions trap pathogens and are another important barrier. Normal bacteria, enzymes, gastric acids, and other body substances destroy many pathogens. Coughing, sneezing, vomiting, and elimination of urine and feces also rid the body of pathogens.

When a pathogen does succeed in invading the body, three things can happen: First, it may multiply and spread, overwhelming the body's defenses. Second, the body and the pathogen may battle to a draw, producing a chronic infection that is kept in check but is not destroyed by the body. Third, the body's defenses, with or without the assistance of medical treatment, may defeat and destroy the pathogen.

The greater the number of body cells invaded or destroyed by a pathogen, the greater the risk of serious or permanent damage to the body. An example would be a localized infection of the hand as compared with widespread peritonitis of the abdominal cavity.

The degree of damage or injury that can be created by a pathogen depends on its numbers, its virulence (or pathogenicity), and the body's ability to contain or destroy it. Virulence is dependent on three factors: first, the pathogen's ability to invade and destroy cells; second, its ability to produce toxins; and third, its ability to produce hypersensitivity (allergic) reactions.

Immunologic/Inflammatory Injury

Protective responses of the body can cause cell injury and even death. The body's responses to cell injury are inflammation and immune responses in which the body attacks invading foreign substances. Sometimes an exaggerated immune response called *hypersensitivity* (allergy), or even a life-threatening *anaphylactic* response, may develop. Any immune response, whether mild or severe, not only attacks foreign cells, but also tends to injure healthy body cells in the same area, in particular damaging or interfering with the function of the cell membrane. Once the foreign cells are destroyed, the injured body cells will generally begin to repair themselves.

Immunological responses will be discussed in greater detail later in this chapter.

Injurious Physical Agents

Cellular damage can be caused by physical agents, such as acids and alkalis. Extreme variances in temperature, whether hot or cold, can cause injury to the epidermis and underlying tissue, as from a burn or frostbite. Electrical burns, including lightning injuries, cause severe cellular damage. Hyperthermia and hypothermia (exposure to unusually warm or cool environmental temperatures) can also cause cell damage by altering body temperature, breathing patterns, and so on.

Other physical agents that can cause cellular damage include atmospheric pressure changes (for example, in a blast injury or deep-sea-diving injury), exposure to ionizing radiation (X-rays, nuclear radiation), illumination (eyestrain from fluorescent lighting, skin cancers from ultraviolet radiation), noise (hearing impairment), and mechanical stresses (blunt or penetrating trauma, irritation to the skin, repetitive-motion injuries, and over-exertion back injuries).

Injurious Nutritional Imbalances

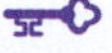

Atherosclerosis is a disease almost solely limited to developed countries that have drifted away from a balanced agrarian diet.

Improper nutrition contributes to one of the most widely publicized forms of cellular injury: atherosclerosis caused by the deposition of lipids, cholesterol, and calcium inside arteries. Many nutritionists identify excessive intake of saturated fats and cholesterol as major contributing causes. Others place the blame on excessive carbohydrate (glucose) intake, which triggers increased insulin secretion, which in turn stimulates production of cholesterol by the liver. Whatever the underlying causes, the result is a narrowing diameter of the arteries, which decreases the amount of oxygenated blood that reaches target cells, increasing the risk of ischemia to vital organs such as the heart and brain.

Problems other than atherosclerosis can also be caused or exacerbated by nutritional imbalances. In diabetic patients, an imbalance between insulin levels and carbohydrate intake causes complex, often severe metabolism problems.

While excessive intake of nutrients may cause problems such as those previously mentioned, insufficient intake of nutrients can cause other problems. The cells require proteins, carbohydrates, lipids, vitamins, and minerals for their metabolism and survival. Deficient intake of any of these nutrients can cause cellular damage and illness.

More commonly in less-developed countries, less commonly in the United States, malnutrition and starvation lead to cellular injury and diseases such as beriberi, scurvy, and rickets, which are all caused by vitamin deficiencies in the diet.

Injurious Genetic Factors

Genes, the basic units of heredity, are composed of DNA. A large number of genes attach to form double-stranded helical molecules of DNA. Molecules of DNA are carried on long threadlike strands called *chromosomes.* The DNA resides in the nucleus of the cells. Some cellular dysfunctions are caused by genetic predisposition, either defective genes or altered chromosomes that the person is born with. Genetic cell injuries can involve alterations to the nucleus or the cell membrane, the shape of the cell, the receptors on the cell membrane, or the transport mechanisms that carry substances across the cell membrane.

A person's genetic makeup is determined at conception, and the interaction of genes and environmental factors determine that person's development. Some diseases are mainly environmental, for example, invasion of the body by bacteria. Other diseases are mainly genetic, for example, sickle cell disease, which is due to a genetic defect. Many diseases result from the combined effects of environmental and genetic factors, including certain metabolic disorders such as diabetes.

Manifestations of Cellular Injury

There are two aspects of the metabolism that take place within cells: anabolism and catabolism. **Anabolism** is the constructive or "building up" phase of metabolism—the processes in which the cell takes in nonliving substances from the blood and the extracellular environment and converts them into the living cytoplasm of the cell. **Catabolism** is the destructive, or "breaking down," phase of metabolism—the processes in which the cell converts complex substances into simpler substances, usually with an accompanying release of energy.

anabolism *the constructive phase of metabolism in which cells convert nonliving substances into living cytoplasm.*

catabolism *the destructive phase of metabolism in which cells break down complex substances into simpler substances with release of energy.*

When cells are injured, metabolism goes awry. A chief consequence is that substances, not all of which are in the cells normally, *infiltrate* or *accumulate* in the cells to an abnormal degree. This can occur from one of three causes: (1) endogenous substances (substances normally found in the cells) are anabolized (produced) in excess; (2) endogenous substances are not properly catabolized (broken down); or (3) harmful exogenous substances (substances from outside the cell, such as heavy metals, mineral dusts, or microorganisms) are taken into and remain in the cells.

When the cells attempt to catabolize the accumulated substances, excessive amounts of metabolites (products of catabolism) are excreted into the extracellular environment. Large numbers of phagocytes (specialized white blood cells) migrate to the area to ingest the excreted metabolites, and this causes swelling of the tissues, as may be seen in enlargement of the liver or spleen.

A variety of substances can accumulate in the cells, including water, lipids, carbohydrates, glycogen, proteins, pigments, calcium, and urate, causing a variety of effects from diabetic disorders to moles and skin color changes to arthritic conditions. Regardless of the type or agent of injury, among the most commonly seen effects of cell injury and accumulation are cellular swelling and fatty change.

Cellular swelling, resulting from a permeable or damaged cellular membrane, is the most frequent result of cellular injury. The cellular swelling is caused by an inability to maintain stable intra- and extracellular fluid and electrolyte levels (which will be explained in more detail later).

cellular swelling *swelling of a cell caused by injury to or change in permeability of the cell membrane with resulting inability to maintain stable intra- and extracellular fluid and electrolyte levels.*

Another response that frequently accompanies cellular swelling is the **fatty change,** in which lipids (small fat vesicles) invade the area of injury. Fatty change with swelling is an ominous sign of impending cellular destruction. The fatty deposits commonly occur in vascular organs such as the kidney and heart, but most commonly in the liver. These deposits begin to cause disruption of the cellular membrane and metabolism and interfere with the vital functions of the affected organs. If the injury does not involve the circulatory system, cellular damage may be contained in the immediate area. If the circulatory system is involved, chemical mediators and lysosomes from the local injury response can enter into the circulatory system, potentially causing systemic injury.

fatty change *a result of cellular injury and swelling in which lipids (fat vesicles) invade the area of injury; occurs most commonly in the liver.*

Systemic signs and symptoms of cellular injury include general feelings of fatigue and malaise, an altered appetite (increased or decreased hunger), fever associated with the inflammatory response, an increased heart rate associated with fever, and pain. Laboratory blood chemistry tests may reveal a high leukocyte (white blood cell) count, resulting from the immune response, as well as the presence of certain cellular enzymes indicating specific sites of cellular injury, such as the skeletal muscle, bone, heart, brain, liver, kidney, or pancreas.

CELLULAR DEATH: APOPTOSIS AND NECROSIS

apoptosis *response in which an injured cell releases enzymes that engulf and destroy itself; one way the body rids itself of damaged and dead cells.*

necrosis *cell death; a pathological cell change. Four types of necrotic cell change are coagulative, liquefactive, caseous, and fatty. Gangrenous necrosis refers to tissue death over a wide area.*

Cellular death leads to one of two processes: apoptosis or necrosis. If the cellular injury or insult is confined to a local region, **apoptosis** may occur. Apoptosis is the body's way of ridding itself of destroyed or nonfunctional cells. It occurs as a result of both normal and pathological tissue changes. The word is Greek, meaning "falling apart." Simply stated, the injured cell releases digestive enzymes that will engulf and destroy itself. By eliminating damaged and dead cells, apoptosis allows tissues to repair and possibly regenerate.

The other process that may follow cellular death is **necrosis.** Unlike apoptosis, necrosis is always a pathological process. Four types of necrotic cell change may occur: coagulative, liquefactive, caseous, and fatty. In *coagulative necrosis,* the transparent viscous albumin of the cell becomes firm and opaque, like a cooked egg white. It generally results from hypoxia and commonly occurs in the kidneys, heart, and adrenal glands. In *liquefactive necrosis,* the cells become liquid and contained in walled cysts. This is common in the ischemic death of neurons and brain cells. In *caseous necrosis,* common in tubercular lung infection, incompletely digested cells take on a cottage-cheese-like consistency. In *fatty necrosis,* commonly occurring in the breast and abdominal structures, fatty acids combine with calcium, sodium, and magnesium ions to create soaps (a process called *saponification*). The dead tissue is opaque and white.

Gangrenous necrosis refers to tissue death over a wide area. *Dry gangrene* results from coagulative necrosis and affects the skin, most commonly of the lower extremities, turning it dry, shrunken, and black. *Wet gangrene* results from liquefactive necrosis and usually affects internal organs. *Gas gangrene* is the result of a bacterial infection of injured tissue, generating gas bubbles in the cells. By attacking red blood cells, gas gangrene can cause death from shock.

Content Review

Results of Cell Death

Apoptosis (usually normal)
Necrosis (always pathological)
— Coagulative
— Liquefactive
— Caseous
— Fatty
Gangrenous necrosis (over a wide area)
— Dry gangrene
— Wet gangrene
— Gas gangrene

There are several key differences between apoptosis and necrosis. In apoptosis, cells shrink. In necrosis, cells swell and rupture. Apoptosis appears to be a form of normal bodily housekeeping. Destroyed cells are cleared away and digested by phagocytes, permitting repair and regeneration. Necrosis is always pathological. Dead cells take on a different physical form (becoming hardened or liquefied) and destroy or interfere with normal physiological processes. Apoptosis has specificity. It occurs in scattered, single cells. Necrosis lacks specificity. It will destroy not only the injured cells but also neighboring cells.

FLUIDS AND FLUID IMBALANCES

Many pathological conditions adversely affect the body's fluid and electrolyte balances.

WATER

Body fluids are mostly water, which is distributed into various compartments. The main compartments are intracellular and extracellular (fluid inside and outside of the body cells). Extracellular fluid is further divided into intravascular (fluid that is part of the blood, mostly plasma) and interstitial (fluid that is neither in the cells nor in the vascular system). Fluid in the interstitial space is generally absorbed into the lymphatic system, which returns it to the vascular system. Fluid moves between body compartments by the mechanisms of osmosis and diffusion.

As described in Chapter 3, movement of water in and out of the vascular system is governed by hydrostatic pressure (blood pressure)—which tends to force water out of the capillaries into the interstitial space—and the countereffect of oncotic force exerted by the large proteins in the plasma—which tends to pull interstitial fluid back into the capillaries. In a healthy person, net filtration of fluid in and out of the capillaries is zero.

EDEMA

Edema is the accumulation of water in the interstitial space, caused by a disruption in the forces that normally keep net filtration at zero. Four mechanisms commonly result in accumulation of water in the interstitial space: (1) a decrease in plasma oncotic force resulting from a decrease in plasma proteins; (2) increased hydrostatic pressure, which may result from venous obstruction, thrombophlebitis, or other causes; (3) increased capillary permeability resulting from mechanisms of inflammation and immune response; and (4) lymphatic channel obstruction, which can result from infection or surgical removal.

Edema can be localized or generalized. There may be local swelling at an injury site or within organ systems such as the lungs or heart or within body areas such as the abdomen or the feet. Edema is not only a sign of an underlying disease or injury. Edema itself causes problems, interfering with the movement of nutrients and wastes between tissues and capillaries and diminishing capillary blood flow. Edema affecting organs such as the brain, lung, heart, or larynx can be life threatening. Little can be done to treat edema in the prehospital setting except elevation of edematous limbs.

edema *excess fluid in the interstitial space.*

Content Review

Blood Components

- Liquid portion (plasma)
- Formed elements (blood cells)

INTRAVENOUS THERAPY

Intravenous (IV) therapy is the introduction of fluids and other substances into the venous side of the circulatory system. It is used to replace blood lost through hemorrhage, for electrolyte or fluid replacement, and for introduction of medications directly into the vascular system.

Blood and Blood Components

To understand IV therapy, it is necessary to understand the function of blood and its components. The blood is the fluid of the cardiovascular system. An adequate amount of blood is required for the transport of nutrients, oxygen, hormones, and heat. Blood consists of the liquid portion, or plasma, and the formed elements, or blood cells (Figure 4-1 ■).

Plasma Plasma is made up of approximately 92 percent water, 6 to 7 percent proteins, and a small portion consisting of electrolytes, lipids, enzymes, clotting factors, glucose, and other dissolved substances.

Formed Elements The formed elements include the red blood cells, or **erythrocytes;** the white blood cells, or **leukocytes;** and the platelets, or **thrombocytes.** More than 99 percent of the blood

plasma *the liquid part of the blood.*

erythrocytes *red blood cells, which contain hemoglobin, which transports oxygen to the cells.*

leukocytes *white blood cells, which play a key role in the immune system and inflammatory (infection-fighting) responses.*

thrombocytes *platelets, which are important in blood clotting.*

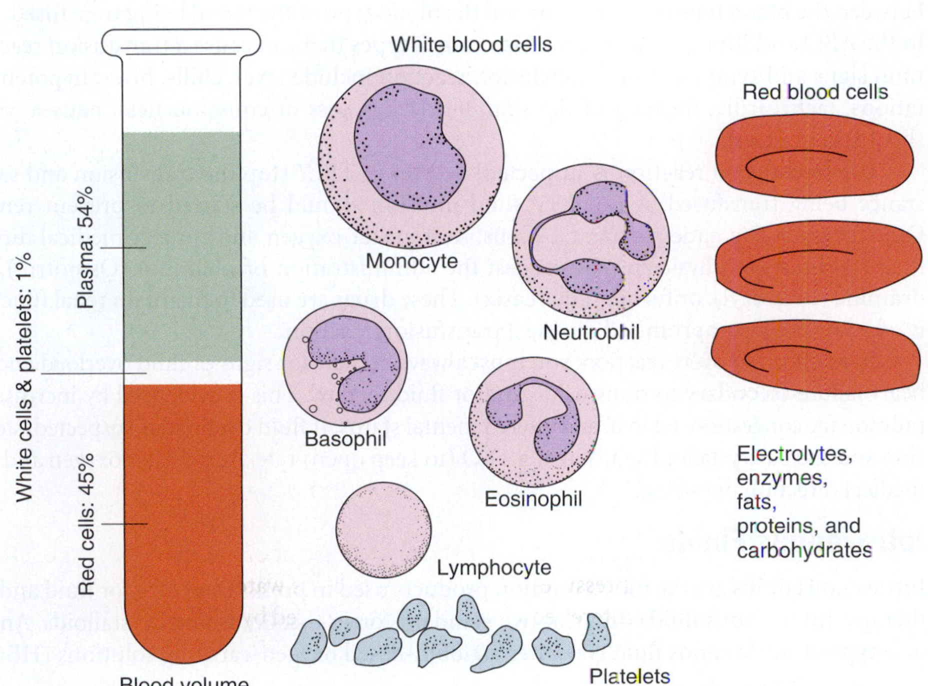

■ Figure 4-1 Blood components.

hemoglobin *an iron-based compound that binds with oxygen and transports it to the cells.*

cells are erythrocytes. Erythrocytes contain hemoglobin and are responsible for transporting oxygen to the body's peripheral cells. **Hemoglobin** is an iron-based compound that binds with oxygen in the pulmonary (lung) capillaries and transports the oxygen to the peripheral tissues where it can be unloaded and taken into the cells. Factors such as pH, oxygen concentration, and exposures to some chemicals affect the amount of oxygen that can be transported by hemoglobin.

The leukocytes are responsible for immunity and fighting infection. The thrombocytes play a major role in blood clotting. The viscosity (thickness) of the blood is determined by the ratio of plasma to formed elements. The greater the proportion of formed elements within the plasma, the greater the viscosity.

hematocrit *the percentage of the blood occupied by erythrocytes.*

The plasma can be separated from the formed elements by centrifugation. That is, blood can be placed in a test tube inside a centrifuge and spun at high speed. The heavier cells, the erythrocytes, will be forced to the bottom of the tube, leaving the plasma portion at the top. Usually, the erythrocytes will account for approximately 45 percent of the blood volume. The percentage of blood occupied by erythrocytes is referred to as the **hematocrit** (Figure 4-2 ■).

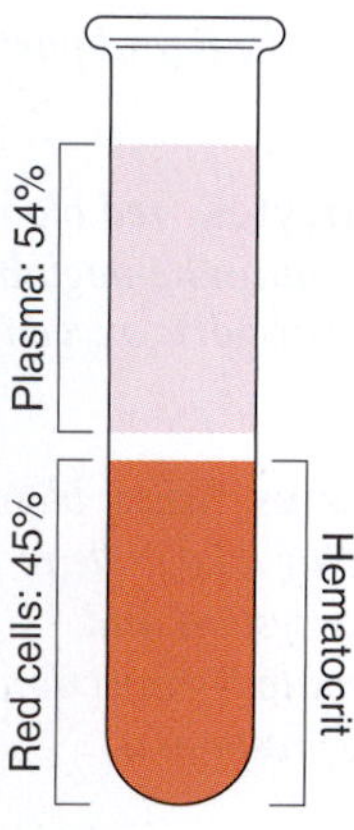

■ Figure 4-2 The percentage of the blood occupied by the red blood cells is termed the hematocrit.

Fluid Replacement

The most desirable fluid for blood loss replacement is whole blood. There are several reasons for this. First, blood contains hemoglobin, which can transport oxygen. In addition, it is the most natural replacement. However, even in the hospital setting, the routine use of whole blood is not practical (Table 4–1). Blood is a precious commodity, and it must be conserved so that it can benefit the most people. Because of this, blood is often fractionated, or separated into parts. The red cells are packaged separately as packed red blood cells. The white cells are used for other purposes. Plasma is packaged as fresh frozen plasma for use when plasma or clotting factors are needed. Thus, with the exception of true hemorrhagic shock (resulting from blood loss), where whole blood is the fluid of first choice, packed red blood cells are now more frequently used.

Before blood, or blood products, can be administered to a patient, they must be typed and crossmatched to prevent a severe allergic reaction. The exception to this is fresh frozen plasma, which does not require crossmatching. If there is not adequate time for typing and crossmatching, O-negative blood (type O, Rh negative), the universal donor, can be administered.

Transfusion Reaction

Blood and blood products are not used in the field. However, on occasion, you may be called upon to transport a patient with blood infusing. Because of this, you must be able to recognize the signs and symptoms of a transfusion reaction. Transfusion reactions occur when there is a discrepancy between the blood type of the patient and the blood type of the blood being transfused. In addition to the ABO and Rh types, there are many minor types that can cause a transfusion reaction. Common signs and symptoms of a transfusion reaction include fever, chills, hives, hypotension, palpitations, tachycardia, flushing of the skin, headaches, loss of consciousness, nausea, vomiting, or shortness of breath.

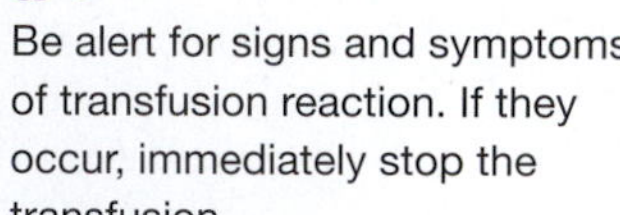

Be alert for signs and symptoms of transfusion reaction. If they occur, immediately stop the transfusion.

If a transfusion reaction is suspected, IMMEDIATELY stop the transfusion and save the substance being transfused. A rapid IV fluid infusion should be started to prevent renal damage. Quickly assess the patient's mental status. Administer oxygen and contact medical direction. The medical direction physician may request the administration of mannitol (Osmotrol), diphenhydramine (Benadryl), or furosemide (Lasix). These drugs are used to maintain renal function, which is often severely compromised during a transfusion reaction.

In addition to overt reaction, you must always be alert for signs of fluid overload and congestive heart failure secondary to transfusion and/or fluid therapy. This is evidenced by increased dyspnea, pulmonary congestion, edema, and altered mental status. If fluid overload is suspected, stop the infusion and start a crystalloid solution at a TKO (to keep open) rate. Administer oxygen and contact the medical direction physician.

Intravenous Fluids

Intravenous fluids are the most common products used in prehospital care for fluid and electrolyte therapy. Intravenous fluids occur in two standard forms—colloids and crystalloids. An important new type of intravenous fluid is the hemoglobin-based oxygen-carrying solutions (HBOCs).

Table 4–1 Resuscitation Fluids

Diagnosis	Resuscitation Fluid Used: 1st Choice	2nd Choice	3rd Choice	4th Choice
Hemorrhagic Shock	Whole blood	Packed RBCs	Plasma or plasma substitute	Lactated Ringer's or normal saline
Shock Due to Plasma Loss (Burns)	Plasma	Plasma substitute	Lactated Ringer's or normal saline	—
Dehydration	Lactated Ringer's or normal saline	—	—	—

Hemoglobin-Based Oxygen-Carrying Solutions (HBOCs) Hemoglobin-based oxygen-carrying solutions (HBOCs) represent a major development in the field of emergency and critical care. These products differ from other intravenous fluids in that they have the capability to transport oxygen. HBOCs contain long chains of *polymerized hemoglobin*. This hemoglobin is obtained from either expired donated human blood or bovine (cow) blood. The hemoglobin is removed from the red blood cells and then repeatedly filtered to remove any infectious substances or antigenic proteins. Finally, the individual hemoglobin molecules are joined together in a large chain through a chemical process known as polymerization. HBOCs are compatible with all blood types and do not require blood typing, testing, or crossmatching.

Initial studies of HBOCs have been disappointing. Further studies are under way.

hemoglobin-based oxygen-carrying solutions (HBOCs) *intravenous fluids with the ability to transport oxygen.*

Colloids Colloids contain proteins, or other high-molecular-weight molecules, that tend to remain in the intravascular space for an extended period of time. In addition, as described earlier, colloids have oncotic force (colloid osmotic pressure), which means they tend to attract water into the intravascular space from the interstitial space and the intracellular space. Thus, a small amount of a colloid can be administered to a patient with a greater-than-expected increase in intravascular volume. The following are examples of colloids:

- *Plasma protein fraction (Plasmanate)* is a protein-containing colloid. The principal protein present is **albumin,** which is suspended along with other proteins in a saline solvent.
- *Salt-poor albumin* contains only human albumin. Each gram of albumin holds approximately 18 milliliters of water in the bloodstream.
- *Dextran* is not a protein, but a large sugar molecule with osmotic properties similar to albumin. It comes in two molecular weights: 40,000 and 70,000 daltons. Dextran 40 has 2–2.5 times the colloid osmotic pressure of albumin.
- *Hetastarch (Hespan),* like dextran, is a sugar molecule with osmotic properties similar to protein. It does not appear to share many of dextran's side effects.

Colloid replacement therapy, at present, does not have a role in prehospital care except under rare circumstances. The colloid products are expensive and have a short shelf life.

colloids *substances, such as proteins or starches, consisting of large molecules or molecule aggregates that disperse evenly within a liquid without forming a true solution.*

albumin *a protein commonly present in plant and animal tissues. In the blood, albumin works to maintain blood volume and blood pressure and provides colloid osmotic pressure, which prevents plasma loss from the capillaries.*

Crystalloids Crystalloids are the primary compounds used in prehospital intravenous fluid therapy. There are multiple fluid preparations. It is often helpful to classify them according to their **tonicity** relative to plasma:

- *Isotonic solutions* have electrolyte composition similar to the blood plasma. When placed into a normally hydrated patient, they will not cause a significant fluid or

crystalloids *substances capable of crystallization. In solution, unlike colloids, they can diffuse through a membrane, such as a capillary wall.*

tonicity *solute concentration or osmotic pressure relative to the blood plasma or body cells.*

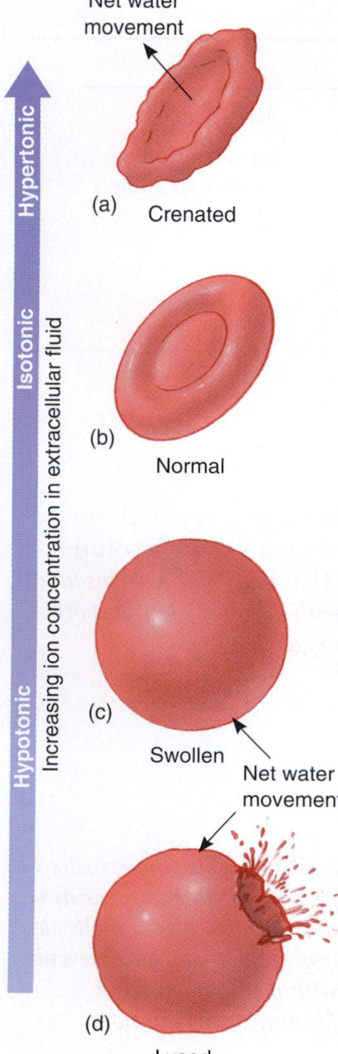

■ Figure 4-3 The effects of hypertonic, isotonic, and hypotonic solutions on red blood cells.

The three most commonly used fluids in prehospital care are lactated Ringer's, normal saline, and D_5W.

electrolyte shift. Examples: normal saline (0.9 percent sodium chloride, also written as 0.9% NaCl), lactated Ringer's.

- ★ *Hypertonic solutions* have a higher solute concentration than the cells. These fluids will tend to cause a fluid shift out of the interstitial space and intracellular compartment into the intravascular space when administered to a normally hydrated patient. Later, there will be a diffusion of solute in the opposite direction. Examples: Plasmanate, dextran.
- ★ *Hypotonic solutions* have a lower solute concentration than the cells. When administered to a normally hydrated patient, they will cause a movement of fluid from the intravascular space into the interstitial space and intracellular compartment. Later, solutes will move in an opposite direction. Example: 5 percent dextrose in water (D_5W).

Intravenous replacement fluids should be chosen based on the needs of the patient and the patient's underlying problem. This is typically guided by laboratory studies obtained in the hospital. However, these studies are not available in the prehospital setting. Hemorrhage occurs so fast that there is usually not time for a significant fluid shift to occur between the intravascular space and interstitial/intracellular spaces. Because of this, isotonic replacement fluids, such as lactated Ringer's and normal saline, should be used (Figure 4-3 ■).

Certain conditions, such as gastroenteritis (characterized by diarrhea, vomiting, and fever) can cause a patient to lose water more rapidly than sodium. These patients will have a deficit in total body water (TBW) due to reduced water intake, excessive water loss, or a combination of both. When water is lost in this manner, the level of sodium in the serum can increase, resulting in hypernatremia (elevated sodium levels). Patients with hypernatremia primarily need water. Because of this, hypotonic intravenous solutions, such as 0.45 percent sodium chloride (half-normal saline), are often chosen, because they provide the needed water with less sodium. However, it is important to point out that, even in cases of hypernatremia, initial fluid replacement therapy should be with an isotonic solution until adequate blood pressure and adequate tissue perfusion have been restored.

Some replacement fluids contain a single element, such as sodium chloride or dextrose, while others contain multiple elements. Solutions such as lactated Ringer's are designed so that the concentration of electrolytes is very similar to that of the plasma. As a result, these solutions are referred to as balanced salt solutions.

The most commonly used solutions in prehospital care are lactated Ringer's solution, 0.9 percent sodium chloride (normal saline), and 5 percent dextrose in water (D_5W).

- ★ *Lactated Ringer's* is an isotonic electrolyte solution of sodium chloride, potassium chloride, calcium chloride, and sodium lactate in water.
- ★ *Normal saline* is an electrolyte solution of sodium chloride in water. It is isotonic with the extracellular fluid.
- ★ *D_5W* is a hypotonic glucose solution used to keep a vein open and to supply calories necessary for cell metabolism. While it will have an initial effect of increasing the circulatory volume, glucose molecules rapidly diffuse across the vascular membrane. Water follows the glucose into the interstitial space, resulting in an increase in interstitial water.

Both lactated Ringer's solution and normal saline are used for fluid replacement, because their administration causes an immediate expansion of the circulatory volume. However, as was noted earlier, due to the movement of electrolytes and water, two-thirds of either of these solutions is lost into the interstitial space within 1 hour.

ACID–BASE DERANGEMENTS

ACIDOSIS AND ALKALOSIS

An increase in hydrogen ion (as occurs, for example, in cardiac arrest) triggers an alteration in acid–base balance. Hydrogen ion is immediately combined with bicarbonate ion. This combination results in the formation of carbonic acid, which then dissociates into carbon dioxide and water with the assistance of carbonic anhydrase. Carbon dioxide is eliminated by the lungs, and water is eliminated through the kidneys. Any change in a component of this equation affects the other components. For example:

$$\Uparrow H^+ + HCO_3^- \Rightarrow \Uparrow H_2CO_3 \Rightarrow H_2O + \Uparrow CO_2$$

Conversely, if the amount of carbon dioxide is increased, the equation is driven in the other direction, resulting in an increase in hydrogen ion (acid).

$$\Uparrow CO_2 + H_2O \Rightarrow \Uparrow H_2CO_3 \Rightarrow \Uparrow H^+ + HCO_3^-$$

Both types of acid–base derangements, alkalosis and acidosis, can be divided into two categories based on the underlying causes. Changes in the concentration of CO_2 result from changes in respiratory function. Thus, an acidosis caused by retained CO_2 is referred to as *respiratory acidosis.* An alkalosis caused by the excess removal of CO_2 is called *respiratory alkalosis.* However, if acidosis results from the production of metabolic acids, such as lactic acid, then *metabolic acidosis* is said to exist. If an alkalosis is caused by the excess elimination of hydrogen ion, it is termed *metabolic alkalosis.*

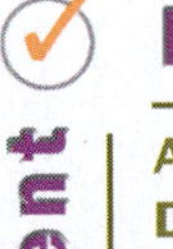

Review

Content

Acid–Base Derangements

- Respiratory acidosis
- Respiratory alkalosis
- Metabolic acidosis
- Metabolic alkalosis

Respiratory Acidosis

Respiratory acidosis is caused by the retention of CO_2. This can result from impaired ventilation due to problems occurring either in the lungs or in the respiratory center of the brain. The CO_2 level is increased and the pH is decreased.

$$\Downarrow \text{RESPIRATION} = \Uparrow CO_2 + H_2O \Rightarrow \Uparrow H_2CO_3 \Rightarrow \Uparrow H^+ + HCO_3^-$$

Treatment is directed at improving ventilation.

respiratory acidosis *acidity caused by abnormal retention of carbon dioxide resulting from impaired ventilation.*

Respiratory Alkalosis

Respiratory alkalosis results from increased respiration and excessive elimination of CO_2. This can occur with anxiety or following ascent to a high altitude. The CO_2 level is decreased and the pH is increased:

$$\Uparrow \text{RESPIRATION} = \Downarrow CO_2 + H_2O \Rightarrow \Downarrow H_2CO_3 \Rightarrow \Downarrow H^+ + HCO_3^-$$

Treatment, if required, consists of increasing the CO_2 level by emotionally supporting the patient and coaching him to reduce his respiratory rate.

respiratory alkalosis *alkalinity caused by excessive elimination of carbon dioxide resulting from increased respirations.*

Metabolic Acidosis

Metabolic acidosis results from the production of metabolic acids such as lactic acid, which consume bicarbonate ion. In addition, it can result from dehydration (as from diarrhea, vomiting), diabetes, and medication usage. The pH is decreased, and the CO_2 level is normal:

$$\Uparrow H^+ + HCO_3^- \Rightarrow \Uparrow H_2CO_3 \Rightarrow H_2O + \Uparrow CO_2$$

In addition to treating the underlying cause, treatment includes ventilation, which causes the elimination of CO_2 and, subsequently, hydrogen ion (Figure 4-4 ■). On rare occasions, an IV bolus of sodium bicarbonate ($NaHCO_3$) may be required.

metabolic acidosis *acidity caused by an increase in acid, often because of increased production of acids during metabolism or from causes such as vomiting, diarrhea, diabetes, or medication.*

Metabolic Alkalosis

Metabolic alkalosis occurs much less frequently than metabolic acidosis. It is usually caused by the administration of **diuretics,** loss of chloride ions associated with prolonged vomiting, or the overzealous administration of sodium bicarbonate. The pH is increased and the CO_2 level is normal:

$$\Downarrow H^+ + HCO_3^- \Rightarrow \Downarrow H_2CO_3 \Rightarrow H_2O + \Downarrow CO_2$$

Treatment consists of correcting the underlying cause.

Usually, both a respiratory and a metabolic component are present in an acid–base derangement. The type of acid–base derangement present can only be determined by arterial blood gas studies. These, of course, are only available in the hospital setting. Arterial blood gases report the pH, $PaCO_2$, PaO_2, bicarbonate concentration, and oxygen saturation.

metabolic alkalosis *alkalinity caused by an increase in plasma bicarbonate resulting from causes including diuresis, vomiting, or ingestion of too much sodium bicarbonate.*

diuretic *an agent that increases urine secretion and elimination of body water.*

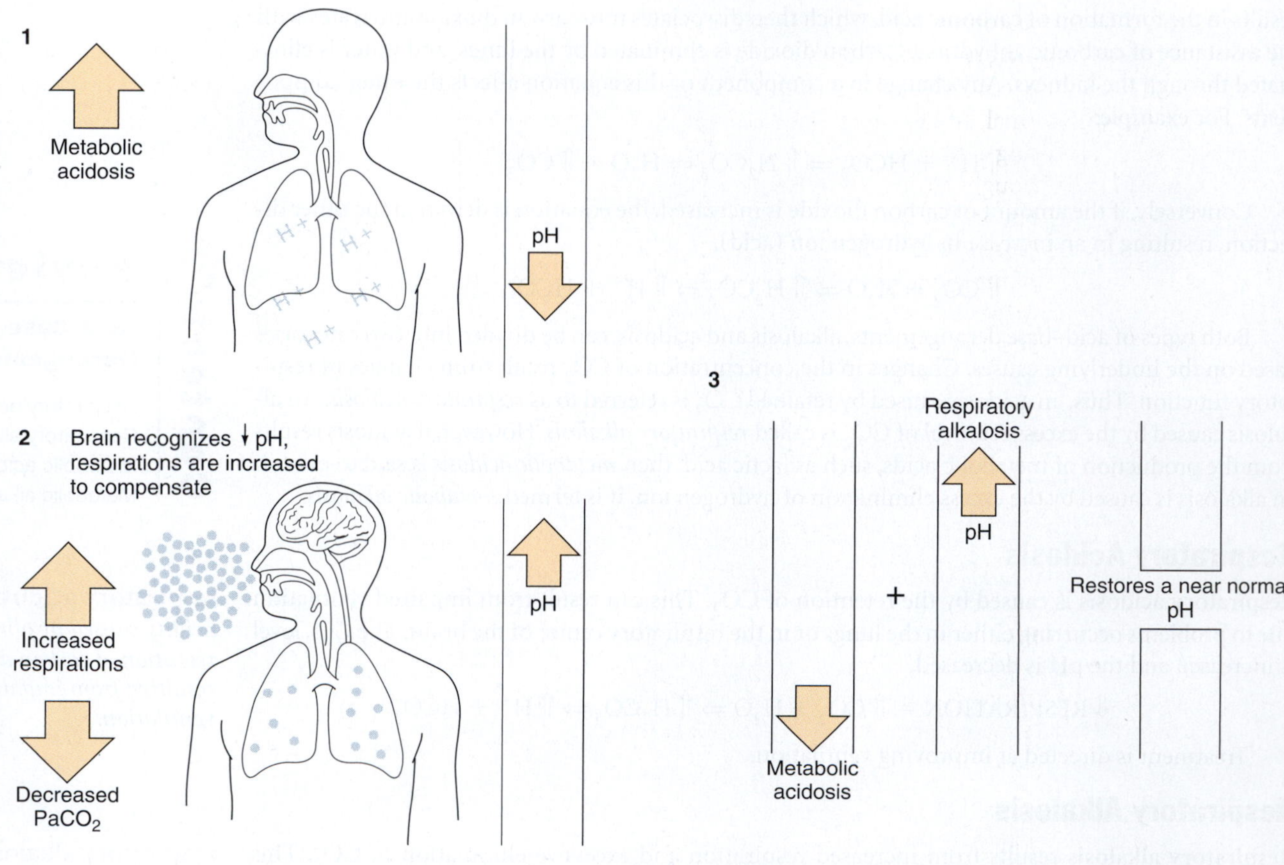

Figure 4-4 Compensation for metabolic acidosis begins with an increase in respirations.

GENETIC AND OTHER CAUSES OF DISEASE

When we think of disease, we are likely to think first of infections caused by pathogens, including bacteria, viruses, fungi, and parasites. In recent years, great strides have been made in the medical treatment of infectious diseases, but many diseases result from genetic causes, which have been far more difficult to identify and treat. The picture is additionally complicated by the fact that many diseases result from a combination of genetic and environmental factors (including lifestyle factors) as well as factors such as age and gender.

Even a family history of a particular disease does not necessarily mean that the disease has a purely genetic origin, because families also share environmental and lifestyle factors that may cause or contribute to the family disease. While family history points to the possibility of genetic causes, these cannot be confirmed, much less treated, until scientists are able to make definitive identifications of the defective genes or chromosomes that cause or contribute to particular diseases.

At present, there is increasing progress in identifying and understanding genetic and other noninfectious causes of disease. Many promising advances toward gene therapies (the replacement of defective genes with normal genes) and other therapies for diseases have been made.

GENETICS, ENVIRONMENT, LIFESTYLE, AGE, AND GENDER

As noted earlier, our inherited traits are determined by molecules of deoxyribonucleic acid, or DNA, which form structures called genes, which reside on larger structures called chromosomes within the nuclei of all our cells. We inherit our genetic structure from our parents. Every one of a person's somatic cells (all the cells except the sex cells) contains 46 chromosomes. The sex cells, however, contain only 23 chromosomes each. The sex cells contribute these 23 chromosomes to the offspring. Thus, the offspring receives 23 chromosomes from the father and 23 chromosomes from the mother, resulting in a total of 46 chromosomes. Occasionally one or more of a person's genes or chromosomes is abnormal, and this may cause a congenital disease (one we are born with) or a propensity toward acquiring a disease later in life.

Every human somatic cell contains 46 chromosomes (23 pairs).

Some diseases are thought to be purely genetic. For example, cystic fibrosis, which affects mainly people of European origin, and sickle cell disease, which affects mainly people of African origin, are known to be caused by disorders of single genes. They affect different populations to a different degree because of the evolutionary history of those populations. A genetic disease may be caused by a single defective gene or by several defective genes or chromosomes. Single-gene causes are, obviously, easier for medical researchers to identify and potentially devise treatments for than are other, more complex genetic causes of disease.

Other diseases are caused by a combination of genetic and environmental factors and are called *multifactorial disorders.* For example, Type II (adult-onset) diabetes has a very high correlation with family history of the disease. However, it is also affected by environmental and lifestyle factors such as a high fat or high carbohydrate diet and lack of exercise, which results in obesity, and with age. (There is a higher incidence of Type II diabetes in overweight people, and the disease tends to appear in middle age or later.) Heart disease, which is highly correlated with family history and age, also has a gender/hormonal factor: Women appear to be somewhat protected from heart disease before menopause, when their bodies are still producing estrogen. Following menopause, women quickly "catch up" with men in the development of heart disease. Estrogen replacement therapy following menopause may afford prolonged protection against heart disease.

Most disease processes are multifactorial in origin.

Content Review

Causative Analysis of Disease

Clinical factors:
Host
Agent
Environment

Epidemiological factors:
Incidence
Prevalence
Mortality

Clinical practitioners and epidemiologists study disease, respectively, from the point of view of their effects on individuals and from the point of view of their effects on populations as a whole.

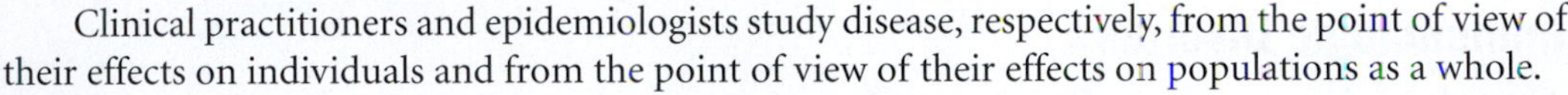

- ★ *Effects on individuals.* Physicians and other clinical practitioners study the effects of diseases on individuals, and find it instructive to view the development of diseases as products of the interactions among three factors: *host, agent,* and *environment.* This establishes a framework for determining how one factor, or a combination of these factors, may precipitate a disease state. Genetic predisposition, gender, and ethnic origin are determinants related to the host. These may interact with a specific agent, in a specific type of environment, to cause illness. The agent may be a bacterium, toxin, gunshot, or other pathophysiological process. The environment may be defined by the local climate, socioeconomic or demographic features, culture, religion, and associated factors. Determination of how the host, agent, and environment interact may yield solutions to curing a disease process. Injury and trauma are now being viewed as "diseases," in the sense of how the interaction of host, agent, and environment may contribute to an understanding of what, heretofore, have been perceived as social problems.
- ★ *Effects on populations.* Epidemiologists, who study the effects of diseases on populations, generally report disease data with three basic measures: *incidence, prevalence,* and *mortality. Morbidity,* a term commonly used in discussing disease statistics, can be more precisely reported as incidence and prevalence. Incidence is the number of new cases of the disease that are reported in a given period of time, usually 1 year. Prevalence is the proportion of the total population who are affected by the disease at a given point in time. (Prevalence is higher than incidence, as those who acquire the disease each year are added to those who already have the disease.) *Mortality* is the rate of death from the disease.

Epidemiologists and clinical practitioners are now collaborating to study risk factors, such as the relationship between smoking and lung cancer. Risk factor analysis is both statistical and complex. Although the correlation of smoking to lung cancer is extremely high, not everyone who smokes develops lung cancer, and not everyone who develops lung cancer has been a smoker. Risk factor analysis would compare the number of smokers to nonsmokers among lung cancer cases, the pack/year (number of packs per day × number of years) history of the smokers with lung cancer, factors that might have aggravated or mitigated the effects of smoking, and so on.

FAMILY HISTORY AND ASSOCIATED RISK FACTORS

It is important for those who have a family history of a particular disease not to conclude that acquiring the disease is their destiny and there is nothing they can do about it. This is not always true. Most diseases with a genetic component that come on during adulthood also have associated risk factors that can be modified to prevent, delay, or reduce the impact of the disease.

Consider the variety of possible risk factors for disease: People who live in less-developed countries are often at higher risk for disease from microorganisms flourishing in their water supply and disease transmission caused by poor sanitation. Physical conditions commonly seen in larger U.S. cities as well as rural areas, such as inadequate housing, poor nutrition, and little or no medical attention, potentiate disease transmission. Chemical factors such as smoke, smog, illicit drug use, occupational chemical exposure, and additives in our food are causative agents for a variety of diseases.

Personal habit is among the most publicized—and controllable—causes of disease in our society. For example, predisposing factors for cardiovascular disease include smoking, excessive alcohol consumption, inactivity, and obesity. Unfortunately, changes in individual lifestyle often occur only after a disease has already manifested itself. As we age, the predisposing factors and causative agents take their toll. The body's ability to defend itself against disease decreases due to the effects of aging on our immunological system and other compensatory mechanisms.

Following is a discussion of some of the most common diseases in which both genetics and other risk factors play a role. You will notice, as you read, that the causation of various diseases varies widely, and that while the causes are known for some diseases, the causes of other diseases are still not clearly understood.

Immunologic Disorders

A number of immunologic disorders, such as rheumatic fever, allergies, and asthma, are more prevalent among those with a family history of the disorder but also involve other risk factors.

Rheumatic fever is an inflammatory reaction to an infection but is not an infection itself. There seems to be a hereditary factor, but inadequate nutrition and crowded living conditions are contributing factors.

Allergies often have a family history factor (and some allergies can be passed from the mother to the fetus during pregnancy). However, allergic reactions are triggered by exposure to allergens and can usually be controlled by avoiding or reducing the presence of allergens as well as with medication.

Asthma sufferers may inherit the propensity for airway-narrowing in response to various stimuli, but other triggering factors may be identified and, perhaps, controlled, including stress, overexertion, exposure to cold air, and stimuli such as pollens, dust mites, cockroach detritus, and smoke.

Cancer

A wide variety of family history and environmental factors are included among the risk factors for cancer. Some kinds of cancer, such as breast and colorectal cancer, tend to cluster in families and seem to have a combination of genetic and environmental causes. Others, such as lung cancer, are more strongly identified with environmental causes.

For *breast cancer,* the greatest risk factor is age, with the majority of cases occurring after age 60 and the greatest risk after age 75. A history of breast cancer in a first-degree relative (mother, sister, or daughter) increases the risk by two or three times. Some progress has been made in identifying genes for certain breast cancers. Lifestyle factors such as lack of exercise and obesity may contribute slightly to the incidence of breast cancer, but this has not been proven.

As with breast cancer, *colorectal cancer* risk factors include age (with the incidence rising after age 40 and peaking between 60 and 75) and family history (incidence in a first-degree relative increases the risk by two or three times). There are gender factors, with rectal cancer being more common in men and colon cancer more common in women. Diet may also be a risk factor, although recent studies have failed to confirm a link between a high-fat, low-fiber diet and colorectal cancer. (However, a high-fat, low-fiber diet has been positively linked to heart disease and other health problems.)

The causes of *lung cancer* are overwhelmingly environmental. Smoking has been identified as the main cause of 90 percent of lung cancers in men and 70 percent of lung cancers in women. Lung cancer can also be caused by inhaling substances such as asbestos, arsenic, and nickel, usually in the workplace.

Endocrine Disorders

The most common endocrine disorder is *diabetes mellitus,* which is a leading cause of blindness, heart disease, kidney failure, and premature death. The causes of diabetes are complex and still not well understood.

There are two major types of diabetes: Type I and Type II. Type I diabetes usually occurs before age 40, sometimes in childhood. Although it is less prevalent than Type II diabetes (accounting for about 20 percent of diabetes cases), it is more severe. In the Type I diabetic, the pancreas produces no or almost no insulin, which is required for the cellular utilization of glucose, the body's chief source of energy. Type I diabetics must take insulin daily. There is some association of Type I diabetes with family history (siblings of Type I diabetics have a 6 percent risk compared to 0.3 percent in the general population), and medical researchers have pinpointed some possible genetic factors. Other causative factors may include autoimmunity disorders and viral infections that invade the pancreas and destroy the insulin-producing cells.

Type II diabetes accounts for about 80 percent of all diabetes cases. It usually occurs after age 40 and the incidence increases with age. It clusters much more strongly in families than does Type I diabetes (siblings have a 10 to 15 percent risk). In contrast to Type I diabetes, in which there is a total lack of insulin, Type II diabetes is associated with a decreased insulin receptor response or a decrease in insulin production. Diet and exercise may also be factors, since the majority of Type II diabetics are obese. Type II diabetes can often be controlled with diet and exercise or with oral medications.

Hematologic Disorders

Hereditary coagulation disorders have been studied by geneticists and physicians in great detail. There are many causes of hereditary hematological disorders such as gene alteration and histocompatibility (tissue interaction) dysfunctions.

Hemophilia is a bleeding disorder that is caused by a genetic clotting factor deficiency. It can be mild, but if severe it can cause not only serious bruising but bleeding into the joints, which can lead to crippling deformities. A slight bump on the head can cause bleeding within the skull, often resulting in brain damage and death. The heredity is sex-linked (associated with the sex chromosomes), inherited through the mother, and affects male children almost exclusively. There is no cure, but administration of concentrated clotting factors can improve the condition.

Hemochromatosis is another genetic disorder, but this time caused by a histocompatibility complex dysfunction. It is marked by an excessive absorption and accumulation of iron in the body, causing weight loss, joint pain, abdominal pain, palpitations, and testicular atrophy in males. It is treated by removing blood from the body at intervals.

Not all blood disorders are genetic. Environmental factors, for example, can cause *anemia* (reduction in circulating red blood cells). For example, some antihypertensive medications and other drugs may cause a drug-induced hemolytic (red-blood-cell-destroying) anemia.

Cardiovascular Disorders

The cardiovascular system can be greatly affected by genetic disorders. Disorders such as *prolongation of the QT interval* (a delay between depolarization and repolarization of the ventricles as revealed in an electrocardiogram) and *mitral valve prolapse* (an upward ballooning of the valve between the left ventricle and atrium that allows blood to regurgitate back into the atrium when the ventricle contracts) tend to cluster in families.

The American Heart Association lists heredity as a major risk factor for cardiovascular disease. Those with parents who have *coronary artery disease* (deposits on the walls of the coronary arteries that reduce blood flow to the heart muscle) have an approximately fivefold risk of developing the disease. This is why it is important to ask about family history of congenital heart disease (CHD), hypertension, and stroke when assessing patients with possible cardiovascular disease. However, environmental factors, such as a diet high in saturated fats and cholesterol (or a diet high in carbohydrates) and lack of exercise, also play a large role in cardiovascular disease.

Hypertension (high blood pressure) is a major risk factor, not only for cardiac disease but also for stroke and kidney disease. Studies of family history show that approximately 20 to 40 percent of the causation of hypertension is genetic. The remaining causative factors, then, are environmental, and may include high sodium ingestion, lack of physical activity, stress, and obesity.

Not all cardiac disorders have a genetic component. For example, *cardiomyopathy* (disease affecting the heart muscle) is thought to occur secondarily to other causes such as infectious disease, toxin exposure, connective tissue disease, or nutritional deficiencies, which may be partially or totally environmental.

Renal Disorders

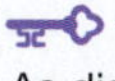

As dialysis treatment shifts from medical centers to homes and community centers, EMS personnel are increasingly being called to deal with complications of dialysis.

Renal (kidney) failure is caused by a variety of factors (primarily hypertension) which may eventually require a patient to receive dialysis treatment several times a week. As the location of dialysis treatment shifts from medical centers to homes and community satellite centers, EMS personnel are increasingly being called to deal with the complications of dialysis. These include problems with vascular access devices (shunts, fistulas), localized infection and sepsis, and electrolyte abnormalities (hyperkalemia), which can result in cardiac arrest.

Rheumatic Disorders

Gout is a condition that may have both genetic and environmental causes. It is characterized by severe arthritic pain caused by deposit of crystals in the joints, most commonly the great toe. The crystals form as the result of an abnormally high level of uric acid in the blood that may be caused when the kidneys do not excrete enough uric acid or by high production of uric acid. High production of uric acid may be caused by a hereditary metabolic abnormality. Although the underlying cause may be genetic, attacks of gout can be triggered by environmental factors such as trauma, alcohol consumption, ingestion of certain foods, stress, or other illnesses. Patients with gout also have a tendency to develop *kidney stones.*

Gastrointestinal Disorders

Gastrointestinal disorders have a variety of causes, and the causes of some are not known. *Lactose intolerance,* for example, is usually identified by the inability of the patient to tolerate milk and some other dairy products. The patient lacks lactase, the enzyme that usually breaks down lactose in the digestive tract. This enzyme deficiency may be congenital (inborn) or may develop later on.

Crohn's disease is a chronic inflammation of the wall of the digestive tract that usually affects the small intestine, the large intestine, or both. The cause is not known, but medical researchers have focused on immune system dysfunction, infection, and diet as the major probabilities. A similar disorder is ulcerative colitis, in which the large intestine becomes inflamed and develops ulcers. As with Crohn's disease, the cause is not known, but an overactive immune response is suspected, and heredity seems to play a role.

Peptic ulcers develop when the normal protective structures and mechanisms, such as mucous production, break down and areas in the lining of the stomach or duodenum are inflamed by stomach acid and digestive juices. Environmental factors, bacterial infection (by *Helicobacter pylori*), diet, stress, and alcohol consumption are thought to play roles in the development of peptic ulcers. Many medications, particularly nonsteroidal anti-inflammatory medications, are associated with ulcer formation.

Cholecystitis is an inflammation of the gallbladder that usually results from blockage by a gallstone. There may be a genetic predisposition for gallstone formation. Gallstones are more prevalent in women and in some groups such as Native Americans and Mexican Americans. Other risk factors include age, a high-fat diet, and obesity.

Obesity can be defined as being more than 20 percent over the ideal body weight. Obesity has both an environmental and familial risk transmission. Research has shown that children whose parents are obese have a much-increased chance of developing obesity. Environmental factors such as proper nutrition and exercise may not be modeled or taught by obese parents, but there also seems to be a genetic factor to many cases of obesity. Obesity has been linked to, or defined as a cause for, diseases such as hypertension, heart disease, and vascular diseases.

Neuromuscular Disorders

Diseases of the nervous and muscular systems also have a variety of causes. *Huntington's disease* (which results in uncontrollable jerking and writhing movements) and muscular dystrophy (which results in progressive muscle weakness) are both known to be caused by genetic defects.

Multiple sclerosis (which affects the nerves of the eye, brain, and spinal cord) seems to have some hereditary factor with clustering among close relatives. Its exact cause is unknown, but it seems to result when the virus-triggered autoimmune response begins to attack the myelin sheath that protects the nerves.

Alzheimer's disease is thought to cause about 50 percent of dementias, or progressive mental deterioration. Its cause is unknown, but it does cluster strongly in families and appears to be either caused or influenced by specific gene abnormalities.

Psychiatric Disorders

Many disease processes have a genetic cause.

Genetic and biological causes of psychiatric disorders are being studied and increasingly understood. An example is *schizophrenia*, which affects about 1 percent of the population worldwide and is more prevalent than Alzheimer's disease, diabetes, or multiple sclerosis. The schizophrenic loses contact with reality and suffers from hallucinations, delusions, abnormal thinking, and disrupted social functioning. People who develop schizophrenia are now thought to be "biologically vulnerable" to the disease, but what makes them vulnerable is not fully understood. The cause may be a genetic predisposition or some problem that occurs before, during, or after birth or a viral infection of the brain.

Another common psychiatric disorder is *manic-depressive illness*, also called *bipolar disorder*, in which the person experiences alternating periods of depression and mania or excitement. It can be mild or severe enough to interfere with the patient's ability to work or function socially. Manic-depressive illness affects about twice as many people as schizophrenia. It is believed to be hereditary, but the exact gene deficit has not yet been discovered.

HYPOPERFUSION

All body cells require a constant supply of oxygen and other nutrients.

All body cells require a constant supply of oxygen and other essential nutrients, while waste products, such as carbon dioxide, must be constantly removed. It is the circulatory system, in conjunction with the respiratory and gastrointestinal systems, that provides the body's cells with these essential nutrients and removal of wastes. This is accomplished by the passage of blood through the capillaries, the small vessels that interface with body cells, while oxygen and carbon dioxide, nutrients and wastes are exchanged by movement across the capillary walls and cell membranes. This constant and necessary passage of blood through the body's tissues is called *perfusion*.

There is some local control of both tissue perfusion and waste removal. When the amounts of metabolic waste products (such as lactic acid) increase, the tissues subsequently become acidotic. This local acidosis causes nearby precapillary sphincters to relax, thus opening the capillaries and increasing perfusion of the affected tissues. This provides increased capacity for waste elimination and response to local metabolic demands.

Inadequate perfusion of body tissues is **hypoperfusion,** which is commonly called shock. Shock occurs first at a cellular level. If allowed to progress, the tissues, organs, organ systems, and ultimately the entire organism is affected. Hypoperfusion is a condition that is progressive (that is, it triggers a self-worsening cycle of pathophysiological events) and fatal if not corrected. It can occur for many reasons, such as trauma, fluid loss, myocardial infarction, infection, allergic reaction, spinal cord injury, and other causes.

hypoperfusion *inadequate perfusion of the body tissues, resulting in an inadequate supply of oxygen and nutrients to the body tissues. Also called shock.*

Although causes differ, all forms of shock have the same underlying pathophysiology at the cellular and tissue levels. As discussed in the next section, shock may be triggered by anything that affects one or more of these components of the cardiovascular system: the pump (the heart), the fluid (the blood), or the container (the blood vessels).

THE PATHOPHYSIOLOGY OF HYPOPERFUSION

Causes of Hypoperfusion

Hypoperfusion (shock) is almost always a result of inadequate cardiac output. A number of factors can decrease effective cardiac output. These include:

- Inadequate pump
  - Inadequate preload

Review

Content

Physiological Classifications of Shock

Inadequate pump (cardiogenic)
Inadequate fluid (hypovolemic)
Inadequate container (distributive/neurogenic)

– Inadequate cardiac contractile strength
– Inadequate heart rate
– Excessive afterload

★ Inadequate fluid
– Hypovolemia (abnormally low circulating blood volume)

★ Inadequate container
– Dilated container without change in fluid volume (inadequate systemic vascular resistance)
– Leak in container

Occasionally, hypoperfusion can develop even when cardiac output is adequate. This can happen when cell metabolism is so excessive that the body cannot increase perfusion enough to meet the cells' metabolic requirements. It can also happen when abnormal circulatory patterns develop, so that circulating blood is bypassing critical tissues.

As mentioned earlier, the conditions that lead to hypoperfusion can result from a number of underlying causes, such as infection, trauma and hemorrhage, loss of plasma through burns, severe cardiac dysrhythmia, central nervous system dysfunction, and many others. But the outcome is always the same: inadequate delivery of oxygen and essential nutrients to, and removal of wastes from, all the tissues of the body, especially the critical tissues (brain, heart, kidneys).

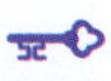

At the simplest level, shock is inadequate tissue perfusion.

Shock at the Cellular Level

Shock is a complex phenomenon. The causes vary, as do the signs and symptoms. At the simplest level, however, shock is inadequate tissue perfusion. Additionally, all types of shock have this in common: The ultimate outcome is impairment of cellular metabolism. Two characteristics of impaired cellular metabolism in any type of shock are impaired oxygen use and impaired glucose use.

Review

Content

Characteristics of Impaired Cellular Metabolism in Shock

Impaired use of oxygen
Impaired use of glucose

aerobic metabolism *the second stage of metabolism, requiring the presence of oxygen, in which the breakdown of glucose (in a process called the Krebs or citric acid cycle) yields a high amount of energy. Aerobic means "with oxygen."*

anaerobic metabolism *the first stage of metabolism, which does not require oxygen, in which the breakdown of glucose (in a process called glycolysis) produces pyruvic acid and yields very little energy. Anaerobic means "without oxygen."*

Impaired Use of Oxygen One characteristic of any type of shock is that the cells are either not receiving enough oxygen or are unable to use it effectively. This may be caused by hypoperfusion resulting from reduced cardiac function, inadequate blood volume, or vasodilation (pump, fluid, or container problems). It may result from insufficient red cells to carry the oxygen, from fever that increases cellular oxygen demand, or from chemical disruption of cellular metabolism.

When the cells don't receive enough oxygen or cannot use it effectively, they change from **aerobic metabolism** to **anaerobic metabolism,** a far less efficient means of producing energy—as explained in the following text.

The primary energy source for the cells is glucose, taken into the cell with the aid of insulin. Glucose does not provide energy until it is broken down inside the cell. The first stage of glucose breakdown, called glycolysis, is anaerobic (does not require oxygen). Glycolysis produces pyruvic acid but yields very little energy. Thus, by itself, glycolysis is an inefficient utilization of glucose. Therefore, in a normal state of metabolism, a second stage of glucose breakdown is required. During this second stage, which is aerobic (requires oxygen), pyruvic acid is further degraded into carbon dioxide, water, and energy in a process termed the Krebs or citric acid cycle. The energy yield of this second-stage aerobic process is much higher than from the first-stage anaerobic process (Figure 4-5 ■).

During shock, or any condition in which the cells do not receive adequate oxygen or cannot use it effectively, glucose breakdown can only complete the first-stage, anaerobic process of glycolysis and cannot enter into the second-stage, aerobic, citric acid cycle. This causes an accumulation of the end product of glycolysis, pyruvic acid. In these cases, pyruvic acid is quickly degraded to lactic acid. If oxygen is promptly restored to the cells, lactic acid will be reconverted to pyruvic acid. However, if time elapses and the cellular hypoxia is not corrected, lactic acid and other metabolic acids will accumulate. One outcome is that the acidic condition of the blood reduces the ability of hemoglobin in red blood cells to bind with and carry oxygen, which compounds the problem of cellular oxygen deprivation.

The energy that is produced during glucose breakdown is in the form of the chemical adenosine triphosphate (ATP), which is essential to all the metabolic processes in the cells. As just noted, the amount of energy, or ATP, produced during first-stage, anaerobic glycolysis is very small. Without oxygen, when the process of glucose breakdown stops after glycolysis (during which very little

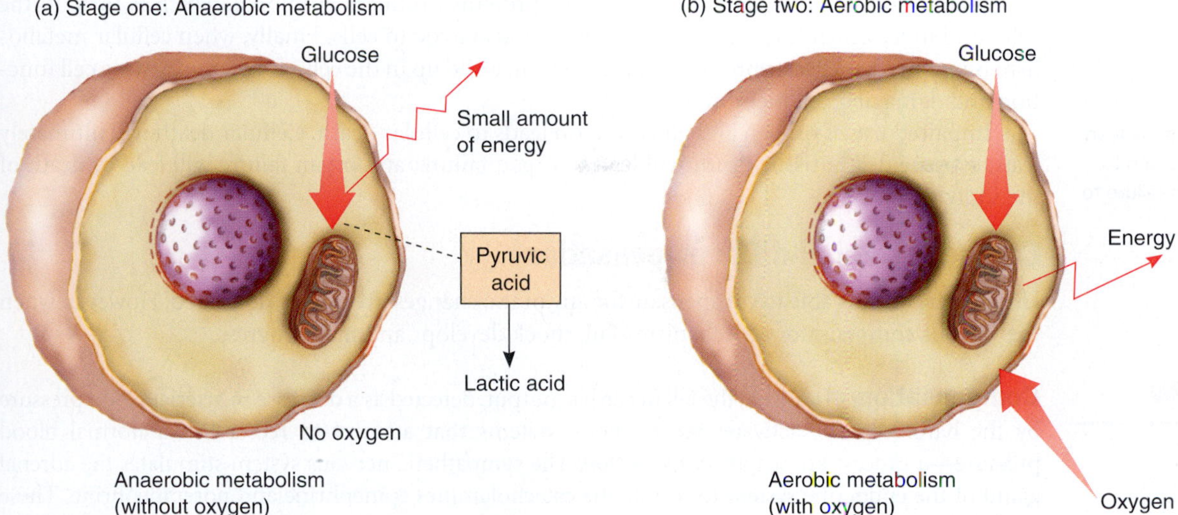

■ **Figure 4-5** Glucose breakdown. (a) Stage one, glycolysis, is anaerobic (does not require oxygen). It yields pyruvic acid, with toxic byproducts such as lactic acid, and very little energy. (b) Stage two is aerobic (requires oxygen). In a process called the Krebs or citric acid cycle, pyruvic acid is degraded into carbon dioxide and water, which produces a much higher yield of energy.

energy has been produced), cellular stores of ATP are used up much faster than they can be replaced, so that all of the processes of cellular metabolism are gravely impaired.

Because of changes to the internal cell and because blood flow has been slowed by the decreased pumping action and vasodilation, sludging of the blood occurs. This further impedes blood flow. Thus, the normal diffusion of nutrients and wastes in and out of the cells is disrupted and the balance of the cellular electrolytes is altered. Lysosomes, the organelles that assist in digestion of nutrients, are normally enclosed by a membrane that prevents the digestive enzymes from damaging other cell components. Now the lysosomes rupture, releasing the lysosomal enzymes into the cell. The sodium-potassium pumping mechanism fails, changing the electrical charge of the cells' internal environment. There is an increase in sodium and water (since water follows sodium) inside the cells, causing cellular edema. The cell membrane then ruptures, allowing lysosomal enzymes and other cellular contents to leak into the interstitial spaces. Cellular death soon follows.

Impaired Use of Glucose The same factors that reduce delivery of oxygen to the cells also reduce delivery of glucose to the cells. In addition, uptake of glucose by the cells may be disrupted by fever, cell damage, or the presence of bacteria, toxins, histamine, or other substances produced or activated by the body's immune and inflammatory responses to disease or injury. Compensatory mechanisms activated by shock may also be responsible for substances that inhibit glucose uptake, including catecholamines and the hormones cortisol and growth hormone.

Glucose that is prevented from entering the cells remains in the blood, resulting in a condition of high serum glucose, or hyperglycemia. Since glucose is the substance from which cells produce energy, the consequences of reduced glucose delivery and uptake are critical.

In the absence of an adequate supply of glucose, certain body cells can create fuel for energy production by converting other substances to glucose. One source is glycogen, the form of glucose that cells store and hold in reserve. Cells convert glycogen to glucose in a process called *glycogenolysis.* However, there is very little stored glycogen in cells other than the liver, kidneys, and muscles. When glycogen reserves are depleted, which typically occurs in 4 to 8 hours, the cells will then derive energy from the breakdown of fats (*lipolysis*) and from the conversion of noncarbohydrate substrates, such as amino acids from proteins, to glucose (*gluconeogenesis*). The energy costs of glycogenolysis and lipolysis are high and contribute to the failure of cells. But the depletion of proteins in gluconeogenesis will ultimately cause organ failure.

For an overview of the pathogenesis of shock, go to www.bradybooks.com and click on the mykit links to access content.

In addition, the anaerobic breakdown of proteins produces ammonia, which is toxic to the cells, and urea, which leads to uric acid, which is also toxic to cells. Finally, when cellular metabolism is impaired, the waste products of metabolism build up in the cells, further impairing cell function and damaging cell membranes.

Cellular death will ultimately lead to tissue death, tissue death to organ failure, and organ failure to death of the individual.

Impaired use of oxygen and glucose soon leads to cellular death. Cellular death will ultimately lead to tissue death; tissue death will lead to organ failure; and organ failure will lead to death of the individual.

Compensation and Decompensation

Usually, the body is able to compensate for any of the changes previously described. However, when the various compensatory mechanisms fail, shock develops and may progress.

Content Review

The Stages of Shock

Compensated
Decompensated (progressive)
Irreversible

Compensation In shock, the fall in cardiac output, detected as a decrease in arterial blood pressure by the baroreceptors, activates several body systems that attempt to reestablish a normal blood pressure—a process known as *compensation.* The sympathetic nervous system stimulates the adrenal gland of the endocrine system to secrete the catecholamines epinephrine and norepinephrine. These chemicals profoundly affect the cardiovascular system, causing an increased heart rate, increased cardiac contractile strength, and arteriolar constriction—all of which serve to elevate the blood pressure.

Another compensatory mechanism, the *renin-angiotensin system,* aids the body in maintaining an adequate blood pressure. When the renin-angiotensin system is activated by a fall in blood pressure, the enzyme *renin* is released from the kidneys into the systemic circulation. Renin acts on a specialized plasma protein called *angiotensin* to produce a substance called *angiotensin I.* Angiotensin I is converted to *angiotensin II* by an enzyme found in the lungs called *angiotensin converting enzyme (ACE).* Angiotensin II is a potent vasoconstrictor. As angiotensin II causes the diameter of the vascular container to decrease, the blood pressure increases. Angiotensin II also stimulates the production of aldosterone, a hormone secreted by the adrenal cortex (outer layer of the adrenal gland) which, in turn, stimulates the kidneys to reabsorb sodium, and, subsequently, water (as noted earlier, "water follows sodium") into peritubular capillaries. The intravascular volume is maintained and elimination of water by the kidneys is reduced.

Another endocrine response by the pituitary gland results in the secretion of antidiuretic hormone (ADH), which also causes the kidneys to reabsorb water, creating an additive effect to that of aldosterone.

The spleen, capable of storing over 300 mL of blood, can expel up to 200 mL of blood into the venous circulation, consequently increasing blood volume, preload, cardiac output, and blood pressure in response to a sudden drop in blood pressure.

Some passive compensatory responses also occur, with beneficial fluid shifts taking place as a result of simple diffusion. With volume loss, the hydrostatic pressure in capillary beds is reduced, and water from the interstitial spaces diffuses into the capillaries.

All of the forementioned mechanisms work to compensate for the shock state, and may be able to restore normal circulatory volume—if excessive bleeding is managed and the shock state has not progressed too far. In this case, the patient is said to be in **compensated shock.**

compensated shock *early stage of shock during which the body's compensatory mechanisms are able to maintain normal perfusion.*

Once normal circulatory function and blood pressure are reestablished, the blood pressure will "feed back" on all of the compensatory mechanisms so that all systems can return to normal. In this way, negative feedback loops work to maintain stability by "signaling" the systems to cease the compensatory responses. In this way, stability and homeostasis are maintained.

Decompensation If the conditions causing shock are too serious, or progress too rapidly, compensatory mechanisms may not be able to restore normal function. In those cases, *decompensation* is said to occur, and the patient is in a state of **decompensated shock,** also called **progressive shock.** During decompensated or progressive shock, medical intervention may still be able to correct the condition.

decompensated shock *advanced stages of shock when the body's compensatory mechanisms are no longer able to maintain normal perfusion; also called* **progressive shock.**

Since all of the "responding" systems have a point at which they can no longer sustain their action (i.e., a limited duration of action), the shock state may progress to a condition where correction, either by the body's own compensatory mechanisms or through medical intervention, is no longer possible. This condition is known as **irreversible shock.**

irreversible shock *shock that has progressed so far that no medical intervention can reverse the condition and death is inevitable.*

A critical factor in the downward spiral of decompensation is cardiac depression. The compensatory mechanisms that increase heart rate and contractile strength create a greatly increased demand for oxygen by the myocardium. When arterial blood pressure has fallen sufficiently, however, coronary blood flow is reduced below the level necessary to adequately perfuse the myocardium. The heart is weakened and cardiac output falls even further.

Depression of the vasomotor center of the brain is another consequence of reduced blood pressure. In early shock, as previously discussed, the sympathetic nervous system is stimulated to cause release of catecholamines that support the function of the circulatory system. But when blood pressure falls to a certain point, in the late stages of shock, reduced blood supply to the vasomotor center results in a slowing, then stoppage, of sympathetic activity.

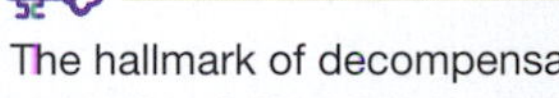

The hallmark of decompensated shock is a fall in blood pressure.

Metabolic wastes, products of anaerobic metabolism, are released into the slower-flowing blood. The blood in the capillary beds becomes acidic, causing formation of minute blood clots ("sludged" blood), which further slows the flow of blood. And a more generalized, systemic acidosis develops, causing further deterioration of cells and tissues, including the capillary walls.

Capillary cells, like other cells, suffer from lack of oxygen and other nutrients, as well as from the ravages of acidosis. This begins to cause permeability of the capillaries and leakage of fluid into the interstitial spaces. This is another self-perpetuating process, as the decreased circulating volume and anaerobic metabolism cause further cell hypoxia and increased permeability.

Cellular deterioration progresses to tissue deterioration, which progresses to organ failure. (See Multiple Organ Dysfunction Syndrome, later in the chapter.) Medical intervention may save the patient if initiated early enough, but when enough damage has been done to cells, tissues, and organs, no known treatment can help the patient to recover. Medical therapies may support function for awhile, but death becomes inevitable.

TYPES OF SHOCK

Content Review

Types of Shock

Cardiogenic
Hypovolemic
Neurogenic
Anaphylactic
Septic
(Alternative classifications of shock: Cardiogenic, Hypovolemic, Obstructive, Distributive)

Shock is usually classified according to the cause. Some newer terminology classifies shock as *cardiogenic* (caused by impaired pumping power of the heart), *hypovolemic* (caused by decreased blood or water volume), *obstructive* (caused by an obstruction that interferes with return of blood to the heart, such as a pulmonary embolism, cardiac tamponade, or tension pneumothorax), and *distributive* (caused by abnormal distribution and return of blood resulting from vasodilation, vasopermeability, or both, as in neurogenic, anaphylactic, or septic shock).

Another, more familiar terminology classifies shock as *cardiogenic, hypovolemic, neurogenic, anaphylactic,* and *septic.* The following discussion of types of shock uses these classifications.

Although all types of shock ultimately have the same effects on the body's cells, tissues, and organs, it is important to try to identify the underlying cause, because correcting the cause is the most important element in reversing the condition and saving the patient's life. Many of the treatments that you, as a paramedic, will provide for the shock patient will be the same, no matter what the cause or type of shock is, but some differ in important ways. For example, providing IV fluid boluses, which may be appropriate to support circulating volume in the hypovolemic patient, would not be indicated for the patient in cardiogenic shock with pulmonary edema.

Try to identify the underlying cause of shock, because correcting the cause is the most important element in reversing the condition and saving the patient's life.

Cardiogenic Shock

An inability of the heart to pump enough blood to supply all body parts is referred to as **cardiogenic shock.** Cardiogenic shock is usually the result of severe left ventricular failure secondary to acute myocardial infarction or congestive heart failure. The reduced blood pressure that accompanies this form of shock aggravates the situation by decreasing coronary artery perfusion. With decreased coronary perfusion, the heart muscle becomes even more damaged, thus establishing a vicious cycle that ultimately results in complete pump failure.

cardiogenic shock *shock caused by insufficient cardiac output; the inability of the heart to pump enough blood to perfuse all parts of the body.*

During cardiogenic shock, as noted earlier, the activation of compensatory mechanisms can actually worsen the situation. When the peripheral resistance increases in an attempt to maintain blood pressure, the myocardial workload increases. This, in turn, increases the myocardial oxygen demand, further aggravating myocardial ischemia and infarction. Cardiac output is further depressed and ejection fraction (the percentage of blood in the ventricle that is ejected with each beat) is decreased.

For an overview of the pathogenesis of cardiogenic shock, go to www.bradybooks.com and click on the mykit links to access content.

While the most common cause of cardiogenic shock is severe left ventricular failure, a number of other factors can have the same result. These include chronic progressive heart disease such as cardiomyopathy, rupture of the papillary heart muscles or interventricular septum, and end-stage valvular disease (mitral stenosis or aortic regurgitation).

Most patients with cardiogenic shock have a normal or increased blood pressure.

Most patients who experience cardiogenic shock will have normal blood volume. However, some patients will be hypovolemic from an excessive use of prescribed diuretics or the severe diaphoresis that accompanies some acute cardiac events. Patients may also experience relative hypovolemia (neurogenic shock) from the vasodilatory (vessel dilation) effects of drugs such as nitroglycerin.

Evaluation and Treatment A major difference between cardiogenic and other types of shock is the presence of pulmonary edema (excess fluid in the lungs), which will probably result in a complaint of difficulty breathing. There may be diminished lung sounds as fluid enters the interstitial spaces of the lungs. As fluid levels rise, wheezes, crackles, or rales may be heard. A productive cough may develop, characterized by white- or pink-tinged foamy sputum. Cyanosis (a dusky blue-gray skin color) is typical, resulting from the decreased diffusion of oxygen across the alveolar/capillary interface, decreasing oxygen delivery to cells that are already hypoxic because of decreased blood pressure and perfusion. Other signs of shock include altered mentation (resulting from reduced perfusion of the brain) and oliguria (diminished urination resulting from compensatory mechanisms that stimulate reabsorption of water by the kidneys to enhance circulating volume).

Provide supportive measures for shock of any origin: Assure an open airway, administer oxygen, assist ventilations, and keep the patient warm.

Treatment of cardiogenic shock includes the supportive measures that should be provided for shock of any origin: Assure an open airway, administer oxygen and assist ventilations if necessary (to support oxygenation of myocardial and other body cells), and keep the patient warm (because impaired cellular metabolism is no longer producing enough energy to keep body temperature normal).

In cardiogenic shock, when pulmonary edema is present, elevate the patient's head and shoulders so that gravity can help isolate fluid and create a clear area where oxygen exchange from the alveoli can take place.

A peripheral intravenous line should be established with normal saline at a TKO rate to provide access for medications, but fluid administration should be kept to a minimum to avoid aggravating the edema. (Some patients with chronic heart failure may be on diuretics and suffering dehydration however, requiring some fluid support.) Since the heart rate may vary from bradycardic (abnormally slow) to tachycardic (abnormally fast), monitoring the heart rate is important. Atropine administration or application of an external pacer may be recommended to manage bradycardia, while extreme tachycardia may be treated by sedation and cardioversion (a type of electric shock) if the patient is awake. Dopamine may be administered to elevate the blood pressure but it will also increase heart rate. Dobutamine may be administered to increase contractile force with little effect on the heart rate. Follow local protocols.

Hypovolemic Shock

hypovolemic shock *shock caused by a loss of intravascular fluid volume.*

Shock due to a loss of intravascular fluid volume is referred to as **hypovolemic shock.** Possible causes of hypovolemic shock include:

- ★ Internal or external hemorrhage (This type of hypovolemic shock is also known as hemorrhagic shock.)
- ★ Traumatic injury
- ★ Long bone or open fractures
- ★ Severe dehydration from vomiting or diarrhea
- ★ Plasma loss from burns
- ★ Excessive sweating
- ★ Diabetic ketoacidosis with resultant **osmotic diuresis**

osmotic diuresis *greatly increased urination and dehydration due to high levels of glucose that cannot be reabsorbed into the blood from the kidney tubules, causing a loss of water into the urine.*

Hypovolemic shock can also be due to internal third-space loss (loss from intracellular or, more commonly, from intravascular spaces into the interstitial spaces). Such a condition can occur with bowel obstruction, peritonitis, pancreatitis, or liver failure resulting in ascites (accumulation of fluid within the abdominal cavity).

For an overview of the pathogenesis of hypovolemic shock, go to www.bradybooks.com and click on the mykit links to access content.

Evaluation and Treatment The signs of hypovolemic shock are considered the "classic" signs of shock. The mental status becomes altered, progressing from anxiety to lethargy or combativeness to unresponsiveness. The skin becomes pale, cool, and clammy (sweaty). The blood pressure may be normal during compensated shock, but then begins to fall. The pulse may be normal in the beginning, then become rapid, finally slowing and disappearing. As the kidneys continue to reabsorb water, urination decreases. Cardiac dysrhythmias may develop in late shock, deteriorating to asystole (absence of heartbeat).

Provide supportive treatment for hypovolemic shock: airway assurance, oxygen, and assisted ventilations, if necessary. Control any severe bleeding. Keep the patient warm. An IV bolus of crystalloid solution (such as normal saline or lactated Ringer's) should be started for fluid replacement. Application of the pneumatic anti-shock garment (PASG) may also be part of your local protocols. While it is accepted practice to administer crystalloid or colloid solutions to replace fluids lost through vomiting, diarrhea, burns, excessive sweating, or osmotic diuresis, the replacement of fluids in trauma patients is quite controversial. It has been demonstrated that the body provides a natural compensation for low-flow states when the systolic pressure is maintained between 70 and 85 mmHg. In a few studies, elevating the systolic blood pressure to greater than 85 mmHg has been associated with worsened outcomes. The worsened outcomes are attributed to the fact that aggressive fluid resuscitation, before the source of bleeding is repaired, causes progressive dilution of the blood, which decreases the oxygen-carrying capacity of the blood. Thus, many surgeons and EMS medical directors are now recommending administering only enough fluid to maintain a systolic blood pressure between 70 and 85 mmHg—a process called "permissive hypotension."

Prehospital care for hypovolemic shock should be guided by local protocols. As a rule, patients suffering from shock from trauma should receive airway management, supplemental oxygenation, assisted ventilations (if necessary), hemorrhage control, and rapid transport. IV access should be obtained immediately or en route. Either lactated Ringer's or normal saline should be administered in small boluses to maintain the systolic blood pressure between 70 and 85 mmHg (enough to restore a radial pulse). Patients with systolic pressures less than 40 mmHg should still receive aggressive fluid resuscitation.

Neurogenic Shock

Neurogenic shock results from injury to either the brain or the spinal cord, resulting in an interruption of nerve impulses to the arteries. The arteries lose tone and dilate, causing a relative hypovolemia. There has been no loss of fluid, but the container has been enlarged. With this inappropriate vasodilation, a disproportionate amount of blood collects in the capillary bed. This reduces venous return, cardiac output, and arterial blood pressure. Sympathetic nerve impulses to the adrenal glands are lost, which prevents the release of catecholamines and their compensatory effects. With injury high in the cervical spine, there may be interruption of impulses to the peripheral nervous system, causing paralysis and loss of sensation. The respiratory and cardiac centers of the brain may also be affected.

neurogenic shock *shock resulting from brain or spinal cord injury that causes an interruption of nerve impulses to the arteries with loss of arterial tone, dilation, and relative hypovolemia.*

The usual cause of neurogenic shock is central nervous system injury. Neurogenic shock is most commonly due to an injury that has resulted in severe spinal cord injury or total transection of the cord (which may be called *spinal shock*) or injury or deprivation of oxygen or glucose to the medulla of the brain.

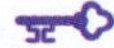

For an overview of the pathogenesis of neurogenic shock, go to www.bradybooks.com and click on the mykit links to access content.

Evaluation and Treatment The vasodilation in neurogenic shock causes warm, red skin, and sweat gland malfunction causes dry skin—in contrast to the cool, pale, sweaty skin associated with hypovolemic shock. Because of the lack of compensatory stimulation from catecholamine release, the patient will have a low blood pressure and a slow pulse even in the early stages—again, in contrast to hypovolemic shock.

Treatment for neurogenic shock or spinal shock is similar to treatment for other types of shock and includes support of the airway, oxygenation, ventilation, maintenance of body temperature, and intravenous access. Spinal shock is characterized by hypotension, reflex bradycardia, and warm, dry skin. Because these symptoms signal a likelihood of spinal injury, cervical spine stabilization must be established on first patient contact, and the patient must be immobilized to a backboard as quickly as possible. A thorough search for other causes of shock (e.g., internal hemorrhage) must be made before concluding that a patient's hypotension is due to spinal shock alone. Treatment of spinal shock should include intravenous fluids (especially if there has been blood or fluid loss) and medications that increase the blood pressure by increasing peripheral vascular resistance. These include norepinephrine (Levophed) and dopamine (Intropin).

Anaphylactic Shock

When a foreign substance enters the body, the immune system responds to rid the body of the invader. (See the discussion of immunity later in this chapter.) This usually happens with no noticeable effects, and the person is not even aware that an immune response is taking place. Some foreign substances (antigens) provoke an exaggerated immune response (allergic response) that will cause noticeable symptoms such as a rash (as from contact with poison ivy) or swollen, irritated airway passages (as with hay fever). In rare cases, an allergic response is very severe and life threatening. This kind of severe allergic response is called **anaphylaxis, or anaphylactic shock.**

anaphylaxis *a life-threatening allergic reaction; also called* **anaphylactic shock.**

An anaphylactic reaction usually occurs very rapidly. Signs and symptoms most often appear within a minute or less, but occasionally may appear an hour or more after exposure. Generally, the faster the reaction develops, the more severe it is likely to be. Death can occur before the patient can get to a hospital, so prompt intervention is critical. This is a situation when the paramedic at the scene can make the difference between life and death.

For an overview of the pathogenesis of anaphylactic shock, go to www.bradybooks.com and click on the mykit links to access content.

Anaphylactic reactions can be triggered by a variety of substances, including foods (especially nuts, eggs, shellfish), venoms, aspirin or nonsteroidal anti-inflammatory drugs (NSAIDS), hormones (animal-derived insulin), preservatives, and others. The most rapid and severe reactions are usually caused by substances injected directly into the bloodstream, which is one reason that penicillin injections and hymenoptera stings (e.g., from bees, wasps, hornets) are the most common causes of fatal anaphylactic reactions.

Evaluation and Treatment

Because the immune responses involved in anaphylaxis can affect different body systems, the signs and symptoms can vary widely. For example:

- ★ Skin
  - Flushing
  - Itching
  - Hives
  - Swelling
  - Cyanosis
- ★ Respiratory system
  - Breathing difficulty
  - Sneezing, coughing
  - Wheezing, stridor
  - Laryngeal edema
  - Laryngospasm
- ★ Cardiovascular system
  - Vasodilation
  - Increased heart rate
  - Decreased blood pressure
- ★ Gastrointestinal system
  - Nausea, vomiting
  - Abdominal cramping
  - Diarrhea

★ Nervous system
  - Altered mental status
  - Dizziness
  - Headache
  - Seizures
  - Tearing

The patient may present with an altered mental status that can progress to unresponsiveness, so gather a brief history as soon as possible, including previous allergic reactions and any information about what the patient may have ingested or been exposed to that could have caused the present reaction. Be sure the patient is no longer in contact with the allergen; if a stinger is in the skin, scrape it away with a fingernail or scalpel blade.

Since laryngeal edema is often a problem, protecting the patient's airway will be your first concern. Administer oxygen by nonrebreather mask or, as necessary, by endotracheal intubation. The anaphylactic response causes depletion of circulatory volume by promoting capillary permeability and leaking of fluid into interstitial spaces, so establish an IV of crystalloid solution (normal saline or lactated Ringer's) for volume support.

The primary treatment for anaphylaxis is pharmacological. In addition to oxygen, epinephrine is usually administered (if the patient has a history of anaphylaxis, he may be carrying a prescribed spring-loaded epinephrine injector), as are antihistamines (diphenhydramine), corticosteroids (methylprednisolone, hydrocortisone, dexamethasone), and vasopressors (dopamine, norepinephrine, epinephrine). Occasionally an inhaled beta agonist (albuterol) may be required. Follow local protocols.

Septic Shock

Septic shock begins with *septicemia* (also called *sepsis*), an infection that enters the bloodstream and is carried throughout the body. The person may have septicemia for some time before septic shock develops, but eventually toxins released by the invading organism overcome the compensatory mechanisms. Unless it is corrected, septic shock will cause the dysfunction of more than one organ system, resulting in multiple organ dysfunction syndrome (discussed in the next section).

septic shock *shock that develops as the result of infection carried by the bloodstream, eventually causing dysfunction of multiple organ systems.*

Evaluation and Treatment The signs and symptoms of septic shock are progressive. In the beginning, cardiac output is increased, but toxins causing vasodilation may prevent an increase in blood pressure. The person may seem to be sick, but not alarmingly so. By the last stages, toxins have increased permeability of the blood vessels to the point where great amounts of fluid are lost from the vasculature and blood pressure falls drastically.

For an overview of the pathogenesis of septic shock, go to www.bradybooks.com and click on the mykit links to access content.

Signs and symptoms can vary widely as the patient progresses from early to late stages of septic shock. Some patients may have a high fever, but others, especially the elderly or the very young, may have no fever or may even be hypothermic. The skin can be flushed, if fever is present, or very pale and cyanotic in the late stages.

The most susceptible organ system is the lungs and respiratory system, so the patient may present with breathing difficulty and altered lung sounds. The brain may be infected, resulting in altered mental status. Suspicion of septic shock is usually based on a history of recent infection or illness.

Treatment includes administration of high-flow, high-concentration oxygen by nonrebreather mask or endotracheal intubation, as necessary. An IV of crystalloid solution (normal saline or lactated Ringer's) should be established, and dopamine may be administered to support the blood pressure. The heart rhythm must be monitored and medications administered to correct any dysrhythmias. Follow local protocols. In the hospital, antibiotic therapy will be initiated.

MULTIPLE ORGAN DYSFUNCTION SYNDROME

In the 1970s, a syndrome of multiple organ failure began to be noticed in hospital intensive care units. Through medical advances, patients survived serious illness and trauma—only to die later of complications of the original disease or injury. The syndrome was described in 1975 as *multisystem organ failure.* In 1991, the American College of Chest Physicians and the Society of Critical Care Medicine named it **multiple organ dysfunction syndrome** (MODS).

multiple organ dysfunction syndrome (MODS) *progressive impairment of two or more organ systems resulting from an uncontrolled inflammatory response to a severe illness or injury.*

MODS is the progressive impairment of two or more organ systems resulting from an uncontrolled inflammatory response to a severe illness or injury. Sepsis and septic shock are the most common causes of MODS, with MODS being the end stage. (The progression from infection to sepsis to septic shock to MODS is known as systemic inflammatory response syndrome, or SIRS.)

Actually, MODS can result from any severe disease or injury that triggers a massive systemic inflammatory response—including trauma, burns, surgery, circulatory shock, acute pancreatitis, acute renal failure, and others. Risk factors include age (>65), malnutrition, and preexisting chronic disease such as cancer or diabetes. With a mortality rate of 60 to 90 percent, MODS is the major cause of death following sepsis, trauma, and burn injuries.

Content Review

Progression to MODS

Infection
↓
Sepsis
↓
Septic shock
↓
MODS
↓
Death (if not corrected early)

Pathophysiology of MODS

MODS occurs in two stages. In primary MODS, organ damage results directly from a specific cause such as ischemia or inadequate perfusion resulting from an episode of shock, trauma, or major surgery. There are stress and inflammatory responses (discussed in detail later in this chapter) to this initial injury, but they may be mild and not readily detectable. However, during this response, neutrophils and macrophages (cells that attack and destroy bacteria, protozoa, foreign cells, and cell debris) as well as mast cells (cells that produce histamine and other components of allergic response) are thought to be "primed" by cytokines (proteins released during an inflammatory or immune response).

The next time there is an insult, such as an additional injury or ischemia or infection—even though the insult may be mild—the primed cells are activated, producing an exaggerated inflammatory response, known as secondary MODS.

Now the inflammatory response enters a self-perpetuating cycle. As inflammatory mediators are released by the injured organ, they enter the circulation, activating inflammatory responses in organ systems throughout the body. These mediators, especially cytokines such as tumor necrosis factor (TNF) and interleukin 1 (IL-1), damage the endothelium (cells that line the blood vessels, the heart, and various body cavities). Gram-negative bacteria, if present, release endotoxins that also damage endothelial cells. The injured endothelial cells release factors that aggravate the inflammation and cause vasodilation. The injured epithelium becomes permeable, allowing leakage of fluid into interstitial spaces, and loses much of its anticoagulation function, which allows formation of tiny blood clots (thrombi) in the microvasculature.

The secondary insult also triggers an exaggerated neuroendocrine response. Catecholamine release causes many of the manifestations of MODS, including tachycardia, increased metabolic rates, and increased oxygen consumption. Release of a variety of hormones contributes to the hypermetabolism and release of endorphins contributes to vasodilation. Additionally, plasma protein systems are activated: specifically, the complement system, the coagulation system, and the kallikrein-kinin system. Plasma proteins are key mediators of the inflammatory response. When activated, each of these systems triggers a cascade of responses with the overall result of increased vasodilation, vasopermeability, cardiovascular instability, endothelial damage, and clotting abnormalities.

As a result of the release of the inflammatory mediators and toxins and the plasma protein cascades, a massive immune/inflammatory and coagulation response develops. Vascular changes (vasodilation, increased capillary permeability, selective vasoconstriction, and microvascular thrombi) continue and worsen. Two metabolites that are released have opposing vascular effects: Prostacyclin, also called prostaglandin I_2 (PGI_2) is a vasodilator, while thromboxane A_2 (TXA_2) is a vasoconstrictor. They are released in differing amounts within different organ tissues, contributing to a maldistribution of blood flow to organs and organ systems.

As noted earlier, the release of catecholamines stimulates hypermetabolism within the body cells, which in turn creates a greatly increased oxygen demand. Because of lung damage, hypoxemia, and hypoperfusion, a severe oxygen supply/demand imbalance develops. As the cells switch from aerobic to anaerobic metabolism, fuel supplies within the cells (ATP and glucose) are used up faster than they can be replenished. Without adequate ATP, the cells lose their ability to operate the sodium-potassium pump, which is essential to cardiac function. The myocardium is profoundly weakened. Cellular lysosomes begin to break down, releasing lysosomal enzymes which damage the cell membrane and the surrounding cells. Large amounts of lactic acid are released, contributing to acidosis, which further damages the cells. The overall response is similar to that seen in septic and anaphylactic shock, except on a larger scale.

Clinical Presentation of MODS

The cumulative effects of MODS at the cellular and tissue levels begin to cause the breakdown of organ systems: The organs that fail first are not necessarily the organs where the initial insult occurred, and there is a lag time between the initial insult and the onset of organ failure. Dysfunction may develop in the pulmonary, gastrointestinal, hepatic, renal, cardiovascular, hematologic, and immune systems. There is decreased cardiac function and myocardial depression, caused by the factors discussed earlier, possibly abetted by release of myocardial depressant factor (MDF) and a decrease in beta-adrenergic receptors in the heart. The smooth muscle of the vascular system fails with consequent release of capillary sphincters and increased vasodilation.

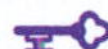

MODS will usually develop over a period of 2, 3, or more weeks.

Survival from MODS is dependent on early recognition and supportive care.

MODS does not occur in one intense crisis. It will usually develop over a period of 2, 3, or more weeks. There is no specific therapy for MODS, and the only chance of rescuing the patient from its self-perpetuating spiral toward death is early recognition and initiation of supportive measures. For this reason, it is important to understand how MODS usually presents in the first 24 hours after initial resuscitation.

Although MODS will usually be detected in the hospital rather than the prehospital setting, there may be occasions when a patient who has not been hospitalized or has returned home from the hospital is the subject of a call to EMS, or when a patient being transported by EMS from one facility to another is suffering from MODS.

The most common presentation of MODS over time is as follows:

24 Hours after Resuscitation

- ★ Low-grade fever
- ★ Tachycardia (rapid heart rate)
- ★ Dyspnea (breathing difficulty)
- ★ Altered mental status
- ★ General hypermetabolic, hyperdynamic state

Within 24 to 72 Hours

- ★ Pulmonary (lung) failure begins

Within 7 to 10 Days

- ★ Hepatic (liver) failure begins
- ★ Intestinal failure begins
- ★ Renal (kidney) failure begins

Within 14 to 21 Days

- ★ Renal and hepatic failure intensify
- ★ Gastrointestinal collapse
- ★ Immune system collapse

After 21 Days

- ★ Hematologic (blood system) failure begins
- ★ Myocardial (heart muscle) failure begins
- ★ Altered mental status resulting from encephalopathy (brain infection)
- ★ Death

Part 2: The Body's Defenses against Disease and Injury

As discussed so far in this chapter, the human body is vulnerable to attack by a variety of diseases and foreign invaders as well as to injury. The major focus of Part 2 will be the body's chief defenses against disease, invaders, and injury—the immune response and the inflammatory response—and the interactions between the immune and inflammatory responses.

In Part 2, we will also examine hypersensitivity, or allergic and anaphylactic responses; that is, what happens when the immune system overresponds to invasive agents to the extent that the body is actually harming itself. Immune deficiencies will also be discussed, including acquired immunodeficiency syndrome, or AIDS.

Finally, we will discuss the interrelationships between stress and disease, including the body's use of the neuroendocrine and immune systems to regulate the stress response. Psychological responses to stress, including various coping mechanisms, are also described.

SELF-DEFENSE MECHANISMS

In Chapter 3, normal body anatomy and physiology were discussed (the normal cell and its environment: fluids and electrolytes, the acid–base balance). In Part 1 of this chapter we discussed how the body may be attacked or injured (cellular injury, infection, genetic and other causes of disease, hypoperfusion, and multiple organ dysfunction syndrome). In the next sections, we will discuss how the body defends itself from infection and injury.

It is important to keep in mind that the body has powerful ways of defending and healing itself (restoring homeostasis) and that medical intervention is needed only when, on occasion, these natural defense mechanisms are unequal to the task and become overwhelmed.

INFECTIOUS AGENTS

Bacteria

bacteria *(singular bacterium) single-cell organisms with a cell membrane and cytoplasm but no organized nucleus. They bind to the cells of a host organism to obtain food and support.*

Content Review

Infectious Agents

- Bacteria
- Viruses
- Fungi
- Parasites
- Prions

antibiotics *substances that destroy or inhibit microorganisms, tiny living bodies invisible to the naked eye. (*Antibiotic *means "destructive to life.")*

Bacteria are single-cell organisms that consist of internal cytoplasm surrounded by a rigid cell wall. Bacteria are prokaryotic cells which, unlike the eukaryotic cells of the human body, lack an organized nucleus and other intracellular organelles. Bacteria can reproduce independently, but they need a host to supply food and other support. Inside the body, they achieve this by binding to host cells.

Bacteria can be cultured and identified readily in most hospital laboratories. Many bacteria are categorized according to their appearance under the microscope after staining with several dyes referred to as *Gram stains.* Some bacteria stain blue, while others stain red. Bacteria that stain blue are referred to as *gram-positive* bacteria. They are somewhat similar to each other in their structure. Bacteria that stain red are referred to as *gram-negative* bacteria. They are also somewhat similar to each other in their structure.

Bacteria can cause many of the common infections in medicine, including middle ear infections in children, many cases of tonsillitis, and meningitis. (These kinds of infections can also be caused by viruses, which are discussed in the next section.) Most bacterial infections respond to treatment with drugs called **antibiotics.** Once administered, antibiotics kill or inhibit the growth of invading bacteria. As mentioned earlier, the bacterial cell membrane is the site of action for many antibiotics. Once the cell membrane is broken down, phagocytes (cells that ingest and destroy pathogens and other foreign and abnormal substances) can begin to destroy the bacterium. A variety of antibiotic drugs have been developed with mechanisms of action tailored to different types of bacteria. However, the broad variety of infectious bacteria, and their ability to develop resistance to drugs, makes developing antibiotics to battle them a difficult job.

Some bacteria protect themselves by forming a capsule outside the cell wall that protects the organism from digestion by phagocytes. Some bacteria, such as *Mycoplasmic* bacteria, have no protective capsule but rely on other mechanisms to survive and attack the body. *Mycobacterium tuberculosis,* which has no protective capsule, can actually survive and be transported by phagocytes.

Other bacteria simply multiply faster than the body's defense systems can respond. Still others overpower the body's defenses by producing enzymes and toxins that attack and injure cells and produce hypersensitivity reactions.

Simple infection is not the only consequence of a bacterial invasion. Many bacteria release poisonous chemicals, or *toxins.* There are two types of toxins produced by bacteria: exotoxins and endotoxins. **Exotoxins** are proteins secreted and released by the bacterial cell during its growth. They travel throughout the body via the blood or lymph, ultimately causing problems. For example, botulism toxin, released by the bacterium *Clostridium botulinum,* blocks the release of cholinergic neurotransmitters at neuromuscular junctions and elsewhere in the autonomic nervous system, causing systemic paralysis. Another example is tetanus, which is caused by the bacterium *Clostridium tetani.* The actual infection by the bacteria themselves is mild and may be limited, for example, to the site of a puncture wound in the foot. Yet, on entering the body, the bacteria release their toxin, *tetanospasmin.* This toxin then travels through the blood to the skeletal muscles, causing the spastic rigidity classically seen in tetanus.

exotoxins *toxic (poisonous) substances secreted by bacterial cells during their growth.*

Endotoxins are complex molecules that are contained in the cell walls of certain Gram-negative bacteria. Endotoxins can be released during the destruction of the bacterial cell by phagocytes or even when the bacterial cell is attacked by an antibiotic, so that antibiotics cannot control the endotoxic effects of bacteria. When released, endotoxins trigger the inflammatory process and produce fever. In the bloodstream, they can cause widespread clotting within the blood vessels, capillary damage, and hypotension, as well as respiratory distress and fever—a condition known as endotoxin shock. Endotoxins can survive even when the cell that produced them is dead.

endotoxins *molecules in the walls of certain gram-negative bacteria that are released when the bacterium dies or is destroyed, causing toxic (poisonous) effects on the host body.*

Depending on their amount and site of release, the effects of toxins can be local or systemic. When a bacterial organism enters the circulatory system, its released toxins can spread throughout the body. The systemic spread of toxins through the bloodstream is known as **septicemia,** or *sepsis,* and is a grave medical illness.

septicemia *the systemic spread of toxins through the bloodstream. Also called sepsis.*

The body counters the bacterial invasion and release of enzymes and toxins through activation of the immune system. The immune system will mobilize foreign-cell-destroying macrophages (a type of white blood cell) to the site of infection in an attempt to rid the body of the foreign pathogen. As the macrophages attempt to destroy the bacteria, they release substances known as pyrogens. Pyrogens are responsible for causing the increase in temperature known as fever. Pyrogens act on the thermoregulation center in the hypothalamus to cause the increased body temperature, which is thought to aid in the destruction of pathogens.

Viruses

Most infections are caused by **viruses.** Viruses are much smaller than bacteria and can only be seen with an electron microscope. In addition, they cannot grow without the assistance of another organism. In fact, viruses are referred to as *intracellular parasites,* since they must invade the cells of the organism they infect.

virus *an organism much smaller than a bacterium, visible only under an electron microscope. Viruses invade and live inside the cells of the organisms they infect.*

A virus has no organized cellular structure except a protein coat (capsid) surrounding the internal genetic material, deoxyribonucleic acid (DNA), or ribonucleic acid (RNA). With no organized cellular structure or cellular organelles, viruses are incapable of metabolism. Once inside a cell, they take over, using the various cellular enzymes to replicate and produce more viruses, which decreases synthesis of macromolecules vital to the host cell.

Some viruses develop a coating in addition to the capsid, called an envelope. The envelope and the protein capsid allow the virus to resist destruction by the phagocytes of the immune system. However, since viruses cannot reproduce outside a host cell, if the virus does not find a host cell, it will die.

The symptoms of a virus may not be readily apparent because it is hidden within the host cell. After replication is complete, the virus will sometimes destroy the host cell. In other cases, a virus will remain dormant within a cell for months or years. An example is the *varicella zoster virus,* which causes childhood chickenpox and may then remain dormant, only to cause shingles in the adult decades later. Some viruses form a long-term symbiotic (living in close association) relationship with the host cell, resulting in a persistent but unapparent infection.

Viruses do not produce toxins, but they can still cause very serious illnesses. Some viruses are capable of altering the host cell to induce a malignancy (cancer). Others, such as the *human immunodeficiency virus (HIV)*, which causes AIDS, can proliferate, attacking cells of the immune system and destroying its ability to ward off infections of all types.

Unlike bacteria, viruses are very difficult to treat. Once a virus infects a cell, it can only be killed by destroying the infected cell. Drugs have not yet been developed that can selectively destroy cells infected by viruses while leaving uninfected cells unharmed. This partially explains the dilemma facing researchers trying to find a cure for AIDS. An additional problem is that some viruses mutate (change) frequently, which is why a new flu vaccine must be developed for every flu season. Fortunately, most viral illnesses are mild and fairly self-limiting. (Because viral agents must spread from cell to cell, the immune system is eventually able to "catch" them outside a host cell and destroy them.) Even so, at present, viruses usually cannot be treated with more than symptomatic care.

Other Agents of Infection

Other biological agents that cause human infection include *fungi* (the plural of *fungus*) and parasites.

Fungi, which includes yeasts and molds, are more like plants than animals. Fungi rarely cause human disease other than minor skin infections such as athlete's foot and some common vaginal infections. Fungus infections are called *mycoses*. Patients with an impaired immune system, such as HIV patients or patients with organ transplants, suffer fungal infection more commonly than healthy people. In such patients, the fungi can invade the lungs, blood, and several organs. Treatment of complicated, deep fungal infections has proven difficult, even in the hospital setting.

Parasites range in size from protozoa (single-cell animals not much larger than bacteria) to large intestinal worms. Parasites tend to be more common in developing nations than in the United States. Treatment depends upon the organism and the location.

Prions are the most recently recognized classification of infectious agents. Initially thought to be slow acting viruses, prions differ from viruses in that they are smaller, are made entirely of proteins, and do not have protective capsids.

For more about infectious diseases, see Chapter 37.

Review Content

Three Lines of Defense

Anatomic barriers
Inflammatory response
Immune response

THREE LINES OF DEFENSE

There are three chief lines of self-defense against infection and injury. One involves anatomical barriers. The other two—the inflammatory response and the immune response—rely on actions of the leukocytes (white blood cells). Each line of defense can be characterized as external or internal, nonspecific or specific (Table 4–2)—characterizations you may want to keep in mind as you read the following sections and compare the ways these defenses protect the body.

Before an infectious agent can attack the body, it has to get past the body's natural anatomical barrier, the epithelium (the skin and the mucous membranes that line the respiratory, gastrointestinal, and genitourinary tracts). The epithelium is more than just a physical barrier; it also provides a chemical defense against infection. The sebaceous glands of the skin secrete fatty and lactic acids, which attack bacteria and fungi. Sweat, tears, and saliva secreted by other glands contain bacteria-attacking enzymes. Various mechanical responses also work to get rid of invading substances. For example, the invader may be coughed or sneezed out of the respiratory tract, flushed out of the urinary tract, or eliminated from the gastrointestinal tract by vomiting or diarrhea.

Table 4–2 Three Lines of Defense against Infection and Injury

	External	Internal	Nonspecific	Specific
Anatomical Barriers	External		Nonspecific	
Inflammatory Response		Internal	Nonspecific	
Immune Response		Internal		Specific

Table 4–3 Characteristics of the Inflammatory and Immune Responses

	Inflammatory Response	Immune Response
Speed	Fast	Slow
Specificity	Nonspecific	Specific
Duration (Memory)	Transient (no memory)	Long-term (memory)
Involving Which Plasma Systems	Multiple plasma protein systems (complement, coagulation, kinin systems)	One plasma protein system (immunoglobulin)
Involving Which Cell Type	Multiple cell types (granulocytes, monocytes, macrophages)	One blood cell type (lymphocytes)

The anatomical defenses are *external* and *nonspecific.* They are considered external because they prevent substances from penetrating the skin or the coverings of internal passageways. They are nonspecific because they defend against all invaders, such as foreign bodies, chemicals, or microorganisms, without targeting any specific type of invader.

If an invading foreign body, chemical, or microorganism penetrates the anatomical barriers and begins to attack internal cells and tissues, two other lines of defense are triggered: the inflammatory response and the immune response. These twin responses of the immune system have contrasting characteristics of speed, specificity, duration (memory), and of the plasma systems and cell types that are involved in the response (Table 4–3).

The *inflammatory response,* or *inflammation,* begins within seconds of injury or invasion by a pathogen. As noted earlier, it is nonspecific, attacking any invader by surrounding it with cells and fluids to isolate, destroy, and eliminate it. Inflammation is mediated by multiple plasma protein systems, especially the complement system, the coagulation system, and the kinin system (which will be explained later) and involves a variety of cell types as it attacks the invader.

The *immune response* develops more slowly (one type of response requires a second exposure after priming by the first exposure to the invader). The immune response is specific, in that it will develop a specialized response for each different invader. It is mediated by just one plasma protein system (immunoglobulin) and attacks the invader mainly with a single cell type (lymphocytes, which are one type of leukocyte, or white blood cell).

Inflammation and the immune response interact in many ways. We will discuss the immune response first, because understanding the immune response is necessary for understanding some parts of the inflammatory response.

THE IMMUNE RESPONSE

HOW THE IMMUNE RESPONSE WORKS: AN OVERVIEW

Most viruses, bacteria, fungi, and parasites—as well as noninfectious substances such as pollens, foods, venoms, drugs, and others that may enter the body—have proteins on their surface called **antigens.** The immune system detects these antigens as being foreign, or "non-self," and responds to produce substances called **antibodies** that combine with antigens to control or destroy them. This is known as the **immune response.** As part of this process, *memory cells* "remember" the antigen and will trigger an even faster and more effective response to destroy the same antigen if it enters the body again. Such long-term protection against specific foreign substances is known as **immunity.**

antigen *a marker on the surface of a cell that identifies it as "self" or "non-self."*

antibody *a substance produced by B lymphocytes in response to the presence of a foreign antigen that will combine with and control or destroy the antigen, thus preventing infection.*

immune response *the body's reactions that inactivate or eliminate foreign antigens.*

immunity *a long-term condition of protection from infection or disease.*

CHARACTERISTICS OF THE IMMUNE RESPONSE AND IMMUNITY

The immune response and immunity can be classified as natural versus acquired immunity or humoral versus cell-mediated immunity.

Natural versus Acquired Immunity

natural immunity *inborn protection against infection or disease.*

acquired immunity *protection from infection or disease that is (1) developed by the body after exposure to an antigen or (2) transferred to the person from an outside source.*

Natural immunity is not generated by the immune response. It is inborn, part of the genetic makeup of the individual or the species. For example, dogs are naturally immune to measles and humans are naturally immune to canine distemper. (Some diseases such as leukemia, however, can affect more than one species.)

Acquired immunity develops as an outcome of the immune response. Acquired immunity can be either active or passive. *Active acquired immunity* is generated by the immune system after exposure to an antigen. *Passive acquired immunity* is transferred to a person from an outside source. For example, a mother may transfer antibodies to the fetus. Or antibodies may be administered as an immune serum against an invader such as rabies, tetanus, or snake venom. Active acquired immunity is long-lasting. Passive acquired immunity is temporary.

Humoral versus Cell-Mediated Immunity

lymphocyte *a type of leukocyte, or white blood cell, that attacks foreign substances as part of the body's immune response.*

B lymphocytes *white blood cells that, in response to the presence of an antigen, produce antibodies that attack the antigen, develop a memory for the antigen, and confer long-term immunity to the antigen.*

humoral immunity *the long-term immunity to an antigen provided by antibodies produced by B lymphocytes.*

T lymphocytes *white blood cells that do not produce antibodies but, instead, attack antigens directly.*

cell-mediated immunity *the short-term immunity to an antigen provided by T lymphocytes, which directly attack the antigen but do not produce antibodies or memory for the antigen.*

A special type of leukocyte (white blood cell) is the **lymphocyte.** Lymphocytes (20 to 35 percent of all leukocytes) are responsible for several critical immune functions, including recognizing foreign antigens, producing antibodies, and developing memory.

As lymphocytes mature, they become one of several types, including B lymphocytes and T lymphocytes. **B lymphocytes** do not attack antigens directly. Instead, they produce the antibodies (immunoglobulins) that attack antigens. B lymphocytes also develop memory, and confer long-term immunity to specific antigens. This type of immunity is called **humoral immunity.** (*Humor* refers to the blood and other fluids of the body; *humoral immunity* refers to the long-lasting antibodies and memory cells present in the blood and lymph.)

T lymphocytes do not produce antibodies. Instead, they recognize the presence of a foreign antigen and attack it directly. This type of immunity is called **cell-mediated immunity.**

INDUCTION OF THE IMMUNE RESPONSE

The immune response must be triggered, or induced. The following sections discuss the role of antigens, immunogens, and blood groups.

Antigens and Immunogens

immunogens *antigens that are able to trigger an immune response.*

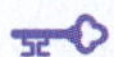

All immunogens are antigens, but not all antigens are immunogens. In other words, only some antigens are capable of triggering an immune response.

Antigens that can trigger the immune response are called **immunogens.** Not every antigen is an immunogen. That is, not every antigen is capable of triggering the immune response. For example, the immune response is not triggered by antigens present on various helpful bacteria in our bodies.

What makes a molecule an antigen is a chemical structure that is capable of reacting with immune system components, such as antibodies and T lymphocytes. However, having this chemical structure, the ability to *react* once the immune system has been triggered, is not enough to *trigger* the immune system in the first place. In order to be immunogenic—able to trigger an immune response—an antigen must have additional characteristics.

Characteristics of Antigenic Immunogenicity

- ★ Sufficient foreignness
- ★ Sufficient size
- ★ Sufficient complexity
- ★ Presence in sufficient amounts

Normally, the immune system is not triggered by self-antigens. In fact, the immune system does not just "tolerate" self-antigens, but it actively protects them through suppression of the immune system.

Blood Group Antigens

HLA antigens do not exist on the surface of erythrocytes (red blood cells), but other antigens, known as the blood group antigens, do. There are more than 80 of these red cell antigens that have been grouped into a number of different blood group systems. The two groups that trigger the strongest immune response are the Rh system and the ABO system.

The Rh System The **Rh blood group** is named for the rhesus monkey in which it was first identified. One of several antigens in this group is known as Rh antigen D, or the **Rh factor.** Rh factor is present in about 85 percent of North Americans (Rh positive), but absent in about 15 percent (Rh negative).

Incompatibility between Rh positive and Rh negative blood can cause harmful immune responses. For example, if a patient with Rh negative blood receives a transplant of Rh positive blood, a primary immune response is triggered. A second transfusion of Rh positive blood may cause a severe transfusion reaction.

Hemolytic disease of the newborn may result from Rh incompatibility between mother and fetus. Problems will usually not occur in a first pregnancy where the mother is Rh negative and the fetus is Rh positive, because few fetal erythrocytes cross the placental barrier to the mother. However, a significant number of fetal erythrocytes do enter the mother's bloodstream at birth when the placenta separates from the uterus. These may (depending on several factors) activate a primary immune response and development of Rh antibodies. If the fetus in her next pregnancy is also Rh positive, the mother's Rh antibodies can cross the placenta and destroy the red blood cells of the fetus. This is actually a rare occurrence. Rh incompatibility occurs in only about 10 percent of pregnancies. Since not all such incompatibilities produce Rh antibodies in the mother, only about 5 percent of women ever have babies with hemolytic disease, even after numerous pregnancies.

Rh blood group *a group of antigens discovered on the red blood cells of rhesus monkeys that is also present to some extent in humans.*

Rh factor *an antigen in the Rh blood group that is also known as antigen D. About 85 percent of North Americans have the Rh factor (are Rh positive) while about 15 percent do not have the Rh factor (are Rh negative). Rh positive and Rh negative blood are incompatible; that is, a person who is Rh negative can experience a severe immune response if Rh positive blood is introduced, as through a transfusion or during childbirth.*

The ABO System The **ABO blood groups** are formed because there are two types of antigens that may be present on the surface of red blood cells. These antigens are named A and B. Persons with blood type A carry only A antigens on their red blood cells. Those with blood type B carry only B antigens. Those with blood type AB carry both, and those with blood type O carry neither.

An immune response will be activated in a person with type A blood who receives a transfusion of type B blood, which is recognized as non-self. The same will happen when a person with type B blood receives type A blood. People with type O blood are known as *universal donors,* because type O blood has no antigens that will trigger an immune response in any other group. Those with type AB blood are known as *universal recipients,* because they have both types of antigens and will not produce antibodies in response to any other blood groups.

Mother-fetus ABO incompatibility is more common than Rh incompatibility, occurring in about 20 to 25 percent of pregnancies, but only 10 percent of ABO incompatibilities will result in hemolytic disease of the infant.

ABO blood groups *four blood groups formed by the presence or absence of two antigens known as A and B. A person may have either (type A or type B), both (type AB), or neither (type O). An immune response will be activated whenever a person receives blood containing A or B antigen if this antigen is not already present in his own blood.*

INFLAMMATION

INFLAMMATION CONTRASTED TO THE IMMUNE RESPONSE

Inflammation, also called the *inflammatory response,* is the body's response to cellular injury. It differs from the immune response in many ways. (Review Tables 4–2 and 4–3.) As you read the following sections, keep in mind that:

- ★ The immune response develops *slowly;* inflammation develops *swiftly.*
- ★ The immune response is *specific* (targets specific antigens); inflammation is *nonspecific* (it attacks all unwanted substances in the same way). In fact, inflammation is sometimes called "the nonspecific immune response."
- ★ The immune response is *long-lasting* (memory cells will remember an antigen and trigger a swift response on reexposure, even years later); inflammation is *temporary,* lasting only until the immediate threat is conquered—usually only a few days to 2 weeks.
- ★ The immune response involves *one type of white blood cell* (lymphocytes); inflammation involves *platelets and many types of white cells* (the granulatory cells called neutrophils, basophils, and eosinophils; the monocytes that mature into macrophages).
- ★ The immune response involves *one type of plasma protein* (immunoglobulins, also called antibodies); inflammation involves *several plasma protein systems* (complement, coagulation, and kinin).

inflammation *the body's response to cellular injury; also called the inflammatory response. In contrast to the immune response, inflammation develops swiftly, is nonspecific (attacks all unwanted substances in the same way), and is temporary, leading to healing.*

However, the immune response and inflammation are interdependent. For example, macrophages that are developed during the inflammatory response must ingest antigens before helper T cells can recognize them and trigger the immune response. Conversely, IgE antibody produced by B cells during an immune response can stimulate mast cells to activate inflammation.

Although inflammation differs from the immune response in many ways, inflammation and the immune response are both considered to be part of the body's immune system.

HOW INFLAMMATION WORKS: AN OVERVIEW

Inflammation is somewhat easier to understand than the immune response, because we have all observed it. The immune response is often hidden; your body's immune system may be knocking out an infectious antigen without your ever being aware of it. However, if you cut your finger, you will probably be acutely aware of the inflammatory process. You will actually see the redness and swelling and feel the pain. You may observe the formation of pus. As days go by, you will see the progress of wound healing and, perhaps, scar formation.

This is not to say that inflammation is simple; in its way, it is as complex as the immune response. There are several phases to inflammation. After each phase, healing may take place, and that will be the end of it. If healing doesn't take place, inflammation moves into its next phase. However, healing is the goal of all the phases.

Phases of Inflammation

Phase 1: Acute inflammation ⇒ healing (If healing doesn't take place, moves to phase 2)

Phase 2: Chronic inflammation ⇒ healing (If healing doesn't take place, moves to phase 3)

Phase 3: Granuloma formation

Phase 4: Healing

During each phase, the components of inflammation work together to perform four functions.

The Four Functions of Inflammation (During All Phases)

Destroy and remove unwanted substances

Wall off the infected and inflamed area

Stimulate the immune response

Promote healing

Content Review

Four Functions of Inflammation

Destroy and remove unwanted substances
Wall off the infected and inflamed area
Stimulate the immune response
Promote healing

ACUTE INFLAMMATORY RESPONSE

Acute inflammation is triggered by any injury, whether lethal or nonlethal, to the body's cells. As discussed earlier in this chapter, cell injury can result from causes such as hypoxia, chemicals, infectious agents (bacteria, viruses, fungi, parasites), trauma, heat extremes, radiation, nutritional imbalances, genetic factors, and even the injurious effects of the immune and inflammatory responses themselves. When cells are injured, the acute inflammatory response begins within seconds (Figure 4-6 ■).

The basic mechanics are always the same: (1) Blood vessels contract and dilate to move additional blood to the site. Then, (2) vascular permeability increases so that (3) white cells and plasma proteins can move through the capillary walls and into the tissues to begin the tasks of destroying the invader and healing the injury site (Figure 4-7 ■).

mast cells *large cells, resembling bags of granules, that reside near blood vessels. When stimulated by injury, chemicals, or allergic responses, they activate the inflammatory response by degranulation (emptying their granules into the extracellular environment) and synthesis (construction of leukotrienes and prostaglandins).*

MAST CELLS

Mast cells, which resemble bags of granules, are the chief activators of the inflammatory response. They are not blood cells. Instead, they reside in connective tissues just outside the blood vessels.

Bacteria enter tissue

Tissue damage occurs

Mediators are released

Chemotaxis

Increased blood flow

Increased vascular permeability

Increased numbers of leukocytes and mediators at site of tissue damage

Bacteria are contained, destroyed, and phagocytized

Bacteria gone

Bacteria remain

Tissue repair

Additional mediators activated

■ **Figure 4-6** The inflammatory response.

Mast cells activate the inflammatory response through two functions: *degranulation* and *synthesis* (Figure 4-8 ■).

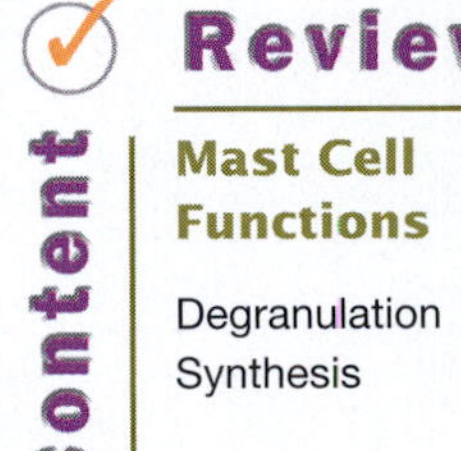

Degranulation

Degranulation is the process by which mast cells empty granules from their interior into the extracellular environment. This occurs when the mast cell is stimulated by one of the following events:

- ★ *Physical injury,* such as trauma, radiation, or temperature extremes
- ★ *Chemical agents,* such as toxins, venoms, enzymes, or a protein released by neutrophils (the latter is an example of inflammatory response causing further cellular injury)
- ★ *Immunologic and direct processes,* such as hypersensitivity (allergic) reactions involving release of IgE antibody or activation of complement components (discussed later)

degranulation *the emptying of granules from the interior of a mast cell into the extracellular environment.*

During degranulation, biochemical agents in the mast cell granules are released, notably vasoactive amines and chemotactic factors.

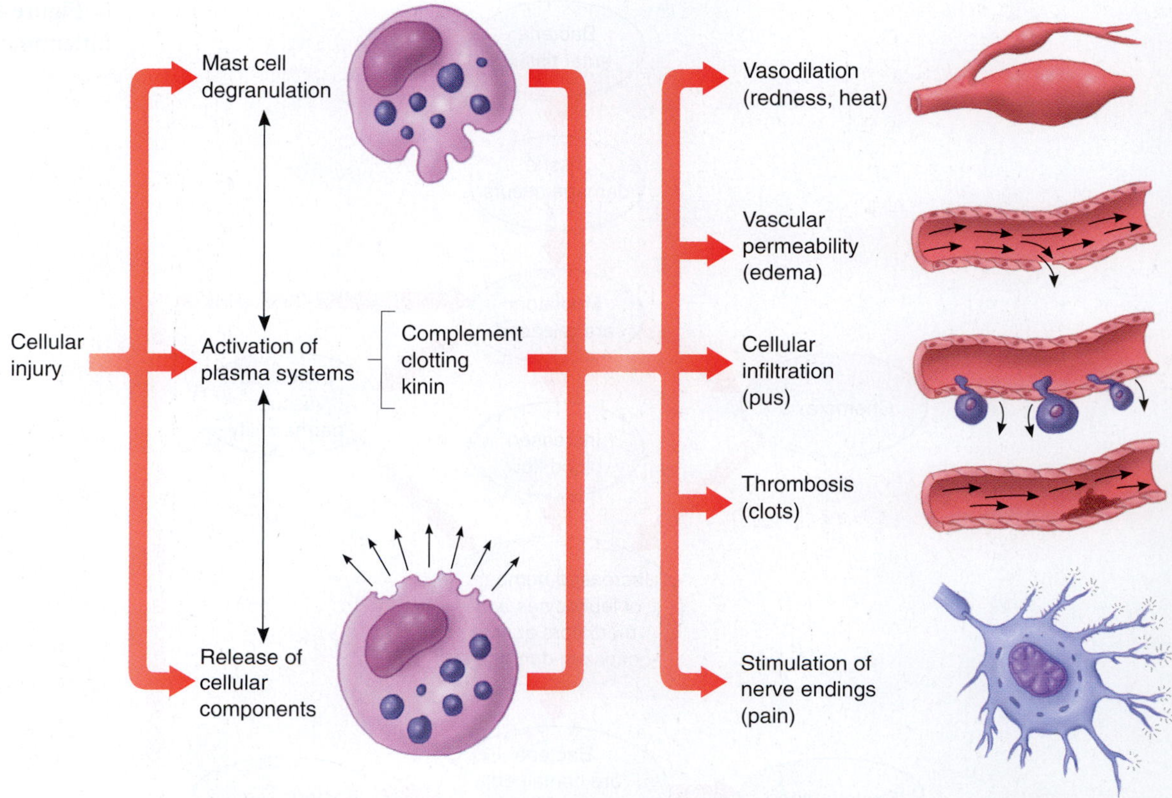

■ **Figure 4-7** The acute inflammatory response.

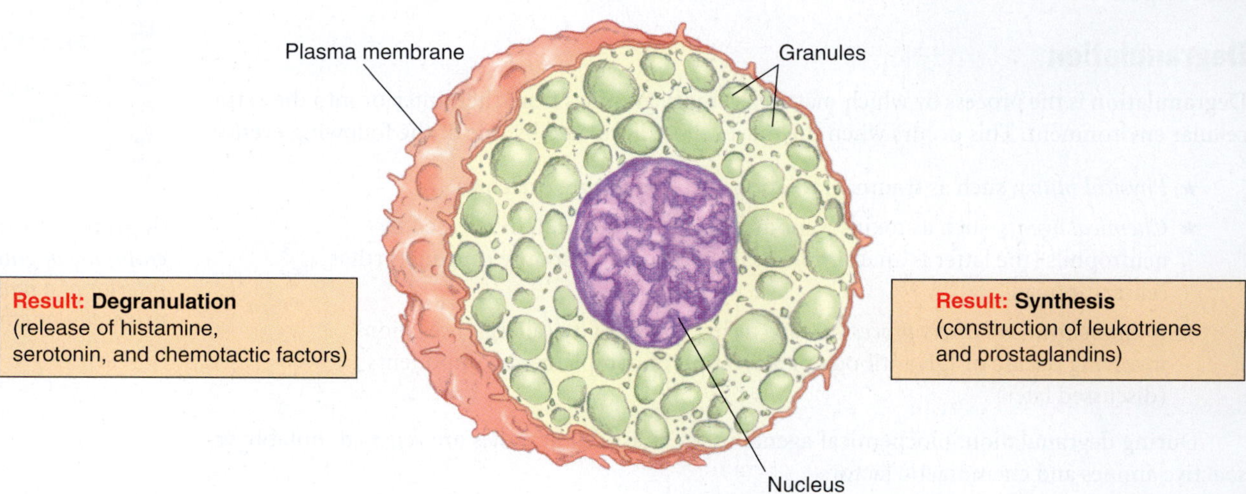

■ **Figure 4-8** Mast cell degranulation and synthesis.

Vasoactive Amines Histamine is a vasoactive amine (organic compound) released during degranulation of mast cells. The effect of vasoactive amines is the constriction of the smooth muscle of large vessel walls and dilation of the postcapillary sphincter, resulting in increased blood flow at the injury site.

Basophils (a type of white blood cell) also release histamine, with the same effect. Additionally, **serotonin,** released by platelets, can have effects of both vasoconstriction and vasodilation that may affect blood flow to the affected site.

Chemotactic Factors Another consequence of degranulation of mast cells is the release of various **chemotactic factors.** Chemotactic factors are chemicals that attract white cells to the site of inflammation. This attraction of white cells is called **chemotaxis.**

Synthesis

When stimulated, mast cells synthesize, or construct, two substances that play important roles in inflammation: leukotrienes and prostaglandins.

Leukotrienes, also known as *slow-reacting substances of anaphylaxis (SRS-A),* have actions similar to histamines—vasodilation and increased permeability—as well as chemotaxis. However, they are more important in the later stages of inflammation because they promote slower and longer-lasting effects than histamines. Like leukotrienes, **prostaglandins** cause increased vasodilation, vascular permeability, and chemotaxis. They are also the substances that cause pain. In addition, they control some inflammation by suppressing release of histamine and lysosomal enzymes from some white cells.

histamine *a substance released during the degranulation of mast cells and also released by basophils that, through constriction and dilation of blood vessels, increases blood flow to the injury site and also increases the permeability of vessel walls.*

serotonin *a substance released by platelets that, through constriction and dilation of blood vessels, affects blood flow to an injured or affected site.*

chemotactic factors *chemicals that attract white cells to the site of inflammation, a process called* **chemotaxis.**

leukotrienes *also called* slow-reacting substances of anaphylaxis (SRS-A); *substances synthesized by mast cells during inflammatory response that cause vasodilation, vascular permeability, and chemotaxis.*

prostaglandins *substances synthesized by mast cells during inflammatory response that cause vasodilation, vascular permeability, and chemotaxis and also cause pain.*

SYSTEMIC RESPONSES OF ACUTE INFLAMMATION

The three chief manifestations of acute inflammation are fever, leukocytosis (proliferation of circulating white cells), and an increase in circulating plasma proteins.

Endogenous pyrogen is a fever-causing chemical that is identical to IL-1 and is released by neutrophils and macrophages. It is released after the cell engages in phagocytosis or to a bacterial endotoxin or is exposed to an antigen-antibody complex. Fever can have both beneficial and harmful effects. On one hand, an increase in temperature can create an environment that is inhospitable to some invading microorganisms. On the other hand, fever may increase susceptibility of the infected person to the effects of endotoxins associated with some gram-negative bacterial infections.

In some infections, the number of circulating leukocytes, especially neutrophils, increases. Several components of the inflammatory response stimulate production of neutrophils, including a component of the complement system. Phagocytes produce a factor that induces production of granulocytes, including neutrophils, eosinophils, and basophils.

Plasma proteins called *acute phase reactants,* mostly produced in the liver, increase during inflammation. Their synthesis is stimulated by various interleukins. Many of these act to inhibit and control the inflammatory response.

CHRONIC INFLAMMATORY RESPONSES

Defined simply, chronic inflammation is any inflammation that lasts longer than 2 weeks. It may be caused by a foreign object or substance that persists in the wound, for example, a splinter, glass, or dirt. Or it may accompany a persistent bacterial infection. This can occur because some microorganisms have cell walls with a high lipid or wax content that resist phagocytosis. Other microorganisms can survive inside a macrophage. Still others produce toxins that persist even after the bacterium is dead, continuing to incite inflammatory responses. Inflammation can also be prolonged by the presence of chemicals and other irritants.

During chronic inflammation, large numbers of neutrophils—the phagocytes that were first on the scene during acute inflammation—degranulate and die. Now, the neutrophils are replaced by components that have taken longer to develop, and there is a large infiltration of lymphocytes from the immune response and of macrophages that have matured from monocytes. In addition to

fibroblasts *cells that secrete collagen, a critical factor in wound healing.*

pus *a liquid mixture of dead cells, bits of dead tissue, and tissue fluid that may accumulate in inflamed tissues.*

granuloma *a tumor or growth that forms when foreign bodies that cannot be destroyed by macrophages are surrounded and walled off.*

attacking foreign invaders, macrophages produce a factor that stimulates **fibroblasts,** cells that secrete collagen, a critical factor in wound healing.

As neutrophils, lymphocytes, and macrophages die, they infiltrate the tissues, sometimes forming a cavity that contains these dead cells, bits of dead tissue, and tissue fluid, a mixture called **pus.** Enzymes present in pus eventually cause it to self-digest, and it is removed through the epithelium or the lymph system.

Occasionally, when macrophages are unable to destroy the foreign invader, a **granuloma** will form to wall off the infection from the rest of the body. The granuloma is formed as large numbers of macrophages, other white cells, and fibroblasts are drawn to the site and surround it. Cells decay within the granuloma, and the released acids and lysosomes break the cellular debris down to basic components and fluid. The fluid eventually diffuses out of the granuloma, leaving a hollow, hard-walled structure buried in the tissues. Some granulomas persist for the life of the individual. Granuloma formation is common in leprosy and tuberculosis, which are caused by mycobacteria, bacteria that resist destruction by phagocytes.

Tissue repair and possible scar formation are the final stages of inflammation and will be discussed in more detail later.

LOCAL INFLAMMATORY RESPONSES

All of the manifestations observed at the local inflammation site result from (1) vascular changes and (2) exudation. Redness and heat result from vascular dilation and increased blood flow to the area. Swelling and pain result from the vascular permeability that permits infiltration of exudate into the tissues.

Exudate has three functions:

- ★ To dilute toxins released by bacteria and the toxic products of dying cells
- ★ To bring plasma proteins and leukocytes to the site to attack the invaders
- ★ To carry away the products of inflammation, (e.g., toxins, dead cells, pus)

The composition of exudate varies with the stage of inflammation and the type of injury or infection. Early exudate (serous exudate) is watery with few plasma proteins or leukocytes, as in a blister. In a severe or advanced inflammation, the exudate may be thick and clotted (fibrinous exudate) as in lobar pneumonia. In persistent bacterial infections, the exudate contains pus (purulent, or suppurative, exudate), as with cysts and abscesses. If bleeding is present, the exudate contains blood (hemorrhagic exudate).

The lesions (infected areas or wounds) that result from inflammation vary, depending on the organ affected. In myocardial infarction, cellular death results in the replacement of dead tissue by scar tissue. An infarction of brain tissue may result in liquefactive necrosis, in which the dead cells liquefy and are contained in walled cysts. In the liver, destroyed cells result in the regeneration of liver cells.

resolution *the complete healing of a wound and return of tissues to their normal structure and function; the ending of inflammation with no scar formation.*

repair *healing of a wound with scar formation.*

Keep in mind that inflammation can only occur in vascularized tissues (tissues to which blood can flow). When perfusion is cut off, as in a gangrenous limb or a limb distal to a tourniquet, inflammation cannot take place—and without inflammation, healing cannot take place.

RESOLUTION AND REPAIR

Content Review

Outcomes of Healing

Resolution—complete restoration of normal structure

Repair—scar formation

Healing begins during acute inflammation and may continue for as long as 2 years. The best outcome is **resolution,** the complete restoration of normal structure and function. This can happen if the damage was minor, there are no complications, and the tissues are capable of *regeneration* through the proliferation of the remaining cells. If resolution is not possible, then **repair** takes place with scarring being the end result. This happens if the wound is large, an abscess or granuloma has formed, or fibrin remains in the damaged tissues.

Both resolution and repair begin in the same way, with the *debridement,* or "cleaning up," of the site. Debridement involves phagocytosis of dead cells and debris and dissolution of fibrin cells (scabs). After debridement, there is a draining away of exudate, toxins, and particles from the site, and vascular dilation and permeability are reversed. At this point, either regeneration and resolution or repair and scar formation will take place. Minor wounds with little tissue loss, like paper cuts, close and heal easily, while more extensive wounds require more complex processes of sealing, filling, and contracting the wound.

hypersensitivity *an exaggerated and harmful immune response; an umbrella term for allergy, autoimmunity, and isoimmunity.*

VARIANCES IN IMMUNITY AND INFLAMMATION

Sometimes the immune and inflammatory systems work "too well" and sometimes not well enough. Hypersensitivity reactions are an example of the former, immune deficiency diseases an example of the latter.

allergy *exaggerated immune response to an environmental antigen.*

autoimmunity *an immune response to self-antigens, which the body normally tolerates.*

isoimmunity *an immune response to antigens from another member of the same species; for example, Rh reactions between a mother and infant or transplant rejections; also called alloimmunity.*

immediate hypersensitivity reaction *a swiftly occurring secondary hypersensitivity reaction (one that occurs after reexposure to an antigen). Immediate hypersensitivity reactions are usually more severe than delayed reactions. The swiftest and most severe such reaction is anaphylaxis.*

delayed hypersensitivity reaction *a hypersensitivity reaction that takes place after the elapse of some time following reexposure to an antigen. Delayed hypersensitivity reactions are usually less severe than immediate reactions.*

HYPERSENSITIVITY

Immune responses are normally protective and helpful. **Hypersensitivity,** however, is an exaggerated and harmful immune response. The word *hypersensitivity* is often used as a synonym for *allergy.* However, *hypersensitivity* is also used as an umbrella term for allergy and two other categories of harmful immune response, which are defined as follows:

Three Types of Hypersensitivity

★ **Allergy**—an exaggerated immune response to an environmental antigen, such as pollen or bee venom

★ **Autoimmunity**—a disturbance in the body's normal tolerance for self-antigens, as in hyperthyroidism or rheumatic fever

★ **Isoimmunity** (also called *alloimmunity*)—an immune reaction between members of the same species, commonly of one person against the antigens of another person, as in the reaction of a mother to her infant's Rh negative factor or in transplant rejections

The exact cause of such pathological immune responses is not known, but at least three factors seem to be involved: (1) the original insult (exposure to the antigen); (2) the person's genetic makeup, which determines susceptibility to the insult; and (3) an immunological process that boosts the response beyond normal bounds.

Hypersensitivity reactions are classified as **immediate hypersensitivity reactions** or **delayed hypersensitivity reactions,** depending on how long it takes the secondary reaction to appear after reexposure to an antigen. The swiftest immediate hypersensitivity reaction is *anaphylaxis,* a severe allergic response that usually develops within minutes of reexposure. (Review anaphylactic shock earlier in this chapter. Also see Volume 3, Chapter 6 on allergies and anaphylaxis.)

Mechanisms of Hypersensitivity

Usually, when a hypersensitivity reaction takes place, inflammation is triggered that results in destruction of healthy tissues. Four mechanisms, or types, of hypersensitivity that cause this destructive reaction have been identified.

Mechanisms of Hypersensitivity Reaction

★ *Type I*—IgE-mediated allergen reactions

★ *Type II*—tissue-specific reactions

★ *Type III*—immune complex-mediated reactions

★ *Type IV*—cell-mediated reactions

In reality, hypersensitivity reactions are not so easy to categorize. Most involve more than one type of mechanism.

Content Review

Four Types of Hypersensitivity Reactions

Type I—IgE reactions
Type II—Tissue-specific reactions
Type III—Immune complex-mediated reactions
Type IV—cell-mediated tissue reactions

Type I—IgE Reactions IgE is the immunoglobulin most involved in allergic reactions. The first exposure to the allergen (antigen that causes allergic reaction) stimulates B lymphocytes to produce IgE antibodies. These bind to receptors on mast cells in the tissues near blood vessels. On reexposure, the allergen binds to the IgE on the mast cell, which causes degranulation of the mast cell, release of histamine, and triggering of the inflammatory response.

Type II—Tissue-Specific Reactions Most tissues contain tissue-specific antigens, so called because they exist on the cells of only some body tissues. An immune response against one of these will affect only the organs or tissues that present that particular antigen.

Type III—Immune Complex-Mediated Reactions These result from antigen-antibody complexes, or immune complexes, formed when antibody meets and binds to a specific antigen. The immune complexes generally circulate for a time before being deposited in vessel walls or other tissues. For this reason, which organs are affected may have very little connection with where or how the antigen or the immune complex originated.

Type IV—Cell-Mediated Tissue Reactions Types I, II, and III hypersensitivity reactions are mediated by antibody. Type IV reactions are activated directly by T cells and do not involve antibody. There are two cell-mediated mechanisms. One involves Td cells, which produce lymphokine that activates other cells such as macrophages. The other involves Tc cells that directly attack and destroy antigen-bearing cells and their toxins.

DEFICIENCIES IN IMMUNITY AND INFLAMMATION

Immune deficiency disorders result from impaired function of some component of the immune system, including phagocytes, complement, and lymphocytes (T cells and B cells), with lymphocyte dysfunction being the primary cause. Immune deficiency can be congenital (inborn) or acquired (after birth). The most common manifestations of immune deficiency are recurrent infections, because the body's ability to ward off invaders has been damaged.

Congenital Immune Deficiencies

Congenital, or primary, immune deficiency develops if the development of lymphocytes in the fetus or embryo is impaired or halted. Different immune-deficiency diseases may develop, depending on whether the T cells, the B cells, or both have been affected.

Review

Content

Two Types of Immune Deficiency

Congenital (inborn)
Acquired (after birth)

In the *DiGeorge syndrome,* there is a lack or partial lack of thymus development, resulting in a severe decrease in T cell production and function. *Bruton agammaglobulinemia* is caused by impaired development of B cell precursors, resulting in B cells that cannot produce IgM or IgD antibodies. In *bare lymphocyte syndrome,* lymphocytes and macrophages are unable to produce Class I or Class II HLA antigens, which disrupts the ability of cells to recognize self or non-self substances, resulting in severe infections that are usually fatal before age 5.

Sometimes there is a defect that depresses the function of just a small portion of the immune system. For example, in *Wiskott-Aldrich syndrome,* IgM antibody production is reduced. *Selective IgA deficiency* is the most common immune deficiency. IgA is the antibody present in mucous membranes. People with IgA deficiency frequently suffer from sinus, lung, and gastrointestinal infections.

Some immune system deficiencies cause a decreased ability to respond to one particular antigen. For example, in *chronic mucocutaneous candidiasis,* the T lymphocytes are unable to respond against candida infections.

Acquired Immune Deficiencies

Acquired, or secondary, immune deficiencies develop after birth and do not result from genetic factors. They can be caused by or associated with pregnancy, infections, and diseases such as diabetes or cirrhosis. The elderly are more prone to acquired immune deficiencies than the young. Among the factors that can severely affect immune function are nutritional deficiencies, medical treatment, trauma, and stress. Of special interest is the fatal acquired immune disorder AIDS.

Nutritional Deficiencies Critical deficits in calorie or protein ingestion can lead to depression of T cell production and function. Complement activity, neutrophil chemotaxis, and the ability of neutrophils to kill bacteria are also seriously affected by starvation. Zinc deficiencies and vitamin deficiencies can affect both B cell and T cell function.

Iatrogenic Deficiencies Iatrogenic deficiencies are those that are caused by medical treatment. Some drugs depress blood cell formation in the bone marrow. Others trigger immune responses that destroy granulocytes. Immunosuppressive drugs administered in the treatment for transplants, cancer, or autoimmune diseases suppress B and T cell function and antibody production. Radiation treatment for cancer exacerbates this effect. Surgery and anesthesia also can suppress B and T cell function, with severely depressed white cell levels persisting for several weeks after surgery. Surgical removal of the spleen depresses humoral response against encapsulated bacteria, depresses IgM levels, and decreases the levels of opsonins.

Deficiencies Caused by Trauma Burn victims are especially susceptible to bacterial infection. Not only has the normal barrier presented by the skin been disrupted, but thermal burns also appear to decrease neutrophil function, complement levels, and other immune functions while increasing immunosuppressive functions, which further depress immune function.

Deficiencies Caused by Stress It has long been suggested that persons undergoing emotional stress (major stresses such as divorce, but also minor stresses such as studying for final exams) are more prone to illness. The speculation was that stress has deleterious effects on immune function. Research into the possible mechanisms of stress-induced immune deficiency are just getting underway. (Stress and susceptibility to disease will be discussed later in the chapter.)

AIDS AIDS is an acronym for *acquired immunodeficiency syndrome,* which has become the best known acquired immune deficiency disorder. AIDS is a syndrome of disorders that develop from infection with **HIV,** the *human immunodeficiency virus.*

HIV is a retrovirus; that is, it carries its genetic information in RNA rather than DNA molecules. As a retrovirus, HIV infects target cells by binding to receptors on their surfaces, then inserting the HIV RNA into the cell. There, the RNA is converted into DNA and becomes part of the infected cell's genetic material. HIV can remain dormant inside the host cell for years; however, once the cell is activated (and the mechanism by which this occurs is not fully understood), HIV proliferates, kills the host cell, and can then infect other cells. The result is a pervasive breakdown of the immune defenses, making the body vulnerable to a wide variety of infections and disorders.

HIV can infect anybody, male or female, homosexual or heterosexual, mostly through the exchange of body fluids during sexual intercourse or through injection. In the United States, most cases to date have involved homosexual men and intravenous drug users. However, preventive measures (safe sex practices, including use of condoms, and clean-needle programs) have reduced the incidence of HIV/AIDS among homosexual populations and drug users. An increasing proportion of new patients are females who have acquired the infection during heterosexual intercourse. In other parts of the world, HIV/AIDS occurs equally among men and women.

The possibility of acquiring HIV/AIDS by contact with patients or accidental needle sticks fostered something of a panic among health care workers when AIDS first spread so alarmingly in the United States in the 1970s. Following recommendations by OSHA, Standard Precautions (body substance isolation practices) have been widely adopted—including the use of disposable gloves, protective eyewear, masks, and gowns, as appropriate, to avoid contact with any body fluids, along with improved techniques for handling needles and other sharps. These measures have proved effective in reducing the fear of HIV/AIDS infection and also in making such infections very rare among health care workers.

Until recently, more than 90 percent of those with AIDS have died within 5 years of the development of severe symptoms. This picture has improved somewhat in developed nations with the initiation of treatments involving multiple chemotherapies (treatment "cocktails") that have shown success in prolonging life, greatly improving feelings of health and well-being, and suppressing measurable blood levels of HIV.

It is not yet known if such treatments can eradicate HIV and cure AIDS. One fear is that the treatments suppress but do not totally destroy the HIV virus, which "hides" somewhere in the body, waiting to proliferate at some later date. Another fear is that HIV will develop strains that are resistant to the treatments that appear to be successful in the short term. Nevertheless, the success of these treatments has caused the first feelings of optimism since AIDS was identified. Preventive

AIDS acquired immunodeficiency syndrome, *a group of signs, symptoms, and disorders that often develop as a consequence of HIV infection.*

HIV human immunodeficiency virus, *a virus that breaks down the immune defenses, making the body vulnerable to a variety of infections and disorders.*

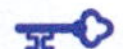

Standard Precautions, including body substance isolation practices, have been effective in relieving fears of HIV/AIDS infection and in making such infections very rare among health care workers.

measures have also helped to greatly reduce the number of new cases reported in the United States. In some parts of the world, however, including Africa and Asia, HIV/AIDS is still spreading at an extremely alarming rate, with seriously inadequate reporting, prevention, and treatment.

Replacement Therapies for Immune Deficiencies

Advances have been made in the treatment of immune deficiencies through the use of replacement therapies, such as those in the following list.

Replacement Therapies

- ★ *Gamma globulin therapy*—Gamma globulin is administered to individuals with B cell deficiencies that cause immunoglobulin (antibody) deficiencies.
- ★ *Transplantation and transfusion*—HLA-matched bone marrow is transplanted into patients suffering *severe combined immune deficiencies (SCID),* which is caused by a lack of the stem cells from which T cells and B cells develop. In patients who lack a thymus or have a defective thymus, fetal thymus tissue may be transplanted. Enzyme deficiencies that cause SCID have been treated with transfusions of red blood cells that contain the needed enzyme. Other substances have been transfused into individuals to help restore T cell function and reactivity against certain antigens.
- ★ *Gene therapy*—Therapies involving identification of defective genes that are responsible for immune disorders, and replacement of these defective genes with cloned normal genes, are in the early stages of development and use.

STRESS AND DISEASE

Stress is a word that is used a lot in modern life. You might have a stressful job, or feel stressed out by too many demands on your job, or be going through a lot of emotional stress in connection with a personal relationship. In some situations, you may be acutely aware of some of the physiological components of stress, for example, sweaty palms and a pounding heart just before you have to get up and give a speech. If so, you already have a basic understanding of stress that can help you grasp the physiological and medical concepts of stress and how stress is related to disease.

CONCEPTS OF STRESS

Mind and body interact. There is a cause-and-effect relationship between stress and disease.

Today, it is commonly understood that mind and body interact. It was not always so. In fact, the concept that psychological states influence physiological states—and particularly that there is a cause-effect relationship between stress and disease—date primarily from the work of Hans Selye, an Austrian-born Canadian physician and educator, in the 1940s.

General Adaptation Syndrome

Dr. Selye was not studying stress when he made his discovery. Instead, he was trying to identify a new sex hormone. He was injecting ovarian extracts into laboratory rats when he discovered the following triad of physiological effects:

Triad of Stress Effects

- ★ Enlargement of the cortex (outer portion) of the adrenal gland
- ★ Atrophy of the thymus gland and other lymphatic structures
- ★ Development of bleeding ulcers of the stomach and duodenum

Dr. Selye soon discovered that this triad of effects was not a response only to the ovarian extracts. The same effects occurred when he subjected the rats to other stimuli, such as cold, surgical injury, and restraint. He concluded that the triad of effects was not specific to any particular stimulus but comprised a nonspecific response to any noxious stimulus, or stressor. (**Stress** is generally defined as a state of physical and/or psychological arousal to a stimulus. Dr. Selye originally intended to use

stress *a state of physical or psychological arousal to stimulus.*

the word *stress* for the stimulus, or cause, but through a mistranslation of his work, *stress* came to mean the arousal, or effect. Dr. Selye then coined the word **stressor** for the stimulus/cause.)

stressor *the stimulus or cause of stress.*

Because the same responses occurred to a wide array of stimuli, Dr. Selye named it the **general adaptation syndrome (GAS).** Later, he identified three stages in the development of GAS:

general adaptation syndrome (GAS) *a sequence of stress response stages: stage I, alarm; stage II, resistance or adaptation; stage III, exhaustion.*

Review

Content

General Adaptation Syndrome (Gas)

Stage I—Alarm
Stage II—Resistance, or adaptation
Stage III—Exhaustion

Stages of GAS

- ★ *Stage I, Alarm*—The sympathetic nervous system is aroused and mobilized in the "fight-or-flight" response syndrome. Pupils dilate, heart rate increases, and bronchial passages dilate. In addition, blood glucose levels rise, digestion slows, blood pressure rises, and the flow of blood to the skeletal muscles increases. At the same time, the endocrine system is aroused, resulting in secretion by the pituitary and adrenal glands of hormones that enhance the body's readiness to meet the challenge.
- ★ *Stage II, Resistance, or Adaptation*—The person begins to cope with the situation. Sympathetic nervous system responses and circulating hormones return to normal. In most situations, this is the last stage; the stress is resolved. If the stress is very severe or prolonged, however, stress is not resolved and stage III occurs.
- ★ *Stage III, Exhaustion*—This is the stage sometimes known as "burnout." During this stage, the triad of physiological effects described by Dr. Selye occurs. The person can no longer cope with or resolve the stress, and physical illness may ensue.

The stages of GAS begin with **physiological stress,** defined by Dr. Selye as a chemical or physical disturbance in the cells or tissue fluid produced by a change, either in the external environment or within the body itself, that requires a response to counteract the disturbance. Selye identified three components of physiological stress: (1) the stressor that initiates the disturbance, (2) the chemical or physical disturbance the stressor produces, and (3) the body's counteracting (adaptational) response.

physiological stress *a chemical or physical disturbance in the cells or tissue fluid produced by a change in the external environment or within the body.*

Psychological Mediators and Specificity

Since Dr. Selye defined GAS, others who have studied adaptation to stress have refined the concept. For example, more attention has been paid to the psychological mediators of stress. Experiments have shown that there isn't a direct correlation between stressor and response. People react differently to the same stressor. One person may take in stride the same situation that greatly upsets another person, and the degree of physiological response may be governed more by the psychological, or emotional, or social response to the stressor than to the stressor itself. In particular, research has demonstrated pituitary gland and adrenal cortex sensitivity to emotional/psychological/social influences.

Another way in which recent research has diverged from Dr. Selye's original hypotheses regards specificity. Dr. Selye postulated that the triad of physiological responses he identified were nonspecific, or the same for any stressor. It is now thought that, while the triad of responses he identified may occur in response to a wide variety of stressors, the total body response to different stressors must be specific, that is, targeted toward correction of the specific disturbance. For example, the body reacts to cold by shivering and to heat through vasodilation and sweating.

Homeostasis as a Dynamic Steady State

An older definition of homeostasis states that the body maintains itself at a "constant" composition. More recently, homeostasis has been described as a **dynamic steady state.** This takes into account the concept of **turnover,** the continual synthesis and breakdown of all body substances (e.g., fats, proteins). Thus, the internal environment of the body is always changing, not constant, but the net effect of all the changes is the dynamic (always changing), yet steady (tending always toward normal balance) state.

dynamic steady state *homeostasis; the tendency of the body to maintain a net constant composition although the components of the body's internal environment are always changing.*

Stressors cause a series of reactions that alter the dynamic steady state. Usually, there is a return to normal, which may be rapid or slow. If a disturbance in the dynamic steady state, for example, a high blood glucose level, is prolonged and a causative stressor is no longer present, it is considered a sign of disease.

turnover *the continual synthesis and breakdown of body substances that results in the dynamic steady state.*

psychoneuroimmunological regulation *the interactions of psychological, neurological/endocrine, and immunological factors that contribute to alteration of the immune system as an outcome of a stress response that is not quickly resolved.*

stress response *changes within the body initiated by a stressor.*

Content Review

Hormones Produced in Response to Stress

- Catecholamines (norepinephrine and epinephrine)
- Cortisol
- Beta endorphins
- Growth hormone
- Prolactin

STRESS RESPONSES

Alteration of the immune system is the ultimate outcome of a stress response that resists quick and successful adaptation. The interactions of psychological, neurological/endocrine, and immunological factors that lead to this outcome are known as **psychoneuroimmunologic regulation.**

The **stress response** is initiated by a stressor. The input of the stressor into the central nervous system, as mediated by the person's psychological response, leads to production of corticotropin-releasing factor (CRF) from the hypothalamus, which in turn stimulates responses by the sympathetic nervous system and the endocrine system (neuroendocrine regulation), which then affect the immune system. This chain of events is outlined in Figure 4-9 ■ and described in the next sections.

Neuroendocrine Regulation

As previously mentioned, when a person encounters a stressor and has a psychological response to the stressor, the sympathetic nervous system is stimulated by *corticotropin-releasing factor (CRF)*. In turn, this stimulates release of catecholamines, cortisol, and other hormones.

Catecholamines Sympathetic nervous system stimulation results in the release of norepinephrine (noradrenalin) and epinephrine (adrenalin), which constitute the category of hormones called *catecholamines.* The nerves of the sympathetic nervous system exit the spine at the thoracic and lumbar levels, and norepinephrine is released into the synaptic spaces (the spaces between the presynaptic ganglia and the postsynaptic nerves).

Additionally, sympathetic nervous system stimulation results in direct stimulation of the adrenal medulla, the inner portion of the adrenal gland. The adrenal medulla, in turn, releases the norepinephrine and epinephrine into the circulatory system. Approximately 80 percent of the hormones released by the adrenal medulla are epinephrine, while norepinephrine constitutes the re-

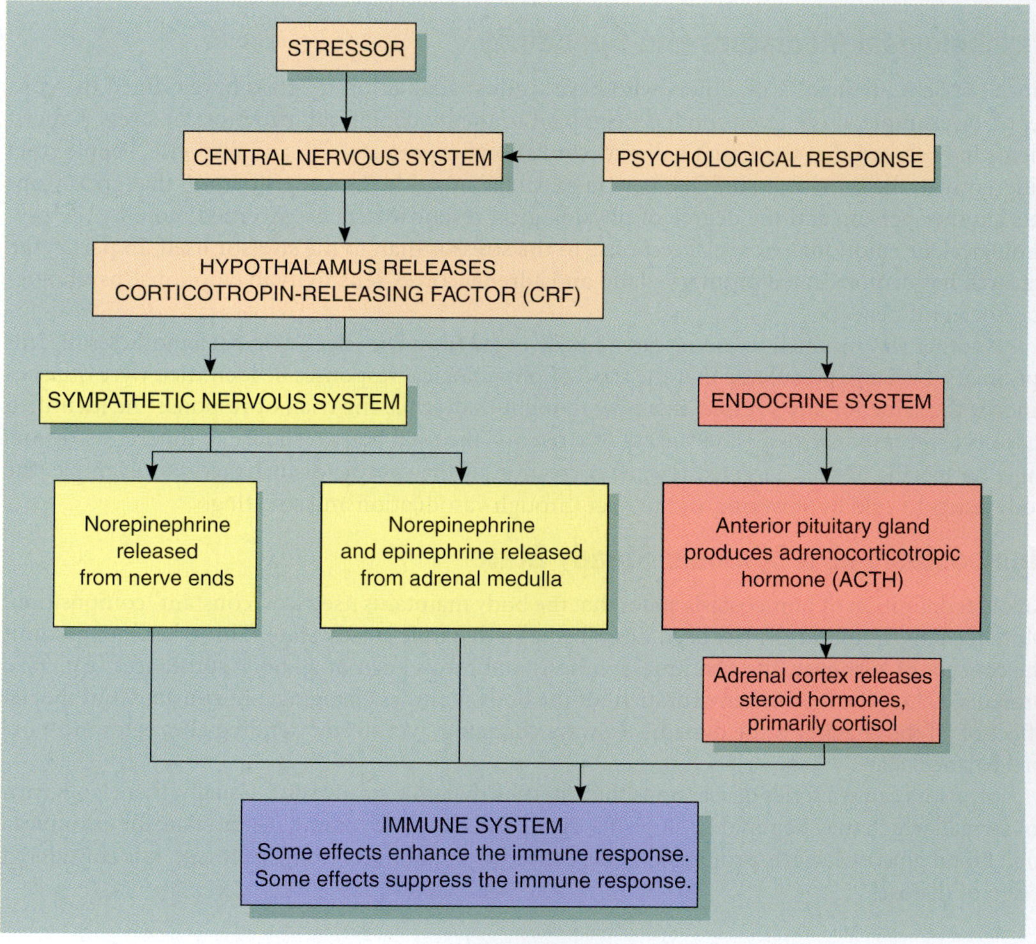

■ **Figure 4-9** The stress response: effects on the sympathetic nervous, endocrine, and immune systems.

maining 20 percent. Once released, these hormones are carried throughout the body where their effects (preparing the body to deal with stressful situations) act on hormone receptors.

Both epinephrine and norepinephrine interact with specialized adrenergic receptors on the membranes of target organs. These receptors are located throughout the body. Once stimulated by the appropriate hormone, they cause a response in the organ or organs they control.

The adrenergic receptors are generally divided into four types, designated alpha 1 (α_1), alpha 2 (α_2), beta 1 (β_1), and beta 2 (β_2). The α_1 receptors cause peripheral vasoconstriction, mild bronchoconstriction, and stimulation of metabolism. The α_2 receptors are found on the presynaptic surfaces of sympathetic neuroeffector junctions. Stimulation of α_2 receptors is inhibitory. These receptors serve to prevent overrelease of norepinephrine in the synapse. When the level of norepinephrine in the synapse gets high enough, the α_2 receptors are stimulated and norepinephrine release is inhibited. Stimulation of β_1 receptors causes increases in heart rate, cardiac contractile force, and cardiac automaticity and conduction. Stimulation of β_2 receptors causes vasodilation and bronchodilation.

All of the effects of the catecholamines prepare the body to "fight-or-flee" in response to a stressor. Their physiological effects are summarized in Table 4–4.

Cortisol Cortisol is another hormone produced in response to stress. The corticotropin-releasing factor (CRF) that stimulates the sympathetic nervous system, as previously discussed, simultaneously stimulates the anterior pituitary gland to produce *adrenocorticotropic hormone (ACTH)*, which in turn stimulates the adrenal cortex to produce a variety of steroid hormones, primarily cortisol.

cortisol *a steroid hormone released by the adrenal cortex that regulates the metabolism of fats, carbohydrates, sodium, potassium, and proteins and also has an antiinflammatory effect.*

One of the primary functions of cortisol is the stimulation of gluconeogenesis. It enhances the elevation of blood glucose by other hormones and also inhibits peripheral uptake and oxidation of glucose by the cells. Because of these functions, it has the overall effect of elevating blood glucose.

Table 4–4 Physiological Effects of Catecholamines

Organ	Effects
Brain	Increased blood flow Increased glucose metabolism
Cardiovascular system	Increased contractile force and rate Peripheral vasoconstriction
Pulmonary system	Increased ventilation Bronchodilation Increased oxygen supply
Liver	Increased glucose production
Gastrointestinal and genitourinary tracts	Increased gluconeogenesis Increased glycogenolysis Decreased glycogen synthesis
Muscle	Decreased protein synthesis Increased glycogenolysis Increased contraction Increased dilation of skeletal muscle vasculature
Skeleton	Decreased glucose uptake and utilization (insulin release decreased)
Adipose (fatty) tissue	Increased lipolysis Increased fatty acids and glycerol
Skin	Decreased blood flow
Lymphoid tissue	Increased protein breakdown (shrinkage of lymphoid tissue)

Cortisol also affects protein metabolism—increasing synthesis of proteins in the liver but increasing breakdown of proteins in the muscle, lymphoid tissue, fatty tissues, skin, and bone. The breakdown of proteins results in increased blood levels of amino acids. Cortisol also promotes lipolysis (fat breakdown) in the extremities and lipogenesis (fat synthesis and deposition) in the face and trunk.

Cortisol acts as an immunosuppressant by inhibiting protein synthesis, including synthesis of immunoglobulins (antibodies). Additionally, it reduces the numbers of lymphocytes, eosinophils, and macrophages in the blood. In large amounts, cortisol can cause lymphoid atrophy. Through a series of actions, cortisol diminishes the actions of helper T cells, which results in a decrease in B cells and antibody production. It inhibits production of interleukin-1 and interleukin-2 and, consequently, blocks cell-mediated immunity and generation of fever. It inhibits the accumulation of leukocytes at the site of inflammation and inhibits release of substances that are critical in the inflammatory response, including kinins, prostaglandins, and histamine. Cortisol also inhibits fibroblast proliferation during inflammatory response, which in turn causes poor wound healing and increased susceptibility to wound infection.

In the gastrointestinal tract, cortisol increases gastric secretions, occasionally enough to cause ulcer formation. Cortisol also suppresses the release of sex hormones, including testosterone and estradiol.

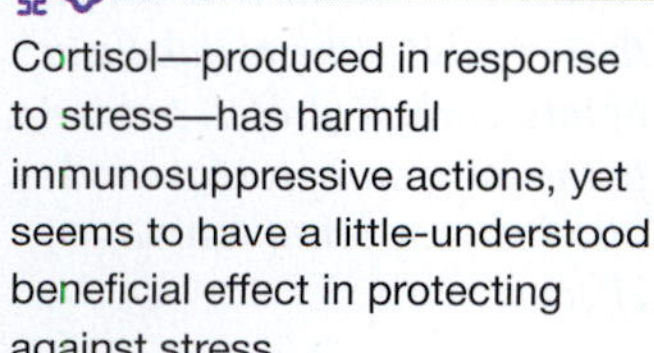

Cortisol—produced in response to stress—has harmful immunosuppressive actions, yet seems to have a little-understood beneficial effect in protecting against stress.

The immunosuppressive actions of cortisol seem clearly harmful, yet its production in response to stress indicates that it is beneficial in protecting against stress. Its beneficial effects in stress, however, are not well understood. It has been suggested that its promotion of gluconeogenesis helps assure an adequate source of glucose as energy for body tissues, especially nerve tissues. Pooled amino acids from protein breakdown may promote protein synthesis in some cells. Its depressive influence on inflammatory responses may play a role in decreasing peripheral blood flow and redirecting blood to critical organs or sites of injury. Suppression of immune function may also help prevent tissue damage that results from prolonged immune responses.

Role of the Immune System in Stress

During a stress response, as noted earlier, there is a complex interaction among the nervous and endocrine systems and the immune system. As a consequence, a variety of immune-related disorders are associated with stress.

The specific mechanisms by which stress leads to immune-related disorders is the subject of ongoing research but is not yet well understood. However, research points to the substances that serve as communicators between the cells of the nervous system, the endocrine system, and the immune system—including hormones, neurotransmitters, neuropeptides, and cytokines—as the pathways of cause and effect.

The pathway is not a straight line. The directional arrows of cause and effect move forward, backward, and in circles. Many components of the immune system can be affected by the factors produced by the neuroendocrine system. Conversely, immune system products can affect components of the neuroendocrine system. Here are two examples:

- *Pathway 1: Central nervous system to immune system*—The central nervous system *stimulates* the hypothalamus to produce CRF ⇒ which *stimulates* the pituitary gland to produce ACTH ⇒ which *stimulates* the adrenal gland to secrete cortisol ⇒ which *suppresses* the development of macrophages, T cells, B cells, and natural killer (NK) cells, a lymphocyte specially adapted to recognize and kill virally infected cells and malignant cells.
- *Pathway 2: Immune system to central nervous system*—During immune system response, macrophages secrete cytokines ⇒ which stimulate the hypothalamus to secrete CRF (which begins Pathway 1 again).

The previous examples are only two examples of the many pathways and interactions that take place among the nervous, endocrine, and immune systems.

The suppression of immune system function that is caused by stress-related products of the sympathetic nervous and endocrine systems—especially catecholamines and cortisol—has been linked to a number of immune-mediated diseases, as listed in Table 4–5.

Table 4–5	Stress- and Immune-Related Diseases and Conditions
Target Organ	**Diseases and Conditions**
Cardiovascular system	Coronary artery disease
	Hypertension
	Stroke
	Dysrhythmias
Muscles	Tension headaches
	Muscle-related backaches
Connective tissues	Rheumatoid arthritis
Pulmonary system	Asthma
	Hay fever
Immune system	Immunosuppression or immune deficiency
Gastrointestinal system	Ulcer
	Irritable bowel syndrome
	Ulcerative colitis
Genitourinary system	Diuresis
	Impotence
Skin	Eczema
	Acne
Endocrine system	Diabetes mellitus
Central nervous system	Fatigue
	Depression
	Insomnia

STRESS, COPING, AND ILLNESS INTERRELATIONSHIPS

Research has shown that the ability to cope with stress has significant effects on associated illnesses. Those who cope positively with stress have a reduced chance of becoming ill in the first place and a better chance of getting better or getting better faster if they do become ill. Conversely, those who don't cope as well with stress have a greater chance of becoming ill or of prolonging the course of illness or of not surviving an illness.

Physiological stress is caused by events that directly affect the body, such as a burn, extreme cold, or starvation. *Psychological stress* consists of the unpleasant emotions caused by life events, such as taking exams or experiencing a divorce. The effects that these stresses will have on the body depend on the individual's ability to cope with them. Some people are "thrown" by events others would perceive as relatively minor, such as a traffic jam or a sprained ankle. Others can take in stride events that others would find very difficult, such as loss of a job or a long-term disability.

The effects of stress, including the degree to which stress causes or affects illness, are moderated by the type, duration, and severity of the stressor in combination with the individual's perception and ability to cope with it. Stressors that are the most likely to have a negative effect on immunity and disease have been characterized as those that are not only undesirable but also are uncontrollable and that overtax the person's ability to cope.

Effective and ineffective coping has been seen to have potentially different effects in healthy persons, symptomatic persons (those who already have some manifestations of disease), and persons who are undergoing medical treatment.

Potential Effects of Stress Based on Effectiveness of Coping

★ *In a healthy person.* Effective coping ⇒ Transient effects, return to normal function
Ineffective coping ⇒ Significant stress effects, illness

★ *In a symptomatic person.* Effective coping ⇒ Little or no effect on symptoms
Ineffective coping ⇒ Exacerbation of symptoms, illness

★ *In a person undergoing medical treatment.* Effective coping ⇒ Person does not perceive the treatment itself as stressful ⇒ Treatment is more likely to have a positive effect on symptoms and the course of illness. Ineffective coping ⇒ Person perceives the treatment itself as stressful ⇒ Treatment is more likely to have a negative effect on symptoms and the course of illness

Because of the importance of coping ability in the interplay between stress and illness, attention is increasingly being paid to providing counseling and support systems—including family members, friends, and other support networks—to assist persons who are ill or in stressful life situations. There is recognition that supporting the patient's ability to cope is a critical adjunct to medical treatment itself.

Summary

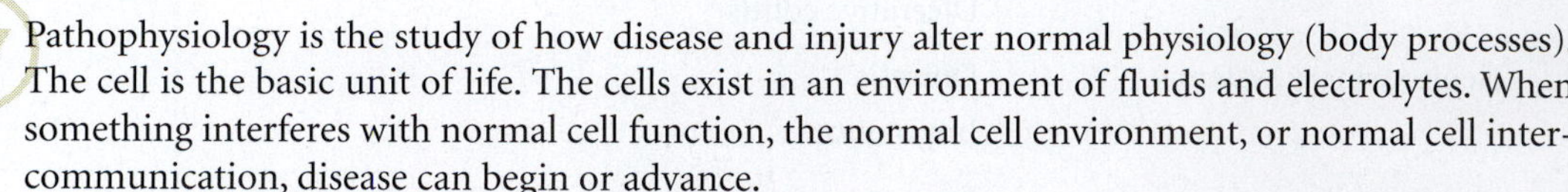

Pathophysiology is the study of how disease and injury alter normal physiology (body processes). The cell is the basic unit of life. The cells exist in an environment of fluids and electrolytes. When something interferes with normal cell function, the normal cell environment, or normal cell intercommunication, disease can begin or advance.

Cells can be injured in a variety of ways, including hypoxia, chemicals, infectious agents, immunological/inflammatory injuries, and others. Diseases can be caused by genetic factors, environmental factors, or a combination of factors (multifactorial diseases).

The body responds to cellular injury in a variety of ways to restore homeostasis, the body's normal dynamic steady state. Cells can adapt through atrophy, hypertrophy, hyperplasia, metaplasia, and dysplasia. Negative feedback mechanisms work to correct, or compensate for, shock—if shock has not progressed too far.

Perfusion of the tissues is necessary to provide essential nutrients to the cells (especially oxygen and glucose) and to remove wastes. Inadequate perfusion, called hypoperfusion or shock, can be caused by a problem in any of the three parts of the cardiovascular system (the heart, the blood vessels, or the blood), sometimes abetted by problems with the respiratory or gastrointestinal system in which the normal intake and transfer of oxygen and glucose may be interrupted. If not corrected, shock continues in a downward spiral toward irreversible shock, possible multiple organ dysfunction syndrome (MODS), and death.

The body's chief means of self-defense is the immune system and the immune and inflammatory responses, which work to attack and destroy infectious agents and other unwanted invaders. Occasionally, the immune response system works "too well," as in hypersensitivity reactions, or not well enough, as in immune deficiency disorders. Stress can also contribute to disease through the interactions of the nerve, endocrine, and immune systems.

Review Questions

1. ____________ is the physiology of disordered function.
   a. Pathology
   b. Anatomy
   c. Physiology
   d. Pathophysiology

2. ___________ is an increase in the number of cells through cell division caused by an increased workload.
   a. Multiplasia
   b. Metaplasia
   c. Dysplasia
   d. Hyperplasia

3. ___________ is the constructive or "building up" phase of metabolism.
   a. Anabolism
   b. Apoptosis
   c. Catabolism
   d. Hyperplasia

4. The mechanisms that most commonly result in accumulation of water in the interstitial space include:
   a. lymphatic obstruction.
   b. an increase in hydrostatic pressure.
   c. increased permeability of the capillary membrane.
   d. all of the above

5. ___________ are secreted by plasma cells in response to antigenic stimulation.
   a. Antigens
   b. Antibodies
   c. Antibiotics
   d. Haptens

6. Progressive impairment of two or more organ systems resulting from an uncontrolled inflammatory response to a severe illness or injury is called:
   a. ALS.
   b. MODS.
   c. ARDS.
   d. AODS.

7. Advanced stages of shock when the body's compensatory mechanisms are no longer able to maintain normal perfusion are called:
   a. reversible shock.
   b. compensated shock.
   c. homeostatic shock.
   d. decompensated shock.

8. The most commonly used fluids in prehospital care are:
   a. D_5W.
   b. normal saline.
   c. lactated Ringer's.
   d. all of the above

9. Every human somatic cell contains ___________ chromosomes.
   a. 48
   b. 46
   c. 24
   d. 23

10. Obstructive shock is caused by an obstruction that interferes with the return of blood to the heart, such as:
   a. cardiac tamponade.
   b. pulmonary embolism.
   c. tension pneumothorax.
   d. all of the above

11. The energy that is produced during glucose breakdown is in the form of the chemical:
    a. ATP.
    b. APT.
    c. TAP.
    d. PTA.
12. With a mortality rate of __________ – __________ percent, MODS is the major cause of death following sepsis, trauma, and burn injuries.
    a. 40–50
    b. 50–60
    c. 60–90
    d. 80–90
13. People with type __________ blood are known as universal donors, because this type of blood has no antigens that will trigger an immune response in any other group.
    a. A
    b. B
    c. O
    d. AB
14. __________ cells are the chief activators of the inflammatory response.
    a. T
    b. Mast
    c. Immune
    d. Histamine
15. The acronym *AIDS* stands for:
    a. acute iatragenic deterioration syndrome.
    b. active immunodefensive system.
    c. acquired immunodeficiency syndrome.
    d. adult inflammatory dilation status.

See Answers to Review Questions at the back of this book.

Chapter 5

Life-Span Development

Objectives

After reading this chapter, you should be able to:

1. Compare and contrast the physiological and psychosocial characteristics of the following life-span development stages:
   - ★ Infant (pp. 292–296)
   - ★ Toddler (pp. 296–298)
   - ★ Preschooler (pp. 296–298)
   - ★ School-aged (pp. 298–299)
   - ★ Adolescent (pp. 299–300)
   - ★ Early adult (pp. 300-301)
   - ★ Middle-aged adult (p. 301)
   - ★ Late-aged adult (pp. 301–305)

Key Terms

anxious avoidant attachment, p. 295
anxious resistant attachment, p. 295
authoritarian, p. 298
authoritative, p. 298
bonding, p. 295
conventional reasoning, p. 299
difficult child, p. 296
easy child, p. 296
life expectancy, p. 301
maximum life span, p. 301
modeling, p. 298
Moro reflex, p. 294
palmar grasp, p. 294
permissive, p. 298
postconventional reasoning, p. 299
preconventional reasoning, p. 299
rooting reflex, p. 294
scaffolding, p. 296
secure attachment, p. 295
slow-to-warm-up child, p. 296
sucking reflex, p. 294
terminal-drop hypothesis, p. 303
trust vs. mistrust, p. 295

INTRODUCTION

People change over the span of a lifetime. Changes in vital signs, body systems, and psychosocial development can necessitate adjustments in your treatment of patients. For example, drug dosages are based on body size, weight, and ability of the patient to process the drug.

Many changes can be associated with development stages. The stages discussed in this chapter are *infancy* (birth to 12 months), *toddlerhood* (12 to 36 months), *preschool age* (3 to 5 years), *school age* (6 to 12 years), *adolescence* (13 to 18 years), *early adulthood* (20 to 40 years), *middle adulthood* (41 to 60 years), and *late adulthood* (61 years and older).

INFANCY

PHYSIOLOGICAL DEVELOPMENT

Vital Signs

The younger the child, the more rapid are the pulse and respiratory rates.

The greatest vital sign changes occur in the pediatric patient (Table 5–1). At birth, the heart rate ranges from 100 to 180 beats per minute but settles to around 120 after the first 30 minutes. An at-birth respiratory rate of 30 to 60 will drop to 30 to 40 after the first few minutes.

Unlike heart and respiratory rates that decrease with age, blood pressure tends to increase with age. An average systolic blood pressure of 60 to 90 at birth rises to a range of 87 to 105 at 12 months.

Weight

Normal birth weight of an infant usually is between 3.0 and 3.5 kg. Because of the excretion of extracellular fluid in the first week of life, the infant's weight usually drops by 5 percent to 10 percent; however, infants usually exceed their birth weight by the second week. During the first month, infants grow

Table 5–1 Normal Vital Signs

	Pulse (beats per minute)	Respiration (breaths per minute)	Blood Pressure (average mmHg)	Temperature	
Infancy:					
At birth	100–180	30–60	60–90 systolic	98°F–100°F	36.7°C–37.8°C
At 1 year	100–160	30–60	87–105 systolic	98°F–100°F	36.7°C–37.8°C
Toddler (12 to 36 months)	80–110	24–40	95–105 systolic	96.8°F–99.6°F	36°C–37.5°C
Preschool age (3 to 5 years)	70–110	22–34	95–110 systolic	96.8°F–99.6°F	36°C–37.5°C
School age (6 to 12 years)	65–110	18–30	97–112 systolic	98.6°F	37°C
Adolescence (13 to 18 years)	60–90	12–26	112–128 systolic	98.6°F	37°C
Early adulthood (19 to 40 years)	60–100	12–20	120/80	98.6°F	37°C
Middle adulthood (41 to 60 years)	60–100	12–20	120/80	98.6°F	37°C
Late adulthood (61 years and older)	+	+	+	98.6°F	37°C

+ Depends on the individual's physical health status.

at approximately 30 grams per day, and they should double their birth weight by 4 to 6 months and triple it at 9 to 12 months (Figure 5-1 ■). The infant's head is equal to 25 percent of total body weight.

Growth charts are good for comparing physical development to the norm, but parents should keep in mind that every child develops at his own rate.

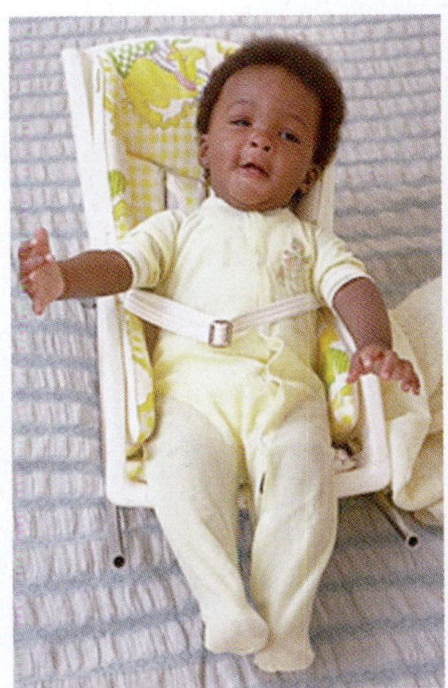

■ Figure 5-1 Infants double their weight by 4 to 6 months old and triple it by 9 to 12 months. (*© Michal Heron*)

The infant's head is equal to 25 percent of total body weight.

Cardiovascular System

As newborns make the transition from fetal to pulmonary circulation in the first few days of life, several important changes occur. Shortly after birth, the *ductus venosus,* a blood vessel that connects the umbilical vein and the inferior vena cava in the fetus, constricts. As a result, blood pressure changes and the *foramen ovale,* an opening in the interatrial septum of the fetal heart, closes. The *ductus arteriosus,* a blood vessel that connects the pulmonary artery and the aorta in the fetus, also constricts after birth. Once it is closed, blood can no longer bypass the lungs by moving from the pulmonary trunk directly into the aorta.

These changes lead to an immediate increase in systemic vascular resistance and a decrease in pulmonary vascular resistance. Although the constriction of the ductus arteriosus may be functionally complete within 15 minutes, the permanent closure of the foramen ovale may take from 30 days to 1 year. The left ventricle of the heart will strengthen throughout the first year.

(You may wish to note that in an adult, the ductus venosus becomes a fibrous cord called the *ligamentum venosum,* which is superficially embedded in the wall of the liver. Also, in an adult, the site of the foramen ovale is marked by a depression called the *fossa ovalis,* and the ductus arteriosus is represented by a cord called the *ligamentum arteriosum.*)

Pulmonary System

The first breath an infant takes must be forceful, because until that moment the lungs have been collapsed. Fortunately, the lungs of a full-term fetus continuously secrete surfactant. Surfactant is a chemical that reduces the surface tension that tends to hold the moist membranes of the lungs together. After the first powerful breath begins to expand the lungs, breathing becomes easier.

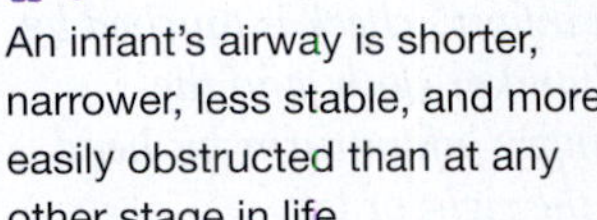

An infant's airway is shorter, narrower, less stable, and more easily obstructed than at any other stage in life.

In general, an infant's airway is shorter, narrower, less stable, and more easily obstructed than at any other stage in life. The infant is primarily a "nose breather" until at least 4 weeks of age; therefore, it is important for the nasal passages to stay clear. A common complaint in infants less than 6 months of age is nasal congestion. This occurs because, as mentioned, young infants are obligate nasal breathers. Even a mild nasal obstruction, as occurs with a viral upper respiratory infection, can cause difficulty breathing, especially during feeding.

An infant's lung tissue is fragile and prone to *barotrauma* (an injury caused by a change in atmospheric pressure). Because of this, prehospital personnel must be careful when applying mechanical ventilation with a bag-valve-mask unit. There are fewer alveoli with decreased collateral ventilation. In addition, the accessory muscles for breathing are immature and susceptible to early fatigue, so they cannot sustain a rapid respiratory rate over a long period of time. Breathing becomes ineffective at rates higher than 60 breaths per minute because air moves only in the upper airway, never reaching the lungs. Rapid respiratory rates also lead to rapid heat and fluid loss.

The chest wall of the infant is less rigid than an adult's, and the ribs are positioned horizontally, causing diaphragmatic breathing. So when you assess respiratory rate and effort in an infant, it is important to observe the abdomen rise and fall. An infant needs less pressure and a lower volume of air for ventilation than an adult does, but the infant has a higher metabolic rate and a higher oxygen-consumption rate than an adult.

Renal System

Usually, the newborn's kidneys are not able to produce concentrated urine, so the baby excretes a relatively dilute fluid with a specific gravity that rarely exceeds 1.0. (Specific gravity is the weight of a substance compared to an equal amount of water. For comparisons, water is considered to have a specific gravity of 1.0.) For this reason, the newborn can easily become dehydrated and develop a water and electrolyte imbalance.

Immune System

During pregnancy, certain antibodies pass from the maternal blood into the fetal bloodstream. As a result, the fetus acquires some of the mother's active immunities against pathogens. Thus, the fetus is said to have naturally acquired passive immunities, which may remain effective for 6 months to a year after birth. A breast-fed baby also receives antibodies through the breast milk to many of the diseases the mother has had.

Nervous System

Sensation is present in all portions of the body at birth, so a young infant feels pain but lacks the ability to localize it and isolate a response to it. As nerve connections develop, the response to pain becomes much more localized. In addition, motor and sensory development are most advanced in the cranial nerves at birth, because of their life-sustaining function and protective reflexes. Since the cranial nerves control such things as blinking, sucking, and swallowing, the infant has strong, coordinated sucking and gag reflexes. The infant also will have well-flexed extremities, which move equally when the infant is stimulated.

Moro reflex *occurs when a newborn is startled, arms are thrown wide, fingers are spread, and a grabbing motion follows. Also called startle reflex.*

palmar grasp *a reflex in the newborn, which is elicited by placing a finger firmly in the infant's palm.*

rooting reflex *occurs when an infant's cheek is touched by a hand or cloth, and the hungry infant turns his head to the right or left.*

sucking reflex *occurs when an infant's lips are stroked.*

Reflexes The infant has several reflexes that disappear over time. These include the Moro, palmar, rooting, and sucking reflexes. The **Moro reflex,** which is sometimes referred to as the "startle reflex," is the characteristic reflex of newborns. When the baby is startled, he throws his arms wide, spreading his fingers and then grabbing instinctively with the arms and fingers. The reflex should be brisk and symmetrical. An asymmetric Moro reflex (in which one arm does not respond exactly like the other) may imply a paralysis or weakness on one side of the body.

The **palmar grasp** is a strong reflex in the full-term newborn. It is elicited by placing a finger firmly in the infant's palm. The palmar grasp weakens as the hand becomes less continuously fisted. Sometime after 2 months, it merges into the voluntary ability to release an object held in the hand.

The **rooting reflex** causes the hungry infant to turn his head to the right or left when a hand or cloth touches his cheek. If the mother's nipple touches either side of the infant's face, above or below the mouth, the infant's lips and tongue tend to follow in that direction. Stroking the infant's lips causes a sucking movement, or the **sucking reflex,** in the infant. Both the rooting and sucking reflexes should be present in all full-term babies and are most easily elicited before a feeding. They usually last until the infant is 3 or 4 months old; however, the rooting reflex may persist during sleep for 7 or 8 months.

Fontanelles Fontanelles allow for compression of the head during childbirth and for rapid growth of the brain during early life. They are diamond-shaped soft spots of fibrous tissue at the top of the infant's skull where three or four bones will eventually fuse together. The fibrous tissue is strong and, generally, can protect the brain adequately from injury. The posterior fontanelle usually closes in 2 or 3 months, and the anterior one closes between 9 and 18 months. You may wish to note that the fontanelles, especially the anterior one, may be used to provide an indirect estimate of hydration. Normally, the anterior fontanelle is level with the surface of the skull, or slightly sunken. With dehydration, the anterior fontanelle may fall below the level of the skull and appear sunken.

Sleep A newborn usually sleeps for 16 to 18 hours daily, with periods of sleep and wakefulness evenly distributed over a 24-hour period. Sleep time will gradually decrease to 14 to 16 hours per day, with a 9- to 10-hour period at night. Infants usually begin to sleep through the night within 2 to 4 months. The normal infant is easily aroused.

Musculoskeletal System

The developing infant's extremities grow in length from growth plates, which are located on each end of the long bones. The infant also has *epiphyseal plates,* or secondary bone-forming centers that are separated by cartilage from larger (or parent) bones. As each epiphysis grows, it becomes part of the larger bone. Bones grow in thickness by way of deposition of new bone on existing bone. Factors affecting bone development and growth include nutrition, exposure to sunlight, growth hormone, thyroid hormone, genetic factors, and general health. Muscle weight in infants is about 25 percent of the entire musculoskeletal system.

Other Developmental Characteristics

Expect rapid changes during an infant's first year of life. At about 2 months of age, he is able to track objects with his eyes and recognize familiar faces. At about 3 months of age, he can move objects to his mouth with his hands and display primary emotions with distinct facial expressions (such as a smile or a frown). At 4 months of age, he drools without swallowing and begins to reach out to people. By 5 months, he should be sleeping through the night without waking for a feeding, and he should be able to discriminate between family and strangers. Teeth begin to appear between 5 and 7 months of age.

At 6 months, the baby can sit upright in a high chair and begin to make one-syllable sounds, such as "ma," "mu," "da," and "di." At 7 months, he has a fear of strangers and his moods can quickly shift from crying to laughing. At 8 months, the infant begins to respond to the word "no," he can sit alone, and he can play "peek-a-boo." At 9 months, he responds to adult anger.

At about 9 months old, the baby begins to pull himself up to a standing position, and explores objects by mouthing, sucking, chewing, and biting them. At 10 months, he pays attention to his name and crawls well. At 11 months, he attempts to walk without assistance and begins to show frustration about restrictions. By 12 months, he can walk with help, and he knows his own name.

PSYCHOSOCIAL DEVELOPMENT

Family Processes and Reciprocal Socialization

The psychosocial development of an individual begins at birth and develops as a result of instincts, drives, capacities, and interactions with the environment. A key component of that environment is the family. The interactions babies have with their families help them to grow and change and help their families do the same. This is called "reciprocal socialization," a model that recognizes the child's active role in its own development.

Raising a baby requires a lot of hard work, but studies show that healthy, happy, and self-reliant children are the products of stable homes in which parents give a great deal of time and attention to their children.

Crying A newborn's only means of communication is through crying. While every cry may seem the same to a stranger, most mothers quickly learn to notice the differences in a basic cry, an anger cry, and a pain cry.

Attachment Infants have their own unique timetables and paths for becoming attached to their parents. **Bonding** is initially based on **secure attachment,** or an infant's sense that his needs will be met by his caregivers. Secure attachment is consistent with healthy development, and leads to a child who is bold in his explorations of the world and competent in dealing with it. It is important for this sense of security to develop within the first 6 months of an infant's life.

When an infant is uncertain about whether or not his caregivers will be responsive or helpful when needed, another type of attachment develops. It is called **anxious resistant attachment.** It leads to a child who is always prone to separation anxiety, causing him to be clinging and anxious about exploring the world.

A third type of attachment is called **anxious avoidant attachment.** It occurs when the infant has no confidence that he will be responded to helpfully when he seeks care. In fact, the infant expects to be rebuffed. This causes him to attempt to live without the love and support of others. The most extreme cases result from repeated rejection or prolonged institutionalization and can lead to a variety of personality disorders from compulsive self-sufficiency to persistent delinquency.

Trust vs. Mistrust Some psychologists believe that human life progresses through a series of stages, each marked by a crisis that needs to be resolved. Each of the crises involves a conflict between two opposing characteristics. From birth to approximately 1½ years of age, the infant goes through the stage called **trust vs. mistrust.** According to psychologists, the infant wants the world to be an orderly, predictable place where causes and effects can be anticipated. When this is true, the

bonding *the formation of a close personal relationship (as between mother and child), especially through frequent or constant association.*

secure attachment *a type of bonding that occurs when an infant learns that his caregivers will be responsive and helpful when needed.*

anxious resistant attachment *a type of bonding that occurs when an infant learns to be uncertain about whether or not his caregivers will be responsive or helpful when needed.*

anxious avoidant attachment *a type of bonding that occurs when an infant learns that his caregivers will not be responsive or helpful when needed.*

trust vs. mistrust *refers to a stage of psychosocial development that lasts from birth to about 1½ years of age.*

scaffolding *a teaching/learning technique in which one builds on what has already been learned.*

easy child *an infant, who can be characterized by regularity of bodily functions, low or moderate intensity of reactions, and acceptance of new situations.*

difficult child *an infant, who can be characterized by irregularity of bodily functions, intense reactions, and withdrawal from new situations.*

slow-to-warm-up child *an infant, who can be characterized by a low intensity of reactions and a somewhat negative mood.*

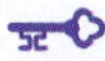

Parental-separation reactions in an infant include protest, despair, and withdrawal.

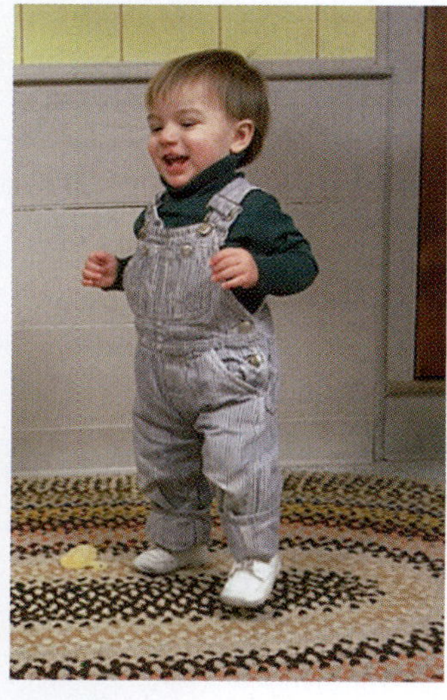

■ **Figure 5-2** Toddlers begin to stand and walk on their own. *(© Michal Heron)*

Remember that toddlers and preschool-age children have immature chest muscles and cannot sustain an excessively rapid respiratory rate for long.

infant develops trust based on consistent parental care. When an infant begins life with irregular and inadequate care, he develops anxiety and insecurity, which have a negative effect on family and other relationships important to the development of trust. This may lead to feelings of mistrust and hostility, which may in turn develop into antisocial or even criminal behavior.

Scaffolding

Infants learn in many ways from their parents and others around them. One way they learn—from infancy and throughout their school years—is through **scaffolding,** or building on what they already know. For example, parents or caregivers usually talk to infants as a natural part of caring for them. With scaffolding, the dialogue is maintained just above the level where the child can perform activities independently. As the baby learns, the parent or caregiver changes the nature of the dialogues so that they continue to support the baby but also give him responsibility for the task. In this way, infants continue to build on what they know.

Temperament

An infant may be classified as an easy child, a difficult child, or a slow-to-warm-up child. An **easy child** is characterized by regularity of bodily functions, low or moderate intensity of reactions, and acceptance of new situations. A **difficult child** is characterized by irregularity of bodily functions, intense reactions, and withdrawal from new situations. A **slow-to-warm-up child** is characterized by a low intensity of reactions and a somewhat negative mood.

Situational Crisis and Parental-Separation Reactions

Infants who have good relationships with their parents usually follow a predictable sequence of behaviors when they experience a situational crisis (a crisis caused by a particular set of circumstances), such as being separated from parents. The first stage of parental-separation reaction is protest; the second stage is despair; and the last is detachment or withdrawal.

Protest may begin immediately upon separation and continue for about 1 week. Loud crying, restlessness, and rejection of all adults show how distressed the infant is. In the second stage, despair, the infant's behavior suggests growing hopelessness marked by monotonous crying, inactivity, and steady withdrawal. In the final stage, detachment or withdrawal, the infant displays renewed interest in its surroundings, even though it is usually a remote, distant kind of interest. This phase is apathetic and may persist even if the parent reappears.

TODDLER AND PRESCHOOL AGE

PHYSIOLOGICAL DEVELOPMENT

Vital signs for toddlers (12 to 36 months, Figure 5-2 ■) and preschool age children (3 to 5 years old, Figure 5-3 ■) are not the same as an infant's. The heart rate for toddlers ranges from 80 to 110 beats per minute. Respiratory rate ranges from 24 to 40 breaths per minute. Systolic blood pressure ranges from 95 to 105 mmHg. For preschoolers, heart rate ranges from 70 to 110 beats per minute, respiratory rate from 22 to 34 breaths per minute, and systolic blood pressure from 75 to 110 mmHg. Normal temperature for both ranges from 96.8°F to 99.6°F (36.3°C to 37.9°C). In addition, the rate of weight gain is slowing dramatically. The average toddler or preschooler gains approximately 2.0 kg per year.

Changes in body systems include the following:

- ★ *Cardiovascular system.* The capillary beds are now better developed and assist in thermoregulation of the body more efficiently. Hemoglobin levels approach normal adult levels at this point. The ability to compensate for blood loss and shock is not yet well developed.
- ★ *Pulmonary system.* The terminal airways continue to branch off from the bronchioles and alveoli increase in number, providing more surfaces for gas exchange to take place in the lungs. However, children have immature chest muscles and cannot sustain an excessively rapid respiratory rate for long. They will tire quickly and their respiratory rate will decrease, indicating the onset of ventilatory failure.

- ★ *Renal system.* The kidneys are well developed by the toddler years. Specific gravity and other characteristics of urine are similar to what would be found in an adult.
- ★ *Immune system.* By this point in life, the passive immunity born with the infant is lost, and the child becomes more susceptible to minor respiratory and gastrointestinal infections. This occurs at the same time the child is being exposed to the infections of other children in child care and preschool. Fortunately, the toddler and preschooler will develop their own immunities to common pathogens as they are exposed to them.
- ★ *Nervous system.* The brain is now at 90 percent of adult weight. Myelination (the development of the covering of nerves) has increased, which allows for effortless walking as well as other basic skills. Fine motor skills, including the use of hands and fingers in grasping and manipulating objects, begin developing at this stage.
- ★ *Musculoskeletal system.* Both muscle mass and bone density increase during this period.
- ★ *Dental system.* All of the primary teeth have erupted by the age of 36 months.
- ★ *Senses.* Visual acuity is at 20/30 during the toddler years. Hearing reaches maturity at 3 to 4 years old.

In addition, though children are physiologically capable of being toilet trained by the age of 12 to 15 months, they are not psychologically ready until 18 to 30 months of age. So, it is important not to rush toilet training. Children will let their parents know when they are ready. The average age for completion of toilet training is 28 months.

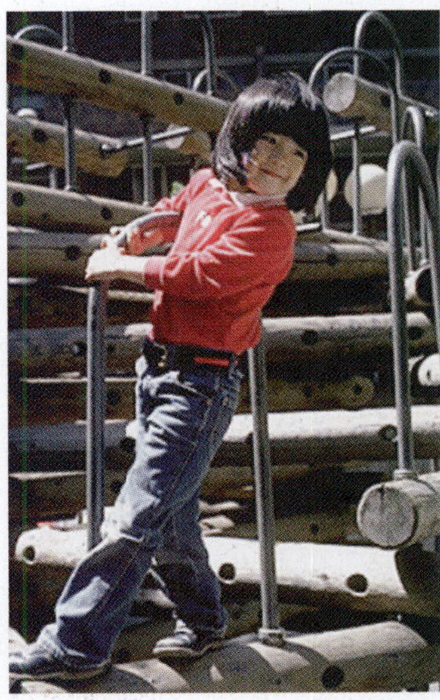

■ Figure 5-3 In the preschool-age child, exploratory behavior accelerates. *(© Michal Heron)*

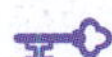

The average age for completion of toilet training is 28 months.

PSYCHOSOCIAL DEVELOPMENT

Cognition

Children begin to use actual words at about 10 months, but they do not begin to grasp that words "mean" something until they are about 1 year of age. Usually, by the time they are 3 or 4 years old, they have mastered the basics of language, which they will continue to refine throughout their childhood. Between 18 and 24 months, they begin to understand cause and effect. Between the ages of 18 and 24 months, they develop separation anxiety, becoming clinging and crying when a parent leaves. Between 24 and 36 months, they begin to develop "magical thinking" and engage in play-acting, such as playing house and similar activities.

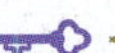

By the age of 3 or 4, children have mastered the basics of language.

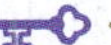

Between the ages of 18 and 24 months, children develop separation anxiety.

Play

Exploratory behavior accelerates at this stage. The child is able to play simple games and follow basic rules, and he begins to display signs of competitiveness. Play provides an emotional release for youngsters, because it lacks the right-or-wrong, life-and-death feelings that may accompany interactions with adults. Therefore, observations of children at play may uncover frustrations otherwise unexpressed.

Sibling Relationships

While there are many positive aspects to growing up with siblings, there also may be negative ones, which can lead to sibling rivalry. The first-born child often finds it very difficult to share the attention of his parents with a younger sibling. If the older child must also help care for the younger ones, he may become even more frustrated. While first-born children usually maintain a special relationship with parents, they also are expected to exercise more self-control and show more responsibility when interacting with younger siblings. Younger children often see only the apparent privileges extended to the older children, such as later bedtimes and more freedom to come and go. Still, when asked if they would be happier if their siblings did not exist, most prefer to keep them around.

Peer-Group Functions

Peers, or youngsters who are similar in age (within 12 months of each other), are very important to the development of toddler and school-age children. In fact, peer groups actually become more important as childhood progresses. Peers provide a source of information about other families and the outside world. Interaction with peers offers opportunities for learning skills, comparing oneself to others, and feeling part of a group.

Parenting Styles and Their Effects

authoritarian *a parenting style that demands absolute obedience without regard to a child's individual freedom.*

authoritative *a parenting style that emphasizes a balance between a respect for authority and individual freedom.*

permissive *a parenting style that takes a tolerant, accepting view of a child's behavior.*

There are three basic styles of parenting: **authoritarian, authoritative,** and **permissive:**

- ★ *Authoritarian* parents are demanding and desire instant obedience from a child. No consideration is given to the child's view, and no attempt is made to explain why. Frequently, the child is punished for even asking the reason for some decision or directive. This parenting style often leads to children with low self-esteem and low competence. Boys are often hostile and girls are often shy.
- ★ *Authoritative* parents respond to the needs and wishes of their children. While they believe in parental control, they attempt to explain their reasons to the child. They expect mature behavior and will enforce rules, but they still encourage independence and actualization of potential. These parents believe that both they and children have rights and try to maintain a happy balance between the two. This parenting style usually leads to children who are self-assertive, independent, friendly, and cooperative.
- ★ *Permissive* parents take a tolerant, accepting view of their children's behavior, including aggressive behavior and sexual behavior. They rarely punish or make demands of their children, allowing them to make almost all of their own decisions. They may be either "permissive-indifferent" or "permissive-indulgent" parents, but it is very difficult to make the distinction. This parenting style may lead to impulsive, aggressive children who have low self-reliance, low self-control, low maturity, and lack responsible behavior.

Divorce and Child Development

Nearly half of today's marriages end in divorce. As a result of divorce, a child's physical way of life often changes (a new home, for example, or a reduced standard of living). The child's psychological life is also touched. The effects on the child's development, however, depend greatly on the child's age, his cognitive and social competencies, the amount of dependency on his parents, how the parents interact with each other and the child, and even the type of child care. Toddlers and preschoolers commonly express feelings of shock, depression, and a fear that their parents no longer love them. They may feel they are being abandoned. They are unable to see the divorce from their parents' perspective, and therefore believe the divorce centers on them. The parent's ability to respond to a child's needs greatly influences the ultimate effects of divorce on the child.

Television

Virtually every family has at least one television in the home. Most children watch television for several hours each day, many with few, if any, parental restrictions. Television violence increases levels of aggression in toddlers and preschoolers, and it increases passive acceptance of the use of aggression by others. Parental screening of the television programs children watch may be effective in avoiding these outcomes.

Modeling

modeling *a procedure whereby a subject observes a model perform some behavior and then attempts to imitate that behavior. Many believe it is the fundamental learning process involved in socialization.*

Toddlers and preschool-age children begin to recognize sexual differences, and, through **modeling,** they begin to incorporate gender-specific behaviors they observe in parents, siblings, and peers.

SCHOOL AGE

PHYSIOLOGICAL DEVELOPMENT

Between the ages of 6 and 12 years, a child's heart rate is between 65 and 110 beats per minute, respiratory rate is between 18 and 30 breaths per minute, and systolic blood pressure ranges from

97 to 112 mmHg. Body temperature is approximately 98.6°F (37°C). The average child of this age gains 3 kg per year and grows 6 cm per year. In most children, vital signs reach adult levels during this period of time, but their lymph tissues are proportionately larger than those of an adult. In addition, brain function increases in both hemispheres, and primary teeth are being replaced by permanent ones. Fine and gross motor skills, which lag slightly behind mental growth, are developed by play.

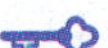

Vital signs in most children reach adult levels during the school-age years.

PSYCHOSOCIAL DEVELOPMENT

School-age children (Figure 5-4 ■) have developed decision-making skills, and usually are allowed more self-regulation, with parents providing general supervision. Parents spend less time with school-age children than they did with toddlers and preschoolers.

The development of a self-concept occurs at this age. School-age children have more interaction with both adults and other children, and they tend to compare themselves to others. They are beginning to develop self-esteem, which tends to be higher during the early years of school than in the later years. Self-esteem may be affected by popularity with peers, rejection, emotional support, and neglect. Negative self-esteem can be very damaging to further development.

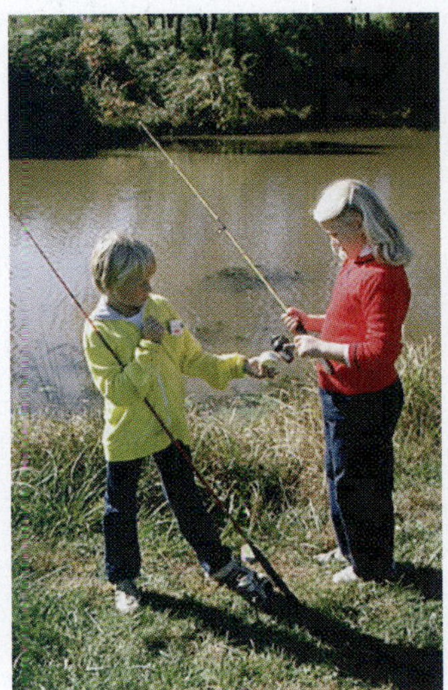

■ Figure 5-4 School-age children are allowed more self-regulation and independence as they grow older. *(© Michal Heron)*

As children mature, moral development begins when they are rewarded for what their parents believe to be right and punished for what their parents believe to be wrong. With cognitive growth, moral reasoning appears and the control of the child's behavior gradually shifts from external sources to internal self-control. According to one theory, there are three levels of moral development: **preconventional reasoning, conventional reasoning,** and **postconventional reasoning,** with each level having two stages:

- ★ *Preconventional reasoning.* Stage one is punishment and obedience; that is, children obey rules in order to avoid punishment. There is no concern about morals. Stage two is individualism and purpose; that is, children obey the rules but only for pure self-interest. They are aware of fairness to others but only as it pertains to their own satisfaction.
- ★ *Conventional reasoning.* In stage three, children are concerned with interpersonal norms, seeking the approval of others and developing the "good boy" or "good girl" mentality. They begin to judge behavior by intention. In stage four, they develop the social system's morality, becoming concerned with authority and maintaining the social order. They realize that correct behavior is "doing one's duty."
- ★ *Postconventional reasoning.* Stage five is concerned with community rights as opposed to individual rights. Children at this level believe that the best values are those supported by law because they have been accepted by the whole society. They believe that if there is a conflict between human need and the law, individuals should work to change the law. Stage six is concerned with universal ethical principles, such as that an informed conscience defines what is right, or people act not because of fear, approval, or law, but from their own standards of what is right or wrong.

According to this theory, individuals will move through the levels and stages of moral development throughout school age and young adulthood at their own rates.

preconventional reasoning *the stage of moral development during which children respond mainly to cultural control to avoid punishment and attain satisfaction.*

conventional reasoning *the stage of moral development during which children desire approval from individuals and society.*

postconventional reasoning *the stage of moral development during which individuals make moral decisions according to an enlightened conscience.*

ADOLESCENCE

PHYSIOLOGICAL DEVELOPMENT

Vital signs in adolescents (13 to 18 years old) are as follows: heart rate is between 60 and 90 beats per minute, respiratory rate is between 12 and 26 breaths per minute, and systolic blood pressure is between 112 and 128 mmHg. Body temperature is approximately 98.6°F (37°C). In addition, the adolescent usually experiences a rapid 2- to 3-year growth spurt, beginning distally with enlargement of the feet and hands followed by enlargement of the arms and legs. The chest and trunk enlarge in the final stage of growth. Girls are usually finished growing by the age of 16 and boys by the age of 18. In late adolescence, the average male is taller and stronger than the average female.

Both males and females reach reproductive maturity during adolescence.

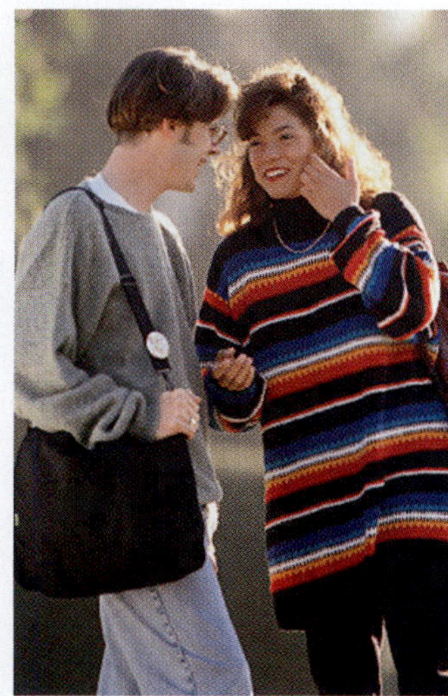

■ **Figure 5-5** Children reach reproductive maturity during adolescence. *(Index Stock Imagery, Inc.)*

At this age, both males and females reach reproductive maturity (Figure 5-5 ■). Secondary sexual development occurs, with noticeable development of the external sexual organs. Pubic and axillary hairs appear and, mostly in males, vocal quality changes. In females, menstruation has begun, breasts and the ductile system of the mammary glands develops, and there is increased deposition of adipose tissue in the subcutaneous layer of the breasts, thighs, and buttocks. In addition, in the female, endocrine system changes include the release of *follicle-stimulating hormone (FSH), luteinizing hormone (LH),* and *gonadrotropin,* which promotes estrogen and progesterone production. In the male, gonadrotropin promotes testosterone production.

Muscle mass and bone growth are nearly complete at this stage. Body fat decreases in early adolescence and increases later. Females require 18 to 20 percent body fat in order for menarche, or the first menstruation, to occur. Blood chemistry is nearly equal to that of an adult, and skin toughens through sebaceous gland activity. (You may wish to note that a disorder of the sebaceous glands is responsible for acne, which is common in adolescence. In acne, the glands become overactive and inflamed, ducts become plugged, and small red elevations containing blackheads or pimples appear.)

PSYCHOSOCIAL DEVELOPMENT

Family

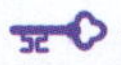

The many biological changes that occur in adolescence cause inner conflict in both the adolescent and parents.

Adolescence can be a time of serious family conflicts as the adolescent strives for autonomy and parents strive for continued control. The many biological changes that occur at this stage cause inner conflict in both the adolescent and parents. Privacy becomes extremely important at this stage of life and, because of modesty, the adolescent prefers that parents not be present during physical examinations. It also is likely that when a patient history is being taken, questions asked in the presence of parents or guardians may not be answered honestly.

Children experience an increase in idealism during adolescence. They believe that adults should be able to live up to their expectations, which of course they cannot always do, which leads to disappointment.

Development of Identity

Adolescents want to be treated like adults.

At this age, adolescents are trying to achieve more independence. They take "time out" to experiment with a variety of identities, knowing that they do not have to assume responsibility for the consequences of those identities. As they attempt to develop their own identity, self-consciousness and peer pressure increase. They become interested in the opposite sex, and they find this somewhat embarrassing. They really do not know how to handle this increased interest. They want to be treated like adults and do not know how to achieve this.

How well and how fast adolescents progress through the various stages of identity development depends on how well they are able to handle crises. Minority adolescents tend to have more identity crises than others. In general, antisocial behavior usually peaks at around the eighth or ninth grade.

Depression and suicide are more common during adolescence than in any other age group.

Body image is a great concern at this point in life. Peers continually make comparisons, and certainly the media lead to unrealistic ideas of what the "perfect" body should look like. This is a time when eating disorders are common. It also is a time when self-destructive behaviors begin, such as the use of tobacco, alcohol, and illicit drugs. Depression and suicide are more common at this age group than in any other.

Ethical Development

As adolescents develop their capacity for logical, analytical, and abstract thinking, they begin to develop a personal code of ethics. Just as they get disappointed when adults do not live up to their expectations, they tend to get disappointed in anyone who does not meet their personal code of ethics.

EARLY ADULTHOOD

Between the ages of 19 and 40 years, heart rate averages 70 beats per minute, respiratory rate averages between 12 and 20 breaths per minute, blood pressure averages 120/80 mmHg, and body temperature averages 98.6°F (37°C). This is the period of life during which adults develop lifelong habits and routines.

Peak physical condition occurs between the ages of 19 and 26 years of age, when all body systems are at optimal performance levels. At the end of this period, the body begins its slowing process. Spinal disks settle, leading to a decrease in height. Fatty tissue increases, leading to weight gain. Muscle strength decreases, and reaction times level off and stabilize. Accidents are a leading cause of death in this age group.

Peak physical condition occurs between the ages of 19 and 26, when all body systems are at optimal performance levels.

Accidents are a leading cause of death in early adulthood.

The highest levels of job stress occur at this point in life, the time in which the young adult strives to find his place in the world. Love develops, both romantic and affectionate. Childbirth is most common in this age group, with new families providing new challenges and stress. In spite of all this, this period is not associated with psychological problems related to well-being.

MIDDLE ADULTHOOD

Between the ages of 41 and 60 years, average vital signs are as follows: heart rate, 70 beats per minute; respiratory rate between 12 and 20 breaths per minute; blood pressure at 120/80 mmHg; and body temperature averages 98.6°F (37°C).

The body still functions at a high level with varying degrees of degradation based on the individual. There are usually some vision and hearing changes during this period. Cardiovascular health becomes a concern, with cardiac output decreasing and cholesterol levels increasing. Cancer often strikes this age group, weight control becomes more difficult, and for women in the late 40s to early 50s, menopause commences.

Cardiovascular health becomes a concern during middle adulthood.

Adults in this age group are more concerned with the "social clock" and become more task oriented as they see the time for accomplishing their lifetime goals recede. Still, they tend to approach problems more as challenges than as threats. This is also the time of life for "empty-nest syndrome," or the time after the last offspring has left home. Some women feel depression or a sense of loss and purposelessness at this time, feelings that are made worse by aging and menopause. Sometimes a father also becomes depressed, but the syndrome seems to affect mothers to a greater extent. Many parents, however, view the period after children have left home as a time of increased freedom and opportunity for self-fulfillment. Unfortunately, adults in this age group often find themselves burdened by financial commitments for elderly parents, as well as for young adult children.

LATE ADULTHOOD

Maximum life span is the theoretical, species-specific, longest duration of life, excluding premature or "unnatural" death. For human beings, maximum life span is approximately 120 years. **Life expectancy,** which is based on the year of birth, is defined as the average number of additional years of life expected for a member of a population. Human beings almost always die of disease or accident before they reach their biological limit.

maximum life span *the theoretical, species-specific, longest duration of life, excluding premature or "unnatural" death.*

life expectancy *based on the year of birth, the average number of additional years of life expected for a member of a population.*

PHYSIOLOGICAL DEVELOPMENT

Vital Signs

At 61 years of age and older, vital signs—heart rate, respiratory rate, and blood pressure—depend on the individual's physical health status. Body temperature still averages 98.6°F (37°C).

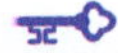

At 61 years of age and older, vital signs—heart rate, respiratory rate, and blood pressure—depend on the individual's physical health status.

Cardiovascular System

During late adulthood, the cardiovascular system changes in ways that affect its overall function. The walls of the blood vessels thicken, causing increased peripheral vascular resistance and reduced blood flow to organs. There is decreased baroreceptor sensitivity and, by 80 years of age, there is approximately a 50 percent decrease in vessel elasticity.

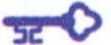

During late adulthood, the cardiovascular system changes in ways that affect its overall function.

In addition, the heart tends to show disease in the heart muscle, heart valves, and coronary arteries. Increased workload causes cardiomegaly (enlargement), mitral and aortic valve changes, and decreased myocardial elasticity. The myocardium is less able to respond to exercise, and the SA node and other cells responsible for producing heartbeats become infiltrated with fibrous connective tissue and fat. Pacemaker cells diminish, resulting in dysrhythmia. Because of prolonged contraction time, decreased response to various medications that would ordinarily stimulate the heart, and increased resistance to electrical stimulation, the heart also becomes less able to contract. Tachycardia (abnormally rapid heart action) is not well tolerated.

Functional blood volume decreases in late adulthood. Decreases also can be expected in platelet count and the number of red blood cells (RBCs), which can lead to poor iron levels.

Respiratory System

The trachea and large airways increase in diameter in late adulthood, and enlargement of the end units of the airway results in a decreased surface area of the lungs. Decreased elasticity of the lungs leads to an increase in lung volume and to a reduction in surface area. The decreased elasticity also causes the chest to expand and the diaphragm to descend. The ends of the ribs calcify to the breastbone, producing stiffening of the chest wall, which increases the workload of the respiratory muscles.

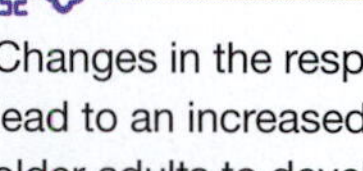

Changes in the respiratory system lead to an increased likelihood for older adults to develop lung disease and progressive declines in lung function.

These changes lead to an increased likelihood for older adults to develop lung disease and progressive declines in lung function. Metabolic changes also may lead to decreased lung function, and because of lifelong exposure to pollutants, diffusion through alveoli is diminished. Coughing also becomes ineffective because of a weakened chest wall and bone structure. Of all the factors that influence lung function, smoking continues to produce the greatest amount of disability.

Endocrine System

During this stage of life, there is a decrease in glucose metabolism and insulin production. The thyroid shows some diminished triiodothyronine (T3) production, cortisol (from the adrenal cortex) is diminished by 25 percent, the pituitary gland is 20 percent less effective, and reproductive organs atrophy in women.

Gastrointestinal System

One way the gastrointestinal system is affected at this stage of life is by way of tooth loss. Age-related dental changes do not necessarily lead to loss of teeth. Usually tooth loss is caused by cavities or periodontal disease, both of which may be prevented by good dental hygiene. With age, the location of cavities in teeth changes and an increasing amount of root cavities and cavities around existing sites of previous dental work are seen. Tooth loss can lead to changes in diet, an increased chance of malnutrition, and serious vitamin and mineral deficiencies.

This is also true when the individual has false teeth, which do not completely restore normal chewing ability and can reduce taste sensation. In addition, alterations in swallowing are more common in older people without teeth because they tend to swallow larger pieces of food. Swallowing takes 50 to 100 percent longer, probably because of subtle changes in the swallowing mechanism. Peristalsis is decreased and the esophageal sphincter is less effective.

In general, the gastrointestinal system shows less age-associated change in function than other body systems. Stomach contractions appear to be normal, but it does take longer to empty liquids from the stomach. The amount of stomach acid secretions decreases, probably because of the loss of the cells that produce gastric acid. There is usually a small amount of atrophy to the lining of the small intestine. In the large intestine, expect to see atrophy of the lining, changes in the muscle layer, and blood vessel abnormalities. Approximately one of every three people over 60 has diverticula, or outpouchings, in the lining of the large intestine resulting from increased pressure inside the intestine. Weakness in the bowel wall also may be a contributing factor.

The number of some opiate receptors increases with aging, which may lead to significant constipation when narcotics are ingested. Changes may occur in the metabolism and in absorption of some sugars, calcium, and iron. Highly fat soluble compounds such as vitamin A appear to be absorbed faster with age. The activity of some enzymes such as lactase—which aids in the digestion of some sugars, particularly those found in dairy products—appears to decrease. The absorption of fat also may change, and the metabolism of specific compounds, including drugs, can be significantly prolonged in elderly people.

Renal System

With aging, there is a 25 to 30 percent decrease in kidney mass. About 50 percent of nephrons are lost and abnormal glomeruli are more common. Reduced kidney function leads to a decreased clearance of some drugs and decreased elimination. The kidney's hormonal response to dehydration is reduced as is the ability to retain salt under conditions when it should be conserved. The ability of the kidneys to modify vitamin D to a more active form may also lessen.

The Senses

Taste buds diminish during this stage of life, which leads to a loss of taste sensation. Smell declines rapidly after the age of 50 and the parts of the brain involved in smell degenerate significantly so that by age 80, the detection of smell is almost 50 percent poorer than it was at its peak. Since taste and smell work together to make enjoyment of food possible, appetite often declines. Response to painful stimuli is diminished as is kinesthetic sense, or the ability to sense movement.

Visual acuity and reaction time is diminished, and there are actual changes in the organs of hearing. The ear canal atrophies, the eardrum thickens, and there may be degenerative and even arthritic changes in the small joints connecting the bones in the middle ear. Significant changes take place in the inner ear. These changes in structure significantly affect hearing. Hearing loss for pure tones, which increases with age in men and women, is called "presbycusis." With presbycusis, higher frequencies become less audible than lower frequencies. Pitch discrimination plays an important role in speech perception so, with age, speech discrimination declines. When exposed to loud background noise or indistinct speech, older people hear less, but at the same time, they may be very sensitive to loud sounds.

Nervous System

With aging, there is a decrease of neurotransmitters and a loss of neurons in the cerebellum, which controls coordination, and the hippocampus, which is involved in some aspects of memory function. The sleep-wake cycle also is disrupted, causing older adults to have sleep problems.

PSYCHOSOCIAL DEVELOPMENT

While disease may reduce physical and mental capabilities, the ability to learn and adjust continues throughout life, and is greatly influenced by interests, activity, motivation, health, and income (Figure 5-6 ■). However, there is a **terminal-drop hypothesis** that there is a decrease in cognitive

terminal-drop hypothesis *a theory that death is preceded by a 5-year period of decreasing cognitive functioning.*

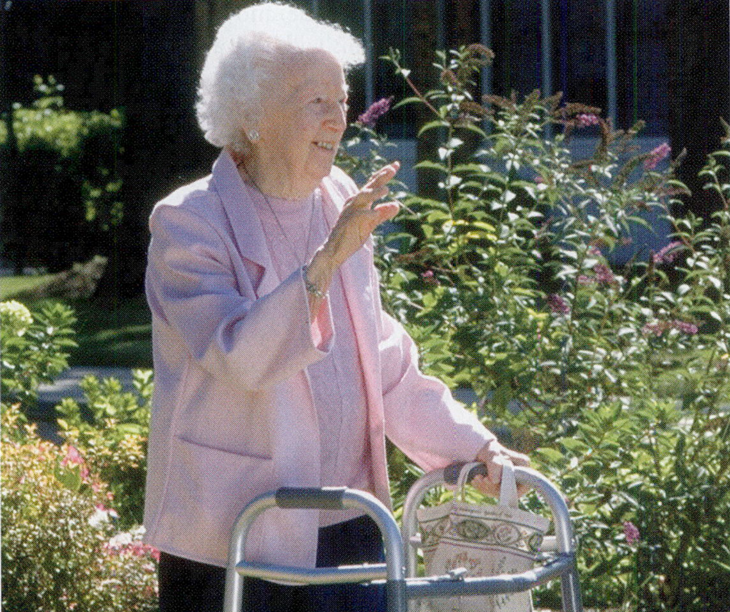

■ **Figure 5-6** The ability to learn and adjust continues throughout life.

functioning over a 5-year period prior to death. The individual may or may not be aware of diffuse changes in mood, mental functioning, or the way his body responds.

Housing

While most older adults would rather stay in their own homes, it is not always possible because home-care services are not affordably available in all communities as a viable alternative to nursing homes. Home-care services usually provide assistance with household chores such as preparing meals, cleaning and laundry, and performing personal care tasks such as feeding and bathing. Health care services in the home are provided by nurses and physical or speech therapists. In order to be eligible for these services under Medicare, the patient must be home-bound, need an intensive level of services, and be expected to benefit from such services over a reasonable amount of time. Home-care services are usually time-limited.

An alternative to home-care services is "assisted living," or living in a facility that offers a combination of home care and nursing home facilities. There is a greater sense of control, independence, and privacy because the older adult has more choices while still being in an institutional setting. Bedrooms and bathrooms can be locked by residents, but dining and recreational facilities are usually shared.

About 95 percent of older adults live in communities, from simple groupings of homes where mostly older adults live to a relatively new type of living arrangement called the "continuing-care retirement community." The appeal of these communities is that future health care needs are covered in a setting that is an attractive residential campus where cultural and recreational activities are available. Entrance fees to this type of community may be as much as $250,000, plus monthly fees which average $1,000.

Challenges

One of the major challenges for the older adult is maintaining a sense of self-worth. Senior citizens are commonly seen as "over the hill," less intelligent than younger adults, and certainly less able to care for themselves. Many older adults are forced into retirement because they are seen as less productive. In reality, although older workers may have slowed down a bit, they are often more concerned than younger workers with producing quality work. Another problem older adults face at this stage of life is a feeling of declining well-being. It is not until adults reach the age of 40 that ill health—as opposed to accidents, homicide, and suicide—becomes the major cause of death. Arteriosclerotic heart disease is the major killer after the age of 40 in all age, sex, and racial groups.

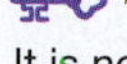

It is not until adults reach the age of 40 that ill health—as opposed to accidents, homicide, and suicide—becomes the major cause of death.

Financial Burdens

The duration of each state in the life cycle, and the ages of family members for each stage, will vary from family to family. Obviously, this will have an effect on the financial status of families. For example, a couple who completes their family while in their early adult years will have a different lifestyle when their last child leaves home than a couple with a "change-of-life" child. Late children can cause serious economic problems for retirees on fixed incomes who are trying to meet the staggering costs of education.

Retirement brings about changes for both spouses, but it seems to be particularly stressful for those wives who are not prepared emotionally or financially. Retirement usually means a decrease in income and in the standard of living, which can be very difficult to handle.

A decreasing level of interest in work is natural as one grows older, but it has a severe impact on the income of older people. Almost 22 percent of all older people live in households below the poverty level. More than 50 percent of all single women above the age of 60 live at or below the poverty level. Older women in the United States make up the single poorest group in our society.

Dying Companions or Death

Whether it is the death of a companion or one's own impending death, fear and grief seem to have a great deal in common. Grief not only follows death, but when there is advance warning, grief may well precede death. Frequently, the death or impending death of a companion leads us to fear for our own lives. Psychiatrist Elisabeth Kübler-Ross believes that regardless of whether it is one's own death or the death of a companion, everyone must go through certain emotions. While the five stages in her theory may sometimes overlap, everyone must deal with each of the stages of death before the grieving process ends. (Review Chapter 1 for Kübler-Ross's five stages.)

Note: Human physiological and psychosocial development will be discussed in more detail in later chapters.

Summary

The changes that take place during the span of a lifetime are innumerable. At some stages, the changes seem to occur almost daily. It is only through experience with patients at all of the various stages of life that you will come to feel comfortable dealing with each of them. Remember that no matter what the stage of development, patience and a sincere desire to help a patient will help you to make the right decisions about emergency care.

Review Questions

1. At birth, the heart rate ranges from ___________ to ___________ beats per minute during the first 30 minutes of life.
   a. 90–120
   b. 100–120
   c. 100–180
   d. 160–240
2. The infant's head is equal to ___________ percent of total body weight.
   a. 10
   b. 15
   c. 20
   d. 25
3. The ___________ ___________, a blood vessel that connects the pulmonary artery and the aorta in the fetus, constricts after birth.
   a. ductus venosus
   b. foramen ovale
   c. ductus arteriosus
   d. ligamentum venosum
4. The ___________ ___________, which is sometimes referred to as the "startle reflex," is the characteristic reflex of newborns.
   a. Moro reflex
   b. rooting reflex
   c. sucking grasp
   d. palmar grasp
5. ___________ parents encourage independence but will enforce rules.
   a. Mutual
   b. Permissive
   c. Authoritative
   d. Authoritarian
6. In this stage of moral development, children are concerned with interpersonal norms, seeking the approval of others, and developing the "good boy" or "good girl" mentality.
   a. permissive reasoning
   b. conventional reasoning
   c. preconventional reasoning
   d. postconventional reasoning

7. The theoretical, species-specific, longest duration of life, excluding premature or "unnatural" death, is:
   a. life expectancy.
   b. early adulthood.
   c. maximum life span.
   d. middle adulthood.
8. As adults reach the age of ____________, ill health—as opposed to accidents, homicide, and suicide—becomes the major cause of death.
   a. 25
   b. 30
   c. 40
   d. 60

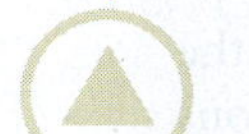

See Answers to Review Questions at the back of this book.

Chapter 6

General Principles of Pharmacology

Please refer to the *Drug Guide for Paramedics* that accompanies this program as a special supplement.

Objectives

Part 1: Basic Pharmacology (begins on p. 309)

After reading Part 1 of this chapter, you should be able to:

1. Describe important historical trends in pharmacology. (p. 309)
2. Differentiate among the chemical, generic (nonproprietary), official (USP), and trade (proprietary) names of a drug. (pp. 309–310)
3. List the four main sources of drug products. (p. 310)
4. List the authoritative sources for drug information. (pp. 310–311)
5. List legislative acts controlling drug use and abuse in the United States. (pp. 311–313)
6. Differentiate among Schedule I, II, III, IV, and V substances and list examples of substances in each schedule. (p. 312)
7. Discuss standardization of drugs. (p. 313)
8. Discuss special considerations in drug treatment with regard to pregnant, pediatric, and geriatric patients. (pp. 314–316)
9. Discuss the paramedic's responsibilities and scope of management pertinent to the administration of medications. (pp. 313–314)
10. Review the specific anatomy and physiology pertinent to pharmacology. (pp. 316–326)
11. List and describe general properties of drugs. (pp. 322–324)
12. List and describe liquid and solid drug forms. (pp. 321–322)
13. List and differentiate routes of drug administration. (pp. 320–321)
14. Differentiate between enteral and parenteral routes of drug administration. (pp. 320–321)
15. Describe mechanisms of drug action. (pp. 322–324)

16. List and differentiate the phases of drug activity, including the pharmaceutical, pharmacokinetic, and pharmacodynamic phases. (pp. 316–326)
17. Describe the processes called pharmacokinetics and pharmocodynamics, including theories of drug action, drug-response relationship, factors altering drug responses, predictable drug responses, iatrogenic drug responses, and unpredictable adverse drug responses. (pp. 316–326)
18. Differentiate among drug interactions. (p. 326)
19. Discuss considerations for storing and securing medications. (p. 322)
20. List the components of a drug profile by classification. (p. 311)

Part 2: Drug Classifications (begins on p. 326)

After reading Part 2 of this chapter, you should be able to:

1. Describe how drugs are classified. (pp. 326–327)
2. Review the specific anatomy and physiology pertinent to pharmacology with additional attention to autonomic pharmacology. (pp. 327–370)
3. List and describe common prehospital medications, including indications, contraindications, side effects, routes of administration, and dosages. (pp. 327–370)
4. Given several patient scenarios, identify medications likely to be prescribed and those that are likely a part of the prehospital treatment regimen. (pp. 327–370)
5. Given various patient medications, assess the pathophysiology of a patient's condition by identifying classifications of drugs. (pp. 326–370)

Key Terms

active transport, p. 317
adjunct medication, p. 328
adrenergic, p. 337
affinity, p. 322
agonist, p. 323
agonist-antagonist (partial agonist), p. 323
analgesia, p. 328
analgesic, p. 328
anesthesia, p. 328
anesthetic, p. 329
antacid, p. 357
antagonist, p. 323
antibiotic, p. 366
anticoagulant, p. 351
antidysrhythmic, p. 343
antiemetic, p. 359
antihistamine, p. 355
antihyperlipidemic, p. 352
antihypertensive, p. 345
antineoplastic, p. 366
antiplatelet, p. 351
antitussive, p. 356
assay, p. 313
autonomic ganglia, p. 337
autonomic nervous system, p. 336
bioassay, p. 313
bioavailability, p. 318
bioequivalence, p. 313
biologic half-life, p. 325
biotransformation, p. 319
blood–brain barrier, p. 319
carrier-mediated diffusion, p. 317
cholinergic, p. 337
competitive antagonism, p. 323
diffusion, p. 317
diuretic, p. 345
dose packaging, p. 314
down-regulation, p. 323
drug, p. 309
drug-response relationship, p. 325
duration of action, p. 325
efficacy, p. 322
enteral route, p. 320
expectorant, p. 356
extrapyramidal symptoms (EPS), p. 333
facilitated diffusion, p. 317
fibrinolytic, p. 351
filtration, p. 317
first-pass effect, p. 319
free drug availability, p. 315
glucagon, p. 362
hemostasis, p. 350
histamine, p. 355
hydrolysis, p. 319
hypnosis, p. 330
immunity, p. 368
insulin, p. 362
ionize, p. 318
irreversible antagonism, p. 323
laxative, p. 358
leukotriene, p. 355
metabolism, p. 319
minimum effective concentration, p. 325
mucolytic, p. 356
neuroeffector junction, p. 337
neuroleptanesthesia, p. 329
neuroleptic, p. 333
neuron, p. 327
neurotransmitter, p. 337
noncompetitive antagonism, p. 323
onset of action, p. 325
osmosis, p. 317
oxidation, p. 319
parasympatholytic, p. 337
parasympathomimetic, p. 337
parenteral route, p. 320
passive transport, p. 317
pathogen, p. 368
pharmacodynamics, p. 317
pharmacokinetics, p. 316
pharmacology, p. 309
placental barrier, p. 319

plasma-level profile, p. 325
postganglionic nerves, p. 337
preganglionic nerves, p. 337
prodrug (parent drug), p. 319
prototype, p. 327
psychotherapeutic medication, p. 333
receptor, p. 322
second messenger, p. 322
sedation, p. 330
serum, p. 368
side effect, p. 324
surfactant, p. 358
sympatholytic, p. 340
sympathomimetic, p. 340
synapse, p. 337
teratogenic drug, p. 314
termination of action, p. 325
therapeutic index, p. 325
up-regulation, p. 323
vaccine, p. 368

INTRODUCTION

The use of herbs and minerals to treat the sick and injured has been documented as long ago as 2000 B.C. Ancient Egyptians, Arabs, and Greeks probably passed formulations down through generations by word of mouth for centuries until they were finally recorded in pharmacopeias. By the end of the Renaissance, pharmacology was a distinct and growing discipline, separate from medicine. During the seventeenth and eighteenth centuries, tinctures of opium, coca, and digitalis were available. The related concept of vaccination with biologic extracts began in 1796 with Edward Jenner's smallpox inoculations. By the nineteenth century, atropine, chloroform, codeine, ether, and morphine were in use. The discoveries of animal insulin and penicillin in the early twentieth century dramatically changed the treatment of endocrine/metabolic and infectious diseases. Now, at the start of the twenty-first century, recombinant DNA technology has produced human insulin and tissue plasminogen activator (tPA). These drugs have markedly changed the treatment of diabetes and cardiovascular disease.

Currently in the United States, the Food and Drug Administration (FDA) is allowing many previously prescription-only drugs to become available over the counter. This is due in part to a growing consumer awareness in health care and also in part to consumer marketing by the pharmaceutical industry. The industry is actively seeking drugs that appeal widely to the consumer for treatments and cures. Pharmaceutical research to limit aging or increase the life span is growing rapidly. The federal government also offers incentives to pharmaceutical companies to research drugs for rare diseases. These so-called "orphan drugs" are often expensive to investigate and have a limited sales potential, making them less profitable to develop and manufacture than others.

General principles of pharmacology are presented in this chapter, which is divided into two parts:

Part 1: Basic Pharmacology
Part 2: Drug Classifications

Part 1: Basic Pharmacology

GENERAL ASPECTS

Part 1 concerns the basics of pharmacology. Drug names (including chemical, generic, official, and brand names) will be explained. The sources of drugs, reference materials for drugs, components of a drug profile, and legal considerations will be described. A major focus of Part 1 will be the safe and effective administration of medications, including the "six rights" (right person, drug, dose, time, route, and documentation) as well as special considerations in medication administration for pregnant, pediatric, and geriatric patients. Finally, basic concepts of pharmacology, specifically pharmacokinetics and pharmacodynamics, will be examined.

NAMES

Drugs are chemicals used to diagnose, treat, or prevent disease. **Pharmacology** is the study of drugs and their actions on the body. To study and converse about pharmacology, health care professionals must have a systematic method for naming drugs. The most detailed name for any drug is its chemical description, which states its chemical composition and molecular structure.

drug *chemical used to diagnose, treat, or prevent disease.*

pharmacology *the study of drugs and their interactions with the body.*

Ethyl-1-methyl-4-phenylisonipecotate hydrochloride, for example, is a chemical name. A generic name is usually suggested by the manufacturer and confirmed by the United States Adopted Name Council. It becomes the Federal Drug Administration's (FDA) official name when listed in the *United States Pharmacopeia* (USP), the official standard for information about pharmaceuticals in the United States. In the case of ethyl-1-methyl-4-phenylisonipecotate hydrochloride, the generic name is meperidine hydrochloride, USP. To foster brand loyalty among its customers, the manufacturer gives the drug a brand name (sometimes called a trade name or proprietary name)—in our example, Demerol. The brand name is a proper name and should be capitalized. Most manufacturers also register the name as a trademark, so the stylized ® or ™ may follow the name, as in Demerol®. Another example is the widely prescribed sedative Valium:

Content Review

Drug Names

- Chemical name
- Generic name
- Official name
- Brand name

- ★ *Chemical name:* 7-chloro-1, 3-dihydro-1-methyl-5-phenyl-2H-1, 4-benzodiazepin-2-one
- ★ *Generic name:* diazepam
- ★ *Official name:* diazepam, USP
- ★ *Brand name:* Valium®

SOURCES

The four main sources of drugs are plants, animals, minerals, and the laboratory (synthetic). Plants may be the oldest source of medications; primitive people probably used them directly as "herbal" medicines. Indirectly, plant extracts such as gums and oils have long been a source of medications. Examples include the purple foxglove, a source of digitalis (a glycoside), and deadly nightshade, a source of atropine (an alkaloid). Animal extracts are another important source of drugs. For many years the primary sources of insulin for treating diabetes mellitus were the extracts of bovine (cow) and porcine (pig) pancreas. Minerals are inorganic sources of drugs such as calcium chloride and magnesium sulfate. Synthetic drugs are created in the laboratory. They may provide alternative sources of medications for those found in nature, or they may be entirely new medications not found in nature.

Content Review

Sources of Drug Information

- *United States Pharmacopeia* (USP)
- *Physicians' Desk Reference*
- *Drug Information*
- *Monthly Prescribing Reference*
- *AMA Drug Evaluation*

REFERENCE MATERIALS

Obtaining information on drugs can be difficult. Using multiple sources of information about drugs is usually a good idea. Every book about drugs, including this one, has a disclaimer regarding doses and current uses, referring the reader to local medical direction for the final word. Using multiple sources and comparing the authors' statements about a drug may lead you to the best available information. EMS providers generally like small, short guides that they can carry in a shirt pocket. These usually include important details about drugs that out-of-hospital providers administer along with a long list of commonly prescribed drugs and their classes. These EMS guides will be useful if you clearly understand the drugs used in your system and have a working knowledge of commonly prescribed drug classes.

It is helpful to carry a pharmaceutical reference in paramedic response vehicles.

Drug inserts, the printed fact sheets that drug manufacturers supply with most medications, contain information prescribed by the United States Food and Drug Administration. The *Physicians' Desk Reference,* a compilation of these drug inserts, also includes three indices and a section containing photographs of drugs. It is among the most popular references, but it contains only factual information and must be interpreted by informed readers. The American Hospital Formulary Service annually publishes *Drug Information* as a service to the American Society of Health System Pharmacists. It contains an authoritative listing of monographs on virtually every drug used in the United States. A less bulky reference to keep in an ambulance might be one of the many drug guides for nurses. They contain information on hundreds of drugs in a format much like the EMS drug guides, but they also offer information on commonly prescribed drugs rather than only on emergency drugs. Also popular is the *Monthly Prescribing Reference.* Designed to assist physicians in prescribing medications, it can also help them determine which medications are available for treating specific diseases. Its information about new medications is especially useful. Most hospitals also maintain a listing of drugs, or formulary, that profiles the particular drugs they have available. The American Medical Association also publishes a useful reference, the *AMA Drug Evaluation*. The Internet provides an enormous amount of information, but you must be especially cautious when using it as a source, because it allows anyone with a computer to be a publisher, with no requirement for accuracy.

COMPONENTS OF A DRUG PROFILE

A drug's profile describes its various properties. As a paramedic student, you will become familiar with drug profiles as you study specific medications. A typical drug profile will contain the following information:

- ★ *Names.* These most frequently include the generic and trade names, although the occasional reference will include chemical names.
- ★ *Classification.* This is the broad group to which the drug belongs. Knowing classifications is essential to understanding the properties of drugs.
- ★ *Mechanism of action.* The way in which a drug causes its effects; its pharmacodynamics.
- ★ *Indications.* Conditions that make administration of the drug appropriate (as approved by the Food and Drug Administration).
- ★ *Pharmacokinetics.* How the drug is absorbed, distributed, and eliminated; typically includes onset and duration of action.
- ★ *Side effects/adverse reactions.* The drug's untoward or undesired effects.
- ★ *Routes of administration.* How the drug is given.
- ★ *Contraindications.* Conditions that make it inappropriate to give the drug. Unlike when the drug is simply not indicated, a contraindication means that a predictable harmful event will occur if the drug is given in this situation.
- ★ *Dosage.* The amount of the drug that should be given.
- ★ *How supplied.* This typically includes the common concentrations of the available preparations; many drugs come in different concentrations.
- ★ *Special considerations.* How the drug may affect pediatric, geriatric, or pregnant patients.

Drug profiles may also include other components, such as its interactions with other drugs or with foods, when appropriate.

LEGAL ASPECTS

Knowing and obeying the laws and regulations governing medications and their administration will be an important part of your career. These laws and regulations come from three distinct authorities: federal law, state laws and regulations, and individual agency regulations.

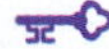

Know and obey the laws and regulations governing medications and their administration.

FEDERAL

Drug legislation in the United States has been aimed primarily at protecting the public from adulterated or mislabeled drugs. The *Pure Food and Drug Act of 1906*, enacted to improve the quality and labeling of drugs, named the *United States Pharmacopeia* as this country's official source for drug information. The *Harrison Narcotic Act of 1914* limited the indiscriminate use of addicting drugs by regulating the importation, manufacture, sale, and use of opium, cocaine, and their compounds or derivatives. The *Federal Food, Drug and Cosmetic Act of 1938* empowered the Food and Drug Administration (FDA) to enforce and set premarket safety standards for drugs. In 1951, the *Durham-Humphrey Amendments* to the 1938 act (also known as the prescription drug amendments) required pharmacists to have either a written or verbal prescription from a physician to dispense certain drugs. It also created the category of over-the-counter medications. The *Comprehensive Drug Abuse Prevention and Control Act* (also known as the Controlled Substances

Content Review

Drug Laws and Regulations

- Federal law
- State laws and regulations
- Individual agency regulations

Table 6–1 Schedules of Drugs According to the Controlled Substances Act of 1970

Schedule	Description	Examples
Schedule I	High abuse potential; may lead to severe dependence; no accepted medical indications; used for research, analysis, or instruction only	Heroin, LSD, mescaline
Schedule II	High abuse potential; may lead to severe dependence; accepted medical indications	Opium, cocaine, morphine, codeine, oxycodone, methadone, secobarbital
Schedule III	Less abuse potential than Schedule I and II; may lead to moderate or low physical dependence or high psychological dependence; accepted medical indications	Limited opioid amounts or combined with noncontrolled substances: Vicodin, Tylenol with codeine
Schedule IV	Low abuse potential compared to Schedule III; limited psychological and/or physical dependence; accepted medical indications	Diazepam, lorazepam, phenobarbital
Schedule V	Lower abuse potential compared to Schedule IV; may lead to limited physical or psychological dependence; accepted medical indications	Limited amounts of opioids; often for cough or diarrhea

Act) of 1970 is the most recent major federal legislation affecting drug sales and use. It repealed and replaced the Harrison Narcotic Act.

The federal government strictly regulates controlled substances because of their high potential for abuse. Since not all drugs cause the same level of physical or psychological dependence, they do not all need to be regulated in the same way. To accommodate their differences, the Controlled Substance Act of 1970 created five schedules of controlled substances, each with its own level of control and record keeping requirements (Table 6–1). Most emergency medical services administer only a few controlled substances, usually a narcotic analgesic such as morphine sulfate and a benzodiazepine anticonvulsant such as diazepam.

The majority of the remaining drugs provided by an EMT are prescription drugs—those whose use the FDA has designated sufficiently dangerous to require the supervision of a health care practitioner (physician, dentist, and in some states, nurse practitioner or certified physician's assistant). For emergency medical services this means the physician medical director is in effect prescribing the drugs in advance, based on the assessments and judgments of EMS providers in the field.

Over-the-counter (OTC) medications are generally available in small doses and, when taken as recommended, present a low risk to patients. Of the few OTC drugs that EMS providers administer, acetaminophen and aspirin are probably the most common. Although laws vary from state to state, they still require most EMS providers to obtain a physician's order (either written, verbal, or standing) to administer OTC drugs.

Consult local protocols, laws, and medical direction for guidance in securing and distributing controlled substances.

Federal drug laws require that certain substances be appropriately secured, distributed, and accounted for. Because of the complexity of this issue and the large variability of drugs used in EMS systems across the country, specific answers to these concerns are not practical here. Consult your local protocols, laws, and most importantly, medical director for guidance in this area.

STATE

State laws vary widely. Some states have legislated which medications are appropriate for paramedics to give, while others have left those decisions to local control. Local control varies as well. In some areas, regional EMS authorities set the local standards; in others the individual medical directors and department directors do. In all cases, however, the physician medical director can delegate to paramedics the authority to administer medications, either by written, verbal, or standing order. You must know the laws of the state where you practice.

LOCAL

In each community, local leaders are responsible for ensuring public safety. Local EMS agencies have the responsibility to create local policies and procedures to ensure the public well-being. An excellent example of a local procedure protecting the patient (and thereby the individual EMS provider and agency) would be a requirement to use a pulse oximeter whenever a patient is sedated or paralyzed. While this requirement would not have the force of law, it would locally help to ensure that local EMS providers do not overlook hypoxia in these patients.

STANDARDS

Because some generic drugs affect patients differently than their brand name counterparts, standardization of drugs is a necessity. Despite FDA standards, drugs sold or distributed by various manufacturers may have biological or therapeutic differences. An **assay** determines the amount and purity of a given chemical in a preparation in the laboratory (in vitro). While two generically equivalent preparations may contain the same amount of a given chemical (drug), they may have different therapeutic effects. This relative therapeutic effectiveness of chemically equivalent drugs is their **bioequivalence.** Bioequivalence is determined by a **bioassay,** which attempts to ascertain the drug's availability in a biological model (in vivo). Again, the *United States Pharmacopeia* (USP) is the official standard for the United States.

assay *test that determines the amount and purity of a given chemical in a preparation in the laboratory.*

bioequivalence *relative therapeutic effectiveness of chemically equivalent drugs.*

bioassay *test to ascertain a drug's availability in a biological model.*

PATIENT CARE: THE SAFE AND EFFECTIVE ADMINISTRATION OF MEDICATIONS

Paramedics are responsible for the standard of care for patients in their charge. They are, therefore, personally responsible—legally, morally, and ethically—for the safe and effective administration of medications. The following guidelines will help you to meet that responsibility:

- ★ Know the precautions and contraindications for all medications you administer.
- ★ Practice proper technique.
- ★ Know how to observe and document drug effects.
- ★ Maintain a current knowledge in pharmacology.
- ★ Establish and maintain professional relationships with other health care providers.
- ★ Understand the pharmacokinetics and pharmacodynamics.
- ★ Have current medication references available.
- ★ Take careful drug histories including:
  - Name, strength, and daily dose of prescribed drugs
  - Over-the-counter drugs
  - Vitamins
  - Herbal medications
  - Folk medicine or folk remedies
  - Allergies
- ★ Evaluate the compliance, dosage, and adverse reactions.
- ★ Consult with medical direction when appropriate.

Content Review

Six Rights of Medication Administration

- Right person
- Right drug
- Right dose
- Right time
- Right route
- Right documentation

SIX RIGHTS OF MEDICATION ADMINISTRATION

No pharmacology chapter would be complete without discussing the six rights of medication administration. They include the right person, the right drug, the right dose, the right time, the right route, and the right documentation.

Right Person As the paramedic's role in health care expands, you will find yourself caring for more people than just "the patient in the back of the truck." You will deal with multiple patients, and the potential for giving medication to the wrong patient will be real. You will have to identify patients by name before administering medications.

Right Drug When following a physician's verbal medication order, repeat the order back to him to confirm that you both intend the same thing for the patient. Inspect the label on the drug at least three times before giving the medication to the patient: first, as you remove the medication from the drug box or cabinet; second, as you draw the medication into the syringe or dole the tablet into a cup; and third, immediately before you administer the medication. Failure to confirm the medication name is one of the most common medication administration errors. If you have any question about a drug, do not administer it without confirmation. Showing the medication container to your partner and asking for confirmation is an easy way to further ensure that you are giving the right drug.

dose packaging *medication packages contain a single dose for a single patient.*

Right Dose To reduce medication errors, many drugs come in unit **dose packaging.** That is, the package contains a single dose for a single patient. Dosages of many emergency drugs, however, are based on patient weight, so a prefilled syringe may not contain the exact amount a patient needs. You will have to calculate the correct dose. One good practice for identifying potential medication errors is to consider the number of unit dose packages needed for a single dose. If your calculations tell you to open 10 vials for one dose of medication, prudence requires you to check the calculation and dose carefully. The package may contain a unit dose of the wrong medication, or you may have miscalculated.

Right Time While paramedics usually give medications in urgent and emergent situations rather than on a schedule, timing can still be very important. Giving nitroglycerin tablets too soon may precipitate hypotension; if epinephrine is not repeated on time during cardiac arrest it may not help to lower the threshold for defibrillation. Take care to give medications punctually and to document their administration promptly.

Right Route You often will have to choose from among several treatments for a particular problem. In these cases, knowing the principles of pharmacokinetics can help greatly in giving your patient the medication via the right route. For example, your knowledge that you should administer epinephrine intravenously rather than subcutaneously to the patient in anaphylactic shock because his blood is being shunted away from the skin will guide you to the proper administration route.

Right Documentation The drugs you administer in the field do not stop affecting your patients when they enter the hospital. As a result, you must completely document all of your care, especially any drugs you have administered and their effects, so that long after you have gone on to your next call, other providers will know what drugs and responses your patient has had.

Content Review

Special Considerations

- Pregnant patients
- Pediatric patients
- Geriatric patients

SPECIAL CONSIDERATIONS

Pregnant Patients Any time you administer drugs to a woman of childbearing years, you must consider the possibility that she is pregnant. Treating pregnant patients clearly means treating two patients. Although emphasis appropriately seems to center on the mother during care, you must understand that many drugs that affect the mother also affect the fetus. A drug's possible benefits to the mother must clearly outweigh its potential risks to the fetus. For example, some situations such as cardiac arrest justify giving the mother medications that may harm the fetus because the drug's possible harm to the fetus is clearly outweighed by the fetus's certain death if the mother dies.

Pregnancy presents two particular pharmacological problems: changes in the mother's anatomy and physiology, and the potential for drugs to harm the fetus. Because the mother is supporting the fetus entirely, her heart rate, cardiac output, and blood volume will increase. This altered maternal physiology can affect the onset and duration of action of many medications. During the first trimester of pregnancy the ingestion of some drugs (**teratogenic drugs**) may potentially deform, injure, or kill the fetus. During the last trimester, drugs administered to the mother may pass

teratogenic drug *medication that may deform or kill the fetus.*

Table 6–2 FDA Pregnancy Categories

Category	Description
A	Adequate studies in pregnant women have not demonstrated a risk to the fetus in the first trimester or later trimesters.
B	Animal studies have not demonstrated a risk to the fetus, *but* there are no adequate studies in pregnant women. OR Adequate studies in pregnant women have not demonstrated a risk to the fetus in the first trimester and there is no risk in the last trimester, *but* animal studies have demonstrated adverse effects.
C	Animal studies have demonstrated adverse effects, *but* there are no adequate studies in pregnant women; however, benefits may be acceptable despite the potential risks. OR No adequate animal studies or adequate studies of pregnant women have been done.
D	Fetal risk has been demonstrated. In certain circumstances, benefits could outweigh the risks.
X	Fetal risk has been demonstrated. This risk outweighs any possible benefit to the mother. Avoid using in pregnant or potentially pregnant patients.

through the placenta to the fetus. Some of these drugs will have unwanted effects on the fetus. Others may not be metabolized and/or excreted, possibly resulting in toxic accumulations. Additionally, a breast-feeding mother's milk may pass some drugs to her infant.

Under some conditions, of course, the health and safety of the mother and fetus demand the use of drugs during the pregnancy. Examples include pregnancy-induced diabetes, hypertension, and seizure disorders. To help health care providers determine when drugs are needed during pregnancy, the FDA has developed the classification system shown in Table 6–2. Always consult medical direction for any questions about drug safety in pregnancy.

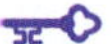

Children are not "small adults." Drug dosages must consider the various physiological differences.

Pediatric Patients Several physiological factors affect pharmacokinetics in newborns and young children. These patients' absorption of oral medications is less than an adult's due to various differences in gastric pH, gastric emptying time, and low enzyme levels. A newborn's skin is thinner than an older patient's and is therefore more permeable to topically administered drugs. This can result in unexpected toxicity. Older children still have less gastric acid than adults do, but their gastric emptying times reach an adult's around the sixth to eighth month of life. Because children up to a year old have diminished plasma protein concentrations, drugs that bind to proteins have higher **free drug availability.** That is, a greater proportion of the drug will be available in the body to cause either desired or undesired effects. Water distribution is different in the neonate as well. Neonates have a much higher proportion of extracellular fluid (nearly 80 percent) than adults (50 to 55 percent). This higher amount of water means a greater volume and, with less-than-expected protein binding, may require higher drug doses. The premature infant is especially susceptible to drugs penetrating the *blood–brain barrier* because his immature connective tissues form a weaker obstacle.

free drug availability *proportion of a drug available in the body to cause either desired or undesired effects.*

The newborn's metabolic rates may be much lower than an adult's, but they rise rapidly and by a few years of age may triple an adult's. These metabolic rates then decline steadily until early adolescence, when they reach adult levels. A newborn's low metabolic rate and incompletely developed hepatic system put him at higher risk for toxic interactions. Neonates' metabolic pathways also are different from an adult's, meaning that some drugs will not have the expected effect or may have other, unexpected effects. Finally, the neonatal renal and hepatic systems' immaturity delays elimination of many drugs and their metabolites. Dosing schedules may have to be adjusted to accommodate longer half-lives until these systems mature at about 6 months to 1 year of age.

■ Figure 6-1 A Broselow tape is useful for calculating drug dosages for pediatric patients.

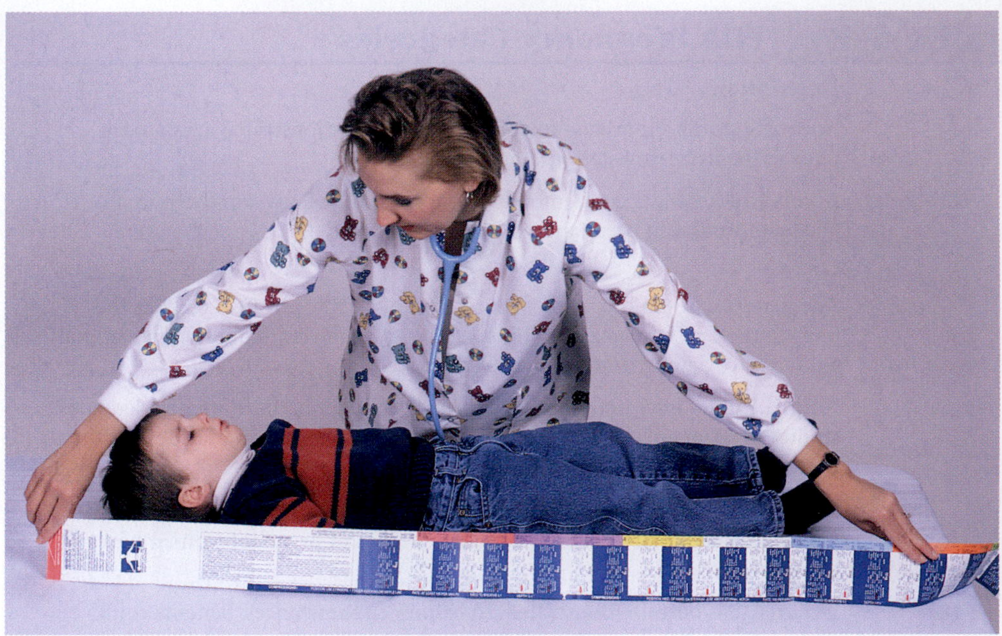

Since dosing for pediatric patients is based on their size and age, dosage ranges vary significantly. It is best to carry a reference containing the various common pediatric dosages.

With all of these factors, a pediatric patient's drug function can differ radically from an adult's. Pediatric drug dosages must be individualized to minimize the risks of toxicity. Body surface area and weight are the two most common factors in calculating dosages. The Broselow tape gives a good approximation for children of average height/weight ratio. It bases its calculations on the child's height (length), and assumes the child's weight is at the fiftieth percentile for his height (Figure 6-1 ■). The Broselow tape primarily addresses drugs administered in the critical care setting.

Geriatric Patients Significant changes in pharmacokinetics may also occur in patients older than about 60 years. They may absorb oral medications slower due to decreased gastrointestinal motility. Decreased plasma protein concentration may alter distribution of drugs in their systems, leaving drugs free that would otherwise have been protein bound. Body fat increases and muscle mass decreases with age; therefore, lipid-soluble drugs may have greater deposition, thereby lowering the amount of available drug. Absorption and distribution of intramuscular injections may change if volumes are inappropriate for the remaining muscle mass. Because the liver primarily handles biotransformation, depressed liver function in an aging patient may delay or prolong drug action. The aging process may also slow elimination by the renal system.

Use caution when administering medications to older patients because they are apt to be on multiple medications.

Older patients are also more likely to be on multiple medications or to have multiple underlying disease processes. Various medication interactions can have a severe impact on patients. For example, sildenafil (Viagra) and nitroglycerin given together may cause severe hypotension. Underlying diseases may affect therapeutics in unexpected ways. Congestive heart failure, for instance, may cause congestion of the gastrointestinal tract's vasculature, delaying the absorption of oral medications. The congestive heart failure patient may also have compromised renal function, delaying his elimination of drugs.

PHARMACOLOGY

pharmacokinetics *how a drug is absorbed, distributed, metabolized (biotransformed), and excreted; how drugs are transported into and out of the body.*

Pharmacology is the study of drugs and their interactions with the body. Drugs do not confer any new properties on cells or tissues; they only modify or exploit existing functions. They may be given for their local action (in which case systemic absorption of the drug is discouraged) or for systemic action. Although generally given for a specific effect, drugs tend to have multiple actions at multiple sites, so they must be thought of in terms of their systemic effects rather than in terms of an isolated single effect. Pharmacology's two major divisions are pharmacokinetics and pharmacodynamics. You have already learned that **pharmacokinetics** addresses how a drug is absorbed, distributed, metabolized (biotransformed), and excreted, that is, how drugs are transported into and out of the body. **Pharmacodynamics** deals with their effects once they reach the target tissues.

pharmacodynamics *how a drug interacts with the body to cause its effects.*

PHARMACOKINETICS

Strictly defined, pharmacokinetics is the study of the basic processes that determine the duration and intensity of a drug's effect. These four processes are absorption, distribution, biotransformation, and elimination.

Content Review

Pharmacokinetic Processes

- Absorption
- Distribution
- Biotransformation
- Elimination

Review of Physiology of Transport

Pharmacokinetics is dependent upon the body's various physiological mechanisms that move substances across the body's compartments. These mechanisms can be broken down into two broad categories based on their energy requirements and then further classified. A mechanism is referred to as **active transport** if it requires the use of energy to move a substance. This energy is achieved by the breakdown of high-energy chemical bonds found in chemicals such as ATP (adenosine triphosphate). ATP is broken down into ADP (adenosine diphosphate) liberating a considerable amount of biochemical energy. A common example of an active transport mechanism is the sodium-potassium (Na^+-K^+) pump. This is a protein pump that actively moves potassium ions into the cell and sodium ions out of the cell. Because this movement goes *against* the ions' concentration gradients, it must use energy.

active transport *requires the use of energy to move a substance.*

Large molecules, such as glucose and most of the amino acids, do not readily pass through the cell membrane because of their size. These molecules are moved across the cell membrane with the help of special "carrier" proteins found on the surface of the target cells. These large molecules are "carried" across the cell membrane in a special transport process called **carrier-mediated diffusion** or **facilitated diffusion.** Once the molecule to be transported binds with the carrier protein, the configuration of the cell membrane changes, allowing the large molecule to enter the target cell. Insulin, an important hormone secreted by the endocrine pancreas, can increase the rate of carrier-mediated glucose transport from 10- to 20-fold. This is the principal mechanism by which insulin controls glucose use in the body.

carrier-mediated diffusion *or* **facilitated diffusion** *process in which carrier proteins transport large molecules across the cell membrane.*

Most drugs travel through the body by means of **passive transport,** the movement of a substance without the use of energy. This requires the presence of concentration gradients in a solution. Diffusion and osmosis are forms of passive transport. **Diffusion** involves the movement of solute in the solution, while **osmosis** involves the movement of the solvent (usually water). In diffusion, the solute's molecules or ions move *down* their concentration gradients from an area of higher concentration to an area of lower concentration. Conversely, in osmosis the solvent's molecules move *up* the concentration gradient from an area of low solute concentration to an area of higher solute concentration. Another way of looking at this is to think of osmosis as simply the diffusion of solvent from an area of high *solvent* concentration to an area of low *solvent* concentration. A final type of passive transport is **filtration.** This is simply the movement of molecules across a membrane down a *pressure* gradient, from an area of high pressure to an area of lower pressure. This pressure typically results from the hydrostatic force of blood pressure.

passive transport *movement of a substance without the use of energy.*

diffusion *movement of solute in a solution from an area of higher concentration to an area of lower concentration.*

osmosis *movement of solvent in a solution from an area of lower solute concentration to an area of higher solute concentration.*

filtration *movement of molecules across a membrane from an area of higher pressure to an area of lower pressure.*

Absorption

When a drug is administered to a patient it must find its way to the site of action. If a drug is given orally or injected into any place except the bloodstream, its absorption into the bloodstream is the first step in this process. (Since drugs given intravenously or intra-arterially enter directly into the bloodstream no absorption needs to occur.) Several factors affect a drug's absorption. The body absorbs most drugs faster when they are given intramuscularly than when they are given subcutaneously. This is because muscles are more vascular than subcutaneous tissue. Of course, anything that slows blood flow will delay absorption. Shock and hypothermia are just two examples. Conversely, processes such as fever and hyperthermia increase peripheral blood flow and speed absorption.

Drugs given orally (enterally) must first survive the digestive processes before being absorbed across the mucosa of the gastrointestinal system. If a drug is not soluble in water, it will have difficulty being absorbed. Time-released medications take advantage of this with an enteric coating that slowly releases the medication. Some drugs have an enteric coating that will not dissolve in the more acidic environment of the stomach, but will dissolve in the alkaline environment of the duodenum. This allows a drug that would irritate the stomach or be destroyed by stomach acid to be passed through the stomach into the duodenum and absorbed there. Besides being able to survive stomach acid, a drug must also be somewhat lipid (fat) soluble in order to cross the cells' lipid two-layered (bilayered) membranes. Many drugs **ionize,** or become electrically charged or polar following administration. Generally speaking, ionized drugs do not absorb across the membranes of cells (lipid bilayers), but fortunately, most drugs do not fully ionize. Instead they reach an equilibrium between their ionized and nonionized forms, and the nonionized form can be absorbed. A drug's pH also affects the extent to which it ionizes. A drug that is a weak acid will ionize much more substantially in an alkaline environment than in an acidic environment; conversely, an alkaline drug will ionize more readily in an acidic environment than in an alkaline environment. For example, aspirin (an acidic drug) does not dissociate well in the stomach (an acidic environment) and is therefore readily absorbed there.

ionize *to become electrically charged or polar.*

The nature of the absorbing surface and the blood flow to the administration site also affect drug absorption. The rate of absorption is directly related to the amount of surface area available for absorption. The greater the area, the faster the absorption. Much of the gastrointestinal system has multiple invaginations, or folds, that increase its surface area. Also, the greater the blood flow is to an area, the faster will be the rate of absorption. Again, the GI tract has a rich vascular system with many capillaries that perfuse its absorbing surfaces, allowing nutrients (and drugs) to diffuse into the bloodstream.

Finally, the drug's concentration affects its absorption. Because drugs diffuse in the body, the higher their concentration, the more rapidly the body will absorb them. This principle is frequently used when giving a "loading dose" of a drug and following it with a "maintenance infusion." The loading dose is typically a larger dose of the same concentration of the drug. On occasion, a more concentrated solution of the drug is used as the loading dose. Regardless, the desired effect is to rapidly raise the amount of the drug in the system to a therapeutic level. This is typically followed by a continuous infusion of the drug at a lower concentration, or slower administration rate, to keep it at the therapeutic level.

bioavailability *amount of a drug that is still active after it reaches its target tissue.*

Bioavailability is the measure of the amount of a drug that is still active after it reaches its target tissue. This is the bottom line as far as absorption is concerned. The goal of administering a drug is to assure sufficient bioavailability of the drug at the target tissue in order to produce the desired effect, after considering all of the absorption factors.

Distribution

Once a drug has entered the bloodstream, it must be distributed throughout the body. Most drugs will pass easily from the bloodstream, through the interstitial spaces, into the target cells. Some drugs, however, will bind to proteins found in the blood, most commonly albumin, and remain in the body for a prolonged time. They thus have a sustained release from the bloodstream and a prolonged period of action. The therapeutic effects of a drug are primarily due to the unbound portion of the drug in the blood. A drug that is bound to plasma proteins cannot cross membranes and reach the target cells. Thus, only the unbound drug is in equilibrium with the target cells and can cross the cell membranes.

Changing the bloodstream's pH can affect the protein-binding action of a drug. Tricyclic antidepressants (TCAs), for instance, are strongly bound to plasma proteins. Making the blood more alkaline increases protein-binding of the TCA molecules. Therefore, in addition to supportive therapy, serious overdoses of TCAs are treated by administering sodium bicarbonate. Sodium bicarbonate makes the blood more alkaline (raises the pH) causing increased binding of the TCA to serum proteins. Cumulatively, this decreases the amount of free drug in the blood, thus decreasing the adverse effects. Sodium bicarbonate administration also facilitates elimination of the drug through the urine.

The presence of other serum protein binding drugs can also affect drug-protein binding. For example, the drug warfarin (Coumadin) is highly protein-bound (99 percent). Its therapeutic effects are due to the 1 percent of the drug that is unbound and circulating in the bloodstream. Aspirin molecules bind to the same binding site on the serum proteins as do warfarin molecules. Thus, when aspirin is administered to a patient on warfarin, it displaces some of the protein-bound warfarin, increasing the amount of free (unbound) warfarin in the blood. Even if it displaces only 1 percent of the total warfarin, it effectively doubles the available warfarin. This can lead to unwanted side effects such as hemorrhage.

Albumin is one of the chief proteins in the blood that is available for binding with drugs. When albumin levels are low (hypoalbuminemia), as occurs in malnutrition, drugs that are normally protein bound rise to much greater blood levels than anticipated. For example, consider a patient who has been taking warfarin without difficulty. If he develops hypoalbuminemia, his normal dose of warfarin will result in much more of the drug being available in the body, possibly leading to dangerous bleeding.

Certain organs exclude some drugs from distribution. For example, the tight junctions of the capillary endothelial cells in the central nervous system (CNS) vasculature form a **blood–brain barrier.** These cells are packed together so tightly that only non-protein-bound, highly lipid-soluble drugs can cross into the CNS. The so-called **placental barrier** can likewise prevent drugs from reaching a fetus, although it is not the solid barrier that its name implies. The fetus is exposed to almost every drug that the mother takes. But because any drug must traverse the maternal blood supply and cross the capillary membranes into the placenta (fetal) circulation, delivering drugs to a fetus requires them to be lipid soluble, nonionized and non-protein-bound. This may slow some drugs or reduce their placental transfer to benign levels.

Other drugs are deposited in specific tissues. Fatty tissue, for example, can serve as a drug depot, or reservoir. Because blood flow is lower in fatty areas than in muscular areas, fatty tissue is a relatively stable depot; it can neither absorb nor release a large amount of drug in a short time. Similarly, bones and teeth can accumulate high amounts of drugs that bind to calcium, especially tetracycline antibiotics.

blood–brain barrier *tight junctions of the capillary endothelial cells in the central nervous system vasculature through which only non-protein-bound, highly lipid-soluble drugs can pass.*

placental barrier *biochemical barrier at the maternal/fetal interface that restricts certain molecules.*

Biotransformation

Like other chemicals that enter the body, drugs are metabolized, or broken down into different chemicals (metabolites). The special name given to the **metabolism** of drugs is **biotransformation.** Biotransformation has one of two effects on most drugs: (1) it can transform the drug into a more or less active metabolite, or (2) it can make the drug more water soluble (or less lipid soluble) to facilitate elimination. Some drugs, such as lidocaine, are totally metabolized before elimination, others only partially, and still others not at all. The body will transform some molecules of most drugs and eliminate others without transformation. Protein-bound drugs are not available for biotransformation. Some so-called **prodrugs** (or parent drugs) are not active when administered, but biotransformation converts them into active metabolites.

Many biotransformation processes occur in the liver. The endoplasmic reticula of hepatocytes (liver cells) contain microsomal enzymes that perform much of the metabolizing. (Smaller quantities of these enzymes are also found in the kidney, lung, and GI tract.) Because the blood supply from the GI tract passes through the liver via the portal vein, all drugs absorbed in the GI tract pass through the liver before moving on through the systemic circulation. The first pass through the liver may partially or completely inactivate many drugs. This **first-pass effect** is why some drugs cannot be given orally but instead must be given intravenously to bypass the GI tract and prevent first-pass hepatic metabolism. It also is why drugs that can be given either orally or intravenously may require a much higher oral dose than IV dose. Because we can observe the extent of first-pass metabolism, we can predict how much to increase a dose of an oral medication to deliver an effective amount of the drug into the general circulation.

The liver's microsomal enzymes react with drugs in two ways: phase I, or nonsynthetic reactions; and phase II, or synthetic reactions. *Phase I reactions* most often **oxidize** the parent drug, although they may reduce it or **hydrolyze** it. These nonsynthetic reactions make the drug more water soluble to ease excretion. A number of drugs and chemicals increase the activity of, or induce, the microsomal enzyme that causes phase I reactions. This means that more enzyme is produced and drugs will be metabolized more rapidly. Because the microsomal enzymes are nonspecific, they can be induced by one drug or chemical and then biotransform other drugs or chemicals. *Phase II reactions,* which are also called conjugation reactions, combine the prodrug or its metabolites with an endogenous (naturally occurring) chemical, usually making the drug more polar and easier to excrete.

metabolism *the body's breaking down chemicals into different chemicals.*

biotransformation *special name given to the metabolism of drugs.*

prodrug *medication that is not active when administered, but whose biotransformation converts it into active metabolites.*

first-pass effect *the liver's partial or complete inactivation of a drug before it reaches the systemic circulation.*

oxidation *the loss of hydrogen atoms or the acceptance of an oxygen atom. This increases the positive charge (or lessens the negative charge) on the molecule.*

hydrolysis *the breakage of a chemical bond by adding water, or by incorporating a hydroxyl (OH^-) group into one fragment and a hydrogen ion (H^+) into the other.*

Elimination

Whether they are unchanged or metabolized before elimination, most drugs (toxins and metabolites) are excreted in the urine. Some are excreted in the feces or in expired air.

Renal excretion occurs through two major processes: glomerular filtration and tubular secretion. Glomerular filtration is a function of glomerular filtration pressure, which in turn results from blood pressure and blood flow through the kidneys. Conditions that affect blood pressure and blood flow can affect renal elimination. Specialized transport systems in the walls of the proximal kidney tubules secrete drugs into the urine. These "pumps" are active transport systems and require energy in the form of adenosine triphosphate (ATP) to function. Some are specialized and transport only specific chemicals, while others can transport a range of similar chemicals. When drugs compete for the same pump, toxicity or other unwanted effects can result; however, combinations of some drugs can take advantage of this specialization to prolong their circulation. For example, probenecid blocks renal tubular pumps and competes for them with many antibiotics, among them penicillin, ampicillin, and oxacillin. Probenecid thus is sometimes given with those antibiotics to increase and prolong their blood levels.

The same factors that affect absorption at any other site also affect reabsorption in the renal tubules. Of particular concern is the urine pH. Lipid soluble and nonionized molecules are readily reabsorbed. Changing the urine pH (usually by administering sodium bicarbonate to make it more alkaline) can affect the reabsorption in the renal tubules. For example, if a drug becomes ionized in a more alkaline environment, then making the urine more alkaline will interfere with reabsorption and cause more of the drug to be excreted. Some drugs and their metabolites can be eliminated in the expired air. This is the basis of the breath test that police use to determine a driver's blood alcohol level. Ethanol is released in the expired air in proportion to its concentration in the bloodstream. Although the liver degrades most ingested ethanol, exhalation releases a measurable quantity. Drugs also can be excreted in the feces. In enterohepatic circulation, if a drug (or its metabolites) is excreted into the intestines from bile, the body may reabsorb the drug and experience a sustained effect. Additionally, drugs may be excreted through sweat, saliva, and breast milk. Excretion through sweat glands is rarely a significant mechanism for elimination. Excretion through mammary glands becomes a concern when nursing mothers take medications.

Review Content

Drug Routes

- Enteral
- Parenteral

Drug Routes

The route of a drug's administration clearly has an impact on the drug's absorption and distribution. The route's impact on biotransformation and elimination may not be so clear. The bloodstream will more quickly absorb and distribute water-soluble drugs if given in more vascular compartments than if given in less vascular compartments. Oral or nasogastric administration of alkaline drugs may allow the gastric acids to neutralize the drug and prevent its absorption. The liver's first-pass effect may biotransform some orally administered drugs and degrade them almost immediately.

enteral route *delivery of a medication through the gastrointestinal tract.*

Enteral Routes **Enteral routes** deliver medications by absorption through the gastrointestinal tract, which goes from the mouth to the stomach and on through the intestines to the rectum. They may be oral, orogastric/nasogastric, sublingual, buccal, or rectal.

Make sure you know the correct route for a specific medication. Some medications that are therapeutic when given by the correct route can be dangerous when given by the wrong route.

- ★ *Oral (PO).* The oral route is good for self-administered drugs. Most home medications are administered by this route. The drug must be able to tolerate the acidic gastric environment and be absorbed. Few emergency drugs are administered through this route.
- ★ *Orogastric/nasogastric tube (OG/NG).* This route is generally used for oral medications when the patient already has the tube in place for other reasons.
- ★ *Sublingual (SL).* This is a good route for self-administration and excellent absorption from the sublingual capillary bed without the problems of gastric acidity or absorption.
- ★ *Buccal.* Absorption through this route between the cheek and gum is similar to sublingual absorption.
- ★ *Rectal (PR).* This route is usually reserved for unconscious or vomiting patients or patients who cannot cooperate with oral or IV administration (small children).

parenteral route *delivery of a medication outside of the gastrointestinal tract, typically using needles to inject medications into the circulatory system or tissues.*

Parenteral Routes Broadly defined, **parenteral** denotes any area outside of the gastrointestinal tract; however, additional, specific criteria apply to parenteral drug administration. Parenteral routes typically use needles to inject medications into the circulatory system or tissues. Consequently, some forms of parenteral drug delivery afford the most rapid drug delivery and absorption.

★ *Intravenous (IV).* With its rapid onset, this is the preferred route in most emergencies.

★ *Endotracheal (ET).* This is an alternative route for *selected* medications (epinephrine, atropine, vasopressin, lidocaine) in an emergency.

★ *Intraosseous (IO).* The intraosseous route delivers drugs to the medullary space of bones. Most often used as an alternative to IV administration in both children and adults.

★ *Umbilical.* Both the umbilical vein and umbilical artery can provide an alternative to IV administration in newborns.

★ *Intramuscular (IM).* The intramuscular route allows a slower absorption than IV administration, as the drug passes into the capillaries.

★ *Subcutaneous (SC, SQ, SubQ).* This route is slower than the IM route, because the subcutaneous tissue is less vascular than the muscular tissue.

★ *Inhalation/nebulized.* This route, which offers very rapid absorption, is especially useful for delivering drugs whose target tissues are in the lungs.

★ *Topical.* Topical administration delivers drugs directly to the skin.

★ *Transdermal.* For drugs that can be absorbed through the skin, the transdermal route allows slow, continuous release.

★ *Nasal.* Useful for delivering drugs directly to the nasal mucosa, the nasal route has an expanding role in delivering systemically acting drugs.

★ *Instillation.* Instillation is similar to topical administration, but places the drug directly into a wound or an eye.

★ *Intradermal.* For allergy testing, intradermal administration delivers a drug or biologic agent between the dermal layers.

Most emergency medications are given intravenously to avoid drug degradation in the liver.

Drug Forms

Drugs come in many forms. Solid forms, generally given orally, include:

★ *Pills.* Drugs shaped spherically to be easy to swallow.

★ *Powders.* Although they are not as popular as they once were, some powdered drugs are still in use.

★ *Tablets.* Powders compressed into a disklike form.

★ *Suppositories.* Drugs mixed with a waxlike base that melts at body temperature, allowing absorption by rectal or vaginal tissue.

★ *Capsules.* Gelatin containers filled with powders or tiny pills; the gelatin dissolves, releasing the drug into the gastrointestinal tract.

Liquid drugs are usually solutions of a solid drug dissolved in a solvent. Some can be given parenterally, while others must be given enterally.

★ *Solutions.* The most common liquid preparations. Generally water based; some may be oil based.

★ *Tinctures.* Prepared using an alcohol extraction process; some alcohol usually remains in the final drug preparation.

★ *Suspensions.* Preparations in which the solid does not dissolve in the solvent; if left alone, the solid portion will precipitate out.

★ *Emulsions.* Suspensions with an oily substance in the solvent, even when well mixed globules of oil separate out of the solution.

★ *Spirits.* Solution of a volatile drug in alcohol.

★ *Elixirs.* Alcohol and water solvent, often with flavorings added to improve the taste.

★ *Syrups.* Sugar, water, and drug solutions.

Some drugs come in a gaseous form. The most common drug supplied this way is oxygen. Paramedics may also find nitrous oxide (N_2O) used as an inhaled analgesic in ambulances and emergency departments.

Drug Storage

Medications are vulnerable to extremes in temperature. It is important that they be stored in conditions where temperature fluctuation is minimized.

Certain guidelines should dictate the manner in which drugs are stored; their properties may be altered by the environment in which they are stored. While some EMS units are parked in heated stations, others are kept outdoors and exposed to the elements. EMS systems must consider the storage requirements of all drugs and diluents when deciding operational issues such as vehicle design and posting policies (as occurs in system status management). This rapidly becomes a clinical issue because the actual potency of most medications is altered if they are not stored in proper conditions. Examples of variables to consider when determining the proper method of drug storage include temperature, light, moisture, and shelf life.

PHARMACODYNAMICS

When we consider a drug's pharmacodynamics, or effects on the body, we are specifically interested in its mechanisms of action and the relationship between its concentration and its effect.

Content Review

Types of Drug Actions

- Binding to a receptor site
- Changing the physical properties of cells
- Chemically combining with other chemicals
- Altering a normal metabolic pathway

Actions of Drugs

Drugs can act in four different ways. They may bind to a receptor site, change the physical properties of cells, chemically combine with other chemicals, or alter a normal metabolic pathway. Each of these actions involves a physiochemical interaction between the drug and a functionally important molecule in the body.

receptor *specialized protein that combines with a drug, resulting in a biochemical effect.*

affinity *force of attraction between a drug and a receptor.*

efficacy *a drug's ability to cause the expected response.*

Drugs That Act by Binding to a Receptor Site Most drugs operate by binding to a **receptor.** Almost all drug receptors are protein molecules on the surfaces of cells. They are part of the body's normal regulatory stimulation/inhibition function, and can be stimulated or inhibited by chemicals. Each different receptor's name generally corresponds to the drug that stimulates it. For example, if an opiate stimulates the receptor, then the receptor is an opioid receptor. When multiple drugs stimulate the same receptor, standard practice is to use the generic name.

The force of attraction between a drug and a receptor is their **affinity.** The greater the affinity, the stronger the bond. Different drugs may bind to the same type of receptor site, but the strength of their bond may vary. The binding site's shape determines its receptivity to other chemicals, whether they are drugs or endogenous substances. These binding sites are relatively specific—a nonopiate drug generally will not affect an opiate binding site, although occasionally a drug with a similar receptor binding site will unexpectedly cross react. Receptors can also have subtypes. At least five subtypes of adrenergic receptors, for example, are important to paramedic practice.

A drug's pharmacodynamics also involve its ability to cause the expected response, or **efficacy.** Just as different drugs may have different affinities for a site, they may also have different efficacies; that is, drug A may cause a stronger response than drug B. Affinity and efficacy are not directly related. Drug A may cause a stronger response than drug B, even though drug B binds to the receptor site more strongly than drug A.

second messenger *chemical that participates in complex cascading reactions that eventually cause a drug's desired effect.*

When a drug binds with its specific type of receptor, a chemical change occurs that ultimately leads to the drug's effect. In most cases, drugs will either stimulate or inhibit the cell's normal biochemical actions. In fact, a drug cannot impart a new function to a cell. Some drugs may interact with a receptor and directly result in the desired effect. Other drugs, however, may interact with a receptor and cause the release or production of a second compound. This secondary compound, or **second messenger,** includes such compounds as calcium or cyclic adenosine monophosphate (cAMP). Cyclic AMP is the most common second messenger. It has a multitude of effects inside the cell. These secondary messengers are particularly important in the endocrine system, as they principally occur in endocrine glands. Once cAMP is formed inside the cell, it activates still other enzymes, usually in a cascading action. That is, the first enzyme activates another enzyme, which activates a third enzyme, and so forth. This is important in that it amplifies the action so that even a small amount of a drug (or hormone) acting on the cell surface can initiate a powerful, cascading, activating force for the entire cell.

The number of receptors on a target cell usually does not remain constant on a daily basis, or even from minute to minute. This is because the receptor proteins are often destroyed during the course of their function. At other times, they are either reactivated or remanufactured by the protein-manufacturing mechanism of the cell. Binding of a drug (or hormone) to a target cell receptor causes the number of receptors to decrease. This process is **down-regulation** of the receptors. It results in a decreased responsiveness of the target cell to the drug or hormone as the number of available active receptors decreases. In other cases, but less commonly, a drug (or hormone) can cause the formation of more receptors than normal. This process, **up-regulation,** increases the target tissue's sensitivity to the particular drug or hormone.

down-regulation *binding of a drug or hormone to a target cell receptor that causes the number of receptors to decrease.*

up-regulation *a drug causes the formation of more receptors than normal.*

Chemicals that stimulate a receptor site generally fall into two broad categories, agonists and antagonists. **Agonists** bind to the receptor and cause it to initiate the expected response. **Antagonists** bind to a site but do not cause the receptor to initiate the expected response. Some drugs, **agonist-antagonists** (also called **partial agonists**), may do both. Nalbuphine (Nubain), for instance, stimulates some of the opioid agonists' analgesic properties but partially blocks others such as respiratory depression.

agonist *drug that binds to a receptor and causes it to initiate the expected response.*

antagonist *drug that binds to a receptor but does not cause it to initiate the expected response.*

agonist-antagonist (partial agonist) *drug that binds to a receptor and stimulates some of its effects but blocks others.*

Receptor-mediated drug actions work like a lock (the receptor) and key (the agonist). If you put the key in the lock and turn it, the lock will open. An antagonist is like a key that fits into the lock but will not turn and cannot open the lock. Target tissues generally have many receptors, so to take the analogy another step, imagine that to get maximal effect a single key (agonist) must move around and open many doors (trigger many biochemical responses). An agonist-antagonist would be a key that unlocks and opens a door but gets stuck in the lock. That is, the drug will cause the expected effect, but that drug will also block another drug from triggering the same receptor. This **competitive antagonism** is considered *surmountable* because a sufficiently large dose of the agonist can overcome the antagonism.

competitive antagonism *one drug binds to a receptor and causes the expected effect while also blocking another drug from triggering the same receptor.*

Noncompetitive antagonism can also occur. Continuing the lock, key, and door analogy, imagine the door is barred. This antagonism would be *insurmountable;* no amount of agonist could overcome it. Noncompetitive antagonism occurs because the binding of the antagonist at a different site causes a deformity of the binding site that actually prevents the agonist from fitting and binding. **Irreversible antagonism** may also occur when a competitive antagonist permanently binds with a receptor site. When this occurs, no amount of agonist will stimulate the receptor. For the effects of such an antagonist to wear off, the body must create new receptors.

noncompetitive antagonism *the binding of an antagonist causes a deformity of the binding site that prevents an agonist from fitting and binding.*

irreversible antagonism *a competitive antagonist permanently binds with a receptor site.*

Two drugs may appear to be antagonists while actually acting independently. This physiologic antagonism can occur when one drug's effects counteract another's. While neither agent chemically affects the other, their net effect is antagonistic. An example of a receptor, agonist, antagonist, and agonist-antagonist can be described using an opiate receptor. These receptors occur naturally in the brain and respond to natural endorphins. Morphine sulfate acts as an agonist. It binds to the opiate receptor and causes the expected response of pain relief. Naloxone (Narcan) acts as an antagonist. It will bind to the opiate receptor, but will not initiate the pain relief. It will prevent morphine sulfate from binding to the site and thus effectively blocks the morphine and its response. If the patient is given nalbuphine (Nubain), an agonist-antagonist, it will bind to the opiate receptor and relieve pain, but it is less efficacious than morphine. The nalbuphine blocks morphine from the receptor like an antagonist, but stimulates the receptor on its own like an agonist, although to a lesser extent.

Drugs That Act by Changing Physical Properties Some drugs change the physical properties of a part of the body. Drugs that change the osmotic balance across membranes are good examples of this type of drug action. The osmotic diuretic mannitol (Osmotrol), for instance, increases urine output by increasing the blood's osmolarity, or osmotic "pull." This increased osmolarity triggers the normal regulatory systems to decrease water reabsorption in the renal tubules, thereby reducing the total amount of water in the body.

Drugs That Act by Chemically Combining with Other Substances Drugs that participate in chemical reactions that change the chemical nature of their substrates (the chemical or substance on which a drug acts) play a large role in paramedic practice. For example, isopropyl alcohol, which is often used to disinfect skin before percutaneous needle insertion for phlebotomy or IV cannulation, denatures the proteins on the surface of bacterial cells. This ruptures the cells, destroying the bacteria. The antacids are another example. They act by chemically neutralizing the hydrochloric acid in the stomach. Sodium bicarbonate given intravenously chemically neutralizes some of the acids in the bloodstream, effectively making the blood more alkalotic.

Drugs That Act by Altering a Normal Metabolic Pathway Some anticancer and antiviral drugs are chemical analogs of normal metabolic substrates. In a process that has been dubbed a counterfeit incorporation mechanism, these drugs can be incorporated into the products of metabolism of cancer cells. Since these drugs are not really the expected substrate, the anticipated product either will not form or, if formed, will be substantially or completely inactive.

Responses to Drug Administration

side effect *unintended response to a drug.*

Always weigh the need for a drug's desired response against the dangers of its side effects.

When a drug is administered, a response is obviously anticipated. The actual response may be the one desired, or it may be an unintended **side effect.** Most, if not all, drugs have at least some minor side effects. Because our knowledge of pharmacology and physiology has not yet arrived at the point where we can engineer the perfect drug, we must weigh the need for the desired response against the dangers of side effects. In essence, every time we give a medication, we must carefully weigh the risks against the benefits. Although undesirable, side effects are predictable. Iatrogenic responses, however, are not predicted. In general, the term *iatrogenic* refers to a disease or response induced by the actions of a care provider. Derived from the Greek *iatros* (physician) and *gennan* (to produce), it literally means *physician produced.* Negligence is not the only cause of iatrogenic responses. Some common unintended adverse responses to drugs include:

- ★ *Allergic reaction.* Also known as hypersensitivity; this effect occurs as the drug is antigenic and activates the immune system, causing effects that are normally more profound than seen in the general population.
- ★ *Idiosyncrasy.* A drug effect that is unique to the individual; different than seen or expected in the population in general.
- ★ *Tolerance.* Decreased response to the same amount of drug after repeated administrations.
- ★ *Cross tolerance.* Tolerance for a drug that develops after administration of a different drug. Morphine and other opioid agents are common examples. Tolerance for one agent implies tolerance for others as well.
- ★ *Tachyphylaxis.* Rapidly occurring tolerance to a drug. May occur after a single dose. This typically occurs with sympathetic agonists, specifically decongestant and bronchodilation agents.
- ★ *Cumulative effect.* Increased effectiveness when a drug is given in several doses.
- ★ *Drug dependence.* The patient becomes accustomed to the drug's presence in his body and will suffer from withdrawal symptoms upon its absence. The dependence may be physical or psychological.
- ★ *Drug interaction.* The effects of one drug alter the response to another drug.
- ★ *Drug antagonism.* The effects of one drug block the response to another drug.
- ★ *Summation.* Also known as an additive effect. Two drugs that both have the same effect are given together, analogous to $1+1=2$.
- ★ *Synergism.* Two drugs that both have the same effect are given together and produce a response greater than the sum of their individual responses, analogous to $1+1=3$.
- ★ *Potentiation.* One drug enhances the effect of another. A common example is promethazine (Phenergan) enhancing the effects of morphine.
- ★ *Interference.* The direct biochemical interaction between two drugs; one drug affects the pharmacology of another drug.

Drug-Response Relationship

To have its optimal desired or therapeutic effects, a drug must reach appropriate concentrations at its site of action. The magnitude of the response therefore depends on the dosage and the drug's course through the body over time. Factors that can affect the drug's concentration may be pharmaceutical (the dosage form's disintegration and the drug's dissolution), pharmacokinetic (the drug's absorption, distribution, metabolism, and excretion), or pharmacodynamic (drug-receptor interaction). To predict how the drug will affect different people, a **drug-response relationship** thus correlates different amounts of drug to the resultant clinical response.

Most of the information needed to describe drug-response relationships comes from **plasma-level profiles,** which describe the lengths of onset, duration, and termination of action, as well as the drug's minimum effective concentration and toxic levels. The **onset of action** is the time from administration until a medication reaches its **minimum effective concentration** (the minimum level of drug necessary to cause a given effect). The length of time the amount of drug remains above this level is its **duration of action. Termination of action** is measured from when the drug's level drops below the minimum effective concentration until it is eliminated from the body.

The ratio of a drug's lethal dose for 50 percent of the population (LD_{50}) to its effective dose for 50 percent of the population (ED_{50}) is its **therapeutic index** (TI) or LD_{50}/ED_{50}. The therapeutic index represents the drug's margin of safety. As the range between effective dose and lethal dose decreases, the value of TI decreases; that is, it becomes closer to 1. TI values of close to one indicate a very small margin of safety. In other words, the effective dose and lethal dose of a drug whose TI value is close to 1 are nearly the same. This drug would be very difficult to effectively dose without causing toxicity.

The last component of the drug-response relationship, the **biologic half-life,** is the time the body takes to clear one-half of the drug. Although the rates of metabolism and excretion both affect it, a drug's half-life ($t_{1/2}$) is independent of its concentration. For example, if the concentration of a drug were 500 mcg/dL after administration and 250 mcg/dL in 10 minutes, then its half-life would be 10 minutes. After another 10 minutes, 125 mcg/dL would remain.

drug-response relationship *correlation of different amounts of a drug to clinical response.*

plasma-level profile *describes the lengths of onset, duration, and termination of action, as well as the drug's minimum effective concentration and toxic levels.*

onset of action *the time from administration until a medication reaches its minimum effective concentration.*

minimum effective concentration *minimum level of drug needed to cause a given effect.*

duration of action *length of time the amount of drug remains above its minimum effective concentration.*

termination of action *time from when the drug's level drops below its minimum effective concentration until it is eliminated from the body.*

therapeutic index *ratio of a drug's lethal dose for 50 percent of the population to its effective dose for 50 percent of the population.*

biologic half-life *time the body takes to clear one-half of a drug.*

Factors Altering Drug Response

Different individuals may have different responses to the same drug given. Factors that alter the standard drug-response relationship include the following:

★ *Age.* The liver and kidney functions of infants are not yet fully developed, so the response to drugs may be altered. Likewise, as we age, the functions of these organs begin to deteriorate. As a result, infants and the elderly are most susceptible to having an altered response to a drug.

★ *Body mass.* The more body mass a person has, the more fluid is potentially available to dilute a drug. A given amount of drug will cause a higher concentration in a person with little body mass than in a much larger person. Thus, most drug dosages are stated in terms of body mass. For example, the standard dose of lidocaine for a patient in cardiac arrest is 1.5 mg/kg. A 100-kg patient will receive 150 mg of lidocaine, while a 50-kg patient will receive only 75 mg.

★ *Sex.* Most differences in drug response due to sex result from the relative body masses of men and women. The different distribution and amounts of body fat also affect the amounts of drug available at any given time.

★ *Environmental milieu.* Various stimuli in a patient's environment affect his response to a given drug. This is most clearly seen with drugs affecting mood or behavior. The same dose of an antianxiety medication such as diazepam (Valium) will have different effects, depending on the patient's mood or surroundings. For example, if the patient were afraid of heights, his usual dose of diazepam would not be likely to help him remain calm while rappelling from the top of a tall building. Surrounding conditions may also affect the distribution or elimination of a drug. Heat, for example, causes vasodilation and increases perspiration, both of which may alter the rate at which the body distributes and eliminates a drug.

Content Review

Factors Affecting Drug-Response Relationship

- Age
- Body mass
- Sex
- Environment
- Time of administration
- Pathology
- Genetics
- Psychology

★ *Time of administration.* If a patient takes a drug immediately after eating, its absorption will be different than if he took the same drug before breakfast in the morning. Some drugs may cause nausea if taken on an empty stomach and must therefore be taken only after eating.

★ *Pathologic state.* Several disease states alter the drug-response relationship. Most notable are renal and hepatic dysfunctions, both of which may lead to excess accumulation of a drug in the body. Renal failure is likely to decrease elimination of drugs, while hepatic failure may decrease or inhibit their metabolism, prolonging their duration of action. Acid–base disturbances may alter a drug's solubility or the extent to which it ionizes, thus changing its absorption rate.

★ *Genetic factors.* Genetic traits such as the lack of specific enzymes or lowered basal metabolic rate alter drug absorption or biotransformation and thus modify the patient's response.

★ *Psychological factors.* A patient's mental state can also affect his response to a drug. The best known example of this is the placebo effect. Essentially, if a patient believes that a drug will have a given effect, then he is much more likely to perceive that the effect has occurred.

The chance of a medication interaction increases significantly the greater the number of medications a patient is taking. Thus, proceed with caution when administering an emergency medication to a patient who routinely takes more than two.

Drug Interactions

Drug interactions occur whenever two or more drugs are available in the same patient. The interaction can increase, decrease, or have no effect on their combined actions. Any number of variables may cause these drug-drug interactions, including:

★ One drug could alter the rate of intestinal absorption.

★ The two drugs could compete for plasma protein binding, resulting in one's accumulation at the other's expense.

★ One drug could alter the other's metabolism, thus increasing or decreasing either's bioavailability.

★ One drug's action at a receptor site may be antagonistic or synergistic to another's.

★ One drug could alter the other's rate of excretion through the kidneys.

★ One drug could alter the balance of electrolytes necessary for the other drug's expected result.

In addition to drug-drug interactions, other types of interactions are possible. They include a drug's effects on the rate of absorption of food and nutrients, alteration of enzymes, and food-initiated alteration of drug excretion. Alcohol consumption and smoking may also cause interactions with drugs. Finally, some drugs are incompatible with each other. As an example, catecholamines such as epinephrine will precipitate in an alkaline solution such as sodium bicarbonate.

Part 2: Drug Classifications

Part 2 begins with a discussion of how drugs are classified, that is, how drugs are organized into groups with common characteristics, most often according to the body system affected. The remainder of Part 2 discusses drugs and subgroups of drugs that are included in the following major classifications:

★ Drugs used to affect the nervous system

★ Drugs used to affect the cardiovascular system

★ Drugs used to affect the respiratory system

★ Drugs used to affect the gastrointestinal system

★ Drugs used to affect the eyes

★ Drugs used to affect the ears

★ Drugs used to affect the endocrine system
★ Drugs used to treat cancer
★ Drugs used to treat infectious diseases and inflammation
★ Drugs used to affect the skin
★ Drugs used to supplement the diet
★ Drugs used to treat poisoning and overdoses

CLASSIFYING DRUGS

The enormous amount of material that you must learn about pharmacology can easily become overwhelming. The best way to surmount this challenge is to break the information into manageable groups. Drugs can be classified many ways. You will often find them listed by the body system they affect, by their mechanism of action, or by their indications. Drugs also can be classified by source or by chemical class. Understanding the properties of drug classes (or the model drug of a class) can increase your understanding of drugs and quicken your learning of new drugs.

Grouping medications according to their uses is a very practical way of classifying them. For example, one class of drugs is used to treat heart dysrhythmias, while another treats hypertension. While the specific dosing regimens and contraindications vary among medications within any class, their general properties are consistent. If you understand those general principles, learning the specific information about individual medications becomes much easier. Thinking in terms of prototypical medications usually helps to describe each classification. A **prototype** is a drug that best demonstrates the class's common properties and illustrates its particular characteristics.

prototype *drug that best demonstrates the class's common properties and illustrates its particular characteristics.*

In the rest of this chapter we will look at specific classifications of medications that as a paramedic you will commonly either administer or encounter. Even though you may not frequently administer medications from every classification, knowing how they work remains important. It will help you to understand the implications of medications your patients may be taking themselves or getting from another caregiver. An example often cited to demonstrate the importance of understanding the classes of medications, even those that you will rarely administer, is the patient who has taken an overdose of tricyclic antidepressants. Based on your knowledge of this classification, you will know to increase your index of suspicion for hypotension and abnormal cardiac rhythms.

DRUGS USED TO AFFECT THE NERVOUS SYSTEM

The two major divisions of the nervous system are the central nervous system and the peripheral nervous system (Figure 6-2 ■). The *central nervous system* includes the brain and spinal cord; all nerves that originate and terminate within either the brain or the spinal cord are considered central. The *peripheral nervous system* comprises everything else. If a **neuron** originates within the brain and terminates outside of the spinal cord, it is part of the peripheral nervous system, which in turn consists of the somatic nervous system and the autonomic nervous system. The *somatic nervous system* controls voluntary, or motor, functions. The *autonomic nervous system*, which controls involuntary, or automatic, functions, is further divided into the sympathetic and parasympathetic nervous systems. The two major groupings of medications used to affect the nervous system are those that affect the central nervous system and those that affect the autonomic nervous system.

neuron *nerve cell.*

CENTRAL NERVOUS SYSTEM MEDICATIONS

Many pathologic conditions involve the central nervous system (CNS). As a result, a great number of drugs have been developed to affect the CNS, including analgesics, anesthetics, drugs to treat anxiety and insomnia, anticonvulsants, stimulants, psychotherapeutic agents (antidepressants and antimanic agents), and drugs used to treat specific nervous system disorders such as Parkinson's disease. Obviously, this is a very broad classification with many different types of agents. Having a firm grasp on the basic physiology involved will help you to understand the various drugs you encounter.

■ **Figure 6-2** Functional organization of the autonomic nervous system.

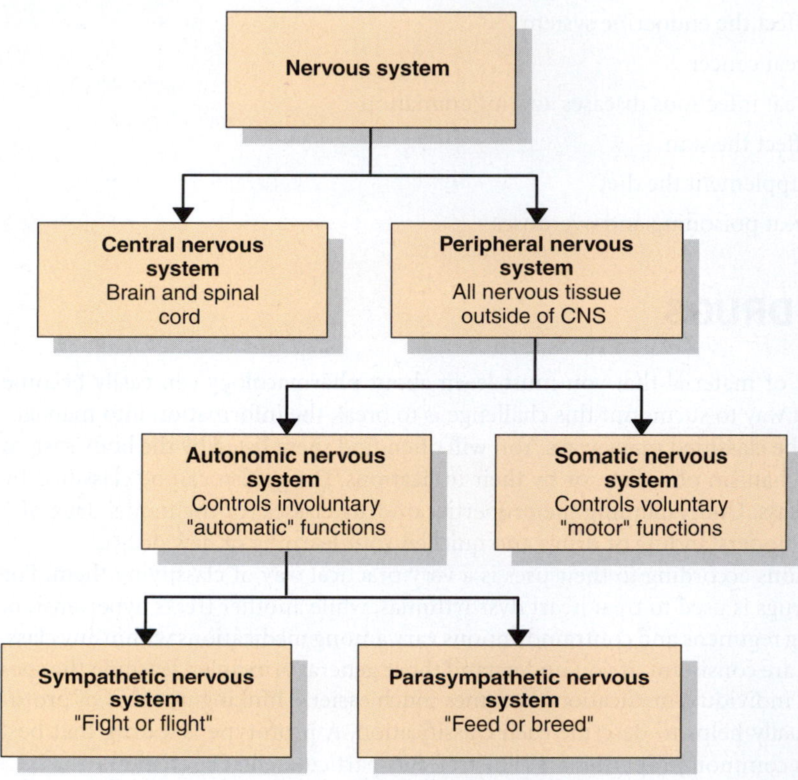

Analgesics and Antagonists

analgesic *medication that relieves the sensation of pain.*

analgesia *the absence of the sensation of pain.*

anesthesia *the absence of all sensations.*

adjunct medication *agent that enhances the effects of other drugs.*

Analgesics are medications that relieve the sensation of pain. The distinction between **analgesia,** the absence of the sensation of *pain,* and **anesthesia,** the absence of *all* sensation, is important. Where an analgesic decreases the specific sensation of pain, an anesthetic prevents all sensation, often impairing consciousness in the process. A frequently used class of medications, analgesics are available by prescription or over the counter. The two basic subclasses of analgesics are opioid agonists and their derivatives and nonopioid derivatives. Opioid antagonists, which we also discuss in this section, reverse the effects of opioid analgesics; **adjunct medications** enhance the effects of other analgesics.

Opioid Agonists An opioid is chemically similar to opium, which is extracted from the poppy plant and has been used for centuries for its analgesic and hallucinatory effects. Opium and all of its derivatives effectively treat pain because of their similarity to natural pain-reducing peptides called *endorphins.* Endorphins and, by extension, opioid drugs work by decreasing the sensory neurons' ability to propagate pain impulses to the spinal cord and brain.

The prototype opioid drug is morphine. Several of morphine's effects make it useful for clinical practice. At therapeutic doses, morphine causes analgesia, euphoria, sedation, and miosis (pupil constriction). It also decreases cardiac preload and afterload, which makes it useful in treating myocardial infarction and pulmonary edema. At higher doses, it may cause respiratory depression and hypotension. Give morphine with caution to patients at high risk for respiratory failure (COPD and asthma) and hypotension (trauma patients with hypovolemia).

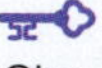

Give morphine with caution to patients at high risk for respiratory failure and hypotension.

Nonopioid Analgesics Three broad types of nonopioid medications also have analgesic properties, several of which also share antipyretic (fever fighting) properties. These are *salicylates* such as aspirin, *nonsteroidal anti-inflammatory drugs (NSAIDS)* such as ibuprofen, and *paraaminophenol derivatives* such as acetaminophen. The drugs in each of these classes affect the production of prostaglandins and cyclooxygenase, important neurotransmitters involved in the pain response.

Opioid Antagonists Opioid antagonists are useful in reversing the effects of opioid drugs. This typically is necessary to treat respiratory depression. Naloxone (Narcan) is the prototype opioid antagonist. It competitively binds with opioid receptors but without causing the effects of opioid bonding. It is commonly used to treat overdoses of heroin and other opioid derivatives; however, it has a shorter half-life than most opioid drugs so repeated doses may be necessary to prevent its unwanted side effects.

Adjunct Medications Adjunct medications are given concurrently with other drugs to enhance their effects. While they may have only limited or no analgesic properties by themselves, combined with a true analgesic they either prolong or intensify its effect. Examples of adjunct medications are benzodiazepines (diazepam [Valium], lorazepam [Ativan], midazolam [Versed]), antihistamines (promethazine [Phenergan]), and caffeine. We will discuss many of these agents in separate sections.

Opioid Agonist-Antagonists An opioid agonist-antagonist displays both agonistic and antagonistic properties. Pentazocine (Talwin) is the prototype for this class. Nalbuphine (Nubain) is commonly used in field care. It is an agonist because, like opioids, it decreases pain response, and it is an antagonist because it has fewer respiratory depressant and addictive side effects. Butorphanol (Stadol) is another common opioid agonist-antagonist.

Anesthetics

Unlike analgesics, an **anesthetic** induces a state of anesthesia, or loss of sensation to touch or pain. Anesthetics are useful during unpleasant procedures such as surgery or electrical cardioversion. At low levels of anesthesia, patients may have a decreased sensation of pain but remain conscious. **Neuroleptanesthesia,** a type of anesthesia that combines this effect with amnesia, is useful in procedures that require the patient to remain alert and responsive.

anesthetic *medication that induces a loss of sensation to touch or pain.*

neuroleptanesthesia *anesthesia that combines decreased sensation of pain with amnesia while the patient remains conscious.*

Anesthetics as a group tend to cause respiratory, central nervous system (CNS), and cardiovascular depression. Different agents affect these systems to different degrees and are typically chosen for their ability to produce the desired effect with minimal side effects. Anesthetic agents are rarely used singly; rather, several different agents are typically given together to achieve a balanced anesthetic result. For example, intubating a conscious patient requires his natural gag reflex to be inhibited. Neuromuscular blocking agents such as succinylcholine are used to induce paralysis. Because this would be a terribly frightening and potentially painful procedure, antianxiety, amnesic, and analgesic agents are also given to produce the desired anesthetic effect.

Anesthetics are given either by inhalation or injection. The gaseous anesthetics given by inhalation include halothane, enflurane, and nitrous oxide. The first clinically useful anesthetic was ether, a gas. Its discovery marked a new generation in surgical care, but it is very flammable. The modern gaseous anesthetics are much less volatile, while still decreasing consciousness and sensation as required. These drugs, by some as yet unidentified mechanism, hyperpolarize neural membranes, making depolarization more difficult. This decreases the firing rates of neural impulses and, therefore, the propagation of action potentials through the nervous system, thus reducing sensation. These effects appear to depend upon the gases' solubility. The rate of onset of anesthesia further depends on several additional factors including cardiac output, inhaled concentration of gas, pulmonary minute volume, and end-organ perfusion. Because these gases clear mostly through the lungs, respiratory rate and depth affect the duration of their effect. While halothane is the prototype of inhaled anesthetics, nitrous oxide is the only medication in this class with which you are likely to have much involvement.

Most anesthetics used outside the operating room are given intravenously. This gives them a considerably faster onset and shorter duration, making them much more useful in emergency care. Paramedics primarily use these agents to assist with intubation in rapid-sequence intubation. They include several pharmacologic classes including ultrashort acting barbiturates (thiopental [Pentothal] and methohexital [Brevital]), benzodiazepines (diazepam [Valium] and midazolam [Versed]), and opioids (fentanyl [Sublimaze], and remifentanil [Ultiva]). We discuss barbiturates' and benzodiazepines' mechanisms of action in the section on antianxiety and sedative-hypnotics.

Anesthetics are also given locally to block sensation for procedures such as suturing and most dentistry. These agents are injected into the skin around the nerves that innervate the area of the procedure. They decrease the nerve's ability to depolarize and propagate the impulse from this area to the brain. Cocaine's first clinical use was as a topical anesthetic of the eye in 1884. The current prototype of this class is lidocaine (Xylocaine). It is frequently mixed with epinephrine. The epinephrine causes local vasoconstriction, decreasing bleeding and systemic absorption of the drug.

Antianxiety and Sedative-Hypnotic Drugs

sedation *state of decreased anxiety and inhibitions.*

hypnosis *instigation of sleep.*

Antianxiety and sedative-hypnotic drugs are generally used to decrease anxiety, induce amnesia, and assist sleeping and as part of a balanced approach to anesthesia. **Sedation** refers to a state of decreased anxiety and inhibitions. **Hypnosis** in this context refers to the instigation of sleep. Sleep may be categorized as either rapid-eye-movement (REM) or non-rapid-eye-movement (non-REM). REM sleep is characterized by rapid eye movements and lack of motor control. Most dreaming is thought to occur during REM sleep. Insomnia, or difficulty sleeping, typically presents with increased latency (the period of time between lying down and going to sleep) or awakening during sleep.

The two main pharmacologic classes within this functional class are benzodiazepines and barbiturates. Alcohol is also in this functional class. Benzodiazepines and barbiturates work in similar ways. Benzodiazepines are frequently prescribed for oral use and are relatively safe and effective for treating general anxiety and insomnia. Barbiturates, which have broader general depressant activities and a higher potential for abuse, are used much less frequently than benzodiazepines. Before the release of benzodiazepines in the 1960s, however, barbiturates were the drug of choice for treating anxiety and insomnia.

Both benzodiazepines and barbiturates hyperpolarize the membrane of central nervous system neurons, which decreases their response to stimuli. Gamma-aminobutyric acid (GABA) is the chief inhibitory neurotransmitter in the central nervous system. GABA receptors are dispersed widely throughout the CNS on proteins that make up chloride ion channels in the cell membrane. When GABA combines with these receptors, the channel "opens" and chloride, which is more prevalent outside of the cell, diffuses through the channel. As chloride is an anion, or negative ion, it makes the inside of the cell more negative than the outside. This hyperpolarizes the membrane and makes it more difficult to depolarize. Depolarization therefore requires a larger stimulus to cause the cell to fire. Both benzodiazepines and barbiturates increase the GABA receptor-chloride ion channel complexes' potential for binding with GABA, and both are dose dependent. At low doses, they decrease anxiety and cause sedation. As the dose increases, they induce sleep (hypnosis) and, at higher doses, anesthesia. Because benzodiazepines only increase the effectiveness of GABA, the amount of GABA present limits their effects. This actually makes benzodiazepines much safer than barbiturates, which at high doses can actually mimic GABA's effects and thus can have unlimited effects. Benzodiazepines and barbiturates are also useful in treating convulsions.

Just as opiates have an antagonist in naloxone (Narcan), benzodiazepines have an antagonist in flumazenil (Romazicon). Flumazenil competitively binds with the benzodiazepine receptors in the GABA receptor-chloride ion channel complex without causing the effects of benzodiazepines. This reverses the sedation from benzodiazepines, but it can occasionally have untoward consequences, specifically if a patient depends upon benzodiazepines for seizure control, is withdrawing from alcohol, or is taking tricyclic antidepressants. In these cases, the patient may develop seizures following the administration of flumazenil.

Antiseizure or Antiepileptic Drugs

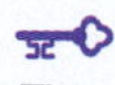

The goal of seizure management is to balance eliminating the seizures against the side effects of the medications used to treat them.

Seizures are a state of hyperactivity of either a section of the brain (partial seizure) or all of the brain (generalized seizure). They may or may not be accompanied by convulsions. Therefore, although the medications in this functional class may be called anticonvulsants, they are more appropriately referred to as antiseizure or antiepileptic drugs. The goal of seizure management is to balance eliminating the seizures against the side effects of the medications used to treat them. Controlling seizures is a lifelong process for most patients and requires diligent compliance with medication dosing regimens.

Partial seizures are those that begin in a focal or discrete area of the brain. This type can be further subdivided into simple partial seizures and complex partial seizures. There is typically no loss of consciousness with simple partial seizures. No change in consciousness occurs. The patient may experience weakness, numbness, and unusual smells or tastes. Twitching of a certain muscle, turning of the head to the side, paralysis, visual changes, or vertigo may occur. A myoclonic seizure is one that is characterized by jerking (myoclonic) movement of a muscle or muscle groups and, like other simple partial seizures, does not involve loss of consciousness. Juvenile myoclonic epilepsy (JME) is one of the most common epilepsy syndromes. Motor symptoms can spread slowly from one part of the body to another. This phenomenon is referred to as an "epileptic march" or "Jacksonian march" and results from spread of the seizure activity across the motor cortex of the brain.

Complex partial seizures, also called temporal lobe seizures, are associated with altered mental status. The patient may have some symptoms similar to those in simple partial seizures but additionally have some change in their ability to interact with the environment. Patients may exhibit automatisms (automatic repetitive behavior) such as walking in a circle, sitting and standing, or lip-smacking. Often these symptoms are accompanied by the presence of unusual thoughts, such as the feeling of *deja vu* (having been someplace before), uncontrollable laughing, fear, visual hallucinations, or experiencing unusual unpleasant odors. These interesting symptoms are thought to be caused by abnormal discharges in the temporal lobe.

Partial seizures sometimes progress and develop into generalized seizures. Generalized seizures involve both hemispheres of the brain and are described in terms of visible motor activity. Generalized tonic-clonic seizures involve periods of muscle rigidity (tonic stage) followed by spasmodic twitching (clonic stage) and then flaccidity and a gradual return to consciousness (postictal stage). Absence seizures are also generalized but do not have obvious convulsions. They involve brief losses of consciousness that may occur hundreds of times a day. They are treated differently than other types of seizures. Finally, status epilepticus is a life-threatening condition characterized by uninterrupted tonic-clonic seizures lasting more than 30 minutes or by two or more tonic-clonic seizures without an intervening lucid interval. The preferred therapy for each type of seizure differs.

Seizures are treated through several general mechanisms. The most common is direct action on the sodium and calcium ion channels in the neural membranes. Phenytoin (Dilantin) and carbamazepine (Tegretol) both inhibit the influx of sodium into the cell, thus decreasing the cell's ability to depolarize and propagate seizures. Valproic acid and ethosuximide act similarly, but they interact with calcium channels in the hypothalamus, where absence seizures typically begin. These two drugs are particularly useful because they are specific to hyperactive neurons and therefore have few side effects. Other medications such as benzodiazepines and barbiturates interact with the GABA receptor-chloride ion channel complex, as explained in the section on antianxiety and sedative-hypnotic drugs.

Antiseizure medications comprise several pharmacologic classes, including benzodiazepines (diazepam [Valium] and lorazepam (Ativan]), barbiturates (phenobarbitol [Luminal]), hydantoins (phenytoin [Dilantin], fosphenytoin [Cerebyx]), succinimides (ethosuximide [Zarontin]), and miscellaneous medications such as valproic acid (Depakote). Table 6–3 lists the preferred medication for treating each type of seizure.

Central Nervous System Stimulants

Stimulating the central nervous system is desirable in certain circumstances such as fatigue, drowsiness, narcolepsy, obesity, and attention deficit hyperactivity disorder. Broadly, two techniques may accomplish this:

- ★ Increasing the release or effectiveness of excitatory neurotransmitters
- ★ Decreasing the release or effectiveness of inhibitory neurotransmitters

Within the functional class of CNS stimulants are three pharmacologic classes, amphetamines, methylphenidates, and methylxanthines.

The amphetamines also include methamphetamine and dextroamphetamine. These drugs all increase the release of excitatory neurotransmitters including norepinephrine and dopamine. Norepinephrine is the primary cause of these drugs' effects, which include an increased wakefulness and

Table 6–3 Antiseizure Medications

Primary Generalized Tonic-Clonic Seizures	
Initial and First-Line Therapy	**Second-Line or Adjunctive Therapy**
Carbamazepine	Phenobarbital
Phenytoin	Primidone
Valproate	
Partial Seizures (with or without secondary generalization)	
Initial and First-Line Therapy	**Second-Line or Adjunctive Therapy**
Carbamazepine	Felbamate*
Phenytoin	Gabapentin
Valproate	Lamotrigine
	Phenobarbital
	Primidone
Absence Seizures	
Initial and First-Line Therapy	**Second-Line or Adjunctive Therapy**
Ethosuximide	
Valproate	
Myoclonic Seizures	
Initial and First-Line Therapy	**Second-Line or Adjunctive Therapy**
Valproate	Clonazepam
Mixed Seizures (myoclonic and tonic-clonic)	
Initial and First-Line Therapy	**Second-Line or Adjunctive Therapy**
Felbamate*	Phenytoin
Valproate	Primidone

*Felbamate (Felbatol) is recommended for use only for patients who respond inadequately to alternative treatments and whose epilepsy is so severe that its benefits are deemed to outweigh a substantial risk of aplastic anemia, liver failure, or both.

awareness as well as a decreased appetite. Amphetamines' most common uses, therefore, are treating drowsiness and fatigue and suppressing the appetite. Most of amphetamines' side effects result from overstimulation; they include tachycardia and other dysrhythmias, hypertension, convulsions, insomnia, and occasionally psychoses with hallucinations and agitation. Examples of this class include amphetamine sulfate (the prototype) and Dexedrine.

Methylphenidate, marketed as Ritalin, is the most commonly prescribed drug for attention deficit hyperactivity disorder (ADHD). While it is chemically different than the amphetamines, its pharmacologic mechanism of action is similar. Also, like the amphetamines, it has a high abuse potential and is therefore listed as a Class II controlled substance. While treating hyperactivity with a stimulant may seem odd, it is quite effective. Frequently, the cause of inappropriate behavior in a child with ADHD is his inability to concentrate or focus. Ritalin's stimulant effects increase this ability, and the unwanted behavior often diminishes.

The methylxanthines include caffeine, aminophylline, and theophylline. While caffeine, the prototype drug in this class, has few clinical uses, it is frequently ingested in coffee, colas, and chocolates. Theophylline's relaxing effects on bronchial smooth muscle make it helpful in treating asthma. The methylxanthines' mechanism of action is unclear, but it seems to block adenosine receptors. Adenosine is an endogenous neurotransmitter which is used clinically for certain types of tachycardias. Because methylxanthines block the adenosine receptors, larger than normal doses may be needed to achieve the desired result. This class's side effects are similar to the amphetamines', but they have a much lower potential for abuse and are not controlled drugs.

Psychotherapeutic Medications

Psychotherapeutic medications treat mental dysfunction. Unlike other disease states, we do not thoroughly understand the pathophysiology of mental dysfunction; therefore, we base much of our pharmacologic treatment of these conditions on our limited knowledge and on clinical correlation (scientific observation that these medications are indeed effective, even if we do not fully understand their mechanism). Medications are typically only one tactic in a balanced strategy for treating mental illness. Depending on the specific disorder, physicians will use other treatments such as psychotherapy and electroconvulsive therapy in conjunction with pharmaceutical interventions.

psychotherapeutic medication *drug used to treat mental dysfunction.*

While we do not completely understand these diseases' specific pathologies, they seem to involve the monoamine neurotransmitters in the central nervous system. These neurotransmitters (norepinephrine, dopamine, serotonin) have been implicated in the control and regulation of emotions. Imbalances in these neurotransmitters, especially dopamine, appear to be at least involved with, if not responsible for, most mental disease. Regulating these and other excitatory and inhibitory neurotransmitters forms the basis for psychopharmaceutical therapy. Schizophrenia appears to be related to an increased release of dopamine, so treatment is aimed at blocking dopamine receptors. Depression seems to be related to inadequate amounts of these neurotransmitters, so treatment is aimed at increasing their release or duration.

Content Review

Major Diseases Treated with Psychotherapeutic Medications

- Schizophrenia
- Depression
- Bipolar disorder

The major diseases treated with psychotherapeutic medications are schizophrenia, depression, and bipolar disorder. The *Diagnostic and Statistical Manual*, fourth edition (*DSM-IV*), published by the American Psychiatric Association, gives schizophrenia's chief characteristics as a lack of contact with reality and disorganized thinking. Its many different manifestations include delusions, hallucinations (auditory more frequently than visual), disorganized and incoherent speech, and grossly disorganized or catatonic behavior. Schizophrenia is typically treated with antipsychotic medications, frequently in conjunction with medications from other classes such as antianxiety drugs or antidepressants. **Extrapyramidal symptoms (EPS)**, a common side effect of antipsychotic medications, include muscle tremors and parkinsonism-like effects. As a result, antipsychotic medications are also known as **neuroleptic** (literally, *affecting the nerves*) drugs.

extrapyramidal symptoms (EPS) *common side effects of antipsychotic medications, including muscle tremors and parkinsonism-like effects.*

neuroleptic *antipsychotic (literally, affecting the nerves).*

The two chief pharmaceutical classes of antipsychotics and neuroleptics are phenothiazines and butyrophenones. Both have been mainstays of psychiatry since the mid-1950s and are considered traditional antipsychotic drugs. Medications in this group block dopamine, muscarinic acetylcholine, histamine, and alpha$_1$-adrenergic receptors in the central nervous system. These medications' therapeutic effects appear to come from blocking the dopamine receptors; their side effects are fairly well understood to originate in blocking the other receptors. The phenothiazines' and butyrophenones' mechanisms of action are the same; they differ only in potency and pharmacokinetics. The distinction between potency and strength is important. Strength refers to the drug's concentration, while potency is the amount of drug necessary to produce the desired effect. While the phenothiazines are considered low-potency and the butyrophenones are considered high-potency, they both produce the same effect. The differences in potency and pharmacokinetics determine which class of medication will be prescribed. Chlorpromazine (Thorazine) is the prototype phenothiazine; haloperidol (Haldol) is the prototype of the butyrophenones.

Content Review

Major Classes of Antipsychotic Medications

- Phenothiazines
- Butyrophenones
- Atypicals

Since the phenothiazines' and the butyrophenones' mechanisms of action are identical, their common side effects are also similar: extrapyramidal symptoms from cholinergic blockade in the basal ganglia of the cerebral hemispheres; orthostatic hypotension from blockage of alpha$_1$-adrenergic receptors; sedation; and sexual dysfunction. Treatment for these side effects typically involves modifying the drug dose. Diphenhydramine (Benadryl), an antihistamine with anticholinergic properties, is indicated for treating acute dystonic reactions (manifestations of EPS), which often present with tongue and neck spasm. Patients with a newly prescribed antipsychotic may experience these effects and contact EMS. Fortunately, treatment with diphenhydramine is effective and rapid. Orthostatic hypotension is treated in the usual fashion described in Chapter 19 on hemorrhage and shock.

Other medications used to treat psychotic conditions are considered atypical antipsychotics. While their mechanisms of action are similar to those of the traditional antipsychotics, the atypical

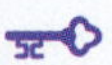

Be alert for the development of extrapyramidal symptoms any time you administer phenothiazine.

antipsychotics block more specific receptors. This specificity allows them to function much like traditional antipsychotics, but without causing the prominent extrapyramidal symptoms. These drugs include clozapine (Clozaril), risperidone (Risperdal), ziprasidone (Geodon), and olanzapine (Zyprexa).

Another functional class of psychotherapeutic medications includes the antidepressants. The *DSM-IV* characterizes major depressive episodes as causing significantly depressed mood, loss of interest in things that normally give the patient pleasure, weight loss or gain, sleeping disturbances, suicide attempts, feelings of hopelessness and helplessness, loss of energy, agitation or withdrawal, and an inability to concentrate. While the specific pathology of this disease is not yet known, it appears to be related to an insufficiency of monoamine neurotransmitters (norepinephrine and serotonin). Thus, the pharmaceutical interventions for this disease appear to increase the number of neurotransmitters released in the brain. The several ways of doing this include increasing the amount of neurotransmitter produced in the presynaptic terminal, increasing the amount of neurotransmitter released from the presynaptic terminal, and blocking the neurotransmitter's reuptake (reabsorption by the presynaptic terminal). This results in a net increase in the neurotransmitter. The antidepressants comprise three pharmacologic classes: tricyclic antidepressants, selective serotonin reuptake inhibitors, and monoamine oxidase inhibitors.

Content Review

Major Classes of Antidepressant Medications

- TCAs
- SSRIs
- MAOIs

Tricyclic antidepressants (TCAs) are frequently used in treating depression because they are effective, relatively safe, and have few significant side effects when taken in therapeutic dosages. TCAs act by blocking the reuptake of norepinephrine and serotonin, thus extending the duration of their action (Figure 6-3 ■). Unfortunately, they also have anticholinergic properties that cause many side effects including blurred vision, dry mouth, urinary retention, and tachycardia. Another frequent side effect, orthostatic hypotension, is likely due to the alpha$_1$-adrenergic blockade. This is commonly seen when patients try to stand up too quickly and become dizzy. Additionally, because TCAs can lower the seizure threshold, patients with existing seizure disorders are at risk for convulsions. Unfortunately, when taken in overdose, TCAs can have very significant cardiotoxic effects that make them a favored means of attempting suicide among depressed patients. These effects include myocardial infarction and dysrhythmias. Partly because of this potential for overdose, TCAs have fallen behind the newer selective serotonin reuptake inhibitors as the drug of choice for depression. Overdoses of these medications also frequently cause marked hypotension. Treatment of TCA overdoses is primarily supportive, with sodium bicarbonate given to increase the excretion of TCAs by alkalinizing the urine. The prototype tricyclic antidepressant, imipramine (Tofranil), was also the first one on the market. Other common examples include amitriptyline (Elavil), desipramine (Norpramin), and nortriptyline (Pamelor).

Selective serotonin reuptake inhibitors (SSRIs) are a recent addition to the antidepressants. The prototype, fluoxetine (Prozac), is one of the most widely prescribed antidepressants in the United States. These drugs' antidepressant effects are comparable to the TCAs', but because the SSRIs selectively block the reuptake of serotonin, they do not affect dopamine or norepinephrine. Nor do they block histaminic or cholinergic receptors, thus avoiding many of the TCAs' side effects. The primary adverse reactions to SSRIs are sexual dysfunction, headache, and nausea. Other selective serotonin reuptake inhibitors include sertraline (Zoloft) and paroxetine (Paxil).

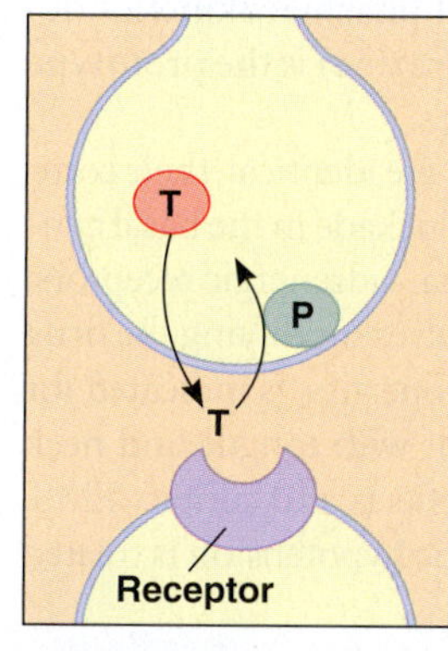

(a) Neurotransmission without TCA

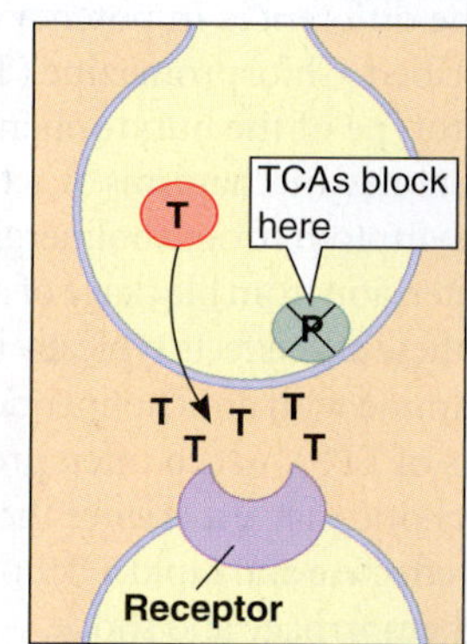

(b) Neurotransmission with TCA

■ **Figure 6-3** Effects of TCAs on reuptake of serotonin and norepinephrine.

A third pharmacologic class of psychotherapeutic medications includes the monoamine oxidase inhibitors (MAOIs). The monoamine neurotransmitters are thought to be insufficient in depression. Monoamine oxidase, an enzyme, metabolizes monoamines into inactive metabolites. MAOIs inhibit monoamine oxidase and block the monoamines' breakdown, thus increasing their availability. Monoamine oxidase is also present in the liver and has a significant role in metabolizing foods that contain tyramine, a substance that increases the release of norepinephrine. The MAOIs' major side effect is hypertensive crisis brought on by the consumption of foods rich in tyramine such as cheese and red wine. By inhibiting monoamine oxidase, these drugs also decrease the body's ability to inactivate tyramine; they therefore promote the release of norepinephrine, a potent vasopressor. Because of this and other unwanted side effects, MAOIs are not commonly used anymore; rather, they are reserved for treating depression that is refractory to TCAs and SSRIs. The prototype of this class is phenelzine (Nardil).

Patients with bipolar disorder (manic depression) exhibit cyclic swings from mania to depression with periods of normalcy in between. According to the *DSM-IV* the manic phases of this disease are characterized by hyperactivity, thoughts of grandeur or inflated self-esteem, decreased need for sleep, increased goal-oriented behavior, increased productivity, flight of ideas (moving from thought to thought with little connection between them), distractibility, and increased risk taking. Lithium is the drug of choice for the management of bipolar disorder. It is frequently given in conjunction with benzodiazepines or antipsychotics. Lithium's mechanism of action is unknown, but it effectively decreases the signs of mania without causing sedation. Adverse reactions include headache, dizziness, fatigue, nausea, and vomiting. Recently, two antiseizure medications—carbamazepine (Tegretol) and valproic acid (Depakote)—have proven successful in treating bipolar disorder.

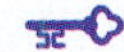

Lithium, widely used in the treatment of bipolar disorder, has a very low therapeutic index.

Drugs Used to Treat Parkinson's Disease

Parkinson's disease is a nervous disorder caused by the destruction of dopamine-releasing neurons in the *substantia nigra,* a part of the basal ganglia, which is a specialized area of the brain involved in controlling fine movements. Dysfunction of parts of the basal ganglia causes the extrapyramidal symptoms (EPS) often seen as a side effect of antipsychotic medications.

Parkinson's disease is characterized by dyskinesia (dysfunctional movements) such as involuntary tremors, unsteady gait, and postural instability. Severe cases also involve bradykinesia (slow movements) and akinesia (the absence of movement). In the later stages, patients frequently present with psychological impairment including dementia, depression, and impaired memory. Parkinson's is a progressive disease that usually begins in middle age with subtle signs and progresses to a state of incapacitation. While no treatments can cure Parkinson's or even slow its progression, treating the symptoms can return some function to the patient. The goal in treating these patients is to restore their ability to function without causing unacceptable side effects. Some remarkably effective drugs are available. Unfortunately, they usually are effective for only several years. After that, signs and symptoms return and often are more severe than before treatment began.

The medications that are effective in treating Parkinson's disease are also effective in treating the extrapyramidal side effects (EPS) of antipsychotics. This is because fine motor control is based in part on a balance between inhibitory and excitatory neurotransmitters. In the basal ganglia, dopamine, an inhibitory transmitter, opposes acetylcholine, an excitatory neurotransmitter. Parkinson's disease and the medications that cause EPS both decrease the number of presynaptic terminals that release dopamine in the basal ganglia. This allows the excitatory stimulus of acetylcholine to dominate, ultimately impeding fine motor control.

Pharmacologic therapy for Parkinson's disease seeks to restore the balance of dopamine and acetylcholine. This may be done either by increasing the stimulation of dopamine receptors or by decreasing the stimulation of acetylcholine receptors. Drugs can do this either through dopaminergic effects or through anticholinergic effects. Dopaminergic effects increase the release of dopamine from the neuron, directly stimulate the dopamine receptors, or decrease the breakdown of however much dopamine is being released. Anticholinergic effects prevent acetylcholine's effects either by reducing the amount of the neurotransmitter released or by directly blocking the acetylcholine receptors.

Dopamine cannot be given directly to Parkinson's disease patients because it cannot cross the blood–brain barrier and consequently would be ineffective in treating the disease while still causing many side effects. The drug of choice in treating Parkinson's disease, therefore, is levodopa, an inactive drug that readily crosses the blood–brain barrier. Levodopa is absorbed by the dopamine-releasing neuron terminals, where the enzyme decarboxylase metabolizes it into dopamine, thus increasing the amount of dopamine available for release. Levodopa is very effective and reduces symptoms in the vast majority of patients. As previously mentioned, however, symptoms will return within a period of years as the disease progresses. Levodopa's side effects include nausea, vomiting, and ironically, for unknown reasons, dyskinesias. Because it is converted to dopamine, levodopa may also have cardiovascular effects, including tachycardias and hypertension.

When given alone, levodopa is metabolized primarily outside of the brain, where it is ineffective. To prevent this, Sinemet, the most popular anti-Parkinson preparation available, combines levodopa with an inactive ingredient, carbidopa. While carbidopa by itself produces no effects, it prevents levodopa's conversion into dopamine in the periphery. Because carbidopa does not cross the blood–brain barrier, however, levodopa can still be metabolized in the CNS. This decreases the incidence of cardiovascular side effects and enables lower doses of levodopa to be effective. Sinemet's side effects are essentially those of levodopa by itself. Nausea and vomiting, stimulated from within the CNS, remain problematic.

Another dopaminergic medication, amantadine (Symmetrel), promotes the release of dopamine from those dopamine-releasing neurons that remain unaffected by the disease. It has a rapid onset but generally becomes ineffective in less than a year. While it can be effective alone, it is usually given in conjunction with Sinemet or levodopa. Several other medications such as bromocriptine directly stimulate the dopamine receptors instead of attempting to increase the amount of dopamine released.

One additional dopaminergic approach is to decrease the breakdown of dopamine after it has been released. The enzyme responsible for breaking down monoamines such as norepinephrine, dopamine, and serotonin is monoamine oxidase. (We have previously described monoamine oxidase inhibitors in our discussion of their role in depression.) One monoamine oxidase inhibitor, selegiline (Carbex), is specific for monoamine oxidase type B. This MAO-B enzyme is involved only in the breakdown of dopamine. (MAO-A is responsible for breaking down norepinephrine and serotonin.) By selectively inhibiting the breakdown of dopamine, selegiline increases the amount available for binding with dopamine receptors, thus promoting the dopamine-acetylcholine balance. This selective blockage avoids increased norepinephrine levels that can lead to undesired tachycardia and hypertension.

As opposed to dopaminergic medications, which act on the dopamine side of the dopamine-acetylcholine balance, anticholinergic medications act on the acetylcholine side to block the acetylcholine receptors. The prototype anticholinergic, atropine, was initially used in this context with success, but it also had the typical peripheral anticholinergic side effects of blurred vision, dry mouth, and urinary hesitancy. More recently developed medications affect the CNS more than they do the peripheral nervous system. The prototype centrally acting anticholinergic medication is benztropine (Cogentin). Another example is diphenhydramine (Benadryl), which is more frequently administered for its antihistaminic properties.

AUTONOMIC NERVOUS SYSTEM MEDICATIONS

autonomic nervous system *the part of the nervous system that controls involuntary actions.*

The **autonomic nervous system** is the part of the nervous system that controls involuntary (automatic) actions. Many medications used in prehospital care directly affect the autonomic nervous system. It is essential that you have a good understanding of this aspect of the nervous system and the ways in which emergency medications affect it.

The two functional divisions of the autonomic nervous system are the sympathetic nervous system and the parasympathetic nervous system. The sympathetic nervous system allows the body to function under stress. It is often referred to as the fight-or-flight aspect of the nervous system. The parasympathetic nervous system, however, primarily controls vegetative functions such as digestion of food. It is often referred to as the feed-or-breed or the rest-and-repose aspect of the nervous system. The parasympathetic nervous system and the sympathetic nervous system work in constant opposition to control organ responses. For example, the sympathetic nervous system stimulates specific receptors in the heart that increase the heart rate. At the same time, the parasympathetic nervous system stimulates specific receptors that decrease the heart rate. The net result is the resting heart rate. When the body's physiologic needs dictate an increased heart rate, the sympathetic stimuli dominate the parasympathetic effects. Conversely, when the body needs to rest (with a decreased heart rate), the parasympathetic stimuli predominate.

Basic Anatomy and Physiology

The autonomic nervous system arises from the central nervous system. The nerves of the autonomic nervous system exit the central nervous system and subsequently enter specialized structures called **autonomic ganglia.** In the autonomic ganglia, the nerve fibers from the central nervous system interact with nerve fibers that extend from the ganglia to the various target organs. Autonomic nerve fibers that exit the central nervous system and terminate in the autonomic ganglia are called **preganglionic nerves.** Autonomic nerve fibers that exit the ganglia and terminate in the various target tissues are called **postganglionic nerves.** The ganglia of the sympathetic nervous system are located close to the spinal cord, while the ganglia of the parasympathetic nervous system are located close to the target organs (see Figure 3-73).

No actual physical connection exists between two nerve cells or between a nerve cell and the organ it innervates. Instead, there is a space, or **synapse,** between nerve cells. The space between a nerve cell and the target organ is a **neuroeffector junction.** Specialized chemicals called **neurotransmitters** conduct the nervous impulse between nerve cells or between a nerve cell and its target organ.

Neurotransmitters are released from presynaptic neurons and subsequently act on postsynaptic neurons or on the designated target organ. When released by the nerve ending, the neurotransmitter travels across the synapse and activates membrane receptors on the adjoining nerve or target tissue. The neurotransmitter is then either deactivated or taken back up into the presynaptic neuron.

The two neurotransmitters of the autonomic nervous system are acetylcholine and norepinephrine. Acetylcholine is utilized in the preganglionic nerves of the sympathetic nervous system and in both the preganglionic and postganglionic nerves of the parasympathetic nervous system. Norepinephrine is the postganglionic neurotransmitter of the sympathetic nervous system. Synapses that use acetylcholine as the neurotransmitter are **cholinergic** synapses. Synapses that use norepinephrine as the neurotransmitter are **adrenergic** synapses.

The anatomy and physiology of the autonomic nervous system were discussed in detail in Chapter 3.

autonomic ganglia *groups of autonomic nerve cells located outside the central nervous system.*

preganglionic nerves *nerve fibers that extend from the central nervous system to the autonomic ganglia.*

postganglionic nerves *nerve fibers that extend from the autonomic ganglia to the target tissues.*

synapse *space between nerves.*

neuroeffector junction *specialized synapse between a nerve cell and the organ or tissue it innervates.*

neurotransmitter *chemical messenger that conducts a nervous impulse across a synapse.*

cholinergic *pertaining to the neurotransmitter acetylcholine.*

adrenergic *pertaining to the neurotransmitter norepinephrine.*

parasympathomimetic *drug or other substance that causes effects like those of the parasympathetic nervous system (also called cholinergic).*

parasympatholytic *drug or other substance that blocks or inhibits the actions of the parasympathetic nervous system (also called anticholinergic).*

Drugs Used to Affect the Parasympathetic Nervous System

The parasympathetic system uses acetylcholine (ACh) as a neurotransmitter. Acetylcholine released by presynaptic neurons activates receptors on the postsynaptic neurons or on the neuroeffector junction.

Receptors that are specialized for acetylcholine are termed cholinergic receptors. Medications that stimulate them are known as cholinergics (**parasympathomimetics**), and those that block them are known as anticholinergics or cholinergic blockers (**parasympatholytics**).

Cholinergics Cholinergic drugs act either directly or indirectly. Direct-acting cholinergics (also called cholinergic esters) simulate the effects of ACh by directly binding with the cholinergic receptors. Drugs in this class generally produce the same effects as cholinergic stimulation, mostly focused on the muscarinic receptors. Their adverse effects are related primarily to decreased heart rate, decreased peripheral vascular resistance resulting in hypotension and excessive salivation, urination, defecation, and sweating. Vomiting and abdominal cramps may also occur. The acronym SLUDGE (***s***alivation, ***l***acrimation, ***u***rination, ***d***efecation, ***g***astric motility, ***e***mesis) is helpful for remembering these effects.

The prototype direct-acting cholinergic is bethanechol (Urecholine). Its pharmacokinetics make it a good clinical substitute for acetylcholine. It is not broken down by cholinesterase, the enzyme responsible for destroying acetylcholine, and therefore it has a longer duration of action. Most of its effects are on muscarinic receptors in the urinary bladder and gastrointestinal tract. It may be given orally or subcutaneously. Thus, it is used primarily to increase micturition (urination) and peristalsis. Adverse effects are rare but are related to its parasympathomimetic effects. Another direct-acting cholinergic medication, pilocarpine, is used as a topical treatment for glaucoma.

Indirect-acting cholinergic drugs affect acetylcholinesterase. By inhibiting its actions in degrading acetylcholine, they prolong the cholinergic response. These drugs affect both muscarinic and nicotinic receptors and therefore have little specificity. Their uses are limited primarily to treating myasthenia gravis, some types of poisoning, and glaucoma as well as for reversing nondepolarizing neuromuscular blockade.

Content Review

SLUDGE Effects of Cholinergic Medications

- Salivation
- Lacrimation
- Urination
- Defecation
- Gastric motility
- Emesis

The two basic types of indirect-acting cholinergic drugs are reversible inhibitors and irreversible inhibitors. Both types bind with cholinesterase (ChE), acting as a substitute for ACh. In doing so, they prevent ChE from destroying ACh. The difference between the reversible and irreversible inhibitors is how long they remain bound with cholinesterase. The reversible inhibitors remain bound with cholinesterase much longer than acetylcholine but eventually release it. The irreversible inhibitors, too, will eventually release cholinesterase, but they remain bound for so long that, from a practical standpoint, they can be considered irreversible.

Neostigmine (Prostigmin) is the prototype reversible cholinesterase inhibitor. It is used to treat myasthenia gravis, an illness characterized by muscle weakness and progressive fatigue. This illness is an autoimmune disease that destroys the nicotinic$_M$ receptors at the neuromuscular junction. With fewer of these receptors, muscles cannot be stimulated as well and weakness occurs. Neostigmine treats the symptoms of myasthenia gravis by blocking the degradation of ACh, thereby prolonging its effects and increasing motor strength. Its primary side effects are due to the stimulation of muscarinic receptors and include the SLUDGE responses. Fortunately, these responses may be treated effectively with a cholinergic blocker. Neostigmine can also reverse a nondepolarizing neuromuscular blockade. This use is fairly uncommon, however, because such blockades typically are administered only intentionally as part of anesthesia or before intubation.

Physostigmine (Antilirium) is another reversible cholinesterase inhibitor. Its mechanism is similar to neostigmine's, with their primary difference being in their pharmacokinetics. While neostigmine is poorly absorbed across the cell membrane, physostigmine crosses rapidly and therefore has a shorter onset and may be given in lower doses. Physostigmine's chief use is for reversing overdoses of atropine, an anticholinergic drug that blocks muscarinic receptors.

Irreversible cholinesterase inhibitors have only one clinical function, the treatment of glaucoma, and only one drug, echothiophate (Phospholine Iodide), has been approved for that purpose. Cholinesterase inhibitors, however, are very useful as insecticides (organophosphates), and unfortunately, their mechanism of action is also very attractive for makers of chemical weapons. They are the chief component in nerve gases such as VX and sarin. They cause extensive stimulation of cholinergic receptors, ultimately resulting in the SLUDGE response. Toxic levels may also affect nicotinic$_M$ receptors, leading to paralysis. Treatment for such toxic exposures involves drugs such as high doses of atropine or pralidoxime (Protopam, 2-PAM) to block the effects of the accumulating acetylcholine. Pralidoxime can encourage irreversible cholinesterase inhibitors to release cholinesterase.

Content Review

Types of Parasympathetic Acetylcholine Receptors

- Muscarinic
- Nicotinic
- Nicotinic$_N$ (neuron)
- Nicotinic$_M$ (muscle)

Anticholinergics Anticholinergic agents oppose the parasympathetic (cholinergic) nervous system. Just as there are multiple types of cholinergic receptors, there are multiple classes of cholinergic receptor antagonists. We will discuss agents that selectively block muscarinic and nicotinic receptors as well as nonselective blockers (ganglionic blockers). A special subclass of nicotinic receptors is neuromuscular blocking drugs.

Muscarinic Cholinergic Antagonists Cholinergic antagonists block the effects of acetylcholine almost exclusively at the muscarinic receptors. They are often called anticholinergics or parasympatholytics. They work by competitively binding with muscarinic receptors without stimulating them. As a result, these receptors cannot bind with acetylcholine.

The prototype anticholinergic drug is atropine, which is widely used to block muscarinic receptors and is commonly administered in the field. Found in the plant *Atropa belladonna,* atropine is one of several drugs classified as belladonna alkaloids (scopolamine is also in this classification). Readily absorbed through both enteral and parenteral routes, it has therapeutic effects at dose dependent levels at most sites with muscarinic receptors. At low doses, atropine decreases secretion from salivary and bronchial glands as well as from the sympathetically innervated sweat glands. At moderate doses, it increases heart rate and causes mydriasis (dilated pupils) and blurry vision. At higher doses, it decreases gastric motility and stomach acid secretion. Atropine is also useful in reversing overdoses of muscarinic agonists (cholinergics or cholinesterase inhibitors). Its side effects, which are predictable, include dry mouth, blurred vision and photophobia, urinary retention, increased intraocular pressure, tachycardia, constipation, and anhidrosis (decreased sweating), which may cause hyperthermia. A helpful mnemonic for remembering the effects of atropine overdose is "hot as hell, blind as a bat, dry as a bone, red as a beet, mad as a hatter."

Content Review

Effects of Atropine Overdose

- Hot as hell
- Blind as a bat
- Dry as a bone
- Red as a beet
- Mad as a hatter

Scopolamine is another belladonna anticholinergic. Its actions are similar to atropine's, but unlike atropine, scopolamine causes sedation and antiemesis. Thus, its primary purpose is to prevent motion sickness. It is available as a transdermal patch.

Several synthetic medications mimic the effects of the belladonna alkaloids while minimizing their side effects. Ipratropium bromide (Atrovent), an inhaled anticholinergic, is effective in treating asthma because it relaxes the bronchial smooth muscle and causes bronchodilation. It is frequently administered along with an inhaled beta-adrenergic agonist. Because it is inhaled and has little systemic effect, ipratropium bromide avoids many of atropine's side effects.

Other anticholinergic drugs include dicyclomine (Bentyl) and benztropine (Cogentin).

Nicotinic Cholinergic Antagonists Nicotinic cholinergic antagonists block acetylcholine only at nicotinic sites. They include ganglionic blocking agents that block the nicotinic$_N$ receptors in the autonomic ganglia and neuromuscular blocking agents that block nicotinic$_M$ receptors at the neuromuscular junction.

Ganglionic Blocking Agents Ganglionic blockade is produced by competitive antagonism with acetylcholine at the nicotinic$_N$ receptors in the autonomic ganglia. This can, in effect, turn off the entire autonomic nervous system. The two drugs in this class are trimethaphan (Arfonad) and mecamylamine (Inversine). Both are used to treat hypertension. The adverse effects of ganglionic blockade include signs associated with antimuscarinic drugs like atropine—dry mouth, blurred vision, urinary retention, and tachycardia. Other adverse effects arising from the vasodilation and decreased preload caused by sympathetic blockage include profound hypotension, with orthostatic hypotension even more evident. Trimethaphan is administered primarily for hypertensive crisis when other treatments are ineffective. These agents are almost never used anymore because they are not selective and many superior agents are available.

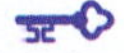

Neuromuscular blockers affect nicotinic$_M$ receptors.

Neuromuscular Blocking Agents Neuromuscular blockade produces a state of paralysis without affecting consciousness. Imagine how terrifying it would be to be fully conscious and aware but completely paralyzed, unable to move or breathe. Neuromuscular blockade is caused by competitive antagonism of nicotinic$_M$ receptors at the neuromuscular junction. This is useful during surgery as part of anesthesia and during electroconvulsive therapy for depression. These agents are most often used in the field to facilitate intubation.

Neuromuscular blocking agents are either depolarizing or nondepolarizing, depending on their mechanism of action. Most are nondepolarizing; only one depolarizing drug, succinylcholine (Anectine), is commonly used in the clinical setting. Tubocurarine, while not frequently used clinically, is the oldest neuromuscular blocker and the prototype nondepolarizing agent. It produces neuromuscular blockade by binding with the nicotinic$_M$ receptor sites without causing muscle depolarization. Succinylcholine acts in the same manner, but like acetylcholine, it does cause muscle depolarization when it binds with the nicotinic$_M$ receptor. It is useful as a neuromuscular blocker because, in contrast to ACh, which rapidly separates from the receptor, it remains bound, preventing the muscle's repolarization. Several nondepolarizing agents are available; the specific agent chosen depends on its rate of onset and duration of action. Succinylcholine has the shortest onset and duration of action because it has a naturally occurring enzyme, pseudocholinesterase, which degrades it.

Ganglionic Stimulating Agents Nicotinic$_N$ receptors reside at the ganglia of both the parasympathetic and sympathetic nervous systems. The alkaloid nicotine stimulates these receptors. Nicotine is found in tobacco and, although it has no therapeutic uses, is of interest for two reasons. Historically, nicotine, along with muscarine, led to a much better understanding of the autonomic nervous system's specific receptors. Also it is one of the most abused drugs in the world.

Nicotine may cause a variety of responses, most of which are dose related. At low doses, like those from smoking, nicotine causes excitation at the autonomic ganglia. This affects both the parasympathetic and sympathetic nervous systems. The parasympathetic response causes increased salivation, peristalsis, and secretion of gastric acid. The sympathetic response causes the release of norepinephrine and epinephrine. These lead to increases in heart rate, myocardial contractility, vasoconstriction, and blood pressure, all of which increase the heart's workload. Sympathetic stimulation also increases awareness and suppresses fatigue and appetite.

Drugs Used to Affect the Sympathetic Nervous System

sympathomimetic *drug or other substance that causes effects like those of the sympathetic nervous system (also called adrenergic).*

sympatholytic *drug or other substance that blocks the actions of the sympathetic nervous system (also called antiadrenergic).*

Medications that stimulate the sympathetic nervous system are **sympathomimetics.** Medications that inhibit the sympathetic nervous system are called **sympatholytics.** Some medications are pure alpha agonists, while others are pure alpha antagonists. Some medications are pure beta agonists, while others are pure beta antagonists. Medications such as epinephrine stimulate both alpha and beta receptors. Other medications, such as the bronchodilators, are termed beta selective, since they act more on beta$_2$ receptors than on beta$_1$ receptors.

The sympathetic nervous system releases norepinephrine from postganglionic end terminals and epinephrine from the adrenal medulla. These neurotransmitters bind with adrenergic receptors. (Epinephrine is also called adrenalin because of its release from the adrenal medulla; hence the term *adren*-ergic.) There are two main types of adrenergic receptors, each with two subtypes. These receptors' effects depend primarily on their locations. Table 6–4 describes the chief locations and primary actions of each receptor.

The primary clinical purpose for medications that stimulate alpha$_1$ receptors is peripheral vasoconstriction. Constriction of the arterioles increases afterload, while constriction of venules increases preload (decreasing venous capacitance or "pooling"). Both of these effects increase systolic and diastolic blood pressure and represent the chief therapeutic indication for alpha$_1$ agonists. Stimulation of alpha$_1$ receptors locally may be useful in combination with local anesthetics. The main reason to add the alpha$_1$ agonist in this context is to cause local vasoconstriction so that the systemic absorption of the anesthetic will decrease, and its duration will increase. Alpha$_1$ agonists are also useful topically to decrease nasal congestion caused by dilation and engorgement of nasal blood vessels. The primary adverse responses to alpha$_1$-agonist agents are hypertension and local tissue necrosis. If a medication with significant alpha$_1$ properties infiltrates the surrounding tissue or distal body parts such as fingers, toes, earlobes, or nose, inadequate local blood flow due to profound vasoconstriction will likely kill the tissue. Also, alpha$_1$ stimulation may cause reflex bradycardia due to the feedback mechanism that regulates blood pressure. As baroreceptors detect a rise in blood pressure, heart rate decreases to compensate.

Table 6–4 Location of Adrenergic Receptors and Effects of Stimulation

Receptor	Response to Stimulation	Location
Alpha$_1$ (α_1)	Constriction	Arterioles
	Constriction	Veins
	Mydriasis	Eye
	Ejaculation	Penis
Alpha$_2$ (α_2)	Presynaptic terminals inhibition*	
Beta$_1$ (β_1)	Increased heart rate	Heart
	Increased conductivity	
	Increased automaticity	
	Increased contractility	
	Renin release	Kidney
Beta$_2$ (β_2)	Bronchodilation	Lungs
	Dilation	Arterioles
	Inhibition of contractions	Uterus
	Tremors	Skeletal muscle
Beta$_3$ (β_3)	Lipolysis of adipose tissues	Fat stores
	Thermogenesis	Skeletal muscle
Dopaminergic	Vasodilation (increased blood flow)	Kidney

*Stimulation of α_2-adrenergic receptors inhibits the continued release of norepinephrine from the presynaptic terminal. It is a feedback mechanism that limits the adrenergic response at that synapse. These receptors have no other identified peripheral effects.

Alpha$_1$ antagonism is indicated almost exclusively for controlling hypertension. By preventing the peripheral vasoconstriction of alpha$_1$ stimulation, these agents decrease blood pressure. They are also useful in treating local tissue necrosis caused by infiltration of alpha$_1$ agonists. Injecting alpha$_1$ antagonists into the area surrounding the infiltration prevents tissue death from excessive vasoconstriction. The effects of pheochromocytoma, a tumor of the adrenal medulla that causes the release of large amounts of catecholamine, may be treated with an alpha$_1$ blocker. The most common adverse effects of alpha$_1$ antagonism are orthostatic hypotension and reflex tachycardia. Just as alpha$_1$ stimulation may increase blood pressure and cause a baroreceptor-mediated bradycardia, the hypotension from alpha$_1$ blockage may lead to reflex tachycardia from the same mechanism. Other side effects include nasal congestion and inhibition of ejaculation. These agents may also increase blood volume. This is ironic, since their primary indication is hypertension. As another feedback mechanism detects hypotension, the kidneys begin to reabsorb sodium and water to increase blood volume. This is typically addressed by use of a diuretic concomitant with the alpha$_1$ antagonist.

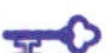

Phentolamine (Regitine), an alpha antagonist, can be used to help minimize tissue necrosis following extravasation of an alpha$_1$ agonist such as dopamine or norepinephrine.

Beta$_1$ stimulation increases heart rate, contractility, and conduction. Its primary indications are cardiac arrest and hypotension resulting from inadequate pumping. During cardiac arrest, beta$_1$ activation may stimulate contractions or increase the force of any existing contractions. Even if the heart is only fibrillating, these agents may increase the effectiveness of electrical defibrillation. In cardiogenic shock, when the heart is not pumping with enough force to overcome the afterload created by peripheral vascular resistance, beta$_1$ agonists can adequately increase the contractions' force. The chief adverse effects of beta$_1$ agonists include tachycardia, dysrhythmias, and chest pain from increasing workload.

Beta$_1$ antagonists are among the most frequently prescribed medications in the United States. Their most common use is to control blood pressure. By blocking the effects of beta$_1$ stimulation, they decrease heart rate (chronotropy) and contractility (inotropy). These agents are also effective in treating supraventricular tachycardias because they decrease the rate of impulse generation at the SA node (negative chronotropic effects) while also slowing conductivity through the AV node (negative dromotropic effects). Blocking beta$_1$ stimulation also helps treat angina pectoris and reduces the recurrence of myocardial infarction. Its main adverse effects are symptomatic bradycardia, hypotension, and AV block.

Beta$_2$ agonists are used to treat asthma and other conditions with excessive narrowing of the bronchioles. By stimulating beta$_2$ receptors in the lungs, these agents relax the bronchial smooth muscle and cause bronchodilation. Beta$_2$ agonists can also cause uterine smooth muscle relaxation, which may help to suppress preterm labor. Their primary adverse effects are muscle tremors and "bleed over" effects on unintended beta$_1$ stimulation such as tachycardias.

While beta$_2$ blockade serves no clinically useful purpose, nonselective beta blockers have side effects of beta$_2$ blockade. Chief among these is bronchoconstriction and inhibition of glycogenolysis, the release of stored glycogen by the liver and skeletal muscles. Beta$_2$ stimulation causes glycogenesis. Antagonizing the beta$_2$ receptors can inhibit this release. While this is not typically a problem for most people, it can be very problematic for diabetics. It not only makes hypoglycemia more likely but also masks one of its common early warning signs, tachycardia.

Adrenergic Agonists Drugs that stimulate the effects of adrenergic receptors work either directly, indirectly, or through a combination of the two. The direct acting agents bind with the receptor and cause the same response as the normal neurotransmitter. In fact, most of the drugs in this category either are synthetically produced versions of the naturally occurring neurotransmitter or are derivatives of those synthetically produced versions. The indirect acting agents stimulate the release of epinephrine from the adrenal medulla and of norepinephrine from the presynaptic terminals. In turn, the epinephrine and norepinephrine stimulate the adrenergic receptors. The mixed actions of direct-indirect acting medications combine these mechanisms.

The most frequently used adrenergic agents are chemically and functionally similar to the endogenous neurotransmitters. These drugs, which are called catecholamines, include norepinephrine, epinephrine, and dopamine. Synthetic catecholamines are also available. They include dobutamine and isoproterenol. Noncatecholamine adrenergic agents, including ephedrine, phenylephrine, and terbutaline, also affect the adrenergic receptors and have useful clinical applications.

Almost all of the drugs in this section act on more than one type of receptor. Their specificity varies and is important in determining their uses. Table 6–5 lists their actions on various receptors.

Review

Content

Common Catecholamines

- Natural
  - Epinephrine
  - Norepinephrine
  - Dopamine
- Synthetic
  - Isoproterenol
  - Dobutamine

Table 6–5 Adrenergic Receptor Specificity

Medication	Receptor: Alpha$_1$	Alpha$_2$	Beta$_1$	Beta$_2$	Dopaminergic
Phenylephrine	✓				
Norepinephrine	✓	✓	✓		
Ephedrine	✓	✓	✓	✓	
Epinephrine	✓	✓	✓	✓	
Dobutamine			✓		
Dopamine*			✓		✓
Isoproterenol			✓	✓	
Terbutaline				✓	

*Receptor specificity is dose-dependent. The higher the dose, the less dopaminergic effects are seen.

Adrenergic Antagonists Unlike most adrenergic agonists, the majority of available adrenergic antagonists are remarkably selective in which receptor they affect. This selectivity, however, occurs only at therapeutic doses. At higher doses, most agents lose their selectivity and begin affecting other receptors as well.

The two basic subcategories of alpha-adrenergic antagonists are "noncompetitive, long-acting" and "competitive, short-acting." They differ chiefly in the stability of their bond with the receptor. The prototype noncompetitive, long-acting alpha antagonist is phenoxybenzamine (Dibenzyline). The prototype competitive, short-acting antagonist is prazosin (Minipress). Prazosin also is the prototype for all alpha-adrenergic antagonists. Phentolamine (Regitine) is an important nonselective alpha antagonist because of its effects in reversing tissue necrosis caused by catecholamine infiltration.

Beta-adrenergic antagonists are more commonly referred to as beta-blockers. Propranolol (Inderal) is the prototype beta-blocker. It is a nonselective antagonist, which means that it blocks both beta$_1$ and beta$_2$ receptors. It is used to treat tachycardia, hypertension, and angina, all results of beta$_1$ blockade. Because it is nonselective, it also has the side effects of beta$_2$ blockade—bronchoconstriction and inhibited glycogenolysis. Propranolol was the first clinically employed beta-blocker, but its use has declined since the development of more selective beta$_1$ antagonists. The prototype of these cardioselective beta-blockers is metoprolol (Lopressor). At normal doses, metoprolol is selective for only beta$_1$ receptors; therefore, it does not cause propranolol's problematic side effects for asthmatics and diabetics. Atenolol (Tenormin) is another commonly used cardioselective beta-blocker.

Skeletal Muscle Relaxants Skeletal muscle relaxants are used to treat muscle spasm from injury and muscle spasticity from CNS injuries or diseases such as multiple sclerosis. Treatment can involve centrally acting agents or direct-acting agents.

The centrally acting muscle relaxants' mechanism is not clear, but it appears to be associated with general sedation. The prototype centrally acting skeletal muscle relaxant is baclofen (Lioresal), which is indicated in the treatment of spasticity. While baclofen is effective in the treatment of muscle spasticity, it is generally ineffective in muscle spasm. Several drugs are effective in treating muscle spasm, including cyclobenzaprine (Flexeril) and carisoprodol (Soma).

The prototype of the direct-acting muscle relaxants is dantrolene (Dantrium). Unlike the centrally acting agents, dantrolene's mechanism is well understood. It decreases the release of calcium from the sarcoplasmic reticulum in response to action potentials propagated from the neuromuscular junction. This calcium is required for the cross-bridge binding of the actin and myosin filaments in the muscle fibers responsible for contraction. Dantrolene is indicated for treating the spasticity associated with multiple sclerosis and cerebral palsy. It is also indicated for treating malignant hyperthermia, which is on rare occasion seen with some anesthetics and succinylcholine. This hyperthermia results from muscular contractions. Since dantrolene decreases these contractions, the heat that they generate also decreases. Dantrolene is not effective in treating muscle spasm.

DRUGS USED TO AFFECT THE CARDIOVASCULAR SYSTEM

Cardiovascular drugs have traditionally comprised one of the largest parts of the paramedic's pharmacologic "tool box." While this is changing with the expansion of paramedic practice, cardiovascular care (and agents used in that care) remains an important and integral part of a paramedic's knowledge base.

CLASSES OF CARDIOVASCULAR DRUGS

The drugs used to treat cardiovascular disease generally fall into the two broad functional classifications of antidysrhythmics and antihypertensives.

Antidysrhythmics

Antidysrhythmic drugs (Table 6–6) are used to treat and prevent abnormal cardiac rhythms. Used inappropriately, these medications can also cause dysrhythmias or deterioration in existing rhythms.

antidysrhythmic *drug used to treat and prevent abnormal cardiac rhythms.*

Sodium Channel Blockers (Class I) All of the medications in this general class affect the sodium influx in phases 0 and 4 of fast potentials. This slows the propagation of impulses down the specialized conduction system of the atria and ventricles, although it does not affect the SA or AV node.

Content Review

Antidysrhythmics are routinely classified in the Vaughn-Williams and Singh Classification System.

- I: Na^+ channel blockers
  - 1A
  - 1B
  - 1C
- II: Beta-blockers
- III: K^+ channel blockers
- IV: Ca^{++} channel blockers
- Miscellaneous

Class IA drugs include quinidine (Quinidex), procainamide (Pronestyl), and disopyramide (Norpace). In addition to slowing conduction, these drugs also decrease the repolarization rate. This widens the QRS complex and prolongs the QT interval. Quinidine is the prototype for this class, but procainamide is administered more frequently in emergency medicine. Procainamide is indicated in the treatment of atrial fibrillation with rapid ventricular response and ventricular dysrhythmias. Quinidine has a similar mechanism of action, but it also has anticholinergic properties that may induce unintended tachycardias.

Class IB drugs include lidocaine (Xylocaine), phenytoin (Dilantin), tocainide (Tonocard), and mexiletine (Mexitil). Unlike Class IA drugs, Class IB drugs increase the rate of repolarization. They also reduce automaticity in ventricular cells, which makes them effective in treating rhythms originating from ectopic ventricular foci. Lidocaine is the drug of choice for treating ventricular tachycardia and ventricular fibrillation. While lidocaine was once used prophylactically for patients with myocardial infarction, its use is now limited to life-threatening dysrhythmias. When given in overdose, lidocaine has significant CNS side effects including tinnitus, confusion, and convulsions.

Class IC drugs include flecainide (Tambocor) and propafenone (Rythmol). They decrease conduction velocity through the atria and ventricles as well as through the bundle of His and the Purkinje network. Like the Class IA drugs, they delay ventricular repolarization. Both of these medications,

Table 6–6 Antidysrhythmic Classifications and Examples

General Action	Class	Prototype	ECG Effects
Sodium Channel Blockers	IA	Quinidine, procainamide*, disopyramide	Widened QRS, prolonged QT
	IB	Lidocaine*, phenytoin, tocainide, mexiletine	Widened QRS, prolonged QT
	IC	Flecainide*, propafenone	Prolonged PR, widened QRS
	I (Misc.)	Moricizine*	Prolonged PR, widened QRS
Beta-Blockers	II	Propranolol*, acebutolol, esmolol	Prolonged PR, bradycardias
Potassium Channel Blockers	III	Bretylium*, amiodarone	Prolonged QT
Calcium Channel Blockers	IV	Verapamil*, diltiazem	Prolonged PR, bradycardias
Miscellaneous		Adenosine, digoxin	Prolonged PR, bradycardias

*Prototype

which are administered orally, are given to prevent recurrence of ventricular dysrhythmias, but both also have prodysrhythmic properties; that is, they are likely to cause dysrhythmias as well as treat them. They also depress myocardial contractility and are therefore reserved for potentially lethal ventricular dysrhythmias that do not respond to any other conventional therapy.

Moricizine (Ethmozine) has additional properties that exclude it from the other Class I subclasses. It blocks sodium influx during fast potential depolarization, thereby decreasing conduction velocity, but it can also depress myocardial contractility. Like the Class IC drugs, it is reserved for the treatment of ventricular dysrhythmias refractory to other conventional therapy.

Beta-Blockers (Class II) The drugs in this class, propranolol (Inderal), acebutolol (Sectral), and esmolol (Brevibloc), are all beta-adrenergic antagonists. Propranolol is nonselective, while acebutolol and esmolol are both selective for the $beta_1$ receptors in the heart. Of the many beta-blockers, these are the only ones approved for the treatment of dysrhythmias. They are indicated in the treatment of tachycardias resulting from excessive sympathetic stimulation. The $beta_1$ receptor in the heart is attached to the calcium channels. Blocking the $beta_1$ receptors thus blocks the calcium channel and prevents the gradual influx of calcium in phase 0 of the slow potential. As a result, the effects of beta-blocker therapy on dysrhythmias are almost identical to those of calcium channel blockers. Propranolol is the prototype Class II drug. Because it is nonselective, it also blocks the effect of $beta_2$ receptors, which leads to many of its side effects.

Potassium Channel Blockers (Class III) Potassium channel blocking drugs are also known as antiadrenergic medications because of their complex actions on sympathetic terminals. They include bretylium (Bretylol) and amiodarone (Cordarone); Bretylium is the prototype. They act on the potassium channels in the fast potentials. By blocking the efflux of potassium, bretylium prolongs repolarization and the effective refractory period. It is indicated in the treatment of ventricular fibrillation and refractory ventricular tachycardia. It causes an initial release, then an inhibition, of norepinephrine at the sympathetic end terminals. This delayed repolarization prolongs the QT interval; consequently, bretylium's primary and frequent side effect is hypotension.

Calcium Channel Blockers (Class IV) Calcium channel blockers' effect on the heart is almost identical to that of beta-blockers. They decrease SA and AV node automaticity, but most of their usefulness arises from decreasing conductivity through the AV node. They effectively slow the ventricular conduction of atrial fibrillation and flutter, and they can terminate supraventricular tachycardias originating from a reentrant circuit. Verapamil (Calan) and diltiazem (Cardizem) are the only two calcium channel blockers that affect the heart. Verapamil is the prototype. Their chief side effect is hypotension and bradycardia.

Miscellaneous Antidysrhythmics Adenosine (Adenocard) and digoxin (Lanoxin) are both effective antidysrhythmics. Magnesium is the drug of choice in *torsades de pointes,* a type of polymorphic ventricular tachycardia. We will briefly discuss each.

Adenosine does not fit any of the previous categories. It is an endogenous nucleoside with a very short half-life (about 10 seconds). It acts on both potassium and calcium channels, increasing potassium efflux and inhibiting calcium influx. This results in a hyperpolarization that effectively slows the conduction of slow potentials such as those found in the SA and AV nodes. It has little effect on the fast potentials in the ventricles and is not particularly effective on ventricular tachycardias or atrial fibrillation or flutter. Because of its short half-life its side effects are short lived, but they can be alarming. They include facial flushing, shortness of breath, chest pain, and marked bradycardias. Adenosine must be given as a rapid IV push, as the drug is rapidly metabolized. Doses should be increased in patients taking adenosine blockers such as aminophylline or caffeine. They should be decreased in patients taking adenosine uptake inhibitors like dipyridamole (Persantine) and carbamazepine (Tegretol).

Digoxin (Lanoxin) is a paradoxical drug. Its many effects on the heart make it both an effective antidysrhythmic and a potent prodysrhythmic (generator of dysrhythmias). While we do not clearly understand its specific actions on the heart's electrical activity, we do understand its effects. Digoxin decreases the intrinsic firing rate in the SA node, whereas it decreases conduction velocity in the AV node. Both of these effects are due to its increasing the strength of the parasympathetic effects on the heart. In the Purkinje fibers and ventricular myocardial cells, it decreases the effective refractory period and increases automaticity, both of which may explain its ability to increase ventricular dysrhythmias. To compound this, by depressing SA node activity, digoxin makes ectopic ventricular beats more likely to assume the pacing activity of the heart. Its side effects include bradycardias, AV blocks, premature ventricular contractions (PVCs), ventricular tachycardia, ventricular fibrillation, and atrial fibrillation. Actually, there are few dysrhythmias that digoxin does not produce. In addition, digoxin has a very narrow therapeutic index, meaning that it is difficult to find a patient's effective dose without producing side effects. Digoxin also increases cardiac contractility. It is indicated for atrial fibrillation with rapid ventricular conduction and chronic treatment of congestive heart failure.

Magnesium is the drug of choice in *torsades de pointes,* a polymorphic ventricular tachycardia, and in other ventricular dysrhythmias refractory to other therapy. Its mechanism of action is not known, but it may act on the sodium or potassium channels or on Na^+K^+ATPase.

Antihypertensives

Hypertension affects more than 50 million people in the United States alone and is a major contributor to coronary artery disease, stroke, and blindness. Fortunately, available drugs can effectively manage blood pressure with limited side effects in the vast majority of patients. Multiple studies have shown conclusively that controlling blood pressure decreases both morbidity and mortality. Blood pressure is equal to cardiac output times the peripheral vascular resistance:

$$\text{Blood pressure} = \text{Cardiac output} \times \text{Peripheral vascular resistance}$$

Cardiac output is equal to the heart rate times the stroke volume:

$$\text{Cardiac output} = \text{Heart rate} \times \text{Stroke volume}$$

Antihypertensive agents can manipulate each of these factors. The primary determinant of peripheral vascular resistance is the diameter of peripheral arterioles, which are affected by alpha$_1$ receptors. Heart rate is affected by both muscarinic receptors of the parasympathetic nervous system and beta$_1$ receptors of the sympathetic nervous system; however, hypertension control typically manipulates only beta$_1$ receptors. Stroke volume is affected by contractility and volume. Recall that Starling's law says that preload and stroke volume are proportionate; that is, as preload increases stroke volume increases (up to a point) and as preload decreases stroke volume decreases. Drugs that affect blood volume control hypertension by manipulating preload.

antihypertensive *drug used to treat hypertension.*

Several pharmacologic classes of medications are used to control blood pressure. The major approaches to dealing with hypertension are diuretics, beta-blockers and other antiadrenergic drugs, angiotensin converting enzyme (ACE) inhibitors, calcium channel blockers, and direct vasodilators. Of these, diuretics and beta-blockers are the most frequently prescribed, and they are effective in many patients. The remaining agents are used when diuretics or beta-blockers are contraindicated or when those approaches are not effective, although ACE inhibitors are gaining increasing popularity. Often, physicians must prescribe multiple drugs to manage hypertension effectively. In these cases, they will pick one drug from two or more classes that complement each other. For example, a physician might prescribe a diuretic with a beta-blocker.

Content Review

Pharmacological Classes of Antihypertensives

- Diuretics
- Beta-blockers and antiadrenergic drugs
- ACE inhibitors
- Calcium channel blockers
- Direct vasodilators

Diuretics Diuretics reduce circulating blood volume by increasing the amount of urine. This reduces preload to the heart, which in turn reduces cardiac output. The main categories of diuretics include loop diuretics (high ceiling diuretics), thiazides, and potassium sparing diuretics. They all affect the reabsorption of sodium and chloride and create an osmotic gradient that decreases the reabsorption of water. These classes differ according to which area of the nephron they affect. In general, the earlier in the nephron the drug works, the more sodium and water will be affected. Almost all electrolytes and other small particles in the blood are filtered through the glomerulus. Most sodium and water (approximately 65 percent) is reabsorbed in the proximal convoluted tubule. Another 20 percent is reabsorbed in the thick portion of the ascending loop of Henle, while only about 1 to 5 percent is recaptured in the distal convoluted tubule and collecting duct.

diuretic *drug used to reduce circulating blood volume by increasing the amount of urine.*

Therefore, a drug that decreases sodium reabsorption in the proximal convoluted tubule will cause the kidneys to excrete more water than will a drug that works on the distal convoluted tubule.

Loop diuretics, particularly furosemide (Lasix), play a major role in the emergency treatment of CHF and acute pulmonary edema.

Loop diuretics profoundly affect circulating blood volume. In fact, they decrease blood volume so well that they are typically considered excessive for treating moderate hypertension. They are, however, one of the primary tools in treating left ventricular heart failure (congestive heart failure). Their use for hypertension is typically because other diuretics have failed. Furosemide (Lasix) is the prototype of this class. Furosemide blocks sodium reabsorption in the thick portion of the ascending loop of Henle (hence, the name *loop diuretic*). In doing so, it decreases the pull of water from the tubule and into the capillary bed, thus decreasing fluid volume. Furosemide's main side effects are hyponatremia, hypovolemia, hypokalemia, and dehydration. Because the decrease in volume is most noticeable as decreased preload, orthostatic hypotension is a problem. Reflex tachycardia may also occur as the baroreceptors detect a decreased blood pressure and attempt to compensate by increasing heart rate. This happens in individuals with hypertension because the homeostatic "thermostat" has been set too high. In other words, the body believes that what is actually hypertension is normal and tries to maintain a higher blood pressure than is healthy. This reflex tachycardia is frequently treated with concurrent administration of a loop diuretic with a $beta_1$ blocker. Hypokalemia is frequently treated by increasing dietary potassium intake (bananas are rich in potassium) or by prescribing potassium supplements. An unexplained side effect of loop diuretics is ototoxicity (tinnitus and deafness). Administering loop diuretics slowly can decrease ototoxicity.

Thiazides have a mechanism similar to loop diuretics. The main difference is that the thiazides' mechanism affects the early part of the distal convoluted tubules and therefore cannot block as much sodium from reabsorption. Thiazides are often the drugs of choice in hypertension treatment because they can decrease fluid volume sufficiently to prevent hypertension but not so much that they promote hypotension. The prototype thiazide is hydrochlorothiazide (HydroDIURIL). This class has essentially the same side effects as loop diuretics. One important distinction is that thiazides depend on the glomerular filtration rate, while loop diuretics do not. Thus, loop diuretics may be preferred for patients with renal disease.

Potassium-sparing diuretics have a slightly different mechanism than other diuretics. Although they still affect sodium absorption, they do so by inhibiting either the effects of aldosterone on the distal tubules (as does spironolactone) or the specific sodium-potassium exchange mechanism (as does triamterene). Acting so late in the nephritic loop, these agents are not very potent diuretics. In fact, they are rarely used alone but instead are typically administered in conjunction with either a loop diuretic or a thiazide diuretic. They are useful as adjuncts to other diuretics because they not only decrease sodium reabsorption (although in small volumes) but also increase potassium reabsorption. This helps to limit the other diuretics' hypokalemic effects. Spironolactone (Aldactone) is the prototype potassium sparing diuretic.

While not used in the treatment of hypertension, osmotic diuretics are important because they alter the reabsorption of water in the proximal convoluted tubule. To do this, they use an osmotically large sugar molecule that is freely filtered through the glomerulus and pulls water after it. Mannitol (Osmitrol), the prototype osmotic diuretic, is used to treat increased intracranial and intraocular pressure.

Adrenergic Inhibiting Agents Inhibiting the effects of adrenergic stimulation can also control hypertension. Several broad mechanisms accomplish this: beta-adrenergic antagonism, centrally acting alpha-adrenergic antagonism, adrenergic neuron blockade, $alpha_1$ blockade, and alpha/beta blockade.

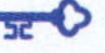

Beta-blockers have proven to decrease both short-term and long-term mortality associated with acute MI.

Beta Adrenergic Antagonists From Table 6–4 in our earlier discussion of $beta_1$ blockers, you will recall that most $beta_1$ receptors are in the heart but some also exist in the juxtaglomerular cells of the kidney. Selective $beta_1$ blockade is useful in treating hypertension for several reasons. It decreases contractility, thereby directly decreasing cardiac output. It also reduces reflex tachycardia by inhibiting sympathetically induced compensatory increases in heart rate. Finally, it represses renin release from the kidneys, which in turn inhibits the vasoconstriction activated by the renin-angiotensin-aldosterone system. The prototype selective $beta_1$ blocker is metropolol (Lopressor); the prototype nonselective beta-blocker is propranolol (Inderal). The section on $beta_1$ blockers discussed these agents' side effects.

Centrally Acting Adrenergic Inhibitors Centrally acting adrenergic inhibitors reduce hypertension by inhibiting CNS stimulation of adrenergic receptors. In effect, they are CNS $alpha_2$ agonists. Recall that $alpha_2$ receptors are located on the presynaptic end terminals in the sympathetic nervous system. When stimulated, they inhibit the release of norepinephrine to counterbalance sympathetic stimulation. By increasing the stimulation of alpha$_2$ receptors in the section of the CNS responsible for cardiovascular regulation, centrally acting adrenergic inhibitors decrease the sympathetic stimulation of both alpha$_1$ and beta$_2$ receptors. The net effect is to decrease heart rate and contractility by decreasing release of norepinephrine at beta$_1$ receptors and to promote vasodilation by decreasing norepinephrine release at alpha$_1$ receptors at vascular smooth muscle. The prototype drug in this category is clonidine (Catapres). While it does have some side effects, notably drowsiness and dry mouth, clonidine is a relatively safe and frequently prescribed antihypertensive agent. Methyldopa (Aldomet) is another centrally acting antihypertensive with a mechanism similar to clonidine.

Peripheral Adrenergic Neuron Blocking Agents Like the centrally acting adrenergic inhibitors, peripheral adrenergic neuron blocking agents work indirectly to decrease stimulation of adrenergic receptors. They do this by decreasing the amount of norepinephrine released from sympathetic presynaptic terminals. These agents are no longer commonly used.

The prototype of this class is reserpine (Serpalan). Reserpine has two actions that decrease the amount of norepinephrine released. First, it decreases the synthesis of norepinephrine. Second, it exposes norepinephrine in the terminal vesicles to monoamine oxidase, an enzyme that destroys it. This decreases stimulation of alpha$_1$ receptors, resulting in peripheral vasodilation, and of beta$_1$ receptors, resulting in decreased heart rate and contractility. The decreased peripheral vascular resistance and cardiac output in turn lower blood pressure.

Reserpine also decreases synthesis of several CNS neurotransmitters (serotonin and other catecholamines). This causes reserpine's primary adverse effect, depression. Reserpine, therefore, is not frequently used as an antihypertensive. Additional side effects include gastrointestinal cramps and increased stomach acid production. Other drugs with similar actions include guanethidine (Ismeline) and guanadrel (Hylorel).

Alpha$_1$ Antagonists This chapter's section on drugs affecting the sympathetic nervous system discusses the alpha$_1$-receptor antagonists in detail. Only their specific action will be repeated here. The prototype selective alpha$_1$ antagonist is prazosin (Minipress). It decreases blood pressure by competitively blocking the alpha$_1$ receptors, thereby inhibiting the sympathetically mediated increases in peripheral vascular resistance. By causing the arterioles to dilate, prazosine directly decreases afterload. By causing the venules to dilate, it promotes venous pooling, which decreases preload. The decreased afterload and preload help to lower blood pressure. Terazosin (Hytrin) is another drug with similar properties.

Combined Alpha/Beta Antagonists Labetalol (Normodyne) and carvedilol (Coreg) competitively bind with both alpha$_1$ and beta$_1$ receptors, increasing their antihypertensive actions. Hypertension is treated by decreasing alpha$_1$ mediated vasoconstriction, which, again, decreases both preload and afterload. Beta$_1$ blockade decreases heart rate, contractility, and renin release from kidneys. By blocking the release of renin, which promotes vasoconstriction, these agents decrease peripheral vascular resistance even further. Labetalol is commonly used to treat hypertensive crisis and is rapidly replacing the use of sublingual nifedipine (Procardia) for this purpose.

Angiotensin-Converting Enzyme (ACE) Inhibitors Agents in this class interrupt the renin-angiotensin-aldosterone system (RAAS) by preventing the conversion of angiotensin I to angiotensin II. Angiotensin II is one of the most potent vasoconstrictors yet discovered. By decreasing the amount of circulating angiotensin II, peripheral vascular resistance can be decreased, which leads to a decrease in blood pressure.

The juxtaglomerular apparatus in the kidneys releases renin in response to decreases in blood volume, sodium concentration, and blood pressure. Renin acts as an enzyme to convert the inactive protein angiotensinogen into angiotensin I. Neither angiotensinogen nor angiotensin I has much pharmaceutical effect, but angiotensin-converting enzyme (ACE) almost immediately converts angiotensin I in the blood into angiotensin II. (ACE is found in the lumen of almost all vessels and is found in the lungs in very high concentrations.) Angiotensin II causes both systemic and local vasoconstriction, with more pronounced effects on arterioles than on venules. It also lessens water loss by decreasing renal filtration secondary to renal vasoconstriction. Finally, angiotensin II also increases the release of aldosterone, a corticosteroid produced in the adrenal cortex. Aldosterone in turn increases sodium and water reabsorption in the distal convoluted tubule of the nephrons.

Angiotensin-converting enzyme inhibitors are very effective in treating hypertension and have also seen success in managing heart failure and renal failure. ACE inhibitors block the conversion of angiotensin I to angiotensin II, thereby providing a host of beneficial effects for patients with hypertension. These include a rapid decrease in arteriolar constriction, which lowers peripheral vascular resistance and afterload. While it does cause some dilation of the venules, this effect is limited. Because of the limited decrease in preload, orthostatic hypotension, common in other antihypertensives, is not a significant concern with ACE inhibitors. These agents also appear to be effective in preventing some of the untoward structural changes in the heart and blood vessels that angiotensin II causes over time.

In addition to their role in the treatment of hypertension, ACE inhibitors play an important role in the treatment of CHF by decreasing afterload.

The prototype ACE inhibitor is captopril (Capoten). Captopril acts like all ACE inhibitors to prevent hypertension. Its main advantage is the absence of side effects common to other antihypertensives. It does not interfere with beta receptors, so it does not decrease the ability to exercise or respond to hemorrhage. It does not cause potassium loss like many diuretics, and it does not cause depression or drowsiness. Because it has no effect on sexual desire or performance, it is much more attractive to many patients who might not comply with other medications. Other common ACE inhibitors include enalapril (Vasotec) and lisinopril (Zestril). These medications are all taken orally. For intravenous use in hypertensive crisis, enalaprilat (Vasotec I.V.) is available.

The most dangerous side effect of ACE inhibitors is pronounced hypotension after the first dose. This can be minimized by reducing initial doses, and it does not reoccur. The main adverse effects of continual use are a persistent cough and angioedema.

Angiotensin II Receptor Antagonists This recently developed classification of antihypertensive drugs also acts on the renin-angiotensin-aldosterone system. Angiotensin II receptor antagonists achieve the same effects as the ACE inhibitors without the side effects of cough or angioedema. The prototype of this new class is losartan (Cozaar).

Calcium Channel Blocking Agents We have already discussed two calcium channel blockers, verapamil and diltiazem, in the section on antidysrhythmics. Another structural subclass of calcium channel blockers is the dihydropyridines. The prototype dihydropyridine is nifedipine (Procardia, Adalat). Nifedipine, as well as the other members of the dihydropyridines, differs from verapamil and diltiazem in that it does not affect the calcium channels of the heart at therapeutic doses. Rather, it acts only on the vascular smooth muscle of the arterioles. These agents act by blocking the calcium channels in the arterioles. Calcium, which is required for muscle contraction, is released from sarcoplasmic reticulum upon activation by an action potential. When it enters the muscle cell through calcium channels, muscle contraction ensues. Blocking the calcium channels prevents the arterioles' smooth muscle from contracting and therefore dilates these vessels. When this occurs, peripheral vascular resistance decreases and blood pressure falls as a result of lower afterload. Because nifedipine has little effect on veins, it does not cause a corresponding drop in preload and consequently avoids orthostatic hypotension. While nifedipine does not affect the cardiac electrical conduction system, it is effective in dilating the coronary arteries and arterioles and thereby helps to increase coronary perfusion. The primary indications for nifedipine are angina pectoris and chronic treatment of hypertension. Its primary side effects include reflex tachycardia (responding to baroreceptor response to decreased blood pressure), facial flushing, dizziness, headache, and peripheral edema. It has been used commonly for the emergent reduction of blood pressure in the field; however, labetalol is replacing it.

Nifedipine was used extensively for emergent reduction of blood pressure. Now, other agents, such as labetalol, are preferred.

Direct Vasodilators We have already discussed several drugs that cause vasodilation. Two specific classes of vasodilators are those that dilate arterioles and those that dilate both arterioles and veins. All of these drugs are used to decrease blood pressure.

Selective dilation of arterioles causes a decrease in peripheral vascular resistance or afterload. This is the resistance that the heart must overcome in order to eject blood. Decreasing peripheral vascular resistance lowers blood pressure, increases cardiac output, and reduces cardiac workload. However, dilating the veins increases capacitance and decreases preload, the amount of blood in the heart prior to contraction. Starling's law tells us that as preload increases, so do stroke volume and cardiac output (up to a point). By decreasing preload, venodilators decrease both blood pressure and cardiac output.

Hydralazine (Apresoline) is the prototype for the selective arteriole dilators. It is effective in decreasing peripheral vascular resistance and afterload and thus lowering blood pressure. Its primary side effects are reflex tachycardia and increased blood volume. Both occur as a compensatory mechanism to lowered blood pressure, and both have the effect of increasing cardiac workload. As a result, hydralazine is almost always prescribed in conjunction with a beta-blocker and a diuretic. It is frequently used in the treatment of pregnancy-induced hypertension.

Hydralazine (Apresoline) is the preferred antihypertensive for the management of pregnancy-induced hypertension.

Minoxidil (Loniten) is another selective arteriole dilator with properties similar to those of hydralazine. One side effect deserves comment. It produces hypertrichosis (excessive hair growth) in about 80 percent of those taking it. While this is particularly irritating when it occurs all over a patient's body, it can become a therapeutic effect when the drug is applied as a topical ointment. Minoxidil is marketed in this form as Rogaine for promoting hair growth in men.

Unlike hydralazine, sodium nitroprusside (Nipride) acts on both arterioles and veins. It is the fastest acting antihypertensive available and is the drug of choice in hypertensive emergencies. It is very potent and is given via controlled IV infusion. Its effects are almost immediate and end within minutes of drug cessation; therefore, blood pressure must be carefully and continuously monitored during infusion, preferably in the ICU. Sodium nitroprusside has several significant side effects. Obviously, hypotension can be a problem when this medication is not carefully administered. Because cyanide and thyocyanate are by-products of nitroprusside metabolism, other adverse effects include cyanide poisoning and thyocyanate toxicity.

Ganglionic Blocking Agents Ganglionic blocking agents are nicotinic$_N$ antagonists. The prototype is trimethaphan (Arfonad). Since nicotinic$_N$ receptors exist at the ganglia of both the sympathetic and the parasympathetic nervous systems, competitive antagonism of these receptors turns off the entire autonomic nervous system, which is obviously not a very selective approach. When this happens, the effects on each organ system are determined by the predominant autonomic tone (the division of the ANS that normally has the greater influence on that organ). Because the arteries and veins have predominant sympathetic control, they dilate in response to trimethaphan administration. This reduces both preload and afterload, and blood pressure drops. Trimethaphan also directly affects vascular smooth muscle, causing dilation and the release of histamine, which is also a vasodilator. Mecamylamine (Inversine) is the other ganglionic blocking drug available in the United States, although it is not commonly used anymore.

Digitalis (Lanoxin) is still frequently used to increase cardiac output in CHF and to control the rate of ventricular response in atrial fibrillation.

Cardiac Glycosides The cardiac glycosides occur naturally in the foxglove plant. The two drugs in the class, digoxin (Lanoxin) and digitoxin (Crystodigin), are chemically related. These drugs are also known as digitalis glycosides. Digoxin is the prototype. One of the 10 most frequently prescribed medications in the country, it is indicated for heart failure and some types of dysrhythmias. Digoxin's mechanism of action is complex. It blocks the effects of Na^+K^+ATPase, an enzyme responsible for returning ion flow to normal levels after muscle depolarization. By interfering with this sodium-potassium pump, digoxin increases the intracellular levels of sodium. Because sodium is also involved in a reciprocal exchange with calcium, a buildup of intracellular sodium leads to a similar buildup of intracellular calcium. These elevated levels of intracellular calcium increase the strength of muscle contraction and are the basis for digoxin's primary indication. Digoxin reduces the symptoms of congestive heart failure by increasing myocardial contractility and cardiac output. This diminishes the dilation of the heart's chambers frequently seen in left heart failure because it enables the heart to effectively pump blood out of its ventricles, thus decreasing the engorgement typical of this condition. Increasing cardiac output decreases the sympathetic discharge mediated by baroreceptor reflexes, resulting in reduced afterload. Furthermore, digoxin indirectly lessens preload by increasing renal blood flow, which results in higher glomerular filtration and decreased blood volume. Digoxin also has antidysrhythmic effects, which we discuss more thoroughly in the section on antidysrhythmic medications.

While digoxin effectively treats the symptoms of heart failure, it also is potentially dangerous. Its therapeutic index is very small, and the individual variability is large. This leads to toxicity in some individuals even though they have normal digoxin levels. Digoxin's chief adverse effects are dysrhythmias. In fact, digoxin frequently induces some of the same dysrhythmias it is used to treat. Other side effects include fatigue, anorexia, nausea and vomiting, and blurred vision with a yellowish haze and halos around dark objects.

Other Vasodilators and Antianginals The drugs discussed in this section have vasodilatory properties that are useful in reducing blood pressure, but they are most commonly used to treat angina. The three basic types of angina pectoris (chest pain) are stable (exertional) angina; unstable angina; and variant, or Prinzmetal's, angina. Stable and unstable angina have the same pathophysiology and differ only by causation: stable angina occurs after exercise as a result of increased myocardial oxygen demand; unstable angina occurs without exertion. Both result from an imbalance between myocardial supply and demand. A buildup of plaque (atherosclerosis) along the walls of coronary arteries decreases these vessels' diameter and, as a result, the amount of blood flow to the heart. The same imbalance causes Prinzmetal's angina but it results from vasospasm instead of plaque buildup. The medications discussed in this section all either increase oxygen supply or decrease oxygen demand.

In addition to their previously discussed use as antihypertensives and antidysrhythmics, calcium channel blockers have a role in the treatment of angina. The three calcium channel blockers most frequently used for this purpose are verapamil (Calan, Isoptin), diltiazem (Cardizem), and nifedipine (Procardia). Recall that calcium is an integral part of both depolarization and muscle contraction. The effects of blocking its entry into the cells are twofold. All of these agents directly affect vascular smooth muscle, leading to dilation of the arterioles and, to a lesser degree, of the venules. This arterial dilation decreases peripheral vascular resistance and, as a result, afterload, which in turn directly decreases the workload of the heart and myocardial oxygen demand. Verapamil and diltiazem also reduce SA and AV node conductivity, which can decrease reflex tachycardia and dysrhythmias. Nifedipine has relatively few effects on the heart and, thus, has limited antidysrhythmic properties. The calcium channel blockers are effective in all forms of angina. A primary side effect of these agents is hypotension.

Nitroglycerin is effective in the management of angina pectoris as it decreases cardiac work.

Organic nitrates are potent vasodilators used to treat all forms of angina. First used clinically in 1879, nitroglycerin (Nitrostat) is the oldest of these drugs and is the category's prototype. Other agents include isosorbide (Isordil, Sorbitrate) and amyl nitrite. Nitroglycerin acts on vascular smooth muscle via a complex series of events to decrease intracellular calcium, thus causing vasodilation. Nitroglycerin primarily dilates veins rather than arterioles. This decreases preload and thus decreases myocardial workload, which is its primary antianginal effect. In Prinzmetal's angina, nitroglycerin reverses coronary artery spasm and increases oxygen supply.

Nitroglycerin is very lipid soluble, which allows it to cross membranes easily. Because of this, it is readily absorbed and can be administered via sublingual, buccal, and transdermal routes. The primary concern with nitroglycerin is orthostatic hypotension, a side effect more common in the presence of right ventricular failure. Other common side effects include headache and reflex tachycardia. Headache is frequently used as an indicator of the effectiveness of nitroglycerin, which rapidly loses its potency when exposed to light. While orthostatic hypotension is a serious concern with the administration of nitroglycerin, this condition typically responds well to fluid infusions.

Hemostatic Agents

hemostasis *the stoppage of bleeding.*

Hemostasis is the stoppage of bleeding. It is a series of events in response to a tear in a blood vessel. Damage to the vessel's intima (innermost layer) exposes the underlying collagen and triggers a release of two naturally occurring substances, adenosine diphosphate (ADP) and thromboxane A_2 (TXA_2). Both ADP and TXA_2 stimulate the aggregation of platelets and vasoconstriction. The vasoconstriction decreases the flow of blood past the tear, thus allowing the newly "sticky" platelets to form a plug that temporarily occludes the bleeding.

While this plug effectively halts bleeding for the short term, it must be reinforced to continue the stoppage until the tear can be permanently repaired. Stabilizing the plug requires a complex cascade of events involving the activation of naturally occurring factors and ending with the conversion of prothrombin into thrombin. The thrombin then converts fibrinogen into fibrin, a strandlike substance that attaches to the vessel's surface and contracts in a mesh web over the platelet plug to form a blood clot. Several of the factors involved need vitamin K to carry out their functions. A vitamin K deficiency inhibits clotting and makes uncontrolled bleeding more likely. Conversely, limiting the clotting cascade to the immediate area of the vessel injury is important for obvious reasons. The protein antithrombin III is key in this process. Antithrombin III binds with several of the factors needed for clotting, thus inhibiting their ability to coagulate.

Once the vessel has been permanently repaired, the fibrin mesh must be broken down. This process, called fibrinolysis, involves another cascading system that ends with the activation of plasminogen into plasmin, which in turn breaks up the clot. Tissue plasminogen activator, a substance in the tissue, activates this last conversion.

Thrombi (blood clots that obstruct vessels or heart cavities) are the primary pathology in several clinical conditions, including myocardial infarction, stroke, and pulmonary embolism. Drugs can effectively treat the causes of these conditions by decreasing platelet aggregation (antiplatelet drugs), by interfering with the clotting cascade (anticoagulants), or by directly breaking up the thrombus (fibrinolytics).

Content Review

Drugs Used to Treat Thrombi

- Antiplatelets
- Anticoagulants
- Fibrinolytics

Antiplatelets **Antiplatelet** drugs decrease the formation of platelet plugs. The prototype antiplatelet drug is aspirin. Aspirin inhibits cyclooxygenase, an enzyme needed for the synthesis of thromboxane A_2 (TXA_2). Remember that TXA_2 causes platelets to aggregate and promotes local vasoconstriction. By inhibiting TXA_2, aspirin decreases the formation of platelet plugs and potential thrombi. Aspirin, as well as other antiplatelet and anticoagulant drugs, has no effect on existing thrombi; it only curbs the formation of new thrombi. Aspirin is indicated in the acute treatment of developing myocardial infarction. It is also useful in preventing the reoccurrence of MI and of ischemic stroke following transient ischemic attacks (TIAs).

antiplatelet *drug that decreases the formation of platelet plugs.*

One of aspirin's primary side effects is bleeding. Aspirin also may lead to an increase in gastric ulcers, which are a frequent source of gastrointestinal hemorrhage. By both stimulating the development of a potential source of bleeding as well as blocking an important mechanism for stopping that bleeding, aspirin can cause dangerous blood loss. Other antiplatelet drugs include dipyridamole (Persantine), abciximab (ReoPro), and ticlopidine (Ticlid).

Anticoagulants **Anticoagulants** interrupt the clotting cascade. The two main types of anticoagulants are parenteral and oral. The prototype parenteral anticoagulant is heparin, a substance derived from the lungs of cattle or the intestines of pigs. Its primary mechanism of action is to enhance antithrombin III's ability to inhibit the clotting cascade. Because heparin is very polar, it is very poorly absorbed and must be given parenterally. Heparin injections and infusions are indicated in treating and preventing deep vein thrombosis, pulmonary embolism, and some forms of stroke. Heparin also is used frequently in conjunction with fibrinolytics to treat myocardial infarction. Finally, it is used to keep rubber-capped IV catheters (Hep-Locks) free from clots. As you would expect, bleeding is heparin's primary side effect. Other untoward effects include thrombocytopenia (decreased platelet counts) and allergic reactions. Heparin is measured in units rather than milligrams. A unit is that amount of heparin necessary to keep 1 mL of sheep plasma from clotting for 1 hour. Using this measurement is necessary because heparin's potency varies greatly when measured in milligrams.

anticoagulant *drug that interrupts the clotting cascade.*

Protamine sulfate is available as a heparin antagonist. Protamine can reverse the effects of heparin in the presence of dangerous and unintended bleeding by binding with heparin. This prevents heparin from binding with antithrombin III and enhancing its anticlotting abilities.

The prototype oral anticoagulant is warfarin (Coumadin). Warfarin's history serves as a useful reminder of its primary side effect. Warfarin was first developed as a rat poison that killed through uncontrolled bleeding. After noticing that a patient who attempted suicide by ingesting warfarin did not, in fact, die, its clinical use was investigated. Needless to say, this drug's primary side effect is bleeding.

Warfarin prevents coagulation by antagonizing the effects of vitamin K, which is needed for the synthesis of multiple factors involved in the clotting cascade. It is prescribed for chronic use to prevent thrombi in high-risk patients such as those who have hip replacements or artificial heart valves or those who are in atrial fibrillation. Because warfarin easily crosses the placental barrier and has dangerous *teratogenic* (capable of causing malformations) properties, it is contraindicated in pregnant patients. It also interacts adversely with many other medications. Like heparin, warfarin may lead to bleeding. In cases of overdose, you may give vitamin K as an antidote.

fibrinolytic *drug that acts directly on thrombi to break them down; also called* thrombolytic.

Fibrinolytics **Fibrinolytics** (also called thrombolytics) act directly on thrombi to break them up. The fibrinolytics share a similar mechanism of action. Through a chemical conversion, these drugs activate enzymes that dissolve thrombi or clots. The prototype drug of this class is streptokinase (Streptase). Other fibrinolytics include alteplase (tPA), reteplase (Retavase), and anistreplase (Eminase). These medications all dissolve clots effectively; they differ primarily in their administration and risk of bleeding side effects.

Streptokinase, which is derived from the streptococci bacterium, is the oldest available fibrinolytic. Its mechanism of action is to promote plasminogen's conversion to plasmin. Since plasmin dissolves the fibrin mesh of clots, it can directly treat the cause of most myocardial infarctions and some strokes, as opposed to antiplatelet agents and anticoagulants, which can only prevent potential future thrombi. Streptokinase also breaks down fibrinogen, the precursor to fibrin. While this action does not serve a clinical purpose (the problematic clot has already been formed), it does play an important role in streptokinase's chief side effect, bleeding. Other side effects include allergic reaction, hypotension, and fever.

Alteplase (Activase) is produced by recombinant DNA technology that is identical to the naturally occurring tissue plasminogen activator (hence its common name, tPA).

The window of opportunity for fibrinolytic therapy is limited. Because of this, some EMS systems administer fibrinolytics in the prehospital setting. Many have chosen to use reteplase (Retavase) because of its ease of administration (two 10-unit boluses administered 30 minutes apart).

Antihyperlipidemic Agents

Elevated levels of low-density lipoproteins (LDLs) have been clearly indicated as a causative factor in coronary artery disease. Lipoproteins are essentially transport mechanisms for lipids (triglycerides and cholesterol). Because lipids are insoluble in plasma, the body coats them in a plasma-soluble shell in order to transport them to their target destinations. Lipoproteins are categorized as very low-density (VLDL), low-density (LDL), intermediate-density (IDL), and high-density (HDL). Low-density lipoproteins contain most of the cholesterol in the blood and are required for transporting cholesterol from the liver to the peripheral tissues. Conversely, high-density lipoproteins (HDLs) carry cholesterol from the peripheral tissues to the liver, where it is broken down.

HDLs have been described as good cholesterol because they lower blood cholesterol levels and decrease the risk of coronary artery disease (CAD). LDLs are known as bad cholesterol because they increase blood cholesterol levels and the risk of CAD. As blood cholesterol levels increase, fatty plaque is deposited under the arteries' endothelial tissues. Atherosclerosis then develops, and coronary arteries decrease in diameter. Coronary vasoconstriction in turn reduces blood flow to the heart and, in times of increased myocardial oxygen demand, may lead to angina. Also, newly deposited plaque is often unstable. Typically, the plaque is under the endothelial tissues, which cap the plaque deposits. As the deposits age, the cap usually becomes fairly stable. In some cases, however, the cap breaks open and exposes the plaque to the blood. When this happens, platelet aggregation and coagulation begin. If the developing clot breaks free of the vessel, it becomes a thrombus and may completely occlude a coronary artery, leading to myocardial infarction.

The goal in lowering LDL levels is to prevent atherosclerosis and subsequent CAD. While raising HDL levels would help accomplish this, no pharmaceutical means of doing so currently exists. By far, the best way to lower LDL levels remains dietary modification. If this is not sufficient, several classifications of **antihyperlipidemic** medications may be used. The most common are drugs that inhibit hydroxymethylglutaryl coenzyme A (HMG CoA) reductase. The liver must have HMG CoA to synthesize cholesterol. By inhibiting this enzyme, HMG CoA agents lower LDL levels; however, they also increase the number of LDL receptors in the liver, causing a further uptake of LDL.

antihyperlipidemic *drug used to treat high blood cholesterol.*

Five HMG CoA reductase inhibitors are available. Because the names of all five end in *–statin*, these agents are also known as statins. They include lovastatin (Mevacor), atorvastatin (Lipitor), and simvastatin (Zocor). Lovastatin is the HMG CoA reductase inhibitors' prototype. Overall, these drugs are well tolerated. Their chief side effects are headache, rash, and flushing. In rare cases, they may cause hepatotoxicity and lead to liver failure.

Bile acid-binding resins can also reduce LDL levels. Inert substances that have no direct biologic activity, these agents pass straight through the GI system without being absorbed and are excreted in feces. They are useful, however, in that they indirectly increase the number of LDL receptors in the liver by binding with bile acids, thus decreasing their availability. Because the liver needs cholesterol to synthesize bile acids, it must have more cholesterol to compensate for the decrease in bile acids. The body therefore increases the LDL receptors on the liver. As more LDLs remain in the liver, their levels in the blood drop. Since the body does not absorb bile acid-binding agents, they have no systemic effects. Their chief untoward effect is constipation. Cholestyramine (Questran) is the prototype.

DRUGS USED TO AFFECT THE RESPIRATORY SYSTEM

Drugs that affect the respiratory system are useful for several purposes. The most obvious is the treatment of asthma, but this class also includes cough suppressants, nasal decongestants, and antihistamines.

ANTIASTHMATIC MEDICATIONS

Asthma is a common disease that decreases pulmonary function and may limit daily activities. It typically presents with shortness of breath, wheezing, and coughing. Its basic pathophysiology has two components, bronchoconstriction and inflammation. Typically a response to some sort of allergen sets both of these processes in motion. Common culprits include pet dander, mold, and dust. In patients with existing asthma, cold air, tobacco smoke, or other pollutants may bring on acute episodes of shortness of breath.

The response to asthma typically begins with an allergen's binding to an antibody on mast cells. This causes the mast cell membrane to rupture and release its contents, including histamine, leukotrienes, and prostaglandins. These cause immediate bronchoconstriction followed by a slower inflammatory response that can lead to mucous plugs and a further decrease in airway size. The inflammation may in turn cause a hyperreactivity to stimuli, and allergens that might not normally produce dyspnea may lead to an acute attack.

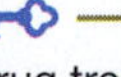

Drug treatment of asthma aims to relieve bronchospasm and decrease inflammation.

Drug treatment of asthma aims to relieve bronchospasm and decrease inflammation. Specific approaches are categorized as $beta_2$ selective sympathomimetics, nonselective sympathomimetics, methylxanthines, anticholinergics, glucocorticoids, and leukotriene antagonists. Cromolyn (Intal), a frequently used anti-inflammatory agent, does not fit neatly into any of those categories. Table 6–7 summarizes these agents.

Early pharmacological intervention in asthma is important in order to minimize inflammation.

$Beta_2$ Specific Agents Drugs that are selective for $beta_2$ receptors are the mainstay in treating asthma-induced shortness of breath. Albuterol (Proventil, Ventolin) is the prototype of this class. In general, these agents relax bronchial smooth muscle, which results in bronchodilation and relief from bronchospasm. Agents from this class are first-line therapy for acute shortness of breath and may also be used daily for prophylaxis. Most are administered via metered-dose inhaler or nebulizer. Albuterol and terbutaline may both be taken orally, and terbutaline may be given by injection. These medications' $beta_2$ specificity is not absolute; some patients may experience $beta_1$ effects such as tachycardia or dysrhythmias. Patients may also experience tremors resulting from the stimulation of $beta_2$ receptors in smooth muscles. Overall, these agents are very safe.

Nonselective Sympathomimetics Medications that stimulate both $beta_1$ and $beta_2$ receptors, as well as alpha receptors, are rarely used to treat asthma because they have the undesired effects of increased peripheral vascular resistance and increased risks for tachycardias and other dysrhythmias. Nonselective drugs include epinephrine, ephedrine, and isoproterenol. Epinephrine is the only nonselective sympathomimetic in common use today, due to the availability of selective agents. It may be given subcutaneously for patients who have severe bronchospasm that does not respond to other treatments.

Methylxanthines The methylxanthines are CNS stimulants that have additional bronchodilatory properties. While they were once first-line therapy for asthma, now they are used only when other drugs such as $beta_2$ specific agents are ineffective. We do not know the methylxanthines' specific action, but they may block adenosine receptors. The prototype methylxanthine, theophylline, is taken orally. Aminophylline, an IV medication, is rapidly metabolized into theophylline and, therefore, has identical effects. These agents' chief side effects are nausea, vomiting, insomnia, restlessness, and dysrhythmias. Aminophylline is still used occasionally in the emergency treatment of acute asthma attacks.

Table 6–7 Drugs Used in the Treatment of Asthma

Mechanism of Action	Medication
Bronchodilators	
Nonspecific agonists	Epinephrine
	Ephedrine
$Beta_2$ specific agonists	
Inhaled (short-acting)	Albuterol (Ventolin, Proventil)
	Metaproterenol (Alupent)
	Levalbuterol (Xopenex)
	Terbutaline (Brethine)
	Bitolterol (Tornalate)
Inhaled (long-acting)	Salmeterol (Serevent)
Methylxanthines	Theophylline (Theo-Dur, Slo-Bid)
	Aminophylline
Anticholinergics	Atropine
	Ipratropium (Atrovent)
Anti-inflammatory agents	
Glucocorticoids	
Inhaled	Beclomethasone (Beclovent)
	Flucticasone (Flovent)
	Triamcinolone (Azmacort)
Oral	Prednisone (Deltasone)
Injected	Methylprednisolone (Solu-Medrol)
	Dexamethasone (Decadron)
Leukotriene Antagonists	Zafirlukast (Accolate)
	Zileuton (Zyflo)
Mast-Cell Membrane Stabilizer	Cromolyn (Intal)

Anticholinergics Ipratropium (Atrovent) is an atropine derivative given by nebulizer. Because stimulating the muscarinic receptors in the lungs results in constriction of bronchial smooth muscle, ipratropium, a muscarinic antagonist, causes bronchodilation. Ipratropium is inhaled and, therefore, has no systemic effects. Ipratropium and $beta_2$ agonists like albuterol act along different pathways, so their concurrent administration has an additive effect. Ipratropium's most common side effect is dry mouth. It results from the local effects of the drug that remains in the oropharynx after administration.

Glucocorticoids Glucocorticoids have anti-inflammatory properties. They lower the production and release of inflammatory substances such as histamine, prostaglandins, and leukotrienes, and they reduce mucus and edema secondary to decreasing vascular permeability. These drugs may be inhaled or taken orally, or they may be given intravenously in emergencies. The prototype inhaled glucocorticoid is beclomethasone; the prototype oral glucocorticoid is prednisone. Primarily preventive, they are taken on a regular schedule as opposed to the as-needed administration of the $beta_2$ agonists. An injectable glucocorticoid (methylprednisolone) is available for use secondary to $beta_2$ agonists in emergencies. When inhaled, glucocorticoids cause few side effects. Those are due mostly to direct exposure on the oropharynx, and gargling after taking the drug can decrease them. Likewise, side effects from the intravenous administrations of methylprednisolone in emergencies are not likely. Given orally or intravenously over long periods, however, glucocorticoids may have profound side effects, including adrenal suppression and hyperglycemia.

Another anti-inflammatory agent used to prevent asthma attacks is cromolyn (Intal), an inhaled powder. While it is not a glucocorticoid, its actions are similar. While the inhaled glucocorticoids are relatively safe, cromolyn is even safer. In fact, it is the safest of all antiasthma agents. Its only side effects are coughing or wheezing due to local irritation caused by the powder. Cromolyn is often used for preventing asthma in adults and children. It is also a useful prophylaxis before activities known to cause shortness of breath such as exercise or mowing grass.

Leukotriene Antagonists **Leukotrienes** are mediators released from mast cells upon contact with allergens. They contribute powerfully to both inflammation and bronchoconstriction. Consequently, agents that block their effects are useful in treating asthma. Leukotriene antagonists can either block the synthesis of leukotrienes or block their receptors. Zileuton (Zyflo) is the prototype of those that block the synthesis of leukotrienes. Zafirlukast (Accolate) is the prototype of those that block their receptors.

leukotriene *mediator released from mast cells upon contact with allergens.*

DRUGS USED FOR RHINITIS AND COUGH

Rhinitis (inflammation of the nasal lining) comprises a group of symptoms including nasal congestion, itching, redness, sneezing, and rhinorrhea (runny nose). Either allergic reactions or viral infections such as the common cold may cause it. Drugs that treat the symptoms of rhinitis and cold are commonly found in over-the-counter remedies. In addition, nasal decongestants, antihistamines, and cough suppressants are available in prescription medications. Although manufacturers of cold medications often combine several drugs in one product intended to treat multiple symptoms, we will discuss each class separately.

Nasal Decongestants Nasal congestion is caused by dilated and engorged nasal capillaries. Drugs that constrict these capillaries are effective nasal decongestants. The main pharmacologic classification in this functional category is alpha$_1$ agonists. Alpha$_1$ agonists may be given either topically or orally. The chief examples of these agents, phenylephrine, pseudoephedrine, and phenylpropanolamine, can be administered either as a mist or in drops. Topical administration reduces systemic effects but has the undesired local effect of rebound congestion, a form of tolerance. Rebound congestion occurs after long-term use (greater than 7 consecutive days). As the drug wears off, congestion becomes progressively worse. This effect ends when the patient stops taking the drug; however, the longer the patient has been using the drug, the more unpleasant stopping becomes.

Nasal decongestants, when overused, can elevate both the pulse rate and the blood pressure.

Antihistamines **Antihistamines** arrest the effects of histamine by blocking its receptors. **Histamine** is an endogenous substance that affects a wide variety of organ systems. It is noted for its role in allergic reaction. In the vasculature, histamine binds with H$_1$ receptors to cause vasodilation and increased capillary permeability. In the lungs, H$_1$ receptors cause bronchoconstriction. In the gut, H$_2$ receptors cause an increase in gastric acid release. Histamine also acts as a neurotransmitter in the central nervous system. Histamine is synthesized and stored in two types of granulocytes; tissue-bound mast cells and plasma-bound basophils. Both types are full of secretory granules, which are vesicles containing inflammatory mediators such as histamine, leukotrienes, and prostaglandins, among others. When these cells are exposed to allergens, they develop antibodies on their surfaces. On subsequent exposures, the antibodies bind with their specific allergen. The secretory granules then migrate toward the cell's exterior and fuse with the cell membrane. This causes them to release their contents. While some available medications stabilize this membrane to prevent the release of these substances, the traditional antihistamines work by antagonizing the histamine receptors.

antihistamine *medication that arrests the effects of histamine by blocking its receptors.*

histamine *an endogenous substance that affects a wide variety of organ systems.*

Commonly thought of as a nuisance, histamines are useful in our immune systems. Only when our immune systems overreact do allergies such as hay fever or cedar fever send us running for the antihistamines. The typical symptoms of allergic reaction include most of those associated with rhinitis. Severe allergic reactions (anaphylaxis) may cause hypotension. While histamines play a major role in mild and moderate allergic reactions, their part in anaphylaxis is minimal; therefore, antihistamines are at best only a secondary drug for treating anaphylaxis. (Epinephrine is the drug of choice.)

Just as there are H$_1$ and H$_2$ histamine receptors, there are H$_1$ and H$_2$ histamine receptor antagonists. When most people refer to antihistamines, they are thinking of H$_1$-receptor antagonists.

These agents were in popular use long before the discovery of the H_2 receptors. (We discuss H_2-receptor antagonists in the section on drugs used to treat peptic ulcer disease.) The chief side effect of antihistamines is sedation, which the early antihistamines all caused to some degree. Now a second generation of antihistamines that do not cause sedation is available.

The first-generation antihistamines comprise several chemical subclasses. Examples include alkylamines (chlorpheniramine [Chlor-Trimeton]), ethanolamines (diphenhydramine [Benadryl], clemastine [Tavist]), and phenothiazines (promethazine [Phenergan]). While the different classes of agents have the same actions, they differ in the degree of sedation they cause and in their ability to block other, nonhistamine receptors. Several antihistamines also have significant anticholinergic properties. In fact, some are used specifically for their anticholinergic effects, notably promethazine and dimenhydrinate (Dramamine), which are used to reduce motion sickness. Other than the sedation that first-generation antihistamines cause, these agents' primary side effects are constipation and the effects of muscarinic blockade, such as dry mouth. Because they can thicken bronchial secretions, antihistamines should not be used in patients with asthma.

Because they can thicken bronchial secretions, you should not use antihistamines in patients with asthma.

The second-generation antihistamines include terfenadine (Seldane), loratadine (Claritin), cetirizine (Zyrtec), and fexofenadine (Allegra). These agents' actions are similar to the first generation's, with the notable exception that they do not cross the blood–brain barrier and therefore do not cause sedation. In addition, their H_1-receptor antagonism is more pronounced, and their anticholinergic actions are greatly diminished. Terfenadine was used widely until the FDA removed it from the market because it had rare but significant side effects of cardiac dysrhythmias in patients with liver dysfunction or taking certain medications. Terfenadine's manufacturer is now marketing fexofenadine (Allegra) as a replacement.

In general, treating a productive cough is not appropriate, as the cough is performing a useful function.

Cough Suppressants Coughing is a complex reflex that depends on functions in the CNS, the PNS, and the respiratory muscles. It is a defense mechanism that aids the removal of foreign particles like smoke and dust. A productive cough is one in which these particles are actually being coughed up. In general, treating a productive cough is not appropriate, as it is performing a useful function. An unproductive cough, however, usually results from an irritated oropharynx and can be troublesome. The three classifications of cough suppressants include one that is supported by evidence and two that are not. **Antitussive** medications suppress the stimulus to cough in the central nervous system. This functional class includes two specific pharmacologic types, opioids and nonopioids. The two most common opioid antitussives are codeine and hydrocodone. Both inhibit the stimulus for coughing in the brain but also produce varying degrees of euphoria. The doses required for cough suppression are not high enough to cause euphoria, but these drugs still have the potential for abuse. The nonopioid antitussives, in contrast, do not have the potential for abuse. Dextromethoraphan is the leading drug in this class. While it is almost never given alone, it is the most common antitussive used in over-the-counter combination products for treating cold and flu symptoms. Diphenhydramine (Benadryl) is also used as a nonopioid antitussive, although its mechanism of action is not clear. Finally, the locally acting anesthetic benzonatate (Tessalon) depresses the cough stimulus by directly reducing oropharyngeal irritation. **Expectorants** are intended to increase the productivity of cough, and **mucolytics** make mucus more watery and, therefore, easier to cough up; however, little data supports the effectiveness of either of these approaches to cough suppression.

antitussive *medication that suppresses the stimulus to cough in the central nervous system.*

expectorant *medication intended to increase the productivity of cough.*

mucolytic *medication intended to make mucus more watery.*

Content Review

Main Indications for Gastrointestinal Drug Therapy

- Peptic ulcers
- Constipation
- Diarrhea and emesis
- Digestion

DRUGS USED TO AFFECT THE GASTROINTESTINAL SYSTEM

The main purposes of drug therapy in the gastrointestinal system are to treat peptic ulcers, constipation, diarrhea, and emesis, and to aid digestion.

DRUGS USED TO TREAT PEPTIC ULCER DISEASE

Peptic ulcer disease (PUD) is characterized by an imbalance between factors in the gastrointestinal system that increase acidity and those that protect against acidity. PUD may manifest as indigestion, heartburn, or more seriously, as perforated ulcers. If the imbalance becomes too severe, parts of the lining of the GI system may be eaten away, exposing the tissue and vasculature underneath to the highly acidic environment of the stomach or duodenum. The GI system's structure fits its function. Many mucus-lined folds surround the GI lumen. The cells of these folds secrete acids needed to help break down foods; they secrete protective mucus that prevents the acid from injuring the underlying tissue; and finally, they secrete bicarbonates, which buffer the effects of acids on the GI system's absorbing surfaces. To absorb the digested nutrients and supply the mucus-producing cells of the lumen wall with oxygen, the entire GI system is very vascular. If the protective lining covering these vessels is removed, hemorrhage may occur.

Several pathologic factors oppose the GI system's defenses. Contrary to popular belief, the most common cause of peptic ulcer disease is not stress or alcohol, but the *Helicobacter pylori* bacterium. *H. pylori* infests the space between the endothelial cells and the mucus lining of the stomach and duodenum. It can remain there for decades, protected against the acid environment by the mucous layer. While we are still uncertain how this bacteria promotes ulcers, it apparently decreases the body's ability to produce the protective mucous lining. *H. pylori* by itself, however, does not cause ulcers. Many people remain infected for years and years without signs of PUD. Evidently, predisposing and contributing factors combine with *H. pylori* to cause ulceration. Some of these factors include smoking and long-term use of nonsteroidal antiinflammatory drugs (NSAIDs) like aspirin and acetaminophen.

The approaches to treating PUD include antibiotics and drugs that block or decrease the secretion of gastric acid. Most often they are used in conjunction with each other. First, and most effective, are antibiotics. When the *H. pylori* infection is eliminated, the signs of PUD resolve and recurrence is low. Typically, three antibiotics will be utilized to assure elimination of the bacteria and prevent resistance. Common medications for this purpose include bismuth (Pepto-Bismol), metronidazole (Flagyl), amoxicillin (Amoxil), and tetracycline (Achromycin V).

Drugs that block or decrease the secretion of gastric acid include H_2-receptor antagonists (H_2RAs), proton pump inhibitors, and anticholinergic agents. Mucosal protectants and antacids are also used.

H_2-receptors occur throughout the gut on the membranes of the parietal cells lining the GI lumen. When stimulated with histamine, they increase the action of H^+K^+ATPase, an enzyme that exchanges potassium for hydrogen, leading to increased gastric acid secretion. Acetylcholine and prostaglandin receptors appear along with H_2 receptors. Stimulating the ACh receptors (muscarinic receptors) increases gastric acid secretion; stimulating the prostaglandin receptors inhibits it.

H_2-Receptor Antagonists H_2RA agents block the H_2-receptors in the gut. This inhibits gastric acid secretion and helps return the balance between protective and aggressive factors. Four approved H_2RAs are in use: cimetidine (Tagamet), ranitidine (Zantac), famotidine (Pepcid), and nizatidine (Axid Pulvules). Cimetidine is the oldest of these and serves as the prototype. These agents' primary therapeutic use is for ulcers, gastroesophageal reflux, heartburn or acid indigestion, and preventing aspiration pneumonia during anesthesia. Most of these agents have few significant side effects, with the exception of cimetidine, which may lead to decreased libido, impotence, and CNS effects in some patients. While these agents could technically be called antihistamines, that name by tradition is reserved for the H_1 antagonists. The H_2RAs have no effect on the H_1 receptors and are of no value in allergic reaction.

Proton Pump Inhibitors Proton pump inhibitors act directly on the K^+H^+ATPase enzyme that secretes gastric acid. Omeprazole (Prilosec) and lansoprazole (Prevacid) are examples. Omeprazole is the prototype. These agents irreversibly block this enzyme, which means that the body must produce new enzyme in order to begin secreting acid again. This gives proton pump inhibitors a long duration of effect. Side effects are minor and rare, occurring in less than 1 percent of patients. They include diarrhea and headache.

Antacids Antacids are alkalotic compounds used to increase the gastric environment's pH. Most available products are either aluminum, magnesium, calcium, or sodium compounds. They are used in conjunction with other approaches to PUD and are available over the counter for relief of acid indigestion and heartburn.

antacid *alkalotic compound used to increase the gastric environment's pH.*

Anticholinergics While it might seem that all muscarinic blocking agents would be effective in decreasing gastric acid secretion, most atropinelike drugs produce too many unwanted effects and, therefore, are not used. The one exception is pirenzepine (Gastrozepine), because of its ability to selectively block the ACh receptors in the gut.

DRUGS USED TO TREAT CONSTIPATION

laxative *medication used to decrease stool's firmness and increase its water content.*

Laxatives decrease the firmness of stool and increase the water content. While an uninformed public frequently uses these agents unnecessarily, they are effective in some situations, specifically with patients for whom excessive strain is inappropriate. These patients include those with recent episiotomy, hemorrhoids, colostomies, or cardiovascular disease (for whom excessive straining may decrease heart rate).

Review

Content

Categories of Laxatives

- Bulk-forming
- Stimulant
- Osmotic
- Surfactant

Laxatives are traditionally grouped into four categories based on their mechanism of action: bulk-forming, surfactant, stimulant, and osmotic. The bulk-forming agents such as methylcellulose (Citrucel) and psyllium (Metamucil) produce a response almost identical to normal dietary fiber intake. Fiber is undigestible and unabsorbable; therefore, it remains in the lumen of the GI system and is passed more or less intact in stool. Most water absorption takes place in the colon. Fiber (or bulk-forming laxatives) in the colon absorbs water, leading to a softer, more bulky stool. Fiber can also provide nutrients for bacteria living in the colon. These bacteria feed and provide even more bulk. The enlarged stool stimulates stretch receptors in the colonic wall, which increases peristalsis. Softening the stool also lessens strain on defecation.

surfactant *substance that decreases surface tension.*

The **surfactant** laxatives include docusate sodium (Colace). They decrease surface tension, which increases water absorption into the feces. They also increase water secretion and limit its reabsorption by the intestinal wall.

Stimulant laxatives increase motility. Like the surfactant laxatives, they also increase water secretion and decrease its absorption. The prototype stimulant laxative is phenolphthalein (Ex-Lax, Correctol). Bisacodyl (Bisacolax) is another example.

The osmotic laxatives are poorly absorbed salts that increase the feces' osmotic pull, thereby increasing their water content. Magnesium hydroxide, the active ingredient in Milk of Magnesia, is the prototype of this class.

DRUGS USED TO TREAT DIARRHEA

Diarrhea is the abnormally frequent passage of soft, liquid stool. It is a symptom of an underlying disease, usually a bacterial infection. It may be caused by an increased gastric motility (the stool does not stay in the colon long enough to have much water absorbed), increased water secretion, or decreased water absorption. While it is a nuisance, diarrhea is often a helpful process because it increases the expulsion of the offending agent. It is usually self-correcting and does not need to be treated. When treatment is necessary, either specific or nonspecific agents may be used. A specific agent directly treats the cause, usually a bacteria. As you would expect, antibiotics are a common specific antidiarrheal medication.

DRUGS USED TO TREAT EMESIS

Emesis is a complex process that involves different parts of the brain as well as receptors and muscles in the stomach and inner ear. The two involved parts of the brain include the vomiting center in the medulla and the chemoreceptor trigger zone (CTZ). The vomiting center stimulates vomiting directly, while the CTZ does so indirectly.

The vomiting center is stimulated by H_1 and ACh receptors in the pathway between itself and the inner ear, by sensory input from the eyes and nose (unpleasant or disturbing sights and smells), and by other parts of the brain in response to anxiety or fear. The CTZ stimulates the vomiting center in response to stimuli from serotonin receptors in the stomach and bloodborne substances such as opioids and ipecac.

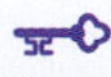

Ipecac is the drug of choice when stimulating emesis is indicated.

Stimulating emesis is rarely desired, but it can be useful in treating certain types of overdoses or poisonings. Ipecac is the drug of choice when stimulating emesis is indicated. It stimulates the CTZ which, in turn, stimulates the vomiting center.

Antiemetics Unlike causing emesis, preventing emesis is frequently desirable. **Antiemetics** are indicated in conjunction with chemotherapy, which may cause violent nausea and vomiting. Antiemetics are also indicated in the prophylactic treatment of motion sickness.

antiemetic *medication used to prevent vomiting.*

Multiple transmitters are involved in the vomiting reflex. They include serotonin, dopamine, acetylcholine, and histamine. Drugs that interfere with any of these transmitters can decrease or prevent nausea and vomiting. This functional class includes several pharmacologic subclasses: serotonin antagonists, dopamine antagonists, anticholinergics, and cannabinoids.

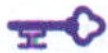

Many of the antiemetics used in emergency care can cause extrapyramidal symptoms. Always be alert for these.

Serotonin Antagonists The prototype serotonin antagonist is ondansetron (Zofran). It blocks the serotonin receptors in the CTZ, the stomach, and the small intestines. It is very effective in the treatment of nausea and vomiting associated with chemotherapy, and unlike the dopamine antagonists, it does not cause extrapyramidal effects like dystonia and ataxia. Its most common side effects are headache and diarrhea.

Dopamine Antagonists Both phenothiazines and butyrophenones effectively block dopamine receptors in the CTZ. (This chapter's section on psychotherapeutic medications discusses both of these medications at length.) The phenothiazines include prochlorperazine (Compazine) and promethazine (Phenergan), while the butyrophenones include haloperidol (Haldol) and droperidol (Inapsine). Agents from both classes cause side effects of extrapyramidal effects and sedation. Another dopamine antagonist, metoclopramide (Reglan), is neither a phenothiazine nor a butyropenone. It is unique in that it blocks both serotonin and dopamine receptors in the CTZ.

Cannabinoids The cannabinoids are derivatives of tetrahydrocannabinol (THC) and are effective antiemetics used to treat chemotherapy-induced nausea and vomiting. The two available agents are dronabinol (Marinol) and nabilone (Cesamet). Because both agents are essentially the same as THC (the active ingredient in marijuana), their side effects include euphoria similar to that of marijuana. While those effects may be desirable for some, they may be intensely unpleasant for others.

DRUGS USED TO AID DIGESTION

Several drugs are available to aid the digestion of carbohydrates and fats. These agents are similar to endogenous digestive enzymes released into the duodenum in response to vagal stimulation. Occasionally, supplemental enzymes are necessary for patients whose vagal stimulus has been surgically severed or whose duodenum has been bypassed. Two of these drugs are pancreatin (Entozyme) and pancrelipase (Viokase). Their chief side effects are nausea, vomiting, and abdominal cramping.

DRUGS USED TO AFFECT THE EYES

Ophthalmic drugs are used to treat conditions involving the eyes, primarily glaucoma and trauma. In addition, some ophthalmic agents are used in diagnosing and examining the eyes.

Glaucoma is a degenerative disease that affects the optic nerve. Its causative factors are not clear; however, correlations are known between it and several risk factors including intraocular pressure, race (its rate is three times higher among African Americans than among whites), and age. The medications used to treat glaucoma are all aimed at reducing intraocular pressure (IOP). Beta-blockers and cholinergics are the most common. Beta blockade decreases IOP by an unknown mechanism. Timolol (Timoptic) and betaxolol (Betoptic) are examples of this class. Pilocarpine (Isopto Carpine) is the prototype cholinergic drug for treating glaucoma. It stimulates muscarinic receptors in the eye to cause miosis (pupil constriction) and ciliary muscle contraction, which indirectly lowers IOP. Drugs from these classes are given topically. Beta-blockers have few side effects, while pilocarpine causes blurred vision and local irritation.

Some diagnostic procedures call for causing mydriasis (pupil dilation) and cycloplegia (paralysis of the ciliary muscles used to focus vision). The two pharmacologic approaches to doing this involve anticholinergics or adrenergic agonists. In this functional class, atropine solutions such as

Atropisol and scopolamine solutions such as Isopto Hyoscine are typical anticholinergics; phenylephrine solution (AK-Dilate) is the class's principal adrenergic agonist. This chapter's sections on anticholinergics and adrenergic agonists discuss these pharmacologic classes in more detail.

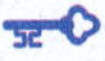

If tetracaine is administered in the field, remind the patient not to rub his eyes, as he can worsen the injury.

Tetracaine (Pontocaine) is a local anesthetic of the ester class. (It is related to cocaine, another ester, but not to lidocaine, an amide.) It is used to decrease pain and sensation in the eye from trauma or during ophthalmic procedures.

DRUGS USED TO AFFECT THE EARS

Most drugs used to treat conditions involving the ear are aimed at eliminating underlying bacterial or fungal infections or at breaking up impacted ear wax. Chloramphenicol (Chloromycetin Otic) and gentamicin sulfate otic solution (Garamycin) are common antibiotics; carbamide peroxide (Auro Ear Drops) and carbamide peroxide and glycerin (Ear Wax Removal System) are both used to treat ear wax. Finally, several drugs are available to treat swimmer's ear, an inflammation/irritation of the external ear. They include isopropyl alcohol (Auro-Dri Ear Drops) and boric acid and isopropyl alcohol (Aurocaine 2).

Some drugs that are used for other purposes have ototoxic (harmful to the organs or nerves that produce hearing or balance) properties if taken in overdose or administered too quickly. The most common ototoxic symptom is tinnitus, or ringing in the ears. Drugs with ototoxic properties include aspirin and other NSAIDs, some antibiotics (including erythromycin and vancomycin), and the diuretic furosemide (Lasix).

DRUGS USED TO AFFECT THE ENDOCRINE SYSTEM

The endocrine system and nervous system together are chiefly responsible for the regulatory activities that maintain homeostasis. The nervous system, with its direct connections between nerves and organs, may be thought of as a "wired" system, while the endocrine system, which releases hormones directly into the bloodstream, may be thought of as "wireless." The endocrine system comprises the following glands: pituitary (anterior and posterior lobes), pineal, thyroid, parathyroid, thymus, adrenal, pancreas, ovaries, and testes. Of these, the pituitary is commonly referred to as the master gland because of its role in controlling the other endocrine glands. (The hypothalamus in turn controls many of the pituitary's functions.) Once in the bloodstream, the hormones from these glands circulate widely throughout the body. To be effective, however, they must bind with very specific receptors. This discussion will focus on the pharmacologic actions of drugs that affect the various endocrine glands.

DRUGS AFFECTING THE PITUITARY GLAND

The pituitary gland has a posterior and an anterior lobe. Anterior pituitary-like drugs are used to treat abnormal growth: dwarfism, acromegaly, and gigantism. The two posterior pituitary hormones are oxytocin and antidiuretic hormone. Oxytocin is discussed in the section on drugs affecting labor and delivery. Antidiuretic hormone (ADH) promotes water retention. ADH analogs are used to treat diabetes insipidus and nocturnal enuresis (bed-wetting). At higher doses, ADH can cause vasoconstriction and increased blood pressure; hence its other name, vasopressin. Vasopressin (Pitressin), desmopressin (Stimate), and lypressin (Diapid) are all available to reverse ADH deficiency.

DRUGS AFFECTING THE PARATHYROID AND THYROID GLANDS

The parathyroid glands are primarily responsible for regulating calcium levels. Hypoparathyroidism leads to decreased levels of calcium and Vitamin D. Treatment, therefore, is through calcium and Vitamin D supplements. Hyperparathyroidism leads to high levels of calcium. Because it usually results from tumors, the treatment of choice is surgical removal of all or part of the parathyroid glands.

The thyroid gland produces thyroid hormones, which play a vital role in regulating growth, maturation, and metabolism. Hypothyroidism can occur in children or adults. When it develops in children, it is known as cretinism and manifests itself as dwarfism and mental retardation with characteristic features. Because most growth and maturation in adults is complete, adult onset of hypothyroidism appears as decreased metabolic rate, weight gain, fatigue, and bradycardia. In some cases, myxedema (facial puffiness) may be present. Treatment is aimed at thyroid hormone replacement. The prototype drug, levothyroxine (Synthroid), is also the most commonly used. A synthetic analogue of T_4 (thyroxine), one of the thyroid hormones, levothyroxine generally has no significant side effects when taken in therapeutic doses. Overdose may lead to thyrotoxicosis or thyroid storm. Thyrotoxicosis is a condition in which hyperthyroidism causes an increase in thyroid hormones. Thyroid storm is a severe form of thyrotoxicosis where the manifestations of the disease increase to life-threatening proportions. Thyroid storm is characterized by tachycardic dysrhythmias, angina, hypertension, and hyperthermia.

Goiters are enlargements of the thyroid gland. They are typically caused by insufficient dietary iodine. In developed countries, goiter is much rarer than in undeveloped countries and is most commonly caused by Hashimoto's disease, a chronic autoimmune disease. Treatment of goiters is aimed at supplementing the inadequate iodine.

Hyperthyroidism is caused by excessive release of thyroid hormones, typically as a result of tumors. The most common cause of hyperthyroidism in the United States is Graves' disease. It presents with tachycardia, hypertension, hyperthermia, nervousness, insomnia, increased metabolic rate, and weight loss. In severe cases, exophthalmos (protrusion of the eyeballs) may occur. Treatment is typically surgical removal of all or part of the thyroid gland. Radioactive iodine (^{131}I) may also be given for radiation therapy. Propylthiouracil (PTU) may be given alone or as adjunct therapy to surgery or radiation in treating hyperthyroidism.

DRUGS AFFECTING THE ADRENAL CORTEX

The adrenal cortex synthesizes and secretes three classes of hormones: glucocorticoids, mineralocorticoids, and androgens. The glucocorticoids and mineralocorticoids are referred to collectively as corticosteroids, adrenocorticoids, or corticoids. As their name implies, glucocorticoids increase the production of glucose by enhancing carbohydrate metabolism, promoting gluconeogenesis, and reducing peripheral glucose utilization. The most important glucocorticoid is cortisol. The mineralocorticoids regulate salt and water balance. The primary mineralocorticoid is aldosterone. The androgens are important hormones in regulating sexual maturation and development.

Two diseases typify the disorders associated with the adrenal cortex: Cushing's disease and Addison's disease. Cushing's disease is characterized by hypersecretion of adrenocorticotropic hormone, an anterior pituitary tropic hormone that increases the synthesis of corticoids, leading to excessive glucocorticoid secretion. Common signs and symptoms include hyperglycemia, obesity, hypertension, and electrolyte imbalances. Addison's disease is characterized by hyposecretion of corticoids as a result of damage to the adrenal gland. Common signs and symptoms include hypoglycemia, emaciation, hypotension, hyperkalemia, and hyponatremia.

Treatment of Cushing's disease is typically surgical. Symptomatic pharmacologic intervention with an antihypertensive (potassium sparing diuretics such as spironolactone [Aldactone] or ACE inhibitors such as captopril [Capoten]) may be necessary. Drugs that may inhibit the synthesis of corticosteroids (antiadrenals) may also be used as an adjunct to surgery or radiation. In high doses, the antifungal agent ketoconazole (Nizoral) is an effective temporary antiadrenal drug. At such doses, however, it may cause liver dysfunction.

Treatment of Addison's disease is aimed at replacement therapy. Cortisone (Cortistan) and hydrocortisone (SoluCortef) are the drugs of choice. Occasionally, a specific mineralocorticoid is necessary. Fludrocortisone (Florinef Acetate) is the only mineralocorticoid available.

DRUGS AFFECTING THE PANCREAS

Diabetes mellitus is the most important disease involving the pancreas. Diabetes mellitus (as opposed to diabetes insipidus, which involves inadequate ADH secretion) involves inappropriate carbohydrate metabolism. Traditionally, the term *diabetes* used alone refers to diabetes mellitus, of which the two main types are, logically, Type I and Type II. Type I diabetes, also known as insulin-dependent diabetes mellitus or IDDM, results from an inadequate release of insulin from the beta cells of the pancreatic islets. Patients with Type I diabetes rely on insulin replacement therapy to survive. Because

IDDM typically manifests itself at an early age (usually before 30 years) it is also commonly called juvenile onset diabetes. Most diabetics have Type II diabetes, which is also referred to as non-insulin-dependent diabetes mellitus (NIDDM) or adult onset diabetes. It results from a decreased responsiveness to insulin and a lack of synchronization between insulin release and blood glucose levels. Type II diabetes typically begins later in life (after 40 years) and almost always occurs in patients with obesity. Because they have functioning beta cells that release insulin, Type II diabetics usually do not depend on insulin replacement. Gestational diabetes, a third type, occurs transitionally during pregnancy. Gestational diabetes is a form of stress-induced diabetes in which the mother cannot effectively manage her blood glucose levels during pregnancy without medical intervention. Gestational diabetes resolves itself within hours to days after delivery.

The two main substances involved with regulating blood glucose are insulin and glucagon. Both are secreted from the pancreas and both are used to manage diabetes. Secreted from the beta cells of the pancreatic islets of Langerhans in response to increased blood glucose levels, **insulin** increases cellular transport of glucose, potassium, and amino acids. It also converts glucose into glycogen for storage in the liver and in skeletal muscle. Finally, insulin promotes cell growth and division.

insulin *substance that decreases blood glucose level.*

glucagon *substance that increases blood glucose level.*

Glucagon, too, is secreted from the pancreatic islets, but by alpha cells rather than by the insulin-producing beta cells. Glucagon's actions are the direct opposite of insulin's; it increases both glycogenolysis (glycogen breakdown into glucose) and gluconeogenesis (the synthesis of glucose from glycerol and amino acids). So, while insulin decreases blood glucose levels, glucagon increases them.

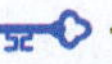

Always consider glucagon in the hypoglycemic patient when an IV cannot be started.

Patients with either Type I or Type II diabetes may experience both hyperglycemia and hypoglycemia. While hyperglycemia more often results from the disease, hypoglycemia is a common side effect of treatment. The main intervention for patients with IDDM is insulin replacement therapy. Several insulin preparations are available. The most effective therapy for patients with NIDDM is usually weight loss through diet modification and exercise. When this is not effective, oral hypoglycemic agents and, occasionally, insulin are used. Finally, glucagon and diazoxide (both can be considered hyperglycemic agents) are occasionally used for treating emergency hypoglycemia.

Insulin Preparations Insulin comes from one of three sources. Initially, it came from either beef or pork intestines. Now, recombinant DNA technology has made human insulin available (that is, insulin synthesized with a human RNA template, not harvested directly from humans). Insulin preparations differ primarily in their onset and duration of action and in their incidence of allergic reaction. Insulin preparations may be short acting, intermediate acting, or long acting, depending on their onset and duration of action. (Table 6–8 lists insulin preparations.)

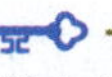

Diabetic ketoacidosis (DKA) is best treated by a continuous insulin infusion accompanied by frequent checks of the blood glucose levels.

Insulin is also classified as natural (regular) or modified. As their name suggests, the natural insulins are used as they occur in nature. The other insulin preparations have been modified to increase their duration of action and thus decrease the frequency of their administration. All insulin preparations are given subcutaneously, with the exception of regular insulin, which may also be given intravenously. Insulin is not available as an oral medication because the digestive enzymes would rapidly render it inactive; therefore, IDDM patients must take multiple injections every day of their lives. This may discourage compliance in some patients.

The modified insulin preparations include neutral protamine Hagedorn (NPH) insulin, which is regular insulin attached to a large protein designed to delay absorption, and the lente series, which is attached to zinc. Two preparations of lente insulin are available by themselves, lente and ultralente. A third, semilente insulin, is available only in a combination product with other insulins.

Insulin preparations are used for lifelong replacement therapy in IDDM and for emergency treatment of hyperglycemia and hyperkalemia in nondiabetics. (Recall that insulin also increases potassium uptake by cells and is therefore useful in lowering potassium levels.) These preparations' primary side effect is unintended hypoglycemia. Because beta$_2$-adrenergic blockers can hide the effects of hypoglycemia, patients may not recognize this condition's signs until they cannot care for themselves. Also, beta-blockers decrease the release of glucagon, so these patients' hypoglycemia may be even worse. Insulin preparations derived from beef or pork, as well as the lentes, may lead to allergic reactions. The natural human insulin preparations do not have this effect.

Oral Hypoglycemic Agents Oral hypoglycemic agents are used to stimulate insulin secretion from the pancreas in patients with NIDDM. These agents are ineffective in people with Type I diabetes since those patients cannot secrete insulin. This functional class comprises four pharmacologic classes:

Table 6–8	**Insulin Preparations**				
Classification	**Trade Name**	**Source**	**Onset (Hrs)**	**Peak (Hrs)**	**Duration (Hrs)**
Rapid-Acting			0.25+	<0.75–2.5	3.5–5.0
Lispro Insulin	Humalog	Human			
Aspart Insulin	NovoRapid	Human			
Short-Acting or Regular			0.5–10	2.0–5.0	5.0–8.0
	Humulin R	Human			
	Novolin R	Human			
	Iletin II R	Pork			
Intermediate-Acting or NPH			1−2	4–12	14–18
	Humulin N	Human			
	Novolin N	Human			
	Iletin II NPH	Pork			
Premixed			0.5–1.0	2–12	14–18
	Humulin 70/30	Human			
	Humulin 50/50	Human			
	Novolin 70/30	Human			
	Novolin 50/50	Human			
Intermediate-Acting			2–4	7–15	12–24
	Humulin L	Human			
	Iletin II Lente	Pork			
Long-Acting			3–4	8–24	24–28
	Humulin U	Human			
	Ultralente				
Insulin Glargine			>1.5	No peak	>20
	Lantus	Human			

sulfonylureas, biguanides, alpha-glucosidase inhibitors, and thiazolidinediones. The sulfonylureas were the first class of oral hypoglycemics available and as such are also known as first-generation or second-generation oral hypoglycemics, depending on when they were released. Drugs in this class include tolbutamide (Orinase), chlorpropamide (Diabinese), glipizide (Glucotrol), and glyburide (Micronase). They work by increasing insulin secretion from the pancreas and may also increase tissue response to insulin. Their major side effect is hypoglycemia.

The only agent in the biguanide class is metformin (Glucophage). It decreases glucose synthesis and increases glucose uptake. It does not stimulate the release of insulin from the pancreas and therefore does not cause hypoglycemia. Its primary side effects are nausea, vomiting, and decreased appetite.

Alpha-glucosidase inhibitors include acarbose (Precose) and miglitol (Glyset). They work by delaying carbohydrate metabolism, which moderates the increase in blood glucose that occurs after meals. These agents' primary side effects are flatulence, cramps, diarrhea, and abdominal distention resulting from colonic bacteria feeding on the increased number of carbohydrates remaining in fecal matter.

Thiazolidinediones are a new class of oral hypoglycemic agents unrelated to the others. The only drug in this class is troglitazone (Rezulin). It works by promoting tissue response to insulin and thus making the available insulin more effective. Troglitazone has no major side effects.

Hyperglycemic Agents Two hyperglycemic agents, glucagon and diazoxide (Proglycem), act to increase blood glucose levels. Glucagon is indicated for the emergency treatment of patients with hypoglycemia. It will frequently be given intramuscularly to hypoglycemic patients in whom an IV line is unobtainable. Occasional side effects are nausea and vomiting and, rarely, allergic reactions. Diazoxide (Proglycem) inhibits insulin release and is typically used only for patients with hyperinsulin secretion resulting from pancreatic tumors; it is more commonly used for hypertension. It is not indicated for treating diabetes-induced hypoglycemia.

Dilute $D_{50}W$ to $D_{25}W$ for administration to pediatric patients.

$D_{50}W$ (50 percent dextrose in water) is a sugar solution given intravenously for acute hypoglycemia. Its primary side effect is local tissue necrosis if infiltration occurs.

DRUGS AFFECTING THE FEMALE REPRODUCTIVE SYSTEM

The main groups of drugs affecting the female reproductive system are estrogens, progestins, oral contraceptives, drugs affecting uterine contraction, and those used to treat infertility.

Estrogens and Progestins Estrogens are produced in females by the ovaries and the ovarian follicles, and in pregnancy, the placenta. Outside of pregnancy, the ovaries are the principal source of estrogens. The principal ovarian estrogen is estradiol, of which there are many commercial preparations. The principal indication for estrogen is replacement therapy in postmenopausal women. After menopause, estrogen levels drop significantly and have been indicated as a major cause of menopausal symptoms such as hot flashes and vaginal dryness and as an increased risk factor for osteoporosis and coronary artery disease. Hormone replacement therapy (HRT) with estrogen has been shown to alleviate menopausal symptoms and reverse the increased risk for osteoporosis; however, it is not without its own risks. Recent studies have shown increased chances of breast cancer and stroke associated with hormone replacement therapy. Side effects include nausea, fluid retention, and breast tenderness. The nausea usually diminishes after several months of therapy. Estrogen is also administered in cases of delayed puberty in girls as a result of hypogonadism.

The progestins' principal noncontraceptive use is to counteract the untoward effects of estrogen on the endometrium in hormone replacement therapy for postmenopausal women. They are also used to treat amenorrhea, endometriosis, and dysfunctional uterine bleeding.

Oral Contraceptives Oral contraception is an effective means of preventing pregnancy. All oral contraceptives' primary mechanism of action is the prevention of ovulation, which makes the endometrium less favorable for implantation and promotes the development of a thick mucous plug that blocks access to sperm through the cervix. These contraceptives are either a combination of estrogen and progestin or, in the case of "mini-pills," progestin only. They may also be classified based on their administration cycle as monophasic, biphasic, or triphasic. These classes differ in how they alter the dose of estrogen or progestin throughout the menstrual cycle. Many different preparations are available, although they all work in similar fashion. In general, these drugs are well tolerated and have few side effects. The oral contraceptives' chief side effects are unintended pregnancy (in less than 3 percent of users), thromboembolism (this risk is much lower with the newer low-estrogen dose preparations), hypertension, and abnormal uterine bleeding. They are in wide use and are one of the most widely prescribed drug classes. They are the second most popular means of birth control after surgical sterilization (male and female combined).

Uterine Stimulants and Relaxants Drugs that increase uterine contraction (uterine stimulants) are oxytocics (oxytocin means rapid birth). Drugs that relax the uterus or inhibit uterine contraction are tocolytics.

The primary indications for administration of an oxytocic are to induce labor and to treat severe postpartum hemorrhage. Oxytocin is available commercially as Pitocin and Syntocinon. The uterus becomes increasingly sensitive to oxytocin throughout gestation, progressing from relatively insensitive before pregnancy to very sensitive around the time of labor. Oxytocin's chief side effect, water retention, is rarely significant and only so if large volumes of fluid have been administered without careful ongoing assessment. Ergonovine (Ergotrate), a derivative of a rye fungus, is a powerful uterine stimulant. It increases both the force and duration of contraction. Because of this increased duration, ergonovine is only used in the treatment of postpartum hemorrhage.

The tocolytics relax uterine smooth muscle by stimulating the $beta_2$ receptors in the uterus. The two $beta_2$ agonists commonly used for this purpose are terbutaline (Brethine) and ritodrine (Yutopar). Terbutaline's primary use is to treat asthma, but it is commonly used to delay labor even though the FDA does not currently approve it for that purpose. Both agents decrease both the force and frequency of contraction. Their chief side effects are the same as those of the other $beta_2$ agonists used to treat asthma: tremors and tachycardia. Occasionally, hyperglycemia may result from glycogenolysis in the liver.

Infertility Agents A number of conditions may cause infertility, which is the inability to become pregnant, and medications can treat only some of them. Most infertility drugs are developed for women and promote maturation of ovarian follicles. Clomiphene (Clomid), urofollitropin (Metrodin), and menotropins (Pergonal) are all within this class, although they each act by a different mechanism. These agents' side effects include ovarian enlargement or cysts, abdominal pain, and menstrual irregularities.

DRUGS AFFECTING THE MALE REPRODUCTIVE SYSTEM

Drugs that affect the male reproductive system include those that treat testosterone deficiency and benign prostatic hyperplasia. Testosterone replacement therapy may be indicated in testosterone deficiency caused by cryptorchidism (failure of one or both of the testes to descend during puberty), orchitis (testicular inflammation), or orchidectomy (testicular removal). It is also used in delayed puberty. Preparations include testosterone enanthate, methyltestosterone (Metandren), and fluoxymesterone (Halotestin).

Benign prostatic hyperplasia is an enlarged prostate. This is a common but problematic age-related disease. By the age of 70, close to 75 percent of men will have symptoms severe enough to seek therapy. These symptoms may include urinary hesitancy and retention. Treatment has traditionally been surgery, but several drugs are available, including finasteride (Proscar), which interferes with the production of an enzyme involved with prostate growth. Side effects may include rash, breast tenderness, headache, impotence, and decreased libido.

DRUGS AFFECTING SEXUAL BEHAVIOR

For centuries, cultures have searched for drugs that would increase libido and sexual potency. Ironically, the reverse has most commonly been found. The largest category of drugs affecting sexual behavior do so as a side effect of their intended purpose. Many drug classifications decrease libido in both sexes and inhibit erection and ejaculation. Examples include antihypertensives (beta-blockers, centrally acting alpha antagonists, and diuretics) and antianxiety/antipsychotic medications (benzodiazepines, phenothiazines, MAO inhibitors, tricyclic antidepressants, and SSRIs).

Many drugs are purported to increase libido. The most notable of these is cantharis (Spanish fly). Despite common belief, no evidence indicates that cantharis actually increases sexual appetite. Indeed, it can produce some very dangerous side effects. Hallucinogens such as LSD and marijuana, as well as alcohol, are also commonly believed to heighten sexuality. Any such effect from these agents is likely an indirect result of decreased inhibitions or anxiety. These drugs all have very different effects, depending on each individual's unique physiology, expectations before use, and surrounding circumstances. They have no proven direct physiologic effect on sexual gratification.

Levodopa (L-dopa), an anti-Parkinson's drug, has demonstrated increased libido and improved erectile ability as a side effect of treatment. Whether this results directly from increased autonomic stimulation or indirectly from improved self-esteem achieved in therapy, any improvement seems to be only temporary. Finally, sildenafil (Viagra) was approved in 1998 for pharmacologic therapy in patients with erectile dysfunction. Several drugs have been developed that aid in erectile dysfunction. Erectile dysfunction becomes more frequent with age or with certain diseases such as diabetes or cardiovascular disease. Drugs that aid in erectile dysfunction increase blood supply to the penis. These include sildenafil (Viagra), vardenafil (Levitra), and tadalafil (Cialis). These drugs act by relaxing vascular smooth muscle, which increases blood flow to the corpus cavernosum, the spongelike tissue on the sides of the penis responsible for erection. These drugs

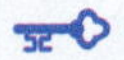

If you treat a patient with chest pain who has taken sildenafil, vardenafil, or tadalafil recently, do not give him nitroglycerin or any other nitrate.

are unique in that they have no effect in the absence of sexual stimulation. Other drugs used to treat impotence have caused prolonged and painful erections (priapism). The chief side effect of sildenafil, vardenafil, or tadalafil is seen when they are used in combination with nitrates. The combined effect of relaxing vascular smooth muscle may lead to a dangerously decreased preload, which may lower blood pressure and lead to myocardial infarction. Prehospital personnel should be aware of this important interaction. If you are called on to treat a patient with chest pain who has taken sildenafil, vardenafil, or tadalafil recently, do not give him nitroglycerin or any other nitrate.

DRUGS USED TO TREAT CANCER

antineoplastic *drug used to treat cancer.*

Drugs used to treat cancer are called **antineoplastic** agents. A detailed discussion of the many different antineoplastic agents is beyond the scope of this text; however, this section will briefly overview their main classes and prototype drugs.

Cancer involves the modification of cellular DNA leading to an abnormal growth of tissues. Of the many known types of cancer, only a few are successfully treated with chemotherapy. In fact, most cancers are best treated by surgical removal of the tumor. Unfortunately, many of the more lethal cancers do not involve a compact growth; rather, they affect the formed elements of the blood, especially leukocytes. Treating these widely dispersed cancers with surgery is not possible, as there is nothing for the surgeon to remove.

Chemotherapy is not nearly as safe or devoid of side effects as antibiotic therapy; however, scientists have yet to identify any unique characteristics of cancer cells that would allow them to develop drugs specific to those cells. Because cancer is the abnormal growth of normal cells, drugs that kill cancerous cells therefore also kill noncancerous cells. Chemotherapy is thus largely a balancing act aimed at maximizing the kill rate of cancer cells while minimizing the death of normal tissue. The one characteristic that most cancer cells share is rapid cell division and replication. Consequently, most antineoplastic agents have their greatest effect on cancer cells during mitosis and on young, small cancers that are undergoing rapid growth.

The agents used to kill cancer cells are grouped according to their mechanism of action. Antimetabolite drugs mimic some of the enzymes and proteins needed for DNA replication but do not have the same effects; therefore, they prevent cells from reproducing. Their prototype is fluorouracil (Adrucil). Alkylating agents that interfere with DNA splitting include cyclophosphamide (Cytoxan) and mechlorethamine (Mustargen). Mitotic inhibitors also interfere with cell division; they include vinblastine (Velban) and vincristine (Oncovin).

Chemotherapy's primary side effects include nausea, vomiting, and other gastrointestinal disturbances, as well as hair loss and weakness. Almost all antineoplastic agents cause severe side effects and are given in conjunction with antiemetics.

DRUGS USED TO TREAT INFECTIOUS DISEASES AND INFLAMMATION

Infectious diseases are typically caused by bacteria, viruses, or fungi and may be treated with antimicrobial drugs developed to fight those particular invaders. We will discuss each broad class.

antibiotic *agent that kills or decreases the growth of bacteria.*

Antibiotics An **antibiotic** agent may either kill the offending bacteria (bactericidal agents) or so decrease the bacteria's growth that the patient's immune system can effectively fight the infection (bacteriostatic agents). In general, all of these agents share one of several mechanisms. Drugs in the penicillin and cephalosporin classes, as well as vancomycin (Vancocin), are bactericidal and act by inhibiting cell wall synthesis. Unlike animal cells, bacteria have hypertonic cell cytoplasm and depend on the rigid and relatively impermeable cell wall to maintain integrity. When cell wall synthesis is inhibited, osmotic pressure pulls water into the cell, and the cell ruptures, killing the bacteria. The macrolide, aminoglycoside, and tetracycline antibiotics inhibit protein synthesis, preventing the bacterial cell from replicating and thus spreading infection. These agents are usually bacteriostatic but can be bactericidal at high doses. Typical side effects from antibiotics include gastrointestinal dysfunction, which commonly results from a decrease in the natural gastrointestinal bacteria that inhabit the colon.

Antifungal and Antiviral Agents Fungi are parasitic microorganisms that cannot synthesize their own food. Fungal infections (mycoses) may be treated with several drugs. The azole antifungals inhibit fungal growth. Their prototype is ketoconazole (Nizoral). Drugs used to treat viruses work by a variety of mechanisms and include acyclovir (Zovirax) and zidovudine (Retrovir), which is commonly known as AZT. Protease inhibitors are one of the more promising classes of drugs for treating viruses such as HIV. Indinavir (Crixivan) is the prototype of this class.

Other Antimicrobial and Antiparasitic Agents While most diseases treated with the medications discussed in this section are uncommon in developed countries, they are leading causes of death in third-world countries. They include malaria, tuberculosis, leprosy, amebiasis, and helminthiasis. Tuberculosis is increasingly appearing in the United States in patients with compromised immune systems.

Malaria is a parasitic infection common in the tropics. It is transmitted by certain types of mosquitoes or, less commonly, by blood transfusion. Drugs used to treat malaria are called schizonticides. They include chloroquine (Aralen), mefloquine (Lariam), and quinine. Treatment is aimed at either preventing infestation (prophylactic treatment for individuals traveling to high-risk areas) or killing the parasites in infected patients.

Tuberculosis is caused by bacteria that are transmitted through airborne droplets from the coughing and sneezing of infected patients. The bacteria can grow only in well-oxygenated areas. Because of the route of infection and the need for oxygen, most patients with tuberculosis have infestations in the lungs. Once in the lungs, the bacteria are typically "walled off," or enclosed in tubercules, and become dormant and noninfective. If the patient's immune system is compromised, the bacteria may become active again and begin to cause symptoms. Drugs commonly used to treat tuberculosis include isoniazid (Nydrazid, INH) and rifampin (Rifadin).

Amebiasis is a parasitic infection of the intestines common in tropical areas. Transmission most frequently occurs via the oral–fecal route from eating poorly cooked food contaminated by cooks who inadequately wash their hands. Drugs used to treat amebiasis include paromomycin (Humatin) and metronidazole (Flagyl).

Helminthiasis is caused by parasitic worms (helminths) including flatworms and roundworms. These worms usually invade the host's intestinal tract and attach themselves to the lumen wall with hooks or suckers. They cause symptoms by depriving the host of nutrients (especially in children); by obstructing the intestinal lumen, which leads to bowel obstruction; and by producing toxins. Treatment is aimed at either killing the organism outright or destroying its ability to latch onto the intestinal wall so it passes with the patient's feces. These drugs include mebendazole (Vermox) and niclosamide (Niclocide).

Leprosy, also known as Hansen's disease, is caused by bacteria. It leads to characteristic lesions, footdrop (plantar flexion), and plantar ulceration. Drugs used to treat it include dapsone (DDS, Avlosulfon) and clofazimine (Lamprene).

Nonsteroidal Anti-inflammatory Drugs NSAIDs are commonly used as analgesics and antipyretics (fever reducers). Many are available over the counter, including acetaminophen and ibuprofen. As a group, these agents interfere with the production of prostaglandins, thereby interrupting the inflammatory process. NSAIDs are indicated for the relief of pain, fever, and inflammation associated with common headache, arthritis, dysmenorrhea, and orthopedic injuries. They are also commonly prescribed to relieve pain following trauma and surgery. Other NSAIDs include ketorolac (Toradol), piroxicam (Feldene), and naproxen (Naprosyn).

Uricosuric Drugs Uricosuric drugs are used to treat and prevent acute episodes of gout. Gout is an inflammatory disease caused by an altered metabolism of uric acid and marked by hyperuricemia (high levels of uric acid in the blood). It may present with acute episodes characterized by pain and swelling of joints. Left untreated, gout may lead to crystal deposits in various parts of the body that can cause kidney stones, nephritis, and atherosclerosis. Drugs used to treat gout include colchicine and allopurinol (Zyloprim).

pathogen *disease-causing organism.*

immunity *the body's ability to respond to the presence of a pathogen.*

serum *solution containing whole antibodies for a specific pathogen.*

vaccine *solution containing a modified pathogen that does not actually cause disease but still stimulates the development of antibodies specific to it.*

Serums, Vaccines, and Other Immunizing Agents The human body has a complex series of systems that help prevent disease. The most important of these are the anatomical barriers such as the skin and mucous membranes that block the entrance of **pathogens** (disease-causing organisms including viruses and bacteria). If pathogens get past these protective barriers, our immune system comes into play. This system consists of the spleen, lymph nodes, thymus, leukocytes, and proteins called antibodies in plasma. The ability to respond to pathogens is called **immunity.**

Immunity may be acquired passively or actively. It is passively acquired when antibodies pass directly into a person, either through artificial routes such as injection or through natural routes such as the placenta or breast milk. Immunity may also be actively acquired in response to the presence of a pathogen.

Actively acquired immunity occurs when T lymphocytes (a type of leukocyte that becomes specialized in the thymus gland) comes in contact with a new pathogen. The body produces an infinite variety of T-cell configurations. When the pathogen comes into contact with a T cell that is specific to it, that T cell begins to rapidly reproduce. Some of these cells become involved in the immune response to the pathogen, while others act as "memory" cells. The cells involved in the immune response either directly attack the pathogen (cell-mediated immunity) or activate the complement system, a complex cascade of events that leads to the immune response. The memory cells remain in the body in higher numbers so that the next time this specific pathogen enters the body, a much faster response is possible. At the same time, B cells (lymphocytes that differentiate or become more specialized in the body, as opposed to the thymus) that are specific for the invading pathogen begin to produce antibodies for that antigen. This process is called humoral immunity or antibody immunity. When an antibody contacts its specific antigen, it forms a complex that triggers the complement system, leading to the immune response.

Serums and vaccines may augment the immune system. A **serum** is a solution containing whole antibodies for a specific pathogen. The antibodies give the recipient temporary, passive immunity. A **vaccine** contains a modified pathogen that does not actually cause disease but still stimulates the development of antibodies specific to it. These pathogens may be either dead or attenuated (having a decreased disease-causing ability).

The best age for vaccination against disease is within the first 2 years of life, as the immune system is fairly immature.

Immune Suppressing and Enhancing Agents Available drugs can either suppress the immune system (immunosuppressants) or enhance it (immunomodulators). Suppressing the immune system is indicated to prevent the rejection of transplanted organs and grafted skin. Azathioprine (Imuran) is a commonly used immunosuppressant that acts by decreasing cell-mediated reactions and suppressing antibody production.

Immunomodulating agents enhance the natural immune reaction in immunosuppressed patients such as those with HIV. Zidovudine (Retrovir), commonly known as AZT, and several protease inhibitors such as ritonavir (Norvir) and saquinavir (Invirase) are examples of these agents.

DRUGS USED TO AFFECT THE SKIN

Dermatologic drugs are used to treat skin irritations. They are common over-the-counter medications. The many different general preparations include baths, soaps, solutions, cleansers, emollients (Lubriderm, Vaseline), skin protectants (Benzoin), wet dressings or soaks (Domeboro Powder), and rubs and liniments (Ben-Gay, Icy Hot). Prophylactic agents such as sunscreens are also available to help prevent skin disease and irritation.

DRUGS USED TO SUPPLEMENT THE DIET

Many disease processes affect the production, distribution, and utilization of essential dietary nutrients. Additionally, the body's intricate balance of fluid (including specific amounts of electrolytes) is a vital component of maintaining homeostasis. Dietary supplements can help to maintain needed levels of these essential nutrients and fluids.

VITAMINS AND MINERALS

Vitamins are organic compounds necessary for many different physiologic processes including metabolism, growth, development, and tissue repair. The body absorbs most vitamins through the gastrointestinal tract following dietary ingestion. Vitamins must be obtained from the diet, as the body cannot manufacture them. In developed countries, healthy adults usually receive adequate amounts of vitamins and do not need supplements. Vitamin supplements may, however, be indicated for special populations including pregnant and nursing women, patients with absorption disorders, the chronically ill, surgery patients, alcoholics, and the malnourished. Additionally, people on a strict vegetarian diet may need supplemental vitamins. Vitamins are either fat soluble or water soluble. The liver stores the fat-soluble vitamins (A, D, E, and K), so the patient will become deficient only after long periods of inadequate vitamin intake. Vitamin D is unique in that the skin produces it with exposure to sunlight. The water-soluble vitamins (C and those in the B complex) must be routinely ingested, as the body does not store them. After short periods of deprivation, patients may begin to experience vitamin deficiency. The B complex vitamins are grouped only because they occur together in foods; otherwise they share no significant characteristics. The individual B vitamins are named for the order in which they were discovered (B_1, B_2, B_3, and so forth). These vitamins also have specific names. For example, B_1 is also known as thiamine, a vitamin that plays a key role in carbohydrate metabolism. Table 6–9 details selected vitamins. Iron is an essential mineral necessary for oxygen transport and several metabolic processes. Iron supplements are the most common mineral supplement. They are indicated for iron deficiency.

FLUIDS AND ELECTROLYTES

Water comprises approximately 60 percent of a person's total body weight. The specific composition and amounts of this fluid are vital to a patient's well-being. The specific amounts of electrolytes such as calcium, potassium, sodium, and chlorine are similarly important. This book's chapter on pathophysiology reviews the physiology of fluids and electrolytes and discusses acid–base balance. The indications and contraindications for administering fluids and electrolytes, as well as these medications' interactions, are covered in Chapter 7 on medication administration and Chapter 19 on hemorrhage and shock.

Table 6–9 Vitamin Sources and Deficiencies

Vitamin	Problems Resulting from Deficiency	Source
Fat Soluble		
A	Night blindness, skin lesions	Butter, yellow fruit, green leafy vegetables, milk
D	Bone and muscle pain, weakness, softening of bones	Fish, fortified milk, exposure to sunlight
E	Hyporeflexia, ataxia, anemia	Nuts, green leafy vegetables, wheat
K	Increased bleeding	Liver, green leafy vegetables
Water Soluble		
B_1 (thiamine)	Peripheral neuritis, depression, anorexia, poor memory	Whole grain, beef, pork, peas, beans, nuts
B_2 (riboflavin)	Sore throat, stomatitis, painful or swollen tongue, anemia	Milk, eggs, cheese, green leafy vegetables
B_2 (niacin)	Skin eruptions, diarrhea, enteritis, headache, dizziness, insomnia	Meat, eggs, milk
B_6 (pyridoxine)	Skin lesions, seizures, peripheral neuritis	Liver, meats, eggs, vegetables
B_9 (folic acid)	Megaloblastic anemia	Liver, fresh green vegetables, yeast
B_{12} (cyanocobalamin)	Irreversible nervous system damage, pernicious anemia	Fish, egg yolk, milk
C	Scurvy	Citrus fruits, tomatoes, strawberries

DRUGS USED TO TREAT POISONING AND OVERDOSES

The treatment for poisoning and overdose depends greatly on the substance involved. In general, therapy aims at eliminating the substance by emptying the gastric contents, by increasing gastric motility in order to decrease the time available for absorption, by alkalinizing the urine with sodium bicarbonate (for tricyclic antidepressant and salicylate overdose), or by filtering the substance from the blood with dialysis. When gastric emptying is indicated, syrup of ipecac is the drug of choice; otherwise, activated charcoal may be used as a gastric absorbent.

Actual antidotes are few; however, some medications are effective in treating certain overdoses or poisonings. General mechanisms for antidote action include receptor site antagonism, blocking enzyme actions involved with metabolism of the substance, and chelation (binding the substance with a stable compound such as iron so that it becomes inactive). Specific antidotes include acetylcysteine (Mucomyst) for acetaminophen overdose and deferoxamine for iron chelation. Organophosphates are a common ingredient in insecticides and herbicides as well as chemical weapons. They are aggressive acetylcholinesterase (AChE) inhibitors that prevent the breakdown of acetylcholine, leading to overstimulation of the parasympathetic nervous system as well as neuromuscular junctions. Signs and symptoms of this overstimulation may be remembered by the acronym SLUDGE (salivation, lacrimation, urination, defecation, gastric motility, and emesis). Other signs include bradycardia, hypotension, bronchospasm, muscle fasciculations, miosis (pupil constriction), and respiratory arrest. The treatments for organophosphate poisoning are atropine and pralidoxime (2-PAM, Protopam). Atropine antagonizes ACh, while pralidoxime breaks the organophosphate-acetylcholinesterase bond, freeing AChE to break down the excess ACh.

Summary

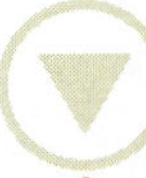

Pharmacology is a cornerstone of paramedic practice. Paramedics must have a solid understanding of its foundations (legal issues, terminology, drug forms, and routes), pharmacokinetics, and pharmacodynamics if they are to practice their profession safely. Additionally, paramedics must understand not only the medications they personally administer, but also the medications that their patients are taking on an ongoing basis. While you are not likely to remember everything in this chapter after your first reading, with diligent study and practice you can master this information. This chapter has barely broken the surface of pharmacology. To continue your education, you should take the time to understand the mechanisms and interactions of the medications your patients are taking. If you do not already know them (you will not in the majority of cases as you begin your career), look them up. Many very useful drug references are available today. Most are small and can be easily carried with you on your unit or in your station.

Finally, pharmacology is a dynamic field with new discoveries being made every day. If you take your responsibilities as a paramedic seriously and remain current on the latest changes in this field, you can be sure that you can give your patients the care they deserve.

Review Questions

1. The study of drugs and their interactions with the body is called:
   a. physiology.
   b. toxicology.
   c. pharmacology.
   d. pharmacopeia.

2. A drug or other substance that blocks the actions of the sympathetic nervous system is called:
   a. adrenergic.
   b. sympatholytic.
   c. sympathomimetic.
   d. anticholinergic.
3. __________ is the preferred antihypertensive for the management of pregnancy-induced hypertension.
   a. Coreg
   b. Apresoline
   c. Captopril
   d. Nifedipine
4. Because they can thicken bronchial secretions, you should not use __________ in patients with asthma.
   a. mucolytics
   b. antitussives
   c. antihistamines
   d. antidysrhythmics
5. The following describes a Schedule __________ drug: High abuse potential; may lead to severe dependence; accepted medical indications.
   a. I
   b. II
   c. III
   d. IV
6. An example of an anticholinergic drug used in the treatment of asthma is:
   a. atropine.
   b. ephedrine.
   c. proventil.
   d. beclovent.
7. The drug name found in the *United States Pharmacopeia* (USP) is its:
   a. official name.
   b. chemical name.
   c. generic name.
   d. trade name.
8. The drug name that is derived from its chemical composition is referred to as its:
   a. official name.
   b. chemical name.
   c. generic name.
   d. trade name.
9. The proprietary name of a drug, such as Valium, is the same as the:
   a. official name.
   b. chemical name.
   c. generic name.
   d. trade name.
10. Drug legislation was instituted in 1906 by the:
   a. Narcotics Act.
   b. Cosmetics Act.
   c. Pure Food and Drug Act.
   d. Pharmacology Act.
11. __________ drug sources may provide alternative sources of medications to those found in nature, or they may be entirely new medications not found in nature.
   a. Plant
   b. Animal
   c. Synthetic
   d. Mineral

12. The six rights of medication administration include the right:
    a. dose.
    b. time.
    c. route.
    d. all of the above
13. Which of the following routes is the least appropriate for medication administration in the pre-hospital setting?
    a. oral
    b. sublingual
    c. subcutaneous
    d. intravenous
14. Drugs manufactured in gelatin containers are called:
    a. pills.
    b. tablets.
    c. capsules.
    d. extracts.
15. A drug's pharmacodynamics involve its ability to cause the expected response, or:
    a. affinity.
    b. efficacy.
    c. side effect.
    d. contraindication.
16. A type of anesthesia that combines decreased sensation of pain with amnesia, while the patient remains conscious, is a(n):
    a. opioid.
    b. nonopioid.
    c. anesthetic.
    d. neuroleptanesthesia.
17. ___________ agents oppose the parasympathetic nervous system.
    a. Cholinergic
    b. Adrenergic
    c. Antiadrenergic
    d. Anticholinergic
18. In antidysrhythmic classifications, Class IA drugs include all of the following except:
    a. quinidine.
    b. lidocaine.
    c. procainamide.
    d. disopyramide.
19. One of aspirin's primary side effects is:
    a. stasis.
    b. bleeding.
    c. headache.
    d. seizures.
20. ___________ are mediators released from mast cells upon contact with allergens.
    a. Histamines
    b. Leukotrienes
    c. Glucocorticoids
    d. Methylxanthines

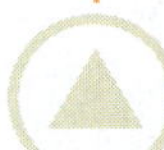

See Answers to Review Questions at the back of this book.

Chapter 7

Intravenous Access and Medication Administration

Objectives

Part 1: Principles and Routes of Medication Administration (begins on p. 375)

After reading Part 1 of this chapter, you should be able to:

1. Review the specific anatomy and physiology pertinent to medication administration. (pp. 378–405)
2. Describe the indications, equipment needed, technique used, precautions, and general principles for the following:
   - A. inhalation routes of medication administration. (pp. 381–395)
   - B. parenteral routes of medication administration. (pp. 390–405)
   - C. percutaneous routes of medication administration. (pp. 378–381)
   - D. enteral routes of medication administration, including gastric tube administration and rectal administration. (pp. 385–390)
3. Describe the indications, contraindications, side effects, dosages, and routes of administration for medications commonly administered by paramedics. (pp. 378–405)
4. Discuss legal aspects affecting medication administration. (pp. 376, 377)
5. Discuss the "six rights" of drug administration and correlate them with the principles of medication administration. (pp. 375–376)
6. Differentiate among the percutaneous routes of medication administration. (pp. 378–381)
7. Discuss medical asepsis and the differences between clean and sterile techniques. (pp. 376–377)
8. Describe uses of antiseptics and disinfectants. (p. 377)
9. Describe the use of Standard Precautions when administering a medication. (p. 376)
10. Describe disposal of contaminated items and sharps. (p. 377)

11. Synthesize a pharmacologic management plan including medication administration. (pp. 375–405)

Part 2: Intravenous Access, Blood Sampling, and Intraosseous Infusion (begins on p. 405)

After reading Part 2 of this chapter, you should be able to:

1. Review the specific anatomy and physiology pertinent to medication administration. (pp. 405–442)
2. Describe the indications, equipment needed, technique used, precautions, and general principles for the following:
   - **A.** peripheral venous or external jugular cannulation. (pp. 405–431)
   - **B.** intraosseous needle placement and infusion. (pp. 435–442)
   - **C.** obtaining a blood sample. (pp. 431–434)

Part 3: Medical Mathematics (begins on p. 442)

After reading Part 3 of this chapter, you should be able to:

1. Review mathematical equivalents. (pp. 442–444)
2. Differentiate temperature readings between the centigrade and Fahrenheit scales. (p. 444)
3. Discuss formulas as a basis for performing drug calculations. (pp. 444–449)
4. Describe how to perform mathematical conversions from the household system to the metric system. (pp. 442–444)

Key Terms

administration tubing, p. 409
air embolism, p. 422
ampule, p. 392
angiocatheter, p. 412
anticoagulant, p. 422
antiseptic, p. 377
asepsis, p. 376
aural medication, p. 380
blood tube, p. 431
blood tubing, p. 412
bolus, p. 390
buccal, p. 379
burette chamber, p. 411
cannula, p. 409
cannulation, p. 405
catheter inserted through the needle (intracatheter), p. 413
central venous access, p. 407
circulatory overload, p. 421
colloid, p. 407
concentration, p. 445
crystalloid, p. 407
desired dose, p. 445
disinfectant, p. 377
dosage on hand, p. 445
drip chamber, p. 410
drip rate, p. 410
drop former, p. 410
drugs, p. 375
embolus, p. 421
enema, p. 390
enteral drug administration, p. 385
extension tubing, p. 411
extravasation, p. 420
extravascular, p. 430
gauge, p. 391
gtts, p. 410
hemoconcentration, p. 434
hemolysis, p. 434
heparin lock, p. 427
hepatic alteration, p. 389
hollow-needle catheter, p. 413
Huber needle, p. 429
hypertonic, p. 408
hypodermic needle, p. 391
hypotonic, p. 408
infusion, p. 397
infusion controller, p. 430
infusion pump, p. 430
infusion rate, p. 448
inhalation, p. 381
injection, p. 381
intradermal, p. 398
intramuscular, p. 400
intraosseous, p. 435
intravenous access, p. 405
intravenous fluid, p. 407
isotonic, p. 408
local, p. 376
Luer sampling needle, p. 434
macrodrip tubing, p. 409
measured volume administration set, p. 411
medically clean, p. 377
medication injection port, p. 411
medicated solution, p. 397
medications, p. 375
metered dose inhaler, p. 382
microdrip tubing, p. 409
Mix-o-Vial, p. 395
nasal medication, p. 380
nebulizer, p. 381
necrosis, p. 422
needle adapter, p. 411
nonconstituted drug vial, p. 395

ocular medication, p. 379
oral drug administration, p. 386
over-the-needle catheter, p. 412
parenteral, p. 390
peripheral venous access, p. 406
peripherally inserted central catheter (PICC), p. 407
prefilled/preloaded syringe, p. 397
pyrogen, p. 421
saline lock, p. 427
sharps container, p. 377
spike, p. 409
Standard Precautions, p. 376
sterile, p. 376
stock solution, p. 444
subcutaneous, p. 399
sublingual, p. 379
suppository, p. 389
syringe, p. 390
systemic, p. 376
thrombophlebitis, p. 422
thrombus, p. 422
topical medications, p. 378
transdermal, p. 378
trocar, p. 436
unit, p. 444
vacutainer, p. 432
venous access device, p. 428
venous constricting band, p. 413
vial, p. 392
volume on hand, p. 445

INTRODUCTION

Medications, or **drugs,** are foreign substances placed into the human body. They serve a variety of purposes such as controlling specific diseases like hypertension or helping the body cure diseases like cancer and infection.

medications/drugs *agents used in the diagnosis, treatment, or prevention of disease.*

Medication administration will be an important part of the medical care you provide as a paramedic. You may have to use medications to correct or prevent many life-threatening situations. You may also use them to stabilize or comfort a patient in distress. In addition to your knowledge of particular medications and their properties from the previous chapter on pharmacology, you must also be thoroughly skilled in drug administration. Specific drugs require specific routes and administration techniques. Their effectiveness depends directly upon their correct route of delivery. Incorrect or sloppy drug administration can have tremendous legal implications for the paramedic. More importantly, it equates to poor care that can harm or even kill the patient.

This chapter discusses the routes and techniques you will use to correctly deliver your patient's medications. It is divided into three parts:

Part 1: Principles and Routes of Medication Administration

Part 2: Intravenous Access, Blood Sampling, and Intraosseous Infusion

Part 3: Medical Mathematics

Part 1: Principles and Routes of Medication Administration

GENERAL PRINCIPLES

As a paramedic, you are responsible for ensuring that all emergency drugs are in place and ready for immediate use. Therefore, you must know your local drug distribution system. You will have to know where to obtain and replace each drug as it expires or is used, as another patient may require it at any time. You also will have to thoroughly document the administration and restocking of narcotics, as many local, state, and federal agencies mandate such record keeping.

Your knowledge of drug indications, dosages, and routes of administration is of paramount importance.

Always be certain that you correctly give all drugs in the right dose. Medication errors may prove disastrous in terms of patient care and legal responsibility. Your knowledge of drug indications, contraindications, side effects, dosages, and routes of administration is crucial to effective patient care.

You can attain effective pharmacologic therapy and eliminate medication errors by following the six rights of drug administration:

- ★ Right person
- ★ Right drug
- ★ Right dose

★ Right time

★ Right route

★ Right documentation

If you ever doubt the use or dosage of a medication, contact medical direction immediately.

In the field, you will be responsible for the safe and appropriate delivery of medications. If you ever doubt the use or dosage of a medication, contact medical direction immediately. You must repeat back, or echo, all drug orders issued by direct medical command. For example, if medical direction ordered you to administer 25 mg of diphenhydramine (Benadryl), you would echo, "Medic 101 copies the medication order for 25 mg of diphenhydramine to be administered slow IV push." By echoing, you confirm your reception and understanding of the order. If medical direction has issued an inappropriate medication or dosage, echoing may bring it to light and elicit an immediate correction. If you still find the order questionable after echoing, diplomatically request clarification or ask about the intent.

Pharmacologic therapy permits you to function as an extension of the physician. No room exists for medication errors, as once a drug is given it is difficult if not impossible to retrieve. In addition, withholding a needed medication can have catastrophic consequences. Concentration and knowledge are the keys to this component of paramedical care.

MEDICAL DIRECTION

Paramedics do not practice autonomously. You will operate under the license of a medical director who is responsible for all of your actions. This responsibility extends to the administration of medications.

The medical director determines which medications you will use and the routes by which you will deliver them. Some states have a "state drug list" whereby the medications a service carries are dictated by law or a legislative or regulatory agency. While some medications can be administered via off-line medical direction (written standing orders), you will need specific authorization for others after consulting on-line or direct medical direction. You must strictly abide by all of your medical director's guidelines.

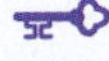

You can ill afford to waste valuable time looking up procedures and directives for the critical patient who requires immediate drug therapy.

Knowing all drug administration protocols is essential, especially which drugs to administer under standing orders and which to deliver only after getting authorization from medical direction. You can ill afford to waste valuable time looking up procedures and directives for the critical patient who requires immediate drug therapy. Furthermore, because inappropriate drug delivery can have serious consequences, you may face severe legal ramifications even if your patient suffers no harm.

STANDARD PRECAUTIONS

Standard Precautions *measures to decrease your risk of exposure to blood and body fluids.*

Establishing routes for drug delivery presents the constant potential for exposure to blood and other body fluids. Always use **Standard Precautions** to decrease your risk of exposure. The type of precautions you use will vary according to the delivery route and your patient's condition. At a minimum, you should wear gloves. Optimally, you will also wear goggles and a mask. Remarkably, the simplest form of minimizing disease transmission is often the most neglected: hand washing. Washing your hands before and after patient contact is one of the most effective ways to decrease your exposure to infectious material. Chapter 1 includes a thorough discussion of Standard Precautions.

MEDICAL ASEPSIS

asepsis *a condition free of pathogens.*

local *limited to one area of the body.*

systemic *throughout the body.*

sterile *free of all forms of life.*

Medical **asepsis** (*a-*, without; *sepsis,* infection) describes a medical environment free of pathogens. Many paramedical procedures, especially those related to drug administration, place the patient at increased risk for infection. The external environment is full of microorganisms, many of them pathogenic. Techniques such as intravenous access or endotracheal intubation can allow pathogens to enter the patient's body, where they may cause **local** or **systemic** complications.

Sterilization

The most aseptic environment is a sterile one. A **sterile** environment is free of all forms of life. Generally, environments are sterilized with extensive heat or chemicals. A sterile environment is difficult to attain in the prehospital setting. Consequently, you must practice medically clean techniques to minimize your patient's risk of infection. **Medically clean** techniques involve the careful handling of sterile equipment to prevent contamination. For example, much of the equipment used for drug administration is packaged sterilely. Once you open the package, you must use a medically clean technique to keep the equipment clean and uncontaminated until you use it. If you drop a piece of equipment on a dirty surface, you should discard it and obtain a new piece. Other medically clean techniques, including hand washing, glove changing, and discarding equipment in opened packages, help to prevent equipment and patient contamination. Remember, too, that many patients have lowered immunity levels or carry infectious diseases. Thus, keeping the ambulance and equipment clean is another essential medically clean procedure.

medically clean *careful handling to prevent contamination.*

Disinfectants and Antiseptics

When administering medications, you must use disinfectants and antiseptics to assure local cleanliness. Do not confuse disinfectants and antiseptics; the distinction is important. **Disinfectants** are toxic to living tissue. You will therefore use them only on nonliving surfaces or objects such as the inside of an ambulance or laryngoscope blades after use. Never use disinfectants on living tissue. **Antiseptics** are not toxic to living tissue. They destroy or inhibit pathogenic microorganisms already on living surfaces and are generally used to cleanse the local area before needle puncture. Common antiseptics include alcohol and iodine preparations used either alone or together. Frequently, antiseptics are diluted disinfectants.

disinfectant *cleansing agent that destroys or inhibits pathogenic organisms and is also toxic to living tissue.*

antiseptic *cleansing agent that destroys or inhibits pathogenic organisms but is not toxic to living tissue.*

DISPOSAL OF CONTAMINATED EQUIPMENT AND SHARPS

Blood and body fluid can harbor infectious material that endangers the health care provider, family, bystanders, or the patient himself. Many times, the patient is infected with pathogenic organisms long before signs and symptoms appear. Therefore, you must treat all blood and body fluids as potentially infectious.

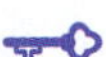

Treat all blood and body fluids as potentially infectious.

Drug administration commonly involves needles in direct contact with the patient's blood and body fluid. Once used, a needle presents a significant risk. Inadvertent needle sticks, the most common accident in health care as a whole, can transmit diseases between the patient and paramedic. Properly handling needles and other sharps before and after patient use can prevent many of these accidental needle sticks. To minimize or eliminate the risk of an accidental needle stick, take these precautions:

- *Minimize the tasks you perform in a moving ambulance.* Use needles as sparingly as possible in the back of a moving ambulance. When appropriate, perform all interventions involving needles on scene. If en route, it may be occasionally necessary to have the driver pull the ambulance to the side of the road and stop briefly. Most paramedics become quite proficient at completing these procedures in a moving ambulance.
- *Immediately dispose of used sharps in a sharps container.* A **sharps container** is a rigid, puncture-resistant container clearly marked as biohazardous. You can deposit whole needles and prefilled syringes in it, thus eliminating the need for bending or cutting. Some sharps containers have adapters that permit the easy removal of needles from blood draw equipment and syringes. You should also dispose of items such as used ampules in the sharps container. Avoid dropping sharps onto the floor for later disposal. In the heat of the moment, you may forget the sharp or mentally misplace it.
- *Recap needles only as a last resort.* If you absolutely must recap a needle, never use two hands to do so. Place the sharp on a stationary surface and replace the cap with one hand. While the one-hand method is still hazardous, it at least reduces the chance for an accidental needle stick.

Content Review

Needle Handling Precautions

- Minimize tasks in a moving ambulance.
- Properly dispose of all sharps.
- Recap needles only as a last resort.

sharps container *rigid, puncture-resistant container clearly marked as a biohazard.*

By law, every medical organization must have a biological hazard exposure plan. Be familiar with yours. If you are exposed to blood or other body substances, follow the plan and immediately notify the appropriate resources. Remember that prevention is the best medicine.

MEDICATION ADMINISTRATION AND DOCUMENTATION

When administering medications, proper and thorough documentation is extremely important. You must record all information concerning the patient and the medication including:

- ★ Indication for drug administration
- ★ Dosage and route delivered
- ★ Patient response to the medication—both positive and negative

Review

Content

Routes of Drug Administration

- Percutaneous
- Pulmonary
- Enteral
- Parenteral

topical medications *material applied to and absorbed through the skin or mucous membranes.*

You must also document the patient's condition and vital signs before medication administration as well as after. In addition to communicating all information to those to whom you transfer care, you must record it on a copy of the patient care report.

In emergent and nonemergent situations alike, you will administer a variety of medications through a variety of delivery routes. The routes of drug administration fall into four basic categories: percutaneous, pulmonary, enteral, and parenteral. Technically, drug deliveries through the rectum and pulmonary system are **topical** applications; however, accepted practice classifies these routes separately. Which route you use will depend on the drug you are administering and your patient's status.

PERCUTANEOUS DRUG ADMINISTRATION

Review

Content

Percutaneous Routes

- Transdermal
- Mucous membrane

Percutaneous medications are applied to and absorbed through the skin or mucous membranes. They are easy to administer and bypass the digestive tract, making their absorption more predictable.

TRANSDERMAL ADMINISTRATION

transdermal *absorbed through the skin.*

Medications given by the **transdermal** (*trans-*, across; *dermal,* skin) route promote slow, steady absorption. Nitroglycerin, hormones, and analgesics are commonly administered transdermally. Transdermal delivery can also produce localized effects, as with anti-inflammatories and other bacteriostatic and softening agents. Applying medication locally avoids passing larger quantities of the medication through the entire body, where it is not needed. Transdermal medications include lotions, ointments, creams, foams, wet dressings, adhesive backed applications, and suppositories.

To administer a transdermal medication, use the following technique:

1. Use Standard Precautions. Always wear gloves to avoid contaminating the medication and inadvertently getting it on your skin.
2. Clean and dry your patient's skin at the administration site.
3. Apply medication to the site as specified by the manufacturer. Avoid overdosing or underdosing when using lotion, ointment, cream, or foam.
4. Leave the medication in place for the required time. Monitor the patient for desirable or adverse effects.

You may need to place a dressing over the medication to protect the site and quantity of drug. Carefully follow all recommendations. Administration may vary subtly, depending upon the form of medication and the specific manufacturer's instructions.

Several factors can affect how quickly the skin absorbs transdermal medications. Thin skin, overdose, or penetrating solvents can increase the absorption rate. Conversely, thick skin, scar tissue, or peripheral vascular disease can decrease the rate. If these factors are present, consider alternative sites or dosage adjustments.

Review

Content

Mucous Membrane Medication Sites

- Tongue
- Cheek
- Eye
- Nose
- Ear

MUCOUS MEMBRANES

The mucous membranes absorb medications at a moderate to rapid rate. Similar to transdermal administration, drug delivery through the mucous membranes avoids the digestive tract and complications associated with that route. You can deliver drugs through the mucous membranes at several sites. However, specific drugs are made for specific sites and generally are not interchangeable.

Sublingual

Sublingual drugs are absorbed through the mucous membranes beneath the tongue (*sub-*, below; *lingual*, tongue). The sublingual region is extremely vascular and permits rapid absorption with systemic delivery. These medications are generally dissolvable tablets or sprays. One commonly administered sublingual medication is nitroglycerin.

sublingual *beneath the tongue.*

To administer a medication via the sublingual route, follow these steps:

1. Use appropriate Standard Precautions.
2. Confirm the indication, medication, dose, sublingual route, and expiration date.
3. Have your patient lift his tongue toward the top and back of his oral cavity.
4. Place the pill or direct spray between the underside of the tongue and the floor of the oral cavity. Have your patient relax his tongue and mouth. If administering a pill, instruct the patient to let the pill dissolve and not to swallow.
5. Monitor the patient for desirable or adverse effects.

Buccal

The **buccal** region lies in the oral cavity between the cheek and gums. Buccal medications are generally tablets. Hormonal and enzyme preparations are typically given buccally.

buccal *between the cheek and gums.*

To administer a medication buccally, follow these steps:

1. Use appropriate Standard Precautions.
2. Confirm the indication, medication, dose, buccal route, and expiration date.
3. Place the medication between the patient's cheek and gum. Instruct the patient to allow the pill or other preparation to dissolve. Ensure that the patient does not swallow the medication.
4. Monitor the patient for desirable or adverse effects.

Ocular

Ocular medications are topical medications that are administered through the mucous membranes of the eye. These are typically local medications for alleviating eye pain, treating infection, decreasing intraocular pressure, or lubricating the eyelid. Medications delivered by way of the eye are labeled for ophthalmic use and packaged as drops or ointments.

ocular medication *drug administered through the mucous membranes of the eye.*

If medication is to be administered only to one eye, be sure to medicate the correct eye. The following abbreviations designate right, left, or both eyes:

o.d.	right eye (*oculus dexter*)
o.s.	left eye (*oculus sinister*)
o.u.	both right and left eyes (*oculus uterque*)

To administer a medication via eyedrops, use the following technique (Figure 7-1 ■):

1. Use gloves and appropriate Standard Precautions.
2. Have your patient lie supine or lay his head back so he looks toward the ceiling.
3. Pull the lower eyelid downward to expose the conjunctival sac. Never touch the eye.
4. Use a medicine dropper to place the prescribed dosage on the conjunctival sac. Never administer medications directly on the eye unless specifically instructed.
5. Instruct the patient to hold his eye(s) shut for 1 to 2 minutes.

Ocular medications may also be packaged as ointments. To apply an ointment, follow the previous procedure, but carefully squeeze the ointment onto the conjunctival sac. If you administer too much medication, carefully blot away the excess drops or ointment with sterile gauze. The ointment will melt as it warms to body temperature and will spread smoothly across the surface of the eye.

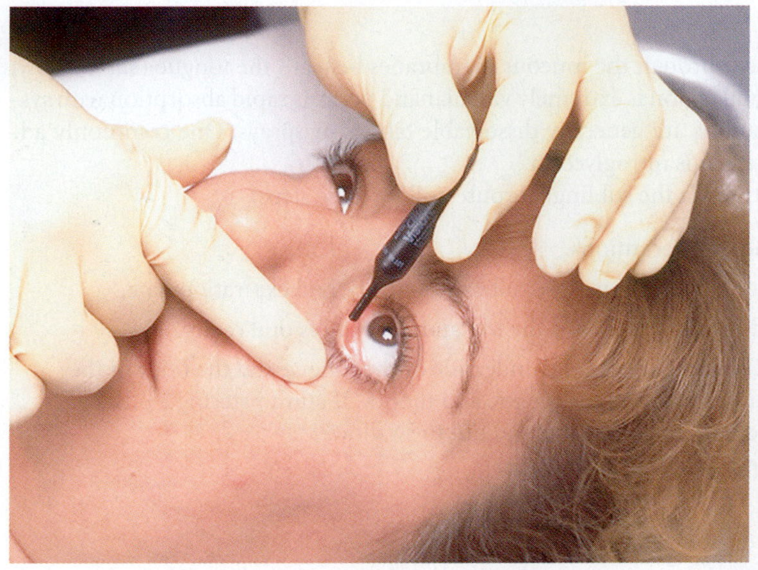

■ **Figure 7-1** Eyedrop administration. Use a medicine dropper to place the prescribed dosage on the conjunctival sac.

Nasal

nasal medication *drug administered through the mucous membranes of the nose.*

The mucous membranes of the nose are another port for topical medication delivery. Given through the nares (nostrils), these **nasal medications** are usually drops or sprays intended for local effect. They commonly treat nasal congestion, hemorrhage, and infection.

To administer a medication via the nose, use the following technique (Figure 7-2 ■):

1. Use gloves and appropriate Standard Precautions.
2. Have the patient blow his nose and tilt his head backwards.
3. Use a medicine dropper or squeezable nebulizer to administer the medication into the appropriate nare(s) according to the manufacturer's instructions.
4. Hold the nare(s) shut and/or tilt the head forward to distribute the medication.
5. Monitor the patient for desirable and undesirable effects.

Aural

aural medication *drug administered through the mucous membranes of the ear and ear canal.*

Some medications are delivered to the mucous membranes of the ear and ear canal through drops or medicated gauze. These **aural medications** primarily treat local infections and ear pain. Use the following technique to administer medicated drops (Figure 7-3 ■):

1. Use gloves and appropriate Standard Precautions.

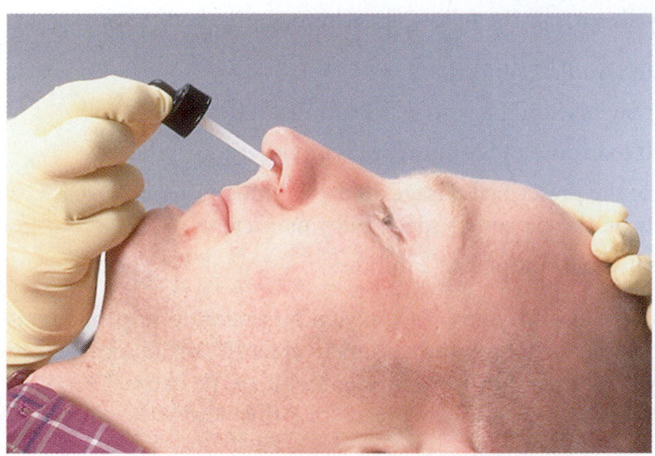

■ **Figure 7-2** Nasal medication administration.

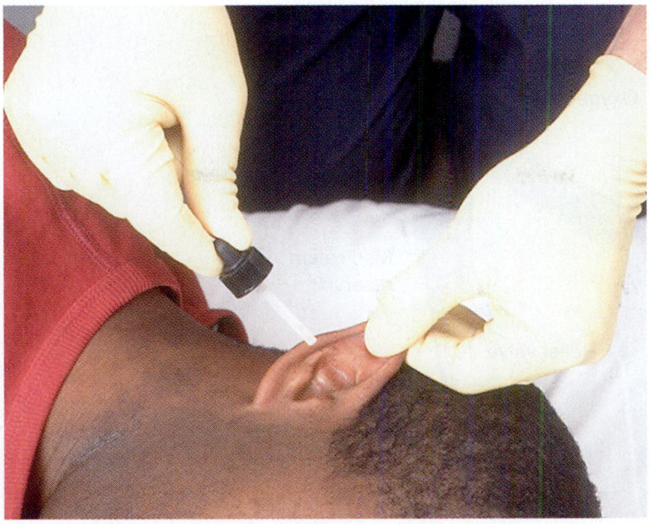

■ Figure 7-3 Aural medication administration. Manually open the ear canal and administer the appropriate dose.

2. Confirm the indication, medication, dose, and expiration date.
3. Determine the correct ear for administration.
4. Have the patient lie in the lateral recumbent position with the affected ear upward.
5. Manually open the ear canal: for adult patients, pull the ear up and back; for pediatric patients, pull it down and back.
6. Administer the appropriate dose of medication with a medicine dropper.
7. Have the patient continue to lie with his ear up for 10 minutes.
8. Monitor the patient for desirable and undesirable effects.

Using medicated gauze or cotton is generally reserved for the hospital setting. If your local protocols permit you to administer these medications, follow the procedure previously outlined, gently inserting the gauze into the ear instead of instilling medicated drops. Avoid tightly packing the ear canal.

PULMONARY DRUG ADMINISTRATION

Special medications can be administered into the pulmonary system via **inhalation** or **injection.** Generally gases, fine mists, or liquids, these drugs include those that promote bronchodilation for respiratory emergencies. Other inhaled drugs are mucolytics, antibiotics, and topical steroids. Inhalation can also be used for humidification and pulmonary decongestion.

inhalation *drawing of medication into the lungs along with air during breathing.*

injection *placement of medication in or under the skin with a needle and syringe.*

NEBULIZER

Typically, drugs administered by inhalation are delivered with the aid of a small volume **nebulizer.** A nebulizer uses pressurized oxygen to disperse a liquid into a fine aerosol spray or mist. Inhalation carries the aerosol into the lungs. Figure 7-4 ■ illustrates a typical nebulizer. The specific design depends upon the manufacturer, but they all work on the same principle and typically have the same parts:

nebulizer *inhalation aid that disperses liquid into aerosol spray or mist.*

- ★ Mouthpiece
- ★ Medication reservoir
- ★ Oxygen port
- ★ Relief valve
- ★ Oxygen tubing
- ★ Oxygen source

Content Review

Pulmonary Medication Mechanisms

- Nebulizer
- Metered-dose inhaler
- Endotracheal tube

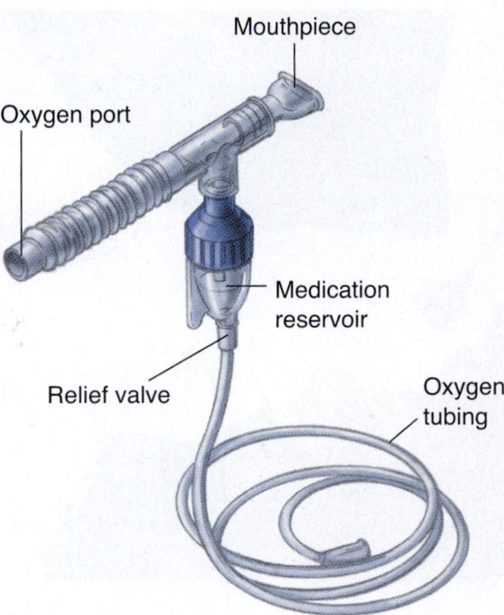

■ **Figure 7-4** Small volume nebulizer.

To administer a drug with a nebulizer, follow these steps:

1. Put the medication in the medication reservoir. If the medication is not diluted, combine it with 3 to 5 mL sterile saline solution. This will allow adequate aerosolization. Screw the reservoir in place.
2. Assemble the nebulizer.
3. Attach oxygen tubing to the oxygen port and oxygen source.
4. Set the oxygen source regulator for 5 to 8 liters per minute.

   Note: Never set the oxygen pressure outside of this range. Less than 5 liters per minute will not create enough pressure to aerosolize the medication. More than 8 liters per minute will create too much pressure and destroy the oxygen tubing or nebulizer at its weakest point. Furthermore, because of pressure restrictions, do not attach the nebulizer to an oxygen humidifier.
5. Place the nebulizer in the patient's mouth. Instruct him to exhale and then seal his lips around the mouthpiece. Now have him hold the nebulizer and slowly inhale as deeply as possible. Upon maximum inhalation, instruct the patient to hold in the medication for 1 to 2 seconds before exhaling. This permits maximum deposition and absorption. Continue this process until the medication is completely gone. Typically, this takes 3 to 5 minutes.

Nebulizers also come preattached to an oxygen face mask in both pediatric and adult sizes (Figure 7-5 ■). Use nebulization face masks for pediatric or adult patients who cannot hold the nebulizer. Nebulizers for those who require long-term therapy may be powered by a battery or other energy source.

For a nebulizer to be effective, the patient must have an adequate tidal volume and respiratory rate. If the tidal volume is shallow or respiratory rate low, the medication will not move from the nebulizer into the lungs. For patients with a poor tidal and/or respiratory rate who cannot pull the medication into their lungs, you can connect nebulizers to a bag-valve mask and/or endotracheal tube.

METERED-DOSE INHALER

metered-dose inhaler *handheld device that produces a medicated spray for inhalation.*

Inhaled medications are also delivered through **metered-dose inhalers** (MDI). These small, handheld devices produce a medicated spray for inhalation. Patients with conditions such as asthma or COPD use metered-dose inhalers to deliver a specific, or metered, dose of medication. A metered-dose inhaler consists of two parts, a medication canister and a plastic shell and

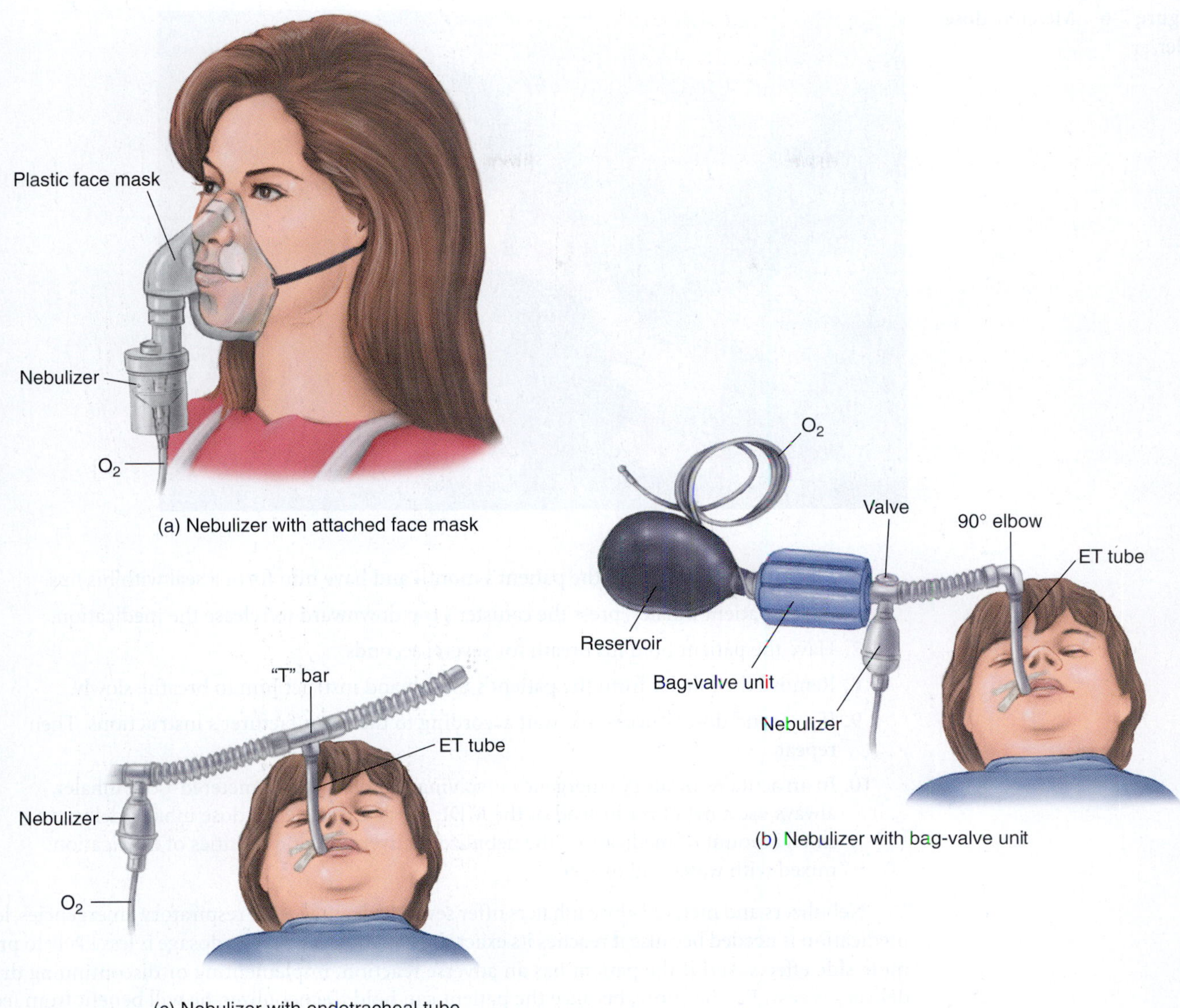

■ **Figure 7-5** Nebulizer with attached face mask, bag-valve mask, and endotracheal tube.

mouthpiece (Figure 7-6 ■). Some metered-dose inhalers come equipped with a spacer, a cylindrical canister between the inhaler and the mouthpiece. Prior to self-administration, the patient will depress the inhaler, sending a measured dose of drug into the spacer. The patient will then breathe in and out of the spacer through the mouthpiece, thus inhaling the drug into the lungs. This system is particularly useful for patients who have a hard time operating and inhaling the metered-dose inhaler. This is common in the elderly and in young children. The spacer, when used in conjunction with a metered-dose inhaler, is very effective.

Metered-dose inhalers are usually self-administered. However, if your patient is incapacitated, you may have to physically assist with the administration or educate the patient or his caregivers in its use. To assist a patient in the use of a metered-dose inhaler, follow this technique:

1. Insert the medication canister into the plastic shell.
2. Remove the cap from the mouthpiece.
3. Gently shake the MDI for 2–5 seconds.
4. Instruct the patient to maximally exhale.

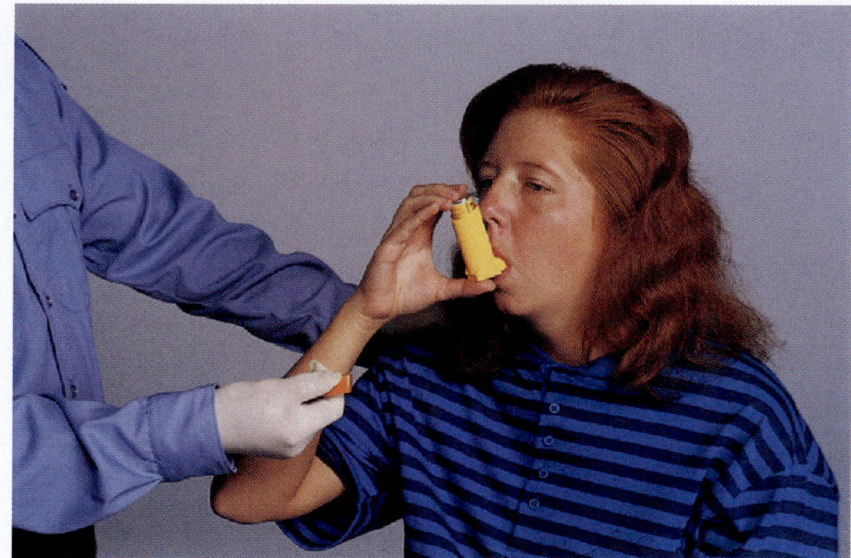

■ Figure 7-6 Metered-dose inhaler.

5. Place the mouthpiece in the patient's mouth and have him form a seal with his lips.
6. As the patient inhales, press the canister's top downward to release the medication.
7. Have the patient hold his breath for several seconds.
8. Remove the inhaler from the patient's mouth and instruct him to breathe slowly.
9. If a second dose is necessary, wait according to the manufacturer's instructions. Then repeat.
10. In an acute respiratory emergency involving a patient with a metered-dose inhaler, always use a nebulizer instead of the MDI. While the metered-dose inhaler delivers a small amount of medication, the nebulizer delivers larger quantities of medication mixed with water and oxygen.

Nebulizers and metered-dose inhalers offer several advantages. In respiratory emergencies, less medication is needed because it reaches its exact site of action. The lower dosage is less likely to promote side effects, and if the patient has an adverse reaction, implementing or discontinuing drug delivery is easy. Furthermore, because the patient can hold the nebulizer, he will benefit from feeling more in control of his overall therapy. Most importantly, if your patient is hypoxic you can administer inhaled medications with supplemental oxygen.

The nebulizer and metered-dose inhaler also have disadvantages. Moving the aerosolized medication into the lungs depends on adequate ventilation. For the patient with a poor tidal and minute volume, nebulized medications are ineffective, as the drug cannot reach its site of action. In these cases, you should use the nebulizer in conjunction with a bag-valve mask and/or endotracheal tube. Additionally, the patient must exhibit an adequate level of consciousness and manual dexterity to hold the nebulizer and follow instructions correctly.

Content Review

Endotracheal Medications

- Lidocaine
- Epinephrine
- Atropine
- Naloxone

ENDOTRACHEAL TUBE

When you have not yet established an IV, you can administer certain medications such as lidocaine (Xylocaine), epinephrine, vasopressin, atropine, and naloxone (Narcan) through an endotracheal tube. Delivering liquid medications into the lungs permits rapid absorption through the pulmonary capillaries. However, recent studies have shown that drugs should be administered through the ET tube only when neither an IV nor an ID can be placed.

When using an endotracheal tube, you must increase conventional IV dosages from two to two and one-half times. You also should dilute the medication in normal saline to create 10 mL of solution and then quickly inject it down the endotracheal tube. Several ventilations must follow to aerosolize the medication and enhance its absorption. Ideally, you can pass a commercially manufactured catheter through the endotracheal tube and inject the medication through it. If CPR is underway, continue compressions while you administer the medication and ventilate for aerosolization.

ENTERAL DRUG ADMINISTRATION

Enteral drug administration is the delivery of any medication that is absorbed through the gastrointestinal tract. The gastrointestinal tract, or alimentary canal, travels from the mouth to the stomach and on through the intestines to the rectum (Figure 7-7 ■). You can administer enteral medications orally, through a gastric tube, or rectally.

enteral drug administration *the delivery of any medication that is absorbed through the gastrointestinal tract.*

Content Review

Enteral Routes

- Oral
- Gastric tube
- Rectal

Several advantages make the gastrointestinal tract the most common route for medication delivery. Aside from sheer convenience, it is the least expensive route, and its use requires little equipment and minimal training. In some instances, after you have delivered a drug you may be able to retrieve it by inducing vomiting, by removing it from the rectum, or simply by having the patient spit it out.

Conversely, enteral drug administration poses several disadvantages. Physical activity, emotions, or food can significantly alter the gastrointestinal tract's chemical and physical environment, making absorption unreliable. In addition, as all blood from the stomach and small intestine must pass through the hepatic circulatory system (portal circulation), the liver's condition can reduce the medication's effectiveness. A dysfunctional liver can significantly alter drug distribution and, in extreme cases, metabolize therapeutic medications into inert or harmful substances. Furthermore, a patient resistant to or *noncompliant* in taking medications makes administration via the enteral route very difficult.

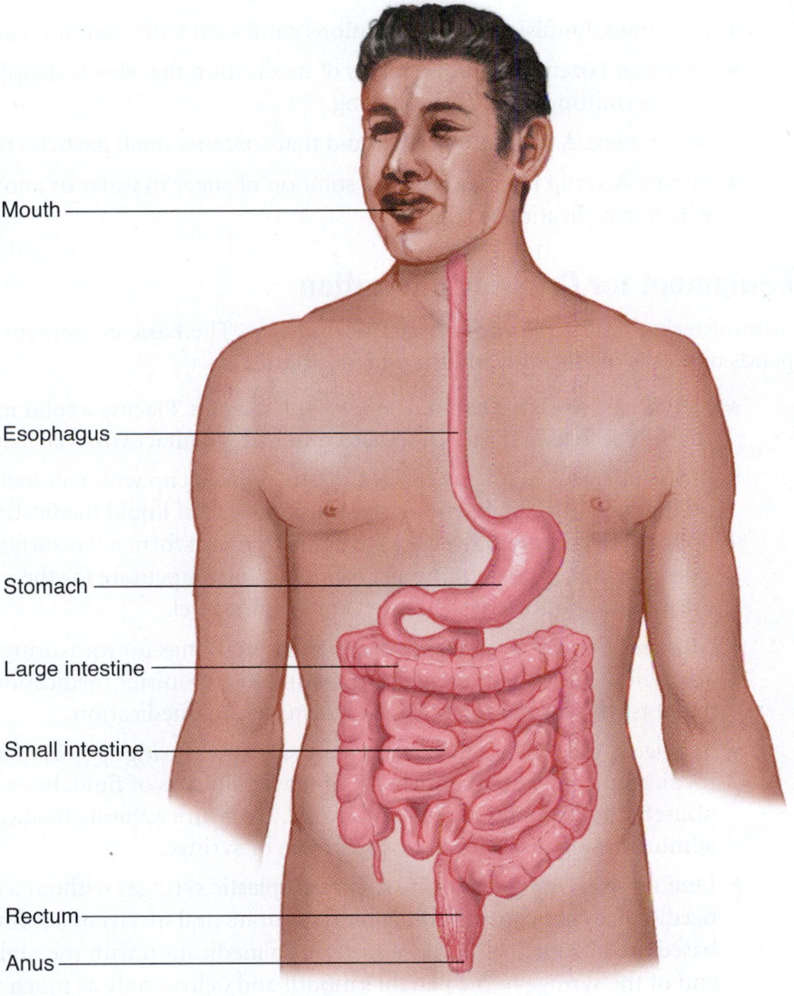

■ Figure 7-7 Gastrointestinal tract.

ORAL ADMINISTRATION

oral drug administration *the delivery of any medication that is taken by mouth and swallowed into the lower gastrointestinal tract.*

Oral drug administration denotes any medication taken by mouth (oral) and swallowed into the gastrointestinal (GI) tract. From the GI tract, the medication is absorbed and distributed throughout the body. When administering a medication by the oral route, you must be sure that the patient has an adequate level of consciousness to support his airway. Administering an oral medication to a patient who cannot support his airway may result in an airway occlusion or aspiration into the lungs. If aspiration into the lungs occurs, aspiration pneumonia and its deadly consequences may occur.

Medications for oral delivery come in a variety of forms, either solid or liquid.

- *Capsules.* Capsules contain liquid, dry, or beaded medication in a soluble casing. For maximum effectiveness, the patient must swallow them whole.
- *Tablets.* Tablets are comprised of medicated powder compressed into a small, solid disk. Typically, tablets may be scored to permit breaking in half or quarters when lesser dosages are required.
- *Pills.* Pills, comprised of medicated powder compressed into a small disk, are the same as tablets. In the past, the term *pill* was used to denote a solid medication taken by mouth. Over time, *tablet* has become the accepted term.
- *Enteric-coated/time-release capsules and tablets.* These forms of medication release the drug gradually as layers of the capsule or tablet slowly erode. Time-release capsules or tablets must be swallowed whole.
- *Elixirs.* Elixirs are liquid medications combined with alcohol or placed in a sweetened fluid.
- *Emulsions.* Emulsions are medications combined with a fat or oil emulsifier.
- *Lozenges.* Lozenges are solid forms of medication that slowly dissolve in the mouth, thus permitting gradual swallowing.
- *Suspensions.* A suspension is a liquid that contains small particles of solid medication.
- *Syrups.* A syrup is a concentrated solution of sugar in water or another liquid to which a medication is added.

Equipment for Oral Administration

Administering oral medications is simple and easy. The basic equipment that you may need depends upon the medication and the patient's status:

- *Soufflé cup.* A soufflé cup is a paper or plastic cup. Placing a solid medication in a soufflé cup makes it easy to see and minimizes contact with the provider's hands.
- *Medicine cup.* A medicine cup is a plastic or glass cup with volumetric measurements on the side. It facilitates giving specific amounts of liquid medication. When you pour medication into the cup, the liquid does not form a flat surface but clings to the sides at a higher level, forming a *meniscus.* To compensate for the meniscus, measure the medication toward the center, at its lowest level.
- *Medicine dropper.* A medicine dropper has markings for measuring liquid volumes. You will use it for special medications and to administer medications to children or patients who cannot tolerate other forms of oral medication.
- *Teaspoon.* You will use these accurately sized measuring spoons to administer liquid medications. A teaspoon normally holds 5 milliliters of fluid; however, the volume of household teaspoons varies significantly. To ensure accurate medication administration, use a measured teaspoon or syringe.
- *Oral syringe.* Oral syringes are calibrated plastic syringes without a hypodermic needle. They are considered the most accurate oral means of administering liquid-based medications. When administering a medication with the oral syringe, place the end of the syringe in the patient's mouth and deliver only as much medication as the

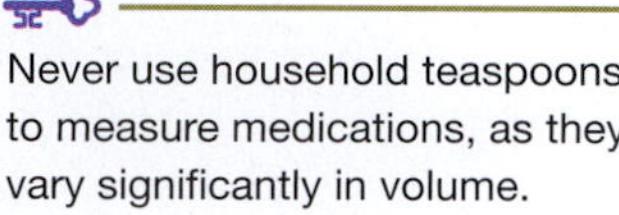

Never use household teaspoons to measure medications, as they vary significantly in volume.

patient can safely swallow. Several administrations may be necessary to deliver a complete dose.

★ *Nipple.* For the neonate or infant, liquid medication can be delivered with a plastic nipple.

General Principles of Oral Administration

To administer medications orally, use the following technique:

1. Use appropriate Standard Precautions.
2. Note whether to administer the medication with food or on an empty stomach.
3. Gather any necessary equipment such as a soufflé cup or teaspoon; mix liquids or suspensions, or otherwise prepare medications as needed.
4. Have your patient sit upright (when not contraindicated).
5. Place the medication into your patient's mouth. Allow self-administration when possible; assist when needed.
6. Follow administration with 4 to 8 ounces of water or other liquid. Swallowing a liquid pushes the medication into the stomach.
7. Ensure that the patient has swallowed the medication and it is not hidden in his mouth. For some pediatric and psychiatric patients, you may have to visually confirm that the patient has swallowed the medication by inspecting the oral cavity.

GASTRIC TUBE ADMINISTRATION

For patients who have difficulty swallowing or whose nutritional status is poor, you may place a *gastric tube* to support or completely supplement nutritional requirements. Gastric tubes are also used in instances of drug overdose, trauma, and upper gastrointestinal bleeding. They may be surgically inserted directly into the stomach through the abdomen or indirectly through the nose (nasogastric tube) or mouth (orogastric tube). Placing a gastric tube through the abdominal wall is reserved for the hospital setting. In some EMS systems, paramedics insert orogastric or nasogastric tubes in the field for emergencies. A properly placed gastric tube allows enteral medication delivery. Activated charcoal for toxic ingestion is commonly administered through a nasogastric or orogastric tube. Other medications, many used in the nonacute setting, also are administered via the gastric tube. With modification, most oral medications can be administered this way. However, you should avoid administering time-release capsules and enteric-coated tablets through a gastric tube, as crushing them for delivery destroys their slow-release mechanism. Also, ensure that the medication has been sufficiently crushed so as not to become trapped and occlude the gastric tube.

To administer a medication via a gastric tube, use the following technique (Procedure 7–1):

1. Confirm proper tube placement. Disconnect the tube from the drainage or suction unit or clamping device. Clamp the tube from the drainage or suction unit to avoid gastric contents spilling from either device. Attach a cone-tipped syringe to the proximal end of the gastric tube. Gently inject air while auscultating over the stomach. Following this, withdraw the plunger while observing for the presence of gastric fluid or contents, which indicates appropriate placement. Leave the tube disconnected from the drainage or suction unit.
2. Irrigate the gastric tube. To irrigate the gastric tube, draw up 50 to 100 mL of normal saline into a cone-tipped syringe. Insert the syringe into the open end of the gastric tube. With the syringe tip pointed at the floor, gently inject the saline into the tube. If the saline encounters resistance, look for problems such as tube kinking. Also, have the patient lie on his left side and reattempt injection. If the saline still meets resistance, reattach the tube to the drainage or suction unit and contact medical direction for further directives.
3. Prepare the medication(s) for delivery. Crush tablets or empty capsules into 30 mL of warm water. Ensure that all particles are small so that they will not occlude the tube. You may administer liquid medications without further preparation.

Procedure 7-1 Medication Administration through a Nasogastric Tube

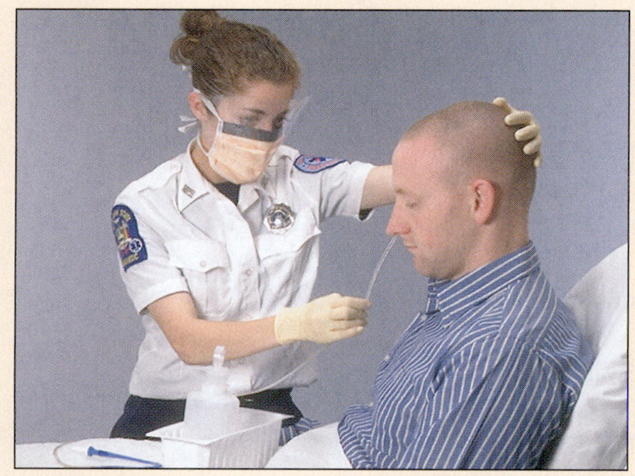

7-1a Confirm proper tube placement.

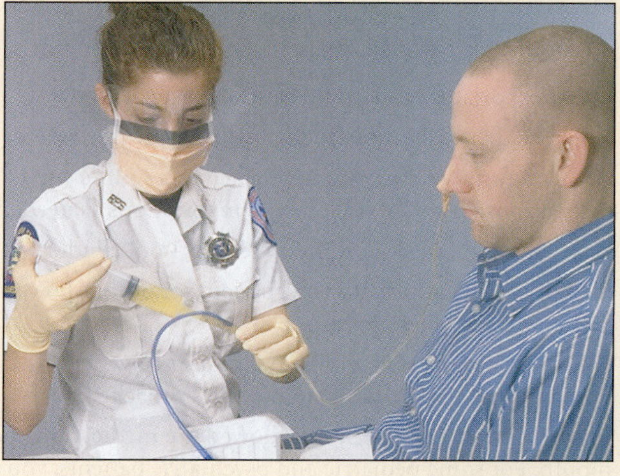

7-1b Withdraw the plunger while observing for the presence of gastric fluid or contents.

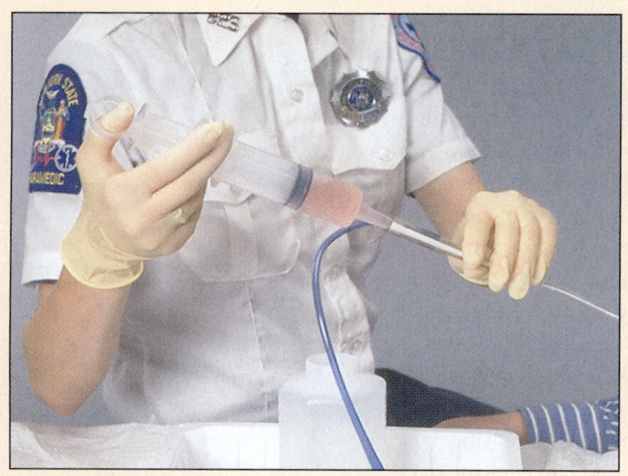

7-1c Instill medication into the gastric tube.

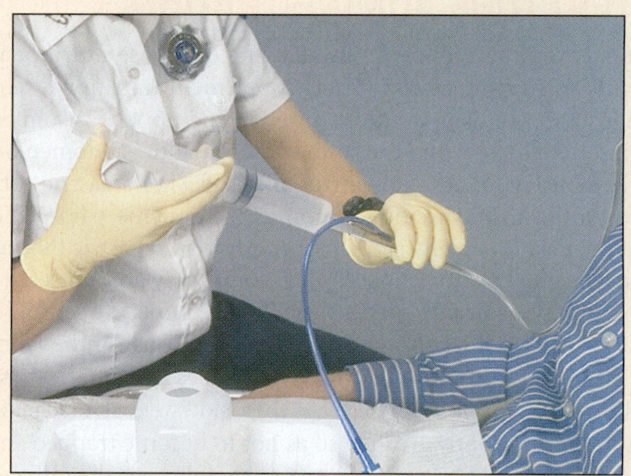

7-1d Gently inject the saline.

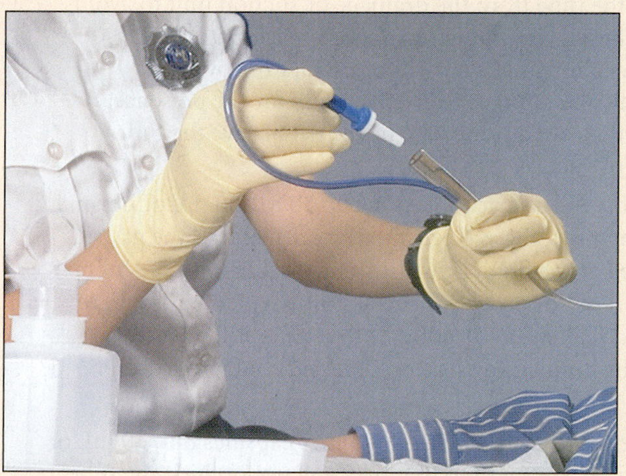

7-1e Clamp off the distal tube.

4. Draw the medication into a 30- to 50-mL cone-tipped syringe and place the tip into the open gastric tube. Gently administer the medication into the gastric tube. Forceful application may create considerable distention and patient discomfort.
5. Draw 50 to 100 mL of warm normal saline into a cone-tipped syringe and attach it to the open end of the gastric tube. Gently inject the saline. This facilitates the medication's passage into the stomach and rinses the tube, ensuring that the patient receives the entire dose. Repeated administrations may be necessary.
6. Clamp off the distal tube. Use a commercially manufactured device or hemostat to clamp shut the distal portion of the gastric tube for approximately 30 minutes after you administer the medication. Do not reattach to the drainage or suction unit. This will prevent the medication's inadvertent removal from the stomach.

If you must refill the syringe in order to administer the full dosage of medication, do not allow the syringe to empty completely before you detach it from the gastric tube. This prevents drawing air into the syringe and then introducing it into the stomach, which causes discomfort.

RECTAL ADMINISTRATION

The rectum's extreme vascularity promotes rapid drug absorption. Additionally, because medications given rectally do not pass through the liver, they are not subject to **hepatic alteration;** thus, their absorption is more predictable.

hepatic alteration *change in a medication's chemical composition that occurs in the liver.*

In the emergency setting, you may give certain drugs rectally if you cannot establish an intravenous line or use the oral route. These include diazepam (Valium) for protracted seizures or aspirin for cardiac or neurologic emergencies. In the nonacute setting, you may administer sedatives, antiemetics, or other specially prepared medications rectally.

Rectal administration may prove advantageous with the unconscious or pediatric patient, or when administering drugs with an objectionable taste or odor. Unfortunately, drug absorption may be erratic if gross fecal matter exists. In addition, some drugs may cause considerable anal or rectal irritation.

Rectal medications come in a variety of forms. In the emergency setting, they are typically liquid, thus permitting easy administration and rapid absorption. To administer a rectal medication in the emergent setting follow this technique:

1. Confirm the indication for administration and dose, and draw the correct quantity of medication into a syringe.
2. Place the hub of a 14-gauge Teflon catheter (removed from the angiocatheter) on the end of a needleless syringe (Figure 7-8 ■).
3. Insert the Teflon catheter into the patient's rectum and inject the medication. Try to keep the medication in the lower part of the rectum. Administration higher in the rectum may result in the medication's being absorbed by veins that deliver the drug to the portal circulation.
4. Withdraw the catheter and hold the patient's buttocks together, thus permitting retention and absorption.

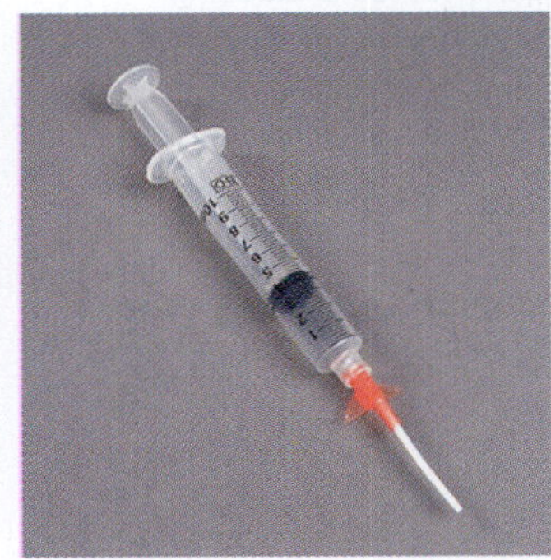

■ Figure 7-8 Catheter placement on needleless syringe.

An alternative technique utilizes a small endotracheal tube instead of the Teflon angiocatheter. Remove the 15/22-mm BVM adapter and connect a syringe to the proximal end of the tube (Figure 7-9 ■). Lubricate the tube and insert it into the rectum. Inject the medication, remove the tube, and hold the buttocks together.

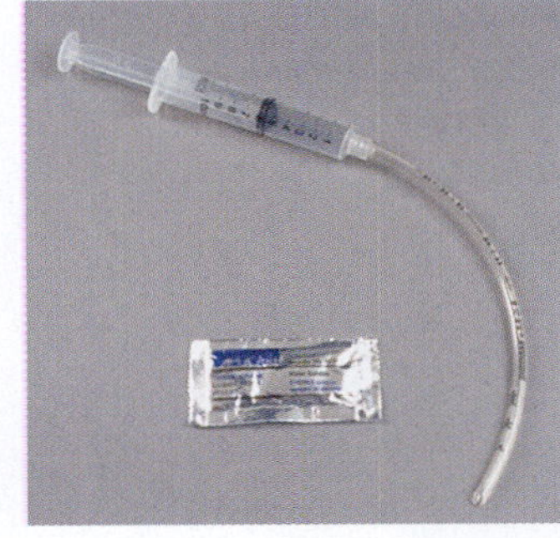

■ Figure 7-9 Syringe attached to endotracheal tube.

In the nonemergent setting, suppositories or enemas are common methods for rectal administration. Because your responsibilities as a paramedic may include nonemergent clinical settings, you should master these techniques. Additionally, the rectal route may prove beneficial for a pediatric patient who resists oral administration or for whom IV access proves impractical.

Suppositories are medications packaged in a soft, pliable form. Generally refrigerated until they are used, they begin to melt at body temperature in the rectum. Some are lubricated to ease insertion. Suppositories can be lubricated by running a small amount of lukewarm tap water over the suppository prior to insertion. To administer a suppository, manually insert it into the rectum. Hold the buttocks shut for 5 to 10 minutes to allow for retention and absorption.

suppository *medication packaged in a soft, pliable form, for insertion into the rectum.*

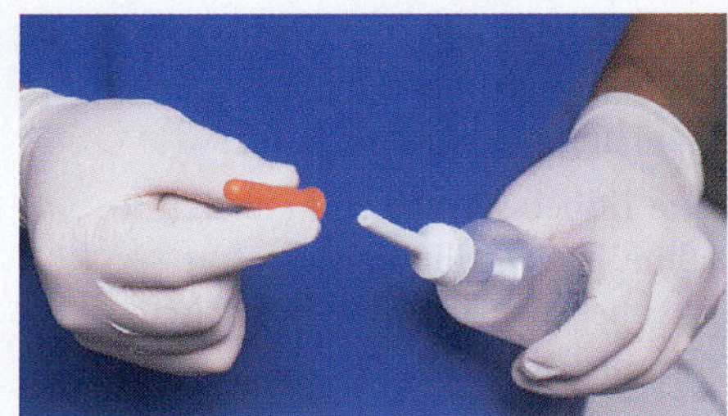

■ **Figure 7-10** Prepackaged enema container.

enema *a liquid bolus of medication that is injected into the rectum.*

bolus *concentrated mass of medication.*

An **enema** is typically a liquid **bolus** of medication that is injected into the rectum. Medications given via this route are typically referred to as small volume enemas. They are typically prepackaged in a squeezable container with a rectal tip (Figure 7-10 ■).

To administer a medicated small volume enema, use the following technique:

1. Apply appropriate Standard Precautions and confirm the need for administration via a small volume enema.
2. Place the patient on his left side. Flex his right leg to expose the anus.
3. Insert the prelubricated rectal tip into the anus and advance 3 to 4 inches.
4. Gently squeeze the medicated solution of the bottle into the rectum and colon.
5. Hold the buttocks together to enhance absorption into the rectal and intestinal tissue.

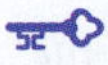

Do not administer rectal medications in the presence of diarrhea, rectal bleeding, hemorrhoids, or any other situation involving severe anal irritation.

Only those medications with specific guidelines for rectal administration should be delivered through this route. Do not administer rectal medications in the presence of diarrhea, rectal bleeding, hemorrhoids, or any other situation involving severe anal irritation.

PARENTERAL DRUG ADMINISTRATION

parenteral *drug administration outside of the gastrointestinal tract.*

Parenteral denotes any drug administration outside of the gastrointestinal tract. Broadly, this encompasses pulmonary and some topical forms of medication delivery; however, additional specific criteria apply to parenteral administration. Typically, the parenteral route involves the use of needles as medications are injected into the circulatory system or tissues. Consequently, some forms of parenteral drug delivery afford the most rapid drug delivery and absorption.

SYRINGES AND NEEDLES

Frequently, giving medications via the parenteral route requires a syringe and hypodermic needle.

Syringe

syringe *plastic tube with which liquid medications can be drawn up, stored, and injected.*

A **syringe** is a plastic tube with which liquid medications can be drawn up, stored, and injected. Syringes range in size from 1 mL to 100 mL and greater. Remember that while medication dosages are generally given by weight (g/mg/mcg), syringes represent volume. Therefore, you must be prepared to mathematically convert these measurements.

A syringe's two major components are a barrel and a plunger (Figure 7-11 ■). The tubelike barrel, or body, functions as a reservoir for medication. Markings on its side calibrate its overall volume. Smaller syringes are calibrated in 0.10-mL intervals, larger syringes in 1.0-mL intervals.

The plunger is a device that fits into the barrel. At one end it has a handle for pulling or pushing. At the opposite end, a rubber stopper fits snugly into the barrel. Pulling on the plunger draws material into the barrel; pushing on it expels material from the barrel. The rubber end forms a tight seal from which the fluid medication cannot escape.

The junction of the fluid and rubber stopper measures the total volume of liquid in the syringe. The barrel's maximum volume should correspond closely to the volume of medication needed. For example, to administer 2 mL of medication, a 3-mL syringe would prove most appropriate.

An adapter at the syringe's distal end is compatible with the hub of an IV catheter or, as many cases will require, a hypodermic needle.

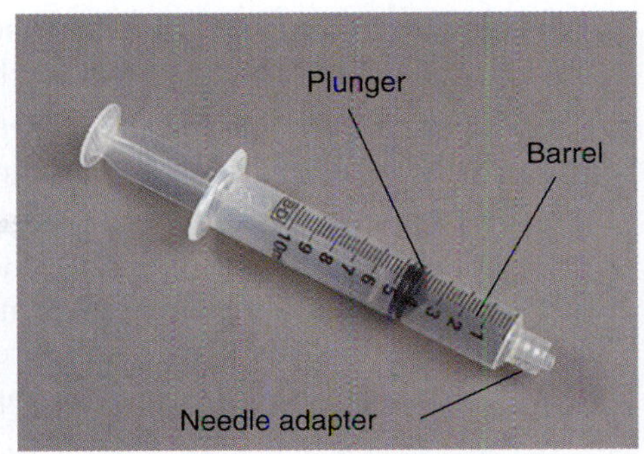

■ Figure 7-11 Syringe.

Hypodermic Needle

The **hypodermic needle** is a hollow metal tube used with the syringe to administer medications. It is sharp enough to easily puncture tissues, blood vessels, or IV medication ports.

hypodermic needle *hollow metal tube used with the syringe to administer medications.*

The hypodermic needle's primary components include a hilt and shaft. The hilt is a threaded plastic tube that screws securely onto the syringe's distal adapter. The shaft is a thin metal tube through which medications can flow from the syringe into the delivery site. A bevel at the shaft's distal end accounts for its sharpness (Figure 7-12 ■).

Hypodermic needles come in a variety of gauges and lengths. A needle's **gauge** describes its diameter. Generally, hypodermic needle gauges range from 18 to 27. The gauge and actual diameter are inversely related: the higher the gauge, the smaller the diameter. Thus, a 25-gauge needle's diameter is smaller than an 18-gauge needle's. Conversely, a 20-gauge needle's diameter is larger than a 22-gauge needle's. Hypodermic needle lengths generally range from ⅜ to 1½ inch. The package label lists the size of the syringe and the gauge and length of the hypodermic needle.

gauge *the size of a needle's diameter.*

Because syringes and hypodermic needles frequently involve invasive procedures, they are packaged sterile. Never use either a syringe or a hypodermic needle from a package that has been opened or tampered with. Used hypodermic needles are sharp and present a biohazard. Dispose of them immediately after you complete any task involving their use.

MEDICATION PACKAGING

All medications delivered by the parenteral route are liquids. They are packaged in a variety of containers with which you must be familiar, as obtaining medication from each type requires a different procedure. The kinds of parenteral drug containers include:

- ★ Glass ampules
- ★ Single and multidose vials
- ★ Nonconstituted drug vials
- ★ Prefilled syringes
- ★ Intravenous medication fluids

You must also be thoroughly familiar with the information included on the labels of all medication containers:

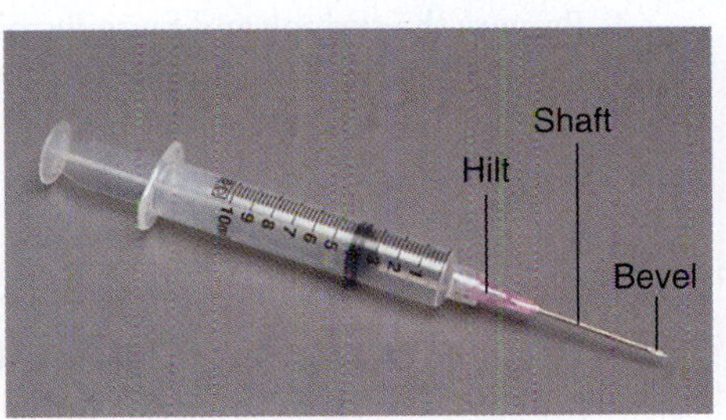

■ Figure 7-12 Hypodermic needle.

★ *Name of medication.* The label lists both the generic and trade name of the medication. Always ensure that you have selected the right medication.

★ *Expiration date.* All medications have an expiration date after which they cannot be used. Never use an expired medication.

★ *Total dose and concentration.* The total dose of drug is the total weight (g/mg/mcg) of medication in the container. The concentration represents the weight of the drug per volume of fluid. For example, if 10 mg of a drug were packaged in 10 mL of fluid, the total dose would be 10 mg, and the concentration would be 10 mg/10 mL or 1 mg/mL. Beware: Identical drugs can be packaged in different dosages and concentrations.

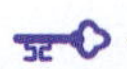

Always use the label printed directly on the container to confirm the correct medication.

These labels are printed directly on the vial, ampule, prefilled syringe, or IV medication bag. Always use them to confirm the correct medication.

Glass Ampules

ampule *breakable glass vessel containing liquid medication.*

An **ampule,** or amp, is a breakable glass vessel containing liquid medication. It has a cone-shaped top, thin neck, and circular tubular base for storing the medication (Figure 7-13 ■). The thin neck is a vulnerable point where you intentionally break the ampule to retrieve its contents. Ampules usually range in volume from 1 to 5 mL. The least expensive form of drug packaging, they contain single doses of medication.

To obtain medication from a glass ampule you will need a syringe and needle. Use the following technique (Procedure 7–2):

1. Confirm medication indications and patient allergies.
2. Confirm the ampule label (medication name, dose, and expiration).
3. Hold the ampule upright and tap its top to dislodge any trapped solution.
4. Place gauze around the thin neck and snap it off with your thumb.
5. Place the tip of a filter needle inside the ampule and withdraw the medication into the syringe. (The filter needle will ensure no glass is drawn into the syringe.) Then replace the filter needle with a hypodermic needle.
6. Reconfirm the indication, drug, dose, and route of administration.
7. Administer the medication appropriately via the indicated route.
8. Properly dispose of the needle, syringe, and broken glass ampule.

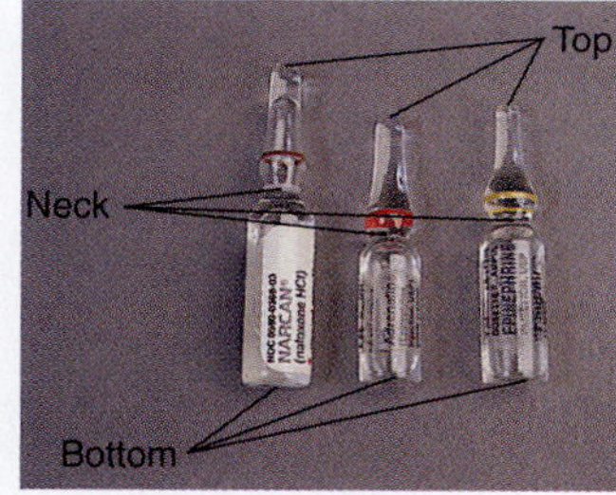

■ Figure 7-13 Ampules.

Single and Multidose Vials

vial *plastic or glass container with a self-sealing rubber top.*

Vials are plastic or glass containers with a self-sealing rubber top (Figure 7-14 ■). Vials may contain single or multiple doses of medication; the self-sealing rubber top prevents leakage from punctures and permits multiple access with a syringe and hypodermic needle. The medication inside the vial is packaged in a vacuum.

To obtain medication from a vial, follow these steps (Procedure 7–3):

1. Confirm medication indications and patient allergies.
2. Confirm the vial label (name, dose, and expiration).
3. Determine the volume of medication to be administered.
4. Prepare the syringe and hypodermic needle. Because the vial is vacuum packed, you will have to replace the volume of medication removed with air in order to maintain equilibrium in the vial. Withdraw the plunger to draw a volume of air into the syringe equal to the volume of medication to be administered. This technique permits easy medication retrieval from the vial.
5. Cleanse the vial's rubber top with an antiseptic alcohol preparation.
6. Insert the hypodermic needle into the rubber top and inject the air from the syringe into the vial. Then withdraw the appropriate volume of medication.

Self-sealing rubber top

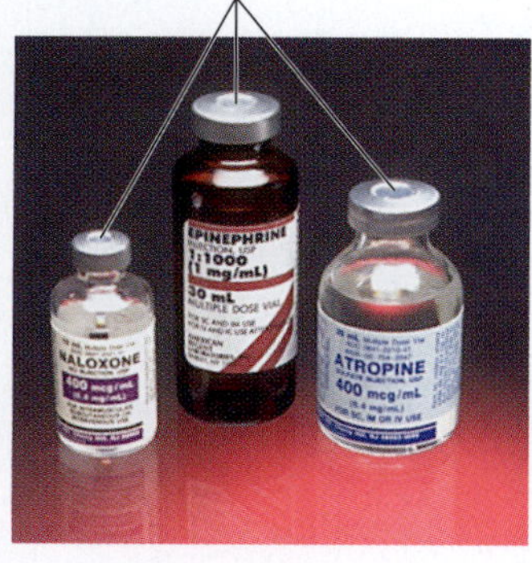

■ Figure 7-14 Vials.

Procedure 7-2 Obtaining Medication from a Glass Ampule

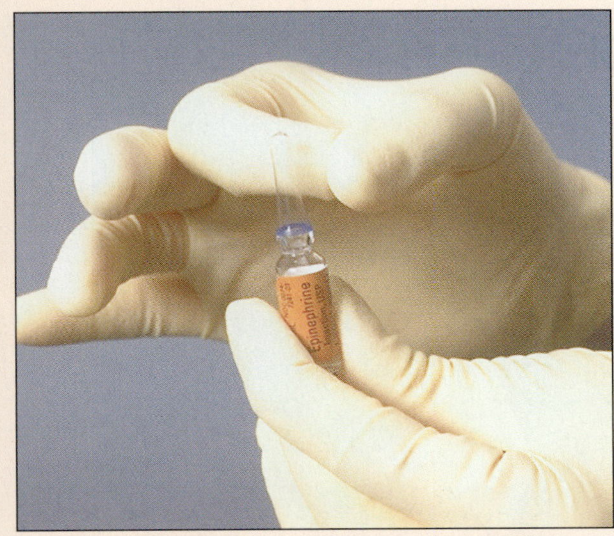

7-2a Hold the ampule upright and tap its top to dislodge any trapped solution.

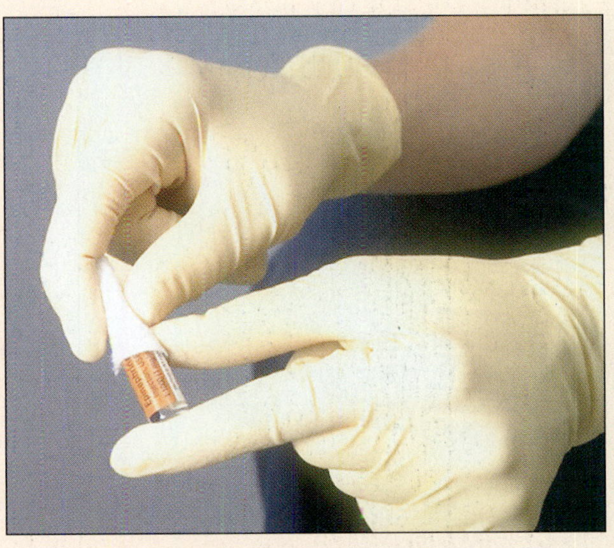

7-2b Place gauze around the thin neck . . .

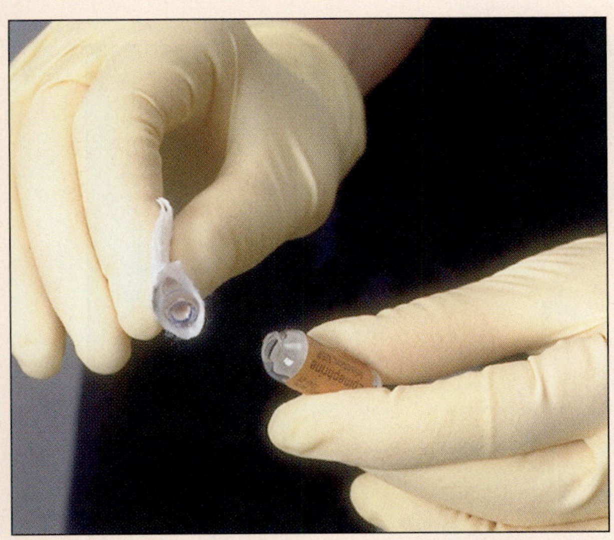

7-2c . . . and snap it off with your thumb.

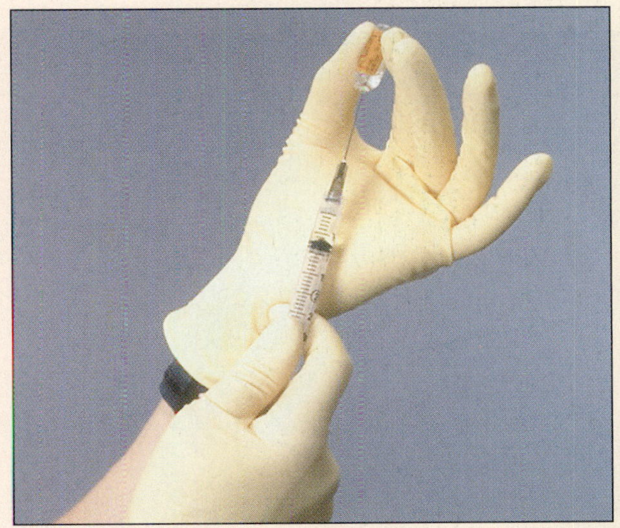

7-2d Draw up the medication.

Procedure 7-3 Obtaining Medication from a Vial

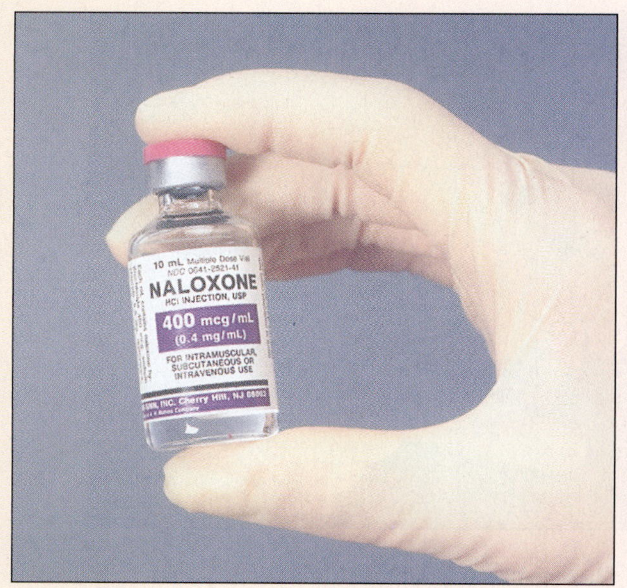

7-3a Confirm the vial label.

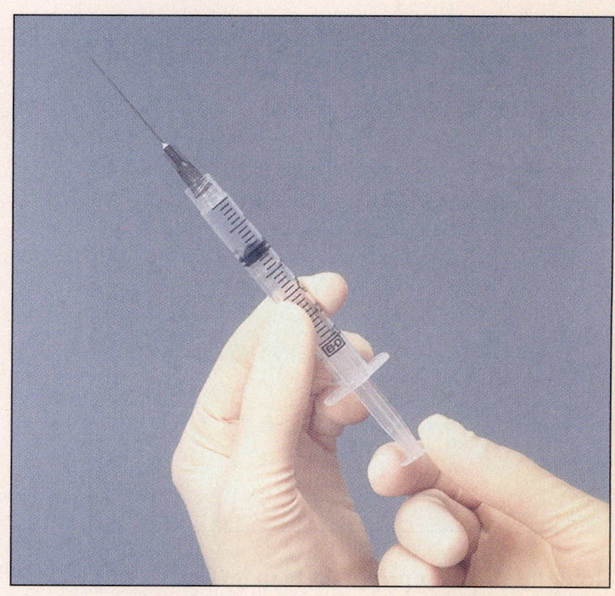

7-3b Prepare the syringe and hypodermic needle.

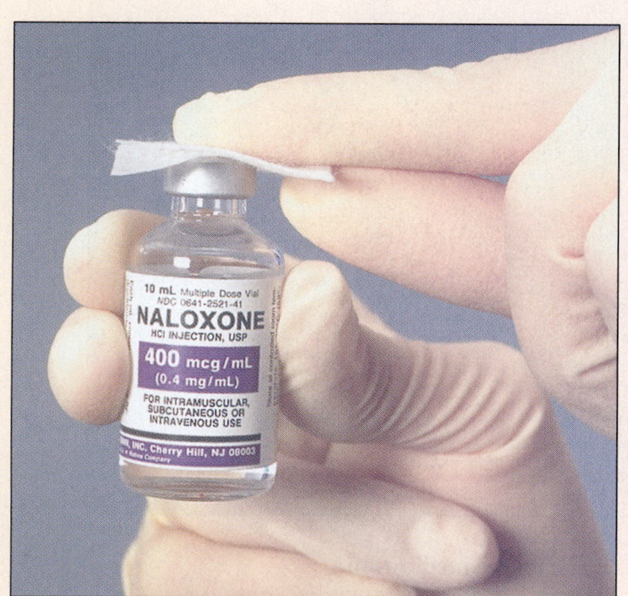

7-3c Cleanse the vial's rubber top.

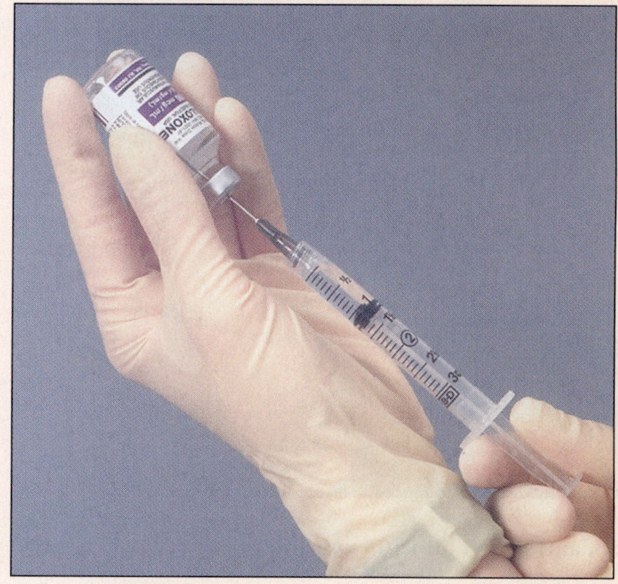

7-3d Insert the hypodermic needle into the rubber top and inject the air from the syringe into the vial.

7. Reconfirm the indication, drug, dose, and route of administration.
8. Administer appropriately via the indicated route.
9. Properly dispose of the needle, syringe, and vial.

Nonconstituted Drug Vial

The **nonconstituted drug vial** extends the viability and storage time of drugs that have a short shelf life or are unstable in liquid form. The nonconstituted drug vial actually consists of two vials, one containing a powdered medication and one containing a liquid mixing solution (Figure 7-15 ■). To prepare the drug you must mix it, or reconstitute it, by withdrawing the liquid solution from its vial and placing it in the powdered medication's vial. In a **Mix-o-Vial** system, the two vials are joined and you must squeeze them together to break the seal and mix.

nonconstituted drug vial/-Mix-o-Vial *vial with two containers, one holding a powdered medication and the other holding a liquid mixing solution.*

To prepare a medication from a nonconstituted drug vial, use the following technique (Procedure 7–4):

1. Confirm medication indications and patient allergies.
2. Confirm the vial's label (name, dose, expiration date).
3. Remove all solution from the vial containing the mixing solution, using the same procedure as you would to withdraw medication from a single or multidose vial.
4. With an alcohol preparation, cleanse the top of the vial containing the powdered drug and inject the mixing solution.
5. Gently agitate or shake the vial to ensure complete mixture.
6. Determine the volume of newly constituted medication to be administered.
7. Prepare the syringe and hypodermic needle. Because the vial is vacuum packed, you will have to replace the volume of medication removed with air in order to retain equilibrium in the vial. By withdrawing the plunger, place into the syringe a volume of air equal to the volume of medication that will be removed. This technique permits easy medication retrieval from the vial.
8. Cleanse the medication vial's rubber top with an antiseptic alcohol preparation.
9. Insert the hypodermic needle into the rubber top and withdraw the appropriate volume of medication.
10. Reconfirm the indication, drug, dose, and route of administration.
11. Administer appropriately via the indicated route.
12. Monitor the patient for the desired effects.
13. Properly dispose of the needle and syringe.

In some instances you may have to place multiple medications into one syringe for a single delivery. For example, meperidine (Demerol) and promethazine (Phenergan) may be delivered in this manner. Meperidine, an analgesic, can cause nausea and vomiting when administered. To decrease the incidence of nausea and vomiting, you can simultaneously administer promethazine, an antiemetic. To perform this task, draw all medications in the appropriate order according to the

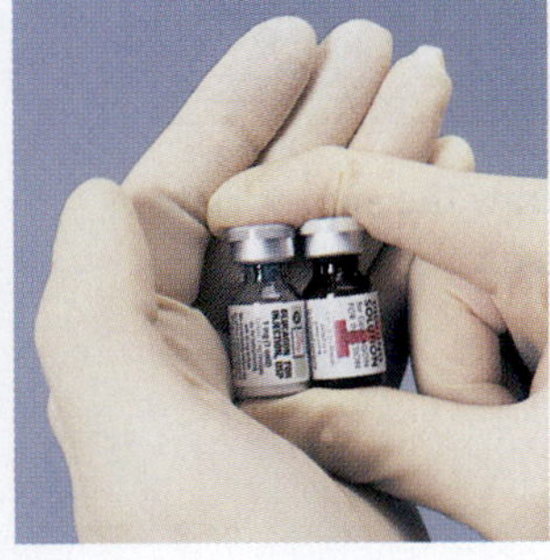

■ Figure 7-15 The nonconstituted drug vial actually consists of two vials, one containing a powdered medication and one containing a liquid mixing solution.

Procedure 7-4 Preparing Medication from a Nonconstituted Drug Vial

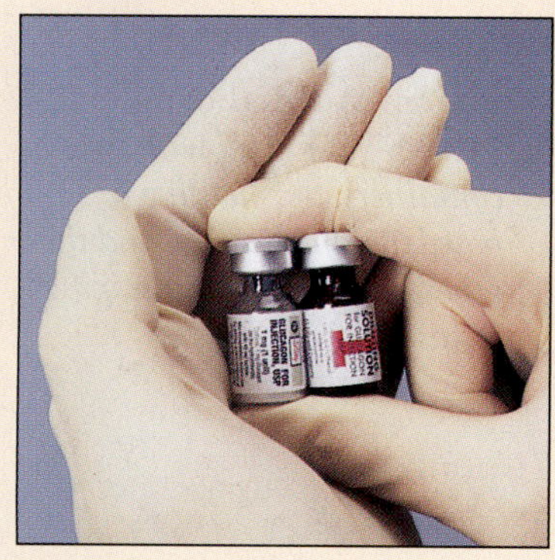

7-4a Nonconstituted drugs come in separate vials. Confirm the labels.

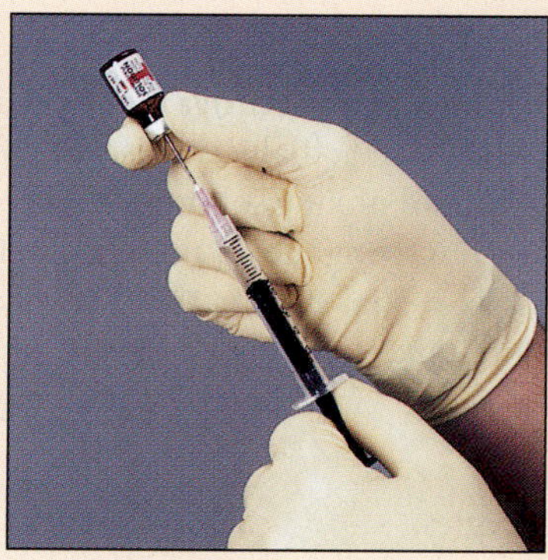

7-4b Remove all solution from the vial containing the mixing solution.

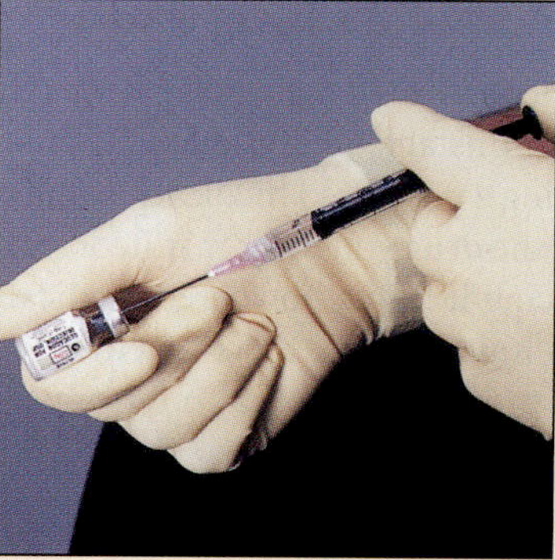

7-4c Cleanse the top of the vial containing the powdered drug and inject the solution.

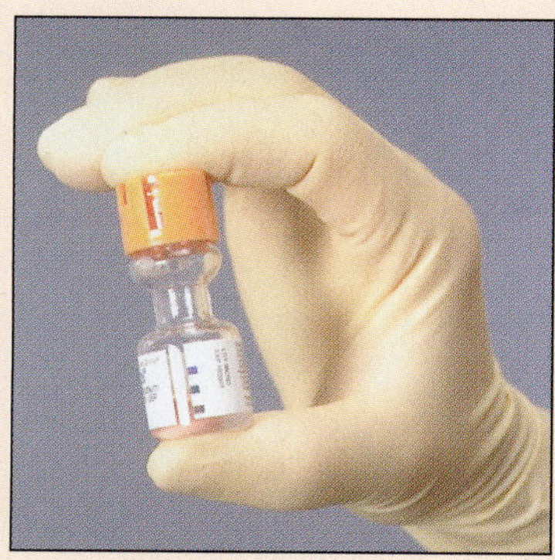

7-4d Agitate or shake the vial to ensure complete mixture.

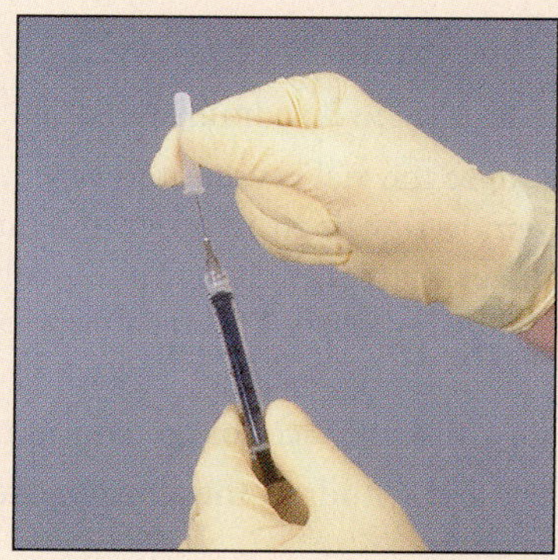

7-4e Prepare a new syringe and hypodermic needle.

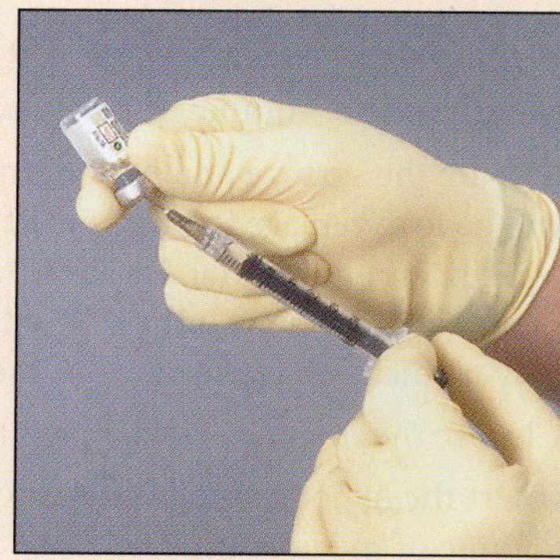

7-4f Withdraw the appropriate volume of medication.

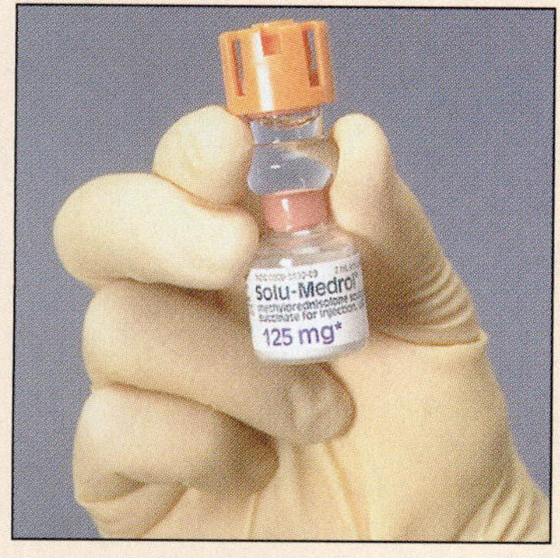

7-4g In the Mix-o-Vial system, the vials are joined at the neck. Confirm the labels.

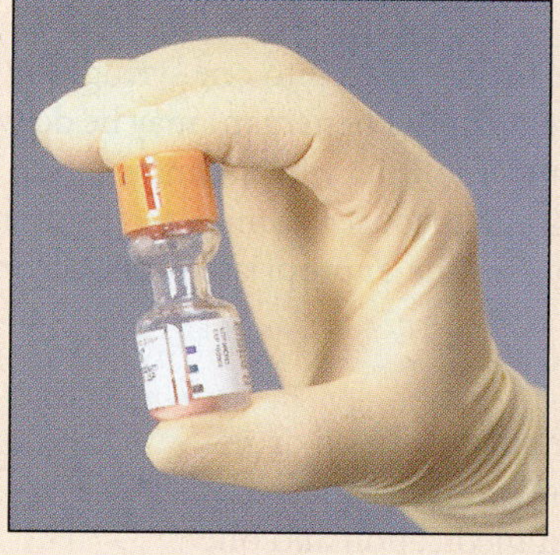

7-4h Squeeze the vials together to break the seal. Agitate or shake to mix completely.

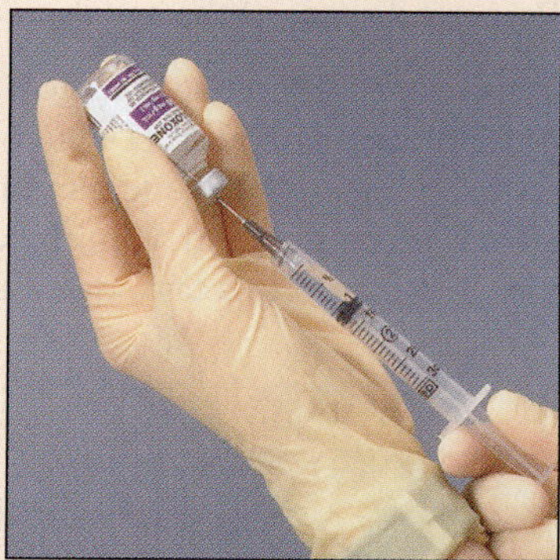

7-4i Withdraw the appropriate volume of medication.

procedures discussed. Always anticipate total volume and select an appropriate syringe size. To avoid complications, you must always be aware of drug incompatibilities.

Prefilled or Preloaded Syringes

Prefilled or **preloaded syringes** are packaged in tamper-proof containers with the medication already in the syringe. Because the syringe is prefilled, you do not need to draw the medication from another source. Generally, prefilled syringes contain standard dosages, thus decreasing the chance of dosage error.

prefilled/preloaded syringe *syringe packaged in a tamper-proof container with the medication already in the barrel.*

The prefilled syringe consists of two parts, a syringe and a glass tube prefilled with liquid medication. The plastic syringe is similar to those described earlier; however, it does not have a plunger. Rather, you screw the prefilled glass tube into the syringe barrel and secure it (Figure 7-16 ■). Pushing the glass container into the syringe barrel expels the medication through the attached hypodermic needle.

Follow these steps to administer a medication from a prefilled syringe:

1. Confirm medication indications and patient allergies.
2. Confirm the prefilled syringe label (name, dose, and expiration date).
3. Assemble the prefilled syringe. Remove the pop-off caps and screw together.
4. Reconfirm the indication, drug, dose, and route of administration.
5. Administer appropriately via the indicated route.
6. Properly dispose of the needle and syringe.

Intravenous Medication Solutions

Medicated solutions are another form of parenteral medication. They are packaged in an IV bag and administered as an IV **infusion.** IV medication solutions may be premixed or you may have to mix them. The section on intravenous drug infusions later in this chapter discusses their actual preparation and administration.

medicated solution *parenteral medication packaged in an IV bag and administered as an IV infusion.*

infusion *liquid medication delivered through a vein.*

PARENTERAL ROUTES

Parenterally administered drugs can be absorbed locally or systemically. Additionally, depending on the route of administration, their absorption rate may be slow, sustained, or rapid. Parenteral delivery bypasses the digestive tract, thus making the drug's absorption, action, and onset more predictable. Because parenteral routes use hypodermic needles that contact body fluids, the risk of disease transmission is ever present.

Content Review

Parenteral Routes

- Intradermal injection
- Subcutaneous injection
- Intramuscular injection
- Intravenous access
- Intraosseous infusion

Parenteral drug delivery employs the following routes:

- Intradermal injection
- Subcutaneous injection
- Intramuscular injection
- Intravenous access
- Intraosseous infusion

Specific medications require specific routes of parenteral delivery; therefore, you must be competent with every route. In this section we will discuss the specialized equipment, medications, and

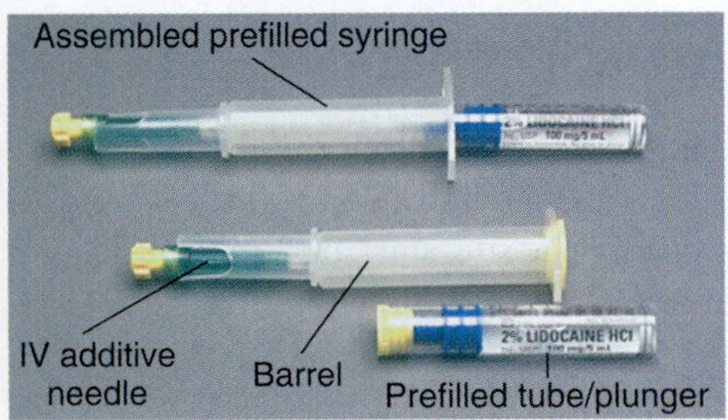

■ Figure 7-16 Prefilled syringes.

■ Figure 7-17 Intradermal injection.

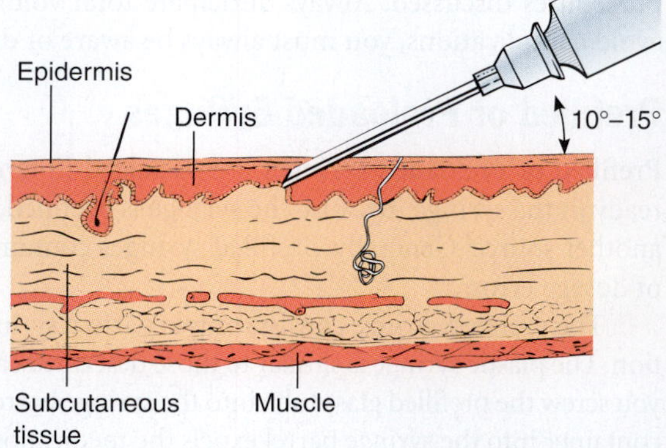

routes for intradermal, subcutaneous, and intramuscular injections. Because of their complexity, we will discuss intravenous access and intraosseous infusions separately in the following sections.

Whether you are administering a parenteral injection or an IV bolus or infusion, you should explain the entire procedure to the patient to help alleviate his anxiety. Finally, remember that hypoperfusion (hypovolemia or peripheral vascular disease, for instance) may significantly reduce parenteral absorption.

Intradermal Injection

intradermal *within the dermal layer of the skin.*

Capillaries in the dermis afford a very slow rate of absorption, with little or no systemic distribution.

Using a syringe and hypodermic needle, **intradermal** injections deposit medication into the dermal layer of the skin (*intra-*, within; *derma*, skin). The amount of medication placed in the dermal layer is quite small, typically less than 1 mL (Figure 7-17 ■).

Capillaries in the dermis afford a very slow rate of absorption, with little or no systemic distribution. Rather, the bulk of medication remains localized in the area of administration. Intradermal delivery proves useful for allergy testing and tuberculin skin testing and for administering local anesthetics during suturing, wound debridement, and IV establishment.

The forearm and upper back are preferred sites for intradermal injections. They have little hair and are highly visible. Additionally, you should look for sites free of superficial blood vessels, which increase the chance for systemic absorption.

To administer an intradermal injection, you will need the following equipment:

- ★ Standard Precautions
- ★ Alcohol or Betadine antiseptic preparations
- ★ Packaged medication
- ★ Tuberculin syringe (1 mL)
- ★ 25 to 27-gauge needle, ⅜ to 1 inch long
- ★ Sterile gauze and adhesive bandage

To administer an intradermal injection, follow these steps:

1. Assemble and prepare the needed equipment.
2. Apply Standard Precautions and confirm the drug, indication, dosage, and need for intradermal injection.
3. Draw up medication as appropriate.
4. Prepare the site with alcohol or Betadine. The intended site must be cleansed of pathogens, therein decreasing the likelihood of infection. Generally, you will use alcohol or Betadine antiseptics. To appropriately cleanse the site, start at the site itself and work outward with an expanding circular motion. This motion will push pathogens away from the intended site of puncture.
5. Pull the patient's skin taut with your nondominant hand.

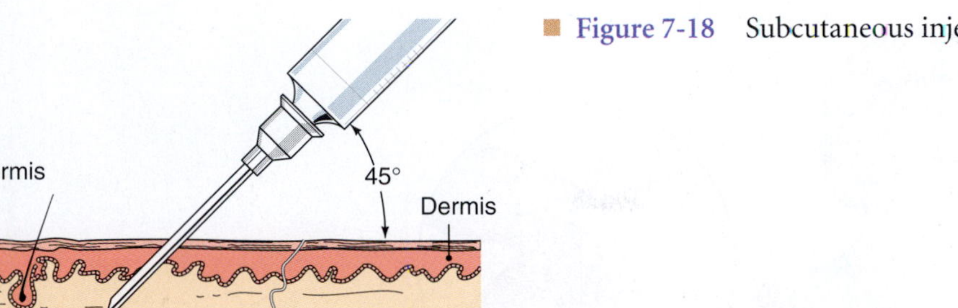

■ Figure 7-18 Subcutaneous injection.

6. Insert the needle, bevel up, just under the skin, at a 10° to 15° angle.
7. Slowly inject the medication, and look for a small bump or wheal to form as medication is deposited and collects in the intradermal tissue.
8. Remove the needle and dispose of it in the sharps container.
9. Place the adhesive bandage over the site; use the gauze for hemorrhage control if needed.

Do not rub or massage the injection site. This promotes systemic absorption and nullifies the advantage of localized effect.

Subcutaneous Injection

Subcutaneous injections place medication into the subcutaneous tissue (*sub-*, below; *cutaneous*, skin). The subcutaneous layer consists of loose connective tissue between the skin and muscle (Figure 7-18 ■). The subcutaneous tissue has few blood vessels and thus promotes slow, sustained absorption, which prolongs a drug's effect on the body. Like intradermal injections, no more than 1.0 mL of medication is administered subcutaneously. Administering more than 1.0 mL of medication can cause irritation and, possibly, an abscess.

subcutaneous *relating to the layer of loose connective tissue between the skin and muscle.*

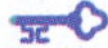

The subcutaneous tissue has few blood vessels and thus promotes slow, sustained absorption, which prolongs a drug's effect on the body.

Administer subcutaneous injections where you can easily pinch the skin on the upper arms, thighs, or occasionally the abdomen (Figure 7-19 ■). Easily pinched skin contains more subcutaneous tissue and readily separates from the muscle. All sites should be free of superficial blood vessels, nerves, and tendons. Additionally, avoid areas with tattoos or bruising.

To perform a subcutaneous injection, you will need the following equipment:

★ Standard Precautions
★ Alcohol or Betadine antiseptic preparations
★ Packaged medication
★ Syringe (1 to 3 mL)
★ 24- to 26-gauge hypodermic needle, ⅜ to 1 inch long
★ Sterile gauze and adhesive bandage

To administer a subcutaneous injection, use the following technique (Procedure 7–5):

1. Assemble and prepare equipment.
2. Apply Standard Precautions and confirm the drug, indication, dosage, and need for subcutaneous injection.
3. Draw up the medication as appropriate.
4. Prepare the site with alcohol or Betadine as described for an intradermal injection.
5. Gently pinch a 1-inch fold of skin.

■ Figure 7-19
Subcutaneous injection sites (injection sites shown in red).

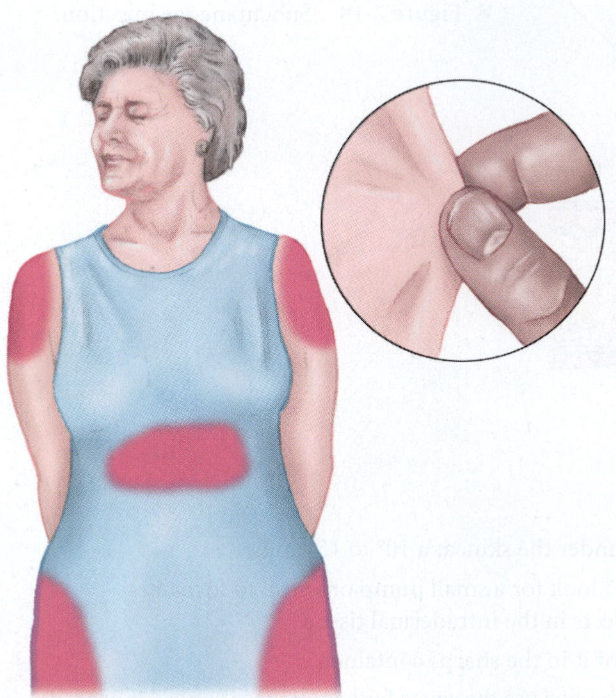

6. Insert the needle just into the skin at a 45° angle with the bevel up.
7. Pull the plunger back to aspirate tissue fluid.
8. If blood appears, the hypodermic needle is in a blood vessel and absorption will be too rapid. Start the procedure over with a new syringe.
9. If no blood appears, proceed with step 10.
10. Slowly inject the medication.
11. Remove the needle and dispose of it in a sharps container.
12. Place an adhesive bandage over the site; use the gauze for hemorrhage control if needed.
13. Monitor the patient.

After you give the injection, gently rubbing or massaging the site will help initiate systemic absorption.

Some authorities recommend using an air plug in the syringe. This is approximately 0.1 mL of air that follows the injection and pushes the medication further into the subcutaneous tissue, thus preventing leakage or medication loss. To place an air plug in the syringe, aspirate approximately 0.1 mL of air into the barrel after you have drawn up the medication. Pointing the needle downward and perpendicular to the ground, tap the syringe with your finger to dislodge the air pocket. It will float to the top of the plunger, and from there it will follow the medication into the subcutaneous tissue.

You can also deliver a subcutaneous injection into the sublingual region, or fleshy tissue below the tongue. To administer a subcutaneous injection, you place the hypodermic needle of a small, medication-filled syringe into the sublingual tissue and then inject the medication as appropriate. Epinephrine can be administered in this manner in severe cases of asthma or anaphylaxis.

intramuscular *within the muscle.*

Content Review

Intramuscular Injection Sites

- Deltoid
- Dorsal gluteal
- Vastus lateralis
- Rectus femoris

Intramuscular Injection

Intramuscular injections deposit medication into muscle (*intra-*, within; *muscular,* muscle). Muscle is extremely vascular and permits systemic delivery at a moderate absorption rate. Drug absorption through muscle is also relatively predictable. To reach the muscle, a needle must penetrate the dermal and subcutaneous tissue (Figure 7-20 ■).

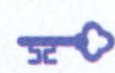

Muscle is extremely vascular and permits systemic delivery at a moderate absorption rate.

Procedure 7-5 Subcutaneous Administration

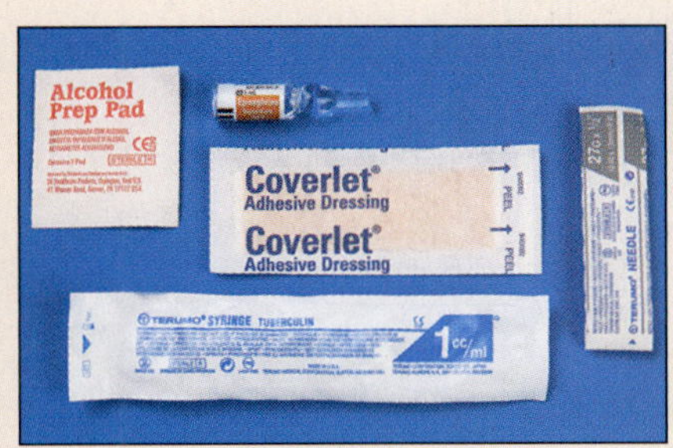

7-5a Prepare the equipment.

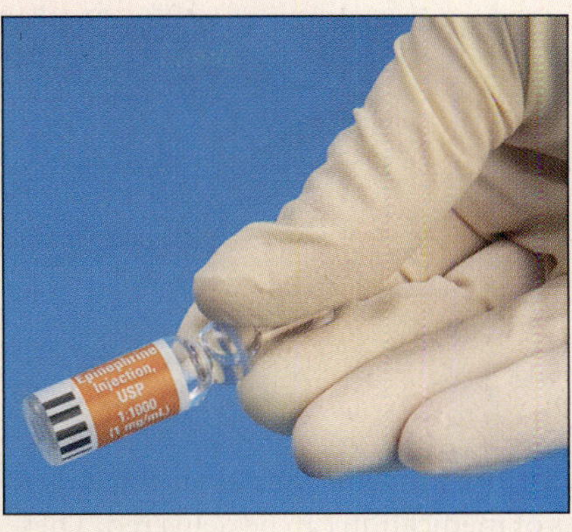

7-5b Check the medication.

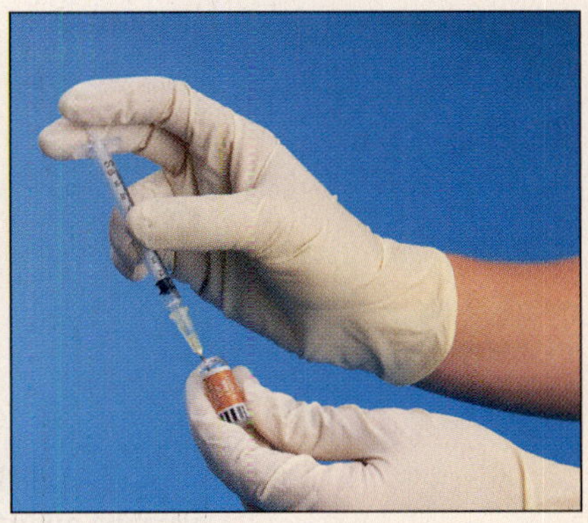

7-5c Draw up the medication.

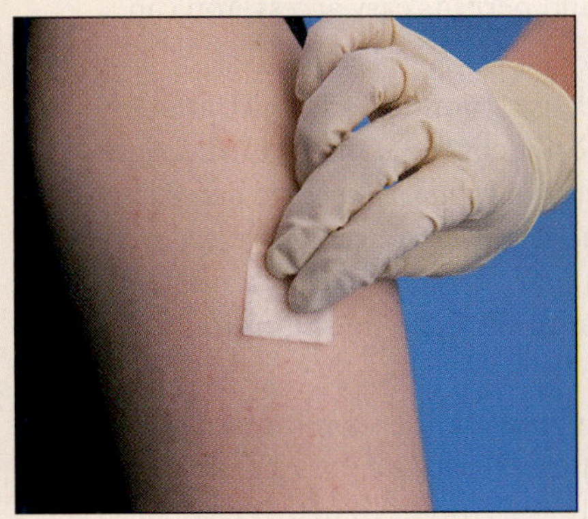

7-5d Prep the site.

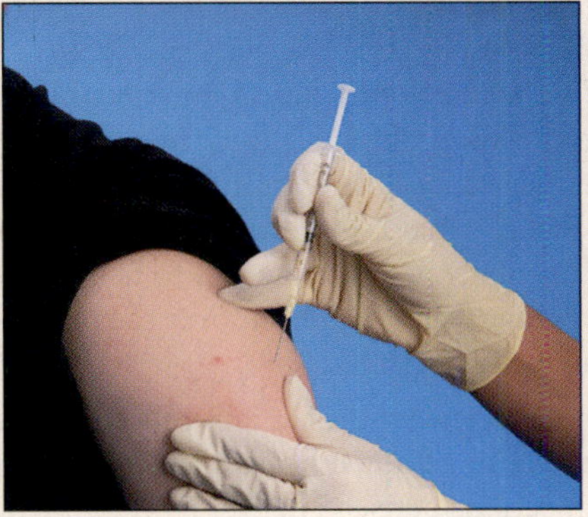

7-5e Insert the needle at a 45° angle.

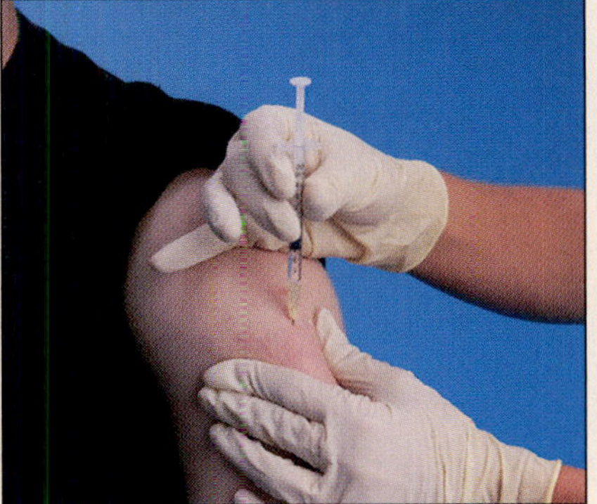

7-5f Remove the needle and cover the puncture site.

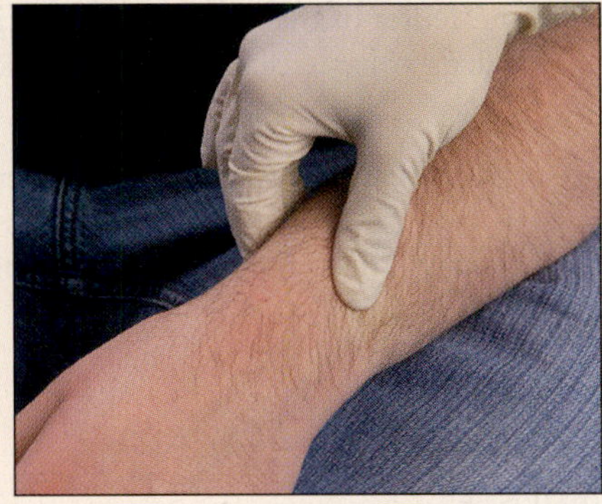

7-5g Monitor the patient.

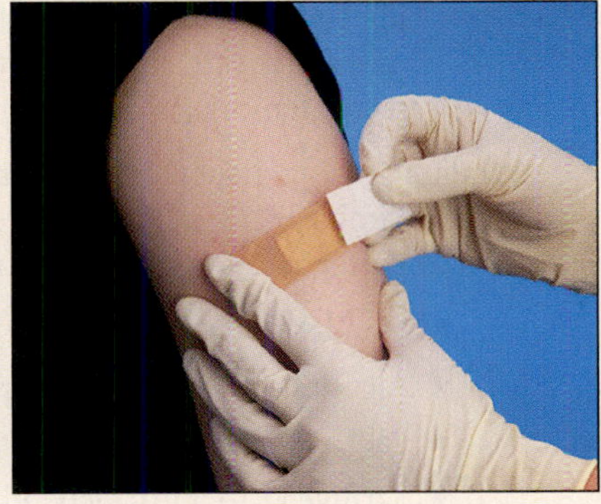

7-5h Apply an adhesive bandage to the injection site.

(Photos © Scott Metcalfe)

■ **Figure 7-20**
Intramuscular injection.

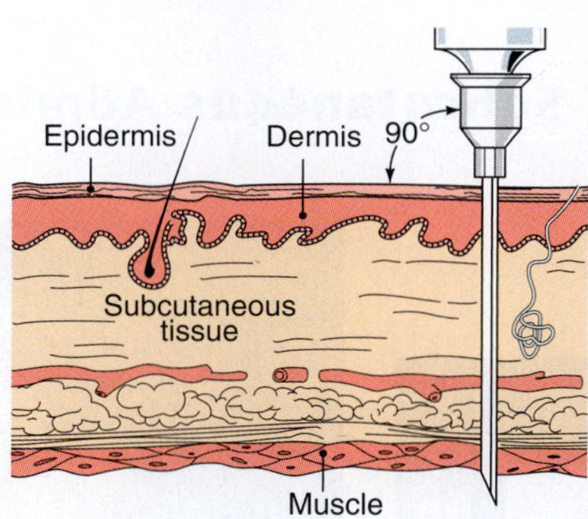

Several sites are used for intramuscular injections (Figure 7-21 ■). Depending upon the site, varying quantities of medication can be delivered. These sites and their correlating volumes of medication include:

★ *Deltoid.* The deltoid muscle is 3 to 4 finger-breadths below the acromial process (the bony bump on the shoulder). It is highly vascular and permits easy access. You can deliver up to 2.0 mL into this muscle.

★ *Dorsal gluteal.* The dorsal gluteal muscle, or buttock, is a common administration point for intramuscular injections. Injections here can deliver 5.0 mL of medication or more. They cause little discomfort, but you must avoid the large sciatic nerve, which is the leg's major motor nerve. Damage to the sciatic nerve can decrease mobility or totally paralyze the leg. To help prevent neurological complication, envision an imaginary quadrant over the buttock; administer all injections in the upper and outer portion.

★ *Vastus lateralis.* The vastus lateralis muscle of the thigh is another common site for intramuscular injection, especially for pediatric patients. As at the dorsal gluteal muscle, injections here can deliver 5 mL of medication or more. To deliver medication at this site, imagine a grid of nine boxes. Administer injections in the middle, outer box, or anterolateral part of the muscle.

★ *Rectus femoris.* The rectus femoris lies over the femur and is closely associated with the vastus lateralis muscle. When utilizing the rectus femoris for intramuscular injection, place the medication into the center of the muscle at approximately midshaft of the femur. Up to 5 mL of drug volume can be administered into the rectus femoris.

When choosing a site, avoid bruised or scarred areas. Areas free of superficial blood vessels are most desirable.

To perform an intramuscular injection, you will need the following equipment:

★ Standard Precautions
★ Alcohol or Betadine antiseptic preparation
★ Packaged medication
★ Syringe (1 to 5 mL, depending on dosage)
★ 21- to 23-gauge hypodermic needle, ⅜ to 1 inch long
★ Sterile gauze and adhesive bandage

Follow these steps to administer an intramuscular injection (Procedure 7–6):

1. Assemble and prepare the needed equipment.
2. Apply Standard Precautions and confirm the drug, indication, dosage, and need for intramuscular injection.

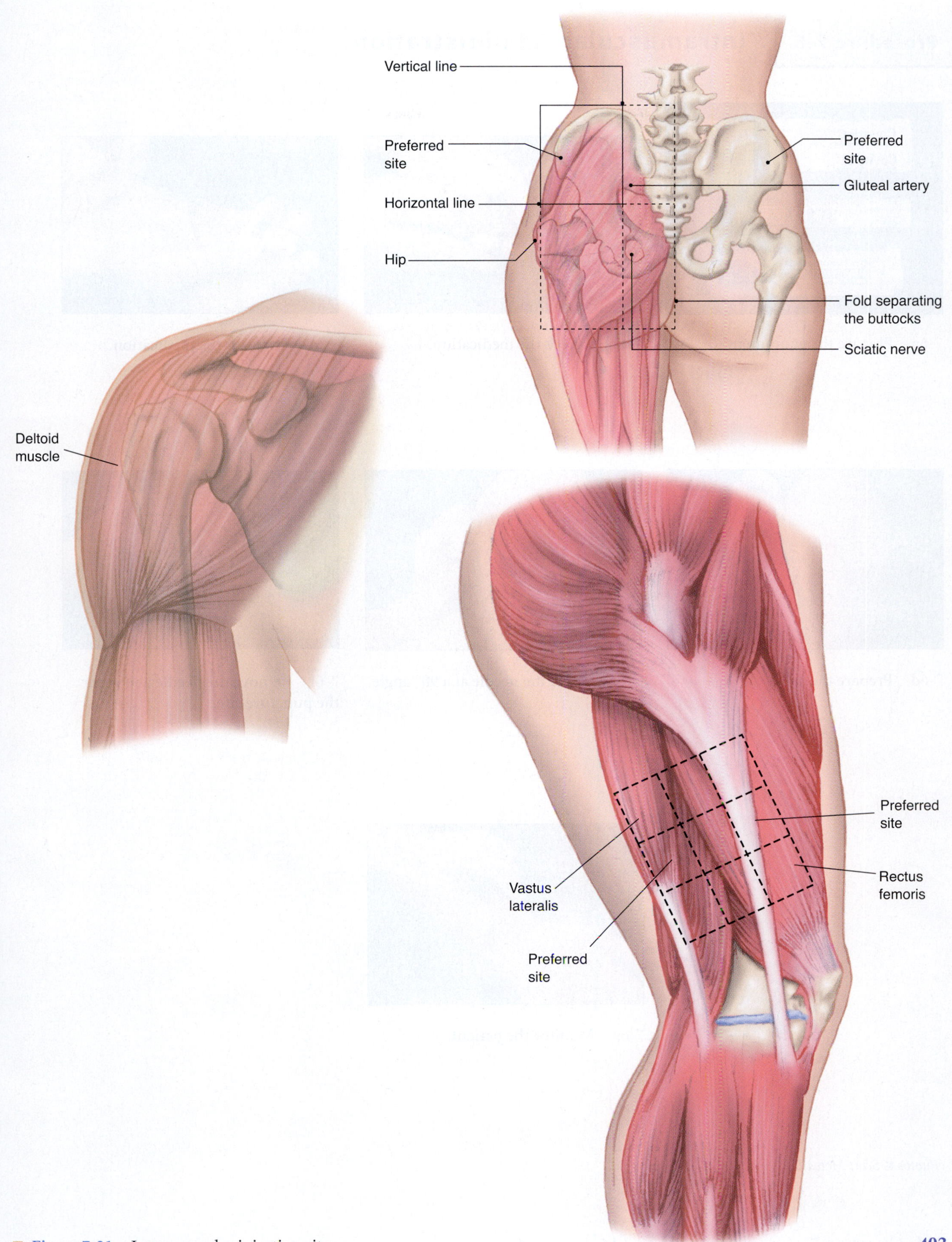

■ Figure 7-21 Intramuscular injection sites.

Procedure 7-6 Intramuscular Administration

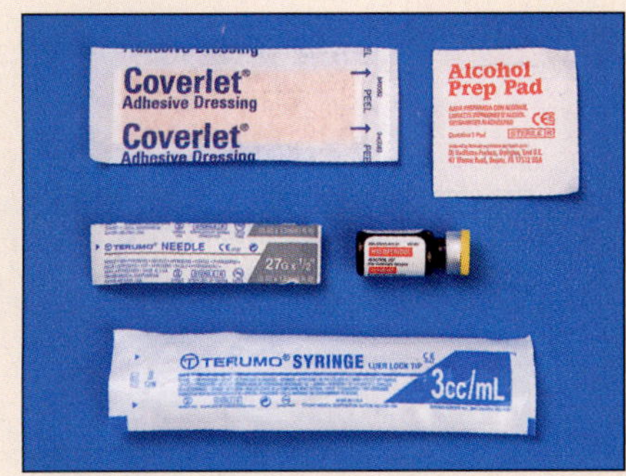

7-6a Prepare the equipment.

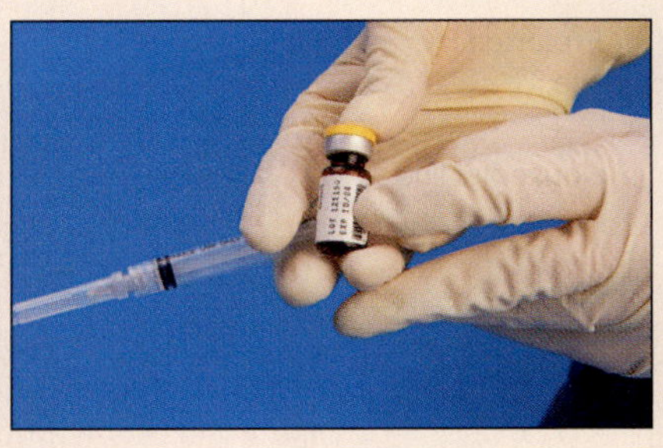

7-6b Check the medication.

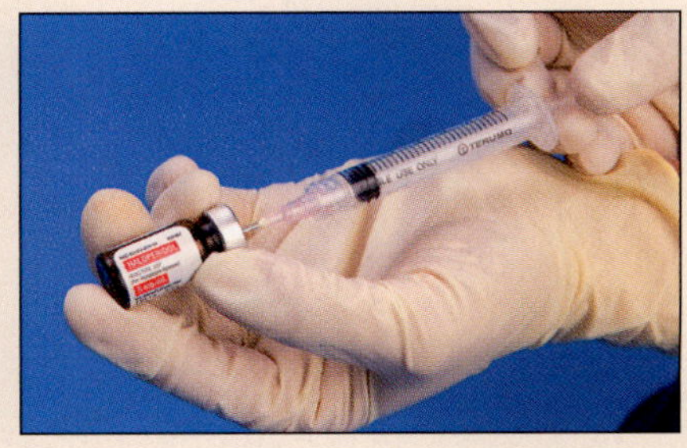

7-6c Draw up the medication.

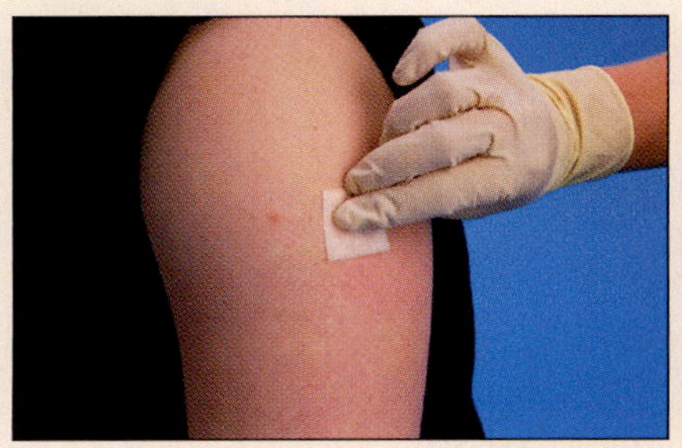

7-6d Prepare the site.

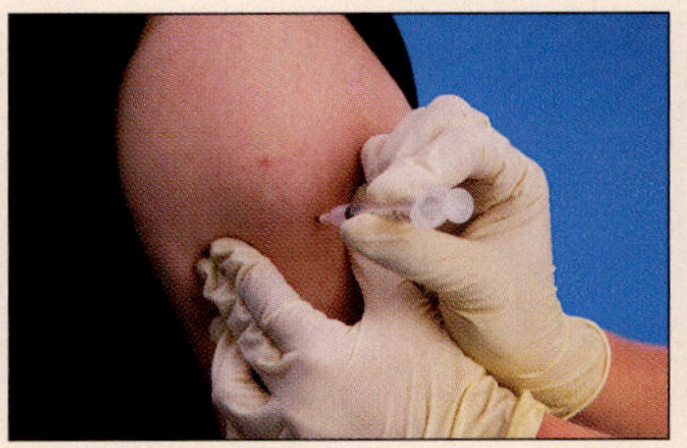

7-6e Insert the needle at a 90° angle.

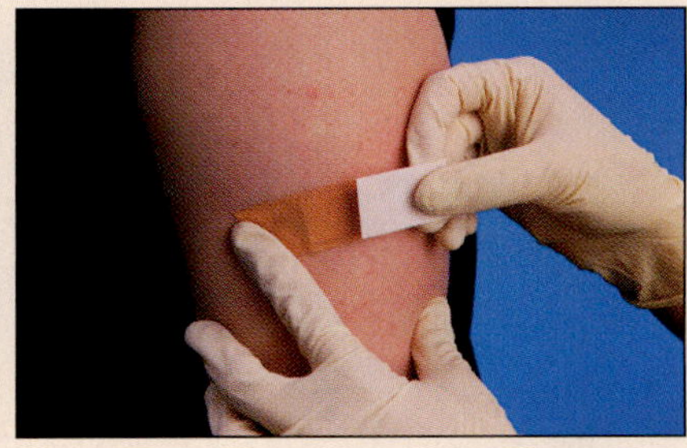

7-6f Remove the needle and cover the puncture site.

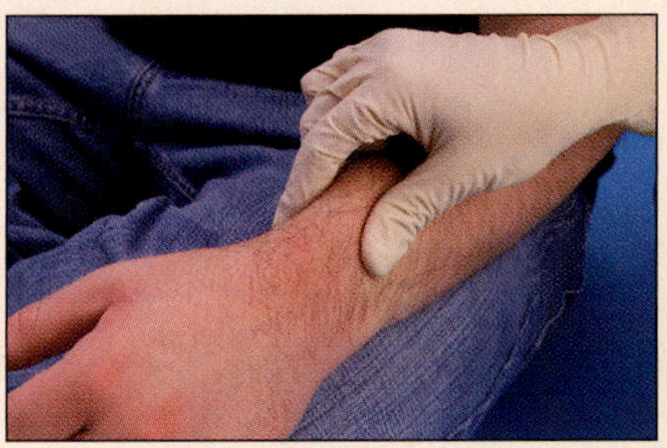

7-6g Monitor the patient.

(Photos © Scott Metcalfe)

3. Draw up medication as appropriate.
4. Prepare the site with alcohol or Betadine as described for an intradermal injection.
5. Stretch the skin taut over the injection site with your nondominant hand.
6. Insert the needle just into the skin at a 90° angle with the bevel up.
7. Pull back the plunger to aspirate tissue fluid.
   —If blood appears, the hypodermic needle is in a blood vessel, and absorption of the medication will be too rapid. Start the procedure over with a new syringe.
   —If no blood appears, proceed with step 8.
8. Slowly inject the medication.
9. Remove the needle and dispose of it in the sharps container.
10. Place an adhesive bandage over the site; use gauze for hemorrhage control if needed.
11. Monitor the patient.

After administration, gently rub or massage the site to help to initiate systemic absorption. Do not massage the site, however, if you have administered heparin or another anticoagulant. Again, some authorities recommend a 0.1-mL air plug as described under Subcutaneous Injection.

Intravenous and Intraosseous Routes

Two important parenteral drug administration routes—intravenous access and intraosseous infusion—are discussed in detail in Part 2.

Part 2: Intravenous Access, Blood Sampling, and Intraosseous Infusion

In this part, we will discuss intravenous access, including types of venous access and the variety of equipment required, where and how to establish intravenous access, flow rates, and possible complications. We will also detail intravenous administration of medications (bolus and infusion). Venous blood sampling techniques will also be covered.

Additionally, this part of the chapter provides information on intraosseous medication administration, including techniques, possible complications, and contraindications. Intraosseous administration is a route most often used in pediatric patients under 5 years of age.

INTRAVENOUS ACCESS

intravenous access (cannulation) *surgical puncture of a vein to deliver medication or withdraw blood.*

Intravenous (*IV*) **access** (*intra-*, within; *venous*, vein) or **cannulation** is a routine paramedic procedure. Circulating blood transports chemicals, proteins, and fluids throughout the body. Venous circulation can likewise deliver medications and fluids into the body and provides an invaluable tool for treating the sick and injured.

The following situations indicate intravenous access:

★ Fluid and blood replacement
★ Drug administration
★ Obtaining venous blood specimens for laboratory analysis

Since veins are easier to locate and penetrate, venous access is preferable to arterial access. Additionally, venous circulation pressure is lower than arterial and presents fewer hemorrhage control complications.

TYPES OF INTRAVENOUS ACCESS

Medical care providers use two types of intravenous access, peripheral and central. As a paramedic, you will most often perform peripheral intravenous access. Central venous access is rarely, if ever, performed in the prehospital setting.

Peripheral Venous Access

peripheral venous access *surgical puncture of a vein in the arm, leg, or neck.*

Although challenging, **peripheral venous access** is relatively easy to master. As its name implies, it uses peripheral veins. Common sites include the arms and legs and, when necessary, the neck. Figure 7-22 ■ illustrates the specific veins commonly accessed on the hand, forearm, and leg.

As some patients' veins may not be readily visible, you must know venous topography. In these cases, you will have to locate veins based on anatomical layout and palpation. Exhaust all possibilities on the arms before trying to locate the veins of the legs. Leg veins are more difficult to access and present complications more frequently. For neonates and infants, you may access veins in the scalp. Chapter 42 on pediatrics explains that technique.

When establishing a peripheral IV, start at the distal end of the extremity and work proximally. Once you have attempted cannulation, the disruption in blood flow hinders using veins distal to that site. However, the purpose of access also determines site selection. For example, rapid fluid administration requires larger veins like the antecubital fossa, as opposed to the smaller veins of the hand. The external jugular vein is considered a peripheral vein and can be accessed when other peripheral sites are not available.

The major advantage of peripheral venous access is that it is relatively simple to perform because visualizing and accessing the veins is usually easy. Additionally, you can access peripheral veins while simultaneously doing other life-sustaining procedures such as CPR or endotracheal intubation. Conversely, peripheral veins collapse in hypovolemia or circulatory failure, thus becoming difficult to locate and access. Furthermore, the peripheral veins of geriatric patients, pediatric patients, or those with peripheral vascular disease may be fragile and difficult to cannulate. Finally, peripheral veins may roll and elude IV placement.

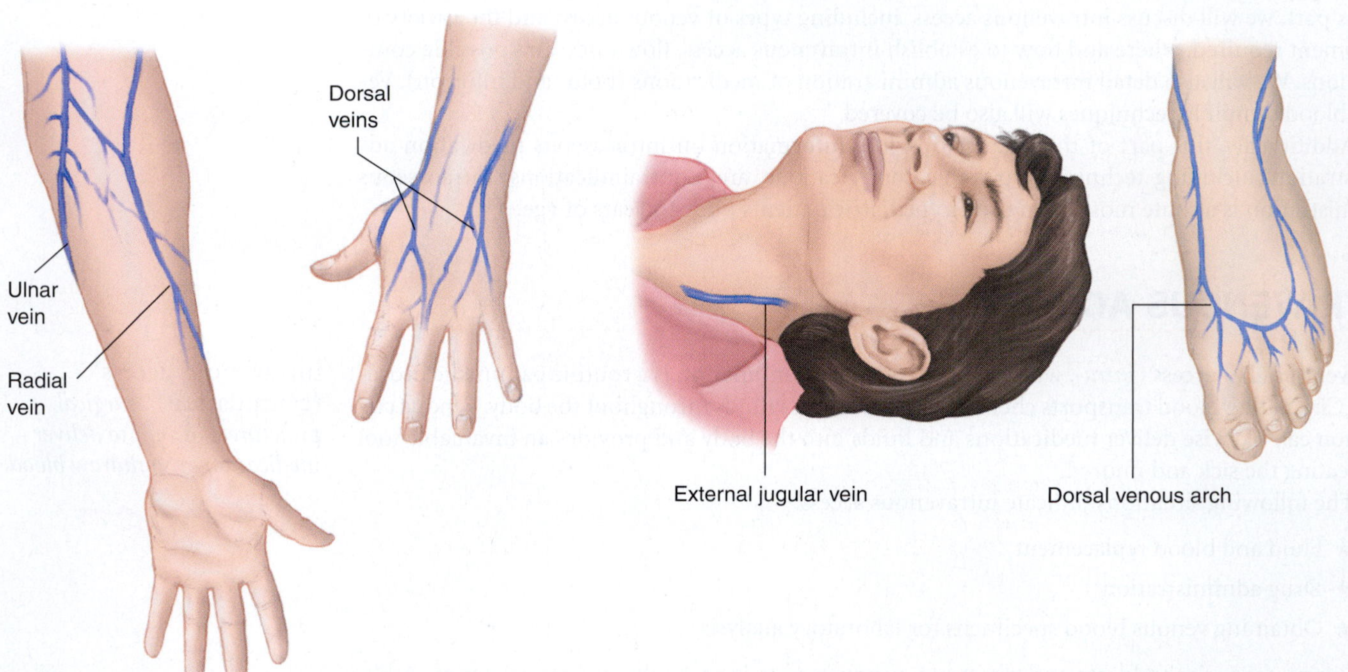

■ Figure 7-22 Peripheral IV access sites: veins of the arm, hand, neck, and foot.

Central Venous Access

Central venous access utilizes veins located deep within the body. These include the internal jugular, subclavian, and femoral veins. They are larger than peripheral veins and will not collapse in shock. Central IV lines are placed near the heart for long-term use. Typically, they are used when medical conditions require repeated access for medication and/or fluid delivery. They also are used for transvenous pacing or for monitoring central venous pressure.

A special type of central line is the **peripherally inserted central catheter,** or PICC, line. PICC lines are smaller than those routinely used for central access and are threaded into the central circulation via a peripheral site. PICC lines are most often used in infants and children requiring long-term care.

Central venous access is typically restricted to the hospital setting because of its invasive nature and high risk of complications such as arterial puncture, pneumothorax, and air embolism. Central veins cannot be accessed during procedures such as CPR, and they often require a chest X-ray for placement confirmation. You may nonetheless encounter a central line during interfacility transports or in a chronically ill homebound patient. Protocols in some EMS systems allow paramedics to access existing central lines during emergency care. Still other systems allow their paramedics to place certain central lines. Always follow local protocols regarding central line access and insertion. For more information about central venous access, consult a text on advanced venipuncture techniques.

central venous access *surgical puncture of the internal jugular, subclavian, or femoral vein.*

peripherally inserted central catheter (PICC) *line threaded into the central circulation via a peripheral site.*

EQUIPMENT AND SUPPLIES FOR VENOUS ACCESS

To establish intravenous access, you will need the following specialized equipment and supplies.

Intravenous Fluids

Intravenous fluids are chemically prepared solutions tailored to the body's specific needs. They replace the body's lost fluids and/or aid the delivery of IV medications. They also can keep a vein patent when no fluid or drug therapy is required.

Intravenous fluids come in four different forms: colloids, crystalloids, blood, and oxygen-carrying fluids.

intravenous fluid *chemically prepared solution tailored to the body's specific needs.*

Colloids

Colloids contain large proteins that cannot pass through the capillary membrane. Consequently, they remain in the circulatory system for a long time. In addition, colloids have osmotic properties that attract water into the circulatory system. A small quantity of colloid can significantly increase intravascular volume (volume of blood and fluid contained within the blood vessels). Common colloids include:

colloids *intravenous solutions containing large proteins that cannot pass through capillary membranes.*

- ★ *Plasma protein fraction (Plasmanate).* Plasmanate is a protein-containing colloid. Its principal protein, albumin, is suspended with other proteins in a saline solvent.
- ★ *Salt-poor albumin.* Salt-poor albumin contains only human albumin. Each gram of albumin will retain approximately 18 milliliters of water in the bloodstream.
- ★ *Dextran.* Dextran is not a protein but a large sugar molecule with osmotic properties similar to albumin's. It comes in two molecular weights: 40,000 and 70,000 daltons. Dextran 40 has from two to two and one-half times the colloid osmotic pressure of albumin. Anaphylactic reaction is a possible side effect.
- ★ *Hetastarch (Hespan).* Like dextran, hetastarch is a sugar molecule with osmotic properties similar to protein's. Hetastarch does not appear to share dextran's side effects.

Although colloids help maintain vascular volume, using them in the field is not practical. Their high cost, short shelf life, and specific storage requirements suit them better to the hospital setting. However, the paramedic who works in an emergency department, aeromedical service, or at a mass casualty incident may have to administer colloids.

crystalloid *intravenous solutions that contain electrolytes but lack the larger proteins associated with colloids.*

Content Review

Crystalloid Classes

- Isotonic
- Hypertonic
- Hypotonic

Crystalloids

Crystalloids are the primary prehospital IV solution. Crystalloids contain electrolytes and water but lack colloids' larger proteins and larger molecules. The many preparations of crystalloid solutions are classified by their tonicity (number of particles per unit volume) relative to that of body plasma:

isotonic *state in which solutions on opposite sides of a semipermeable membrane are in equal concentration.*

hypertonic *state in which a solution has a higher solute concentration on one side of a semipermeable membrane than on the other side.*

hypotonic *state in which a solution has a lower solute concentration on one side of a semipermeable membrane than on the other side.*

- *Isotonic solutions.* **Isotonic** solutions have a tonicity equal to blood plasma's. In a normally hydrated patient, they will not cause a significant fluid or electrolyte shift.
- *Hypertonic solutions.* **Hypertonic** solutions have a higher solute concentration than do the cells. When administered to the normally hydrated patient, they cause fluid to shift out of the intracellular compartment and into the extracellular compartment. Later, solute will diffuse in the opposite direction.
- *Hypotonic solutions.* **Hypotonic** solutions have a lower solute concentration than do the cells. When administered to a normally hydrated patient, they cause fluid to move from the extracellular compartment and into the intracellular compartment. Later, the solutes will move in the opposite direction.

The particular type of IV solution you select depends on your patient's needs. The three most commonly used IV fluids in prehospital care are:

- *Lactated Ringer's.* Lactated Ringer's solution is an isotonic electrolyte solution. It contains sodium chloride, potassium chloride, calcium chloride, and sodium lactate in water.
- *Normal saline solution.* Normal saline is an isotonic electrolyte solution containing 0.90 percent sodium chloride in water.
- *5 percent dextrose in water (D_5W).* D_5W is a hypotonic glucose solution used to keep a vein patent and to supply calories needed for cellular metabolism. While D_5W initially increases circulatory volume, glucose molecules rapidly diffuse across the vascular membrane and increase the free water.

Both lactated Ringer's and normal saline solution are used for fluid replacement because of their immediate ability to expand the circulating volume. However, due to the movement of electrolytes and water, two-thirds of either solution will be lost to the extravascular space within 1 hour. Crystalloids such as normal saline mixed with D_5W or half-strength normal saline (0.45 percent) are combinations or modifications of the previously mentioned solutions.

Occasionally, you will have to warm or cool the IV fluid. A hypothermic patient may benefit from having a crystalloid warmed before and during fluid administration. Warm fluids assist in elevating the patient's core temperature. Conversely, cool fluids may benefit the patient with an increased core temperature. You can cool or warm fluids by storing them in a special temperature-controlled compartment or by using the heater or air conditioner in the ambulance, helicopter, or mobile intensive care unit. Commercial fluid heaters are available. Their use is detailed later in this chapter. Some fluids, such as blood and some colloids, require constant storage in a cool environment.

Blood The most desirable fluid for replacement is whole blood. Unlike colloids and crystalloids, the hemoglobin in blood carries oxygen. Blood, however, is a precious commodity and must be conserved so that it can be of benefit to the most people. Its use in the field is generally limited to aeromedical services or mass casualty incidents. O-negative blood's universal compatibility makes it ideal for administration in the field. Chapter 35 on hematology discusses blood in detail.

Oxygen-Carrying Solutions Considerable research has been devoted to the development of solutions that can carry oxygen and off-load it for cellular use. These fluids, which remain experimental at present, show promise for treating hypovolemia in the field. There are two general classes of oxygen-carrying solutions: perfluorocarbons and hemoglobin-based oxygen-carrying solutions (HBOCs). These agents provide a significant advantage over standard colloids and crystalloids because, as their name indicates, in addition to replacing volume they can transport oxygen.

- *Perfluorocarbons.* Perfluorocarbon compounds are in various stages of research and testing. These agents are denser than water and have a high capacity to dissolve large quantities of gases such as oxygen. Products in development include LiquiVent and Oxygent.

★ *Hemoglobin-based oxygen-carrying solutions (HBOCs).* HBOCs represent a major development in the field of emergency and critical care. These products differ from other intravenous fluids in that they have the capability to transport oxygen. HBOCs contain long chains of *polymerized hemoglobin.* This hemoglobin is obtained from either expired donated human blood or bovine (cow) blood. The hemoglobin is removed from the red blood cells and then repeatedly filtered to remove any infectious substances or antigenic proteins. Finally, the individual hemoglobin molecules are joined together in a large chain through a chemical process known as polymerization. HBOCs are compatible with all blood types and do not require blood typing, testing, or crossmatching.

- *PolyHeme,* derived from expired donated human blood, contains 50 grams of hemoglobin per unit, which is the same as human blood. PolyHeme must be refrigerated and the shelf life is 1 year.
- *Hemopure,* derived from bovine (cow) blood, has been widely used in South Africa. Hemopure does not require refrigeration and has a shelf life of 3 years.

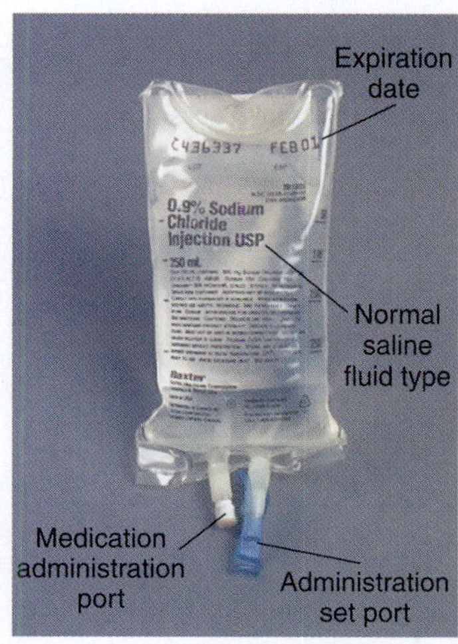

■ Figure 7-23 IV solution containers.

Packaging of Intravenous Fluids Most intravenous fluids and blood are packaged in soft plastic or vinyl bags of various sizes (50, 100, 250, 500, 1,000, 2,000, and 3,000 mL) (Figure 7-23 ■). Some contain medication that is incompatible with plastic or vinyl and must be packaged in glass bottles.

The IV-fluid container provides important information.

★ *Label.* A label on every IV bottle or bag lists the fluid type and expiration date. Like any other medication, intravenous solutions have a shelf life; do not use them after their expiration date. Discard any fluid that appears cloudy, discolored, or laced with particulate. Additionally, avoid using any fluid whose sealed packaging has been opened or tampered with.

★ *Medication administration port.* A medication port on IV-solution bags or bottles permits you to inject medication into the fluid for infusion.

★ *Administration set port.* The administration set port is where you place the spike from the IV administration tubing.

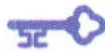

Do not use any IV fluids after their expiration date; any fluids that appear cloudy, discolored, or laced with particulate; or any fluid whose sealed packaging has been opened or tampered with.

Administration Tubing

Intravenous **administration tubing** connects the solution bag to the IV **cannula** that is inserted into the patient's vein. Administration tubing is made of very flexible clear plastic. You must select from several types of administration tubing according to your patient's need. All tubing is packaged in a sterile container. If the container is opened or appears damaged, select another administration set. Any pathogens on the tubing will enter the patient, possibly causing long-term complications.

administration tubing *flexible, clear plastic tubing that connects the solution bag to the IV cannula.*

cannula *hollow needle used to puncture a vein.*

Microdrip and Macrodrip Tubing **Microdrip** administration tubing delivers relatively small amounts of fluid to the patient. It is more appropriate when you need to restrict the overall fluid volume a patient will receive. **Macrodrip** administration tubing delivers relatively large amounts of fluid. It is more appropriate when volume replacement is necessary, as in shock, fluid replacement, or hypotension.

To effectively deliver intravenous fluids, you must be thoroughly familiar with the microdrip and macrodrip administration sets, their components, and their subtle differences (Figure 7-24 ■).

★ *Spike.* The **spike** is a sharp-pointed plastic device that you insert into the administration set port on the IV solution bag. A plastic sheath covering the spike keeps it sterile. When the sheath is removed, you must use a medically clean technique to avoid contaminating the spike. If the spike becomes contaminated, discard the administration set and start over with new tubing.

microdrip tubing *administration tubing that delivers a relatively small amount of fluid.*

macrodrip tubing *administration tubing that delivers a relatively large amount of fluid.*

spike *sharp-pointed device inserted into the IV solution bag's administration set port.*

■ Figure 7-24 Macrodrip and microdrip administration sets.

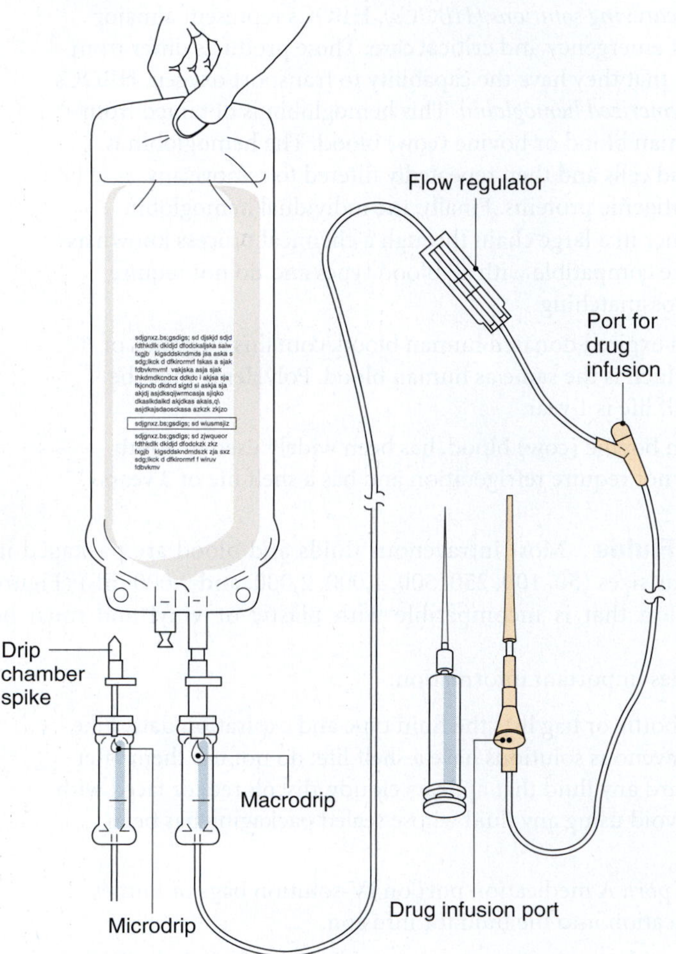

drip chamber *clear plastic chamber that allows visualization of the drip rate.*

drip rate *pace at which the fluid moves from the bag into the patient.*

drop former *device that regulates the size of drops.*

gtts *drops (Latin* guttae, *drops [*gutta, *drop]).*

★ *Drip chamber.* The **drip chamber** is a clear plastic chamber that allows you to view the **drip rate.** The drip chamber is squeezable; when compressed, it collects fluid from the IV solution bag and acts as a reservoir for administration. For optimal fluid delivery, the drip chamber should be about one-third full; a line on the chamber marks the correct fluid level.

★ *Drop former.* Inside the drip chamber is a **drop former.** In microdrip administration tubing, the drop former is a hollow metal stylet. In macrodrip tubing, it is a large circular opening at the top of the drip chamber. The drop former regulates each drop's size. The narrow metal stylet in the microdrip tubing creates smaller drops; the wider opening in the macrodrip tubing creates larger drops. In either case, the drop former's precise calibration allows you to calculate fluid volumes by counting drops, or **gtts:**

Microdrip	60 gtts = 1 mL
Macrodrip	10 gtts = 1 mL

Depending upon the manufacturer, macrodrip sets may equate 15 or 20 gtts to 1 mL. You must know drops per milliliter to calculate flow rates or medicated infusion dosages.

★ *Tubing.* Intravenous administration tubing is clear and very flexible. Thus, you can watch the solution flow through the administration set, and you can manipulate the tubing in tight situations. Some medications such as intravenous nitroglycerin are chemically incompatible with regular tubing and require special tubing.

- ★ *Clamp.* IV administration tubing has a simple plastic clamp. When slid over the tubing, the clamp completely stops the flow of solution from the IV bag to the patient. It prevents both the entrainment of air into the tubing when changing IV bags and the backflow of medication when administering medications. You can also use it to stop infusion without disturbing the flow-regulator setting.
- ★ *Flow regulator.* The flow regulator is a dial enclosed in a triangular plastic casing. It allows infinite control of flow rates ranging from a continuous stream to completely stopped. Rolling the dial toward the IV solution bag increases the drip frequency; rolling the dial toward the patient decreases the drip frequency.
- ★ *Medication injection ports.* The **medication injection ports** have a self-sealing membrane into which you can insert a hypodermic needle for drug administration. Their design varies, depending upon the manufacturer. When possible, use the medication port nearest the patient.
- ★ *Needle adapter.* The **needle adapter** is a rigid plastic device at the administration tubing's distal end. It is specifically constructed to fit into the hub of an intravenous cannula. Similar to the spike, the needle adapter is sterile and covered by a protective cap. If it becomes contaminated at any time, start over with a new administration set.

medication injection port *self-sealing membrane into which a hypodermic needle is inserted for drug administration.*

needle adapter *rigid plastic device specifically constructed to fit into the hub of an intravenous cannula.*

IV Extension Tubing **Extension tubing** is IV tubing used to extend the original macrodrip or microdrip setup. Its packaging clearly marks it as such. Like administration sets, extension tubing is sterile and must be handled accordingly.

extension tubing *IV tubing used to extend a macrodrip or microdrip setup.*

Extension tubing also permits the paramedic to change the original administration tubing or the IV solution bag with little difficulty. For example, if you have to switch from a macrodrip set to a microdrip set, you can close the clamp on the extension and detach the primary tubing. Once you have flushed the new tubing with fluid, you place the needle adapter into the receiving port on the extension tubing and release the clamp. You can now resume fluid therapy without risking complications or having to painfully reinitiate a second IV line.

Electromechanical Pump Tubing Mechanical infusion devices may require specially manufactured pump tubing. Typically, pump tubing has special components that attach directly to the pump. Additionally, bladders and relief points permit you to void possible air bubbles. Many specific models of electromechanical infusion pumps require specific pump tubing. When using a mechanical infusion pump, be sure to have the appropriate tubing on hand.

Measured Volume Administration Set The **measured volume administration set** can deliver specific volumes of fluid with or without medication. It is especially advantageous for pediatrics, renal failure, or other patients who cannot tolerate fluid overload.

measured volume administration set *IV setup that delivers specific volumes of fluid.*

The measured volume administration set consists of either micro- or macrodrip tubing, with the addition of a large **burette chamber** marked in 1.0-mL increments. The burette chamber holds between 120 and 150 mL of fluid. The components of the measured volume administration set include:

burette chamber *calibrated chamber of Berutrol IV administration tubing that enables precise measurement and delivery of fluids and medicated solutions.*

- ★ Flanged spike
- ★ Clamp
- ★ Airway handle
- ★ Medication injection port
- ★ Burette chamber
- ★ Float valve
- ★ Drip chamber
- ★ Flow regulator
- ★ Medication injection port
- ★ Needle adapter

When opened, the airway handle on top of the burette chamber permits air to be displaced or replaced as fluid enters or exits the chamber. If a medication must be mixed in a specific amount of IV solution, you can add it through the medication administration port after correctly filling the chamber.

blood tubing *administration tubing that contains a filter to prevent clots or other debris from entering the patient.*

Blood Tubing

Administering whole blood or blood components requires **blood tubing,** which contains a filter that prevents clots and other debris from entering the patient. Without exception, all blood must be filtered. Blood that is stored or delivered over an extended period is prone to form fibrin clots or to accumulate other debris. If these clots or debris enter the circulatory system, they can travel in the form of an embolus.

Many aeromedical and facility-based paramedics administer blood and must be familiar with blood tubing. Although most ambulances do not carry blood, paramedics may initiate normal saline with blood tubing in anticipation that whole blood or blood products will be required immediately in the emergency department.

Blood tubing comes in two configurations, straight and Y. Y tubing has two administration ports, one for blood and one for IV normal saline solution. Typically, blood is administered with normal saline. Fluids like lactated Ringer's increase the potential for blood coagulation. The two-port design permits immediate access to normal saline if the blood supply is exhausted or must be shut down, as for a transfusion reaction. When you use Y blood tubing, establish a traditional IV by connecting a bag of normal saline to the tubing. Attach the blood to the second port when needed, while maintaining strict medical asepsis. Using the flow regulator, discontinue the normal saline while opening the clamp regulating the flow of blood. Straight blood tubing has only one reservoir. Therefore, only blood is attached to the tubing. A medication administration port close to the needle adapter allows you to piggyback a secondary line of normal saline into the tubing.

Miscellaneous Administration Sets

Some tubing now has a manual dial that can set drops per minute or specific flow rates. Some manufacturers have created a single drip chamber that can create either microdrips or macrodrips.

Intravenous Cannulas

The intravenous cannula permits actual puncture and access into a patient's vein. The distal portion of the administration tubing connects to the IV cannula. The three basic types of IV cannulas are:

- ★ Over-the-needle catheter
- ★ Hollow-needle catheter
- ★ Plastic catheter inserted through a hollow needle

over-the-needle catheter/angiocatheter *semiflexible catheter enclosing a sharp metal stylet.*

Over-the-Needle Catheter

Often called an **angiocatheter,** the semiflexible **over-the-needle catheter** encloses a sharp metal stylet (needle) (Figure 7-25 ■).

- ★ *Metal stylet (needle).* The metal stylet punctures the skin and blood vessel. Blood flows through the hollow stylet to the flashback chamber.
- ★ *Flashback chamber.* Blood in the clear plastic flashback chamber confirms placement of the stylet in the vein.
- ★ *Teflon catheter.* The Teflon catheter slides over the metal stylet into a successfully punctured vein.
- ★ *Hub.* Located on the back of the Teflon catheter, the hub receives the needle adapter of the administration tubing once removed from the metal stylet.

For peripheral venous access, the over-the-needle catheter is preferred since it is easy to place and anchor and permits freer patient movement.

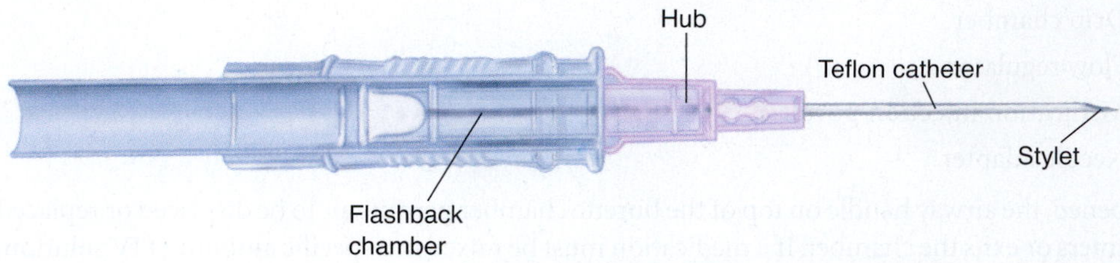

■ Figure 7-25 Over-the-needle catheter.

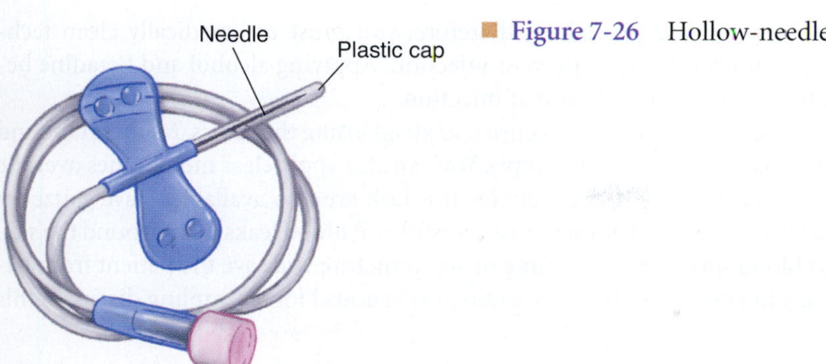

■ Figure 7-26 Hollow-needle catheter.

Hollow-Needle Catheter For pediatrics or other patients with tiny, delicate veins, use **hollow-needle catheters** (Figure 7-26 ■). These catheters do not have a Teflon tube; rather, the metal stylet itself is inserted into the vein and secured there. Because the sharp metal stylet can easily damage the vein, you must insert it very carefully. Some hollow-needle catheters have wings to guide and secure them into a vein. These hollow-needle catheters are referred to as winged catheters or butterfly catheters.

hollow-needle catheter *stylet that does not have a Teflon tube but is itself inserted into the vein and secured there.*

Catheter Inserted through the Needle The **catheter inserted through the needle** is also called an **intracatheter.** It consists of a Teflon catheter inserted through a large metal stylet (Figure 7-27 ■). Used in the hospital setting to implement central lines, its proper placement requires great skill, as discussed previously.

catheter inserted through the needle (intracatheter) *Teflon catheter inserted through a large metal stylet.*

The size of an intravenous cannula is expressed as its gauge. The *larger* the gauge, the *smaller* the diameter of the stylet and catheter. For example, a 22-gauge cannula is smaller than a 14-gauge cannula. The larger diameter, 14-gauge catheter allows greater flow rates than the smaller diameter 22-gauge cannula. When establishing venous access, choose the cannula size most appropriate for the patient condition. Typical uses for the various sizes of cannulas are:

- ★ *22-gauge.* Small gauges are used for *fragile* veins such as those of the elderly or children.
- ★ *20-gauge.* Moderate gauges are used for the average adult who does not need fluid replacement.
- ★ *18-gauge, 16-gauge, or 14-gauge.* Larger gauge cannulas are used to increase volume or to administer viscous medications such as dextrose. Blood can be administered only through a cannula that is 16 gauge or larger.

Intravenous access is painful and causes discomfort not only to those receiving it but also to family members watching a loved one in distress.

The largest gauge cannula that will fit into a vein is not always appropriate. A cardiac patient with large veins should not receive a 14-gauge cannula for medication administration, just as a multisystems trauma patient with good veins should not receive a 22-gauge cannula for fluid administration. Remember that intravenous access is painful and causes discomfort not only to those receiving it but also to family members watching a loved one in distress.

Miscellaneous Equipment

The **venous constricting band** is a flat rubber band applied proximal to the intended puncture site. It impedes venous return, thereby engorging veins and making them easier to see. This helps you to select the best site and makes venipuncture easier. Never restrict arterial blood flow with the constricting band, and never leave it in place longer than 2 minutes.

venous constricting band *flat rubber band used to impede venous return and make veins easier to see.*

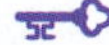

To minimize the chances of a catheter shear reaching the patient's central circulation, always leave the venous constricting band in place until you have completely removed the needle from the catheter. However, never leave the constricting band in place more than 2 minutes.

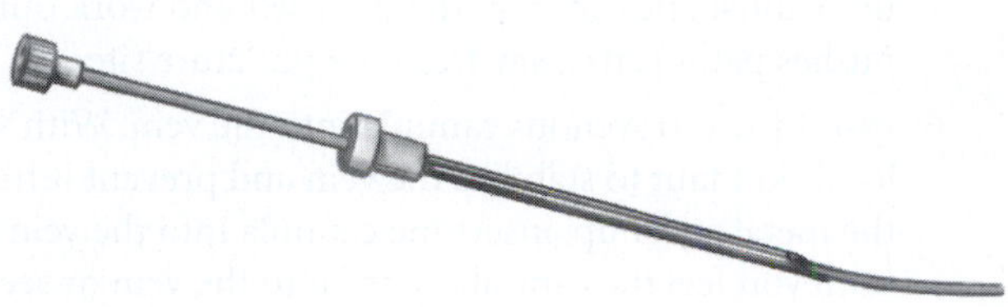

■ Figure 7-27 Catheter inserted through the needle.

Intravenous access is an invasive procedure; therefore, you must use medically clean techniques, including antiseptic preparations, to prevent infection. Applying alcohol and Betadine before and after venipuncture decreases the chance of infection.

Once you have established an IV, you must secure it to avoid losing the access. Medical tape and an adhesive bandage are inexpensive and easy to apply. You can also apply clear membranes over the site. Commercial devices manufactured specifically for this task are also available. Have gauze on hand for hemorrhage control if IV cannulation is unsuccessful or if blood leaks from around the site.

Obtaining a venous blood specimen at the time of venipuncture will save the patient from being stuck with a needle again later. This chapter's section on venous blood sampling discusses this technique in detail.

INTRAVENOUS ACCESS IN THE HAND, ARM, AND LEG

As a paramedic you will most often establish peripheral IVs in the hand, arm, or leg. The veins in these places are relatively easy to locate and accessing them causes the patient less pain. In addition, the likelihood of complications is less with these veins than with the external jugular vein (discussed later) or central IV initiation. Therefore, the veins of the hand, arm, and leg are the primary sites for IV initiation.

To establish a peripheral IV in the hand, arm, or leg, use the following technique (Procedure 7–7):

1. Confirm indication and type of IV setup needed. Gather and arrange all supplies and equipment beforehand to make the process easy and accessible.
   —IV fluid
   —Administration set
   —Intravenous cannula
   —Tape or commercial securing device
   —Venous blood drawing equipment
   —Venous constricting band
   —Antiseptic swab (Betadine/alcohol)
   When appropriate, explain the entire process to the patient. Apply Standard Precautions—gloves and goggles, as IV access is invasive and presents the potential for blood exposure.
2. Prepare all needed equipment. Examine the IV fluid for clarity and expiration date. Insert the administration tubing spike in the IV solution bag's administration set port. Squeeze fluid from the IV fluid container into the drip chamber until it reaches the fill line. Open the clamp and/or flow regulator to flush the solution through the administration tubing and expel trapped air bubbles. Shut down the flow regulator and replace the cap over the needle adapter. Remember that the IV administration set is sterile; if any contamination occurs you must replace the set with a new one.
3. Select the venipuncture site. Acceptable sites have clearly visible veins and are free of bruising or scarring. Straight veins are easier to cannulate than crooked ones.
4. Place the constricting band proximal to the intended site of puncture. Tighten it enough to impede venous blood flow without restricting arterial blood passage. Never leave the constricting band in place more than 2 minutes, as intrinsic changes will occur in the slowed venous blood.
5. Cleanse the venipuncture site. You must cleanse the intended site of pathogens to decrease the likelihood of infection. Alcohol and Betadine are the most commonly used antiseptics. Start at the site itself and work outward in an expanding circle. This pushes pathogens away from the puncture site.
6. Insert the intravenous cannula into the vein. With your nondominant hand, pull all local skin taut to stabilize the vein and prevent it from rolling. With the distal bevel of the metal stylet up, insert the cannula into the vein at a 10° to 30° angle. Continue until you feel the cannula "pop" into the vein or see blood in the flashback chamber.

Procedure 7-7 Peripheral Intravenous Access

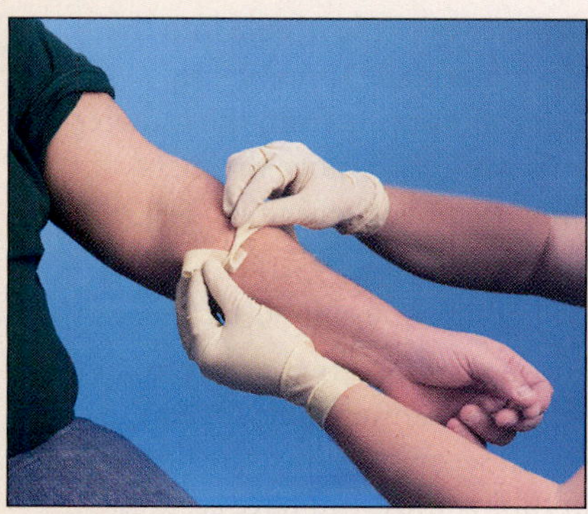

7-7a Place the constricting band.

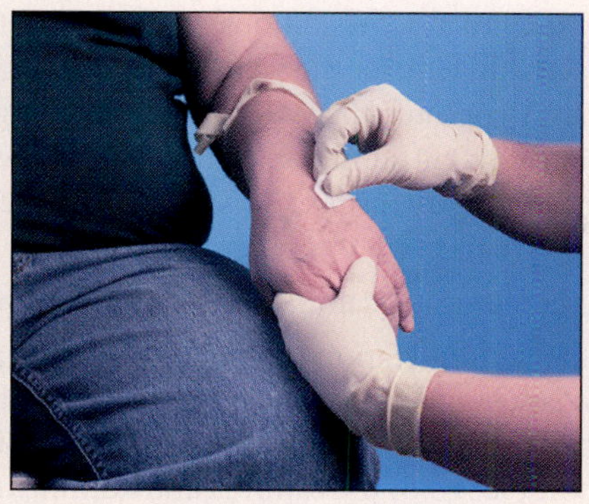

7-7b Cleanse the venipuncture site.

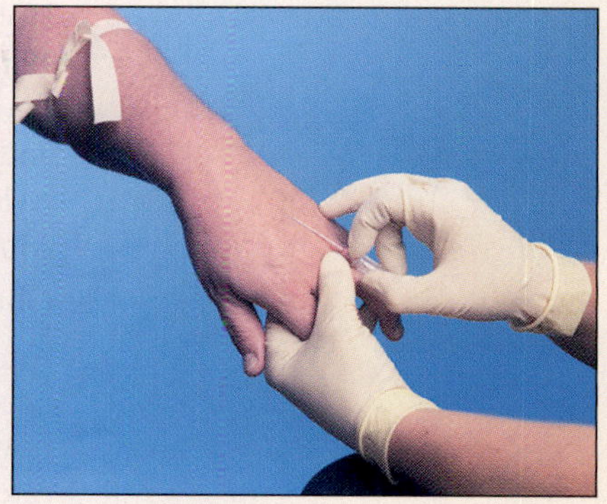

7-7c Insert the intravenous cannula into the vein.

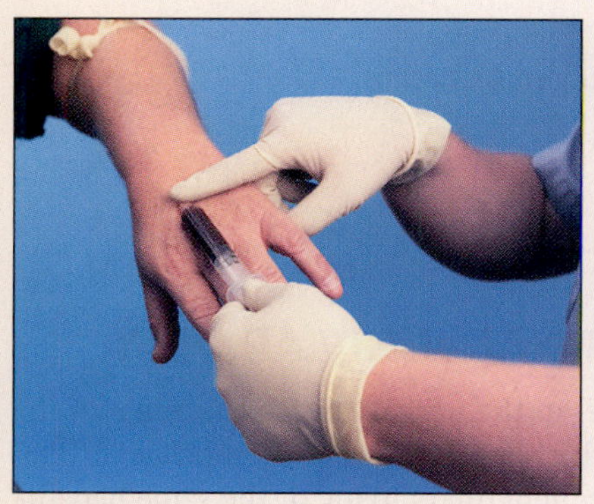

7-7d Withdraw any blood samples needed.

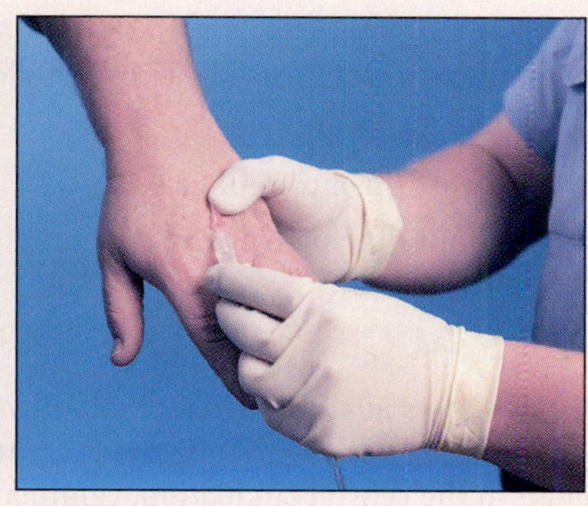

7-7e Connect the IV tubing.

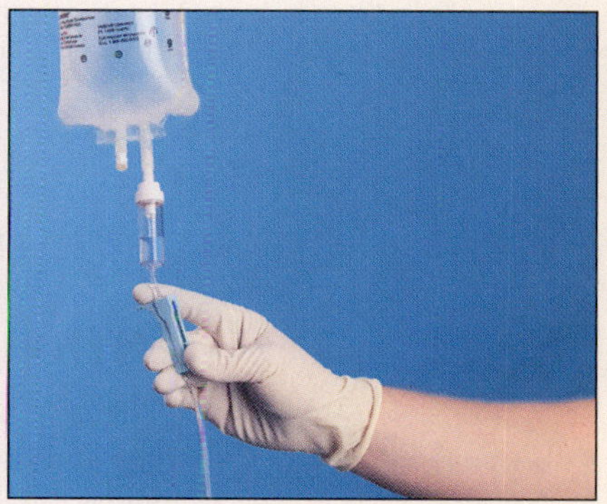

7-7f Turn on the IV and check the flow.

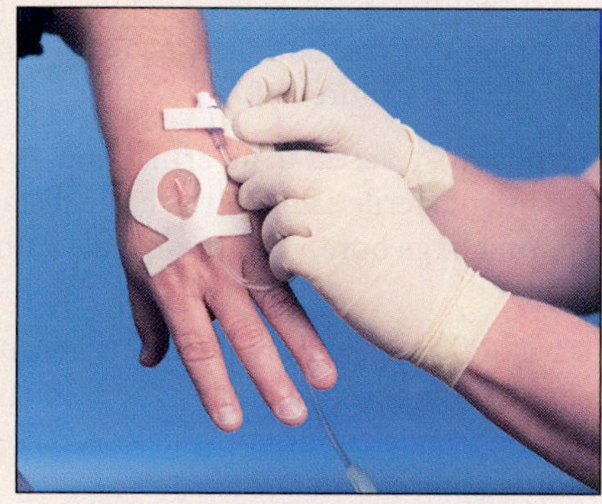

7-7g Secure the site.

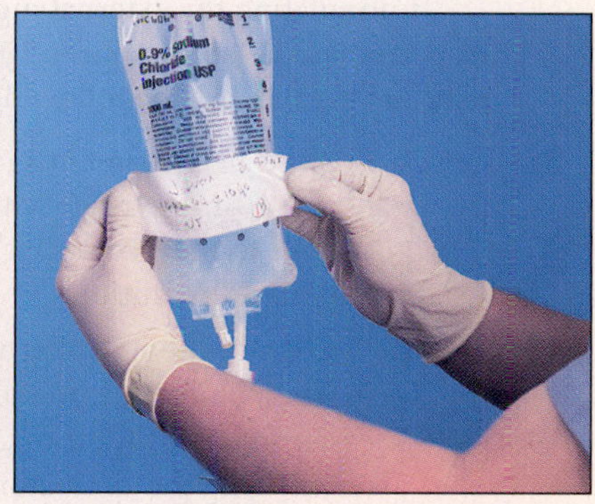

7-7h Label the intravenous solution bag.

(Photos © Scott Metcalfe)

The metal stylet is now in the vein; however, the Teflon catheter is not. To place the catheter into the vein, carefully advance the cannula approximately 0.5 cm further. (If you are using a butterfly cannula, it has no Teflon catheter, and you must carefully advance the needle itself.)

7. Holding the metal stylet stationary, slide the Teflon catheter over the needle into the vein. Place a finger over the vein at the catheter tip and tamponade (press gently downward to occlude the vein), thus preventing blood from flowing from the catheter and/or air from entraining into the circulatory system. Carefully remove the metal stylet and promptly dispose of it in the sharps container. Remove the venous constricting band.
8. Obtain venous blood samples as discussed in the section on venous blood sampling.
9. Attach the administration tubing to the cannula. Remove the protective cap from the needle adapter and tightly secure the needle adapter into the cannula hub. Open the flow regulator and allow the fluid to run freely for several seconds. Adjust the flow rate. Do not let go of the cannula and administration tubing until you have secured them as explained in step 10.
10. Apply antibiotic ointment to the site and cover it with an adhesive bandage or other commercial device. Loop the distal tubing and secure with tape. This makes the medication administration port more accessible and attaches the device to the patient more securely. Continue by taping the administration tubing to the patient, proximal to the venipuncture site.
11. Label the intravenous solution bag with the following information:
    —Date and time initiated
    —Person initiating the intravenous access
12. Continually monitor the patient and flow rate.

INTRAVENOUS ACCESS IN THE EXTERNAL JUGULAR VEIN

The external jugular vein is a large peripheral blood vessel in the neck, between the angle of the jaw and the middle third of the clavicle. It connects into the central circulation's subclavian vein. Since it lies so close to the central circulation, cannulation here offers many of the same benefits afforded by central venous access. Fluids and medications rapidly reach the core of the body from this site.

Consider accessing the external jugular only after you have exhausted other means of peripheral access or when a patient requires immediate fluid administration.

Consider accessing the external jugular only after you have exhausted other means of peripheral access or when a patient requires immediate fluid administration. This is an extremely painful site to access, so you typically will reserve its use for patients with a decreased or total loss of consciousness.

Cannulating the external jugular vein requires essentially the same equipment as other forms of peripheral IV access, plus a 10-mL syringe. You will not need a constricting band. To access the external jugular, use the following technique (Procedure 7–8):

1. Prepare all equipment as for peripheral IV access in an arm, hand, or leg. In addition, fill the 10-mL syringe with 3 to 5 mL of sterile saline. Attach the distal part of the syringe to the flashback chamber of a large bore, over-the-needle catheter. Apply Standard Precautions.
2. Place the patient supine and/or in the Trendelenburg position. This position will increase blood flow to the chest and neck, thus distending the vein and making it easier to see. In addition, the supine-Trendelenburg position decreases the chance of air entering the circulatory system during cannulation.
3. Turn the patient's head to the side opposite of access. This maneuver makes the site easier to see and reach; do not perform it if the patient has traumatic head and/or neck injuries.
4. Cleanse the site with antiseptics. Start at the site of intended puncture and work outward 1 to 2 inches in ever increasing circles.

Procedure 7-8 Peripheral Intravenous Access in an External Jugular Vein

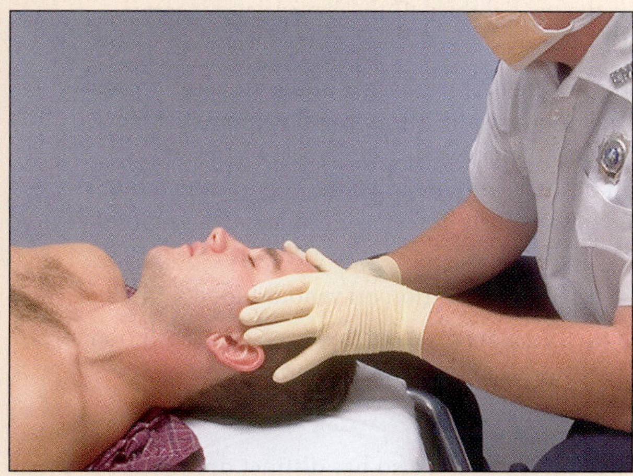

7-8a Place the patient supine or in the Trendelenburg position.

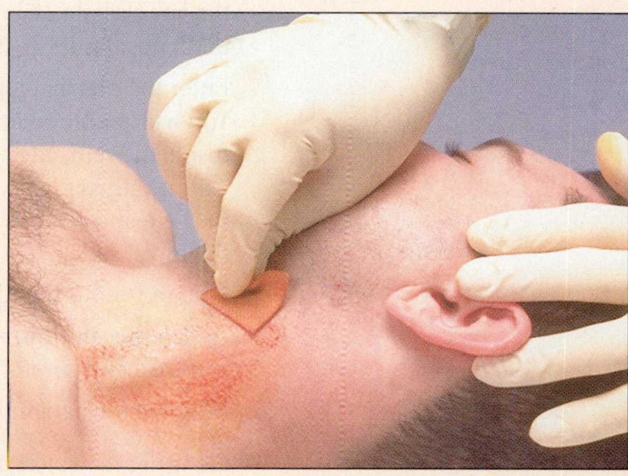

7-8b Turn the patient's head to the side opposite of access and cleanse the site.

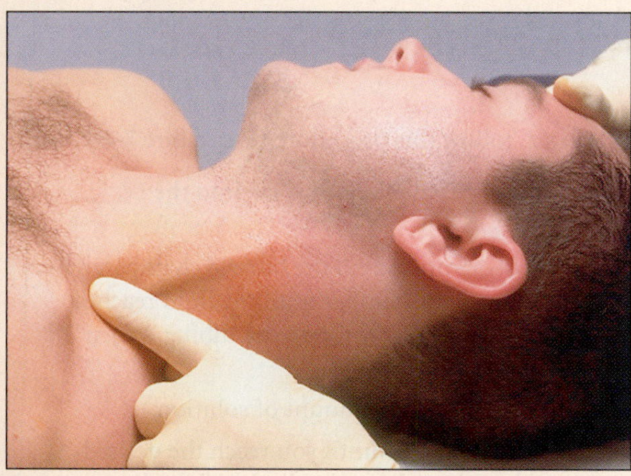

7-8c Occlude venous return by placing a finger on the external jugular just above the clavicle.

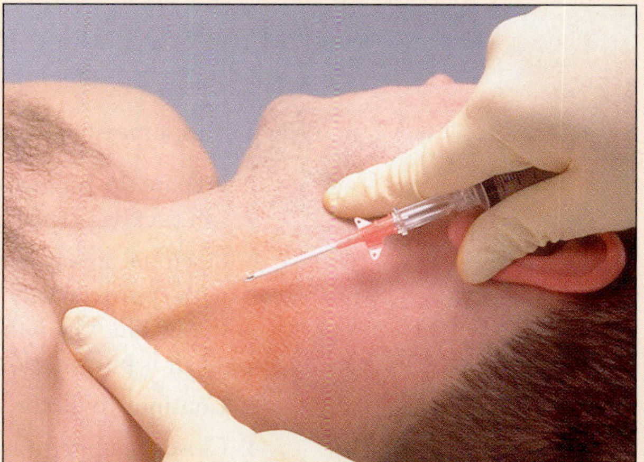

7-8d Point the catheter at the medial third of the clavicle and insert it, bevel up, at a 10°–30° angle.

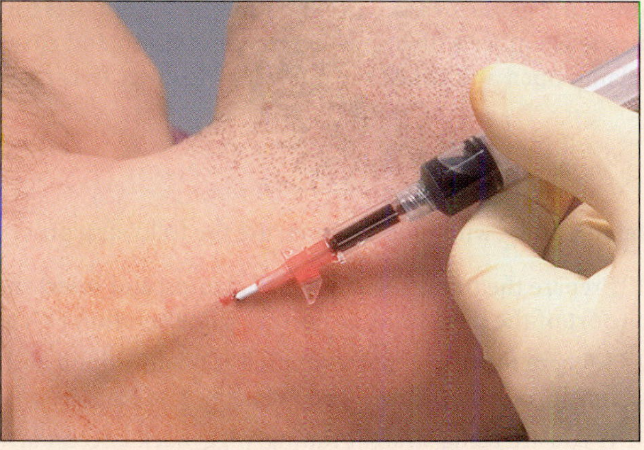

7-8e Enter the external jugular while withdrawing on the plunger of the attached syringe.

5. Occlude venous return by placing a finger on the external jugular just above the clavicle. This should distend the vein, again allowing greater visualization and ease of puncture. Never apply a venous constricting band around the patient's neck.
6. Position the intravenous cannula parallel with the vein, midway between the angle of the jaw clavicle. Point the catheter at the medial third of the clavicle and insert it, bevel up, at a 10° to 30° angle.
7. Enter the external jugular while withdrawing on the plunger of the attached syringe. You will see blood in the syringe or feel a pop as the cannula enters the vein. Once inside the vein, advance the entire angiocatheter another 0.5 cm so the tip of the Teflon catheter lies within the lumen of the vein. Then slide the Teflon catheter into the vein and remove the metal stylet as previously described. Immediately dispose of the metal stylet.
8. Obtain venous blood samples as discussed in the section on venous blood sampling.
9. Attach the administration tubing to the IV catheter. Allow the intravenous solution to run freely for several seconds. Set the flow rate and secure as appropriate.
10. Monitor the patient for complications.

While using the external jugular vein has advantages, it also has distinct drawbacks. You may inadvertently puncture the airway or damage the nearby arterial vessels. Additionally, this is a painful entry site for the conscious patient. To minimize risks, perform the procedure very carefully.

INTRAVENOUS ACCESS WITH A MEASURED VOLUME ADMINISTRATION SET

When using a measured volume administration set, follow this procedure (Procedure 7–9):

1. Prepare the tubing by closing all clamps, and insert the flanged spike into the IV solution bag's spike port.
2. Open the airway handle. Open the uppermost clamp and fill the burette chamber with approximately 20 mL of fluid. Squeeze the drip chamber until the fluid reaches the fill line. Open the bottom flow regulator to purge air through the tubing. When all air is purged, close the bottom flow regulator.
3. Continue to fill the burette chamber with the designated amount of solution.
4. Close the uppermost clamp and open the flow regulator until you reach the desired drip rate. Leave the airway handle open, so that air replaces the displaced fluid.

To refill the burette chamber, open the uppermost clamp until you have delivered the desired volume; then repeat step 4.

You can also use measured volume administration sets for continuous fluid administration. Fill the burette chamber with at least 30 mL of solution and close the airway handle. Leave the uppermost clamp open and adjust the rate with the lower flow regulator.

INTRAVENOUS ACCESS WITH BLOOD TUBING

To establish an IV with blood tubing, use the following procedure:

1. Prepare the tubing by closing all clamps, and insert the flanged spike into the spike port of the blood and/or normal saline solution (Y-configured tubing).
2. Squeeze the drip chamber until it is one third full and blood covers the filter. Repeat for the normal saline if you are using Y tubing.
3. If you are using straight tubing, piggyback a secondary line of normal saline into the blood tubing, unless you plan to piggyback the straight blood tubing into a large bore primary line.

Procedure 7-9

Intravenous Access with a Measured Volume Administration Set

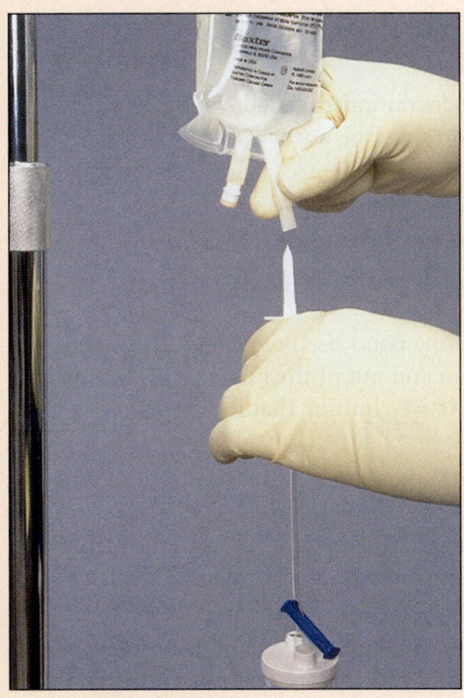

7-9a Spike the solution bag.

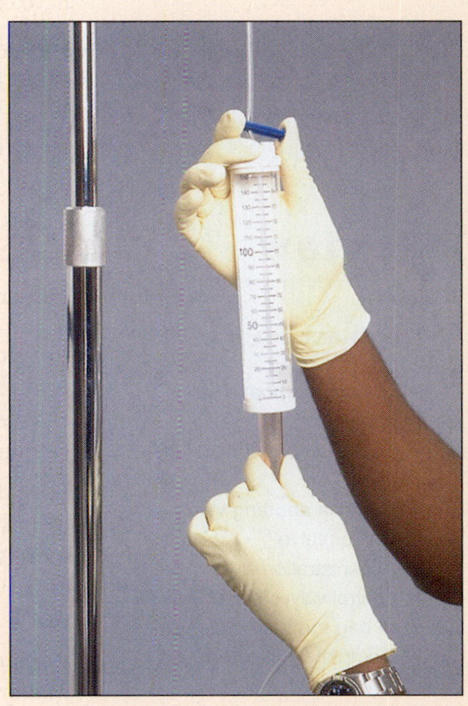

7-9b Open the uppermost clamp and fill the burette chamber with the desired volume of fluid.

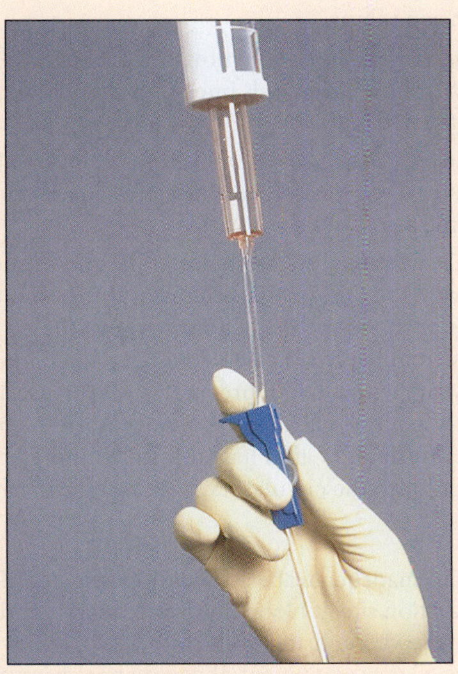

7-9c Close the uppermost clamp and open the flow regulator.

4. Flush all tubing with normal saline and blood as appropriate.
5. Attach blood tubing to the intravenous cannula or into a previously established IV line.
6. Ensure patency by infusing a small amount of normal saline. Shut down when you have confirmed patency.
7. Open the clamp(s) and/or flow regulator(s) that allows blood to move from the bag to the patient. Adjust the flow rate accordingly.
8. When blood therapy is complete or must be discontinued, shut down the flow regulator from the blood supply and open the regulator(s) for the normal saline solution.

Content Review

IV Troubleshooting

- Constricting band still in place?
- Edema at puncture site?
- Cannula abutting vein wall or valve?
- Administration set control valves closed?
- IV bag too low?
- Completely filled drip chamber?

extravasation *leakage of fluid or medication from the blood vessel that is commonly found with infiltration.*

FACTORS AFFECTING INTRAVENOUS FLOW RATES

If an IV does not flow properly, check for the following problems and correct them as appropriate.

★ *Constricting band.* Has the venous constricting band been removed? This is probably the most common mistake both in and out of the hospital. Additionally, ensure that the patient is not wearing restrictive clothing that interferes with venous blood flow.

★ *Edema at the puncture site.* Swelling at the IV site indicates fluid collection caused by infiltration. This **extravasation** occurs if you accidentally puncture the vein more than once, thus allowing IV solution and blood to escape from the second puncture and accumulate in the surrounding tissue. An infiltrated IV site is not usable.

★ *Cannula abutting the vein wall or valve.* If the distal tip of the cannula butts against a wall or valve, carefully reposition it. You may have to untape and retape the cannula once you have achieved an adequate flow rate. Additionally, you may need to use an arm board to keep the patient's extremity straight, as flexion may kink the vein at the site and impede the solution's flow.

★ *Administration set control valves.* Ensure that the flow regulator is open. Be sure to check the flow regulator and clamps of both the primary and any secondary or extension tubing.

★ *IV bag height.* When you move the patient, you may raise the cannulation site above the IV solution bag. This interrupts the solution's gravitational flow from the bag into the patient.

★ *Completely filled drip chamber.* Is the drip chamber completely filled? You can easily correct this by inverting the bag and squeezing the fluid from the drip chamber back into the bag.

★ *Catheter patency.* A blood clot at the end of the Teflon catheter or needle may obstruct the flow of solution from the IV solution bag into the body. If the flow slows, increase the IV drip rate to keep the catheter or needle clear. If the flow stops completely, cleanse the medication administration port closest to the IV entry site with alcohol preparations and insert a syringe and hypodermic needle. Gently aspirate back on the syringe until the blood clot is pulled into the syringe. Never flush an IV that has stopped running because of a clot. Flushing will force the clot into the circulatory system and can cause occlusions in the heart or lungs.

If flow remains inadequate after you have eliminated all of these possible causes, lower the IV bag below the insertion site. If blood flows into the IV administration tubing, the site is patent and the problem lies elsewhere. If the problem persists, remove the IV and reestablish it on another extremity, using all new equipment. If you do not observe blood return, the site is inoperable.

COMPLICATIONS OF PERIPHERAL INTRAVENOUS ACCESS

Even though it is a routine procedure, intravenous access is not trouble free. It can cause a number of complications.

Pain

Pain at the puncture site occurs during needle penetration or with extravasation. To minimize pain, use a smaller gauge catheter or use a 1 percent lidocaine solution (without epinephrine) to anesthetize the overlying skin before insertion.

Local Infection

Local infection occurs if you do not properly cleanse the site and thus introduce pathogens through the puncture. This complication does not become apparent until after the IV has been established for several hours.

Pyrogenic Reaction

Pyrogens (foreign proteins capable of producing fever) in the administration tubing or IV solution can cause a pyrogenic reaction. The abrupt onset of fever (100°F to 106°F), chills, backache, headache, nausea, and vomiting characterize these reactions. Cardiovascular collapse may also result.

Typically, a pyrogenic reaction will occur within one half to one hour after you initiate an IV. If you suspect a pyrogenic reaction, immediately terminate the IV and reestablish access in the opposite side with new equipment and fluid.

Typically, pyrogenic reactions occur secondary to the use of intravenous solutions that have been contaminated with a microorganism or other foreign matter. Pyrogenic reactions underscore the need to discard any fluid that is cloudy or any equipment that has been opened.

Allergic Reaction

A patient receiving IV therapy may develop an allergic reaction. Most often allergic reactions accompany the administration of blood or colloid (protein containing) solutions. In addition, some patients may react to the latex in some types of IV administration tubing.

The sudden onset of hives (urticaria), itching (pruritis), localized or systemic edema, or shortness of breath may signify an allergic reaction. If you suspect an allergic reaction, stop the IV infusion and remove the IV catheter. Treat the patient as discussed in Chapter 31 on allergies and anaphylaxis.

Catheter Shear

A catheter shear can occur if you pull the Teflon catheter through or over the needle after you have advanced it into the vein. The soft plastic catheter will easily snag on the metal stylet's sharp point and shear off, thus forming a plastic **embolus.** Therefore, never draw the Teflon catheter over the metal stylet after you have advanced it.

Inadvertent Arterial Puncture

Because arteries may lie close to veins, accidental arterial puncture may occur. Arterial blood is bright red and characteristically spurts with each contraction of the heart. When an arterial puncture occurs, immediately remove the catheter and apply direct pressure to the site for at least 5 minutes. Do not release the pressure until the hemorrhage has stopped.

Circulatory Overload

Circulatory overload occurs if you administer too much fluid for the patient's condition. You must monitor flow rates carefully, especially for patients with medical conditions such as kidney failure or heart failure who are intolerant of excessive fluid. Continually examine the patient for

Content Review

IV Access Complications

- Pain
- Local infection
- Pyrogenic reaction
- Allergic reaction
- Catheter shear
- Inadvertent arterial puncture
- Circulatory overload
- Thrombophlebitis
- Thrombus formation
- Air embolism
- Necrosis
- Anticoagulants

pyrogen *foreign protein capable of producing fever.*

embolus *foreign particle in the blood.*

circulatory overload *an excess in intravascular fluid volume.*

signs of circulatory overload (crackles, tachypnea, dyspnea, and jugular venous distention, as discussed in Chapter 11 on physical exam techniques). If you encounter circulatory overload, adjust the flow rate.

Thrombophlebitis

thrombophlebitis *inflammation of the vein.*

Thrombophlebitis, or inflammation of the vein, is particularly common in long-term intravenous therapy. Redness and edema at the puncture site are typical signs of thrombophlebitis. This complication may also present as pain along the course of the vein, sometimes accompanied by inflammation and tenderness. Typically, thrombophlebitis does not occur until several hours after IV initiation. When you suspect thrombophlebitis, terminate the IV and apply a warm compress to the site.

Thrombus Formation

thrombus *blood clot.*

A **thrombus,** or blood clot, can form if IV access injures the vessel wall. A thrombus may form around the catheter and occlude the movement of fluid between the IV and the blood vessel. If you suspect a thrombus, restart the IV using new equipment. Do not attempt to dislodge the clot with a fluid bolus, as this may create an embolus that causes neurological or pulmonary complications.

Air Embolism

air embolism *air in the vein.*

Air embolism occurs when air enters the vein. Air embolus is most likely to occur during central venous access or when administration tubing has not been properly flushed. Failure to tamponade larger veins during cannulation may allow air into the vein.

Necrosis

necrosis *the sloughing off of dead tissue.*

Necrosis, or the sloughing off of dead tissue, occurs later in IV therapy as medication has extravasated into the interstitial space.

Anticoagulants

anticoagulant *drug that inhibits blood clotting.*

Anticoagulant drugs such as aspirin, Coumadin, or heparin increase the chance of bleeding and impede hemorrhage control during IV establishment. They drastically increase the complications of hematoma or infiltration.

CHANGING AN IV BAG OR BOTTLE

You may sometimes have to change an IV bag or bottle. This generally occurs when only 50 mL of solution remains and you must continue therapy after those 50 mL are depleted. Changing the solution bag or bottle is a sterile process. If the equipment becomes contaminated you should dispose of it.

To change the IV solution bag or bottle, use the following technique:

1. Prepare the new IV solution bag or bottle by removing the protective cover from the IV tubing port.
2. Occlude the flow of solution from the depleted bag or bottle by moving the roller clamp on the IV administration tubing.
3. Remove the spike from the depleted IV bag or bottle. Be careful not to drop or contaminate the spike in any way.
4. Insert the spike into the new IV bag or bottle. Ensure that the drip chamber is filled appropriately.
5. Open the roller clamp to the appropriate flow rate.

If air becomes entrained within the administration tubing during this process, cleanse the medication administration port below the trapped air and insert a hypodermic needle and syringe. Pull the plunger back to aspirate the trapped air into the syringe. After you have removed the air, adjust the IV flow rate as needed.

INTRAVENOUS DRUG ADMINISTRATION

Medications can be delivered through an existing IV line. As the IV line is seated directly into a vein, the blood rapidly absorbs these medications and distributes them throughout the body. Intravenous administration avoids many of the barriers to drug absorption in other routes. For example, drugs given via the gastrointestinal tract face enzymes and other chemicals that may deactivate, exacerbate, or in some other way alter the medication being administered. Likewise, local tissues can absorb drugs administered via the subcutaneous or intramuscular routes, thus preventing the total dosage from reaching the bloodstream for delivery. The two methods for administering drugs through an IV line are intravenous bolus and intravenous infusion.

Intravenous Bolus

An intravenous bolus involves injecting the circulatory system with a concentrated dose of drug through the medication administration port of an established IV. This procedure requires the following equipment:

- ★ Standard Precautions
- ★ Alcohol antiseptic preparation
- ★ Packaged medication
- ★ Syringe (size depends upon the volume of drug you will administer)
- ★ 18- to 20-gauge hypodermic needle, 1 to 1½ inch long
- ★ Existing intravenous line with medication port

To administer an intravenous medication bolus, use the following technique (Procedure 7–10):

1. Assure that the primary IV line is patent.
2. Confirm the drug, indication, dosage, and need for an IV bolus.
3. Draw up the medication or prepare a prefilled syringe as appropriate.
4. Cleanse the medication port nearest the IV site with an alcohol antiseptic preparation.
5. Insert a hypodermic needle through the port membrane.
6. Pinch the IV line above the medication port. This prevents the medication from traveling toward the fluids bag, forcing it instead toward the patient.
7. Inject the medication as appropriate.
8. Remove the hypodermic needle and syringe and release the tubing.
9. Open the flow regulator to allow a 20-mL fluid flush. The fluid will push the medication into the patient's circulatory system.
10. Dispose of the hypodermic needle and syringe as appropriate. Monitor the patient for desired or undesired effects.

Intravenous Drug Infusion

Many cardiac drugs and antibiotics are given as intravenous infusions (IV piggybacks). Intravenous drug infusions deliver a steady, continual dose of medication through an existing IV line. You may give them either as an initial dosage or to maintain drug levels after delivering an initial bolus.

Piggybacking IV infusions through an existing intravenous line gives you greater control over medication delivery and allows you to easily discontinue the infusion when therapy is complete or must be stopped. Never administer intravenous infusions as a primary IV line.

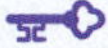

Never administer intravenous infusions as a primary IV line.

IV infusions are contained in bags or bottles of intravenous solution. If the IV infusion is premixed, read the label on the bag for the following information:

- ★ Name of medication
- ★ Total dosage in weight mixed in bag
- ★ Concentration (weight per single mL)
- ★ Expiration date

Procedure 7-10 Intravenous Bolus Administration

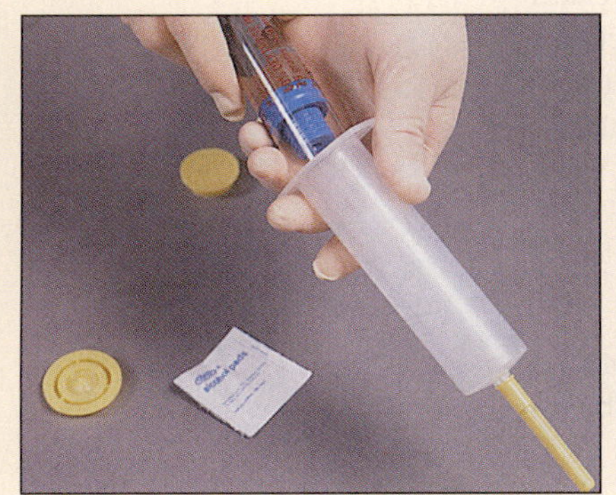

7-10a Prepare the equipment.

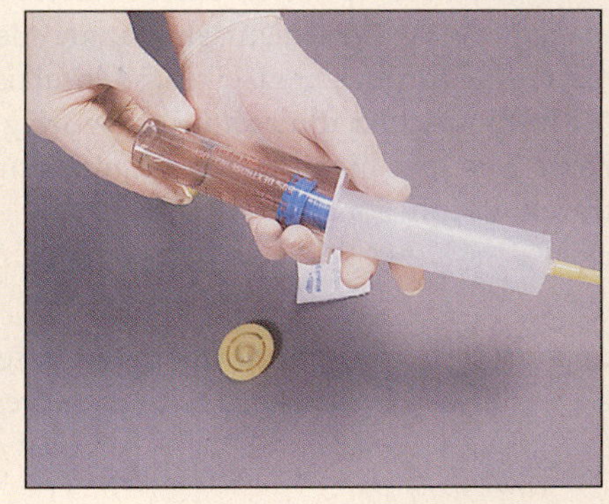

7-10b Prepare the medication.

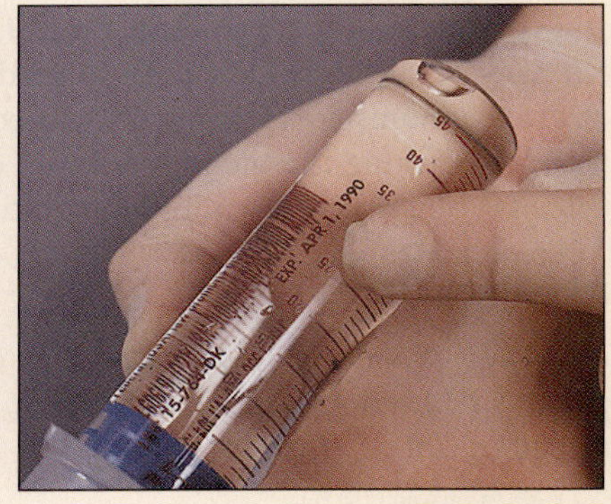

7-10c Check the label.

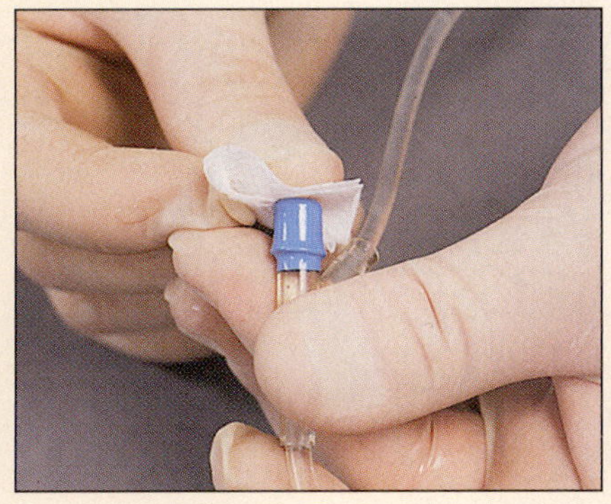

7-10d Select and clean an administration port.

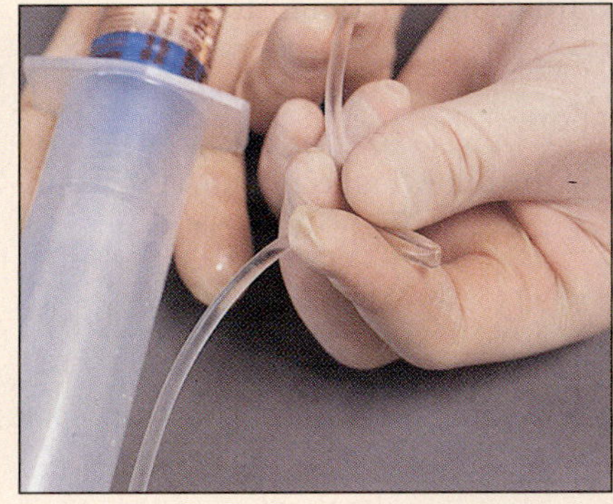

7-10e Pinch the line.

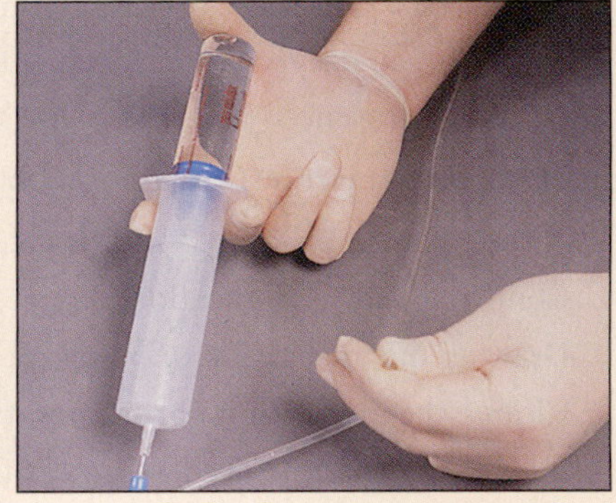

7-10f Administer the medication.

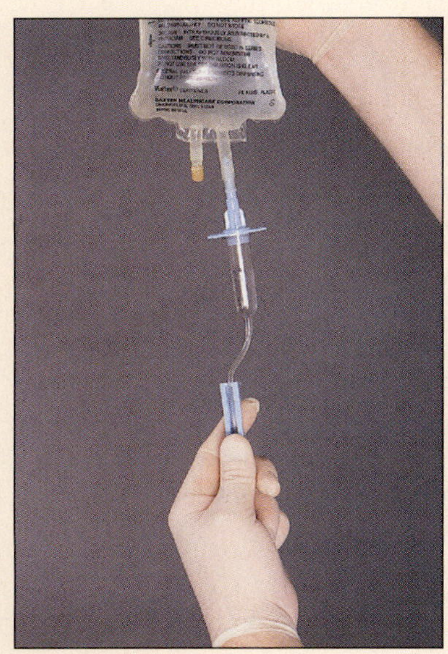

7-10g Adjust the IV flow rate.

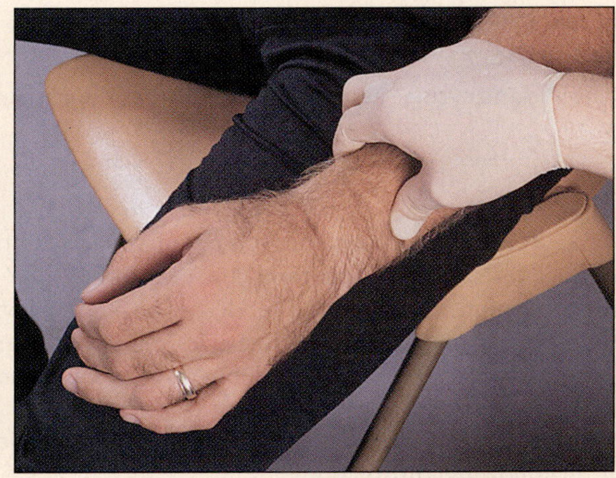

7-10h Monitor the patient.

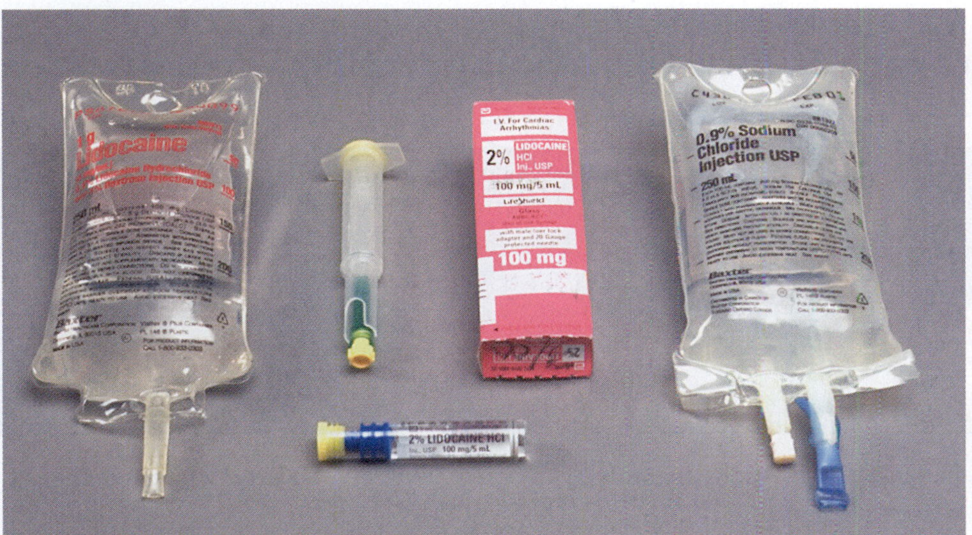

■ **Figure 7-28** If an IV solution is not premixed, you will have to mix and label it yourself.

If the infusion is not premixed, make a label listing this information and attach it to the bag (Figure 7-28 ■). Additionally, note the date and time you mixed the infusion, and initial it.

Use the following technique to administer a medication as an IV infusion (Procedure 7–11):

1. Establish a primary IV line and assure patency.
2. Confirm administration indications and patient allergies.
3. Prepare the infusion bag or bottle. (If the infusion is premixed, continue to step 4.)
   a. Draw up the appropriate quantity of medication from its source with a syringe.
   b. Cleanse the IV bag or bottle's medication port with an alcohol antiseptic wipe.
   c. Insert the hypodermic needle into the medication port and inject the medication.
   d. Gently agitate the bag or bottle to mix its contents.
   e. Label the bag or bottle.
4. Connect administration tubing to the medication bag or bottle and fill the drip chamber to the fluid line. Most infusions require microdrip tubing. If you use a mechanical infusion pump, you may need to use special tubing.
5. Place the hypodermic needle on the administration tubing's needle adapter and flush the tubing with solution. (The needle adapter typically accepts a 20-gauge needle.)
6. Cleanse the medication administration port on the primary line with alcohol and insert the secondary line's hypodermic needle. Secure the hypodermic needle and the secondary administration line with tape or another securing device.
7. Reconfirm the indication, drug, dose, and route of administration.
8. Shut down the primary line so that no fluid will flow from the primary solution bag.
9. Adjust the secondary line to the desired drip rate. If you are using a mechanical infusion pump set it accordingly.
10. Properly dispose of the needle and syringe.

When the infusion is complete, shut down the secondary line with the flow regulator or a clamp. Open the primary line and adjust it to the indicated drip rate. Remove the hypodermic needle from the medication administration port and properly dispose of all contents. If required by your local protocols, retain the medication bag to verify administration and for quality assurance.

You can also use measured volume administration tubing to administer medicated infusions. First, fill the burette chamber of a measured volume administration device with a specific volume of fluid. Then you can inject the drug through the medication injection site on top of the burette chamber. You

Procedure 7-11 Intravenous Infusion Administration

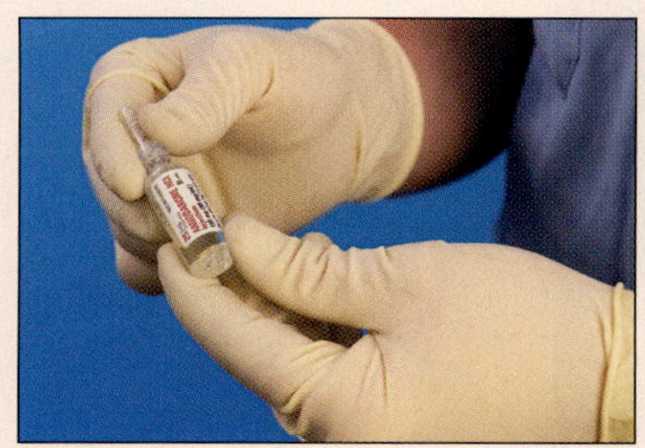

7-11a Select the drug.

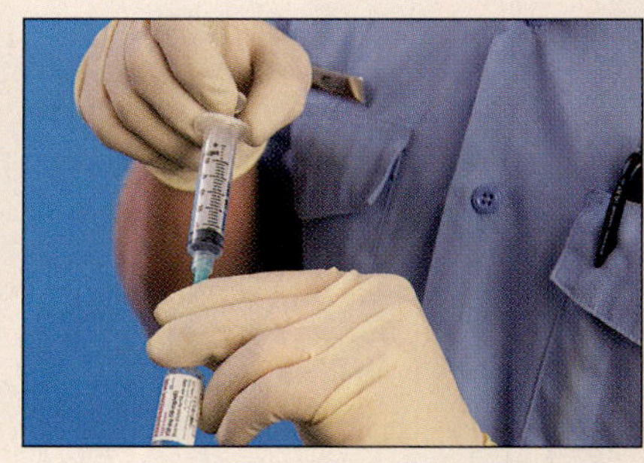

7-11b Draw up the drug.

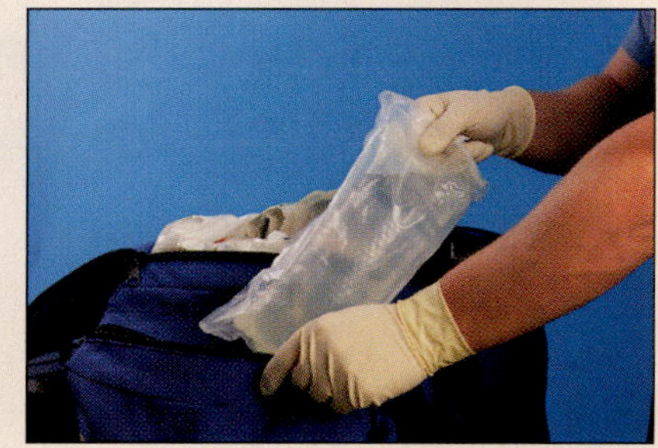

7-11c Select IV fluid for dilution.

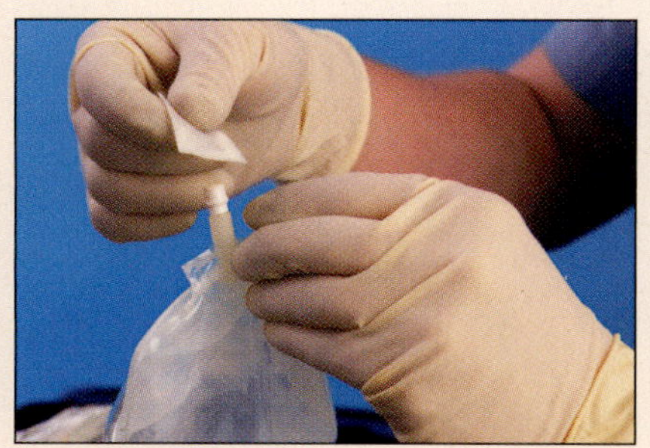

7-11d Clean the medication addition port.

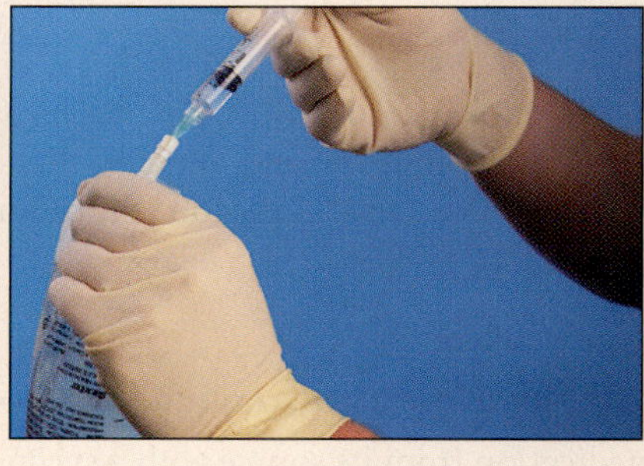

7-11e Inject the drug into the fluid.

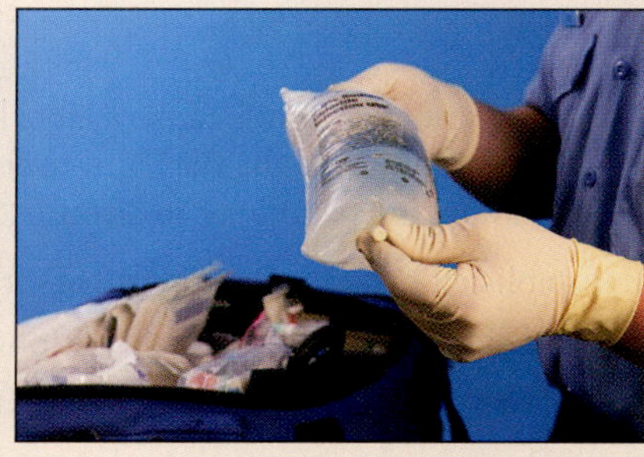

7-11f Mix the solution.

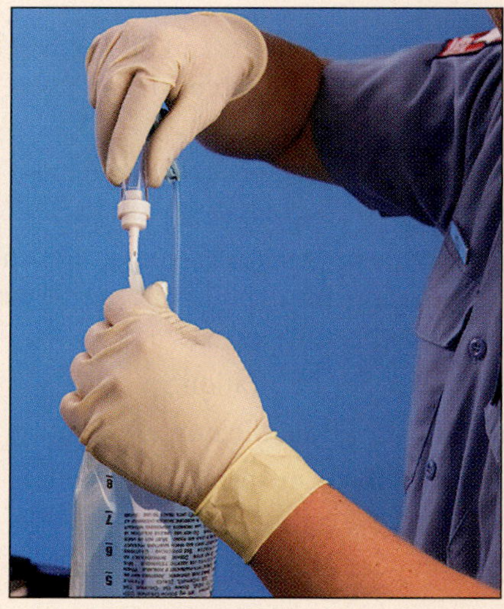

7-11g Insert an administration set and connect to the main IV line with needle.

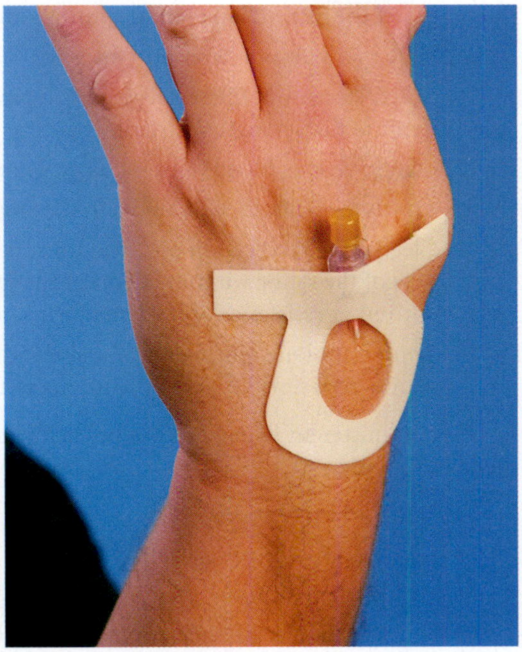

■ Figure 7-29 Heparin lock. (*© Scott Metcalfe*).

must adjust the flow rate to deliver the precise amount of medication required. In addition, you can mix the medication within the IV bag or bottle as previously described and use the measured volume administration tubing solely for administering the infusion rather than for mixing it.

Heparin Lock and Saline Lock

When a patient requires occasional IV medication drips or boluses but does not need continuous fluid, heparin locks are used. A **heparin lock** is a peripheral IV port that does not use a bag of fluid. Like a typical IV start, it places an IV cannula into a peripheral vein; however, instead of IV administration tubing, it has attached short tubing with a clamp and a distal medication port (Figure 7-29 ■). A heparin lock decreases the risk of accidental fluid overload and electrolyte derangement. You also may withdraw blood samples from the lock if it is in a suitable vein. For short-term use, **saline locks** may be used. Sterile saline is injected following the drug. Saline remains in the lock to keep it open. For long-term use, a heparin lock is preferred. Although it functions the same as a saline lock, a heparin lock is filled with a low-concentration solution of heparin, which aids in keeping any blood that gets into the device from clotting. Typically, a drug will be administered through the heparin lock. This is followed by a saline flush to assure that no drug remains in the lock or hub. Then, the lock and hub are filled with a heparin solution. This aids in keeping the IV site open for a long period of time.

heparin lock *peripheral IV port that does not use a bag of fluid.*

saline lock *peripheral IV cannula with a distal medication port used for intermittent fluid or medication infusions. Saline is injected into the device to maintain its patency.*

Initiating a heparin lock requires the following equipment:

- IV cannula
- Heparin lock
- Syringe with 3 to 5 mL sterile saline or commercial saline injection device
- Tape or commercial securing device
- Venous blood drawing equipment
- Venous constricting band
- Antiseptic swab (Betadine/alcohol)

To place a heparin lock, follow these steps:

1. Select the venipuncture site.
2. Place the constricting band proximal to the puncture site.
3. Cleanse the venipuncture site with alcohol or Betadine antiseptics.

4. Insert the intravenous cannula into the vein.
5. Slide the Teflon catheter into the vein.
6. Carefully remove the metal stylet and promptly dispose of it in the sharps container. Remove the venous constricting band.
7. Obtain venous blood samples, as explained under Venous Blood Sampling.
8. Attach the heparin lock tubing to the angiocatheter hub.
9. Cleanse the medication port and inject 3 to 5 mL of sterile saline into the lock. Easy flow of the saline without edema at the puncture site indicates patency. If you encounter resistance or if edema forms, restart the procedure with new equipment.
10. Apply antibiotic ointment to the site and cover with an adhesive bandage or other commercial device. Secure the tubing to the patient.

To administer an IV medication bolus through a heparin lock, assemble the following equipment and supplies:

- ★ Standard Precautions
- ★ Alcohol antiseptic preparation
- ★ Packaged medication
- ★ Syringe (the size depends on the volume being administered)
- ★ 18- to 20-gauge hypodermic needle 1 to 1½ inch long

After you have gathered all equipment and supplies, use the following technique to administer an IV medication bolus with a heparin lock:

1. Confirm the drug, indication, dosage, and need for an IV bolus.
2. Draw up the medication or prepare a prefilled syringe as appropriate.
3. Cleanse the medication port nearest the IV site with alcohol antiseptic preparation.
4. Ensure that the plastic clamp is open.
5. Insert the hypodermic needle through the port membrane.
6. Inject the medication as appropriate.
7. Remove the hypodermic needle and dispose of it in the sharps container.
8. Follow the medication administration with a 10- to 20-mL saline flush from another syringe.
9. Properly dispose of the hypodermic needle and syringe. Monitor the patient for desired or undesired effects.

If fluid administration becomes necessary, you can unscrew the medication port and insert IV administration tubing. Periodically flush with sterile saline or heparin to prevent clot formation and occlusion at the Teflon catheter's distal end.

Venous Access Device

venous access device *surgically implanted port that permits repeated access to central venous circulation.*

A **venous access device** is a surgically implanted port that permits repeated access to the central venous circulation. Implanted just under the skin, venous access devices are constructed of a plastic or stainless steel injection port and flexible catheter. The injection port, which lies just beneath the skin, contains a self-sealing septum that allows repeated penetration and access into the venous circulation. The self-sealing septum is connected to a flexible catheter that is placed within the lumen of a central vein, most often the superior vena cava.

Typically, patients with venous access devices have chronic illnesses that require repeated intravenous access for medication administration, long-term intravenous therapy, or blood sampling. Generally, venous access devices are placed on the anterior chest near the third or fourth rib lateral to the sternum. A venous access device is apparent as a raised circle just beneath the skin.

Use of an indwelling central venous access device requires special training. Delivering a medication through the venous access device requires a special needle specific for the venous access device in question. A common needle, the **Huber needle,** has an opening on the side of its shaft instead of at the tip. When placed into the injection port, this configuration allows easy administration of medication into the venous access device. Never access a venous access device unless you have the specific needle unique for the particular device. Always ask the patient, family, or nursing staff about the type of venous access device. Often, they will have a supply of needles for the device.

Huber needle *needle that has an opening on the side of the shaft instead of the tip.*

To administer fluids, medication, or blood through a venous access device, you must first prepare the site using the following technique:

1. Use Standard Precautions.
2. Fill a 10-mL syringe with approximately 7 mL of normal saline.
3. Place a 21- or 22-gauge Huber needle (or other specialized needle) on the end of the syringe.
4. Cleanse the skin over the injection port with povidone-iodine or alcohol preparations.
5. Stabilize the site with one hand while inserting the Huber needle at a 90° angle. Gently advance it until it meets resistance. This signals that the needle has contacted the floor of the injection port.
6. Pull back on the plunger and observe for blood return. The presence of blood confirms placement.
7. Slowly inject the normal saline to assure patency.

To administer the medication by intravenous bolus, use the following technique:

1. Prepare the medication, fluid, or blood for administration.
2. Attach a 21- or 22-gauge Huber needle (or other specialized needle) to the end of the syringe.
3. Cleanse the skin over the injection port with povidone-iodine or alcohol preparations.
4. Insert the needle into the injection port at a 90° angle until the needle cannot be further advanced. Pull back on the plunger of the syringe and observe for the return of blood. The presence of blood confirms proper placement.
5. Inject the medication as appropriate.
6. Remove and dispose of the syringe appropriately.
7. With another syringe and attached specialized needle, administer a bolus of heparinized saline to clear the catheter of any blood clots or other obstruction.

If the venous access device is not patent or access proves difficult, contact medical direction for further directives.

To administer IV fluids, use the following technique:

1. Prepare a primary IV line. Be sure to prime or flush the air from the administration tubing.
2. Attach a 21- or 22-gauge Huber needle (or other specialized needle) to the primary IV administration tubing. Insert a 10-mL syringe and hypodermic needle filled with 7 mL of normal saline solution into the tubing medication delivery port nearest the venous access device.
3. Cleanse the skin over the injection port with povidone-iodine or alcohol preparations.
4. Insert the needle into the injection port at a 90° angle until it encounters resistance.
5. Pinch the administration tubing above the medication administration port and pull back on the syringe plunger. Observe for the return of blood. The presence of blood confirms proper placement.
6. Gently inject the 7 mL of normal saline solution.
7. Set the primary line to the appropriate flow rate.

If administering a secondary medicated infusion, continue as follows:

1. Prepare a secondary line containing the fluid, blood, or medicated solution for infusion.
2. Attach a hypodermic needle to the needle adapter of the secondary line. Insert the secondary line into a medication administration port on the primary tubing.
3. Shut down the primary line and infuse the medicated solution as appropriate. Look for ease of administration as a sign of patency.
4. When infusion is complete, administer a bolus of heparinized saline to clear the catheter of any blood clots or other obstruction.

Using a venous access device is a very sterile procedure. You must take care to clean the site before delivering medications. Other complications of using a venous access device include infection, thrombus formation, and dislodgment of the catheter tip from the vein.

Electromechanical Infusion Devices

Electromechanical infusion devices permit the precise delivery of fluid and/or medications through electronic regulation. Anytime that intravenous infusion occurs, electromechanical infusion pumps provide optimal delivery. Infusion devices are classified as either infusion controllers or infusion pumps.

infusion controller *gravity-flow device that regulates fluid's passage through an electromechanical pump.*

extravascular *outside the vein.*

infusion pump *device that delivers fluids and medications under positive pressure.*

Infusion Controllers Infusion controllers are gravity-flow devices that regulate the fluid's passage through the pump. Because infusion controllers do not use positive pressure, they will not force fluids into the **extravascular** space if you infiltrate the vein.

Infusion Pumps Infusion pumps deliver fluids and medications under positive pressure (Figure 7-30 ■). This pressure can cause complications such as hematoma or extravasation if you infiltrate the vein. Some infusion pumps contain a pressure monitor and will warn you if they encounter the increased resistance that occurs with infiltration.

Syringe-type infusion pumps are gaining popularity for medical transport. Syringe pumps deliver their medications from a medical syringe without a hypodermic needle instead of from IV solution bags, fluids, or liquid medications (Figure 7-31 ■). You place the syringe containing the medications in the pump, which uses computerized mechanics to gradually depress the plunger at the correct rate. These compact pumps prove advantageous during transport.

Manufacturers make many different electromechanical infusion pumps. Depending on the maker, pump compatibility may require specialized administration tubing. With some computerized pumps, you can enter the basic information and then the pump will perform all medical calculations internally and automatically set the drip rate. Most infusion pumps contain internal

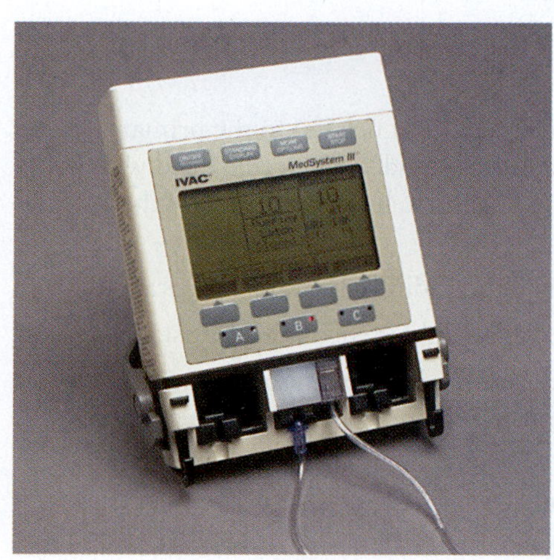

■ **Figure 7-30** Infusion pump.

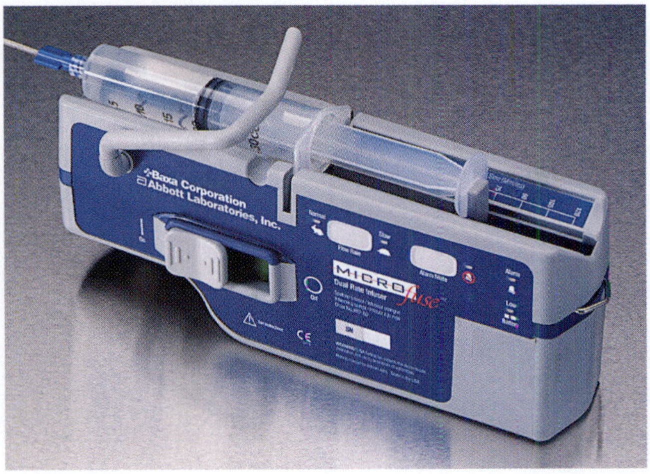

■ Figure 7-31 Syringe-type infusion pump.

monitoring devices that sound an alarm for problems such as infiltration, occlusion, or fluid source depletion. Electronic devices are prone to malfunction, so you must be prepared to perform all calculations and set the drip rate manually.

VENOUS BLOOD SAMPLING

The laboratory analysis of blood can provide valuable information about the sick and/or injured patient. The concentrations of electrolytes, gases, hormones, or other chemicals in blood can often shed light on the underlying causes of vague complaints such as dizziness or generalized weakness. Additionally, blood evaluation can confirm suspected conditions. For example, elevated cardiac enzymes in a patient's blood can confirm a suspected myocardial infarction.

In the field, you often will be the first to assess and treat an ill or injured patient. Many of your interventions can alter the blood's composition and erase important information. If you obtain venous blood samples before performing those interventions, they will enable the physician to evaluate the patient's original status.

Venous blood is commonly obtained via venipuncture. Thus, paramedics, who routinely initiate intravenous access, can simultaneously obtain blood samples. Doing so saves considerable hospital time and avoids multiple needle sticks.

You should obtain venous blood in the following situations:

- ★ During peripheral access
- ★ Before drug administration
- ★ When drug administration may be needed

Never stop to draw blood if it will delay critical measures such as drug administration in cardiac arrest or transport in a multisystems trauma.

Never stop to draw blood if it will delay critical measures.

Equipment for Drawing Blood

You will need the following equipment to obtain venous blood.

Blood Tubes **Blood tubes** are made of glass and have color-coded, self-sealing rubber tops. Blood tube sizes for adults generally range from 5 to 7 mL; for pediatrics, from 2 to 3 mL (Figure 7-32 ■). They are vacuum packed, and some contain a chemical anticoagulant. The different colored tops correspond to specific anticoagulants. A label on every blood tube identifies the type of additive and its expiration date. Do not use a blood tube after its expiration date, as both the anticoagulant and the vacuum lose their effectiveness.

blood tube *glass container with color-coded, self-sealing rubber top.*

■ Figure 7-32 Blood tubes.

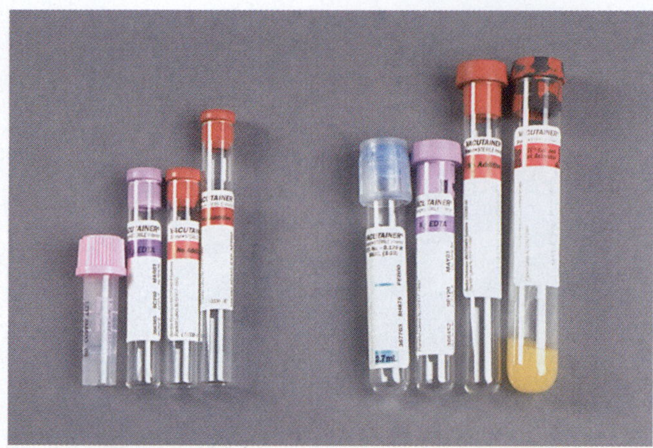

Using blood tubes in their correct order is essential. If you do not follow the proper sequence, the various anticoagulants will cause cross contamination, skewing the results and rendering the blood useless. Table 7–1 lists anticoagulants, the order in which you should use them, and the colors of their tops.

Miscellaneous Equipment Depending upon the technique you use to obtain venous blood, you will also need syringes, hypodermic needles, and commercially manufactured plastic sleeves called vacutainers.

Obtaining Venous Blood

Obtaining venous blood is a simple process; however, if the blood is to remain usable, you must pay strict attention to detail. You can obtain blood either from an angiocath or directly from the vein. Which technique you use will depend on the situation. In either case, venous blood samples are best obtained from sturdy veins such as the cephalic, basilic, or median. Smaller veins such as those on the back of the hand are more likely to collapse during retrieval, making the procedure difficult to complete.

Obtaining Venous Blood from an IV Angiocath The most convenient way to obtain venous blood is through an angiocath at the time of peripheral vascular access. In addition to blood tubes, you will need a tube holder (Figure 7-33 ■). The tube holder is commonly referred to as a **vacutainer.** A special needle called a multi-draw needle fits into the tube holder. The multi-draw needle has a rubber-covered needle used to puncture the self-sealing top of the blood tube. The remaining portion of the multi-draw needle protrudes from the tube holder and fits snugly into the hub of the angiocath.

vacutainer *device that holds blood tubes.*

To obtain blood directly from the angiocath, use the following procedure:

1. Assemble and prepare all equipment. Inspect the blood tubes for expiration or damage and insert the multi-draw needle into the vacutainer.

   Note: Never place blood tubes into the assembled vacutainer and multi-draw needle until you are ready to draw blood. This will destroy the vacuum and render the blood tube useless.

Table 7–1 Blood Tube Sequence

	Anticoagulant	Color of Top
1.	none	red
2.	citrate	blue
3.	heparin	green
4.	EDTA	purple
5.	fluoride	gray

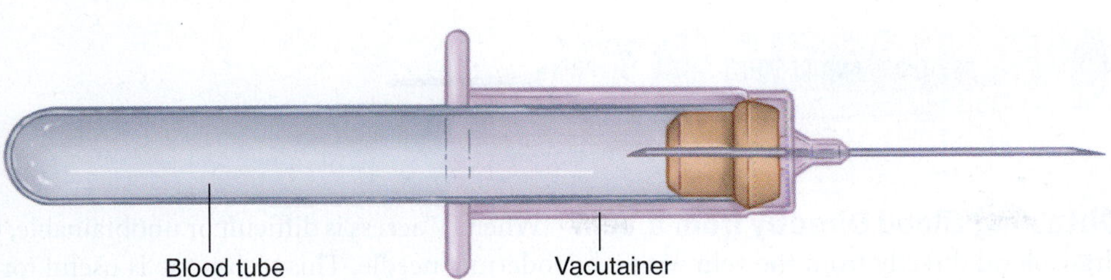

■ Figure 7-33 Vacutainer with Luer sampling needle.

2. Establish IV access with the angiocatheter. Do not connect IV administration tubing.
3. Attach the end of the multi-draw needle adapter to the hub of the cannula.
4. In correct order, insert the blood tubes so that the rubber-covered needle punctures the self-sealing rubber top. Blood should be pulled into the blood tube.
5. Fill all blood tubes completely, as the amount of anticoagulant is proportional to the tube's volume. Gently agitate the tubes to mix the anticoagulant evenly with the blood.
6. Tamponade the vein and remove the vacutainer and multi-draw needle. Attach the IV and assure patency.
7. Properly dispose of all sharps.
8. Label all blood tubes with the following information:
   —Patient's first and last name
   —Patient's age and gender
   —Date and time drawn
   —Name of the person drawing the blood

If commercial equipment is not available, use a 20-mL syringe (Figure 7-34 ■). Attach the syringe's needle adapter to the angiocath hub and gently pull back the plunger. Blood will fill the syringe. When the syringe is full, remove it from the angiocath and place the IV line into the angiocath. Carefully attach a hypodermic needle to the syringe to puncture the tops of the blood tubes. In the appropriate order, place the collected blood into the blood tubes and gently agitate. When finished, properly dispose of all sharps and label the blood tubes.

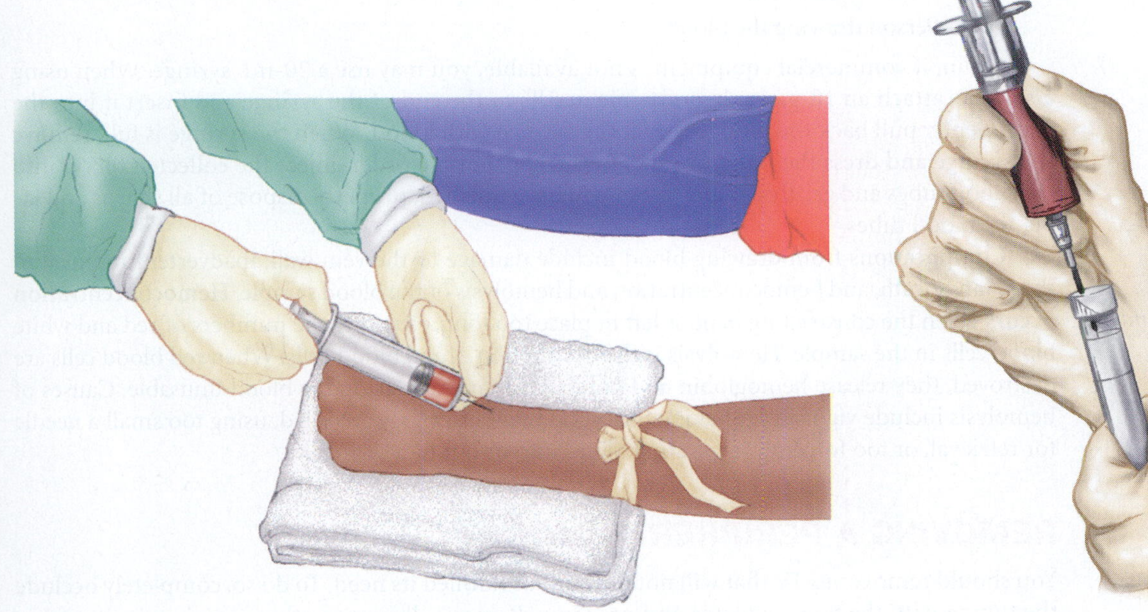

■ Figure 7-34 Obtaining a blood sample with a 20-mL syringe.

■ Figure 7-35 Luer sampling needle.

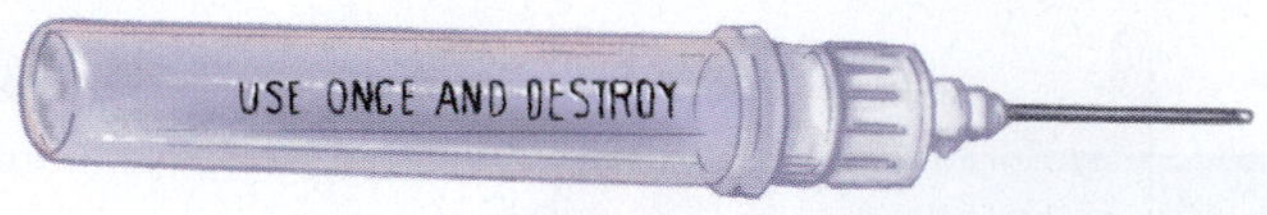

Luer sampling needle *long, exposed needle that screws into the vacutainer and is inserted directly into the vein.*

Obtaining Blood Directly from a Vein When IV access is difficult or unobtainable, you may draw blood directly from the vein with a hypodermic needle. This technique is useful for routine sampling that will not require further IV access. To draw blood directly from a vein, you will need the same equipment as for obtaining blood from an angiocath, but you will use a **Luer sampling needle** (Figure 7-35 ■). A Luer sampling needle is similar to a multi-draw needle, but instead of an angiocath adapter it has a long, exposed needle. The Luer sampling needle screws into the vacutainer, and you insert the exposed needle directly into the vein. You will also need a constricting band and antiseptic wipes.

To obtain blood directly from a vein, use the following procedure:

1. Assemble and prepare all equipment. Inspect the blood tubes for expiration or damage, and insert the needle into the vacutainer.
2. Apply the constricting band and select an appropriate puncture site.
3. Cleanse the site with alcohol or betadine.
4. Insert the end of the Luer sampling needle into the vein and remove the constricting band.
5. In the correct order, insert each blood tube so that the rubber-covered needle punctures the self-sealing rubber top. Blood should be pulled into the tube.
6. Gently agitate the tube to evenly mix the anticoagulant with the blood. Completely fill all blood tubes, as the anticoagulant is proportional to the volume of the tube.
7. Place sterile gauze over the site and remove the sampling needle. Properly dispose of all sharps.
8. Cover the puncture site with gauze and tape or an adhesive bandage.
9. Label all blood tubes with the following information:
   —Patient's first and last name
   —Patient's age and gender
   —Date and time drawn
   —Person drawing the blood

Again, if commercial equipment is not available, you may use a 20-mL syringe. When using a syringe, attach an 18-gauge hypodermic needle to the end of the syringe and insert it into the vein. Gently pull back the plunger to fill the syringe with blood. When the syringe is full, remove the syringe and dress the puncture site. In the appropriate order, inject the collected blood into the blood tubes and gently agitate. When you have finished, properly dispose of all sharps and label the blood tubes.

hemoconcentration *elevated numbers of red and white blood cells.*

hemolysis *the destruction of red blood cells.*

Complications from drawing blood include damage to the vein wall, inadvertent removal of the IV angiocath, and hemoconcentration and hemolysis of the blood sample. **Hemoconcentration** occurs when the constricting band is left in place too long, elevating the numbers of red and white blood cells in the sample. **Hemolysis** is the destruction of red blood cells. When red blood cells are destroyed, they release hemoglobin and potassium, thus rendering the blood unusable. Causes of hemolysis include vigorously shaking the blood tubes after they are filled, using too small a needle for retrieval, or too forcefully aspirating blood into or out of a syringe.

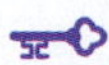

Remove any IV that will not flow or has fulfilled its need.

REMOVING A PERIPHERAL IV

You should remove any IV that will not flow or has fulfilled its need. To do so, completely occlude the tubing with the flow regulator and/or clamp. Remove all tape or other securing devices from the tubing and patient. Place a sterile gauze pad over the puncture site. Apply pressure to the gauze with the fingers or thumb of your nondominant hand. With your dominant hand, grasp the cannula at its hub and swiftly remove it, pulling straight back. The site may bleed, so apply direct pressure with the gauze for 5 minutes. Immediately dispose of all materials in the appropriate biohazard container. Apply an adhesive bandage or tape clean gauze over the site to protect against infection.

INTRAOSSEOUS INFUSION

Intraosseous (IO) infusions involve inserting a rigid needle into the cavity of a long bone or into the sternum (*intra-*, within; *os*, bone). The bone marrow contains a network of venous sinusoids that drain into the nutrient and emissary veins. These sinusoids accept fluids and drugs during intraosseous infusion and transport them to the venous system. Any solution or drug that can be administered intravenously, either bolus or infusion, can be administered by the intraosseous route.

intraosseous *within the bone.*

Generally, you will use IO infusions for the critical patient less than 5 years old when you cannot establish peripheral IV access. Less commonly, you may use intraosseous infusions in adult patients. These patients have different access sites than pediatric patients, and rapid volume administration may not be as effective. Situations that might require an intraosseous insertion include shock, status epilepticus, trauma, and cardiac arrest, as well as critical pediatric patients where rapid IV access cannot be obtained. Initiate intraosseous lines only after 90 seconds or three unsuccessful attempts to establish peripheral IV access.

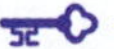

Initiate intraosseous lines only after 90 seconds or three unsuccessful attempts to establish peripheral IV access.

ACCESS SITE

The bone most commonly used for intraosseous access is the tibia. For pediatric access, the proximal tibia is most commonly used. The tibia (both proximal and distal) and sternum can also be used for IO access in the adult patient. To properly locate appropriate sites and avoid complications, you must understand the anatomy and physiology of the tibia (Figure 7-36 ■) and sternum. The three main sections of the tibia are the diaphysis, which comprises the middle, and the two epiphyses, one at either end. Epiphyseal disks, or growth plates, between the diaphysis and the epiphyses allow the tibia to grow and develop and are present in children. Damage to these disks during intraosseous access can cause long-term growth complications or abnormalities in children.

On either side of the proximal tibia are the medial and lateral condyles. You can identify the proximal epiphysis by palpating the condyles. Within the diaphysis, the medullary canal contains the bone marrow. When placed correctly, the distal part of the intraosseous needle will lie in the medullary canal.

Between the condyles, on the top of the anterior tibial crest, is a palpable bump called the tibial tuberosity. The tibial tuberosity lies at the level of the epiphyseal growth plate. Consequently, the tibial tuberosity is extremely important in locating the appropriate pediatric intraosseous access site.

At the distal end of the leg lie the lateral malleolus and the medial malleolus. These aid in location of the distal epiphyseal portion of the tibia and are important landmarks for intraosseous placement in the adult patient.

For the pediatric patient (under 5 years old), you will establish intraosseous access on the medial aspect of the proximal tibia (Figure 7-37a ■). This site is from two to three finger-breadths below the tibial tuberosity. At this level, place the needle on the flat area medial to the anterior tibial crest. For adult or geriatric patients, place the needle at the distal part of the tibia, one to two finger-breadths above the medial malleolus (Figure 7-37b).

EQUIPMENT FOR INTRAOSSEOUS ACCESS

Intraosseous placement requires a specially designed needle and a 10-mL syringe. Manufactured specifically for intraosseous access, an intraosseous needle is a 14- to 18-gauge hollow cannula

■ Figure 7-36 Tibia.

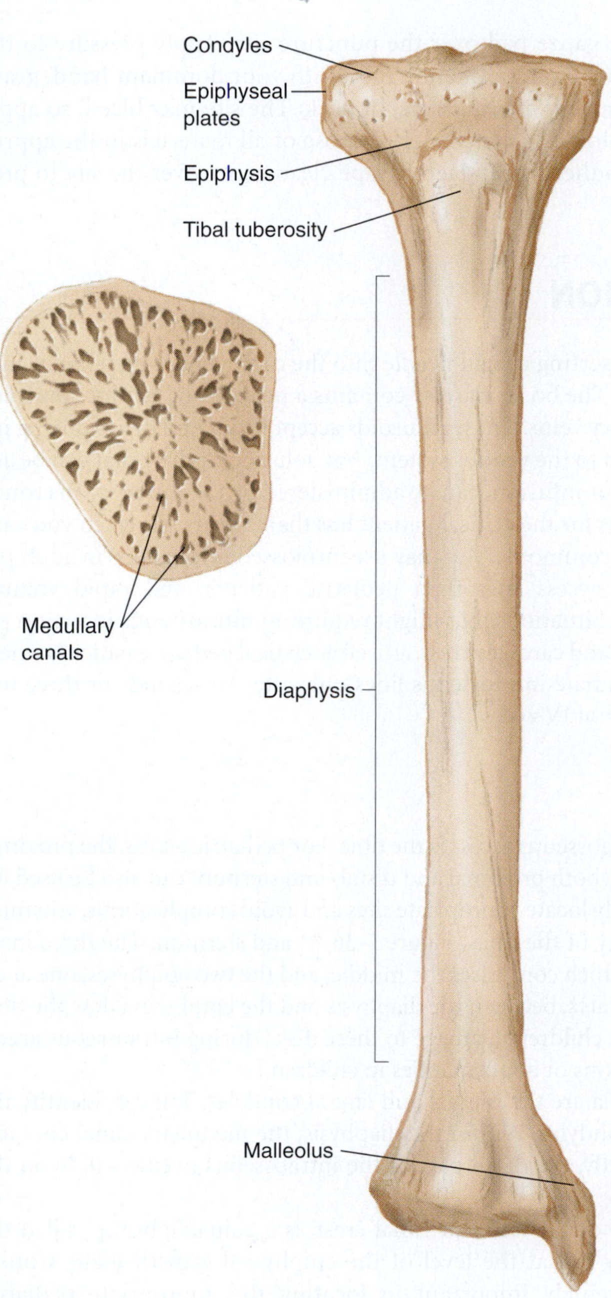

trocar *a sharp, pointed instrument.*

with a sharp metal **trocar** inside (Figure 7-38 ■). The trocar gives strength for puncture and prevents occlusion during insertion. Upon placement, the trocar is removed. The intraosseous needle has a plastic handle for insertion and an adjustable plastic disk to stabilize the needle once it is in place. You will attach a 10-mL syringe containing 3 to 5 mL of sterile saline to the intraosseous needle. The syringe and saline are used similarly to IV access of the external jugular vein. A large-bore spinal needle with a trocar in place is an acceptable substitute for an intraosseous needle.

Other equipment for intraosseous placement is similar to that for a peripheral intravenous access line (fluid, administration tubing, tape, antiseptics, and gauze). A pressure infuser is often needed for IO fluid administration. Some IO devices require a specialized adapter for flushing or using a pressure infuser. Depending upon the specific intraosseous needle, you may need an adapter to connect the administration tubing and the needle.

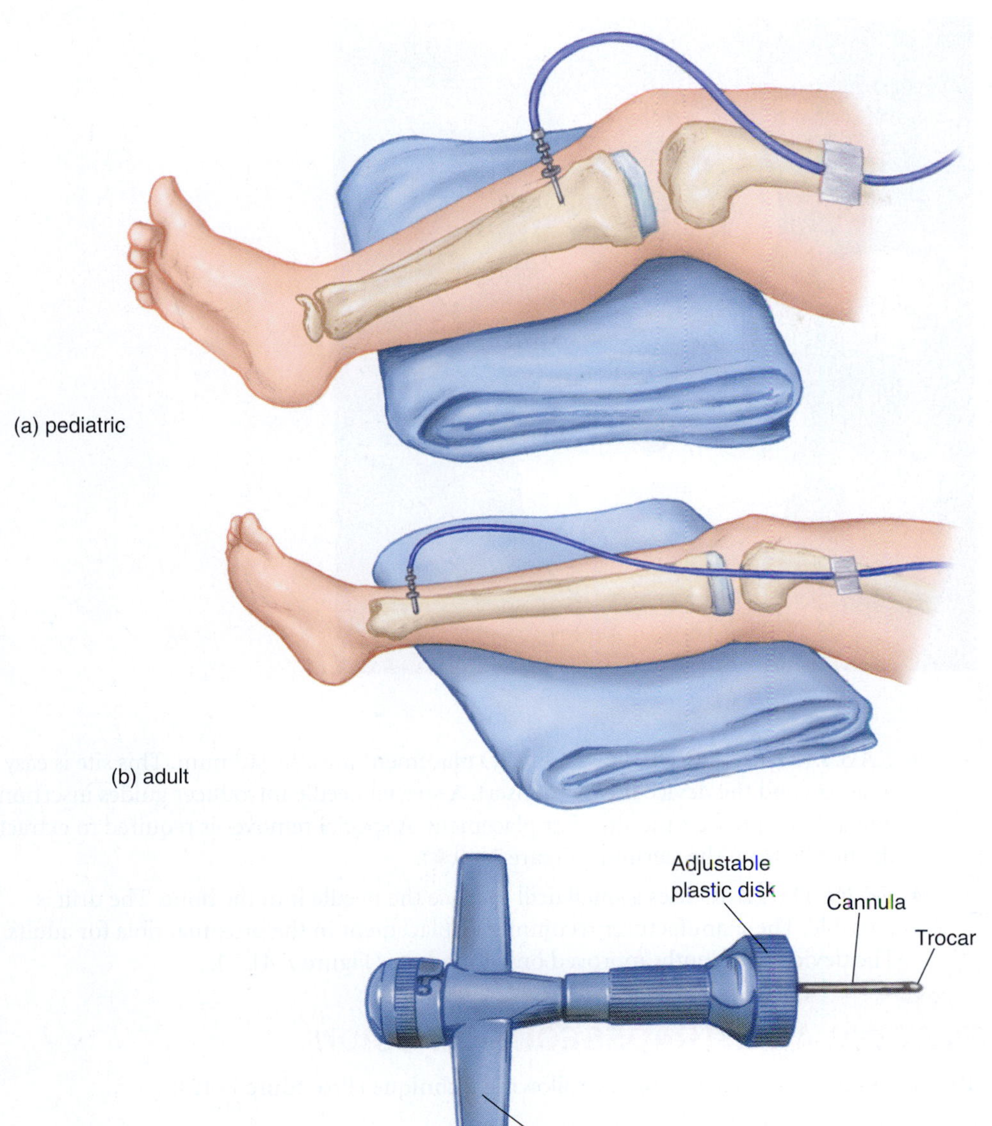

■ **Figure 7-37** Pediatric and adult intraosseous needle placement sites.

■ **Figure 7-38** Intraosseous needle.

Several commercial devices are available for both pediatric and adult intraosseous access. While these devices differ in their mechanism and location, they still must be placed through the cortex of a bone and into the marrow cavity where fluids and medications can be administered. Examples of commercial IO access devices include:

★ *Bone Injection Gun (B.I.G.).* The Bone Injection Gun (B.I.G.) was developed in Israel and is available in an adult and a pediatric model. (Figures 7-39 a and b ■).

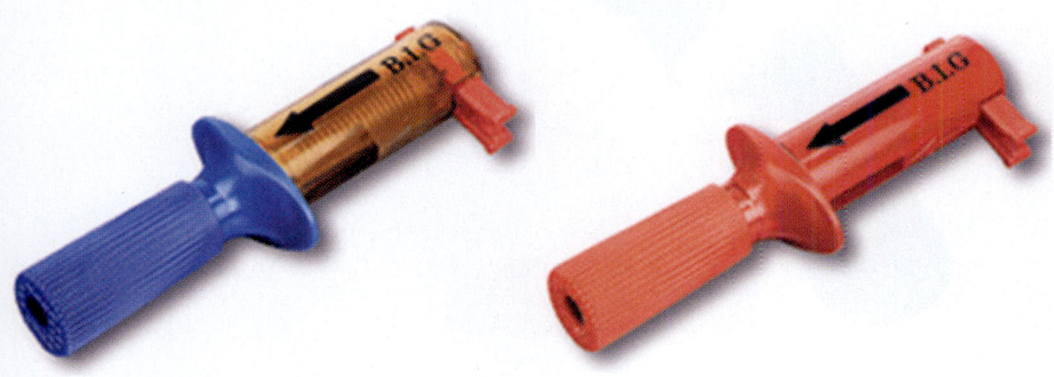

■ **Figure 7-39** The Bone Injection Gun (B.I.G.): (a) adult model (b) pediatric model. (*Both: WAISMed, Ltd.*)

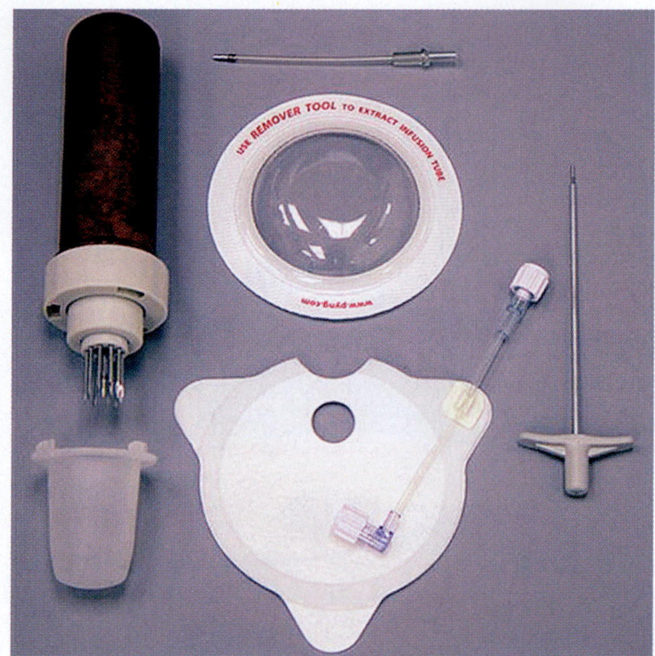

■ **Figure 7-40** The F.A.S.T.1 allows IO placement in the sternum of an adult. (*Pyng Technologies Corp.*)

- ★ *F.A.S.T.1.* The F.A.S.T.1 allows adult IO placement into the sternum. This site is easy to access and the device is easy to insert. A special needle introducer guides insertion, and a dome protects the site after placement. A special remover is required to extract the needle from the sternum (Figure 7-40 ■).
- ★ *EZ-IO.* The EZ-IO uses a small drill to place the needle into the bone. The drill is reusable. The manufacturer recommends placement in the proximal tibia for adults. The device is presently approved only for adults (Figure 7-41 ■).

PLACING AN INTRAOSSEOUS INFUSION

To place an intraosseous line use the following technique (Procedure 7–12):

1. Determine the indication for intraosseous access.
2. Assemble and check all equipment.
3. Position the patient. Rotate the leg toward the outside to expose the medial, proximal aspect of the tibia.

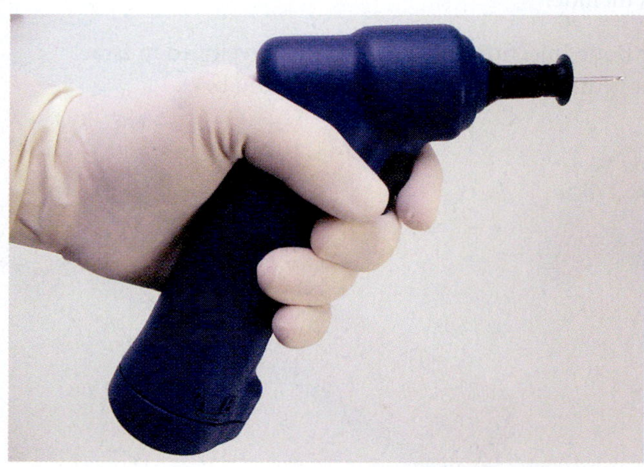

■ **Figure 7-41** The EZ-IO, which uses a small drill to place the needle into the bone, is presently approved only for adults. *(Vida-Care Corporation)*

Procedure 7-12 Intraosseous Medication Administration

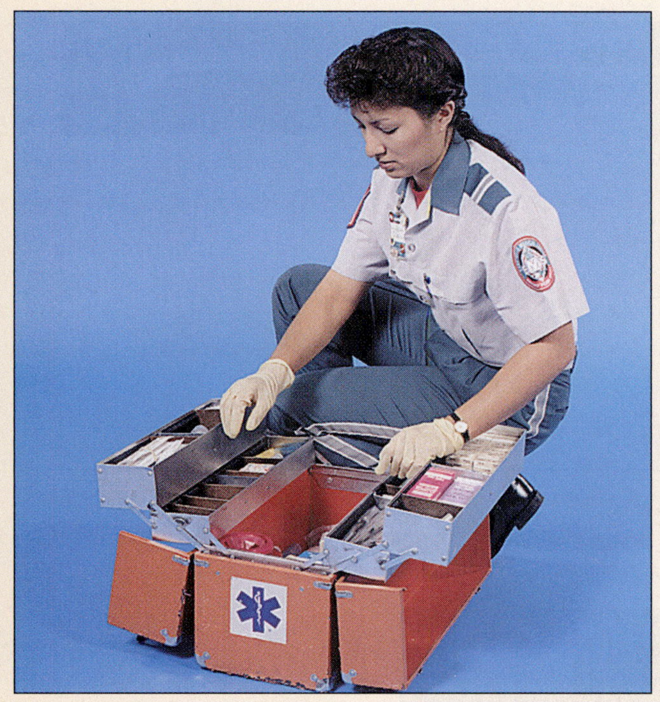

7-12a Select the medication and prepare the equipment.

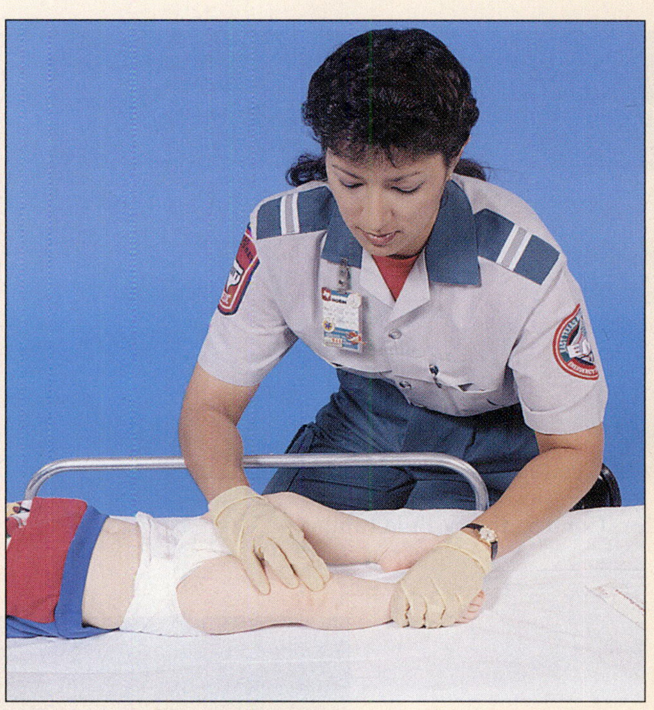

7-12b Palpate the puncture site and prep with an antiseptic solution.

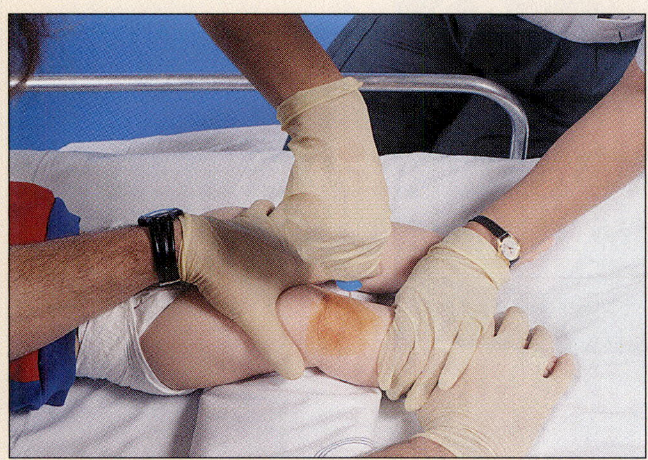

7-12c Make the puncture.

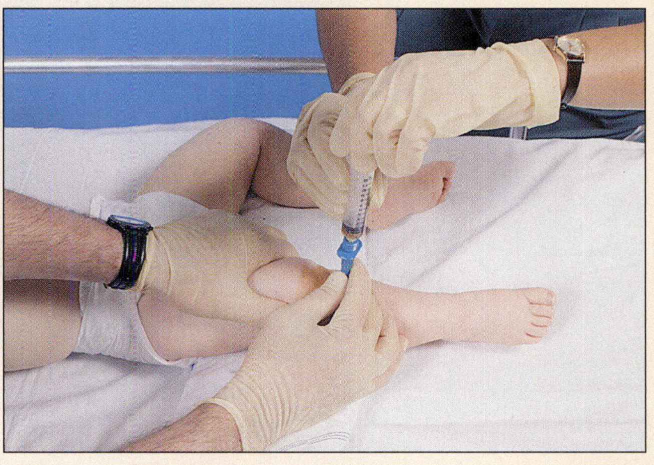

7-12d Aspirate to confirm proper placement.

continued on next page

Procedure 7-12 Intraosseous Medication Administration *(continued)*

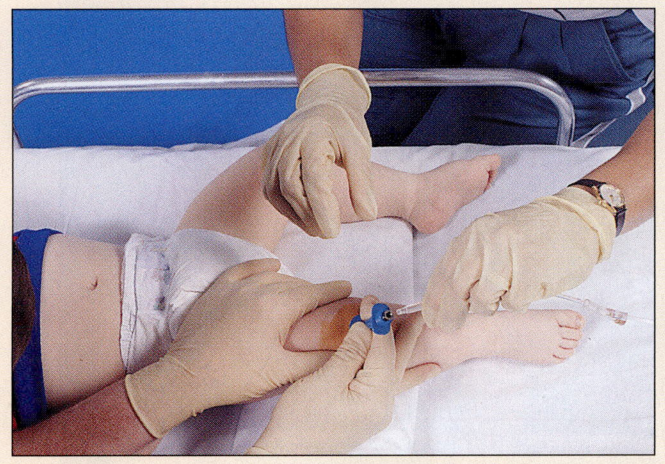

7-12e Connect the IV fluid tubing.

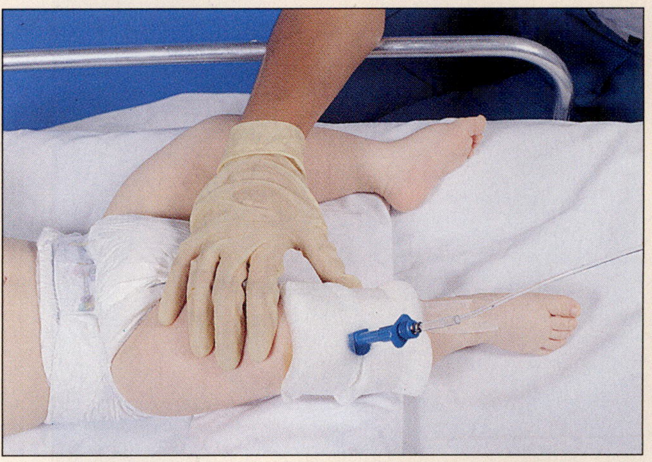

7-12f Secure the needle appropriately.

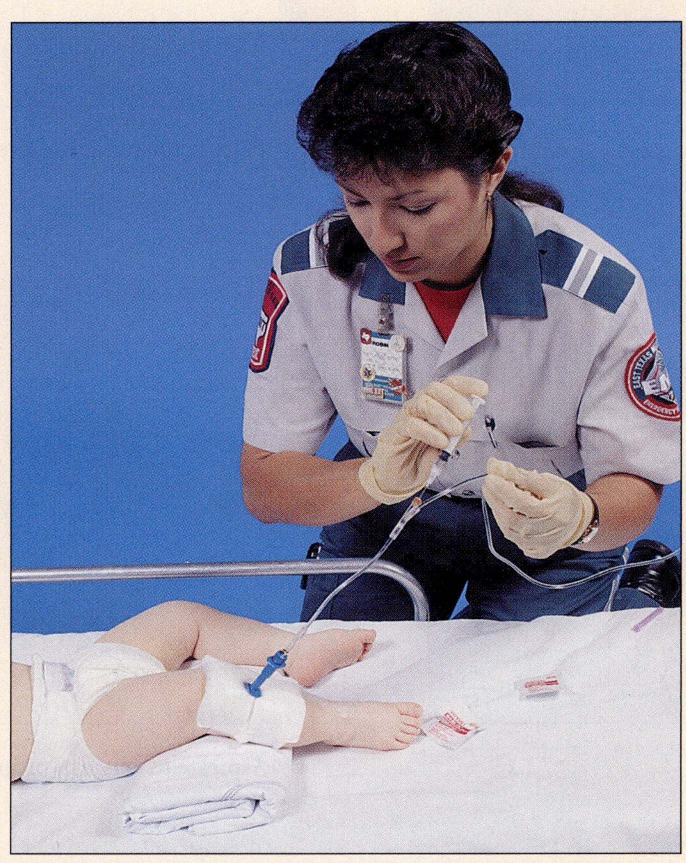

7-12g Administer the medication. Monitor the patient for effects.

4. Locate the access site. Palpate the tibia and use all landmarks.
   —*Pediatric.* Locate the tibial tuberosity. Move from one to two finger-breadths below the tibial tuberosity and find the flat expanse medial to the anterior tibial crest.
   —*Adult.* Find the medial malleolus. Move from one to two finger-breadths above the medial malleolus and locate the flat expanse medial to the anterior tibial crest.
5. Cleanse the site with alcohol or Betadine. Start at the puncture site and work outward in an expanding circular motion.
6. Perform the puncture. Holding the needle perpendicular to the puncture site, insert it with a twisting motion until you feel a decrease in resistance or a "pop." When this occurs, the needle is in the medullary canal. Do not advance it any further. Generally, you will need to insert the needle only 2 to 4 mm for entry.
7. Remove the trocar and attach the saline-filled syringe. Slowly pull back the plunger to attempt aspiration into the syringe. Easy aspiration of bone marrow and blood confirms correct medullary placement.
8. Once you have confirmed placement, rotate the plastic disk toward the skin to secure the needle.
9. Remove the syringe and attach the prepared administration tubing and solution. Set the appropriate flow rate.
10. Secure the needle as if securing an impaled object by surrounding it with bulky dressings and taping them securely in place. Commercial devices are available.
11. Periodically flush the needle to keep it patent.

Any solution or drug that can be administered by IV bolus or continuous infusion can also be delivered by the intraosseous route. Use the medicinal administration port on the primary administration tubing with the techniques as described under Intravenous Drug Administration.

When an intraosseous infusion is complete, shut down the secondary line with the flow regulator or a clamp. Open the primary line and adjust it to the indicated drip rate. Remove the hypodermic needle from the medication administration port and properly dispose of all contents if the infusion has been exhausted.

INTRAOSSEOUS ACCESS COMPLICATIONS AND PRECAUTIONS

Intraosseous access poses serious potential complications similar to those of peripheral access: local infection, thrombophlebitis, air embolism, circulatory overload, and allergic reactions, plus the following:

- ★ *Fracture.* Too large a needle or too forceful an insertion can fracture the tibia, particularly in very young children.
- ★ *Infiltration.* Infiltration occurs when IV solution collects in the local tissues instead of in the intramedullary canal. Infiltration may occur if you run fluids through an incorrectly placed needle or if a fracture has occurred. An infusion that does not run freely or the formation of an edema at the puncture site indicates infiltration. If infiltration occurs, immediately discontinue infusion and restart on the other leg.
- ★ *Growth plate damage.* An improperly located puncture may damage the growth plate and result in long-term growth complications.
- ★ *Complete insertion.* To avoid complete puncture (needle passing through both sides of the tibia), stop advancing the needle once you feel the pop. If complete puncture occurs, remove the needle with a reverse twisting motion and start again on the other leg. Apply direct pressure and a sterile dressing over the site(s) for at least 5 minutes.
- ★ *Pulmonary embolism.* If bone, fat, or marrow particles make their way into the circulatory system, pulmonary embolism may result. Use proper technique and watch for signs associated with pulmonary embolism (sudden onset of chest pain or shortness of breath).

Review

Content

Intraosseous Access Complications

- Fracture
- Infiltration
- Growth plate damage
- Complete insertion
- Pulmonary embolism
- Infection

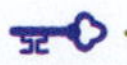

You must continually refresh your intraosseous access skills so that you can perform this technique properly when needed.

CONTRAINDICATIONS TO INTRAOSSEOUS PLACEMENT

Do not attempt intraosseous placement in the following situations:

- ★ Fracture to the tibia or femur on the side of access
- ★ Osteogenesis imperfecta—a congenital disease causing fragile bones
- ★ Osteoporosis
- ★ Establishment of a peripheral IV line

Part 3: Medical Mathematics

Proper drug administration requires basic mathematical proficiency. Because drug dosages are not always standardized, you may have to calculate amounts according to your patient's age, weight, or other medically related criteria. To properly prepare and administer medications, you must understand roman numerals and be proficient in multiplication, division, fractions, decimal fractions, proportions, and percentages. If you are deficient in one or more of these areas, refer to any text on basic and intermediate math.

Content Review

Fundamental Metric Units

- Grams—mass
- Meters—distance
- Liters—volume

METRIC SYSTEM

The metric system's three fundamental units are grams, meters, and liters. Prefixes denote values greater or less than the basic unit. Table 7–2 lists metric prefixes.

The most commonly used prefixes in pharmacology are *kilo-*, *centi-*, *milli-*, and *micro-*. The prefix *milli-* (*m*) refers to 1/1,000. Thus, a *milliliter* equals 1/1,000 of a liter. Similarly, a milligram is 1/1,000 of a gram. The prefix *micro-* expresses 1/1,000,000. A *microgram* is 1/1,000,000 of a gram.

CONVERSION BETWEEN PREFIXES

If you know the prefixes and their numeric equivalents, you can easily convert measurements to smaller or larger units. To convert a measurement to a smaller unit, multiply the original measurement by the numerical equivalent of the smaller measurement's prefix.

Example 1: Convert 3 grams to milligrams.

Milligrams (1/1,000) are smaller than grams; therefore, multiply 3 by 1,000:

$$3 \text{ (grams)} \times 1{,}000 \text{ (milli)} = 3{,}000$$

$$3 \text{ grams} = 3{,}000 \text{ milligrams}$$

Table 7–2 Metric Prefixes

Prefix	Multiplier	Abbreviation
kilo	1,000	(k)
hecto	100	(h)
deka	10	(D)
deci	1/10 or 0.1	(d)
centi	1/100 or 0.01	(c)
milli	1/1,000 or 0.001	(m)
micro	1/1,000,000 or 0.000001	(mcg or µg)

Example 2: Convert 2.67 liters to milliliters.

Milliliters (1/1,000) are smaller than a liter; therefore multiply 2.67 by 1,000:

2.67 liters × 1,000 (milli) = 2,670
2.67 liters = 2,670 milliliters

To convert a measurement to a larger unit, divide the original measurement by the numerical equivalent of the smaller measurement's prefix.

Example 3: Convert 1,600 micrograms to grams.

A microgram is 1/1,000,000 the size of a gram; therefore, divide 1,600 by 1,000,000:

1,600/1,000,000 = 0.0016 grams
1,600 micrograms = 0.0016 grams

When converting a measurement to or from a prefix that is not the fundamental unit, first convert the *existing* measurement to the *fundamental* measurement. Then convert the fundamental measurement to the desired unit.

Example 4: Convert 5.6 milligrams to micrograms.

First, convert the 5.6 milligrams to grams:

5.6 milligrams/1,000 = 0.0056 grams (g)
5.6 milligrams = 0.0056 grams

Now, convert 0.0056 grams to micrograms as previously described:

0.0056 (grams) × 1,000,000 = 5,600 micrograms
5.6 milligrams = 5,600 micrograms

For the beginner, this technique avoids confusion. The more experienced provider will be able to make a direct conversion from milligrams to micrograms.

HOUSEHOLD AND APOTHECARY SYSTEMS OF MEASURE

In the past, pharmacology traditionally used the household and apothecary systems to measure drug dosages. Gradually, the metric system has replaced those systems, but you may occasionally encounter their remnants. Table 7–3 gives the metric equivalents of the household and apothecary units you will most likely confront.

WEIGHT CONVERSION

Some medications' dosages are calculated according to kilograms of body weight. To convert pounds to kilograms use the following formula:

kilograms = pounds/2.2

Table 7–3 Metric Equivalents

Household	Apothecary	Metric
1 gallon	4 quarts	3.785 liters
1 quart	1 quart	0.946 liters
16 ounces	approximately 1 pint	473 milliliters
1 cup	approximately 1/2 pint	approximately 250 milliliters
1 tablespoon		approximately 16 milliliters
1 teaspoon		approximately 4–5 milliliters

Example 5: How many kilograms does a 182 lb person weigh?

kilograms = 182 lbs/2.2
kilograms = 82.7

TEMPERATURE

The international thermometric scale measures temperature in degrees Celsius. While degrees Celsius is often cited interchangeably with degrees centigrade, the two scales are slightly different. For practical purposes, however, you can think of them both as dividing the interval between the freezing and boiling points of water into 100 equal parts, with 0° being the freezing point and 100° being the boiling point. The household measurement system, in contrast, divides the interval between the freezing and boiling points of water into 180 equal parts, with 32° being the freezing point and 212° being the boiling point. When taking a body temperature, use the following formulas to convert between degrees Fahrenheit and degrees Celsius:

$$°F = 9/5° C + 32$$
$$°C = 5/9 (° F - 32)$$

Example 6: Convert 98.2° F to °C

$$°C = 5/9 (98.2 - 32)$$
$$°C = 5/9 (66.2)$$
$$°C = 36.8$$
$$36.8° C = 98.2° F$$

Example 7: Convert 28.4° C to °F

$$°F = 9/5 (28.4) + 32$$
$$°F = 51.12 + 32$$
$$°F = 83.1$$
$$83.1° F = 28.4° C$$

Continually practice all mathematical conversions throughout your career in the emergency medical services.

Converting between the different prefixes and between different systems of measurement is crucial in calculating drug dosages. You should continually practice all conversions, not only during your formal education but throughout your career in the emergency medical services.

UNITS

unit *predetermined amount of medication or fluid.*

Some medications are measured in **units.** Penicillin, heparin, and insulin are administered in units. Units do not convert between the metric, household, and apothecary systems.

MEDICAL CALCULATIONS

Frequently you will have to apply basic mathematical principles to calculate specific quantities before administering medications and fluids. In prehospital care, the following forms of medications often require calculation:

- ★ Oral medications
- ★ Liquid parenteral medications
- ★ Intravenous fluid administration
- ★ Intravenous medication infusions

stock solution *standard concentration of routinely used medications.*

Most medications are provided in **stock solution.** Therefore, you must calculate the exact amount of medication to remove from the stock for administration. To calculate basic drug dosage, you will need three facts:

- ★ Desired dose
- ★ Dosage on hand
- ★ Volume on hand

DESIRED DOSE

The **desired dose** is the specific quantity of medication needed. Most dosages are expressed as a weight (grams, milligrams, or micrograms). Dosages may be standard or calculated according to body weight or age.

desired dose *specific quantity of medication needed.*

DOSAGE AND VOLUME ON HAND

All liquid medications are packaged as concentrations. ***Concentration*** refers to weight per volume. A liquid medication's concentration is the drug's weight (grams, milligrams, or micrograms) per volume of liquid (mL) in which it is dissolved. For example, 50 percent dextrose (D_{50}) is packaged as a concentration of 25 grams (weight) dextrose in 50 mL (volume) of water. From the concentration, you can determine the **dosage on hand** (weight) and the **volume on hand.** For 50 percent dextrose, the dosage on hand is 25 grams and the volume on hand is 50 mL. Concentrations are identified on all drug packaging and labels.

concentration *weight per volume.*

dosage on hand *the amount of drug available in a solution.*

volume on hand *the available amount of solution containing a medication.*

Because you cannot see the desired dose dissolved in liquid, you must convert its weight to volume, a readily visible measurement, using the following formula:

$$\text{Volume to be administered} = \frac{\text{Volume on hand (desired dose)}}{\text{Dosage on hand}}$$

To use this formula, you must express all weight and volume measurements with the same metric prefix. For example, if the desired dose is expressed in *milli*grams, the dosage on hand must also be expressed in *milli*grams, volume on hand in *milli*liters.

CALCULATING DOSAGES FOR ORAL MEDICATIONS

The following example illustrates how to calculate the volume of a specific drug dosage:

> **Example 1:** A physician orders you to administer 90 mg of acetaminophen to a pediatric patient. The liquid acetaminophen is packaged as a concentration of 500 mg in 8 mL of solution. How much of the medication will you administer?

Because you cannot see the 90 mg of acetaminophen, you must convert this weight to a volume. To do so you need these facts:

$$\text{Desired dose} = 90\text{ mg}$$
$$\text{Dosage on hand} = 500\text{ mg}$$
$$\text{Volume on hand} = 8\text{ mL}$$

Use the formula to calculate the dosage's volume:

$$\text{Volume to be administered} = \frac{\text{Volume on hand (8 mL)} \times \text{Desired dose (90 mg)}}{\text{Dosage on hand (500 mg)}}$$
$$\text{Volume to be administered} = (8 \times 90)/500$$
$$\text{Volume to be administered} = 720/500$$
$$\text{Volume to be administered} = 1.44$$

Administer 1.44 mL of solution to deliver 90 mg of acetaminophen.

Another way to calculate drug dosages is the ratio (fraction) and proportion method. A ratio (fraction) illustrates a relationship between two numbers. A proportion is the comparison of two numerically equivalent ratios. Using the variable *x*, the previous problem can be stated:

$$8\text{ mL}/500\text{ mg} = x\text{ mL}/90\text{ mg}$$

To solve the problem, cross-multiply the numerals:

$$8/500 = x/90$$
$$720/500 = x$$
$$1.44 = x$$
$$x = 1.44\text{ mL}$$

Math Summary 1

$$x\text{ mL} = \frac{8\text{ mL} \times 90\text{ mg}}{500\text{ mg}}$$
$$x\text{ mL} = \frac{720}{500}$$
$$x\text{ mL} = 1.44$$

Math Summary 2

$$\frac{8\text{ mL}}{500\text{ mg}} = \frac{x\text{ mL}}{90\text{ mg}}$$
$$x\text{ mL} = \frac{720}{500}$$
$$x = 1.44\text{ mL}$$

CONVERTING PREFIXES

The following example shows how to calculate the volume to be administered when the desired dose, the dosage on hand, and the volume on hand are not all expressed in metric units with the same prefix.

> **Example 2:** A physician orders you to give 250 mg of a drug via IV bolus. The multidose vial contains 2 grams of the drug in 10 mL of solution. How much of the medication should you administer?

Because the desired dose is expressed as *milli*grams, the dosage on hand must be converted from grams to milligrams. In the metric system, 2 grams equal 2,000 milligrams. You now know:

$$\text{Desired dose} = 250 \text{ mg}$$

$$\text{Dosage on hand} = 2{,}000 \text{ mg}$$

$$\text{Volume on hand} = 10 \text{ mL}$$

Now you can use the formula to calculate the volume to be administered:

$$\text{Volume to be administered} = \frac{\text{Volume on hand (10 ml)} \times \text{Desired dose (250 mg)}}{\text{Dosage on hand (2,000 mg)}}$$

$$\text{Volume to be administered} = (10 \times 250)/2{,}000$$

$$\text{Volume to be administered} = 2{,}500/2{,}000$$

$$\text{Volume to be administered} = 1.25$$

Administer 1.25 mL of solution to deliver 250 mg of medication.

You can also solve this problem using the ratio proportion as follows:

$$10 \text{ mL}/2{,}000 \text{ mg} = x \text{ mL}/250 \text{ mg}$$

$$2{,}500 = 2{,}000\,x$$

$$2{,}500/2{,}000 = x$$

$$1.25 = x$$

$$x = 1.25 \text{ mL}$$

Math Summary 3

$$x \text{ mL} = \frac{10 \text{ mL} \times 250 \text{ mg}}{2{,}000 \text{ mg}}$$

$$x \text{ mL} = \frac{2{,}500}{2{,}000}$$

$$x \text{ mL} = 1.25$$

Math Summary 4

$$\frac{10 \text{ mL}}{2{,}000 \text{ mg}} = \frac{x \text{ mL}}{250 \text{ mg}}$$

$$x \text{ mL} = \frac{2{,}500}{2{,}000}$$

$$x = 1.25 \text{ mL}$$

Tablets also come in stock doses. If the dosage of one tablet or pill is more than needed, divide the tablet or pill to make the correct dose. Do not divide enteric or time-release capsules.

CALCULATING DOSAGES FOR PARENTERAL MEDICATIONS

You can use the same formula to calculate specific doses and volume for parenteral medication delivery.

> **Example 3:** A physician wants you to administer 5 milligrams of medication subcutaneously. The ampule contains 10 mg of the drug in 2 mL of solvent. How much medication should you use?

$$\text{Desired dose} = 5 \text{ mg}$$

$$\text{Dosage on hand} = 10 \text{ mg}$$

$$\text{Volume on hand} = 2 \text{ mL}$$

$$\text{Volume to be administered} = \frac{\text{Volume on hand (2 mL)} \times \text{Desired dose (5 mg)}}{\text{Dosage on hand (10 mg)}}$$

$$\text{Volume to be administered} = (2 \times 5)/10$$

$$\text{Volume to be administered} = 10/10$$

$$\text{Volume to be administered} = 1 \text{ mL}$$

A bullet may, however, open the chest wall or disrupt larger airways, thus permitting air to escape into the thorax (pneumothorax) or creating a valvelike defect that results in accumulating pressure within the chest (tension pneumothorax). Bullet wounds only infrequently induce an open pneumothorax (sucking chest wound) because the entrance wound diameter is usually limited to the bullet caliber. Close-range shotgun blasts or explosive exit wounds may be large and cause significant disruption of the chest wall integrity. In these cases, a pneumothorax is a more likely outcome.

Suspect the possibility of pneumothorax when there has been a significant disruption of chest wall integrity.

BONE

In contrast to lung tissue, bone is some of the body's densest, most rigid, and nonelastic tissue. When struck by a projectile or its associated pressure wave, bone resists displacement until it fractures, often into numerous pieces. These bone fragments then may distribute the impact energy to surrounding tissue. The projectile's contact with bone may also significantly alter the projectile's path through the body.

GENERAL BODY REGIONS

Several body regions deserve special attention regarding projectile wounds. They include the extremities, abdomen, thorax, neck, and head (Figure 18-13 ■). A projectile's passage also has a special effect on the first and last tissue contacted, the sites of the entrance and the exit wounds.

Content Review

Body Regions Deserving Special Attention with Penetrating Trauma

- Extremities
- Abdomen
- Thorax
- Neck
- Head

Extremities

The extremities consist of skin covering muscles and surrounding large long bones. An extremity injury may be debilitating but does not immediately threaten life unless there is severe hemorrhage associated with it. The severity of injury is limited by the resiliency of the skin and muscle, although if the bone is involved, the degree of soft tissue damage may be increased. In recent military experience, extremity injuries account for between 60 and 80 percent of injuries yet result in less than

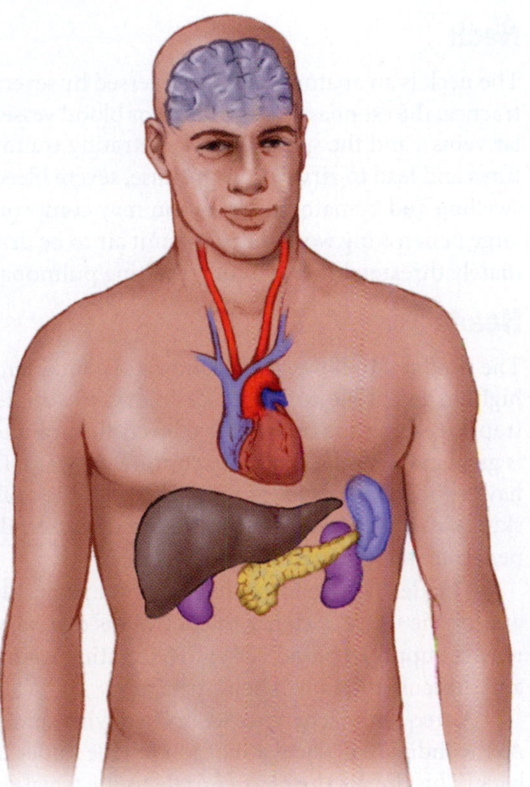

■ Figure 18-13 Critical structures in which the seriousness of a bullet's impact is increased include the brain, great vessels, heart, liver, kidneys, and pancreas.

Some 90 percent of penetrating trauma mortality involves the head, thorax, and abdomen.

10 percent of fatalities. The remaining 20 to 40 percent of penetrating injuries are divided among wounds of the abdomen, thorax, and head and account for more than 90 percent of mortality.

Abdomen

The abdomen (including the pelvic cavity) is the largest body cavity and contains most of the human organs. The area is not well protected by skeletal structures other than the upper pelvic ring, the lower rib cage border, and the lumbar vertebral column. The passage of a projectile through the abdominal cavity can produce a significant cavitational wave. The major occupant of the cavity, the bowel, is very tolerant of compression and stretching, but the liver, spleen, kidneys, and pancreas are highly susceptible to injury and hemorrhage. Since these organs occupy the upper abdominal quadrants, you should consider any penetrating projectile injury to this area to be serious and to have the potential to cause severe internal hemorrhage. Serious consequences should also be anticipated with injuries to the abdominal aorta and inferior vena cava, which are located along the spinal column in the posterior and central abdomen.

Consider any penetrating projectile injury to the abdomen to be serious and to have the potential to cause severe internal hemorrhage.

If a projectile perforates the small or large bowel, those organs may spill their contents into the abdominal cavity. This spillage results in serious peritoneal irritation due to chemical action or infection, although the signs and symptoms take some time to develop. If the injury process disrupts the blood vessels, the free blood will result in only limited abdominal irritation.

Thorax

Within the chest is a cavity formed by the ribs, spine, sternum, clavicles, and the diaphragm's strong muscle. This thoracic cavity houses the lungs, heart, and major blood vessels as well as the esophagus and part of the trachea. The impact of a bullet with the ribs may induce an explosive energy exchange that injures the surrounding tissue with numerous bony fragments. Lung tissue can absorb much of the cavitational energy while sustaining limited injury itself. However, the heart and great vessels, as fluid-filled containers, may suffer greatly from the energy of the bullet's passage. The damage to these structures and the associated massive hemorrhage may cause almost instant death. Because of the pressure-driven dynamics of respiration, any large chest wound may compromise breathing. Air may pass through a wound instead of the normal airway (pneumothorax) or may build up under pressure within the chest wall (tension pneumothorax).

Neck

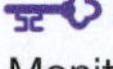
Monitor the airway closely in any patient with a penetrating wound to the neck.

The neck is an anatomical area traversed by several critical structures. These include the larynx, the trachea, the esophagus, several major blood vessels (the carotid and vertebral arteries and the jugular veins), and the spinal cord. Penetrating trauma in this area is very likely to damage vital structures and lead to airway compromise, severe bleeding, and/or neurological dysfunction. Associated swelling and hematoma formation may compromise circulation and the airway. Additionally, any large penetrating wound may permit air to be drawn into an open external jugular vein and immediately threaten life due to the resulting pulmonary emboli.

Head

Bullet wounds to the head, particularly those that penetrate the skull, are especially lethal.

The skull is a hollow, strong, and rigid container, housing the brain's delicate semisolid tissue. It is highly susceptible to projectile injury. If a bullet penetrates the skull, its cavitational energy is trapped within the cavity and subjects the brain to extreme pressures. If the released kinetic energy is great enough, the skull may rupture outward. In some cases, a bullet may enter the skull and not have enough energy to exit; in such a case, the bullet may continue to travel along the interior of the skull, disrupting more and more brain matter. Bullet wounds to the head, particularly those that penetrate the skull, are especially lethal.

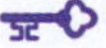
Suspect the possibility of airway compromise in patients with projectile wounds to the head and face.

The destructive forces released by a projectile wound to the head may also disrupt the airway and/or the victim's ability to control his own airway. The head and face are also areas with an extensive supply of blood vessels. Penetrating trauma may damage these vessels and result in serious and difficult-to-control hemorrhage.

A frequent occurrence associated with suicide attempts is severe damage to the facial region. As the individual places a shotgun or rifle under the chin and pulls the trigger, the head tilts up and back. This directs the blast entirely to the facial region, but the projectile(s) may not enter the cranium or strike any immediately life-threatening structures. There is, however, serious bleeding. The

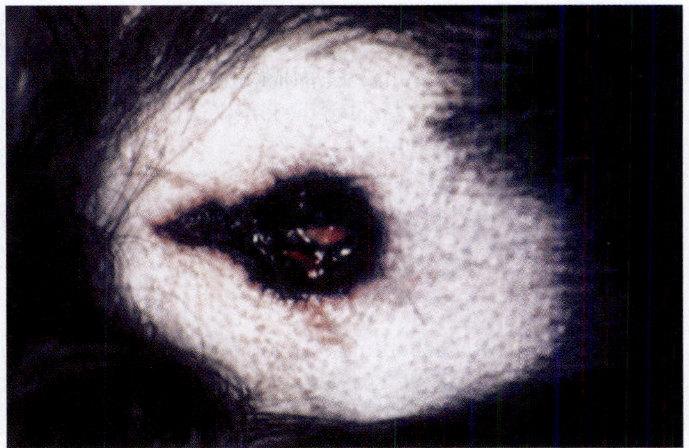

■ Figure 18-14 The entrance wound is often the same size as the projectile's profile and may demonstrate some bruising on the inner border of the wound. *(Hamilton County, NY Coroner's Office, Dorothy E. Dean, MD)*

bleeding and the associated damage can make the airway very hard to control. In these cases, use of an endotracheal tube to secure the airway can be difficult because many airway structures and landmarks are often obliterated by the blast.

Entrance Wound

Entrance wounds are usually the size of the bullet's profile. At this point, cavitational wave energy has not had time to develop and contribute to the wounding process (Figure 18-14 ■). The situation is different, however, with bullets that deform or tumble during flight. With these projectiles, the initial impact can be especially violent, producing a much larger and more disrupted entry wound than the caliber of the bullet alone would suggest.

Bullet entry wounds sustained at close range, a few feet or less, display special characteristics. Such wounds may be marked by elements of the barrel exhaust and bullet passage. Tattooing from the propellant residue may form a darkened circle or an oval (if the gun is held at an angle) around the entry wound and contaminate the wound itself. At the wound site, you may notice a small (usually 1- to 2-mm) ridge of discoloration around the entrance caused by the spinning bullet. If the gun barrel is held very close or against the skin as the weapon is fired, it may push the barrel exhaust into the wound producing subcutaneous emphysema (air within the skin's tissue) and crepitus to the touch. If the barrel is held a few inches from the skin, you may notice some burns caused by the hot gases of the barrel exhaust.

Exit Wound

The exit wound is caused by the physical damage from both the passage of the bullet itself and from the cavitational wave. Since the pressure wave is moving forward and outward, the wound may have a "blown outward" appearance. The exit wound may appear as stellate, referring to the tears radiating outward in a starlike fashion (Figure 18-15 ■). Because the cavitational wave has had time to develop,

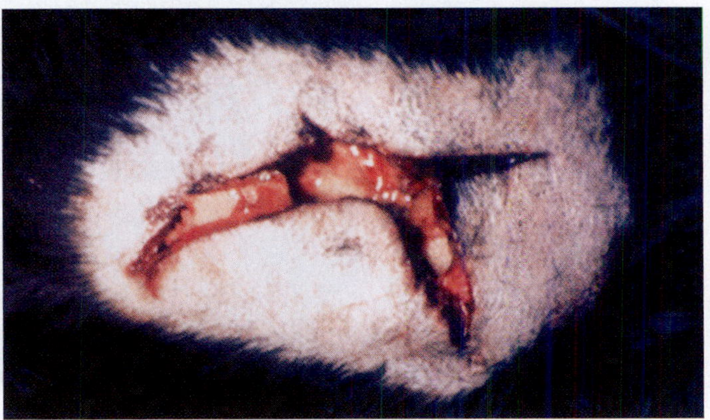

■ Figure 18-15 A bullet's exit wound often has a "blown outward" appearance, with stellate tears. *(Hamilton County, NY Coroner's Office, Dorothy E. Dean, MD)*

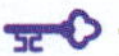

An exit wound may more accurately reflect the potential damage caused by a bullet's passage through the body than an entrance wound.

the exit wound may more accurately reflect the potential for damage caused by the bullet's passage than the entrance wound. If the bullet expends all its kinetic energy before it can exit the body, there is no exit wound and the bullet remains within the body. If the bullet does exit, the kinetic energy expended within the body is equal to the kinetic energy before impact minus the energy that remains in the bullet as it leaves the body.

SPECIAL CONCERNS WITH PENETRATING TRAUMA

SCENE SIZE-UP

In cases involving shootings or stabbings, always be sure that police have secured the scene before you enter it.

The scene size-up for a shooting or stabbing raises special concerns not associated with most other emergency care situations. The very nature of these injuries should suggest the possibility of danger from further violence and potential injury to you and your crew. Do not approach a shooting or stabbing scene unless and until law-enforcement personnel arrive and secure it and direct you to enter and provide care. If law enforcement personnel are not yet on the scene when you arrive, stage your vehicle at least a block away and out of sight of the scene. Once police or other law-enforcement personnel arrive, bring your vehicle closer to the scene but keep the police and their vehicles between you and the shooting or stabbing site. Wait there for the police to indicate that it is safe to approach the patient (Figure 18-16 ■).

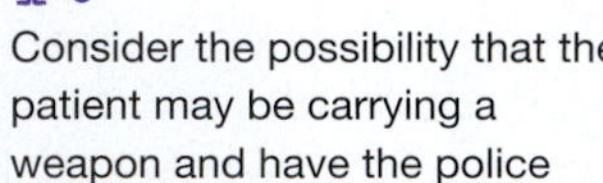

Consider the possibility that the patient may be carrying a weapon and have the police search him if necessary.

Once you reach the patient, survey carefully to determine that there are no weapons within the patient's reach. Consider the possibility that the victim may be carrying a knife or other weapon. If you have any doubts, request that the police search the victim for weapons before you begin to provide care.

As you carefully survey the scene of a shooting, try to reconstruct the event. Attempt to determine the victim's original position and his or her angle to and distance from the shooter. This helps you determine the angle at which the bullet entered the patient (which may not otherwise be revealed by the entrance wound) and whether the wound was received at point blank range or from a distance. Also try to determine the caliber of weapon and its type—handgun, rifle, or shotgun.

If the call involves a knifing injury, attempt to determine the gender and approximate weight of the attacker and the length of the blade. (You probably will not be able to determine the wound depth.) This information will help the emergency department determine the potential severity of the wound.

Make every effort to preserve evidence at a crime scene, but remember that care of the patient takes priority.

As you move on to your assessment of the patient, do all that you can to preserve the crime scene while providing any needed patient care. Disturb only those materials around the patient that you must move in order to render care. Cut around any bullet or knife holes in clothing and give the clothing to police for use as evidence. If there is ever any doubt about what to do, however, err on the side of providing patient care. (See Chapter 48, the section on "Crime Scene Awareness.") If

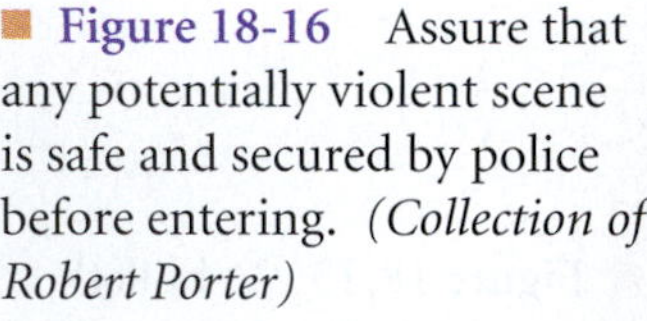

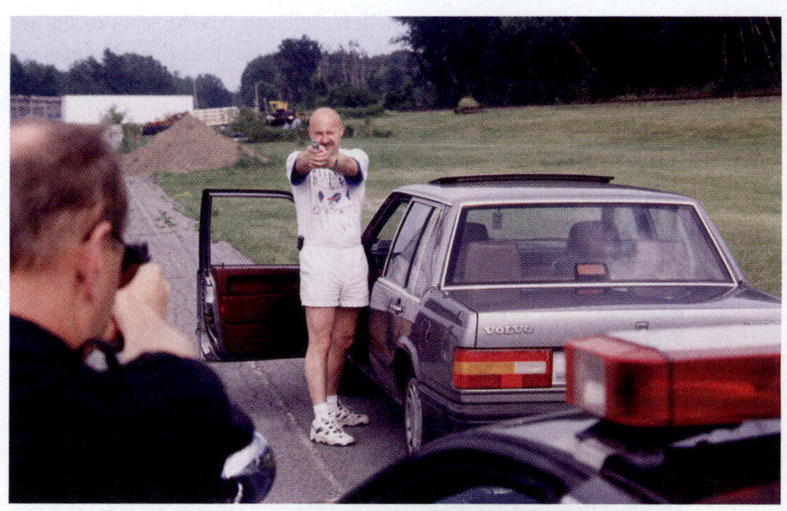

■ **Figure 18-16** Assure that any potentially violent scene is safe and secured by police before entering. *(Collection of Robert Porter)*

the victim is obviously dead, employ your jurisdiction's protocols for handling the body, but try to do so without disturbing evidence that may be crucial in determining what happened.

During assessment, you may identify an entrance or exit wound, but do not denote it in your report since an erroneous identification may confound the crime investigation.

PENETRATING WOUND ASSESSMENT

When assessing the victim of penetrating trauma, try to determine the pathway of the penetrating object and the organs that may have been affected by the wounding process. Anticipate the impact of potential organ injury and use this determination in setting priorities for on-scene care or rapid transport of the victim. Remember, however, that a bullet may not travel in a straight line between entrance and exit wounds. Often, a very small shift in a bullet's pathway may mean the difference between tearing open a large blood vessel or missing critical organs completely. The human body is also a dynamic place. The diaphragm moves the kidneys, pancreas, liver, spleen, and heart during respirations, so whether or not these organs are injured may be somewhat dependent on the phase of respiration in which the injury occurs.

It is often hard to anticipate the severity of a projectile wound. Injuries to the large blood vessels, heart, and brain may be immediately or rapidly fatal, while injuries to solid organs (liver, pancreas, kidneys, or spleen) may also be deadly but take more time in working their effects. Consequently, always suspect the worst with bullet wounds that involve the head, chest, or abdomen. Provide rapid transport in these cases, and treat shock aggressively.

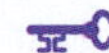

Provide rapid transport for patients with bullet wounds to the head, chest, or abdomen and treat aggressively for shock.

PENETRATING WOUND CARE

Certain penetrating wounds need special attention. These include wounds of the face and chest and those involving impaled objects. Their care is described in the following sections; care for other penetrating injuries and shock is discussed in later chapters.

If endotracheal intubation cannot be accomplished in a patient whose airway landmarks have been destroyed by a gunshot wound, emergency cricothyrotomy or cricothyrostomy may be necessary to create a route for ventilations.

Facial Wounds

Some facial gunshot wounds destroy many airway landmarks (Figure 18-17 ■). With wounds like these, endotracheal intubation is extremely difficult. You might find it helpful to visualize the larynx with the laryngoscope while another rescuer gently presses on the chest. Look for any bubbling during the chest compression, and try to pass the endotracheal tube through the bubbling tissue. Then, very carefully assure that the endotracheal tube is properly placed in the trachea and that lung ventilation is adequate. Capnography can be very helpful here.

If this approach is not effective, two related techniques may restore the airway, at least for long enough to reach more definitive care. These techniques are the **cricothyrotomy** and the **cricothyrostomy.** These emergency surgical or needle airway procedures perforate the membrane between the thyroid and cricoid cartilages, providing a route for ventilation directly into the lower airway. (These techniques are discussed in detail in Chapter 23, "Head, Facial, and Neck Trauma.")

cricothyrotomy *a surgical incision into the cricothyroid membrane, usually to provide an emergency airway.*

cricothyrostomy *the introduction of a needle or other tube into the cricothyroid membrane, usually to provide an emergency airway.*

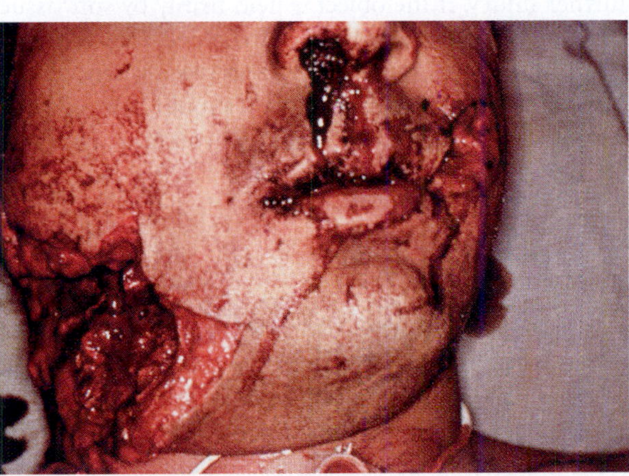

■ **Figure 18-17** Facial wounds may distort or destroy airway landmarks. *(Collection of Robert Porter)*

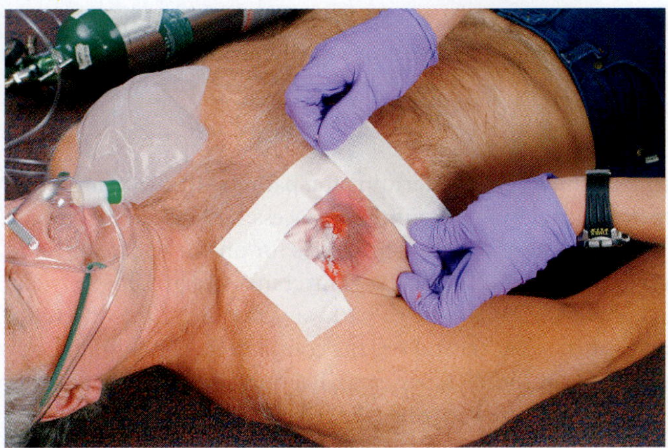

■ Figure 18-18 Seal open chest wounds and assure adequate respirations.

Chest Wounds

The chest wall is rather thick and resilient. It requires a large wound to create an opening big enough to permit free air movement through the chest wall, an open pneumothorax. Wounds caused by small-caliber handguns usually result in no air movement, while wounds caused by shotgun blasts and exiting high-velocity bullets more commonly cause such injuries. If frothy blood is associated with a chest wound, anticipate a developing tension pneumothorax, in which air builds up under pressure within the thorax. Remember, it takes pressure to push air through the wound and froth the blood. If you completely seal the chest wound, you may stop any outward air flow. This can increase both the speed of development of the tension pneumothorax and its severity. Cover any open chest wound with an occlusive dressing sealed on three sides (Figure 18-18 ■). If dyspnea is significant, assess for tension pneumothorax and perform needle decompression as indicated (see Chapter 25, "Thoracic Trauma").

Anticipate a developing tension pneumothorax if your assessment reveals frothy blood in a patient with a bullet wound to the chest.

Always consider the possibility of heart and great vessel damage with a penetrating chest wound. These injuries may lead rapidly to severe internal hemorrhage and death. Another serious complication of penetrating chest trauma is pericardial tamponade. This condition occurs when an object or projectile perforates the heart and permits blood to leak into the pericardial sac. As blood accumulates in the sac, the heart no longer fully fills with blood and circulation slows. If pericardial tamponade is uncorrected, the **prognosis** for the patient is very poor. However, a needle introduced into the pericardial space, a procedure available at the emergency department, can quickly alleviate the life threat. Therefore, if you suspect this condition, arrange for rapid transport. The assessment of pericardial tamponade is discussed in Chapter 25, "Thoracic Trauma."

prognosis *the anticipated outcome of a disease or injury.*

Impaled Objects

If an object that causes a low-velocity wound lodges in the body, removal of the object may be dangerous for the patient. If the object bent as it hit a bone upon entry, attempts at removal may cause further injury. If the object is held firmly by soft tissue, it may obstruct blood vessels, thereby restricting blood loss; removal of the object may then increase hemorrhage.

Immobilize impaled objects in place where and as they are found and transport the patient. The only impaled objects that you should remove are those lodged in the cheek or trachea that interfere with the airway or those that you must remove to provide CPR.

Immobilize impaled objects in place. Only remove those that have lodged in the cheek, interfere with the airway, or prevent CPR.

Summary

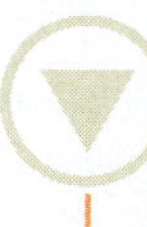

Penetrating injuries, especially those associated with gunshot wounds, are responsible for a high incidence of prehospital trauma and death. Your understanding of the mechanisms of injury that produce these wounds and an understanding of the types of injuries caused by these mechanisms (index of suspicion) can help you rapidly identify serious life threats and assure these patients receive rapid transport to a trauma center. Special prehospital care techniques such as sealing an open pneumothorax and managing a difficult airway can also help you stabilize the patient in the field and help assure that he safely reaches definitive care.

Review Questions

1. The tissue displacement caused by the pressure wave that accompanies a bullet as it travels through human tissue is called:
   a. drag.
   b. cavitation.
   c. trajectory.
   d. ballistics.
2. Which of the following would you expect to cause the greatest cavitation?
   a. arrow
   b. ice pick
   c. rifle bullet
   d. handgun bullet
3. Which of the following is considered a high-velocity weapon?
   a. arrow
   b. rifle
   c. shotgun
   d. handgun
4. The characteristics of a bullet determine how much damage it creates as it strikes its target. Which of the following would create the most damage?
   a. a bullet that does not tumble
   b. a bullet that mushrooms when it hits
   c. a small-profile bullet
   d. a full-metal-jacket bullet
5. Which of the following abdominal organs is the most tolerant of the cavitational wave associated with penetrating trauma?
   a. liver
   b. bowel
   c. spleen
   d. kidneys
6. In a puncture wound resulting from a knife or gunshot injury, the paramedic must always examine the patient for:
   a. an exit wound.
   b. epistaxis.
   c. powder burns.
   d. tattooing.
7. Powder burns and crepitus around the entrance generally suggest:
   a. a gun used at close range.
   b. a high-powered rifle.
   c. a handgun.
   d. the use of a black powder.
8. Penetrating trauma is dangerous when it involves the neck because it may cause problems with:
   a. severe hemorrhage.
   b. the airway.
   c. the cervical spine.
   d. all of the above

9. The path a bullet follows once it is fired is called:
   a. yaw.
   b. drag.
   c. caliber.
   d. trajectory.
10. The forces acting on a bullet to slow it down are called:
   a. yaw.
   b. drag.
   c. profile.
   d. caliber.

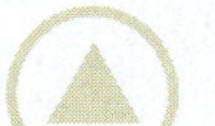

See Answers to Review Questions at the back of this book.

Chapter 19

Hemorrhage and Shock

Objectives

After reading this chapter, you should be able to:

1. Describe the epidemiology, including the morbidity/mortality and prevention strategies, for shock and hemorrhage. (pp. 829–831, 837–841)
2. Discuss the anatomy, physiology, and pathophysiology of the cardiovascular system. (see Chapters 3 and 4)
3. Define shock based on aerobic and anaerobic metabolism. (see Chapter 4)
4. Describe the body's physiological response to changes in blood volume, blood pressure, and perfusion. (pp. 837–841)
5. Describe the effects of decreased perfusion at the capillary level. (pp. 838–839)
6. Discuss the cellular ischemic, capillary stagnation, and capillary washout phases related to hemorrhagic shock. (pp. 838–839)
7. Discuss the various types and degrees of shock and hemorrhage. (pp. 829–831, 837–841)
8. Predict shock and hemorrhage based on mechanism of injury. (pp. 832, 841–842)
9. Identify the need for intervention and transport of the patient with hemorrhage or shock. (pp. 831–834, 841–843)
10. Discuss the assessment findings and management of internal and external hemorrhage and shock. (pp. 831–834, 841–843)
11. Differentiate between the administration rate and volume of IV fluid in patients with controlled versus uncontrolled hemorrhage. (pp. 844–846)
12. Relate pulse pressure and orthostatic vital sign changes to perfusion status. (pp. 834, 843)
13. Define and differentiate between compensated and decompensated hemorrhagic shock. (pp. 839–840)
14. Discuss the pathophysiological changes, assessment findings, and management associated with compensated and decompensated shock. (pp. 839–840)
15. Identify the need for intervention and transport of patients with compensated and decompensated shock. (pp. 841–849)
16. Differentiate among normotensive, hypotensive, or profoundly hypotensive patients. (pp. 841–849)

17. Describe differences in administration of intravenous fluid in the normotensive, hypotensive, or profoundly hypotensive patients. (pp. 844–846)
18. Discuss the physiologic changes associated with application and inflation of the pneumatic anti-shock garment (PASG). (pp. 846–847)
19. Discuss the indications and contraindications for the application and inflation of the PASG. (pp. 846–847)
20. Given several preprogrammed and moulaged hemorrhage and shock patients, provide the appropriate scene size-up, primary assessment, secondary assessment (rapid trauma or focused physical exam, detailed exam), and reassessments and provide appropriate patient care and transportation. (pp. 822–849)

Key Terms

aggregate, p. 824
anaerobic, p. 825
anemia, p. 829
catecholamine, p. 830
clotting, p. 823
coagulation, p. 824
compensated shock, p. 839
decompensated shock, p. 839
direct pressure, p. 825
epistaxis, p. 828
esophageal varices, p. 828
fascia, p. 826
fibrin, p. 824
hematochezia, p. 834
hematoma, p. 826
hemorrhage, p. 822
homeostasis, p. 822
hydrostatic pressure, p. 839
irreversible shock, p. 841
ischemia, p. 838
lactic acid, p. 825
melena, p. 828
metabolism, p. 838
orthostatic hypotension, p. 834
overdrive respiration, p. 844
platelet phase, p. 824
pneumatic anti-shock garment (PASG), p. 846
pulse pressure, p. 830
rouleaux, p. 839
shock, p. 822
tilt test, p. 834
tourniquet, p. 825
vascular phase, p. 823
washout, p. 839

hemorrhage *an abnormal internal or external discharge of blood.*

homeostasis *the natural tendency of the body to maintain a steady and normal internal environment.*

shock *a state of inadequate tissue perfusion.*

INTRODUCTION

The loss of the body's most important and dynamic medium, blood, is called **hemorrhage.** Acute and continuing loss of blood adversely impacts the body's ability to provide oxygen and essential nutrients to the cells, while at the same time removing carbon dioxide and other waste products from the body's elemental building blocks, the cells. In the absence of an adequate volume of circulating blood, the cells and the organs begin to function less effectively and can ultimately fail. If allowed to progress untreated, the organism itself may die. The transition between normal function (**homeostasis**) and death is called **shock.** The ability to recognize hemorrhage and shock and to care for these conditions are critical skills for the paramedic and are essential to reducing mortality and morbidity in trauma patients. This chapter provides you with an understanding of the cardiovascular system as it relates to hemorrhage and shock and then describes how to recognize and care for these life-threatening assaults on the human body.

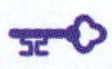

The paramedic must be able to recognize hemorrhage and shock in trauma patients in order to reduce mortality and morbidity.

HEMORRHAGE

As noted previously, hemorrhage is loss of blood from the closed vascular system because of injury to the blood vessels. Hemorrhage is usually classified based on the injured vessel from which it flows: capillary, venous, or arterial.

Content Review

Types of Hemorrhage

- Capillary
- Venous
- Arterial

Capillary hemorrhage generally oozes from the wound, normally an abrasion, and clots quickly on its own. The blood is usually bright red because it is well oxygenated.

Venous hemorrhage flows more quickly, though it, too, generally stops in a few minutes. Bleeding associated with venous hemorrhage is generally dark red because the blood has already given up its oxygen as it passes though the capillary beds.

Bleeding associated with arterial hemorrhage flows very rapidly, often spurting from the wound. This blood is well oxygenated and appears bright red as it escapes from the wound. The blood volume lost can be extreme because of the pressure behind arterial bleeding. The spurting nature of arterial hemorrhage results from the variations in the blood pressure driving the blood loss.

While it is convenient to determine the type of hemorrhage, the nature and depth of a wound may make it hard to differentiate between heavy venous and arterial bleeding. Internal hemorrhage cannot be classified by type with the diagnostic techniques available to paramedics providing prehospital care.

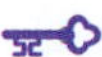

It may be hard to differentiate between heavy venous and arterial bleeding in the field; likewise, paramedics cannot classify internal hemorrhage by type when providing prehospital care.

clotting *the body's three-step response to stop the loss of blood.*

vascular phase *step in the clotting process in which smooth blood vessel muscle contracts, reducing the vessel lumen and the flow of blood through it.*

CLOTTING

The body's response to local hemorrhage is a complex three-step process called **clotting** (Figure 19-1 ■). As a blood vessel is torn and begins to lose blood, its smooth muscle contracts. This reduces its lumen and the volume and strength of blood flow through it. This is called the **vascular phase.**

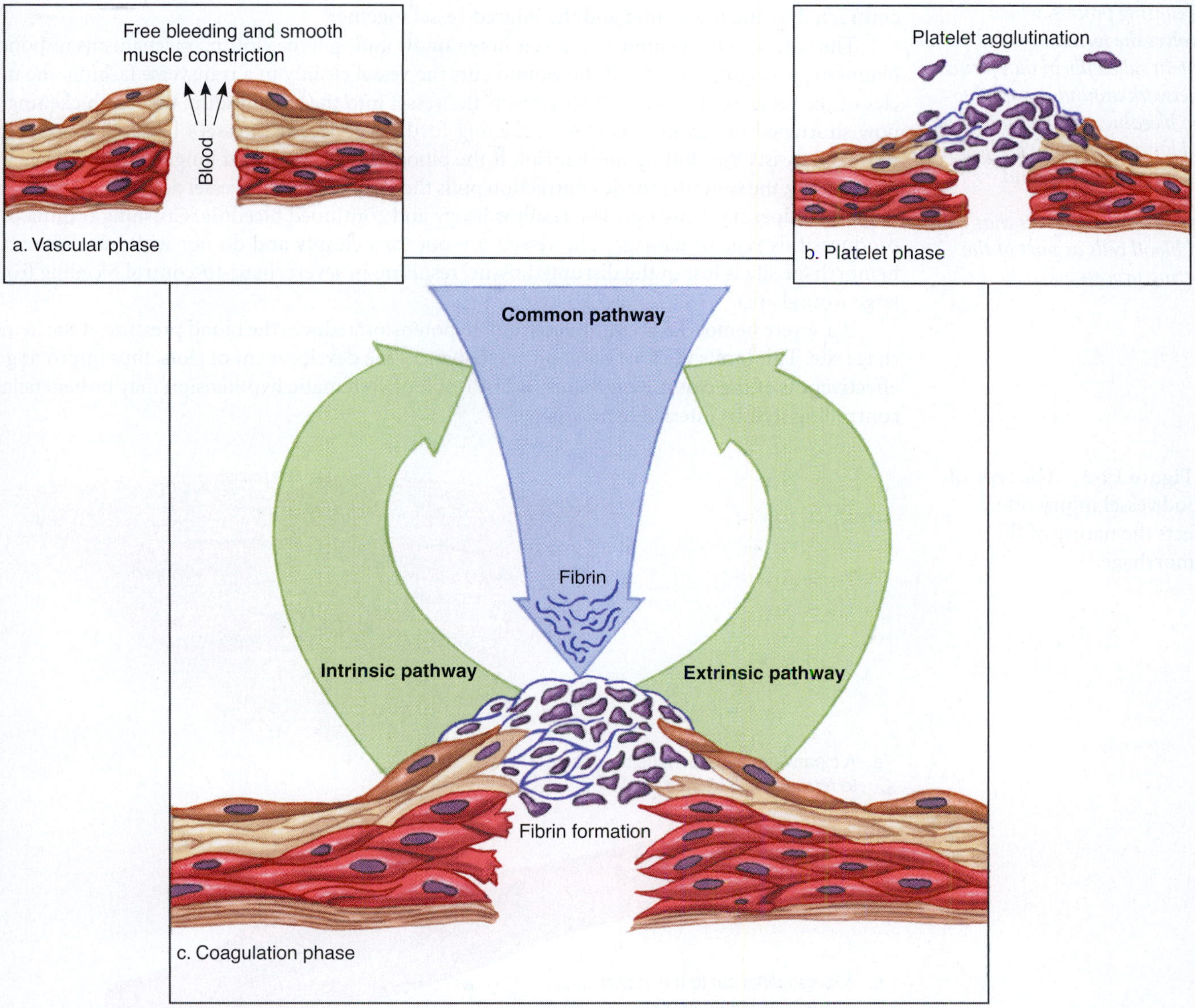

■ **Figure 19-1** The three steps of the clotting process are the vascular phase, the platelet phase, and coagulation.

Review

Content

Phases of the Clotting Process

- Vascular phase
- Platelet phase
- Coagulation

aggregate *to cluster or come together.*

platelet phase *second step in the clotting process in which platelets adhere to blood vessel walls and to each other.*

coagulation *the third step in the clotting process, which involves the formation of a protein called fibrin that forms a network around a wound to stop bleeding, ward off infection, and lay a foundation for healing and repair of the wound.*

fibrin *protein fibers that trap red blood cells as part of the clotting process.*

At the same time, the vessel's smooth interior lining (the tunica intima) is disrupted, causing a turbulent blood flow. The turbulent blood flow within the vessel attracts platelets. Factors released at the time of hemorrhage make the platelets "sticky," or adherent. Platelets then stick to collagen, a protein fiber found in connective tissue, on the vessel's injured inner surface, and to other injured tissue in the area. The blood vessel walls also become adherent. If they are small enough, like capillaries, they may stick together, further occluding blood flow. As platelets adhere to the vessel walls, they **aggregate,** or collect, other platelets. This is the **platelet phase,** the second step of the clotting process. These events occur almost immediately after injury and effectively halt hemorrhage from capillaries and small venous and arterial vessels. While this is a rapid method of hemorrhage control, the resulting clot is unstable.

As time passes, the wound initiates the third and final step of the process, **coagulation.** In this phase, clotting factors are activated and released into the bloodstream, initiating a complex sequence of events. These clotting factors come from the damaged blood vessel and surrounding tissue (the extrinsic pathway), from the damaged platelets (the intrinsic pathway), or from both. The release of the clotting factors triggers a series of chemical reactions that result in the formation of strong protein fibers, or **fibrin.** These fibers entrap red blood cells and form a stronger, more durable clot. This further collection of cells halts all but the most severe hemorrhage. Coagulation normally takes from 7 to 10 minutes. Over time, the cells trapped in the clot protein matrix slowly contract, drawing the wound and the injured vessel together.

The nature of the wound also affects how rapidly and well the clotting mechanisms respond to hemorrhage (Figure 19-2 ■). If the wound cuts the vessel cleanly in a transverse fashion, the muscles of the vessel wall contract. This retracts the vessel into the surrounding tissues, thickening the now shortened tunica media. This thickening further reduces the vessel's lumen, reduces blood flow, and assists the clotting mechanism. If the blood vessel is lacerated longitudinally rather than transversely, the smooth muscle contraction pulls the vessel open. The vessel does not withdraw and the lumen does not constrict. The result is heavy and continued bleeding. Crushing trauma often produces this type of damage. The vessels are not torn cleanly and do not withdraw. The actual hemorrhage site is lost in the disrupted tissue, resulting in severe, hard-to-control bleeding from a large wound area.

If a severe hemorrhage continues, frank hypotension reduces the blood pressure at the hemorrhage site. This limits the flow of blood and enhances the development of clots, thus improving the effectiveness of the clotting mechanism. The result of systematic hypotension may be beneficial in controlling serious internal hemorrhage.

■ **Figure 19-2** The type of blood vessel injury often affects the nature of the hemorrhage.

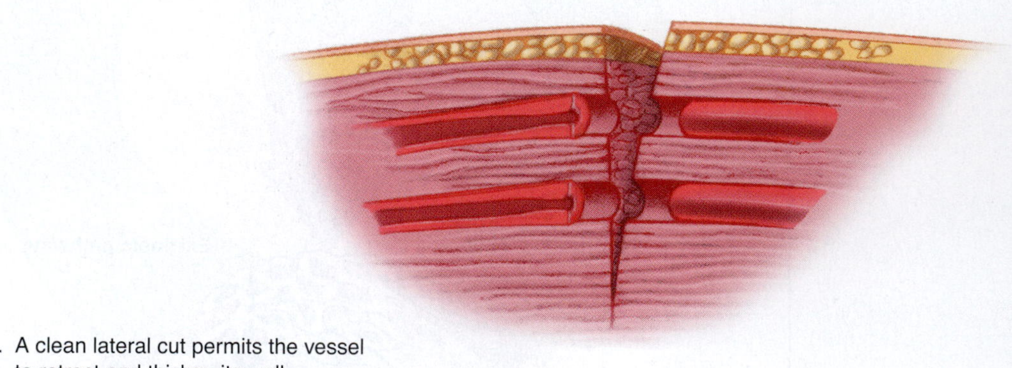

a. A clean lateral cut permits the vessel to retract and thicken its wall.

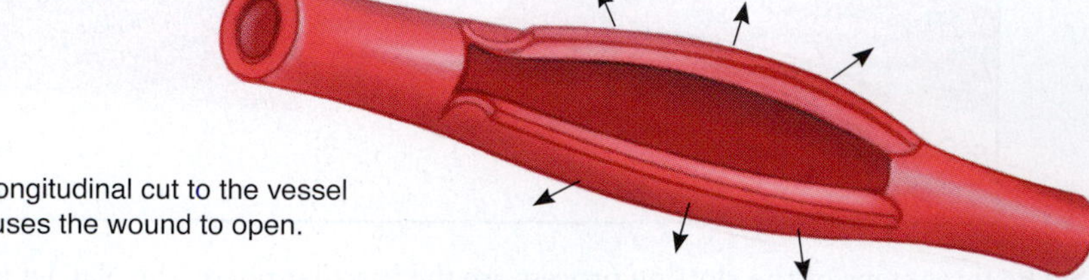

b. A longitudinal cut to the vessel causes the wound to open.

FACTORS AFFECTING THE CLOTTING PROCESS

The clotting process can be either helped or hindered by a variety of factors. For example, movement at or around the wound site, as in the manipulation of a fracture, may break the developing clot loose and disrupt the forming fibrin strands. For this reason, immediate wound immobilization (splinting) is beneficial.

Aggressive fluid therapy, which is sometimes provided in cases of severe hemorrhage, may adversely impact the effectiveness of clotting mechanisms. Aggressive fluid resuscitation may increase blood pressure, which in turn increases the pressure pushing against the developing clots. In addition, the water and salts used in fluid therapy dilute the clotting factors and platelets, further inhibiting the clotting process.

The patient's body temperature also has an effect on the clotting process. As the body temperature begins to fall, as it may in shock states, clot formation is neither as rapid nor as effective as when the body temperature is 37°C (98.6°F). Thus, it is important to keep a patient with severe hemorrhage warm.

Medications may interfere with the body's ability to form a clot and halt both internal and external hemorrhage. Aspirin modifies the enzymes on the surface of platelets that cause them to aggregate after an injury. Ibuprofen (Tylenol) and other NSAIDs (nonsteroidal anti-inflammatory drugs) may have a similar but temporary effect. Heparin and warfarin (Coumadin) interfere with the normal generation of protein fibers that produce a stable clot. While these drugs may prevent thrombosis and emboli in patients with heart disease, they may prolong or worsen hemorrhage when that patient is injured. Try to gather information on whether the patient uses such medications when taking the patient history.

Content Review

Factors Hindering the Clotting Process

- Movement of the wound site
- Aggressive fluid therapy
- Low body temperature
- Medications such as aspirin, heparin, or Coumadin

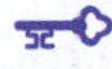

Immediate immobilization (splinting) of the wound site aids the clotting process.

HEMORRHAGE CONTROL

Hemorrhage is either internal or external. While there are a number of steps you can take to control external hemorrhage in the field, prehospital care of internal hemorrhage is more limited.

External Hemorrhage

External hemorrhage is easy to identify and care for. It presents with blood oozing, flowing, or spurting from the wound. Bleeding from capillary and venous wounds is easy to halt because the pressure driving it is limited (Figure 19-3 ■). Usually **direct pressure** on the wound or a combination of direct pressure and elevation work quite well in stopping the bleeding. Bleeding from an arterial wound, however, is powered by the arterial blood pressure and escapes from the blood vessel with significant force. The normal control and clotting mechanisms help reduce blood loss but do not stop it if the injured vessel is large. To stop bleeding from such a wound, pressure on the bleeding site must exceed the arterial pressure. Direct digital pressure on the site of blood loss, maintained by a dressing and pressure bandage, is most effective. Elevation of the wound area and use of pressure points may also be necessary if the bandage cannot apply enough pressure directly to the hemorrhage site.

Be extremely cautious if you consider using a **tourniquet.** Employ the device *only* to halt persistent, life-threatening hemorrhage. If you apply the tourniquet at a pressure less than the arterial pressure, blood continues to flow into the limb, while the tourniquet restricts venous flow out. The limb's arterial and venous pressures then rise, as does the rate of hemorrhage. If the tourniquet meets its objective and halts all blood flow to the limb, blood loss stops, but so does circulation to the distal extremity. During this absence of perfusion, **lactic acid,** potassium, and other **anaerobic** metabolites accumulate in the stagnant blood. When the tourniquet is released, the resumption of blood flow may transport these toxins into the central circulation with devastating results (Figure 19-4 ■). Once you apply the tourniquet, therefore, leave it in place until the patient is in the emergency department or some other facility where the negative effects of reperfusion can be addressed. If you must apply a tourniquet, use a wide cravat or belt or a blood pressure cuff. A thin or narrow constricting device may damage tissue beneath the tourniquet. Despite these hazards, the tourniquet may be essential in halting life-threatening arterial hemorrhage.

direct pressure *method of hemorrhage control that relies on the application of pressure to the actual site of the bleeding.*

Use a tourniquet only as a last resort to halt persistent, life-threatening hemorrhage.

tourniquet *a constrictor used on an extremity to apply circumferential pressure on all arteries to control bleeding.*

lactic acid *compound produced from pyruvic acid during anaerobic glycolyis.*

anaerobic *able to live without oxygen.*

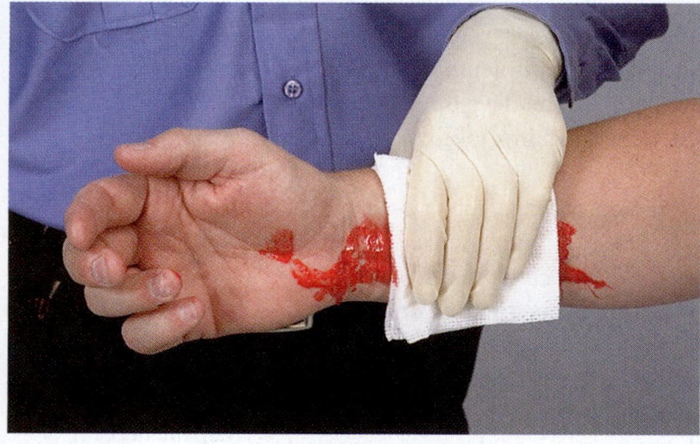

■ **Figure 19-3a** Hemorrhage control: apply direct pressure.

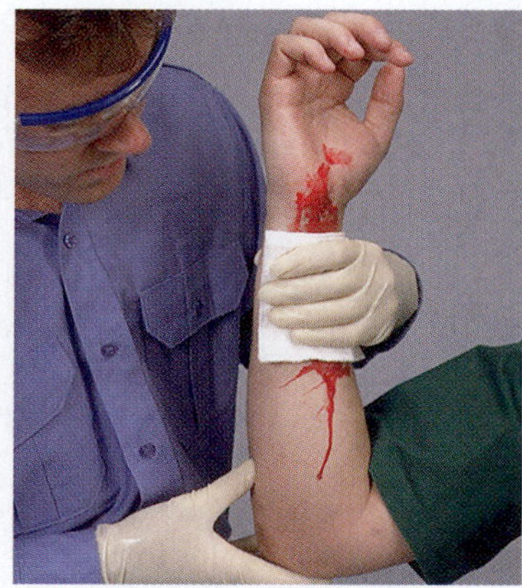

■ **Figure 19-3b** Hemorrhage control: elevate the extremity above the level of the heart.

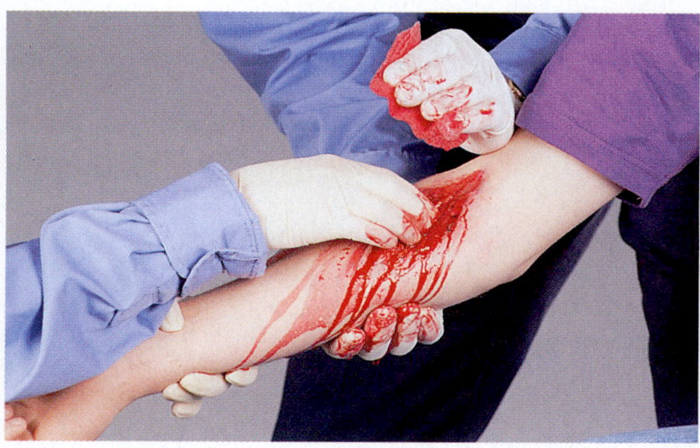

■ **Figure 19-3c** Hemorrhage control: if bleeding does not stop, apply direct fingertip pressure.

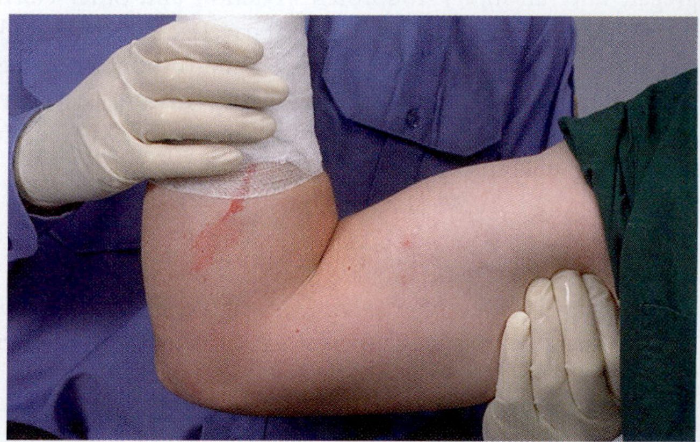

■ **Figure 19-3d** Hemorrhage control: if bleeding continues, apply pressure to a pressure point.

Internal Hemorrhage

Internal hemorrhage is associated with almost all serious blunt and penetrating trauma. As with external hemorrhage, internal hemorrhage can involve capillary, venous, or arterial blood loss. The blood can accumulate in the tissue itself, forming a visible or hidden contusion, or it can be forced between **fascia** and form a pocket of blood called a **hematoma.** In most of these cases, the hemorrhage is self-limiting because the pressure within the tissue or fascia controls the blood loss. However, large contusions, massive soft-tissue injuries, and large hematomas, especially those affecting large muscle masses like the thighs or buttocks, can account for moderate blood and body fluid loss. Fractures of the humerus and tibia/fibula may account for 500 to 750 mL of loss, while femur fractures may account for up to 1,500 mL of loss.

fascia *a fibrous membrane that covers, supports, and separates muscles and may also unite the skin with underlying tissue.*

hematoma *collection of blood beneath the skin or trapped within a body compartment.*

In body cavities such as the chest and the abdominal, pelvic, and retroperitoneal spaces, the resistance to continuing blood loss does not develop. With bleeding in these areas, loss continues unabated until the normal clotting process is effective, the blood pressure drops significantly, or surgical intervention is provided. The best indicators of significant internal hemorrhage are the mechanism of injury (MOI), local signs and symptoms of injury, and the early signs and symptoms of blood loss and shock. If a patient has sustained significant trauma to the chest, abdomen, or pelvis, anticipate significant, continuing, and uncontrolled blood loss. Such a patient requires rapid transport to a trauma center or hospital for surgical repair of any damaged vessels or organs. Recent evidence suggests that

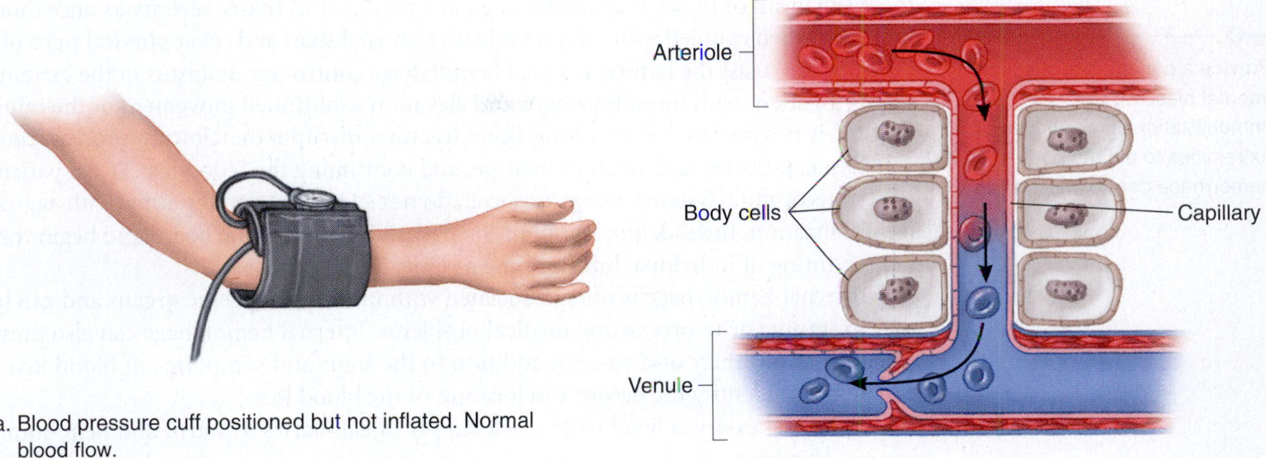

a. Blood pressure cuff positioned but not inflated. Normal blood flow.

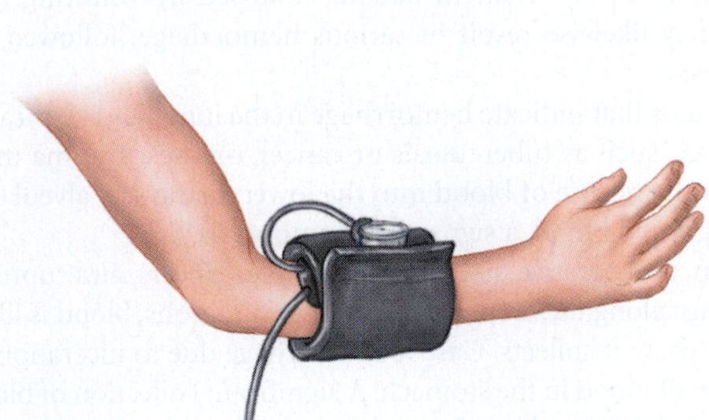

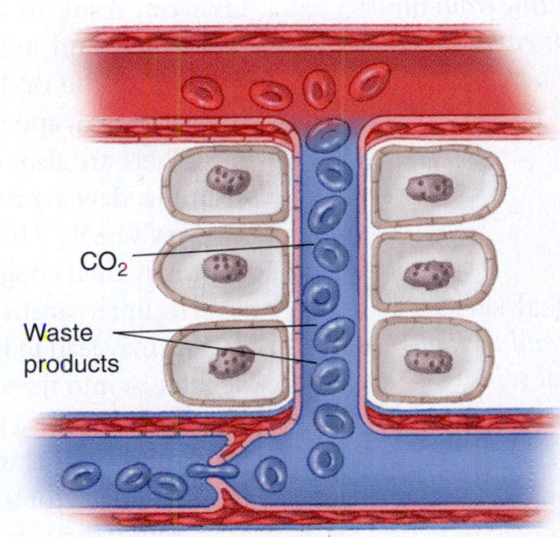

b. Inflation of B/P cuff as a tourniquet cuts off circulation. Blood flow stagnates and metabolic by-products accumulate.

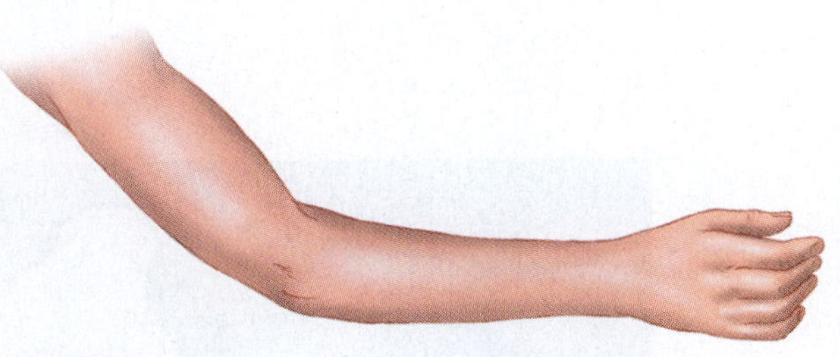

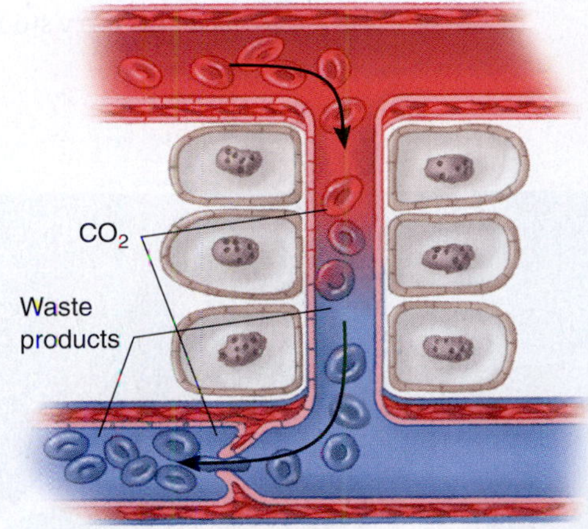

c. Release of cuff restores circulation. Returning blood flow pushes acidic by-products back into the central circulation.

■ **Figure 19-4** Release of a tourniquet may send accumulated toxins into the central circulation with devastating results for the patient.

Provide a patient with suspected internal bleeding with immobilization and elevation of extremities to aid the body's hemorrhage control mechanisms.

the mechanism of injury may not be as good a predictor of injury severity as once thought. MOI is best used when coupled with careful evaluation of vital signs and other physical signs of injury.

You can assist the natural internal hemorrhage control mechanisms in the extremities by providing a patient with immobilization and elevation. Continued movement of the injury site, especially if it is associated with a long-bone fracture, disrupts the clotting process, causing further soft-tissue, nervous, and vascular damage, and continuing the blood loss. If the patient is a victim of serious or multisystem trauma, however, do not spend time on the scene with aggressive skeletal immobilization. Instead, quickly splint the patient to a long spine board and begin transport. Provide splinting of individual limbs if time permits during transport.

Internal hemorrhage is often associated with injuries to specific organs and can be related either to trauma or to preexisting medical problems. Internal hemorrhage can also present with external signs of injury or disease in addition to the signs and symptoms of blood loss. These signs can help you identify the nature and location of the blood loss.

epistaxis *bleeding from the nose resulting from injury, disease, or environmental factors; a nosebleed.*

The nasal cavity is lined with a rich supply of capillaries to warm and help humidify incoming air. Hypertension, a strong sneeze, or direct trauma may rupture the vessels supplying these capillary beds and produce the moderate to severe hemorrhage called **epistaxis.** Prolonged epistaxis can result in hypovolemia, while blood flowing down the posterior nasal cavity, down the esophagus, and into the stomach may result in nausea, followed by vomiting (Figure 19-5 ■). Trauma to the oral cavity may likewise result in serious hemorrhage, followed by ingestion of blood, nausea, and then emesis.

There are also outward signs that indicate hemorrhage in the lungs and respiratory system. For example, degenerative diseases, such as tuberculosis or cancer, or chest trauma may rupture pulmonary vessels. This leads to the release of blood into the lower airways or alveolar space. The patient may then cough up bright red blood, a sign called hemoptysis.

esophageal varices *enlarged and tortuous esophageal veins.*

Trauma, caustic ingestion, degenerative disease (for example, cancer), and rupturing **esophageal varices** may lead to hemorrhage along the esophagus. In these conditions, blood is likely to travel, via peristalsis, into the stomach, where it collects. Gastric hemorrhage due to ulceration or trauma may also result in the accumulation of blood in the stomach. A significant collection of blood acts as a gastric irritant, inducing vomiting. If the blood is evacuated early, it is bright red in color. If blood remains in the stomach for some time, emesis resembles coffee grounds in both color and consistency.

melena *black, tarlike feces due to gastrointestinal bleeding.*

Hemorrhage in the small or large bowel can be associated with trauma, degenerative disease, or diverticulosis (small pouches in the walls of the bowel begin to hemorrhage). Bowel hemorrhage may present as bleeding from the rectum, or the blood may be digested before release, producing a black and tarry stool called **melena.**

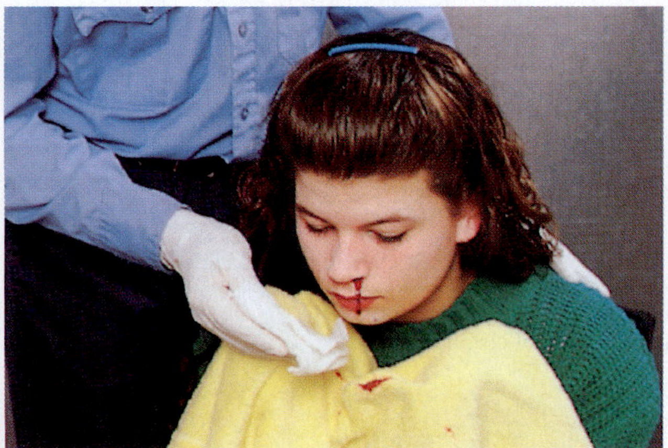

■ Figure 19-5a To control nosebleed, have the patient sit leaning forward.

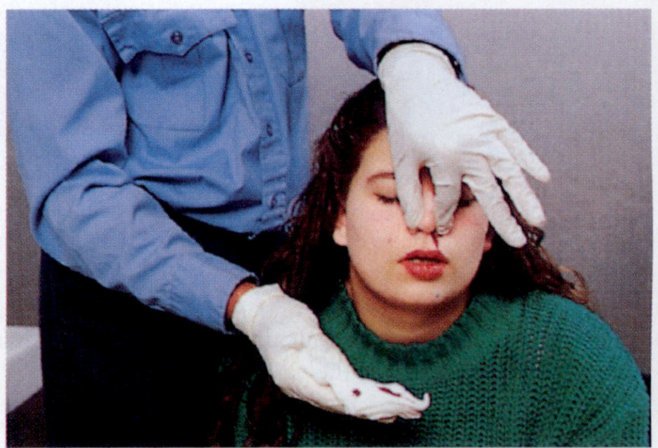

■ Figure 19-5b Pinch the fleshy part of the patient's nostrils firmly together.

Rectal injury may be caused by pelvic fracture or direct trauma. This presents with bleeding, which may be severe.

Vaginal hemorrhage may be associated with trauma, degenerative disease, menstruation, ectopic pregnancy, placenta previa, and potential or actual miscarriage. Urethral hemorrhage is generally minor and may reflect damage to the prostate or urethra. Blood in the urine may indicate injury to the genitourinary tract.

Nontraumatic forms of hemorrhage may be either acute or chronic. Acute hemorrhage moves the victim rapidly toward shock and is quickly recognizable. Chronic hemorrhage is likely to be rather limited in volume, but it does continue over time. The resulting loss depletes the body of red blood cells and leads to **anemia.** This condition reduces the blood's oxygen-carrying capacity, and the patient experiences fatigue and lethargy. Clotting factors may likewise be depleted, which reduces the blood's ability to coagulate and makes any secondary hemorrhage more difficult to control.

anemia *a reduction in the hemoglobin content in the blood to a point below that required to meet the oxygen requirements of the body.*

STAGES OF HEMORRHAGE

Fluid accounts for about 60 percent of the body's weight and is distributed among the cellular, interstitial, and vascular spaces. The cells contain about 62 percent of the total fluid volume, while the interstitial (nonvascular) space holds 26 percent. Between 4 and 5 percent of body fluid is found in other spaces such as the ventricles of the brain and meninges (cerebrospinal fluid). The remaining 7 percent of fluid volume resides in the vascular space. This fluid, called plasma, and the blood cells account for 7 percent of the average adult male's body weight (about 6.5 percent in the female). Fluid in the vascular space is distributed among the heart, arteries, veins, and capillaries and accounts for 5 liters (10 units) of blood volume in the healthy 70-kg adult male.

The effects of hemorrhage can be categorized into four progressive stages as blood volume is lost. These stages relate to the volume of blood lost in acute hemorrhage and that result in "classic" signs and symptoms. Remember, however, that each individual's response to blood loss may vary as may the rate and progress of the loss. Use these categories to help determine the relative severity of the loss and the need for intervention. It is also important to identify the following: the length of time elapsed since the incident that caused the trauma; the stage of hemorrhage the victim is in when you arrive at his side; and how quickly the patient is moving from one stage to another (Table 19–1).

With hemorrhage patients, determine the relative severity of blood loss, the need for aggressive intervention, the length of time since the incident that caused the trauma, the current stage of hemorrhage, and how quickly the patient is moving from one stage to another.

Stage 1 Hemorrhage

Stage 1 hemorrhage is a blood loss of up to 15 percent of the circulating blood volume. In the 70-kg male that is approximately 500 to 750 mL of blood, about the amount you might give during a blood drive. The healthy human system can easily compensate for such a blood loss volume by constricting the vascular beds, especially on the venous side. In this stage, the blood pressure remains

Table 19–1 Patient Signs Associated with Stages of Hemorrhage

Stage	Blood Loss	Vasoconstriction	Pulse Rate	Pulse (Pressure) Strength	Blood Pressure	Respiratory Rate	Respiratory Volume
1	<15%	↑	↑	→	→	→	→
2	15–25%	↑↑	↑↑	↓	→	↑	↑
3	25–35%	↑↑↑	↑↑↑	↓↓	↓	↑↑	↓
4	>35%	↓↓	Variable	↓↓↓	↓↓↓	↓	↓↓

pulse pressure *difference between the systolic and diastolic blood pressures.*

catecholamine *a hormone, such as epinephrine or norepinephrine, that strongly affects the nervous and cardiovascular systems, metabolic rate, temperature, and smooth muscle.*

constant as do the **pulse pressure,** respiratory rate, and urine output. The central venous pressure may drop slightly, but it returns to normal quickly. The pulse rate elevates slightly, and the patient may display some signs of **catecholamine** (epinephrine and norepinephrine) release, notably nervousness and marginally cool skin with a slight pallor.

Stage 2 Hemorrhage

Stage 2 hemorrhage occurs as 15 to 25 percent (750 to 1,250 mL) of the blood volume is lost. The body's first-line compensatory responses can no longer maintain blood pressure, and secondary mechanisms are now employed. Tachycardia becomes very evident, and the pulse strength begins to diminish (the pulse pressure is noticeably narrowed). A strong release of catecholamines increases peripheral vascular resistance. This maintains systolic blood pressure but results in peripheral vasoconstriction and cool, clammy skin. Anxiety increases, and the patient may begin to display restlessness and thirst. Thirst is present as fluid leaves the intracellular and interstitial spaces and the osmotic pressure of the blood changes. Renal output remains normal, but the respiratory rate increases.

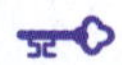

Without rapid intervention, survival of a stage 3 hemorrhage patient is unlikely.

Stage 3 Hemorrhage

Stage 3 hemorrhage occurs when blood loss reaches 25 to 35 percent of blood volume (1,250 to 1,750 mL). The body's compensatory mechanisms are unable to cope with the loss, and the classic signs of shock appear. Rapid tachycardia is present as the blood pressure begins to fall. The pulse is barely palpable as the pulse pressure remains very narrow. The patient experiences air hunger and tachypnea. Anxiety, restlessness, and thirst become more severe. The level of responsiveness decreases, and the patient becomes very pale, cool, and diaphoretic. Urinary output declines. Without rapid intervention, this patient's survival is unlikely.

Content Review

Stages of Hemorrhage

- Stage 1—blood loss of up to 15 percent; patient may display some nervousness and marginally cool skin with slight pallor
- Stage 2—blood loss of 15 to 25 percent; patient displays thirst, anxiety, restlessness, cool, clammy skin, increased respiratory rate
- Stage 3—blood loss between 25 and 35 percent; patient experiences air hunger, dyspnea, severe thirst, anxiety, restlessness; survival unlikely without rapid intervention
- Stage 4—blood loss greater than 35 percent; pulse barely palpable, respirations ineffective; patient lethargic, confused, moving toward unresponsiveness; survival unlikely

Stage 4 Hemorrhage

Stage 4 hemorrhage occurs with a blood loss of greater than 35 percent of the body's total blood supply. The patient's pulse is barely palpable in the central arteries, if one can be found at all. Respirations are very rapid, shallow, and ineffective. The patient is very lethargic and confused, moving rapidly toward unresponsiveness. The skin is very cool, clammy, and extremely pale. Urinary output ceases. Even with aggressive fluid resuscitation and blood transfusions, patient survival is unlikely.

These descriptions of the stages of hemorrhage presume that the patient is a normally healthy adult. Any preexisting condition may affect the volume of blood loss required for movement from one stage to another as well as the speed at which the patient moves through the stages. The patient's state of hydration, from dehydrated to fluid-rich, may also affect how quickly and to what degree compensation takes place.

The rate of the blood loss also has a profound effect on how quickly a patient moves from stage 1 to stage 4. If the blood loss is very rapid, the compensatory mechanisms may not work as effectively. However, a small wound bleeding uncontrollably but very slowly for days may not move the patient from stage 1 to stage 2, even with a loss much greater than 750 mL.

Certain categories of patients—pregnant women, athletes, obese patients, children, and the elderly—react differently to blood loss. The blood volume of a woman in late pregnancy is 50 percent greater than normal. This patient may lose rather large volumes of blood before progressing through the various stages of hemorrhage. Although the mother in this circumstance appears to be somewhat protected from the effects of serious hemorrhage, the fetus is deprived of good circulation early in the blood loss and is more susceptible to harm.

A well-conditioned athlete often has greater fluid and cardiac reserves than a typical patient. This means that he may move more slowly through the early stages with greater percentages of loss needed to advance from one stage to another.

The obese patient, however, has a blood volume close to 7 percent of ideal body weight, but not actual body weight. Thus, the blood volume as a percentage of actual body weight is lower than 7 percent. This means that what appears to be only a small blood loss may have a more serious effect in such a patient.

In infants and young children, blood volumes approximate 8 to 9 percent of body weight, volumes that are proportionally about 20 percent greater than those of adults. However, compensatory mechanisms in infants and children are neither as well developed nor as effective as those in adults. These young patients may not show early signs and symptoms of compensation as clearly as adults. They may instead move quickly into the later stages of shock. Suspect hemorrhage early with child and infant trauma and treat it aggressively.

Suspect hemorrhage early in cases of child and infant trauma and treat it aggressively.

The elderly are likewise more adversely affected by blood loss. They have lower volumes of fluid reserves, and their compensatory systems are less responsive to fluid losses. These patients may also be on medications such as beta-blockers that further reduce the body's ability to respond to blood loss and varying blood pressures or on medications such as aspirin, warfarin, and heparin that interfere with the body's natural hemorrhage control system. Often, elderly patients do not experience the tachycardia associated with blood loss, and their blood pressures drop before those of healthy adults. Signs of blood loss and shock may be masked by reduced perceptions of pain in the elderly and by lowered levels of mental acuity due to disease. The elderly also do not tolerate periods of inadequate tissue perfusion well because of chronic cardiovascular inefficiency.

Be aware that signs and symptoms of blood loss in elderly patients may be masked by use of medications, bodily changes, reduced perception of pain, and the effects of disease.

HEMORRHAGE ASSESSMENT

The assessment of various types of trauma patients will be the subject of the next few chapters. In these chapters, only the aspects of assessment that are pertinent to those pathologies will be addressed. Please refer to the patient assessment chapters (Chapter 10, "History Taking"; Chapter 11, "Physical Exam Techniques"; Chapter 12, "Patient Assessment in the Field"; Chapter 13, "Clinical Decision Making") for a more complete discussion of trauma assessment.

The assessment of the hemorrhage patient is directed at identifying the source of the hemorrhage and halting any serious and controllable loss. During assessment, you should also examine the circumstances of injury to approximate the volume of blood lost and the rate of past and continuing hemorrhage. This process begins with the scene size-up and continues throughout transport and care.

The assessment of the hemorrhage patient is directed at identifying the source of the hemorrhage and halting any serious and controllable loss.

Scene Size-up

Remember that Standard Precautions are essential during the assessment of trauma patients. A patient's blood and other body fluids may contain pathogens capable of transmitting HIV, hepatitis, and other diseases to you. Conversely, you may transmit infectious agents to the wounds of the patients you assess and care for. In fact, the risk of your transmitting disease or infection to a patient with open wounds or burns is probably much greater than the risk that he will transmit disease or infection to you. For these reasons, always observe Standard Precautions with all trauma patients. These precautions include the use of gloves and a mask when you inspect or palpate any injured area, especially one with open wounds (Figure 19-6 ■). If there is spurting blood, as with arterial hemorrhage; if a patient is combative; or if there is airway trauma with or without bleeding; also wear eye protection and a disposable gown to protect your uniform. Be sure to wash your hands before each ambulance call and do so immediately afterward as well. Scrub vigorously when washing to remove as much of the bacterial load as possible.

Standard Precautions protect the patient as well as the caregiver.

If your gloves become contaminated with earth, debris, blood, or body fluids while caring for a patient, change them immediately. If you will be assessing or treating multiple patients, consider double gloving. This means that you put on two or more sets of gloves and remove a set each time you complete assessment of one patient and move on to the next. Place any contaminated gloves, clothing, dressings, or other materials in a biohazard bag and assure proper disposal.

The handling of needles presents special problems for prehospital personnel. Once a needle is used, it carries the potential of introducing a patient's blood directly into a caregiver's or bystander's tissues. This greatly increases the likelihood of disease transmission. When dealing with needles, always ensure that they are not recapped, but rather placed in a properly marked and secure, puncture-resistant sharps container. Should you be stuck with a needle, continue your care, but document the incident immediately upon arrival at the emergency department. Wash and cover the wound, then report the incident to your service's infection control officer or other designated officer. There are several prophylactic regimens available that may protect against the transmission of some infectious diseases. Even more important, you can guard against some diseases, such as hepatitis, by obtaining immunizations before you begin your career as a care provider.

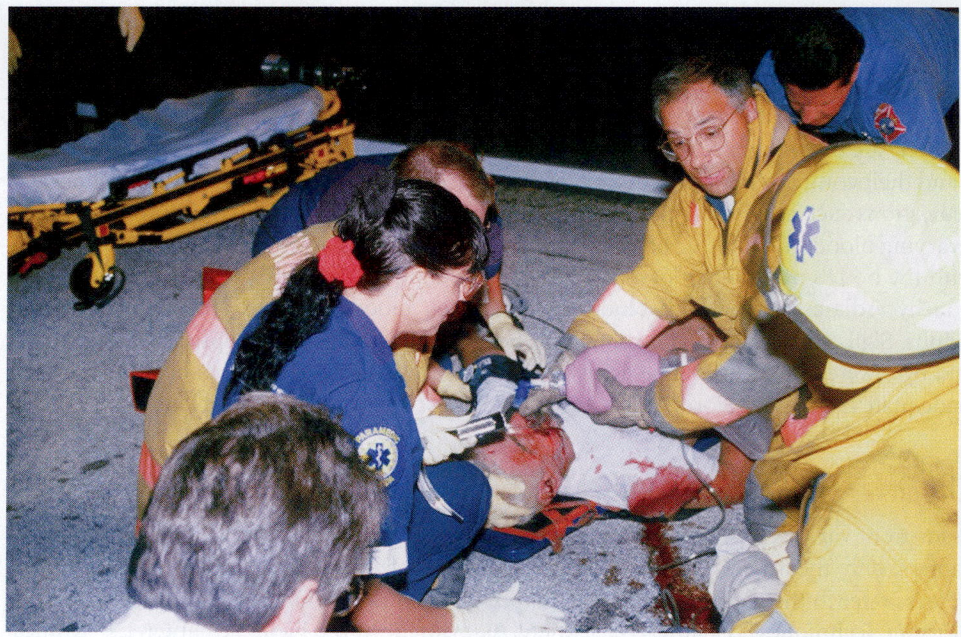

Figure 19-6 When caring for a hemorrhaging patient, employ appropriate body substance isolation procedures. *(© Eddie Sperling Photography)*

Patients may see your gloves and then feel uncomfortable about being treated by someone who is "afraid to touch them." Assure those patients that the gloves and other precautions are for their protection as well as yours.

When appropriate Standard Precautions have been taken, continue with the scene size-up. Evaluate the mechanism of injury to anticipate sites of both external and internal hemorrhage. Anticipating external hemorrhage sites focuses your subsequent assessment and care, while anticipating internal hemorrhage affects your decision on whether to provide rapid transport.

When evaluating the mechanism of injury (MOI), also attempt to determine the amount of time that has elapsed between the injury and your evaluation of it. Knowing the length of this time period is very important in determining the amount and rate of blood loss. For example, if you arrive on a scene 3 minutes after an injury-producing incident and find a patient losing 150 mL of blood per minute, you can estimate that 450 mL of blood have been lost. You would not expect the patient to display the signs and symptoms of stage 1 hemorrhage. If, however, you arrive 10 minutes after the incident, the same patient, losing blood at the same rate, will have lost 1,500 mL of blood and is likely to have reached stage 3. In both these cases, the patient is suffering serious, life-threatening hemorrhage. Good assessment and recognition assures provision of a proper course of care. However, the earlier you arrive at the patient's side, the harder it is to identify serious hemorrhage. For this reason, you must be aware of and appreciate the progressive effects of blood loss and use both the MOI analysis and the time since an incident to increase your suspicions of a problem. Remember, the sooner the signs of later stages of hemorrhage appear, the greater the rate and volume of blood loss.

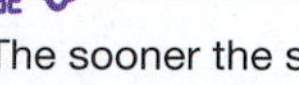

The sooner the signs of the later stages of hemorrhage appear, the greater the rate and volume of blood loss.

Primary Assessment

As you begin the primary assessment, form a general impression of the patient. Be especially alert for any signs and symptoms of internal hemorrhage. These early signs are very subtle and may go unnoticed unless you deliberately look for them. Provide in-line immobilization and correct any immediate life threats if you suspect spinal injury. Assess the patient's initial mental status to determine alertness, orientation, and responsiveness. Be alert for any signs of anxiety, confusion, or combativeness. Any central nervous system deficit may be secondary to hemorrhage, so be suspicious.

Assess both airway and breathing carefully, noting any tachypnea or air hunger. Administer oxygen via nonrebreather mask at a rate of 15 L/minute. When assessing circulation, pay special attention to the pulse strength (the pulse pressure) and rate. Remember that the pulse pressure narrows well before the systolic pressure begins to drop. The pulse rate, too, may suggest developing shock. A fast—and especially a fast, weak (thready)—pulse may be the first noticeable sign of serious internal blood loss. Note also skin color and condition. Pale or mottled skin is an early sign of shock, while cool and clammy skin is also an indicator of potential blood loss and shock.

Complete the primary assessment by establishing patient priorities. Decide, based on your findings to this point, whether the patient is to receive a rapid trauma assessment or a focused history and exam. If any indication, mechanism of injury, sign, or symptom suggests serious internal hemorrhage or uncontrolled external hemorrhage, consider the rapid trauma assessment and then immediate transport for the patient.

Secondary Assessment

Your primary assessment findings and the evaluation of the mechanism of injury determine how you will proceed with the secondary assessment. For trauma patients who have a significant MOI, continue spinal immobilization, and perform a rapid secondary assessment. Then obtain baseline vital signs and a patient history.

For trauma patients who have no significant MOI and who have revealed no critical findings during primary assessment, perform an assessment focused on the area of injury, then obtain baseline vital signs and gather a patient history. Finally, provide care as appropriate and transport.

With both these types of trauma patients, perform reassessments during transport. If time and the patient's condition permit, you may also perform a detailed physical exam. However, you should never delay transport to perform the detailed examination.

Rapid Secondary Assessment For trauma patients with a significant MOI, you should perform a rapid secondary assessment, inspecting and palpating the patient in an orderly fashion from head to toe. Pay particular attention to areas where critical trauma has occurred and areas where the MOI suggests forces were focused.

Carefully and quickly observe the head for serious bleeding. Internal head injury rarely accounts for the classic signs of shock. However, the scalp bleeds profusely because the vessels there are large and do not constrict as well as peripheral vessels do elsewhere. If any external bleeding appears serious, halt it immediately.

Next, examine the neck. The carotid arteries and jugular veins are located close to the skin's surface. Injury to them can produce rapid and fatal exsanguination. An added danger is the aspiration of air directly into an open jugular vein. At times, venous pressure, due to deep inspiration, can be less than atmospheric pressure. Air may then be drawn into the vein, traveling to the heart and forming emboli, which then lodge in the pulmonary circulation. Quickly control any serious hemorrhage from neck wounds with sterile occlusive dressings. If spinal injury is suspected, apply a rigid cervical collar when assessment of the neck is complete, but maintain in-line manual immobilization until the patient is immobilized to a spine board.

Visually sweep the chest and abdomen for any serious external hemorrhage, though such bleeding is infrequent there. You are more likely to note signs of blunt or penetrating trauma, suggesting internal injury and hemorrhage within. Look to the abdomen for signs of soft-tissue injury, contusions, abrasions, rigidity, and guarding and tenderness that suggest internal injury.

Quickly examine the pelvic and groin region. Test the integrity of the pelvic ring by pressing gently on the iliac crest. Remember that pelvic fracture can account for blood loss of more than 2,000 mL. Lacerations to the male genitalia may also account for serious external hemorrhage.

Assess the extremities and rule out fractures of the femur, tibia/fibula, or humerus. Keep in mind that femur fracture can account for up to 1,500 mL of blood loss, while each tibia/fibula or humerus fracture may contribute an additional 500 to 750 mL of blood loss. Hematomas and large contusions may account for up to 500 mL of blood loss in the larger muscle masses. Quickly check distal pulse strength and muscle tone in the extremities, comparing findings in the opposing extremities.

Finally, visually sweep the body, including the posterior, for any external hemorrhage that may have gone unnoticed in your examination to this point.

At the end of the rapid secondary assessment, assess the patient's vital signs, obtain a patient history if possible, and inventory the injuries that may contribute to shock. Provide rapid transport for any patient with an MOI and physical findings that meet trauma triage criteria (see Chapter 16, "Trauma and Trauma Systems"). Any patient with injuries likely to induce hemorrhage at the level of stage 2 or greater should likewise receive immediate transport. If travel time to the trauma center will exceed 30 minutes, consider requesting air medical transport. Be sure to record the results

Content Review

Injuries That Can Cause Significant Blood Loss

- Fractured pelvis (2,000 mL)
- Fractured femur (1,500 mL)
- Fractured tibia (750 mL)
- Fractured humerus (750 mL)
- Large contusion (500 mL)

Content Review

Signs and Symptoms of Internal Hemorrhage

Early

- Pain, tenderness, swelling, or discoloration of suspected injury site
- Bleeding from mouth, rectum, vagina, or other orifice
- Vomiting of bright red blood
- Tender, rigid, and/or distended abdomen

Late

- Anxiety, restlessness, combativeness, or altered mental status
- Weakness, faintness, or dizziness
- Vomiting of blood the color of dark coffee grounds
- Thirst
- Melena
- Shallow, rapid breathing
- Rapid, weak pulse
- Pale, cool, clammy skin
- Capillary refill greater than 2 seconds (most reliable in infants and children under 6)
- Dropping blood pressure
- Dilated pupils sluggish in responding to light
- Nausea and vomiting

of your assessment carefully. Compare this information with signs and symptoms you discover during the ongoing assessment to identify trends in the patient's condition.

Perform a detailed physical exam only when all immediate life threats have been addressed. Normally, this would be when you are en route to the hospital or trauma center or when transport has been delayed for some reason.

Focused Physical Exam Employ the focused secondary assessment for patients without a significant MOI; for example, a patient who has lacerated his finger with a knife. In such cases, the hemorrhage can be controlled on the scene and the MOI does not suggest additional problems. With such patients, focus your exam on the area injured, inspecting and palpating the area thoroughly, looking for additional injuries beyond the one that prompted the call. Control the hemorrhage, if you have not already done so. Obtain baseline vital signs and a patient history, and prepare and transport the patient.

In some cases, you may wish to perform a rapid secondary assessment, even though the patient does not have a significant MOI. This would be the case, for example, if you suspect the patient has more injuries than he has complained of or if his condition suddenly begins to deteriorate. With such patients, it may be necessary to perform a rapid head-to-toe examination, inspecting and palpating all body regions.

Additional Assessment Considerations In the trauma patient with a significant MOI or the medical patient showing signs and symptoms of blood loss and shock, it is important to search for evidence of internal hemorrhage. This evidence may be in the form of blood, or material suggestive of blood, flowing from the body orifices. Bright red blood from the mouth, nose, rectum, or other orifice suggests direct bleeding. The vomiting of material that looks like coffee grounds is associated with partially digested blood in the stomach, suggestive of a long-term and slow hemorrhage. A black, tarry stool called melena suggests blood has remained in the bowel for some time. **Hematochezia** is stool with frank blood in it and reflects active bleeding in the colon or rectum.

hematochezia *passage of stools containing red blood.*

In the patient with nonspecific complaints—general ill feeling, anxiousness, restlessness—or a lowered level of responsiveness, suspect and look for other signs of internal hemorrhage. Watch for an increasing pulse rate, rising diastolic blood pressure (narrowing blood pressure), and cool and clammy skin.

Also observe for dizziness or syncope when the patient moves from a supine to a sitting or standing position. This condition is called **orthostatic hypotension** and is suggestive of a volume loss, possibly attributable to internal hemorrhage. This phenomenon is the basis of the **tilt test,** which can be employed to determine blood or fluid loss and the body's reduced ability to compensate for normal positional change. Perform this test only on patients who do not already display signs and symptoms of shock. Prepare for the test by obtaining blood pressure and pulse rates from the patient in a supine or seated position. Then have the supine patient move to a seated position or the seated patient stand up and obtain another set of blood pressure and pulse rates. If the systolic blood pressure drops more than 20 mmHg, the pulse rate rises more than 20 beats per minute, or the patient experiences light-headedness, the test is considered positive, indicating hypovolemia.

orthostatic hypotension *a decrease in blood pressure that occurs when a person moves from a supine or sitting to an upright position.*

tilt test *drop in the systolic blood pressure of 20 mmHg or an increase in the pulse rate of 20 beats per minute when a patient is moved from a supine to a sitting position; a finding suggestive of a relative hypovolemia.*

Reassessment

Once you have rendered all appropriate lifesaving care, perform reassessments frequently—at least every 5 minutes with unstable patients and every 15 minutes with stable ones. Reevaluate your general impression, and reassess the patient's mental status, airway, breathing, and circulation, and obtain additional sets of vital signs. Compare each set of findings with earlier ones to determine if the patient's condition is stable, deteriorating, or improving. Pay special attention to the pulse pressure because it is a clear indicator of the body's efforts to compensate for hypovolemia. Also pay particular attention to changes in patient symptoms or mental status, noting any increasing anxiety or restlessness.

HEMORRHAGE MANAGEMENT

The management of hemorrhage is an integral part of care for the trauma patient, one that begins during the primary assessment and is shaped by findings of the rapid or focused secondary assessment.

First, ensure that the airway is patent, that the patient is breathing adequately, and that you have administered high-flow, high-concentration oxygen. If you have not, establish and maintain the airway and provide the necessary ventilatory support. Be prepared to provide endotracheal intubation if necessary to secure the airway.

Assure that the patient has a pulse. If not, initiate CPR, attach a monitor-defibrillator, and employ advanced cardiac life support measures. Rule out pericardial tamponade and tension pneumothorax as possible causes of cardiac dysfunction. Understand that cardiac arrest in trauma cases due to hypovolemia carries an extremely poor prognosis. When resources are scarce, your efforts may be better utilized caring for other salvageable patients.

During the primary assessment, care for serious hemorrhage only after any airway and breathing problems are corrected.

During the primary assessment, care for serious (arterial and heavy venous) hemorrhage only after any airway and breathing problems are corrected. Quickly apply a pressure dressing held in place by self-adherent bandage material or a firmly tied cravat. Return to provide better hemorrhage control after you complete the primary and rapid secondary assessments and set priorities for care of the hemorrhages and other trauma you discover. If the patient displays early signs of shock, consider applying a PASG and initiating fluid therapy; do not, however, delay transport in order to carry out these measures.

Once you have completed the secondary assessment, begin caring for injuries, including hemorrhage, as you have prioritized them. As you work down your injury priority list and come to a wound, inspect the site to identify the type and exact location of bleeding. This helps you apply pressure—either digitally or with dressings and bandages—most effectively to halt the blood flow. With cases of external hemorrhage, it is important to identify the exact source and type of bleeding and to be sure to look at the wound site.

Document your findings on the prehospital care report. If you document and convey this information clearly to the emergency department staff, you will reduce the need for others to open the wound (thus disrupting the clotting process) to determine and describe its nature.

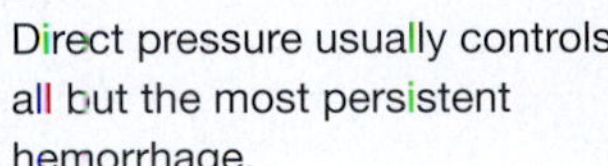

Direct pressure usually controls all but the most persistent hemorrhage.

Direct pressure controls all but the most persistent hemorrhage (Figure 19-7 ■). Although systolic blood pressure drives arterial hemorrhage, you can stop such a hemorrhage with simple finger pressure properly applied to the source of the bleeding. If a wound looks as though it may pose a problem, insert a wad of dressing material over the site of the heaviest bleeding and apply a bandage over the dressing. This focuses pressure on the site and away from the surrounding area. If bleeding saturates the dressing, cover it with another dressing and apply another bandage to keep pressure on the wound. Removing the soaked bandage and dressing disrupts the clotting process and prolongs the hemorrhage. If, however, the wound continues to bleed through your layers of dressings and bandages, consider removing the dressing materials you have applied, directly visualizing the exact site of bleeding, and then reapplying a wad of dressing and firm direct pressure to the precise hemorrhage site.

If direct pressure alone does not halt the blood flow to an extremity, consider elevation. Elevation reduces the systolic blood pressure because the heart has to push the blood against gravity and

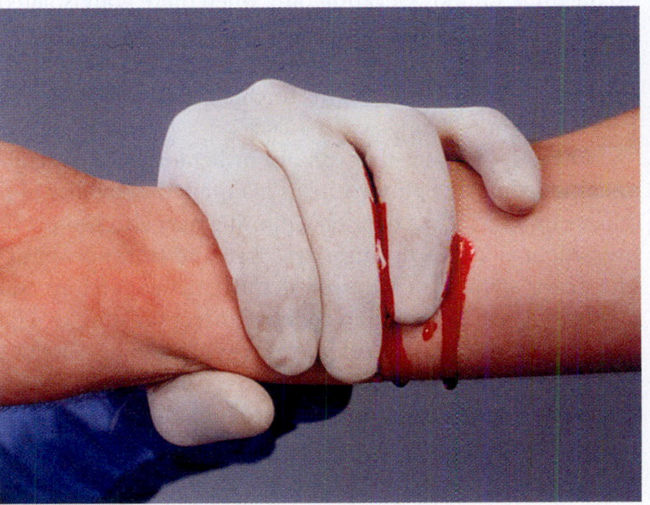

■ **Figure 19-7** In most cases of moderate to severe external hemorrhage, direct pressure, maintained by a bandage and dressing, will control bleeding.

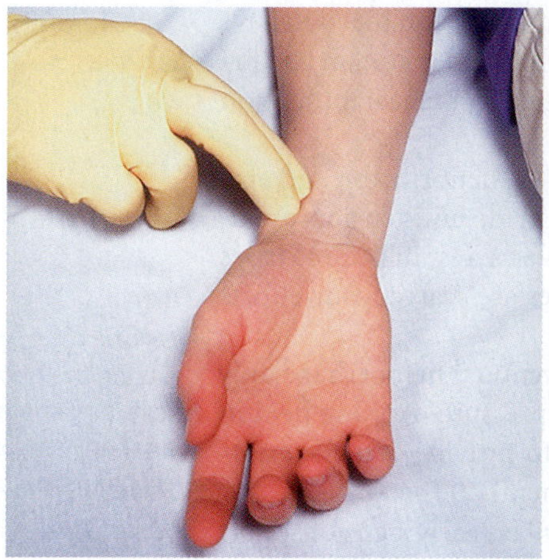

a. Radial artery for hand.

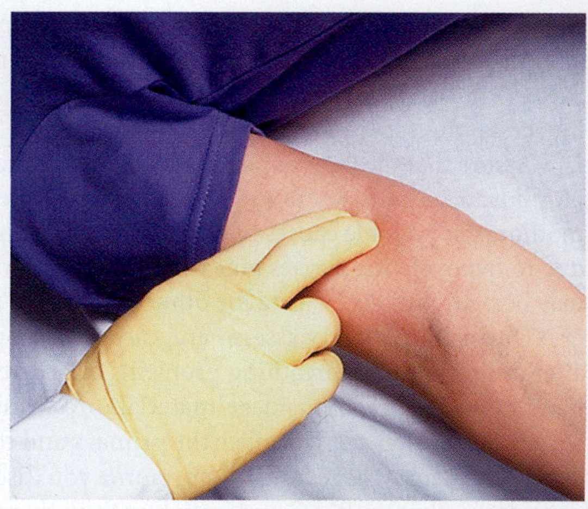

b. Brachial artery for forearm.

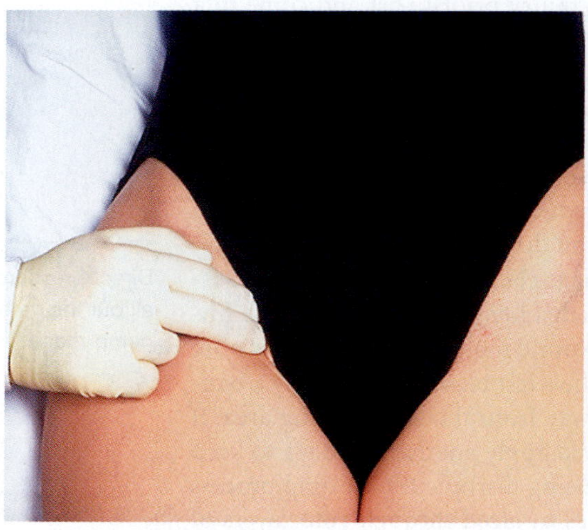

c. Femoral artery for thigh.

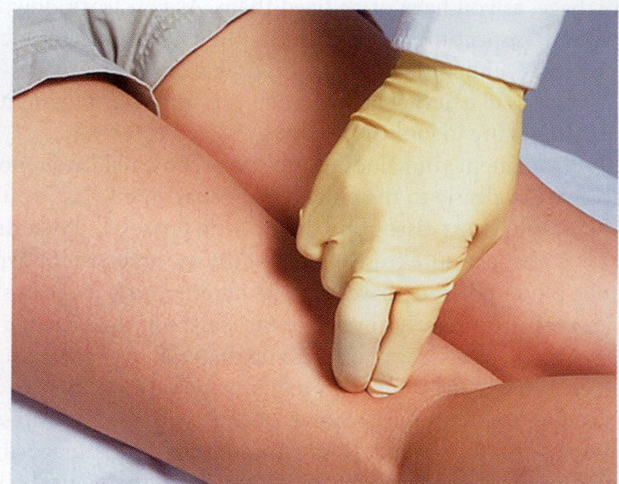

d. Popliteal artery for leg and foot.

■ **Figure 19-8** Common pressure points for hemorrhage control.

up the limb. Employ elevation only when there is an isolated bleeding wound on a limb and movement will not aggravate any other injuries.

If bleeding still persists, find an arterial pulse point proximal to the wound and apply firm pressure there (Figure 19-8 ■). This further reduces the blood pressure within the limb and should reduce the hemorrhaging.

Other techniques that can aid in hemorrhage control include limb splinting and the use of pneumatic splints. Splinting helps maintain the stability of the wound site, thus assisting the mechanisms by which clots develop. Splinting may also protect the site from injuries that might occur if the patient is jostled during extrication and transport or as you assess and care for other wounds. Pneumatic splints can also prevent movement of an injured limb. They may also be helpful in holding dressings in place and in applying direct pressure to a limb circumferentially.

Consider using a tourniquet only as a last resort when hemorrhage is prolonged and persistent. As mentioned earlier, there are hazards associated with tourniquet use. Apply a blood pressure cuff just proximal to the hemorrhage site and inflate it to apply a pressure 20 to 30 mmHg greater than the systolic blood pressure. Assure there is no continued bleeding after you apply the tourniquet, and mark the patient's forehead with the letters "TQ" and the time of application.

Specific Wound Considerations

Several types of wounds require special attention for hemorrhage control. They include head wounds, neck wounds, large gaping wounds, and crush injuries.

Head injuries raise some special concerns regarding hemorrhage control. Head wounds may be associated with both severe hemorrhage and the loss of skull integrity (fracture). Control bleeding with such wounds very carefully, using gentle direct pressure around the wound site and against the stable skull. Fluid drainage from the ears and nose may be secondary to skull fracture. Cerebrospinal fluid, as it escapes the cranial vault, relieves building intracranial pressure. Halting the flow of fluid would end this relief mechanism and compound the increase in pressure. In addition, stopping the flow may provide a pathway for pathogens to enter the meninges and cause serious infection (meningitis). Cerebrospinal fluid quickly regenerates as the injury heals. Thus, if there is hemorrhage from either the nose or ear canal, simply cover the area with a soft, porous dressing and bandage it loosely.

With head injury patients, do not attempt to stop the flow of blood or fluid from the nose or ear canal, but cover the area with porous dressing to collect the material and bandage loosely.

Neck wounds carry the risk of air being drawn into the venous circulation with life-threatening results. Cover any open neck wound with an occlusive dressing held firmly in place. Do not employ circumferential bandages to create direct pressure with neck wounds. Digital pressure controls most, if not all, neck bleeding. It may, however, be necessary to apply and maintain this manual pressure continuously during the patient's prehospital care.

Cover any open neck wound with an occlusive dressing held firmly in place.

Gaping wounds often present hemorrhage control problems. With such wounds, bleeding originates from many sites and their open nature prevents application of uniform direct pressure. To manage bleeding from such a wound, create a mass of dressing material approximating the volume and shape of the wound. Place the material with the sterile, nonadherent side against the wound and bandage it firmly in place.

Controlling hemorrhage associated with crush injuries can be particularly challenging. The source of hemorrhage in such cases is frequently difficult to determine, and the vessels are damaged in such a way that the normal hemorrhage control mechanisms may be ineffective. Place a dressing around and over the crushed tissue, place a pneumatic splint over that, and inflate the splint to apply pressure and hold the dressing in place. If bleeding is heavy and persistent, consider using a tourniquet but keep in mind the precautions discussed previously.

Transport Considerations

Consider rapid transport for any patient who experiences serious external hemorrhage that you cannot control and for any patient with suspected serious internal hemorrhage. Be vigilant for any signs of compensation for blood loss and for the early signs of shock. Monitor your patient's mental status, pulse rate, and blood pressure (for narrowing pulse pressure). When in doubt, transport.

Consider rapid transport for any patient who experiences serious external hemorrhage that you cannot control and for any patient with suspected serious internal hemorrhage.

Understand that serious hemorrhage can have a significant psychological impact on patients. Stress triggers the "fight-or-flight" response, increases heart rate and blood pressure, increases the body's metabolic demands, works against the body's hemorrhage control mechanisms, and contributes to the development of shock. Do what you can to ease the anxieties of such patients. Communicate freely with them, and explain what care measures you are taking and why. Be especially alert to their comfort needs and address them as appropriate. If possible, keep these patients from seeing their injuries or the serious injuries affecting friends and other accident victims.

SHOCK

A simple medical definition of shock is "a state of inadequate tissue perfusion." Beyond that simple definition, however, shock is the transitional stage between normal life, called homeostasis, and death. It is the underlying killer of all trauma patients and often presents with only subtle signs and symptoms until the body can no longer compensate. Then the patient moves quickly, and often irreversibly, toward death. Because of this, you, as a paramedic, must understand the process of shock and recognize its earliest signs and symptoms.

Shock is the underlying killer of all trauma patients and often presents with only subtle signs and symptoms.

Cells are the microscopic building blocks of the human body. When cells cease to function—and if the process is not reversed—the result is cell death, which leads to tissue death, then to organ failure, and ultimately to the death of the organism. In order for cells to function, they must be continually perfused by blood, as carried through the capillaries, in order to receive a constant supply of oxygen and other nutrients and to eliminate waste products.

Shock is a tissue perfusion problem affecting the individual body cells. There are many causes of shock, though all are commonly manifested by signs and symptoms of cardiovascular system compensation followed by decompensation and, ultimately, collapse. The best way to understand shock and how body systems compensate for it is to look at the cell and its functions and then to examine how the body provides for the cells' metabolic needs and how this process can fail. Normal cell **metabolism** is discussed in Chapter 3, while the pathophysiology of shock is discussed in Chapter 4.

metabolism *the total changes that take place in an organism during physiological processes.*

THE BODY'S RESPONSE TO BLOOD LOSS

The sympathetic nervous system and the hormones it releases begin progressive responses as hemorrhage causes blood to leave the cardiovascular system. As the draw down of the vascular volume reaches the heart, the ventricles do not completely engorge. Cardiac contractility therefore suffers as the ventricular myocardium does not stretch (Starling's law of the heart). The stroke volume drops, and there is an immediate drop in the systolic blood pressure. This reduced pressure reduces the cardiovascular system's ability to drive blood through the capillary beds (tissue perfusion). The carotid and aortic baroreceptors recognize this decrease in blood pressure and signal to the cardiovascular center of the medulla oblongata. The vasomotor center increases peripheral vascular resistance and venous tone while the cardioacceleratory center increases heart rate. With the reduced venous capacitance and an increase in heart rate and peripheral vascular resistance, the blood pressure returns to normal, as does tissue perfusion. These actions normally compensate for small blood losses. If the blood loss stops, the body reconstitutes the volume of loss from the interstitial fluid and replaces the lost red blood cells gradually, without noticeable or ill effects.

Cellular Ischemia

If blood loss continues, the venous system constricts to its limits in order to maintain cardiac preload. However, it becomes more and more difficult for the venous system to compensate because its limited musculature tires and relaxes. Peripheral vascular resistance also continues to increase to maintain the systolic blood pressure. As it does, the diastolic blood pressure rises, the pulse pressure narrows, and the pulse weakens. The constriction of arterioles means that less and less blood is directed to the noncritical organs, and those organs' supply of oxygen is reduced. The skin, the largest of the noncritical organs, receives reduced circulation and becomes cool, pale, and moist. If the hemorrhage continues, some noncritical organ cells begin to starve for oxygen. Anaerobic metabolism is their only energy source, and carbon dioxide and lactic and other acids begin to accumulate. Cellular hypoxia begins, followed by **ischemia.** The heart rate increases, but slowly, because the other compensatory mechanisms are still effectively maintaining preload.

ischemia *a blockage in the delivery of oxygenated blood to the cells.*

As the volume of blood loss increases, more and more body cells are deprived of their oxygen and nutrient supplies, and more and more waste products accumulate. The bloodstream becomes acidic, and the body's chemoreceptors stimulate an increase in depth and rate of respirations. Hypoxia causes alterations in the level of consciousness, and circulating catecholamines cause the patient to become anxious, restless, and possibly combative. Ischemia now affects not only noncritical organs but also the arterioles. These vessels, which also require oxygen, become hypoxic and relax. Meanwhile, the coronary arteries provide a decreasing amount of oxygenated blood to the laboring heart.

If the blood loss stops, the blood draws fluid from within the interstitial space, at a rate of up to 1 L per hour, to restore its volume, and erythropoietin accelerates the production of red blood cells. The kidneys reduce urine output to conserve water and electrolytes, and a period of thirst provides the stimulus for the patient to drink liquids and replace the lost volume on a more permanent basis. Transfusion with whole blood may be required at this point. While some signs of circulatory compromise and fatigue are present, the patient's recovery is probable with a period of rest.

Capillary Microcirculation

If blood loss continues, sympathetic stimulation and reduced perfusion to the kidneys, pancreas, and liver cause the release of hormones. Angiotensin II further increases peripheral vascular resistance and reduces the blood flow to more of the body's tissues. If the blood loss continues, circulation is further limited to only those organs most critical to life. This further decrease in circulation leads to an increase in cellular hypoxia in noncritical tissues, and more cells begin to use anaerobic metabolism for energy in a desperate attempt to survive. The buildup of lactic acid and carbon dioxide relaxes the precapillary sphincters. The circulating blood volume is diminished both by the continued hemorrhage and by fluid loss as the capillary beds engorge. Postcapillary sphincters remain closed, forcing fluids into the interstitial spaces by **hydrostatic pressure.** The circulatory crisis worsens as the compensatory mechanisms begin to fail. Interstitial edema reduces the ability of the capillaries to provide oxygen and nutrients to, and remove carbon dioxide and other waste products from, the cells. The capillary and cell membranes also begin to break down. Red blood cells begin to clump together, or agglutinate, in the hypoxic and stagnant capillaries forming columns of coagulated cells called **rouleaux.**

hydrostatic pressure *the pressure of liquids in equilibrium; the pressure exerted by or within liquids.*

rouleaux *group of red blood cells that are stuck together.*

Capillary Washout

The building acidosis from the accumulating lactic acid and carbon dioxide (carbonic acid) finally causes relaxation of the postcapillary sphincters. With relaxation, those by-products along with potassium (released by the cells to maintain a neutral environment in the presence of building acidosis) and the columns of coagulated red blood cells are dumped into the venous circulation. This **washout** causes profound metabolic acidosis and releases microscopic emboli. Cardiac output drops toward zero; peripheral vascular resistance drops toward zero; blood pressure drops toward zero; cellular perfusion, even to the most critical organs, drops toward zero. The body moves quickly and then irreversibly toward death.

washout *release of accumulated lactic acid, carbon dioxide (carbonic acid), potassium, and rouleaux into the venous circulation.*

compensated shock *hemodynamic insult to the body in which the body responds effectively. Signs and symptoms are limited, and the human system functions normally.*

STAGES OF SHOCK

The shock process, as previously described, can be divided into three stages based on presenting signs and symptoms. The stages are progressively more serious and include compensated, decompensated, and irreversible shock (Table 19–2).

Compensated Shock

Compensated shock is the initial shock state. In this stage, the body is still capable of meeting its critical metabolic needs through a series of progressive compensating actions (Figure 19-9). This progressive compensation creates a series of signs and symptoms that range from the subtle to the obvious. The compensated shock stage ends with the precipitous drop in blood pressure. Compensated shock is the shock stage in which prehospital interventions and rapid transport are most likely to meet with success.

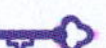

Compensated shock is the shock stage in which prehospital interventions and rapid transport are most likely to meet with success.

The body's first recognizable response to serious blood loss is probably an increase in pulse rate. However, a rate increase due to blood loss may be difficult to differentiate from tachycardia due to excitement and the "fight-or-flight" response. The first sign usually attributable to shock is a narrowing pulse pressure and weakening pulse strength (weak and rapid pulse). As the condition becomes more serious, vasoconstriction causes the patient's skin to become pale, cyanotic, or ashen as blood is directed away from the skin and toward the more critical organs. The skin becomes cool and moist (clammy), and capillary refill times begin to exceed 3 seconds. As compensation becomes more acute, the victim becomes anxious, restless, or combative and complains of thirst and weakness. Near the end of the compensated shock stage, the patient may experience air hunger and tachypnea.

Content Review

Stages of Shock

- Compensated
- Decompensated
- Irreversible

Decompensated Shock

Decompensated shock begins as the body's compensatory mechanisms become unable to respond to a continuing blood loss. Mechanisms that initially compensated for blood loss now fail, and the body

decompensated shock *continuing hemodynamic insult to the body in which the compensatory mechanisms break down. The signs and symptoms become very pronounced, and the patient moves rapidly toward death.*

Table 19–2 The Stages of Shock

Compensated Shock

Initial stage of shock in which the body progressively compensates for continuing blood loss.

- Pulse rate increases
- Pulse strength decreases
- Skin becomes cool and clammy
- Patient feels progressing anxiety, restlessness, combativeness
- Patient experiences thirst, weakness, eventual air hunger

Decompensated Shock

Begins when the body's compensatory mechanisms can no longer maintain preload.

- Pulse becomes unpalpable
- Blood pressure drops precipitously
- Patient becomes unconscious
- Respirations slow or cease

Irreversible Shock

Shortly after the patient enters decompensated shock, the lack of circulation begins to have profound effects on body cells. As they are irreversibly damaged, the cells die, tissues dysfunction, organs dysfunction, and the patient dies.

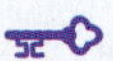

Entry into decompensated shock is indicated by a precipitous drop in systolic blood pressure.

moves quickly toward complete collapse. Entry into decompensated shock is indicated by a precipitous drop in systolic blood pressure. Despite all compensatory mechanisms, venous return is inadequate, and the heart no longer has enough blood volume to pump. Even extreme tachycardia produces little cardiac output. No amount of vascular resistance can maintain blood pressure and circulation. Even the most critical organs of the body are hypoperfused. The heart, already hypoxic because of poor perfusion and the increased oxygen demands created by tachycardia, begins to fail. This state may be indicated by the presence of a bradycardia. In this stage, the brain is extremely hypoxic. This means that the patient displays a rapidly dropping level of responsiveness. The brain's control over bodily functions, including respiration, ceases, and the body takes on a deathlike appearance.

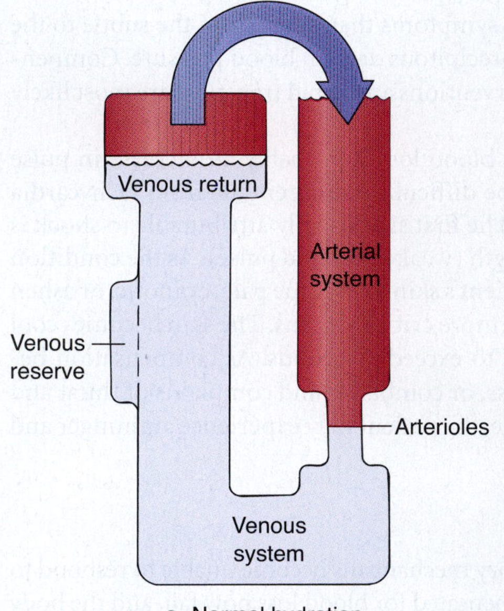

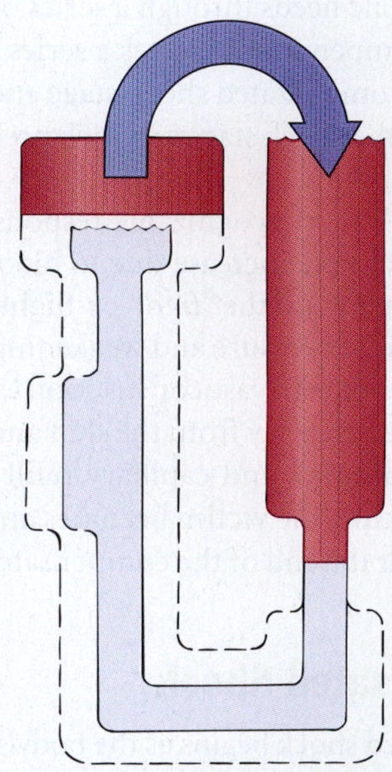

■ **Figure 19-9** In compensated shock, the body reduces venous capacitance in response to blood loss.

Irreversible Shock

Irreversible shock exists when the body's cells are badly injured and die in such quantities that the organs cannot carry out their normal functions. While aggressive resuscitation may restore blood pressure and pulse, organ failure ultimately results in organism failure. The transition to irreversible shock is very difficult to identify in the field. Clearly, the longer a patient is in decompensated shock, the more likely it is that he has moved to irreversible shock.

irreversible shock *final stage of shock in which organs and cells are so damaged that recovery is impossible.*

The transition between decompensated and irreversible shock is very difficult to identify in the field.

SHOCK ASSESSMENT

You must be able to recognize shock as early as possible in your patient assessment and begin to provide care just as promptly. You must search out the signs and symptoms of shock in each phase of the assessment process: the scene size-up, the primary assessment, the rapid or focused secondary assessment, and—when appropriate—the detailed physical exam. Further, you must carefully monitor for the development or progression of shock with frequent ongoing assessments during care and transport of the trauma patient.

Scene Size-up

Anticipate shock during the scene size-up. Analyze the forces that caused the trauma and their impacts on your patient for the possibility of both external and internal injury and hemorrhage. Look especially for injury mechanisms that might result in internal chest, abdominal, or pelvic injuries or in external hemorrhage from the head, neck, and extremities. Apply trauma triage criteria as early as practical to identify the patients who are most likely to require immediate transport to the trauma center and access to air medical transport, if appropriate.

Primary Assessment

The primary assessment directs your attention to the body systems/patient priorities that present the early signs of shock. Determine the patient's level of consciousness, responsiveness, and orientation. Any mental deficit or restlessness, anxiety, or combativeness may be due to blood loss and hypovolemia. As you assess the airway and breathing, apply high-flow, high-concentration oxygen. Watch for tachypnea and air hunger, which are late signs of shock. When assessing circulation, recall that tachycardia suggests hypovolemia. Baseline rates suggestive of tachycardia are about 160 in the infant, 140 in the preschooler, 120 in the school-age child, and 100 in the adult. An increase of 20 beats per minute above any of these rates suggests a significant blood loss. The weaker the pulse, the more the patient is compensating for blood loss.

During assessment, be aware that any mental deficit or restlessness, anxiety, or combativeness may be due to blood loss and hypovolemia.

Carefully observe the patient's body surface and be quick to anticipate potential shock, either as a cause of or a contributing factor to the patient's condition. Look also to the general condition of the skin. It should be warm, pink, and dry. If it is cyanotic, gray, ashen, pale, and cool and moist (clammy), suspect peripheral vasoconstriction, an early sign of shock.

Watch the pulse oximeter for the saturation value and keep it above 95 percent, if possible. As compensation increases and the pulse strength diminishes, the pulse oximeter readings will become more and more unreliable. If you note erratic or intermittent readings with the device, suspect increasing cardiovascular compensation and progressing shock as the reason.

Capnography can be a valuable assessment tool during the resuscitation of the trauma patient and is rapidly becoming the standard of care. Waveform analysis and evaluation of the end-tidal CO_2 ($ETCO_2$) may assure proper initial and continuing endotracheal tube placement and guide artificial ventilation. The capnograph measures the partial pressures of CO_2 in exhaled air, reflecting the status of both ventilation and circulation. Decreased $ETCO_2$ levels reflect cardiac arrest, shock, pulmonary embolism, or incomplete airway obstruction (bronchospasm, mucous plugging). Increased $ETCO_2$ levels reflect hypoventilation, respiratory depression, or hyperthermia. $ETCO_2$ readings above 40 mmHg suggest the need for increased ventilatory support. Readings below 30 mmHg suggest hyperventilation or the need for circulatory support. Capnography may not recognize intubation of a mainstem bronchus, so assure breath sounds are equal while an endotracheal tube is in place.

Capnography is especially important in head injury, as an abnormally low alveolar CO_2 level may produce severe cerebral vasoconstriction. Normal expiratory CO_2 levels are between 35 and

40 mmHg and should not drop below 30 mmHg, especially in head trauma patients. An expiratory CO_2 level above 40 mmHg suggests hypoventilation and the need for faster or deeper ventilations.

Conclude the primary assessment by establishing patient priorities. If any indication, MOI, sign, or symptom suggests serious internal hemorrhage or uncontrolled external hemorrhage, consider rapid trauma assessment and expeditious transport. If the patient has minor and isolated injuries, move to the focused history and physical exam.

Secondary Assessment

The focused physical exam is performed on a trauma patient with an expected, isolated, non-serious injury.

As noted earlier, the order in which the steps of the secondary assessment are performed vary with the patient's MOI. For trauma patients who have no significant mechanism, perform an assessment focused on the area of injury, then obtain baseline vital signs and gather a patient history. For trauma patients who have a significant MOI, continue spinal immobilization and perform a rapid trauma assessment and then obtain baseline vital signs and a patient history. Remember that trauma patients with significant mechanisms of injury are the most likely to suffer from shock.

The rapid secondary assessment is performed on a patient with a significant MOI or signs of shock or serious injury.

Rapid Secondary Assessment When you have a trauma patient with a significant MOI, perform a rapid secondary assessment, inspecting and palpating the patient from head to toe (Figure 19-10 ■). Immediately control any significant hemorrhage. Put a dressing and bandage over the wound and apply direct pressure. Provide more complete hemorrhage control once you attend to the other priorities.

Be sure to examine areas of the body where you expect to find serious injury, as suggested by your scene size-up. Pay special attention to the areas most likely to produce serious, life-threatening injury: the head, neck, chest, abdomen, and pelvis. Minor reddening may be the only sign of a developing contusion and serious internal injury. Also examine the neck veins. In the supine, normovolemic patient, they should be full. If they are flat, suspect hypovolemia.

During your rapid secondary assessment, rule out the possibility of obstructive shock. Assess the chest to identify any tension pneumothorax. Look for dyspnea, a hyperinflated chest, distended jugular veins, resonant percussion, and diminished or absent breath sounds on the affected side, lower tracheal shift to the opposite side, and any subcutaneous emphysema. Consider pleural decompression if the signs suggest tension pneumothorax (see Chapter 25, "Thoracic Trauma"). Also suspect and search for pericardial tamponade. Look for penetrating injury, distended jugular veins, muffled or distant heart tones, tachycardia, and progressive and extreme hypotension. Pericardial tamponade is treated with IV fluids in the field and requires immediate and rapid transport to a trauma center. If the patient received significant anterior chest trauma, suspect myocardial contusion. Apply an ECG monitor and analyze the cardiac rhythm.

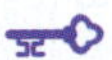

During assessment, be alert to the possibility that hemorrhagic shock is not the problem or is not the only problem affecting your patient.

During the assessment, be alert to the possibility that hemorrhagic shock is not the problem or is not the only problem affecting your patient. Conditions such as stroke, epilepsy, or heart attack

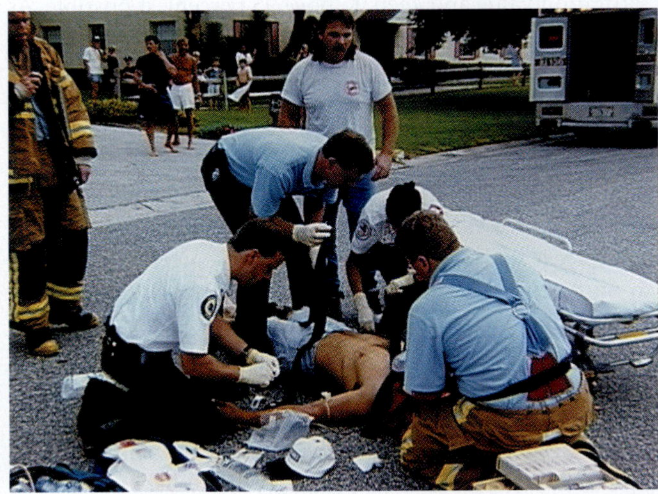

■ **Figure 19-10** The rapid trauma assessment focuses on potential shock-inducing injuries to the head, neck, and torso.

can lead to auto crashes and other traumatic events. Be careful to rule out cardiogenic shock by questioning the patient about crushing substernal chest pain and looking for pulmonary edema, jugular vein distention, and cardiac dysrhythmias (see Chapter 28, "Cardiology"). Also suspect and check for neurogenic shock (see Chapter 24, "Spinal Trauma"). Ask about neck or back pain and evaluate for tenderness along the spine. Look for the presence of pink and warm skin below the point of nervous system injury, while the skin above the injury is pale, cool, and clammy. Other shock states such as anaphylactic, septic, and diabetic shock are not likely unless the patient history suggests them.

Take a quick set of vital signs, keying in on both the pulse rate and pulse pressure. If the pulse is weak, its rate is elevated, or the pulse pressure is diminished, suspect serious hemorrhage. Gauge your findings against the MOI and the time from the injury to your assessment. The shorter the time and the more pronounced the signs and symptoms, the more rapidly the patient is moving toward decompensation and then irreversible shock.

Complete this step of the assessment process by gathering a patient history. Listen to any patient complaints of weakness, thirst, or nausea, which may be further signs of shock. Be especially alert for patient complaints suggestive of a myocardial infarction. Be prepared to monitor the heart for dysrhythmias.

At the end of the rapid or focused secondary assessment, inventory your findings. Set the patient's priority for transport, and set priorities for the order in which you will care for injuries. Again, if any indication, MOI, sign, or symptom suggests serious internal hemorrhage or uncontrolled external hemorrhage, consider rapid transport for the patient. Approximate the probable volume of blood lost to fractures, large contusions, and hematomas. Also note the probable locations of internal hemorrhage and attempt to approximate blood loss from them. Identify all significant injuries and assign each a priority for care. While you may not complete care for all the injuries, setting priorities assures that you quickly address those injuries most likely to contribute to the patient's hypovolemia and shock.

Detailed Physical Exam

Consider performing a detailed physical exam on a potential shock patient only after all priorities have been addressed and the patient is either en route to the trauma center or circumstances such as a prolonged extrication prevent immediate transport. If you have the time, assess the patient from head to toe and look for any additional signs of injury. Remember that your early arrival at the patient's side may mean that the ecchymosis (black-and-blue discoloration) associated with injuries has not had time to develop. Therefore, be very careful to look for reddening (erythema) and areas of local warmth, suggestive of trauma.

Reassessment

After completing the primary assessment and the rapid or focused secondary assessment, perform serial reassessments. Reassess mental status, airway, breathing, and circulation. Reestablish patient priorities and reassess and record the vital signs. This reassessment allows you to identify any trends in the patient's condition. Pay particular attention to the pulse rate and pulse pressure. If the pulse rate is increasing and the difference between the diastolic and systolic pressures is decreasing, suspect increasing compensation and worsening shock. Perform a focused assessment for any changes in symptoms the patient reports. Also, check the adequacy and effectiveness of any interventions you have performed. Provide this reassessment every 5 minutes for the seriously injured patient or for any patient who displays any of the signs or symptoms of shock.

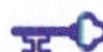

A primary principle of shock care is to ensure the best possible chance for tissue oxygenation and carbon dioxide off-load; do this by providing supplemental high-flow, high-concentration oxygen or positive-pressure ventilation.

SHOCK MANAGEMENT

Airway and Breathing Management

Management of the shock patient begins with corrective actions taken during the primary assessment. One of the primary principles of shock care is to ensure the best possible chance for tissue oxygenation and carbon dioxide off-load. Accomplish this by assuring or providing good ventilations with supplemental high-flow, high-concentration oxygen (15 L/min via nonrebreather mask). If the patient is moving air ineffectively (at a breathing rate less than 12/min or with inadequate respiratory volume), provide positive-pressure ventilations.

overdrive respiration *positive-pressure ventilation supplied to a breathing patient.*

Positive-pressure ventilation to the breathing patient, called **overdrive respiration,** is coordinated with the patient's breathing attempts if possible (Figure 19-11 ■). However, assure that the ventilations provide both a good respiratory volume (at least 500 mL) and an adequate respiratory rate (at least 12 to 16 per minute). Overdrive respiration may be indicated in patients with rib fractures, flail chest, spinal injury with diaphragmatic respirations, head injury, or any condition in which the patient, because of bellows system or respiratory control failure, is not breathing adequately on his own.

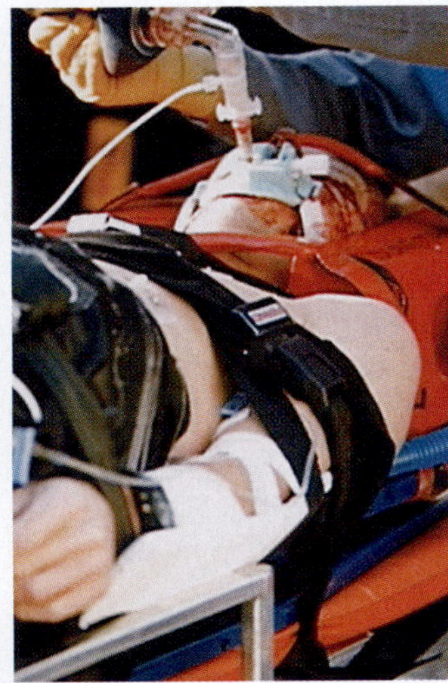

■ **Figure 19-11** Assure that the potential shock patient receives adequate ventilation, using overdrive respiration, if necessary.

Two techniques to improve ventilatory efficiency are positive end-expiratory pressure (PEEP) and continuous positive airway pressure (CPAP). PEEP uses a restrictive valve on the endotracheal tube or mask of the bag-valve unit. There it resists exhalation, maintaining a positive pressure and keeping the patient's airway open longer during exhalation. CPAP uses special ventilation equipment that increases pressure during both inspiration and expiration. This keeps the airway open during more of the respiratory cycle.

If necessary, protect the airway with endotracheal intubation. If the patient is unresponsive or somewhat unresponsive and unable to protect his airway, be aggressive in your care. Rapid-sequence intubation may be required. Shock patients frequently vomit, and gastric aspiration presents a serious, possibly fatal, consequence. Capnography may help assure proper endotracheal tube placement, help you guide your ventilatory rate and volume, and confirm that the endotracheal tube remains in the trachea.

If there is any sign of tension pneumothorax, confirm it and provide pleural decompression either at the second intercostal space, midclavicular line or at the fifth intercostal space, midaxillary line (see Chapter 25, "Thoracic Trauma"). Continue to monitor the patient because it is common for the catheter to clog and the tension pneumothorax to reappear. Insert another needle close to the first to relieve any subsequent buildup of pressure.

Hemorrhage Control

Provide rapid control of any significant external hemorrhage. Use direct pressure, direct pressure and elevation where practical, and pressure points as needed. Apply a tourniquet to control serious and continuing hemorrhage only if it is absolutely necessary. Remember, there are serious consequences with both proper and improper use of a tourniquet.

Fluid Resuscitation

The field treatment of choice for significant blood loss in trauma cases is blood transfusion. Blood has red blood cells to carry oxygen, has clotting factors and platelets to assist in hemostasis, and remains in the bloodstream once it is infused. Blood, however, must be refrigerated, typed, and cross-matched. (O-negative blood may be given in emergency circumstances.) Blood also has a short shelf life and is costly for field use. The most practical fluid for prehospital administration, then, is an isotonic crystalloid like lactated Ringer's solution or normal saline.

The most practical choice for prehospital fluid resuscitation is lactated Ringer's solution.

Some hypertonic and synthetic solutions may have some applications for fluid resuscitation. None of these, however, has been identified as superior to isotonic electrolyte solutions for prehospital use. Hypertonic crystalloid solutions can mobilize the interstitial and cellular fluid volumes to replace lost blood volume but, like other crystalloids, they are not able to carry either the oxygen or the clotting factors essential for hemorrhage control. The biggest advantage of hypertonic solutions is their low volume and weight—an advantage in wilderness, remote, and military applications.

Another category of new solutions with possible indications for prehospital care are the polyhemoglobins. These solutions are either animal or human hemoglobin that has been processed to exclude antigens and microorganisms that would cause disease or adverse reaction in the recipient. Polyhemoglobins have a prolonged shelf life, are relatively inexpensive, and can effectively carry oxygen from the lungs to the tissues. Prehospital studies are being conducted and, if successful, these agents may be very useful in combating hypovolemia due to hemorrhage.

When administering fluids to a trauma patient or to any patient who may need large fluid volumes, consider the internal lumen size of both the catheter and the administration set. Fluid flow is proportional to the fourth power of the internal diameter. This means that if you double the lu-

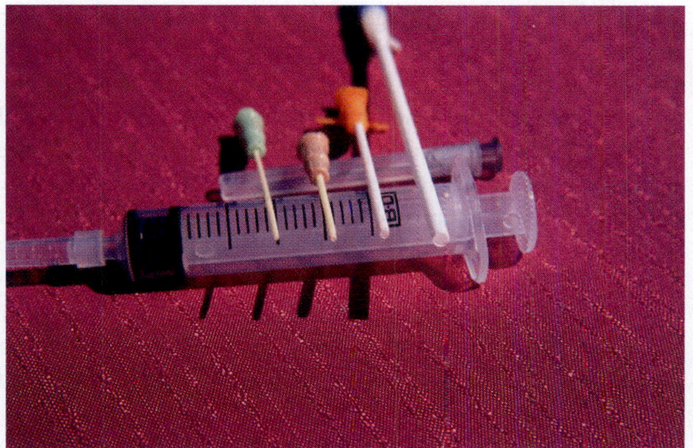

■ Figure 19-12 Catheter size greatly influences fluid flow. Shown here are 22-, 18-, 14-, and 8-gauge catheters.

men's diameter, the same fluid under the same pressure will flow 16 times more quickly. Hence, use the largest catheter you can introduce into the patient's vein and use a large-bore trauma or blood administration set (Figure 19-12 ■).

Catheter length and fluid pressure also influence fluid flow. The longer the catheter, the greater the resistance to flow. The ideal catheter for the shock patient is relatively short, 1½ inch or shorter. An increase in pressure increases fluid flow. This means that the higher you position the bag or the greater the pressure differential between the solution and the venous system, the faster the fluid flow. If you cannot elevate the fluid bag, position it under the patient or place it in a pressure infuser or a blood-pressure cuff inflated to 100 or 200 mmHg.

Electrolyte administration is indicated for the patient with the classic signs and symptoms of shock and isolated external hemorrhage that has been halted. Employ aggressive fluid resuscitation using lactated Ringer's solution or normal saline via two lines running wide open until the blood pressure returns to 100 mmHg and the level of consciousness increases (Figure 19-13 ■). Use large-bore catheters (14 or 16 gauge) connected to trauma or blood tubing to assure unimpeded flow and a non-flow-restrictive saline lock if your system so requires. This fluid resuscitation approach is also prudent for the patient with continuing (internal or uncontrolled external) hemorrhage with absent peripheral pulses or a systolic BP below 80 mmHg. Run the two lines wide open until 350 to 500 mL of solution is infused. Then evaluate for the return of peripheral pulses or rise of the systolic blood pressure to just under 80 mmHg—sometimes referred to as permissive hypotension. If the patient's conditions do not improve, consider repeating the fluid bolus.

If penetrating trauma to the chest exists and/or you cannot control other hemorrhage, be more conservative with fluid administration. Cautiously control fluid volume, remembering that your goal is maintaining vital signs, not improving them. Increases in blood pressure can dislodge developing clots and disrupt the normal clotting processes. The result may be further hemorrhage with further dilution of the clotting factors and hemoglobin. Closely monitor your patient's vital signs,

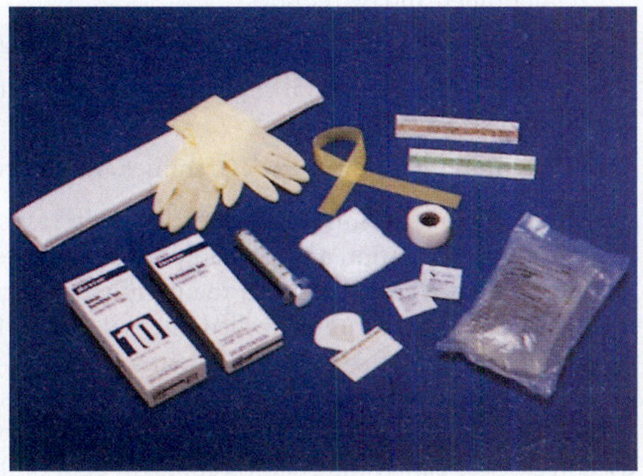

■ Figure 19-13 Supplies for initiating IV therapy.

and administer lactated Ringer's solution to keep the patient's mental status and pulse pressure at a steady level. Maintain the blood pressure at a steady level even if it has dropped below 100 mmHg; studies suggest that a blood pressure of 88 mmHg may be optimal for the patient with continuing internal hemorrhage. Head injury patients (Glasgow Coma Scale [GCS] of 8 or less) may require a slightly higher systolic blood pressure (90 mmHg) to assure cerebral perfusion. Note, however, that prehospital fluid resuscitation is an area of much research and controversy. Consult with your medical director and local protocols to determine your system's parameters for prehospital fluid resuscitation of the shock patient.

Prehospital fluid resuscitation is an area of much research and controversy. Consult with your medical director and local protocols regarding fluid resuscitation of the shock patient.

In children, infuse 20 mL/kg of body weight rapidly when you see any signs and symptoms of shock. Administer a second fluid bolus if the vital signs do not improve after the first bolus or if, at some later time, the patient again begins to deteriorate. The objective of fluid resuscitation in the field is not the return of normal vital signs but the stabilization of vital signs until the patient reaches the trauma center.

During fluid resuscitation, cautiously control fluid volume, remembering that your goal is maintaining vital signs, not improving them. Increases in blood pressure can dislodge developing clots and disrupt the normal clotting processes. The result may be further hemorrhage with further dilution of the clotting factors and hemoglobin. Closely monitor your patient's vital signs, and administer lactated Ringer's solution or normal saline to keep the patient's mental status and pulse pressure steady. Maintain the blood pressure at a steady level once it has dropped below 80 mmHg. Do not, however, let the pressure drop below 50 mmHg, nor below 90 mmHg for head injury patients with a GCS of 8 or less.

Temperature Control

Trauma and blood loss deal serious blows to the mechanisms that normally adjust the body's core temperature. Reduced body activity reduces heat production to subnormal levels. Cutaneous vasoconstriction decreases the skin's ability to act as part of the body's temperature control system. The result is a patient highly susceptible to fluctuations in body temperature. In cases of trauma, patients commonly lose heat more rapidly than normal and heat production is low. At the same time, the heat-generating reflexes, like shivering, are ineffective and, in fact, are counterproductive to the shock care process.

In all but the warmest environments, cover the hemorrhage or shock patient with a blanket and keep the patient compartment of the ambulance very warm.

In all except the warmest environments, help conserve body temperature by covering the patient with a blanket and keeping the patient compartment of the ambulance very warm. If you infuse fluids, assure that they are well above room temperature—ideally at body temperature or slightly above (no more than 104° F). Use fluid warmers or keep IV solutions in a compartment that is warmer than the rest of the ambulance. Be very sensitive to any patient complaints about being cold, and provide whatever assistance you can to assure that heat loss is limited.

Pneumatic Anti-shock Garment

pneumatic anti-shock garment (PASG) *garment designed to produce uniform pressure on the lower extremities and abdomen; used with shock and hemorrhage patients in some EMS systems.*

The **pneumatic anti-shock garment (PASG),** sometimes referred to as the medical anti-shock trouser (MAST), is a device designed to apply firm circumferential pressure around the lower extremities, pelvis, and lower abdomen. The device is intended to compress the vascular space, thereby accomplishing four objectives:

- ★ To increase peripheral vascular resistance by pressurizing the arteries of the lower abdomen and extremities.
- ★ To reduce the vascular volume by compressing venous vessels.
- ★ To increase the central circulating blood volume with blood returned from areas under the garment.
- ★ To immobilize the lower extremities and the pelvic region.

Research has determined that the garment is responsible for a return of about 250 mL of blood to the central circulation and probably reduces the venous capacitance by the same volume. The PASG also does seem to increase the peripheral vascular resistance, although this may be detrimental to patients with uncontrolled internal hemorrhage.

Research has further revealed potential problems with PASG use. The abdominal component of the PASG pressurizes the abdominal cavity, increasing the work associated with breathing and, in some cases, reducing chest excursion. Application of the garment also increases mortality when used in cases of penetrating chest trauma. In light of this information, it is imperative that you understand the limitations of the device and comply with your local protocols and medical direction when considering use of the PASG.

The PASG is a puncture-resistant, easy to clean, three-compartment trouser attached to the patient circumferentially around the lower abdomen and extremities with Velcro closures. The compartments can be inflated either independently or all together with a foot- or electric-powered pump. However, the abdominal segment should be inflated with the leg segments or after them, never before. A PASG may or may not come with pressure gauges, although all models should be equipped with pop-off valves to prevent inflation above 110 mmHg.

Indications for PASG use include shock patients with controlled hemorrhage, patients with pelvic fracture and instability with hypotension, patients with possible neurogenic shock, and any shock patients with uncontrolled hemorrhage below the mid-abdomen. Penetrating chest trauma, pulmonary edema, and cardiogenic shock are contraindications to PASG application and inflation. Use the PASG with caution for patients in late pregnancy, patients with suspected diaphragmatic ruptures, and patients with objects impaled in the abdomen or with abdominal eviscerations. In these cases, do not inflate the abdominal section because doing so increases intra-abdominal pressure.

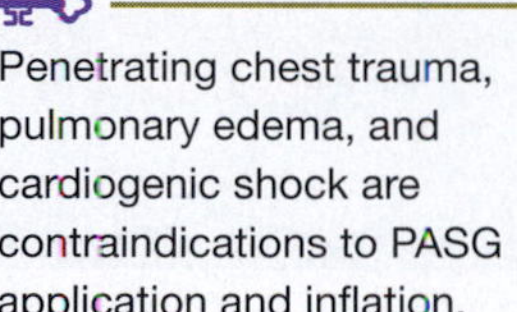

Penetrating chest trauma, pulmonary edema, and cardiogenic shock are contraindications to PASG application and inflation.

Begin application of the PASG by removing the patient's clothing, although you may leave on the undergarments for patient modesty if they are not bulky (Procedure 19–1). Assess areas of the patient's body that will lie beneath the garment, as these regions will be hidden from view and inaccessible once the PASG is applied. Then move the patient onto a spine board or other patient-carrying device with an opened garment positioned for application. One application technique calls for securing the garment's Velcro attachments at the ends of their travel and having a caregiver at the patient's feet put one arm through each of the garment's leg sections from the foot ends. That caregiver then grasps the patient's toes while another caregiver pulls the garment off the first caregiver's arms, onto the patient's legs, and up to the small of the patient's back. Alternatively, you may slide the device under the patient from the feet with the extra garment and the anterior abdominal segment folded between the legs. Position the PASG so that the upper portion of the abdominal segment is just below the rib margin. Secure the abdominal and leg segments with the Velcro strips, assuring that they hold the segments firmly around the limbs and abdomen. This reduces the air volume necessary to inflate the PASG.

Quickly take baseline vital signs, and be especially alert for breath sounds. If there are no crackles or other suggestions of pulmonary edema, then inflate the PASG slowly. Watch for any change (improvement) in your patient's mental status, skin color, or pulse rate. If you notice such a change, stop the inflation and reassess vital signs and level of responsiveness. The intent of PASG use is to stabilize the patient's condition, not to return the blood pressure and circulation to normal levels. As with too-aggressive fluid resuscitation, inflation of PASG to a point where blood pressure increases can interfere with the clotting process or even increase internal hemorrhage, thus moving the patient more quickly toward decompensation and death. If vital signs and the level of responsiveness deteriorate, continue PASG inflation until you regain the level of your baseline findings. Once the pop-off valves release, stop inflation. Then inflate the garment every few minutes until the pop-off valves release to assure that the PASG maintains its maximum pressure.

Carefully monitor respirations during PASG inflation. The device may put pressure on the diaphragm, thus increasing the work of respiration as well as reducing respiratory excursion. Also listen carefully for breath sounds. The PASG may increase blood pressure and respiratory congestion as well. If you hear any crackles in the chest or if the patient complains of difficulty breathing, halt the PASG inflation.

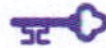

The PASG should not be deflated in the prehospital setting.

The PASG should not be deflated in the prehospital setting. The release of circumferential pressure reduces peripheral vascular resistance, expands the size of the vascular space, and removes about 250 mL of blood from the active circulation. This could seriously harm the healthy patient and have devastating effects on one who is compensating for shock.

Pharmacological Intervention

In shock, pharmacological interventions are generally limited, especially in hypovolemic patients. The sympathetic nervous system efficiently compensates for low volume, and no agent has been shown effective in the prehospital setting, other than intravenous fluid and, in some cases, blood and blood products. For cardiogenic shock, fluid challenge, vasopressors like dopamine, and the

Procedure 19-1 Application of the Pneumatic Anti-shock Garment

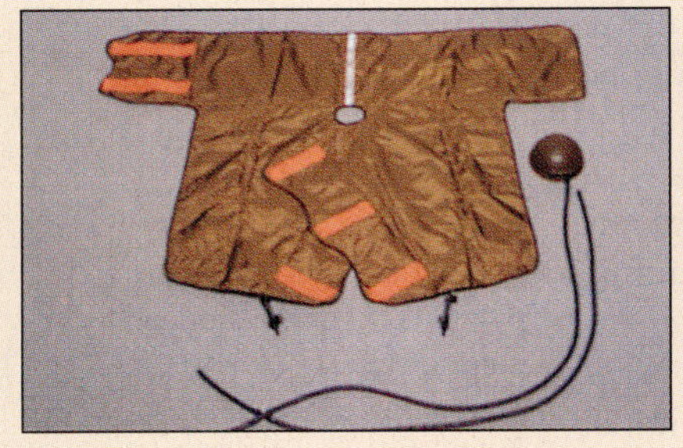

19-1a Prepare the PASG.

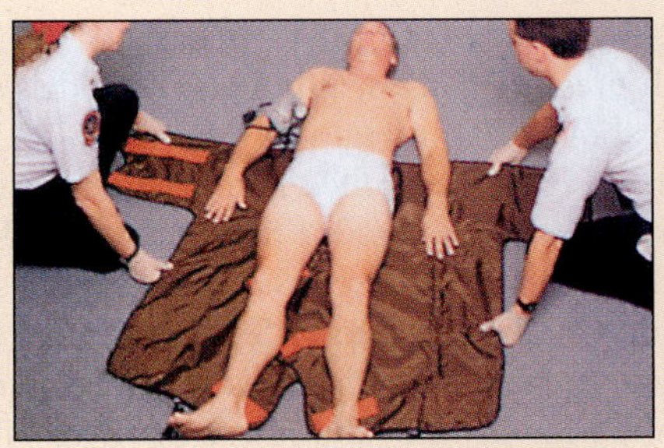

19-1b Position the patient.

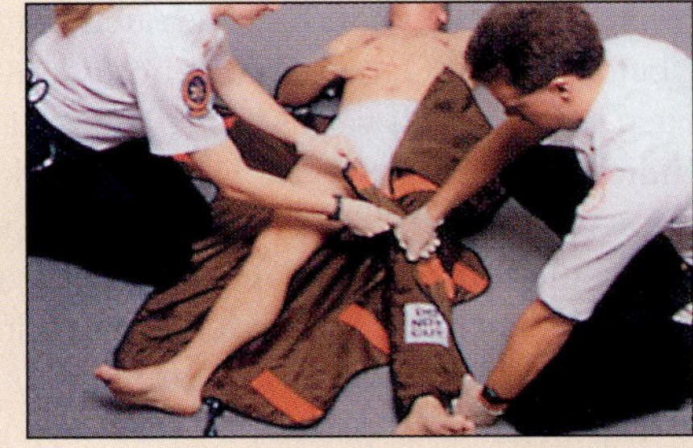

19-1c Following the manufacturer's recommendations, wrap one leg.

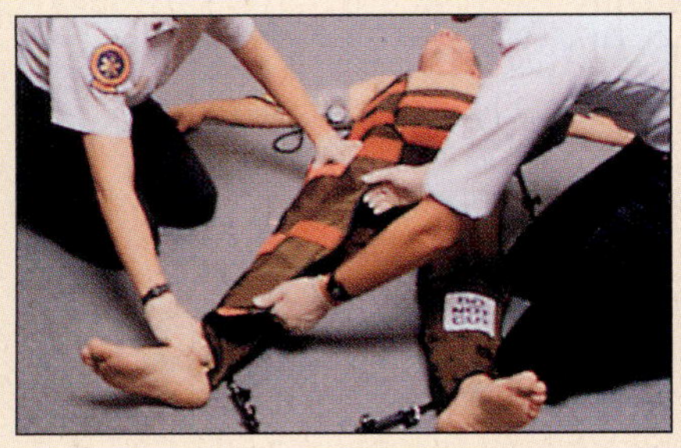

19-1d Wrap the other leg.

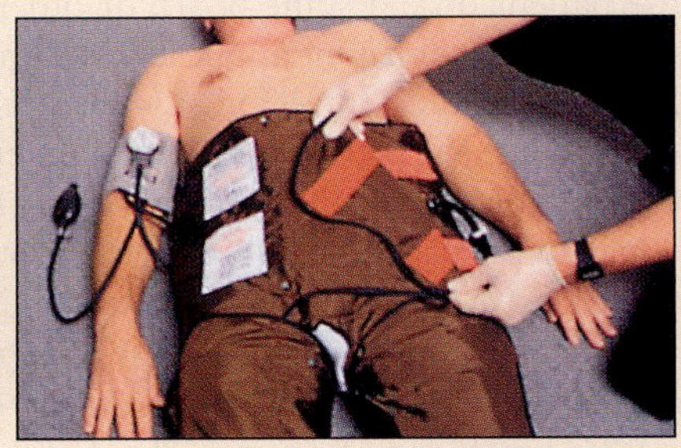

19-1e Wrap the abdomen last.

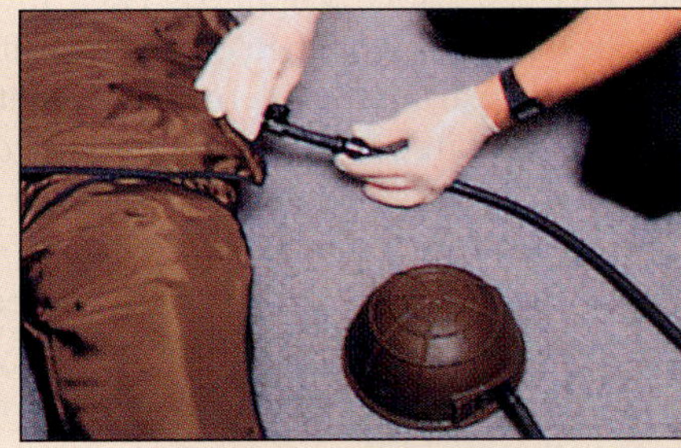

19-1f Connect the tubing.

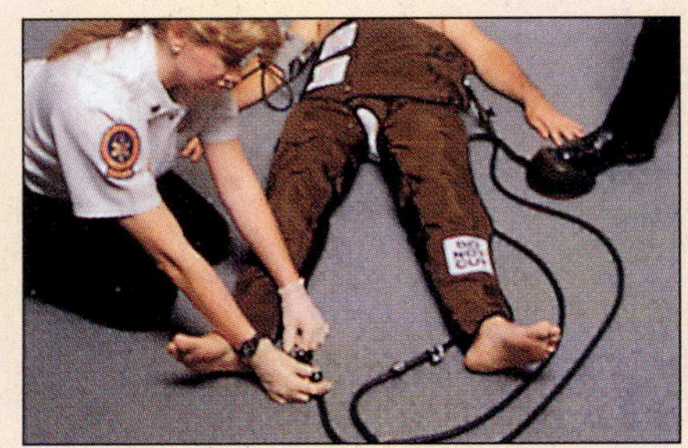

19-1g Inflate the PASG, both legs first.

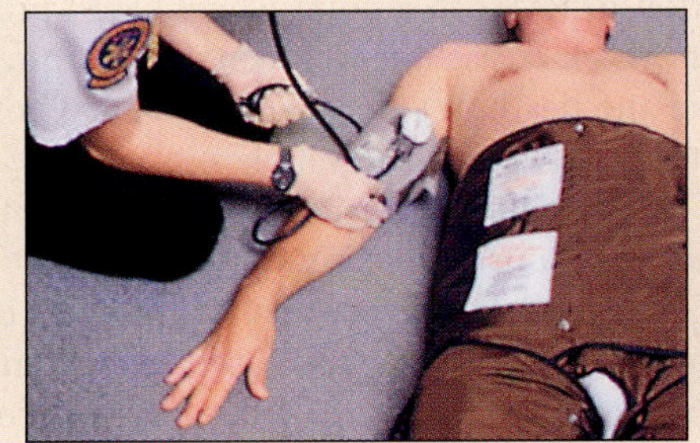

19-1h Monitor the patient.

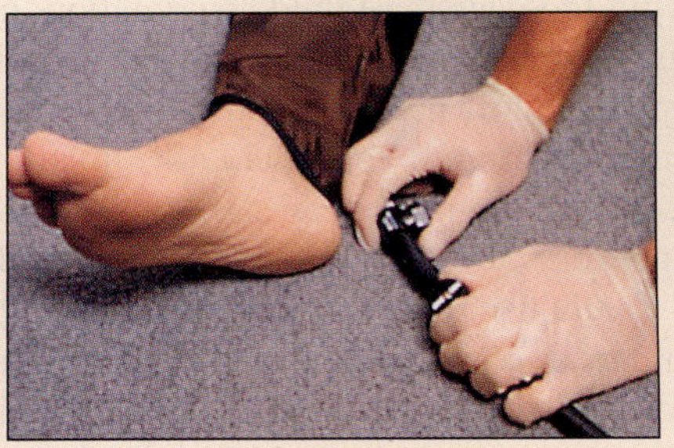

19-1i Close the stopcock valve.

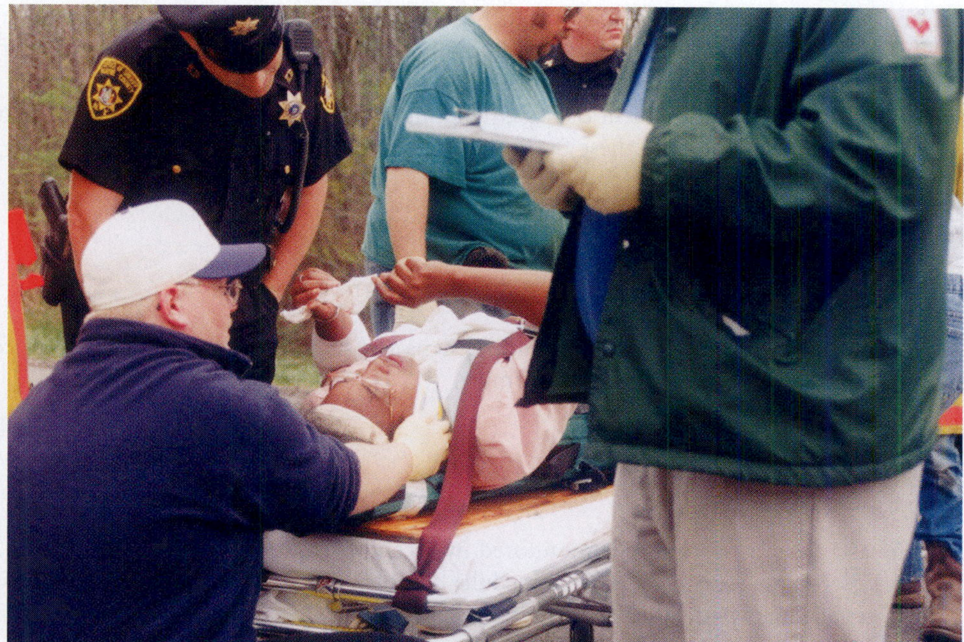

■ **Figure 19-14** Emotional support for the seriously injured trauma patient is an important part of shock patient care.

other cardiac drugs are indicated (see Chapter 28, "Cardiology"). For spinal and obstructive shock, consider intravenous fluids like normal saline and lactated Ringer's solution. For distributive shock, consider IV fluids, dopamine, and use of the PASG.

The patient who has experienced trauma sufficient to induce hemorrhage and hypovolemia will be anxious and bewildered. As the care provider at the patient's side, it is your responsibility to be calm and reassuring, thus counteracting the natural "fight-or-flight" response (Figure 19-14 ■). By acting in this manner, you not only help your patient deal with the event's emotional trauma but also combat some of the negative effects of sympathetic stimulation.

Summary

Significant hemorrhage and its serious consequence, shock, are genuine threats to the trauma patient's life. The signs of these threats are often subtle or hidden, especially if bleeding is internal. Only through careful analysis of the mechanism of injury during the scene size-up and careful evaluation of the patient during the assessment process can you recognize and then treat these life-threatening problems. Treatment often involves rapidly bringing the patient to the services of a trauma center and, while doing so, providing aggressive care—supplemental oxygen, positive-pressure ventilations, fluid resuscitation, and use of a PASG as necessary—aimed at maintaining vital signs, not necessarily improving them. With this approach, you afford your patient the best chance for survival.

Review Questions

1. The initial signs of compensated shock accompanying external hemorrhage include all of the following except:
   a. unconsciousness.
   b. thirst.
   c. combativeness.
   d. weakness.

2. You and your crew respond to a motor vehicle collision where a 20-year-old female has received several cuts over her body. You determine that her airway is patent and she is breathing adequately. Her blood pressure is maintaining at a stable level, and you estimate that she has lost approximately 15 percent of her circulating blood volume. She is alert and oriented but seems a bit nervous. From these findings, you determine that your patient is in __________ hemorrhage.
   a. stage 4
   b. stage 1
   c. stage 3
   d. stage 2
3. In a patient with no suspected trauma, and signs and symptoms of shock, you can perform the tilt test. This test is performed to determine:
   a. cardiogenic shock.
   b. septic shock.
   c. orthostatic hypertension.
   d. orthostatic hypotension.
4. The arterial blood pressure is monitored by receptors in the aortic arch and carotid sinuses. These receptors send signals to the medulla oblongata to help maintain a blood pressure that assures adequate perfusion. These receptors are the:
   a. chemoreceptors.
   b. baroreceptors.
   c. cardioinhibitory centers.
   d. cardioacceleratory centers.
5. When the body is working to counteract the effects of hemorrhage and cardiovascular insufficiency, it constricts arterioles and increases the heart rate and contractility. The most rapid hormonal response occurs with the release of:
   a. angiotesin II.
   b. glucocorticoids.
   c. antidiuretic hormone.
   d. catecholamines.
6. You are called to the scene where a man is very nearly unconscious. His vital signs indicate a falling blood pressure and bradycardia as well as cool, clammy skin. Based on these assessment findings, you conclude that the patient is most likely in:
   a. neurogenic shock.
   b. irreversible shock.
   c. decompensated shock.
   d. compensated shock.
7. Rapid transport to a trauma facility is indicated in which of the following patients?
   a. a patient in stage 1 hemorrhage
   b. a patient with suspected serious internal hemorrhage
   c. a patient who is vomiting coffee-ground material
   d. a patient with external hemorrhage that is controlled on the scene
8. The PASG is contraindicated for which of the following types of shock?
   a. neurogenic
   b. respiratory
   c. hypovolemic
   d. cardiogenic
9. Your patient is determined to be in decompensated shock. Fluid therapy is indicated. The most practical fluid for prehospital administration is:
   a. D_5W.
   b. blood plasma.
   c. lactated Ringer's.
   d. D_5W in half normal saline.

10. A patient develops shock secondary to hypovolemia. You understand that the reduced flow of oxygen to the cells leads to a buildup of lactic acid and other by-products. You further understand that ___________ metabolism causes this process to occur.
    a. Krebs
    b. aerobic
    c. glycolysis
    d. anaerobic

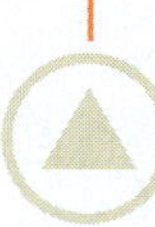

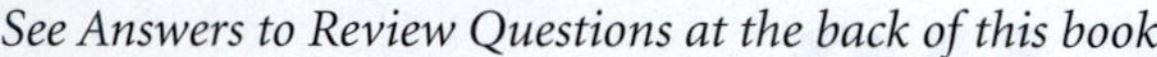

See Answers to Review Questions at the back of this book.

Chapter

20

Soft-Tissue Trauma

Objectives

After reading this chapter, you should be able to:

1. Describe the incidence, morbidity, and mortality of soft-tissue injuries. (p. 854)
2. Describe the anatomy and physiology of the integumentary system, including epidermis, dermis, and subcutaneous tissue. (see Chapter 3)
3. Identify the skin tension lines of the body. (pp. 857–858)
4. Predict soft-tissue injuries based on mechanism of injury. (pp. 872–874)
5. Discuss blunt and penetrating trauma. (pp. 854–860)
6. Discuss the pathophysiology of soft-tissue injuries. (pp. 854–860)
7. Differentiate among the following types of soft-tissue injuries:
   - A. Closed (pp. 855–856)
     - i. Contusion
     - ii. Hematoma
     - iii. Crush injuries
   - B. Open (pp. 857–860)
     - i. Abrasions
     - ii. Lacerations
     - iii. Incisions
     - iv. Avulsions
     - v. Impaled objects
     - vi. Amputations
     - vii. Punctures
8. Discuss the assessment and management of open and closed soft-tissue injuries. (pp. 871–888)
9. Discuss the incidence, morbidity, and mortality of crush injuries. (pp. 856, 884–886)
10. Define the following conditions:
    - A. Crush injury (pp. 856, 867–868, 884–886)
    - B. Crush syndrome (pp. 856, 868, 884–886)
    - C. Compartment syndrome (pp. 866–867, 886)
11. Discuss the mechanisms of injury, assessment findings, and management of crush injuries. (pp. 856, 867–868, 884–886)
12. Discuss the effects of reperfusion and rhabdomyolysis on the body. (pp. 868, 885–886)

13. Discuss the pathophysiology, assessment, and care of hemorrhage associated with soft-tissue injuries, including: (pp. 861, 875–878)
    A. Capillary bleeding
    B. Venous bleeding
    C. Arterial bleeding
14. Describe and identify the indications for and application of the following dressings and bandages: (pp. 869–871)
    A. Sterile/nonsterile dressing
    B. Occlusive/nonocclusive dressing
    C. Adherent/nonadherent dressing
    D. Absorbent/nonabsorbent dressing
    E. Wet/dry dressing
    F. Self-adherent roller bandage
    G. Gauze bandage
    H. Adhesive bandage
    I. Elastic bandage
15. Predict the possible complications of an improperly applied dressing or bandage. (pp. 869–871, 881–882)
16. Discuss the process of wound healing, including:
    A. Hemostasis (pp. 862–863)
    B. Inflammation (p. 863)
    C. Epithelialization (p. 863)
    D. Neovascularization (p. 863)
    E. Collagen synthesis (p. 864)
17. Discuss the assessment and management of wound healing. (pp. 861–868)
18. Discuss the pathophysiology, assessment, and management of wound infection. (pp. 864–866)
19. Formulate treatment priorities for patients with soft-tissue injuries in conjunction with:
    A. Airway/face/neck trauma (pp. 886–887)
    B. Thoracic trauma (open/closed) (pp. 887–888)
    C. Abdominal trauma (p. 888)
20. Given several preprogrammed and moulaged soft-tissue trauma patients, provide the appropriate scene size-up, primary assessment, secondary assessment (rapid trauma or focused physical exam, detailed exam), and reassessments and provide appropriate patient care and transportation. (pp. 854–888)

Key Terms

abrasion, p. 857
amputation, p. 860
avulsion, p. 859
chemotactic factors, p. 863
collagen, p. 864
compartment syndrome, p. 866
contusion, p. 855
crush injury, p. 856
crush syndrome, p. 856
degloving injury, p. 860
ecchymosis, p. 855
epithelialization, p. 863
erythema, p. 855
fibroblasts, p. 864
gangrene, p. 865
granulocytes, p. 863
hematoma, p. 856
hemostasis, p. 862
impaled object, p. 859
incision, p. 858
inflammation, p. 863
integumentary system, p. 854
keloid, p. 867
laceration, p. 857
lymphangitis, p. 864
macrophage, p. 863
necrosis, p. 868
neovascularization, p. 863
phagocytosis, p. 863
puncture, p. 858
remodeling, p. 864
rhabdomyolysis, p. 868
serous fluid, p. 866
tension lines, p. 857

INTRODUCTION

The skin is one of the largest, most important organs of the human body, comprising 16 percent of total body weight. It provides a protective envelope that keeps invading pathogens out while containing body substances and fluids. It is also a key organ of sensation as well as a radiator of excess body heat in warm weather and a conservator of heat in cold conditions. Even as it accomplishes these various functions, the skin remains a durable, pliable, and accommodating tissue, and one that is very able to repair itself.

integumentary system *skin, consisting of the epidermis, dermis, and subcutaneous layers.*

Known collectively as the **integumentary system,** the skin is the first tissue of the human body to experience the effects of trauma. Because skin covers the entire body surface, any penetrating injury or the kinetic forces of blunt injury must pass through it before impacting on other vital organs. Often, the signs of this energy transmission can only be observed with very careful examination of the skin. Therefore, the skin is of great significance at all stages of the patient assessment process.

Trauma to the skin may present as open injuries—abrasions, lacerations, incisions, punctures, avulsions, and amputations—or as closed injuries—contusions, hematomas, and crush injuries. Such injuries infrequently threaten life but may endanger blood vessels, nerves, connective tissue, and other important internal structures. Uncontrolled blood loss may lead to hypovolemia and shock, while the wound may provide a pathway for infection.

EPIDEMIOLOGY

Soft-tissue injuries are the most common type of trauma.

Soft-tissue injuries are by far the most common form of trauma. Over 10 million patients present to emergency departments annually with soft-tissue wounds, many of which require closure. Most, but not all, open wounds require only simple care and limited suturing. A significant minority, however, damage arteries, nerves, or tendons and can lead to permanent disability. Uncontrolled external hemorrhage of an otherwise uncomplicated open wound is a very rare but completely preventable situation that sometimes occurs with this type of injury and can result in death. Of the open wounds presenting to emergency departments, up to 6.5 percent will eventually become infected, resulting in significant morbidity.

Closed wounds share a similar epidemiology, except that they are probably even more common than open injuries. Most minor "bumps and bruises" never reach the paramedic, as most patients elect to self-treat all but the most serious cases. Despite their frequency and usually minor nature, closed injuries *can* result in significant pain, suffering, and morbidity. Infection, however, is not usually a complication with closed wounds. Risk factors for soft-tissue wounds include age (especially school-age children and the elderly), alcohol or drug abuse, and occupation. Laborers, machine operators, and others whose hands and body parts are exposed to heavy objects, machines, or tools are at great risk.

Simple measures can reduce risks and prevent soft-tissue injuries. For example, locating playgrounds on grass, sand, gravel, or other forgiving surfaces and padding the equipment in them can cut injury rates among children. In factories, machine guards, fail-safe switches, and similar engineering controls can reduce injuries. Protective clothing such as steel-toed boots and leather gloves also provide simple methods of reducing the incidence and severity of soft-tissue injuries.

PATHOPHYSIOLOGY OF SOFT-TISSUE INJURY

Although we often take the skin's functions for granted, soft-tissue injury can seriously affect health, causing severe blood and fluid loss, infection, hypothermia, and other problems.

Trauma is a violent transfer of energy that produces an open or closed wound to the skin and possible injury to the structures underneath. Wounds can be either blunt or penetrating (Figure 20-1 ■). While all penetrating wounds are open, blunt trauma can, on occasion, create open wounds. Common soft-tissue injuries include closed wounds—contusions, hematomas, and crush injuries—and open wounds—abrasions, lacerations, incisions, punctures, avulsions, and amputations. Each type of wound is different and deserves special consideration.

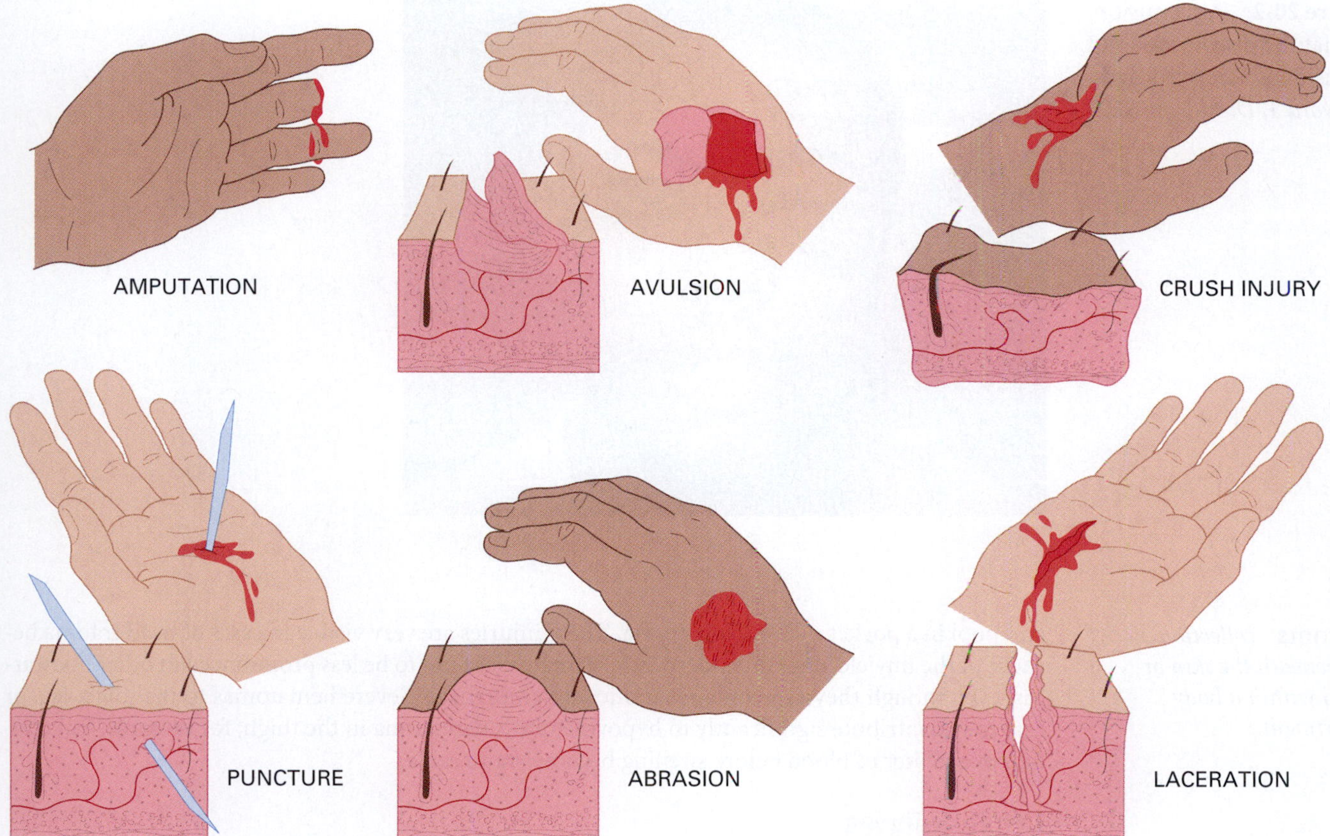

■ Figure 20-1 Types of open soft-tissue injuries.

CLOSED WOUNDS

Contusions

Contusions are blunt, nonpenetrating injuries that crush and damage small blood vessels (Figure 20-2 ■). Blood is drawn to the inflamed tissue, causing a reddening called **erythema.** Blood also leaks into the surrounding interstitial spaces through damaged vessels. As the hemoglobin within the free blood loses its oxygen, it becomes dark red and then blue, resulting in the black-and-blue discoloration called **ecchymosis.** Because the development of ecchymosis is a progressive process, the discoloration may not be evident during prehospital care.

Contusions are more pronounced in areas where the mechanism causing the injury (for example, a steering wheel) and skeletal structures (such as the ribs or skull) trap the skin. Occasionally, a chest injury displays an erythematous or ecchymotic outline of the ribs and sternum, reflecting an impact with the auto dashboard or some other blunt object. Early signs of such an injury may be difficult to identify, but they will become more evident as time passes and discoloration increases.

Hematomas

Soft-tissue bleeding can occur within the tissue and at times can be quite significant. When the injury involves a larger blood vessel, most commonly an artery, the blood can actually separate tissue

contusion *closed wound in which the skin is unbroken, although damage has occurred to the tissue immediately beneath.*

erythema *general reddening of the skin due to dilation of the superficial capillaries.*

ecchymosis *blue-black discoloration of the skin due to leakage of blood into the tissues.*

Content Review

Types of Closed Wounds

- Contusions
- Hematomas
- Crush injuries

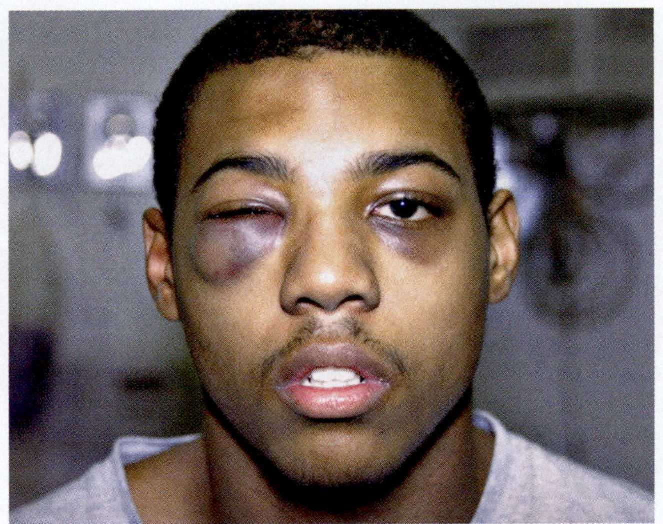

■ Figure 20-2 A contusion. Note that the discoloration of a contusion is a delayed sign. *(© Edward T. Dickinson, MD)*

hematoma *collection of blood beneath the skin or trapped within a body compartment.*

and pool in a pocket called a **hematoma.** These injuries are very visible in cases of head trauma because of the unyielding skull underneath. Hematomas tend to be less pronounced in other body areas, even though they can contain significant hemorrhage. Severe hematomas to the thigh, leg, or arm may contribute significantly to hypovolemia. A hematoma in the thigh, for example, can contain over a liter of blood before swelling becomes noticeable.

Crush Injuries

crush injury *mechanism of injury in which tissue is locally compressed by high pressure forces.*

crush syndrome *systemic disorder of severe metabolic disturbances resulting from the crush of a limb or other body part.*

The term **crush injury** describes a collection of traumatic insults that includes both crush injury itself and crush syndrome. In crush injury, a body part that is compressed, possibly by a heavy object, sustains deep injury to the muscles, blood vessels, bones, and other internal structures (Figure 20-3 ■). Damage can be massive, despite minimal signs displayed on the skin itself. **Crush syndrome** is the term used to describe the systemic effects of a large crush injury. If the pressure that causes a crush injury remains in place for several hours, the resulting destruction of skeletal muscle cells leads to the accumulation of large quantities of myoglobin (a cell protein), potassium, lactic acid, uric acid, and other toxins. When the pressure is released, these products enter the bloodstream. They circulate, causing a severe metabolic acidosis. These materials are also toxic to the kidneys and heart. Crush syndrome is thus a potentially life-threatening trauma event. It will be discussed in more detail later in this chapter.

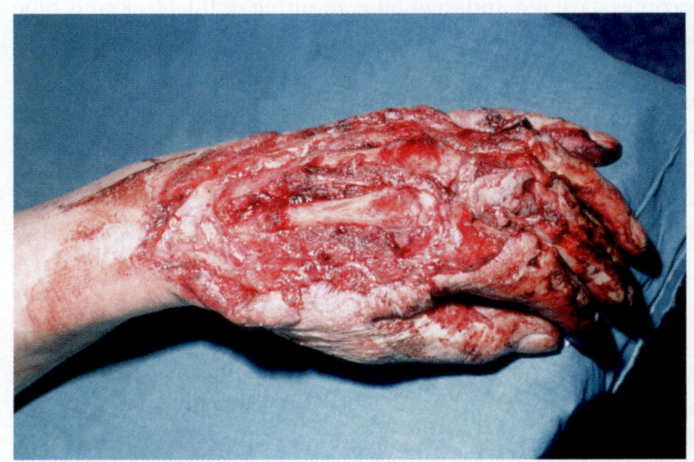

■ Figure 20-3 A crush injury.

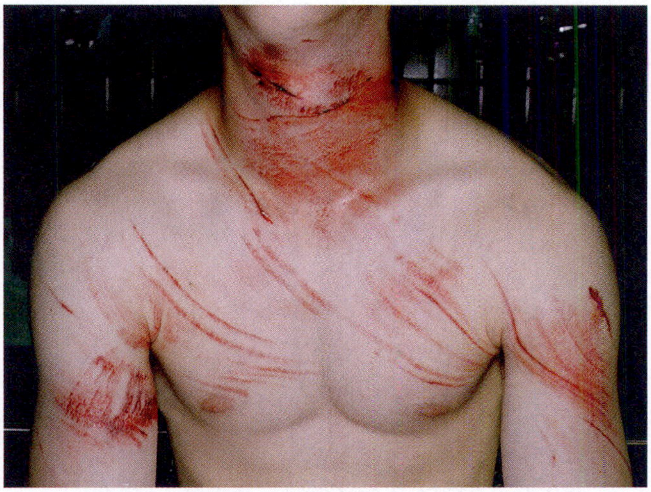

■ Figure 20-4 Abrasions. *(© Charles Stewart, MD)*

OPEN WOUNDS

Abrasions

Abrasions are typically the most minor of injuries that violate the protective envelope of the skin. They involve a scraping or abrasive action that removes layers of the epidermis and the upper reaches of the dermis (Figure 20-4 ■). Bleeding can be persistent but is usually limited because the injury involves only superficial capillaries. If the injury compromises a large area of the epidermis, it carries the danger of serious infection.

abrasion *scraping or abrading away of the superficial layers of the skin; an open soft-tissue injury.*

Content Review

Types of Open Wounds

- Abrasions
- Lacerations
- Incisions
- Punctures
- Impaled objects
- Avulsions
- Amputations

Lacerations

A **laceration** is an open wound that penetrates more deeply into the dermis than an abrasion (Figure 20-5 ■). A laceration tends to involve a smaller surface area, being limited to the tissue immediately surrounding the penetration. It endangers the deeper and more significant vasculature—arteries, arterioles, venules, and veins—as well as nerves, muscles, tendons, ligaments, and perhaps some underlying organs. As with an abrasion, the injury breaks the skin's protective barrier and provides a pathway for infection.

Note that the skin does not merely hang on the flesh, but rather is spread over the body and attached to fit the contours of the underlying structures. This creates natural stretch or tension in the skin. The orientation of tension in the skin is revealed in characteristic patterns called **tension lines** (Figure 20-6 ■). The effects of tension on the skin become evident when the skin is transected, as with a laceration. Lacerations cutting across the tension lines have a tendency to be pulled apart and thus spread widely or gape. Lacerations parallel to the tension lines tend to gape very little. Wounds

laceration *an open wound, normally a tear with jagged borders.*

tension lines *natural patterns in the surface of the skin revealing tensions within.*

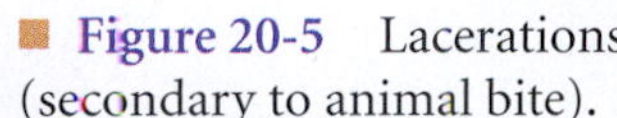

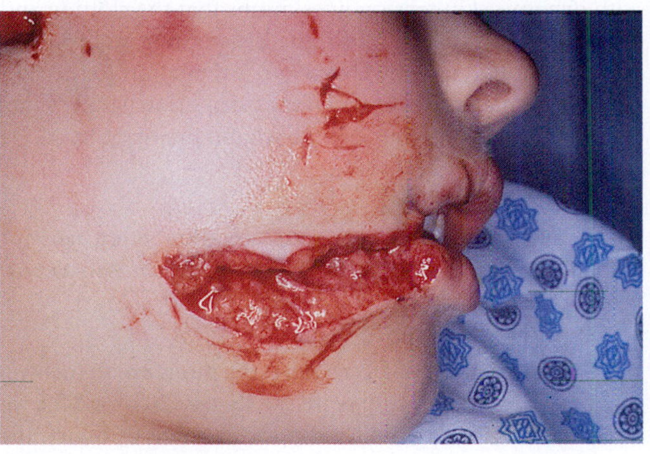

■ Figure 20-5 Lacerations (secondary to animal bite).

■ Figure 20-6 Tension lines of the skin.

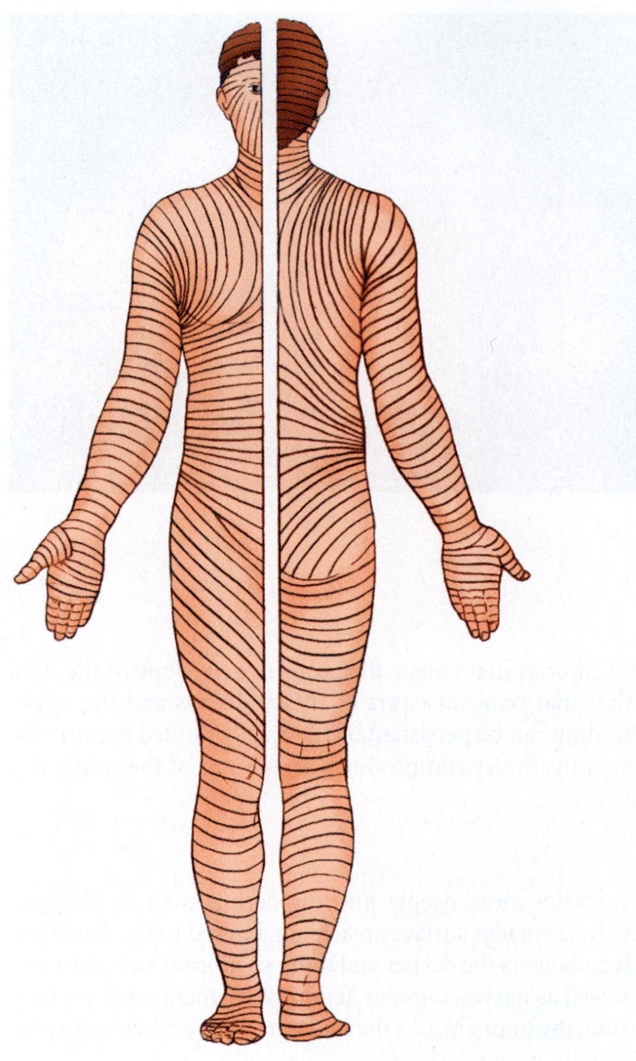

that spread widely tend to bleed more than those with minimal gaping. Large gaping wounds heal more slowly and are more likely to leave noticeable scars than wounds that spread less.

The tension represented by skin tension lines can be either static or dynamic. Static tension is noted in areas with limited movement of the tissue and structures beneath, as in the anterior abdomen or between joints in the extremities. Dynamic tension lines occur in areas subject to great movement, as in the skin over joints like the elbow, wrist, or knee. The increased motion in areas with dynamic skin tension lines means that the clotting and tissue mending processes in these areas are more frequently interrupted, disrupting and complicating skin repair.

You should note the laceration's orientation to the skin tension lines during your assessment of the patient. Remember that if the orientation parallels those lines, the wound may remain closed. If it is perpendicular to them, the wound may gape open.

incision *very smooth or surgical laceration, frequently caused by a knife, scalpel, razor blade, or piece of glass.*

puncture *specific soft-tissue injury involving a deep, narrow wound to the skin and underlying organs that carries an increased danger of infection.*

Incisions

An **incision** is a surgically smooth laceration, often caused by a sharp instrument such as a knife, straight razor, or piece of glass. Such a wound tends to bleed freely. In all other ways, it is a laceration.

Punctures

Another special type of laceration is the **puncture.** It involves a small entrance wound with damage that extends into the body's interior (Figure 20-7 ■). The wound normally seals itself and presents in a way that does not reflect the actual extent of injury. If the puncture penetrates deeply, it may

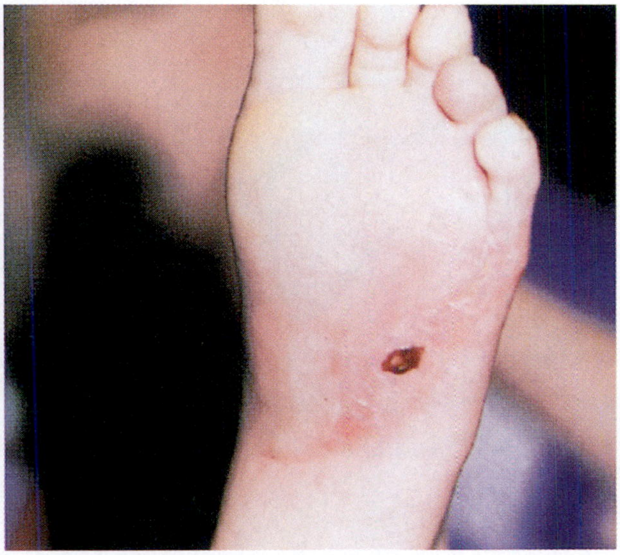

■ Figure 20-7 A puncture wound.

involve not just the skin but underlying muscles, nerves, bones, and organs. A puncture additionally carries an increased danger of infection. A penetrating object introduces bacteria and other pathogens deep into a wound. There, the disrupted tissue and blood vessels, along with a reduced oxygen level, create a warm and moist environment that is ideal for the colonization of bacteria.

Impaled Objects

An **impaled object** is not a wound itself, but rather a wound complication often associated with a puncture or laceration. Impaled objects are important for the damage they may cause if withdrawn. Frequently, embedded objects are irregular in shape and may become entangled in important structures such as arteries, nerves, or tendons (Figure 20-8 ■). Their removal in the field can result in further damage. Perhaps more critically, the embedded object may have lacerated a large blood vessel and the object's presence temporarily blocks, or tamponades, blood loss. Removal of the object may cause an uncontrollable flow of blood. This situation is particularly dangerous when the object is impaled in the neck or trunk, where the application of effective direct pressure is difficult or impossible.

impaled object *foreign body embedded in a wound.*

Avulsions

Avulsion occurs when a flap of skin, although torn or cut, is not torn completely loose from the body (Figure 20-9 ■). Avulsion is frequently seen with blunt trauma to the skull, where the scalp is torn and folds back. It may also occur with animal bites and machinery accidents. The seriousness of the avulsion depends upon the area involved, the condition of the circulation to (and distal to) the injury site, and the degree of contamination.

avulsion *forceful tearing away or separation of body tissue; an avulsion may be partial or complete.*

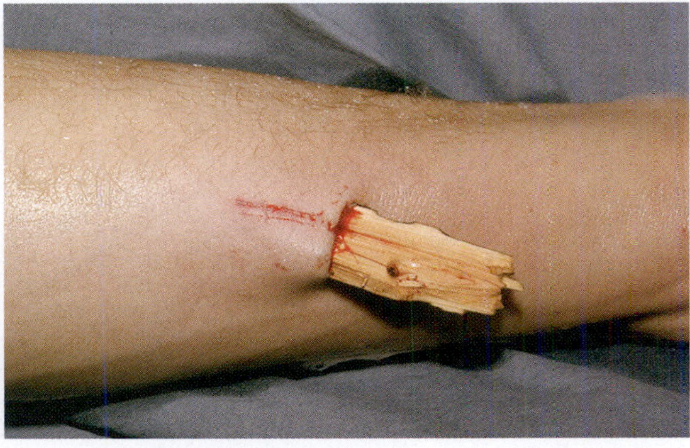

■ Figure 20-8 An impaled object. *(© Charles Stewart, MD)*

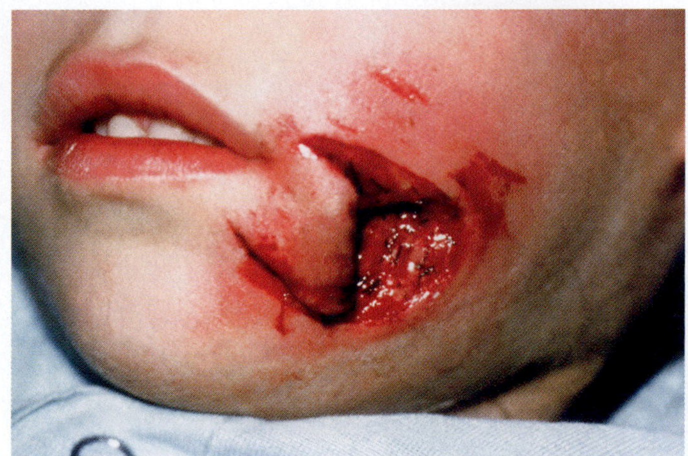

■ Figure 20-9 An avulsion.

degloving injury *avulsion in which the mechanism of injury tears the skin off the underlying muscle, tissue, blood vessels, and bone.*

A special type of avulsion is the **degloving injury.** In this wound, the mechanism of injury tears the skin off the underlying muscle, connective tissue, blood vessels, and bone. It is a particularly gruesome injury, occurring occasionally with farm and industrial machinery. The device pulls the skin off with great force as the skeletal tissue underneath is held stationary. The wound exposes a large area of tissue and is often severely contaminated. The injury carries with it a poor prognosis. If, however, the vasculature and innervation remain intact, there may be some hope for future use of the digit or extremity.

A variation of the degloving process is the ring injury (Figure 20-10 ■). As a person jumps or falls, the ring is caught, pulling the skin of the finger against the weight of the victim. The force may tear the upper layers of tissue away from the phalanges, exposing the tendons, nerves, and blood vessels. Although the ring injury involves a smaller area, it is otherwise a degloving injury.

Amputations

amputation *severance, removal, or detachment, either partial or complete, of a body part.*

The partial or complete severance of a digit or limb is an **amputation** (Figure 20-11 ■). It often results in the complete loss of the limb at the site of severance. The hemorrhage associated with the amputation may be limited if the limb or digit is cut cleanly or may be severe and continuing if the wound is a jagged or crushing one. The surgeon may attempt to replant the amputated part or use its skin for grafting as the remaining limb is repaired. If this skin is unavailable, the surgeon may have to cut the bone and musculature back further to close the wound. This reduces the length of the limb as well as its future usefulness. When amputation is considered, great care is used to ensure that the stump will be as functional as possible and suitable for prosthetic devices.

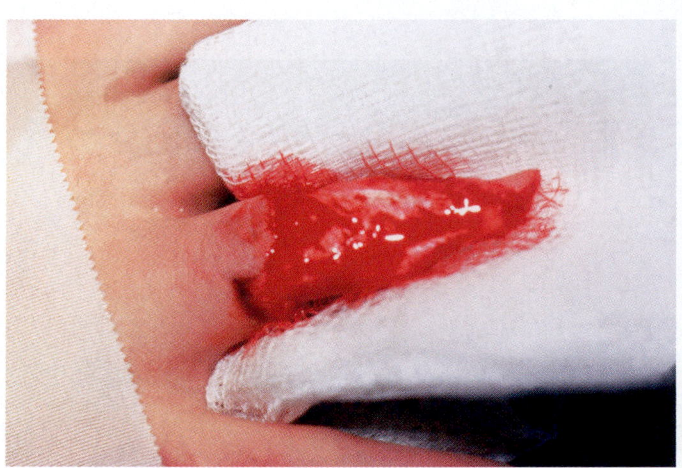

■ Figure 20-10 A ring-type degloving injury.

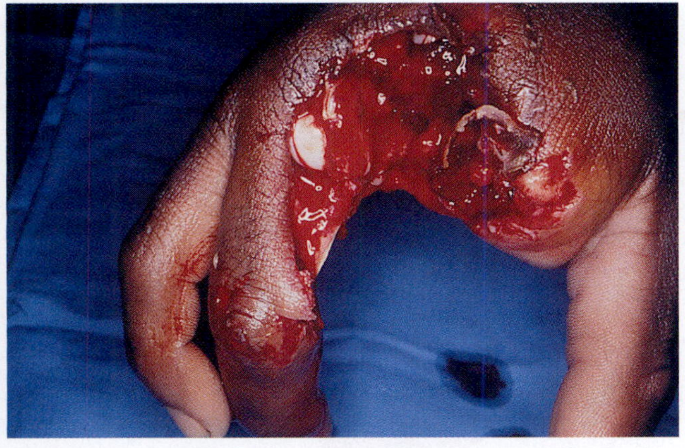

■ Figure 20-11 An amputation of the first two fingers.

HEMORRHAGE

Soft-tissue injuries frequently cause blood loss, ranging in severity from inconsequential to life threatening. The loss can be arterial, venous, or capillary (Figure 20-12 ■). Bleeding can be easy or almost impossible to control. Hemorrhage is usually dark red with venous injury, red with capillary injury, and bright red with arterial injury. The rate of hemorrhage also varies from oozing capillary, to flowing venous, to pulsing arterial bleeding. In practice, it may be hard to differentiate among the types and origins of hemorrhage. It is important, however, to determine the rate and quantity of blood loss. This information helps you to decide upon the most effective means of stopping the blood flow and prioritizing the patient for care and transport.

During assessment, it is important to determine the rate and quantity of hemorrhage.

Often the nature of the soft-tissue wound may be more important than the size or type of vessel involved in determining the severity of the blood vessel injury. If a moderately sized vein or artery is cut cleanly, the muscles in the vessel wall will tend to contract. This constricts the vessel's lumen and retracts the severed vessel into the tissue. As the muscle is drawn back from the wound, it thickens and further restricts the lumen. This restricts blood flow, reduces the rate of loss, and assists the clotting mechanisms. Therefore, clean lacerations and amputations generally do not bleed profusely. If, however, the vessel is not severed cleanly but is laid open instead, muscle contraction opens the wound, thereby increasing and prolonging blood loss.

WOUND HEALING

Wound healing is a complex process that begins immediately following injury and can take many months to complete. Wound healing is an essential component of homeostasis, the process whereby

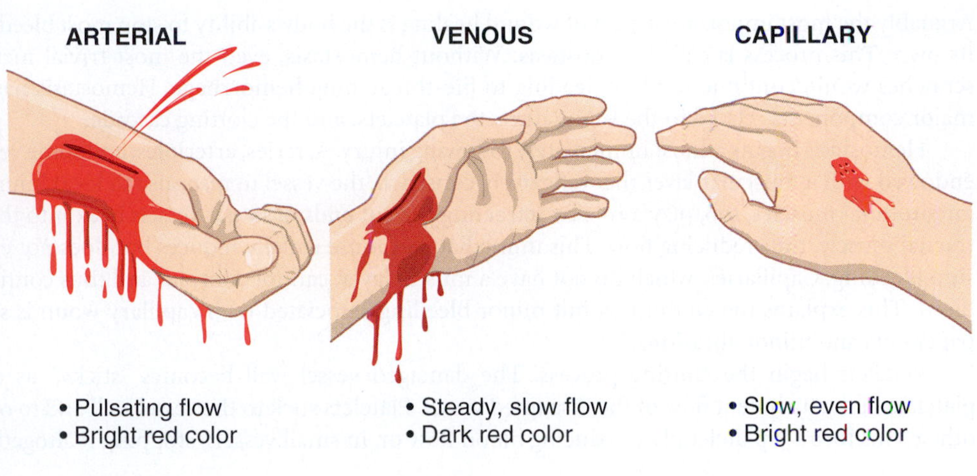

■ Figure 20-12 Hemorrhage. Arterial hemorrhage is bright red and flows rapidly from a wound. Venous hemorrhage is darker red and flows slowly. Capillary hemorrhage is also bright red and flows slowly.

■ Figure 20-13 The wound healing process.

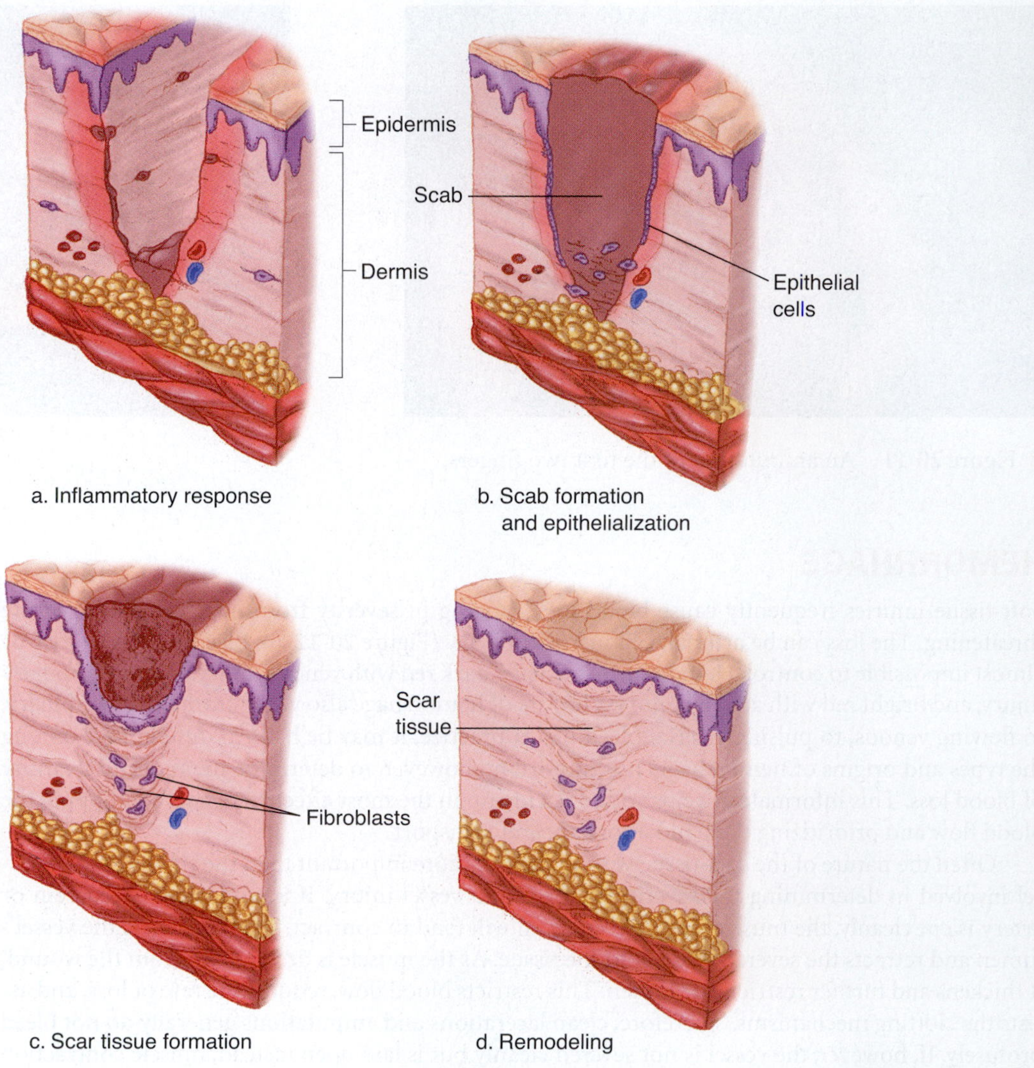

Content Review

Stages of Wound Healing

- Hemostasis
- Inflammation
- Epithelialization
- Neovascularization
- Collagen synthesis

hemostasis *the body's natural ability to stop bleeding; the ability to clot blood.*

the body maintains a uniform environment for itself. Although it is useful to divide the wound healing process into stages or parts, it is important to note that these phases overlap considerably and are intertwined physiologically (Figure 20-13 ■).

Hemostasis

Arguably the most important aspect of wound healing is the body's ability to stop most bleeding on its own. This process is called **hemostasis.** Without hemostasis, even the most trivial nicks and scratches would continue to bleed, leading to life-threatening hemorrhage. Hemostasis has three major components related to the vasculature, the platelets, and the clotting cascade.

Hemostasis begins almost immediately following injury. Arteries, arterioles, and some veins are endowed with a muscular layer that reflexively constricts the vessel in response to local injury. The longitudinal muscles, too, play a role by retracting the cut ends of larger vessels back into the contracted muscle, thus reducing flow. This immediate response usually reduces but does not entirely stop bleeding. Capillaries, which do not have a muscle layer, cannot contract and thus continue to bleed. This explains the continuing but minor bleeding associated with capillary wounds such as paper cuts and minor abrasions.

Platelets begin the clotting process. The damaged vessel wall becomes "sticky," as do the platelets in the turbulent flow of the disrupted vessel. Platelets stick to the vessel wall and to one another. This forms a platelet plug, reducing blood flow or, in small vessels, stopping it altogether.

When a blood vessel is injured, the disrupted tunica intima exposes collagen and other structural proteins to the blood. These proteins activate a complicated series of enzyme reactions that change certain blood proteins into long fibrin strands. These strands then entrap erythrocytes and produce a gelatinous mass that further occludes the bleeding vessel. This complex process, called coagulation, stops all but the most severe and persistent hemorrhage. With time, the clot shrinks or contracts, bringing the wound margins closer together, further facilitating wound healing. When the clot is no longer needed, it is reabsorbed by the body and any superficial scab merely drops off.

Inflammation

Shortly after hemostasis begins, the body sets in motion a very complex process of healing called **inflammation.** The inflammatory process involves a host of elements including various kinds of white blood cells, proteins involved in immunity, and hormone-like chemicals that signal other cells to mobilize.

Cells damaged by direct trauma or by invading pathogens release a number of proteins and chemicals into the surrounding tissue and blood. These agents, called **chemotactic factors,** recruit cells responsible for consuming cellular debris, invading bacteria, or other foreign or damaged cells and for beginning the inflammatory process. The first cells to arrive are specialized white blood cells called **granulocytes** and **macrophages.** These cells (also called phagocytes) are capable of engulfing bacteria, debris, and foreign material, digesting them, and then releasing the by-products in a process called **phagocytosis.** Other white blood cells called lymphocytes, in combination with immunoglobulins or immune proteins, are also mobilized. Lymphocytes attack invading pathogens directly or through an antibody response.

The injury process, the material released from injured cells, and the debris released as the phagocytes destroy invading cells cause mast cells to release histamine. Histamine dilates precapillary blood vessels, increases capillary permeability, and increases blood flow into and through the injured or infected tissue. This brings much-needed oxygen and more phagocytes to the injured area and draws away the by-products of cell destruction and repair. The increasing blood flow and local tissue metabolism also increase tissue temperature, which may in turn denature pathogen membranes. This response produces a swollen (edematous), reddened (erythematous), and warm region, characteristic of inflammation in response to local infection or injury. The result of the inflammation stage is the clearing away of dead and dying tissue, removal of bacteria and other foreign substances, and the preparation of the damaged area for rebuilding.

inflammation *complex process of local cellular and biochemical changes as a consequence of injury or infection; an early stage of healing.*

chemotactic factors *chemicals released by white blood cells that attract more white blood cells to an area of inflammation.*

granulocytes *white blood cells charged with the primary purpose of neutralizing foreign bacteria.*

macrophage *immune system cell that has the ability to recognize and ingest foreign pathogens.*

phagocytosis *process in which a cell surrounds and absorbs a bacterium or other particle.*

Epithelialization

Epithelialization is an early stage in wound healing in which epithelial cells migrate over the surface of the wound. The stratum germinativum cells rapidly divide and regenerate, thus restoring a uniform layer of skin cells along the edges of the healing wound. In clean, surgically prepared wounds, complete epithelialization may take place in as little as 48 hours. Except in minor, superficial wounds, the new epithelial layer is not a perfect facsimile of the original, undamaged skin. Instead, the new skin layer may be thinner, pigmented differently, and devoid of normal hair follicles. However, the new skin is usually quite functional and cosmetically similar to the original. If the wound is very large, epithelialization may be incomplete, and collagen will show through as a shiny, pinkish line of tissue called a scar.

epithelialization *early stage of wound healing in which epithelial cells migrate over the surface of the wound.*

Neovascularization

For healing to take place, new tissue must grow and regenerate. That requires blood rich in oxygen and nutrients. The body responds to this increased demand by generating new blood vessels in a process called **neovascularization.** These vessels bud from undamaged capillaries in the wound margins and then grow into the healing tissue. Neovascularized tissue is very fragile and has a tendency to bleed easily. It takes weeks to months for the newly formed blood vessels to become fully resistant to injury and for the surrounding tissue to strengthen enough to protect the new and delicate circulation.

neovascularization *new growth of capillaries in response to healing.*

Collagen Synthesis

collagen *tough, strong protein that comprises most of the body's connective tissue.*

fibroblasts *specialized cells that form collagen.*

Collagen is the body's main structural protein. It is a strong, tough fiber forming part of hair, bones, and connective tissue. Scar tissue, cartilage, and tendons are almost entirely collagen. Specialized cells called **fibroblasts** are brought to the wound area and synthesize collagen as an important step in rebuilding damaged tissues. Collagen binds the wound margins together and strengthens the healing wound. It is important to note that as the wound heals, it is not "as good as new." Regenerated skin has only about 60 percent of the tensile strength of undamaged skin at 4 months, when the scar is fully mature. This accounts for the occasional reinjury and reopening of wounds weeks or months after healing. The fibroblasts continue to reshape the scar tissue and shrink the wound for months after the scab falls off. This **remodeling** involves reorganizing collagen fibers into neat, parallel bands, strengthening the healing tissue still more. Remodeling can continue for up to 6 to 12 months after the initial injury, so the final cosmetic outcome of the healing process may not be evident until then.

remodeling *stage in the wound healing process in which collagen is broken down and relaid in an orderly fashion.*

INFECTION

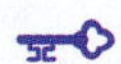

Infection is the most common complication of open wounds.

Infection is the most common and, next to hemorrhage, the most serious complication of open wounds. Approximately 1 in 15 wounds seen at the emergency department results in a wound infection. These infections delay healing. They may also spread to adjacent tissues and endanger cosmetic appearances. Occasionally, they cause widespread or systemic infection, called sepsis.

The most common causes of skin and soft-tissue infections are the Staphylococcus and Streptococcus bacterial families. These bacteria are gram-positive (Gram staining is a procedure to differentiate between types of bacteria), aerobic, and very common in the environment. Staphylococcus bacteria frequently colonize on the surface of normal skin, so it is not surprising to find them driven into wounds by the forces of trauma. Less commonly, wound infections are caused by other bacteria such as gram-negative rods, including *Pseudomonas aeruginosa* (diabetics and foot puncture wounds) and *Pasteurella multocida* (cat and dog bites).

It takes bacteria a few days to grow into numbers sufficient to cause noticeable signs or symptoms of infection. Infections appear at least 2 to 3 days following the initial wound and commonly present with pain, tenderness, erythema, and warmth. Infection earlier than that is very unusual. Pus, a collection of white blood cells, cellular debris, and dead bacteria, may be visible draining from the wound. The pus is usually thick, pale yellowish-to-greenish in color, and has a foul smell. Visible red streaks, or **lymphangitis,** may extend from the wound margins up the affected extremity proximally. These streaks represent inflammation of the lymph channels as a result of the infection. The patient may also complain of fever and malaise, especially if the infection has begun to spread systemically.

lymphangitis *inflammation of the lymph channels, usually as a result of a distal infection.*

Infection Risk Factors

Risk factors for wound infections are related to the host's health, the type and location of the wound, any associated contamination, and the treatment provided. Diabetics, the infirm, the elderly, and individuals with serious chronic diseases such as chronic obstructive pulmonary disease are at greater risk for infection and heal more slowly and less efficiently than healthy individuals. Patients with any significant disease or preexisting medical problem such as cancer, anemia, hepatic failure, or cardiovascular disease have difficulty mobilizing the immune and tissue-repair response necessary for good wound healing. HIV and AIDS attack the body's immune system and seriously impair its ability to ward off infection, increasing risk significantly. Smoking constricts blood vessels and robs healing tissues of needed oxygen and nutrients, while also increasing infection risk.

Several drugs detract from the body's ability to fight infection. Persons on immunosuppressant medications such as prednisone or cortisone (corticosteroids) are also at increased risk for serious infection. Colchicine, a drug used to treat gout, and nonsteroidal anti-inflammatory drugs (NSAIDS) such as ibuprofen also reduce the body's inflammation response. Neoplastic agents, which are used to combat rapidly reproducing cells in cancer patients, also disrupt cell regeneration at an injury site.

The wound type strongly affects the likelihood of a wound infection. A puncture wound traps contamination deep within tissue where there is a perfect environment for bacterial growth. Avulsion tears away blood vessels and supporting structures, robbing the damaged tissue of its blood supply, a critical factor in preventing or reducing infection. Crush injuries and other wounds that produce large areas of injured or dead (devitalized) tissue provide an excellent environment for bacterial growth and are at great risk for wound infection.

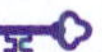

The type of wound—for example, a puncture or an extensive crush injury—may influence the likelihood of infection.

In a similar fashion, wound location influences infection risk. Well-vascularized areas such as the face and scalp are very resistant to infection. Distal extremities, the feet in particular, are at greater risk.

Clean objects, such as uncontaminated sheet metal or a clean knife, usually leave only small amounts of bacteria in a wound and, consequently, do not often cause infections. However, objects contaminated with organic matter and bacteria, such as a nail on a barnyard floor, a knife used to clean raw meat, or a piece of wood, pose much greater risks of infection. The infection risk associated with bites caused by mammals, and carnivores in particular, is very great. Bites by humans, cats, and dogs are among the most common and most serious types of bites.

The type of treatment provided for a wound affects the risk of infection. Use of sterile dressings and clean examination gloves minimizes wound contamination during prehospital treatment. Gloves protect not only the rescuer but also the patient from contaminants on the rescuer's hands. Irrigation of wounds with sterile saline using a pressurized stream device has been shown to reduce bacterial loads and reduce infection rates. Closing wounds (with sutures or staples, for example) increases infection risks as compared to leaving wounds open. However, the risks associated with wound closure are frequently accepted in order to achieve the best possible cosmetic outcome and more rapid healing.

In most cases, routine use of antibiotics with wounds does not help reduce infection rates and, in fact, may increase the likelihood of infection with antibiotic-resistant microorganisms. Antibiotics may be helpful if given within the first hour or so after deep major wounds, such as those from gunshots or stabbings, puncture wounds to the feet, and wounds where retention of a foreign body is suspected.

Infection Management

Despite the potential problems previously noted, the mainstay in treatment for infections is the use of chemical bactericidals, also known as antibiotics. Antibiotics for the treatment of gram-positive infections include the antistaphylococcal penicillins, cephalosporins. Erythromycin (and similar agents) can be used in patients allergic to penicillin. The pharmacalogical approach against *Pseudomonas* often requires the use of two drugs, while *Pasteurella* can be adequately treated with penicillin.

On occasion, a wound forms a collection of pus called an abscess and requires a minor incision and drainage to correct. Surgical removal of this material helps the body return to normal more quickly.

Gangrene One of the rarest and most feared wound complications is **gangrene.** Gangrene is a deep space infection usually caused by the anaerobic bacterium *Clostridium perfringens.* These bacteria characteristically produce a gas deep within a wound, causing subcutaneous emphysema and a foul smell whenever the gas escapes. Once they have become established, the bacteria are particularly prolific and can rapidly involve an entire extremity. Left unchecked, gangrene frequently leads to sepsis and death. In the days before antibiotics, amputation was frequently necessary to stop the spread of the disease. Modern treatment with a combination of antibiotics, surgery, and hyperbaric oxygenation effectively arrests most cases of gangrene early in their course.

gangrene *deep space infection usually caused by the anaerobic bacterium* Clostridium perfringens.

Tetanus Another highly feared but, fortunately, rare complication of wound infections is tetanus, or lockjaw. Tetanus is caused by the bacterium *Clostridium tetani,* and like its cousin *Clostridium perfringens,* it is anaerobic. Tetanus presents with few signs or symptoms at the local wound site, but the bacteria produce a potent toxin that causes widespread, painful, involuntary muscle contractions. Early observers noted mandibular trismus, or jaw-clenching ("lockjaw"). There is an antidote for the tetanus toxin, but it only neutralizes circulating toxin molecules, not those already bound to the motor endplates. Thus, treatment is slow and recovery prolonged.

Fortunately, tetanus is preventable through immunization. Widespread immunization has reduced incidence to a very few cases. The standard immunization is a series of three shots in childhood, with boosters every 10 years thereafter. It is common practice in emergency departments to provide boosters to wound patients if they have not been immunized in the past 5 years. Immigrants from Third World countries often have never completed a tetanus vaccine series. In these cases, it is prudent to administer tetanus immune globulin (TIG) in addition to the tetanus vaccine to prevent development of the disease while the body gears up to make new antibodies.

OTHER WOUND COMPLICATIONS

Several circumstances or conditions can interfere with normal wound healing processes. These conditions include impaired hemostasis, rebleeding, and delayed healing.

Impaired Hemostasis

Some medications, such as aspirin, warfarin, and heparin, can interfere with the clotting process.

Several medications can interfere with hemostasis and the clotting process. Aspirin is a powerful inhibitor of platelet aggregation, and it is used clinically to help prevent clot formation in the coronary and cerebral arteries of patients at risk for myocardial infarction or stroke. Thus, a side effect of aspirin use is a prolongation of clotting time, an important consideration in a patient who has sustained significant trauma or is undergoing major surgery. Likewise, anticoagulants, such as warfarin (Coumadin) and heparin, and fibrinolytics, such as tPA and streptokinase, interfere with or break down the protein fibers that form clots and are used to prevent or destroy obstructions at critical locations. They also adversely affect clot development in soft-tissue wounds. Penicillins may increase clotting times and interfere with blood cell production. Additionally, abnormalities in proteins involved in the fibrin formation cascade may result in delayed clotting, as is the case in hemophiliacs.

Rebleeding

Despite treatment that provides adequate initial control of bleeding, rebleeding is possible from any wound. Movement of underlying structures, such as muscles or bones, or of the bandage or dressing material may dislodge clots and reinstitute hemorrhage.

Also, hemorrhage that appears to have been stopped may actually be bleeding into an oversized dressing until it saturates the dressing and pushes through it. Monitor your dressings and bandages frequently to ensure that blood loss is not continuing.

Partially healed wounds are also at risk for rebleeding. Postoperative wounds in particular can start bleeding again with life-threatening results. Because patients are discharged from hospitals more quickly today than in the past and return home sooner after surgery, be wary of this potential complication.

Delayed Healing

In some patients, the wound repair process may be delayed or even arrested, resulting in incomplete wound healing. Persons at greatest risk for this complication are diabetics, the elderly, the chronically ill, and the malnourished. Nutrition must be adequate for wound healing to occur. Patients with multiple injuries often require significantly more calories during the healing phase than normal. Seriously or chronically infected wounds and wounds in locations with limited blood flow (distal extremities) are also at risk for incomplete healing. Incompletely healed wounds remain tender and are easily reinjured. A pale yellow or blood-tinged **serous fluid** may drain from them. Prehospital treatment of incompletely healed wounds includes frequent changes of sterile, nonadherent dressings and protection of the wound.

serous fluid *a cellular component of blood, similar to plasma.*

Compartment Syndrome

compartment syndrome *muscle ischemia that is caused by rising pressures within an anatomical fascial space.*

Compartment syndrome is a complication of closed and, occasionally, open wounds. In compartment syndrome, an extremity injury causes significant edema and swelling in the deep tissues. Because the extremity muscles are encapsulated in tough, inflexible fasciae, the swollen tissue has "nowhere to go," and the pressure in the compartment rises (Figure 20-14 ■). When the pressure

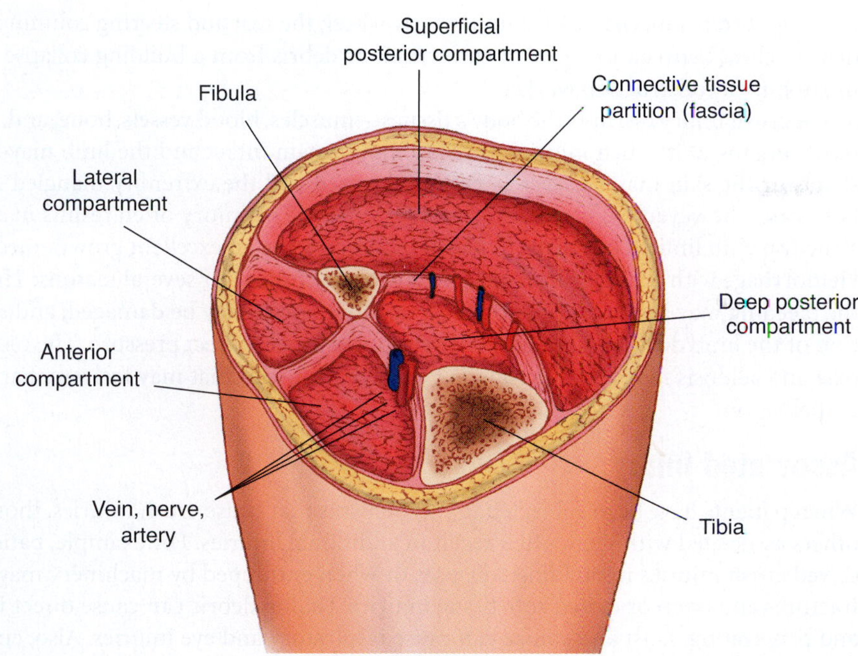

Figure 20-14 Musculoskeletal compartments segregated by fascia.

rises above 45 to 60 mmHg, the blood flow to that muscle group or compartment is compromised and ischemia ensues. If the condition continues for more than a few hours, irreversible damage and permanent disability may result. The muscle mass may die and its contribution to limb function may be lost. Frequently, the resulting scar tissue shortens the length of the muscle strand and produces what is called Volkmann's contracture, thus further reducing the usefulness of the limb after compartment syndrome. All extremities may experience compartment syndrome, but the lower extremities, especially the calves, are at greatest risk because of their bulk and fascial anatomy.

Abnormal Scar Formation

During the healing process, scar tissue sometimes develops abnormally. A **keloid** is excessive scar tissue that extends beyond the boundaries of a wound. It develops most commonly in darkly pigmented individuals and develops on the sternum, lower abdomen, upper extremities, and ears. Another healing abnormality is hypertrophic scar formation. This is an excessive accumulation of scar tissue, usually within the injury border, that is often associated with dynamic skin tension lines, like those at flexion joints.

keloid *a formation resulting from overproduction of scar tissue.*

Pressure Injuries

A special type of soft-tissue injury is the pressure injury, which is caused by prolonged compression of the skin and tissues beneath. This may occur in the chronically ill (bedridden) patient, the patient who falls and remains unconscious for hours (due to alcohol intoxication, stroke, or drug overdose), or the patient who is entrapped with no crushing mechanism. The patient's weight against the ground or other surface compresses tissue and induces hypoxic injury. The injury is similar to a crush injury, although the mechanism is more passive and more likely to go unnoticed. Pressure injury may also occur when a long spine board, PASG, air splint, or rigid splint remains on a patient for an extended period of time.

Pressure injuries may occur if a long spine board, splint, or PASG is left on a patient for an extended period.

CRUSH INJURY

Crush injury involves a trauma pattern in which body tissues are subjected to severe compressive forces. A crush injury can be relatively minor—for example, one that involves only a finger or part of an extremity—or it can be massive—one that affects much or all of the body. The mechanisms of injury can be varied. A packing machine might compress a worker's finger or extremity; a collapsed jack might trap a mechanic's leg under a car wheel; the seat and steering column might compress a driver's chest between them in an auto crash; or debris from a building collapse or trench cave-in might bury a construction worker.

A crush injury disrupts the body's tissues—muscles, blood vessels, bone, and, in some cases, internal organs. With such injuries, the skin may remain intact and the limb may appear normal in shape, or the skin may be severely cut and bruised and the extremity mangled and deformed. In both cases, however, the damage within is extensive. The injury often results in a large area of destruction with limited effective circulation, thus creating an excellent growth medium for bacteria. Hemorrhage with crush injuries may be difficult to control for several reasons: The actual source of the bleeding may be hard to identify; several large vessels may be damaged; and the general condition of the limb does not support effective application of direct pressure. The resulting tissue hypoxia and acidosis may result in muscle rigor, with muscles that may feel very hard and "woodlike" on palpation.

Associated Injury

When patients have been subjected to mechanisms that cause crush injuries, those mechanisms or others associated with them often result in additional injuries. For example, patients who have received crush injuries in building collapses or when entrapped by machinery may suffer additional fractures and open or closed soft-tissue injuries. Falling debris can cause direct injury, both blunt and penetrating. Dust and smoke can cause respiratory and eye injuries. Also, entrapment for any length of time leads to dehydration and hypothermia. You should consider all these possibilities when assessing and providing emergency care to victims of crush injury.

Crush Syndrome

necrosis *tissue death, usually from ischemia.*

rhabdomyolysis *acute pathologic process that involves the destruction of skeletal muscle.*

Crush syndrome occurs when body parts are entrapped for 4 hours or longer. Shorter periods of entrapment may result in direct body part damage, but they usually do not cause the broad, systemic complications of crush syndrome. The crushed skeletal muscle tissue undergoes **necrosis** and cellular changes with resultant release of metabolic by-products. This degenerative process, called traumatic **rhabdomyolysis** (skeletal muscle disintegration), releases many toxins. Chief among these by-products of cellular destruction are myoglobin (a muscle protein), phosphate and potassium (from cellular death), lactic acid (from anaerobic metabolism), and uric acid (from protein breakdown). These by-products accumulate in the crushed body part but, because of the entrapment and the resulting minimal circulation through the injured tissue, do not reach the systemic circulation. Once the limb or victim is extricated and the pressure is released, however, the accumulated by-products and toxins flood the central circulation.

High levels of myoglobin can lodge in the filtering tubules of the kidney, especially with patients who are in hypovolemic (shock) states, leading to renal failure, a leading cause of delayed death in crush syndrome. More immediate problems include hypovolemia and shock from the flow of sodium, chloride, and water into the damaged tissue. Increased blood potassium (hyperkalemia) can reduce the cardiac muscle's response to electrical stimuli, induce cardiac dysrhythmias, and lead to sudden death. Rising phosphate levels (hyperphosphatemia) can lead to abnormal calcifications in the vasculature and nervous system, compounding problems for the patient. In addition, as oxygenated circulation returns to the cells the aerobic process by which uric acid is produced can operate again, thus increasing cellular acidity and injury.

INJECTION INJURY

A unique type of soft-tissue injury is the injection injury. A bursting high-pressure line, most commonly a hydraulic line, may inject fluid through a patient's skin and into the subcutaneous tissues. If the pressure is strong enough, the fluid may push between tissue layers and travel along the limb (Figure 20-15 ■). The fluid thus injected—for example, a petroleum-based hydraulic fluid—may then chemically damage the surrounding tissue. The body's repair mechanisms are unprepared to remove the great quantities of injected material, and the resulting damage is severe. A limb may be lost due to the direct physical damage from the injection process, from the chemical damage done by the injected material, or from infection that develops after the injection.

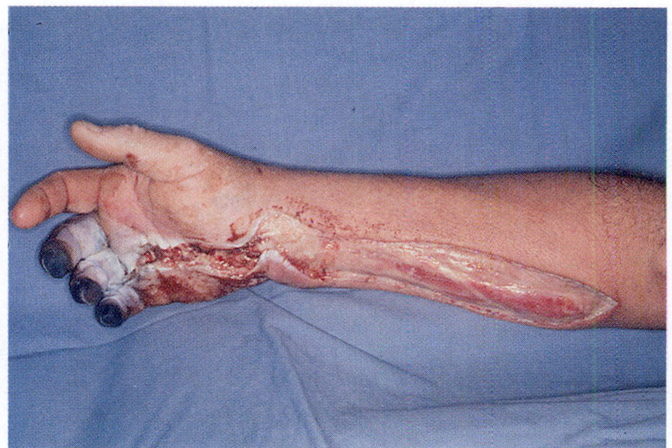

■ **Figure 20-15** An injection injury resulting from the pressurized injection of grease.

DRESSING AND BANDAGE MATERIALS

TYPES OF DRESSINGS AND BANDAGES

Several types of dressings and bandages are effective in prehospital care. A dressing is the material placed directly on the wound to control bleeding and maintain wound cleanliness (Figure 20-16 ■). A bandage is the material used to hold a dressing in place and to apply direct pressure to control hemorrhage (Figure 20-17 ■). Dressings and bandages have various designs and are used for a variety of purposes in emergency care.

Content Review

Types of Bandaging and Dressing Materials

Dressings

- Sterile/nonsterile
- Occlusive/nonocclusive
- Adherent/nonadherent
- Absorbent/nonabsorbent
- Wet/dry

Bandages

- Self-adherent roller
- Gauze
- Adhesive
- Elastic
- Triangular

Sterile/Nonsterile Dressings

Sterile dressings are cotton or other fiber pads that have been specially prepared to be without microorganisms. They are usually packaged individually and remain sterile for as long as the package is intact. Once the packaging is opened, sterile dressings become contaminated by airborne dust and particles that harbor bacteria and other microorganisms. Sterile dressings are designed to be used in direct contact with wounds.

Nonsterile dressings are clean—that is, free of gross contamination—but are not free of microscopic contamination and microorganisms. Nonsterile dressings are not intended to be applied directly to a wound, but rather to be placed over a sterile dressing to add bulk or absorptive power.

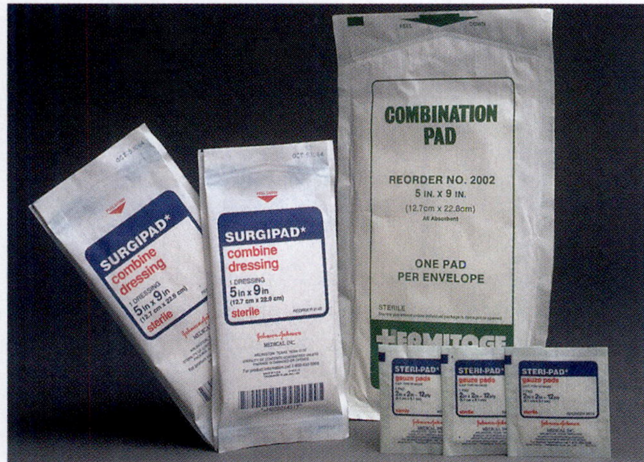

a. A variety of sterile dressings.

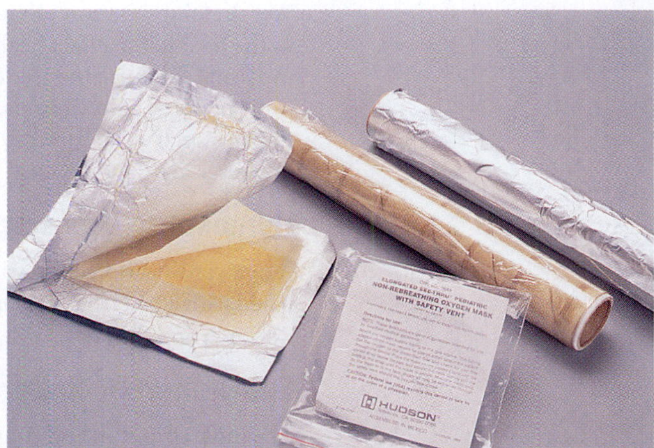

b. Occlusive dressings.

■ **Figure 20-16** Assorted dressings used in the care of soft-tissue injuries.

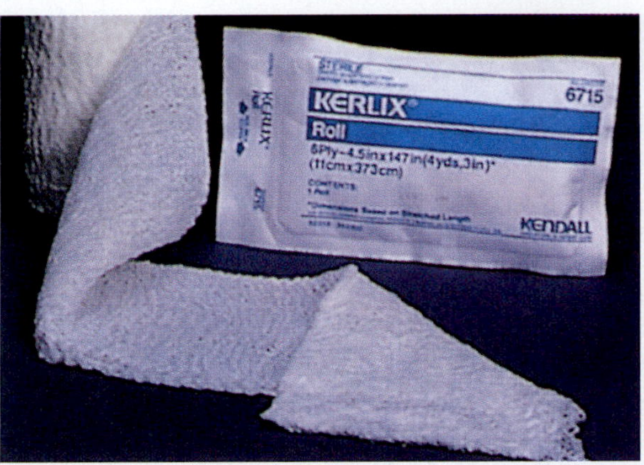

■ **Figure 20-17** Kerlix®, a type of self-adherent roller bandage.

Occlusive/Nonocclusive Dressings

Some dressings, such as sterilized plastic wrap and petroleum-impregnated gauze, are designed to prevent the movement of fluid and air through them. These dressings are called occlusive and are helpful in preventing air aspiration into chest wounds (open pneumothorax) and open neck wounds (air emboli into the jugular vein). Most dressing material is nonocclusive.

Adherent/Nonadherent Dressings

Adherent dressings are untreated cotton or other fiber pads that will stick to drying blood and fluid that has leaked from open wounds. Adherent dressings have the advantage of promoting clot formation and thus reducing hemorrhage, but their removal from wounds can be quite painful. Removal or disturbance of an adherent dressing is also likely to break the clot and cause rebleeding. Nonadherent dressings are specially treated with chemicals such as polymers to prevent the wound fluids and clotting materials from adhering to the dressing. Nonadherent dressings are preferred for most uncomplicated wounds.

Absorbent/Nonabsorbent Dressings

Absorbent dressings readily soak up blood and other fluids, much as a sponge soaks up water. This property is helpful in many bleeding situations. Nonabsorbent dressings absorb little or no fluid and are used when a barrier to leaking is desired. The clear membrane dressings frequently placed over intravenous puncture sites are good examples of nonabsorbent dressings. Most other dressings used in prehospital care are absorbent dressings.

Wet/Dry Dressings

Wet dressings are sometimes applied to special types of wounds such as burns. They are also used in the hospital to effect healing in some complicated postoperative wounds. Sterile normal saline is the usual fluid used to wet dressings. Wet dressings provide a medium for the movement of infectious material into wounds, however, and are not commonly used in prehospital care, except with injuries such as abdominal eviscerations or burns involving only a limited body surface area. Dry dressings are the type most often employed for wounds in prehospital care.

Hemostatic Dressings

A new classification of dressings now available is the hemostatic dressings. These are dressings impregnated with agents that potentiate the clotting mechanisms, causing more rapid and aggressive clotting. Research and field trials will determine the ultimate usefulness of these dressings in prehospital care.

Self-Adherent Roller Bandages

The most common and convenient bandage material is the soft, self-adherent, roller bandage (Kling or Kerlix). It has limited stretch and resists unraveling as it is rolled over itself. It conforms well to body contours and is quick and easy to use. This bandage is most appropriate for injuries located where it can be wrapped circumferentially. It comes in rolls from 1 to 6 inches wide.

Gauze Bandages

Like soft, self-adherent bandages, gauze bandages are a convenient material for securing dressings. They do not stretch, however, and thus do not conform as well to body contours as the self-adherent material, but they are otherwise functional for bandaging. Since gauze bandages do not stretch, they may increase the pressure associated with tissue swelling at injury sites. Gauze usually comes in rolls from 1/2 to 2 inches wide.

Adhesive Bandages

An adhesive bandage (or adhesive tape) is a strong plastic, paper, or fabric material with adhesive applied to one side. It can effectively secure a small dressing to a location where circumferential wrapping is impractical. When used circumferentially, an adhesive bandage does not allow for any swelling and permits pressure to accumulate in the tissues beneath it. Adhesive bandages usually come in widths that range from 1/4 to 3 inches.

Elastic (or Ace) Bandages

Elastic bandages stretch easily and conform to the body contours. Elastic bandages provide stability and support for minor musculoskeletal injuries, but they are not commonly used in prehospital care. When you do use these bandages, however, remember that it is very easy to apply too much pressure with them. Each consecutive wrap applied will contain and add to pressure on the wound site. Swelling associated with the wound may increase the pressure until blood flow through and out of the affected limb is reduced or stopped.

Triangular Bandages

Triangular bandages, or cravats, are large triangles of linen or cotton fabric. They are strong, nonelastic bandages commonly used to make slings and swathes and, in some cases, to affix splints. They can also be used to hold dressings in place, but they do not conform as well to body contours as soft, self-adherent bandages and do not maintain pressure or immobilize wound dressings very well.

ASSESSMENT OF SOFT-TISSUE INJURIES

Proper evaluation of the skin can tell you more about the body's condition after trauma than any other aspect of patient assessment. Not only is the skin the first body organ to experience the effects of trauma, but it is the first and often the only organ to display them. Therefore, assessment of the skin and its injury must be deliberate, careful, and complete. While the processes that cause soft-tissue injuries and the manifestations of those injuries vary, prehospital assessment is a simple, well-structured process. Follow the assessment process carefully and completely to ensure that you establish the nature and extent of each injury. Doing so enables you to assign soft-tissue injuries, and other injuries associated with them, the appropriate priorities for care.

Wound assessment must be comprehensive to ensure that care of each injury can be assigned an appropriate priority.

Assessment of patients with soft-tissue wounds follows the same general progression as the assessment of other trauma patients. First, size-up the scene, ruling out potential hazards, identifying the mechanism of injury, and determining the need for additional medical and rescue resources. Next, perform a quick primary assessment and identify and care for any immediately life-threatening injuries. For the patient with a mechanism of injury or signs and symptoms that suggest serious trauma, you will perform a rapid secondary assessment and use trauma triage criteria to determine the need for rapid transport. For a patient with no significant mechanism of injury and no indication from the primary assessment of a serious injury or life threat, perform a focused trauma assessment and gather vital signs and patient history at the scene. Perform a detailed physical exam only if conditions warrant and time permits. Provide serial ongoing assessments to track your patient's response to his injuries and your care.

SCENE SIZE-UP

During the scene size-up, look for evidence that will help you determine the mechanism of injury and anticipate the likely injuries and their severity. While soft-tissue injuries are not usually life

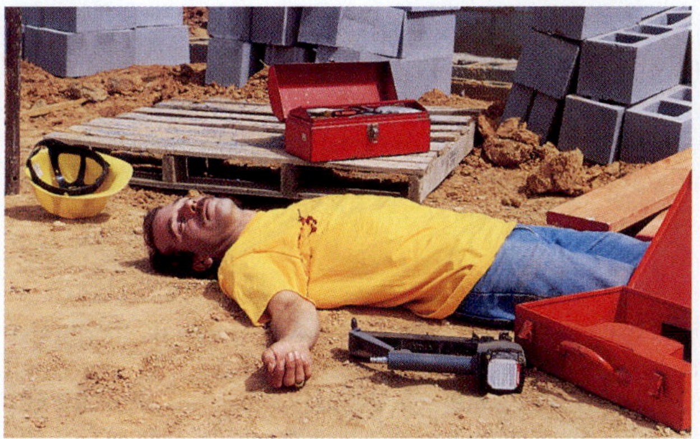

■ **Figure 20-18** During the scene size-up, rule out hazards, don gloves, and analyze the mechanism of injury.

No mechanism of injury can impact the human body without first traveling through the skin.

threatening, they can suggest other, serious life threats. Remember: No injury mechanism can impact the human body without first traveling through the skin. Identify where injury is likely and be prepared to carefully examine the skin for evidence that suggests internal injury. Consider mechanisms of injury that could cause entrapment and either crush injury or crush syndrome.

Be alert to the fact that the mechanisms that injured the patient may still be present and pose threats to you and other rescuers. Rule out or eliminate any threats to yourself or fellow care providers before entering the scene (Figure 20-18 ■).

Because trauma and injuries that penetrate the skin are likely to expose you to the hazards of contact with a patient's body fluids, don sterile gloves and observe other Standard Precautions as you approach the patient. Recognize that arterial bleeding and hemorrhage associated with the airway can cause blood to splatter at the scene. If you suspect these injuries, don splash protection for your eyes and clothing.

PRIMARY ASSESSMENT

Begin your primary assessment by establishing manual cervical in-line immobilization if you suspect significant head or spine injury and forming a general impression of the patient. Determine the patient's level of consciousness and assess the airway, breathing, and circulation. Assess perfusion by noting skin color, temperature, and condition and by assessing capillary refill.

During this assessment, pay particular attention to the location and types of visible wounds to gain further understanding of the mechanism of injury and whether it produced blunt or penetrating trauma. If responsive, the patient may be able to give you critical information about how the wound occurred. If the patient is unable to speak, First Responders or bystanders may be able to provide this information. Correct any immediate threats to the patient's life as you discover them.

SECONDARY ASSESSMENT

Use the information you have gathered through the primary assessment to determine how to proceed in the assessment process. Patients with serious trauma, suggested by a significant mechanism of injury or the findings of the initial assessment, will receive a rapid secondary assessment. All other patients will receive a focused trauma assessment.

Significant Mechanism of Injury—Rapid Secondary Assessment

In the rapid secondary assessment, you will perform a swift evaluation of the patient's head, neck, chest, abdomen, pelvis, extremities, and posterior body. Examine these areas for signs of internal or life-endangering injuries. Quickly investigate any discolorations, deformities, temperature variations, abnormal muscle tone, or open wounds.

Ensure that any wounds that you discover, or the injuries suggested beneath them, do not involve or endanger the airway or breathing or contribute significantly to blood loss. Focus your immediate care during the rapid secondary assessment on continuing to ensure the patient's airway and breathing and then on controlling severe blood loss.

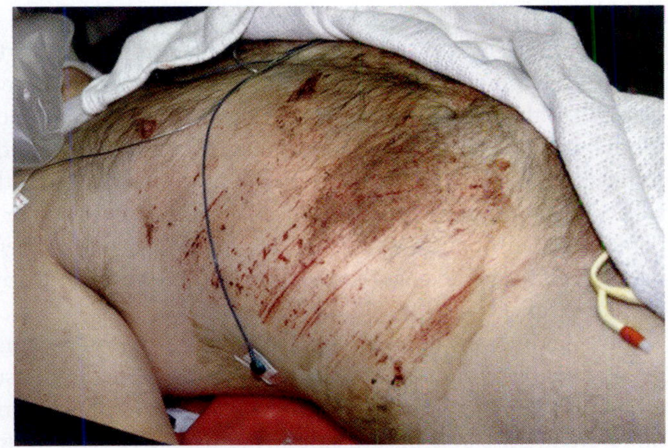

■ Figure 20-19 Often the only signs of serious internal injury are external soft-tissue injuries. *(© Edward T. Dickinson, MD)*

Inspect and palpate areas where the mechanism of injury suggests serious injuries may exist. Again, look for discoloration, temperature variation, abnormal muscle tone, and deformity suggestive of trauma (Figure 20-19 ■). If the mechanism of injury suggests open wounds, sweep body areas hidden from sight with gloved hands; this will rule out the possibility of unseen blood loss and pooling. Control moderate to severe hemorrhage immediately. Hemorrhage control need not be definitive, but should stop continuing significant blood loss. Once more serious injuries are cared for, you can return and dress and bandage wounds more carefully.

Survey all bleeding wounds to determine the type of hemorrhage—arterial, venous, or capillary. Attempt to approximate the volume of blood lost since the time of the accident, which suggests the rate of blood loss.

Carry out your exam using the methods described in "Assessment Techniques" later in this chapter. Apply a cervical spinal immobilization collar once you have completed the rapid assessment of the head and neck. Continue to provide manual immobilization, however, until the patient is fully immobilized to a backboard, orthopedic stretcher, or vacuum mattress.

When the rapid secondary assessment is complete, obtain a set of baseline vital signs and a patient history. Be sure to maintain manual in-line immobilization while the signs and history are being gathered. If you have enough personnel, the vital signs and history may be obtained simultaneously as the rapid trauma assessment is performed.

When obtaining the history, be sure to question the patient about medications, especially those that may have some direct relevance to soft-tissue injuries. For example, the patient's tetanus history is important with any penetrating trauma. Determine if the patient has had a tetanus booster and how long ago it was given. Note that a patient's routine use of aspirin or blood thinners—for example, heparin or warfarin for stroke or MI risk—may impact the body's ability to halt even minimal hemorrhage. Ask about the use of anti-inflammatory medications, such as prednisone, because those medications reduce the inflammatory response and slow the normal healing process. Question the patient about any preexisting diseases. Note that certain diseases, especially HIV, AIDS, or anemia, increase the risks of infection and the problems of hemorrhage control.

At the conclusion of the rapid secondary assessment, confirm the decision either to transport the patient immediately with further care provided en route to the hospital or to remain at the scene and complete treatment of non-life-threatening injuries. Consider the rate and volume of any blood loss and any uncontrollable bleeding in this decision.

If your patient's condition merits care at the scene, prioritize the soft-tissue wounds you have identified to establish an order of care to follow. The few moments taken to sort out injuries and to plan the management process save valuable time in the field. They also ensure that you provide early care for injuries with the highest priority.

No Significant Mechanism of Injury—Focused Secondary Assessment

When a patient has a soft-tissue injury but neither a significant mechanism of injury nor an indication of a serious problem from the primary assessment—for example, a cut finger or a knee abrasion from a fall—the sequence of assessment steps is different than for a patient with a significant injury mechanism. Begin this phase of the assessment with a focused trauma assessment, which is an exam directed at the injury site—the finger or the knee in the examples previously noted. A full head-to-toe rapid secondary assessment is not necessary in most such cases.

Direct the focused assessment at the chief complaint and any area of injury suggested by the mechanism of injury. Use the examination techniques of inquiry, inspection, and palpation (described in the following sections) to evaluate the injury and the surrounding area. In the case of a wound to an extremity, be sure to check the distal extremity for pulses, capillary refill, color, and temperature. Then, obtain a set of baseline vital signs and a history from the patient. If any of your findings suggest the patient has more serious injuries, perform a rapid secondary assessment and consider rapid transport.

Depending on the nature of the patient's injury, you may decide to provide transport or to refer/release the patient. If you are treating an isolated injury such as a cut finger, your system's protocols may prescribe whether you may release/refer the patient or transport the patient. More and more often, EMS systems are employing release/referral protocols to increase system efficiency. If you do transport, provide reassessment.

DETAILED PHYSICAL EXAM

Once the rapid or focused secondary assessment has been completed, vital signs and history have been gathered, and necessary emergency care steps have been taken, you may perform a detailed physical exam. Like the rapid secondary assessment, this head-to-toe evaluation of the skin (and the rest of the body) involves the techniques of inquiry, observation, and palpation. The detailed exam should follow a planned and comprehensive process, ideally progressing from head to toe although the order is not critical. The main purpose of the detailed assessment is to pick up any additional information regarding the patient's condition and to search for any unsuspected or subtle injuries. Manage any additional injuries you discover during the examination. The detailed physical exam is usually performed during transport or on scene if transport has been delayed. Never delay transport to perform it, and only perform it if the patient's condition permits.

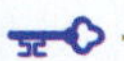

The detailed head-to-toe examination should be performed at the scene only if significant and life-threatening bleeding can be ruled out.

ASSESSMENT TECHNIQUES

The assessment techniques that follow can be used during both the rapid secondary assessment and the detailed physical exam.

Inquiry

Question the patient about the mechanism of injury, any pain, pain on touch or movement, and any loss of function or sensation specific to an area. Additionally, attempt to determine the exact nature of the pain or sensory or motor loss. Question the patient about signs and symptoms before touching an area.

Inspection

Continue the exam by carefully observing a particular body region. Identify any discolorations, deformities, or open wounds in those regions.

Determine if any discoloration is local, distal, or systemic, reflecting local injury, circulation compromise, or systemic complications such as shock. Contusions, blood vessel injuries, dislocations, and fractures may cause local discoloration, including erythema or ecchymosis. Distal discoloration may present as a pale, cyanotic, or ashen-colored limb distal to the point of circulation loss. You may also notice systemic discoloration, such as pale, ashen, or grayish skin in all limbs, suggestive of hypovolemia and shock.

Examine any deformities you find to determine their cause. Is the deformity due to a developing hematoma, to the normal swelling associated with the inflammatory process, or to underlying injuries?

Inspect any wounds you discover in detail. Study the wound to determine its depth and evaluate its potential for damage to underlying muscles, nerves, blood vessels, organs, or bones. If possible, identify the object that caused the wound and determine the amount of force transmitted by it to the body's interior. Ascertain if there are any foreign bodies, contamination, or impaled objects in the wound. Finally, identify the nature and location of any hemorrhage.

The wound should be observed in such a way that it can later be described to the attending physician.

Observe each wound carefully so you can describe it to the attending physician after you dress and bandage the injury. This information will help the emergency department staff prioritize the patient's injuries. Careful observation will also aid you in preparation of your prehospital care report. Adequate lighting is crucial for evaluating wounds. If necessary, defer this portion of the detailed physical exam until better lighting is available, as in the back of the ambulance.

If a patient's limb or digit has been amputated, have other rescuers conduct a brief but thorough search for the amputated part. If the part cannot be located immediately or remains entrapped, do not delay transport. Instead, leave someone at the scene to continue the search. Ensure that once the body part is retrieved, it is properly handled, packaged, and brought to the same hospital as the patient.

Palpation

In addition to questioning the patient and inspecting the body regions, you should palpate the body's entire surface. Be alert for any deformity, asymmetry, temperature variation, unexpected mass, or localized loss of skin or muscle tone. Gently palpate all apparent closed wounds for evidence of tenderness, swelling, crepitus, and subcutaneous emphysema. Avoid palpating the interior of open wounds, which may introduce contamination and disturb the clotting process. Ascertain the presence or absence of distal pulses and capillary refill time with any extremity injury. Also, check motor and sensory function distal to any extremity wound and compare findings with those from the opposite limb.

REASSESSMENT

During transport, provide a reassessment, reassessing the patient's mental status, airway, breathing, and circulation, gathering additional sets of vital signs, and evaluating the sites of the patient's injuries. Also inspect any interventions you have performed. Provide a reassessment at least every 5 minutes with unstable patients and every 15 minutes with stable patients. If you note any change in the patient's condition, modify your priorities for transport and care accordingly.

MANAGEMENT OF SOFT-TISSUE INJURY

Once you complete your patient assessment, take steps to manage the soft-tissue injury, either in the field or en route to the hospital. Control of blood loss, prevention of shock, and decontamination of affected areas take priority. The following sections describe some of the most important of these care steps.

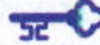

The management of minor wounds is a late priority in the care of the trauma patient, unless extensive bleeding is noted.

Unless you note extensive bleeding, wound management by dressing and bandaging is a late priority in the care of trauma patients. Dress and bandage wounds whose bleeding does not represent a life threat only after you stabilize your patient by caring for higher priority injuries.

OBJECTIVES OF WOUND DRESSING AND BANDAGING

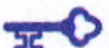

The three objectives of bandaging are to control hemorrhage, to keep the wound clean, and to immobilize the wound site.

The dressing and bandaging of a wound has three basic objectives. These are to control all hemorrhaging, to keep the wound as clean as possible, and to immobilize the wound (Procedure 20–1). The appearance of the final dressing and bandage is not as critical as the achievement of these three objectives.

Hemorrhage Control

The primary method—and the most effective one—of controlling hemorrhage associated with soft-tissue injury is direct pressure. In cases of serious hemorrhage flowing from a wound with some force, place a small dressing directly over the site of the bleeding and apply pressure directly to it with a finger. When the bleeding is the more commonly encountered slow-to-moderate type, use a dressing that has been sized to cover and pad the wound. Then simply wrap the dressing with a soft, self-adherent bandage using moderate pressure to halt the blood loss. Monitor the wound frequently to ensure bleeding has stopped.

A combination of techniques for hemorrhage control may be effective when bleeding is resistant to direct pressure.

Procedure 20-1 Hemorrhage Control

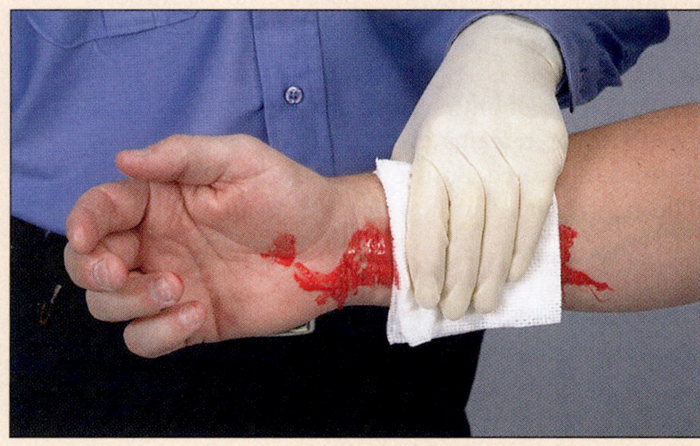

20-1a Apply direct pressure with a dressing to the site of hemorrhage.

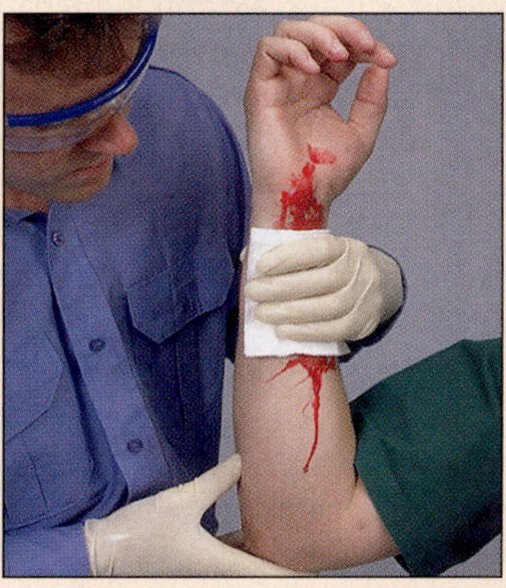

20-1b Elevate the hemorrhage site if there is no serious musculoskeletal injury.

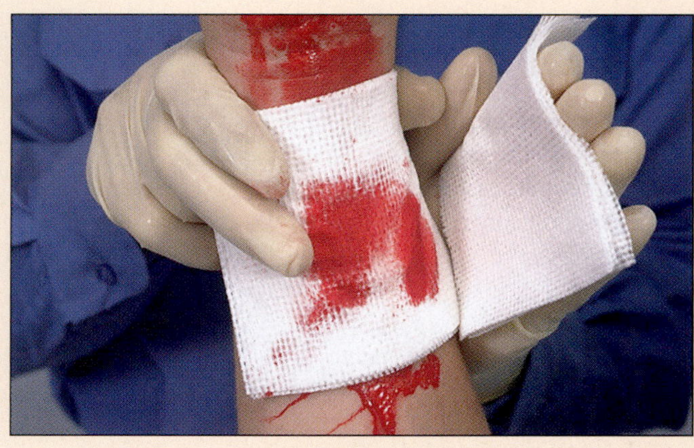

20-1c Apply additional dressings as needed.

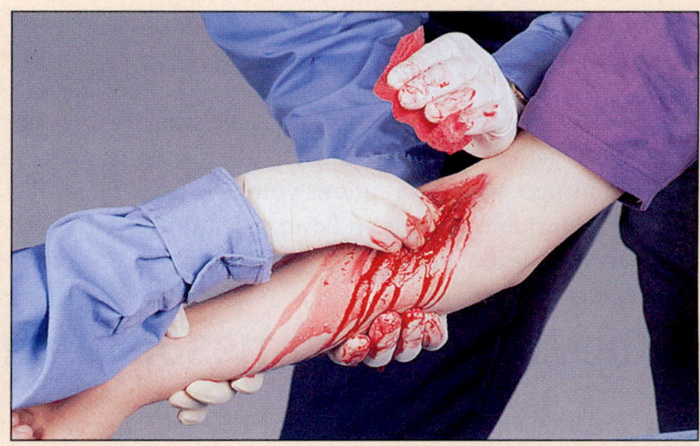

20-1d If serious hemorrhage persists, expose the wound and place digital pressure with a gloved hand on the site of bleeding.

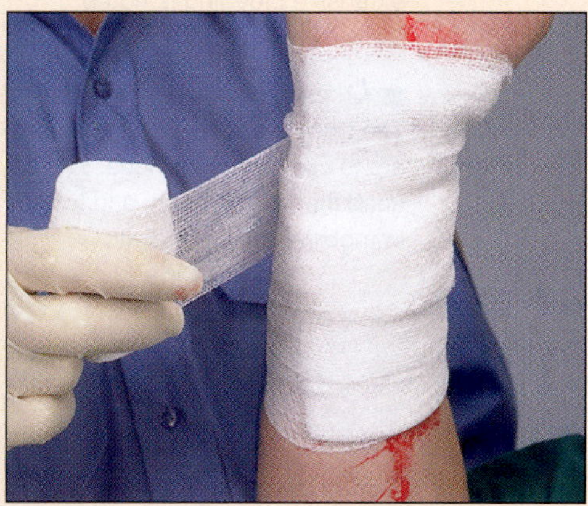

20-1e Bandage the dressing in place, maintaining pressure on the wound.

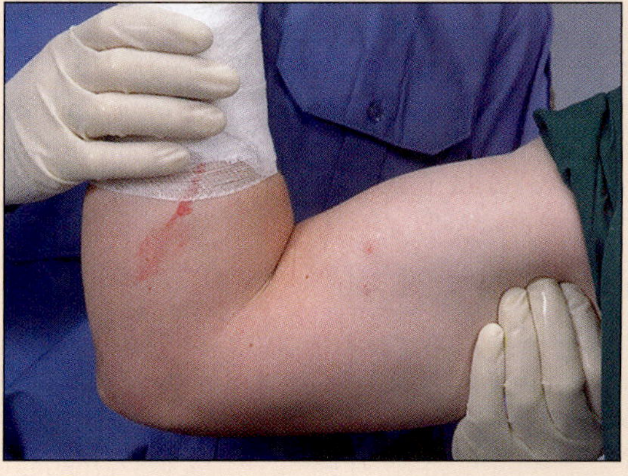

20-1f Apply digital pressure to a proximal artery if the hemorrhage persists.

Elevation can assist in the control of hemorrhage, although it is generally not as effective as direct pressure. Elevation reduces arterial pressure in the extremity and increases venous return. Elevation can thus reduce edema and increase blood flow through the wound and injured extremity. This promotes good oxygenation and wound healing. Do not elevate a limb, however, if doing so will cause any further harm as would be the case if the patient has a suspected spinal or associated musculoskeletal injury or if there is an object impaled in the limb.

Use pressure points to assist with bleeding control and the clotting process when direct pressure and elevation together do not control it. Locate a pulse point immediately proximal to the wound and above a bony prominence. Apply firm pressure and maintain it for at least 10 minutes. Ensure that the hemorrhage does not continue.

To halt hemorrhage, apply firm pressure to the site for at least 10 minutes.

Occasionally, bleeding from a soft-tissue injury can be difficult to control. If the bleeding continues despite the use of direct pressure, elevation, and pressure points, reassess the wound to be sure you have determined the exact site of blood loss. Then reapply direct digital pressure to that precise point. Too often, hemorrhage continues because the bandaging technique distributes pressure over the entire wound site rather than focusing it directly on the source of the bleeding. The force driving the hemorrhage is no greater than the patient's systolic blood pressure, and properly applied digital pressure can thus easily provide a pressure greater than this to compress the vessel and halt any blood loss.

In certain circumstances, the use of direct pressure, elevation, and a pressure point may not control hemorrhage. Crush injuries and amputations are situations in which normal bleeding control measures may be ineffective. With these traumatic injuries, several blood vessels are jaggedly torn, confounding the body's normal hemorrhage control mechanisms and making it difficult to pinpoint the source of bleeding. Even if the source of bleeding can be found, applying firm direct pressure to it may be difficult. In such cases, the application of a tourniquet may be useful. The tourniquet should be considered the last option for controlling hemorrhage. If properly applied, the tourniquet will stop the flow of blood; however, its use has serious associated risks. Keep the following precautions in mind whenever you consider using a tourniquet:

1. If the pressure applied is insufficient, the tourniquet may halt venous return while permitting continued arterial blood flow into the extremity, increasing the rate and volume of blood loss.
2. When the tourniquet is applied properly, the entire limb distal to the device is without circulation. Hypoxia, ischemia, and necrosis may permanently damage the tissue distal to the tourniquet.
3. When circulation is restored, the blood flows and pools in the extremity, adding to any hypovolemia. In addition, any blood that returns to the central circulation is highly hypoxic, acidic, and toxic. This blood can cause shock, lethal dysrhythmias, renal failure, and death. The return of circulation may also restart hemorrhage and introduce emboli into the central circulation.

Do not use a tourniquet unless you cannot control bleeding by any other means.

Do not use a tourniquet unless you cannot control severe bleeding by any other means. Place it just proximal to the wound site, but stay away from the elbow or knee joints (Figure 20-20 ■). Apply the tourniquet in a way that will not injure the tissue beneath. For example, do not use very narrow material, like rope or wire, for a tourniquet; applying great pressure to a limb with such material may cause serious injury in the compressed tissue. Instead, select a 2-inch or wider band for compression.

A readily available, effective, and easily controllable tourniquet is the sphygmomanometer (regular for the upper extremity and thigh for the lower). It is wide, simple to apply, rapid to inflate, and easy to monitor. Inflate it to a pressure 30 mmHg above the patient's systolic blood pressure and beyond the pressure at which the patient's hemorrhage ceases.

Once applied, a tourniquet should be left in place until the patient arrives at the emergency department.

Once you apply a tourniquet, leave it in place until the patient arrives at the emergency department. Monitor the tourniquet during transport to ensure that it does not lose pressure, and watch for signs of renewed bleeding. If bleeding starts again, increase the tourniquet pressure. Alert the hospital staff to your use of the tourniquet during transport as well as upon arrival. Mark the patient's forehead clearly with the letters "TQ," and note the time the tourniquet was applied.

■ Figure 20-20 The steps of tourniquet application.

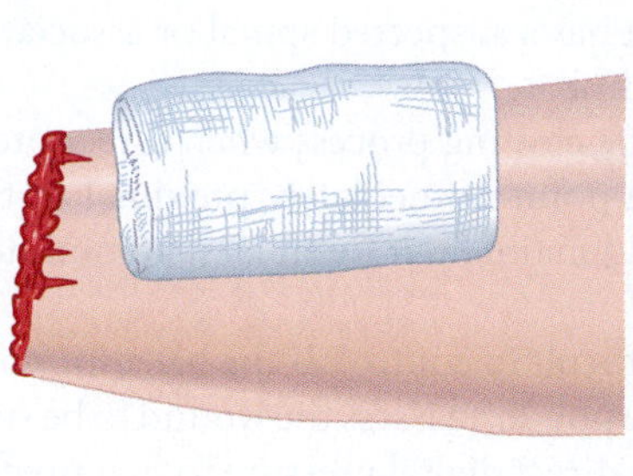

a. Place a bulky dressing over the distal artery.

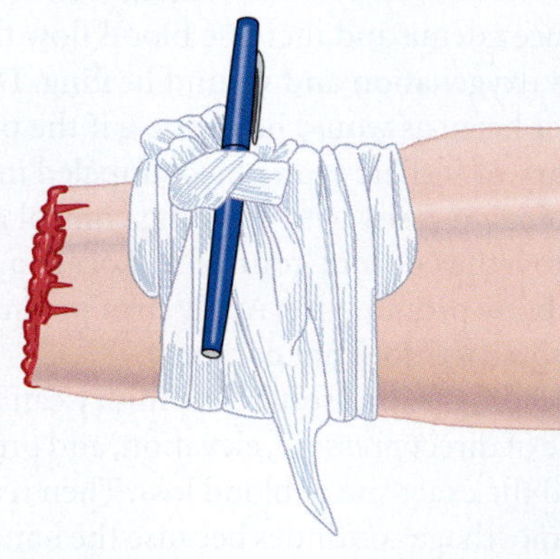

b. Apply a pressure exceeding the systolic pressure.

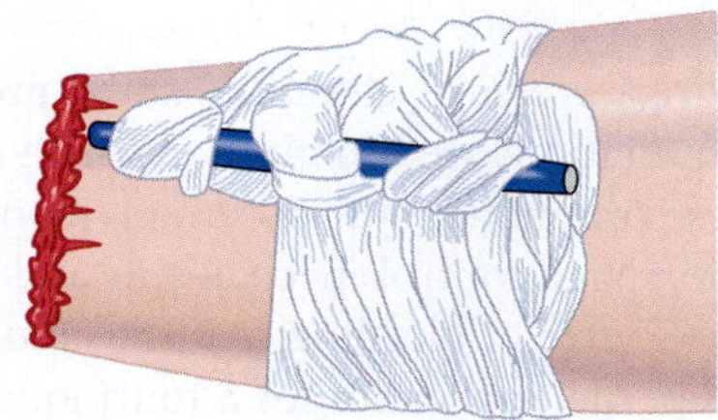

c. Secure the tourniquet and monitor the wound site for continuing hemorrhage.

Do not release a tourniquet in the field except under exceptional circumstances and then only during consultation with medical direction. Be prepared to provide vigorous fluid resuscitation, ECG monitoring, dysrhythmia treatment, and rapid transport if a tourniquet release is attempted.

Sterility

Once you halt severe bleeding, keep the wound as sterile as possible. Under field conditions, this may simply mean keeping the wound as clean as reasonably possible. With very small open wounds, like an IV start or a small laceration, you may consider the application of an antibacterial ointment to help with infection control. However, the effectiveness of such ointments on larger wounds is limited, and ointments are not generally applied to these wounds.

Under normal conditions, you need not cleanse the wound. If a wound is grossly contaminated, however, irrigate it with normal saline or lactated Ringer's solution. A 1,000-mL bag of saline, connected to a macrodrip administration set and pressurized by squeezing the bag under your arm, may allow rapid and gentle wound cleansing. Try to move any contamination from the center of the wound outward. You may also carefully remove larger particles—glass, gravel, debris, and so forth—if you can do this swiftly and without inducing further injury.

Apply a bandage to make the dressing appear as neat as time and the conditions under which you are working will allow. Often, this is as easy as covering the entire dressing with wraps of soft, self-adherent roller bandage. The neat appearance calms and reassures the patient, while the bandaging reduces contamination and the chances of post-trauma infection.

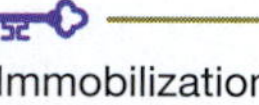

Immobilization is an important, but frequently overlooked, component of hemorrhage control.

Immobilization

The last objective of bandaging is immobilization. The stability of the wound site helps the natural clotting mechanisms operate and reduces the patient's discomfort. Maintaining gentle pressure with the bandage may reduce pain and local swelling. With bandaging material, immobilize the limb to the patient's body or to a rigid surface such as a padded board or ladder splint.

When immobilizing a limb, do not use elastic bandaging material or apply the bandage too tightly. The edema that develops rapidly with an injury puts increasing pressure on underlying tissue. This pressure may quickly reduce or halt circulation.

Frequently monitor any limb that you bandage circumferentially to ensure that the distal pulse remains strong and that the distal extremity maintains good color and does not swell. If you cannot locate the distal pulse, monitor capillary refill, skin color, and temperature. If signs or symptoms suggest that the distal circulation is compromised, elevate the extremity, if possible, and check and consider loosening the bandage.

Pain and Edema Control

Treat painful soft-tissue injuries or those likely to cause large debilitating edema with the application of cold packs and moderate-pressure bandages. Cold reduces inflammatory response and local edema. It also dulls the pain associated with serious soft-tissue trauma. Use a commercial cold pack or ice in a plastic bag wrapped in a dry towel and apply it to the wound. Do not use a cold pack directly against the skin as it cools beyond any therapeutic value. Direct application of a cold pack may also cause tissue freezing, especially in areas with reduced circulation.

Some moderate pressure over the wound area may also help reduce pain and wound edema. In cases where the patient reports severe pain, consider use of morphine sulfate, fentanyl, or other analgesics for patient comfort. Administer morphine in 2-mg increments titrated to pain relief every 5 minutes (up to a total of 10 mg). Fentanyl may be administered in a 25–50 mcg dose, followed by 25-mcg doses, titrated to relieve pain.

ANATOMICAL CONSIDERATIONS FOR BANDAGING

Each area of the body has specific anatomical characteristics. Your application of bandages and dressings should take these characteristics into account to provide effective prehospital wound care (Figure 20-21 ■).

Scalp

The scalp has a rich supply of vessels that can bleed heavily when injured. It's commonly said that head wounds rarely account for shock, but scalp hemorrhage can be severe and difficult to control and can lead to the loss of moderate to large volumes of blood.

In scalp hemorrhage uncomplicated by skull fracture, direct pressure against the skull is effective in the control of bleeding. To hold a dressing in place and maintain pressure, wrap a bandage around the head, capturing the occiput or brow or, in some cases, passing the bandage under the chin (while still allowing for jaw movement).

If a head wound is complicated by fracture, be very careful in your application of pressure. Apply gentle digital pressure around the wound and attempt to locate the small scalp arteries that feed it to use as pressure points. Then simply hold a dressing on the wound without much pressure.

Face

Facial wounds are frequently gruesome and bleed heavily. Gentle direct pressure to these wounds can effectively control hemorrhage. You can maintain this pressure by wrapping a bandage around the head. Be careful to ensure a clear airway and use your bandaging to splint any facial instability.

Remember, blood is a gastric irritant and swallowed blood may induce emesis. Be ready to provide suctioning in patients with oral or nasal hemorrhage because unexpected emesis may compromise the airway.

Ear or Mastoid

Wounds to the ear region can be easily bandaged by wrapping the head circumferentially. Use open gauze to collect, not stop, any bleeding or fluids flowing from the ear canal. These materials may contain cerebrospinal fluid and halting their flow may add to any increasing intracranial pressure.

Neck

Minor neck wounds may be lightly wrapped circumferentially with bandages or taped to hold dressings in place. If bleeding is moderate to severe, however, direct manual pressure may be necessary because the amount of pressure applied by circumferential wrapping may compromise both

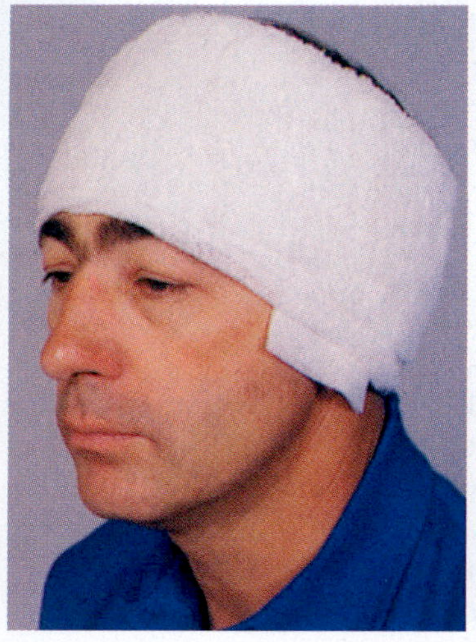

a. Head and/or ear bandage.

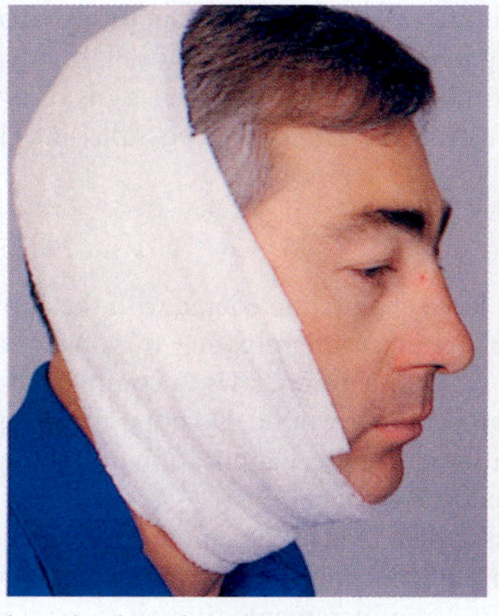

b. Cheek and ear bandage (be sure mouth will open).

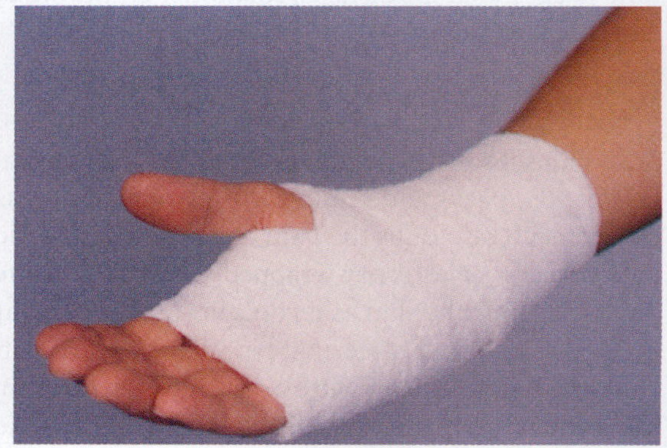

c. Hand bandage.

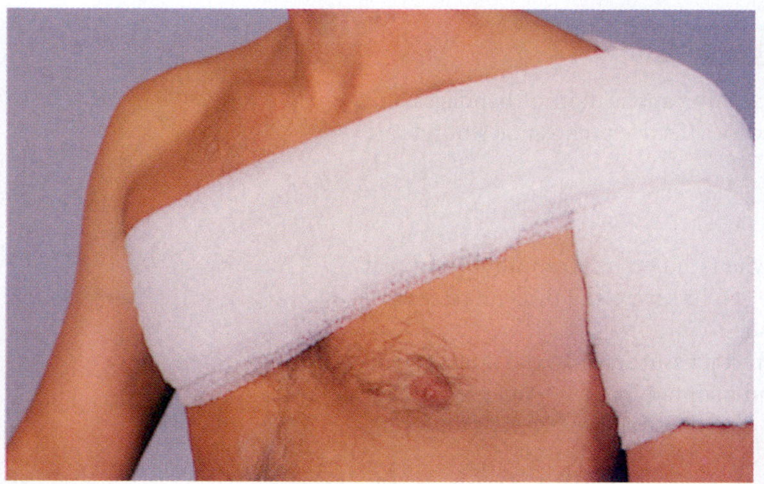

d. Shoulder bandage.

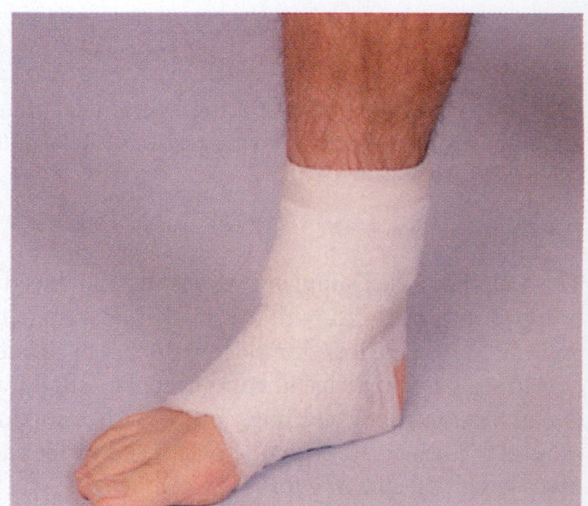

e. Foot and/or ankle bandage.

■ **Figure 20-21** Good bandaging uses the natural body curves and the self-adherent characteristics of bandages to hold dressings firmly in place.

the airway and circulation to and from the head. In cases of large wounds or moderate to severe bleeding, also consider using an occlusive dressing to prevent aspiration of air into a jugular vein.

Shoulder

The shoulder is an easy area to bandage as soft, self-adherent roller bandages readily conform to body contours. Use the axilla, arm, and neck as points of fixation, but be careful not to put pressure on the anterior neck and trachea.

Trunk

For minor trunk wounds, adhesive tape may be sufficient to hold dressings in place. With larger wounds, bandaging can be more difficult because you must wrap the patient's body circumferentially to apply direct pressure to a wound. Applying a bandage in this way may require moving the patient unnecessarily and risk causing or worsening an injury. Consider instead using a ladder splint that is negotiated beneath the patient's torso, folded to the curve of the back, and then folded out-

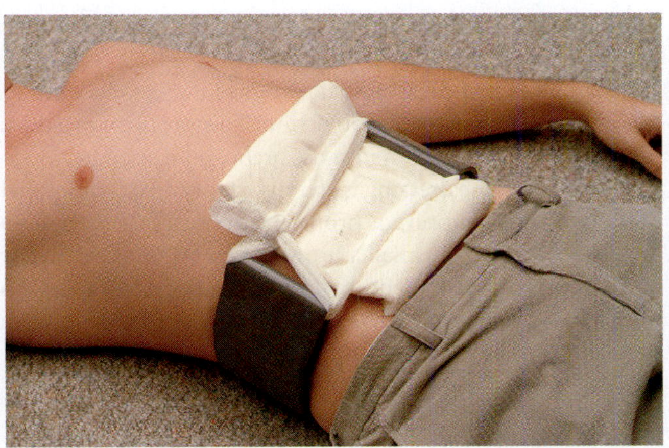

■ Figure 20-22 Affixing the bandaging material to a ladder splint may help in circumferential bandaging of a wound to the trunk.

ward sharply at each end to serve as a bandaging fixation point. You then wrap the bandage between the ends of the ladder splint to hold the dressing in place (Figure 20-22 ■).

Groin and Hip

The groin and the hip are easy places to affix a dressing. Bandage by following the contours of the upper thighs and waist, similar to the technique of bandaging a shoulder. Be careful here, though. Any movement of the patient is likely to affect the tightness of the bandage and the amount of pressure over the dressing. With these injuries, therefore, bandage after the patient is in final position for transport.

Elbow and Knee

Joints, especially the elbow and knee, are difficult to bandage. Bandage using circumferential wraps and then splint the area to ensure that the bandage does not loosen with movement. If possible, place the joint in a position halfway between flexion and extension. This position, called the position of function, relaxes the muscles controlling the joint and the skin tension lines, and is most comfortable for the patient during long transports or periods of immobilization.

Hand and Finger

Hand and finger injuries are easy to bandage by simple circumferential wrapping. Again, consider placing the hand or digit in the position of function, halfway between flexion and extension. Accomplish this by placing a large, bulky dressing in the palm of the patient's hand and then wrapping around it. You may use a malleable finger splint to obtain the position of function and then wrap circumferentially to splint the finger. If possible, before bandaging, carefully remove any jewelry from the wrist and fingers, as swelling may restrict distal circulation and also make it difficult to remove the jewelry later.

Ankle and Foot

Ankle and foot wounds are also easy to bandage by wrapping circumferentially and by using the natural body contours. If strong direct pressure is needed to maintain hemorrhage control, start your wrapping from the toes and work proximally. This ensures that the pressure of bandaging does not form a venous tourniquet and compromise circulation to this very distal injury.

COMPLICATIONS OF BANDAGING

Bandaging can lead to some complications, although such occurrences are infrequent. If a bandage—particularly a circumferential bandage—is too tight, the area beneath it may continue to swell, increasing pressure in the area of the wound. This can lead to decreased blood flow and ischemia distal to the bandage. Pressure can build to such an extreme that the bandage acts like a tourniquet. Pain, pallor, tingling, a loss of pulses, and prolonged capillary refill time are typical signs of developing pressure and ischemia. Avoid this complication by making bandages snug but

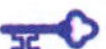

Frequently check the pressure beneath a bandage to ensure good distal circulation.

not too tight. A useful technique is to wrap a bandage only so tight that one finger can still be easily slipped beneath it.

Bandages and dressings left on too long can become soaked with blood and body fluids and then serve as incubators for infection. This problem usually takes at least 2 to 3 days to develop and is not a common concern in most prehospital settings.

The size of the dressing is an important consideration in bandaging. An unnecessarily large and bulky dressing can prevent proper inspection of a wound and hide contamination and continued serious bleeding. Too small a dressing can become lost in a wound and become, in effect, a foreign body. This is most frequently a problem with large, gaping wounds and deep wounds that penetrate the thoracic or abdominal body cavities. When dressing a wound, choose a dressing just larger than the wound yet not so small as to become lost in it.

CARE OF SPECIFIC WOUNDS

Some circumstances—amputations, impaled objects, and crush syndrome cases—deserve special attention during the patient management process. These injuries can challenge even the seasoned paramedic to provide the most appropriate care.

Amputations

Amputations may bleed either heavily or minimally. Attempt to control hemorrhage with direct pressure by applying a large, bulky dressing to the wound. If this fails to control hemorrhage, consider using a tourniquet just above the point of severance. If there is a crushing wound associated with the limb loss, apply the tourniquet just above the crushed area. Do not delay patient transport while locating or extricating the amputated body part. Transport the patient immediately, and then have other personnel transport the part once it is located or released from entrapment.

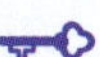

Current recommendations for managing amputated body parts includes dry cooling and rapid transport.

Current recommendations for managing separated body parts include dry cooling and rapid transport. Place the amputated part in a plastic bag and immerse the bag in cold water (Figure 20-23 ■). The water may have a few ice cubes in it, but avoid direct contact between the ice and the injured part. Even if the amputated part cannot be totally reattached, skin from it may be used to cover the limb end (Figure 20-24 ■).

Impaled Objects

When possible, immobilize all impaled objects in place (Figure 20-25 ■). Position bulky dressings around the object to stabilize it, and tape over the dressings to hold them in place. Try to make

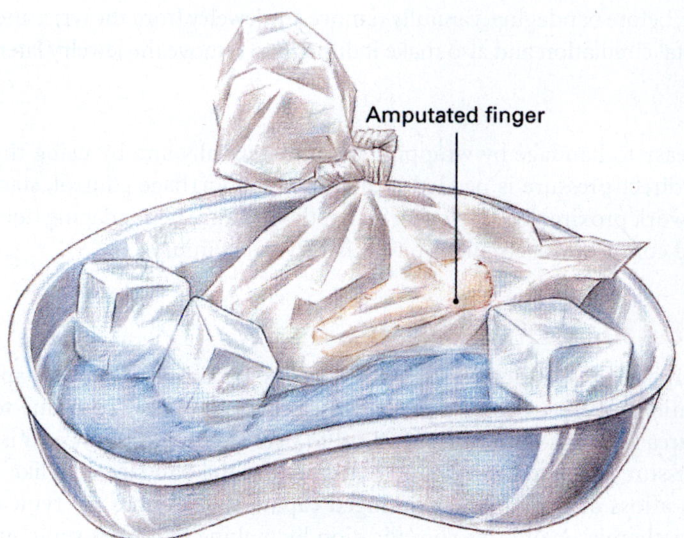

■ Figure 20-23 Amputated parts should be put in a plastic bag, sealed, and placed in cool water that contains a few ice cubes.

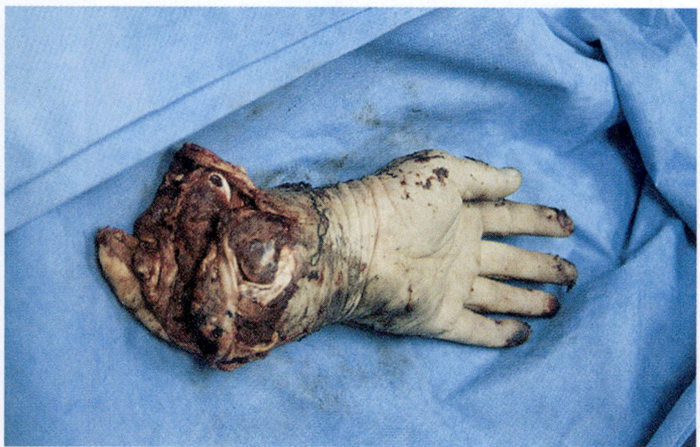

a. An amputated hand.

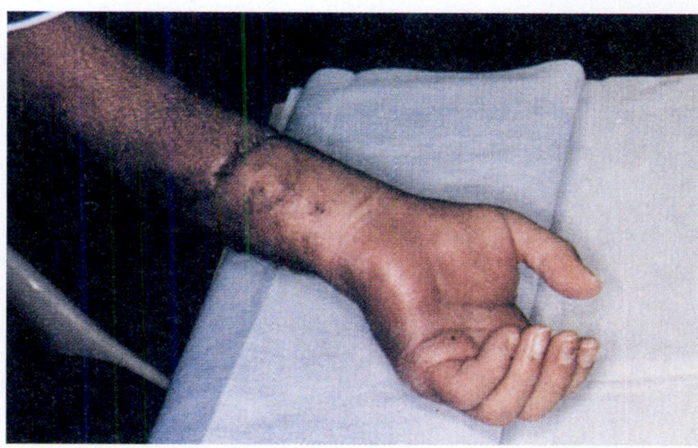

b. A successfully replanted hand.

■ Figure 20-24 Amputated parts should be located and transported with the patient to the hospital for possible replantation.

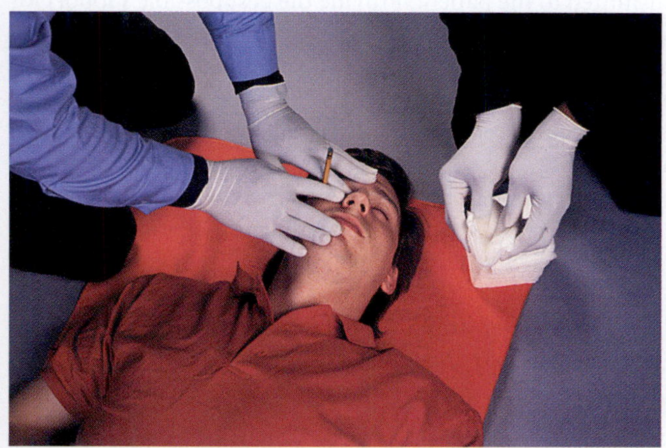

a. Manually stabilize any impaled object.

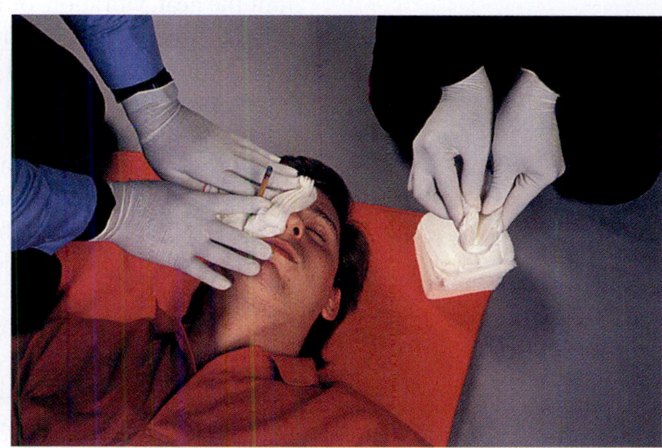

b. Use bulky padding or dressing to immobilize the object.

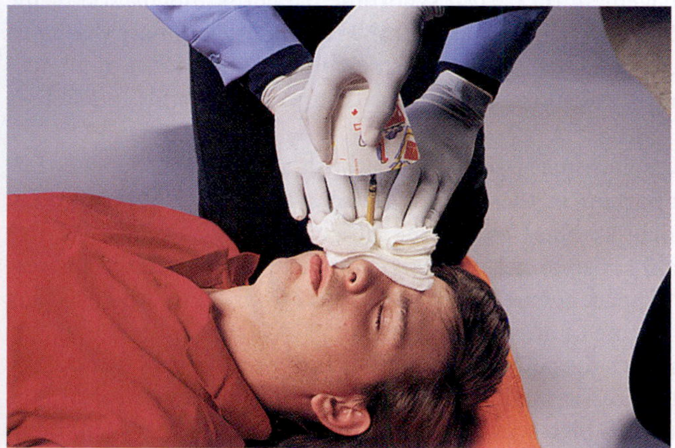

c. If the object protrudes, cover it with a paper cup.

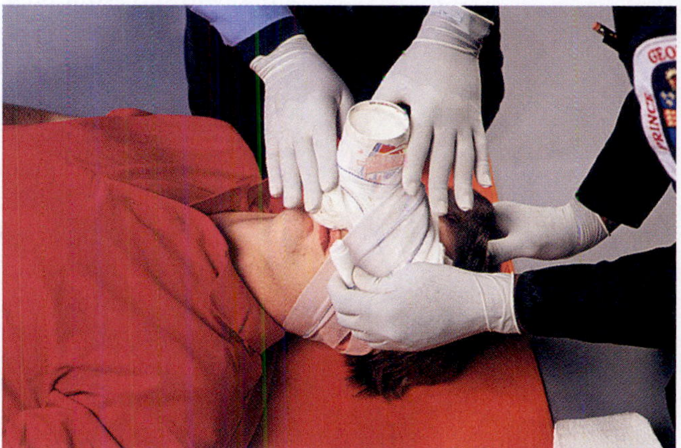

d. Bandage the cup and padding securely in place.

■ Figure 20-25 Stabilization of an impaled object.

■ Figure 20-26 Objects impaled in the cheek may be removed because the sites of hemorrhage can be controlled and the object may interfere with airway control.

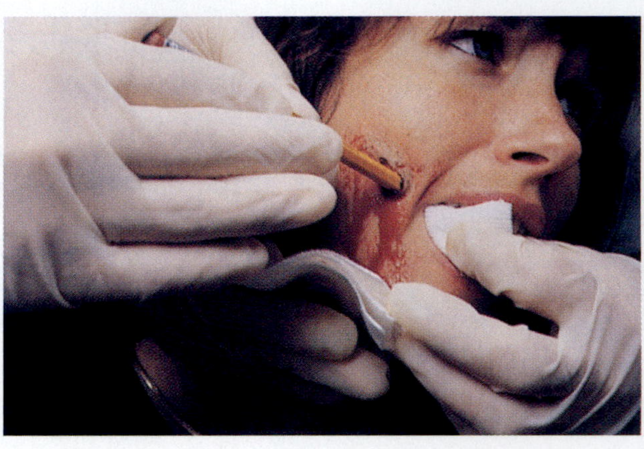

Do not remove impaled objects because of the risk of serious, uncontrollable bleeding.

movement of the patient to the ambulance and transport to the emergency department as smooth and nonjarring as possible. Remember that any movement of the impaled object is likely to cause continued internal bleeding and additional tissue damage.

If the impaled object is too large to transport or is affixed to something that cannot be moved, such as a reinforcing rod set in concrete, consider cutting it. Use appropriate techniques and tools depending on the circumstances of the impalement. A hand or power saw, an acetylene torch, or bolt cutters might be employed. Whatever tools and techniques are used, be sure to take steps to limit the heat, vibration, or jolting transmitted to the patient. Provide the best possible support for both the object and the patient during the cutting procedure.

Only remove impaled objects that obstruct the airway or prevent CPR.

There are some special circumstances in which you *should* remove an impaled object. For example, you may remove an object impaled in the cheek if the removal is necessary to maintain a patent airway (Figure 20-26 ■). In this case, be prepared to apply direct pressure to the wound both from inside the cheek (intraorally) and externally.

Another object that would require removal is one impaled in the central chest of a patient who needs CPR. In such a circumstance, the risk associated with not performing resuscitation outweighs the risk of removing the object. Be aware, however, that a trauma patient who needs CPR has a very poor prognosis.

Another complication associated with an impaled object occurs when a patient is impaled on an object that cannot be cut or moved. In such a case, contact medical direction for advice and guidance. If the object is impaled in a limb, bleeding may be controllable. If it has entered the head, neck, chest, or abdomen, it may not be.

Crush Syndrome

The key to successful prehospital management of a crush syndrome patient is anticipation of the problem and prevention of its effects. Since, by definition, all crush syndrome patients are victims of prolonged entrapment, cases can be identified before extrication is complete. The focus of prehospital crush injury care is on rapid transport, adequate fluid resuscitation, diuresis, and—possibly—systemic alkalinization.

The prehospital approach to crush syndrome is similar to that with other trauma patients. Ensuring scene safety is particularly important in these cases. Crush syndrome victims are often buried in heavy rubble or other large debris, and access may be difficult (Figure 20-27 ■). You may need to request the assistance of specialized personnel and their equipment—urban search and rescue teams, or trench, heavy, or confined space rescue teams. Never place yourself or other rescuers in unreasonable danger when providing care or attempting a rescue.

Once the scene is safe and you can reach the patient, conduct a primary assessment. Remove debris from around the head, neck, and thorax to minimize airway obstruction and restriction of ventilation. Control any reachable and obvious bleeding. Perform as much of the primary and rapid secondary assessment as possible, keeping in mind that portions of the patient's body will be inaccessible as a result of the entrapment. The dark, dusty, and cramped conditions of many confined space rescues may force you to improvise. Be alert for signs and symptoms of associated injuries such as dust inhalation, dehydration, and hypothermia.

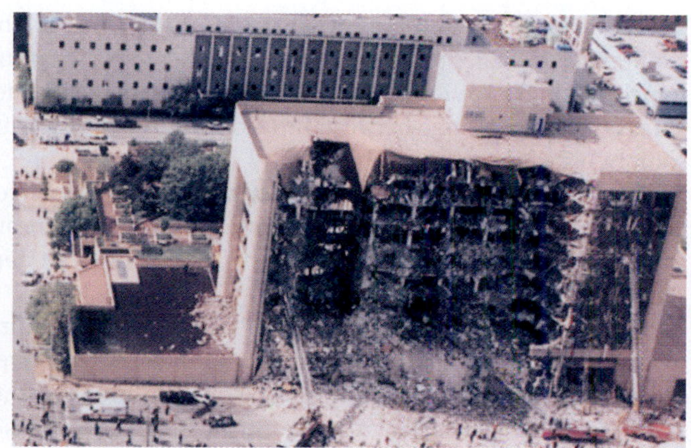

■ **Figure 20-27** Explosion and structural collapse frequently produce crush injury and crush syndrome. *(Pool/Gamma Liaison/Getty Images)*

Remember that the greater the body area compressed and the longer the time of entrapment, the greater the risk of crush syndrome. Initially, a trapped patient will usually complain only of entrapment symptoms: pain, lack of motor function, tingling, or loss of sensation in the affected limb. The patient may also experience flaccid paralysis and sensory loss in the limb unrelated to the normal distribution of peripheral nerve control and sensation.

As long as the body part is still trapped and the metabolic by-products of the crush injury are confined to the entrapped part, the patient will not experience the full effects of crush syndrome. With extrication, however, toxic by-products are released into the circulation, and the patient may rapidly develop shock and die. If the patient survives the initial release of the by-products, he remains at great risk of developing renal failure with serious morbidity or delayed death. Note, too, that a crush injury may also induce compartment syndrome (explained later), especially with prolonged entrapment.

Once you have ensured the patient's ABCs (airway, breathing, circulation), turn your attention to obtaining IV access. Intravenous fluids and selected medications are important in treating crush syndrome. Initiate two large-bore IVs if possible. Because of the entrapment, it may be necessary to consider alternative IV sites such as the external jugular vein or the veins of a lower extremity. Avoid any site distal to a crush injury.

When you encounter crush syndrome, it is unlikely that your protocols will address it. Contact the trauma center for medical direction and communicate, on-line, with the emergency physician. Expect to provide frequent vital sign and patient updates, and be prepared to administer large fluid volumes and, possibly, alkalizing agents.

Alkalinization of the blood and urine is a consideration for preventing and treating crush syndrome. In combination with fluid resuscitation, alkalinization can correct acidosis, help prevent renal failure, and help correct hyperkalemia. Administer sodium bicarbonate 1 mEq/kg initially, followed by 0.25 mEq/kg/hr thereafter. It is preferable to add the bicarbonate to the normal saline bag rather than administering it as a bolus or IV push.

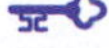

Note: The milliequivalent (mEq) is a means of measuring electrolytes in a standard solution and is based upon the molecular weight and valence of the electrolyte in question.

Diuretics may help keep the kidneys well perfused and more resistant to failure during crush syndrome. Mannitol, an osmotic diuretic, is the drug of choice because it draws interstitial fluid into the vascular space and eliminates it, as mannitol is excreted by the kidneys. Furosemide, a loop diuretic, inhibits the reabsorption of both sodium and chloride. Its use is not advisable in hypovolemic states because it may add to the electrolyte imbalance and volume loss.

Consider applying a tourniquet before the entrapping pressure is released if you have been unable to medicate the patient and provide fluid resuscitation. The tourniquet will sequester the toxins and prevent reperfusion injury. Tourniquet use, however, will continue the development of crush syndrome and worsen its effects.

In cases where the entrapping object may not be moved for many hours or days, medical direction may consider field amputation. This operation will likely be performed by a physician responding to the scene but, in dire circumstances, may be performed by a paramedic under the on-line direction of the emergency physician.

Cardiac (ECG) monitoring is important with all crush syndrome patients. Dysrhythmias may develop at any time but are most likely to occur immediately following the release of pressure upon extrication. Sudden cardiac arrest should be treated in the usual fashion with defibrillation and cardiac drugs as appropriate. Consider 500 mg calcium chloride IV push (in addition to the sodium bicarbonate) to counteract life-threatening dysrhythmias induced by hyperkalemia. Watch for the tenting, or peaking, of the T-wave, a prolonged PR interval, and ST segment depression. Be sure to flush the IV line between infusions or to use different lines because calcium chloride and sodium bicarbonate precipitate.

Once the crush injury patient is freed from entrapment, anticipate the rapid development of shock.

Once the patient is freed from entrapment, be prepared to treat rapidly progressing shock. Continue the normal saline infusions at 30 mL/kg/hr and provide additional boluses of sodium bicarbonate as needed. Rapidly transport the patient to an appropriate hospital (usually a trauma center) for all cases of suspected crush syndrome.

Prehospital care of the crushed limb or body parts requires no special techniques. Cover open wounds and splint fractures, keeping in mind that progressive swelling will necessitate ongoing reassessment, with monitoring of distal circulation and the tightness of bandages, straps, and splints. Handle all crushed limbs gently because the ischemic tissue is prone to injury. Elevation of severely crushed extremities is not indicated in the prehospital setting.

Care at the hospital for crush injury is aggressive and may use techniques such as debridement and hyperbaric oxygenation. During hyperbaric oxygenation, the patient is placed in a chamber with artificially high concentrations of oxygen under several atmospheres of pressure. This drives oxygen into poorly oxygenated tissue to help with the destruction of anaerobic bacteria and to increase tissue oxygenation for repair and regeneration, ultimately reducing tissue necrosis and edema. Hyperbaric oxygenation is most effective when provided early in the course of care.

Hospital care for crush injuries also includes administration of several medications as well as hemodialysis to help salvage the kidneys from the ravages of myoglobin and other toxic agents. Allopurinol, a xanthine oxidase inhibitor, interferes with the production of uric acid, a by-product of skeletal muscle destruction, and may help reperfusion of both the kidneys and the skeletal muscles. It is most effective if administered immediately before release of the compression. Amiloride hydrochloride is a potassium-sparing diuretic that inhibits the sodium/calcium exchange. Mannitol, tetanus toxoid (if needed), and prophylactic antibiotics may also be administered in the hospital to treat crush syndrome.

Compartment Syndrome

The most prominent symptom of compartment syndrome is pain out of proportion with the physical findings.

The most prominent symptom of compartment syndrome is severe pain, often out of proportion to the physical findings. Other signs are often subtle or absent, or they may be overshadowed by the original injury such as a fracture or contusion. Some people suggest using the six Ps—pain, paresthesia, paresis, pressure, passive stretching pain, pulselessness—to identify compartment syndrome, but many of these signs are not dependable or they appear very late in the course of the injury. (Passive stretching pain is pain or an increase in pain noted by a patient as a muscle is extended by a care provider.) Motor and sensory functions are usually normal with compartment syndrome, as are distal pulses. Even capillary refill shows little change. It is important to note that compartment syndrome rarely occurs within the first 4 hours after an acute injury. It is more likely to appear 6 to 8 hours (or as much as a day or more) after the initial injury. Recognition of compartment syndrome can be challenging and requires a healthy suspicion for the problem.

The first step in prehospital treatment for compartment syndrome is care of the underlying injury. Splint and immobilize all suspected fractures, and use traction as appropriate for femur fractures. Apply cold packs to severe contusions. Elevation of the affected extremity is the single most effective prehospital treatment for compartment syndrome. This reduces edema, increases venous return, lowers compartment pressure, and helps prevent ischemia. In the hospital, compartment syndrome is treated surgically, through a procedure that incises the restrictive fascia, a fasciotomy.

SPECIAL ANATOMICAL SITES

Several anatomical sites provide challenges to the care of soft-tissue injuries. These include the face and neck, the thorax, and the abdomen.

Face and Neck

Soft-tissue injuries to the face and neck present potential challenges owing to the anatomical relationships of the airway and great vessels. Injuries to the face may result in blood and tissue debris

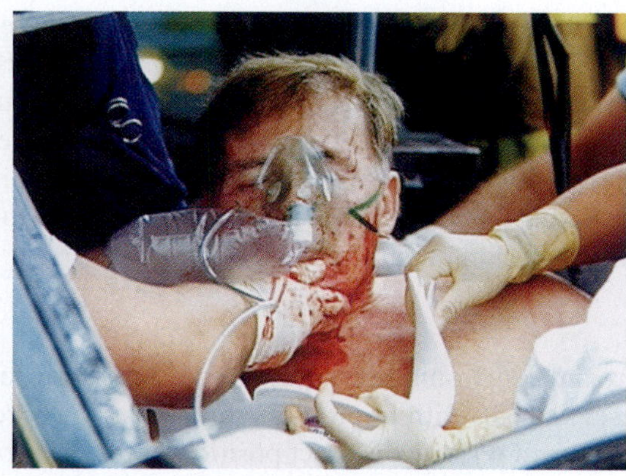

Figure 20-28 Severe facial soft-tissue injuries may interfere with airway control and distort landmarks used for intubation. *(© Eddie Sperling Photography)*

in the airway, posing risks of airway obstruction, asphyxia, and aspiration (Figure 20-28). Pooled secretions and tissue edema may add to airway problems. Trauma to the face or neck may also distort the anatomical structures of the upper airway, leading to airway compromise, and complicating attempts at endotracheal intubation.

Emergency treatment of face and neck injuries can be challenging and may tax your skills. First, gain control of the airway. Open the airway using manual maneuvers. If you suspect the possibility of spinal injury, use the jaw-thrust maneuver in conjunction with in-line manual immobilization. Aggressively suction blood, saliva, and debris from the pharynx, but avoid stimulating the gag reflex in the patient or inducing emesis. Insert an oro- or nasopharyngeal airway as needed.

Direct visualization of the endotracheal tube passing through the cords is the gold standard for securing the airway, but achieving it is fraught with complications in cases of face and neck trauma. Secretions and blood may prevent adequate visualization even with aggressive suctioning. Airway edema can distort the anatomy beyond recognition, and even prevent passage of the ET tube. In all cases, meticulous and absolute confirmation of tube placement is mandatory to avoid fatal hypoxia.

In desperate circumstances, needle or surgical cricothyrotomy may be lifesaving. Avoid placing the needle or making the incision through neck hematomas to avoid life-threatening bleeding.

Once you have secured the airway, focus your attention on any serious facial or neck bleeding. Direct pressure is usually successful for bleeding control, but be certain to avoid compressing or occluding the airway. Pressure points and tourniquets should not be used because of the risks they present of cerebral ischemia and strangulation. Open neck wounds also carry the danger of air aspiration and emboli. Cover any open neck wound with an occlusive dressing, which should then be held or bandaged firmly in place. Because of the neck's anatomy, you may have to maintain digital pressure throughout the course of prehospital care to ensure effective bleeding control.

Thorax

Superficial soft-tissue injury to the thorax may suggest more serious intrathoracic injuries. The pleural space extends superiorly to the supraclavicular fossa and inferiorly to include the entire rib cage both anteriorly and posteriorly. Trauma to this area is likely to injure both the pleura and lungs. Small "lacerations" may actually be deep, penetrating stab or gunshot wounds with resultant hemothorax, pneumothorax, pericardial tamponade, penetrating heart trauma, or injury to the great vessels, esophagus, bronchi, or diaphragm. A seemingly minor "rib bruise" may be the only visible sign of serious lung or cardiac contusions beneath.

Perform a thorough physical examination to detect any signs of internal bleeding, pulmonary edema, dysrhythmias, or shock. However, never explore a thoracic wound beyond the skin edges. Probing deeper can convert a minor wound to a pneumothorax or a bleeding disaster. Consider all thoracic wounds to be potentially life threatening until evidence proves otherwise. See Chapter 25, "Thoracic Trauma," for detailed care procedures.

Never explore a thoracic open wound beyond its edges. Probing may create a pneumothorax or induce serious bleeding.

Dress all open thoracic wounds with sterile dressings in the usual fashion. Be alert, however, for the presence of air bubbling, subcutaneous emphysema, crepitus, or other hints of open pneumothorax. Be extremely cautious about making an airtight seal on any thoracic wound because doing so can rapidly lead to tension pneumothorax and death. Instead, use an occlusive dressing sealed on three sides and be prepared to assist ventilations. Auscultate the chest and monitor respirations frequently. Watch the occlusive dressing so that it does not seal with blood against the chest wall and convert a simple pneumothorax into a tension pneumothorax.

Watch any patient with an open chest wound for the development of a pneumothorax or tension pneumothorax.

Abdomen

The peritoneal cavity extends approximately from the symphysis pubis inferiorly to the diaphragm superiorly. Since the diaphragm rises and falls with respiration, so too does the border between the abdominal and thoracic cavities. You cannot know the exact position of the diaphragm at the time the injury occurred, so suspect associated injuries to both abdominal and thoracic organs if the soft-tissue injury involves the region between the rib margin and the fifth rib anteriorly, the seventh rib laterally, and the ninth rib posteriorly.

Blunt or penetrating trauma to the abdomen can injure both hollow and solid organs, penetrate or rupture the diaphragm, and cause serious internal bleeding. Anteriorly and just underlying the rib margin are the liver on the right and the spleen on the left. Posteriorly, the kidneys (not true abdominal organs since they lie retroperitoneally) are located in the costovertebral angle region. Hollow organs—the bowel, stomach, and urinary bladder—may rupture. In addition to bleeding copiously, these organs may release their contents and inflame the peritoneum.

Consider any soft-tissue wound in the abdominal region as potentially damaging to the underlying organs. Signs and symptoms of internal damage can be subtle, particularly early on. Eviscerations and other massive injuries are obvious, but other internal injuries that are just as serious may not be apparent. Prehospital treatment is primarily supportive and includes ensuring adequate oxygenation, preventing shock, and dressing open wounds (see Chapter 26, "Abdominal Trauma").

WOUNDS REQUIRING TRANSPORT

Transport any patient with a wound that involves a structure beneath the integument for emergency department evaluation. This includes wounds involving, or possibly involving, nerves, blood vessels, ligaments, tendons, or muscles. Also transport any patient with a significantly contaminated wound, a wound involving an impaled object, or a wound that was received in a particularly unclean environment. Also transport any patient with a wound with likely cosmetic implications, such as facial wounds or large gaping wounds.

SOFT-TISSUE TREATMENT AND REFERRAL/RELEASE

In some EMS systems, paramedics are permitted to treat and release patients with minor and superficial soft-tissue injuries or treat and refer them to their personal physicians. This generally occurs under on-line medical direction or according to strict protocols.

In such circumstances, you must evaluate and dress the wound. Then explain to the patient the steps to follow for continuing care of the injury. Tell the patient of the need to change the dressing and to monitor the injury site for further hemorrhage or developing infection. Provide the patient with simple written instructions (approved and/or published by medical direction) explaining wound care, monitoring, protection, dressing change, cleansing, and the signs of problems such as infection or hemorrhage.

Instruct the patient to contact a physician if certain signs and symptoms appear and describe those signs and symptoms thoroughly. Ensure that the patient has the means to obtain physician or health care provider follow-up and again stress the circumstances in which such follow-up care should be sought. During any referral or release, if the patient's tetanus immunization history is unclear or it has been longer than 5 years since the last immunization, instruct the patient to obtain a tetanus booster.

Document all refer/release incidents carefully in the prehospital care report. The report should include a description of the nature and extent of the wound and of the care provided for it. Note in the report all instructions and materials provided to the patient and any medical direction you received.

Summary

Soft-tissue injury may compromise the skin—the envelope that protects and contains the human body. Any trauma must penetrate the skin before it can harm the interior organs and threaten life. Any damage to the skin may interfere with its ability to contain water and blood and to prevent damaging agents from entering. For these reasons, the assessment and care of soft-tissue injuries are important parts of prehospital care.

Assess wounds carefully since they may provide the only overt signs of serious internal injury. Realize that discoloration and swelling take time to develop and may not be as apparent in the field as when you present the patient at the emergency department. Look carefully for the early signs of wounds, and use the mechanism of injury to locate potential trauma sites. When caring for soft-tissue injuries, keep in mind the basic goals: controlling hemorrhage, keeping the wound as clean as possible, and immobilizing the injury site.

Review Questions

1. How does the integumentary system prevent pathogens from attacking the body?
   a. The skin provides a pathway out of the body for pathogens.
   b. Leukocytes in the skin attack pathogens.
   c. Antibodies in the skin attack and destroy pathogens.
   d. The skin provides a protective barrier against pathogens.
2. Of the open wounds presenting to emergency departments, up to ___________ percent will eventually become infected, resulting in significant morbidity.
   a. 8
   b. 6.5
   c. 10
   d. 15
3. When an artery is ruptured but the skin is not broken, blood can separate the tissues and pool in a pocket. This pocket of blood is known as a(n):
   a. contusion.
   b. abrasion.
   c. hematoma.
   d. crush injury.
4. ___________ are typically the most minor of injuries that violate the protective envelope of the skin.
   a. Incisions
   b. Avulsions
   c. Abrasions
   d. Lacerations
5. Specialized white blood cells capable of engulfing bacteria are called:
   a. granulocytes.
   b. macrophages.
   c. phagocytes.
   d. all of the above
6. The anaerobic bacterium *Clostridium perfringens* causes a deep space infection called:
   a. gangrene.
   b. tetanus.
   c. collagen.
   d. lockjaw.

7. You have been called to a scene where a patient has caught one of his hands between two pieces of machinery. As the hand is removed from the machinery, there is no visible injury. You should expect the internal injuries to be:
   a. extensive.
   b. unimportant.
   c. life-threatening.
   d. minimally significant.
8. As you begin to bandage a soft-tissue injury, you should continue to check distal pulses to ensure proper tissue perfusion. This is primarily because the bandage may fit properly at first but later become too tight and reduce circulation as a result of the:
   a. shrinking of the bandage.
   b. development of shock.
   c. toxins entering central circulation.
   d. damaged tissue swelling.
9. When bandaging the foot and ankle to create pressure and control bleeding, wrap in a:
   a. distal-to-proximal fashion to avoid forming a venous tourniquet.
   b. proximal-to-distal fashion to avoid forming a venous tourniquet.
   c. proximal-to-distal fashion to help maintain gentle traction.
   d. distal-to-proximal fashion to help maintain gentle traction.
10. When a soft-tissue injury occurs, a process to stop bleeding starts almost immediately; in addition, the vessels constrict, platelets clot, and the blood coagulates. This process is called:
   a. inflammation.
   b. hemostasis.
   c. epithelialization.
   d. neovascularization.

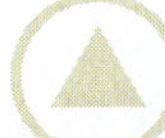

See Answers to Review Questions at the back of this book.

Chapter 21

Burns

Objectives

After reading this chapter, you should be able to:

1. Describe the anatomy and physiology of the skin and remaining human anatomy as they pertain to thermal burn injuries. (see Chapter 3)
2. Describe the epidemiology, including incidence, mortality, morbidity, and risk factors, for thermal burn injuries as well as strategies to prevent such injuries. (p. 892)
3. Describe the local and systemic complications of a thermal burn injury. (pp. 893–894, 904–906)
4. Identify and describe the depth classifications of burn injuries, including superficial burns, partial-thickness burns, and full-thickness burns. (pp. 902–903)
5. Describe and apply the "rule of nines" and the "rule of palms" methods for determining body surface area percentage of a burn injury. (pp. 903–904)
6. Identify and describe the severity of a burn including a minor burn, a moderate burn, and a critical burn. (pp. 909–912)
7. Describe the effects age and preexisting conditions have on burn severity and a patient's prognosis. (pp. 905–906, 910–911)
8. Discuss complications of burn injuries caused by trauma, blast injuries, airway compromise, respiratory compromise, and child abuse. (pp. 901–902, 906–909, 914–915)
9. Describe thermal burn management including considerations for airway and ventilation, circulation, pharmacological and non-pharmacological measures, transport decisions, and psychological support/communication strategies. (pp. 906–915)
10. Describe special considerations for a pediatric patient with a burn injury and describe the criteria for determining pediatric burn severity. (pp. 903–904, 905–906, 910–911)
11. Describe the specific epidemiologies, mechanisms of injury, pathophysiologies, and severity assessments for inhalation, chemical, and electrical burn injuries and for radiation exposure. (pp. 914–921)
12. Discuss special considerations that impact the assessment, management, and prognosis of patients with inhalation, chemical, and electrical burn injuries and with exposure to radiation. (pp. 914–921)
13. Differentiate between supraglottic and subglottic inhalation burn injuries. (pp. 901–902)
14. Describe the special considerations for a chemical burn injury to the eye. (p. 919)
15. Given several preprogrammed, simulated thermal, inhalation, electrical, and chemical burn injury and radiation exposure patients, provide the appropriate scene size-up, primary assessment, secondary assessment (rapid trauma or focused physical exam, detailed exam), and reassessments and provide appropriate patient care and transportation. (pp. 892–921)

Key Terms

ampere, p. 894
blepharospasm, p. 919
body surface area (BSA), p. 903
coagulation necrosis, p. 896
current, p. 894
denature, p. 893
emergent phase, p. 893
eschar, p. 905
extravascular space, p. 894
fluid shift phase, p. 894
full-thickness burn, p. 902
Gray (Gy), p. 899
half-life, p. 897
hypermetabolic phase, p. 894
intravascular space, p. 894
ionization, p. 897
ionizing radiation, p. 897
Jackson's theory of thermal wounds, p. 893
Joule's law, p. 895
liquefaction necrosis, p. 896
ohm, p. 894
Ohm's law, p. 894
partial-thickness burn, p. 902
radiation absorbed dose (rad), p. 899
radioactive substance, p. 897
resistance, p. 894
resolution phase, p. 894
roentgen equivalent in man (rem), p. 899
rule of nines, p. 903
rule of palms, p. 903
subglottic, p. 902
superficial burn, p. 902
supraglottic, p. 901
voltage, p. 894
zone of coagulation, p. 893
zone of hyperemia, p. 893
zone of stasis, p. 893

INTRODUCTION

The incidence of burn injuries in the United States and other developed countries has been declining for several decades. Despite the decline, an estimated 1.25 to 2 million Americans are treated for burns annually and 50,000 are hospitalized. Some 3 to 5 percent of these burns are considered life threatening. Persons at greatest risk for serious burns include the very young and old, the infirm, and workers, such as firefighters, metal smelters, and chemical workers. Burn injuries remain the second leading cause of death in children under 12 years of age and the fourth overall cause of trauma death.

Much of the national decline in burn mortality is attributed to improved building codes, safer construction techniques, sprinkler systems, and the use of smoke detectors. Smaller but still important effects are attributed to educational campaigns aimed primarily at school children. Other simple and inexpensive measures that have helped prevent burns include keeping cigarette lighters and matches away from children and reducing household hot-water temperatures to below scalding levels.

Burns are a specific subset of soft-tissue injuries with a specific pathologic process. While the term *burn* suggests combustion, the actual process that produces burn injuries is much different. The human body is predominantly water and does not support combustion. Instead, body tissues change chemically, evaporating water and denaturing the proteins that make up cell membranes. The result can be widespread damage to the skin, or integumentary system.

Although the skin and its functions are often taken for granted, burn injury to this organ can cause severe fluid loss, infection, hypothermia, and other injuries.

PATHOPHYSIOLOGY OF BURNS

Burns result from the disruption of proteins in the cell membranes. Burns can be caused by several different mechanisms including thermal, electrical, chemical, or radiation energies as well as a combination of these. Being able to understand the mechanism of a burn and to determine the degree and area of burn helps you assess the seriousness of the burn and thus guide your care.

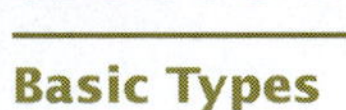

Content Review

Basic Types of Burns

- Thermal
- Electrical
- Chemical
- Radiation

TYPES OF BURNS

Soft-tissue burns can occur from thermal (heat), electrical, chemical, or radiation insults to the body. While the resulting burns are much the same, the damage process differs with the various mechanisms. The following sections describe each of these four types of burns.

Thermal Burns

A thermal burn causes damage by increasing the rate at which the molecules within an object move and collide with each other. We measure the energy of this molecular motion as temperature. At a temperature greater than absolute zero, the molecules of any object move about. As the object's temperature increases, so does the speed of the molecules and the incidences of their collisions with other molecules. These changes in internal energy cause many substances—for example, steel—to expand with increasing temperature. Heat energy may also cause chemical changes. As temperature increases, substances such as gasoline may combine with oxygen. The nature of matter may change as well. Water, for example, may change into ice (with decreasing heat energy) or steam (with increasing heat energy). In addition, the chemical structure of proteins can be affected by heat. An egg changes its nature as the proteins break down, or **denature,** in a hot frying pan. This is why cooked eggs have a rubbery consistency.

denature *alter the usual substance of something.*

Content Review

Effects of Heat According to Jackson's Theory of Thermal Wounds

- Zone of coagulation—most damaged area nearest heat source; cell membranes rupture and are destroyed, blood coagulates, structural proteins denature
- Zone of stasis—adjacent to most-damaged region; inflammation present, blood flow decreased
- Zone of hyperemia—area farthest from heat source; limited inflammation and changes in blood flow

Similar changes also take place in burned tissue. As molecular speed increases, the cell components, especially membranes and proteins, begin to break down just like the egg in a frying pan. The result of exposure to extreme heat is progressive injury and cell death.

The extent of burn injury relates to the amount of heat energy transferred to the patient's skin. The amount of that heat energy in turn depends upon three components of the burning agent: its temperature, the concentration of heat energy it possesses, and the length of its contact time with the patient's skin.

Obviously, the greater the temperature of an agent, the greater is the potential for damage. However, it is also important to consider the amount of heat energy possessed by the object or substance. Receiving a blast of heated air from an oven at 350°F is much less damaging than contact with hot cooking oil at the same temperature. In general, water, oils, and other liquids tend to have a high heat energy content. This content is roughly related to the density of the material. In a similar fashion, solids also usually have a high heat content. Gases, however, usually have less capacity to hold heat owing to their less dense nature.

The duration of exposure to the heat source is also obviously important in determining the severity of a burn. A patient's momentary contact with hot oil would result in less damage than if the oil were poured into his shoe with his foot in it.

A burn is a progressive process, and the greater the heat energy transmitted to the body, the deeper the wound. Initially, the burn damages the epidermis through the increase in temperature. As contact with the substance continues, heat energy penetrates further and deeper into the body tissue. Thus, a burn may involve the epidermis, dermis, and subcutaneous tissue as well as muscles, bone, and other internal tissue.

At the level of local tissues, thermal burns cause a number of effects collectively termed **Jackson's theory of thermal wounds.** This theory helps us understand the physical effects of high heat and helps explain a number of clinical effects (Figure 21-1 ■).

Jackson's theory of thermal wounds *explanation of the physical effects of thermal burns.*

With a burn, the skin nearest the heat source suffers the most profound changes. Cell membranes rupture and are destroyed, blood coagulates, and structural proteins denature. This most damaged area is the **zone of coagulation.** If the zone of coagulation penetrates the dermis, the resulting injury is termed a full-thickness or third-degree burn. Adjacent to this area is a less damaged yet still inflamed region where blood flow decreases that is called the **zone of stasis.** More distant from the burn source is a broader area where inflammation and changes in blood flow are increased. This is the **zone of hyperemia;** this zone accounts for the erythema (redness) associated with some burns.

zone of coagulation *area in a burn nearest the heat source that suffers the most damage and is characterized by clotted blood and thrombosed blood vessels.*

zone of stasis *area in a burn surrounding the zone of coagulation that is characterized by decreased blood flow.*

zone of hyperemia *area peripheral to a burn that is characterized by increased blood flow.*

Large burns have profound pathological effects on the body as a whole. In general, these effects are important in any burn that covers more than 15 to 20 percent of the patient's body surface area. To understand these effects and the resulting burn shock, you must first learn a little about the progression of burns.

The body's response to burns occurs over time and can usefully be classified into four stages. The first stage occurs immediately following the burn and is called the **emergent phase.** This is the body's initial reaction to the burn. This phase includes a pain response as well as the outpouring of catecholamines in response to the pain and the physical and emotional stress. During this stage, the patient displays tachycardia, tachypnea, mild hypertension, and mild anxiety.

emergent phase *first stage of the burn process that is characterized by a catecholamine release and pain-mediated reaction.*

■ Figure 21-1 The zones of injury commonly caused by a thermal burn.

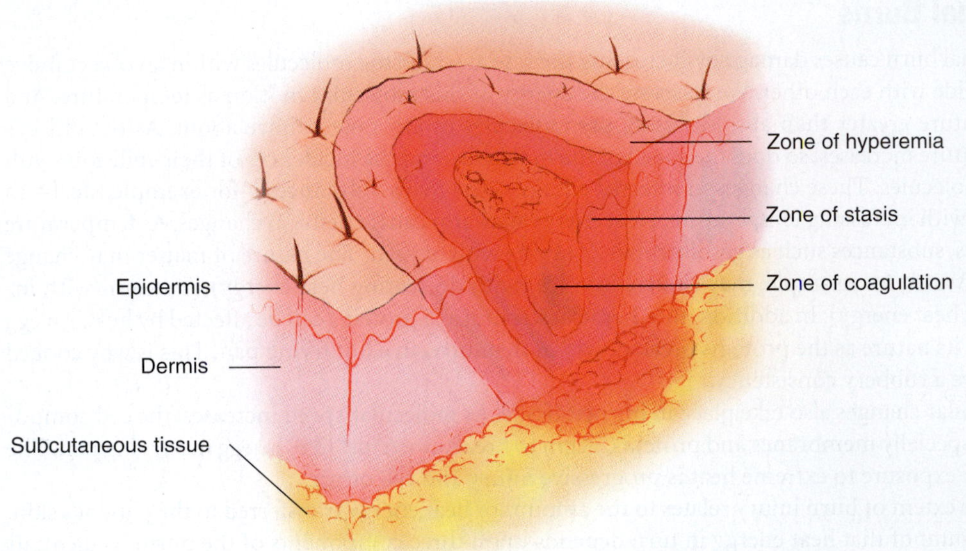

fluid shift phase *stage of the burn process in which there is a massive shift of fluid from the intravascular to the extravascular space.*

intravascular space *the volume contained by all the arteries, veins, capillaries, and other components of the circulatory system.*

extravascular space *the volume contained by all the cells (intracellular space) and the spaces between the cells (interstitial space).*

hypermetabolic phase *stage of the burn process in which there is increased body metabolism in an attempt by the body to heal the burn.*

resolution phase *final stage of the burn process in which scar tissue is laid down and the healing process is completed.*

voltage *the difference of electric potential between two points with different concentrations of electrons.*

current *the rate of flow of an electric charge.*

ampere *basic unit for measuring the strength of an electric current.*

resistance *property of a conductor that opposes the passage of an electric current.*

ohm *basic unit for measuring the strength of electrical resistance.*

Ohm's law *the physical law identifying that the current in an electrical circuit is directly proportional to the voltage and inversely proportional to the resistance.*

The **fluid shift phase** follows the initial phase and can last for up to 24 hours. It occurs in those with thermal burns larger than 15 to 20% total body surface area and is unlikely to occur in those with smaller burns. The fluid shift phase begins shortly after the burn and reaches its peak in 6 to 8 hours. You are therefore likely to see the beginning of it in the prehospital setting. In this phase, damaged cells release agents that initiate an inflammatory response in the body. This increases blood flow to the capillaries surrounding the burn and increases the permeability of the capillaries to fluid. The response results in a large shift of fluid away from the **intravascular space** into the **extravascular space** (massive edema). Note that the capillaries leak fluid (water, electrolytes, and some dissolved proteins) and not blood cells. Blood loss from burns uncomplicated by other trauma is usually minimal.

After the fluid shift phase comes the **hypermetabolic phase,** which may last for many days or weeks, depending on the burn severity. This phase is characterized by a large increase in the body's demands for nutrients as it begins the long process of repairing damaged tissue. Gradually this phase evolves into the **resolution phase,** in which scar tissue is laid down and remodeled, and the burn patient begins to rehabilitate and return to normal function.

Electrical Burns

Electricity's power is the result of an electron flow from a point of high concentration to one of low concentration. The difference between the two concentrations is called the **voltage.** It is helpful to envision voltage as the "pressure" of the electric flow. The rate or the amount of flow in a given time is termed the **current** and is measured in **amperes.** With direct current, the electrons flow in one direction, while alternating current reverses the flow in short intervals. Standard house current is alternating at 60 cycles per second.

Another factor that affects the flow of electricity is **resistance,** which is measured in **ohms.** Copper electrical wire has very little resistance and allows a free flow of electrons. Tungsten (the filament in a light bulb) is moderately resistant and heats, glows, and emits light as more and more current is applied to it.

The relationship between current (I), resistance (R), and voltage (V) is well-known as **Ohm's law:**

$$V = IR \text{ or } I = V/R$$

Like tungsten, the internal parts of the human body are moderately resistant to the flow of electricity. The skin, however, is highly resistant to electrical flow. Moisture or sweat on the skin lowers this resistance. If the human body is subjected to voltage, the body initially resists the flow. If the voltage is strong enough, the current begins to pass into and through the body. As it does, heat en-

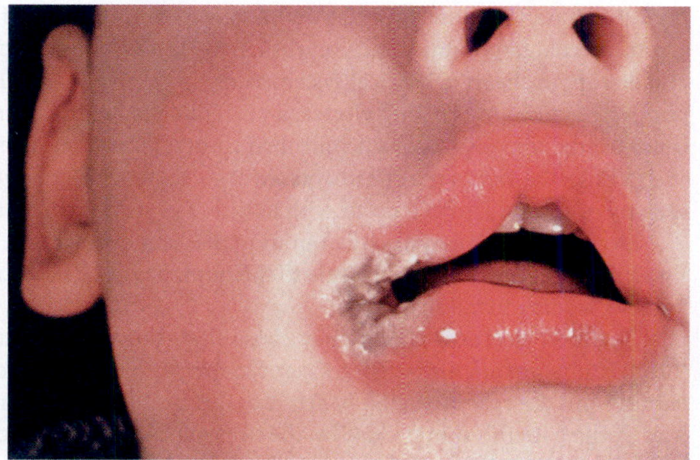

■ Figure 21-2 Electrical burns to a child's mouth caused by chewing on an electrical cord.

ergy is created. The heat produced is proportional to the square of the current flow, is related to power, *P*, and increases with exposure time, *t*, as expressed in **Joule's law:**

$$P = I^2Rt$$

Joule's law *the physical law stating that the rate of heat production is directly proportional to the resistance of the circuit and to the square of the current.*

The highest heat occurs at the points of greatest resistance, often at the skin. This accounts for the severe "entry" and "exit" wounds sometimes seen in electrical injuries. Dry, callused skin can have enormous resistance values, ranging from 500,000 to 1,000,000 ohms/cm. Wet skin, particularly the thin skin on the palm side of the arm or on the inner thigh, can have values as low as 300 to 10,000 ohms/cm. Mucous membranes have very low resistance (100 ohms/cm) and allow even small currents to pass. This accounts for the relative ease with which household current can cause lip and oral burns in children who accidentally bite electrical cords (Figure 21-2 ■).

With small currents, the heat energy produced is of little consequence. But if the voltage or current is high, profound body damage can occur. The longer the duration of contact, the greater will be the potential for injury. Electrical burns can be particularly damaging because the burn heats the victim from the inside out, causing great damage to internal organs and structures while possibly leaving little visible damage on the surface, save for the entry and exit wounds (Figure 21-3 ■).

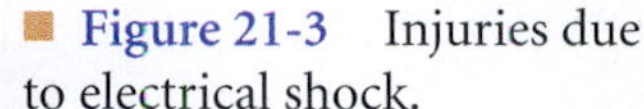

Electrical burns can be particularly damaging because the current burns the victim from the inside out.

Thermal injury due to electrical current occurs as energy travels from the point of contact to the point of exit. At both these points, the concentration of electricity is great, as is the degree of damage you might expect. The smaller the area of contact, the greater will be the concentration of current flow and the greater the injury. Between the entrance and exit points, the energy spreads out over a larger cross-sectional area and generally causes less injury. Electrical current may follow blood vessels and nerves because they offer less resistance than muscle and bone. This may lead to serious vascular and nervous injury deep within the involved limbs or body cavity.

Electrical contact also interferes with the control of muscle tissue. The passage of current, especially alternating current, severely disrupts the complicated electrochemical reactions that control muscles. If contact with a current as small as 20 to 50 milliamperes (mA) is maintained for a

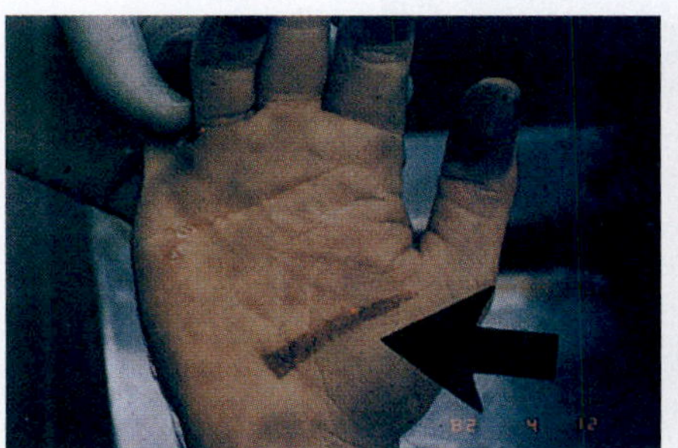

a. Entrance wound

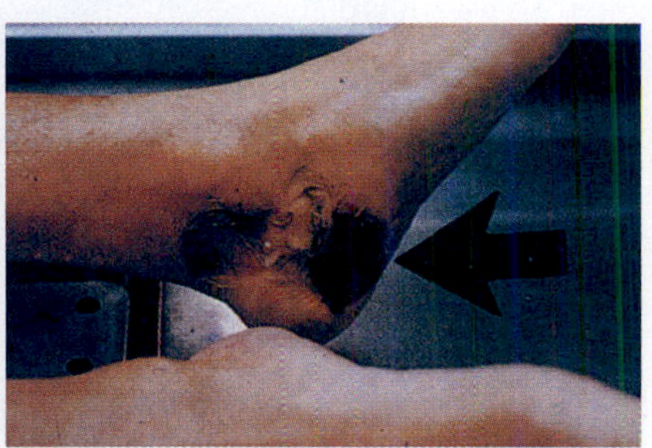

b. Exit wound

■ Figure 21-3 Injuries due to electrical shock.

period of time, the muscles of respiration may be immobilized. The result is prolonged respiratory arrest, anoxia, hypoxemia, and—eventually—death. Electrical currents greater than 50 mA may also disrupt the heart's electrical system, causing ventricular fibrillation accompanied by ineffective pumping action. Alternating electrical current such as that found in household current can also cause tetanic convulsions or uncontrolled contractions of muscles. If the victim is holding a wire at such a time, the victim may be unable to let go, thereby prolonging the exposure and increasing the severity of injury. This can occur with as little as 9 mA of current.

Electrical injury may also disrupt muscular and other tissue, leading to its degeneration. As the tissue dies, it releases materials toxic to the human body. These materials may damage the liver and kidneys, leading to failure.

At times, electrical energy may cause flash burns secondary to the heat of current passing through adjacent air. Air is very resistant to the passage of electrical current. If the current is strong enough and the space through which it passes is small, the electricity arcs, producing tremendous heat. If the patient's skin is close by, the heat may severely burn or vaporize tissue. In addition, the heat may ignite articles of clothing or other combustibles and produce thermal burns.

Content Review

Processes of Chemical Burns

- Acids—usually form a thick, insoluble mass where they contact tissue through coagulation necrosis, limiting burn damage
- Alkalis—usually continue to destroy cell membranes through liquefaction necrosis, allowing them to penetrate underlying tissue and causing deeper burns

Chemical Burns

Chemical burns denature the biochemical makeup of cell membranes (primarily the proteins) and destroy the cells. Such injuries are not transmitted through the tissue as are thermal injuries. Instead, a chemical burn must destroy the tissue before it can chemically burn any deeper. This fact generally limits the "burn" process unless very strong chemicals are involved (Figure 21-4 ■). Agents that can cause chemical burns are too numerous to mention. However, the most common causes of these burns are either strong acids or alkalis (bases).

Both acids and alkalis burn by disrupting cell membranes and damaging tissues on contact. As they cause damage, acids usually form a thick, insoluble mass, or coagulum, at the point of contact. This process is called **coagulation necrosis** and helps to limit the depth of acid burns. Alkalis, however, do not form a protective coagulum. Instead, the alkali continues to destroy cell membranes, releasing the intercellular and interstitial fluid, destroying tissue in a process called **liquefaction necrosis.** This process allows the alkali to rapidly penetrate the underlying tissue, causing progressively deeper burns. For this reason, alkali burns can be quite serious.

coagualtion necrosis *the process in which an acid, while destroying tissue, forms an insoluble layer that limits further damage.*

liquefaction necrosis *the process in which an alkali dissolves and liquefies tissue.*

Radiation Injury

Nuclear radiation has bombarded Earth since long before recorded time. It is a daily, natural phenomenon. Radiation becomes a danger when people are exposed to synthetic sources that greatly increase its intensity. Deaths from exposure to radiation are extremely rare as are serious injuries because of the safety measures commonly used with the handling of nuclear materials. The risk of injury typically comes from accidents associated with improper handling, either on-site or during transport. The incidence of radiation emergencies has increased in recent years because of the ex-

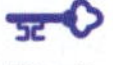

Radiation emergencies should be handled only by those with proper protective equipment and adequate training.

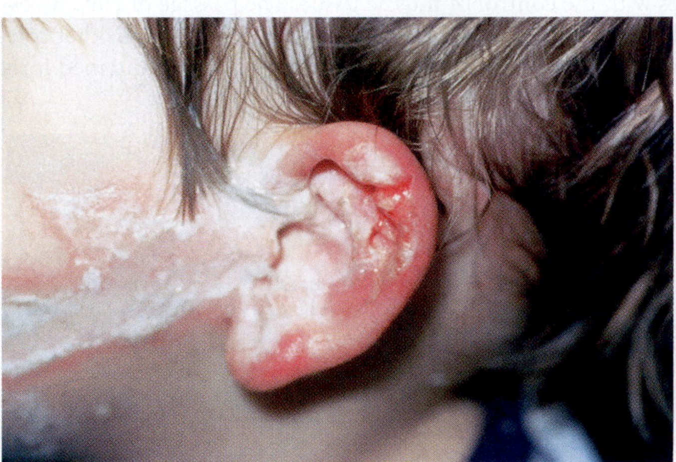

■ Figure 21-4 A chemical burn to the ear.

pansion of nuclear medicine procedures and commercial nuclear facilities. In addition, the possibility of large-scale exposure to radiation from terrorist acts is considered to be increasing.

Keep in mind that radiation emergencies should be handled only by those with proper protective equipment and adequate training.

Basic Nuclear Physics *Radiation* is a general term applied to the transmission of electromagnetic or particle energy. This energy can include nuclear energy, ultraviolet light, visible light, infrared, and X-ray. To understand nuclear radiation, look at the structure of an atom and become familiar with some of the basic terms associated with nuclear physics.

The atom consists of various subatomic particles, which include:

★ *Protons.* Positively charged particles that form the nucleus of hydrogen and that are present in the nuclei of all elements. The atomic number of the element indicates the number of protons present.

★ *Neutrons.* Subatomic particles that are approximately equal in mass to a proton but lack an electrical charge. As a free particle, a neutron has an average life of less than 17 minutes.

★ *Electrons.* Minute particles with negative electrical charges that revolve around the nucleus of an atom. When emitted from radioactive substances, electrons are called beta particles.

You should also be familiar with the following two basic terms associated with nuclear medicine:

★ *Radioactive isotopes (radioisotopes).* Atoms in which the nuclear composition is unstable and that, consequently, give off **ionizing radiation.**

★ *Half-life.* **Half-life** is the time required for half the nuclei of a radioactive substance to lose their activity due to radioactive decay.

Ionization is the process by which radiation causes damage (Figure 21-5 ■). A radioactive energy particle travels into a substance and changes an internal atom. In the human body, the affected cell either repairs the damage, dies, or goes on to produce other damaged cells (cancer). The cells most sensitive to radiation injury are the cells that reproduce most quickly, such as those responsible for erythrocyte, leukocyte, and platelet production (bone marrow), cells lining the intestinal tract, and cells involved in human reproduction.

A substance that emits ionizing radiation is a **radioactive substance,** also referred to as a *radionuclide* or *radioisotope.* Following are the four types of ionizing radiation.

★ *Alpha radiation.* Alpha particles are slow-moving, low-energy particles that can travel only a short distance through the air and that can usually be stopped by such things as clothing and paper. When they contact the skin, the particles penetrate only a few cells deep. Because they can be absorbed (stopped) by a layer of clothing, a few inches of air, or the outer layer of skin, alpha particles usually constitute a minor hazard. However, they can produce serious effects if taken internally by ingestion or inhalation.

★ *Beta radiation.* Smaller than alpha particles, beta particles are higher in energy. Although beta particles can travel 6 to 10 feet through the air, they can be stopped by aluminum and similar materials. Beta particles can penetrate the first few millimeters of the skin but generally cause less local damage than alpha particles; however, like alpha particles, they can be harmful if inhaled or ingested.

★ *Gamma radiation.* Gamma rays, which are related to X-rays, are more highly energized and penetrating than alpha and beta particles. Gamma radiation is extremely dangerous, carrying high levels of energy capable of penetrating thick shielding. Gamma rays easily pass through clothing and the entire body, inflicting extensive cell damage. They also create indirect damage by causing internal tissue to emit alpha and beta particles. Many feet of concrete or many inches of lead are needed to shield against the highest energy gamma rays. Fortunately, high-energy gamma ray exposure occurs only to individuals who are exposed to nuclear blasts, are

ionizing radiation *electromagnetic radiation (e.g., X-ray) or particulate radiation (e.g., alpha particles, beta particles, and neutrons) that ionizes materials that absorb the radiation. Ionizing radiation can penetrate the body cells, depositing an electrical charge that, when sufficiently intense, kills the cells.*

half-life *time required for half of the nuclei of a radioactive substance to lose activity by radioactive decay. In biology and pharmacology, the time required by the body to metabolize and inactivate half of a substance taken in.*

ionization *the changing of a substance into separate charged particles (ions).*

radioactive substance *a substance that emits ionizing radiation; also called a* radionuclide *or* radioisotope.

Content Review

Types of Radiation

- Alpha—very weak, stopped by paper, clothing, or the epidermis
- Beta—more powerful than alpha; can travel 6–10 feet through air; can penetrate some clothing and the first few millimeters of skin
- Gamma—most powerful ionizing radiation; great penetrating power; protection requires thick concrete or lead shielding
- Neutron—great penetrating power, but uncommon outside nuclear reactors and bombs

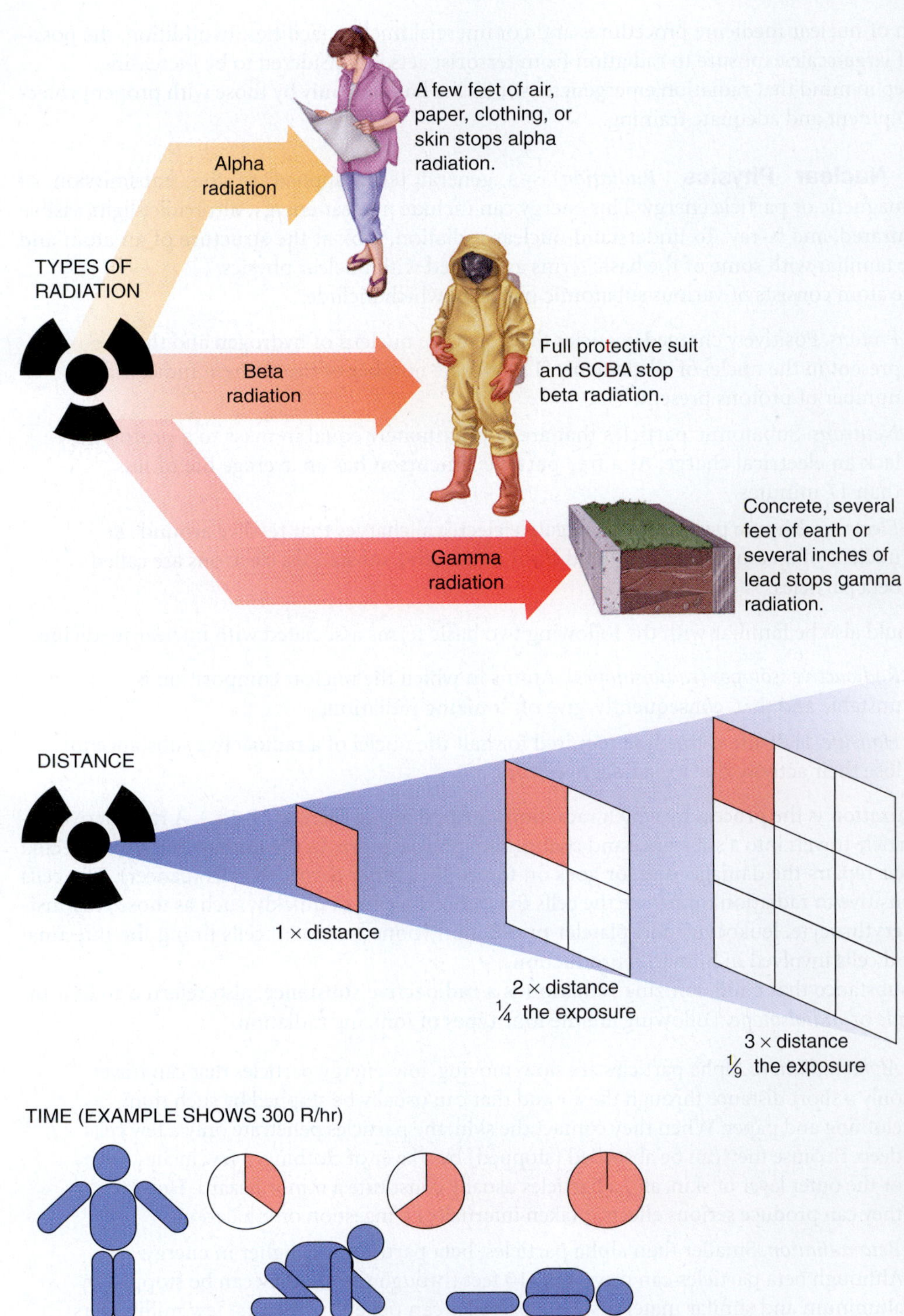

■ **Figure 21-5** The injury considerations associated with nuclear radiation.

near the cores of nuclear reactors, or are very close to highly radioactive materials. More modest amounts of concrete, steel, or lead can provide shielding from more common and lower-energy X-rays and gamma rays.

- *Neutron radiation.* Neutrons are more penetrating than the other types of radiation. The penetrating power of neutrons is estimated to be three to ten times greater than the penetrating power of gamma rays, but neutrons present less internal hazard than ingested alpha or beta particles. Exposure to neutrons causes direct tissue damage. However, in nuclear accidents, neutron exposure is not normally a problem for paramedics because neutrons tend to be present only with a nuclear bomb explosion or near a reactor core.

Effects of Radiation on the Body Exposure to radiation and the effects of ionization can occur through two mechanisms. In the first, an unshielded person is directly exposed to a strong radioactive source, for example, an unstable material such as uranium. The second mechanism of exposure is contamination by dust, debris, or fluids that contain very small particles of radioactive material. These contaminants give off weaker radiation than a direct radioactive source like uranium. However, the proximity of these contaminants to the body and their longer contact times with the body may result in greater exposure and contamination. Note that most substances, including human tissue, do not give off radiation. The patient himself is not the danger in a radiological exposure incident. Any danger comes from the radioactive source such as the contaminated material on the patient.

The two basic types of ionizing radiation accidents are often called "clean" and "dirty." In a *clean accident,* the patient is exposed to radiation but is not contaminated by the radioactive substance, particles of radioactive dust, or radioactive liquids, gases, or smoke. If he is properly decontaminated before arrival of rescue personnel, there will be little danger, provided the source of the radiation is no longer exposed at the scene. After exposure to ionizing radiation, the patient is not radioactive. Therefore, he poses no hazard to rescue personnel.

In contrast, the *dirty accident,* often associated with fire at the scene of a radiation accident, exposes the patient to radiation and contaminates him with radioactive particles or liquids. The scene may be highly contaminated, although the primary source of radiation is shielded when rescue personnel arrive. Unless you are properly trained in dealing with this type of emergency, you may have to delay rescue procedures until properly trained technical assistance arrives.

Ionizing radiation cannot be seen, felt, or heard. Therefore, a detection instrument is required to measure the radiation given off by the radiation source. The most commonly used device is the Geiger counter (Figure 21-6a ■). The rate of radiation is measured in roentgens per hour (R/hr) or milliroentgens per hour (mR/hr) (1,000 mR = 1 R).

Cumulative exposure is measured by a device called a dosimeter (Figure 21-6b ■), which records units of radiation expressed as either the **radiation absorbed dose (rad)** or the **Gray (Gy),** with 1 Gray equal to 100 rads. **Roentgen equivalent in man (rem)** provides a gauge of the likely injury to the irradiated part of an organism. For all practical purposes, rad and rem are equal in clinical value. When neutrons or other high-energy radiation sources are used, a *quality factor (qf)* is applied to determine the equivalent dose.

Different tissues are sensitive to different levels of absorbed radiation. As little as 0.2 Gy can cause cataracts in exposed eyes and damage the blood-cell-producing bone marrow (hematopoietic) tissue. The radiation dose that is lethal to about 50 percent of exposed individuals is approximately 4.5 Gy.

With whole-body exposure, and as the radiation dose increases, the signs and symptoms of exposure appear earlier and become more severe. The first signs of serious exposure are slight nausea and fatigue, occurring between 4 and 24 hours after exposure. As the radiation dose moves into the lethal range, the severity of the nausea increases and is joined by anorexia, vomiting, diarrhea, and malaise. Erythema of the skin may be present, and fatigue becomes more intense. These signs appear within 2 to 6 hours. With exposure to even higher, fatal doses, the patient displays all the signs

Content Review

"Clean" Radiation Accidents

Patient is exposed to radiation but not contaminated by radioactive particles, liquids, gases, or smoke.

"Dirty" Radiation Accidents

Patient is contaminated by radioactive particles, liquids, gases, or smoke.

radiation absorbed dose (rad) *basic unit of absorbed radiation dose.*

Gray (Gy) *a unit of absorbed radiation dose equal to 100 rads.*

roentgen equivalent in man (rem) *a gauge of the likely injury to the irradiated part of an organism.*

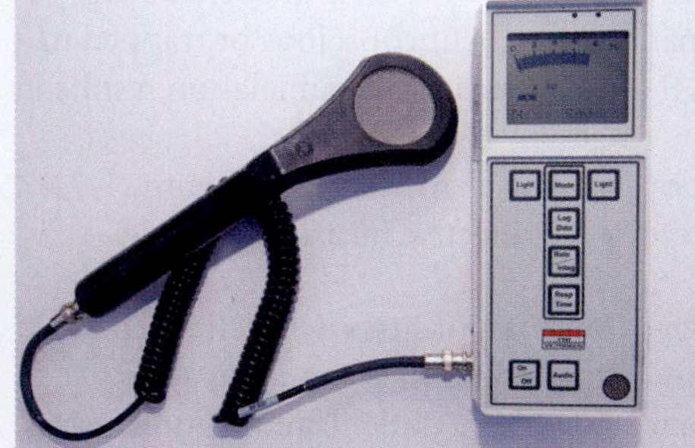

■ **Figure 21-6a** A Geiger counter measures the radiation exposure level. *(© Jeff Forster)*

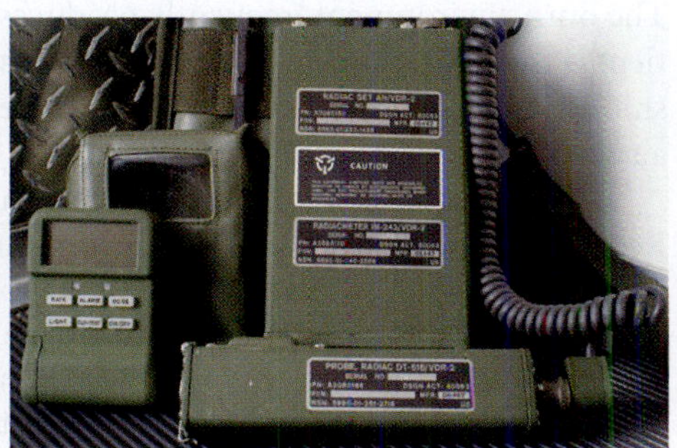

■ **Figure 21-6b** A dosimeter records cumulative exposure. *(Ogunquit, Maine Fire-Rescue)*

of radiation exposure almost immediately and soon thereafter experiences confusion, watery diarrhea, and physical collapse. Note that the signs and symptoms of radiation exposure and the injuries associated with it vary because individual sensitivity to radiation exposure varies greatly.

Prolonged exposure to even small amounts of radiation may produce long-term and delayed problems. Infertility is a potential injury, because the cells producing eggs and sperm are very susceptible to ionization damage, or there may be birth defects in offspring. Cancer is another delayed and severe side effect. It may occur years or even decades after a radiation exposure.

Simply stated, ionizing radiation causes alterations in the body's cell, primarily the genetic material (DNA). Depending on the dosage received, the changes can be in cell division, cell structure, and cellular biochemical activities. Cell damage due to ionizing radiation is cumulative over a lifetime.

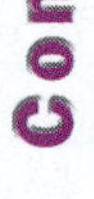

Content Review

Factors Affecting Exposure to Radiation

- Time (duration) of exposure
- Distance from the source
- Shielding from the source

Principles of Safety Three factors are important to keep in mind whenever you are called to incidents of radiation exposure. They are time (duration of exposure), distance (from the radioactive source), and shielding (between you, the patient, and the source). (Review Figure 21-5.) Knowledge of these three factors can limit your exposure and potential for injury.

- ★ *Time.* Radiation exposure is an accumulative danger. The longer you or the patient remain exposed to the source, the greater the potential for injury.
- ★ *Distance.* Radiation strength diminishes quickly as you travel farther from the source. The effect is similar to that of a light bulb's intensity. At a few feet, you can easily read by it, while at a few hundred feet the light barely casts a shadow. Mathematically, the relationship is inverse and squared. As you double your distance from the radioactive source, its strength drops to one-fourth of the original strength. As you triple the distance, its strength diminishes to one-ninth, and so on.
- ★ *Shielding.* The more material between you and the source, the less radioactive exposure you experience. With alpha and beta radiation, shielding is very easy to provide and reasonably effective. With gamma and neutron sources, dense objects such as earth, concrete, metal, and lead are needed to provide any real protection.

The amount of radiation received by a person depends on the source of radiation, the length of time exposed, the distance from the source, and the shielding between the exposed person and the source. For example, the amount of radiation at the patient's initial location may be 300 R/hr. If exposure is for 20 minutes, this is the same radiation equivalent as working for 1 hour at a 100 R/hr scene. (Again review Figure 21-5.) Determining exposure, absorption, and damage done by radiation requires specialized training.

The amount of radiation may drop off rapidly as the patient is decontaminated and moved away from the exposure. The distance from an ionizing radiation source is crucial since, as noted earlier, exposure is determined by the inverse square relationship. Doubling the distance away from a radiation source reduces the exposure by a factor of 4. Conversely, halving the distance to a radiation source increases exposure by a factor of 4.

Inhalation Injury

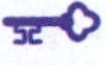

Inhalation injury may be associated with burns, especially if the injury occurred in an enclosed space.

The burn environment frequently produces inhalation injury. This, however, is only true if the patient is trapped or unconscious in an enclosed space. A patient who is unconscious or trapped in a smoke-filled area will eventually inhale gases, heated air, flames, or steam. The inhalation results in airway and respiratory injury.

You can expect to find the following inhalation conditions in a burn environment (Figure 21-7 ■). Keep them in mind as you survey the scene and take the necessary protective measures.

Toxic Inhalation Modern residential and commercial construction uses synthetic resins and plastics that release toxic gases as they burn. Combustion of these materials can form agents such as cyanide, hydrogen sulfide, and other toxic or caustic substances. If a patient inhales these gases, the gases either react with the lung tissue, causing internal chemical burns, or they diffuse across the alveolar-capillary membrane, enter the bloodstream, and interfere with the delivery of or with the cell's use of oxygen. The signs and symptoms of these injuries may present immediately following

Extreme heat
Carbon monoxide
Toxic gases
Airway burns from thermal injuries, toxic gases.
Systemic poisoning from CO, cyanide, other toxic gases.

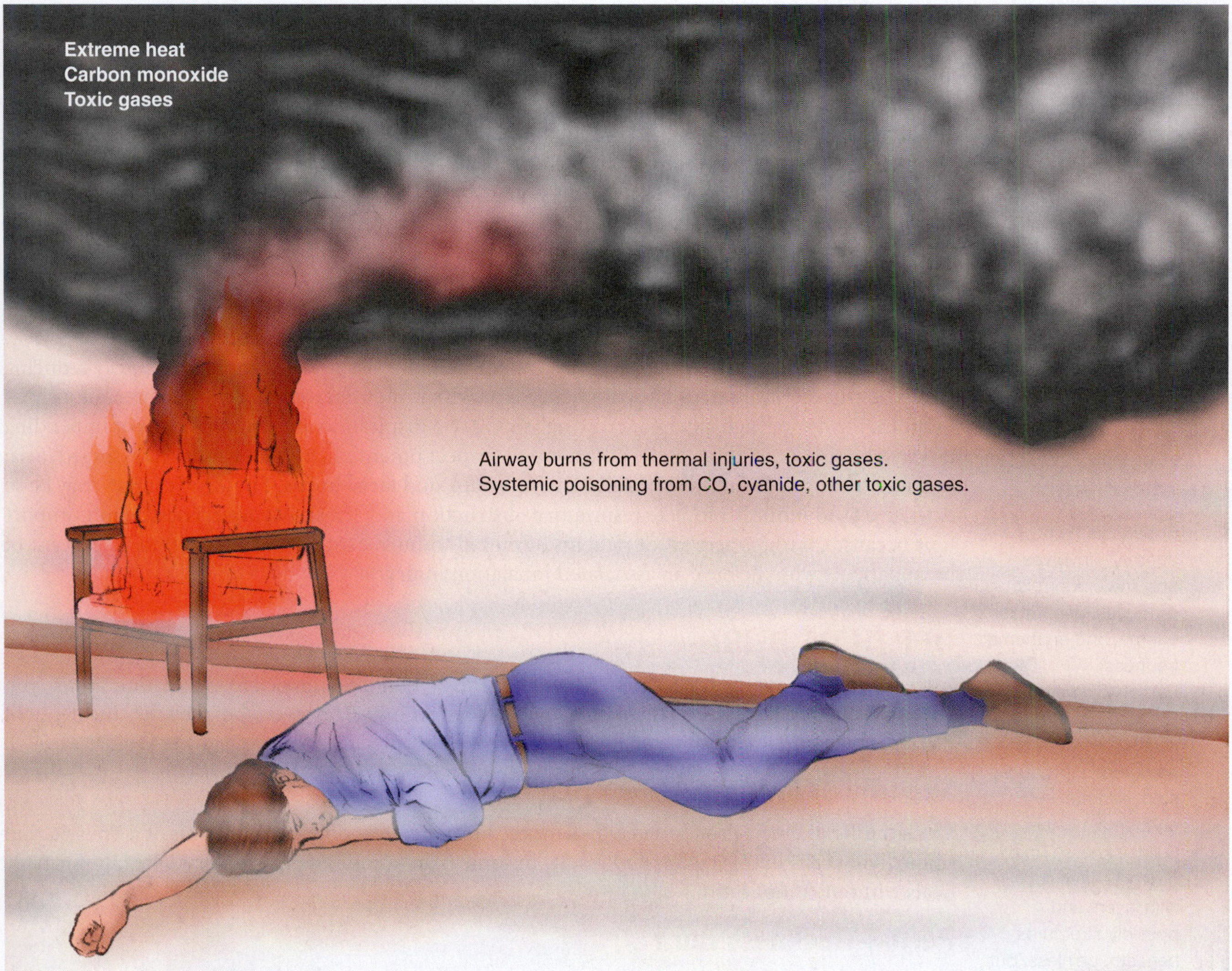

■ **Figure 21-7** Hazards of fire in an enclosed environment.

exposure or their onset may be delayed for an hour or two after inhalation. Toxic inhalation injury occurs more frequently than thermal inhalation burns.

Carbon Monoxide Poisoning An additional concern associated with the burn environment is carbon monoxide (CO) poisoning. Suspect it in any patient who has been within an enclosed space during combustion. Carbon monoxide is created during incomplete combustion, like that which may occur with a faulty heating unit or when someone tries to heat a room with an unvented device like a barbecue grill. Poisoning occurs because carbon monoxide has an affinity for hemoglobin more than 200 times greater than oxygen. If your patient inhales carbon monoxide, even in the smallest quantities, the carbon monoxide displaces oxygen in the hemoglobin and remains there for hours. The result is hypoxemia. Hypoxemia, which is difficult to detect, subtly compromises the delivery of oxygen to the patient's vital organs. If carbon monoxide inhalation is associated with airway burns, the respiratory compromise will be further compounded.

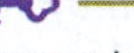

Suspect carbon monoxide poisoning in any patient who was in an enclosed space during combustion.

Airway Thermal Burn Another, though less frequent, injury is the airway thermal burn. Very moist mucosa lines the airway and helps insulate it against heat damage. Because of this mucosa, **supraglottic,** or upper airway, structures may absorb the heat and prevent lower airway burns. High levels of thermal energy are required to evaporate the fluid and injure the cells. Inspiration of hot air or flame rarely produces enough heat to cause significant thermal burns to the lower airway.

supraglottic *referring to the upper airway.*

subglottic *referring to the lower airway.*

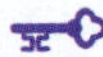

Superheated steam is a common cause of airway burns.

Superheated steam has greater heat content than hot, dry air and can cause **subglottic,** or lower airway, burns. Superheated steam is created under great pressure and can have a temperature well above 212° F. A common hazard to firefighters, superheated steam develops when a stream of water strikes a hot spot and vaporizes explosively. The blast can dislodge the mask of a firefighter's self-contained breathing apparatus, exposing him to superheated steam inhalation. The steam contains enough heat energy to severely burn the upper airway. It also may damage the lower respiratory tract, although this happens less frequently.

Risk factors for inhalation injuries associated with burns include standing in the burn environment (hot gases rise), screaming or yelling there (the open glottis allows toxic gases to enter the lower airway), and being trapped in a closed burn environment.

With any thermal or smoke-related chemical burn injury to the respiratory tract, there is the danger of airway restriction, severe dyspnea, and possible respiratory arrest. The airway is a narrow tube, lined with extremely vascular tissue. If damaged, this tissue swells rapidly, seriously reducing the size of the airway lumen. The patient presents with minor hoarseness, followed precipitously by dyspnea. Stridor or high-pitched "crowing" sounds on inspiration are ominous signs of impending airway obstruction. Other clues leading you to suspect potential airway burns include singed facial and nasal hair, black-tinged (carbonaceous) sputum, and facial burns. The airway injury may be so extensive as to induce complete respiratory obstruction and arrest. Accurate assessment is important because 20 to 35 percent of patients admitted to burn centers and some 60 to 70 percent of burn patients who die have an associated inhalation injury.

Content Review

Depth of Burn

- Superficial (First degree)—involves only the epidermis; produces pain, minor edema, and erythema (redness)
- Partial thickness (Second degree)—involves epidermis and dermis; produces pain, edema, erythema, blisters
- Full thickness (Third degree)—involves all skin layers and possibly structures beneath; painless, but tissue is destroyed; white, brown, or charred, leatherlike appearance

DEPTH OF BURN

After you determine the burn source and assess the possibility of associated inhalation injury, you need to assess the burn's severity. One element in determining the severity of a burn is the depth of damage it causes. Depth of burn damage is normally classified into three categories (Figure 21-8 ■).

Superficial Burn

superficial burn *a burn that involves only the epidermis; characterized by reddening of the skin; also called a first-degree burn.*

The **superficial burn,** also termed a first-degree burn, involves only the epidermis. It is an irritation of the living cells in this region and results in some pain, minor edema, and erythema. It normally heals without complication.

Partial-Thickness Burn

partial-thickness burn *burn in which the epidermis is burned through and the dermis is damaged; characterized by redness and blistering; also called a second-degree burn.*

The **partial-thickness burn,** also termed a second-degree burn, penetrates slightly deeper than a superficial burn and produces blisters. Heat energy travels into the dermis, involving more of the tissue and resulting in greater destruction. The partial-thickness burn is similar to a superficial burn in that it is reddened, painful, and edematous. You can differentiate it from the superficial burn only after blisters form. Because there are many nerve endings in the dermis, both superficial and partial-thickness burns are often very painful. With both superficial and partial-thickness burns, the dermis is still intact and complete skin regeneration is very likely.

The sunburn is a common, but specialized type of burn. Ultraviolet radiation causes the burn rather than normal thermal processes. The radiation penetrates superficially and damages the uppermost layers of the dermis. Sunburn can present as either a superficial or partial-thickness burn.

Another similar type of burn occurs as someone watches an arc welder without proper protection. In this injury, called ultraviolet keratitis, the outermost parts of the eye (cornea) absorb the ultraviolet radiation, causing injury to the layer. This results in delayed eye pain and, possibly, transient blindness. The injury usually heals completely within 24 hours.

Full-Thickness Burn

full-thickness burn *burn that damages all layers of the skin; characterized by areas that are white and dry; also called third-degree burn.*

The **full-thickness burn,** or third-degree burn, penetrates both the epidermis and the dermis and extends into the subcutaneous layers or even deeper, into muscles, bones, and internal organs. These burns destroy the tissue's regenerative properties and the peripheral nerve endings. The injury is painless because of the nerve destruction, but the margins of the full-thickness burn are frequently partial-thickness burns, which can be quite painful. The full-thickness burn takes on various colorations depending on the nature of the burning agent and the damaged, dying, or dead tissue.

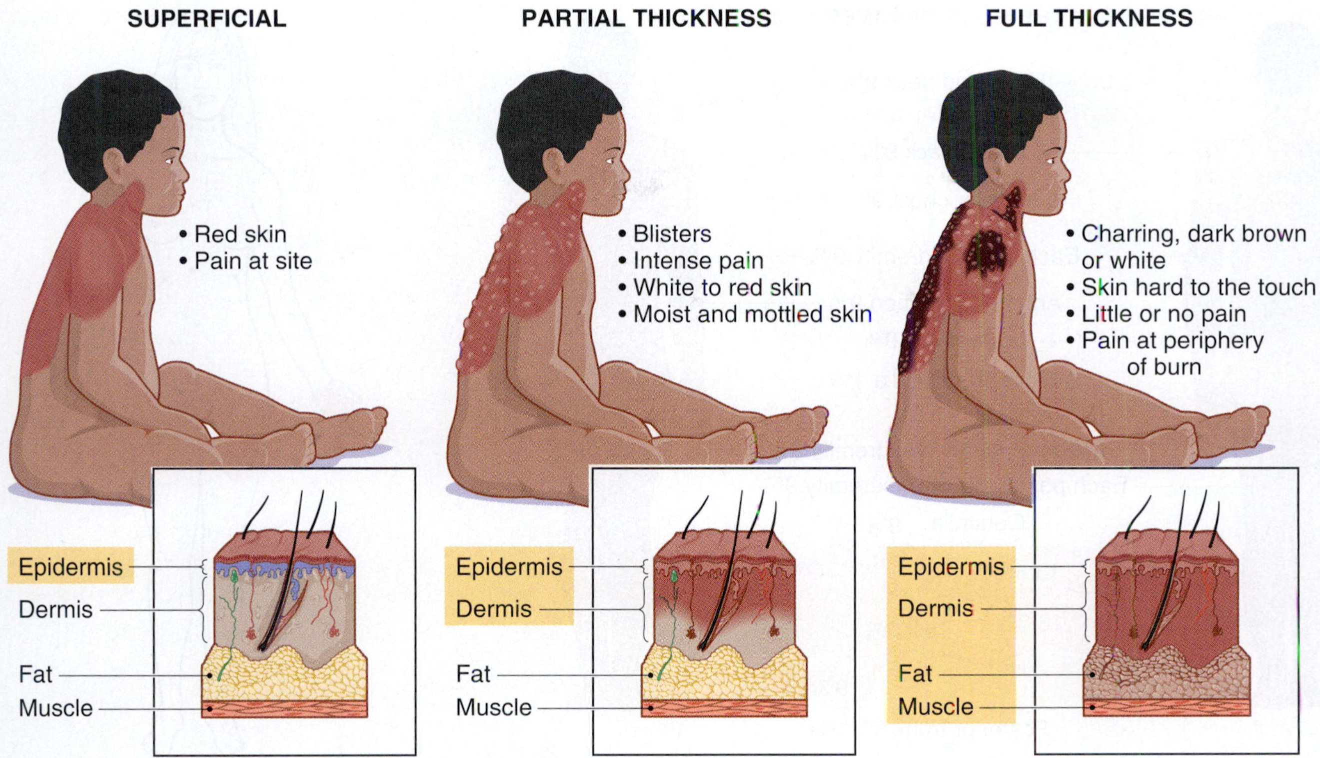

■ Figure 21-8 Classification of burns by depth.

They can be white, brown, or a charred color and typically have a dry, leatherlike appearance. Because the burn destroys the entire dermis, healing is difficult unless the wound is small or skin grafting is possible.

BODY SURFACE AREA

Another factor affecting burn severity is how much of a person's **body surface area (BSA)** the burn involves. There are two approaches to estimating the BSA involved in a burn. The first, the rule of nines, is useful in estimating large burn areas. The second method, the rule of palms, is helpful in assessing smaller wounds more accurately.

body surface area (BSA) *amount of a patient's body affected by a burn.*

Rule of Nines

The **rule of nines** identifies 11 topographical adult body regions, each of which approximates 9 percent of the patient's BSA (Figure 21-9 ■). These regions include the entire head and neck; the anterior chest; the anterior abdomen; the posterior chest; the lower back (the posterior abdomen); the anterior surface of each lower extremity; the posterior surface of each lower extremity; and each upper extremity. The genitalia make up the remaining 1 percent of BSA.

rule of nines *method of estimating amount of body surface area burned by a division of the body into regions, each of which represents approximately 9 percent of total BSA (plus 1 percent for the genital region).*

Because infant and child anatomy differs significantly from that of adults, you must modify the rule of nines to maintain an accurate approximation of BSA. Divide the head and neck area into the anterior and posterior surface and award 9 percent for each. Reduce the surface area of each lower extremity by 4½ percent to ensure the total body surface area remains at 100 percent. The rule of nines is at best an approximation of the area burned. It is, however, an expedient and useful tool to help measure the burn's extent.

Rule of Palms

The **rule of palms,** an alternative system for approximating the extent of a burn, uses the palmar surface as a point of comparison in gauging the size of the affected body area (Figure 21-10 ■). The patient's palm (the hand less the fingers) represents about 1 percent of the BSA, whether the patient

rule of palms *method of estimating amount of body surface area burned that sizes the area burned in comparison to the patient's palmar surface.*

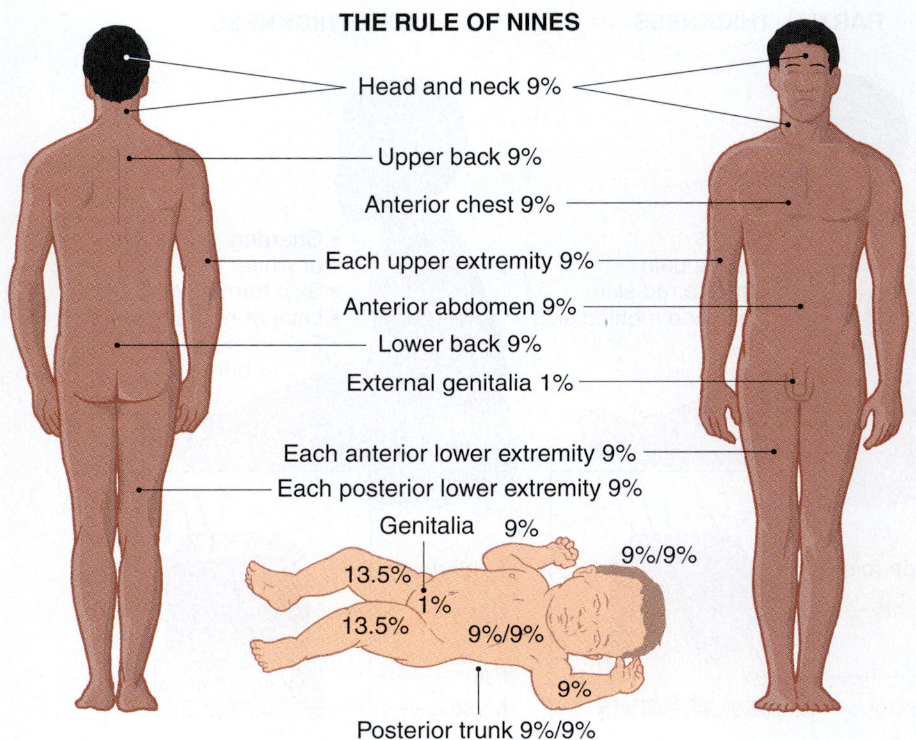

Figure 21-9 The rule of nines.

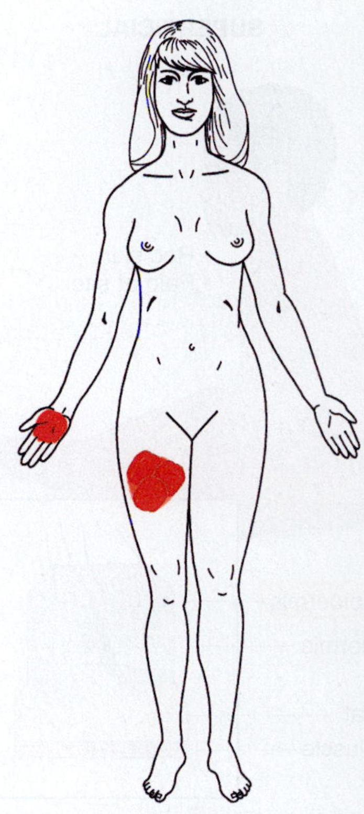

Figure 21-10 Using the rule of palms, the surface of the patient's palm represents approximately 1 percent of BSA and is helpful in estimating the area of small burns.

is an adult, a child, or an infant. If you can visualize the palmar surface area and apply it to the burn area mentally, you can then obtain an estimate of the total BSA affected.

The rule of palms is easier to use for local burns of up to about 10 percent BSA, while the rule of nines is simpler and more appropriate for larger burns. Many other burn approximation techniques exist that are both more specific to age and, in general, more accurate. However, these techniques are more complicated and time-consuming to use. Both the rule of nines and the rule of palms provide reasonable approximations of BSA when used properly in the field.

SYSTEMIC COMPLICATIONS

Burns cause several systemic complications. These can affect the overall severity of a burn. Typical complications include hypothermia, hypovolemia, eschar formation, and infection.

Hypothermia

A burn may disrupt the body's ability to regulate its core temperature. Tissue destruction reduces or eliminates the skin's ability to contain the fluid within. The burn process releases plasma and other fluids, which seep into the wound. There they evaporate and rapidly remove heat energy. The injured skin has increased blood flow, enhancing the heat loss, and the burn injury does not have the reflex vasoconstriction that normally protects against excessive heat loss. If the burn is extensive, uncontrolled body heat loss induces rapid and severe hypothermia.

Hypovolemia

Hypovolemia also may complicate the severe burn. The inability of damaged blood vessels to contain plasma causes a shift of proteins, fluid, and electrolytes into the burned tissue. Additionally, the loss of plasma protein reduces the blood's ability, via osmosis, to draw fluids from the uninjured tissues. This in turn compromises the body's natural response to fluid loss and may produce a profound hypovolemia. Although this is a serious complication of the extensive burn, it takes hours to develop. Modern aggressive fluid resuscitation can effectively counteract this aspect of the burn process.

A related complication is electrolyte imbalance. With the massive shift of fluid to the interstitial space, the body's ability to regulate sodium, potassium, and other electrolytes becomes overwhelmed. In addition, large thermal and electrical burns can lead to massive tissue destruction with a resultant release of breakdown products into the bloodstream. Potassium is one such breakdown product and its oversupply, or hyperkalemia, can lead to life-threatening cardiac dysrhythmias. Careful ECG monitoring and appropriate fluid resuscitation can help prevent hyperkalemic complications.

Eschar

Skin denaturing further complicates full-thickness thermal burns. As the burn destroys the dermal cells, they become hard and leathery, producing what is known as an **eschar.** The skin as a whole constricts over the wound site, increasing the pressure of any edema beneath and restricting the flow of blood (Figure 21-11 ■). If the extremity burn is circumferential, the constriction may be severe enough to occlude all blood flow into the distal extremity. In the case of a thoracic burn, eschar may drastically reduce chest excursion and respiratory tidal volume.

eschar *hard, leathery product of a deep full-thickness burn; it consists of dead and denatured skin.*

Infection

Although infection is the most persistent killer of burn victims, its effects do not appear for several days following the acute injury. Pathogens invade the wound shortly after the burn occurs and continue to do so until the wound heals. These pathogens pose a hazard to life when they grow to massive numbers, a process that takes days or weeks. To reduce the patient's exposure to infectious pathogens, carefully employ Standard Precautions, use sterile dressings and clean equipment, and avoid gross contamination of the burn.

Organ Failure

As previously noted, the burn process releases material from damaged or dying body cells into the bloodstream. Myoglobin from the muscles clogs the tubules of the kidneys and, with hypovolemia, may cause kidney failure. Hypovolemia and the circulating byproducts of cellular destruction may also induce liver failure. In addition, the release of cellular potassium into the bloodstream affects the heart's electrical system, causing dysrhythmias and possible cardiac arrest.

Special Factors

Certain factors involving the burn patient's overall health and age will also affect the patient's response to a burn and should influence your field decisions regarding treatment and transport. Geriatric and pediatric patients and patients who are already ill or otherwise injured have greater difficulty coping with burn injuries than do healthy individuals. The pediatric patient has a high body surface area to body weight ratio, which means the fluid reserves needed for dealing with the

Consider any patient with a preexisting illness or disease or any pediatric or geriatric patient as having a more serious burn injury.

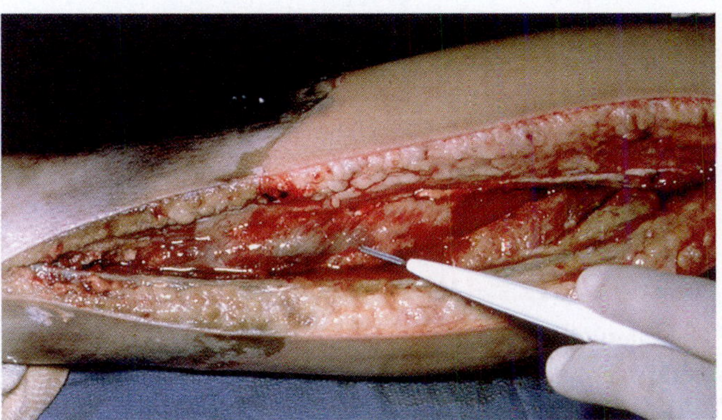

■ **Figure 21-11** The constriction created by an eschar can limit chest excursion or cut off blood flow to and from a limb.

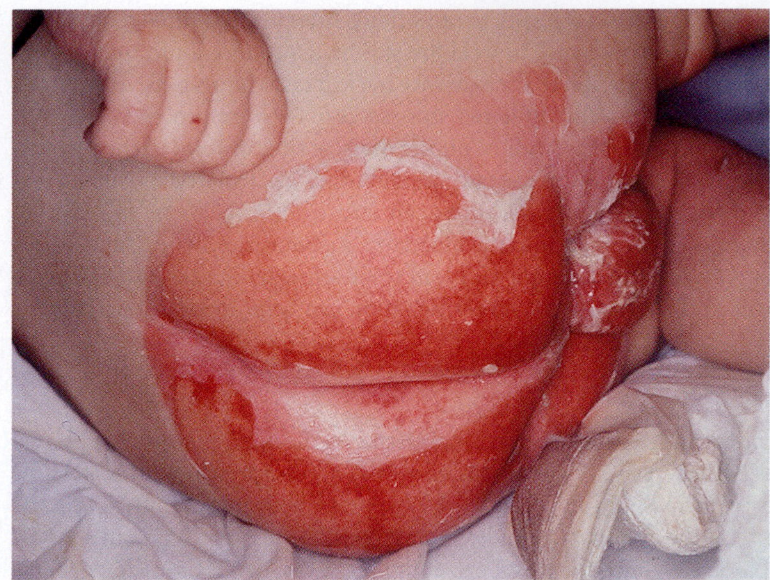

■ **Figure 21-12** Burn injury from placing a child's buttocks in hot water as punishment.

effects of a burn are low. Geriatric patients have reduced mechanisms for fluid retention and lower fluid reserves. They are also less able to combat infection and more apt to have underlying diseases. Ill patients are already using body energy to fight their diseases; with burns, these patients have additional medical stresses to combat. The fluid loss that accompanies a burn also compounds the effects of blood loss in a trauma patient. This patient now must recover from two injuries.

Physical Abuse

When assessing any burn, particularly in a child or an elderly and infirm adult, be alert for any signs of potential physical abuse. Look for mechanisms of injury that don't make sense, such as stove burns on an infant who cannot yet stand or walk. Certain burn patterns should also give rise to suspicion. Multiple circular burns each about a centimeter in diameter may reflect intentional cigarette burns. Infants who have been dipped in scalding hot water will have characteristic circumferential burns to their buttocks as they raise their feet and legs in an attempt to avoid the burning water (Figure 21-12 ■). Branding is an unusual form of abuse and is sometimes seen in ritualistic or hazing ceremonies in some organizations. In all cases of suspected abuse, document your findings objectively and accurately, report them to the person assuming patient care in the emergency department, and notify the proper authorities as state and local laws require.

ASSESSMENT OF THERMAL BURNS

Skin evaluation tells more about the body's condition than any other aspect of patient assessment. Not only is the skin the first body organ to experience the effects of burns, but it is the first and often the only organ to display them. Therefore, assessment of the skin and the associated burns must be deliberate, careful, and complete.

While the burn process varies, assessment is simple and well structured. Assess burn patients carefully and completely to assure that you establish the nature and extent of each injury. This helps you to assign burns the appropriate priority for care.

The assessment of thermal burns follows established procedures for performing the scene size-up, the primary assessment, the rapid secondary assessment or focused history and physical exam, the detailed physical exam, and the reassessment.

SCENE SIZE-UP

The safety of your patients, fellow rescuers, and yourself depends upon a complete and thorough scene size-up. Look around carefully as you arrive at the scene to ensure there is no continuing dan-

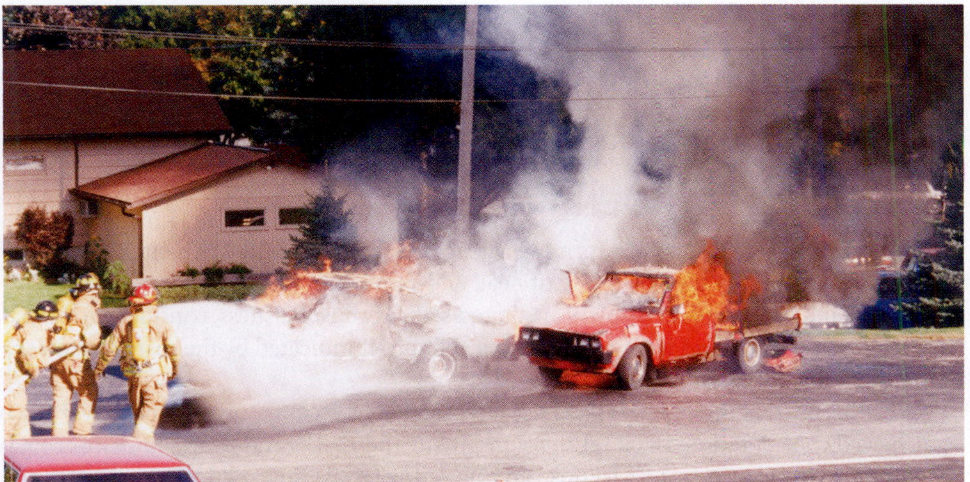

■ **Figure 21-13** Never enter a fire scene until it has been safely contained by appropriately trained personnel.

ger to you or your patient. Examine the scene to ensure it is safe for you to enter. If there is any doubt, do not enter until the scene is made safe by appropriate emergency personnel (Figure 21-13 ■).

Be wary of entering any enclosed space associated with a fire because of the dangers of flashover and toxic gases.

On calls involving burn patients, be wary of entering enclosed spaces, such as a bedroom or a garage, if there is recent evidence of a fire. Even small fires can cause intense heat in small, enclosed spaces. This can rapidly lead to a near explosive process (called flashover) in which the contents of a room rise in temperature to the point of rapid ignition. Flashover is frequently fatal to victims caught in the immediate area.

Another significant hazard at fire-ground scenes is the buildup of toxic gases. Carbon monoxide, cyanide, and hydrogen sulfide are common by-products of combustion and can be produced in large quantities in some fires. Cyanide, in particular, can kill after as little as 15 seconds of exposure, a time short enough to fell any would-be rescuer without proper protection.

Never enter any potentially hazardous scene. Instead, ensure that the fire is thoroughly extinguished or that the patient is brought to you by persons skilled in working in hazardous environments who are using proper personal protective equipment. Ensure that the area where you will be caring for the patient is free from dangers such as structural collapse, contamination, electricity, and any other hazards.

Once at the burn patient's side, stop the burning process so it no longer threatens you or the patient. Extinguish any overt flame using copious irrigation, as water is available. As an alternative, a heavy wool or cotton blanket (avoid most synthetics such as nylon or polyester) will smother flames.

Look for and extinguish smoldering shoes, belts, or watchbands early in the assessment of burn patients.

Quickly survey the patient for other materials he is wearing that may continue the burn process. Remember that burn patients may be an actual hazard both to themselves and to you. Leather articles, such as shoes, belts, or watchbands, can smolder for hours and continue to induce thermal injury. Watches, rings, and other jewelry may also hold and transmit heat or may restrict swelling tissue and occlude distal circulation. Synthetics (such as a nylon windbreaker) produce great heat as they burn and leave a hot, smoldering residue once the overt flames are out. Remove materials like those previously described as soon as possible. Be careful as you check for and remove these items. They may be hot enough to burn you.

Once the scene is safe and there are no further dangers to you or others, consider the burn mechanism. Ask yourself: "Is there any possibility that the patient was unconscious during the fire or trapped within the building?" If so, be ready to place a special emphasis upon your assessment and management of the patient's airway and breathing. Watch for any signs of airway restriction, and be alert to possible poisoning from carbon monoxide or other toxic gases.

Also consider and examine for other mechanisms of injury associated with the burn. Remember that the victim, in attempting to escape the flames, may have fallen down a flight of stairs or jumped from a second- or third-story window. Anticipate skeletal and internal injuries. In cases of electrical burns, consider the possibility that muscle spasms caused by contact with high voltage may also have caused skeletal fractures. Be aware that trauma injuries will increase the severity of the burn's impact on your patient.

Conclude the scene size-up by considering the need for other resources to manage the scene and treat the patient. Request additional EMS, police, and fire personnel and equipment as necessary. If you suspect serious airway involvement or carbon monoxide poisoning, consider requesting air medical service to reduce transport time to the hospital or burn/trauma center.

PRIMARY ASSESSMENT

Start your primary assessment by forming a general impression of the patient. Rule out any danger of associated trauma or the possibility of head and spine injury. Evaluate the patient's level of consciousness, and, if the patient displays an altered state of consciousness, consider toxic inhalation as a cause. Protect the patient from further cervical injury if indicated by the suspected mechanism of injury or by the patient's symptoms.

Next, ensure that the airway is patent. If it is not, protect it. You must give the airway of a burn patient special consideration. Look for the signs of any thermal or inhalation injury during your initial airway exam (Figure 21-14 ■). Look carefully at the facial and nasal hairs to see if they have been singed. Examine any sputum and the areas around the mouth and nose for carbonaceous residue or any other evidence of inhalation. Listen for airway sounds, such as stridor, hoarseness, or coughing, that indicate irritation or inflammation of the mucosa. Such sounds should alert you to the possibility that the airway has been injured and that progressive swelling of the airway is likely. Stridor, in particular, is a serious finding. Consider a patient with any signs of respiratory involvement as a potential acute emergency, and provide immediate care and transport.

With patients in whom respiratory involvement is suspected, provide high-flow, high-concentration oxygen, and prepare the equipment for endotracheal intubation. High-concentration oxygen (at levels approaching 100 percent) is especially important for burn patients because they may be suffering from carbon monoxide poisoning. Very high oxygen percentages more effectively provide oxygen to body cells and may reduce the half-life of carbon monoxide on the hemoglobin molecule by up to two-thirds.

Pulse oximetry is a very useful tool in evaluating respiratory and cardiovascular effectiveness in the burn patient. However, carbon monoxide replaces oxygen in the red blood cell and colors it much as oxygen does. This leads the oximeter to display high saturation readings when the blood actually has greatly reduced oxygen-carrying capacity. Do not rely on pulse oximetry readings alone for the patient who is suspected of suffering carbon monoxide poisoning, who has been burned in an enclosed space, or who has inhaled significant amounts of smoke.

Burn patients may progress rapidly from mild dyspnea to total respiratory arrest. While the intubation of a respiratory burn patient may be difficult in the field, there are distinct advantages to performing it early. The edema is progressive and rapidly reduces the airway lumen. If intubation

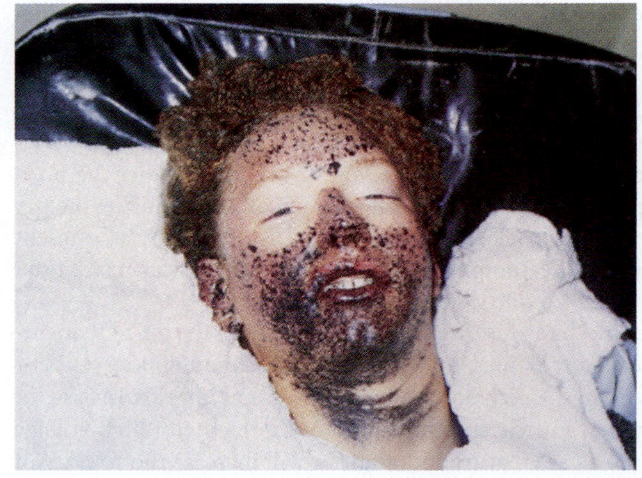

■ **Figure 21-14** Facial burns or carbonaceous material around the mouth and nose suggest the potential for chemical and thermal burns to the airway.

is delayed until the patient becomes extremely dyspneic or goes into respiratory arrest, the airway may be so edematous that it will be difficult, if not impossible, to intubate.

If you elect field intubation for the burn patient (and medical direction approves), perform it quickly and carefully. The airway is already narrowing, and the normal trauma associated with intubation could make matters worse. Intubation can be more complicated if the patient is conscious and fights the process. Consider using rapid-sequence intubation techniques and pharmacological adjuncts including sedatives and paralytics. Use succinylcholine (see Chapter 23, "Head, Facial, and Neck Trauma") cautiously, if at all, since it may worsen the hyperkalemia sometimes associated with severe burns. You may also find nasotracheal intubation useful. In any case, select the crew member with the most experience to ensure that intubation is completed quickly and with the least amount of associated airway trauma.

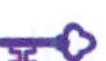

In cases of severe airway burns, intubate early. If intubation is delayed until the patient arrives at the emergency department, the airway may be so edematous that it may be difficult or impossible to intubate.

As with all intubation, it is best to maintain an airway using the largest endotracheal tube possible. Be sure, however, to have several tubes smaller than you would normally use ready, because edema may have reduced the size of the airway. Select the largest tube that you think will easily pass through the cords. In extreme cases, creation of a surgical airway by either cricothyrotomy or needle cricothyrostomy may be a lifesaving necessity; in such cases follow local protocols or on-line medical direction. Confirm tube placement with capnography.

Ensure that the patient's breathing is adequate in both volume and rate. Carefully assess tidal volume if there are circumferential burns of the chest, because the developing eschar may restrict chest excursion. Ventilate as necessary via bag-valve mask using the reservoir and high-flow, high-concentration oxygen.

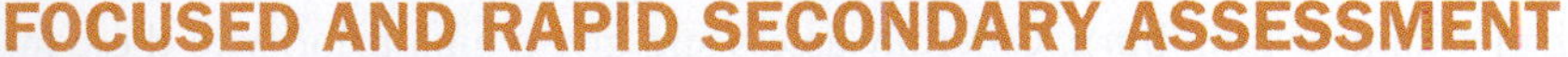

FOCUSED AND RAPID SECONDARY ASSESSMENT

The secondary assessment for the burn patient are much the same as for any other trauma patient, beginning with a rapid or focused secondary assessment and proceeding to the taking of baseline vital signs and a patient history. With a burn patient, however, you must also accurately approximate the area of the burn and its depth. This approximation guides your care and helps emergency department personnel prepare for patient arrival.

Except in cases of very localized burns, examine the patient's entire body surface, both anterior and posterior. Remove any clothing that was or could have been involved in the burn. If any of the clothing adheres to the burn or resists removal, cut around it as necessary.

Apply the rule of nines to determine the total body surface area (BSA) burned. Add 9 percent if the burn involves an entire "rule of nines" region. If it only involves a portion, add that proportion of 9 percent. For example, if one third of the upper extremity is burned, the surface area approximation is 3 percent (1/3 of 9 percent = 3 percent). For small burns, use the rule of palms to approximate the affected BSA.

The depth of a burn injury is also an important consideration. Identify areas of painful sensation as partial-thickness burns (Figure 21-15 ■). Consider those that present with limited or absent

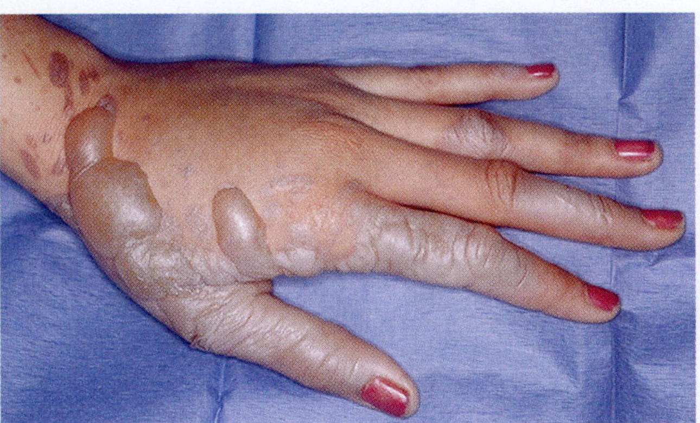

■ **Figure 21-15** A partial-thickness burn.

■ Figure 21-16 A deep full-thickness burn.

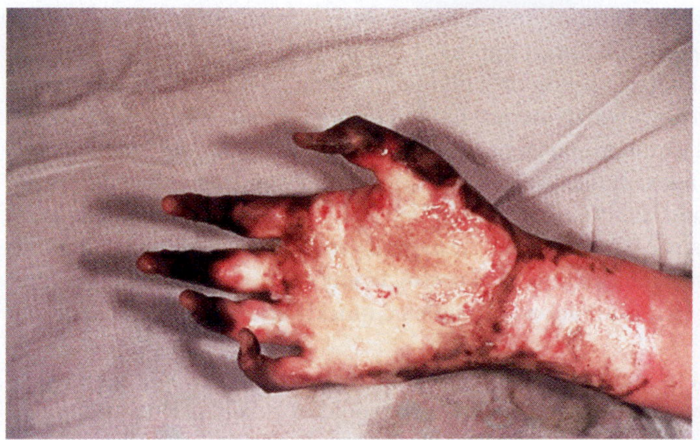

pain as probable full-thickness burns (Figure 21-16 ■). This differentiation is difficult because partial-thickness injury and its associated pain commonly surrounds the full-thickness burn (Figure 21-17 ■). See Table 21–1 for the characteristics of the different types of burns.

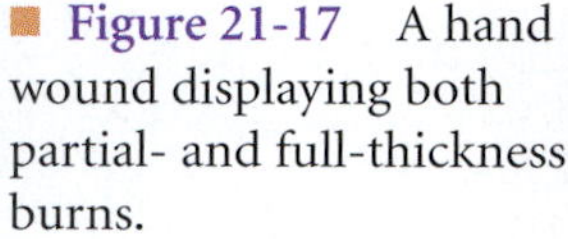

Burns to the face, hands, feet, joints, genitalia, and circumferential burns are of special concern.

A third consideration in determining the severity of a burn is the area of the body affected. The face, hands, feet, joints, genitalia, and circumferential burns deserve particular consideration. Each presents with special problems to patients and their recovery.

You have already assessed the face for burns to eliminate respiratory involvement. But this area also needs special consideration for aesthetic reasons. Facial damage and scarring may be more socially debilitating than a joint or limb burn. Carefully assess and give a high priority to these injuries, even if you do rule out respiratory involvement.

Consider burns involving the feet or the hands as serious. These areas are critical for much of the patient's daily activities. Serious burns and the associated scar tissue make thermal hand or foot injuries very debilitating. Assess these areas and communicate the precise location of the injury and the degree of the burn to the receiving physician. Joint burns can likewise be debilitating for patients. Scar tissue replaces skin, leading to loss of joint flexibility and mobility. Give any burn assessed as full thickness that involves the hands, feet, or joints a higher priority than a burn of equal surface area and depth elsewhere.

Also pay particular attention to burns that completely ring an extremity, the thorax, the abdomen, or the neck. Due to the nature of a full-thickness burn, the area underneath the burn may be drastically compressed as an eschar forms. The resulting constriction may hinder respirations, restrict distal blood flow, or cause hypoxia of the tissues beneath. Carefully assess any burn encircling a part of the body for distal circulation or other signs of vascular compromise. Once you note such an injury, perform ongoing assessments to monitor distal circulatory status.

Finally, assign a higher priority to any burns affecting pediatric or geriatric patients or patients who are ill or otherwise injured. Serious burns cause great stress for these patients. The massive fluid

■ Figure 21-17 A hand wound displaying both partial- and full-thickness burns.

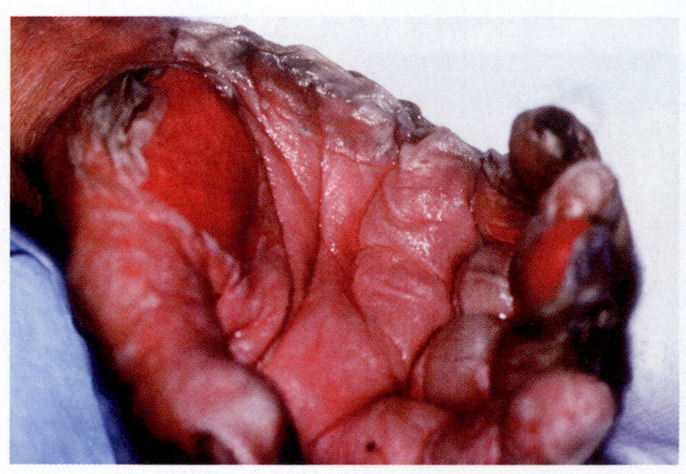

Table 21–1	Characteristics of Various Depths of Burns		
	Superficial (First Degree)	Partial Thickness (Second Degree)	Full Thickness (Third Degree)
Cause	Sun or minor flame	Hot liquids, flame	Chemicals, electricity, hot metals, flame
Skin color	Red	Mottled red	Pearly white and/or charred, translucent, and parchment-like
Skin	Dry with no blister	Blisters with weeping	Dry with thrombosed blood vessels
Sensation	Painful	Painful	Anesthetic
Healing	3–6 days	2–4 weeks	May require skin grafting

and heat loss as well as the infection often associated with burns challenge the ability of body systems to perform adequately. Consider a burn more serious whenever it is accompanied by any other serious patient problem.

Once you determine the depth, extent, and other factors that contribute to burn severity, categorize the patient as having either minor, moderate, or severe burns. Use the criteria in Table 21–2 as a guide.

The severity of a burn should be increased one level with pediatric and geriatric patients and patients suffering from other trauma or acute medical problems. Also consider burns as critical with a patient who shows any signs or symptoms of respiratory involvement. Such patients require immediate transport to a burn (or trauma) center, if possible (see Table 21–3).

The burn center is a hospital with a commitment to providing specialty treatment to burn patients. That commitment includes measures necessary to reduce the risk of infection presented by serious burns. The center must also have the resources to perform delicate skin grafts necessary to replace destroyed skin. Because serious burns leave scar tissue that covers joints and other important areas and affects movement, the center can provide rehabilitation programs requiring prolonged patient stays and intensive nursing care. While immediate transport to a burn center is not as critically time dependent as transport for other seriously injured patients to a trauma center, the burn center's resources can optimize a patient's recovery prospects. Review your local protocols for criteria regarding patient transport to a burn center.

Table 21–2 Burn Severity

Minor

Superficial: BSA < 50 percent (sunburns, and so on)

Partial thickness: BSA < 15 percent

Full thickness: BSA < 2 percent

Moderate

Superficial: BSA > 50 percent

Partial thickness: BSA < 30 percent

Full thickness: BSA < 10 percent

Critical

Partial thickness: BSA > 30 percent

Full thickness: BSA > 10 percent

Inhalation injury

Any partial- or full-thickness burns involving hands, feet, joints, face, or genitalia

Source: American Burn Association.

Table 21–3	Injuries That Benefit from Burn Center Care
Partial-thickness (second-degree) burn greater than 15 percent of BSA	
Full-thickness (third-degree) burn greater than 5 percent BSA	
Significant burns to the face, feet, hands, or perineal area	
High-voltage electrical injuries	
Inhalation injuries	
Chemical burns causing progressive tissue destruction	
Associated significant injuries	

Source: American Burn Association.

Conclude the focused history and physical exam by prioritizing the patient for transport. Rapidly transport any patient with full-thickness burns over a large portion of the BSA. Patients with associated injuries to the face, joints, hands, feet, or genitalia are also candidates for immediate transport. Other cases needing rapid transport include patients who have experienced smoke, steam, or flame inhalation, or any geriatric, pediatric, otherwise ill, or trauma patient. Direct these patients to the nearest burn center as described by your local protocols or by on-line medical direction.

The head-to-toe examination should continue at the scene only if significant and life-threatening burns can be ruled out.

REASSESSMENT

Conduct reassessments for all burn patients, every 15 minutes for minor burns and every 5 minutes for moderate or critical burns. Although the burn injury mechanism has been halted, the nature of the burn will continue to affect the patient. In addition to monitoring vital signs, watch for early signs of hypovolemia and airway problems. Also be cautious of aggressive fluid therapy. Monitor for lung sounds and respiratory effort suggestive of pulmonary edema, and slow the fluid resuscitation if any signs develop. Also carefully monitor distal circulation and sensation with any circumferential burn. Finally, monitor the ECG to identify any abnormalities, which may be caused by electrolyte imbalances secondary to fluid movement and tissue destruction.

MANAGEMENT OF THERMAL BURNS

Once you complete your burn patient assessment and correct or address any immediate life threats, you can begin certain burn management steps, either in the field or en route to the hospital. These include the prevention of shock, hypothermia, and any further wound contamination.

Thermal burn management can be divided into two categories: that for local and minor burns and that for moderate to severe burns.

LOCAL AND MINOR BURNS

Use local cooling to treat minor soft-tissue burns involving only a small proportion of the body surface area at a partial thickness. Provide this care only for partial-thickness burns that involve less than 15 percent of the BSA or very small full-thickness burns (less than 2 percent BSA). Cooling of larger surface areas may subject the patient to the risk of hypothermia. Cold or cool water immersion has some effect in reducing pain and may limit the depth of the burning process if applied immediately (within 1 or 2 minutes) after the burn.

Cool water immersion of minor localized burns may be effective if accomplished in the first few minutes after a burn.

If you have not already done so, remove any article of clothing or jewelry that might possibly act to constrain edema. As body fluids accumulate at the injury site, the site begins to swell. If the swelling encounters any constriction, it increases pressure on other tissue and may, in effect, serve as a tourniquet. This pressure may result in the loss of pulse and circulation distal to the injury. Evaluate distal circulation and sensation frequently during care and transport.

Also provide the burn patient with comfort and support. Even rather minor burns can be very painful. Calm and reassure the patient; in severe cases, consider fentanyl or morphine sulfate analgesia.

Standard in-hospital treatment for minor burns can be varied depending on the clinical circumstances. Therapies may include the application of topical (not systemic) antibiotic ointments and sterile dressings. In addition, there are other options such as biologic dressings that may be appropriate. This is why it is important to cover the burns only with a clean sheet until a definitive management decision has been reached. For example the early use of silver sulfadiazine may preclude the use of biologic dressings. Encourage the patient, as much as possible, to keep the burn elevated. Provide analgesia in either oral or parenteral form as burns can be quite painful. Full-thickness burns are open wounds, so any patient without an up-to-date tetanus immunization is given a booster of tetanus-diphtheria toxoid.

MODERATE TO SEVERE BURNS

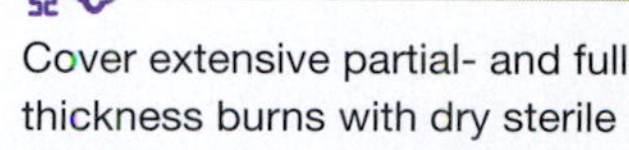

Cover extensive partial- and full-thickness burns with dry sterile dressing, keep the patient warm, and initiate fluid resuscitation.

Use dry, clean (not necessarily sterile) dressings to cover partial-thickness burns that involve more than 15 percent BSA or full-thickness burns involving more than 5 percent of the BSA. Dressings keep air movement past the sensitive partial-thickness burn to a minimum, and thereby reduce pain. Bulky sterile dressings also provide padding against minor bumping and other trauma. In full-thickness burns, they provide a barrier to possible contamination.

Keep the patient warm. When burns involve large surface areas, the patient loses the ability to effectively control body temperature. If the burn begins to seep fluid, as in a full-thickness burn, evaporative heat loss can be extreme. Cover such an area with dry sterile dressings, cover the patient with a blanket, and maintain a warm environment.

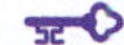

Use soft, nonadherent dressings between areas of full-thickness burns, as between the fingers and toes, to prevent adhesion.

When treating full-thickness burns to the fingers, toes, or other locations where burned surfaces may contact each other, place soft, nonadherent bandages between the burned skin areas (Figure 21-18 ■). Without this precaution, the disrupted and wet wounds would stick together and cause further damage when pulled apart for care at the emergency department.

If the surface area of the burn is great, medical direction may ask you to provide aggressive fluid therapy during prehospital care. While hypovolemia is not an early development after a burn, fluid migration into the wound later during the burn cycle eventually leads to serious fluid loss. Early and aggressive fluid therapy can effectively reduce the impact of this fluid loss.

If burns cover all the normal IV access sites, you may place the catheter through tissue with partial-thickness burns, proximal to any more serious injury. (Full-thickness burns usually damage the blood vessels or coagulate the blood, making intravenous cannulation difficult and possibly impeding effective fluid flow.) Be careful with insertion. The skin may be leathery, but the tissue underneath is very delicate. Adhesive tape may not stick to the burn tissue or may injure the skin when it is removed. Try to secure the intravenous needle and lines by alternate means, when possible.

Establish intravenous routes in any patient with moderate to severe burns. Introduce two large-bore catheters and hang 1,000-mL bags of either normal saline or lactated Ringer's (preferred) solution. Current fluid resuscitation formulas recommend 4 mL of fluid for every kilogram of patient weight multiplied by the percentage of body surface area burned:

$$4 \text{ mL} \times \text{Patient weight in kg} \times \text{BSA burned} = \text{Amount of fluid over 24 hours}$$

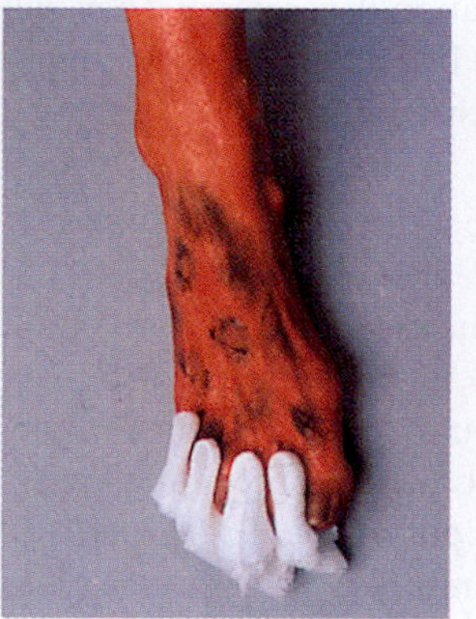

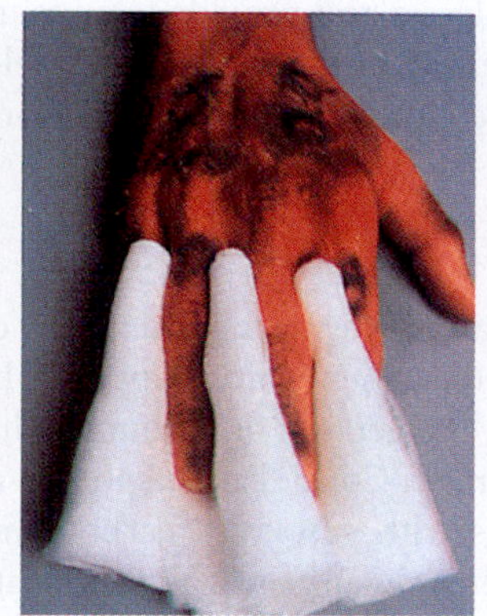

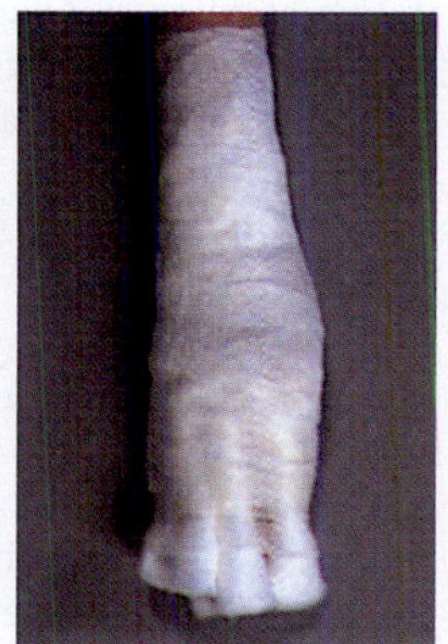

■ **Figure 21-18** Separate burned toes and fingers with dry sterile gauze.

Thus, for a 70-kg patient with 30 percent BSA burned, the calculation is:

$$4 \times 70 \times 30 = 8{,}400 \text{ mL}$$

The patient needs half this amount of fluid in the first 8 hours after the burn. This particular fluid resuscitation protocol is known as the Parkland formula. Other variations exist and may be in use in your local area. In most prehospital situations where transport time is short (less than 1 hour), an initial fluid bolus of 0.25 mL of fluid for every kilogram of patient weight multiplied by the percentage of BSA burned is reasonable:

$$0.25 \text{ mL} \times \text{Patient weight in kg} \times \text{BSA burned} = \text{Amount of fluid}$$

Thus, for an 80-kg patient with 20 percent BSA burned, the calculation is:

$$0.25 \times 80 \times 20 = 400 \text{ mL}$$

Be cautious and conservative when administering fluids to the burn patient with inhalation injury.

You may repeat this infusion once or twice during the first hour or so of care.

Be cautious and conservative when administering fluids to the burn patient if there is any possibility of airway or lung injury. Rapid fluid administration may worsen airway swelling or the edema that accompanies toxic inhalation. Carefully monitor the airway and auscultate for breath sounds frequently whenever you administer fluid to a burn patient.

Burns are quite painful, yet the pain is often paradoxical to the burn severity. Less severe superficial and partial-thickness (first- and second-degree) burns are very uncomfortable, while extensive full-thickness (third-degree) burns are often almost without pain. Provide patients in severe pain with narcotic analgesia. Fentanyl or morphine should be administered as needed. Consider morphine in 2-mg IV increments every 5 minutes until suffering is relieved. Use morphine with caution as it may depress the respiratory drive and increase any existing hypovolemia. With fentanyl, start with a loading dose of 25 to 50 mcg IV and administer repeat doses of 25 mcg IV as needed.

Infection is another classic and deadly problem associated with extensive soft-tissue burns. This life-threatening condition does not develop until well after prehospital care is concluded. However, proper field care can significantly reduce mortality and morbidity. Providing a clean environment and dressings can lessen the bacterial load for the patient. Avoid prophylactic antibiotics because their early use has been shown to actually worsen outcomes for burn patients.

In dire circumstances medical direction may request you to perform an emergency escharotomy. To do this, you incise the burned tissue through the eschar, perpendicular to the constriction. Be certain to incise about 1 cm deeper than the developing eschar to ensure the release of pressure. If adequate respirations or distal pulses do not return after the escharotomy, medical direction may request you to repeat the procedure a short distance from the first incision.

Emergency department personnel will continue fluid resuscitation for serious burn patients according to the Parkland or another suitable formula. They will perform arterial blood gas evaluation to determine oxygen tension, carbon monoxide concentration, and cyanide poisoning levels. Urine output and cardiac monitoring are instituted as well. The staff will ensure adequate administration of parenteral narcotic analgesia and provide tetanus immunization if necessary. They will closely evaluate severe circumferential burns for eschar development. If the blood flow in an extremity or respirations are impaired, the physician may perform an escharotomy.

INHALATION INJURY

Early intubation can be lifesaving for the inhalation injury patient.

If you suspect thermal (or chemical) airway burns and airway compromise is imminent, intubation can be lifesaving. Once you ensure the patient's airway, provide high-flow, high-concentration oxygen by nonrebreather mask at 15 lpm. Oxygen not only counters hypoxia but is also therapeutic in carbon monoxide and cyanide poisoning. Consider transport to a center capable of providing hyperbaric oxygen therapy for patients with suspected carbon monoxide poisoning. The hyperbaric chamber provides oxygen under the pressure of two or more atmospheres. This pushes oxygen into the patient's bloodstream, carrying it directly to the body's cells. Hyperbaric oxygenation also drives

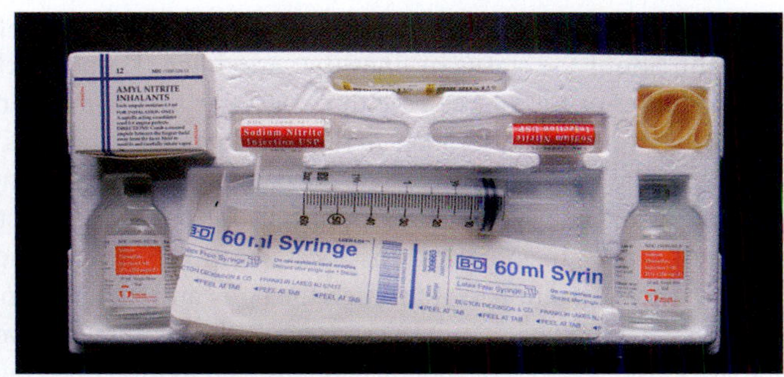

■ **Figure 21-19** A cyanide antidote kit. *(© Jeff Forster)*

carbon monoxide from the hemoglobin, shortening the time to recovery. If hyperbaric oxygen therapy is available in your area, any smoke inhalation or suspected carbon monoxide poisoning patient should be considered for treatment at the facility.

Suspect cyanide toxicity in patients with severe symptoms such as dyspnea, chest pain, altered mental status, seizures, and unconsciousness. To be effective, antidotal treatment of serious cyanide poisoning must be started early. Vapor exposures are likely to result in severe respiratory distress or apnea in addition to unconsciousness. Rapid airway intervention with endotracheal intubation and ventilatory support with a bag-valve mask are initial priorities. However, a rapid shift to antidotal therapy is essential to save the patient.

Administration of the antidote for cyanide is a two-stage process, first using a nitrite compound, followed by a sulfur-containing compound (Figure 21-19 ■). The nitrite acts by converting the hemoglobin (the primary oxygen-carrying protein in the blood) to methemoglobin. Methemoglobin then binds the cyanide, removing it from the cytochrome$_{a3}$ (an enzyme necessary for oxygen processing by cells). The sulfur-containing antidote then removes the cyanide by forming a nontoxic compound, excreted in the urine. The administration of the cyanide antidote should be reserved for patients with a history of acute cyanide inhalation and frank signs and symptoms of serious exposure. The administration of the nitrites is not without risk because they bind to the hemoglobin molecule and produce an effect similar to carbon monoxide poisoning.

Ambulances serving industrial areas with high cyanide use may carry antidote kits containing amyl nitrite, sodium nitrite, and sodium thiosulfate. If an IV is already established, administer 300 mg sodium nitrite over 2 to 4 minutes for adults. If an IV is not yet established, crush one amyl nitrite ampule for the patient to inhale. If the patient has spontaneous respirations, place the ampule under an oxygen mask with high-flow, high-concentration oxygen running. In patients needing ventilatory support, place the ampule in the bag or oxygen reservoir of the bag-valve mask. Do not let the ampule fall into the patient's mouth or down the endotracheal tube. Always follow inhaled amyl nitrite with intravenous sodium nitrite, and do not use amyl nitrite if the patient has already received sodium nitrite. Use care in the administration of sodium nitrite or amyl nitrite as they may induce hypotension. They also bind to the hemoglobin, reducing its ability to carry oxygen. In addition to antidotal therapy, keep the patient supine and administer high-flow, high-concentration oxygen.

Following administration of IV sodium nitrite, administer 12.5 g of sodium thiosulfate for the adult. Avoid sodium thiosulfate unless the patient has received IV sodium nitrite, as it does not work well by itself. A highly effective and much safer antidote (related to vitamin B_{12}) is on the horizon, but is not yet available for general use in the United States.

ASSESSMENT AND MANAGEMENT OF ELECTRICAL, CHEMICAL, AND RADIATION BURNS

ELECTRICAL INJURIES

Be certain that the power has been shut off before you approach the scene of a suspected electrical injury. Until it is, do not allow anyone to approach the patient or the proximity of the electrical source. Remember that an energized power line need not spark or whip around to be deadly; a power line simply lying on the ground can still present a significant danger. Note also that some utility lines

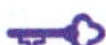

Until the power is off, no one should be allowed to approach the electrical burn patient.

have breakers that will try to reestablish power periodically. Establish a safety zone if there is any question about the status of lines that are down. Keep vehicles and personnel at a distance from downed lines or the source pole that is greater than the distance between the power poles. Also be aware that downed power lines may energize metal structures such as buildings, vehicles, or fences.

Once the scene is secure, assess the patient and prepare him for transport. Search for both an entrance and an exit wound. Look specifically for possible contact points with both the ground and the electrical source. In some circumstances, multiple entrance and exit wounds are present. Remember that electrical current passes through the body and therefore may result in significant internal burns, especially to blood vessels and nerves, while the assessment reveals only minimal superficial findings. Rapidly progressive cardiovascular collapse can follow contact with an electrical source. Also, examine the patient for any fractures resulting from forceful muscle contractions caused by the current's passage.

As with thermal burns, look for smoldering shoes, belts, or other items of clothing. Such items may continue the burning process well after the current is shut off. Also remove rings, watches, and any other constrictive items from the fingers, limbs, and the neck.

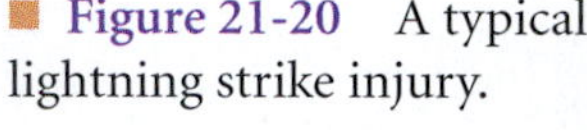

Monitor the electrical burn patient for abnormalities in the ECG.

Perform ECG monitoring for possible cardiac disturbances in victims of electrical burns. Electrical current may induce dysrhythmias including bradycardias, tachycardias, ventricular fibrillation, and asystole. Ensure that emergency department personnel examine any patient who has sustained a significant electrical shock. The damage the current causes may be internal and not apparent to you or your patient during assessment. Consider any significant electrical burn or exposure patient as a high priority for immediate transport.

Lightning strikes to humans occur more than 300 times each year in the United States and result in over 100 deaths. Strikes to people riding tractors, on open water, on golf courses, and under trees are most common, and men are the victims of 75 percent of all strikes. A lightning strike is a high-voltage (up to 100,000 volts), high-current (10,000 amperes), and high-temperature (50,000° F) event that lasts only a fraction of a second. A direct strike will impart this energy to the patient (Figure 21-20 ■). However, the lightning will often strike a nearby object with some current traveling sideways (sideflash) or the current may radiate outward in alternate pathways from the strike point, thus diminishing the voltage (step voltage).

By the time anyone reaches the victim of a lightning strike, the electricity has long since dissipated. (There will be, however, a continued risk of further strikes as long as the storm remains nearby.) There is no danger of electrical shock from touching someone who has been struck by lightning. The person's clothing, however, may continue to smolder, so remove it as necessary. Among

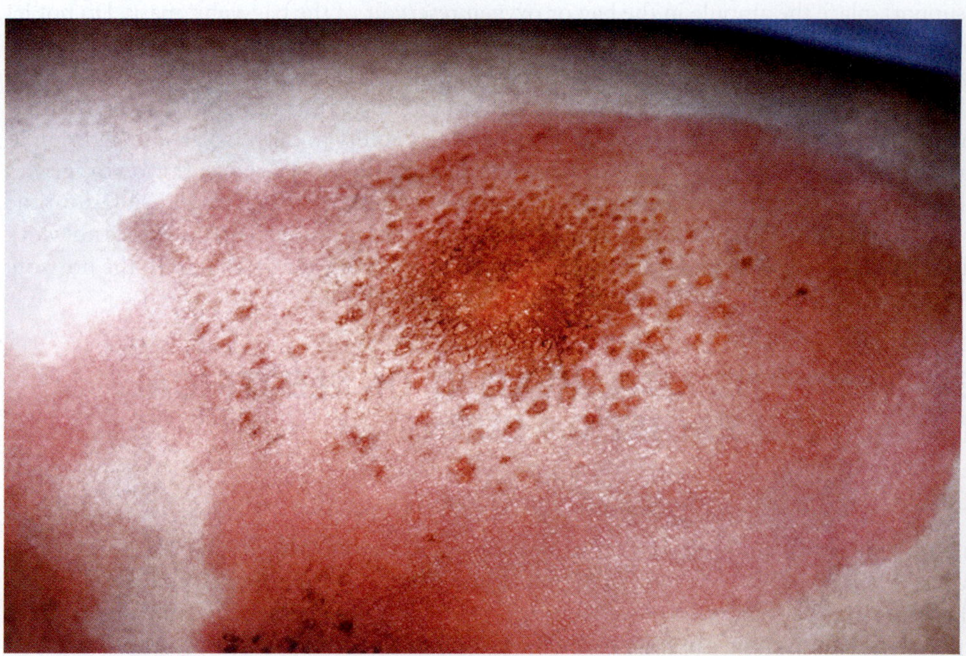

■ **Figure 21-20** A typical lightning strike injury.

other serious effects, lightning can produce a sudden cessation of breathing. Despite being apneic and perhaps pulseless, these patients frequently survive with prompt prehospital intervention.

Treat visible burns ("entrance" and "exit" wounds) just as any thermal burn with cooling, if necessary, followed by the application of dry sterile dressings. Do not focus too much on the visible burns, but instead recognize that the electricity has passed through the body, possibly causing widespread internal effects.

Treat cardiac or respiratory arrest in electrical burn patients with aggressive airway, ventilatory, and circulatory management. Patients in cardiac arrest because of contact with electrical current have a high survival rate if prehospital intervention is prompt. Check immediately for ventricular fibrillation and defibrillate if necessary. Secure the airway with an endotracheal tube and begin ventilations and chest compressions. The usual resuscitative procedures for cases of cardiac arrest apply equally when the cause of the arrest is electrical injury; they might include the use of vasopressors and antidysrhythmics.

For serious electrical burn injuries, initiate at least two large bore IVs and administer 1,000 mL of fluid per hour in 0.20 mL/kg boluses. Consider the use of sodium bicarbonate and mannitol, usually at the discretion of medical direction, to prevent the complications of rhabdomyolysis (discussed in Chapter 20, "Soft-Tissue Trauma") and hyperkalemia. The usual starting dose is 1 mEq/kg for sodium bicarbonate and 10 g for mannitol.

CHEMICAL BURNS

As you perform the scene size-up, identify the nature of the chemical spill/contamination and, if possible, approach from uphill and upwind. Identify the location of the chemical and ensure that it poses no hazard to you, other rescuers, or the public. Be wary of toxic fumes and cross-contamination from the patient and the surrounding environment. If necessary, have hazardous material team members evacuate and decontaminate the victim before you begin assessment and care. Seek out personnel on the scene who are familiar with the agent and consult with them regarding dangers posed by the agent and any specific medical care and patient handling procedures required with it.

During your assessment and care, always wear medical examination (preferably tyvex) gloves, but never presume that they will protect you from the agent. Take appropriate protective action against airborne dust, toxic fumes, and splash exposure for both yourself and the patient (goggles and mask as needed). Wear a disposable gown if there is danger of the agent contacting your clothing. Make certain the agent is isolated and no longer a danger to the patient or others. Have any of the patient's clothing that you suspect may be contaminated removed, and isolate it from accidental contact. Save the clothing and ensure that it is disposed of properly. Identify the type of agent, its exact chemical name, the length of the patient's contact time with it, and the precise areas of the patient's body affected by it.

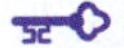

In dealing with a chemical burn, take all precautions to ensure that no one else becomes contaminated.

As you begin your primary assessment, ensure that the patient is alert and fully oriented and that airway and breathing are unaffected by the contact. If there is any airway restriction or respiratory involvement, consider early intubation. As airway tissue swells, the obstruction worsens and intubation becomes more difficult. Monitor the patient's heart rate and consider ECG monitoring, because many chemicals (for example, organophosphates) may affect the heart. If the patient is stable, begin the rapid trauma assessment.

Examine any chemical burn carefully to establish the depth, extent, and nature of the injury. If you suspect the involvement of phenol, dry lime, sodium, or riot agents, then treat as indicated below.

- ★ *Phenol.* A gelatinous caustic called phenol is used as a powerful industrial cleaner. Phenol is very difficult to remove because it is sticky and insoluble in water. Alcohol, which dissolves it, is frequently available in places where phenol is regularly used. You can use the alcohol to remove the phenol and follow removal with irrigation using large volumes of cool water.
- ★ *Dry lime.* Dry lime is a strong corrosive that reacts with water. It produces heat and subsequent chemical and thermal injuries. Brush dry lime off the patient gently, but as completely as possible. Then rinse the contaminated area with large volumes of cool to cold water. While the water reacts with any remaining lime, it cools the

contact area and removes the rest of the chemical. By rinsing with water, you ensure that the lime reacts with that water rather than with the water contained within the patient's soft tissues.

- ★ *Sodium.* Sodium is an unstable metal that reacts destructively with many substances, including human tissue. It reacts vigorously with water, creating extreme heat, explosive hydrogen gas, and possible ignition. Sodium is normally stored submerged in oil because the metal reacts with moisture in the air. If a patient is contaminated with sodium, decontaminate him quickly by gentle brushing. Then cover the wound with the oil used to store the substance.
- ★ *Riot control agents.* These agents, which include CS, CN (Mace), and oleoresin capsicum (OC, pepper spray), deserve special mention because people are targets of their intended use and because that use is frequent. These agents cause intense irritation of the eyes, mucous membranes, and respiratory tract. In general, they do not cause permanent damage when properly deployed. Patients who have contacted them typically present with eye pain, tearing, and temporary "blindness." Coughing, gagging, and vomiting are not uncommon. Treatment is supportive and most patients recover spontaneously within 10 to 20 minutes of exposure to fresh air. Irrigate the patient's eyes with normal saline if you suspect that any riot agent particles remain in the eye.

Irrigation with copious amounts of cool water is indicated for burns from an unknown chemical agent.

If it has not been done earlier, decontaminate the patient who has come in contact with any other chemical capable of causing tissue damage. Stop the damage by irrigating the site with large volumes of water (see Figure 21-21 ■). Water rinses away the offending material and dilutes any water-soluble agents. The water also reduces the heat and rate of the chemical reaction and, ultimately, the chemical's effects upon the patient's skin. If the contamination is widespread, douse the patient with large volumes of water. Use a garden hose or low-pressure water from a fire truck. Ensure that the water is neither too warm nor too cold.

When the patient has been thoroughly rinsed for a few minutes, have the patient remove any remaining clothing to avoid contaminating the rescuers. If the agent is dangerous, save all clothing

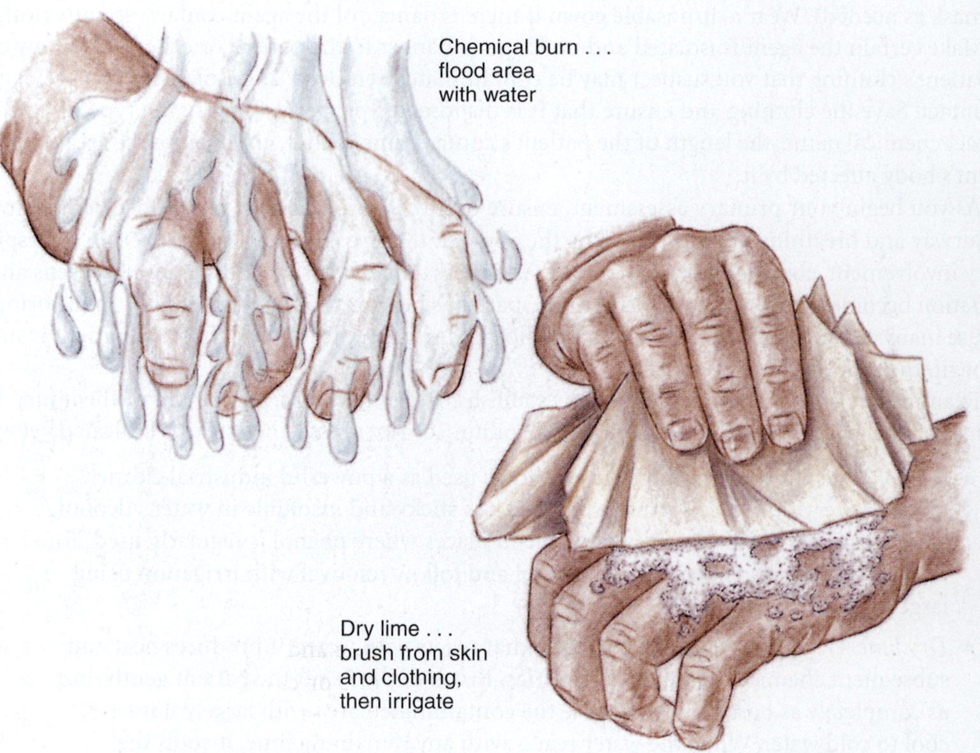

■ **Figure 21-21** Chemical burns should be flushed with large quantities of water. Dry lime should be first brushed away before applying cool water.

and contain the rinse water for proper disposal at a later time. Next, gently wash the burn with a mild soap (such as ordinary dish detergent) and a gentle brush or sponge. Be careful not to cause further soft-tissue damage. After washing, gently irrigate the wound with a constant flow of water. While the pain and the burning process may appear to subside, it is important to continue the irrigation until the patient arrives at the emergency department. If practical, transport the label from the corrosive's container, the product's Material Safety Data Sheet (MSDS), or a sample of the agent (safely contained and marked) along with the patient. On arrival at the hospital, be sure to describe to emergency department personnel, and enter in your prehospital care report, any first aid given prior to your arrival.

Do not use any antidote or any neutralizing agent on chemical burns.

Do not use any antidote or neutralizing agent. Neutralizing agents often react violently with contaminants and may increase the heat of the reaction and induce thermal burns. In some cases, the antidote or neutralizing agent is more damaging to the skin than the contaminant.

With chemical burns, pay particular attention to the patient's eyes. Eyes are very sensitive to chemicals and can easily be damaged, even by weak agents. Prompt treatment of chemical eye injury is critical and can reduce damage and preserve eyesight. Ask the patient about chemical contact with the eyes, eye pain, vision changes, and contact lens use. Examine the eyes for eyelid spasm (**blepharospasm**), conjunctival erythema, discoloration, tearing, and other evidence of burns or irritation.

blepharospasm *twitching of the eyelids.*

Irrigate all alkali burns to the eye for at least 15 minutes.

Irrigate chemical splashes that involve the eye with large volumes of water. Alkali burns are especially damaging and with them you should flush the eye for at least 15 minutes. Irrigate acid burns for at least 5 minutes. Flush splashes of an unknown agent for up to 20 minutes. Do not, however, delay transport while irrigating.

A useful technique for irrigation is to hang a bag of normal saline (lactated Ringer's is an acceptable substitute) and use the flow regulator to control the flow of fluid into the nasal corner of the eye. Turn the patient's head to the side to facilitate drainage and avoid cross-contaminating the other eye with the waste fluid. Be alert for contact lenses in cases where chemicals are splashed into the eyes. Chemicals may become trapped under the lenses, preventing adequate irrigation. Gently remove the lenses, continuing irrigation.

RADIATION BURNS

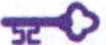

Because radiation can be neither seen nor felt, it can endanger EMS personnel unless proper precautions are taken.

An incident involving potential radiation exposure or burns must be a concern during both dispatch and response phases of the emergency call. Because radiation can neither be seen nor felt, it can endanger EMS personnel unless the hazard has been anticipated and proper precautions taken. If you suspect radiation exposure, do not approach the scene until personnel trained and equipped for radiation emergencies arrive. If the incident occurs at a power generation plant or in an industrial or a medical facility, seek out personnel knowledgeable about the radioactive substance being used. Such persons are always on staff and frequently on-site at these facilities. Stay a good distance from the scene and ensure that bystanders, rescuers, and patients remain remote from the source of the exposure. Remember that potential exposure is reduced by distance and the nature of the materials, like concrete or earth, between you and the radiation source. Be aware of the wind direction and always try to stay upwind from the contamination. Always approach from and remain upwind of the radiation source.

In radiation exposure incidents, ensure that personnel trained in radiation hazards isolate the source, contain it, and test the scene for safety. If this is impossible, move the patient to a site remote from the radioactivity source where you can give care without danger to either yourself or the patient. Plan the removal carefully. Use as much shielding as possible and keep exposure times to a minimum. Remember, the dose of radiation received is related to three primary factors: time, distance, and shielding.

If there is a risk that patients are contaminated, ensure that they are properly decontaminated before you begin assessment and care. If available for this task, use persons knowledgeable in decontamination and monitoring techniques who have the appropriate protective gear. If this is not possible, don goggles, a mask, gloves, and a disposable gown. Direct the evacuation team to place the patients in a decontamination area remote from your vehicle and other personnel and where any contamination can be contained. Have the patients disrobe or carefully disrobe them, rinse them with large volumes of water, then wash them with a soft brush and rinse again. Ordinary dish detergent is effective as a cleansing agent. Scrub, or cut off and then scrub, any areas of body hair.

As in incidents of chemical contamination, save all clothing and decontamination water and dispose of them safely. Perform decontamination before moving the patients to the ambulance.

Carefully document the circumstances of the radioactive exposure. If possible, identify the source and strength of the agent. Determine the patient's proximity to the source during the exposure as well as the length of exposure.

Once properly decontaminated, the radiation injury patient presents no radiation danger to caregivers.

Once he is decontaminated, treat a radiation exposure patient as you would any other patient. Remember that the human body by itself cannot be a source of ionizing radiation, so the decontaminated patient poses no threat to you or your crew. Also remember, however, that any contaminated material remaining on the patient or any contamination transferred to you does provide a source of radiation exposure and may contaminate you and your vehicle.

The actual assessment of a patient exposed to radiation is quite simple and usually reveals minimal signs or symptoms of injury. Only extreme exposures result in the classical presentation of nausea, vomiting, and malaise. Burns are rare, although they may occur if the exposure is extremely intense. Even though a patient seems well, the delayed consequences of high-dose radiation exposure can be devastating. If you note any early patient complaints, record the findings in the patient's own words and include the time the complaint first was made. This information is helpful in determining the patient's degree of radiation exposure (Table 21–4).

Treat the symptoms of the radiation injury patient, make the patient as comfortable as possible, and offer psychological support. Cover any burns with sterile dressing and, if general symptoms are noticeable, provide oxygen and initiate an IV. Maintain the patient's body temperature and provide transport to the emergency department.

To summarize: If you find yourself involved in a radioactive emergency, take the following precautionary steps:

★ Park the rescue vehicle upwind to minimize contamination.

★ Look for signs of radiation exposure. Radioactive packages are marked by clearly identifiable color-coded labels (Figure 21-22 ■).

Table 21–4 Dose-Effect Relationships to Ionizing Radiation

Whole Body Exposure Dose (RAD)	Effect
5–25	Asymptomatic. Blood studies are normal.
50–75	Asymptomatic. Minor depressions of white blood cells and platelets in a few patients.
75–125	May produce anorexia, nausea, vomiting, and fatigue in approximately 10–20 percent of patients within 2 days.
125–200	Possible nausea and vomiting. Diarrhea, anxiety, tachycardia. Fatal to less than 5 percent of patients.
200–600	Nausea and vomiting. Diarrhea in the first several hours. Weakness, fatigue. Fatal to approximately 50 percent of patients within 6 weeks without prompt medical attention.
600–1,000	"Burning sensation" within minutes. Nausea and vomiting within 10 minutes. Confusion, ataxia, and collapse within 1 hour. Watery diarrhea within 1 to 2 hours. Fatal to 100 percent within short time without prompt medical attention.
Localized Exposure Dose (RAD)	**Effect**
50	Asymptomatic
500	Asymptomatic (usually). May have risk of altered function of exposed area.
2,500	Atrophy, vascular lesion, and altered pigmentation.
5,000	Chronic ulcer, risk of carcinogenesis.
50,000	Permanent destruction of exposed tissue.

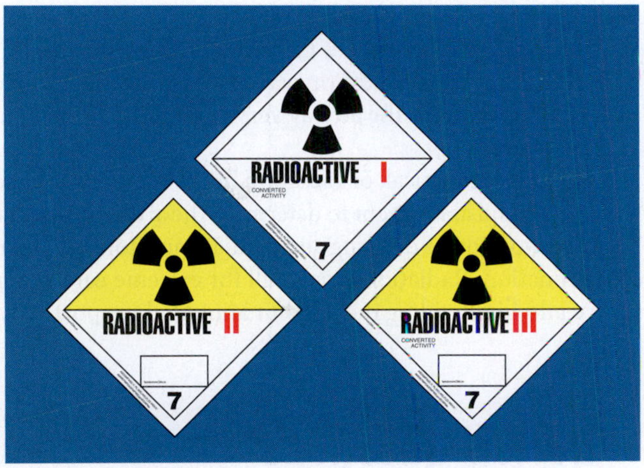

Figure 21-22 Warning labels may indicate the presence of radioactive materials.

- ★ If you are trained and equipped with appropriate gear, consider using portable instruments to measure the level of radioactivity. If dose estimates are significant, rotate rescue personnel.
- ★ Apply normal principles of emergency care, for example, ABCs, shock management, and trauma care.
- ★ Once they are decontaminated as necessary, externally radiated patients pose little danger to rescue personnel. Initiate normal care procedures for injuries other than radiation.
- ★ Internally contaminated patients (who have ingested or inhaled radioactive particles) pose little danger to rescue personnel. Normal care procedures should be undertaken. Collect body wastes. If assisted ventilation is required, use a bag-valve-mask unit or demand valve. If radioactive particles are inhaled, swab the nasal passages and save the swabs.
- ★ Externally contaminated patients (liquids, dirt, smoke) require decontamination. Following decontamination, initiate normal emergency care procedures. Decontamination of paramedic personnel and equipment is required after the call is completed.
- ★ Patients with open, contaminated wounds require normal emergency care procedures. Avoid cross-contamination of wounds.

REASSESSMENT

Monitor patients with inhalation, chemical, and electrical burns and radiation exposure for signs of increasing complications associated with their burn mechanisms. Also monitor blood pressure, pulse, and respirations and note any changes or trends. Perform these evaluations every 15 minutes in stable patients and every 5 minutes in unstable patients.

Summary

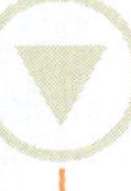

Burn injuries may compromise the skin—the protective envelope that protects and contains the human body. Burn damage to the skin may interfere with its ability to contain water within the body and to prevent damaging agents from entering. For these reasons, assessment and care of these soft-tissue injuries are important.

Assess the burn to determine its depth and the extent of the body surface area it involves. Be sensitive to any respiratory, joint, hand, foot, or circumferential regions affected by the burn.

Give special consideration to pediatric and geriatric burn patients and to burn patients who are also ill or otherwise injured. Consider all these factors in determining the overall severity of a burn. If the patient's condition warrants, institute aggressive care. Anticipate airway compromise and fluid loss. Secure the airway very early in prehospital care. Initiate IV access, and begin fluid administration.

Electrical, chemical, or radiation burns require special care and assessment. An electrical burn requires careful assessment to determine the area and depth of burn involvement and should be followed by wound site dressing and cardiac monitoring. Chemical burns need rapid and effective decontamination. Radiation burns call for extreme care in removing the patient from the radiation source and in providing decontamination and supportive care.

Review Questions

1. During the healing process for burns, scar tissue is laid down and remodeled, and the patient begins to rehabilitate and return to normal function. This is called the:
   a. fluid shift phase.
   b. resolution phase.
   c. emergent phase.
   d. hypermetabolic phase.
2. Chemical burns caused by __________ usually continue to destroy cell membranes through liquefaction necrosis, allowing them to penetrate underlying tissue and causing deeper burns.
   a. acids
   b. alkalis
   c. electricity
   d. coagulation
3. The type of radiation that can travel through 6 to 10 feet of air, penetrate a few layers of clothing, and cause both external and internal injuries is:
   a. gamma radiation.
   b. alpha radiation.
   c. beta radiation.
   d. neutron radiation.
4. Airway edema is a major concern when dealing with inhalation injuries. To provide the best protection and prevent patient deterioration, it is important to initiate early:
   a. cardiac monitoring.
   b. endotracheal intubation.
   c. intravenous cannulation.
   d. rapid fluid replacement.
5. To reduce the patient's exposure to infectious pathogens, the paramedic must carefully:
   a. employ body substance isolation.
   b. use sterile dressings and clean equipment.
   c. avoid gross contamination of the burn.
   d. all of the above
6. For pediatric or geriatric patients and patients suffering from other trauma or medical conditions, always:
   a. increase burn severity one level.
   b. initiate immediate intubation.
   c. reduce administered fluids.
   d. initiate immediate transport.

7. Your patient is experiencing airway compromise due to an inhalation injury. You elect to perform rapid-sequence intubation to protect the patient's airway. Which of the following paralytics should you use with caution, if at all, because it may worsen hyperkalemia?
   a. morphine
   b. vecuronium
   c. succinylcholine
   d. pancuronium
8. Which of the following burns would be classified as a moderate burn?
   a. full-thickness burns < 2 percent body surface area
   b. superficial burns < 50 percent body surface area
   c. partial-thickness burns > 30 percent body surface area
   d. partial-thickness burns < 30 percent body surface area
9. Fluid replacement is indicated in the care of patients with moderate to severe burns greater than 15 to 20% total body surface area. The Parkland formula sets up a calculation for determining the amount of fluid to infuse over 24 hours. Which of the following accurately depicts the Parkland formula?
   a. 4 mL × patient weight in kilograms × BSA involved
   b. 4 mL × patient weight in pounds × BSA involved
   c. 6 mL × patient weight in kilograms × BSA involved
   d. 8 mL × patient weight in pounds × BSA involved
10. In general, how should dry lime be removed from the skin?
    a. Flush with vinegar, then with water.
    b. Brush dry lime away and then flush with water.
    c. Apply baking soda and a sterile dressing.
    d. Cover the wound as is, flush with water, and transport.
11. Your 45-year-old male patient was working on his roof, came into contact with power lines, and has experienced possible electrocution. The patient has an irregular pulse of 124 BPM and his respiratory rate is 22 and irregular. The patient's blood pressure is 106/76. You note both entrance and exit wounds. You immediately manage the airway and decide to start an IV. You realize that you should administer an initial fluid bolus of:
    a. 20 mL/kg.
    b. 10 mL/kg.
    c. 10 mg/kg.
    d. 20 mg/kg.
12. The burn patient's injured tissue will swell. Therefore, with this knowledge, you realize that it is important to:
    a. start IV therapy early.
    b. remove restrictive jewelry.
    c. administer high-flow, high-concentration oxygen.
    d. cover the injury with a burn sheet.
13. All of the following are basic principles that allow rescue personnel and patients to limit exposure to ionizing radiation *except:*
    a. time.
    b. distance.
    c. weight.
    d. shielding.

See Answers to Review Questions at the back of this book.

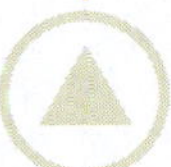

Chapter

22

Musculoskeletal Trauma

Objectives

After reading this chapter, you should be able to:

1. Describe the incidence, morbidity, and mortality of musculoskeletal injuries. (p. 925)
2. Discuss the anatomy and physiology of the muscular and skeletal systems. (see Chapter 3)
3. Predict injuries based on the mechanism of injury, including: (pp. 926–931, 933)
   - ★ Direct
   - ★ Indirect
   - ★ Pathologic
4. Discuss the types of musculoskeletal injuries, including:
   - ★ Fractures (open and closed) (pp. 928–931)
   - ★ Dislocations/fractures (pp. 927–928)
   - ★ Sprains (p. 928)
   - ★ Strains (p. 927)
5. Describe the six "Ps" of musculoskeletal injury assessment. (p. 935)
6. List the primary signs and symptoms of extremity trauma. (pp. 933–937)
7. List other signs and symptoms that can indicate less obvious extremity injury. (pp. 935–937)
8. Discuss the need for assessment of pulses, motor function, and sensation before and after splinting. (p. 940)
9. Identify the circumstances requiring rapid intervention and transport when dealing with musculoskeletal injuries. (pp. 933–934)
10. Discuss the general guidelines for splinting. (pp. 938–942)
11. Explain the benefits of the application of cold and heat for musculoskeletal injuries. (p. 944–945)
12. Describe age-associated changes in the bones. (p. 931)
13. Discuss the pathophysiology, assessment findings, and management of open and closed fractures. (pp. 928–931, 933–948)
14. Discuss the relationship between the volume of hemorrhage and open or closed fractures. (pp. 934, 945–946)

15. Discuss the indications and contraindications for use of the pneumatic antishock garment (PASG) in the management of fractures. (pp. 945–946)
16. Describe the special considerations involved in femur fracture management. (pp. 945–947)
17. Discuss the pathophysiology, assessment findings, and management of dislocations. (pp. 928, 948–949, 949–950, 951)
18. Discuss the out-of-hospital management of dislocations/fractures, including splinting and realignment. (pp. 942–952)
19. Explain the importance of manipulating a knee dislocation/fracture with an absent distal pulse. (pp. 949–950)
20. Describe the procedure for reduction of a shoulder, finger, or ankle dislocation/fracture. (pp. 950, 951, 952)
21. Discuss the pathophysiology, assessment findings, and management of sprains, strains, and tendon injuries. (pp. 927, 928, 952)
22. Differentiate among musculoskeletal injuries based on the assessment findings and history. (pp. 933–938)
23. Given several preprogrammed and moulaged musculoskeletal trauma patients, provide the appropriate scene size-up, primary assessment, secondary assessment (rapid trauma or focused physical exam, detailed exam), and reassessments and provide appropriate patient care and transportation. (pp. 925–955)

Key Terms

arthritis, p. 932
bursitis, p. 932
callus, p. 932
closed fracture, p. 929
comminuted fracture, p. 930
cramping, p. 927
dislocation, p. 928
epiphyseal fracture, p. 931
fatigue, p. 927
fatigue fracture, p. 930
gout, p. 933
greenstick fracture, p. 931
hairline fracture, p. 930
impacted fracture, p. 930
Lyme disease, p. 933
oblique fracture, p. 930
open fracture, p. 929
osteoarthritis, p. 932
osteoporosis, p. 931
reduction, p. 944
rheumatoid arthritis, p. 933
spasm, p. 927
spiral fracture, p. 930
sprain, p. 928
strain, p. 927
subluxation, p. 928
tendonitis, p. 932
transverse fracture, p. 930

INTRODUCTION

In trauma, incidences of musculoskeletal injury are second in frequency only to soft-tissue injuries. They usually result from application of significant direct or transmitted blunt kinetic forces. Skeletal or muscular injuries may also occasionally result from penetrating mechanisms of injury. Millions of Americans sustain musculoskeletal injuries each year from a variety of sources including sports injuries, motor vehicle crashes, falls, and acts of violence. These incidents can cause a variety of injuries to the body's bones, cartilage, ligaments, muscles, or tendons. While injuries to the upper extremities can be painful and sometimes debilitating, they rarely threaten life. Lower extremity injuries, however, are generally associated with a greater magnitude of force and greater secondary blood loss and, thus, more often constitute threats to life or limb. In addition, the same forces responsible for a musculoskeletal injury may damage the spine, internal organs, nerves, and blood vessels, causing serious problems throughout the body. In fact, most patients (up to 80 percent) who suffer multisystem trauma experience significant musculoskeletal injuries.

Incidences of musculoskeletal injury are second in frequency only to soft-tissue injuries in trauma.

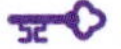

Up to 80 percent of patients who suffer multisystem trauma experience significant musculoskeletal injuries.

PREVENTION STRATEGIES

Stopping injury before it occurs—injury prevention—is the optimal way of dealing with musculoskeletal injuries. Strategies for preventing musculoskeletal injuries include application of modern vehicle and highway designs and safe driving practices, including the use of restraint systems. Auto crashes are the greatest single cause of musculoskeletal injuries, and improved vehicle safety has done much to reduce injury incidence and severity. Workplace safety standards developed by the National Institutes of Safety and Health (NIOSH) and enforced by the Occupational Safety and Health Administration (OSHA) have done much to reduce on-the-job injuries. These standards include criteria for proper footwear, scaffolding, fall protection devices, and the like. Sports injuries, which most commonly affect the musculature, joints, and long bones, account for a significant number of traumas. While protective gear, improved equipment design, and better conditioning of athletes has reduced injuries, the very nature of contact sports means that these activities remain a significant cause of injury. Household accidents and falls also account for many musculoskeletal injuries, and use of good safety practices—for example, proper footwear, well-designed railings, proper use of stepladders—can reduce injury incidence at home.

PATHOPHYSIOLOGY OF THE MUSCULOSKELETAL SYSTEM

Bone is alive and requires a constant supply of oxygenated circulation.

The musculoskeletal injury process is a complicated one, resulting in much more damage than the disruption of an inert structural element of the body. Bone is alive and requires a continuous supply of oxygenated circulation. Bone lies deep within muscle tissue, and major nerves and blood vessels parallel it as they travel to the distal extremity. At points of articulation, there is a complex arrangement of ligaments, cartilage, and synovial fluid that holds the joint together while permitting a wide range of movement. Finally, the muscles attach and direct skeletal movement through the collections of fibers, fasciculi, and muscle bodies connected to the skeletal system by tendons. This complex arrangement of connective, skeletal, vascular, nervous, and muscular tissue is endangered whenever significant kinetic forces are applied to the extremities. If the forces are severe enough, they are likely to cause muscular, joint, or skeletal injury.

Review

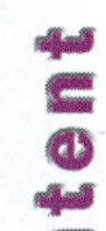

Types of Muscular Injuries

- Contusion
- Compartment syndrome
- Penetrating injury
- Muscle fatigue
- Muscle cramp
- Muscle spasm
- Muscle strain

MUSCULAR INJURY

Muscular injuries may result from direct blunt or penetrating trauma, overexertion, or problems with oxygen supply during exertion. These injuries include contusions, compartment syndrome, penetrating injuries, fatigue, sprains, cramps, spasms, and strains. Muscular problems usually do not contribute significantly to hypovolemia and shock, with the exceptions of severe contusions with large associated hematomas and penetrating injuries with extensive hemorrhage.

Contusion

Severe trauma frequently crushes muscles between a blunt force and the skeletal structure beneath. This damages both the muscle cells and the blood vessels that supply them. Small blood vessels rupture, leaking blood into the interstitial spaces and causing pain, erythema, and then ecchymosis. Blood in the interstitial spaces and muscle cell damage set off the body's inflammatory response. Capillary beds engorge with blood, and fluid shifts to the interstitial space, leading to tissue edema. The injury may also cause blood to pool beneath tissue layers in a hematoma. In more massive body muscles, like those of the thigh, buttocks, calf, or arm, large volumes of blood may accumulate, contributing significantly to hypovolemia. A large hematoma or significant muscular edema will increase the diameter of the injured limb, especially as compared to the opposing uninjured limb. For the most part, however, signs of muscle injury remain hidden beneath the skin.

Compartment Syndrome

The muscular configuration of the extremities, and especially the leg and forearm, are prone to a specific injury called compartment syndrome. The muscle bodies of these regions are contained in strong inelastic envelopes of fascia. When injury damages the soft tissue within the compartment, localized swelling results. Contained by the fascia, this swelling increases the pressure within the compartment, reducing capillary blood flow to the muscle and nerve tissues. The reduced capillary flow causes the release of histamine, which increases capillary permeability and worsens the swelling and pressure. As the pressure builds, the blood flow to the tissues all but stops. However, the pressure necessary to halt capillary blood flow is much less than that needed to stop arterial blood flow to the distal extremity. The patient still has a distal pulse, capillary refill, and venous return from the distal limb. The leg is the most common location associated with this syndrome, although it has also been reported with arm, thigh and hand injuries.

The patient with compartment syndrome most commonly complains of a deep and burning pain that appears out of proportion to the apparent injury. The pain is not reduced by positioning. An increase in pain when you (not your patient) move the extremity and stretch the muscles involved is a related finding. The patient may also report pain when he flexes the foot. Distal pulses and capillary refill may be normal, although the patient may report increased distal sensitivity or numbness due to nerve compression and injury.

Penetrating Injury

Deep lacerations may penetrate skin and subcutaneous tissues, thus affecting muscle masses and tendons below. Massive wounds involving a large percentage of a muscle body or those injuring or severing a tendon may reduce the distal limb's strength or render muscular control ineffective. When a tendon or muscle is cut, contraction of the opposing muscle moves the limb while the injured muscle/tendon is unable to return the limb toward the neutral position. Such injuries call for surgical intervention to identify and rejoin the damaged tendon or muscle body. These wounds may also introduce infectious agents, damage muscle tissue, and affect the muscle's blood supply. The resulting infection, ischemia, or a combination of the two may result in further tissue injury and poor healing.

Fatigue

fatigue *condition in which a muscle's ability to respond to stimulation is lost or reduced through overactivity.*

Muscle **fatigue** occurs as the muscles reach their limit of performance. Exercise draws down the muscle's oxygen and energy reserves and causes accumulation of metabolic by-products. The cell environment becomes hypoxic, toxic, and energy deprived. Fewer and fewer muscle fibers are able to contract. The strength of the muscle mass diminishes, and further exertion becomes painful. Until adequate circulation restores oxygen and the muscle cells can replenish energy sources, the muscle fibers and muscle body remain weakened.

Muscle Cramp

cramping *muscle pain resulting from overactivity, lack of oxygen, and accumulation of waste products.*

Cramping is not really an injury, but a painful spasm of the muscle tissue. Muscle pain results when exercise consumes the available oxygen and energy sources and the circulatory system fails to remove metabolic waste products. The pain begins during or immediately after vigorous exercise or after the limb has been left in an unusual position for a period of time (obstructing circulatory flow). Cramping usually presents with a continuous muscle contraction (spasm). Changing the limb's position or massaging it may help return the circulation and reduce the pain. Once rest and adequate circulation restore the metabolic balance, the pain of muscle cramp usually subsides.

Muscle Spasm

spasm *intermittent or continuous contraction of a muscle.*

In muscle **spasm,** the affected muscle goes into an intermittent (clonic) or continuous (tonic) contraction. The spasm may be firm enough to feel like the deformity associated with a fracture and can confound assessment. (The extreme of muscle spasm is rigor mortis, an anoxic, rigid, whole-body muscle spasm that occurs after death.) As with the cramp, the spasm usually subsides uneventfully with rest.

Strain

strain *injury resulting from overstretching of muscle fibers.*

A **strain** occurs when muscle fibers are overstretched by forces that exceed the strength of the fibers. The muscle fibers then stretch and tear, causing pain that increases with any use of the muscle. The injury may occur with extreme muscle stress, as during heavy lifting or sprinting, or at times of fatigue, when only a limited number of fibers are in contraction. With a strain, the fibers are damaged without internal bleeding, edema, or discoloration. The site of injury is generally painful to palpation, and patients normally report pain that limits use of the affected muscle.

Content Review

Types of Joint Injury

- Sprain
- Subluxation
- Dislocation

JOINT INJURY

Joint injuries include sprains, subluxations, and dislocations. The following sections detail the pathologies behind each of these injuries.

Sprain

sprain *tearing of a joint capsule's connective tissues.*

A **sprain** is a tearing of a joint capsule's connective tissues, specifically a ligament or ligaments. This injury causes acute pain at its site, followed shortly by inflammation and swelling. Ecchymotic discoloration occurs over time, but not usually during prehospital care. The tearing of ligaments weakens the joint. Continued use of the joint may lead to its complete failure. Sprains are classified, or graded, according to their severity, using the following criteria:

- *Grade I.* Minor and incomplete tear. The ligament is painful, and swelling is usually minimal. The joint is stable.
- *Grade II.* Significant but incomplete tear. Swelling and pain range from moderate to severe. The joint is intact but unstable.
- *Grade III.* Complete tear of the ligament. Due to severe pain and spasm, the sprain may present as a fracture. The joint is unstable.

Content Review

Types of Sprains

- Grade I—minor and incomplete capsule tear; painful, but minimal swelling; joint stable.
- Grade II—significant but incomplete tear; moderate to severe pain, swelling; joint intact but unstable.
- Grade III—complete tear; severe pain and spasm; joint unstable.

Subluxation

subluxation *partial displacement of a bone end from its position in a joint capsule.*

A **subluxation** is a partial displacement of a bone end from its position within a joint capsule. It occurs as the joint separates under stress, stretching the ligaments. The subluxation differs from the sprain in that it more significantly reduces the joint's integrity. The injured joint is painful and swells quickly, its range of motion is limited, and the joint is unstable. Hyperflexion, hyperextension, lateral rotation beyond the normal range of motion, or application of extreme axial force are common causes of subluxations.

Dislocation

dislocation *complete displacement of a bone end from its position in a joint capsule.*

A **dislocation** is a complete displacement of bone ends from their normal joint position (Figure 22-1 ■). The joint then fixes in an abnormal position with noticeable deformity. The site is painful, swollen, and immobile. This type of injury carries with it the danger of entrapping, compressing, or tearing blood vessels and nerves. Dislocation occurs when the joint moves beyond its normal range of motion with great force. By its nature, a dislocation has serious associated ligament damage and may involve injury to the joint capsule and articular cartilage.

BONE INJURY

The fracture is an involved process that ultimately disrupts the continuity of the bone. When extreme compressional forces or significant lateral forces exceed the tensile strength of a bone, the bone fractures.

A fracture may be caused by direct injury—for example, an auto bumper impacts a patient's femur or a high-powered rifle bullet slams into a patient's thigh and, then, femur. The cause of

■ **Figure 22-1** Knee dislocation. *(Edward T. Dickinson, MD)*

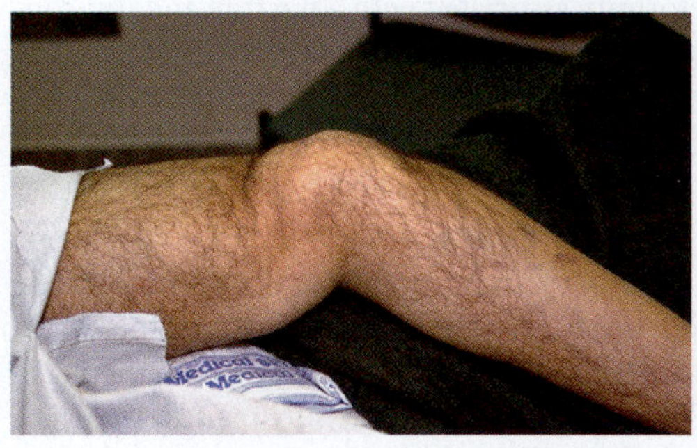

a. Presentation of a knee dislocation.

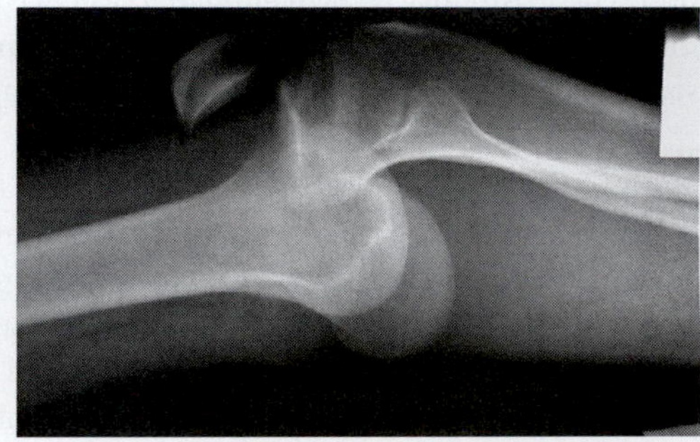

b. X-ray of the dislocation.

the fracture may also be indirect. This might occur when a bike rider is thrown over the handlebars and braces the fall with an outstretched upper extremity. In this case, the energy of impact is transmitted from the hand to the wrist, to the forearm, to the arm, to the shoulder, to the clavicle. The transmitted force fractures the clavicle and may cause internal injury to blood vessels and the upper reaches of the lung. For this reason, always analyze the mechanism of injury carefully, recognizing that kinetic forces may be transmitted and cause injury far from the point of impact. Remember, 80 percent of multisystem trauma cases have associated serious musculoskeletal injury.

Recognize that kinetic forces may be transmitted through the skeletal system and cause injury remote from the impact site.

Review

Content

Types of Fractures

- Open
- Closed
- Hairline
- Impacted
- Transverse
- Oblique
- Comminuted
- Spiral
- Greenstick
- Epiphyseal

As kinetic energy is transmitted to the bone and the bone fractures, the collagen, osteocytes, salt crystals, blood vessels, nerves, and medullary canal of the bone, as well as its periosteum and endosteum (the inner lining of the medullary canal), are disrupted. If the broken bone ends displace, they may further injure surrounding muscles, tendons, ligaments, veins, and arteries. The result is a serious insult to the limb structure.

Vascular damage may restrict blood flow to the distal limb, increasing capillary refill time, diminishing pulse strength and limb temperature, and causing discoloration and paresthesia (a "pins-and-needles" sensation). Nerve injury may result in distal paresthesia, anesthesia (loss of sensation), paresis (weakness), and paralysis (loss of muscle control). Muscle or tendon damage may interfere with the victim's ability to move the limb. If muscle tissue is badly damaged where fasciae firmly contain it, compartment syndrome may develop.

If the bone does not seriously displace and the forces causing fracture do not penetrate, the surrounding skin remains intact and the resulting injury is termed a **closed fracture.** If the sharp bone ends displaced by the forces causing the fracture or other subsequent motion of the limb lacerate through the muscle, subcutaneous tissue, and skin, the result is termed an **open fracture** (Figure 22-2 ■). An open fracture may also occur when any object such as a bullet travels through the limb and fractures the bone. Open fractures carry the risk of associated infection within the disrupted soft, bone, and medullary tissues. Such an infection may seriously reduce the bone's ability to heal. Where bones are located very close to the skin, as with the tibia (the shin), an open fracture can occur with relatively minimal bone displacement.

closed fracture *a broken bone in which the bone ends or the forces that caused the fracture do not penetrate the skin.*

open fracture *a broken bone in which the bone ends or the forces that caused the fracture penetrate the surrounding skin.*

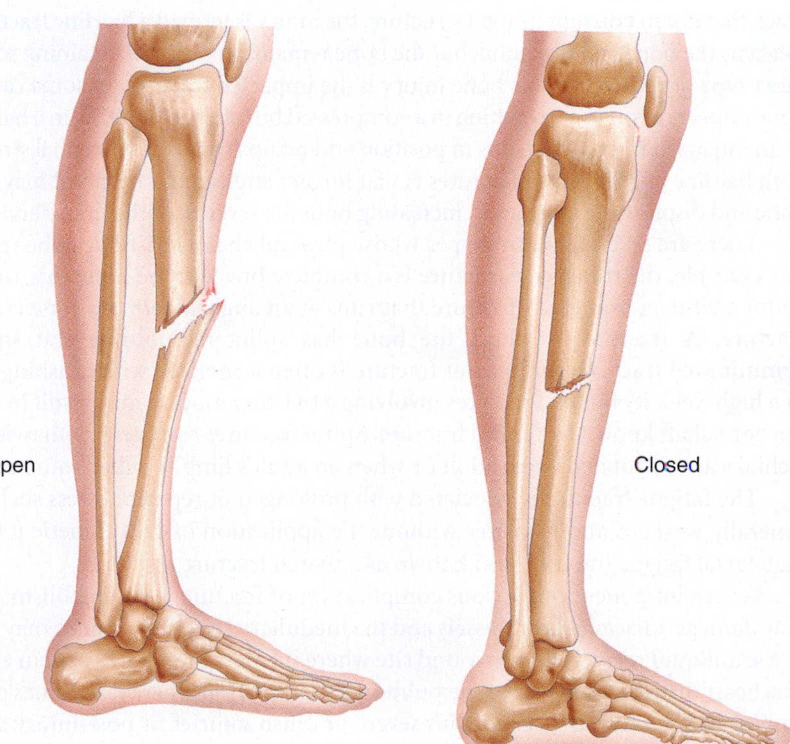

■ Figure 22-2 Open and closed fractures.

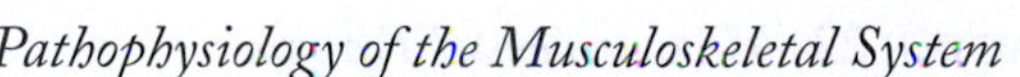

■ **Figure 22-3** Types of fractures.

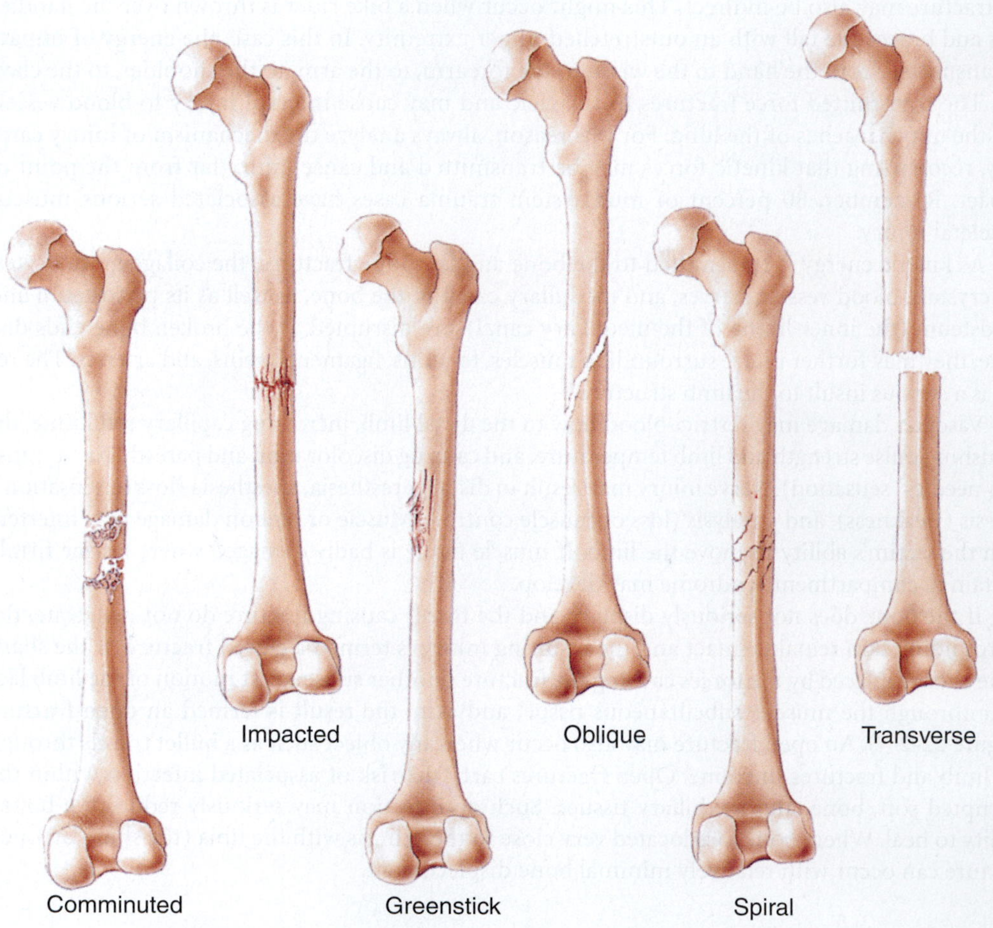

hairline fracture *small crack in a bone that does not disrupt its total structure.*

impacted fracture *break in a bone in which the bone is compressed on itself.*

transverse fracture *a break that runs across a bone perpendicular to the bone's orientation.*

oblique fracture *break in a bone running across it at an angle other than 90 degrees.*

comminuted fracture *fracture in which a bone is broken into several pieces.*

spiral fracture *a curving break in a bone as may be caused by rotational forces.*

fatigue fracture *break in a bone associated with prolonged or repeated stress.*

Surprisingly, some fractures may be relatively stable (Figure 22-3 ■). When the bone suffers a small crack that doesn't disrupt its total structure, the injury is termed a **hairline fracture.** This type of injury weakens the bone and is painful, but the bone remains in position, retaining some of its strength. Another type of relatively stable bone injury is the **impacted fracture.** In some cases of compression, the bone impacts upon itself, resulting in a compressed but aligned bone. As in a hairline fracture, the bone in an impacted fracture remains in position and retains some of its original strength. The danger with both hairline and impacted fractures is that further stress and movement may fracture the remaining bone and displace the bone ends, increasing both the severity of the injury and its healing time.

There are several fracture types whose physical characteristics can be revealed only by X-rays. For example, the **transverse fracture** is a complete break in the bone that runs straight across it at about a 90-degree angle. A fracture that runs at an angle across the bone is considered an **oblique fracture.** A fracture in which the bone has splintered into several smaller fragments is a **comminuted fracture;** this type of fracture is often associated with crushing injuries or the impact of a high-velocity bullet. Fractures involving a twisting motion may result in a curved break around the bone shaft known as a **spiral fracture.** Spiral fractures can occur with twisting motions, as when a child's arm is rotated by an adult or when an adult's limb is pulled into machinery like an auger.

The **fatigue fracture** is associated with prolonged or repeated stress such as walking. The bone generally weakens and fractures without the application of great kinetic force. An example is the metatarsal fatigue fracture, also known as a march fracture.

A very infrequent but serious complication of fracture is fat embolism. The bone's disruption may damage adjacent blood vessels and the medullary canal. The injury may then release fat, stored in a semiliquid form, into the wound site where it enters the venous system and travels to the heart. The heart distributes the fat to the pulmonary circulation where it becomes pulmonary emboli. Fat embolism is usually associated with severe or crush injuries or post-injury manipulation of larger long-bone fractures.

Pediatric Considerations

The bones of infants, young children, and, to a degree, older children contain a greater percentage of cartilage than those of adults and are still growing from the epiphyseal plate. Pediatric patients thus often sustain different types of fractures than adults do.

The flexible nature of pediatric bones is responsible for the **greenstick fracture,** a type of partial fracture. The injury disrupts only one side of the long bone and remains angulated, resisting alignment due to the disrupted bone fibers on the fracture side. During the bone repair process, the injured side experiences more rapid growth than the other side. This results in increasing angulation of the bone as it heals. Surgeons often complete a greenstick fracture by breaking the bone fully, thereby ensuring proper healing.

greenstick fracture *partial fracture of a child's bone.*

A child's bone grows at the epiphyseal plate, which forms a weak spot in the long bone. In pediatric trauma, this is a common site of the long-bone disruption called an **epiphyseal fracture.** If the growth plate is disrupted, the disruption may lead to a reduction or halt in bone growth, a condition most commonly involving the proximal tibia.

epiphyseal fracture *disruption in the epiphyseal plate of a child's bone.*

Geriatric Considerations

The aging process causes several changes to the musculoskeletal system. A gradual, progressive decrease in bone mass and collagen structure begins at about the age of 40 and results in bones that are less flexible, more brittle, and more easily fractured. The bones also heal more slowly. The aging adult also loses some muscle strength and coordination, increasing the likelihood of skeletal injury. Fractures of the lumbar spine and femoral neck occur because of stress, often without a history of significant trauma.

Another age-related and more significant problem secondary to poor bone remodeling is called **osteoporosis.** Osteoporosis is an accelerated degeneration of bone tissue due to loss of bone minerals, principally calcium. It typically affects women more than men and becomes most serious after menopause. The condition leads to increases in bone structure degeneration, spinal curvature, and incidences of fractures.

osteoporosis *weakening of bone tissue due to loss of essential minerals, especially calcium.*

Pathological Fractures

Pathological fractures result from disease pathologies that affect bone development or maintenance. Such problems may be caused by tumors of the bone, periosteum, or articular cartilage or by diseases that release agents that increase osteoclast activity and osteoporosis. Other diseases and infections can have the same impact on bone tissue and result in fracture, especially in older patients. Radiation treatment may also kill bone cells, resulting in localized bone degeneration, weakened bones, and fractures. These fractures are not likely to heal well, if they heal at all. Providers should be suspicious of pathological fractures in patients with a PMH of cancer, or low-energy mechanisms that cause fractures in young, otherwise healthy patients or non-osteoporitic elderly patients.

GENERAL CONSIDERATIONS WITH MUSCULOSKELETAL INJURIES

The potential effects of trauma can be better anticipated when the skeletal structure and the musculature are examined together. It is important to note that long bones are smallest through the diaphysis and largest at the epiphyseal area, or joint. However, the external extremity diameter is greatest surrounding the midshaft due to the placement of skeletal muscle. This anatomical relationship is significant when looking at the potential for nervous or vascular injury.

Since there is limited soft tissue surrounding joints, joint fractures, dislocations, and—to a lesser degree—subluxations and sprains may cause severe problems beyond the direct injury. Any swelling, deformity, or displacement may compromise the nerve and vascular supply to the distal extremity. Fractures near a joint are more likely to compress or sever blood vessels or nerves. With shaft fractures, neurovascular injury is less likely, although manipulation of the fracture site or gross deformity may still endanger vessels and nerves running along the bone.

Because there is limited soft tissue surrounding joints, injuries there may cause severe problems beyond the direct injury because blood vessels and nerves may be affected.

Areas around the joints are further endangered because blood vessels supplying the epiphysis enter the long bone through the diaphysis. If a fracture close to the epiphysis displaces the bone ends, it may compromise this blood supply with devastating results. The distal bone tissue may die without adequate circulation, destroying the joint and its function.

Once injury occurs, the stability of the extremity is reduced. Any additional movement can increase pain, damage to soft tissues, and the possibility of vascular or nerve involvement. Even slight manipulation can cause internal trauma. For example, a fractured femur has bone ends that are about the size of a broken broom handle. If, during extrication, splinting, and patient transport, the bone ends move about within the soft tissue, the resulting damage may be much more severe than that which initially occurred with the fracture. Manipulation of the injury site may also increase the likelihood of introducing bone fragments or fat emboli into the venous system, causing pulmonary embolism.

Another complication associated with long-bone fracture is muscle spasm induced by pain. In a long-bone fracture, pain causes the surrounding muscles to contract. This contraction forces the broken bone ends to override the fracture site. The result, in the case of the femur, is two broom-handle-sized bones driven into the muscles of the thigh, causing a cycle of more pain, more spasm, and more damage.

BONE REPAIR CYCLE

The bone repair cycle is a complex process that results in almost complete healing. When trauma fractures a bone, the periosteum tears, as do local blood vessels, soft tissues, and the endosteum. Blood fills the injured area and congeals, establishing a red blood cell and collagen clot. This hemorrhagic clot is not very stable, but does begin the bone repair process. Osteocytes from the bone ends begin to multiply rapidly and produce osteoblasts. These osteoblasts lay down salt crystals within the collagen clot fibers. This establishes lengthening and widening regions of skeletal tissue from each disrupted bone end. Over time, the two growing ends join and form a large knob of cancellous bone, called the **callus,** that encapsulates the fracture site.

callus *thickened area that forms at the site of a fracture as part of the repair process.*

As the process continues, the deposition of salts and the increasing collagen fiber matrix strengthen the callus and stabilize the bone to near-normal strength. Then osteoclasts dissolve salt crystals and collagen in areas where stress is minimal, while osteoblasts lay down new collagen and salts in high-stress areas. Through this process, the bone is remodeled until it looks very much like it did before the injury. If a fracture occurs when a patient is young and the bone ends are well aligned, there may be little evidence to suggest an injury ever occurred. If the bone ends are misaligned or if the bone experiences stress, infection, or movement before it has a chance to heal properly, the injury site may never return to normal and may leave the person with some disability. Conditions such as smoking, infection, poor health, diabetes, and the use of NSAIDs and immunosuppressive drugs may impair the healing process. In some cases pre-existing conditions may disrupt the bone healing process to the degree that the two broken bone ends do not rejoin (non-union).

INFLAMMATORY AND DEGENERATIVE CONDITIONS

Patients suffering from inflammatory and degenerative conditions may complain of joint pain, tenderness, and fatigue. These patients may also have difficulty walking and moving, may require additional assistance with their normal daily activities, and may be prone to musculoskeletal injuries. Common inflammatory diseases of the musculoskeletal system include bursitis, tendonitis, and arthritis.

bursitis *acute or chronic inflammation of the small synovial sacs.*

tendonitis *inflammation of a tendon and/or its protective sheath.*

arthritis *inflammation of a joint.*

osteoarthritis *inflammation of a joint resulting from wearing of the articular cartilage.*

Bursitis is an acute or chronic inflammation of the bursae, the small synovial sacs that reduce friction and cushion ligaments and tendons from trauma. Bursitis may result from repeated trauma, gout, infection, and, in some cases, unknown etiologies. A patient with bursitis experiences localized pain, swelling, and tenderness at or near a joint. Commonly affected locations include the olecranon (elbow), the area just above the patella, and the shoulder.

Tendonitis is characterized by inflammation of a tendon and its protective sheath and has a presentation similar to that of bursitis. Repeated trauma to a particular muscle group is a common cause of the condition, which usually affects the major tendons of the upper and lower extremity.

Arthritis is literally an inflammation of a joint, frequently due to damage or destruction of the joint's cartilage. Three of the most common types of arthritis are osteoarthritis, rheumatoid arthritis, and gout (more formally known as gouty arthritis).

Osteoarthritis, which is also known as degenerative joint disease, is the most common type of connective tissue disorder. It is characterized by a general degeneration, or "wear-and-tear," of articular cartilage that results in irregular bony overgrowths. Signs and symptoms include pain, stiffness, and diminished movement in the joints. Joint enlargement may be visible, especially in the fingers. Predisposing factors for osteoarthritis include trauma, obesity, and aging.

Rheumatoid arthritis is a chronic, systemic, progressive, and debilitating disease resulting in deterioration of peripheral joint connective tissue. It is characterized by inflammation of the synovial joints, which causes immobility, pain, increased pain on movement, and fatigue. The disease occurs two to three times more frequently in women than in men. In extreme cases, flexion contractures may develop due to muscle spasms induced by inflammation.

rheumatoid arthritis *chronic disease that causes deterioration of peripheral joint connective tissue.*

Gout is an inflammation in joints and connective tissue produced by an accumulation of uric acid crystals. It occurs most frequently in males who often have high concentrations of uric acid in the blood. Uric acid is a metabolism end-product that is not easily dissolved. Signs and symptoms of gout include peripheral joint pain, swelling, and possible deformity. Pseudogout is a gout-like disease caused by the deposition of a crystalline substance similar to uric acid.

gout *inflammation of joints and connective tissue due to buildup of uric acid crystals.*

Lyme disease is a joint inflammation caused by a tick-introduced infectious agent (*Borrelia burgdorferi*). The infection causes small red lesions and the patient develops symptoms such as fever, fatigue, headache, and muscle and joint pain. Untreated, the disease commonly leads to arthritis.

Lyme disease *joint inflammation caused by a tick-introduced infectious agent* (Borrelia burgdorferi).

MUSCULOSKELETAL INJURY ASSESSMENT

With the majority of patients, fractures, dislocations, or muscular injuries only infrequently threaten life or seriously contribute to the development of shock. In most circumstances, a patient with an isolated fracture, dislocation, or trauma to muscular or connective tissue will receive complete assessment and management at the scene.

However, serious musculoskeletal injury is common in a patient who presents with other serious injuries. As you read earlier, energy is often transmitted from the point of impact along the skeletal system to the internal organs. Thus, when you discover a skeletal injury, always look for indications of the severity of the trauma forces and the possibility that the forces also caused internal injuries.

When you discover a skeletal injury, always look for indications of the severity of the trauma forces and the possibility that the forces also caused internal injuries.

As with any trauma patient, the assessment process progresses through the scene size-up, the primary assessment, either the rapid secondary assessment or focused exam and history, the detailed physical examination when appropriate, and serial reassessments. You will usually focus your attention on musculoskeletal injuries during the rapid secondary assessment or focused exam and history and then as part of the detailed physical exam.

SCENE SIZE-UP

Remember to ensure scene safety and don the appropriate personal protective equipment before approaching any scene. Gloves are mandatory when dealing with open musculoskeletal wounds, but those wounds, by themselves, do not usually suggest the need for protective eyewear, mask, or gown. Since most musculoskeletal injuries result from trauma, analyze the mechanism of injury to anticipate the nature and severity of those injuries. Enhance your analysis of the mechanism of injury by talking with the patient, family members, and bystanders to identify what happened and how.

PRIMARY ASSESSMENT

It is imperative that assessment of the trauma patient begin with an evaluation of the patient's mental status and ABCs. During this primary assessment, you must also identify the potential for spinal injury and the need for spinal precautions. Remember, any serious musculoskeletal injury suggests kinetic energy forces sufficient to cause spinal injury, so always take spinal precautions with such an injury. Proceed with the primary assessment and ensure that any life-threatening injuries are addressed before moving on in the assessment process. Never let the gruesome nature of a musculoskeletal injury distract you from performing a proper primary assessment and identifying and caring for life-threatening injuries first (Figure 22-4 ■).

Any serious musculoskeletal injury suggests kinetic energy forces sufficient to cause spinal injury, so always take spinal precautions.

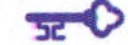

Never let the gruesome nature of a musculoskeletal injury distract you from identifying and caring for more subtle, but life-threatening injuries first.

Patients with musculoskeletal injuries are classified into four categories:

- ★ Patients with life- and limb-threatening injuries
- ★ Patients with life-threatening injuries and minor musculoskeletal injuries

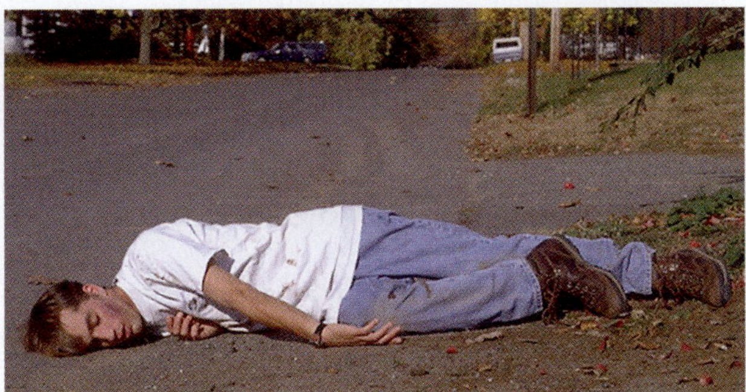

Figure 22-4 As you begin assessment, examine the patient quickly for musculoskeletal injuries, but remember that they are not often life-threatening.

Review

Content

Classification of Patients with Musculoskeletal Injuries

- Life- and limb-threatening injuries
- Life-threatening injuries, minor musculoskeletal injuries
- Non-life-threatening injuries, serious limb-threatening injuries
- Non-life-threatening injuries, isolated minor musculoskeletal injuries.

★ Patients with non-life-threatening injuries but serious limb-threatening musculoskeletal injuries

★ Patients with non-life-threatening injuries and only isolated minor musculoskeletal injuries

Perform a rapid secondary assessment for those patients with possible life- or limb-threatening injuries. A patient without life threat but with serious musculoskeletal injury may receive the rapid secondary assessment or the focused exam and history, depending upon the mechanism of injury and the information you discover during the primary assessment. Provide patients presenting with isolated and simple musculoskeletal injuries with a focused exam and history, though you must remain watchful for any sign or symptom of more serious injury and the need for both a rapid secondary assessment and rapid patient transport to a trauma center.

RAPID SECONDARY ASSESSMENT

The rapid secondary assessment is performed on any patient with any sign, symptom, or mechanism of injury that suggests serious injury. While musculoskeletal injuries do not often cause life-threatening hemorrhage, remember that 80 percent of patients with serious multisystem trauma have associated musculoskeletal injury. When you have evidence of serious musculoskeletal injury, maintain a high index of suspicion for serious internal injury.

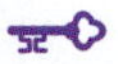

A pelvic fracture may account for hemorrhage of more than 2 liters.

Perform the rapid trauma assessment in a carefully ordered way, progressing through an evaluation of the head, neck, chest, and abdomen, and arriving at the pelvis. Pay particular attention to the possibility of pelvic fracture, because such an injury may account for hemorrhage of more than 2 liters. If no other signs of pelvic fracture exist, check the stability of the pelvic ring by directing firm pressure downward, then inward on the iliac crests, and then directing gentle downward pressure on the symphysis pubis. If the pressure reveals any instability or crepitus or elicits a response of pain from the patient, suspect pelvic fracture. Crepitus is a grating sensation felt as bone ends rub against one another. If you feel crepitus once, presume that bone injury exists and do not attempt to recreate the sensation. Consider the patient a candidate for rapid transport with fluid resuscitation initiated en route.

A femur fracture may account for as much as 1,500 mL of blood loss.

In assessing the thighs, look for signs of tissue swelling and femur fracture. Each femur fracture may account for as much as 1,500 mL of blood loss. Evidence of this loss may be hidden within the tissue and muscle mass of the thigh, so compare one thigh to the other to evaluate swelling. If you find evidence of either pelvic or bilateral femur fracture, apply the pneumatic anti-shock garment (PASG), and inflate all compartments to a pressure that immobilizes the pelvis and the lower extremities. Monitor for the signs that the patient is compensating for blood loss, and consider both rapid transport and fluid resuscitation.

While fractures and muscular injuries of the extremities may not by themselves produce shock, they may significantly contribute to hypovolemia. Consider the effects of these injuries in your decision on whether to provide rapid transport or on-scene care. Further, fractures and dislocations may entrap or damage blood vessels or nerves, thus seriously threatening the future use of a limb. Quickly survey each limb and check the distal pulses, temperature, sensation (if the patient is conscious), motor function, and muscle tone.

Complete the rapid secondary assessment by gathering a patient history and a baseline set of vital signs (which may be done at the same time the physical assessment is being performed). If the rapid trauma assessment reveals a serious threat to life or limb, rapidly transport the patient to the nearest appropriate facility.

FOCUSED HISTORY AND PHYSICAL EXAM

The focused history and physical exam directs your attention to the injuries found or suggested during the primary assessment by the mechanism of injury and the patient's signs and symptoms. This step of the assessment process is performed for patients without life-threatening injuries and permits both assessment and care focused on isolated injuries.

Begin the focused physical exam by observing and inquiring carefully for signs and symptoms of fracture, dislocation, or other musculoskeletal injury in each limb with suspected injury (Figure 22-5 ■). Expose and visualize the entire limb by removing any restrictive clothing or cutting it away carefully. In doing so, avoid manipulation of any potential injury site. Inspect the injury site carefully to locate any deformities (angulation or swelling), discolorations (unlikely in the first minutes after the incident), and indications of soft-tissue wounds that suggest injury beneath. Any unusual limb placement, asymmetry, or inequality in limb length (when compared to the opposing limb) should also arouse suspicion of musculoskeletal injury. Consider the possibility that any open wounds communicate with an associated fracture or dislocation. Observe for any contamination or sign of the bone protruding. Question the patient about pain, pain with attempted movement, discomfort, or unusual feeling or sensation. Also inquire about weakness, paralysis, paresthesia, or anesthesia. It may be helpful to think of the "six Ps" as a way to remember the key elements to be alert for when evaluating an extremity:

- ★ *Pain.* The patient may report this upon palpation (tenderness) or movement.
- ★ *Pallor.* The patient's skin may be pale or flushed, and capillary refill may be delayed.
- ★ *Paralysis.* The patient may have inability or difficulty in moving an extremity.
- ★ *Paresthesia.* The patient may report numbness or tingling in the affected extremity.
- ★ *Pressure.* The patient reports a feeling of tension within the extremity.
- ★ *Pulses.* These may be diminished or absent in the extremity.

If you do not identify a specific injury, palpate the extremity for instability, deformity (swelling or angulation), crepitus, unusual motion (jointlike motion where a joint doesn't exist), muscle tone (normal, flaccid, or spasming), or any regions of unusual warmth or coolness. Palpate the entire anterior and posterior surfaces, then the lateral and medial surfaces. Your assessment must be gentle,

Content Review

The Six Ps in Evaluating Limb Injury

- Pain
- Pallor
- Paralysis
- Paresthesia
- Pressure
- Pulses

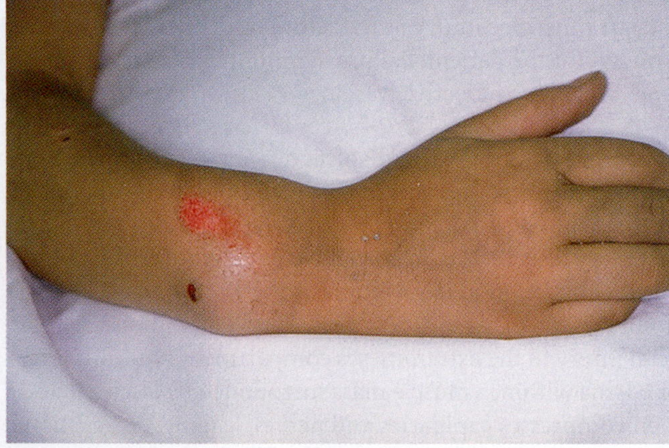

a. A fracture will often present with deformity.

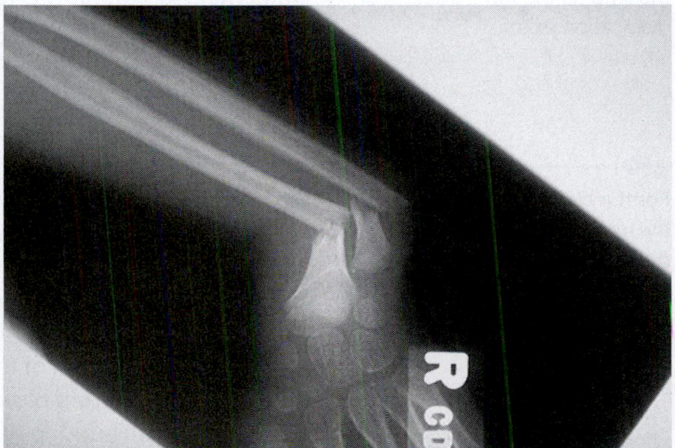

b. An X-ray of the fracture.

■ **Figure 22-5** Presentation of a forearm fracture.

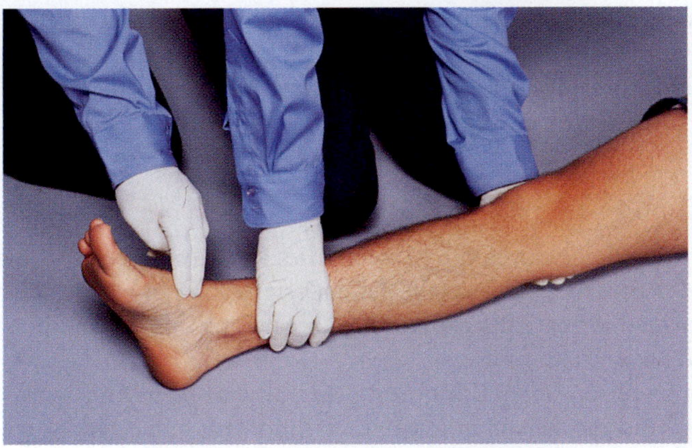

■ **Figure 22-6** Evaluate the distal extremity for pulse, temperature, color, sensation, and capillary refill.

yet complete. Record any abnormal signs. When assessing the feet, carefully evaluate the distal circulation. Assess pulses for presence and relative strength, and then compare bilaterally. Test the skin for humidity and warmth. Suspect circulatory compromise if capillary refill time is prolonged compared to the uninjured limb. Observe the skin for discoloration, noting any erythema, ecchymosis, or any abnormal hue (pale, ashen, or cyanotic). Approximate the level at which any deficit begins, and note any relation to possible extremity injury.

In a conscious and responsive patient, evaluate sensation and muscle strength distal to the injury (Figure 22-6 ■). Check tactile (touch) response by touching or stroking the bottom of the foot with the blunt end of a bandage scissors or other similar instrument. Ask the patient to describe the feeling. If the patient is responsive and if there is no indication that the limb is injured, ask the patient to push down with the balls of both feet (plantar flexion) against your hands. Then ask the patient to pull upward with the top of the feet (dorsiflexion), again against your hands. If you feel any unilateral or bilateral weakness or the patient reports any pain, document the finding on the prehospital care report and look for the cause. Check abnormal sensation and the patient's ability to wiggle the toes or fingers.

Assess for potential upper extremity injury in a manner similar to your assessment of the lower extremity. Expose, observe, question about, and then palpate the limb as previously described. Determine tactile response by using the back of the patient's hand. Test muscular strength by having the patient squeeze two of your fingers. Compare strength and sensation bilaterally, identify any deficit, and attempt to locate the cause. Evaluate the upper extremity and ensure it is uninjured before you use it for blood pressure determination.

When the assessment of an extremity suggests injury, treat the limb as though a fracture or dislocation exists.

When the assessment of an extremity suggests injury, treat the limb as though a fracture or dislocation exists because the only definitive way to rule out these injuries is X-ray examination. Also note that splinting protects strains, sprains, and subluxations as well as fractures and dislocations from further injury. Treating a soft-tissue or muscular injury as a fracture or dislocation produces nothing more harmful than slight discomfort for the patient. Failure to immobilize an injury properly, however, may lead to additional soft, skeletal, connective, vascular, or nervous tissue damage and possibly cause permanent harm.

Form a clear mental picture of the injury site and be able to describe it to the emergency physician.

If possible, find the exact site of injury and determine if it involves a joint area or a long-bone shaft. Form a clear visual image of the injury site in your mind so that you can describe the injury in the patient care report and to the receiving physician. Remember that the splinting device (e.g., a padded board splint for a wrist fracture) may hide the site from view, leaving the attending physician unable to determine what exists beneath it. A good description of the wound may delay the need to remove the splint to view the injury.

One complication of musculoskeletal injury to the extremities is compartment syndrome. This condition results from bleeding into, or edema within, a muscle mass surrounded by fasciae that do not stretch. The buildup of pressure then compresses capillaries and nerves, leading to local tissue ischemia and then necrosis, with some loss of distal sensation. A pulse deficit may be a very late finding in compartment syndrome. Suspect compartment syndrome in any patient who has any paraesthesia, especially in the webs between the medial toes or fingers; who has an extremity injury with a firm mass or increased skin tension at the injury site; or who has pain out of proportion to the nature of the injury or pain that increases when you move the limb (passive stretching). Also suspect compartment syndrome in any unconscious patient with a swollen limb. Compartment syndrome most often occurs in the forearm or leg.

During the physical exam, question the patient about the symptoms of injury. Ensure that your verbal investigation is detailed and complete. Determine the nature and location of pain and tenderness or dysfunction. The patient's description of the fracture or dislocation event may also be helpful. The patient may state that he felt the bone "snap" or the joint "pop out." Determine if the bone snapped, thus causing the fall, or whether the fall caused the fracture. Evaluate for the amount of pain and discomfort the patient is experiencing with the injury. For example, an elderly patient may present with a fractured hip and limited pain, a presentation usually related to a degenerative disease and secondary fracture. These findings may suggest that you adopt a less aggressive approach to care for this patient, focusing upon the patient's comfort rather than upon traction splinting and shock care. Also identify the signs and symptoms of injury as well as pertinent patient allergies, medications, past medical history, last oral intake, and events leading up to the incident.

Compare the findings of your assessment to the index of suspicion for injury you developed during the scene size-up. If you have found less significant injury than you suspected, consider reevaluating the patient to assure that no injury has been overlooked. If you find a more significant injury, suspect other severe injury may have occurred elsewhere and expand your focused exam.

As you conclude the focused history and physical exam, identify all injuries found, prioritize them, and establish the order of care for them. Identify the extent to which each injury may contribute to hemorrhage and shock. Then prioritize the patient for transport. Taking these few moments to sort out what is wrong with the patient and to plan care steps will increase the efficiency of your patient care, reduce on-scene time, and ensure that the patient receives the proper care at the right time.

Content Review

Early Indicators of Compartment Syndrome

- Feelings of tension within limb
- Loss of distal sensation (especially in webs of fingers and toes)
- Complaints of pain
- Condition more severe than mechanism of injury would indicate
- Pain on passive extension of extremity
- Pulse deficit (late sign)

At the conclusion of the rapid secondary assessment or the focused exam, identify all injuries and prioritize them for care.

DETAILED PHYSICAL EXAM

After you have ruled out or addressed potential threats to the patient's life or limbs, attended to any serious problems, and assessed any suspected injuries, you may perform a detailed physical exam. You will most likely perform the detailed physical exam on the patient who is unconscious or has a lowered level of consciousness. The exam may be performed at the scene or, more likely, while en route to the hospital. The detailed physical exam is a search for the signs and symptoms of further injury. It is performed as a head-to-toe evaluation, looking specifically where you have not looked before and with enough care to identify any subtle indications of injury. Be alert for the signs and symptoms of internal or external injury or hemorrhage. Use the same assessment techniques for evaluating musculoskeletal injuries during the detailed physical exam that you employed during the rapid secondary assessment and focused history and physical exam.

REASSESSMENT

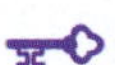

During the reassessment, be sure to ask about the patient's complaints and description of the musculoskeletal injury, because over time, the patient may display more significant and specific symptoms of injury and complain of other injuries masked earlier by the chief complaint.

The reassessment focuses on serial measurement of the patient's vital signs, level of consciousness, and the signs and symptoms of the major trauma affecting the patient. For patients with musculoskeletal injuries, monitor distal sensation and pulses frequently. Remember to ask about the patient's complaints and description of the musculoskeletal injury, watching for any changes in the responses. As time passes and the effects of the "fight-or-flight" response wear off, the patient may display more significant and specific symptoms of injury. The patient may also begin to complain of other injuries masked earlier by the chief complaint and of other major pain or discomfort. If this occurs, provide a focused assessment on the area of complaint and modify your patient priorities as additional injuries are found.

SPORTS INJURY CONSIDERATIONS

Many of the musculoskeletal injuries you attend as an EMT-Paramedic are associated with sports activities. Activities such as football, basketball, soccer, baseball, in-line skating, skiing, snowboarding, bicycling, wrestling, hiking, and rock climbing often lead to injury for participants. When you are called to the scene of a sports injury, assess the mechanism of injury and determine whether there was a major kinetic force involved, a hyperextension or flexion injury, or a fatigue-type injury. Athletic injuries often affect major body joints like the shoulder, elbow, wrist, knee, and ankle. Injuries in these areas are especially troubling for patients because serious ligament damage might preclude future participation in a sport and limit limb usefulness. It is imperative that any potentially significant sports injury be attended to by an emergency department physician. The competitive natures of players, teammates, coaches, and athletic trainers may lead them to downplay injuries in order to keep an injured athlete in competition. Allowing an injured athlete to keep playing, however, places additional stress on the injury and may result in further, and more debilitating, damage.

Any potentially significant sports injury should be attended to by an emergency department physician.

MUSCULOSKELETAL INJURY MANAGEMENT

Management of musculoskeletal injuries is not normally a high priority in trauma patient care. It usually does not occur until after you have completed the primary assessment; stabilized the airway, breathing, and circulation; and finished the rapid secondary assessment. While the focus of care for the serious trauma patient is the current life threats, some protection for serious musculoskeletal injuries is provided by moving the patient as a unit (with axial alignment) and by packaging the patient for transport using the long spine board (see Chapter 24, "Spinal Trauma"). These techniques help you reduce the risks of aggravating musculoskeletal injuries, increasing hemorrhage, and worsening shock and patient outcome. However, do not let gruesome musculoskeletal injury distract you from the priorities of trauma management.

Fractures of the pelvis and, to a lesser degree, the femur can significantly contribute to hypovolemia and shock. These injuries deserve a high priority in patient care. Other musculoskeletal injuries that merit a priority for care include those that threaten a limb, such as injuries with loss of distal circulation or sensation (most commonly joint injuries), and those that cause compartment syndrome (most likely leg or forearm injuries). You may prioritize other injuries by the relative size of the bone fractured or the body area involved and by the energy that was required to cause injury. Prioritize the patient's musculoskeletal injuries for care, then proceed with splinting and transport.

GENERAL PRINCIPLES OF MUSCULOSKELETAL INJURY MANAGEMENT

The objectives of musculoskeletal injury care are to reduce the possibility of any further injury during patient care and transport and to reduce the patient's discomfort. Accomplish these goals by protecting open wounds, positioning the extremity properly, immobilizing the injured extremity, and monitoring neurovascular function in the distal limb. In some cases, care involves manipulating the injury to reestablish distal circulation and sensation or simply to restore normal anatomical position for the patient expecting prolonged extrication or transport. In most cases, care for musculoskeletal injuries will also include application of a splinting device.

As you begin to care for a patient with musculoskeletal injuries, talk to him and explain what you are doing, why, and what impact it will have on the patient. Alignment and splinting will likely first cause an increase in pain followed by a significant reduction in it. By telling the patient of this in advance, you will increase confidence in both your intent to help and your ability to provide care.

Review

Content

Basics of Musculoskeletal Injury Care

- Protecting open wounds
- Exposure of the injury
- Proper positioning
- Immobilizing the injury
- Monitoring of neurovascular function

Protecting Open Wounds

If there is any open wound in close proximity to the fracture or dislocation, consider the fracture or dislocation to be an open one. Carefully observe the wound and note any signs of muscle, tendon, ligament, or vascular injury and be prepared to describe the wound in your report and at the emergency department. Cover the wound with a sterile dressing held in place with bandaging or a splint. Frequently, the attempts to align a limb, the splinting process, or the application of traction will draw protruding bones back into the wound. This is an expected consequence of proper care but must be brought to the attention of the attending emergency department physician.

Positioning the Limb

Proper limb positioning is essential to ensure patient comfort, to reduce the chances of further limb injury, and to encourage venous drainage. Proper positioning is different with fractures and dislocations, although splinting with the limb in a normal anatomical position, the position of function, is beneficial for both.

Limb alignment is appropriate for any fractures of the midshaft femur, tibia/fibula, humerus, or radius/ulna. Alignment can be maintained by using the air splint, padded rigid splint, PASG, vacuum, or traction splint. Proper alignment of a fracture enhances circulation and reduces the potential for further injury to surrounding tissue. It is also very difficult to immobilize a limb with a fracture in an unaligned, angulated position because the fracture segments are short and buried in soft tissue. Perform any limb alignment with great care so as not to damage the tissue surrounding the fracture site. During the process, the proximal limb should remain in position while you bring the distal limb to the position of alignment using gentle axial traction. Stop the process when you detect any resistance to movement or when the patient reports any significant increase in pain.

Stop realignment attempts when you detect any resistance to movement or when the patient reports any significant increase in pain.

Generally, you should not attempt alignment of dislocations and serious injuries within 3 inches of a joint. Only attempt to manipulate such injury sites if the distal circulation is compromised. In such a case, try to move the joint while another care provider palpates the distal pulse. If the pulse is restored, if you meet significant resistance to movement, or if the patient complains of greatly increased pain, stop the manipulation and splint the injured limb as it is. Be sure to transport the patient quickly, because a loss of circulation can endanger the future usefulness of the limb.

Do not attempt alignment of dislocations and serious injuries within 3 inches of a joint.

If you suspect a limb will remain dislocated for an extended period, as during lengthy transports or prolonged patient entrapments, consider reducing the dislocation. Apply a firm and progressive traction to the limb, which draws the dislocated ends away from each other and moves the joint toward normal positioning. When (and if) the bone ends "pop" back into position, ensure there is a distal pulse and immobilize the limb in the position of function.

Proper positioning of injured limbs is important for maintaining distal circulation and sensation and increasing patient comfort. Deformities and extremes of flexion or extension put pressure on the soft tissues and may compress nerves and blood vessels. These positions also fatigue the surrounding muscles and increase the pain associated with the injury. By placing the uninjured joints of the limb halfway between flexion and extension in what is called the position of function, you place the least stress on the joint ligaments and the muscles and tendons surrounding the injury. Place the limb in the position of function whenever possible (Figure 22-7 ■). Note, however, that some injuries and some splinting devices commonly used for musculoskeletal injuries may preclude this positioning.

When possible, place injured limbs in the position of function or neutral position.

When practical, elevate the injured limb. This will assist with venous drainage and reduce the edema associated with musculoskeletal injury.

Immobilizing the Injury

The aim in immobilizing musculoskeletal injuries is to prevent further injury caused by the movement of broken bone ends and bone ends dislodged from a joint and by further stress placed on

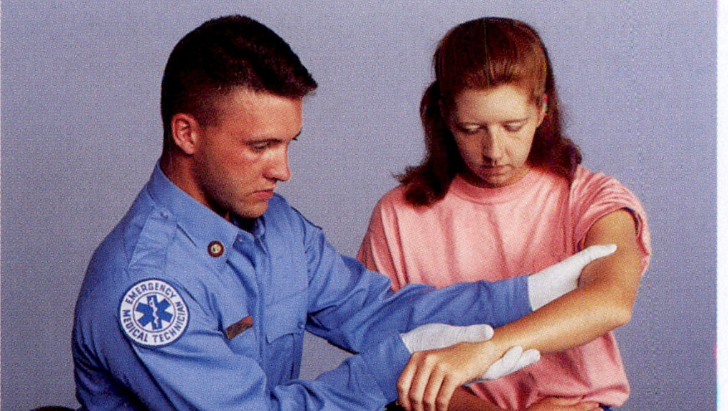

■ **Figure 22-7** Gently position the limb in the position of function, unless your attempts meet with resistance or a significant increase in pain or the injury is within 3 inches of a joint.

muscles, ligaments, or tendons already injured by a strain, sprain, subluxation, dislocation, or fracture. This immobilization is usually accomplished through the use of a splinting device.

Since most long bones lie buried deep within the musculature of the extremities, it is very difficult to immobilize them directly. Hence, we immobilize the joint above and the joint below the injury, regardless of whether the injury occurs at a joint or midshaft in a long bone. This ensures that no motion is transmitted through the injury site as might occur, for example, with the rotation (supination/pronation) of the radius against the ulna at the elbow when the wrist turns.

Wrap any splinting device or associated bandage from a distal point to a proximal one. This ensures that the pressure of bandaging moves any blood into the systemic circulation and does not trap it in the distal limb. This method of wrapping thus assists venous drainage and the healing process. Apply firm pressure when wrapping, but be sure you can easily push a finger beneath the wrapping.

Checking Neurovascular Function

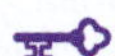

Always check pulses, motor function, and sensation in the distal extremity before, during, and after splinting.

It is imperative that you identify the status of the circulation, motor function, and sensation distal to the injury site before, during, and after splinting of all musculoskeletal injuries. The check before splinting identifies a baseline condition and establishes that the initial injury has not disrupted circulation. The check during splinting ensures that inadvertent limb movement or circumferential pressure does not compromise distal circulation. The check after splinting identifies any restriction caused by progressive swelling of the injured area against the splinting device. Clearly identify and document these evaluations whenever you apply a splint.

To perform this evaluation, first palpate for a pulse and ensure it is equal in strength to that of the opposing limb. If the pulse cannot be located or is weak, check capillary refill and skin temperature, color, and condition. Again compare your findings to the opposing limb. Ask the patient to describe the sensation when you rub or pinch the bottom of the foot or back of the hand and ask him to move the fingers or toes. The patient response establishes your baseline circulation, sensory, and motor findings. Reevaluate pulse, motor function, and sensation frequently during the remaining care and transport. If a care provider is holding the limb while you apply the splint, have him monitor both pulse and skin temperature. That care provider can then immediately note any compromise in circulation.

The pulse oximeter can be used to monitor the distal pulse during the splint process. Affix the probe to a free finger or toe and ensure a good reading. Then monitor the oximeter, watching for any change, especially the readings becoming erratic or the device becoming unable to obtain a reading at all. This suggests a compromise in distal circulation (loss of the pulsing necessary to obtain a reading) and the need to reassess the distal pulse, skin temperature, and capillary refill.

SPLINTING DEVICES

An essential part of managing any musculoskeletal system injury is the use of devices to immobilize a limb and permit patient transport without causing further injury. These devices, called splints, are designed to help you reduce or eliminate any movement of the injured extremity. Splints come in several forms that can assist in immobilizing common fractures and dislocations associated with musculoskeletal trauma (Figure 22-8 ■). They include rigid, formable, soft, traction, and other splints.

Rigid Splints

Rigid splints, as the name implies, are firm and durable supports for the injured limb. They can be constructed of cardboard, plastic, metal, synthetic products, or wood. Such devices very effectively immobilize injury sites but require adequate padding to lessen patient discomfort. This padding may be built into the splint or may simply be a bulky dressing affixed to the splint with soft bandaging. Several types of commercially available rigid splints are used in prehospital care. They are usually flat and rigid devices and are about 3 inches wide and from 16 to 48 inches long. The injured limb that is in alignment is immobilized to the splint by circumferential wrapping, while an angulated limb may be held in position by cross-wrapping at two locations.

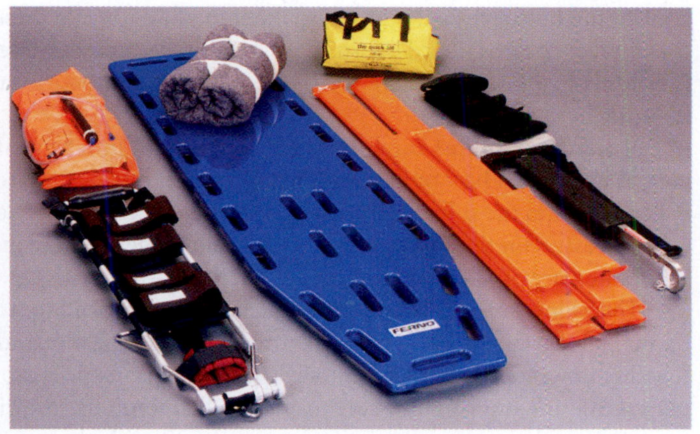

■ Figure 22-8 A variety of splints are available for musculoskeletal injuries.

A special form of rigid splint is the preformed splint. It is usually a stamped metal or preformed plastic or fiberglass device shaped to the contours of the distal limbs. These splints are usually available for the ankles and hands.

Formable Splints

Another type of rigid splint is the formable, or malleable, splint. It is made up of a material that you can easily shape to match the angulation of a limb. You then affix the formed splint to the limb with circumferential bandaging. Formable splints include both the ladder splint, which is a matrix of soft metal wires soldered together, and the metal sheet splint, which is made up of thin aluminum or another easily shaped metal.

Vacuum splints are now available and sized for almost all long-bone fractures. The device is an airtight fabric bag filled with small plastic particles. The splint is applied to the injured limb and formed and secured around it. As the air is withdrawn from the device, the small particles lock in position, creating a firmly fixed form around the limb (Figure 22-9 ■). The splint firmly and comfortably secures the limb in position, although there is a small amount of shrinkage with the evacuation of air.

Soft Splints

Soft splints use padding or air pressure to immobilize an injured limb in place. Varieties of soft splints include air splints, which include the PASG, pelvic sling, and pillow splints.

The air splint provides immobilization as air pressure fills the splint and compresses the limb. Since the splint is a formed cylinder, and may include shaping for the foot, it immobilizes the limb in an aligned position. Air splints should not be used with long-bone injuries at or above the knee or elbow because they cannot prevent movement of hip or shoulder joints and are thus unable to immobilize the proximal joints of the limb. Air splints also apply a pressure that may be helpful in

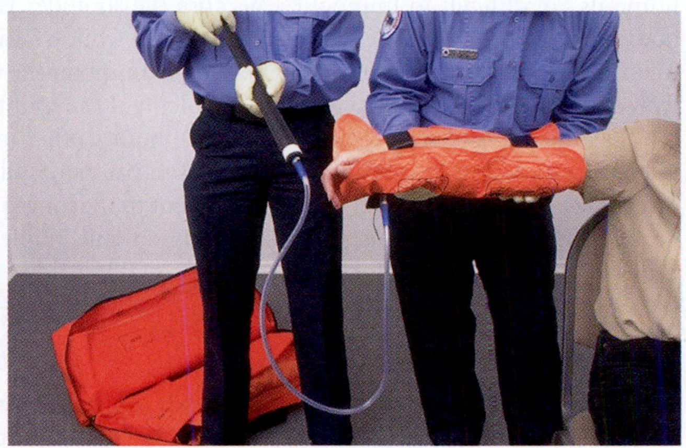

■ Figure 22-9 Suction the air out of a vacuum splint until the device is rigid. Reassess pulse, motor function, and sensation in the extremity after application.

controlling both external and internal hemorrhage. While these devices may limit assessment of the distal extremity, they do permit observation because they are transparent. (Note that the PASG is not transparent, so carefully assess the patient from the rib cage to the feet before applying and inflating it.)

Monitor pressure within the air splint or PASG, as it may change with changes in altitude or temperature.

Monitor air splints carefully with any changes in temperature or atmospheric pressure. Increases in ambient heat or decreases in pressure, as during an ascent in a helicopter, will increase the pressure within the splint. Conversely, decreases in temperature or a descent in a helicopter will decrease pressure in the splint. Constantly monitor the pressure in the air splint and PASG to ensure it does not rise or fall during your care.

The pillow splint is a comfortable splint for ankle and foot injuries. The foot is simply placed on the pillow while the outer fabric is drawn around the foot and pillow. The outer fabric is pinned together or wrapped circumferentially with bandage material around the injury site. This device applies gentle and uniform pressure to effectively immobilize the distal extremity. Using a bulky blanket or two and wrapping them firmly may also provide the same type of immobilization.

Traction Splints

The traction splint was developed during World War I and used extensively during World War II. This splint dramatically reduced both mortality and limb loss from femur fractures caused by projectile wounds, blast injuries, and other traumas. Today, the traction splint is the mainstay of prehospital care for the isolated traumatic femur fracture.

The traction splint is a frame that applies a pull (traction) on the injured extremity and against the trunk. The application of traction is useful when splinting the femur, which is surrounded by very heavy musculature. Frequently, the pain of fracture initiates muscle spasm that causes the bone ends to override each other, causing further pain and muscle spasm and aggravating the original injury. The traction splint prevents overriding of the bone ends, lessens patient pain, and may help relax any muscle spasm.

There are basically two styles of traction splint, the bipolar frame device and the unipolar device (Figure 22-10 ■). The bipolar (Fernotrac or Thomas) traction splint has a half ring that fits up and against the ischial tuberosity of the pelvis. A distal ratchet connects to a foot harness and pulls traction from the foot and against the pelvis. The frame lifts and supports the limb and a foot stand suspends the injured limb above the ground. This construction helps prevent motion of the limb during movement of the patient, while the elevation supplied by the stand enhances venous drainage. The unipolar (Sager or Kendrick) traction splint uses a single lengthening shaft to pull a foot harness against pressure applied to the pubic bone. The unipolar splint does not elevate or stabilize the extremity, so you must observe greater care whenever you move the patient. You can use the unipolar splint in conjunction with the PASG.

Other Splinting Aids

Cravats or Velcro straps can augment the effectiveness of rigid splints. You can secure the lower extremities, one to the other, to help the patient control the musculoskeletal injury site or you can use a sling and swathe to help immobilize a splinted upper extremity to the chest. Fractures of the humerus are difficult to immobilize because the shoulder is such a large and mobile part of the body. A sling may hold the elbow at a fixed angle, while a swathe secures the limb against the body to limit further shoulder motion. By holding a thumb in the fold of the elbow, the patient can easily reduce any motion of the limb and complement the splinting process.

In some cases of serious musculoskeletal injury, other injuries preclude the splinting of individual fractures and dislocations. In such cases, you may splint the limbs to the body with cravats or bandage material and immobilize the patient to the long spine board. Simply strap the body and limbs to the board and transport the patient as a unit. While this is not definitive splinting, it will provide reasonable protection for musculoskeletal injuries.

FRACTURE CARE

Consider any injury within 3 inches of a joint to be a joint injury.

For prehospital care purposes, consider a joint injury to be any muscular or connective tissue injury or dislocation or fracture within 3 inches of a joint. Fractures are then defined as shaft injuries

a. A bipolar frame traction splint.

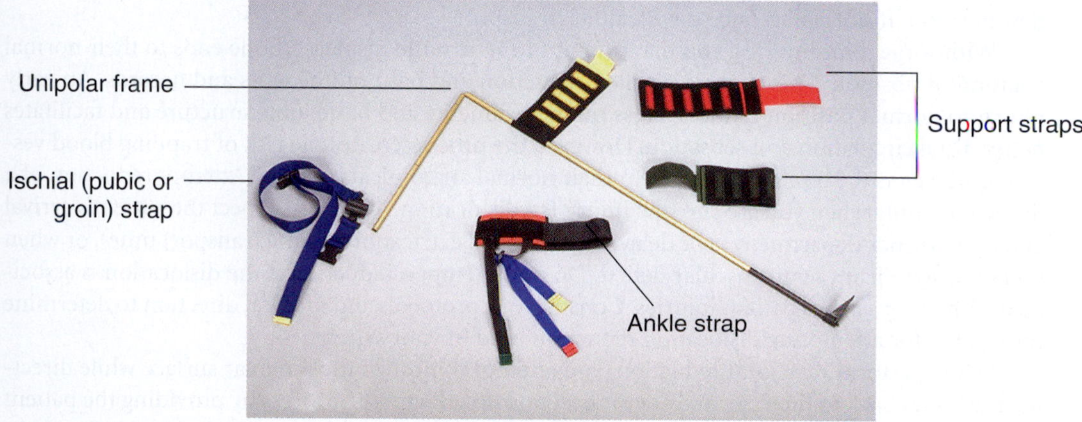

b. A unipolar frame traction splint.

■ **Figure 22-10** Traction splints.

at least 3 inches away from the joint. These definitions are essential because injury near the joint carries a higher incidence of blood vessel and nerve involvement and requires a different approach to positioning and splinting.

Begin fracture care by ensuring distal pulses, sensation, and motor function. Then align the limb for splinting. Quickly recheck the circulation and motor and sensory function below the injury. If you identify any neurovascular deficit, attempt to correct the problem by gentle repositioning, even if the limb is relatively aligned. Also consider aligning the limb if the bone end is close to the skin and in danger of converting a closed fracture into an open one. If the limb is angulated, proceed with realignment. Remember that most splinting devices are designed to immobilize aligned limbs and that alignment provides the best chance for ensuring good neurovascular function distal to the injury.

To move an injured limb from an angulated position into alignment, use gentle distal traction applied manually. Have an assisting EMT immobilize the proximal limb in the position found. Grasp the distal limb firmly and apply traction along the limb's axis, gently moving it from the angulated to an aligned position. Should you feel any resistance to movement or notice a great increase in patient discomfort, stop the alignment attempt and splint the limb as it lies. Once you complete alignment, recheck the distal neurovascular function. If it is adequate, proceed with splinting. If function is inadequate, move the limb around slightly while another care provider monitors for a pulse. If one attempt at gentle manipulation does not reestablish a pulse, splint and transport the patient quickly.

Proceed with splinting by selecting an appropriate device and secure the limb to it in a way that ensures you immobilize both the fracture site and the adjacent joints. Have the care provider who is holding the limb apply a gentle traction to stabilize the limb (and monitor the distal pulse) during splinting. If you apply your splint properly, the device may maintain this traction and provide greater stabilization of the limb and greater patient comfort. Secure the limb to the body (upper extremity) or to the opposite limb (lower extremity) to protect it and to give the patient some control over the limb.

JOINT CARE

Unless you identify a neurovascular deficit, immobilize joint injuries as you find them.

Joint care, too, begins with exposing the injury and assessing for distal neurovascular function. If you find pulse, sensation, and motor function to be adequate, immobilize the joint in the position found. Use a ladder, vacuum, or other malleable splint, shaped to the limb's angle, or cross-wrap with a padded rigid splint to immobilize the joint in place. Ensure that your splinting immobilizes the injured joint and both the joint above and the joint below the injury. If not, secure the limb firmly to the body to immobilize these joints.

If circulation or motor or sensory function is lost below the joint injury, consider moving the limb to reestablish it. While you gently move the limb, have another care provider monitor the circulation and sensation. If you can reestablish neurovascular function quickly, splint the limb in the new position. If not, splint and provide quick transport.

reduction *returning of displaced bone ends to their proper anatomical orientation.*

With some joint injuries, you may attempt to return the displaced bone ends to their normal anatomical position. This process is called **reduction** and has both benefits and hazards. An early return to normal position reduces stress on the ligaments and basic joint structure and facilitates better distal circulation and sensation. However, the process creates the risk of trapping blood vessels or nerves as the bone ends return to their normal anatomical position. Attempt reduction of a dislocation only when you are sure the injury *is* a dislocation, when you expect the patient's arrival at the emergency department to be delayed (prolonged extrication or long transport time), or when there is a significant neurovascular deficit. Do not attempt a reduction if the dislocation is associated with other serious patient injuries. Consult your protocols and medical direction to determine the criteria for attempting dislocation reduction used in your system.

When performing a joint reduction, you attempt to protect the articular surface while directing the bones back to their normal anatomical position. Begin the process by providing the patient with analgesic therapy to reduce pain associated with the injury and the reduction itself. Then have an assisting care provider hold the proximal extremity in position and provide a countertraction during the reduction. You then apply traction to pull the bone surfaces apart, reducing the pressure between the nonarticular surfaces. Slowly increase traction and direct the displaced limb toward its normal anatomical position. Successful relocation is indicated when you feel the joint "pop" back into position, the patient experiences a lessening of pain, and the joint becomes mobile within at least a few minutes of the procedure. Carefully evaluate the distal circulation, sensation, and motor function after the reduction. If the procedure does not meet with success within a few minutes, splint the limb as it is and provide rapid transport for the patient. If the reduction is successful, splint the limb in the position of function and transport.

MUSCULAR AND CONNECTIVE TISSUE CARE

Injuries to the soft tissues of the musculoskeletal system deserve special care. While such injuries are not usually life threatening, they can be very painful and, in some cases, threaten limbs. For example, compartment syndrome can restrict capillary blood flow, venous blood return, and nerve function beyond the site of the injury. If such an injury is not discovered and relieved, it may produce severe disability. Deep contusions and especially large hematomas can also contribute to blood loss and hypovolemia. Once you care for life threats, fractures, joint injuries, and other limb threats, give injuries to muscular and connective tissues your attention.

To manage these muscle, tendon, and ligament injuries, immobilize the region surrounding them. Doing so will reduce the associated internal hemorrhage and pain. Provide gentle circumferential bandaging (loose enough to let you slide a finger underneath) to further reduce hemorrhage, edema, and pain, but be sure to monitor distal circulation and loosen the bandage further if there are any signs of neurovascular deficit. Application of local cooling will reduce both edema and patient discomfort. Be careful to wrap any cold or ice pack in a dressing to prevent too drastic a cooling and any consequent injury. You may apply heat to the wound after 48 hours to enhance both circulation and healing. If possible, place the limb in the position of function and elevate the extremity to ensure good venous return, limit swelling, and reduce patient discomfort. Monitor distal neurovascular function to ensure your actions do not compromise circulation, sensation, or motor function.

CARE FOR SPECIFIC FRACTURES

Pelvis

Pelvic fractures involve either the iliac crest or the pelvic ring. While iliac crest fractures may reflect serious trauma, they do not represent the patient life threat suggested by ring fractures. Iliac crest fractures are often isolated and stable injuries that you can care for by simple patient immobilization.

Pelvic ring fractures, however, are often serious, life-threatening events. The ring shape of the pelvis provides strength to the structure, but when it breaks, two fracture sites usually result. The kinetic forces necessary to fracture the pelvic ring are significant and are likely to produce fractures and internal injuries elsewhere. In addition, the pelvis is actively involved in blood cell production, has a rich blood supply, and its interior surface is adjacent to major blood vessels serving the lower extremities. Injury to the pelvic ring, therefore, can result in heavy hemorrhage that is likely to empty into the pelvic and retroperitoneal spaces and account for blood loss in excess of 2 liters. Such injury may also result in circulation loss to one or both lower extremities. Pelvic fractures may also be associated with hip dislocations and injuries to the bladder, female reproductive organs, the urethra, the prostate in the male, and the end of the alimentary canal (anus and rectum). Clearly, pelvic ring fractures are very serious injuries.

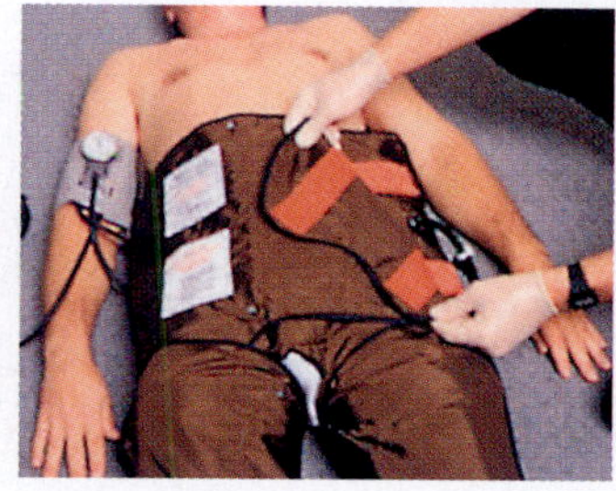

■ **Figure 22-11** The PASG is an effective splint for traumatic pelvic fractures and helps control internal hemorrhage.

The objectives of pelvic injury care are to stabilize the fractured pelvis, support the patient hemodynamically, and provide rapid transport to a trauma center. Because of the potential for severe blood loss and the difficulty of immobilizing the broken pelvic ring, application of the PASG is sometimes recommended for pelvic fractures (Figure 22-11 ■). Inflate the PASG until it stabilizes the pelvis and hip joint. If the patient is hypotensive, start two large-bore IVs, and hang two 1,000-mL bags of lactated Ringer's solution or normal saline. Set up using trauma tubing, and administer fluid boluses as needed to maintain a systolic blood pressure of at least 80 mmHg. Always consider a pelvic fracture patient to be a candidate for rapid transport.

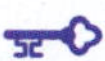

Always consider a pelvic fracture patient to be a candidate for rapid transport.

Another effective technique to immobilize an unstable pelvis is application of a pelvic sling. The sling is a wide band, either commercially available or made from a sheet. To apply, fold a sheet to about 10 inches wide and gently negotiate it under the patient, or move the patient to the spine board with the device in place. The band should engage the pelvis with the band's upper border just below the iliac crests. Secure the commercial device or tie the sheet firmly to immobilize the pelvis with firm but not excessive pressure. Place a folded blanket between the patient's lower extremities and tie them together. If necessary for comfort, place a pillow under the patient's knees. A commercial pelvic sling is now available.

Femur

Femur fractures may be traumatic, resulting from the application of very strong and violent forces, or atraumatic, resulting from degenerative diseases. Patients with disease-induced fractures usually are of advancing age and present with a history of a degenerative disease, a clouded or limited history of trauma, and only moderate discomfort. Care for such patients by immobilizing them as found and then providing gentle transport. Generally, you can provide effective splinting by placing the patient on a long spine board and padding with pillows and blankets for patient comfort. Use of a traction splint is not essential because pain is not inducing the spasms that cause broken bone ends to override.

Atraumatic femur fractures may be splinted by gently placing the patient on a long spine board.

A patient who has suffered a traumatic femur fracture usually experiences extreme discomfort and is often writhing in pain. In such a case, providing distal traction immobilizes both bone ends, relieves muscle spasms, and reduces the associated pain. Traction splinting is the best avenue for care of the hemodynamically stable patient with an isolated femur fracture. However, the traction splint is not indicated if the patient has concurrent serious knee, tibia, or foot injuries.

Proximal fractures (surgical neck and intertrochanteric fractures) are frequently caused by hip injuries, transmitted forces, or the degenerative effects of aging. Midshaft fractures often result from high-energy, lateral traumas and are associated with significant blood loss. Injuries to the distal femur (condylar and epicondylar fractures) can be extensive and are likely to involve blood vessels, nerves, and connective tissue. The energy necessary to fracture the femur may be sufficient to dislocate the hip and cause serious internal injuries elsewhere in the body.

If the femur fracture is accompanied by a severe pelvic fracture, you may best achieve limb immobilization and hemodynamic stability by using the PASG alone or by simply immobilizing the patient on a backboard, pelvic sling, vacuum splint, or vacuum mattress. If a pelvic fracture is suspected, do *not* apply a traction splint, which may apply pressure to the fractured pelvis, thereby causing further bone displacement and hemorrhage. Also, if the early signs of shock are present or if the history suggests that the patient has sustained trauma severe enough to induce shock, the PASG may be a better choice because it effectively splints the entire region and contributes to hemodynamic stability.

You may find it difficult to differentiate between proximal fractures of the femur (hip fractures) and anterior hip dislocations. Generally, a femur fracture presents with the foot externally rotated (turned outward) and the injured limb shortened when compared to the other. This difference may be slight and may be unnoticeable if the patient's legs are not straight and parallel. An anterior dislocation presents similarly to the femur fracture, but with the head of the femur protruding in the inguinal region. In either case, treat as a dislocation. Traction splints should not be used if a joint injury (hip or knee) is suspected.

If you suspect femur fracture, align the limb, determine the status of circulation and sensory and motor function, and apply the traction splint (Figure 22-12 ■). (If you use manual traction to align the femur, maintain it until the splint is applied and continues the traction.) Adjust the length of the splint to the uninjured extremity, position the device against the pelvis, and secure it in position with the inguinal strap. With a bipolar splint, apply the ankle hitch, provide gentle traction, and elevate the distal limb to place the splint's ring against the ischial tuberosity. With a unipolar splint, position the T-shaped support against the pubic bone and simply apply the ankle hitch. Ensure that hitch and splint hold the foot and limb in an anatomical position as you apply firm traction. Position and secure the limb to the splint with straps, then gently move the patient and splint to the long spine board. Firmly secure the patient and limb for transport.

Guide your application of traction by the patient's response. Ask the patient how the limb feels as you initiate and increase the amount of traction. Stop the application of traction when the limb is immobilized and patient discomfort decreases. Remember, as the traction splint prevents the overriding of bone ends, the pain of injury decreases. This reduces the strength of muscle spasm and lets the limb return toward its initial length. This, in turn, reduces the traction provided by the splint, which means that the bone ends will no longer be as well immobilized. Check the amount of traction frequently to ensure that it does not lessen during your care. If the patient reports increasing pain, consider increasing traction gradually until some reduction in pain is noted.

When the need for rapid transport or other patient injuries preclude the use of the traction splint, consider using the long spine board for immobilizing and transporting the femur fracture

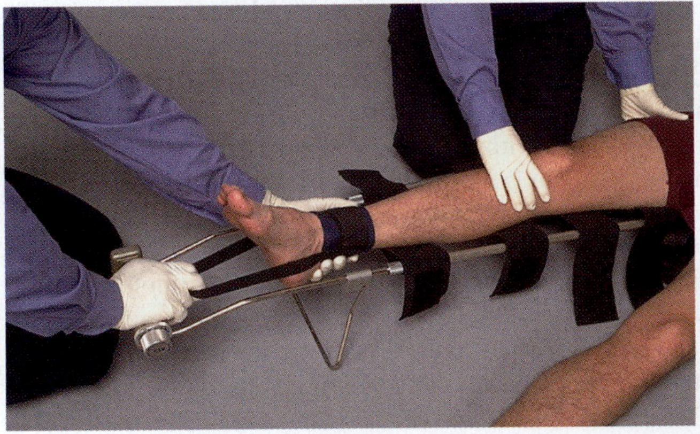

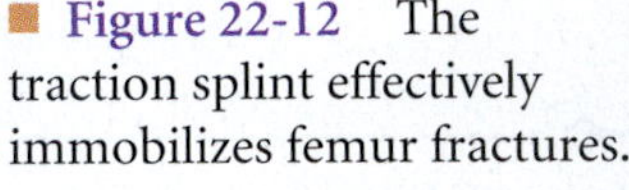

■ **Figure 22-12** The traction splint effectively immobilizes femur fractures.

patient. Use long padded rigid splints, one medial and one lateral, to quickly splint the injured limb, and then tie that limb to the uninjured one. Use an orthopedic stretcher or another device or movement technique to transfer the patient to a long spine board and secure the patient firmly on it.

Tibia/Fibula

Fractures of the leg bones, the tibia and the fibula, can occur separately or together. The tibia is the most commonly fractured leg bone and may be broken by direct force, crushing injury, or twisting forces. Tibial fracture is likely to cause an open wound. Fibular fractures are often associated with damage to the knee or ankle. If the tibia is fractured and the fibula is intact, the extremity may not angulate, but it is not able to bear weight. If only the fibula is broken, the limb may be relatively stable. Injuries to either bone may result in compartment syndrome. Direct trauma suffered during an auto crash or athletic impact frequently causes these tibia and fibula injuries.

Fibular fractures are relatively stable, while tibial fractures are not.

Align the injured limb; assess circulation, sensation, and motor function; and then immobilize the limb with gentle traction. A full-leg air splint (one that accommodates the foot), vacuum, or lateral and medial padded rigid splints will provide effective immobilization (Figure 22-13 ■). You may also use a cardboard splint as long as it accommodates the full limb and is rigid enough to maintain immobilization. After you splint the injured limb, secure it to the uninjured leg. This affords some protection against uncontrolled movement and may reassure the patient that he still has some control over the extremity.

Clavicle

The clavicle is the most frequently fractured bone in the human body. Fractures to it usually result from transmitted forces directed along the upper extremity that cause relatively minor skeletal injury. The clavicle, however, is located adjacent to both the upper reaches of the lung and the vasculature that serves the upper extremity and head. Hence, an injury to the clavicle has the potential to cause serious internal injury, especially if very powerful mechanisms of injury are involved. The clavicular fracture patient often presents with pain and the shoulder shifted forward with palpable deformity along the clavicle. Accomplish splinting either by immobilizing the affected limb in a sling and swathe or by wrapping a figure-eight bandage around the shoulders, drawing the shoulders back, and then securing the bandage tension. Monitor the patient carefully for any sign of internal hemorrhage or respiratory compromise.

Humerus

A fractured humerus is very difficult to immobilize at its proximal end. The proximal humerus is buried within the shoulder muscles, and the shoulder joint is very mobile atop the thoracic cage. The axillary artery runs through the axilla, making it difficult to apply any mechanical traction to the limb without compromising circulation. Hence, the most effective techniques for splinting this fracture are to apply a sling and swathe to immobilize the bent limb against the chest or to tie the extended and splinted limb to the body.

The preferred technique is to use the sling and swathe. Apply a short padded rigid splint to the lateral surface of the arm to distribute the pressure of the swathing and better immobilize the arm. Sling the forearm with a cravat, catching just the wrist region and not the elbow. This permits some

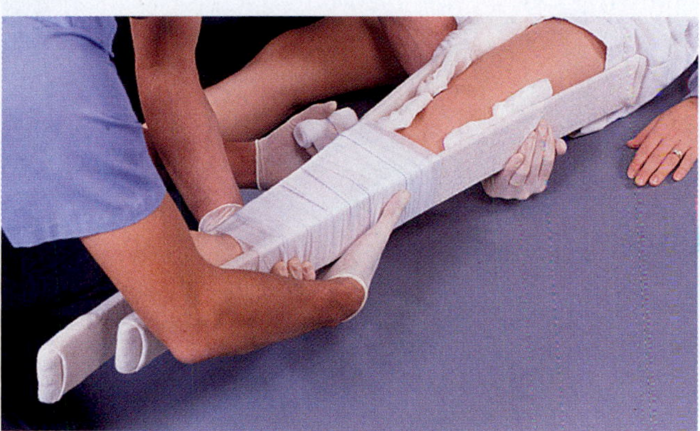

■ **Figure 22-13** Placement of long padded board splints laterally and medially can effectively splint tibia/fibula fractures.

gravitational traction in the seated patient and prevents inadvertent application of pressure by the sling, which could push the limb together. Then use several cravats to gently swathe the arm and forearm to the chest. If the patient is conscious, have him place the thumb of the uninjured extremity in the fold of the elbow to help control the injured limb's motion. This gives the patient control over the limb, decreases limb movement, and increases patient comfort.

You may also immobilize the limb by using a long padded rigid splint affixed to the extended limb. Place the splint along the medial aspect of the upper extremity and ensure that it does not apply pressure to the axilla. Such pressure disrupts axillary artery blood flow to the limb and is uncomfortable for the patient. Secure the splint firmly to the limb, wrapping from the distal end toward the proximal end. Then secure the splint to the supine patient's body, and move the patient and splint to a long spine board.

Radius/Ulna

The forearm may fracture anywhere along its length and the fracture may involve the radius, the ulna, or both. Most commonly, fracture occurs at the distal end of the radius, just above the articular surface. This is known as a Colles' fracture, and it presents with the wrist turned up at an unusual angle. Another term for this injury is the "silver fork deformity" because it is contoured like a fork and the distal limb often becomes ashen. As with most joint fractures, the major concern here is for distal circulation and innervation. If you find a neurovascular injury, use only slight adjustments to restore nervous or circulatory function because movement in this area is likely to cause further injury.

When possible, leave a distal digit exposed to evaluate capillary refill and skin color and temperature.

Splint forearm fractures with a short, padded rigid splint affixed to the forearm and hand. Secure the hand in the position of function by placing a large wad of dressing material in the palm to maintain a position like that of holding a large ball. Place the rigid splint along the medial forearm surface and wrap circumferentially from the fingers to the elbow. Leave at least one digit exposed to permit checking for capillary refill. Bend the elbow across the chest and use a sling and swathe to hold the limb in position. This provides relative elevation and improved venous drainage in both seated and supine patients.

The air splint or long padded rigid splint, tied firmly to the body, may also adequately immobilize forearm fractures (Figure 22-14 ■). When using these devices, remember to place the hand in the position of function to increase patient comfort.

CARE FOR SPECIFIC JOINT INJURIES

Hip

The hip may dislocate anteriorly or posteriorly. The anterior dislocation presents with the foot turned outward, the hip and knee flexed, and the head of the femur sometimes palpable in the inguinal area. The posterior dislocation is most common and presents with the knee flexed and the foot rotated in-

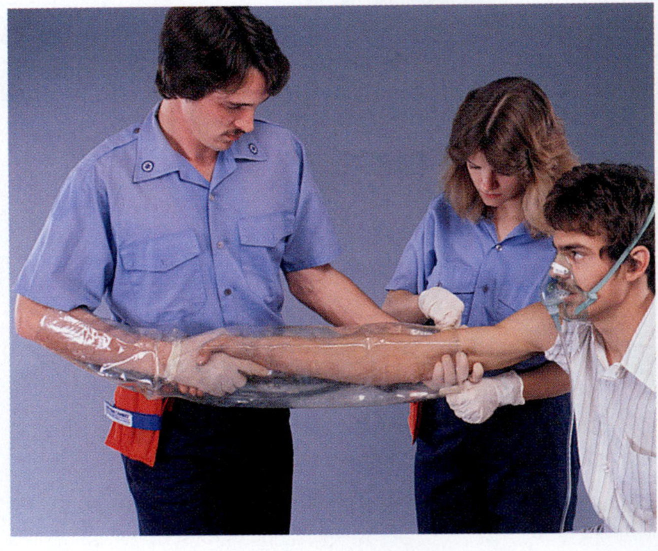

■ **Figure 22-14** A full-arm air splint can effectively splint fractures of the radius and/or ulna.

ternally. The displaced head of the femur is buried in the muscle of the buttocks. Immobilize a patient with either type of dislocation on a long spine board using pillows and blankets as padding to maintain the patient's position and provide comfort. If distal circulation, sensation, or motor function is severely compromised, consider one attempt at reduction of a posterior dislocation. (Consult local protocols and medical direction to identify criteria for reduction attempts.) However, do not attempt reduction if there are other serious injuries, like a pelvic fracture. Anterior dislocations cannot be reduced in the prehospital setting.

For reduction of a posterior hip dislocation, have a care provider hold the pelvis firmly against the long spine board or other firm surface by placing downward pressure on the iliac crests. Flex both the patient's hip and knee at 90 degrees and apply a firm, slowly increasing traction along the axis of the femur. Gently rotate the femur externally. It takes some time for the muscles to relax, but when they do the head of the femur will "pop" back into position. If you feel this "pop" or if the patient reports a sudden relief of pain and is able to extend the leg easily, the reduction has likely been a success. Immobilize the patient in a comfortable position, either in flexion (not to exceed 90 degrees) or fully supine with the hip and leg in full extension. Reevaluate sensation, motor function, and circulation. If the femur head does not move into the acetabulum after a few minutes of your attempted reduction, immobilize the patient as found and consider rapid transport.

Knee

Knee injuries may include fractures of the femur, the tibia, or both; patellar dislocations; or frank dislocations of the knee. Because the knee is such a large joint and bears such a great amount of weight, an injury to it is serious and threatens the patient's future ability to walk. Another concern with knee injury is possible injury to the major blood vessel traversing the area, the popliteal artery. This artery is less mobile than blood vessels in other joints, which leaves it more subject to injury and distal vascular compromise.

Immobilize knee joint fractures and patellar dislocations in the position found unless distal circulation, sensation, or motor function is disrupted. If the limb is flexed, splint it with two medium rigid splints, placing one medially and one laterally (Figure 22-15 ■). Cross-wrap with bandage material to secure the limb in position. You may also use ladder or malleable splints, conformed to the angle of the limb and placed anteriorly and posteriorly, or a vacuum splint to immobilize the knee. If the limb is extended, simply apply two padded rigid splints or a full-leg air splint.

Immobilize knee injuries in the position found unless you discover significant distal circulation, sensation, or motor deficit.

Dislocation of the patella is more common than dislocation of the knee joint and usually leaves the knee in a flexed position with a lateral displacement of the patella. The injured knee appears significantly deformed, though patellar dislocation has a lower incidence of associated vascular injury than does knee dislocation.

Anterior dislocations of the knee produce an extended limb contour that lifts at the knee (moving from proximal to distal) while posterior dislocations produce a limb that drops at the knee. (Ensure that the injury is not a patellar dislocation.) If there is neurovascular compromise, have another care provider immobilize the femur. You should then grasp the limb just above the ankle and at the calf muscle and apply a firm and progressive traction, first along the axis of the tibia and then pulling the limb toward alignment with the femur. With posterior dislocations, a third care provider

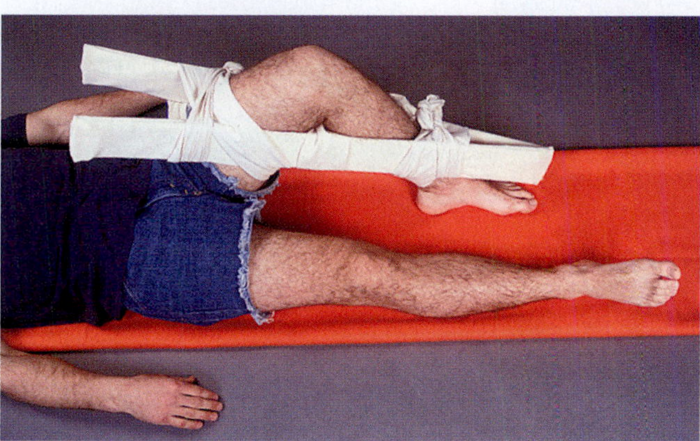

■ **Figure 22-15** Angulated knee dislocations can be immobilized with two padded rigid splints.

may provide moderate downward pressure on the distal femur and upward pressure on the proximal tibia to facilitate the reduction. As with most dislocations, success is measured by feeling the bone end "pop" back into place, hearing the patient report a dramatic reduction in pain, and noting a freer movement of the limb at the knee joint. Once you reduce the knee dislocation, immobilize the joint in the position of function and transport the patient. If you cannot reduce the dislocation with a few minutes of distal traction, immobilize the extremity in the position found and transport quickly. Perform a knee dislocation reduction even if the patient has good distal circulation and nervous function when the time to definitive care will exceed 2 hours.

Ankle

Ankle injuries often produce a distal lower limb that is grossly deformed, either due to malleolar fracture, dislocation, or both. Sprains are also injuries of concern, although with them the limb remains in anatomical position. Splint sprains or nondisplaced fractures with an air splint (shaped to accommodate the foot) or with long rigid splints positioned on either side of the limb, padded liberally, and wrapped firmly. You may also use a pillow splint, especially if there is any ankle deformity (Figure 22-16 ■). Apply local cooling to ease the pain and reduce swelling.

Ankle dislocation may occur in any of three directions: anteriorly, posteriorly, or laterally. The anterior dislocation presents with a dorsiflexed (upward-pointing) foot that appears shortened. The posterior dislocation appears to lengthen the plantar flexed (downward-pointing) foot. The lateral dislocation is most common and presents with a foot turned outward with respect to the ankle. If distal neurovascular compromise indicates the need for reduction, have a care provider grasp the calf, hold it in position, and pull against the traction you apply. You then grasp the heel with one hand and the metatarsal arch with the other. Pull a distal traction to disengage the bone ends and protect the articular cartilage during the relocation. For anterior dislocations, move the foot posteriorly with respect to the ankle; with lateral dislocations, rotate the foot medially; with posterior dislocations, pull the heel toward you and the foot toward you, then away. The joint should return to the normal position with a "pop," a reduction in patient pain, and an increase in the mobility of the joint. Apply local cooling and immobilize the limb. If the procedure does not result in joint reduction within a few minutes, splint the joint as found and provide rapid transport.

Foot

Injuries to the foot include dislocations and fractures to the calcanei (heel bones), metatarsals, and phalanges. Injuries to the calcanei generally result from falls and can cause significant pain and swelling. Injuries to the metatarsals and phalanges can result from penetrating or blunt trauma or the typical "stubbing" of a toe. Fatigue fractures of the metatarsal bones, or "march fractures," are relatively common. These injuries are reasonably stable, even though the extremity cannot bear weight. When foot or ankle injury is suspected, anticipate both bilateral foot injuries and lumbar spinal injury.

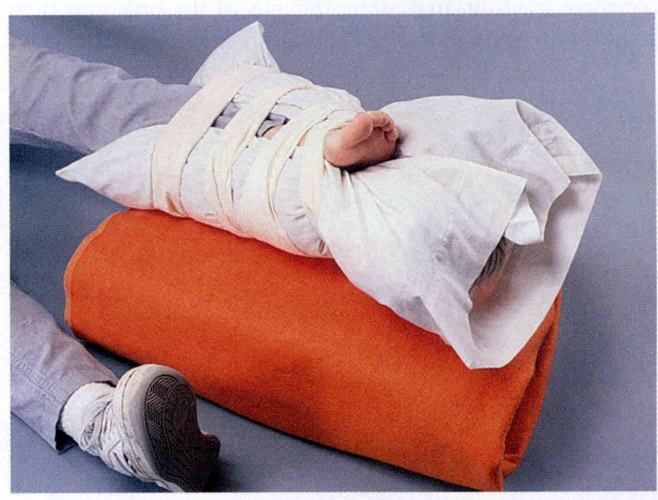

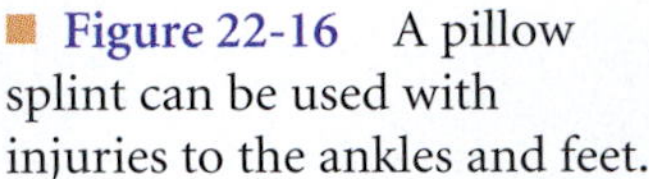

■ **Figure 22-16** A pillow splint can be used with injuries to the ankles and feet.

Immobilize foot injuries in much the same way you do with ankle injuries. Use pillow, vacuum, ladder, or air splints (with foot accommodation). If possible, leave some portion of the foot accessible so you can monitor distal capillary refill or, at least, skin temperature and color.

Shoulder

Fractures to the shoulder most commonly involve the proximal humerus, lateral scapula, and distal clavicle. Dislocations can include anterior, posterior, and inferior displacement of the humeral head. Anterior dislocations displace the humeral head forward, resulting in a shoulder that appears "hollow" or "squared-off," with the patient holding the arm close to the chest and forward of the midaxillary line. Posterior dislocations rotate the arm internally, and the patient presents with the elbow and forearm held away from the chest. Inferior dislocations displace the humeral head downward, with the result that the patient's arm is often locked above the head.

You should immobilize shoulder injuries, like all joint injuries, as found, unless pulse, sensation, or motor function distal to the injury is absent. Immobilize anterior and posterior dislocations with a sling and swathe and, if needed, place a pillow under the arm and forearm. Immobilization of any inferior dislocation (with the upper extremity fixed above the head) will call for ingenuity on your part in splinting. In such cases, immobilize the extended arm in the position found. Using cravats, tie a long, padded splint to the torso, shoulder girdle, arm, and forearm to immobilize the arm above the head. Gently move the patient to the long spine board and secure both splint and patient to the spine board.

Begin reduction of anterior and posterior shoulder dislocations by placing a strap across the patient's chest, under the affected shoulder (through the axilla), and across the back. Have a care provider prepared to pull countertraction across the chest and superiorly using the strap. You, meanwhile, should flex the patient's elbow, drawing the arm somewhat away from the body (abduction) and pull firm traction along the axis of the humerus. Some slight internal and external rotation of the humerus may facilitate reduction. For reduction of inferior dislocations, have one care provider hold the thorax while you flex the elbow. Gradually apply firm traction along the axis of the humerus and gently rotate the arm externally. If the joint does not relocate in a few minutes, immobilize it as it lies and transport the patient. If reduction is successful, immobilize the upper extremity in the normal anatomical position with a sling and swathe.

Elbow

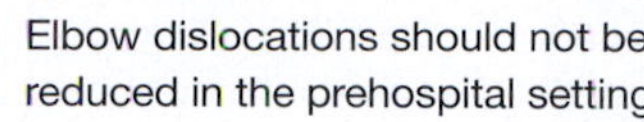

Elbow dislocations should not be reduced in the prehospital setting.

Elbow injuries display a high incidence of nervous and vascular involvement, especially in children. As in the knee, the blood vessels running through the elbow region are held firmly in place. The probability is good, therefore, that any fracture or dislocation will involve the brachial artery and the medial, ulnar, and radial nerves. Assess the distal neurovascular function and, if you detect a deficit, move the joint very carefully and minimally to restore distal circulation. Then splint the elbow with a single padded rigid splint, providing cross-strapping as necessary, or use a ladder splint bent to conform to the angle of the limb (Figure 22-17 ■). Keeping the wrist slightly elevated above the elbow, secure the limb to the chest using a sling and swathe. This position increases venous return and reduces the swelling and pain associated with the injury.

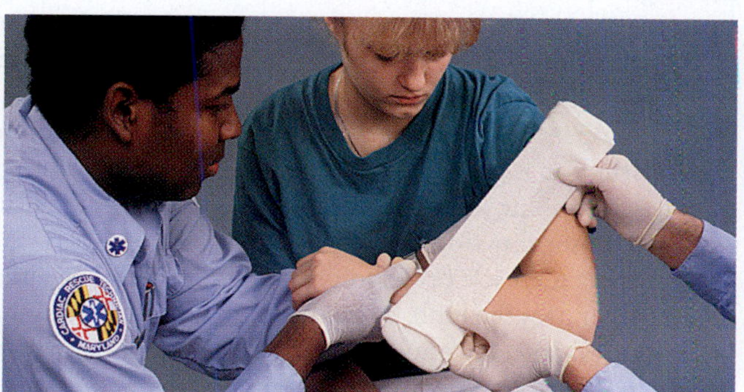

■ **Figure 22-17** Use a padded board splint to immobilize angulated fractures or dislocations of the elbow.

Wrist/Hand

Fractures of the hand and wrist are commonly associated with direct trauma. They present with very noticeable deformity and significant pain reported by the patient. These fractures are of serious concern to the patient. Since the hand and wrist bones are small, any fracture is in close proximity to a joint. Exercise concern when you care for these injuries because of the possibility of vascular and neural involvement.

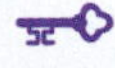

When splinting the distal upper extremity, place padding in the palm of the hand to maintain the position of function.

You can effectively immobilize musculoskeletal injuries of the forearm, wrist, hand, or fingers with a padded rigid, vacuum, or air splint. Place a roll of bandaging, a wad of dressing material, or some similar object in the patient's hand to maintain the position of function. Then secure the extremity to the padded board or inflate the air splint. Be sure to leave some portion of the distal extremity accessible so that you can monitor the adequacy of perfusion and sensation. Place the wrist above the elbow to assist venous return and reduce distal swelling.

Hand and wrist injuries are very common, particularly among athletes and children. A particular type of wrist fracture is the Colles' fracture in which the wrist has a "silver fork" appearance. Fortunately, such injuries are seldom serious and can be managed in the prehospital setting quite easily.

Finger

Forces may displace the phalanges from their joints, resulting in deformity and pain. Displacement usually occurs between the phalanges or between the proximal phalanx and the adjacent metacarpal and moves the bone either anteriorly or posteriorly. (Amputations are multisystem injuries that severely damage the musculoskeletal system. They are addressed in depth in Chapter 20, "Soft-Tissue Trauma.")

Splint finger fractures using tongue blades or small, malleable splints designed for the purpose that you shape to the contour of the injured finger. The finger may also be taped to the adjoining fingers to limit additional motion. The hand is then placed in the position of function and further immobilized.

Finger dislocations usually involve the proximal joint (and sometimes the distal joint) with the digit commonly displacing posteriorly. If reduction is indicated, grasp the distal finger and apply a firm distal traction. Then direct the digit toward the normal anatomical position by moving its proximal end. You should feel the finger "pop" into place, and the digit should resume its normal alignment when compared to the uninjured finger. Splint the finger with a slight bend (10 to 15 degrees) and immobilize the hand in the position of function.

SOFT AND CONNECTIVE TISSUE INJURIES

Tendon, ligament, and muscle injuries are rarely life threatening.

Care for muscular injuries with immobilization, gentle compression with snug dressings, and local cooling to suppress edema and pain.

Tendon, ligament, and muscle injuries are rarely, if ever, life threatening. Massive muscular contusions and hematomas can, however, contribute to hypovolemia, while ligament and tendon injuries can endanger the future function of a limb. Be careful about permitting the patient to put further stress on a limb, especially with higher grades of sprains. The weakened ligaments may fail completely, resulting in dislocation or complete joint instability. For the purpose of care, treat these injuries as you would dislocations and immobilize the adjacent joints. Monitor distal neurovascular function because tissue swelling within the circumferential wrapping of a splint may compress blood vessels and nerves. Care for muscular injuries with immobilization, gentle compression with snug (but not overly tight) dressings, and local cooling to suppress edema and pain using cold packs or ice wrapped in dressing material. Be watchful for signs of compartment syndrome, especially in the calf and forearm regions.

Open wounds involving the muscles, tendons, and ligaments can be severe and debilitating. Carefully evaluate such wounds for signs of connective tissue involvement. Be especially watchful with deep open injuries close to the joints. With such wounds, the likelihood of tendon and ligament disruption is great and may affect the use of the joint, the muscles controlling the joint, or the muscles controlling joint movement distal to the injury. Carefully evaluate for circulation, sensation, and motor function below these injuries.

Injury to a muscle or tendon may limit its ability to either extend or flex the limb. The opposing muscle moves the limb, while the injured muscle cannot return it to the normal position. With limb injuries, note any unusual limb position, especially if the patient is unable to return the limb to a neutral position. At any sign of pain or dysfunction, splint the limb.

MEDICATIONS

Medications are frequently administered to the patient with musculoskeletal injury to relieve pain and to premedicate before the relocation of a dislocation. Medications used include nitrous oxide, diazepam, morphine, fentanyl, and nalbuphine.

Sedatives/Analgesics

Nitrous Oxide Nitrous oxide (Nitronox) is a nitrogen and oxygen compound in a gas state. It is administered in the prehospital setting for its anesthetic properties, specifically to reduce the perception of pain in cases of musculoskeletal injuries. For prehospital care, it is administered in a 50 percent nitrous oxide and 50 percent oxygen mixture via a special regulator and a self-administration mask. Self-administration of nitrous oxide prevents overmedication because the patient will drop the mask when too heavily sedated.

Nitrous oxide is nonexplosive, and its analgesic effects dissipate within 2 to 5 minutes of discontinuing administration. High concentrations of nitrous oxide may lead to hypoxia and may cause respiratory depression and vomiting. These side effects are minimized, however, because the gas is premixed with oxygen by the administration set during prehospital delivery.

The chief concern with the use of nitrous oxide is that it diffuses easily into air-filled spaces in the body, increasing the pressure within them. This diffusion is especially dangerous in patients with pneumothorax or tension pneumothorax, bowel obstruction, and middle ear obstruction. Rule out COPD and these pathologies before you administer nitrous oxide in the prehospital setting.

The nitrous oxide administration device consists of two cylinders of equal size, one holding oxygen (green) and the other, nitrous oxide (blue). The gases are mixed in a special blender/regulator and distributed to the patient when his inspiration generates a less-than-atmospheric pressure. (In other countries, both gases are premixed in one cylinder, reducing the weight and size of the administration device.) The patient must hold the administration mask firmly to the face to trigger administration, thus preventing administration in a patient who is heavily sedated. Nitrous oxide is a controlled substance and its use is carefully monitored for provider abuse.

Diazepam Diazepam (Valium) is a benzodiazepine with both antianxiety and skeletal muscle relaxant qualities. Although it does not have any pain-relieving properties, diazepam does reduce the patient's perception and memory of pain. It is used with musculoskeletal injuries and to premedicate patients before painful procedures such as cardioversion and dislocation reduction. It is administered in a slow IV bolus of 5 to 15 mg, not to exceed 5 mg/minute, into a large vein. Diazepam is rather fast acting, with IV effects occurring almost immediately and reaching peak effectiveness in 15 minutes. Its duration of effectiveness is from 15 to 60 minutes. Do not mix diazepam with any other drugs, and flush the IV line before and after administration. Administer diazepam as close to the IV catheter as possible, and do not inject it into a plastic IV bag. Diazepam is readily absorbed by plastic, which quickly reduces its concentration.

Diazepam is usually supplied in single-use vials or preloaded syringes containing 2 mL of a 5 mg/mL solution (10 mg). Administer 5 to 15 mg IV and repeat in 10 to 15 minutes if necessary.

The effects of diazepam may be reversed by the administration of flumazenil. Usually, 2 mL of a 0.1 mg/mL solution is given IV (over 15 seconds) with a second dose repeated at 60 seconds.

Morphine Morphine sulfate (Duramorph, Astramorph) is an opium alkaloid used to relieve pain (narcotic analgesic), to sedate, and to reduce anxiety. It is used with musculoskeletal injuries for its ability to reduce pain perception. Morphine may reduce vascular volume and cardiac preload by increasing venous capacitance and may thus decrease blood pressure in the hypovolemic patient. It should not be administered to a patient with hypovolemia or hypotension. Its major side effects are respiratory depression and possible nausea and vomiting.

Morphine is available in 10-mL single-use vials or Tubex units of a 1 mg/mL solution or as 1 mL of a 10-mg/mL solution vial for dilution with 9 mL normal saline. Administer a 2-mg bolus slowly IV, repeating as necessary every few minutes to effect.

Naloxone hydrochloride (Narcan) is a narcotic antagonist that can quickly reverse the effects of narcotics (morphine, fentanyl, and nalbuphine) and should be available anytime you use any of these drugs. Naloxone is administered as an IV bolus of 0.4 to 2 mg, repeated every 2 to 3 minutes until effective. Naloxone is a shorter-acting drug than morphine, so repeat doses may be necessary.

Fentanyl Fentanyl is an opiate narcotic, chemically unrelated to morphine, that provides immediate and effective pain control. Fentanyl's onset of action is more rapid than morphine's and it is considerably more potent, thus requiring lower doses. Fentanyl does not cause hypotension to the same degree as does morphine, which makes it an ideal agent for trauma.

Fentanyl is supplied in various doses. The typical starting dose is 25 to 50 mcg IV. Repeat doses of 25 mcg IV can be provided as needed. As with all opiates, continuously monitor the patient's vital signs.

Nalbuphine Nalbuphine hydrochloride (Nubain) is a synthetic narcotic analgesic with properties much like those of morphine. It is equivalent on a milligram-to-milligram basis to morphine, although it antagonizes some of the actions of that drug. Recent studies have questioned the effectiveness of nalbuphine as a prehospital analgesic, and it has fallen into relative disuse. Nalbuphine does not generally decrease blood pressure, although it may produce respiratory depression and bradycardia. Unlike morphine and meperidine, it is not a controlled substance. It is a rapid acting—within 2 to 3 minutes—drug with a long duration of effectiveness—3 to 6 hours.

Nalbuphine is supplied in ampules or preloaded syringes containing 1 mL of a 10 or 20 mg/mL solution. It is administered IV in a dose of 5 mg, then 2 mg repeated as needed up to 20 mg. Narcan will reverse its effects.

OTHER MUSCULOSKELETAL INJURY CONSIDERATIONS

Other areas for special consideration with musculoskeletal injuries include pediatric injuries, athletic injuries, patient refusals and referrals, and the psychological support for the patient with musculoskeletal injury.

Pediatric Musculoskeletal Injury

Children are at higher risk than adults for musculoskeletal injuries due to their activity levels and incompletely developed coordination. Special injuries affecting them include greenstick fractures and epiphyseal fractures.

The incomplete nature of the greenstick fracture produces a stable but angulated limb in the young child. The injured limb is painful and will not bear weight. In these cases, do not attempt to realign the limb and understand that the orthopedic specialist will probably complete the fracture to permit proper healing.

Epiphyseal fractures disrupt the child's growth plate and endanger future bone growth. This injury is likely with fractures within a few inches of the joint because the epiphyseal plate is a point of skeletal weakness. Treat these fractures as you would for an adult, but recognize that they are potentially limb-threatening injuries.

Athletic Musculoskeletal Injuries

Athletes, especially those involved in contact sports like football, soccer, basketball, and wrestling, have a higher incidence of musculoskeletal injuries than the general public. Injuries to the joints, often serious knee and ankle sprains, are common reasons for calls to EMS. Such injuries are especially important because they occur in individuals who are at least moderately well conditioned and result from the application of significant kinetic forces. When you are called to the side of an injured athlete, be especially sensitive to the potential for residual disability caused by these injuries and be predisposed to transport instead of permitting the patient to remain at the scene.

Knowing the athletic trainers in your area may help your on-scene operations run more smoothly and efficiently.

Knowing the athletic trainers in your area may help your on-scene operations run more smoothly and efficiently. In many cases, the athletic trainer works under the supervision of a local physician much as you work under medical direction. It is important for trainers to understand that, once you are called to the scene, the injured athlete becomes a patient of the EMS system and will be treated under the system's medical direction and protocols. Also, as the representative of that system, you are likely to assume responsibility for decisions about care and transport of the patient. Ensuring that trainers understand these facts may eliminate confrontations over care of injured athletes.

Athletic trainers use the acronym RICE to identify the recommended treatment for sprains, strains, and other soft-tissue injuries. RICE stands for: *R*est the extremity, *I*ce for the first 48 hours, *C*ompress with an elastic bandage, and *E*levate for venous drainage. This is consistent with standard emergency care for sprains and strains. (Note, however, that the application of the elastic bandage in this case is to strengthen the limb for further activity and is not recommended for prehospital care.)

Content Review

RICE Procedure for Strains, Sprains, and Soft-Tissue Injuries

- *R*est the extremity
- *I*ce for first 48 hours
- *C*ompress with elastic bandage
- *E*levate extremity

Patient Refusals and Referral

In some situations, you may encounter a patient suffering from an isolated sprain or strain with no significant mechanism of injury and no other signs, symptoms, or complaints. This patient may refuse your assistance or be a candidate for on-scene treatment and referral for follow-up medical care. Evaluate the need for immobilization and X-rays and determine if the patient should seek immediate care in an emergency department or see a personal physician. Any referral to a personal physician must be done in conjunction with medical direction and following local protocol.

Contact medical direction and follow local protocols with patient refusals and referrals. Document such cases thoroughly.

Psychological Support for the Musculoskeletal Injury Patient

Regardless of the specific type of injury sustained, patients need psychological as well as physiological support. Too often, we concentrate all efforts on the patient's injuries, forgetting the emotional impact that the incident and the emergency care measures employed have on the patient. Keep in mind that patients are not frequently exposed to injuries. They do not know what effects injuries will have on their lives or what to expect from medical care in the prehospital, emergency department, or in-hospital settings. Remember that you can have a significant impact on a patient's emotional response to trauma. Displaying a concerned attitude and a professional demeanor and communicating frequently and compassionately with patients will go far to calm and reassure them. Simple attention paid to the patient may make the experience with prehospital emergency medical service one that is remembered positively.

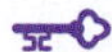

Psychological support provided by the paramedic can have a significant impact on a patient's emotional response to trauma.

Summary

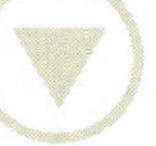

Injuries to the bones, ligaments, tendons, and muscles of the extremities rarely threaten your patient's life. Major exceptions to this statement are pelvic and serious or bilateral femur fractures, in which associated hemorrhage can contribute significantly to hypovolemia and shock. In addition, serious musculoskeletal trauma suggests the possibility of other, life-threatening trauma and, in fact, occurs in about 80 percent of cases of major multisystem trauma. The presence of serious musculoskeletal trauma should increase your index of suspicion for other serious internal injuries.

Care for isolated musculoskeletal trauma is usually delayed until the ABCs and other patient life threats are stabilized. The goals of the care are to protect any open wounds, position affected limbs properly, immobilize the area of injury, and carefully monitor distal extremities to ensure neurovascular function.

Pelvic and bilateral femur fractures are immobilized through application of the PASG. This device both provides splinting for the pelvis and upper portion of the lower extremity and helps control internal blood loss in the region. Manage other fractures by aligning the extremity with gentle traction and immobilizing it by splinting. In cases where you discover a loss of distal neurovascular function, move the extremity slightly to restore distal neurovascular function and then splint.

Joint injuries carry a greater risk of damage to distal circulation, sensation, and motor function. Splint these injuries as you find them unless there is distal neurovascular compromise. If that is the case, employ gentle manipulation to restore circulation, motor function, or sensation. If gentle manipulation is unsuccessful and transport is to be delayed, attempt reduction of dislocations for the hip, knee, ankle, shoulder, or finger as permitted by local protocol.

Care for injuries to connective and muscular tissues by immobilizing the area of injury in the position of function. Evaluate distal extremities for pulse, capillary refill, color, temperature, sensation, and motor function before, during, and after any immobilization or movement of a limb and provide frequent monitoring thereafter.

Review Questions

1. Overexertion can cause which of the following muscle injuries?
   a. muscle fatigue
   b. muscle cramp
   c. muscle strain
   d. all of the above
2. Joints can move beyond their normal range of motion with a great enough applied force. This movement causes a complete displacement of bone ends from their normal position, is known as a(n) ___________, and is characterized by___________.
   a. oblique fracture; pain, edema, and possibly bleeding
   b. dislocation; pain, edema, and immobility
   c. grade III sprain; severe pain and spasm without joint instability
   d. subluxation; pain, rapid edema, and an unlimited range of motion
3. A grade ___________ sprain may present as a fracture.
   a. I
   b. II
   c. III
   d. IV
4. A small crack in a bone that does not disrupt its total structure is called a(n) ___________ fracture.
   a. open
   b. closed
   c. fatigue
   d. hairline
5. A break in a bone in which the bone is compressed on itself is known as:
   a. compartment syndrome.
   b. dislocation.
   c. impacted fracture.
   d. comminuted fracture.
6. A common disintegration of the articular joints often associated with the aging process describes degenerative joint disease. Another disorder, characterized by inflammation of the synovial joints and causing immobility, pain, and fatigue, is known as:
   a. osteoarthritis.
   b. costrochondritis.
   c. inflammatory gout.
   d. rheumatoid arthritis.
7. A thickened area that forms at the site of a fracture is called a(n):
   a. crystal.
   b. disphysis.
   c. bursa.
   d. callus.
8. A femur fracture may account for as much as ___________ mL of blood loss.
   a. 1,000
   b. 1,500
   c. 2,000
   d. 2,500
9. You should stop attempts to realign a limb with a suspected fracture if:
   a. there is no resistance to movement.
   b. the patient reports a significant increase in pain.
   c. the injury is within 3 inches of the midshaft.
   d. all of the above

10. Ladder splints, metal sheet splints, and vacuum splints are examples of:
    a. formable splints.
    b. soft splints.
    c. rigid splints.
    d. pneumatic anti-shock garments.
11. Your patient has been involved in a motor-vehicle collision. You suspect concurrent femur and pelvic fractures. Treatment of this patient would best be provided by:
    a. traction device, long board, transport to trauma center.
    b. long board, one IV line, transport to emergency department.
    c. traction device, PASG, transport to trauma center.
    d. PASG, supportive oxygen and fluid therapies, transport to trauma center.
12. The term *reduction* refers to:
    a. straightening an angulated fracture.
    b. returning displaced bone ends to normal position.
    c. a stage of the bone repair cycle.
    d. application of warm packs to an area of swelling.

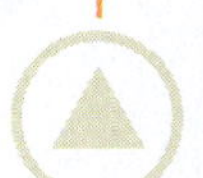

See Answers to Review Questions at the back of this book.

Chapter

23

Head, Facial, and Neck Trauma

Objectives

After reading this chapter, you should be able to:

1. Describe the incidence, morbidity, and mortality of head, facial, and neck injuries. (pp. 959–960)
2. Explain head and facial anatomy and physiology. (see Chapter 3)
3. Differentiate between the following types of facial injuries, highlighting the defining characteristics of each:
   - A. Eye (pp. 975–977)
   - B. Ears (pp. 974–975)
   - C. Nose (pp. 973–974)
   - D. Throat (pp. 977–978)
   - E. Mouth (p. 973)
4. Predict head, facial, and other related injuries based on mechanism of injury. (pp. 960–961)
5. Differentiate between facial injuries based on the assessment and history. (pp. 972–977)
6. Explain the pathophysiology, assessment, and management for patients with eye, ear, nose, throat, and mouth injuries. (pp. 972–997)
7. Explain anatomy and relate physiology of the CNS to head injuries. (pp. 966–972)
8. Distinguish between facial, head, and brain injury. (pp. 961–977)
9. Explain the pathophysiology of head/brain injuries. (pp. 960–972)
10. Explain the concept of increasing intracranial pressure (ICP). (pp. 969–970)
11. Explain the effect of increased and decreased carbon dioxide on ICP. (pp. 969–970)
12. Define and explain the process involved with each of the levels of increasing ICP. (pp. 969–970)
13. Relate assessment findings associated with head/brain injuries to the pathophysiologic process. (pp. 961–972)

14. Classify head injuries (mild, moderate, severe) according to assessment findings. (pp. 966–970)
15. Identify the need for rapid intervention and transport of the patient with a head/brain injury. (pp. 978, 984)
16. Describe and explain the general management of the head/brain injury patient, including pharmacological and nonpharmacological treatment. (pp. 985–996)
17. Analyze the relationship between carbon dioxide concentration in the blood and management of the airway in the head/brain injured patient. (pp. 969–970)
18. Explain the pathophysiology, assessment, and management of a patient with:
    A. Scalp injury (pp. 961–962, 980–981, 985–996)
    B. Skull fracture (pp. 962–965, 980–981, 985–996)
    C. Cerebral contusion (pp. 966–967, 985–996)
    D. Intracranial hemorrhage (including epidural, subdural, subarachnoid, and intracerebral hemorrhage) (pp. 967–968, 985–996)
    E. Axonal injury (including concussion and moderate and severe diffuse axonal injury) (pp. 968, 985–996)
    F. Facial injury (pp. 972–977, 985–996)
    G. Neck injury (pp. 977–978, 982, 985–996)
19. Develop a management plan for the removal of a helmet for a head-injured patient. (p. 979)
20. Differentiate between the types of head/brain injuries based on the assessment and history. (pp. 960–985)
21. Given several preprogrammed and moulaged head, face, and neck trauma patients, provide the appropriate scene size-up, primary assessment, secondary assessment (rapid trauma or focused physical exam, detailed exam), and reassessments and provide appropriate patient care and transportation. (pp. 959–997)

Key Terms

acute retinal artery occlusion, p. 976
anterograde amnesia, p. 970
bilateral periorbital ecchymosis, p. 964
Cheyne-Stokes respirations, p. 971
concussion, p. 968
consensual reactivity, p. 981
contrecoup injury, p. 966
coup injury, p. 966
Cushing's reflex, p. 971
Cushing's triad, p. 971
diffuse axonal injury (DAI), p. 968
diplopia, p. 973
epidural hematoma, p. 967
fasciculations, p. 993
Glasgow Coma Scale (GCS), p. 972
hyphema, p. 975
intracerebral hemorrhage, p. 967
Le Fort criteria, p. 973
retinal detachment, p. 976
retroauricular ecchymosis, p. 964
retrograde amnesia, p. 970
subdural hematoma, p. 967

INTRODUCTION

Head, facial, and neck injuries are common with major trauma. Approximately 4 million people experience a significant head impact each year, with 1 in 10 requiring hospitalization. While most of these hospitalizations are due to relatively minor injuries, severe head injury is the most frequent cause of trauma death. It is especially lethal in auto crashes and frequently produces significant long-term disability in patients who survive them. Gunshot wounds that penetrate the cranium result in a mortality of about 75 to 80 percent. Injuries to the face and neck threaten critical airway structures as well as the significant vasculature found in these regions.

Severe head injury is the most frequent cause of trauma death.

The populations most at risk for serious head injury are males between the years of 15 and 24, infants and young children, and the elderly. Education programs promoting safe practices in many different fields and the use of head protection, seat belts, and air bags have had major effects on reducing head injury mortality and morbidity. The use of helmets for bicycling, rollerblading, and motorcycling and in contact sports such as football has also significantly reduced the incidence of serious head injury. In motorcycle crashes, for example, helmet use reduces serious head injury by more than 50 percent. Once a head injury occurs, however, time becomes a critical consideration. Intracranial hemorrhage and progressing edema can increase the intracranial pressure, hypoxia, and the internal and permanent damage done.

PATHOPHYSIOLOGY OF HEAD, FACIAL, AND NECK INJURY

Head, facial, and neck injuries are difficult to assess in the prehospital setting, yet they commonly threaten life or may expose victims to lifelong disability. A clearer appreciation of the anatomy of these regions, of the various mechanisms of injury affecting them, and of the specific pathological processes related to head, facial, and neck injury can help you better anticipate, assess, and then manage these injuries and their effects on the human system.

MECHANISMS OF INJURY

Injuries to the head, neck, and face are divided by mechanisms of injury into blunt (closed) and penetrating (open).

Blunt Injury

The structures of the head, face, and neck protect very well against most blunt trauma. At times, however, the forces producing blunt trauma are of such magnitude as to compromise the body's well-designed protective mechanisms. For example, head injuries most frequently result from auto and motorcycle crashes and account for more than half of vehicle crash deaths. Sports-related impacts, falling objects, falls, and acts of violence, like assault with a club, are less common, but still significant mechanisms of head injury (Figure 23-1 ■).

The face is another area frequently subjected to blunt trauma. Significant facial injury occurs less frequently than head injury in auto impacts because the head's frontal or parietal regions are more likely to impact the windshield than the face. The same holds true for falls, as the arms, chest,

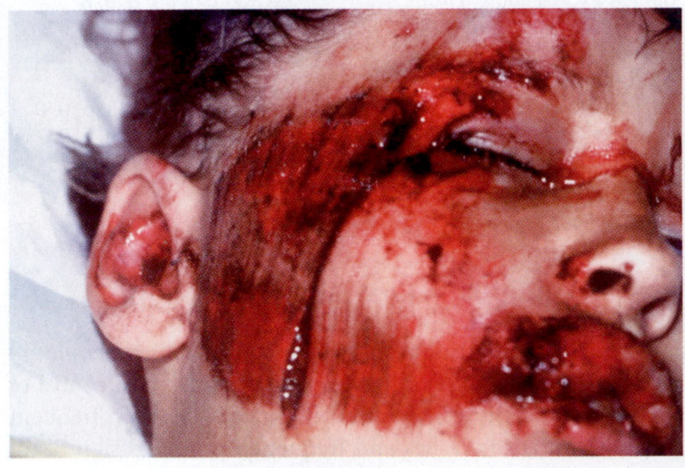

■ **Figure 23-1** Blunt injury to the facial region can produce hemorrhage, soft-tissue injuries, internal fractures, and brain injuries.

or head absorb energy as the conscious victim tries to protect the facial area from injury. Intentional violence is less likely to spare the facial region. The face is often the target of blows from a fist or from impact-enhancing objects like sticks or clubs. The middle and inner ears and the eyes are very well protected against most blunt trauma, though ear injury may be caused by compressional forces associated with diving or explosions. The eyes may occasionally be injured by impacts from smaller blunt objects like a racquetball, baseball, or tennis ball.

The neck is anatomically well protected from most blunt trauma because the head and chest protrude more anteriorly. Laterally, the neck is protected as the shoulders protrude a significant distance from the neck. The neck is, however, a point of impact in special situations. For example, during an auto crash the neck may strike the steering wheel or be injured by a shoulder strap that is worn without a lap belt. The region may also be impacted by objects during fights or traumatically constricted or distracted during an attempted suicide by hanging.

Penetrating Injury

Penetrating injuries to the head, face, and neck are not as common as those resulting from blunt trauma, but they can be just as severe and potentially life threatening. In addition, a penetrating injury to the head suggests the meninges have been opened, producing a route for potentially serious infection.

Penetrating injuries to the head, face, and neck usually result from either gunshots or stabbings. Gunshot wounds are most common and especially hideous because bullets release tremendous energy as they slow during collision with skeletal and central nervous tissue. Similarly, explosions propel projectiles, either intrinsic to the explosive device or from debris produced by the blast, that may penetrate and damage this region. Knife wounds to the head and face tend to be superficial because of the region's extensive skeletal components. The anterior and lateral neck, however, are not as well protected, and wounds there may compromise both the airway and major blood vessels, quickly threatening the patient's life.

There are many other types of penetrating injuries that may involve the head, face, and neck. Some examples include the "clothesline" impact with a wire fence while a victim is riding an all-terrain vehicle or snowmobile; bites from humans, dogs, and other animals; or a tongue bitten when the victim traps it between the teeth during an impact. Infrequently, a fall may impale a person on a fixed object such as a concrete reinforcing bar, producing a penetrating injury.

Blunt and penetrating injury mechanisms have different impacts depending on the structures they involve. The following sections discuss the pathological processes of injuries as they affect the head, face, and neck.

HEAD INJURY

Head injury is defined as a traumatic insult to the cranial region that may result in injury to soft tissues, bony structures, and the brain. Let us look at head injury as it progresses from the exterior to the interior, examining scalp, cranial, and brain injuries.

Scalp Injury

The most superficial head injuries involve the scalp (Figure 23-2 ■). A scalp injury may also be the only overt indication of deeper, more serious injury beneath. The scalp overlies the firm cranium and is very vascular. Its blood vessels lack the ability to constrict as effectively as those elsewhere in the body; hence, scalp wounds tend to bleed heavily. Some people believe that head injuries do not result in shock. This, however, assumes that the hemorrhage they cause is easy to control. In fact, any serious blood loss from scalp wounds can contribute to shock and, if left uncontrolled, may itself cause hypovolemia and shock. Scalp wounds further provide a route for infection because emissary veins drain from the dural sinuses, through the cranium, and into the superficial venous circulation. Because of rich circulation to the area, scalp wounds tend to heal well.

■ **Figure 23-2** Scalp wounds can bleed heavily.

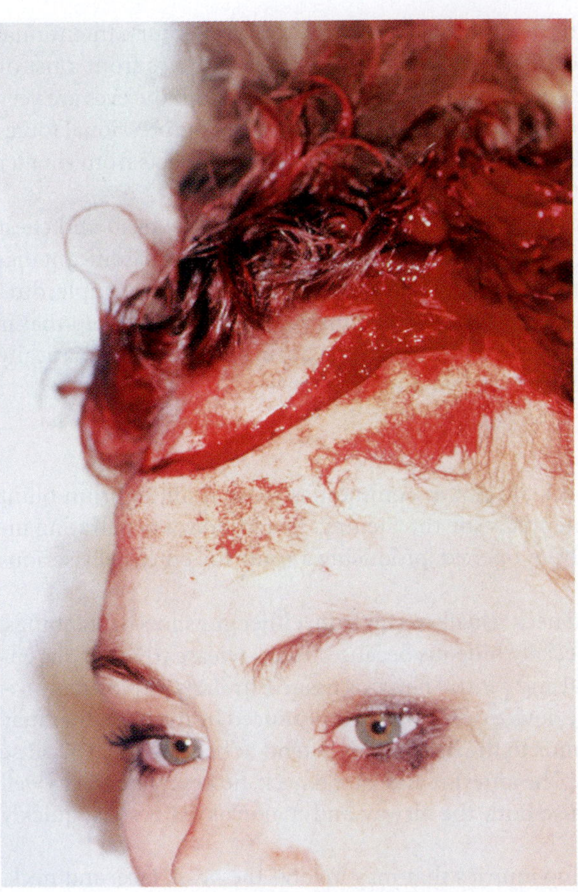

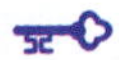

The presentation of scalp wounds may make them difficult to assess.

Scalp wounds may present in a manner that confounds assessment (Figure 23-3 ■). Usually, blunt trauma creates a contusion that, because of the firm skull underneath, expands outwardly in a very rapid and noticeable way. However, blunt trauma may also tear underlying fascia and areolar tissue, causing it to separate. This can leave an elevated border surrounding a depression, mimicking the contour of a depressed skull fracture. However, the scalp's blood vessels may bleed into a depressed skull fracture, fill any depression, and conceal the injury's true nature.

A common and special type of scalp wound is the avulsion. Areolar tissue is only loosely attached to the skull, and glancing blows can create a shearing force against the scalp's border. Such blows frequently tear a flap of scalp loose and fold it back against the uninjured scalp, exposing a portion of the cranium. The mechanism of injury may also seriously contaminate the wound and may cause moderate hemorrhage unless the avulsed tissue folds back sharply, compressing the blood vessels.

Cranial Injury

The temporal bone is one of the thinnest and most frequently fractured cranial bones.

Because of its spherical shape and skeletal design, the skull does not fracture unless trauma is extreme. Such fractures may present as linear, depressed, comminuted, or basilar in nature (Figure 23-4 ■). Linear fractures are small cracks in the cranium and represent about 80 percent of all skull fractures. The temporal bone is one of the thinnest and most frequently fractured cranial bones. If there are no associated intracranial injuries, a linear fracture poses very little danger to the patient. In contrast, a depressed fracture represents an inward displacement of the skull's surface and results in a greater likelihood of intracranial damage. Comminuted fractures involve multiple skull fragments that may penetrate the meninges and cause physical harm to the structures beneath.

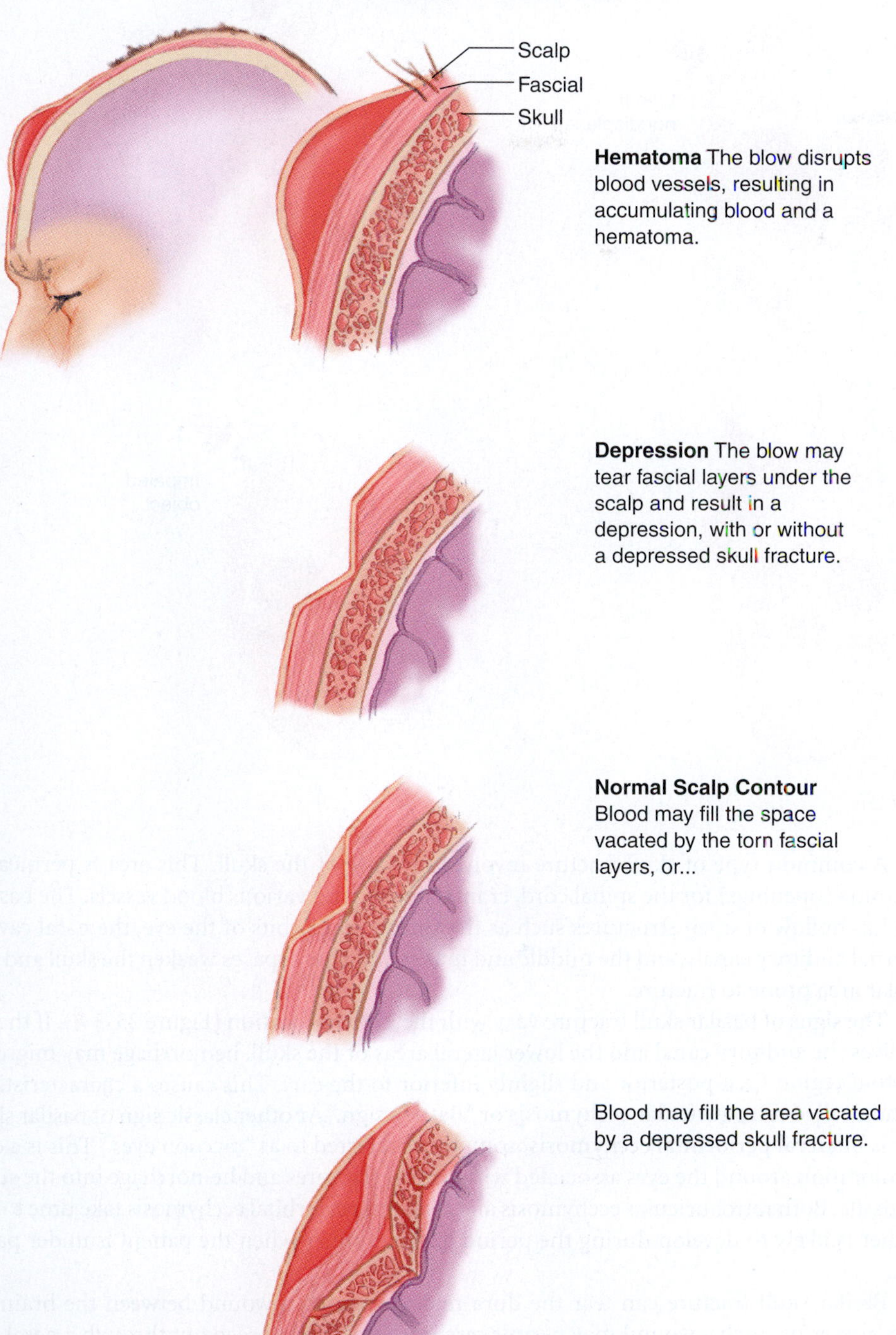

■ Figure 23-3 Scalp/head injuries can present as a raised hematoma, a depression, or be disguised by a normal scalp contour.

■ Figure 23-4 Various types of skull fractures may occur.

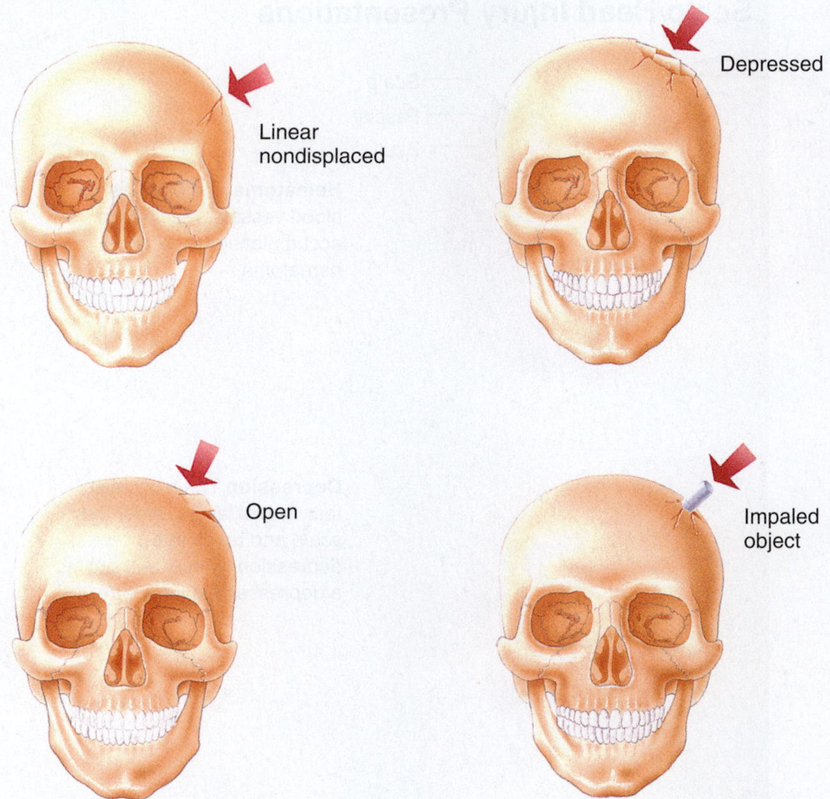

retroauricular ecchymosis *black-and-blue discoloration over the mastoid process (just behind the ear) that is characteristic of a basilar skull fracture (also called Battle's sign).*

bilateral periorbital ecchymosis *black-and-blue discoloration of the area surrounding the eyes. It is usually associated with basilar skull fracture (also called raccoon eyes).*

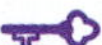

The "halo" sign is most reliable when associated with fluid leaking from the ear.

The glucose level of CSF is normally half that of the blood. If you are unsure whether a clear fluid is water or CSF, check the glucose level of the fluid and compare it to the patient's blood glucose level.

A common type of skull fracture involves the base of the skull. This area is permeated with foramina (openings) for the spinal cord, cranial nerves, and various blood vessels. The basilar skull also has hollow or open structures such as the sinuses, the orbits of the eye, the nasal cavities, the external auditory canals, and the middle and inner ears. These spaces weaken the skull and leave the basilar area prone to fracture.

The signs of basilar skull fracture vary with the injury's location (Figure 23-5 ■). If the fracture involves the auditory canal and the lower lateral areas of the skull, hemorrhage may migrate to the mastoid region (just posterior and slightly inferior to the ear). This causes a characteristic discoloration called **retroauricular ecchymosis** or "Battle's sign." Another classic sign of basilar skull fracture is **bilateral periorbital ecchymosis,** sometimes referred to as "raccoon eyes." This is a dramatic discoloration around the eyes associated with orbital fractures and hemorrhage into the surrounding tissue. Both retroauricular ecchymosis and bilateral periorbital ecchymosis take time to develop; neither is likely to develop during the period after an injury when the patient is under paramedic care.

Basilar skull fracture can tear the dura mater, opening a wound between the brain and the body's exterior. Such a wound may permit cerebrospinal fluid to seep out through a nasal cavity or an external auditory canal and also provide a possible route for infection to enter the meninges.

This type of wound may also provide an escape for cerebrospinal fluid in the presence of increasing intracranial pressure. Escaping cerebrospinal fluid may mediate the rise in ICP and somewhat limit damage to the brain. (While cerebrospinal fluid is an important medium, the body can regenerate it quite rapidly.) Blood mixed with cerebrospinal fluid and flowing from the nose, mouth, or ears will demonstrate the target or "halo" sign (a dark red circle surrounded by a lighter yellowish one) when dropped on a pillow or towel (Figure 23-6 ■). Normal blood demonstrates a narrow concentric ring of yellowish coloration surrounding the red circle produced by the less mobile erythrocytes. If cerebrospinal fluid is mixed with the blood, this outer ring is much larger. Be aware, however, other fluids, like lacrimal or nasal fluids or saliva, may cause a similar response. Hence, the halo sign is most reliable when associated with fluid leaking from the ear.

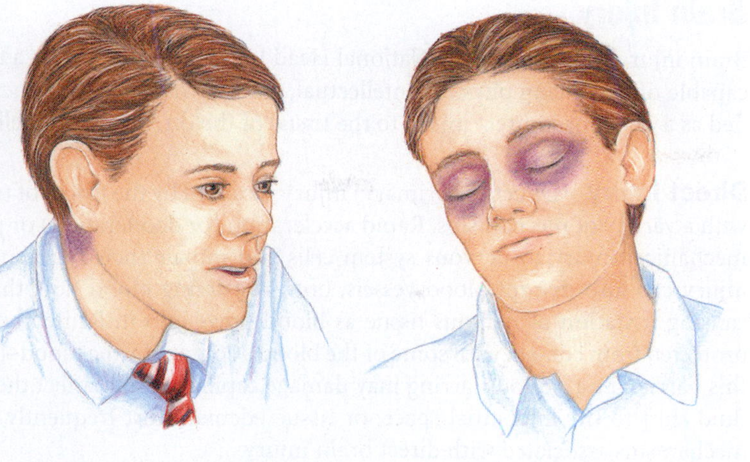

Retroauricular ecchymosis (Battle's sign).

Bilateral periorbital ecchymosis (raccoon eyes).

■ **Figure 23-5** Retroauricular or periorbital ecchymosis may indicate a basilar skull fracture.

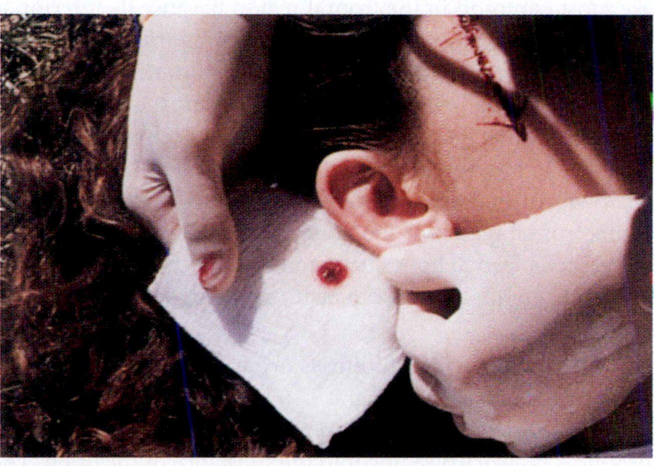

■ **Figure 23-6** The "halo test" can detect the presence of cerebrospinal fluid. If CSF is present, it will diffuse faster across a paper towel or gauze because it is thinner than blood.

Bullet impacts induce specific types of cranial fracture. The entrance wound often produces a comminuted fracture and sends bone fragments into the brain. Often the bullet's kinetic energy is sufficient to permit the bullet to exit from the cranium and cause a second fracture. This exit wound site is blown outward and is often more severe in appearance than the entrance wound.

In many cases, the energy of the projectile's passage through the cranium causes a cavitational wave of extreme pressure, which is contained and enhanced by the rigid container of the skull. The result is extreme damage to the cranial contents, and, if the transmitted kinetic energy is strong enough, the skull may fracture and "explode" outward.

Another type of wound occurs when a bullet enters the cranium at an angle, is deflected within, and continues to move along the cranium's interior until its energy is completely exhausted. This process does devastating damage to the cerebral cortex and is rarely survivable.

A special type of cranial injury involves an impaled object. As is the case with objects impaled in most other regions of the body, any further motion of the object may cause additional hemorrhage and tissue damage. When the object is impaled in the cranium, the situation is especially serious. Brain tissue is much more delicate than other body tissue, does not immobilize the object as well, and is easily injured by the object's motion. As with objects impaled elsewhere, removal of the impaled object from the cranium may cause further injury and increase blood accumulation.

Note that a cranial fracture, by itself, is a skeletal injury that will heal with time; it does not, by itself, threaten the brain. Rather, it is the possibility of injury beneath and suggested by the skull fracture that is of greatest concern. The forces necessary to fracture the cranium are extreme and likely to cause injury within.

A cranial fracture, by itself, is a skeletal injury that will heal with time. However, the forces necessary to fracture the skull are often sufficient to induce brain injury.

Brain Injury

Brain injury is defined by the National Head Injury Foundation as "a traumatic insult to the brain capable of producing physical, intellectual, emotional, social, and vocational changes." It is classified as a direct or indirect injury to the tissue of the cerebrum, cerebellum, or brainstem.

coup injury *an injury to the brain occurring on the same side as the site of impact.*

contrecoup injury *occurring on the opposite side; an injury to the brain opposite the site of impact.*

Content Review

Types of Direct Brain Injury

Focal

- Cerebral contusion
- Intracranial hemorrhage
- Epidural hematoma
- Subdural hematoma
- Intracerebral hemorrhage

Diffuse

- Concussion (mild to moderate diffuse axonal injury)
- Moderate diffuse axonal injury
- Severe diffuse axonal injury (formerly, brainstem injury)

Direct Injury Direct (or primary) injury is caused by the forces of trauma and can be associated with a variety of mechanisms. Rapid acceleration (or deceleration) or penetrating injury can cause mechanical injury to nervous system cells and impair their function. The forces causing direct injury can also disrupt blood vessels, both restricting blood flow through the injured area and causing irritation of nervous tissue as blood flows into it. Remember that the brain is specially protected from contact with some of the blood's content by the blood–brain barrier. Injury disrupts this barrier. Last, serious jarring may damage capillary walls, affect their permeability, and cause a fluid shift to the interstitial space, or tissue edema. Most frequently, there is a mixture of these mechanisms associated with direct brain injury.

Two specific types of direct brain injury are coup and contrecoup injury (Figure 23-7 ■). **Coup injuries** are tissue disruptions that occur directly at the point of impact. These injuries are inflicted as the brain displaces toward the impact surface and collides with the interior of the cranium. They are most common in the frontal region because its interior surface is rough and irregular. In contrast, the occipital areas are smooth; coup injuries occur there less frequently. Coup injury may also occur as the brain slides along the rough contours at the base of the skull.

Contrecoup injuries produce tissue damage away from the impact point as the brain, floating in cerebrospinal fluid inside the cranium, "sloshes" toward the impact, then away from it, again impacting the interior of the skull. For example, a blow to the forehead might result in injury to the occipital region (visual center) and produce visual disturbances (seeing stars). Contrecoup injury to the frontal region of the brain is most common (from an impact to the occipital region) again because the frontal bones have an irregular inner surface.

Direct brain injuries can be further assigned to one of two specific categories—focal or diffuse.

Focal Injuries Focal injuries occur at a specific location in the brain and include contusions and intracranial hemorrhages.

Cerebral Contusion A cerebral contusion is caused by blunt trauma to local brain tissue that produces capillary bleeding into the substance of the brain. The contusion is relatively common with blunt head injuries and often produces prolonged confusion or other types of neurologic deficit. This pathology may result from a coup or contrecoup mechanism and may occur at one or several sites in the brain. The localized form of the injury manifests with dysfunctions related to the site of the injury.

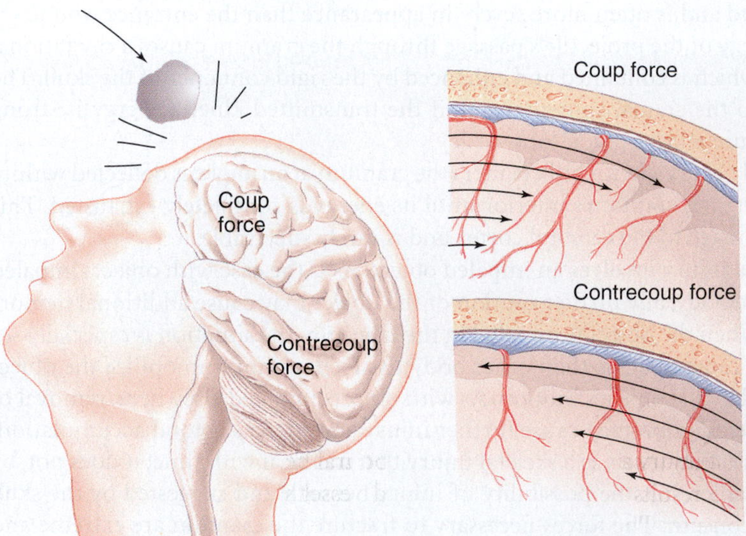

■ **Figure 23-7** Coup and contrecoup movement of the brain.

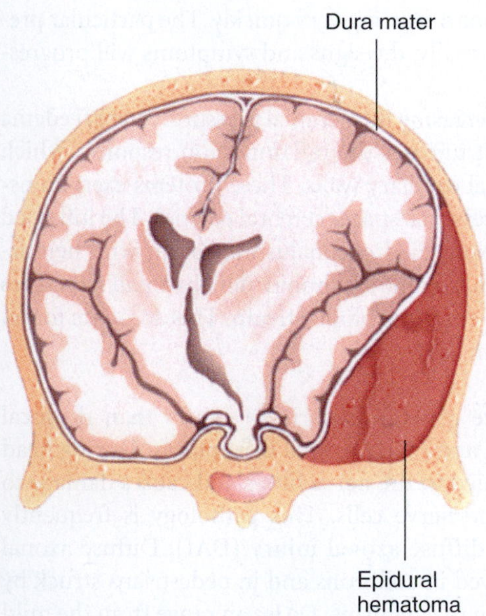

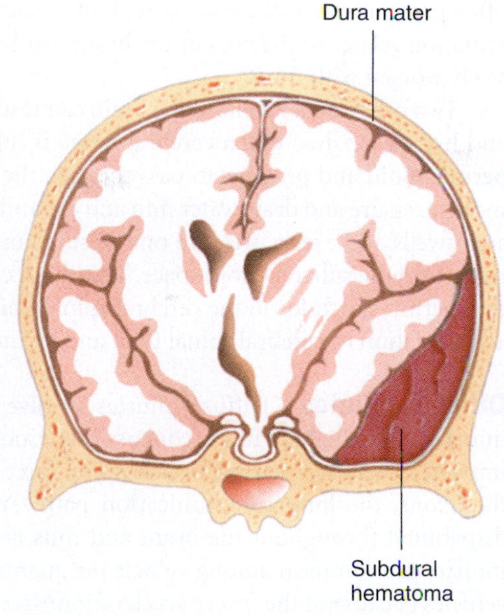

■ **Figure 23-8** Epidural hematoma.

■ **Figure 23-9** Subdural hematoma.

For example, a patient who suffers a contusion of the frontal lobe after trauma to the forehead may experience personality changes. (Remember, the frontal lobe is the most commonly injured lobe.)

Intracranial Hemorrhage Bleeding can occur at several locations within the brain, each presenting with a different pathological process. These injuries—proceeding from the most superficial to the deepest—are epidural, subdural, and intracerebral hemorrhages. In contrast to patients with concussions and contusions, expect the intracranial hemorrhage patient to deteriorate during your assessment and care because of associated indirect injury such as increasing intracranial pressure.

Bleeding between the dura mater and the skull's interior surface is called **epidural hematoma** (Figure 23-8 ■). It usually involves arterial vessels, often the middle meningeal artery in the temporal region. Because the bleeding is from a relatively high-pressure vessel, intracranial pressure builds rapidly, compressing the cerebrum and increasing the pressure within the skull. As pressure builds, the patient moves quickly toward unresponsiveness. The hemorrhage-induced increase in intracranial pressure reduces oxygenated circulation to the nerve cells (indirect injury). Bleeding may be so extensive that it displaces the brain away from the injury site, pushing it toward the foramen magnum. Although the progression is both rapid and life threatening, immediate surgery can frequently reverse it.

epidural hematoma *accumulation of blood between the dura mater and the cranium.*

Bleeding within the meninges, specifically beneath the dura mater and within the subarachnoid space, is called **subdural hematoma** (Figure 23-9 ■). This type of bleeding occurs very slowly and may have a subtle presentation because blood loss is usually due to rupture of a small venous vessel, often one of those bridging to the dural sinuses. The vessel most commonly involved is the superior sagittal sinus. Because the subdural hemorrhage occurs above the pia mater, it does not cause the cerebral irritation associated with intracerebral hemorrhage. The free blood in the cerebrospinal fluid may clog the structures responsible for the fluid's reabsorption, which can result in an increasing intracranial pressure. The patient usually does not show overt signs and symptoms until hours or even days after the injury. Because of this delay, subdural hemorrhage is difficult to detect in the prehospital setting.

subdural hematoma *collection of blood directly beneath the dura mater.*

Suspect subdural hematoma in a medical (nontrauma) patient who demonstrates neurologic signs and symptoms. Careful history taking may uncover a recent mechanism of injury, such as a fall, that could cause this presentation. You occasionally encounter such pathologies with the elderly or with chronic alcoholics. Because both the aging process and chronic alcoholism reduce the size of the brain, head impact causes greater and less controlled motion of the brain within the cranium. This increases the likelihood of injury and, specifically, the subdural hematoma.

Suspect subdural hematoma in a medical (nontrauma) patient who demonstrates neurologic signs and symptoms.

Intracerebral hemorrhage results from a ruptured blood vessel within the substance of the brain. Although blood loss is generally minimal, it is particularly damaging. Tissue edema results because free blood, outside the blood vessels, irritates the nervous tissue. Intracerebral hemorrhage

intracerebral hemorrhage *bleeding directly into the tissue of the brain.*

often presents much like a stroke with the manifestations occurring very quickly. The particular presentation relates to the area of the brain involved. Normally, the signs and symptoms will progressively worsen with time.

Two other local insults to the brain can result in increasing intracranial pressure: cerebral edema and hydrocephalus. When cerebral tissue is injured, it initiates the inflammation response, which permits fluid and proteins to pass through the cerebral capillary walls. These proteins exert an osmotic pressure and draw water into and expand the interstitial space (cerebral edema). The inflamed area swells and exerts pressure on the surrounding tissue. Hydrocephalus may occur with hemorrhage into the subarachnoid space. The blood cells then clog the arachnoid villi, the small structures that permit the fluids in the cerebral spinal fluid to re-enter the blood stream. This accounts for an accumulation of cerebral spinal fluid and an increase in ICP.

Diffuse Injuries Diffuse injuries involve a more general scenario of injury than do focal injuries. They include mild (concussions), moderate, and severe axonal disruptions. During head impact, a shearing, tearing, or stretching force is applied to the nerve fibers and causes damage to the axons, the long communication pathways of the nerve cells. This pathology is frequently distributed throughout the brain and thus is called **diffuse axonal injury (DAI).** Diffuse axonal injuries are common among vehicle occupants involved in collisions and in pedestrians struck by vehicles because of the severe acceleration/deceleration mechanisms. DAIs can range from the mild (a concussion) to the severe and life threatening (a brainstem injury).

diffuse axonal injury (DAI) *type of brain injury characterized by shearing, stretching, or tearing of nerve fibers with subsequent axonal damage.*

concussion *a transient period of unconsciousness. In most cases, the unconsciousness will be followed by a complete return of function.*

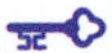

A concussion disrupts the electrical activities of the brain without causing detectable injury to the brain itself.

Concussion A **concussion** is a mild to moderate form of DAI and is the most common outcome of blunt head trauma. It represents nerve dysfunction without substantial anatomic damage (i.e., a normal head CT scan). Concussion results in a transient episode of neuronal dysfunction (confusion, disorientation, event amnesia), followed by a rapid return to normal neurologic activity. Prehospital management of concussion consists of frequent neurologic assessments with attention to the airway, to respiratory effort, and to subtle changes in the level of consciousness. Most patients survive with no neurologic impairment.

A concussion, contusion, intracerebral hemorrhage, subdural hematoma, and epidural hematoma may occur alone or in combination with one another. For example, an injury may cause a patient to sustain a concussion and an epidural hematoma concurrently. The concussion results in immediate unconsciousness, which resolves after only a few minutes. The patient becomes conscious and alert, but then later exhibits a deteriorating level of consciousness. This interim period of consciousness, called a lucid interval, occurs while the epidural hematoma expands.

Moderate Diffuse Axonal Injury Here again, shearing, stretching, or tearing of the axons occurs, but now there is minute bruising of brain tissue. This type of injury is often referred to as the "classic concussion." If the cerebral cortex or reticular activating system of the brainstem is involved, the patient may be rendered unconscious. This type of injury is more severe than a mild concussion, occurs in 20 percent of all severe head injuries, and comprises 45 percent of all DAI cases. Moderate DAI is commonly associated with basilar skull fracture. Although most patients survive this injury, some degree of residual neurologic impairment is common.

Short- and long-term signs and symptoms associated with moderate DAI include immediate unconsciousness, followed by persistent confusion, inability to concentrate, disorientation, and retrograde and anterograde amnesia. The patient may also complain of headache, focal neurologic deficits, light sensitivity (photophobia), and disturbances in smell and other senses. Anxiety may be present, and the patient may experience significant mood swings.

Severe Diffuse Axonal Injury Severe DAI (previously known as brainstem injury) is a significant mechanical disruption of many axons in both cerebral hemispheres with extension into the brainstem. Approximately 16 percent of all severe head injuries and 36 percent of all cases of DAI are classified as severe. Many patients do not survive this type of injury; those that do have some degree of permanent neurologic impairment. The patient experiencing severe DAI is unconscious for a prolonged period of time and displays the signs of increased ICP (Cushing's response and decerebrate or decorticate posturing).

Indirect Injury Indirect (or secondary) injuries are the result of factors that occur because of, though after, the initial (or primary) injury. These processes are progressive and cause the patient deterioration often associated with serious head injuries. The indirect injuries may be as or more damaging than the initial injury because of the unique design of the skull and the especially delicate nature of central nervous system tissue.

Indirect injuries are caused by two distinct pathological processes. The first process is a diminishing circulation to brain tissue (intracranial perfusion) due to an increasing intracranial pressure and possibly exacerbated by hypoxia, hypercarbia, and systemic hypotension. The second process is progressive pressure against, or physical displacement of, brain tissue secondary to an expanding mass within the cranium. Both these pathologies continue and expand the nervous tissue injury and cause some of the specific and progressive signs and symptoms associated with head injury.

Intracranial Perfusion The brain is one of the body's most perfusion-sensitive organs. Any injury that affects perfusion has a rapid and devastating effect on the brain and its control of body systems. Cerebral, cerebellar, and brainstem perfusion may be disrupted both by increasing intracranial pressure and by low systemic blood pressure (hypotension).

As discussed in Chapter 3, the cranial volume is fixed and does not vary. The cerebrum, cerebellum, and brainstem account for 80 percent (1,200 mL) of this volume. Venous, capillary, and arterial blood account for most of the remaining space, or about 12 percent (150 mL), while cerebrospinal fluid accounts for roughly the remaining 8 percent (90 mL). Any increase in the size of one internal component must be matched by a similar reduction in another component. If it is not, the intracranial pressure (ICP) will rise.

As a mass expands within the cranium, the first means of compensating for the expansion is compression of the venous blood vessels. If the mass continues to expand, the next intracranial volume affected is the cerebrospinal fluid, which is pushed out of the cranium and into the spinal cord. These mechanisms respond very quickly and maintain an ICP very close to normal. However, once they reach their compensatory limits, the intracranial pressure rises quickly and begins to restrict arterial blood flow. The reduction in cerebral blood flow triggers a rise in the systemic blood pressure in an attempt to ensure adequate cerebral perfusion, a process known as autoregulation. The greater the pressure of arterial blood flow, the greater the ICP. This increase in ICP further increases the resistance to cerebral blood flow, producing more hypoxia and hypercarbia. The resulting additional increase in systolic blood pressure, and then ICP, leads to a worsening, eventually deadly, cycle (Figure 23-10 ■). If the mass, injury (edema), or hemorrhage continues to expand, the ICP becomes so high that cerebral circulation all but stops.

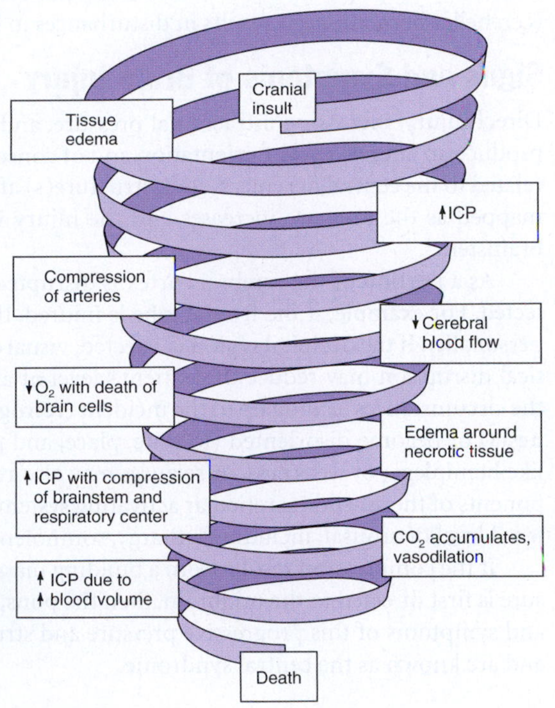

■ **Figure 23-10** Pathway of deterioration following central nervous system insult.

Another factor affecting ICP and circulation through the brain is the level of carbon dioxide in the cerebrospinal fluid. As the carbon dioxide level rises, the cerebral arteries dilate to encourage greater blood flow and reduce the hypercarbia. In the presence of an already high ICP, this process can have devastating results. The brain's response to high carbon dioxide concentrations and the increasing ICP causes the classical hyperventilation and hypertension associated with head injury. Low levels of carbon dioxide, however, can also have dire effects, triggering cerebral arterial constriction. In extreme cases, the resulting constriction can all but stop circulation through the brain. This is the reason that capnography is a valuable tool in the reassessment of head injury patients, especially if you are ventilating them.

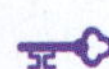

Low blood pressure and poor respiratory exchange seriously compound any existing head injury.

Two systemic problems frequently associated with trauma and sometimes related to brain injury are low blood pressure and poor ventilation. These problems seriously compound any existing head injury through a tertiary injury mechanism.

Hypotension, especially in the brain-injured patient with increasing ICP, may contribute to poor cerebral perfusion pressure. In turn, diminished cerebral circulation causes increasing acidosis (retained carbon dioxide) and anaerobic metabolism. This induces further neural cell injury due to hypoxia and acidosis. At the same time, vasodilation (in response to increasing acidosis and carbon dioxide levels) elevates any existing intracranial pressure.

Review

Content

Signs and Symptoms of Brain Injury

- Altered level of consciousness
- Altered level of orientation
- Alterations in personality
- Amnesia
  - Retrograde
  - Anterograde
- Cushing's triad
  - Increasing blood pressure
  - Slowing pulse rate
  - Irregular respirations
- Vomiting (often without nausea)
- Body temperature changes
- Changes in reactivity of pupils
- Decorticate posturing

Hypoxia, secondary to shock or respiratory injury, increases the severity of any head injury. The reduced blood oxygen levels increase the cellular hypoxia at and around the injury site. Since central nervous tissue is extremely dependent upon good cellular oxygenation, neural cell damage becomes more severe.

Pressure and Structural Displacement As hemorrhage accumulates or edema increases in a region of the brain, this expansion pushes uninjured tissue away from the injury site. Even in the absence of increased ICP, such expansion puts pressure on adjacent brain cells, most commonly along the brainstem. As the mass continues to increase in size, it may physically compress brainstem components. With further expansion, it may push the brain tissue against and around the falx cerebri and the tentorium cerebelli. Because these are basically immobile structures within the skull, the displacement results in a process called herniation. With herniation, a portion of a brain structure is pushed into and through an opening, physically disrupting the structure and compromising its blood supply. If the displacement affects the upper brainstem by pushing it through the tentorium incisura (uncal herniation), it causes vomiting, changes in the level of consciousness, and pupillary dilation. If the displacement affects the medulla oblongata by pushing it into the foramen magnum (cerebellar herniation), it results in disturbances in breathing, blood pressure, and heart rate.

Signs and Symptoms of Brain Injury

Direct injury, increasing intracranial pressure, and compression and displacement of brain tissue produce an altered level of orientation and of consciousness as well as specific signs and symptoms related to the central nervous system structure(s) affected. The actual process of brain injury can be mapped as the pressure increases and the injury moves from the cortical surface and down the brainstem.

As a portion of the cerebral cortex is disrupted by injury, the specific activity it controls is affected. For example, if the frontal lobe is injured, the patient will likely present with alterations in personality. If the occipital region is affected, visual disturbances are expected. A large region of cortical disruption may reduce the patient's level of awareness. The patient may become unaware of the circumstances leading up to the incident (**retrograde amnesia**) or following it (**anterograde amnesia**) or become disoriented (to time, place, and person), confused, or combative. Focal deficits, like hemiplegia or weakness, or seizures may also result. When intracranial injury extends to components of the ascending reticular activating system in the brainstem, the patient may display an altered level of arousal, including lethargy, somnolence, or coma.

retrograde amnesia *inability to remember events that occurred before the trauma that caused the condition.*

anterograde amnesia *inability to remember events that occurred after the trauma that caused the condition.*

If the compression results from a building mass along the central region of the cerebrum, pressure is first directed to the midbrain, then the pons, and finally to the medulla oblongata. The signs and symptoms of this progressive pressure and structural displacement are somewhat predictable and are known as the central syndrome.

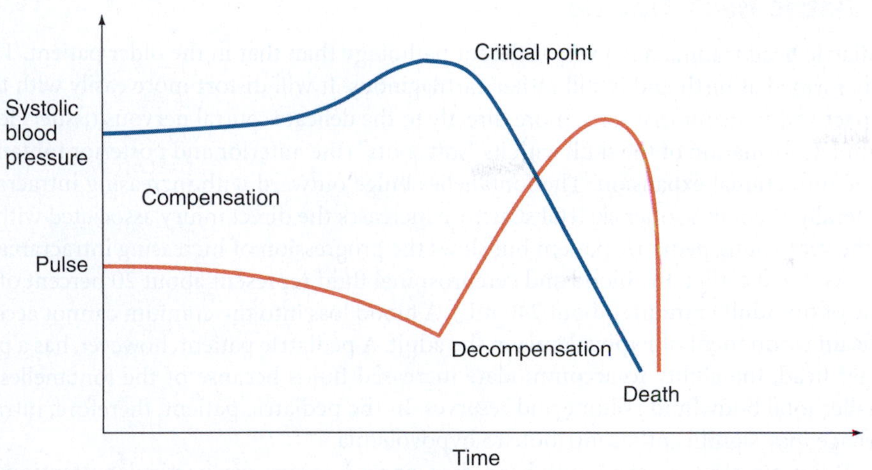

■ **Figure 23-11** How systolic blood pressure and pulse rate respond to increasing intracranial pressure.

In this syndrome, upper brainstem compression produces an increase in blood pressure to maintain cerebral perfusion pressure (called **Cushing's reflex**) and a reflex decrease in heart rate in response to vagus nerve (parasympathetic) stimulation of the SA node and AV junction. The patient may also exhibit a characteristic cyclic breathing pattern called **Cheyne-Stokes respirations.** This consists of increasing, then decreasing, respiratory volumes, followed by a period of apnea. The combination of an increasing blood pressure, slowing pulse, and irregular respirations is a classical sign of brainstem pressure or injury called **Cushing's triad** (Figure 23-11 ■). If the brain injury involves the hypothalamus, the patient may experience vomiting, frequently without nausea, and body temperature changes. The pupils remain small and reactive. Decorticate posturing (body extension with arm flexion) in response to painful stimuli may occur as the neural pathways through the upper brainstem are disrupted.

Cushing's reflex *response due to cerebral ischemia that causes an increase in systemic blood pressure, which maintains cerebral perfusion during increased intracranial pressure.*

Cheyne-Stokes respirations *respiratory pattern of alternating periods of apnea and tachypnea.*

Cushing's triad *the combination of increasing blood pressure, slowing pulse, and erratic respirations in response to increased intracranial pressure.*

As the middle brainstem becomes involved the pulse pressure widens and the heart rate becomes bradycardic. Respirations now may be deep and rapid (central neurologic hyperventilation). Increasing intracranial pressure may also induce pupil sluggishness or nonreactivity (bilaterally since the pathology involves compression from above) as the oculomotor nerve (CN III) is compressed. The patient develops extension (decerebrate) posturing. Few patients ever function normally again once they have reached this ICP level.

Finally, as the pressure reaches the lower brainstem the pupils become fully dilated and unreactive. Respirations become ataxic (erratic with no characteristic rhythm) or may even cease altogether. The pulse rate is often very irregular with great swings in rate. ECG conduction disturbances become apparent, including QRS complex, ST segment, and T wave changes. As control over blood pressure is disrupted, the patient becomes hypotensive. The patient no longer responds to painful stimuli, and the skeletal muscles become flaccid. Patients rarely survive once the ICP rises to this level.

If the mass causing the compression is located more laterally than in the central syndrome just described, the signs and symptoms occur in a less predictable sequence. The pupillary responses, sluggishness, nonreactivity, and dilation, are usually ipsilateral (on the same side) to the expanding mass.

Recognition of Herniation

The recognition of cerebral herniation is essential in the patient with head injury because it directs your care. The patient with herniation has a history of head trauma and is likely to display an increasing blood pressure, decreasing pulse rate, and respirations that become irregular (Cushing's triad). They also may have a lowering level of consciousness (Glasgow Coma Scale < 9 and dropping), singular or bilaterally dilated and fixed pupils, and posturing (decerebrate or decorticate) or no movement with noxious stimuli.

The recognition of cerebral herniation is essential in the patient with head injury because it directs your care.

Pediatric Head Trauma

Pediatric head trauma has a very different pathology than that in the older patient. The skull is not fully formed at birth and is still rather cartilaginous. It will distort more easily with the force of an impact and transmit that force more directly to the delicate central nervous tissue. However, the incomplete formation of the skull with its "soft spots" (the anterior and posterior fontanelles) permits some intracranial expansion. The fontanelles bulge outward with increasing intracranial pressure. Generally, then, this softer skeletal structure increases the direct injury associated with head trauma in the very young pediatric patient but slows the progression of increasing intracranial pressure.

As noted earlier, the blood and cerebrospinal fluid represent about 20 percent of the total volume of the adult cranium (about 240 mL). A blood loss into the cranium cannot account for a significant component of hypovolemia in the adult. A pediatric patient, however, has a proportionally larger head, the ability to accommodate increased fluids because of the fontanelles, and a much smaller total body fluid volume and reserves. In the pediatric patient, therefore, intracranial hemorrhage may significantly contribute to hypovolemia.

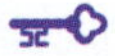

In the pediatric patient, intracranial hemorrhage may significantly contribute to hypovolemia.

When treating an infant with head, face, or neck injury, pay particular attention to the airway. Infants are obligate nasal breathers and must have a patent nasal passage and pharynx to ensure a clear airway. Hyperextension of the head will obstruct the airway as the tongue pushes the soft palate closed. Ensure proper head positioning, and ventilate using both the mouth and nose.

Glasgow Coma Scale

Glasgow Coma Scale (GCS) *scoring system for monitoring the neurologic status of patients with head injuries.*

The **Glasgow Coma Scale** (GCS) is a standardized evaluation tool used to measure a patient's level of consciousness. The scale assesses the best eye opening, verbal, and motor response and awards points for the various responses. Responses must be determined for both sides of the patient and any side-to-side differences noted. (A more detailed discussion of the scale is found later in this chapter.)

Eye Signs

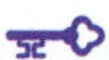

Evaluation of the eyes is very important in patients with suspected head injury.

Pay close attention to the eyes when evaluating a patient with possible head trauma. The eyes are a very specialized body tissue (like central nervous system tissue) and a very visible special sense organ. The eyes can give indications of problems with cranial nerves CN II, III, IV, and VI and with perfusion associated with cerebral blood flow. The surface of the eye is very dependent on good perfusion and lacrimal fluid flow. If perfusion is diminished, the eyes lose their luster quickly. The eyes also give quick, highly visible signs of the patient's demeanor—anxiety, fear, anger, and so forth.

Pupil size and reactivity also give clues to underlying conditions. Depressant drugs or cerebral hypoxia will reduce pupillary responsiveness, while extreme hypoxia causes them to dilate and fix. An expanding cranial lesion places progressive pressure on the oculomotor nerve (CN III), causing the ipsilateral (same side) pupil to become sluggish, then dilated, then fixed. This occurs because the outer oculomotor nerve contains parasympathetic fibers. As increasing pressure interferes with these nerve fibers, the pupil dilates and is unable to constrict. If one pupil is fixed yet shows some response to consensual stimulation (light variations in the other eye), the problem most likely lies with the oculomotor nerve.

FACIAL INJURY

Facial injury is a serious trauma complication, not only because of the cosmetic importance people place on facial appearance, but also because of the region's vasculature and the location of the initial airway and alimentary canal structures and the organs of sight, smell, taste, and hearing present there. Remember, too, that serious facial injuries suggest associated head and spinal injuries.

Facial Soft-Tissue Injury

Facial soft-tissue injury is common and can threaten both the patient's airway and physical appearance. Because of the ample supply of arterial and venous vessels, injuries in the region may bleed heavily, contributing to hypovolemia. Facial injuries are often the result of violence from, for instance, bullet or knife wounds. Superficial injuries and hemorrhage rarely affect the airway. With deep lacerations, however, blood may accumulate and endanger the airway or enter the digestive tract and induce vomiting. Serious blunt or penetrating injury to the soft tissues and skeletal structures supporting the pharynx may reduce the patient's ability to control the airway, increasing the likelihood of foreign body or fluid aspiration and airway compromise. Hypoxia caused by aspiration is more likely caused by blood than by other fluids or physical obstruction.

Remember, the process of inspiration creates a less-than-atmospheric pressure in the lungs to draw air in. This reduction in pressure may collapse damaged structures along the airway that are normally held open by bony or cartilaginous formations. Soft-tissue swelling may also rapidly restrict the airway or close it completely. Swelling and deformity from trauma may distort the facial region so landmarks are hard to recognize, making airway control even more difficult. In serious facial soft-tissue injury, always consider the likelihood of associated injury, especially basilar skull fracture and spine injury.

Patients with serious facial soft-tissue injuries are likely to have associated injury, especially basilar skull fractures and spine injuries.

Facial Dislocations and Fractures

Trauma may result in open or closed facial fractures with significant associated pain, swelling, deformity, crepitus, and hemorrhage. Common injuries include mandibular, maxillary, nasal, and orbital fractures and dislocations.

Mandibular dislocation occurs as the condylar process displaces from the temporomandibular joint, just anterior to the ear. This dislocation may result in the malocclusion of the mouth, misalignment of teeth, deformity of the facial region at or around the joint, immobility of the jaw, and pain. The patient's ability to control the airway may be decreased, but dislocation is not usually a significant airway or breathing threat.

Fractures of the mandible are painful, present with deformity along the jaw's surface, and may result in the loosening of a few teeth. An open mandibular fracture may produce blood-stained saliva. Mandibular fracture may represent a serious life threat if the patient is placed supine. With such a fracture, the tongue is no longer supported at its base and may displace posteriorly, blocking the airway even in a conscious patient. Always look for a second fracture site when you encounter a patient with a mandibular fracture.

Maxillary fractures are classified according to **Le Fort criteria** (Figure 23-12 ■). A slight instability involving the maxilla alone usually presents with no associated displacement and is classified as a Le Fort I fracture. A Le Fort II fracture results in fractures of both the maxilla and nasal bones. Le Fort III fractures characteristically involve the entire facial region below the brow ridge, including the zygoma, nasal bone, and maxilla. The Le Fort II and III fractures usually result in cerebrospinal fluid leakage and may endanger the patency of the nasal and oral portions of the airway.

Le Fort criteria *classification system for fractures involving the maxilla.*

Review

Content

Le Fort Facial Fractures

- I—slight instability to maxilla; no displacement
- II—fracture of both maxilla and nasal bones
- III—fracture involving entire face below brow ridge (zygoma, nasal bone, maxilla)

Dental injury is commonly associated with serious blunt facial trauma. Teeth may chip, break, loosen, or dislodge from the mandible or maxilla. They may then become foreign objects drawn (aspirated) into the airway. Note that a dislodged tooth may be reimplanted if fully intact and handled properly during prehospital care.

Orbital (blowout) fractures most commonly involve the zygoma or maxilla of the inferior shelf. Zygomatic arch fractures are painful and present with a unilateral depression over the prominence of one cheek. The fracture may entrap the extraocular muscles, reducing the eye's range of motion and can cause blurred or double vision (**diplopia**). Zygomatic fracture may also entrap the masseter muscle and limit jaw movement. With maxillary bone fracture, the patient often experiences significant swelling and pain in the maxillary sinus region. Although these injuries are not life threatening, they warrant evaluation by emergency department staff.

A special type of facial injury is that associated with a suicide attempt using a rifle or shotgun. The victim places the barrel under the chin but in an effort to push the trigger, stretches and tilts the head back. The gunshot blast is directed under the chin and at the facial region but may be deflected from entering the cranium. The result is a very disrupted facial region with most of the structures of, and supporting, the airway destroyed. The patient may still be conscious, there is usually heavy bleeding, and the remains of the airway are hard to locate. With such a patient, the airway is in serious danger of obstruction and attempts to secure it are very challenging.

With a Le Fort II injury, the mid-face and zygoma move concurrently. This results in the "dish-face" description often given to this injury.

diplopia *double vision.*

Nasal Injury

Nasal injuries are painful and often create a grossly deformed appearance, but they are not usually life threatening. While dislocation or fracture of the cartilage and nasal bone may interfere with

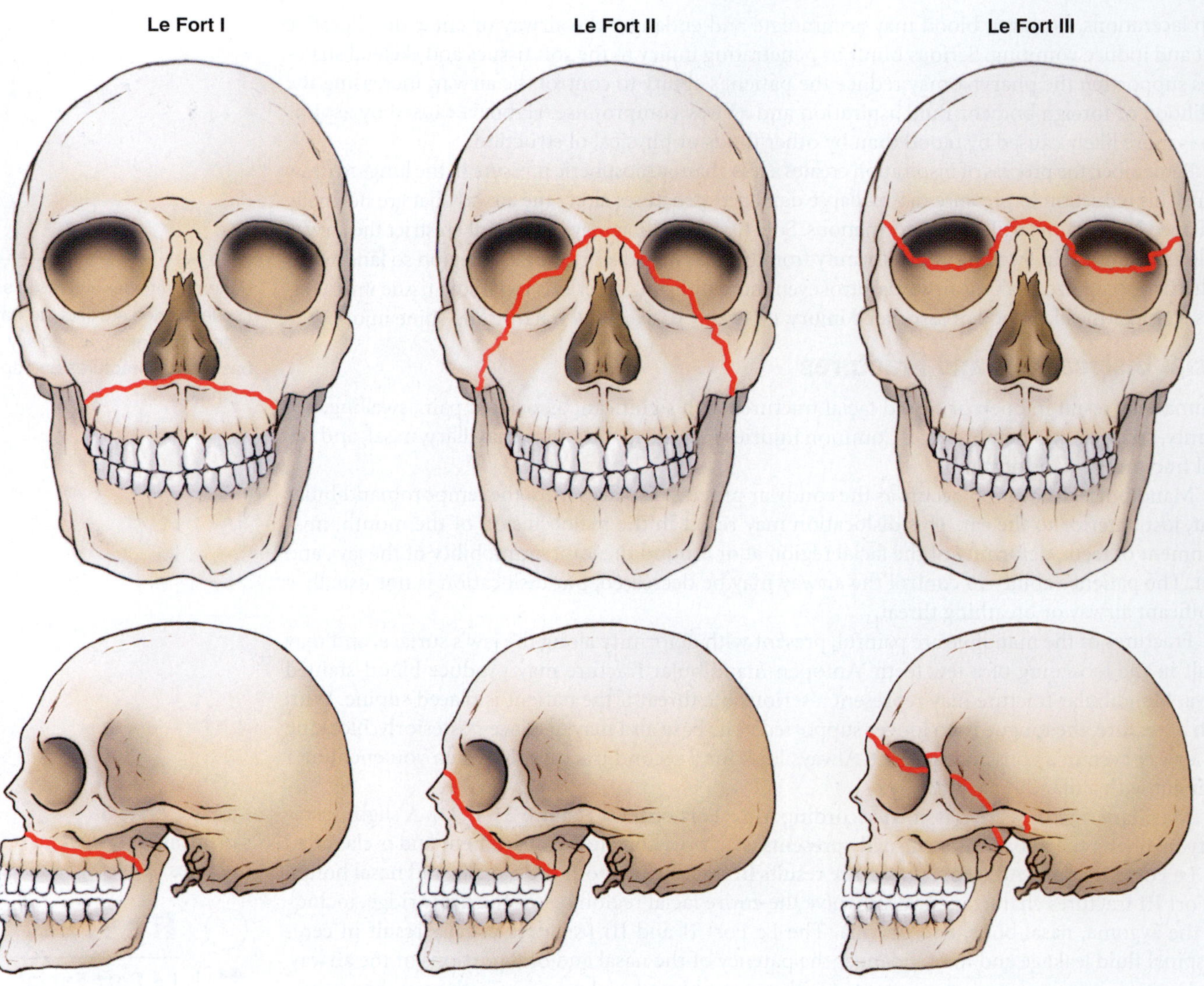

Figure 23-12 Le Fort facial fracture classification.

nasal air movement, the swelling and associated hemorrhage are more likely threats to the airway. However, the conscious and alert patient is usually very able to control the airway.

Epistaxis (nosebleed) is a common nasal problem. Bleeding can be spontaneous as well as traumatic and can be further classified as either anterior or posterior. Anterior hemorrhage comes from the septum and is usually due to bleeding from a network of vessels called Kiesselbach's plexus. Such hemorrhage bleeds slowly and is usually self-limiting. Posterior hemorrhage may be severe and cause blood to drain down the back of the patient's throat. In epistaxis secondary to severe head trauma with likely basilar skull fracture, the integrity of the nasal cavity's posterior wall may be compromised. Attempts at nasal airway, nasogastric tube, or nasotracheal tube insertion may permit the tube to enter the cerebral cavity and directly damage the brain.

Ear Injury

The external ear, or pinna, which is exposed to the environment, is frequently subjected to trauma. It has a minimal blood supply and does not often bleed heavily when lacerated. In glancing blows, the pinna may be partially or completely avulsed. In a folding type of injury, the cartilage may separate. Due to the poor blood supply, external ear injuries do not heal as well as other facial wounds.

The internal portions of the ear—the external auditory canal and the middle and inner ear—are well protected from trauma by the structure of the skull. Injury only results from objects forced into the ear or from rapid changes in pressure as in diving accidents or explosions. With an explosion—even with repeated small arms fire—the pinna focuses the rapidly changing air pressure and directs it into the external auditory canal. This enhanced pressure irritates or ruptures the tympanum and, if strong enough, fractures the small bones of hearing (the ossicles). The result can be temporary or permanent hearing loss. In a diving injury, the changing pressure is not equalized by the eustachian tube (also called the pharyngotympanic passage) and eventually builds until the eardrum ruptures. Water floods the middle ear and interferes with the function of the semicircular canals. The patient experiences vertigo, an extremely dangerous sensation when near weightless under water.

Basilar skull fracture may also disrupt the external auditory canal and tear the tympanum. If the dura mater is torn, cerebrospinal fluid may flood the middle ear and seep outward through the torn tympanum (Figure 23-13 ■). As with the other mechanisms described earlier, hearing loss may result.

Tympanic injuries are not life threatening and, in many cases, repair themselves, even with a rupture that tears as much as half the tympanum. However, a victim with an acute hearing loss can be quite apprehensive and anxious. The patient may be frustrated when unable to hear and understand questions or instructions. Such a patient may also be unable to hear sounds of approaching danger such as traffic noise.

Eye Injury

Although the orbit is a very effective protective housing for the eye, penetrating and some blunt trauma may cause serious injury. The anterior eye structures are extremely specialized and, like most specialized tissues, do not regenerate effectively. If significant penetrating injury occurs, especially if accompanied by loss of the eye's fluids—aqueous or vitreous humor—the patient's sight is threatened, possibly with permanent loss. A penetrating object is likely to disturb the integrity of the anterior and possibly the posterior chamber. In addition, removal of the object may allow fluids to leak from the chambers and further threaten the patient's vision. Penetrating injuries may be caused by foreign bodies so small that they are difficult to see with the naked eye. Suspect the presence of such bodies if the patient reports a history of sudden eye pain and the sensation of an impaled foreign body after using a power saw or grinder, especially when working with metal.

Similarly, small foreign particles that land on the eye's surface can also cause ocular injury. The object may embed in the surface of the eyelid and then drag across the cornea as the eye blinks. Corneal abrasions or lacerations result, often causing intense and continuing pain even after the object is cleared from the eye. These lacerations are usually superficial but can be deep (Figure 23-14 ■).

Blunt trauma may result in several ocular presentations. Hemorrhage may occur in the anterior chamber pools, displaying a collection of blood in front of the iris and pupil. This condition, called **hyphema,** is a potential threat to the patient's vision and requires evaluation by an ophthalmologist and may result in hospital admission.

hyphema *blood in the anterior chamber of the eye, in front of the iris.*

A hyphema is a sight-threatening injury.

Occasionally, blood will completely fill the anterior chamber, resulting in what is called an "eight-ball" hyphema. This can easily be missed without close examination.

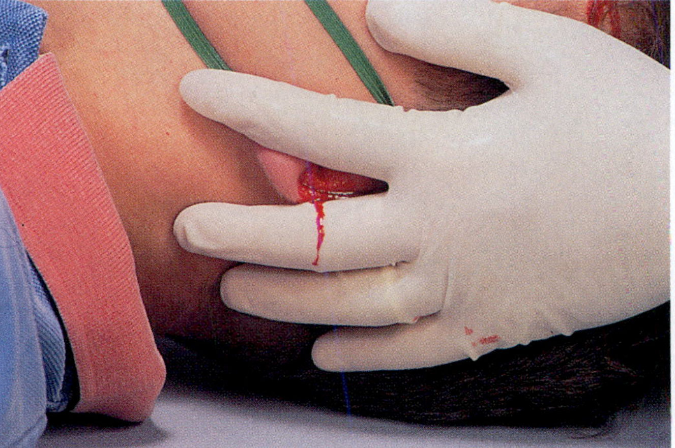

■ Figure 23-13 Blood or fluid draining from a patient's ear suggests basilar skull fracture.

■ Figure 23-14 Laceration of the eyelid.

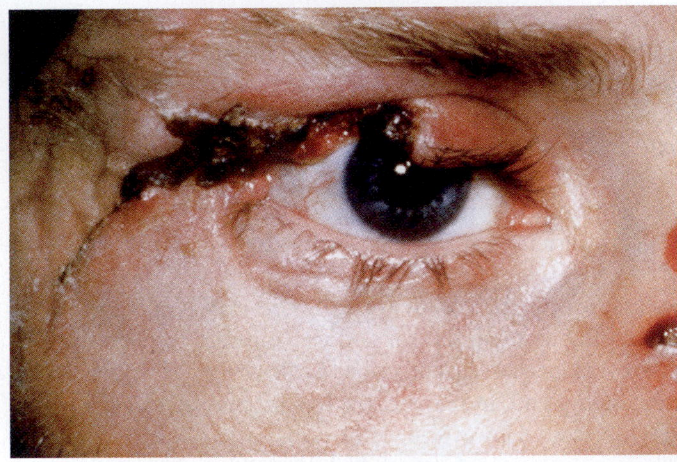

A less serious, but equally dramatic, eye injury is a subconjunctival hemorrhage. This may occur after a strong sneeze, vomiting episode, or direct eye trauma, such as orbital fracture. It occurs when a small blood vessel in the subconjunctival space bursts, leaving a portion of the eye's surface blood red (Figure 23-15 ■). Subconjunctival hemorrhage often clears without intervention and rarely causes any residual scars or impairment.

Blunt trauma may fracture the orbital structures surrounding the eye and produce an injury called eye avulsion. In such a case, the eye is not really avulsed but appears to protrude from the wound as the structure of the orbit is crushed and depressed. If the eye as well as the nerves and vasculature remain intact, sight in the eye can usually be salvaged.

acute retinal artery occlusion *a nontraumatic occlusion of the retinal artery resulting in a sudden, painless loss of vision in one eye.*

retinal detachment *condition that may be of traumatic origin and presents with patient complaint of a dark curtain obstructing a portion of the field of view.*

Two other, more serious ocular problems involve the retina. **Acute retinal artery occlusion** is not an injury but rather a vascular emergency caused when an embolus blocks the blood supply to one eye. The patient complains of sudden and painless loss of vision in the eye. In **retinal detachment,** which may be traumatic in origin, the retina separates from the eye's posterior wall. The patient complains of a dark curtain obstructing part of the field of view. Both of these conditions are true emergencies in which the patient's eyesight is at risk.

Soft-tissue lacerations can occur around the eye and involve the eyelid. If not properly identified and repaired, such an injury may disrupt the function of the lacrimal duct and interrupt lu-

■ Figure 23-15 Subconjunctival hemorrhage.

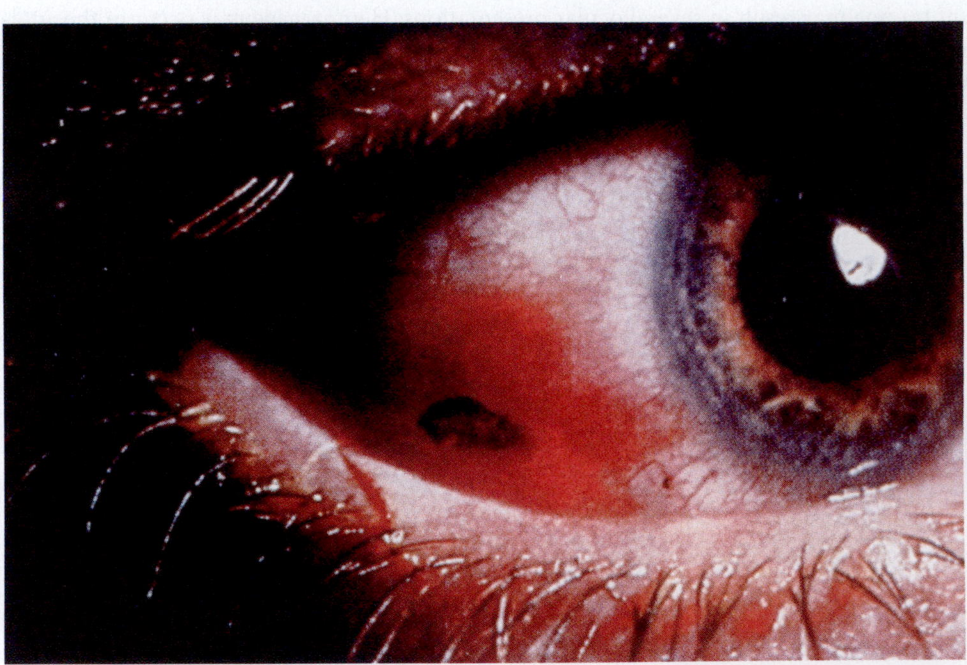

brication and oxygenation of the cornea. Another soft-tissue problem may occur if a contact lens is left in the eye of an unconscious patient. The contact lens will then obstruct the normal lacrimal fluid flow across the eye. This loss of circulation may dry out the eye's surface and cause hypoxic injury. The result is usually severe eye pain and possible damage to the cornea.

NECK INJURY

The neck is protected from impact by the more anterior head and chest and by its own skeletal and muscular structures. The neck's major skeletal component is the cervical vertebral column, which is strengthened by interconnecting ligaments. The neck muscles provide additional protection to the vital structures in the neck. They include the muscles that support and move the head through a large range of motion as well as the shoulder muscles that help move the upper extremities and act as auxiliary breathing muscles. The skeletal structures and muscles of the neck protect the airway, carotid and jugular blood vessels, and the esophagus very well from all but anterior blunt trauma and deep penetrating trauma. Such trauma may result in serious injuries to the airway, cervical spine, blood vessels, and other structures in the region.

Most trauma surgeons feel that any neck injury that penetrates the most superficial muscle (platysma) should be surgically explored.

Blood Vessel Trauma

Blunt trauma to a blood vessel may produce a serious and rapidly expanding hematoma. This hematoma may be trapped within the fascia of the region and apply restrictive pressure to the jugular veins. Laceration of the external jugular vein, or deep laceration involving the internal jugular vein or the carotid arteries, may result in severe hemorrhage due to the large size of the vessels and the volume of blood they carry (Figure 23-16 ■). Their laceration and subsequent hemorrhage can rapidly lead to hypovolemia and shock. Arterial interruption may cause subsequent brain hypoxia and infarct, mimicking the signs and symptoms of a stroke. An open neck wound affecting the external jugular vein may permit formation of an air embolism as the venous pressure drops below atmospheric pressure with deep respirations.

Airway Trauma

Trauma may also injure the larynx and trachea. Severe blunt or penetrating trauma may separate the larynx from the trachea, fracture or crush either of these two structures, or open the trachea to the environment. These injuries may result in serious hemorrhage that threatens the airway, vocal cord contusion or swelling, destruction of the integrity of the airway and collapse on inspiration, disruption of normal airway landmarks, and restrictive soft-tissue swelling.

Cervical Spine Trauma

Severe blunt trauma and, in some cases, gunshot wounds to the neck may cause vertebral fracture and cervical spine instability. The wounds may cause pressure on the spinal cord, cord contusion,

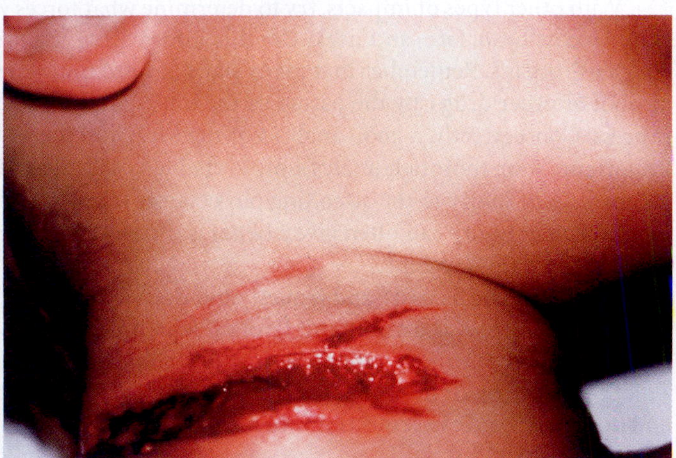

■ **Figure 23-16** Laceration to the neck.

or severing of the cord. Such injuries will likely cause bilateral paresthesia, anesthesia, weakness (paresis), or paralysis, generally at and below the dermatome controlled by the peripheral nerve branch leaving the spinal column at the level of the injury. Neurogenic shock from these injuries may cause hypotension from vasodilation. (This is discussed in Chapter 24, "Spinal Trauma.") Blunt trauma may disrupt and injure the muscles and connective tissues of the region and result in serious pain and limited motion.

Other Neck Trauma

The neck may also demonstrate subcutaneous emphysema due to tension pneumothorax (air pushed into the skin from intrathoracic pressure that migrates to the neck) or from tracheal injury in the neck. Penetrating trauma may involve the esophagus, perforating it and permitting gastric contents or undigested material to enter the fascia. Since the fascia communicates with the mediastinum, this foreign material can physically harm mediastinal structures or provide the medium for infection, which may have devastating results. Deep penetrating trauma may disrupt the vagus nerve, causing tachycardia and gastrointestinal disturbances. More anterior and superficial injuries may damage the thyroid and parathyroid glands.

ASSESSMENT OF HEAD, FACIAL, AND NECK INJURIES

As with all trauma patients, assessment of head, facial, and neck injury patients follows the standard format, including the scene size-up, primary assessment, rapid secondary assessment/focused exam and history, and the detailed assessment as appropriate. Perform reassessments frequently on these patients. With head, facial, and neck injuries, pay special attention to ensuring airway patency and monitoring breathing, level of consciousness and orientation, pupillary signs, and blood pressure. With these patients, be sure to consider the need for rapid transport to a trauma center specializing in neurologic care.

SCENE SIZE-UP

Analysis of the mechanism of injury is a key part of the assessment of the patient with a possible head, face, or neck injury. During the scene size-up, consider the circumstances of injury and identify the nature and extent of forces that caused the injury. In a vehicle crash, for example, look for evidence of head impact such as the characteristic spider-web windshield. Look also for deformity of the upper steering wheel, which suggests head or neck trauma or the use of the shoulder belt without the lap belt. Identify the direction of the forces causing injury and anticipate what body structures the forces may have damaged. In motorcycle impacts, remember that helmet use reduces head injury by about 50 percent but does not spare the neck from cervical spine injury. In shootings, try to determine the caliber and type of weapon, the distance from the gun to the patient, and the approximate angle of the bullet's entry into the patient's body.

With other types of impacts, try to determine what forces were involved and how they were directed to the head, face, and neck. Use this information to anticipate injuries to the brain, airway, and sense organs. Remember that many signs of head injury may be masked by the patient's use of alcohol or other drugs, by the nature of the injury, and/or by the slow development of the wound process. Consequently, a good analysis of the MOI and the resulting indexes of suspicion are very important. Your thorough analysis must enable you to describe both the incident scene and the mechanism of injury to the attending physician at the emergency department. Remember that the mechanism of injury can often give a better indication of the seriousness of the injury than the patient's signs and symptoms.

Rule out scene hazards, and request any additional resources needed at the scene as soon as you can. Use of gloves is the minimum level of Standard Precautions when approaching the potential head, face, and neck injury patient. Serious head injuries pose real risks of exposure to blood or other fluids propelled by air movement or by arterial or heavy venous bleeding. Anticipate such exposures, and don splash and eye protection when contacting any patient with significant trauma to the head, face, or neck.

PRIMARY ASSESSMENT

Although determining the patient's level of orientation may add a few seconds to the initial assessment, assessing trends in orientation can be critical to rapid identification of a brain injury patient.

As you approach, form an initial impression of the patient's condition. Is the patient alert? Does the patient show any signs of anxiety? If there is any reason to suspect that the head or neck sustained serious impact, provide immediate manual immobilization of the head and cervical spine (Figure 23-17 ■). Quickly determine the patient's level of consciousness and then orientation to time, place, and person early in the primary assessment. While determining the patient's level of orientation may add a few seconds to the primary assessment, assessing trends in orientation can be critical to rapid identification of a brain injury patient. Be alert to the patient's facial skin color, respiratory effort, and to pupil luster and level of responsiveness throughout the primary assessment, as these factors can help you recognize internal head injury. As you gather information about the patient, continue to build and modify your general patient impression and your index of suspicion for head injury.

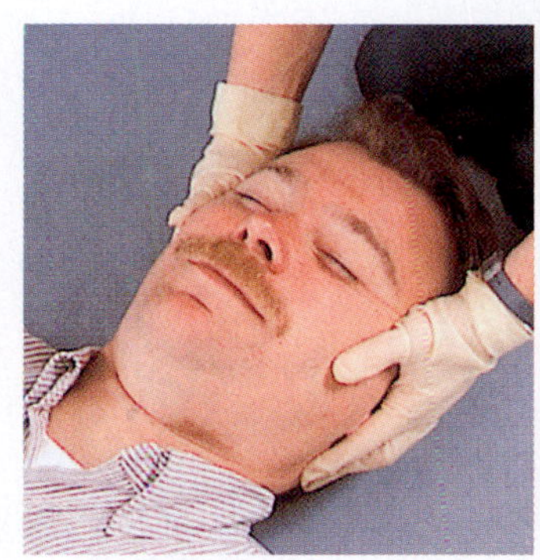

■ Figure 23-17 If spinal injury is suspected, immediately immobilize the head and neck manually.

Apply a cervical collar at the end of the primary assessment and maintain manual head immobilization until the patient is fully immobilized to a short spine board, KED, or long spine board with a cervical immobilization device. If there are any significant injuries to the neck, do not apply the collar until you complete the assessment and provide needed care. While the cervical collar provides some neck stabilization, it does not completely immobilize the region, and its placement may be delayed so long as manual immobilization is continued.

If the patient is wearing a helmet, consider whether or not to remove it as described in Chapter 24, "Spinal Trauma." A patient's use of a helmet reduces the likelihood of soft-tissue injury and skull and facial fracture. Helmet use can also significantly reduce the incidence of brain injury, but do not be lulled into a false sense of security by the absence of outward signs of trauma. Be watchful for the early signs of internal brain injury, and be sure to inform the emergency department staff that the patient was wearing a helmet. Also alert them to any signs of impact or helmet damage suggestive of the forces of trauma that the patient experienced.

Always be sure to inform the emergency department staff if a patient was wearing a helmet.

Airway

Move quickly to evaluate the airway. Examine the face and neck for any deformity, swelling, hemorrhage, foreign bodies, or other signs of injury that may threaten the airway. Suction and insert an oral or nasal airway as necessary. Listen for unusual or changing voice patterns as they may be indicative of airway injury and developing edema. Swelling can quickly occlude the airway, and any hemorrhage can complicate airway maintenance as the patient loses consciousness and the gag reflex. Anticipate vomiting, possibly without warning. Ensure that the airway is structurally sound and that the mandible supports the tongue well enough to keep it out of the airway. Have a large-bore suction catheter and strong suction ready to remove any fluids, and consider positioning the patient to enhance airway drainage (left lateral recumbent position) if doing so is not contraindicated by injuries. If the patient does not display a protective airway reflex or if he has an altered level of consciousness, consider early insertion of an endotracheal tube. Note that any manipulation of the airway may increase ICP. Use deep suctioning, oral airway insertion, and endotracheal intubation as last resorts and have an experienced provider accomplish them quickly.

If there is a serious neck injury, check the structural integrity of the trachea. If the trachea is open to the environment, keep the wound clear of blood to prevent aspiration, and seal the wound unless the patient's upper airway is blocked. If an impaled object obstructs the airway, remove it, anticipating that heavy bleeding may then threaten the airway. Blunt wounds may crush the cartilage of the trachea, permitting it to close with the reduced pressure during inspiration. This type of crushing injury may require surgical opening of the trachea by needle or surgical cricothyrotomy to ensure air exchange.

Breathing

Closely monitor breathing to ensure that the patient is moving an adequate volume of air. Determine the rate of respirations and their rhythm. Estimate the amount of air moved with each breath, and from those numbers determine the minute volume:

$$\text{Minute volume} = \text{Tidal volume} \times \text{Respiratory rate}$$

If the patient is breathing fewer than 10 times per minute, moving significantly less than 500 mL of air with each breath, or has a minute volume of less than 5 liters, consider ventilating the patient.

Remember that head injury is likely to produce irregular breathing patterns and that hypoxia and carbon dioxide retention both contribute to morbidity and mortality with brain injury. Ventilate at 12 to 20 full breaths per minute with a volume of between 800 and 1,200 mL. Do not hyperventilate the patient if you suspect brain injury. Hyperventilation will blow off carbon dioxide and cause vasoconstriction, further decreasing cerebral perfusion.Ventilations for the serious head injury patient (GCS ≥8) are guided by capnography. For the head injury patient without signs of herniation, adjust ventilation rates to maintain an end-tidal CO_2 reading of between 35 and 40 mmHg (adults at about 10 breaths per minute, children at about 20 breaths per minute, and infants at about 25 breaths per minute). For patients with suspected herniation, the end-tidal CO_2 reading should range between 30 and 35 mmHg, using ventilation rates about 10 breaths per minute faster than for patients without herniation. Also ensure the oxygen saturation level is at least 95 percent for any serious head injury patient.

Ventilations for the serious head injury patient (GCS ≤ 8) are guided by capnography.

For a patient who is breathing adequately on his own, apply oxygen via nonrebreather mask with a flow of 15 liters per minute, to ensure inspiration of high concentrations. It is advisable to apply pulse oximetry to monitor oxygenation. Attempt to keep oxygen saturation above 95 percent.

Circulation

Begin to monitor the patient's pulse rate and its rhythm early in your care and continue to do so frequently thereafter. A slow and strong (bounding) pulse may be an early sign of building intracranial pressure. Apply an ECG monitor and watch for rhythm disturbances. Quickly look for any hemorrhage from the head, face, and neck and control any moderate to severe bleeding with direct pressure and bandaging. Be cautious of open neck wounds because they may present a risk for air embolism. Cover any such wounds quickly with occlusive dressings and secure them in place. Hypotension in the patient with an increased intracranial pressure carries a very high mortality and morbidity rate. Maintain a blood pressure of at least 90 mmHg with aggressive fluid resuscitation as necessary.

A slow and strong (bounding) pulse may be an early sign of building intracranial pressure.

At the end of the primary assessment, you must determine whether to perform a rapid secondary assessment followed by gathering of vital signs and the patient history or to perform a focused history and physical exam followed by gathering of vital signs. With most head, face, and neck injury patients, you will perform a rapid secondary assessment because of the high likelihood of airway, vascular, special sense organ, or central nervous system injuries in these regions. If there is no significant mechanism of injury and injuries appear minor and superficial, perform an exam focused on the specific area(s) of injury.

RAPID SECONDARY ASSESSMENT

The rapid secondary assessment calls for performance of a quick and directed head-to-toe examination of a patient with a significant mechanism of injury. When head, facial, or neck injury is suggested in such a patient, pay particular attention to the procedures described in the following sections as you carry out the assessment. Manage any life-threatening injuries and conditions as you find them during the rapid secondary assessment. If the patient shows any signs of pathology within the cranium, consider rapid transport. Brain injury patients can deteriorate quickly, but rapid neurosurgical intervention can frequently alleviate life-threatening problems.

Head

Look at, then sweep, each region of the skull, feeling for deformity and bleeding with the more sensitive tips of your fingers. Interlock your fingers to sweep the posterior head, and look at your gloves to check for any blood that indicates hemorrhage there. If you find any moderate or serious hemorrhage, apply direct pressure unless you suspect skull fracture. Control the hemorrhage with gentle pressure around the wound and place a loose dressing over it. Palpate gently for any deformities, being careful, however, not to palpate the interior of open wounds (Figure 23-18 ■).

Shine a penlight into the external auditory canal and look for signs of escaping cerebrospinal fluid. This fluid loss may be difficult to notice early during assessment, so observe carefully. If blood or fluid drains from the auditory canal, cover the ear with a gauze dressing to permit fluid to move outward while providing a barrier to keep contaminants from entering. If the fluid drains on a gauze dressing or other fabric, look for the halo sign. However, you should presume (regardless of the presence or absence

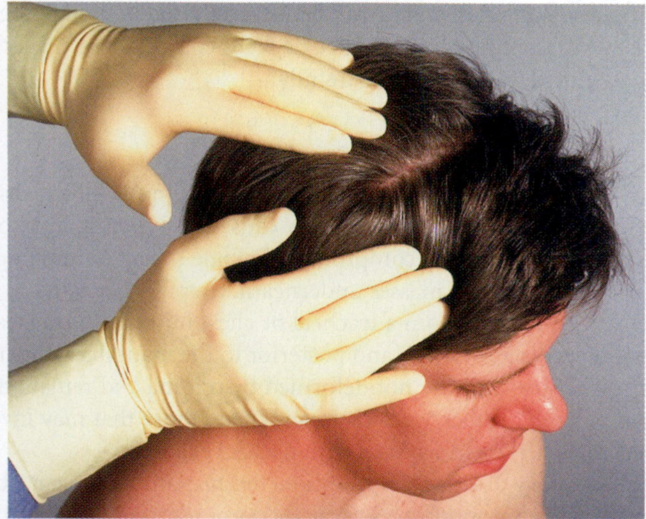

■ Figure 23-18 Carefully inspect and palpate the head for bleeding and other signs of injury.

of halo sign) that any fluid draining from the ear contains cerebrospinal fluid. Examine the pinnae for injury and, after you complete the rapid secondary assessment, bandage and dress as needed.

If you observe a skull deformity, palpate such a closed wound very gently. Try to determine the probability of skull fracture before swelling makes this determination more difficult. Cover any open wounds with dressings to restrict blood flow and prevent further contamination. The signs of basilar skull fracture—bilateral periorbital ecchymosis and retroauricular ecchymosis (raccoon eyes and Battle's sign)—are very late indications of this injury and are not likely to be recognizable during field assessment and care.

Raccoon eyes and Battle's sign are very late signs of basilar skull fracture and are not likely to be recognizable during field assessment and care.

Head injury may cause patient seizures. Seizures are serious complications because they may compromise the airway and respirations, increase the intracranial pressure, and exacerbate any existing brain injury. If you observe a seizure or the patient or bystanders describe one as you gather the history, find out as much about the episode as you can and be prepared to describe the seizure in detail, including its origin and progression, to the attending physician. Protect the seizing patient from further injury and be especially watchful of the airway. Consider the administration of diazepam, which reduces electrical impulse transmission across the cerebrum and may limit seizure activity.

Face

Study the patient's facial features carefully, looking for asymmetry, swelling, discoloration, or deformity. Palpate the facial region including the brow ridge, nasal region, cheek, maxilla, and mandible searching for any deformity, instability, or crepitus that suggest fracture and for any signs of soft-tissue swelling (Figure 23-19 ■). Palpate the maxilla and attempt, gently, to move it from left to right. It should be firmly attached to the facial bones and should display no crepitus. Do likewise with the mandible. It should be solid yet very mobile from left to right and up and down. Note and investigate any patient report of pain during your palpation and movement. Open the mouth and examine for any signs of trauma, excessive secretions and bleeding, or swelling. All teeth should be firmly in place (loose teeth may suggest mandibular fracture). Find any displaced teeth and prepare them for transport with the patient or suspect that missing teeth may have been aspirated. Ensure that the mandible is intact and supports the airway.

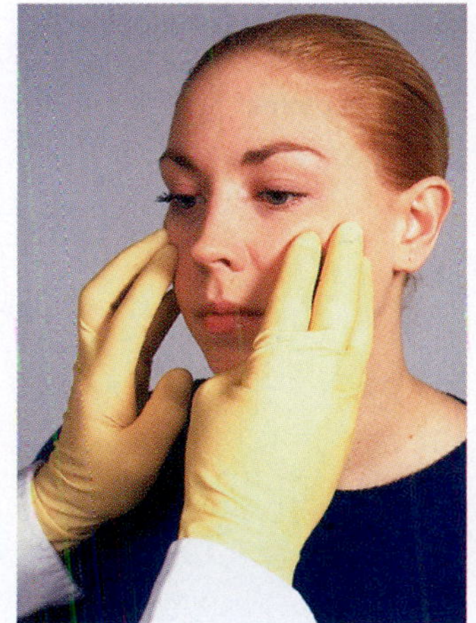

■ Figure 23-19 Carefully palpate the facial bones.

consensual reactivity *the response of both eyes to changes in light intensity that affect only one eye.*

Carefully examine the eyes. In general, eye reactivity and luster reflect the oxygenation status of the brain. Watch for bright and sparkling eyes and briskly reactive pupils. Shine a bright light into the eyes—or in bright sunlight, shade them—and watch for sluggishness, nonreactivity, and constriction (or dilation). Ensure that reactivity is bilateral. Note that both eyes should respond to changes in light intensity affecting only one eye (**consensual reactivity**). Both eyes should gaze together and, at rest, directly forward. Watch for a down and out gaze. Usually, an affected pupil is on the same side (ipsilateral) as a head injury. If the patient is conscious and alert, have him follow your finger up and down, left and right, with each eye. Watch for and note any limited eye movement. Restricted eye movement suggests eye muscle entrapment and nerve compression or injury and paralysis.

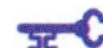

Restricted eye movement suggests eye muscle entrapment, nerve compression, or injury and paralysis.

Carefully examine the pupil, iris, and conjunctiva. The pupil and iris should be round, the anterior chamber clear, and the sclera free of accumulating blood. Check for contact lenses, especially in the unconscious patient. If they are noted, remove them carefully.

Neck

Examine the anterior, lateral, and posterior neck for signs of injury including swelling, discoloration, wounds, blood loss, or frothy blood. Frothy blood is likely caused by bleeding in association with a tracheal injury and suggests serious airway compromise. Palpate the region, feeling for any changes in skin tension, deformities, or unusual masses underneath. Crepitus beneath the skin may be associated with subcutaneous emphysema from a tracheal or chest injury or a tracheal or laryngeal fracture. Identify the thyroid cartilage, beneath and posterior to the mandible. Palpate it, the cricoid cartilage, then the trachea. Ensure they are not deformed by trauma and remain midline in the neck. Visually examine the depth of neck wounds to anticipate those that may involve jugular or carotid blood vessels, and cover any open wounds with occlusive dressings.

Any penetration of the lateral neck muscles should heighten your index of suspicion for a serious neck injury.

While carrying out the rapid secondary assessment, question the responsive patient about headaches and increased light sensitivity (photophobia), which are common symptoms of head injury. Also question the patient about his memory of the events preceding and following the injury to identify retrograde and anterograde amnesia. Note any repetitive questioning by the patient (inability to establish short-term memory) and any unusual behavior or confusion. Ask if the patient has any unusual fullness in the throat and any difficulty swallowing. Ask about any visual disturbances such as double vision (diplopia) and blurred vision that may indicate eye muscle entrapment. Inquire about visual acuity (the ability to distinguish objects) both near and far, and note reports of any restriction to vision, which the patient might describe as a curtain drawn across the field of view. Patient complaints of eye pain are also important and may suggest conjunctival or corneal injury. You may also note patient complaints about focal deficits. Examine any area of facial paresthesia, anesthesia, weakness, or paralysis, noting the borders of the area and whether it is unilateral or bilateral. Question the patient frequently to identify any increase or decrease in awareness and any changes in injury symptoms.

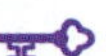

Question the head, face, or neck injury patient frequently to identify any increase or decrease in awareness and any changes in injury symptoms.

Complete the rapid secondary assessment by examining the rest of the body, paying particular attention to any region where the mechanism of injury suggests serious injury and in which the patient complains of serious symptoms. While examining the extremities, look for any signs of decreased muscle tone, flaccid muscles, diminished sensation or muscle strength, and determine if any unusual findings are bilateral or unilateral and where the deficit begins. Then gather the balance of the patient history, determine the patient's Glasgow Coma Scale score, and take a set of the patient's vital signs.

Glasgow Coma Scale Score

Determine the patient's best eye opening, motor, and verbal responses using the Glasgow Coma Scale (GCS). The Glasgow Coma Scale awards the patient points for different responses, with a total score that will range between 3 and 15 points (see the adult GCS in Table 23–1, the pediatric GCS in Table 23–2). The scale is a moderately good predictor of head injury severity. A patient with a score of between 13 and 15 is considered to have a mild head injury. A score between 9 and 12 indicates moderate injury, while a score of 8 or less represents severe head injury. Most patients with GCS of 8 or less are in a coma.

Patients with a Glasgow Coma Scale score of 8 or less should be immediately intubated.

When assessing eye-opening response, award 1 point for no response, 2 points for eye opening in response to pain, 3 points for response to verbal command, and 4 points for spontaneous eye opening. With verbal response, award 1 point for no sound or response; 2 points for incomprehensible, garbled sounds; 3 points for inappropriate words or speech that makes no sense; 4 points for confused or disoriented speech; and 5 points for clear and oriented speech. With motor response, award 1 point for no movement or response, 2 points for decerebrate posturing, 3 points for decorticate posturing, 4 points for purposeful motion (withdrawal of a body part from pain), 5 points for purposeful movement (of the hand) to localize pain, and 6 for following simple verbal commands. The lowest GCS value is 3, which represents a completely unresponsive patient. The maximum GCS value is 15, which represents the fully conscious and alert patient.

Table 23–1 Glasgow Coma Scale

Eye Opening		*Motor Response*	
Spontaneous	4	Obeys verbal commands	6
To verbal command	3	Localizes pain	5
To pain	2	Withdraws from pain (flexion)	4
No response	1	Abnormal flexion in response to pain (decorticate rigidity)	3
Verbal Response		Extension in response to pain (decerebrate rigidity)	2
Oriented and converses	5	No response	1
Disoriented and converses	4		
Inappropriate words	3		
Incomprehensible sounds	2		
No response	1		

Table 23–2 Pediatric Glasgow Coma Scale

		> 1 Year	< 1 Year	
Eye Opening	4	Spontaneous	Spontaneous	
	3	To verbal command	To shout	
	2	To pain	To pain	
	1	No response	No response	
		> 1 Year	< 1 Year	
Best Motor Response	6	Obeys		
	5	Localizes pain	Localizes pain	
	4	Flexion-withdrawal	Flexion-withdrawal	
	3	Flexion-abnormal (decorticate rigidity)	Flexion-abnormal (decorticate rigidity)	
	2	Extension (decerebrate rigidity)	Extension (decerebrate rigidity)	
	1	No response	No response	
		>5 Years	2–5 Years	0–23 Months
Best Verbal Response	5	Oriented and converses	Appropriate words and phrases	Smiles, coos, cries appropriately
	4	Disoriented and converses	Inappropriate words	Cries
	3	Inappropriate words	Cries and/or screams	Inappropriate crying and/or screaming

Record the best response for each of the GCS criteria (for example, as E_3, V_4, M_5) and note any differences, either from side-to-side or in the upper versus lower extremities. Also note the eye signs along with the Glasgow Coma Scale score results because they help identify the existence and nature of the patient's brain injury. Determine the GCS score every 5 minutes (with the ongoing assessment) in the patient with any GCS less than 15. The pediatric patient is a special challenge to Glasgow Coma Score assessment. To arrive at an accurate value, you must modify your evaluation of the child's best verbal response as appropriate for the developmental age. See the criteria identified in the pediatric Glasgow Coma Scale (review Table 23–2).

Vital Signs

Carefully monitor the vital signs for evidence of increasing intracranial pressure. Identify and record the pulse rate and strength. Note the blood pressure and especially the pulse pressure. Lastly, note the respiratory pattern. The vital signs change with increasing ICP or injury to the brainstem. Be watchful for a slowing pulse rate, increasing systolic blood pressure, and the development of irregular respirations (Cheyne-Stokes, central neurologic hyperventilation, or ataxic respirations), which together are known as Cushing's triad.

At the conclusion of the rapid secondary assessment, determine the need for rapid transport.

At the conclusion of the rapid secondary assessment, determine the need for rapid transport. A history of head trauma coupled with any history of unconsciousness, a degradation in the level of orientation or consciousness, or any vital sign suggestive of brain injury requires rapid transport to the closest appropriate facility. If such signs and symptoms of brain injury exist, begin rapid transport and contact medical direction for approval to transport to the nearest neurocenter. Significant airway threats and uncontrolled hemorrhage are also indicators for rapid transport. Carefully monitor other head, face, and neck injury patients during further assessment and care for any signs of increasing intracranial pressure or expanding lesions. Identify the wounds and other injuries you have found or suspect and prioritize them for care.

FOCUSED SECONDARY ASSESSMENT

If your head, face, or neck injury patient has no significant mechanism of injury and no other indications of serious injury, perform a focused secondary assessment, concentrating on the area of injury. During your assessment, however, carefully observe for any signs of a diminished level of consciousness or orientation or any evidence of previous unconsciousness or airway or vascular restriction or compromise. If you discover any of these things, complete a rapid secondary assessment and consider the patient for rapid transport to the appropriate facility. Remember, the signs of significant brain injury may not develop for some time or may be masked by drug or alcohol use or by the patient's anxiety. It is always better to err on the side of more intensive patient care.

Direct the focused secondary assessment to the areas of specific patient complaint and to areas where the mechanism of injury suggests injury. Use the assessment techniques—inspection, palpation, and so forth—suggested for the rapid secondary assessment.

When you have completed the focused assessment, obtain a set of baseline vital signs and gather a patient history. Then provide emergency care for the injuries you have found and prepare the patient for transport.

With superficial wounds to the head, face, and neck, apply dressings and bandages as for minor soft-tissue injuries but be alert for hemorrhage into the airway and vomiting that may follow it and for any signs of progressive swelling that may restrict the airway. Watch also for open neck wounds that may permit air to enter the jugular vein. Cover such wounds with occlusive dressings held firmly in place.

Inspect any soft-tissue head, facial, or neck injury very carefully before bandaging it and be prepared to describe the injury to the attending emergency department physician or nurse so they do not have to remove and replace dressings and bandages unnecessarily.

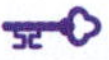

Of special concern for the head injury patient is the blood glucose level.

Of special concern for the head injury patient is the blood glucose level. Research has found that depressed glucose levels (hypoglycemia) increase the morbidity and mortality in these patients. It may be prudent to perform a quick blood glucose check to ensure the glucose level is above 60 mg/dL. If not, administer IV glucose ($D_{50}W$).

DETAILED ASSESSMENT

You will normally perform a detailed assessment for the head, face, and neck injury patient during transport and only if and when you have cared for all other serious injuries. The detailed assessment is an in-depth, head-to-toe assessment searching for any other signs or symptoms suggestive of injury. Use your skills of questioning, inspection, palpation, and—as appropriate—auscultation to search out these additional injuries. Look for signs of neurologic deficit in the extremities, including flaccidity, paresthesia, anesthesia, weakness, and paralysis. Remember that early in the course of trauma, serious injuries may be masked by other more painful ones, by patient anxiety, and by drug and alcohol use. Careful evaluation is required to identify injuries at this stage of patient care.

REASSESSMENT

Perform reassessments every 5 minutes for patients with potentially serious injuries. Be especially alert for slowing of the pulse, increasing systolic blood pressure (an increasing pulse pressure), and development of deeper, more rapid, or erratic respirations. Carefully observe the patient for changes in the level of consciousness and orientation as well. Finally, watch the eyes for signs of cerebral hypoxia—they become dull and lackluster—or of increasing intracranial pressure—one pupil becomes sluggish, nonreactive, then dilated. Note any changes in any element of patient presentation, and track any trends to identify whether the patient's condition is deteriorating, improving, or remaining the same.

A slowing pulse rate, increasing systolic blood pressure, and the development of erratic respirations are signs of increasing intracranial pressure.

If the patient's eyes become dull and lackluster, it is a sign of cerebral hypoxia; if one pupil becomes sluggish, nonreactive, then dilated, that indicates intracranial injury.

Watch pulse oximetry and blood pressure readings to ensure that the patient becomes neither hypoxic nor hypovolemic. Both of these conditions are associated with increased mortality and morbidity when associated with brain injury. If you notice any sign of deterioration, provide rapid transport. Monitor the $PaCO_2$ reading on your capnography device to ensure the carbon dioxide level remains between 35 and 40 mmHg.

HEAD, FACIAL, AND NECK INJURY MANAGEMENT

The management priorities for the patient sustaining head, face, or neck trauma include care directed at maintaining the patient's airway and breathing, ensuring circulation through hemorrhage control, addressing or taking steps to avoid hypoxia and/or hypovolemia, and providing appropriate medications. Once these priorities have been attended to, you may dress and care for minor head, facial, and neck wounds.

AIRWAY

The airway is one of the most important care priorities with head, face, and neck injury patients. Head, face, and neck injury can leave patients unable to control the airway due either to an altered level of consciousness or to damaged airway structures. In addition, soft-tissue trauma to the airway may cause edema that can quickly progress from restriction of the airway to its complete obstruction. Vigilant attention to the airway and aggressive airway care are the only means of ensuring that the airway of these patients remains protected and patent. Airway management techniques appropriate for such patients include suctioning, patient positioning, oral and nasal airway insertion, endotracheal intubation, and cricothyrotomy. (You can review these techniques in Chapter 8, "Airway Management and Ventilation.")

Vigilant attention to the airway and aggressive airway care are vital with head, facial, and neck injury patients.

Sellick Maneuver

In the time between determining the need for endotracheal intubation and its successful insertion, consider using the Sellick maneuver. Apply pressure directed posteriorly to the cricoid ring with the thumb and index finger, moving it downward toward the vertebral column. This compresses the esophagus, thus reducing the likelihood of vomitus entering the upper airway during intubation. Exercise caution to prevent the pressure from flexing the cervical spine. If the patient should actively vomit, release the pressure immediately and suction the airway. Continuing to hold the esophagus closed may result in its rupture. *Be aware that the Sellick maneuver may not align the airway enough to permit visualized oral intubation.*

Suctioning

Airway tissues are extremely vascular, bleed profusely, and swell quickly. Soft-tissue injury may cause significant hemorrhage that can compromise the airway in two ways. First, the sheer volume of blood may block the airway. Note that aspiration of blood is more often responsible for hypoxia than physical obstruction of the airway, so be certain to suction as necessary in order to remove blood from the airway.

Secondly, blood is a gastric irritant that frequently induces emesis. If a large volume of blood is swallowed, the patient may vomit, thus endangering the airway. In addition, vomiting is common with head injury patients because emesis is a frequent result of brain injury or increasing intracranial pressure. Vomiting often occurs without warning (without nausea) and can be projectile in nature. Vomiting is especially dangerous with head injury patients because they commonly have a depressed or absent gag reflex. Gastric contents are very acidic and will quickly damage the tissues of the lower airway if aspirated. Aspiration of gastric contents is associated with a high patient mortality. Be ready to suction aggressively as needed in any patients with nasal, oral, or head trauma. Use a large-bore catheter or a suction hose without a tip to clear the airway of any blood or emesis.

Patient Positioning

Consider placing the patient in a position that protects the airway early in your care (during the primary assessment). The best position for the patient with suspected head injury is on the left side with the head turned slightly and facing downward, the left lateral recumbent position. Remember, of course, that head injury patients require spinal precautions. Maintain manual immobilization until the patient is secured to a long spine board, and then be prepared to turn the patient and board as a unit to facilitate airway drainage.

It is unlikely that suction alone will evacuate all emesis from the oral cavity before the unconscious or semiconscious patient attempts an inspiration. If the patient experiencing serious oral, nasal (epistaxis), or facial bleeding is conscious and alert and no serious spinal injury is suspected, have the patient sit leaning forward to promote drainage and keep fluids from flowing into the posterior airway. If the patient has sustained an open neck injury with the danger of air embolism, place the patient on a spine board in the Trendelenburg position, with the lower part of the patient's body elevated about 12 inches. Otherwise, position the patient with potential brain injury by elevating the head of the spine board to about 30 degrees to reduce both external hemorrhage and intracranial pressure.

Oropharyngeal and Nasopharyngeal Airways

Oro- and nasopharyngeal airways each have advantages and disadvantages when used with head, face, and neck injury patients. The nasal airway does not trigger the gag reflex as easily as the oral airway and is better tolerated by the semiconscious patient. Because there is less stimulation of the gag reflex, there is also a reduction in transient increases in intracranial pressure and in the chances of increasing the severity of head injury. One hazard of nasal airway use is the possible insertion of the tube directly into the cranium through a fracture of the posterior nasal border. Always insert the nasal airway straight back, through the largest of the nares (nostrils), and use only gentle force in its introduction. If you suspect basilar skull fracture, use an oral airway or endotracheal intubation to establish and maintain the airway.

While the oral and nasal airways help to keep the respective pharynxes open, they can represent threats to the airway. The ends of the tubes sit just superior to the opening of the larynx. If a patient vomits, which frequently happens with brain injury, the vomitus is blocked from exiting the patient's mouth through the airway and remains just at the laryngeal opening. With the next breath, the patient can aspirate the gastric contents, which may have serious consequences. Whenever an oral or nasal airway is in place, monitor the patient's airway carefully and be prepared to remove the airway and evacuate any emesis.

Endotracheal Intubation

Intubate early in the care of the unresponsive patient, and consider intubation for any patient with a reduced level of consciousness.

Endotracheal intubation is the most definitive method of ensuring a clear and patent airway in the head injury patient. Intubate early in the care of the unresponsive patient, and consider intubation for any patient with a reduced level of consciousness. Techniques useful in caring for head injury patients include orotracheal, digital, nasotracheal, retrograde, directed, and rapid-sequence intubation.

Orotracheal Intubation Orotracheal, or oral, intubation is the most common and usually the most successful technique for placing an endotracheal tube (Figure 23-20 ■). It does, however, pose some hazards for head, face, and neck injury patients. All patients who sustain serious injuries in these regions require spinal immobilization. Immobilization, however, limits the movement of the patient's head during intubation attempts, restricting you from manually bringing the oral opening, pharynx, and trachea in line. The result is often an inability to visualize the vocal folds and watch the endotracheal tube pass into the trachea, seriously reducing the chances of a successful oral intubation.

To improve visualization during oral intubation (and especially with patients in need of spinal immobilization), employ a technique called the BURP maneuver. Using your thumb and first finger, displace the larynx **B**ackward (posteriorly), **U**pward (cephalid), and just slightly to the patient's **R**ight with slight **P**ressure. This maneuver is likely to move the laryngeal opening into better view for endotracheal intubation.

Attempts at endotracheal intubation can increase the parasympathetic (vagal) tone. This, in turn, may increase intracranial pressure and lower the heart rate or increase the severity of other cardiac dysrhythmias already induced by the brain injury. Therefore, carry out the intubation rapidly. If possible, have the most experienced care provider attempt the procedure to reduce both intubation time and vagal stimulation. Also consider use of a pharmacologic agent, such as a topical anesthetic spray, to reduce both vagal stimulation and the retching associated with stimulation of the gag reflex.

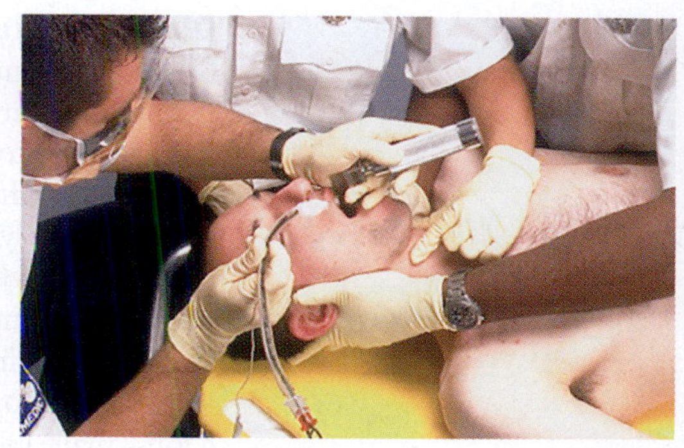

■ **Figure 23-20** Oral intubation is difficult in the patient with facial trauma because landmarks may be distorted, blood may flow into the airway, and the head must remain in the neutral position.

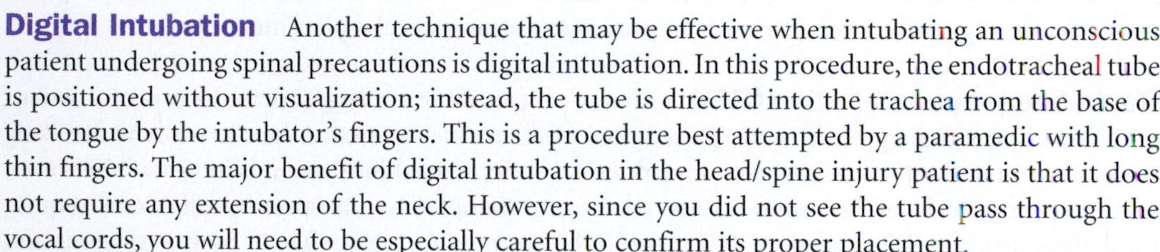

Digital Intubation Another technique that may be effective when intubating an unconscious patient undergoing spinal precautions is digital intubation. In this procedure, the endotracheal tube is positioned without visualization; instead, the tube is directed into the trachea from the base of the tongue by the intubator's fingers. This is a procedure best attempted by a paramedic with long thin fingers. The major benefit of digital intubation in the head/spine injury patient is that it does not require any extension of the neck. However, since you did not see the tube pass through the vocal cords, you will need to be especially careful to confirm its proper placement.

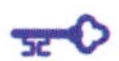

If possible, have the most experienced care provider attempt intubation to reduce both the length of the procedure and vagal stimulation.

A slightly smaller-diameter-than-usual endotracheal tube is shaped by a stylet into a "J" configuration. The patient's mouth is held open with a bite block while you insert the first two fingers of one hand and "walk" them back along the tongue to its base. Use these fingers to locate and lift the epiglottis. Advance the tube with your other hand along the back of the tongue and direct it with your fingers past the epiglottis and toward the tracheal opening. Continue to advance the endotracheal tube with slight anterior pressure along the posterior surface of the epiglottis for about 1½ to 2½ inches. Remove the stylet and carefully confirm tube placement in the trachea, not the esophagus.

Nasotracheal Intubation A third procedure for intubation of the patient with possible spinal injury is nasotracheal, or nasal, intubation. Insert the endotracheal tube into the largest of the nares. Then direct it posteriorly, curving it toward the floor of the nasal cavity. Advance the tube the length of an oral airway (the distance between the earlobe and the corner of the mouth). At this point, slowly continue insertion while you, with your ear at the endotracheal tube opening, listen for the sounds of respirations. Gently manipulate the tube until the respiratory sounds are loudest and then advance it during inspiration. The tube should pass directly into the trachea. The technique can be made somewhat easier using an endotracheal tube with a directable tip (such as an Endotrol). With this device, a small cord connected to the tube's end permits the user to increase or decrease the tube's curve.

The disadvantages to nasal intubation include the necessity of having a breathing patient and a quiet environment, and the danger of inserting the tube through a fractured cribriform plate and into the skull. The procedure has a lower rate of success than either oral or digital intubation. Nasal intubation also tends to raise intracranial pressure more than oral intubation because it generally takes longer and more aggressively stimulates the posterior nasal and oral pharynxes.

Retrograde Intubation Retrograde intubation is a process in which a wire is introduced through the cricothyroid membrane into the larynx, then the pharynx, and then out through the mouth. The process begins with the placement of a catheter through the cricothyroid membrane, directed superiorly. A flexible wire is advanced through the catheter toward the oral opening. A laryngoscope may be inserted to visualize the oral cavity and identify the advancing wire. When you see the wire, use the McGill forceps to retrieve it. Then advance an endotracheal tube over the wire down to the thyroid cartilage. When the tube reaches the larynx, withdraw the wire and advance the tube into the trachea.

Retrograde intubation may be the only effective technique for intubation when the normal landmarks are disrupted by severe facial and airway trauma.

Directed Intubation In some cases of serious facial or upper neck trauma, as in a shotgun blast, the landmarks of the upper airway are disrupted or destroyed. In such cases, obtaining and maintaining an airway may be extremely difficult. Use strong suction over the area, and use the laryngoscope to attempt to visualize the elements of the oro- and laryngopharynx. If you cannot see airway landmarks themselves, look for bubbling air escaping from the trachea with expirations. If you believe you are close to the tracheal opening and can visualize the area, have an assistant compress the chest to induce bubbling. Attempt to pass the endotracheal tube along the route of bubbles and into the trachea. With this technique, it is critically important to confirm proper placement of the endotracheal tube.

Another form of directed intubation uses a device called the gum elastic bougie. The bougie is a long, malleable, gum rubber stylet you insert into the trachea while visualizing it with the laryngoscope. You then insert the endotracheal tube over the bougie and into the trachea. The bougie is withdrawn and the patient is ventilated through the endotracheal tube. The bougie can be placed by the digital intubation techniques, with the endotracheal tube then introduced. However, you must then be especially careful to confirm proper endotracheal tube placement.

Rapid-Sequence Intubation (RSI) Airway protection is a critical skill in the care of a patient with serious head injury. Head injury patients are often unable to care for their airway and are likely to vomit. If they are unconscious and unresponsive, endotracheal intubation is indicated. However, if they are unable to protect their airway yet are not completely unresponsive, they may require intubation using an RSI procedure. RSI may also be required for patients with airway concerns and whose teeth are clenched (trismus) and patients with serious oral trauma with the risk of swelling and progressive airway obstruction. RSI is a medication-facilitated procedure that paralyzes the conscious or semiconscious patient to permit intubation. A sedative/amnestic is administered to sedate the patient and reduce anxiety. A quick-acting paralytic agent is then given to induce muscle relaxation, including the muscles of the oral and pharyngeal cavities. The patient must then be intubated and positive-pressure ventilations provided quickly because the paralytic agent paralyzes all skeletal muscles, including those associated with breathing. The paralytic also eliminates the gag reflex and the patient's ability to maintain the airway.

The drugs most commonly used for this procedure are the paralytics succinylcholine, atracurium, and vecuronium and the sedatives etomidate, diazepam, midazolam, fentanyl, and morphine. Sedative antagonists are frequently used to reverse the effects of these drugs when given and include flumazenil (for diazepam or midazolam) and naloxone (for morphine or fentanyl). (See Chapter 8, "Airway Management and Ventilation," and the discussion later in this chapter.)

The process for RSI begins with reconfirmation of the indications: a patient experiencing muscle spasm (trismus) or who has an altered level of consciousness (Glasgow Coma Scale < 8) and who needs a protected airway. Apply the Sellick maneuver and ventilate or be ready to ventilate the patient as needed. Premedicate the patient with the sedative and then administer the paralytic quickly. When the muscles relax and/or the gag reflex ceases, have the most experienced care provider attempt oral or digital intubation.

The role of RSI in the prehospital management of a head injury patient remains controversial. Some studies have shown that prehospital RSI actually causes a worse outcome when compared to routine airway management. Other studies seem to support its use. RSI may be best suited for services that encounter a great deal of head trauma or who have a limited number of paramedics who perform the procedure to ensure that the provider remains competent in the skill. Above all, the decision to use prehospital RSI rests with the system medical director, and local protocols should be followed.

Confirmation of tube placement is especially important when the tube has been placed blindly.

If you hear good breath sounds bilaterally, detect no epigastric sounds, and see the chest wall move equally with each breath, the tube is most likely in the trachea.

Confirmation of Tube Placement Once the endotracheal tube is inserted using one of the techniques previously described, confirm its proper placement in the trachea. This is especially important when the tube has been placed blindly. Auscultate, at a minimum, the axillae and over the epigastrium. (Good breath sounds at the axillae reflect good ventilation to the distal alveoli.) Watch carefully for adequate, symmetrical chest wall excursion with each ventilation. If you hear good breath sounds bilaterally, detect no epigastric sounds, and see the chest wall move equally with each breath, the tube is most likely in the trachea. Inflate the cuff of the tube and hyperventilate the patient for a short period of time. Use capnography, pulse oximetry, and observation of the patient's skin color to help confirm and monitor proper and continuing endotracheal tube placement.

Remember that the endotracheal tube may dislodge from the trachea during any movement of the patient, as from the ground to the stretcher or as the stretcher is loaded into the ambulance. Reconfirm proper tube placement frequently. Confirm (and document) proper endotracheal tube placement using at least three methods with the initial intubation and after every time you move the patient (visualize the tube passing through the vocal cords, auscultate bilateral breath sounds, observe symmetrical chest rise, and obtain capnography and oxygen saturation readings).

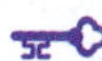

Use of waveform capnography is highly recommended.

The use of continuous waveform capnography provides a graphic and almost irrefutable record of endotracheal tube placement. It also provides information about tube placement and ventilation on a breath-to-breath basis. Waveform capnography is rapidly becoming the gold standard for confirmation of initial and continuing endotracheal tube placement.

Cricothyrotomy

In some cases of face and neck trauma, the region may be so distorted or blocked that oral and nasal intubation are impossible. Here the only potential for providing a lifesaving airway may be opening a surgical pathway for the air. There are two forms of this procedure: the needle cricothyrostomy and the open cricothyrotomy. Consult your protocols and medical direction to identify whether these advanced airway procedures or the other procedures already described may be used in your system.

With needle cricothyrostomy, one or more large-bore catheters are inserted into the cricothyroid membrane to provide a temporary airway. This technique permits only limited air exchange and does not sustain the patient (a temporizing measure). Inspirations can be enhanced by oxygen-powered ventilation (termed *transtracheal jet insufflation*); however, exhalations through the needle are not adequate and the patient cannot be sustained by the technique for more than several minutes. Devices such as the Quick-Trak and Pertrach are variations of the needle cricothyrostomy. These commercially available large-bore devices, designed specifically for ventilation, are relatively easy to insert and their large bore permits adequate ventilation with a bag-valve-mask. They may require prolonged exhalation times to ensure adequate air exchange.

With open cricothyrotomy, an incision and opening is made in the cricothyroid membrane to provide an emergency airway. The soft tissue covering the membrane that separates the thyroid and cricoid cartilages is then held open by a tracheostomy tube or a shortened #6 or #7 endotracheal tube. The chief dangers associated with surgical cricothyrotomy are serious bleeding from the soft tissue surrounding the site (and that bleeding's threat to the airway) and damage to the thyroid and parathyroid glands just below the incision site.

To begin either the needle or open cricothyrotomy, don gloves, goggles, and gown. Then briskly cleanse the upper anterior neck with an alcohol swab in concentric circles outward from the base of the thyroid cartilage. Set out the needed equipment including a large-bore (16-gauge or larger) over-the-needle catheter and a syringe for the needle procedure or a sharp scalpel and a tracheostomy tube or shortened endotracheal tube for the surgical cricothyrotomy. Palpate upward along the trachea from the sternal notch. The first slightly larger and firm ring you feel is the cricoid cartilage. Immediately above it and before the next firm and even larger cartilage (the thyroid cartilage) is the cricothyroid membrane. It is found in the depression between the two cartilages (Figure 23-21 ■).

For the needle cricothyrostomy, attach the catheter to the syringe and perforate the cricothyroid membrane by inserting the needle at a 45-degree angle into the skin and membrane until you feel a "pop." Aspirate air to ensure you are in the trachea. Advance the catheter 1 centimeter over the needle and then withdraw the needle. When using a single large-bore catheter, remove the tube from a 6.0 pediatric endotracheal tube and connect it to the catheter hub. If spontaneous respirations are absent, use a high-flow transtracheal jet insufflation device to ventilate the patient. Use of a bag-valve-mask or demand valve is not acceptable since the pressure of their airflow is insufficient to adequately ventilate the patient through the needle. Give the patient a very long time to exhale as the airway is now extremely restricted. Normally, expiration through the catheter takes about four times longer than inspiration. Watch carefully for chest rise and good breath sounds. When using a commercially available cricothyrostomy device, follow the manufacturer's listed procedure for insertion and ventilation.

Give the patient who has received a needle cricothyrostomy a very long time to exhale because the airway is now extremely restricted.

Placing a second needle adjacent to the first needle will help facilitate exhalation.

For the open cricothyrotomy, insert the blade of a sterile scalpel into the skin over the cricothyroid membrane and make a 1- to 2-cm ventrical incision. Then again locate the membrane and make a 1-cm horizontal incision along its midline (being careful to avoid the adjacent vasculature and nerves). Insert a curved hemostat and open the incisions to enlarge the opening and permit the insertion of the endotracheal or tracheostomy tube. Insert the tube into the trachea. Ventilate the patient with a bag-valve-mask

■ Figure 23-21 Anatomical landmarks associated with the cricothyroid membrane.

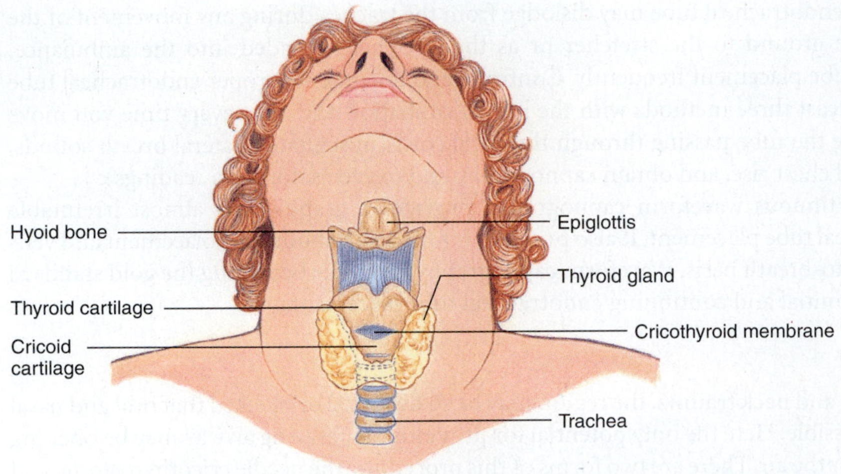

device connected to the endotracheal tube and seal the area with sterile dressings as necessary. You may have to close the patient's mouth and nose or otherwise seal the upper airway opening to ensure that the air reaches the lungs. If the airway obstruction is partial, open the mouth and nose during expiration to enhance the flow of air outward, especially when using needle cricothyrotomy.

BREATHING

Assurance of breathing is an important priority with any patient, but it becomes extremely critical with the head injury patient. Not only is reduced air exchange a problem, but excessive air exchange and the excessive depletion of carbon dioxide can also endanger the patient. Providing supplemental oxygenation and appropriate ventilation are essential with such patients.

Oxygen

Any patient who has sustained a significant head injury or who displays any indication of lowered level of consciousness, orientation, or arousal is a candidate for high-flow, high-concentration oxygen.

Any patient who has sustained a significant head injury or who displays any indication of lowered level of consciousness, orientation, or arousal is a candidate for high-flow, high-concentration oxygen. Administer oxygen at a rate of 15 liters per minute via a nonrebreather mask with a patient who is moving an adequate respiratory volume. If the patient is not breathing adequately, supplement any positive-pressure ventilations with oxygen via reservoir, again flowing at 15 liters per minute.

Ventilation

Provision of a good supply of oxygen is critical to the head injury patient, but so too is the removal of carbon dioxide. Hyperventilation removes too much carbon dioxide and causes profound cerebral vasoconstriction and reduced cerebral perfusion. Hyperventilation also may increase intrathoracic pressure, decreasing venous return and the effectiveness of circulation. Hypoventilation increases the circulating CO_2 levels, causing cerebral vasodilation and an increase in ICP. Either condition can be very dangerous for the head injury patient. Use both capnography and pulse oximetry to guide your ventilations. Assess the patient's respiratory status and, if the patient is not moving a normal volume of air, ventilate. Ventilations for the serious head injury patient (GCS $\leq$ 8) are guided by capnography. For the head injury patient without signs of herniation (increasing blood pressure, decreasing heart rate, and irregular respirations), adjust ventilation rates to maintain an end-tidal CO_2 reading of between 35 and 40 mmHg (adults at about 10 breaths per minute, children at about 20 breaths per minute, and infants at about 25 breaths per minute). For patients with suspected herniation (increasing blood pressure, decreasing heart rate, and irregular respirations), the capnography reading should range between 30 and 35 mmHg, using ventilation rates about 10 breaths per minute faster than for patients without herniation. Also ensure the oxygen saturation with pulse oximetry to maintain a level of at least 95 percent or greater for any serious head injury patient. *If you will be ventilating a patient who does have some ventilations on his own (sometimes referred to as overdrive ventilation), consider RSI, as the patient's fighting your ventilation attempts may increase intracranial pressure.*

CIRCULATION

Your care of the patient with head, facial, and neck injury includes both control of any serious hemorrhage and support of the body's attempts to maintain blood pressure and cerebral circulation.

Hemorrhage Control

Head and facial hemorrhage is usually easy to control because most of these injuries are to the tissues that lie over facial and cranial bones. Direct pressure is commonly an effective means of controlling such bleeding, though you should take care not to put pressure directly on suspected skull or facial fractures. Wrap bandaging circumferentially, but be careful to keep the airway clear and give the patient the freedom to rid himself of vomitus should emesis occur. Watch the airway and be prepared to suction aggressively to limit danger from aspiration. Suctioning can also ensure that the patient does not swallow large volumes of blood, stimulating emesis. Permit the conscious and alert patient with no suspected spinal injury who is suffering epistaxis to sit leaning forward, allowing the blood to drain. This positioning keeps blood from flowing down the pharynx and entering the esophagus.

An open neck injury carries the risk of air entering the external jugular during strong inspiration, leading to cerebral embolism with strokelike symptoms. Seal any open neck wound with an occlusive dressing held firmly in place by bandaging and tilt the patient's body and head down on a backboard or stretcher, if possible. Carefully evaluate any other open wounds for frothy blood suggestive of tracheal involvement, seal those wounds with occlusive dressings, and monitor respirations.

Blunt trauma to the neck may produce the equivalent of compartment syndrome. Fasciae in the region compartmentalize muscle and anatomical structures and permit pressures to rise with rapid edema or blood accumulation. Any sign of neck edema or hematoma is an indication for rapid transport. Monitor the patient's skin tension and level of consciousness while en route to the hospital.

Severe hemorrhage associated with open neck wounds can lead quickly to hypovolemia and shock. Control the blood loss by using a dressing and gloved fingers to apply direct pressure to the source of bleeding. You may have to maintain digital pressure throughout prehospital care because application of circumferential bandaging may restrict the airway and circulation.

Blood Pressure Maintenance

Another component of circulation care for the head, face, and neck injury patient is guarding against hypotension. The brain is very dependent upon receiving a continuous supply of oxygenated blood. Any interruption of the supply, such as might be caused by hypotension in response to increasing intracranial pressure, will rapidly prove fatal. Care for the patient in whom you suspect increased intracranial pressure with fluid resuscitation, even though the patient's other injuries might not suggest that step. For example, the patient with penetrating chest trauma might not receive aggressive fluid resuscitation until the systolic blood pressure drops to below 80 mmHg. If that patient also has a head injury with increasing intracranial pressure, waiting for the blood pressure to drop to that level would be life threatening. Hence, provide rapid fluid (electrolyte) administration, application of a PASG, and other shock care measures to maintain a systolic blood pressure of 90 mmHg.

HYPOXIA

It is very important to monitor the patient with a head injury at all times in order to quickly identify and correct any hypoventilation. Hypoxia can further damage central nervous system tissue already affected by direct injury. If someone else is delivering ventilations, frequently monitor both that person's performance as well as the patient's oxygen saturation levels. Care providers often find it difficult to determine accurate ventilation rates while using a bag-valve-mask unit during the emergency. Assure that the patient is well oxygenated before any intubation attempt and hyperventilated (at 20 times per minute) for a short time after intubation. Also be watchful for interruptions in ventilations that might occur during patient movement or when changing ventilation providers.

HYPOVOLEMIA

Like hypoxia, hypovolemia and any associated hypotension reduce oxygen transport to the brain. This condition also reduces both circulation through the brain and the blood's ability to remove the products of metabolism. Since brain tissue is especially sensitive to oxygen deprivation, with head injury patients who have already suffered some damage to brain tissue, any further circulatory loss might prove devastating. The problems of hypovolemia and hypotension are compounded if there is any increase in intracranial pressure, which further restricts cerebral blood flow. The body's autoregulatory mechanisms cannot compensate in a preexisting state of hypotension.

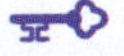

Provide aggressive fluid resuscitation for any patient with significant head injury in whom you suspect brain injury and who shows signs of shock compensation.

Provide fluid resuscitation for any patient with significant head injury in whom you suspect brain injury and who shows signs of shock compensation—rapid, thready pulse, slowed capillary refill, lowered level of consciousness, anxiety, or restlessness. Insert two large-bore catheters and administer lactated Ringer's solution or normal saline at a wide-open rate through nonrestrictive trauma IV tubing. Administer 1,000 mL of an isotonic solution, followed by additional fluids as needed to maintain a systolic blood pressure of 90 mmHg. In the child (6–12 years), young child (2–5 years), and infant (0–1 year), maintain a systolic blood pressure of at least 80, 75, or 65 mmHg, respectively. Periods of hypotension, as well as hypoxia, are associated with a poor outcome from serious head injury.

In serious head injury, the blood pressure remains above 90 mmHg or may rise. This elevation in blood pressure is a reflex response to increasing intracranial pressure and represents an attempt by the body to maintain perfusion of the brain. In the patient with probable brain injury, do not treat hypertension.

MEDICATIONS

Several medications may be useful in the care of the head injury patient. These medications include oxygen, diuretics (mannitol), paralytics (succinylcholine, atracurium, vecuronium), sedatives (diazepam, etomidate, midazolam, morphine, fentanyl), atropine, dextrose, thiamine, and topical anesthetic sprays.

Oxygen

Oxygen is the primary first-line drug used in the care of the patient with suspected head injury.

Oxygen is the primary first-line drug used in the care of the patient with suspected head injury. Administration of high-flow, high-concentration oxygen provides a high inspired oxygen level and facilitates both diffusion through the alveolar and capillary walls and the highest oxygen uptake by the hemoglobin of the red blood cells. Oxygen saturation is important for the head injury patient because the brain is acutely dependent upon a good supply of oxygen. There are no contraindications nor side effects of concern for use of oxygen during prehospital emergency care. (Note, however, that hyperventilation is contraindicated in head injury patients—unless the patient exhibits signs or symptoms of herniation—because it reduces circulating CO_2 levels.)

Administer oxygen via a nonrebreather mask at a flow rate of 15 liters per minute for the patient who is breathing adequately. If the patient is receiving positive-pressure ventilations, supplement the ventilations with 15 liters per minute of oxygen flowing into the reservoir. Monitor oxygen administration using the pulse oximeter, and keep the saturation level above 95 percent. Also monitor skin color, respiratory excursion, orientation, and anxiety to ensure the patient is well oxygenated.

Diuretics

Mannitol Mannitol is an osmotic diuretic that draws water from the interstitial space and into the cardiovascular system. The water is then eliminated, with sodium, by the kidneys. In head injury, this draws fluid from the cerebrum and may reduce cerebral edema and ICP. It is indicated in severe head injury with elevated ICP and/or the signs of herniation. However, use with caution in patients with reduced kidney function, as mannitol may induce hypertension; do not use in patients with hypotension (SBP below 90), as it will further reduce blood pressure. Mannitol is administered as a slow IV bolus of 0.25 to 1 g/kg over 10 to 20 minutes.

Paralytics

Paralytics are drugs that paralyze the skeletal muscles, permitting intubation in patients with whom the procedure would otherwise be impossible. Administration is a part of the RSI procedure, in which you must quickly sedate, paralyze, then intubate the patient while ensuring the patient is well oxygenated and the airway remains clear. RSI uses etomidate, diazepam, midazolam, fentanyl, or morphine sulfate to sedate the patient; in some cases, atropine sulfate to limit muscle fasciculations; and succinylcholine chloride, atracurium, or vecuronium to paralyze the patient.

Succinylcholine Succinylcholine (Anectine) is an ultra-short-acting depolarizing skeletal muscle relaxant. It acts upon cholinergic receptors to cause the muscles to contract (depolarize). This action produces **fasciculations,** individual muscle contractions seen beneath the skin. Succinylcholine induces complete paralysis in 30 to 60 seconds and persists for about 2 to 3 minutes with IV administration. Onset of paralysis occurs in 75 seconds to 3 minutes with IM administration. Succinylcholine is frequently administered to achieve temporary paralysis for the intubation of patients with muscle tone, spasms, or seizures that may otherwise prevent the procedure. Succinylcholine paralyzes the muscles of respiration, so care providers must be immediately ready to intubate and ventilate the patient when the drug takes effect. Succinylcholine does not affect the patient's level of consciousness, cerebration, anxiety, or pain perception, so its use should follow the administration of a sedative/amnestic agent. Succinylcholine increases ICP, may induce vomiting, and should be used with caution, if at all, in cases of head injury. Because it slightly increases intraoccular pressure, it is contraindicated for patients with penetrating eye injuries and should be used with caution in patients who are taking digitalis because of the risk of hypokalemia.

fasciculations *involuntary contractions or twitchings of muscle fibers.*

It is important to remember that neuromuscular blockers do not affect the patient's level of consciousness. All conscious patients should be sedated before administration of one of these agents.

Succinylcholine is administered rapidly in a dosage of 1 to 1.5 mg/kg IV. It may be given IM if necessary. In that case, it is usually supplied in a single-use vial with 10 mL of a 20 mg/mL solution. Storage of succinylcholine requires refrigeration. If the patient is conscious, succinylcholine is given after a sedative/amnestic to sedate the patient during the procedure. Frequently 0.5 mg of atropine is administered prior to succinylcholine to halt the fasciculations and reduce secretions.

Atracurium and Vecuronium Atracurium (Tracrium) and vecuronium (Norcuron) are nondepolarizing skeletal muscle relaxants. They induce paralysis without causing muscle contractions and fasciculations. Both are effective agents with a more rapid onset (less than 1 minute) and shorter duration (25 to 40 minutes) than other nondepolarizing blockers. They also have fewer cardiovascular side effects than succinylcholine. Like succinylcholine, atracurium and vecuronium are used to paralyze patients with muscle tone, spasms, or seizures in order to permit endotracheal intubation. They also do not have any effect on the level of consciousness, cerebration, anxiety, or pain perception, so their use should follow administration of a sedative/amnestic agent.

Atracurium comes in single-use vials containing 10 mg/mL. It is administered by rapid IV bolus of 3 to 6 mg/kg. Atracurium must be refrigerated. Vecuronium is administered rapidly in a dose of 0.08 to 0.1 mg/kg IV. Vecuronium comes as 10-mg vials of powder that must be reconstituted with saline (either 5 or 10 mL) prior to administration.

Sedatives

Diazepam Diazepam (Valium) is a benzodiazepine with both anti-anxiety and muscle relaxant qualities. In prehospital care, it is often used to premedicate patients to facilitate intubation. Diazepam is also a potent anticonvulsant. It is administered in a slow IV bolus of 5 to 10 mg, not to exceed 5 mg/minute, into a large vein. Diazepam is rather fast acting, with IV effects occurring almost immediately and reaching peak effectiveness in 15 minutes. Its duration is from 15 to 60 minutes. Do not mix diazepam with any other drugs, and flush the IV line before and after administration. Administer it as close to the IV catheter as possible. Do not inject it into a plastic IV bag because diazepam is readily absorbed by plastic, which quickly reduces its concentration.

Diazepam is usually supplied in single-use vials or preloaded syringes containing 2 mL of a 5 mg/mL solution (10 mg). Administer 5 to 10 mg IV every 10 to 15 minutes to a maximum of 30 mg. When an IV line is not immediately available, diazepam may be administered rectally for seizures with effects occurring quickly.

The effects of diazepam (and midazolam) may be reversed by the administration of flumazenil. Usually, 2 mL of a 0.1 mg/mL solution is given IV (over 30 seconds) with a second dose repeated at 60 seconds. Be careful in its administration as flumazenil may precipitate seizures in the head injury patient.

Etomidate Etomidate (Amidate) is a very rapid-acting, short-duration, nonbarbiturate hypnotic with no analgesic properties. Etomidate lowers cerebral blood flow and oxygen consumption and has minimal cardiovascular and respiratory effects. Etomidate is of special interest for head injury patients as it somewhat lowers intracranial pressure. An IV administration of etomidate induces hypnosis within 1 minute that lasts for 3 to 5 minutes.

Etomidate is supplied in a preloaded syringe at a concentration of 2 mg/mL and administered in a dose of 0.1 to 0.3 mg/kg over 15 to 30 seconds. It is not recommended for use in children under 10 years of age. Use with caution in hypotensive patients or those with severe asthma. Flumazenil is not effective in reversing the actions of etomidate.

Midazolam Midazolam (Versed) is a benzodiazepine similar to diazepam though it is three to four times more potent. Onset of its effects occurs within 3 to 5 minutes. Administration of midazolam may cause cardiorespiratory arrest and hypotension, and the drug does not protect against increasing intracranial pressure that follows succinylcholine and pancuronium administration. Midazolam is frequently paired with vecuronium to achieve rapid sedated paralysis. It may cause vomiting and nausea and many of the signs and symptoms of head injury.

Administer midazolam very slowly in small increments (at no more than 1 mg/min) titrated to the desired effect or the maximum administration of 2.5 mg. Midazolam is supplied in 2-, 5-, and 10-mL vials of a 1 mg/mL concentration and may be mixed in the same syringe with morphine, meperidine, or atropine or diluted with normal saline.

Morphine Morphine (Duramorph, Astramorph) is an opium alkaloid used to relieve pain (narcotic analgesic), to sedate, and to reduce anxiety. It may mask the signs and symptoms of head injury and mildly increase intracranial pressure. It also reduces cardiac preload by increasing venous capacitance and thus may decrease blood pressure in the hypovolemic patient. Its major side effects are respiratory depression and possible nausea and vomiting.

Morphine is available in 10-mL single-use vials or Tubex units of a 1-mg/mL solution or as 1 mL of a 10-mg/mL solution vial for dilution with 9 mL normal saline. Administer a 5- to 10-mg bolus, slowly IV, and repeat as necessary every few minutes until effective.

Fentanyl Fentanyl is an opiate narcotic, chemically unrelated to morphine, that provides immediate and effective pain control. Fentanyl's onset of action is more rapid than morphine's and it is considerably more potent, thus requiring lower doses. Fentanyl does not cause hypotension to the same degree as does morphine, which makes it an ideal agent for trauma.

Fentanyl is supplied in various doses. The typical starting dose is 25 to 50 mcg IV. Repeat doses of 25 mcg IV can be provided as needed. As with all opiates, continuously monitor the patient's vital signs.

Naloxone (Narcan) is a narcotic antagonist that can quickly reverse the effects of narcotics and should be available anytime you use morphine sulfate or fentanyl. Naloxone is administered IV bolus of 0.4 to 2 mg, repeated every 2 to 3 minutes until effective (up to 10 mg). Naloxone is a shorter acting drug than morphine, so repeat doses may be necessary.

Atropine

Atropine is an anticholinergic (parasympatholytic) agent sometimes administered as part of a rapid-sequence intubation routine. It has the ability to reduce parasympathetic (vagal) stimulation associated with intubation attempts and the resultant decrease in heart rate. Atropine may reduce oral and airway secretions and limit the fasciculations associated with administration of succinylcholine. Atropine may cause pupillary dilation and other CNS signs frequently associated with head injury—headache, nausea, vomiting, and blurred vision.

Atropine is available in many concentrations, from 0.05 and 0.1 mg/mL preloaded syringes to 10-mL vials of 1 mg/mL solution. For emergency administration, its usual form is 10-mL preloaded syringes of 0.1 mg/mL concentration. Atropine is usually administered as a 0.5-mg bolus for rapid-sequence intubation. The pediatric dose is 0.01 mg/kg IV (this dose should be administered to all pediatric patients undergoing RSI and under 3 years of age).

Dextrose

In general, both hypoglycemia and hyperglycemia are detrimental to the patient with head injury. In the past, dextrose was given routinely to patients who were unresponsive with an undetermined cause. However, current practice calls for identifying the blood glucose level on all unresponsive patients, especially those with a possible history of chronic alcoholism or diabetes. If significant hypoglycemia is found, administer 25 mg of glucose and 100 mg of thiamine.

The empiric use of dextrose in the head injury patient is contraindicated.

Dextrose is supplied in preloaded syringes containing 50 mL of a 0.5 mg/mL (50 percent) solution ($D_{50}W$). It is to be administered slowly through a large vein because it is a very hypertonic solution. In severe cases of hypoglycemia, a second dose may be administered.

Thiamine

Thiamine, more commonly known as vitamin B_1, is a substance obtained from diet and needed for body metabolism. Thiamine is essential for the processing of glucose through the Krebs cycle, from which the body gains its life-sustaining energy. In malnourished patients (like the chronic alcoholic), thiamine is depleted and the body tissue cannot obtain energy from glucose. The brain is especially affected since it does not store energy sources.

Thiamine is supplied in 1-mL single-use ampules, vials, and preloaded syringes containing a 100 mg/mL solution. Most commonly, 100 mg are administered IV bolus or IM. It should be administered before or with glucose.

Topical Anesthetic Spray

Topical sprays use an anesthetic agent, such as xylocaine or benzocaine, to anesthetize the oral and pharyngeal mucosa. This reduces the gag reflex, making endotracheal intubation easier and reducing the impact retching has on intracranial pressure. The agent is sprayed into the oral pharynx where it is rapidly absorbed by mucosal tissue. It inhibits nerve sensation, thereby reducing the gag reflex. The effects of the agent are immediate (within 15 seconds), remain local, and last for about 15 minutes. These agents are usually supplied in 2-ounce aerosol spray cannisters with long, hollow extension tubes to direct the spray down the throat. The agent is applied by directing a spray of the material into the posterior oral cavity and pharynx. While topical anesthetic sprays permit easier intubation and reduce the associated vagal effects, they also reduce the patient's ability to remove fluids from the airway and increase the danger of aspiration.

TRANSPORT CONSIDERATIONS

There are special considerations to observe when transporting the patient with serious head injury to the hospital. Some suggest that the use of red lights, siren, rough ride (high speed), and other patient stimulation may agitate the patient, increase intracranial pressure, and induce seizures. While there is little evidence to support this claim, it is probably prudent to reduce speed and use red lights and siren sparingly.

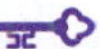

When transporting head injury patients, limit external stimulation, such as the use of red lights and sirens, and try to provide a smooth ride.

Be cautious in considering the head injury patient as a candidate for air medical service transport. While the time saved by helicopter transport may be very important, the head injury patient is prone to seizures, especially with the physical stimulation (noise and vibration) associated with this mode of transport. Seizures aboard any type of aircraft are very dangerous. If you elect to transport by air, ensure that the patient is firmly secured to a long spine board (including feet and hands) and that his airway is protected by endotracheal intubation.

EMOTIONAL SUPPORT

Identify someone to remain with the patient with the specific role of calming and reassuring him during care and transport. Have that person continuously reorient the patient to his environment. Remember, head injury patients may have trouble remembering events preceding and immediately following the incident as well as have difficulty laying down short-term memory. The person assigned the role should describe what happened to the patient and help the patient remain oriented to the current location and what is happening. This simple step aids greatly in reducing the patient's anxiety and in helping to return to a normal level of orientation.

Head injury patients may be very confused, distressed, abusive, or even combative. Do not take their behavior personally. Maintain a professional demeanor and provide emotional support during assessment, care, and transport.

SPECIAL INJURY CARE

There are certain types of head, face, and neck trauma that deserve special care. They include scalp avulsion, injury to the pinna of the ear, eye injury, dislodged teeth, and impaled objects.

Scalp Avulsion

Avulsion occurs when a glancing blow tears the scalp's border and releases a flap of scalp. The flap may remain in anatomical position, fold back exposing the cranium, or may be torn completely free. If the avulsion uncovers the cranium, cover both the open wound and the undersurface of the exposed scalp flap with a large bulky dressing. Also place padding under the fold of the scalp to prevent a sharp kinking along its border. If the region is seriously contaminated, remove gross contamination and rinse the area with normal saline before applying the dressings. Scalp avulsions tend to heal very well unless grossly contaminated or the circulation to the flap is severely disrupted.

Pinna Injury

Serious injury to the pinna, or exposed portion of the ear, often results from glancing blows and trauma, like a tearing or avulsion injury, that disrupts its structure. Such an injury is best treated by placing the pinna in as close to its anatomical position as possible. Then place a dressing between the head and medial surface of the injured ear and cover the exposed ear with a sterile dressing. Finally, bandage the dressed injury firmly to the head.

Eye Injury

Care for eye injuries involves careful assessment and protective care. Most eye wounds or injuries are best cared for by applying soft dressings to cover the closed, injured eye. The other eye, even if uninjured, is also dressed and the dressings on both eyes are held in place with gentle bandaging. This technique prevents sympathetic motion (one eye moving with the other) which may cause additional damage to the injured eye. If the eye injury is an open wound or torn eyelid, consider using a sterile dressing soaked in normal saline to reduce the pain and discomfort and prevent evaporative loss of lacrimal fluid. Place the patient in the supine position if other injuries do not prevent it.

If the patient complains of eye pain without apparent injury, suspect corneal abrasion or laceration, possibly caused by an object embedded in the conjunctiva or sclera. Gently evert the eyelid and examine for any small embedded objects (Figures 23-22a and 23-22b ■). If you observe one, you may attempt to remove it with a saline-moistened cotton swab. Even if you successfully remove the object, the patient is likely to continue reporting pain and the sensation of the foreign body. As with apparent wounds, cover both eyes with soft dressings and loose bandaging.

If the eye is avulsed or has an impaled object in it, cover the eye and the object with a cup or other protective material and again dress and bandage both eyes. If the patient is combative or has a significantly reduced level of consciousness, secure his hands, first together, and then to his waist or belt. This prevents accidental dislodging of the protective dressing and possible aggravation of the eye injury.

Eye injuries and the loss of eyesight in one or both eyes can create anxiety in most patients. Be sure to calm and reassure the patient and explain in advance your actions as you move the patient from the scene to the ambulance and to the hospital.

If, during the assessment, you observe that the patient is wearing contact lenses and there is any risk that he may become unresponsive, have the patient remove the lenses. If the patient is already unresponsive, try removing the lenses yourself with a contact removal suction cup (Figure 23-22c ■). This miniature suction cup seals against the contact lens and allows easy removal. Alternatively, lift the

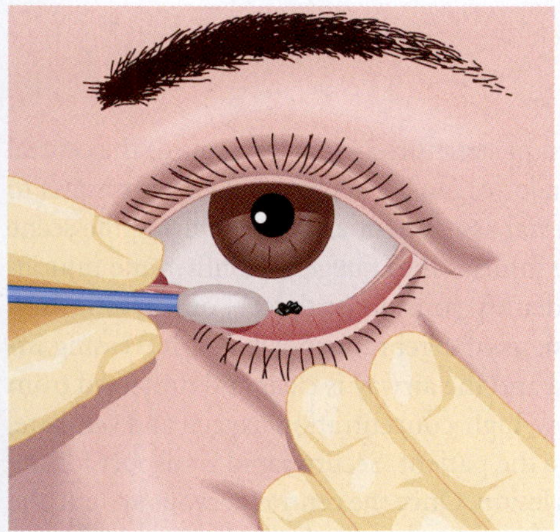

(a)

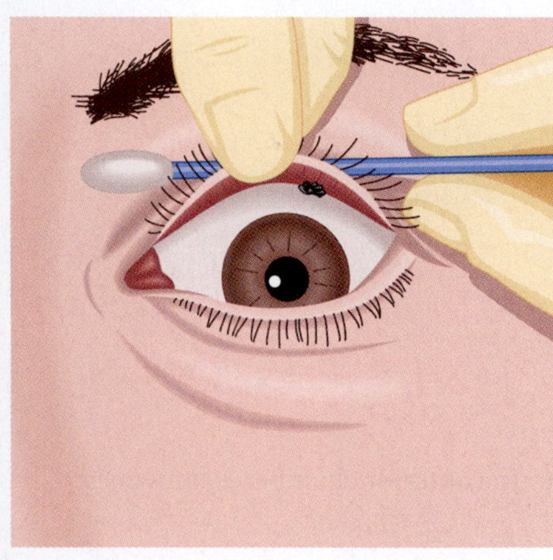

(b)

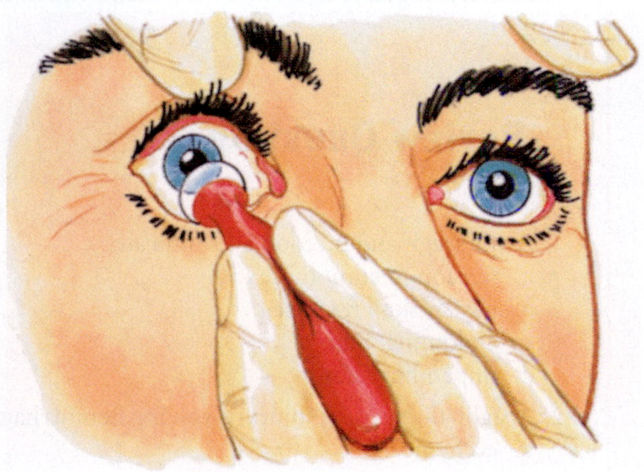

(c)

■ **Figure 23-22** To remove particles from the white of the eye, (a) pull down the lower lid while the patient looks up or (b) pull up the upper lid while the patient looks down. (c) You can use a moistened suction cup to remove hard lenses.

eyelid, which may cause the lens to dislodge, or, with the eye closed, gently push the lens into the corner of the eye. Keep the lens you remove in a contact lens case where it should be soaked in a contact lens or sterile saline solution.

Dislodged Teeth

Locate any teeth that may have been dislodged by trauma and transport them to the hospital with the patient. Rinse the teeth in normal saline and wrap them in saline-soaked gauze for transport to the emergency department. If a tooth is largely intact, it may be successfully replanted.

Impaled Objects

Any object impaled in the head, face, or neck should be left in place and dressed and bandaged to ensure that it does not move about during care and transport. Use bulky dressings to stabilize the object. Secure the patient's hands if there is a danger that he may dislodge the object. Only if the object obstructs or seriously threatens the airway should you consider its removal. In such cases, removal will likely increase the associated hemorrhage and possibly damage adjoining structures, but the patency of the airway is essential.

Removal of objects that pass through the patient's cheek pose the least danger for removal. With such a wound, you have ready access to both of its sides, and the wound involves no critical structures or organs. Nevertheless, expect increased hemorrhage from the wound, have dressings ready, and be prepared to apply direct pressure as soon as the object is removed.

Summary

The head, face, and neck contain very special and important structures—key elements of the central nervous system, the airway, the alimentary canal, and major organs of sensation. Serious trauma to the region endangers these structures and demands special assessment and care. During the scene size-up, identify possible mechanisms of injury and the injuries they suggest. Confirm the injuries during the primary and rapid secondary assessments. Identify your patient's level of consciousness and orientation early, and watch the eyes carefully for signs of cerebral hypoxia and increasing intracranial pressure. Ensure that the spine is immobilized and the airway is clear and protected from aspiration and physical obstruction. Administer high-flow, high-concentration oxygen and ventilate, as necessary, being careful not to under- or overventilate the patient. Secure rapid transport for the patient with possible intracranial hemorrhage or serious lesion. Once the central nervous system, the airway, and breathing are protected, address skeletal structure fractures, minor bleeding, and open wounds. During all your care for the patient with injury to the head, face, or neck, provide emotional support.

Review Questions

1. Battle's sign and raccoon eyes indicate:
   a. tension pneumothorax.
   b. basilar skull fracture.
   c. abdominal injury.
   d. impending shock.
2. A sight-threatening injury, involving hemorrhage into the anterior chamber is known as:
   a. ecchymosis.
   b. blepharospasm.
   c. erythema.
   d. hyphema.
3. Patients with a Glasgow Coma Scale score of ___________ or less should be immediately intubated.
   a. 8
   b. 10
   c. 12
   d. 14
4. Your patient has been involved in an accident and has received open trauma to the neck and blood vessels therein. Your concern should be directed toward the danger of exsanguination and:
   a. pulmonary edema.
   b. tension pneumothorax.
   c. air embolism.
   d. subcutaneous emphysema.
5. Sudden painless loss of sight in one eye is most generally associated with:
   a. ocular trauma.
   b. acute retinal artery occlusion.
   c. retinal detachment.
   d. increasing intracranial pressure.
6. A classic sign of increasing intracranial pressure, which includes increasing blood pressure, slowing pulse, and irregular respirations, is referred to as:
   a. Cheyne-Stokes.
   b. Cushing's triad.
   c. Kernig's sign.
   d. medullary syndrome.

7. The inability to remember events that occurred after a traumatic event is known as:
   a. anterograde amnesia.
   b. retrograde amnesia.
   c. transient amnesia.
   d. morbid amnesia.
8. Which of the following drugs may cause fasciculations and raises ICP?
   a. succinylcholine
   b. Solu-Medrol
   c. mannitol
   d. furosemide
9. For the head injury patient without signs of herniation, you should adjust ventilation rates to maintain an end-tidal CO_2 reading of between:
   a. 20 and 25.
   b. 25 and 30.
   c. 30 and 35.
   d. 35 and 40.
10. Your patient has presented with a facial injury secondary to blunt trauma. You note left facial abrasions and lacerations, depression over the prominence of the left cheek, diminished movement of the left ocular muscles, and diplopia. This injury pattern is consistent with:
    a. Le Fort I fracture.
    b. mandibular dislocation.
    c. basilar skull fracture.
    d. orbital fracture.

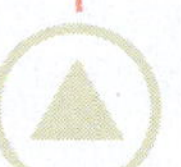

See Answers to Review Questions at the back of this book.

Chapter 24

Spinal Trauma

Objectives

After reading this chapter, you should be able to:

1. Describe the incidence, morbidity, and mortality of spinal injuries in the trauma patient. (p. 1001)
2. Describe the anatomy and physiology of spinal structures and structures related to the spine, including the cervical spine, thoracic spine, lumbar spine, sacrum, coccyx, spinal cord, nerve tracts, and dermatomes. (see Chapter 3)
3. Predict spinal injuries based on mechanism of injury. (pp. 1001–1004)
4. Describe the pathophysiology of spinal injuries. (pp. 1004–1007)
5. Identify the need for rapid intervention and transport of the patient with spinal injuries. (pp. 1007–1012)
6. Describe the pathophysiology of traumatic spinal injury related to:
   - ★ Spinal shock (p. 1006)
   - ★ Neurogenic shock (p. 1006)
   - ★ Quadriplegia/paraplegia (p. 1005)
   - ★ Incomplete and complete cord injury (pp. 1005–1006)
   - ★ Cord syndromes:
     - —Central cord syndrome (p. 1006)
     - —Anterior cord syndrome (p. 1005)
     - —Brown-Séquard syndrome (p. 1006)
7. Describe the assessment findings associated with and management for traumatic spinal injuries. (pp. 1007–1027)
8. Describe the various types of helmets and their purposes. (p. 1019)
9. Relate the priorities of care to factors determining the need for helmet removal in various field situations including sports-related incidents. (pp. 1019–1020)
10. Given several preprogrammed and moulaged spinal trauma patients, provide the appropriate scene size-up, primary assessment, secondary assessment (rapid trauma or focused physical exam, detailed exam), and reassessments and provide appropriate patient care and transportation. (pp. 1001–1027)

Key Terms

anterior cord syndrome, p. 1005
autonomic hyperreflexia syndrome, p. 1006
Brown-Séquard syndrome, p. 1006
cauda equina syndrome, p. 1006
central cord syndrome, p. 1006
transection, p. 1005

INTRODUCTION

A spinal cord injury can both threaten life and induce serious, lifelong disability. Each year more than 11,000 permanent spinal cord injuries occur, most commonly in men aged from 16 to 30. Auto and other vehicle crashes account for almost half these spinal cord injuries (48 percent), with falls (21 percent), intentional injuries (15 percent), and sports-related injuries (14 percent) also contributing significantly to the total. Further, of all patients who suffer neurologic deficit from trauma, some 40 percent have experienced cord injury. The remaining patients with neurologic deficits have suffered injuries that disrupt the spinal or peripheral nerve roots along their course.

Of all patients who suffer neurologic deficit from trauma, some 40 percent have experienced spinal cord injury.

Spinal cord injury is an especially devastating type of trauma. The spinal cord consists of highly specialized central nervous system tissue and does not repair itself when seriously injured. Permanent injury to it affects the body's major communications pathways and control over the lower extremities (paraplegia) or both upper and lower extremities (quadriplegia). Spinal cord injuries also affect the body's control over internal organs and the body's internal environment (homeostasis). A patient with a serious spinal injury is left less able to care for himself, will have a significantly altered lifestyle, and will face increased expenses associated with care and support. In fact, lifelong care costs for the victim of a permanent spinal cord injury may well exceed 1 million dollars. This figure does not include the patient's lost earning power due to the disability.

As with most trauma, the best form of care is prevention. Recent advances in motor vehicle and highway design have helped reduce the incidence of spine injury in its most common category, motor vehicle trauma. Proper use of lap and shoulder belts further reduces the incidence of spinal cord injury, as do programs to reduce drinking and driving. Education programs aimed at teaching safe practices also reduce the potential for spinal cord injury. These programs can foster such behaviors as not diving into unknown waters, developing good physical conditioning, and wearing protective equipment in sports. Following good safety practices in the workplace and in the home can also reduce both temporary and permanent spinal column and cord injury.

PATHOPHYSIOLOGY OF SPINAL INJURY

If you understand how the events of trauma impact the spinal cord and body systems, you will be better prepared to anticipate and recognize spinal column and cord injuries. Traumatic events may cause immediate and devastating injury to the cord with no chance for the patient's recovery. Such events may also cause damage to bones or ligaments, resulting in spinal column instability and providing the potential for cord injury during patient care and transport. By understanding the mechanism of injury and the spinal problems it may produce (the pathophysiology), you can more quickly recognize and better protect the patient with spinal cord trauma.

MECHANISMS OF SPINAL INJURY

The mechanisms of injury that affect the spinal column and cord include extremes of normal motion such as flexion, extension, rotation, and lateral bending (Figure 24-1 ■). Damaging mechanisms also include stresses along the axis of the spine: axial loading and distraction. Finally, spinal injury may occur as a direct result of either blunt or penetrating trauma or as an indirect effect of trauma, when an expanding mass (edema or hematoma) compresses the cord or when a disruption in the blood supply damages it.

Extremes of Motion

Hyperextension or hyperflexion bends the spine forcibly, most commonly in the cervical or lumbar regions. A classic example of an extension injury mechanism is a rear-impact auto crash. The patient's head remains stationary while the upper torso moves rapidly and abruptly forward with the auto. The heavy head moves backwards and hyperextends the neck. The hyperextension places compressing forces on the posterior vertebral structures (the spinous processes, laminae, and pedicles)

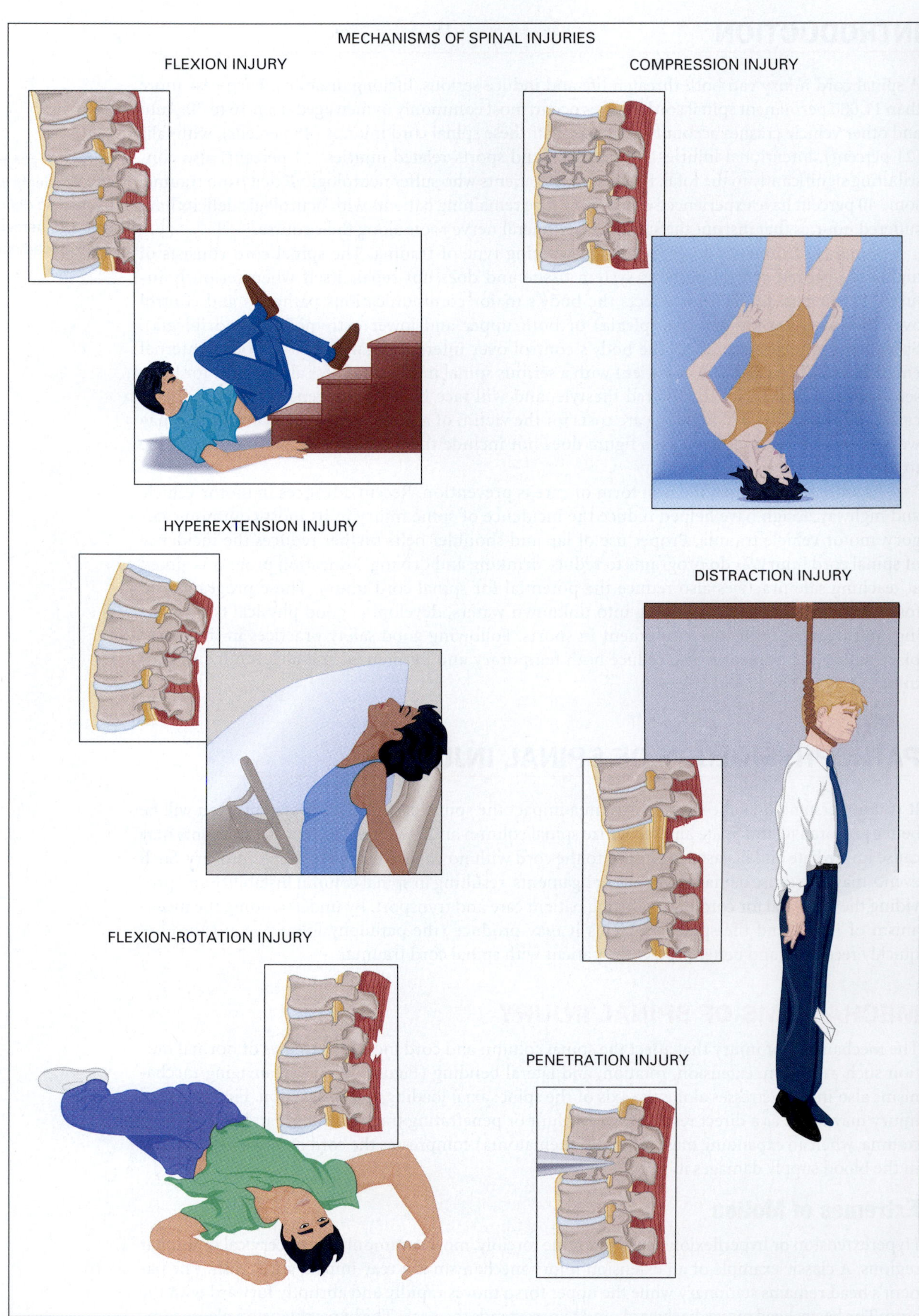

■ **Figure 24-1** Mechanisms causing spinal injury.

and stretching forces on the anterior vertebral ligaments. Extremes of extension may cause disk disruption, compression of the interspinous ligaments, and fracture of the posterior vertebral elements. If the forces are great enough, ligaments may tear or the vertebra may fracture, resulting in instability and bone displacement.

In frontal impact crashes, the shoulder strap may restrain the body while the head continues its forward travel. The attachment of the neck restrains the head and flexes the spine with the movement. The process is frequently forceful enough to cause a patient to literally "kiss the chest" (sometimes demonstrated by the patient's lipstick print on the shirt front). Extreme flexion may lead to wedge fractures of the anterior vertebral bodies, stretching or rupture of the posterior longitudinal and interspinous ligaments, compression injury to the cord, fracture of the pedicle(s), and disruption of the intervertebral disks with dislocation of the vertebrae.

Excessive rotation may occur both in the cervical and lumbar spine. Anatomically, the head is attached to the vertebral column at the foramen magnum, located well posterior of the midline and the head's center of mass. With lateral impact, the head turns toward the impacting force as the body moves out from under it. The cervical spine attachment restrains its motion and turns the head violently. Rotation injury normally affects the upper reaches of the cervical region, but may also be transmitted to the lumbar spine as, for example, when a tackled football player's thorax twists while his feet are firmly planted. The result is a rotational injury that may include stretching or tearing of the ligaments, rotational subluxation or dislocation, and vertebral fracture.

Lateral bending may take place along the entire vertebral column, though it is most common and likely to cause injury in the cervical and lumbar regions. As one portion of the body moves sideways and the remaining portion remains fixed, the spine absorbs the energy. The movement may compress the vertebral structures inducing compression fracture on one side of the column (toward the impact) while it tears ligaments on the opposite side. The result may be compression of the vertebral pedicles with bone fragments driven into the spinal foramen, torn ligaments, and vertebral instability. An example of this mechanism is a lateral-impact auto crash in which the forces of the crash move the thorax to the side and out from under the head, placing severe lateral stress on the cervical spine. Because of the structure of the spine, the forces necessary to induce injury from lateral bending are generally less than those needed to cause flexion/extension injury.

Because of the structure of the spine, the forces necessary to induce injury from lateral bending are generally less than those needed to cause flexion/extension injury.

Axial Stress

Axial loading occurs as compressional stress is brought to bear along the axis of the spine. It may occur when a person lifts a weight too great for the strength of his lumbar spine or when a person falls and lands on his heels. The resulting force is transmitted up the lower extremities to the pelvis, the sacrum, and the lumbar spine. Another frequent mechanism of axial loading injury is the shallow water dive. In this case, the diver impacts the pool bottom with the head while the weight of the lower portion of the body drives the thorax into the head, crushing the cervical spine. This mechanism also occurs in auto crashes, when an occupant is propelled into the windshield by the crash forces. With these mechanisms, impact is likely to compress, fracture, and crush the vertebrae and herniate (rupture) disks, releasing their semiliquid centers into the vertebral foramina and compressing the spinal cord. The most common sites of axial loading injuries are between T-12 and L-2 (for lifting injuries and heel-first falls) and the cervical region (for head impacts).

Distraction is the opposite of axial loading. A force, such as gravity applied during hanging or at the end of a bungee jumper's travel, stretches the spinal column and tears ligaments. The process may also stretch and damage the spinal cord without causing physical damage to the spinal column. The upper cervical region is most commonly affected by this mechanism of injury.

Often the actual spinal injury process involves complicated combinations of the various injury mechanisms previously mentioned. Hanging may suspend the victim from the side of the head, causing injury from distraction and severe lateral bending directed at the C-1/C-2 region (causing a hangman's fracture). The lateral-impact auto crash may produce both lateral bending and rotational injury mechanisms affecting the cervical spine. The shallow water dive may result in both axial loading and hyperflexion as the body pushes against and bends the neck. (Note that the cervical spine is posterior to the midline of both the head and chest. In-line impacts frequently cause the head and neck to flex as the body pushes forward.)

Often the spinal injury process involves a combination of mechanisms.

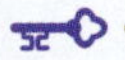

Connective tissue and skeletal injuries represent potential instability of the spinal column and the danger that any subsequent motion may result in spinal cord injury.

Be aware of the distinctions among connective tissue, skeletal, and spinal cord injuries. Connective tissue and skeletal injuries do not necessarily result in spinal cord injuries. They do, however, represent potential instability of the spinal column and the danger that any subsequent motion, even normal motion, may result in spinal cord injury. Spinal cord injury can also occur without noticeable injury to the ligaments, disks, and vertebra of the spinal column. This is why, whenever a patient shows any sign of spine injury or has experienced a mechanism that suggests the possibility of spine injury, you must provide immediate manual immobilization and full mechanical immobilization as soon as possible. Maintain immobilization during all of your assessment, care, and transport.

Other Mechanisms of Injury

Other mechanisms of spine injury can involve both direct blunt and penetrating trauma. Kinetic forces may be directed at the spine when objects strike the spine posteriorly (or laterally in the neck) or when a person falls on or is thrown against an object (as in a blast). Penetrating injuries caused by objects like knives and ice picks or by missiles like blast fragments and bullets may also apply the forces of trauma directly to the spinal column. The penetrating object may harm vertebral ligaments, fracture vertebral structures, drive bone fragments directly into the spinal cord, or directly damage the cord itself. However, unlike blunt trauma, penetrating injury rarely results in ligamentous instability of the vertebral column.

As a result of trauma, tissues adjacent to the spinal cord may swell or otherwise encroach upon the vertebral foramen. With the close tolerance between the interior surfaces of the vertebral foramen and the cord, this swelling may place pressure on the cord, producing direct compression injury and halting blood flow through the compressed tissues. Such injury may also involve the spinal nerve roots that exit the vertebral column close to the injury.

Electrocution, on rare occasions, can cause spinal injury. The extreme and uncontrolled muscular contractions associated with it can tear tendons and ligaments and fracture vertebrae, resulting in column instability and possible spinal cord injury.

A direct injury to the spinal or vertebral blood vessels or any soft-tissue or skeletal injury and the swelling associated with them may decrease the circulation to portions of the cord. This will likely result in tissue ischemia and compromise of cord function.

The coccygeal region of the spinal column can also be injured. Although it contains neither the spinal cord nor many peripheral nerve roots, injury to the region can be painful. Such injuries are usually related to direct blunt trauma, for example, "falling on one's tailbone."

RESULTS OF TRAUMA TO THE SPINAL COLUMN

Spinal injuries may damage the musculoskeletal components of the spinal column, injure the spinal cord, or both. Spinal column injury alone may damage the ligaments and skeletal elements of the column, damaging its integrity and endangering the spinal cord. Injury to the cord may endanger or destroy the ability of the central nervous system to communicate with the body distal to the injury.

Column Injury

The spine is subject to numerous types of injury. The forces of trauma or the stresses of heavy lifting may tear tendons, muscles, and ligaments, resulting in pain and a reduction in the stability of the vertebral column. Those forces may cause movement of the vertebrae from their normal position, a subluxation (partial or incomplete dislocation), or dislocation. The injury process may fracture the spinous or transverse processes, the pedicles, the laminae, or the vertebral bodies. Trauma, especially axial loading, may damage the intervertebral disks. These injuries are to the connective or skeletal tissues of the vertebral column. They may or may not be associated with injury to the spinal cord itself.

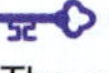

The cervical spine accounts for over half of all spinal injuries.

Several sites along the spinal column are especially subject to injury. The cervical region accounts for over half of all spinal injuries, with the atlas/axis (C-1/C-2) joint being most frequently involved. This is due to the very delicate nature of the two vertebrae, the mobility of the joint, and the great weight of the head it supports. C-7 is also injured frequently because it is located at the transition between the flexible cervical spine and the more rigid thoracic spine.

Similar injuries occur at the transition point between the thoracic and lumbar vertebrae (T-12/L-1), again due to the differences between the rigid thoracic spine and the flexible lumbar spine. The lumbosacral area (L-5/S-1) likewise is injured because the pelvis immobilizes the sacral spine. Spinal injuries not associated with the cervical spine are about equally divided between the thoracolumbar and lumbosacral regions.

Remember that the spinal cord ends at the L-1/L-2 region. Below this point, the spinal nerve roots extend until they exit the spinal column. These spinal nerve roots are more mobile than the cord and less likely to be injured within the spinal foramen during spinal column injury.

Cord Injury

The spinal cord can be injured through the mechanisms discussed earlier. Those injuries can be further described as either primary or secondary. A primary injury is one directly associated with the insult and its effects occur immediately. For example, a primary injury may be caused by cord compression, stretching, or a direct injury. A secondary injury results, as the initial injury causes swelling or ischemia, further injuring the cord tissue. It may also occur as an unstable spinal column is moved about and causes physical injury to the spinal cord. Primary and secondary injuries to the spinal cord can include concussion, contusion, compression, laceration, hemorrhage, and transection.

Review Content

Types of Primary and Secondary Spinal Cord Injuries

- Concussion
- Contusion
- Compression
- Laceration
- Hemorrhage
- Transection

Concussion Concussion of the cord, like a cerebral concussion (see Chapter 23, "Head, Facial, and Neck Trauma"), causes a temporary and transient disruption of cord function. Without associated injuries, cord concussion generally does not produce any residual deficit.

Contusion Spinal cord contusion is simply a bruising of the cord. It is associated with some tissue damage, vascular leakage, and swelling. If blood crosses the blood–brain barrier, more significant edema may occur. But, in general, this injury is likely to repair itself with limited residual effects or none at all. The resolution of a cord contusion and its associated signs and symptoms is likely to take longer than is the case with a concussion.

Review Content

Signs and Symptoms of Spinal Injury

- Paralysis of the extremities
- Pain with and without movement
- Tenderness along the spine
- Impaired breathing
- Spinal deformity
- Priapism
- Posturing
- Loss of bowel or bladder control
- Nerve impairment to extremities

Compression Spinal cord compression may occur secondary to the displacement of a vertebra, through herniation of an intervertebral disk, from displacement of a vertebral bone fragment, or from swelling of adjacent tissue. The pressure caused by these mechanisms results in restricted circulation, ischemic damage, and possibly physical damage to the cord.

Laceration Cord laceration can occur as bony fragments are driven into the vertebral foramen or the cord is stretched to the point of tearing. Laceration is likely to result in hemorrhage into the cord tissue, swelling due to the injury, and disruption of some portions of the cord and their associated communication pathways. In very minor lacerations, some recovery may be expected. Severe lacerations usually result in permanent neurologic deficit.

Hemorrhage Spinal cord hemorrhage, often associated with a contusion, laceration, or stretching injury, produces injury by disruption of the blood flow, application of pressure from accumulating blood, and irritation by blood passing across the blood–brain barrier. Some of the arteries supplying the cord may affect circulation distant from the injury and result in ischemic injury above the level of physical injury.

Transection A cord **transection** is an injury that partially or completely severs the spinal cord. In a complete transection, the cord is totally cut and the potential to send and receive nerve impulses below the site of injury is lost. With transection injuries below the beginning of the thoracic spine, the results include incontinence and paraplegia, while injuries to the cervical spine cause quadriplegia, incontinence, and partial or complete respiratory paralysis.

transection *a cutting across a long axis; a cross-sectional cut.*

Incomplete cord transection involves only a portion of the cord, and some spinal tracts remain intact. There is potential for some recovery of function. There are three particular types of incomplete spinal cord transection: anterior cord syndrome, central cord syndrome, and Brown-Séquard syndrome.

Anterior cord syndrome is caused by bony fragments or pressure compressing the arteries that perfuse the anterior cord. The cord is damaged by vascular disruption and its potential for recovery is poor. The injury generally involves loss of motor function and of sensation to pain, light touch, and temperature below the injury site. The patient is likely to retain motion, positional, and vibration sensation.

anterior cord syndrome *condition that is caused by bony fragments or pressure compressing the arteries of the anterior spinal cord and resulting in loss of motor function and sensation to pain, light touch, and temperature below the injury site.*

central cord syndrome *condition usually related to hyperextension of the cervical spine that results in motor weakness, usually in the upper extremities and possible bladder dysfunction.*

Brown-Séquard syndrome *condition caused by partial cutting of one side of the spinal cord resulting in sensory and motor loss to that side of the body.*

cauda equina syndrome *condition occurring when nerve roots at the lower end of the spinal cord are compressed, interrupting sensation and movement.*

Spinal shock is a temporary form of neurogenic shock that presents with hypotension, bradycardia, and the signs and symptoms of cord injury.

Central cord syndrome is usually related to hyperextension of the cervical spine, as might occur with a forward fall and facial impact. It is often associated with a preexisting degenerative disease, such as arthritis, that has narrowed the vertebral canal. This syndrome results in motor weakness, more likely affecting the upper rather than the lower extremities, and possible bladder dysfunction. Of the three syndromes, central cord syndrome has the best prognosis for recovery.

Brown-Séquard syndrome is usually caused by a penetrating injury that affects one side of the cord (hemitransection). The damage to one side results in sensory and motor loss to that side (ipsilateral) of the body. Pain and temperature perception are lost on the opposite (contralateral) side of the body because of the switching of the associated nerves that occurs as they enter the spinal cord. This injury is rare and is usually associated with some recovery, except in cases of direct penetrating trauma.

Another form of spinal injury is the **cauda equina syndrome**. The cauda equina syndrome occurs when the nerve roots at the lower end of the spinal cord are compressed, interrupting sensation and movement. The nerve roots that control the function of the bladder and bowel are especially vulnerable to injury. A cauda equina syndrome may result from a herniated disk, tumor, infection, fracture, or narrowing of the spinal canal. Signs and symptoms include bowel or bladder dysfunction and progressive weakness in the lower extremities. In addition, there is often a loss of or altered sensation between the legs and over the buttocks, inner thighs and back of legs (saddle area), and feet/heels. Because of the pain, numbness or weakness, the patient may stumble or have difficulty getting up from a chair.

Spinal Shock

Spinal shock is a temporary insult to the cord that affects the body below the level of injury. The affected area becomes flaccid and without feeling, and the patient is unable to move the extremities or other musculature (flaccid paralysis). There is frequently a loss of bowel and bladder control and, in the male, priapism (a prolonged, nonsexual penile erection). Body temperature control is affected, and hypotension is often present due to vasodilation. Spinal shock is often a transient problem if the cord is not seriously damaged.

Neurogenic Shock

Neurogenic (or spinal-vascular) shock results when injury to the spinal cord disrupts the brain's ability to exercise control over the body. The interruption of signals limits vasoconstriction, most noticeably in the skin below the level of injury. Lack of sympathetic tone permits the arteries and veins to dilate, expanding the vascular space, resulting in a relative hypovolemia. With the reduced cardiac preload, the atria fail to fill adequately, and their contraction does not stretch the walls of the ventricles. This reduces the strength of contraction (Frank-Starling reflex) and cardiac output. The problem is further compounded as the autonomic nervous system loses its sympathetic control over the adrenal medulla. It can then no longer control the release of epinephrine and norepinephrine. These hormones are responsible for increasing the heart rate against direct parasympathetic stimulation. Their absence restricts the increase in heart rate that normally follows reduced cardiac preload and falling blood pressure. The result of all these factors is a patient in relative hypovolemia. In addition, it is difficult for the patient to maintain blood pressure with a reduced cardiac output when the body is unable to increase peripheral vascular resistance through vasoconstriction. The patient in neurogenic shock is thus likely to present with a slow heart rate, low blood pressure, and shocklike symptoms (cool, moist, and pale skin) above the cord injury, and warm, dry, and flushed skin below the injury, as well as with priapism in the male.

Autonomic Hyperreflexia Syndrome

autonomic hyperreflexia syndrome *condition associated with the body's adjustment to the effects of neurogenic shock; presentations include sudden hypertension, bradycardia, pounding headache, blurred vision, and sweating and flushing of the skin above the point of injury.*

Autonomic hyperreflexia syndrome is associated with the body's resolution of the effects of neurogenic shock. It occurs in patients well after the initial spinal injury as the body begins to adapt to the problems associated with loss of neurologic control below the injury. After a time, the vascular system adjusts to the lack of sympathetic stimulation and the blood pressure moves toward normal. However, the body now does not respond to increases in blood pressure with vasodilation below the cord injury so only bradycardia results. Autonomic hyperreflexia syndrome is most commonly associated with injuries at or above T-6. The syndrome presents with sudden hypertension, as high as 300 mmHg, bradycardia, pounding headache, blurred vision, and sweating and flushing of the skin above the point of injury. Nasal congestion, nausea, and bladder and rectum distention are also frequently present in autonomic hyperreflexia syndrome. The patient is at risk of developing seizures, stroke, or death. Autonomic hyperreflexia syndrome is a medical emergency and must be treated immediately.

Other Causes of Neurologic Dysfunction

Not all injuries that result in neurologic dysfunction affecting a dermatome or myotome are related to spinal cord injuries. An injury may occur anywhere along a nerve impulse's path of travel. For example, the C-7 nerve root travels from just below the seventh cervical vertebra through the shoulder, arm, and forearm before innervating the little finger. It may be injured by a vertebral fracture; soft-tissue injury and swelling; a shoulder, arm, or forearm fracture; penetrating trauma; or compartment syndrome.

Any of the injuries previously described will interrupt sensory impulses to the brain from the little finger region and motor signals to the region from the brain (to initiate movement and maintain muscle tone). The most obvious difference between nerve root injury and spinal cord injury is the size of the region affected. Remember, however, that an injury that is currently affecting only a single dermatome may have created a vertebral column instability that threatens the entire cord.

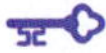

The obvious difference between nerve root and spinal cord injury is that in the former a single dermatome is affected while in the latter multiple dermatomes are affected.

There are also several nontraumatic processes that affect the spinal cord. Refer to Chapter 29, "Neurology," for further information on them.

ASSESSMENT OF THE SPINAL INJURY PATIENT

Assessment and care for the patient with a potential spinal injury begins with special emphasis on the analysis of the mechanism of injury. During this analysis, consciously try to identify or rule out the likelihood of spinal injury. This is important because the patient who has suffered serious trauma may have other injuries that are much more painful and more obvious and that may distract you and the patient from the less obvious signs and symptoms of spinal injury. Also, a seriously injured trauma patient may have a reduced level of consciousness due to intoxication or to other processes such as shock or head injury and thus be an unreliable reporter of the symptoms of spinal injury. For these reasons, you should consider the mechanism of injury to be the most critical indicator of spinal injury.

Put special emphasis on your analysis of the mechanism of injury with a potential spinal injury patient.

SCENE SIZE-UP

Analyze the mechanism of injury very carefully to identify what forces were transmitted to the patient and from which direction they came (Figure 24-2 ■). Identify the likely movements of the spine during the crash or impact and determine if severe flexion, extension, lateral bending, rotation, axial loading,

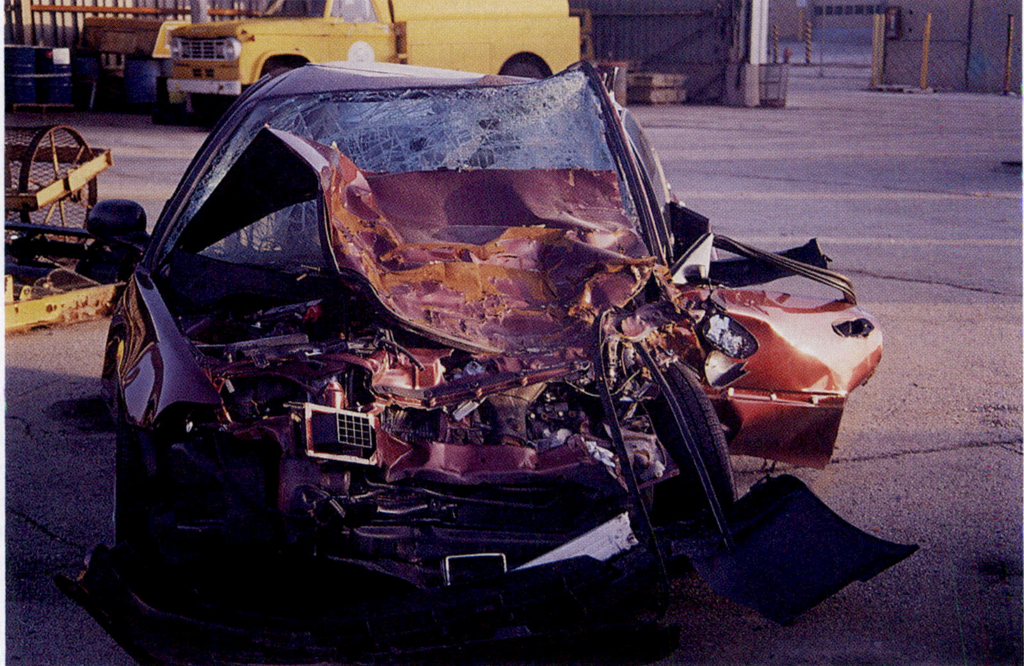

■ **Figure 24-2** Often the mechanism of injury will suggest the potential for spinal column injury.

or distraction was likely. Also, ensure that direct forces of blunt or penetrating trauma did not involve the spine. Be especially concerned about high-speed motor vehicle crashes (including motorcycles, ejections, and pedestrian collisions), any fall (especially in the elderly), any diving or shallow-water injury, any serious blunt injuries above the shoulders, and any penetrating wounds close to or directed toward the spine. Also maintain a high level of suspicion regarding athletic injuries, in which blunt and twisting forces are often transmitted to the spine. If there is any reason to suspect spinal injury, be prepared to employ immediate cervical immobilization as you begin the primary assessment.

Examine the scene to determine whether the patient used a helmet or other protective gear. Remember that helmets reduce the likelihood of head injury but neither increase nor decrease the likelihood of neck injury. Whenever a patient wearing a helmet sustains moderate or severe head impact, suspect spine injury and employ spinal precautions. Bring the helmet to the emergency department with the patient or relate the damages it displayed to the emergency department physician. Also keep in mind that while seat belt use prevents some injuries, it does not preclude spinal injury.

Even if the incident does not appear to involve a significant mechanism of injury or forces directed at the spine, look for and ensure that there are no signs or symptoms of spinal injury during your early assessment. If you are unclear about the mechanism of injury or the potential for spinal involvement, always err on the side of protecting the patient. Full spinal precautions cause some patient discomfort and extend your time at the scene, but failure to provide needed immobilization may result in an unnecessary, devastating, and lifelong patient disability or even death. Generally, a patient sustaining any serious injury receives immediate manual spinal immobilization, thereafter maintained by mechanical immobilization from your first moments at his side until arrival at the emergency department.

If you are unclear about the mechanism of injury or the potential for spinal involvement, always err on the side of overprotecting the patient.

Provide any patient sustaining a serious injury with immediate manual spinal immobilization, followed by full mechanical immobilization from your first moments at his side until arrival at the emergency department.

Recent research is demonstrating that we can reliably identify patients who are likely to have spinal injury. The decision to continue spinal precautions is predicated on an evaluation of the injury mechanism and of patient signs or symptoms of injury. If the patient has a mechanism of injury suggestive of spinal injury you will employ spinal precautions until you can determine that the patient is a reliable reporter of injury symptoms, that there are no distracting injuries, and that there are no signs or symptoms of spinal injury. If you cannot rule out spinal injury, you will provide the patient with full spinal precautions: in-line manual immobilization of the head and spine until the patient is fully immobilized to the long spine board or full-body vacuum mattress.

PRIMARY ASSESSMENT

As you approach the patient and begin your primary assessment, first manually immobilize the head and neck of the patient who has a mechanism of injury likely to cause spinal injury and then determine the patient's mental status. Initial spinal precautions are required to ensure that any spinal injury is not compounded during assessment and care. If the likelihood of spinal injury can be excluded (after the rapid secondary assessment), you may release immobilization of the head—as permitted by your local protocols.

The mental status evaluation is essential in determining the patient's reliability to report symptoms of spinal injury and your ability to rule out the need for spinal precautions. Ensure that the patient is fully conscious, alert, and oriented. If the potential spinal injury patient is found to be intoxicated by drugs or alcohol, to have an altered level of consciousness (Glasgow Coma Scale of less than 15), or seems to be significantly affected by the "fight-or-flight" response, employ full and continuing spinal precautions. You will also employ full and continuing spinal precautions whenever the patient is distracted by a serious injury, such as an open wound, or a symptom, such as dyspnea.

When evaluating a patient for possible spinal injury and the need for spinal precautions, also take into account the patient's age. The elderly often have a reduced sensitivity to pain and may not report an injury or claim it as significant. The elderly are also more likely to have sustained injury with a less significant mechanism of injury. Young children may not be able to localize or accurately report their symptoms. Therefore, whenever presented with an elderly or a very young patient with a mechanism of injury suggestive of spinal injury, be suspicious of injury and provide spinal precautions unless you can confidently rule out spinal injury.

Firmly apply manual immobilization to hold the patient's head in the neutral, in-line position before proceeding with the remaining assessment and care. (Prehospital medicine currently uses terms such as *immobilization, stabilization,* and *spinal motion restriction* [*SMR*] to describe the objective of care techniques used for the spinal injury patient. To limit confusion, we use the term *immobilization* throughout this text. With time, however, *spinal motion restriction,* or a similar term or phrase, may become the standard used to describe the optimal handling of the spinal injury patient. When that becomes evident, we will adopt that term or phrase in subsequent editions.)

Manual immobilization should continue from the moment you arrive at the patient's side and suspect spinal injury until the patient receives full mechanical immobilization to a long spine board with a cervical immobilization device or vest-type immobilization device or is immobilized in a full-body vacuum mattress or until you can determine that spinal precautions are no longer indicated. It is best if the caregiver responsible for the overall assessment and care of the patient does not hold the manual immobilization. A well-trained EMT-Basic or First Responder may best provide this manual immobilization.

Neutral, in-line positioning is very important in the care of a spinal injury patient because it maintains the best orientation of the spinal column and the greatest clearance between the cord and the interior of the spinal foramen. This positioning permits the best circulation and thus lessens the impact of local injury and edema. As your assessment progresses, gently and smoothly move any body segment that is out of alignment toward alignment as you examine it. If the patient feels any increase in pain or if you feel resistance to movement, immobilize the head and neck or other portion of the body in the position achieved. Do not continue movement as doing so may compromise the spinal cord. Maintain the patient's head and body position using manual immobilization until you can secure the position with full mechanical immobilization using the spine board, firm padding, and a cervical immobilization device or full-body vacuum mattress.

Once you assess the neck, consider applying a cervical collar. While the collar does not prevent flexion/extension, rotation, or lateral bending, it does limit cervical motion. However, manual immobilization of the head and neck is adequate until time and patient priorities permit you to apply the collar. Manual immobilization must continue even after a cervical collar has been applied until full mechanical immobilization is achieved.

Manual immobilization must continue even after a cervical collar has been applied and until it is maintained with mechanical immobilization.

As you move on to assess the airway, be sure that the patient's head remains in the neutral, in-line position. The airway is more difficult to control when you are required to observe spinal precautions. Be ready to carefully log roll the patient if he vomits or if necessary to drain the upper airway of fluids. Have adequate suction ready and anticipate the possible need to clear the airway during transport should vomiting occur. To prepare for this, secure the patient firmly to a spine board and immobilize him well enough to permit 90-degree rotation of the board.

If advanced airway procedures are indicated, consider either orotracheal intubation with spinal precautions or digital intubation. Have the patient's head held firmly in the neutral, in-line position as you attempt to identify airway features and insert the endotracheal tube. Anticipate that landmarks will be hard to visualize because the head cannot be brought into the sniffing position and the upper airway aligned. During the procedure, be careful not to displace the jaw anteriorly beyond the point at which it begins to lift the neck (extension) or to permit any rotation of the head. Digital intubation has the benefit of not requiring any displacement of the head and neck, although it requires a completely unconscious patient and takes a provider skilled in the procedure and who has long fingers to direct the tube properly.

After using any modified or blind intubation technique like those just described, be very careful to ensure proper tube placement by assessing for the presence of good chest excursion and bilaterally equal breath sounds and the absence of epigastric sounds with ventilation. Check the depth of tube placement by noting the number on the side of the tube and secure the tube firmly. Monitor both the tube's depth and the breath sounds frequently during your care and transport. Using the pulse oximeter or capnography is essential to ensure proper tube placement and effective oxygenation.

Quickly evaluate your patient's respiratory effort. In the potential spinal injury patient, watch the motion of the chest and abdomen carefully. They should rise and fall together. Exaggerated movement of the abdomen and limited chest excursion with motion opposite to that of the abdomen suggest diaphragmatic breathing. For such a patient, immediately provide positive-pressure ventilation coordinated with the patient's respiratory effort (overdrive ventilation) while maintaining spinal precautions. Your assistance will make breathing more effective and less energy consuming. Use pulse oximetry to continuously evaluate the effectiveness of respirations.

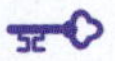

Be very watchful of patients with bradycardia, especially when it is likely that they may be experiencing hypovolemia and shock.

During your check of the patient's circulation status, monitor the pulse carefully. Be very watchful of patients with bradycardia, especially when it is likely that they may be experiencing hypovolemia and shock. This bradycardia may be relative—for example, if a patient has a normal heart rate in the presence of low blood pressure and hypovolemia when a tachycardia might be expected. As you scan the body for other signs of vascular injury or shock, watch for warm and dry skin in the lower extremities while the upper portions of the body show the cool, clammy skin associated with hypovolemic compensation. This is an indication of neurogenic injury and possible shock secondary to spinal cord damage. Spinal cord injury may also induce paralysis and anesthesia below the lesion, reducing the pain or other symptoms of blood loss into an abdominal or extremity injury.

RAPID SECONDARY ASSESSMENT

Once the primary assessment is complete, determine the need for the rapid secondary assessment or the focused physical exam and history. For patients with suspected or likely spinal column or cord injury, move directly to the rapid secondary assessment (Figure 24-3 ■). Even if such patients are otherwise stable, consider rapid secondary assessment, expeditious employment of spinal precautions, and immediate transport to the trauma center. These patients are likely to deteriorate and to need neurologic intervention.

During the rapid secondary assessment, palpate the entire posterior spine. Feel for any deformity, pain, crepitus, unusual warmth, or tenderness from C-1 through L-5. It may be beneficial to repeat palpation of the spine from L-5 to C-1 as pain or tenderness may be difficult to identify in

SIGNS AND SYMPTOMS OF POSSIBLE SPINAL INJURY

- PAIN Unprovoked pain in area of injury, along spine, in lower legs.
- TENDERNESS Gentle touch of area may increase pain.
- DEFORMITY (rare) There may be abnormal bend or bony prominence.
- SOFT-TISSUE INJURY Injury to the head, neck, or face may indicate cervical spine injury. Injury to shoulders, back, and abdomen may indicate thoracic or lumbar spine injury. Injury to extremities may indicate lumbar or sacral spine injury.
- PARALYSIS Inability to move or inability to feel sensation in some part of body may indicate spinal fracture with cord injury.
- PAINFUL MOVEMENT Movement may cause or increase pain. Never try to move the injured area.
- ALSO Loss of bowel or bladder control, priapism, impaired breathing.

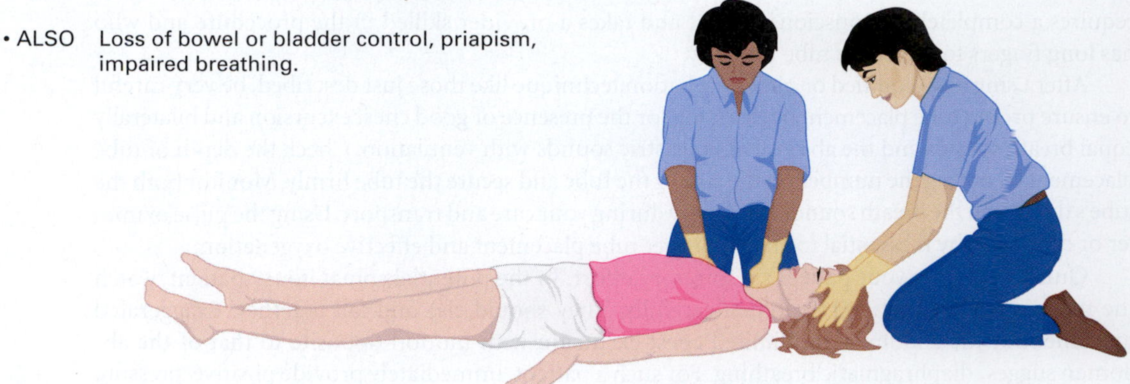

■ **Figure 24-3** Provide immediate and continuing manual immobilization of the patient with possible spine injury while assessing for additional signs and symptoms.

the presence of other painful injuries when minor tenderness may be the only symptom of significant vertebral column instability.

Continue your exam, inspecting each distal extremity and evaluating both motor and sensory function. If there is any limb injury, perform what spinal assessment you can while working around the injuries and ensuring that you do not cause further harm to the limb.

For each upper extremity, test finger abduction/adduction (T-1) by having the patient spread the fingers of the hand while you squeeze the second, third, and fourth fingers together. You should meet with bilaterally equal and moderate resistance to your effort. Test finger or hand extension (C-7) by having the patient hold the fingers and/or wrists fully extended. Place pressure against the back of the fingers while you hold the forearm immobile. Again, you should meet bilaterally equal and moderate resistance. Finally, have the patient squeeze your first two fingers in his hand and ensure that the grip is firm and bilaterally equal (Figure 24-4 ■).

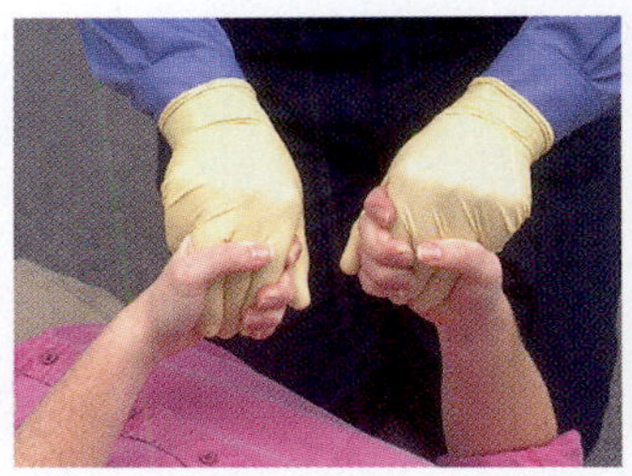

■ **Figure 24-4** Compare grip strength bilaterally.

To assess for limb sensation, first ask about any abnormal feelings in the limb—inability to move (paralysis), weakness, numbness (anesthesia), tingling (paresthesia), or pain. Have the patient close both eyes and check the ability to distinguish between sensations of pain and light touch. To check pain reception (the spinothalamic tract), use the retracted tip of a ballpoint pen or another pointed object not likely to cause injury to induce slight point pain. To check for light touch (involving several tracts), use a cotton swab or a gentle touch with the pad of a finger. Responses to both pain and touch stimulation should be bilateral and equal.

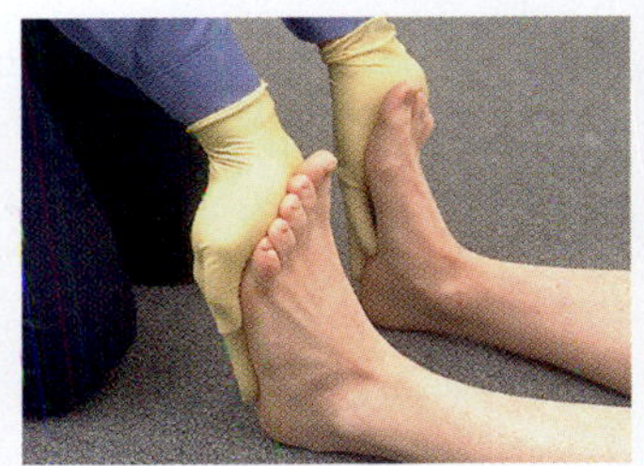

■ **Figure 24-5** Compare lower limb strength bilaterally.

Also test motor and sensory function for the lower extremities (Figure 24-5 ■). Place your hand against the ball of the patient's foot and have him push firmly against it (plantar flexion, S-1 and S-2). Then place your hand on top of the toes and have the patient pull the toes and foot upwards (dorsiflexion, L-5). To evaluate pain sensation, use the same techniques you used in testing the upper extremities. Lower limb strength and sensations should be present and bilaterally equal.

During the full body exam, look for any line of demarcation between normal sensation and paresthesia or anesthesia and any differences in muscle tone. Begin the exam with the feet, and work up the body toward the head. Try not to alarm the patient because if he recognizes that your touch is not felt, his anxiety may increase. Use a sharp object not likely to cause injury, like a ballpoint pen with tip retracted, and move upward. Note the level at which the patient first identifies sensation or pain and relate it to the dermatomes. You might mark the level at which sensation is first noticed on the patient with a pen so that you can compare the results of later tests with your initial results.

Also evaluate the myotomes to determine the level of muscular control. Suspect muscle flaccidity if a body area has muscle masses with a more relaxed tone than the rest of the body. These neurologic signs give you a good indication of the level of spinal cord disruption. Examine both sides of the body as there may be differences from side to side both in sensation and in levels of voluntary and involuntary (muscle tone) motor activity.

You may also perform a test for Babinski's sign (Figure 24-6 ■). Stroke the lateral aspect of the bottom of the foot and watch for the movement of the toes and great toe. Fanning of the toes and

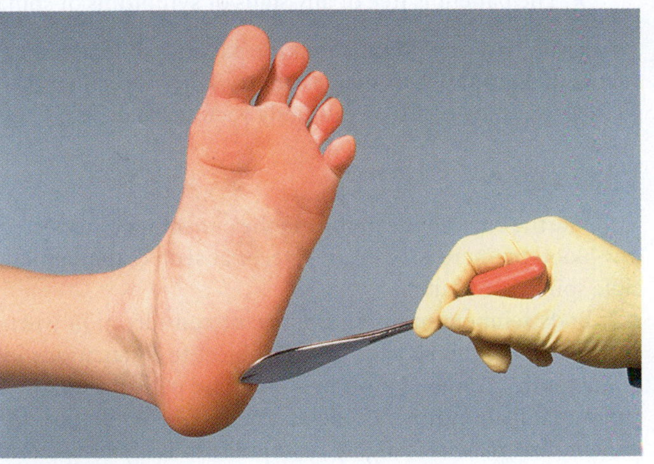

■ **Figure 24-6** Test for Babinski's sign.

dorsiflexion (lifting) of the great toe is a positive sign and suggests injury along the pyramidal (descending spinal) tracts.

If discrete areas of nervous deficit exist, relate them to an injury along the nerve pathway or suspect injury to the spinal nerve root as it emerges from the spinal column. A nerve root injury suggests the possibility of a vertebral column injury and the need for spinal immobilization. Also consider that the source of a deficit may be peripheral nerve damage related to soft-tissue or skeletal damage along its pathway to the affected area. Again, try to identify the associated dermatome and myotome and, thus, the likely location of the lesion along the spinal column, spinal root, or peripheral nerve.

Another sign of spinal injury is priapism. This prolonged, possibly painful erection of the male genitalia is due to unopposed parasympathetic stimulation. Disruption of the sympathetic (thoracolumbar) pathways during a cervical spinal injury can produce this sign. In many cases, the pain sensation is lost due to disruption of the sensory pathways to the brain.

Occasionally, the patient with midcervical spine injury presents with the "hold-up" position. Left on his own, the patient's arms rise to a position above the shoulders and head. This occurs because the injury paralyzes the adductor and extensor muscles while the patient maintains control over the abductors and flexors. Without the opposition of the adductors and extensors, normal muscle tone impulses or any attempt by the patient to move the limb cause it to move toward the flexed position. With such cases, simply secure the patient's wrists to his belt to hold the limbs down for transport.

If the patient is a reliable reporter of injury and does not show any signs or symptoms of spinal injury or the mechanism of injury does not suggest spinal injury, ask the patient to gently move his neck. If the patient experiences any pain or discomfort or shows any neurologic deficit, employ spinal precautions and consider transport to a neurocenter for further evaluation. Also continue to examine the extremities for signs of neurologic impairment. If any are found, immediately employ spinal precautions.

Various spinal clearance protocols have been developed and validated. Among the first of these was the Maine protocol. Some of these spinal clearance protocols were based on a protocol used in emergency departments to determine whether X-rays are required. The study, termed the National Emergency-X-Radiography Utilization Study (NEXUS), was proposed and validated and used by emergency physicians to determine which patients need spinal X-rays and which do not. It seemed intuitive that if a patient did not meet criteria for emergency department spinal X-rays, prehospital spinal immobilization of these patients is probably unwarranted. The NEXUS criteria are essentially the same criteria used in the Maine protocol. International Trauma Life Support (ITLS) recommends a similar protocol. There are several derivations of these protocols (see Figure 24-7 ■), but all have common features. Spinal precautions may be discontinued if all of the following three criteria are met:

- The patient is alert and fully oriented; is not intoxicated or under the influence of drugs, including alcohol; has a Glasgow Coma Scale of 15; and is not significantly affected by the "fight-or-flight" response.
- The patient is free of significant distracting injuries or symptoms such as a fracture, joint injury, abdominal pain, or dyspnea.
- The patient is free of any signs or symptoms of spinal injury.

If you have any doubt about the patient's potential for spinal injury or his ability to accurately report the symptoms of such an injury, continue spinal precautions including full immobilization to the long spine board or full-body vacuum mattress.

Any signs of abnormally low blood pressure, slow heart rate, or absent, diaphragmatic, or shallow respirations suggest possible spinal cord injury.

Vital Signs

Evaluate the vital signs carefully in the patient with suspected spinal injury. Any signs of abnormally low blood pressure, slow heart rate, or absent, diaphragmatic, or shallow respirations indicate possible spinal cord injury.

Body temperature is an important consideration when evaluating the potential spinal injury patient. Spinal injury patients are subject to fluctuations in body temperature related to ambient temperature changes. This is because those patients lose the ability to control the skin's heat conservation/dissipation function below the lesion. While this does not result in an obvious sign in the patient, that patient is highly susceptible to body temperature fluctuations. Cover the patient with blankets in all but the warmest environments and monitor the patient's temperature carefully.

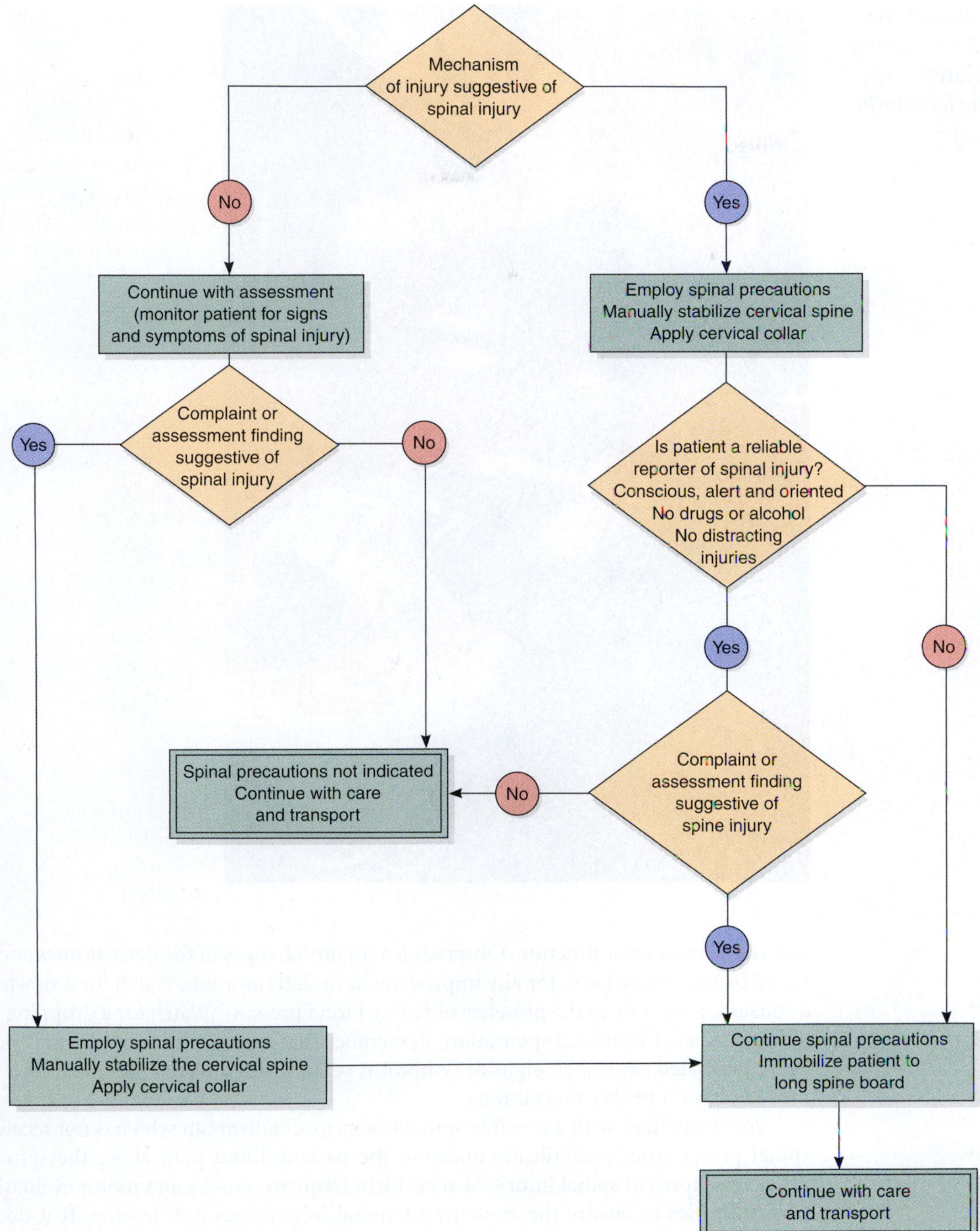

■ Figure 24-7 A spinal clearance protocol.

At the conclusion of the rapid secondary assessment, consider the patient with any sign, symptom, or mechanism of injury suggestive of vertebral column or spinal cord injury, not otherwise excluded, for rapid transport to a nearby neurocenter or trauma center. Employ full spinal precautions, monitor for neurogenic shock, and perform frequent patient reassessments.

REASSESSMENT

During the reassessment, repeat the elements of the primary assessment, take vital signs, and reevaluate any signs or symptoms of spinal cord injury every 5 minutes (Figure 24-8 ■). Monitor carefully for any changes in neurologic signs, including the levels of orientation, responsiveness,

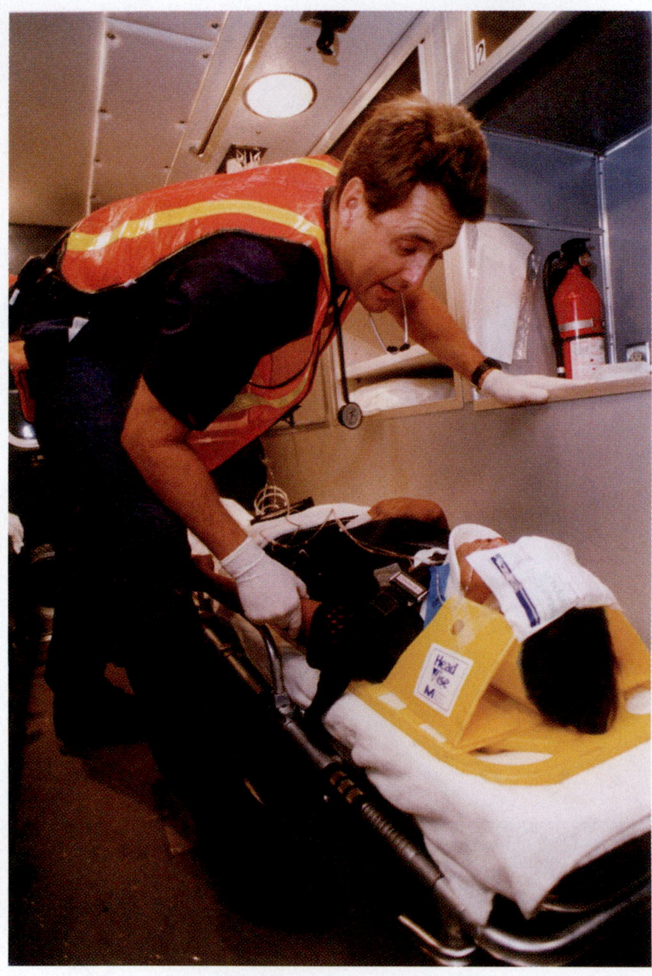

■ **Figure 24-8** Repeat the reassessment every 5 minutes with seriously injured patients. *(© Craig Jackson/In the Dark Photography)*

sensation, and motor function. Observe also for any changes in the dermatomes and myotomes affected by the injury. Look for any improvement or deterioration. Watch for a slowing pulse rate or a constant pulse rate in the presence of falling blood pressure. Watch for a dropping blood pressure without signs of shock compensation. Remember that spinal column injury may not produce any overt associated neurologic signs or symptoms yet may still threaten the spinal cord if the patient is moved without proper precautions.

For the patient with a possible spinal injury mechanism but who has not received continuing spinal precautions, periodically question the patient about pain along the spinal column and other symptoms of spinal injury. Also perform frequent sensory and motor evaluations of the distal extremities to ensure the evidence of spinal injury does not develop. If it does, employ full spinal precautions.

MANAGEMENT OF THE SPINAL INJURY PATIENT

Spinal injury care steps (spinal precautions) performed during the primary assessment include moving the patient to the neutral, in-line position; maintaining that position with manual immobilization until the patient is fully immobilized by mechanical means; and applying the cervical collar once the neck assessment is complete. The remaining steps in management of the spinal injury patient are related to maintaining the neutral, in-line position while moving the patient to the long spine board and then firmly securing him to the board for transport to the hospital.

These skills have but one major objective: maintaining the neutral, in-line position. Although this might seem a simple objective, it is not. Remember that the spine is a chain of 33 small, rather delicate bones, which is attached to other skeletal members only at the head, thorax, and pelvis. These skeletal attachments may transmit forces that attempt to flex, extend, rotate, compress, distract, and laterally bend the spine during any patient movement. The procedures and devices discussed in the following text are intended to ensure that the patient remains in the neutral, in-line position throughout care, movement, and transport.

Spinal precautions have one major objective: maintaining the patient in a neutral, in-line position.

Constantly calm and reassure the patient with suspected spinal injury. Spinal injury can produce extreme anxiety in patients because of the severity of its effects and their potentially lifelong implications. The application of spinal precautions can compound this anxiety. The patient must endure complete immobilization on a rigid and relatively uncomfortable device, the long spine board. He will be unable to move and protect himself during the processes of immobilization, assessment, care, and transport to the hospital. To alleviate some of the anxiety, be sure to communicate frequently with the patient. Tell the patient why you are employing spinal precautions and explain, in advance, what you will be doing in each step of the process. Do what you can to make the patient comfortable and to provide assurance that you and your team are caring for his needs.

SPINAL ALIGNMENT

The first step of the spinal precautions process is to bring the patient from the position in which he is found into a neutral, in-line position adequate for assessment, airway maintenance, and spinal immobilization. This process involves moving the patient to the supine position with the head facing directly forward and elevated 1 to 2 inches above the ground. Remember that the spine curves in an "S" shape through its length. This leaves the head displaced forward when the posterior thorax and buttocks (supporting the pelvis) rest on a firm, flat surface. Also remember that the neutral position (also known as the position of function) is generally with the joints halfway between the extremes of their motion. In spinal positioning, this means the hips and knees should be somewhat flexed for maximum comfort and minimum stress on the muscles, joints, and spine. For complete spinal immobilization, consider placement of a rolled blanket under the knees.

It is also important to ensure there are no distracting or compressing forces on the spine. If the patient is seated or standing, support the head to leave only a portion of the head's weight on the spine. Be careful not to lift the entire head as this places a distracting force on the spine. Lastly, bring the spine into line by aligning the nose, navel, and toes to ensure that there is no rotation along the spine's length. The head must face directly forward and the shoulders and pelvis must be in a single plane with the body. This neutral, in-line positioning allows for the greatest spacing between the cord and inner lumen of the spinal foramen. Neutral, in-line positioning both reduces pressure on the cord and increases circulation to and through it, an especially important consideration in the presence of injury. There are many techniques for moving and immobilizing the potential spine injury patient; whichever you employ, always focus on obtaining and then maintaining neutral, in-line positioning. Doing this assures you the best opportunity to protect the vertebral column and the spinal cord of the patient during your time at his side.

The only contraindications to moving the potential spine injury patient from the position in which he is found to the neutral, in-line position are as follows: when movement causes a noticeable increase in pain; when you meet with noticeable resistance during the procedure; when you identify an increase in neurologic signs as you move the head; or when the patient's spine is grossly deformed. Pain and resistance both suggest that the alignment process may be moving the injury site and thus may be causing further injury. When you meet with resistance or increased pain during any positioning of the head or spine, immobilize the patient as he lies. The same rule applies when you note an increase in the signs of neurologic injury in the patient with movement of the spine. Finally, in cases of severe deformity of the spine, do not move the patient because any movement will further compromise the column and cord. Use whatever padding and immobilization devices are necessary to accommodate the patient's positioning and ensure that no further movement occurs.

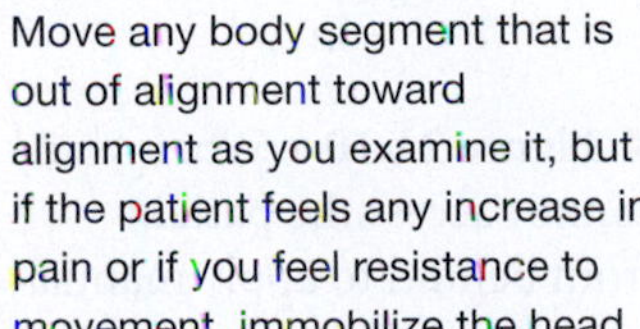

Move any body segment that is out of alignment toward alignment as you examine it, but if the patient feels any increase in pain or if you feel resistance to movement, immobilize the head and neck or other portion of the body in the position achieved.

Ensure that any movement of the patient during assessment or care is toward alignment. If, for example, the patient is lying twisted on the ground when you find him, assess the exposed areas, then move the patient toward alignment. If the patient is found prone, assess the patient's posterior surfaces before you log roll him (to a long spine board) for further assessment and care. Never move a patient twice before you complete your mechanical immobilization, if possible.

MANUAL CERVICAL IMMOBILIZATION

The typical trauma patient is found either seated (as in an auto) or lying on the ground. For the seated patient, initially approach from the front and carefully direct the patient not to move or turn his head. It is an almost reflexive act to turn to listen when we hear someone speak to us from behind. Such movement is dangerous in the potential spine injury patient. Ask your patient to keep his head immobile and explain to the patient that a caregiver is going to position him- or herself behind the patient to immobilize the spine.

The assigned caregiver should then move behind the patient and bring his hands up along the patient's ears, using the little fingers to catch the mandible and the medial aspect of the heels of the hand to engage the mastoid region of the skull (Figure 24-9 ■). Gentle pressure inward engages the head and prevents it from moving. A gentle lifting force of a few pounds helps takes some of the weight of the head off the cervical spine, but care should be taken not to lift the head or apply any traction to this critical region. The patient's head should then be moved slowly and easily to a position in which the eyes face directly forward and along a line central to and perpendicular to the shoulder plane.

If there is no access to the seated patient from behind, employ the same techniques of movement and immobilization from in front with the little fingers engaging the mastoid region while the heels of the hand support the mandible. When approaching from the patient's side, place one hand under the mandible while using the other to support the occiput (Figure 24-10 ■).

If the patient is supine, support the head by placing your hands along the lateral and inferior surfaces of the head. Position the little fingers and heels of the hands just lateral to the occipital region of the skull to support the head. With gentle inward pressure, hold the patient's head immobile and prevent flexion/extension, rotation, and lateral bending motion. Lift the head gently off the ground to approximate the neutral position, usually 1 to 2 inches for the adult. (If the surface on which the patient is found is not flat, adjust the height accordingly.) Position a small adult's or a large child's head at about ground level. Elevate the shoulders of infants or very small children be-

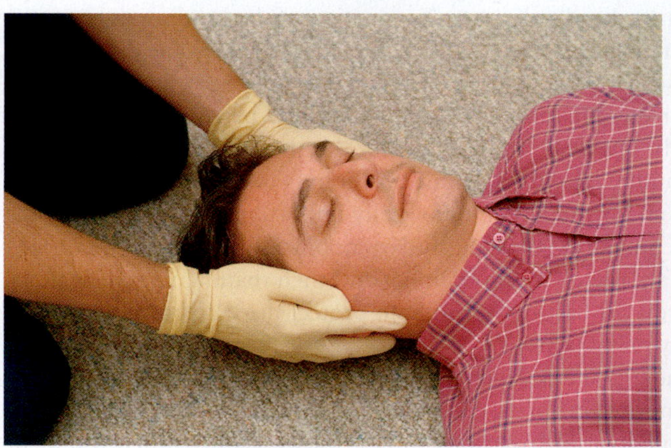

■ **Figure 24-9** Bring the head to the neutral in-line position and maintain manual immobilization until the head, neck, and spine are mechanically immobilized.

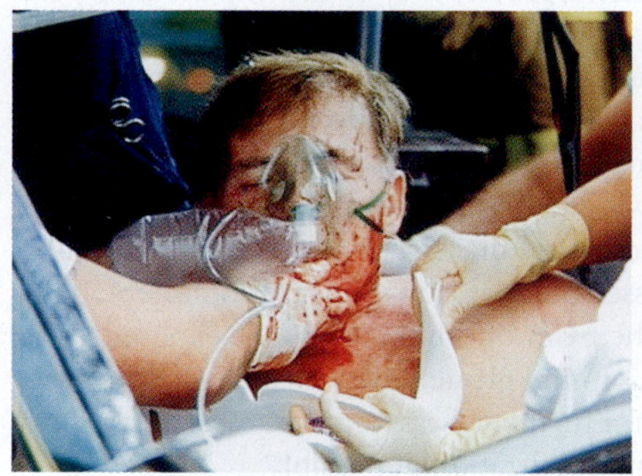

■ **Figure 24-10** When you cannot access the patient from behind to apply manual immobilization, use alternative hand placement.

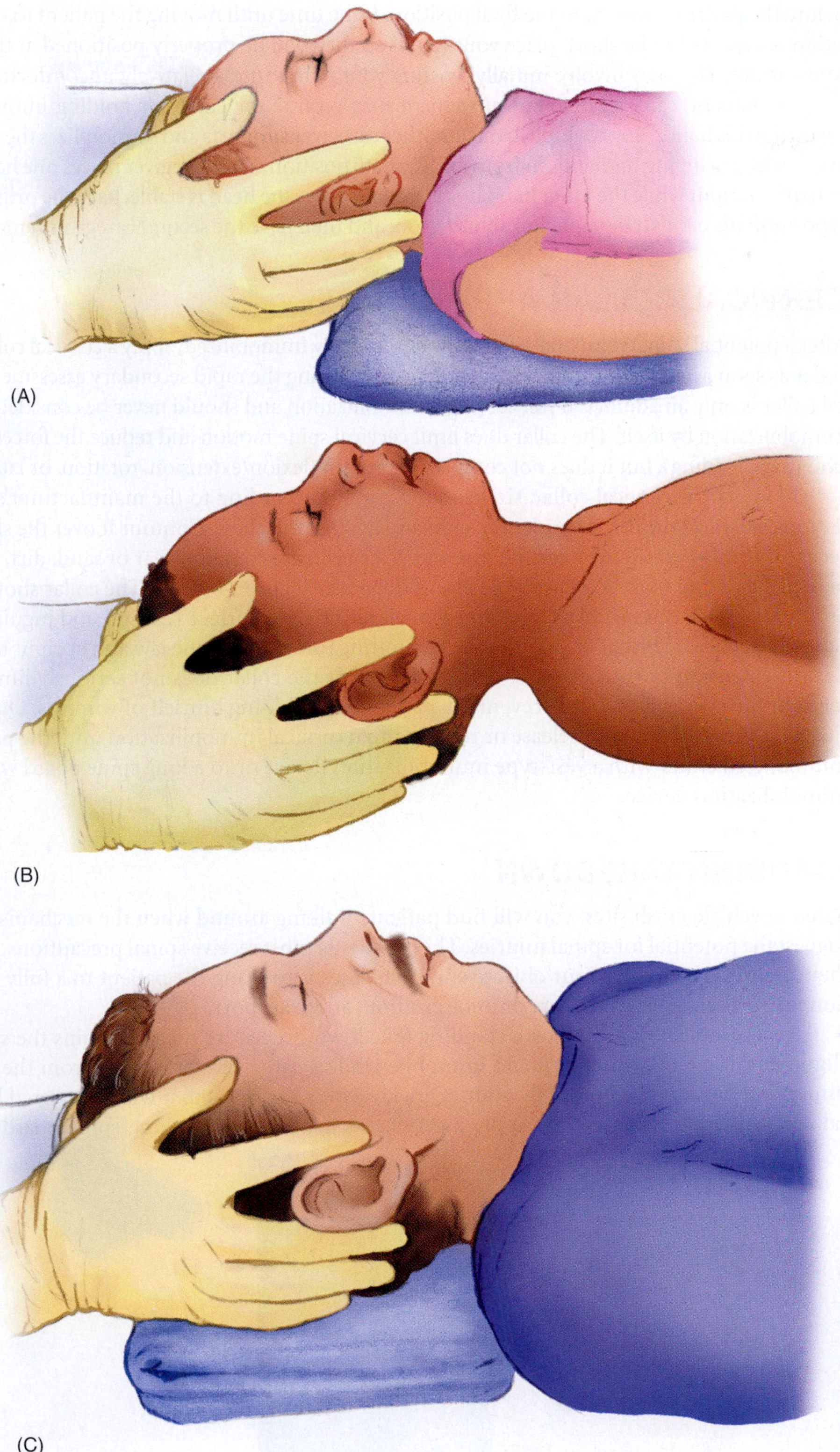

■ Figure 24-11 Neutral spinal positioning for infant, child, and adult patients. (a) Due to the large heads of infants and small children, you may need to raise the shoulder with padding. (b) In older children or small adults, obtain neutral positioning with the shoulders and head on a flat firm surface. (c) With adults, elevate the head 1 to 2 inches with firm padding.

cause of their proportionally larger heads (Figure 24-11 ■). Apply no axial pressure; neither push nor pull the head toward or away from the body.

If a patient is found prone or on the side, position your hands according to the patient's position. If it will be some time until the patient can be moved to the supine position, place your hands so that they are comfortable during cervical immobilization. You should then reposition your hands just before the patient is moved to the final position. If the time until moving the patient to the supine position is expected to be short, place your hands so they will be properly positioned at the conclusion of the move. This may involve initially twisting your hands into a relatively uncomfortable position.

Assessment, care, and patient movement may require the caregiver holding immobilization to reposition his hands. To accomplish this, another caregiver supports and immobilizes the patient's head and neck by bringing his hands in from an alternate position. This caregiver places one hand under the patient's occiput while the other hand holds the jaw. Once the head is stable, have the original caregiver reposition his hands, reassume immobilization, and then have the second caregiver remove his hands.

CERVICAL COLLAR APPLICATION

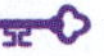

A cervical collar by itself does not immobilize the cervical spine.

Always ensure that the cervical collar is correctly sized for the patient or choose another one.

After a potential spinal injury patient has been manually immobilized, apply a cervical collar. Apply the collar as soon as the neck is fully assessed, generally during the rapid secondary assessment. The cervical collar is only an adjunct to full cervical immobilization and should never be considered to provide immobilization by itself. The collar does limit cervical spine motion and reduce the forces of compression (axial loading), but it does not completely prevent flexion/extension, rotation, or lateral bending.

To apply the cervical collar, size it to the patient according to the manufacturer's recommendations. Position the device under the chin and against the chest. Contour it over the shoulders and secure it firmly behind the neck. Be sure the Velcro closures remain clear of sand, dirt, fabric, or the patient's hair and make a secure seal behind the neck (Figure 24-12 ■). The collar should fit snugly around the neck but not place pressure against its anterior surface (carotid and jugular blood vessels and trachea). The collar should direct a limiting force against the jaw and occiput to restrict any flexion/extension of the head and neck. Ensure that the collar does not seriously limit the movement of the jaw, as this could prevent the patient from ridding himself of vomitus. Once the cervical collar is in place, do not release or relax manual cervical immobilization until the patient is fully immobilized either with a vest-type immobilization device or to a long spine board with a cervical immobilization device.

STANDING TAKEDOWN

Often at vehicle crash sites, you will find patients walking around when the mechanisms of injury suggest the potential for spinal injuries. These patients must receive spinal precautions, even though they are found standing. Your objective in such cases is to bring the patient to a fully supine position for further assessment, care, immobilization, and transport.

To accomplish this, employ a standing takedown procedure that maintains the spine in axial alignment. Have the patient remain immobile while a caregiver approaches from the rear and assumes manual cervical immobilization. Quickly assess any areas that will be covered by the cervical collar or long spine board. Apply a cervical collar and place a long spine board behind and

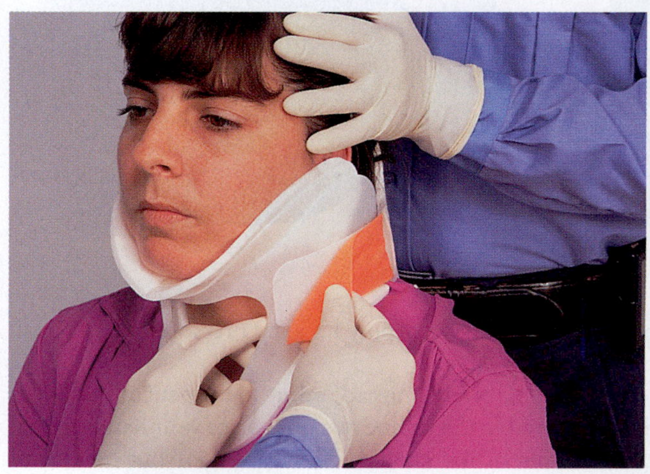

■ **Figure 24-12** Properly place and secure the cervical collar on suspected spinal injury patients.

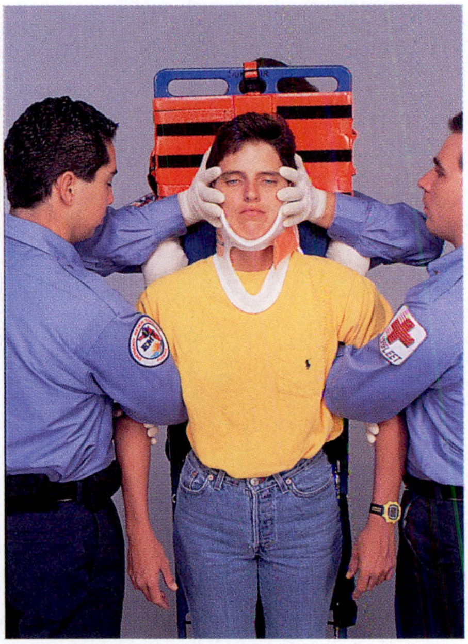

■ **Figure 24-13** The standing takedown.

against the patient, with the caregiver holding immobilization spreading his arms to accommodate the board. Position two other caregivers, one on each side of the spine board, and have each place a hand under the patient's axilla and with it grasp the closest (preferably next higher) handhold on the board. The team should then move the patient and spine board backward, tilting the patient on his heels until the patient and board are supine (Figure 24-13 ■).

During the move, the hands in the handholds support the thorax while the caregiver holding cervical immobilization rotates his hands against the patient's head without either flexing or extending the head and neck as the patient moves from standing to supine. During this maneuver, the hands holding the patient's head must move from grasping the mastoid and mandible (standing) to grasping the lateral occiput (supine). This is not easy, because the head must rotate while the caregiver's hands remain in the same relative position. As with all movement procedures, the caregiver at the patient's head should be in control and direct the process.

Once the patient and board are on the ground, continue to maintain manual immobilization while assessing and caring for the patient. Then provide mechanical immobilization to the long spine board before moving the patient to the ambulance.

HELMET REMOVAL

Helmet use in contact sports, bicycling, skateboarding, in-line skating, and motorcycling has increased over the past decade. While these devices offer significant protection for the head during impact, they have not been proven to reduce spine injuries. Their use also complicates spinal injury care for prehospital care providers. Many helmets are of the partial variety (such as those worn while bicycling and skateboarding) and are easy to remove at the trauma scene. Some motorcycle and sports helmets, however, fully enclose the head and are very difficult to remove in the field. These helmets are also very difficult to secure to the spine board because of their spherical shapes. Further, most full helmets do not hold the head firmly within, so even fixing the helmet securely to the spine board does not result in effective cervical immobilization. Some newer contact sport helmets contain air bladders that expand and firmly hold the head in position within the helmet. These helmets immobilize the head well, but they are still difficult to firmly secure to a spine board. Consequently, most full-enclosure helmets must be removed to ensure adequate spinal immobilization.

Helmet removal may be a tricky endeavor. You should familiarize yourself with the types of helmets used by sporting teams in your area (e.g., high-school football).

The helmet must be removed if you find any of the following conditions:

★ The helmet does not immobilize the patient's head within.

★ You cannot securely immobilize the helmet to the long spine board.

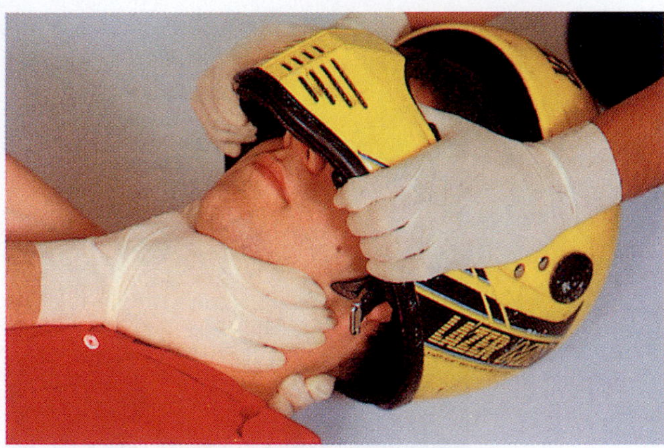

■ **Figure 24-14** Helmet removal.

★ The helmet prevents airway care.

★ The helmet prevents assessment of anticipated injuries.

★ There are, or you anticipate, airway or breathing problems.

★ Helmet removal will not cause further injury.

During helmet removal, have a caregiver initially stabilize the cervical spine by manually immobilizing the helmet. Remove the face mask, if present, either by unscrewing it or by cutting it off, if possible. Remove or retract any eye protection or visor and unfasten or cut away any chin strap as well. Be careful not to manipulate the helmet or otherwise transmit movement to the patient through the helmet. Then have another caregiver immobilize the head by sliding his hands under the helmet and placing them along the sides of the head, supporting the occiput, or by placing one hand on the jaw and the other on the occiput. This caregiver should choose the hand placement that works best for him and can be accommodated by the helmet. The caregiver holding the helmet should then grasp the helmet and spread it slightly to clear the ears by pulling laterally just below and anterior to the ear enclosure. That caregiver then rotates the helmet to clear the chin, counter-rotates it to clear the occiput, and then rotates it to clear the nose and brow ridge (Figure 24-14 ■). The clearance is usually very tight with a well-fitted helmet.

Execute the previous procedure slowly and carefully to prevent head and neck motion and to minimize patient discomfort. For helmets with air bladders, use the same procedure, but empty the bladder after someone stabilizes the head and before you begin the removal. Helmet removal is a complicated skill that you must practice frequently before you can employ it successfully in the field.

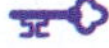

Recent design improvements in the orthopedic stretcher have made it a rigid movement device. It can now be considered an acceptable alternative to the long spine board.

MOVING THE SPINAL INJURY PATIENT

Once you assess and provide the essential care for a patient with a potential spinal injury, plan the movement to the long spine board carefully. If any step of assessment or patient care requires patient movement, consider moving the patient onto the long spine board. Movement techniques suitable for moving the spinal injury patient to the long spine board include the log roll, straddle slide, rope-sling slide, orthopedic stretcher lift, application of a vest-type device (or short spine board), and rapid extrication. Choose a technique that affords the least spinal movement for the conditions and equipment at hand. Also select your movement technique and adjust its steps to accommodate the patient's particular injuries.

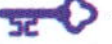

Choose a patient movement technique that affords the least spinal movement.

A key factor in all movement techniques for the patient with potential spinal injury is the coordination of the move. It is essential that you move the patient as a unit with his head facing forward and in a plane with the shoulders and hips. This can best be accomplished if the caregiver at the head controls and directs the move. He is able to see the other rescuers and has a focused and limited function (holding the head), which permits that person to evaluate what the other caregivers are doing. The caregiver at the head directs the move by counting a cadence such as, "Move

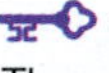

The caregiver at the head directs and controls the movement of the patient with a suspected spinal injury.

on four—one, two, three, four." A four-count is preferable because it gives the other caregivers a good opportunity to anticipate the actual start of movement. All moves must be slowly executed and well coordinated among caregivers.

A four-count is a preferable cadence as it gives a good opportunity to anticipate the start of the move.

Consider what the final positioning of the patient will be when you choose a spinal movement technique. Most spinal injury patients are best served with supine positioning on a long spine board. However, a patient with a thoracic spine injury is frequently placed in a prone position on a soft stretcher. With this patient, other positioning, such as supine on a firm spine board, puts pressure on the injury site from the body's weight and any movement is more likely to cause motion of the injury site and compound any damage.

Log Roll

The log roll can be used to rotate the patient 90 degrees, insert the long spine board, and then roll the patient back. It can also be used to roll the patient 180 degrees from prone to supine or vice versa.

As you begin the 90-degree roll, ensure manual spinal immobilization and apply a cervical collar. Notice that anatomically the shoulders are wider than the hips and legs. To provide a uniform roll, extend the patient's arm above his head. Then place a rolled bulky blanket between the legs (with its bulkiest portion between the feet) and tie the legs together. This reduces pelvic movement and lateral bending of the lumbar spine.

It takes four caregivers to properly perform the log roll for a spinal injury patient (Figure 24-15 ■). One caregiver holds the head, while one kneels at the patient's shoulder with the knees tight against the patient's chest. The third caregiver kneels at the patient's hip with the knees tight against the patient's hip. The last caregiver kneels at the patient's knees with the knees tight against the patient's knees.

The caregivers reach across the patient and around the opposite shoulder, hip, and knee, respectively, and grasp the patient firmly. On a count initiated by the caregiver at the head, the team, in unison, rolls the patient against their knees and up to a 90-degree angle. With a free hand, the caregiver at the knees (or an additional caregiver) slides a long spine board under the patient from the patient's side or the foot end. The board should be positioned tightly against the patient so that the head, torso, and pelvis will eventually rest solidly on the board. Then, at the count of the caregiver at the head, the team rolls the patient back 90 degrees onto the board.

The 180-degree log roll begins with placement of the long spine board between the caregivers and the patient, with the board resting at an angle on the caregivers' thighs. The caregivers reach across the board and grasp the patient as for the 90-degree log roll. The caregiver at the head must be careful to anticipate the turning motion and position his hands so they will be comfortably positioned at the end of the roll. On the count of the caregiver at the head, the team rolls the patient past 90 degrees until he is positioned against the tilted long spine board. Then they reposition their hands against the other (lower) side of the patient and slowly back their thighs out from under the patient until the board rests on the ground.

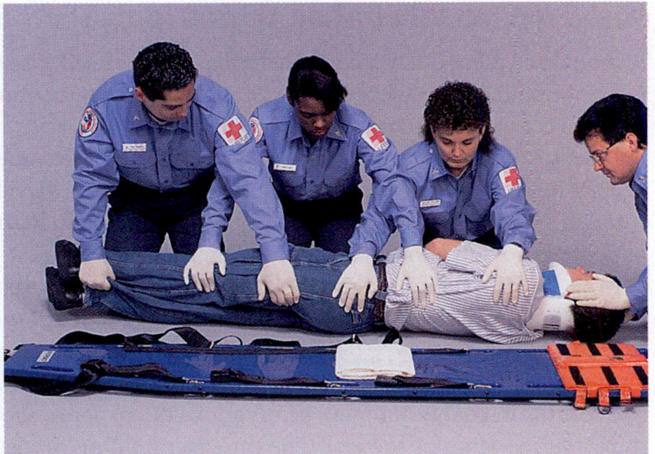

■ **Figure 24-15** The four-person log roll.

Straddle Slide

Another technique effective for moving the patient with potential spinal injury is the straddle slide. In this procedure, three caregivers are positioned at the patient's head, shoulders, and pelvis, while a fourth prepares to insert the long spine board from either the patient's head or feet. The caregiver at the head holds cervical immobilization and guides the lift with a cadence. The second caregiver straddles the patient (facing the patient's head) and grasps the shoulders. The third caregiver straddles the patient (facing the head) and grasps the pelvis. All the caregivers keep their feet planted widely enough apart to permit the insertion of the long spine board. At the direction of the caregiver at the head, the three caregivers lift the patient just enough to permit the fourth caregiver to negotiate the long spine board underneath the patient. (Note: If the board is to be inserted from the patient's feet, the caregiver inserting the board lifts the patient's feet with one hand and slides the board into place with the other.) On a signal from the caregiver at the head, the team gently lowers the patient to the long spine board.

Rope-Sling Slide

A continuous ring or length of thick rope or other material can be used to help slide a supine patient, using axial traction, onto a long spine board. One caregiver holds cervical immobilization, while another places the rope across the patient's chest and under his arms. The rope is tied together (with a cravat) behind the patient's neck and brought out between the legs of the first caregiver. A long spine board is placed between the legs of the caregiver holding cervical stabilization. The second caregiver positions him- or herself at the head end of the spine board with the board resting on his thighs (this provides a small angle to more easily drag the patient onto the board). The second caregiver then pulls on the two strands of rope, guiding the patient onto the spine board as directed by the caregiver at the head. The caregiver holding cervical immobilization moves backwards as the patient is moved onto the spine board. (The caregiver at the head may crouch or kneel to the patient's side to hold immobilization.) The caregiver at the head must be careful to move smoothly with the caregiver pulling axial traction. That person must ensure that the head moves with the body and does not pull against it.

Orthopedic Stretcher

The orthopedic stretcher, also known as the scoop stretcher, is a valuable device for positioning the patient on the spine board or helping to secure the patient to the long spine board. To apply the device, lengthen it to accommodate the patient's height and then separate it into its two halves. Maintain cervical immobilization while you gently negotiate each half of the stretcher under the patient from the sides and connect them at the top, then bottom. Be careful not to entrap the patient's skin or body parts while positioning the stretcher, especially on uneven ground. Once the device is connected, you may use the stretcher to lift the patient to the waiting spine board. Recent design improvements in the orthopedic stretcher have made it a rigid movement device, effective in immobilizing the patient with potential spine injury. It can now be considered an acceptable alternative to the long spine board.

Vest-Type Immobilization Device (and Short Spine Board)

A specialized piece of EMS equipment that may be used with some spinal injury patients is the vest-type immobilization device (Figure 24-16 ■). This device immobilizes the patient's head, shoulders, and pelvis to a rigid board so that you can move the patient from a seated position, as in an automobile, to a fully supine position. The vest-type device comes as a commercially made device that usually has the needed strapping already attached. The device is usually constructed of thin, rigid wood or plastic strips embedded in a vinyl or fabric vest. It is then wrapped and secured around the patient to provide immobilization. An alternative to the vest-type device is the short spine board, a cut-out piece of rigid plywood to which you attach strapping and padding. The basic principles of application are the same with both short-board and vest-type devices.

To apply the vest-type device, manually immobilize the patient's cervical spine and apply a cervical collar while the device is being readied for application. If the patient is positioned against a soft seat (as in an automobile), gently move the patient's shoulders and head a few inches forward to permit insertion of the vest. The caregiver holding cervical immobilization directs and coordi-

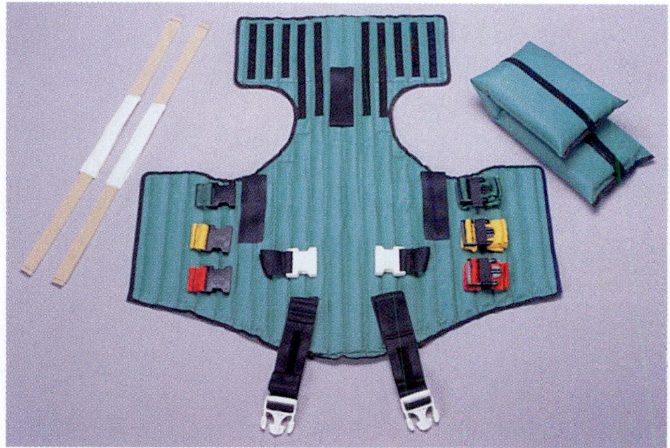

■ Figure 24-16 A vest-type immobilization device.

iates the move, while a second caregiver guides and controls shoulder motion. Negotiate the device behind the patient by either inserting the head portion under and through the arms of the caregiver providing cervical immobilization, or angling it, base first, then moving it behind the patient's back. Position the device vertically so the chest appendages fit just under the arms. This positioning permits you to fasten the straps and secure the shoulders without any upward or downward movement of the device. First, secure the device to the chest and pelvis with strapping and ensure that the vest is immobile. Tighten the straps firmly, but be sure that they do not inhibit respiration. Secure the thigh straps as they hold the hips and thighs in the flexed position, limiting lumbar motion. Then fill the space between the occiput and the device with noncompressible padding to ensure neutral positioning. Secure both the brow ridge and chin to the device with straps, but be very careful to allow for vomiting by the patient and subsequent clearing of the airway or be prepared to release the chin strap immediately if vomiting occurs. Tie the patient's wrists together.

The vest-type immobilization device is not meant to allow lifting the patient but rather to facilitate rotating him on the buttocks and then to tilt the patient to the supine position for further spinal immobilization (Figure 24-17 ■). Once the patient is positioned on the long spine board, gently and carefully release the thigh straps and slowly and gently extend the hips and knees. If after transfer to the spine board the patient's head remains firmly affixed to the vest-type device, leave the vest on the patient and secure the vest to the long spine board since doing this effectively secures both head and torso. If the head becomes loose during the transfer, reapply manual cervical immobilization, secure the torso with strapping, and secure the head with a cervical immobilization device.

The vest-type device is not meant to allow lifting the patient but rather to facilitate rotating and tilting the patient to the supine position.

Rapid Extrication

Applying a vest-type immobilization device is a time-consuming process. Often the circumstances of the emergency, either issues of scene safety or the need for rapid transport to the trauma center,

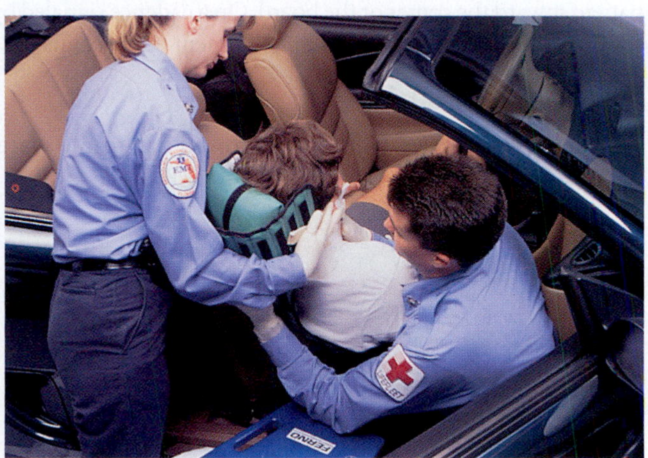

■ Figure 24-17 The vest-type immobilization device is not intended for lifting the patient, but for pivoting him.

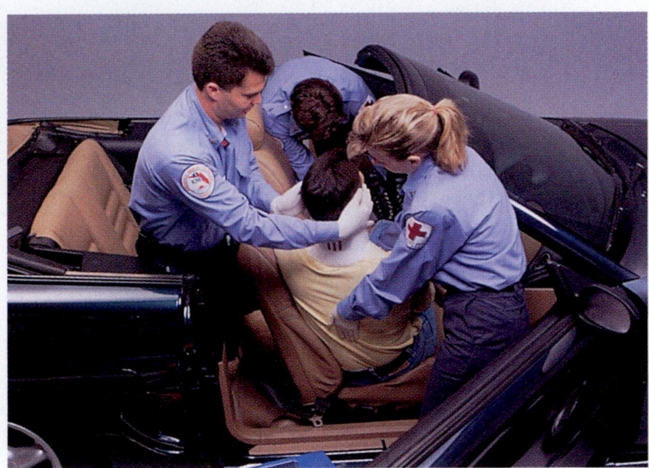

■ **Figure 24-18** Rapid extrication of a patient with a spinal injury.

preclude spending the time required for standard spinal immobilization. In such cases, use a rapid extrication procedure.

With whatever personnel are available, stabilize the patient's spine, shoulders, pelvis, and legs with the patient's nose, navel, and toes kept in line. Ensure that caregivers are coordinated and understand what movement is to take place. One caregiver, usually at the patient's head, should direct the move, counting a cadence to permit the crew to work together (Figure 24-18 ■). Ensure that personnel involved in the extrication move the patient while maintaining the alignment of the patient's nose, navel, and toes. Then, on the leader's count, they should move the patient from a seated or other position to a waiting spine board.

During all movement of a spinal injury patient, keep the spine in the neutral, in-line position by keeping the patient's eyes facing directly forward, and the shoulders, pelvis, and toes in the same plane.

Remember the objectives of spinal movement and stabilization: Keep the spine in the neutral, in-line position by keeping the patient's eyes facing directly forward and keeping the shoulders and pelvis in a plane perpendicular to that of the gaze. Be sure to prevent any flexion/extension, rotation, or lateral bending.

While the technique of rapid extrication does not provide maximum protection for the spine, it does permit rapid movement of the patient with a spinal injury when other considerations demand it. Use the procedure only when your patient cannot afford the time it would take for normal spinal movement techniques. Rapid extrication from the confined space of a wrecked automobile is difficult at best. Plan your move carefully and execute the rapid extrication by carefully explaining the process and individual responsibilities to your team members.

Final Patient Positioning

Centering the patient on the board is essential to ensuring that the patient's spine remains in-line and he is effectively immobilized. Accomplish this by placing team members at the patient's head, shoulders, pelvis, and feet. The caregivers then place one hand on each side of the patient and prepare to move the patient toward the center of the board. On a cadence signaled by the caregiver at the head, they slide the portion of the patient that is out of alignment to an in-line position, centered on the long spine board.

Long Spine Board

The long spine board is simply a reinforced flat, firm surface designed to facilitate immobilization of a patient in a supine or prone position (Figure 24-19 ■). While the board may immobilize pa-

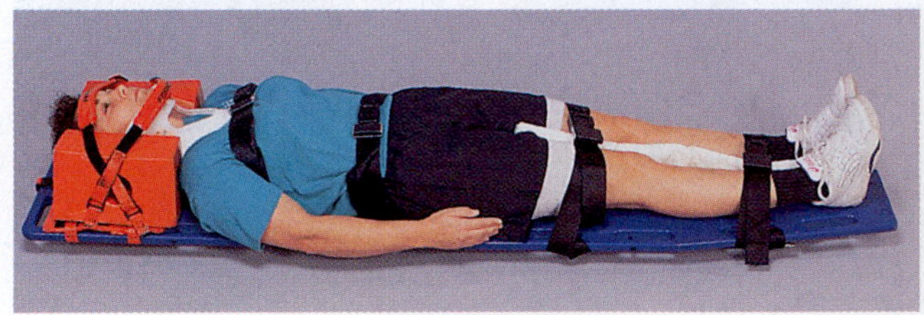

■ **Figure 24-19** Immobilization of a spinal injury patient to a long spine board with a cervical immobilization device in place.

tients with multisystem trauma, pelvic and lower limb fractures, and many other types of trauma, it is primarily designed for patients with spine injuries. The board has several hand and strap holes along its lateral borders. Using nylon web strapping, you can immobilize a patient with almost any combination of injuries to the board firmly enough to permit rotating the patient and board 90 degrees to clear the airway in case of vomiting.

Secure the patient to the board with the strapping, immobilizing and holding the shoulders and pelvis firmly to the board. Such strapping may cross the body and capture the shoulder and pelvic girdles. Ensure that you firmly immobilize the patient to prevent lateral motion as well as cephalad (head-ward) and caudad (tail-ward) motion. Be sure that the pressure created by strapping does not come to bear on the central abdomen. That would cause forced extension of the lumbar spine. Immobilize the lower legs and feet with strapping or cravats. Tie the legs together, and place a rolled blanket under the patient's knees to immobilize them in a slightly flexed position.

Long spine board immobilization is made more effective by use of the cervical immobilization device (CID). This device is made up of two soft, padded lateral pieces that bracket the patient's head, maintaining its position, and a base plate that permits you to easily secure the device to the board. The base plate is affixed to the long spine board before the patient is moved to it. Once you position the patient on the board, fill the void between the occiput and the CID base plate with firm, noncompressible padding. Use no padding for the small adult or older child, and pad the shoulders in the young child or infant to ensure proper spinal positioning. While a caregiver maintains manual immobilization of the head, bring the lateral components of the CID against the sides of the patient's head. Use medial pressure to hold them against the head and keep the head in position. Then affix the lateral CID components to the Velcro of the CID base plate. Secure the head in position and to the long spine board using forehead and chin straps or tape. Make sure the strapping catches the brow ridge and the mandible or the upper portion of the collar. The properly secured CID must hold the patient's head in the neutral position without movement while not placing undue pressure on the neck or restricting jaw movement (in case of vomiting). Be careful that the straps do not flex, extend, or rotate the head. Bulky blanket rolls, placed on each side of the head and secured both to the head and the board, will also effectively immobilize the head to the long spine board.

The long spine board does have drawbacks. Its firm surface places extreme pressure on the skin and tissues covering the ischial tuberosities and the shoulder blades. If a patient remains immobilized to the board for more than a couple of hours, ulceration injuries are likely to result.

Immobilize the adult patient to the long spine board with the head elevated 1–2 inches, the knees slightly flexed, and with limited padding at the small of the back and the space behind the neck.

The board also tends to encourage caregivers to immobilize the patient directly to it in a nonneutral position. In a proper neutral position, the head should be elevated about 1 to 2 inches above the board's surface and the knees should be bent at 15 to 30 degrees. This positioning relieves pressure on the cervical spine, lumbar spine, hips, and knees and increases patient comfort. You can obtain proper knee positioning by placing folded blankets under the patient's knees. Also pad under the curves of the back. Do not overpad; just fill the voids at the small of the back and neck with bulky soft dressing material.

Full-Body Vacuum Mattress

A device that is now showing merit for spinal immobilization is the full-body vacuum mattress (Figure 24-20 ■), also known as a full-body vacuum splint. Like the vacuum splints for the limbs discussed in Chapter 22, "Musculoskeletal Trauma," the full-body vacuum mattress uses small plastic beads that maintain their position in the reduced pressure after air is evacuated from the splint. To apply the vacuum mattress, place the patient on the flattened device and shape it around him. Evacuating the air causes the device to form to the contours of the patient's body and maintain immobilization.

Diving Injury Immobilization

Patients injured in shallow water dives are often paralyzed from the impact. They must rely on others to protect their airways and remove them from the water. When carried out by untrained bystanders, however, these activities may compound any spinal injury. If you are present when such an incident occurs, be sure to carefully control any patient motion while he is still in the water. If necessary, turn him to a supine position, ensuring that the nose, navel, and toes remain in a single plane and that the eyes face directly forward. You may accomplish this by sandwiching the patient's

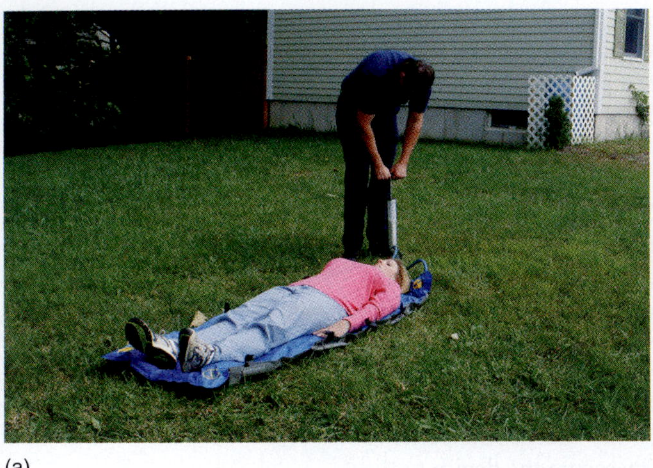

(a)

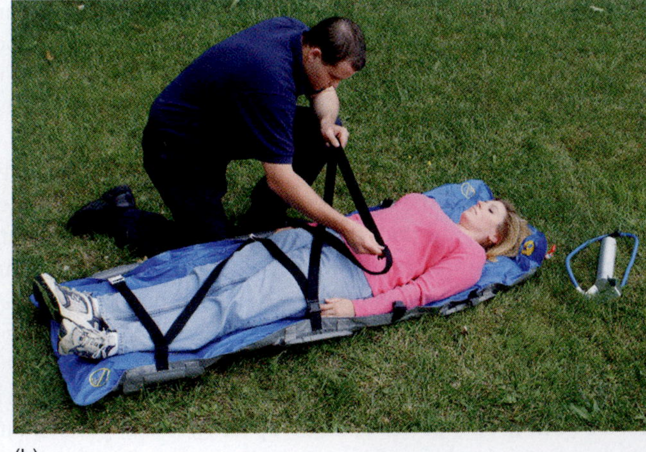

(b)

■ **Figure 24-20** A full-body vacuum mattress can adequately immobilize the spine injury patient. (a) The device is shaped around the patient and air is withdrawn. (b) The patient is then secured to the rigid, conforming vacuum mattress.

chest between your forearms while your arms and shoulders cradle the head. Once the patient is in the supine position, water provides an almost neutral buoyancy and, if the water is calm, helps to immobilize the patient. Move the patient by pulling on the shoulders while you cradle the head, in the neutral position, with the forearms. Float a long spine board under the patient, strap him firmly to the board, and then lift and carry him from the water.

MEDICATIONS

There are several conditions that merit the use of medications for the patient with spine injury. These conditions include neurogenic shock and the combative patient. As noted in the following sections, recent research has changed views about administering steroids for spinal cord injury.

Medications and Spinal Cord Injury

Routine use of steroids for spinal injury is no longer recommended.

In the past, steroids have been used to combat the inflammation frequently associated with spinal cord injury. Recent research and other information now suggest that this treatment is not as effective as once thought, and high-dose steroid treatment is not without significant side effects. Hence, the routine use of steroids for the treatment of spinal injury is no longer recommended. Consult your medical director and protocols for any system-specific recommendations regarding the use of medications in the treatment of spinal injury.

Medications and Neurogenic Shock

The loss of sympathetic control leads to both a relaxation of the blood vessels (vasodilation) below the level of the lesion and the inability of the body to increase the heart rate. This expanded vascular system leads to a relative hypovolemia and lower blood pressure. The problem is further compounded as the heart, without sympathetic stimulation and in the presence of this relative hypovolemia, displays a normal or bradycardic heart rate. Frequently, the hypovolemia is treated with a fluid challenge, followed by careful use of a vasopressor such as dopamine. The slow heart rate is treated with atropine to reduce any parasympathetic stimulation.

The use of the PASG to combat the relative hypovolemia of neurogenic shock is somewhat controversial. The compression of the lower extremities and abdomen may counteract the vasodilation associated with the shock state, but research has not yet proven the garment's use contributes to a better outcome. Follow local protocols and consult with medical direction before using the device.

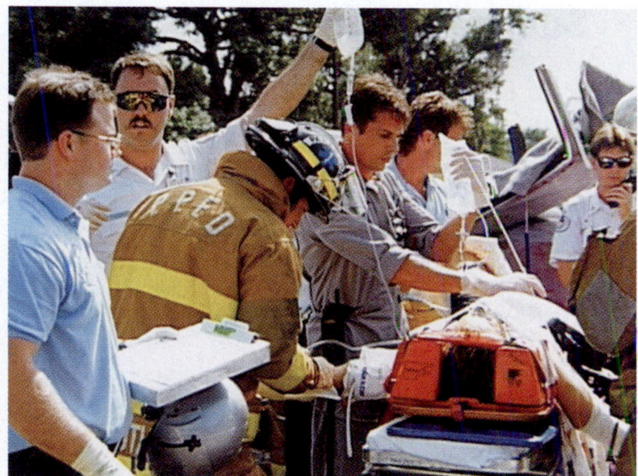

■ **Figure 24-21** Aggressive fluid resuscitation may be necessary for the patient in neurogenic shock.

The initial treatment for hypovolemia from suspected neurogenic shock is by fluid challenge (Figure 24-21 ■). Establish an IV with a 1,000-mL bag of lactated Ringer's solution or normal saline, a nonrestrictive administration set, and a large-bore IV catheter. Administer 250 mL of solution quickly, monitor the blood pressure and heart rate, and auscultate the lungs for signs of developing pulmonary edema (crackles). If the patient responds with an increasing blood pressure, a slowing heart rate, and signs of improved perfusion, consider a second bolus, or monitor the patient and administer a second bolus if the patient's signs and symptoms begin to deteriorate. If the patient does not improve with the fluid challenge, consider vasopressor therapy, as allowed by your protocols.

Dopamine (Intropin) is a naturally occurring catecholamine that, in addition to its own actions, causes the release of norepinephrine. Dopamine increases cardiac contractility and hence cardiac output and, at higher doses, increases peripheral vascular resistance, venous constriction, cardiac preload, and blood pressure. While there are no contraindications for dopamine use in the emergency setting, its common side effects include tachydysrhythmias, hypertension, headache, nausea, and vomiting.

Interruption of the sympathetic pathways by spinal cord injury causes unopposed parasympathetic stimulation and bradycardia (or at least prevents the compensatory tachycardia that occurs with decreased cardiac preload). The net result is a decrease in cardiac output. Atropine is administered to block the parasympathetic impulse that might contribute to slow the heart rate.

Atropine is an anticholinergic agent most frequently used for symptomatic bradycardia and heart blocks in the myocardial infarction patient. It is sometimes helpful in increasing the heart rate of patients with upper spinal cord injury due to unopposed vagal stimulation. It acts by inhibiting the actions of acetylcholine, the major parasympathetic neurotransmitter.

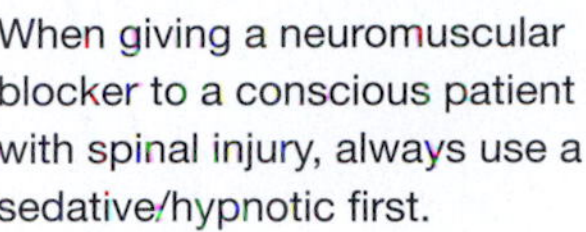

When giving a neuromuscular blocker to a conscious patient with spinal injury, always use a sedative/hypnotic first.

Medications and the Combative Patient

Frequently the patient who has sustained potentially serious spinal injury has also sustained head injury, is intoxicated, or is otherwise very uncooperative or combative. In some of these cases, sedatives may be indicated to reduce anxiety and because the patient actively resists spinal precautions. Consider using fentanyl, morphine, diazepam, or midazolam to calm the patient. In extreme circumstances, consider use of the paralytics mentioned in Chapter 23, "Head, Facial, and Neck Trauma," in the discussion of facilitated intubation to paralyze the patient. Whenever you use these agents, you must carefully monitor the patient's level of consciousness and respirations. With use of paralytics, you must provide continuing ventilation for the patient during the action of the drug. Sedatives and paralytics should only be administered as permitted by your system's protocols and under the close and direct supervision of an on-line medical direction physician.

Summary

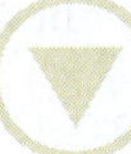

Spinal injury is a frequent consequence of serious trauma and is likely to induce serious disability or death. Injury to the spinal column may occur with only minimal signs and patient symptoms. Therefore, prehospital care for any patient with a significant mechanism of injury or any trauma patient with a reduced level of consciousness must include spinal precautions. Throughout patient care, provide emotional support and calming reassurance to help alleviate your patient's anxiety.

Review Questions

1. The most common sites of axial loading for lifting injuries and heel-first falls are located between:
   a. T-12 and L-2.
   b. C-1 and C-7.
   c. C-5 and T-4.
   d. L-3 and L-5.
2. During a trauma assessment you notice that a patient has no sensation below the lower border of the rib cage. This would suggest spinal pathology between which vertebral areas?
   a. C-1 and C-3
   b. C-3 and T-4
   c. T-4 and T-10
   d. T-10 and S-1
3. Which of the following vital signs would most likely indicate a potential spinal cord injury?
   a. hypotension, bradycardia, and shallow respirations
   b. hypertension, bradycardia, and shallow respirations
   c. hypotension, tachycardia, and deep respirations
   d. hypertension, tachycardia, and deep respirations
4. For which of the following patients would the anticholinergic agent atropine be best suited? A patient:
   a. in early spinal shock.
   b. with an injury to the upper spinal cord.
   c. with an injury to the lower spinal cord.
   d. with autonomic hyperreflexia syndrome.
5. The primary management objective in a patient with a suspected spinal cord injury is to:
   a. administer medications to prevent further paralysis.
   b. apply a cervical collar independent of spinal stabilization.
   c. initiate mechanical stabilization followed by manual immobilization.
   d. maintain the patient in a neutral, in-line position.
6. Priapism is defined as:
   a. a sustained erection of the penis.
   b. clear discharge from the nose.
   c. an occasional variant of angina.
   d. always associated with paralysis.
7. Which of the following statements regarding cervical collars is true?
   a. They serve as an adjunct to full cervical immobilization.
   b. They serve to accentuate axial loading and prevent flexion/extension.
   c. They serve to immobilize the cervical, thoracic, and lumbar spine.
   d. They serve to prevent axial loading when utilized before manual stabilization.

8. All of the following are signs or symptoms of spinal shock except:
   a. priapism.
   b. hypertension.
   c. loss of bladder control.
   d. flaccid paralysis.
9. Which of the following best defines spinal shock?
   a. a permanent insult to the cord that affects the body above the level of the injury
   b. a permanent insult to the cord that affects the body through extravasation of blood volume
   c. a permanent insult to the cord that affects the body above and below the level of the injury
   d. a temporary insult to the cord that affects the body below the level of the injury
10. When a neuromuscular blocker is to be given to a patient, a(n) __________ should be administered first.
    a. sedative/hypnotic
    b. catecholamine
    c. anticholinergic agent
    d. glucocorticoid

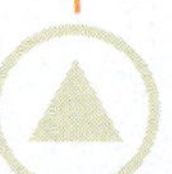

See Answers to Review Questions at the back of this book.

Chapter

25

Thoracic Trauma

Objectives

After reading this chapter, you should be able to:

1. Describe the incidence, morbidity, and mortality of thoracic injuries in the trauma patient. (pp. 1031–1032)
2. Discuss the anatomy and physiology of the thoracic organs and structures. (see Chapter 3)
3. Predict thoracic injuries based on mechanism of injury. (pp. 1032–1034)
4. Discuss the pathophysiology of, assessment findings with, and the management and need for rapid intervention and transport of the patient with chest wall injuries, including:
   - **A.** Rib fracture (pp. 1035–1036, 1054–1055)
   - **B.** Flail segment (pp. 1037–1038, 1055)
   - **C.** Sternal fracture (pp. 1036–1037)
5. Discuss the pathophysiology of, assessment findings with, and management and need for rapid intervention and transport of the patient with injury to the lung, including:
   - **A.** Simple pneumothorax (pp. 1038–1039)
   - **B.** Open pneumothorax (pp. 1039–1040, 1055–1056)
   - **C.** Tension pneumothorax (pp. 1040–1041, 1056–1057)
   - **D.** Hemothorax (pp. 1041–1042, 1057)
   - **E.** Hemopneumothorax (pp. 1041–1042)
   - **F.** Pulmonary contusion (pp. 1042–1043)
6. Discuss the pathophysiology of, findings of assessment with, and management and need for rapid intervention and transport of the patient with myocardial injuries, including:
   - **A.** Myocardial contusion (pp. 1043–1044, 1057–1058)
   - **B.** Pericardial tamponade (pp. 1044–1045, 1058)
   - **C.** Myocardial rupture (p. 1046)
7. Discuss the pathophysiology of, findings of assessment with, and management and need for rapid intervention and transport of the patient with vascular injuries, including injuries to:
   - **A.** Aorta (pp. 1046–1047, 1058)
   - **B.** Vena cava (p. 1047)
   - **C.** Pulmonary arteries/veins (p. 1047)

8. Discuss the pathophysiology of, findings of assessment with, and management and need for rapid intervention and transport of patients with diaphragmatic, esophageal, and tracheobronchial injuries. (pp. 1047–1048, 1058)
9. Discuss the pathophysiology of, findings of assessment with, and management and need for rapid intervention and transport of the patient with traumatic asphyxia. (pp. 1048, 1058)
10. Differentiate between thoracic injuries based on the assessment and history. (pp. 1048–1053)
11. Given several preprogrammed and moulaged thoracic trauma patients, provide the appropriate scene size-up, primary assessment, secondary assessment (rapid trauma or focused physical exam, detailed exam), and reassessments and provide appropriate patient care and transportation. (pp. 1031–1058)

Key Terms

aneurysm, p. 1046
comorbidity, p. 1031
electrical alternans, p. 1045
flail chest, p. 1037
hemopneumothorax, p. 1041
hemoptysis, p. 1043
hemothorax, p. 1041
pericardial tamponade, p. 1044
pneumothorax, p. 1038
precordium, p. 1044
pulsus paradoxus, p. 1045
tension pneumothorax, p. 1040
tracheobronchial tree, p. 1031

INTRODUCTION

The thoracic cavity contains many vital structures including the heart, great vessels, esophagus, **tracheobronchial tree,** and lungs. Trauma to any one of these structures could lead to a life-threatening event. Twenty-five percent of all motor vehicle deaths are due to thoracic trauma (about 12,000 per year in the United States). The majority of these deaths are secondary to injury to the heart and great vessels. In addition, abdominal injuries are also common in patients with traumatic chest injury and can cause significant **comorbidity.**

tracheobronchial tree *the structures of the trachea and the bronchi.*

comorbidity *associated disease process.*

Twenty-five percent of all motor vehicle deaths are due to thoracic trauma (about 12,000 per year in the United States).

The incidence of blunt thoracic trauma has increased with the development of the modern automobile (Figure 25-1 ■). Together with the development of a national highway system, more people are traveling greater distances, at greater speeds, and roadways are becoming more congested. This allows for an increased incidence of motor vehicle collisions (MVCs) and thus an increase in the incidence of thoracic injuries and subsequent deaths, as most blunt thoracic trauma deaths are MVC related. An increase in penetrating trauma has also been observed in urban areas associated with violent crime. The weapons used in violent crime in years past were likely to be of the "Saturday night special" variety: cheap small-caliber revolvers often producing just single wounds. The weapons of choice now are more likely to be large-caliber semiautomatic or automatic weapons that increase the likelihood of multiple missile injuries. With multiple wounds, there is a higher likelihood of injury to vital structures and therefore a higher mortality. Many advances in the treatment of penetrating thoracoabdominal trauma have been made during military conflicts, and the incidence of mortality from these wounds, which was 8 to 40 percent during World War II, has decreased to 3 to 18 percent today.

Penetrating trauma is increasing in urban areas.

Prevention efforts include gun control legislation, firearm safety courses, seat belt laws, and better design of automobiles including passive restraint systems such as air bags. Statistics indicate that these efforts have already decreased the incidence of these injuries and the related morbidity and mortality.

In this chapter, we will discuss thoracic trauma in relation to penetrating and blunt injury. These mechanisms have more clinical significance than simple injury categories. Certain injuries are almost exclusively associated with one type of chest trauma but unlikely with the other. For example, pericardial tamponade is almost exclusively associated with penetrating thoracic trauma

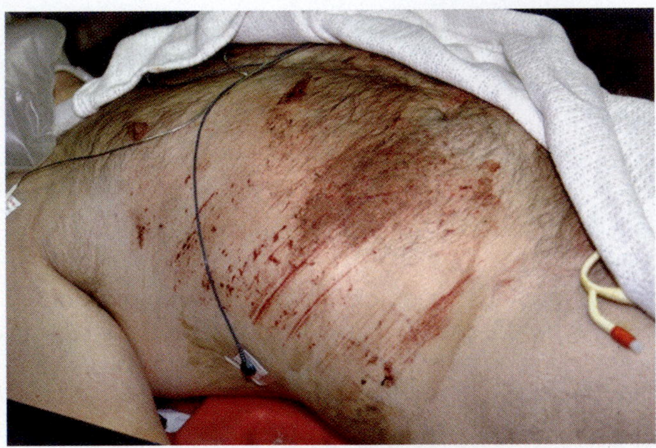

■ Figure 25-1 An example of blunt trauma to the chest. *(Edward T. Dickinson, MD)*

while cardiac rupture is almost exclusively caused by blunt thoracic trauma. By considering the mechanism of injury, understanding the pathology of the various injuries, and by being aware of the patient's physical signs of injury and symptoms, you will be better able to predict, identify, and treat potential life threats.

PATHOPHYSIOLOGY OF THORACIC TRAUMA

Thoracic trauma is classified into two major categories by mechanism: blunt and penetrating. It is important to examine these injury mechanisms and their effects on the organs of the thorax.

BLUNT TRAUMA

Blunt thoracic trauma is injury resulting from kinetic energy forces transmitted through the tissues. These injuries may be further subdivided by mechanism into blast, crush (compression), and deceleration injuries.

Blast injuries result from an explosive chemical reaction that creates a pressure wave traveling outward from the epicenter. This pressure wave causes tissue disruption by dramatic compression and then decompression as the wave passes. In the thorax, this action may tear blood vessels and disrupt the alveolar tissue. These injuries may lead to hemorrhage, pneumothoraces, and air embolism (air entering the disrupted pulmonary vasculature and subsequently returning to the central circulation). Other injuries associated with a blast mechanism can include disruption of the tracheobronchial tree and traumatic rupture of the diaphragm. When the blast occurs in a confined space, the pressure wave may be contained and accentuated. The result is an increase in the incidence and severity of the associated injuries.

Crush injuries occur when the body is compressed between an object and a hard surface. This leads to direct injury or disruption of the chest wall, diaphragm, heart, or tracheobronchial tree. If the victim remains pinned between two objects, significant restriction in ventilation and venous return may occur, which is also known as traumatic asphyxia.

Deceleration injuries occur when the body is in motion and impacts a fixed object, such as when the chest impacts the steering column in a front-end collision (Figure 25-2 ■). This impact causes a direct blunt injury to the chest wall while the internal organs of the thoracic cavity continue in motion. The organs and structures then impact with the internal surface of the thoracic cavity and may be compressed as more posterior structures collide with them. If the organ or structure has points of fixation, as with the aorta at the ligamentum arteriosum, the force of the organ moving against this point of fixation (shear force) can lead to a traumatic disruption. These sudden deceleration and shear forces can cause disruption of the myocardium, great vessel, lung, trachea, and bronchi. The rapid compression of the chest, especially against a closed glottis, may also cause alveolar and tracheobronchial rupture and pneumothorax.

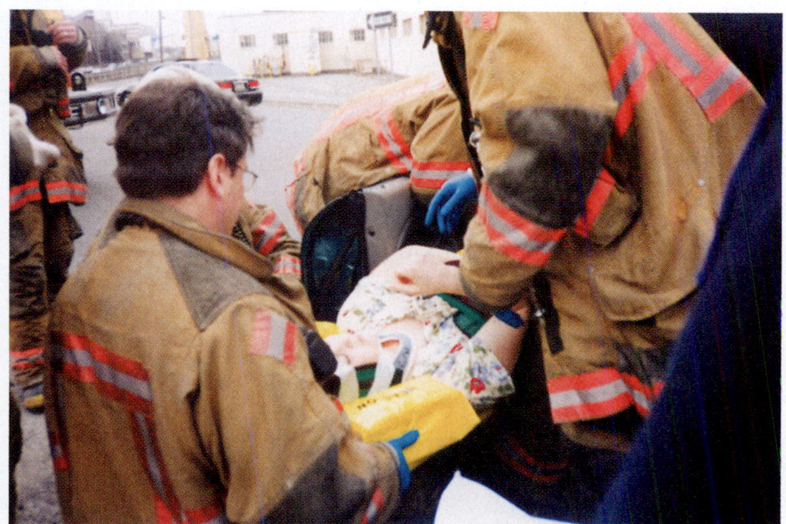

■ Figure 25-2 Frontal impact auto crashes frequently result in chest trauma.

The age of the blunt trauma victim may affect the trauma received and its seriousness. The cartilaginous nature of the pediatric thorax spares the infant or child from rib fractures but more easily transmits the energy of trauma to the vital organs below. This results in less significant signs of injury, few rib fractures, and a greater incidence of serious internal injury than in adults. The geriatric patient responds very differently to blunt chest trauma. That patient will suffer more frequent rib fracture than the younger adult due to calcification of the skeletal system. Though the greater incidence of rib fracture may somewhat protect the underlying organs, preexisting disease and the progressive reduction of respiratory and cardiac reserves result in a greater morbidity and mortality from serious chest trauma.

The age of the blunt trauma victim may affect the seriousness of the trauma received.

PENETRATING TRAUMA

Penetrating thoracic trauma induces injury as an object enters the chest and causes either direct trauma or secondary injury from transmitted kinetic energy forces related to the cavitational wave of high-velocity projectiles. Penetrating chest trauma can be subdivided into three categories: low energy, high energy, and shotgun wounds.

Low-energy wounds are those caused by arrows, knives, hand guns, and other relatively slow-moving objects (Figure 25-3 ■). They cause injury by direct contact or very limited creation of temporary cavities. The injury that occurs from this type of wound is related to the direct path that the missile or object takes.

High-energy wounds are caused by military and hunting rifles (and some high-powered hand guns at close range) that fire missiles at very high velocity. Their velocity gives the projectile very high kinetic energy. As the projectile passes through tissue, it creates a shock wave, tissue movement (including compression and stretching), and a large temporary cavity. These wounds cause extensive tissue damage perpendicular to the track of the projectile.

Shotgun wounds are classified according to the distance between the victim and the shotgun. A smaller gauge (a larger caliber) of shotgun and a larger size of shot also increase the effective range and penetrating power of the weapon and its potential to cause tissue damage. Type I injuries are those where the target is greater than 7 meters from the gun barrel at discharge. The pellets usually penetrate the skin and subcutaneous tissue but rarely penetrate the deep fascia to cause body cavity penetration. Type II injuries occur at a distance of 3 to 7 meters and often permit the pellets to penetrate the deep fascia with internal organ injury possible. Type III injuries occur at a distance of less than 3 meters and usually involve massive tissue destruction and life-threatening injury.

Shotgun wounds within 3 meters of the discharging barrel cause serious tissue destruction and are frequently life threatening.

Penetrating thoracic trauma is often related to the structures involved. Lung tissue is very resilient when impacted by high-energy projectiles. The "spongy" nature of the air-filled alveoli absorbs the energy of cavitation and reduces the size of the temporary cavity and injury associated

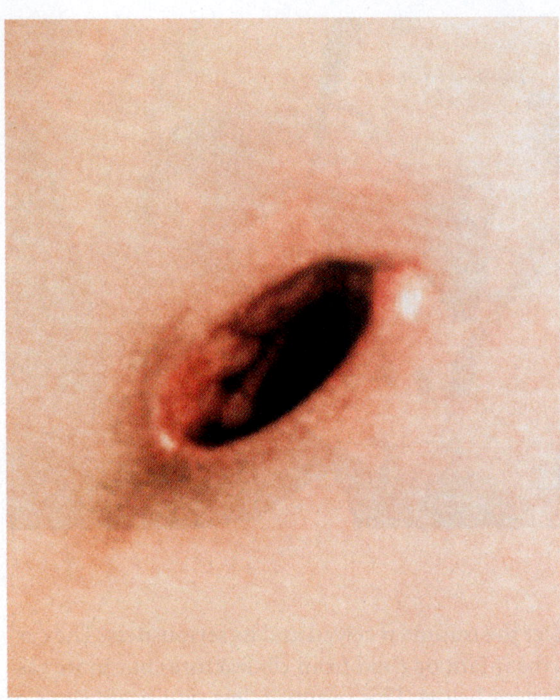

■ **Figure 25-3** Penetrating (stab) wound to the chest.

with the compression and stretching. The great vessels and heart (if it is distended with blood) respond much differently. The fluid transmits the kinetic energy very well and may result in cardiac or vessel rupture. With slower-moving projectiles or if the heart is struck while in diastole, the result may be a simple penetration. While a projectile tends to move in a straight line, it is easily deflected by contact with a rib, clavicle, scapula, or the spinal column. Contact with skeletal structures may also fragment the projectile (as well as the skeletal structure), increasing the rate of energy exchange and the seriousness of injury. Penetrating trauma frequently leads to pneumothorax, which may be bilateral, depending on the track of the missile or knife. Table 25–1 lists common injuries associated with penetrating thoracic trauma.

Table 25–1	Injuries Associated with Penetrating Thoracic Trauma
Closed pneumothorax	
Open pneumothorax (including sucking chest wound)	
Tension pneumothorax	
Pneumomediastinum	
Hemothorax	
Hemopneumothorax	
Laceration of vascular structures, including the great vessels	
Tracheobronchial tree lacerations	
Esophageal lacerations	
Penetrating cardiac injuries	
Pericardial tamponade	
Spinal cord injuries	
Diaphragmatic penetration/laceration/rupture	
Intra-abdominal penetration with associated organ injury	

CHEST WALL INJURIES

Chest wall injuries are by far the most common injuries encountered in blunt chest trauma. As previously discussed, an intact and moving chest wall is necessary to develop the pressures essential for air movement into and out of the lungs (the bellows effect). Chest wall injury may disrupt this motion and result in respiratory insufficiency. Closed injuries of the chest wall include contusions, rib fractures, sternal fractures/dislocations, and flail chest. Open injuries to the chest wall are almost entirely due to penetrating trauma and are often associated with deep structure injury in addition to disruption of the changing intrathoracic pressure necessary for respiration.

Chest wall injuries are by far the most common injuries encountered in blunt chest trauma.

Chest Wall Contusion

Chest wall contusion is the most common result of blunt injury to the thorax. The injury damages the soft tissue covering the thoracic cage and causes pain with respiratory effort. Like contusions elsewhere, contusion of the chest wall may present with erythema initially, then ecchymosis. The discoloration may outline the object that caused the trauma, may outline the ribs as the soft tissue is trapped between the ribs and the offending agent, or may outline a combination of both. The most noticeable symptom of chest wall contusion is pain, made worse with deep breathing and possibly resulting in reduced chest expansion. The area will be tender at the contusion site, and you may observe decreased chest wall movement due to pain. You may auscultate limited breath sounds because of decreased air movement due to limited chest expansion.

The pain of chest wall contusion and associated limiting of deep inspiration may lead to hypoventilation. Hypoventilation may not be apparent in a young, otherwise healthy individual and may not pose a significant life threat due to the individual's significant pulmonary reserves. The aged patient, however, often has preexisting medical problems, little pulmonary reserve, and does not tolerate this injury as well. Such a patient quickly becomes hypoxemic (low oxygen levels in the blood) without proper respiratory support. In a pediatric patient, the ribs are very flexible, resist fracture, and easily transmit the forces of trauma. The result may be chest wall contusion and internal injury without rib fracture.

Chest wall contusion is the most common result of blunt injury to the thorax.

Review

Content

Signs and Symptoms of Chest Wall Injuries

- Blunt or penetrating trauma to chest
- Erythema
- Ecchymosis
- Dyspnea
- Pain on breathing
- Limited breath sounds
- Hypoventilation
- Crepitus
- Paradoxical motion of chest wall

Rib Fracture

Rib fractures are found in more than 50 percent of cases of significant chest trauma from blunt mechanisms. Rib fractures are likely to occur at the point of impact or along the border of the object that impacts the chest (Figure 25-4 ■). Fractures may also occur at a location remote from the injury site. The thoracic cage is a hollow cylinder that has some flex to it. As the compressional force of blunt trauma deforms the thorax, the ribs flex and may fracture at their weakest point, the posterior angle (along the posterior axillary line).

Rib fractures are found in more than 50 percent of cases of significant chest trauma from blunt mechanisms.

Ribs 4 through 8 are the most commonly fractured as they are least protected by other structures and are firmly fixed at both ends (to the spine and sternum). It takes great force to fracture ribs 1 through 3 because the shoulder, scapula, and the heavy musculature of the upper chest protect them. Their fracture is more likely to be associated with severe intrathoracic injuries (tracheobronchial tree injury, aortic rupture, and other vascular injuries), especially if multiple ribs are involved. Ribs 9 through 12 are less firmly attached to the sternum, are relatively mobile, and are thus less likely to fracture. However, they better transmit the energy of trauma to internal organs and may permit intra-abdominal injury without fracture. Fractures of ribs 9 through 12 are frequently associated with serious trauma and splenic or hepatic injury.

Ribs 4 through 8 are the most commonly fractured.

The incidence and significance of rib fracture varies with age. The pediatric patient has very cartilaginous ribs that bend easily. The ribs resist fracture and transmit kinetic forces to the thoracic and abdominal structures underneath. The pediatric patient hence has a decreased incidence of rib fracture and an increase in the incidence of underlying injury. The geriatric patient, however, has ribs that are calcified, less flexible, and more easily fractured. The geriatric patient is also more likely to have comorbidity like COPD, which reduces respiratory reserves and compounds the effects of rib injury. If multiple rib fractures are noted in a young adult, they are probably associated with severe trauma and may lead to significant pain, splinting, hypoventilation, and inadequate cough. They also are likely to be associated with significant internal injuries. The mortality associated with rib fractures increases with the number of fractures,

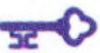

In pediatric patients, more flexible ribs permit more serious internal injury before fracture occurs.

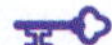

Rib fracture mortality increases with the number of fractures, extremes of age, and associated disease.

Figure 25-4 Rib fractures.

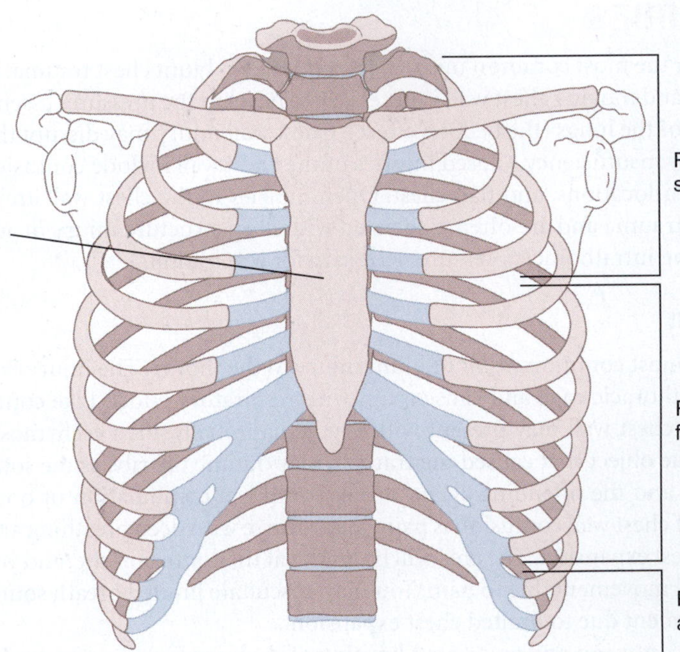

extremes of age (the very young or very old), and associated chronic respiratory or cardiac problems, especially in the elderly trauma victim.

The rib fracture is likely to be associated with an overlying chest wall contusion and presents with those signs and symptoms. The fracture site may also demonstrate a grating sensation (crepitus) as the bone ends move against each other, either during chest wall movement or during direct palpation. The pain associated with rib fracture is greater than that with chest wall contusion and will more greatly limit respiratory excursion. This reduced chest wall excursion frequently leads to hypoxia, hypoventilation, and muscle spasms at the fracture site. Hypoventilation can result in a progressive collapse of alveoli called atelectasis. This collapse reduces the lung surface available for gas exchange and contributes to hypoxia. These atelectatic segments also may become filled with blood or tissue fluid due to the injury and set the stage for secondary infection such as pneumonia. While pneumonia does not develop in the emergency setting, it is the cause of a significant mortality in blunt chest injury patients. Serious internal injuries may also result as the jagged rib ends move about and lacerate structures beneath them. Laceration of the intercostal arteries may result in hemothorax, while damage to the intercostal nerves may result in a neurologic deficit. Fracture and displacement of the lower ribs may injure the liver (right) or spleen (left).

Sternal Fracture and Dislocation

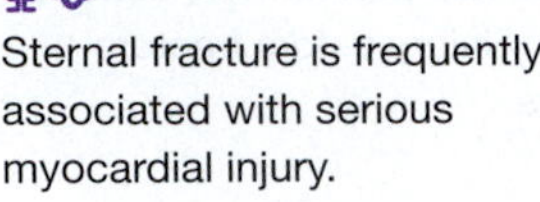

Sternal fracture is frequently associated with serious myocardial injury.

Sternal fractures and dislocations are usually associated with blunt anterior chest trauma. Sternal fracture results only from severe impact, as this region of the chest is well supported by the ribs and clavicles. The most likely mechanism is a direct blow, a fall against a fixed object, or the blunt force of the sternum against the steering wheel or dashboard in a motor vehicle crash. The overall incidence of sternal fracture in thoracic trauma patients is between 5 and 8 percent. However, the mortality associated with it is between 25 and 45 percent due to underlying myocardial contusion, cardiac rupture, pericardial tamponade, and pulmonary contusion. If the surrounding ribs or costochondral joints are disrupted, the injury may result in a flail chest. The injury results in a noticeable deformity and possible crepitus with chest wall movement or palpation.

Dislocation at the sternoclavicular joint is uncommon and also requires significant force. It too may occur with blunt trauma to the anterior chest or with a lateral compression mechanism, as in side-impact collisions or falls with the patient landing on the shoulder. The clavicle may dislocate from the sternum in one of two ways, anteriorly or posteriorly. The anterior dislocation creates a

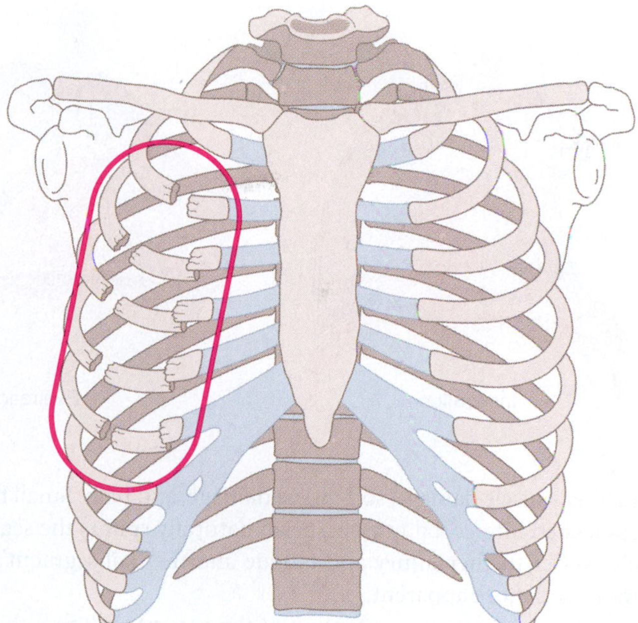

■ Figure 25-5 Flail chest occurs when one or more ribs fracture in two or more places.

noticeable deformity anterior to the manubrium. The posterior dislocation displaces the head of the clavicle behind the sternum where it may compress or lacerate underlying great vessels or compress or injure the trachea and esophagus. Tracheal compression may result in stridor and voice change, though any deformity is more difficult to identify except that the shoulder may noticeably displace anteriorly and medially.

Flail Chest

flail chest *defect in the chest wall that allows for free movement of a segment. Breathing will cause paradoxical chest wall motion.*

Flail chest is a segment of the chest that becomes free to move with the pressure changes of respiration. The condition occurs when one or more ribs fracture in two or more places (Figure 25-5 ■). It is one of the most serious chest wall injuries because it is often associated with severe underlying pulmonary injury (contusion) and it reduces the volume of respiration and increases the effort associated with it. This underlying injury adds to mortality in serious thoracic trauma (between 20 and 40 percent), as does age, head injury, shock, and other associated injuries. The most common mechanisms of injury causing flail chest are blunt traumas from falls, motor vehicle crashes, industrial injuries, and assaults.

The flail segment created by this injury is no longer a controlled component of the chest wall and bellows system. Increasing intrathoracic pressure associated with expiration moves the flail segment outward while the rest of the chest moves inward, pushing air under the moving segment that would normally be exhaled. This reduces the change in chest volume caused by the breathing effort as well as the volume of air expired and draws the mediastinum toward the injury. During inspiration, the intrathoracic pressure falls as the respiratory muscles move the chest wall outward and the diaphragm drops caudally (tail-ward). The reduced pressure draws the flail segment inward. The lung beneath it moves away from the inward-moving segment, reducing the volume of air moving into the thorax and displacing the mediastinum away from the injury. In summary, the injury produces a segment of the chest wall that moves in opposition to the chest's normal respiratory effort (paradoxical movement), it reduces the volume of air moved with each breath, and it displaces the mediastinum toward and then away from the injury site with each breath (Figure 25-6 ■). In flail chest, the patient takes more energy to move less air and the respiratory volume is further reduced as the rib fracture pain produces a natural splinting of the chest.

It takes tremendous energy to create these six fracture sites (three or more ribs fractured in two or more places) and, accordingly, flail chest is often associated with serious internal injury. In addition, the movement of the flail segment, which is opposite to the rest of the chest wall, is damaging to surrounding tissue. With each breath, the bone fracture sites move against one another causing

■ Figure 25-6 Paradoxical movement of the chest wall seen in flail chest.

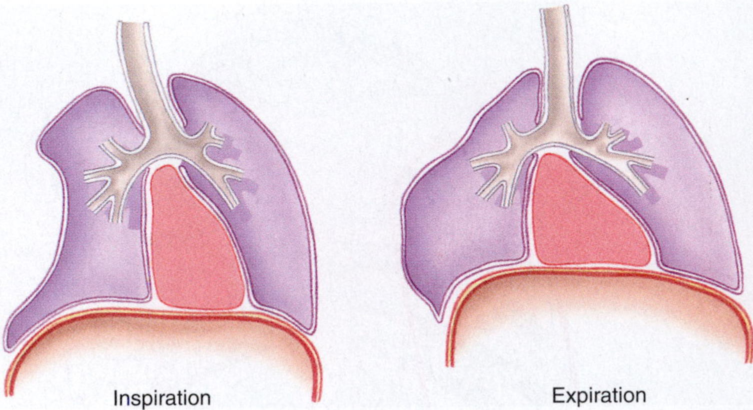

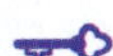

Over time, the muscles splinting the flail segment will fatigue, and paradoxical respiration will become more evident.

further muscle damage, soft-tissue damage, and pain. Small flail segments may go undetected as the associated intercostal muscle spasm naturally splints the segment. With time, however, these muscles suffer further injury and fatigue and the flail segment's paradoxical movement may become more and more apparent.

Positive-pressure ventilation of the patient with flail chest reverses the mechanism that causes the paradoxical chest wall movement, restores the tidal volume, and reduces the pain of chest wall movement. It accomplishes this by pushing the chest wall and the flail segment outward with positive pressure. Passive expiration then may cause both the flail segment and the rest of the chest to move inward, again, together. However, in the presence of underlying injury, positive-pressure ventilation may induce pneumothorax.

PULMONARY INJURIES

Pulmonary injuries are injuries to lung tissue or injuries that damage the system that holds the lung to the interior of the thoracic cavity. They include the simple pneumothorax, open pneumothorax, tension pneumothorax, hemothorax, and pulmonary contusion.

Simple (Closed) Pneumothorax

pneumothorax *air in the pleural space.*

Pneumothorax occurs when lung tissue is disrupted and air leaks into the pleural space. With simple pneumothorax (also known as closed pneumothorax), there may be an external, and possibly penetrating, wound, but there is no communication between the pleural space and the atmosphere (Figure 25-7 ■). The pressure within the thorax does not exceed normal expiratory pressures and there is no associated mediastinal shift. As more and more air accumulates in the pleural space, the lung collapses. With lung collapse, the alveoli collapse (atelectasis) and blood flowing past the collapsed alveoli does not exchange oxygen and carbon dioxide. As more and more of the alveoli collapse, this condition, called ventilation/perfusion mismatch, becomes more pronounced and begins to lower the blood oxygen level (hypoxemia). This soon becomes life endangering, especially if there are other associated injuries or shock.

Simple pneumothorax can occur with penetrating and blunt mechanisms. Blunt trauma may cause a pneumothorax when a rib fracture directly punctures the lung. Another mechanism may cause alveolar rupture from a sudden increase in intrathoracic pressure as the chest impacts the steering column with fully expanded lungs and a closed glottis (the "paper bag syndrome"—like clapping an air-filled paper bag between two hands). The incidence of pneumothorax in serious thoracic trauma is between 10 and 30 percent and its morbidity is related to the amount of atelectasis and the degree of perfusion mismatch. Penetrating trauma to the chest is frequently associated with simple pneumothorax, or with an injury that allows air to enter the pleural space through an external wound (open pneumothorax).

A simple pneumothorax reduces the efficiency of respiration and quickly leads to hypoxia. The hypoxia and increase in blood levels of CO_2 cause the medulla to increase the respiratory rate (tachypnea) and volume. If only a very small portion of the lung is involved, there may be no apparent signs or symptoms. A larger pneumothorax may cause mild dyspnea, or complete lung col-

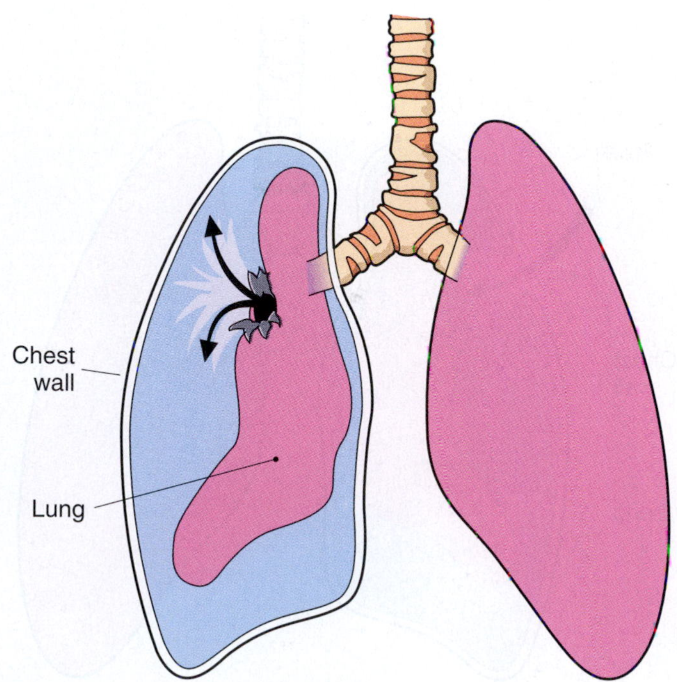

■ **Figure 25-7** Simple (closed) pneumothorax.

lapse may result in severe dyspnea and hypoxia. The signs, symptoms, and significance of simple pneumothorax increase with preexisting disease. Pneumothorax may produce local chest pain with respiration as the pleurae become irritated (respirophasic pain). The pathology may cause the chest to hyperinflate and breath sounds to diminish on the affected side (usually in the extremes of the upper and lower lung first). A small pneumothorax involving collapse of less than 15 percent of the affected lung may be difficult to detect clinically and requires only supportive measures. Often the small pneumothorax will seal itself and the air in the pleural cavity will be absorbed. A larger pneumothorax is often clinically apparent and requires more aggressive therapy such as high-flow, high-concentration oxygen and chest tube placement (in the emergency department).

Content Review

Signs and Symptoms of Pneumothorax

- Trauma to chest
- Chest pain on inspiration
- Hyperinflation of chest
- Diminished breath sounds on affected side

Open Pneumothorax

Open pneumothorax is most commonly noted in military conflicts when a high-velocity bullet creates a significant wound in the chest wall (usually the exit wound). Recently use of high-velocity assault weapons has become more common in civilian settings and thus the frequency of these injuries is on the increase. Another cause of open pneumothorax is a shotgun blast at close range with an associated large wound to the chest wall. This chest wall disruption leads to the free passage of air between the atmosphere and the pleural space (Figure 25-8 ■). Air is drawn into the wound as the chest moves outward and the diaphragm moves downward during inspiration. The internal thoracic pressure drops and air rushes through the wound and into the chest cavity. This air replaces the lung tissue, permits lung collapse, and results in a large functional dead space. The inspiratory effort of the intact side of the chest draws the mediastinum toward it and away from the injury. This prevents the uninjured lung from fully inflating. On exhalation, the contracting chest wall and rising diaphragm increase the internal pressure and force air outward through the wound. This movement of air into and out of the chest through the wound is the cause of the “sucking” sound that leads to the wound’s common name, “sucking chest wound.”

For air movement to occur through the opening in the chest wall, the opening must be at least two-thirds the diameter of the trachea. Remember, the size of the trachea is about the size of the patient’s little finger. This must be the size of the opening into the chest, not the size of the wound. The thickness and resiliency of the chest wall often closes the wound to air movement unless it is quite large. Then the remaining defect may permit the free movement of air and create an open pneumothorax.

Content Review

Signs and Symptoms of Open Pneumothorax

- Penetrating chest trauma
- Sucking chest wound
- Frothy blood at wound site
- Dyspnea
- Hypovolemia

For air movement to occur through the opening in the chest wall, the opening must be at least two-thirds the diameter of the trachea.

■ Figure 25-8 Open pneumothorax (sucking chest wound).

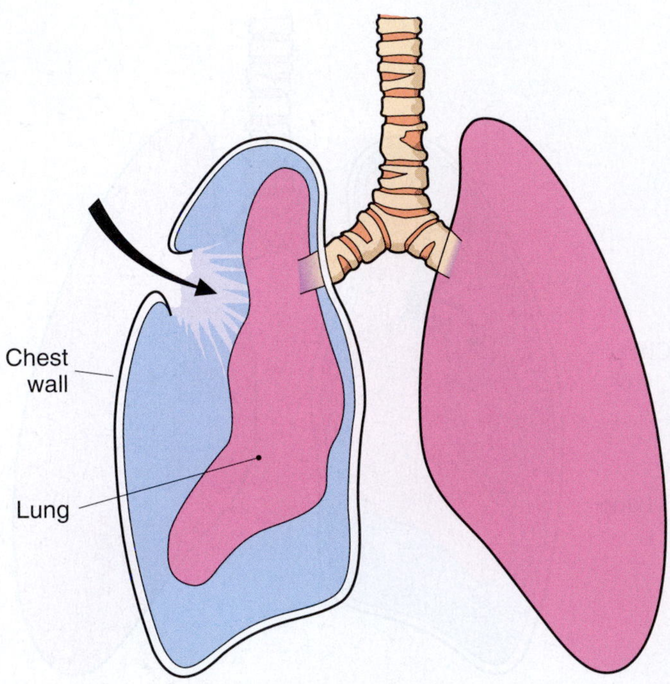

The open pneumothorax can be recognized by the large open wound to the thorax and the characteristic air movement (or sound) it produces. Air passage through the wound and the wound's associated hemorrhage may produce frothy blood around the opening, another characteristic of the open pneumothorax. The patient is likely to experience severe dyspnea, and possibly hypovolemia from associated injury and hemorrhage. The patient's condition is further compromised because the reduced intrathoracic pressures developed during inspiration do not complement venous return to the heart as they do with the intact thorax and respiratory effort.

tension pneumothorax *buildup of air under pressure within the thorax. The resulting compression of the lung severely reduces the effectiveness of respirations.*

Tension Pneumothorax

Tension pneumothorax is an open or simple pneumothorax that generates and maintains a pressure greater than atmospheric pressure within the thorax. It may be caused by a traumatic mechanism and injury or possibly by positive-pressure ventilation of a patient with chest trauma or congenital defect affecting the respiratory tree. Tension pneumothorax may also occur as an open pneumothorax is sealed and an internal injury or defect permits the buildup of pressure.

Tension pneumothorax occurs because the mechanism of injury (either the external wound, or the internal injury) forms a one-way valve. Air flows into the pleural space through the defect during inspiration as the pressure within the pleural space is less than atmospheric. With expiration, the increasing pleural pressure closes the defect and does not permit air to escape. With each breath, the volume of air and the pressure within the pleural space increase. The increasing intrapleural pressure collapses the lung on the ipsilateral (same or injury) side, causes intercostal and suprasternal bulging, and begins to exert pressure against the mediastinum. As the pressure continues to build, it displaces the mediastinum, compressing the uninjured lung and crimping the vena cava as it enters the thorax through the diaphragm or where it attaches to the heart. This reduces venous return (which reduces cardiac output), results in an increase in venous pressure, causes the jugular veins to distend (JVD), and narrows the pulse pressure. Tracheal shift may occur as the mediastinal structures are pushed away from the increasing pressure. This is a very late and rare finding and is more commonly seen in the young trauma victim as the pediatric mediastinum is more mobile than the adult's. Atelectasis occurs in the ipsilateral side from the initial lung collapse and on the contralateral (uninjured or opposite) side from the mediastinal shift and compression of that lung. These mechanisms lead to ventilation/perfusion mismatch, further hypoxemia, and systemic hypoxia.

Content Review

Signs and Symptoms of Tension Pneumothorax

- Chest trauma
- Severe dyspnea
- Ventilation/perfusion mismatch
- Hypoxemia
- Hyperinflation of affected side of chest
- Hyperresonance of affected side of chest
- Diminished, then absent, breath sounds
- Cyanosis
- Diaphoresis
- Altered mental status
- Jugular venous distention
- Hypotension
- Hypovolemia

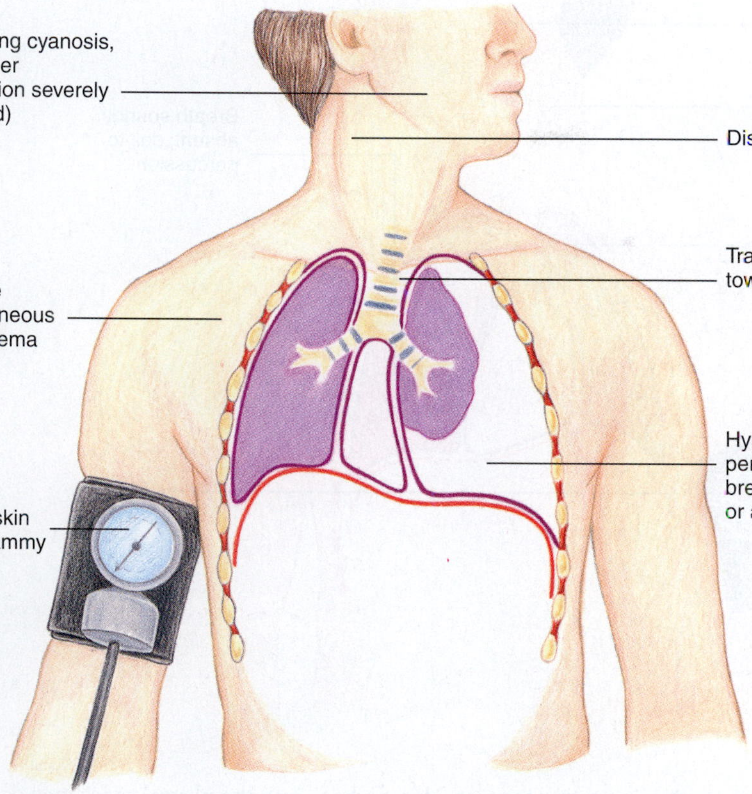

Apprehension, agitation

Increasing cyanosis, air hunger (ventilation severely impaired)

Distended neck veins

Tracheal displacement toward uninjured side

Possible subcutaneous emphysema

Hyperresonant percussion note; breath sounds ↓ or absent

Shock; skin cold, clammy

■ **Figure 25-9** Physical findings of tension pneumothorax.

Tension pneumothorax begins with the presentation of a simple or open pneumothorax (Figure 25-9 ■). As the pressure in the pleural space begins to increase, dyspnea, ventilation/perfusion mismatch, and hypoxemia develop. The ipsilateral side of the chest becomes hyperinflated, hyperresonant to percussion, and respiratory sounds become very faint, then absent. The pressure may cause the intracostal tissues to bulge. The opposite or contralateral side of the chest becomes somewhat dull to percussion, with progressively fainter respiratory sounds as the tension pneumothorax becomes worse. Severe hypoxia results in cyanosis, diaphoresis, and an altered mental status while the increased intrathoracic pressure reduces venous return and may cause JVD and hypotension. If the condition is not quickly recognized and promptly treated, it may lead to death.

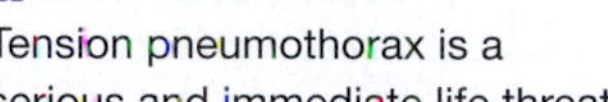

Tension pneumothorax is a serious and immediate life threat.

Tension pneumothorax is a serious and immediate life threat. It is corrected by relieving the intrapleural pressure by inserting a needle through the chest wall to convert the tension pneumothorax to an open pneumothorax. If a valve is added to the decompression needle, it may permit only the escape of air during expiration. If there is no continuing internal defect, this may progressively reexpand the collapsed lung and return effective respiration.

Hemothorax

hemothorax *blood within the pleural space.*

Hemothorax is simply the accumulation of blood in the pleural space due to internal hemorrhage. It can be very minor and not detectable in the field or, when associated with serious or great vessel injury, may result in rapid patient deterioration. Serious hemorrhage may displace a complete lung, accumulate over 1,500 mL of blood quickly, and produce a mortality rate of 75 percent, with most (two-thirds) of those dying at the scene. Hemothorax is primarily a blood loss problem as each side of the thorax may hold up to 3,000 mL of blood (or half the total blood volume). However, the blood lost into the thorax reduces the tidal volume and efficiency of respiration in a patient who has already suffered trauma and is likely to move quickly into shock.

hemopneumothorax *condition where air and blood are in the pleural space.*

Hemothorax is frequently associated with rib fractures and can be associated with either blunt or penetrating mechanisms. It often accompanies pneumothorax (a **hemopneumothorax**) and occurs

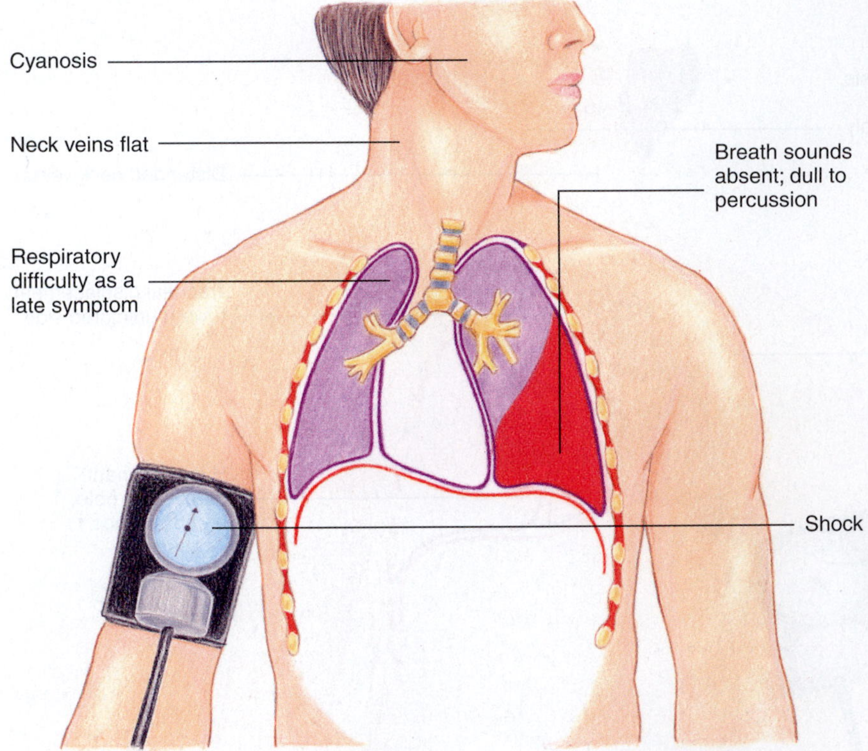

■ **Figure 25-10** Physical findings of massive hemothorax.

Content Review

Signs and Symptoms of Hemothorax

- Blunt or penetrating chest trauma
- Signs and symptoms of shock
- Dyspnea
- Dull percussive sounds over site of collecting blood

25 percent of the time with penetrating trauma. Hemorrhage into the pleural space may occur from a lung laceration (most common) or laceration of the intercostal arteries, pulmonary arteries, great vessels, or internal mammary arteries. The intercostal arteries can bleed at a rate of 50 mL/min. The bleeding into the chest is more rapid than would occur elsewhere because the pressure within the chest is often less than atmospheric pressure (law of Laplace). The blood lost into the hemothorax contributes to hypovolemia and displaces lung tissue. If the accumulation is significant, it may cause significant hypovolemia and shock, hypoxemia, respiratory distress, and respiratory failure.

The patient with hemothorax will have either a blunt or penetrating injury like those associated with open or simple pneumothorax. The patient may also display the signs and symptoms of shock and some respiratory distress (Figure 25-10 ■). The blood pools in the lower chest in the seated patient or posterior chest in the supine patient. The lungs present with normal percussion and breath sounds except directly over the accumulating fluid. There the lung percussion is very dull and breath sounds are very distant, if they can be heard at all.

Pulmonary Contusion

Pulmonary contusions are simply soft-tissue contusions affecting the lung. They are present in 30 to 75 percent of patients with significant blunt chest trauma and are frequently associated with rib fracture. Pulmonary contusions range in severity from very limited, minor, and unrecognizable injuries, to those that are extensive and quickly life threatening. They result in a mortality rate of between 14 and 20 percent of serious chest trauma patients.

There are two specific mechanisms of injury that allow the transfer of energy to the pulmonary tissue and result in pulmonary contusions. They are deceleration and the pressure wave associated with either passage of a high-velocity bullet or explosion. Deceleration injury occurs as the moving body strikes a fixed object. A common example of this mechanism is chest impact with the steering wheel during an auto crash. As the chest wall contacts the wheel and stops, the lungs continue forward, compressing and stretching the alveolar tissue or shearing it from the relatively fixed tracheobronchial tree. This causes disruption at the alveolar/capillary membrane leading to microscopic hemorrhage and edema. The second mechanism, the pressure wave of an explosion or bullet's passage, dramatically compresses and stretches the lung tissue. Due to the nature of the lung tissue (air-filled sacs surrounded by delicate and vascular membranes), the passage of this pressure is partially reflected at the gas/fluid (alveolar/capillary) interface. This leaves small, flame-shaped areas of disruption throughout the membrane leading to microhemorrhage and edema (called the Spalding effect). Pulmonary contusion is not generally associated with low-speed penetration of the chest and laceration of the lung tissues and structures.

The overall magnitude of pulmonary injury depends on the degree of deformity or stretch, and the velocity at which it occurs. Similar pulmonary contusions may result from different mechanisms. For example, an AK-47 round fired at 2,300 ft/sec striking body armor and deforming the chest wall instantaneously by 1 to 2 cm (high velocity) may cause pulmonary contusions similar to chest impact during an MVA where the chest is deformed 50 percent as it strikes the steering wheel at 50 ft/sec (low velocity).

Microhemorrhage into the alveolar tissue associated with pulmonary contusion may be extensive and result in up to 1,000 to 1,500 mL of blood loss. This hemorrhage into the tissue of the alveoli also causes irritation, initiates the inflammation process, and causes fluid to migrate into the region. The accumulation of fluid in the alveolar/capillary membrane (pulmonary edema) progressively increases its dimension and decreases the rate at which gases, and especially oxygen, can diffuse across it. The fluid accumulation also stiffens the membrane, makes the lung less compliant, and increases the work necessary to move air in and out of the affected tissue.

The thickening wall reduces the efficiency of respiration and results in hypoxemia, while the stiffening makes respiration more energy consuming. The development of edema also increases the pressure necessary to move blood through the capillary beds. This increases the pressure within the pulmonary vascular system (pulmonary hypertension) and the workload of the right heart. In combination, these effects lead to atelectasis, hypovolemia, ventilation/perfusion mismatch, hypoxemia, hypotension, and, possibly, respiratory failure and shock. Although isolated pulmonary contusions can occur, they are frequently associated with chest wall injury and injuries elsewhere (87 percent of the time).

The patient with pulmonary contusion presents with a mechanism of injury and evidence of blunt or penetrating chest impact. While the associated injuries may display immediate signs and symptoms (as in the pain of a rib fracture), the signs and symptoms of the pulmonary contusion take time to develop. The patient will likely complain of increasing dyspnea, demonstrate increasing respiratory effort, and show the signs of hypoxia. Oxygen saturation may gradually fall as the pathology develops. Careful auscultation of the chest may reveal increasing crackles and fainter breath sounds. Serious pulmonary contusion may cause **hemoptysis** (coughing up blood) and the signs and symptoms of shock.

Review

Content

Signs and Symptoms of Pulmonary Contusion

- Blunt or penetrating chest trauma
- Increasing dyspnea
- Hypoxia
- Increasing crackles
- Diminishing breath sounds
- Hemoptysis
- Signs and symptoms of shock

hemoptysis *coughing of blood that originates in the respiratory tract.*

CARDIOVASCULAR INJURIES

Cardiovascular injuries are the subset of thoracic trauma that leads to the most fatalities. They include myocardial contusion, pericardial tamponade, myocardial aneurysm or rupture, aortic aneurysm or rupture, and other vascular injuries.

Cardiovascular injuries are the subset of thoracic trauma that leads to the most fatalities.

Myocardial Contusion

Myocardial contusion is a frequent result of trauma and may occur in 76 percent of all serious chest trauma. It carries a high mortality rate and occurs most commonly with severe blunt anterior chest trauma. Here, the chest is struck by or strikes an object. The heart, which is relatively mobile within the chest, impacts the inside of the anterior chest wall and then may be compressed between the sternum and the thoracic spine as the thorax flexes with impact. The resulting contusion will most likely affect the right atrium and right ventricle (Figure 25-11 ■). This is related to the heart's position in the chest, rotated somewhat counterclockwise and presenting the right atrium and ventricle surfaces toward the sternum.

The cardiac contusion is similar to a contusion in any other muscle tissue. The injury disrupts the muscle cells and microcirculation, resulting in muscle fiber tearing and damage, hemorrhage, and edema. The injury may reduce the strength of cardiac contraction and reduce cardiac output. Because of the automaticity and conductivity of the cardiac muscle, contusion may also disturb the cardiac electrical system. If the injury is serious, it may lead to hematoma, hemoperitoneum (blood

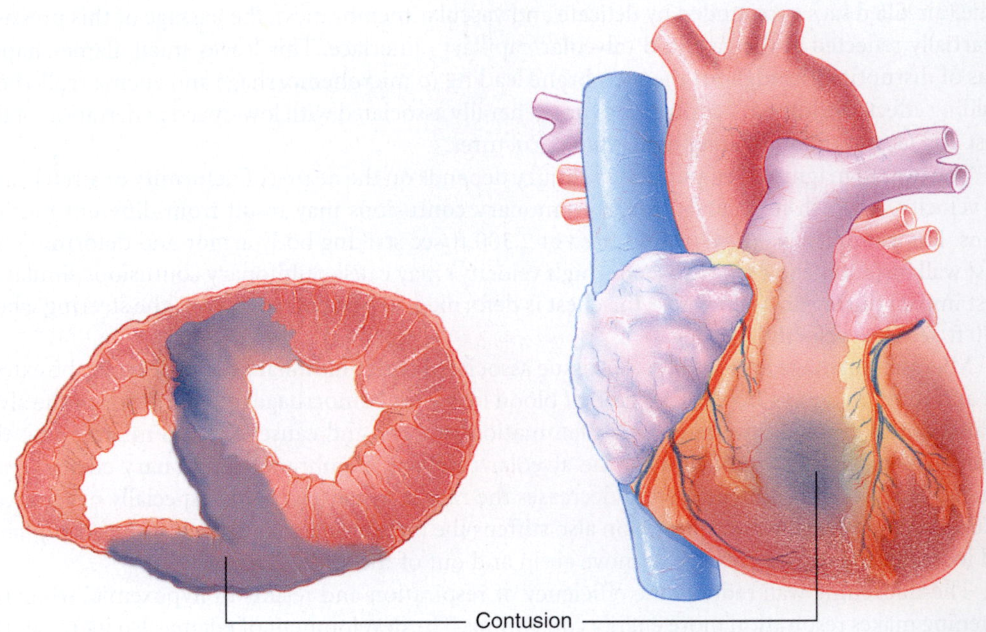

■ **Figure 25-11** Myocardial contusion most frequently affects the right atrium and ventricle as they collide with the sternum.

in the peritoneal sac), and necrosis and may result in cardiac irritability, ectopic (of abnormal origin) beats, and conduction system defects such as bundle branch blocks and dysrhythmias. If the injury is very extensive, it may lead to tissue necrosis (death), decreased ventricular compliance, congestive heart failure, cardiogenic shock, myocardial aneurysm, and acute or delayed myocardial rupture. In contrast to a myocardial infarction from coronary artery disease, the cellular damage from myocardial contusions heals with less scarring and there is no progression of the injury in the absence of associated coronary artery disease.

The patient experiencing myocardial contusion will have a history of significant blunt chest trauma, most likely affecting the anterior chest. The patient will likely complain of chest or retrosternal pain, very much like that of myocardial infarction and may have associated chest injuries such as anterior rib or sternal fractures. Cardiac monitoring most frequently reveals sinus tachycardia (though it may be caused by pain, hypovolemia, or hypoxia from associated chest injury). Other dysrhythmias associated with myocardial contusions are atrial flutter or fibrillation, premature atrial or ventricular contractions, tachydysrhythmias, bradydysrhythmias, bundle branch patterns, T wave inversions, and ST segment elevations. A pericardial friction rub and murmur may be auscultated over the **precordium** but is more likely to occur weeks after the injury and is associated with the development of an inflammatory pericardial effusion.

Content Review

Signs and Symptoms of Cardiac Contusion

- Blunt injury to chest
- Bruising of chest wall
- Rapid heart rate—may be irregular
- Severe nagging pain not relieved with rest but may be relieved with oxygen

precordium *area of the chest wall overlying the heart.*

Pericardial Tamponade

Pericardial tamponade is a restriction to cardiac filling caused by blood (or other fluid) within the pericardial sac. It occurs in less than 2 percent of all serious chest trauma patients and is almost always related to penetrating injury. Gunshot wounds are the most frequent mechanism and carry a high overall mortality, though they often result in rapid hemorrhage through the myocardial wall and then out the defect in the pericardium. The frequency of gunshot wound mortality is probably related to the depth of injury, the degree of cardiac tissue damage caused by the cavitational wave, and a more rapid progression of the pathology.

pericardial tamponade *a restriction to cardiac filling caused by blood (or other fluid) within the pericardial sac.*

The pathology of pericardial tamponade begins with a tear in a superficial coronary artery or penetration of the myocardium. Blood seeps into the pericardial space and accumulates (Figure 25-12 ■). The fibrous pericardium does not stretch and the accumulating blood exerts pressure on the heart. The pressure limits cardiac filling, first affecting the right ventricle where the pressure of filling is the lowest. This restricts venous return to the heart, increases venous pressure, and causes jugular vein distention. The reduced right ventricular output limits outflow to the pulmonary arteries and then venous return to the left heart. The result is a decreasing cardiac output and systemic

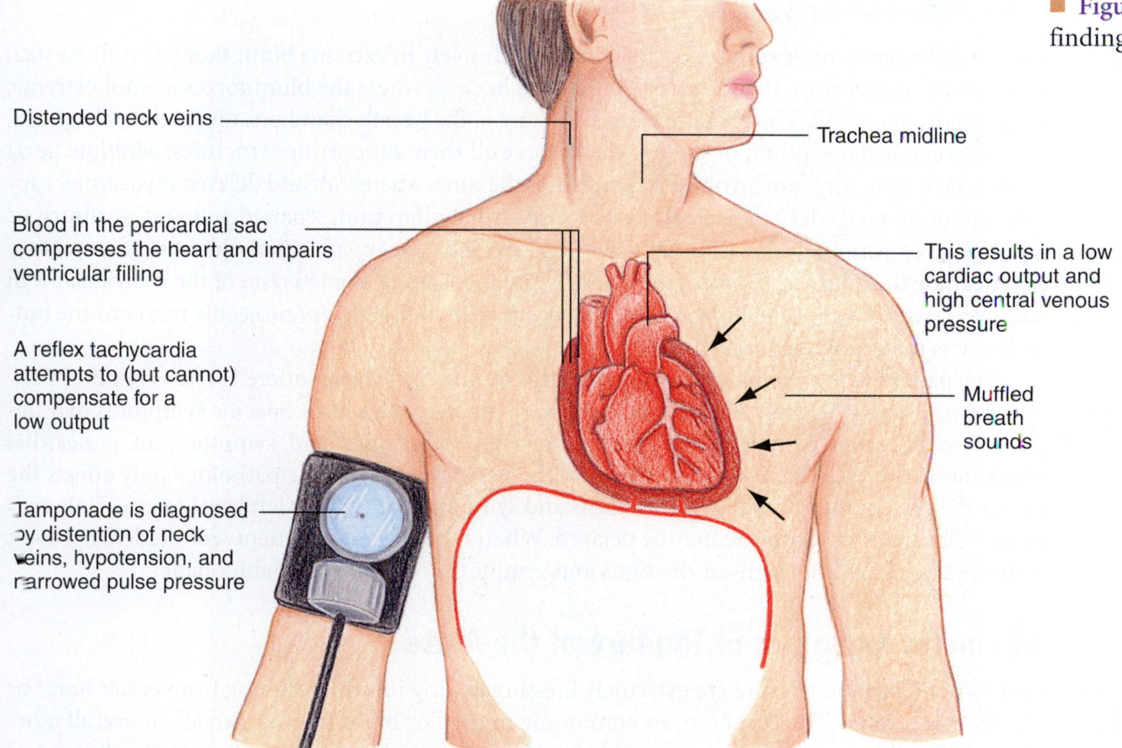

■ **Figure 25-12** Physical findings of cardiac tamponade.

hypotension. The pressure exerted by the blood in the pericardium also restricts the flow of blood through the coronary arteries and to the myocardium. This may result in myocardial ischemia and infarct. It takes about 150 to 300 mL of blood to exert the pressure necessary to induce frank tamponade, while removing as little as 20 mL may provide significant relief. The progression of pericardial tamponade depends on the rate of blood flow into the pericardium. It may occur very rapidly and result in death before the arrival of emergency medical services or may gradually progress over hours.

The patient experiencing pericardial tamponade will likely have penetrating trauma to the anterior or posterior chest, though blunt trauma can also cause this problem. While the trajectories of missiles and knife blades are difficult to predict, consider pericardial tamponade with any thoracic or upper abdominal penetrating wound, especially if it is over the precordium (central lower chest). Pericardial tamponade will diminish the strength of pulses, decrease the pulse pressure, and distend the jugular veins (JVD). The patient will likely be agitated, tachycardic, diaphoretic, and ashen in appearance. Cyanosis may be noted in the head, neck, and upper extremities. Heart tones may be muffled or distant sounding. Beck's triad (JVD, distant heart tones, and hypotension) is indicative of pericardial tamponade but may not be recognized early in the injury's progression. Another sign of pericardial tamponade is Kussmaul's sign, the decrease or absence of JVD during inspiration. As the patient inspires, the reduced intrathoracic pressure increases venous return and decreases the pressure the accumulating pericardial fluid exerts on the heart. This then translates to a better venous return and cardiac output during inspiration and the effect then seen in the jugular veins

Other findings during pericardial tamponade may include pulsus paradoxus and electrical alternans. **Pulsus paradoxus** is a drop in systolic blood pressure of greater than 10 mmHg as the patient inspires during the normal respiratory cycle. (Normally the systolic blood pressure drops just slightly with each inspiration.) Pulsus paradoxus results because cardiac output increases with the minimal relief of the tamponade associated with the reduced intrathoracic pressure of inspiration. **Electrical alternans,** which is only rarely seen in acute pericardial tamponade, is noted on the cardiac rhythm strip as the P, QRS, and T amplitude decreasing with every other cardiac cycle. In profound pericardial tamponade, the heart displays a rhythm without producing a pulse (PEA).

Content Review

Signs and Symptoms of Pericardial Tamponade

- Dyspnea and possible cyanosis
- Jugular venous distention
- Weak, thready pulse
- Decreasing blood pressure
- Shock
- Narrowing pulse pressure

pulsus paradoxus *drop of greater than 10 mmHg in the systolic blood pressure during the inspiratory phase of respiration that occurs in patients with pericardial tamponade.*

electrical alternans *alternating amplitude of the P, QRS, and T waves on the ECG rhythm strip as the heart swings in a pendulumlike fashion within the pericardial sac during tamponade.*

Myocardial Aneurysm or Rupture

aneurysm *a weakening or ballooning in the wall of a blood vessel.*

Myocardial **aneurysm** or rupture occurs almost exclusively in extreme blunt thoracic trauma such as automobile collisions. It also has been reported in cases where the blunt forces are not extreme, such as a result of CPR. The condition can affect any of the heart's chambers, the interatrial septum, the interventricular septum, or involve the valves and their supporting structures. Multiple heart chambers or structures are involved 30 percent of the time. Aneurysm and delayed myocardial rupture also occur secondary to necrosis from a myocardial infarction, repaired penetrating injury, or myocardial contusion. Necrosis usually develops around 2 weeks after the injury as inflammatory cells degrade the injured cells, weakening the tissue, and leading to aneurysm of the ventricular wall and/or subsequent rupture. Rupture can also occur with high-velocity projectile injury as the bullet impacts the engorged heart chamber.

The patient who experiences myocardial rupture will likely have suffered serious blunt or penetrating trauma to the chest and may have severe rib or sternal fracture. Specific symptoms may depend on the actual pathology. The victim may have the signs and symptoms of pericardial tamponade if the rupture is contained within the pericardial sac. If the pathology only affects the valves, the patient may present with the signs and symptoms of right or left heart failure. If there is myocardial aneurysm, rupture may be delayed. When it happens, the patient will suddenly present with the absence of vital signs or the signs and symptoms of pericardial tamponade.

Traumatic Aneurysm or Rupture of the Aorta

Traumatic rupture of the thoracic aorta is almost always fatal.

Aortic aneurysm and rupture are extremely life-threatening injuries resulting from either blunt or penetrating trauma. The aorta is most commonly injured by blunt trauma, carries an overall mortality of 85 to 95 percent, and is responsible for 15 percent of all thoracic trauma deaths. Aneurysm and rupture are usually associated with high-speed automobile crashes (most commonly lateral impact) and in some cases with high falls. Unlike myocardial rupture, a significant number, possibly as high as 20 percent, of these victims will survive the initial insult and aneurysm. Some 30 percent of these initial survivors will die in 6 hours if not treated, increasing to about 50 percent at 24 hours, and just under 70 percent by the end of the first week. It is this subset of patients that survive the initial impact and are alive at the scene that you can benefit the most by recognizing the potential injury and then by rapidly extricating, packaging, and transporting the patients to the trauma center.

The aorta is a large high-pressure vessel that provides outflow from the left ventricle for distribution to the body. It is relatively fixed at three points as it passes through the thoracic cavity and, because of this, experiences shear forces secondary to severe deceleration of the chest. The areas of fixation are the aortic annulus where the aorta joins the heart, the aortic isthmus where it is joined by the ligamentum arteriosum, and the diaphragm where it exits the chest (Table 25–2). Traumatic dissecting aneurysm occurs infrequently to the ascending aorta and, most commonly, to the descending aorta. With severe deceleration, shear forces separate the layers of the artery, specifically the interior surface (the tunica intima) from the muscle layer (the tunica media). This allows blood to enter and, because it is under great pressure, it begins to dissect the aortic lining like a bulging inner tube. It is likely to rupture if it is not surgically repaired.

The patient with aortic rupture will be severely hypotensive, quickly lose all vital signs, and die unless moved into surgery immediately. Dissecting aortic aneurysm progresses more slowly, though

Table 25–2 Incidence and Anatomic Location of Traumatic Aortic Rupture

Location	Incidence
Aortic annulus	9%
Aortic isthmus	85%
Diaphragm	3%
Other	3%

the aneurysm may rupture at any moment. The patient will probably have a history of a high fall or severe auto impact and deceleration. Lateral impact is an especially high risk factor for aortic aneurysm. The patient may complain of severe tearing chest pain that may radiate to the back. The patient may have a pulse deficit between the left and right upper extremities and/or reduced pulse strength in the lower extremities. Blood pressure may be high (hypertension) due to stretching of sympathetic nerve fibers present in the aorta near the ligamentum arteriosum, or the pressure may be low due to leakage and hypovolemia. Auscultation may reveal a harsh systolic murmur due to turbulence as the blood exits the heart and passes the disrupted blood vessel wall.

Serious lateral chest impact carries a high incidence of dissecting aortic aneurysm.

OTHER VASCULAR INJURIES

The pulmonary arteries and vena cava are other thoracic vascular structures that can sustain injury during chest trauma. Their injury, and the resulting hemorrhage, may cause significant hemothorax, possibly leading to hypotension and respiratory insufficiency. The blood may also flow into the mediastinum and compress the great vessels, esophagus, and heart. Penetrating trauma is the primary cause of injury to the pulmonary arteries and vena cava.

The patient with pulmonary artery or vena cava injuries will likely have a penetrating wound to the central chest or elsewhere with a likelihood of central chest involvement. These injuries present with the signs and symptoms of hypovolemia and shock and result in hemothorax or hemomediastinum and the signs and symptoms associated with those pathologies.

OTHER THORACIC INJURIES

Traumatic Rupture or Perforation of the Diaphragm

Traumatic rupture or perforation of the diaphragm can occur in both high-speed blunt thoracoabdominal trauma as well as in penetrating trauma. Incidence is estimated from 1 to 6 percent of all patients with multiple trauma. It is more common in patients sustaining penetrating trauma to the lower chest, which has as much as a 30 to 40 percent incidence of abdominal organ and tissue involvement. Remember that during expiration the diaphragm may move superiorly to the level of the fourth intercostal space (nipple level) anteriorly and the sixth intercostal space posteriorly. Any penetrating injuries at these levels or below may penetrate the diaphragm. Diaphragmatic perforation and herniation occur most frequently on the left side because assailants are most frequently right handed and the size and solid nature of the liver protect the diaphragm on the right. The liver is also unlikely to herniate through the torn diaphragm unless the injury is sizable.

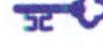

Suspect diaphragmatic perforation with any penetrating injury to the lower thorax.

If traumatic diaphragmatic rupture occurs, the abdominal organs may herniate through the defect into the thoracic cavity causing strangulation or necrosis of the bowel, restriction of the ipsilateral lung, and displacement of the mediastinum. Mediastinal displacement occurs when the displaced abdominal contents place pressure on the lung and mediastinal structures, moving them toward the contralateral side through much the same mechanism as is seen in tension pneumothorax.

Diaphragmatic rupture presents with signs and symptoms similar to tension pneumothorax, including dyspnea, hypoxia, hypotension, and JVD. The patient will have a history of blunt abdominal trauma or penetrating trauma to the lower thorax or upper abdomen. The abdomen may appear hollow, and bowel sounds may be noted in one side of the thorax (most commonly the left). The patient may be hypotensive and hypoxic if the herniation is extensive. The patient may complain of upper abdominal pain, though this symptom is often overshadowed by other injuries. Diaphragmatic rupture may be recognized at the time of injury or may be missed if not extensive. A patient may then present with delayed herniation months to years later.

Traumatic Esophageal Rupture

Traumatic esophageal rupture is a rare complication of blunt thoracic trauma. The incidence of it related to penetrating trauma of the thorax is somewhat higher but still only about 0.4 percent. Since the esophagus is rather centrally located within the chest, its injury usually coincides with other mediastinal injuries. (Esophageal rupture may also be the result of medical problems such as violent emesis, carcinoma, anatomical distortion, or gastric reflux.) Esophageal rupture carries a

30 percent mortality, even if quickly recognized, and mortality is much greater if this injury is not diagnosed promptly. The life threat from esophageal rupture is related to material entering the mediastinum as it passes down the esophagus or as emesis comes up. This results in serious infection or chemical irritation and serious damage to the mediastinal structures. Air may also enter the mediastinum through an esophageal rupture, especially during positive-pressure ventilations.

The patient with esophageal rupture will probably have deep penetrating trauma to the central chest and may complain of difficult or painful swallowing, pleuritic chest pain, and pain radiating to the mid back. The patient may also display subcutaneous emphysema around the lower neck.

Tracheobronchial Injury (Disruption)

Tracheobronchial injury is a relatively infrequent finding in thoracic trauma with an incidence of less than 3 percent in patients with significant chest trauma. It may occur from either a blunt or a penetrating injury mechanism and carries a relatively high mortality similar to esophageal rupture of 30 percent. In contrast to patients with esophageal rupture who usually die days after injury, 50 percent of patients with tracheobronchial injury die within 1 hour of injury. Disruption can occur anywhere in the tracheobronchial tree but is most likely to occur within 2.5 cm of the carina.

The patient with disruption of the trachea or mainstem bronchi is generally in respiratory distress with cyanosis, hemoptysis, and, in some cases, massive subcutaneous emphysema. The patient may also experience pneumothorax and, possibly, tension pneumothorax. Intermittent positive-pressure ventilation drives air into the pleura or mediastinum and makes the condition worse.

Traumatic Asphyxia

Traumatic asphyxia occurs when severe compressive force is applied to the thorax and leads to a reverse flow of blood from the right heart into the superior vena cava and into the venous vessels of the upper extremities. (Traumatic asphyxia is not as much a respiratory problem as it is a vascular problem.) Traumatic asphyxia engorges the veins and capillaries of the head and neck with desaturated venous blood, turning the skin in this region a deep red, purple, or blue. The backflow of blood damages the microcirculation in the head and neck, producing petechiae (small hemorrhages under the skin) and stagnating blood above the point of compression. The backflow may damage cerebral circulation, resulting in numerous small strokes in the older patient whose venous vessels are not very elastic. If flow restriction continues, toxins and acids accumulate in the blood and may have a devastating effect when they return to the central circulation with the release of pressure. If the thoracic compression continues, it restricts venous return and may prevent the victim from ventilating. This results in hypotension, hypoxemia, and shock. Death may follow rapidly. Extrication of the patient may result in rapid hemorrhage from the injury site with release of the pressure. Release of the compression may likewise result in rapid patient deterioration and death.

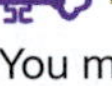

You must be ready to immediately handle the complications of traumatic asphyxia as soon as the patient is released from entrapment.

The traumatic asphyxia patient will have suffered a severe compression force to the chest that is likely to continue until extrication. The result of the compression, the backflow of blood and restricted blood flow, will be dramatic and cause the classical discoloration of the head and neck regions. The face appears swollen, the eyes bulge, and there are numerous conjunctival hemorrhages. The patient may have severe dyspnea related to the compression and injuries associated with severe chest impact. Once the pressure is released, the patient may show the signs of hypovolemia, hypotension, and shock as well as signs related to any coexisting respiratory problems.

ASSESSMENT OF THE CHEST INJURY PATIENT

The proper assessment of the patient with a severe chest injury mechanism is critical to anticipating injury and providing the correct interventions. While the approach to this patient follows the standard format for assessment, special considerations regarding chest trauma occur during the scene size-up, primary assessment, and especially during the rapid secondary assessment. The reassessment is also critical for monitoring the thoracic trauma patient for the progression of injuries sustained during serious chest trauma.

SCENE SIZE-UP

Chest injury care, like that for any other serious trauma, requires Standard Precautions with gloves as a minimum. Consider a face shield if you will be attending to the airway and a gown for splash protection with serious penetrating thoracic trauma. Ensure that the scene is safe, including protection from the assailant, if penetrating trauma is suspected.

Examine the mechanism of injury carefully and try to determine if the central chest (heart, great vessels, trachea, and esophagus) might be in the pathway of penetrating trauma. In gunshot injuries, determine the type of weapon, caliber, distance between the gun barrel and the victim, and the probable pathway of the projectile. Determine the direction of blunt trauma impact as it may also have a bearing on which organs sustain injury. Anterior impact may rupture lung tissue and contuse the lung and heart. Lateral impact may tear the aorta as the heart displaces laterally and stresses the aorta's ligamentous attachments.

PRIMARY ASSESSMENT

During the primary assessment, determine the patient's mental status and the status of the airway, breathing, and circulation. Intervene as necessary to correct life-threatening conditions. It is during the primary assessment that you will first identify the signs and symptoms of serious chest trauma. Be especially watchful for any dyspnea; asymmetrical, paradoxical, or limited chest movement; hyperinflation of the chest; or an abdomen that appears hollow. Notice any general patient color reflective of hypoxia such as cyanosis or an ashen discoloration. Look for distended jugular veins, costal or suprasternal retractions, and the use of accessory muscles of respiration.

Ensure that ventilation is adequate and administer high-flow, high-concentration oxygen by nonrebreather mask. Administer any positive-pressure ventilations with care as thoracic injury may weaken the lung tissue and make the patient prone to pneumothorax or tension pneumothorax. Aggressive (or even cautious) ventilations may induce these problems. Be suspicious of internal hemorrhage and initiate at least one large-bore intravenous catheter and line in anticipation of hypovolemia, hypotension, and shock. With anterior blunt or penetrating trauma that may involve the heart, attach the ECG electrodes and monitor for dysrhythmias. Attach a pulse oximeter and monitor oxygen saturation to evaluate the effectiveness of respiration. If there is any mechanism suggesting serious trauma to the chest or any physical signs of either hypoventilation or hypovolemia compensation, perform the rapid secondary assessment with a special focus on the chest and prepare for rapid patient transport to the trauma center.

Administer ventilations with care in the patient with chest trauma.

RAPID SECONDARY ASSESSMENT

During the rapid secondary assessment you will examine the patient's chest in detail, carefully observing, questioning about, palpating, and auscultating the region.

Observe

Observe the chest for evidence of impact. Look for the erythema that develops early in the contusion process, especially as it outlines the ribs or forms a pattern reflecting the contours of the object the chest hit. Look carefully for penetrating trauma and try to determine the angle of entry and depth of penetration. Also look for exit wounds. Lateral chest injury is likely to involve the lungs, while a pathway of energy through the central chest is likely to involve the heart, great vessels, trachea, or esophagus. Injury to the mediastinal structures is also likely to result in serious hemorrhage, hypovolemia, and shock. Look for intercostal and suprasternal retractions as well as external jugular vein distention. Remember, JVD is present in supine normotensive patients and may be exaggerated in them or may continue when the patient is moved to the seated position if venous pressure is elevated.

Watch chest movement carefully during respiration. The chest should rise and the abdomen should fall smoothly with inspiration and return to their positions during expiration. Any limited motion, either bilaterally or unilaterally, suggests a problem. Watch for the paradoxical motion of flail chest. That movement will be limited due to muscle spasm during early care, but continued motion will further damage the surrounding soft tissue and the intracostal muscles will fatigue.

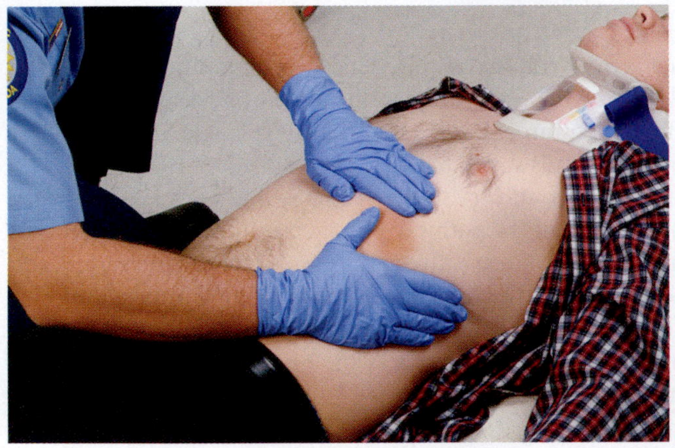

■ **Figure 25-13** Carefully palpate the thorax of a patient with a suspected injury to the region. *(Maria A. H. Lyle)*

This will lead to a more obvious paradoxical motion and greater respiratory embarrassment with time. Look, too, for any hyperinflation of one side of the chest and any deformity that may exist from rib fracture, sternal fracture or dislocation, or subcutaneous emphysema. Assess the volume of air effectively moved with each breath and ensure that the minute volume is greater than 6 liters. If not, consider overdrive ventilation with the bag-valve mask. Examine any open wound for air movement in or out, which is indicative of an open pneumothorax. Observe the patient's general color. If a patient's skin is dusky, ashen, or cyanotic, suspect respiratory compromise. If the head and neck are red, dark red, or blue, suspect traumatic asphyxia.

Question

Question the patient about any pain, pain on motion, pain with breathing effort (pleuritic pain), or dyspnea. Note if the pain is crushing, tearing, or is described otherwise by the patient. Have the patient describe the exact location of the pain, its severity, and any radiation of the pain. Question about other sensations and carefully monitor the patient's level of consciousness and orientation.

You may have to rely on your palpation skills to assess chest injuries when scene noise is excessive.

Palpate

Palpate the thorax carefully, feeling for any signs of injury (Figure 25-13 ■). Feel for any swelling, deformity, crepitus, or the crackling of subcutaneous emphysema. Compress the thorax between your hands with pressure directed inward. Then apply downward pressure on the midsternum. Such pressure will flex the ribs and should elicit pain from any fracture site along the thorax. (Apply pressure only if you have found no signs or symptoms of chest injury. If you suspect rib or sternal fracture, provide appropriate care but do not aggravate the injury.) Rest your hands on the lower thorax; let the chest lift your hands with inspiration and let them fall with expiration (Figure 25-14 ■). The motion should be smooth and equal. If not, determine the nature of any asymmetry.

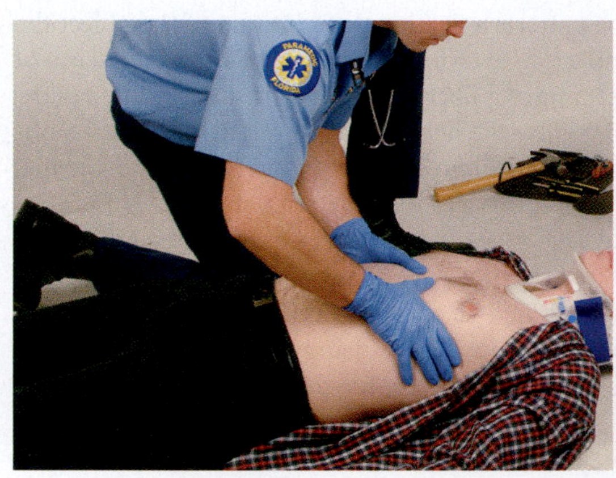

■ **Figure 25-14** Place your hands on the lower thorax and let them rise and fall with respiration. *(Maria A. H. Lyle)*

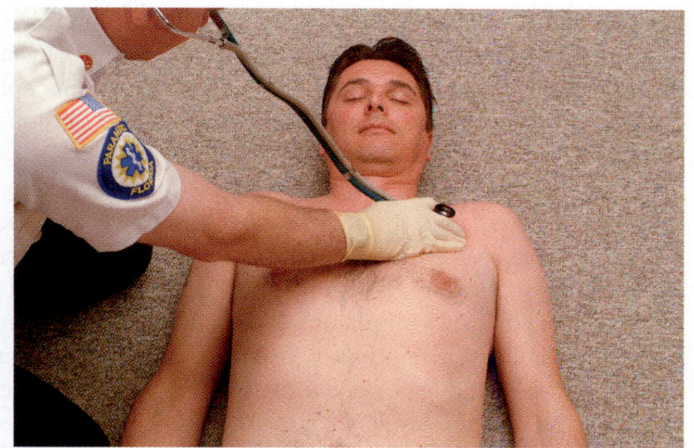

■ Figure 25-15 Auscultate all lung lobes, both anteriorly and posteriorly.

Auscultate

Auscultate all lung lobes, both anteriorly and posteriorly (Figure 25-15 ■). Listen for both inspiratory and expiratory air movement and note any crackles, indicating edema from contusion or congestive heart failure, or any diminished breath sounds, suggesting hypoventilation. Compare one side to the other and one lobe to another. Be sensitive for distant or muffled respiratory or heart sounds.

Percuss

Percuss the chest and note the responses (Figure 25-16 ■). Determine if the area percussed is normal, hyperresonant, or dull. A dull response suggests collecting blood or other fluid, while hyperresonance suggests air or air under pressure as in a pneumothorax or tension pneumothorax.

Your findings from the rapid secondary assessment may suggest an injury or multiple injuries. Identify the likely cause of the signs and symptoms you find and suspect and anticipate the worst. You are likely to note clear evidence of chest wall injury and some signs of internal injuries if they exist. As mentioned earlier, blunt and penetrating trauma present with different typical injuries.

Blunt Trauma Assessment

In blunt trauma, you commonly find slight discoloration of the surface of the chest reflective of contusions. The contusions also cause the patient pain, generally in an area or region, and somewhat limit respiration. As the impact energy increases, it may cause fractures of ribs 4 through 8 and a greater possibility of underlying injury. If the upper ribs or ribs 9 through 12 fracture, suspect serious underlying injury. Sternal fracture takes great energy and is also associated with a higher incidence of internal injury. Rib fractures generate a point-specific pain (at the fracture site) and crepitus upon deep breathing or your flexing of the patient's chest during the rapid trauma assessment. That

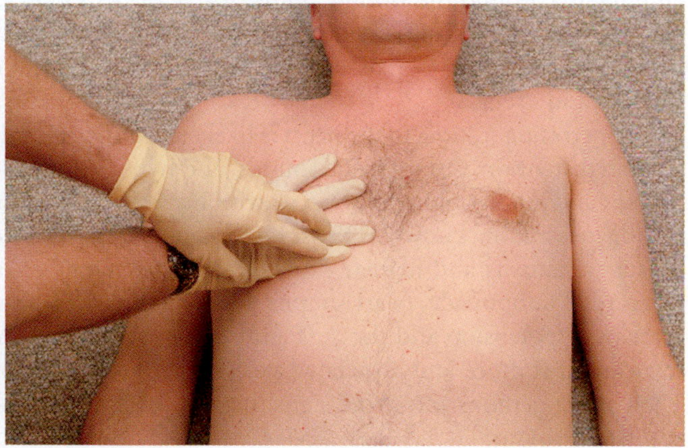

■ Figure 25-16 Percuss all lung lobes, listening for a dull response or hyperresonance.

pain may further limit chest excursion during respiration. As the energy of trauma and the seriousness of chest trauma increase, more ribs may fracture, causing a flail chest. Remember that a flail chest's paradoxical motion is initially limited by muscular splinting; it grows more noticeable and causes more respiratory distress as the time since the collision increases.

In blunt injury to the chest, you must anticipate and assess for additional signs suggesting internal injury. Signs specific for lung injury include increasing dyspnea, signs of hypoxemia, accessory muscle use, and intracostal and suprasternal retractions. Auscultation will help you differentiate between pulmonary contusion and pneumothorax. Contusions demonstrate progressively increasing crackles, while pneumothorax presents with diminished breath sounds on the ipsilateral side. Further, with pneumothorax the affected side may be hyperinflated and resonant to percussion. If the pneumothorax progresses to tension pneumothorax, you will likely note progressing dyspnea and hypoxia, use of accessory muscles, distended jugular veins, tracheal shift toward the contralateral side (a late finding), and hyperresonance of the ipsilateral chest on percussion. Subcutaneous emphysema may develop, especially if the lung defect was caused by or is associated with a rib fracture that disturbs the integrity of the parietal pleura. Hemothorax is noticeable due to the vascular loss, more so than for the respiratory component of the pathology. Suspect it if you find the signs of hypovolemia associated with blunt chest trauma. Hemothorax, when sizable, may cause dyspnea and a lung field that is dull to percussion.

Blunt mediastinal injury will probably affect the heart, great vessels, and trachea. Heart injury may present with chest pain similar to that of the myocardial infarction and, if serious enough, with the signs of heart failure or cardiogenic shock. The ECG may reveal tachycardia, bradycardia, cardiac irritability, and in cases of severe cardiac contusion, may demonstrate ST elevation. Cardiac rupture presents with the signs of sudden death, while pericardial tamponade is unlikely in blunt chest trauma. Injury to the great vessels (aneurysm) is most frequently associated with lateral impacts or feet-first high falls and may produce a tearing chest pain and pulse deficits in the extremities. If the aneurysm ruptures, rapidly progressing hypovolemia, hypotension, shock, and death ensue. Tracheobronchial injury results in rapidly developing pneumomediastinum or pneumothorax and possible subcutaneous emphysema, hemoptysis, dyspnea, and hypoxia. Positive-pressure ventilations may increase the development and severity of signs. Traumatic asphyxia presents with jugular vein distention, discoloration of the head and neck, severe dyspnea, and possibly the signs of hypovolemia and shock.

Penetrating Trauma Assessment

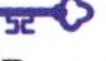

Remember, the severity of internal injury associated with penetrating trauma may be great despite seemingly minor entrance and/or exit wounds.

Penetrating injury displays a different set of signs associated with different injuries. Inspect a chest wound for frothy blood or sounds of air exchange with respirations (open pneumothorax). Remember that a wound needs to be rather large (high-velocity bullet exit wound or close-range shotgun blast) for these signs to occur. A penetrating wound, however, commonly induces a simple pneumothorax with its associated signs and symptoms. A hyperinflated chest, distended jugular veins, tracheal shift away from the injury, distant or absent breath sounds, hyperresonance to percussion, and severe dyspnea and hypotension suggest tension pneumothorax. The pressure of tension pneumothorax may push air outward through a penetrating wound or cause subcutaneous emphysema around the wound. Some degree of hemothorax is likely to be associated with penetrating chest trauma and, if extensive, may reveal diminished or absent breath sounds and a chest region that is dull to percussion. Hemothorax also causes or significantly contributes to hypovolemia and shock.

Penetrating trauma to the heart is likely to cause pericardial tamponade and present with jugular vein distention, distant heart sounds, and hypotension (Beck's triad). Pulsus paradoxus may be present and jugular filling may occur with inspiration (due to a paradoxical rise in venous pressure during inspiration, known as Kussmaul's sign, that is associated with pericardial tamponade). Both pulsus paradoxus and jugular filling are indicative of pericardial tamponade. Additionally, with pericardial tamponade, heart sounds are distant, pulses are weak, and the patient experiences increasing hypotension and shock (Figure 25-17 ■). Penetrating trauma to the heart may also cause myocardial rupture and associated pericardial tamponade or immediate death (Figure 25-18 ■). The patient demonstrates vital signs that fall precipitously as the vascular volume is pumped into the mediastinum.

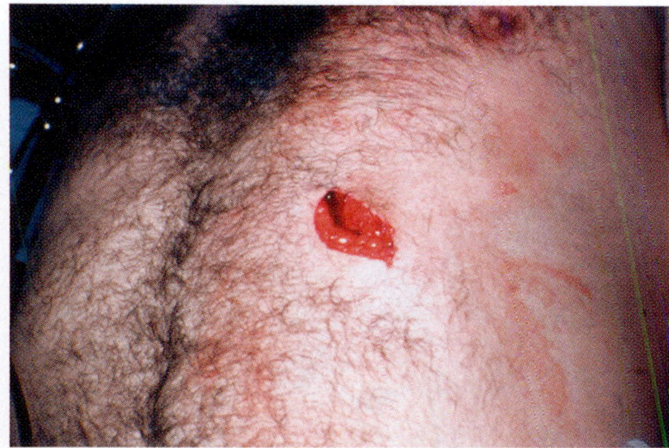

■ **Figure 25-17** Penetrating stab wound to the chest involving the heart.

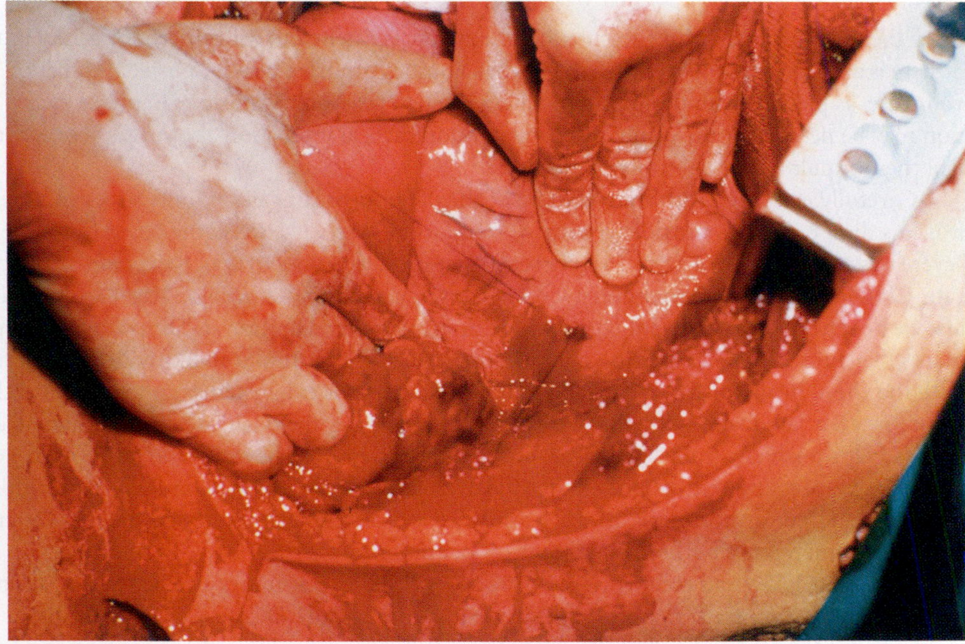

■ **Figure 25-18** Stab wound that penetrated the pericardium.

REASSESSMENT

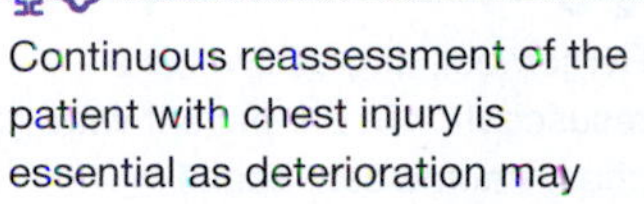

Continuous reassessment of the patient with chest injury is essential as deterioration may occur within a matter of seconds.

While the reassessment simply repeats elements of the primary assessment, the taking of vital signs, and examination of any injury signs discovered during earlier assessment, it takes on great importance for the patient with chest trauma. With any serious chest impact or any penetrating injury to the chest, observe the respiratory depth, rate, and symmetry of effort. Auscultate the lung fields for equality and crackles and monitor the distal pulses, oxygen saturation, skin color, and blood pressure for signs of progressing hypovolemia (Figure 25-19 ■). If any signs change between assessments, search out the cause and rule out progressing chest injury. Be especially suspicious of developing tension pneumothorax, pericardial tamponade, extensive and evolving pulmonary contusion, and hypovolemia associated with hemothorax. If any of these is found, institute the appropriate management steps.

MANAGEMENT OF THE THORACIC TRAUMA PATIENT

General management of the patient with serious chest trauma requires assurance of good oxygenation and adequate respiratory volume and rate.

The general management of the patient with significant chest injury focuses on ensuring good oxygenation and adequate respiratory volume and rate. Administer high-flow, high-concentration oxygen

Figure 25-19 With pulse oximetry, you can continuously monitor the percentage of the patient's oxygen saturation.

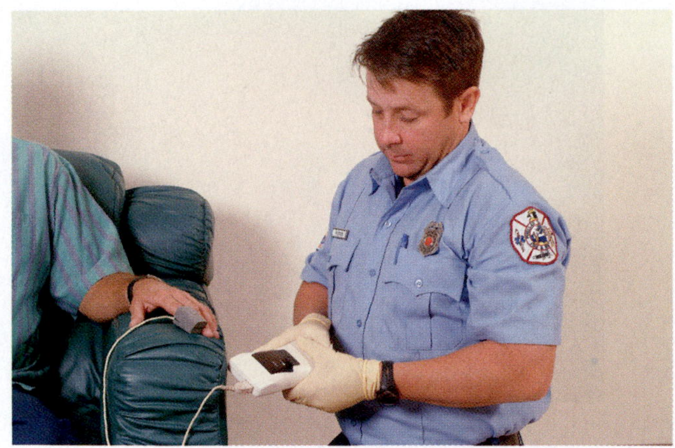

using the nonrebreather mask. Ensure that the airway is patent and consider endotracheal intubation if there is any significant loss in the level of consciousness or orientation. Consider intubation early in your care, as patients with thoracic trauma are likely to get worse with time. Rapid-sequence intubation may be needed for the combative patient. Endotracheal intubation also makes ventilation of the flail chest or pulmonary contusion patient easier.

Carefully evaluate the minute volume of the patient (breaths per minute times volume) and if it is less than 6,000 mL consider overdrive ventilation. Bag-valve mask the conscious patient with severe dyspnea at a rate of 12 to 16 full breaths per minute, trying to match the patient's respiratory rate. Closely monitor pulse oximetry, level of consciousness, and skin color. Bag-valve masking may also be beneficial for the patient with serious rib fractures and flail chest. The positive pressure displaces the chest outward, reducing the movement of the fracture site and moving the flail segment with the chest. It may also be beneficial to the patient who is exhausted from the increased breathing effort associated with pulmonary contusion. In this case, the positive pressure of assisted ventilations helps push any fluids back into the vascular system to relieve edema. Remember, however, that positive-pressure ventilations change the dynamics of respiration from a less than atmospheric to a greater than atmospheric process and may exacerbate respiratory problems like tracheobronchial injury, pneumothorax, and tension pneumothorax.

Anticipate heart and great vessel compromise with thoracic injury and be ready to support the patient's cardiovascular system. Initiate at least one large-bore IV site if the patient has a serious mechanism of chest trauma and place two lines if there are any signs of hypovolemia or compensation. Be prepared to administer fluids quickly (in 250- to 500-mL boluses) if the patient's systolic blood pressure is below 80 mmHg. Use of the PASG is contraindicated for penetrating chest trauma as it may increase the rate and volume of blood loss and disrupt the clotting process.

Remember, aggressive fluid resuscitation in the patient with chest trauma can result in hemodilution and loss of clotting factors.

The IV fluid infusion for the patient with chest trauma should be conservative. Rapid fluid administration may increase the rate of hemorrhage and dilute the clotting factors, further adding to the problem. Additional fluid also increases the edema associated with pulmonary contusion, increasing the rate and extent of its development. Anytime you administer fluids to the chest trauma patient, auscultate all lung fields carefully and reduce the fluid resuscitation rate whenever you hear respiratory crackles or the patient's dyspnea increases.

Care is specific for thoracic injuries including rib fractures, sternoclavicular dislocation, flail chest, open pneumothorax, tension pneumothorax, hemothorax, cardiac contusion, pericardial tamponade, aortic aneurysm, tracheobronchial injury, and traumatic asphyxia.

RIB FRACTURES

Rib fractures, either isolated or associated with other respiratory injuries, may produce pain that significantly limits respiratory effort and leads to hypoventilation. In these patients you may consider administering analgesics to grant greater patient comfort and improve chest excursion. Ensure that the patient is hemodynamically stable, that there is no associated abdominal or head injury, and that the patient is fully conscious and oriented. Consider administration of diazepam, morphine sulfate, or meperidine as described in Chapter 22, "Musculoskeletal Trauma." Note that use of nitrous oxide is contraindicated in chest trauma because the nitrous oxide may migrate into a pneumothorax or tension pneumothorax.

STERNOCLAVICULAR DISLOCATION

Supportive therapy with oxygen is usually all that is required for an isolated sternoclavicular dislocation. However, hemodynamic instability indicates associated injuries requiring rapid transport to the trauma center with aggressive resuscitation measures instituted en route. If you suspect posterior sternoclavicular dislocation and note the patient to be in significant respiratory distress that is not effectively treated with initial airway maneuvers and high-flow, high-concentration oxygen, then consider dislocation reduction. Place the patient in the supine position with a sandbag between the shoulder blades. The sandbag helps to pull the shoulders backward and moves the head of the clavicle laterally and away from the trachea. Do not perform this procedure for the multiple-trauma patient due to the probability of spine injury. An alternative reduction method is to place the patient supine and grasp the clavicle near the sternum. Pull it upward and laterally, directly perpendicular to the sternum. This distracts the clavicle forward, alleviating its impingement of the airway.

FLAIL CHEST

Place the patient on the side of injury if spinal immobilization is not required, or secure a large and bulky dressing with bandaging against the flail segment to stabilize it (Figure 25-20 ■). Employ high-flow, high-concentration oxygen therapy; monitor oxygen saturation with pulse oximetry; and monitor cardiac activity with the ECG. If there is significant dyspnea, evidence of underlying pulmonary injury, or signs of respiratory compromise, these measures will not suffice. Then consider endotracheal intubation, positive-pressure ventilations, and high-flow, high-concentration oxygen. Positive-pressure ventilations internally splint the flail segment, expand atelectatic areas of the lung, and also treat underlying pulmonary contusion. Use of sandbags to support the flail segment is not indicated because it may diminish chest movement, adding to hypoventilation, atelectasis, and subsequent hypoxemia. Rapid transport to the trauma center is indicated as this injury, its complications, and associated injuries are often life threatening.

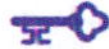

Consider early intubation of the patient with flail chest, especially when oxygenation remains impaired despite the provision of high-flow, high-concentration oxygen.

OPEN PNEUMOTHORAX

Support the patient with open pneumothorax by administering high-flow, high-concentration oxygen and monitoring oxygen saturation and respiratory effort. If you find a penetrating injury, cover it with a sterile occlusive dressing (sterile plastic wrap) taped on three sides (Figure 25-21 ■). This process converts the open pneumothorax into a closed pneumothorax, prevents further aspiration of air, and relieves any building pressure (tension pneumothorax) through the valvelike dressing. If the dyspnea diminishes somewhat but still continues, provide positive-pressure ventilations and intubate as indicated. Carefully monitor the patient when you employ intermittent positive-pressure ventilation because its use may lead to a tension pneumothorax. If, after the dressing has been applied, the patient has progressive breathing difficulty, appears to be hypoventilating and hypoxemic,

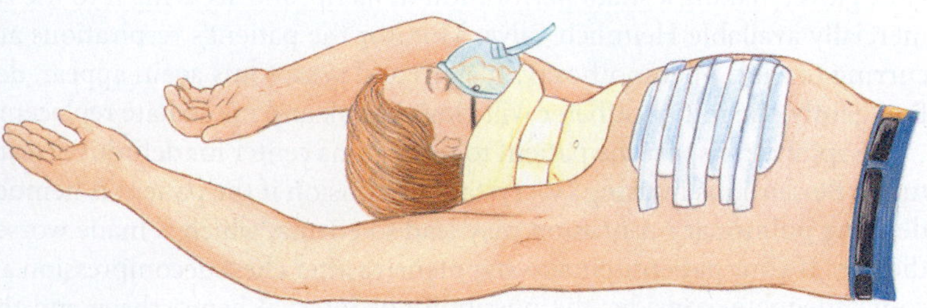

■ **Figure 25-20** Flail chest should be treated with administration of oxygen and gentle splinting of the flail segment with a pillow or pad.

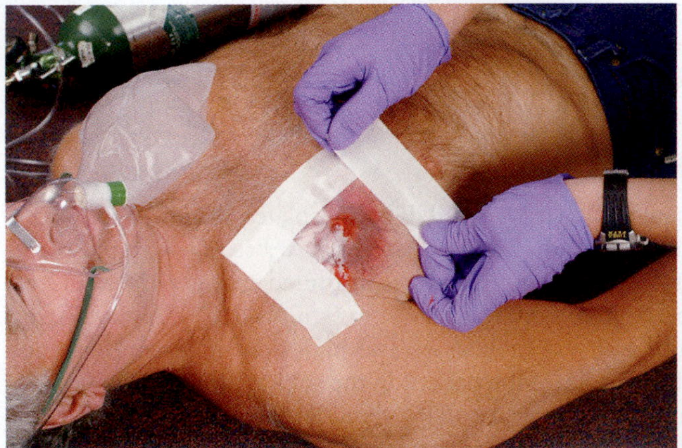

■ Figure 25-21 By taping the occlusive dressing on three sides, you create a flutter valve that helps to prevent tension pneumothorax.

has decreasing breath sounds on the injured side, and has increasing jugular distention, remove the occlusive dressing. If you hear air rush out and the patient's respirations improve, reseal the wound, monitor breathing carefully, and again remove the dressing if any respiratory signs or symptoms redevelop. If removing the dressing does not relieve the increasing signs and symptoms, suspect and treat for tension pneumothorax.

TENSION PNEUMOTHORAX

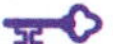

Tension pneumothorax is an occasional complication of multiple trauma. Always assess for it and decompress the chest when indicated.

Pleural decompression should only be employed if the patient demonstrates significant dyspnea and distinct signs and symptoms of tension pneumothorax.

Confirm possible tension pneumothorax by auscultating the lung fields for diminished breath sounds, percussing for hyperresonance, and observing for severe dyspnea, hyperinflation of the chest, and jugular vein distention. Successful treatment depends on rapid recognition of this condition and then pleural decompression. As you prepare to decompress the affected (ipsilateral) side, apply high-flow, high-concentration oxygen if the airway is intact and the patient is able to demonstrate adequate ventilatory effort. Pleural decompression should be employed only if the patient demonstrates significant dyspnea and distinct signs and symptoms of tension pneumothorax.

Provide ventilations with the bag-valve mask and supplemental oxygen and intubate if the patient is unable to maintain an airway or continues to show signs/symptoms of hypoxemia on high-flow, high-concentration oxygen. Perform needle thoracentesis by inserting a long 14-gauge intravascular catheter into the second intercostal space, midclavicular line on the side of the thorax with decreased breath sounds and hyperinflation (Figure 25-22 ■). Attach a syringe filled with sterile water or saline to the needle hub of the catheter. Then advance the catheter through the chest wall while maintaining gentle traction on the syringe plunger. Ensure you enter the thoracic cavity by passing the needle just over the rib. The intercostal artery, vein, and nerve pass just under each rib and may be injured if the needle's track is too high. As you enter the pleural space, you will feel a pop and note bubbling air through the fluid in the syringe. Advance the catheter into the chest and then withdraw the needle and syringe.

If the patient remains symptomatic, place a second or third catheter to more rapidly facilitate decompression. Secure the catheter in place with tape, being careful not to block the port or kink the catheter. Leaving the catheter open to air converts the tension pneumothorax into a simple pneumothorax and stabilizes the patient. You may create a flutter valve by cutting the finger off a latex glove, making a small perforation in its tip, and securing it to the catheter hub, or use a commercially available Heimlich valve. Monitor the patient's respirations and breath sounds for a recurring tension pneumothorax. If signs and symptoms again appear, decompress the chest again. Frequently, the initial catheter will clog or kink and necessitate replacement by another.

Rapidly transport the patient to the trauma center for definitive treatment (usually with a chest tube). Be cautious in using IV crystalloid infusion if the patient is hemodynamically stable. An underlying pulmonary contusion may lead to edema, which is made worse with overaggressive fluid therapy. If your patient remains hypotensive after chest decompression and respirations do not become adequate, consider the possibility of internal hemorrhage and the need for (conservative)

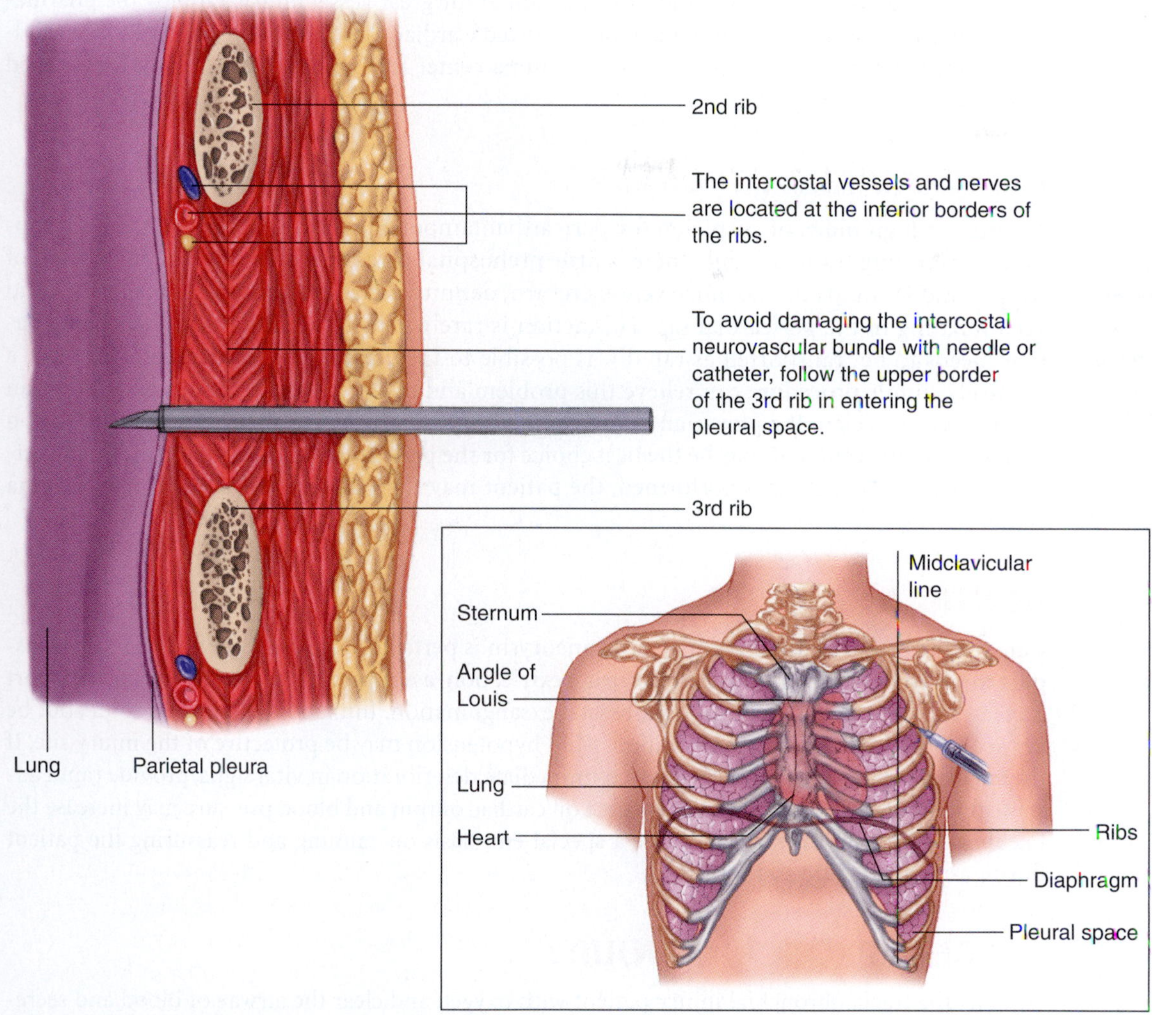

■ **Figure 25-22** Needle decompression of a tension pneumothorax.

fluid resuscitation. If respirations do not dramatically improve, assess for a contralateral tension pneumothorax or pericardial tamponade as the cause.

HEMOTHORAX

Treat the patient with suspected hemothorax with oxygen administration and ventilatory support, as needed. Initiate two large-bore intravenous catheters, readied to infuse large volumes of fluid. Be conservative in fluid administration. Maintain a blood pressure of 80 mmHg, but do not attempt to return it to preinjury levels. Carefully listen to breath sounds during any infusion because the increasing vascular volume may increase the edema and congestion of pulmonary contusion. It may also increase the pressure, rate, and volume of internal hemorrhage. If the pulmonary contusion is extensive and the patient cannot be adequately oxygenated by high-flow, high-concentration oxygen, positive-pressure ventilations are indicated and may limit further edema that contributes to the injury.

MYOCARDIAL CONTUSION

In serious frontal impact collisions, suspect myocardial contusion and administer high-flow, high-concentration oxygen. Monitor cardiac electrical activity and watch for tachycardias, bradycardias, ectopic beats, and conduction defects. Establish an IV line in the event that antidysrhythmics (such as amiodarone) are needed, and monitor the patient for great vessel injury. Employ the pharmacological care measures recommended for Advanced Cardiac Life Support (Chapter 28, "Cardiology"). Rapidly transport the patient to the trauma center for further evaluation and continued monitoring.

PERICARDIAL TAMPONADE

Maintain a high index of suspicion for pericardial tamponade in the patient with central thoracic penetrating trauma. While there is little prehospital care other than the administration of oxygen and IV fluids to maximize venous return, definitive care is to remove some of the fluid accumulating in the pericardial sac. This action is rarely permitted in the field; hence, the patient needs to be transported as rapidly as possible to the emergency department. Note that a relatively simple procedure can relieve this problem and can be adequately administered by an emergency physician. If a physician-staffed emergency department is significantly closer to you than the trauma center, it may be the best choice for the patient with pericardial tamponade. After the pericardiocentesis is performed, the patient may then be directed to the closest trauma center.

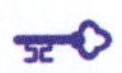

If pericardial tamponade is suspected, consider diverting to the closest hospital with a physician-staffed emergency department where emergency pericardiocentesis can be performed.

AORTIC ANEURYSM

Care for the patient with dissecting aortic aneurysm is performed through gentle but rapid transport to the trauma center. Any jarring during extrication, assessment, care, packaging, or transport increases the risk of rupture and rapidly fatal exsanguination. Initiate IV therapy en route, but be very conservative in fluid administration. Mild hypotension may be protective of the injury site. If the aneurysm ruptures, as indicated by an immediate deterioration in vital signs, provide rapid administration of fluids. Anxiety and its effect on cardiac output and blood pressure may increase the likelihood of aneurysm rupture. Place a special emphasis on calming and reassuring the patient during very gentle care and transport.

TRACHEOBRONCHIAL INJURY

Support the tracheobronchial injury patient with oxygen and clear the airway of blood and secretions. If you are unable to maintain a patent airway or adequately oxygenate the patient, then intubate the trachea and provide positive-pressure ventilations. Observe the patient carefully for the development of a tension pneumothorax, which may result as a complication of positive-pressure ventilations, and treat as previously prescribed. Provide rapid transport as soon as the patient can be extricated and stabilized. This is important because these patients can rapidly destabilize and then require emergency surgical intervention.

TRAUMATIC ASPHYXIA

Administer oxygen and support the airway and respiration of the traumatic asphyxia patient. This may require using positive-pressure ventilations with the bag-valve mask to ensure adequate ventilation during the entrapment and possibly thereafter. Establish two large-bore IV lines for rapid infusion of crystalloid in anticipation of rapidly developing hypovolemia with chest decompression. Once the compressing force is removed, the direct effects of traumatic asphyxia spontaneously resolve; however, serious internal hemorrhage may begin. Prepare to transport immediately after release from entrapment because the patient will likely have severe coexisting injuries.

If the patient remains entrapped for a prolonged time, consider the administration of sodium bicarbonate. Prolonged stagnant blood flow and a hypoxic cellular environment may cause accumulation of metabolic acids. As the compression is released, this blood returns to the central circulation, much as it does with entrapped limbs during crush injury. Consider the administration of 1 mEq/kg of sodium bicarbonate just before or during decompression of the chest if entrapment has lasted more than 20 minutes. Employ this therapy as discussed in Chapter 20, "Soft-Tissue Trauma."

Summary

Thoracic trauma by either blunt or penetrating mechanisms has a great potential for posing a threat to a patient's life. In fact, 25 percent of all traumatic deaths are secondary to injuries in this region. In assessing these patients, the mechanism of injury, when considered along with the clinical findings, may help in differentiating among the many possible injuries. The assessment, in turn, helps guide your interventions and determines the need for rapid extrication and transport. Aggressive airway management, oxygenation, ventilation, and fluid resuscitation, when indicated, can mean the difference between the patient's survival or death. Specific interventions, such as pleural decompression or stabilization of a flail segment, can also affect mortality and morbidity from chest trauma. Understanding the pathological processes affecting the chest during trauma and employing proper assessment and care measures will ensure the best possible outcome for your patients.

Review Questions

1. The structures of the trachea and the bronchi, together, are called the:
   a. lungs.
   b. pulmonary system.
   c. mediastinum.
   d. tracheobronchial tree.
2. During a football game, a 17-year-old male is tackled and knocked to the ground. Although he reports hearing a "bone crack," he initially appears to be stable. The team manager summons the paramedics. By the time they arrive, the patient states that he is "feeling funny" and having difficulty breathing. Upon primary assessment, a rapid, weak pulse and a low BP are noted. The patient's appearance suggests that he may be developing shock. You suspect a fractured rib and possibly:
   a. traumatic asphyxia.
   b. pericardial tamponade.
   c. tension pneumothorax.
   d. traumatic aortic rupture.
3. Which of the following signs/symptoms is most commonly seen in association with a severe chest wall contusion?
   a. retractions
   b. hypoventilation
   c. deep, gasping respirations
   d. use of accessory muscles
4. You have elected to apply an occlusive dressing to your patient who has sustained a stab wound to the chest. You realize that you should secure the dressing:
   a. on two sides.
   b. on four sides.
   c. on three sides.
   d. loosely over the wound.
5. Your patient has received significant deceleration trauma to his chest. He presents with absent radial and brachial pulses in the left upper extremity and severe hypotension. He reported that he felt a tearing sensation in his chest before quickly losing consciousness. He most likely has experienced a:
   a. severe rib fracture.
   b. pericardial tamponade.
   c. pulmonary contusion.
   d. traumatic aortic aneurysm.

6. The type of crash impact most commonly associated with aortic rupture when the patient has been involved in a motor vehicle collision is:
   a. lateral.
   b. frontal.
   c. rollover.
   d. rotational.
7. The following mechanism of injury most likely to cause traumatic asphyxia is:
   a. blunt trauma, low impact.
   b. penetrating trauma, low velocity.
   c. penetrating trauma, high velocity.
   d. blunt trauma, compressive force.
8. You and your partner are called to the scene of a motor vehicle collision. When you arrive, you note that a car has struck a parked vehicle. Your 30-year-old female patient complains of difficulty breathing and you note that breath sounds are diminished bilaterally. The patient states that, at the last minute, she anticipated the impending accident and held her breath. You suspect "paper-bag syndrome" in which the sudden pressure exerted on her expanded lungs, with closed glottis preventing the escape of air, caused the rupture of:
   a. alveoli.
   b. arteries.
   c. the spleen.
   d. the diaphragm.
9. The most appropriate prehospital management for a patient with a flail segment and no other suspected underlying injury is:
   a. chest tube insertion.
   b. positive-pressure ventilation.
   c. needle decompression.
   d. sandbag placed on the injured side.
10. The most appropriate prehospital management for a patient with a traumatic rupture of the aorta is to:
   a. initiate two large-bore IVs prior to transport.
   b. delay transport to complete application of the PASG garment.
   c. begin a rapid IV drip of plasma expanders bilaterally, prior to transport.
   d. expedite transport to a trauma center; administer conservative IV fluids en route.

See Answers to Review Questions at the back of this book.

Chapter 26

Abdominal Trauma

Objectives

After reading this chapter, you should be able to:

1. Describe the epidemiology, including morbidity/mortality, for patients with abdominal trauma as well as prevention strategies to avoid the injuries. (p. 1062)
2. Apply the epidemiologic principles to develop prevention strategies for abdominal injuries. (p. 1062)
3. Describe the anatomy and physiology of the abdominal organs and structures. (see Chapter 3)
4. Predict abdominal injuries based on blunt and penetrating mechanisms of injury. (pp. 1062–1069)
5. Describe open and closed abdominal injuries. (pp. 1062–1065)
6. Identify the need for rapid intervention and transport of the patient with abdominal injuries based on assessment findings. (pp. 1069–1074)
7. Explain the pathophysiology of solid and hollow organ injuries, abdominal vascular injuries, pelvic fractures, and other abdominal injuries. (pp. 1065–1069)
8. Describe the assessment findings associated with and the management of solid and hollow organ injuries, abdominal vascular injuries, pelvic fractures, and other abdominal injuries. (pp. 1069–1077)
9. Differentiate between abdominal injuries based on the assessment and history. (pp. 1069–1075)
10. Given several preprogrammed and moulaged abdominal trauma patients, provide the appropriate scene size-up, primary assessment, secondary assessment (rapid trauma or focused physical exam, detailed exam), and reassessments and provide appropriate patient care and transportation. (pp. 1062–1077)

Key Terms

abruptio placentae, p. 1069
evisceration, p. 1064
guarding, p. 1067
hematemesis, p. 1065
hematochezia, p. 1065
hematuria, p. 1065
peritonitis, p. 1067
rebound tenderness, p. 1067

INTRODUCTION

Injury to the abdomen does not always present as dramatically as it does elsewhere in the body and often occurs without overt signs.

The abdominal cavity is one of the body's largest cavities and contains many organs essential to life. Serious direct or secondary injury may damage these vital organs. In addition, large volumes of blood can be lost in the cavity before the loss becomes evident. In the abdomen, however, injury does not always present as dramatically as it does elsewhere in the body. Injury often occurs without overt signs because few skeletal structures protect the abdomen. The signs of transmitted injury—deformity, swelling, and the discoloration of contusions—take time to develop and are not often seen in the prehospital setting. These considerations make the anticipation of possible abdominal injuries and careful abdominal assessment critical for the patient with trauma to this region.

Over the past decade, the relative mortality and morbidity for the various abdominal injuries has declined due to improved surgical and critical care techniques. Reduced injury-to-surgery times have also contributed to this decline as EMS systems have recognized the necessity of rapid surgical intervention. The severity of injuries and the number of deaths associated with blunt trauma have also decreased thanks to improvements in highway design and vehicle structure and to a greater use of seat belts and other safety practices. However, the overall mortality and morbidity from penetrating trauma is on the rise due to the increasing violence in our society, most specifically in the growing use and power of hand guns. Penetrating trauma is approaching trauma associated with auto collisions as the number-one trauma killer. Nowhere is this more apparent than with injuries to the abdomen.

Prevention of abdominal injuries, as with most other types of trauma, is the best way to reduce mortality and morbidity. As noted, highway and vehicle design improvements and the following of safety practices at home and in the workplace play important roles in reducing both the incidence and seriousness of abdominal injury.

There remains room for further improvements in safety practices, however. For example, many people still do not use seat belts. Failure to use the seat belt increases the incidence of abdominal injury secondary to impact with the steering wheel, dash, or other parts of the auto's interior and of impact after ejection. (Side-impact air bags have the potential to reduce the incidence of pelvic fracture and internal abdominal injuries frequently associated with this mechanism of injury.)

One area of special concern is the proper application of the auto lap belt. If the belt rides too high on the abdomen, with deceleration the belt directs forces both to the contents of the abdominal cavity and to the lumbar spine. Severe compression may result in serious associated abdominal injury. Proper placement, in which the belt rests on the iliac crests, transmits the forces of severe deceleration to the pelvis and the body's skeletal structure, thus sparing the abdominal contents and the spine from injury. Proper positioning of seat belts is especially important with children.

Mortality and morbidity associated with penetrating trauma can also be reduced by reducing violence in society and by reducing the availability of hand guns.

PATHOPHYSIOLOGY OF ABDOMINAL INJURY

MECHANISM OF INJURY

Because the abdomen is bound by muscles rather than skeletal structures, there is a freer transmission of the energy of trauma to the internal organs and structures.

Unlike the other major body containers (skull, spine, and thorax), the abdomen is bound by muscles rather than skeletal structures. This results in a freer transmission of the energy of trauma to the internal organs and structures. Concurrently, the overt physical signs of this energy transmission are limited.

Penetrating Trauma

Penetrating trauma imparts its energy directly to the tissues touched by the offending object (Figure 26-1 ■) or, as with high-velocity projectiles (from hand guns, shotguns, and rifles), transmits energy and injury some distance from the projectile pathway. The bullet injury process causes damage as the projectile contacts tissue, sets that tissue and surrounding tissue in motion, then compresses and stretches surrounding tissue. The projectile adds to the damage as it draws debris

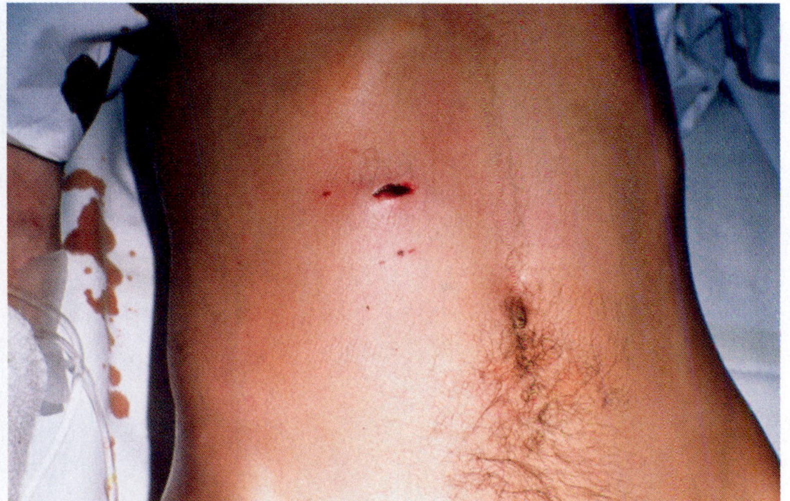

■ Figure 26-1 Stab wound to the right upper quadrant.

and contaminants into the wound, causing wound infection and poor healing. The disruption of tissue from penetrating trauma may permit uncontrolled hemorrhage, organ damage, the spillage of hollow organ contents, and, eventually, irritation of the abdominal lining, the peritoneum. Gunshot wounds to the abdomen, especially those from rifles, high-powered hand guns, and shotguns at close range, impart tremendous energy to the tissue and organs of the region and tend to cause a mortality and morbidity about 10 times greater than that associated with the lower velocity stab wounds. When penetrating trauma induces injury, it affects the liver 40 percent of the time, the small bowel about 25 percent of the time, and the large bowel about 10 percent of the time. Injuries to the spleen, kidneys, and pancreas follow in decreasing order of incidence.

Penetrating trauma most frequently involves the liver and small bowel.

A special type of penetrating trauma is induced by a blast from a shotgun. The shotgun delivers numerous round pellets (called shot) through the hollow gun barrel. The aerodynamics of the shot and the rapid expansion of their distribution (the pattern) cause the energy of impact to decrease rapidly the farther the projectiles move from the barrel. Generally, shotgun blasts at short range (under 3 yards) are extremely lethal. Between 3 and 7 yards, the penetration of the projectiles is great but often survivable. At distances greater than 7 yards, the depth of penetration and subsequent injury fall off quickly. These parameters change somewhat with the decreasing gauge size (gun barrel diameter) and the size of the projectiles. (See Chapter 18, "Penetrating Trauma.")

Blunt Trauma

Blunt trauma to the abdomen produces the least visible signs of injury and causes trauma through three mechanisms: deceleration, compression, and shear (Figure 26-2 ■). As the exterior of the abdomen decelerates (or accelerates) during impact, its contents slam into one another in a chain reaction. They are first injured by the force changing their velocity, then by the forces of compression, as they are trapped between the impacting energy and the more posterior organs. The entire contents of the cavity may be compressed between the force impacting the anterior abdominal cavity and the spinal column. Shear forces induce damage when one part of an organ is free to move while another part is restricted by the forces of trauma or by ligamentous or vascular attachments. Blunt trauma is responsible for about 40 percent of the incidences of splenic injury and a little more than 20 percent of hepatic (liver) injury. The bowel and kidneys are the next most frequently injured abdominal structures in blunt trauma.

Blunt trauma most frequently involves the spleen and liver.

Blast injuries to the abdomen involve both blunt and penetrating mechanisms. Shrapnel and debris propelled by the blast act as projectiles and create penetrating trauma. However, because of the irregular shapes of the objects and their poor aerodynamic properties, they tend to produce serious injury only in close proximity to the blast's center. The pressure wave generated by the explosion causes blunt trauma as it dramatically compresses and relaxes air-filled organs and is likely to contuse organs or rupture them. Since the stomach and bowel are only occasionally distended with

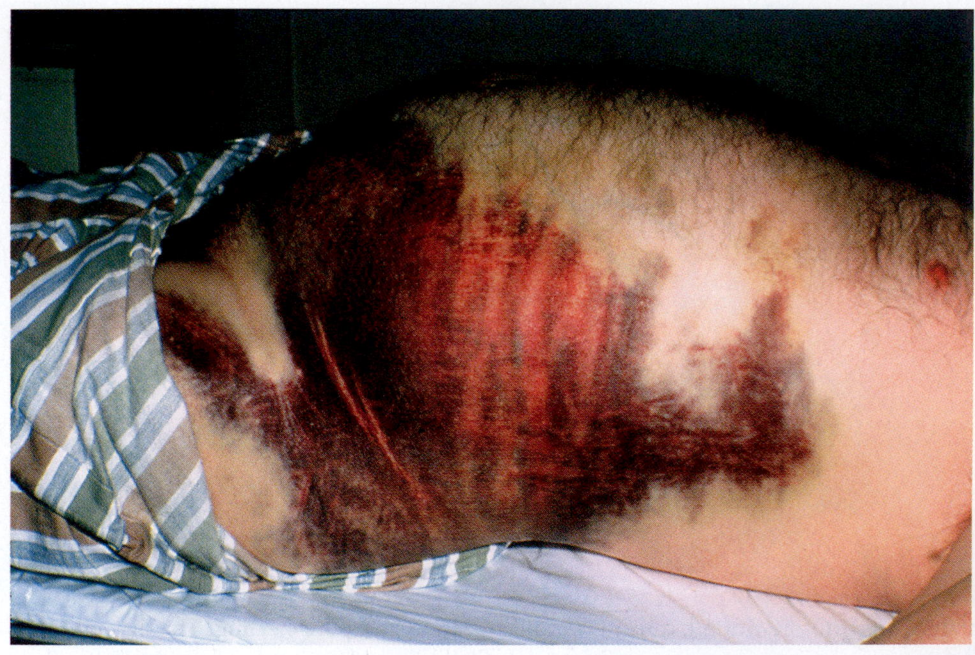

■ **Figure 26-2** Blunt trauma to the left lower quadrant.

air, they are neither as frequently nor as seriously injured as the lungs by the blast pressure wave. Abdominal injury is a secondary concern with blast injury patients.

Careful evaluation of the mechanism of injury, including identification of the force and direction of impact as it relates to the abdomen, is important for anticipating injuries within the region. Pay special attention to the potential for seat belt injury or direct injury as the abdomen impacts the steering wheel in a vehicle crash, impacts with objects or the ground during a fall, or is struck during an assault. Remember that the early presentation of a contusion will likely be a simple reddening (erythema) of the affected area. Hence, it is critically important to carefully analyze the mechanism of injury, identify a high index of suspicion for intra-abdominal injury, and investigate the abdomen for signs and symptoms of injury. The abdominal wall, hollow organs, solid organs, vascular structures, mesentery, and peritoneum all respond differently to trauma.

INJURY TO THE ABDOMINAL WALL

Any injury to the contents of the abdomen must disrupt or be transmitted through the abdominal wall. Since the skin and muscular lining of the abdomen are more resistant to injury than many of the internal organs, they are likely to be uninjured or minimally injured by blunt trauma forces that cause serious injury within. Even when injured, the skin and underlying muscle may only show erythema during the first hour or so. The more visible discoloration of ecchymosis and noticeable swelling require several hours to develop. Penetrating wounds may also be difficult to assess properly because the musculature and skin tension close the wound opening. Bullet and knife wounds look especially small and may appear much less lethal than they are.

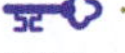

With trauma to the abdomen, the discoloration of ecchymosis and noticeable swelling require several hours to develop.

evisceration *a protrusion of organs from a wound.*

Penetrating abdominal injury may permit abdominal contents to protrude through the opening. This type of injury, called an **evisceration,** occurs most frequently through the anterior abdominal wall and is usually associated with a large and deep laceration. The omentum and/or small bowel are most likely to protrude. The evisceration endangers the protruding bowel because of compromised circulation and the drying of this delicate intra-abdominal tissue. However, replacing the protrusion risks introducing bacteria into the peritoneal space. If the bowel is torn, there is the additional danger of its contents leaking into the peritoneal space if it is replaced.

Penetrating trauma to the thorax, buttocks, flanks, and back may also enter the abdomen and injure its contents. The abdominal organs extend well into the thorax and move up to the nipple line, anteriorly, and to the tips of the scapulae, posteriorly, during deep expiration. Injury to the lower portion of the chest may lacerate the diaphragm and injure the stomach, liver, spleen, or gallbladder. The flank, back, and buttock muscles are thick and resist penetrating trauma very well. However, deep wounds in these locations can penetrate into the abdominal cavity and cause injury to adjacent organs. High-powered projectiles, especially those from hunting or military rifles, may have enough energy to deflect when striking bone and enter the abdomen from as far away as a proximal extremity wound.

Tears in the diaphragm may also disrupt the abdominal container. These tears may occur when the patient holds his breath just before an impact or with penetrating injury to the lower thorax or upper abdomen. Not only may such an injury compromise the important role of the diaphragm in respiration, but it may also permit or force abdominal contents (like those of the stomach, liver, or a portion of the small bowel) to enter the thoracic cavity. This reduces the volume of the thoracic cage available during respiration and compromises the blood supply to the herniated organs. Diaphragmatic injury most frequently occurs from stab injuries on the left side because this is where right-handed assailants strike. Gunshot wounds affect both sides equally. Small tears are unlikely to permit abdominal contents to enter the thorax, and are not likely to greatly affect respiration. Large tears are more likely to do both.

INJURY TO THE HOLLOW ORGANS

Hollow organs like the stomach, small bowel, large bowel, rectum, urinary bladder, gallbladder, and pregnant uterus may rupture with compression from blunt forces, especially if the organ is full and distended. They may also tear as penetrating objects disrupt their structure. (The small bowel is the most frequently injured hollow abdominal organ during penetrating trauma because it rests anteriorly and just beneath the thin anterior abdominal muscles and omentum.) Damage to the hollow organs results in hemorrhage and in the spillage of their contents into the retroperitoneal, peritoneal, or pelvic spaces. The jejunum, ileum, colon, and rectum contain progressively higher bacterial concentrations, and their rupture and the subsequent leakage of material into the abdomen will likely induce severe but delayed infection (called sepsis). The other hollow organs are more likely to release contents that cause a chemical irritation of the abdominal lining. The urinary bladder will release urine; the gallbladder, bile; and the stomach and duodenum, chyme, which is acidic and rich in digestive enzymes. Injury to the hollow organs may result in frank blood in the stool (**hematochezia**), blood in emesis (**hematemesis**), and blood in the urine (**hematuria**).

hematochezia *blood in the stool.*

hematemesis *the vomiting of blood.*

hematuria *blood in the urine.*

INJURY TO THE SOLID ORGANS

Solid organs such as the spleen, liver, pancreas, and kidneys are also subject to blunt and penetrating trauma. These organs are especially dense and are not held together as strongly as the more muscular hollow organs of the body. They are prone to contuse, resulting in organ damage and minimal bleeding, or to rupture. If the organ's capsule remains intact, it will limit the hemorrhage. However, if the capsule is disrupted by penetrating trauma or torn by the mechanism of blunt trauma, unrestricted hemorrhage may result.

The spleen is especially well protected by the lower ribs, the back and flank muscles, and the spinal column. It is not, however, protected by a strong peritoneal capsule and is very fragile in nature. It may be injured with severe abdominal compression, blunt left flank trauma, or penetrating injury to the region (Figure 26-3 ■). The spleen then bleeds profusely, frequently resulting in shock and a life threat to the patient. The blood loss may accumulate against the diaphragm (especially in the supine patient) and result in referred pain to the left shoulder region.

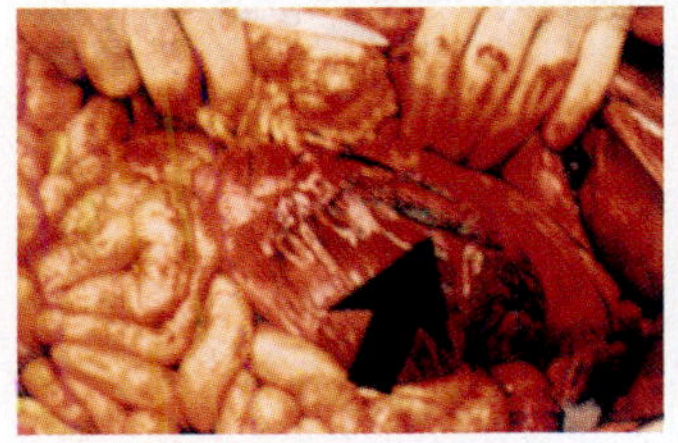

■ **Figure 26-3** Penetrating trauma to the spleen.

The pancreas is central to the upper abdomen, somewhat less delicate than the spleen, and well protected from blunt trauma by its location deep in the central abdominal cavity. Penetrating trauma may lacerate its structure and permit blood and digestive enzymes to flow into the abdominal cavity. These digestive juices may actually begin to digest pancreatic and surrounding tissues, leading to severe internal injury. Pancreatic injury does sometimes result from severe blunt trauma to the upper abdomen that compresses the pancreas between the trauma force and the vertebral column. This may occur when a patient impacts a steering wheel or the handlebars of a motorcycle during a crash. Such a patient frequently complains of upper abdominal pain that may radiate to the back.

The kidneys are equally well protected by their location deep in the abdominal cavity. They are somewhat more resistant to injury than the pancreas, have a more substantial serous capsule, and

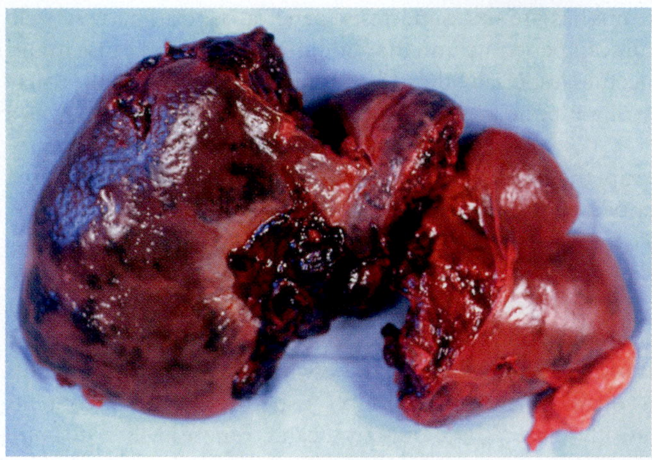

■ **Figure 26-4** Rupture of the liver.

are attached by large renal arteries to the aorta. They are most frequently injured with trauma to the flanks. Renal injury may result in regional (back or flank) pain as well as hematuria.

The liver is the largest single organ within the abdomen. Being a peritoneal organ, it is surrounded by the strong visceral peritoneum, which resists injury and will hold the organ together if injured. The liver is firmer than both the spleen and pancreas and is somewhat protected by the inferior border of the thorax. When the forces of trauma are directed to this region, however, they are likely to damage the liver, especially if they induce lower rib fracture on the right side (Figure 26-4 ■). The liver is restrained from forward motion by the ligamentum teres. During severe deceleration, the weight of the liver forces it into the ligament, causing shear forces, laceration, and hemorrhage. Liver injury often presents with tenderness along the right lower border of the thoracic cage and, as blood accumulates against the diaphragm, pain in the upper right shoulder.

INJURY TO THE VASCULAR STRUCTURES

Most vascular trauma is associated with penetrating injury.

Arteries and veins within the abdomen are prone to injury with serious consequences. The abdominal aorta and its major tributaries can be injured by direct blunt or penetrating trauma or may be injured as abdominal organs decelerate and pull on their vascular attachments during an auto crash or similar impact. Penetrating trauma does not frequently involve the very large vessels of the abdomen, but when the aorta or other major artery is damaged, internal hemorrhage can be severe. The vena cava and its tributaries can likewise be injured. Most vascular injuries (97 percent) are associated with penetrating trauma. As blood accumulates in the abdomen of a supine patient, it will come to rest against the diaphragm. There it irritates the muscular structure and produces a referred pain in the shoulder region. However, other signs of significant hemorrhage may be limited.

Vascular injury in the peritoneal, retroperitoneal, and pelvic spaces can be serious for several reasons. These spaces are easily expandable, and hemorrhage may continue without the increase in pressure exerted by surrounding tissue that would occur if the vascular injury were within a mass of muscle elsewhere in the body. Without this pressure, both the rate and volume of blood loss do not diminish. These spaces also contain organs that require significant circulation supplied by rather large arterial and venous vessels. The dynamic nature of the abdomen and its anatomical size mean that a greater volume of blood can be accommodated there before its presence becomes noticeable. Further, due to vagal stimulation caused by the presence of blood in the peritoneal cavity, an increasing heart rate (a common sign of internal hemorrhage) may not be present.

INJURY TO THE MESENTERY AND BOWEL

The mesentery provides the bowel with circulation, innervation, and attachment. Blunt injury occurs as the mesentery stretches during impact. This type of injury occurs most frequently at points of relative immobility such as the duodenal/jejunal juncture (where the small bowel is affixed by the ligament of Trietz) or where the small bowel joins the large bowel at the ileocecal junction. Injury involving the mesentery may disrupt blood vessels supplying the bowel and eventually cause ischemia, necrosis, and possible rupture. Mesenteric injuries do not usually bleed profusely because the peritoneal layers contain the hemorrhage. Deceleration or compression may tear or rupture the full bowel. With penetrating trauma, the omentum is frequently disrupted and the bowel may be torn anywhere along its length, though tears to the small bowel (jejunum and ileum) are the most likely because of its central and anterior location. Expect a tear to release bowel contents into the peritoneal space, but remember that signs and symptoms of such release are delayed. The duodenum is less frequently injured because of its location deep within the abdomen. Penetrating trauma to the lateral abdomen is likely to injure the large bowel (ascending colon on the right and descending colon on the left).

Expect a tear of the small bowel to release bowel contents into the peritoneal space, but remember that signs and symptoms of such release are delayed.

INJURY TO THE PERITONEUM

The peritoneum is the very delicate and sensitive lining of the anterior abdominal cavity. Its inflammation, called **peritonitis,** can be caused by two major mechanisms, bacterial and chemical irritation. Bacterial peritonitis is an irritation due to infection, which is often released into the space by a torn bowel or open wound. It takes the bacteria between 12 and 24 hours to grow in sufficient numbers to produce the inflammation and hence the condition is usually not apparent during prehospital care. Chemical peritonitis occurs more rapidly than bacterial peritonitis because the caustic nature of digestive enzymes and acids (from the stomach or duodenum), and, to a lesser degree, urine quickly irritate the peritoneum and induce the inflammatory response. Blood induces limited peritoneal inflammation, and hence serious hemorrhage into the peritoneal cavity will not, by itself, cause this condition.

peritonitis *inflammation of the peritoneum caused by chemical or bacterial irritation.*

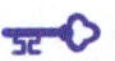

When assessing the abdomen, be aware that local muscle injury caused by trauma may result in local or regional abdominal muscle tenderness and spasm that mimics peritonitis.

Peritonitis is a progressive process that presents with characteristic signs and symptoms. It usually begins with a slight tenderness at the location of injury. Over time, the area of inflammation expands, as does the area of tenderness. Any jarring of the abdomen, as occurs with percussion or when you quickly release the pressure of deep palpation, causes a twinge of pain (**rebound tenderness**). In response to pain induced by any movement of the irritated abdominal tissue, the anterior abdominal muscles contract, even in the unconscious patient. This is called **guarding.** If the pain becomes severe, the abdominal muscles assume an extreme contraction and leave the abdominal wall with a rigid, boardlike feel. When assessing the abdomen, be aware that local muscle injury caused by trauma may result in local or regional abdominal muscle tenderness and spasm that mimics peritonitis. Tenderness or frank pain from the physical injury may coexist with the signs of peritonitis.

rebound tenderness *pain on release of the examiner's hands, allowing the patient's abdominal wall to return to its normal position; associated with peritoneal irritation.*

guarding *protective tensing of the abdominal muscles by a patient suffering abdominal pain; may be a voluntary or involuntary response.*

INJURY TO THE PELVIS

A pelvic fracture represents a serious skeletal injury, serious and often life-threatening hemorrhage, and potential injury to the organs within the pelvic space. These organs—the ureters, bladder, urethra, female genitalia, prostate, rectum, and anus—can all be injured by the severe kinetic forces, the crushing nature of the injury, or by displaced bone fragments. Pelvic fracture can also cause serious injury to the pregnant uterus. Pelvic hemorrhage and fracture have been discussed in Chapter 22, "Musculoskeletal Trauma."

Sexual assault may also injure the reproductive structures located internally in the female and externally in the male. Direct trauma to the external female genitalia or injury caused by objects inserted into the vagina may tear the soft tissues of this region. Since these tissues are both very sensitive and vascular, the injury may bleed heavily and be very painful. The same is true for the male genitalia, though they are more prone to injury because of their more external location.

INJURY DURING PREGNANCY

Trauma is the number one killer of pregnant females. Penetrating abdominal trauma alone accounts for as much as 36 percent of overall maternal mortality. Gunshot wounds to the abdomen of the pregnant female also account for fetal mortality rates of between 40 and 70 percent. In blunt trauma, auto collisions are the leading cause of maternal and fetal mortality and morbidity. Proper

Trauma is the number one killer of pregnant females and penetrating abdominal trauma alone accounts for as much as 36 percent of overall maternal mortality.

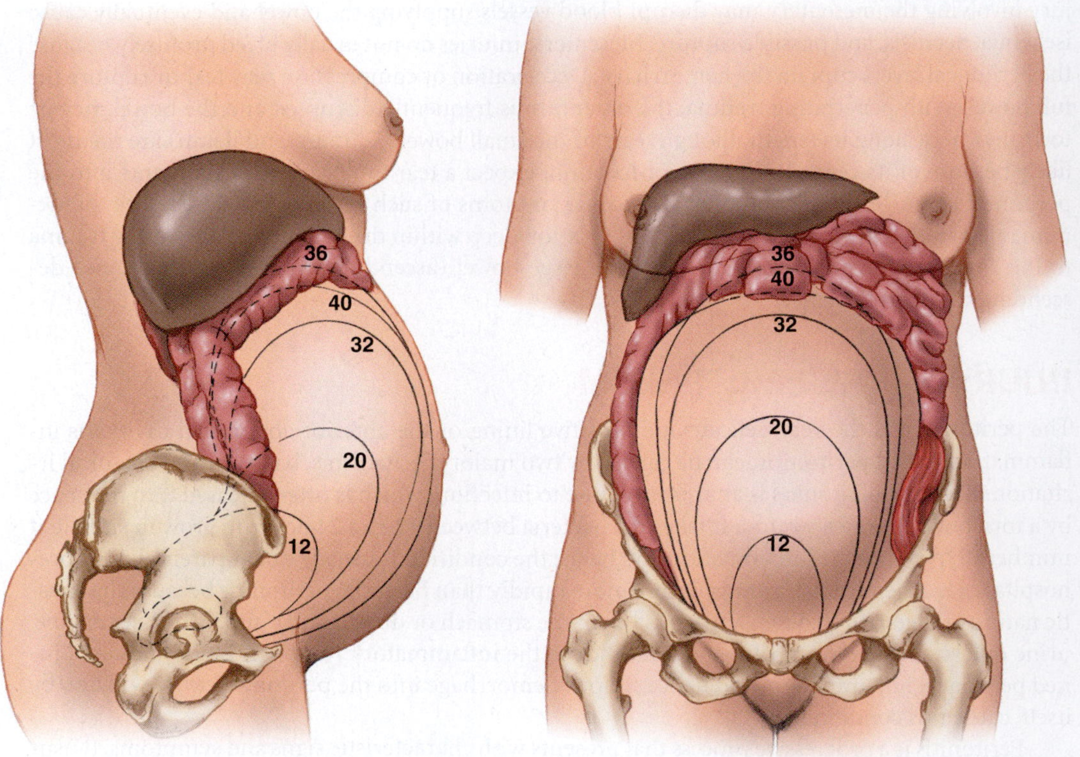

■ **Figure 26-5** Changing dimensions of the pregnant uterus. Numbers represent weeks of gestation.

seat belt placement can significantly reduce injury to the pregnant mother and fetus, while improper placement increases the incidence of both uterine rupture and separation of the placenta from the wall of the uterus. Unrestrained mothers in serious auto collisions are four times more likely to suffer fetal mortality.

The physiological changes associated with pregnancy protect both the mother and her abdominal organs. With the increasing size of the uterus, most of the abdominal organs are displaced higher in the abdomen (Figure 26-5 ■). This generally protects them, unless blunt or penetrating trauma impacts the upper abdomen. If that happens, then the injury may involve numerous organs with increased morbidity and mortality. Direct penetrating injury to the central and lower abdomen of the late pregnancy mother often spares her from serious injury; the resulting injury, however, often damages the uterus and endangers the fetus.

The late-term female is at additional risk of vomiting and possible aspiration. Increasing uterine size increases intra-abdominal pressure, while the hormones of pregnancy relax the cardiac sphincter (the valve that prevents reflux of the stomach contents). The bladder is displaced superiorly early in pregnancy and then becomes more prone to injury and, when injured, bleeds more heavily.

The increasing size and weight of the uterus and its contents have several effects on the mother, especially when trauma strikes. The uterus of a supine patient in late pregnancy may compress the inferior vena cava and reduce the venous return to the heart. This may induce hypotension in the uninjured patient and have severe consequences in the hemorrhaging trauma patient. The increased intra-abdominal pressure along with the compression of the inferior vena cava by the uterus raise venous pressure in the pelvic region and lower extremities. This pressure engorges the vessels and increases the rate of venous hemorrhage from pelvic fracture or lower extremity wounds.

While a pregnant mother is somewhat protected from hypovolemia, the fetus is not so protected.

The increased maternal vascular volume (up by 45 percent) helps protect the mother from hypovolemia. However, this protection does not extend to the fetus because fetal blood flow is affected well before there are changes in the maternal blood pressure or pulse rate. In fact, it may take a maternal blood loss of between 30 and 35 percent before changes in maternal blood pressure or heart rate are evident. Therefore, it becomes very important to ensure early and aggressive resuscitation of the potentially hypotensive pregnant mother.

In the pregnant female, the thick and muscular uterus contains both the developing fetus and amniotic fluid. This container is strong, distributing the forces of trauma uniformly to the fetus and thereby reducing chances for injury. Significant blunt trauma may cause the uterus to rupture or penetrating trauma may perforate or tear it. The dangers of severe maternal hemorrhage and disruption of the blood supply to the fetus present life threats to both. The potential release of amniotic fluid into the abdomen is also of great concern. The risk of uterine and fetal injury increases with the length of gestation and is greatest during the third trimester of pregnancy.

If an open wound to the uterus does occur, there may be added risk to the mother (in addition to hemorrhage) if she is Rh negative and the fetus is Rh positive. (However, this situation does not impact prehospital assessment or care.) Penetrating or severe blunt trauma may permit some fetal/maternal blood mixing and lead to compatibility problems. Frank uterine rupture is a rare complication of trauma, but it does occur with severe blunt impact, pelvic fracture, and—very infrequently—with stab or shotgun wounds.

Blunt trauma to the uterus may cause the placenta to detach from the uterine wall because the placenta is rather inelastic while the uterus is very flexible. This condition, called **abruptio placentae,** presents a life-threatening risk to both mother and fetus because the separation permits both maternal and fetal hemorrhage (Figure 26-6 ■). More frequently than not, this hemorrhage is contained within the uterus and does not extend to the vaginal outlet. Blunt trauma may also cause the premature rupture of the amniotic sac (breaking of the "membranes" or "bag of waters") and may induce an early labor.

abruptio placentae *a condition in which the placenta separates from the uterine wall.*

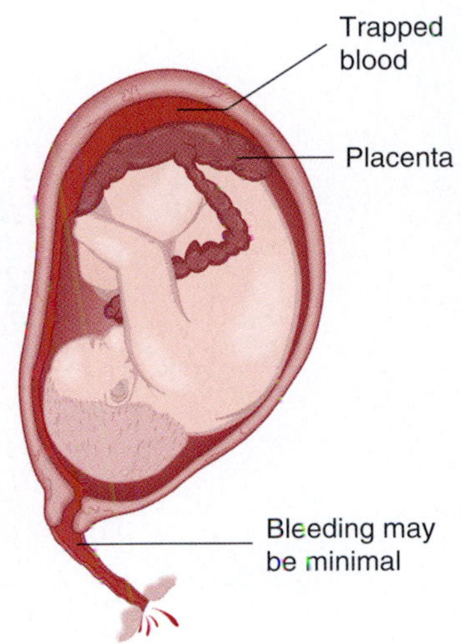

■ Figure 26-6 Abruptio placentae.

INJURY TO PEDIATRIC PATIENTS

Another special patient with regard to abdominal injuries is the child. Children have poorly developed abdominal musculature and a reduced anterior/posterior diameter. The rib cage is more cartilaginous and flexible and more likely to transmit injury to the organs beneath. These factors increase the incidence of pediatric abdominal injury, especially to the liver, spleen, and kidney. Children also compensate very well for blood loss and may not show any signs or symptoms until they have lost over half of their blood volume. This is especially important with abdominal injuries, because a great volume of blood may be lost into the abdomen with little pain or noticeable distention.

ASSESSMENT OF THE ABDOMINAL INJURY PATIENT

Assessment of the patient who has sustained abdominal trauma is somewhat abbreviated because definitive care for such injury is often surgical intervention. Hence, it is imperative that you quickly assess the patient and, if indications of serious abdominal injury exist, you should package and transport him expeditiously. Assessment of the abdominal injury patient is like that for any trauma patient, with pertinent and significant information gained during the scene size-up, primary assessment, rapid secondary assessment (or focused exam and history), and serial reassessments.

SCENE SIZE-UP

Ensure that the scene is safe for you, fellow rescuers, bystanders, and the patient. Be ready to use appropriate Standard Precautions before moving to the patient's side. Also determine the number of expected patients and need for additional EMS, police, fire, and other service personnel.

For the patient who has sustained abdominal injury, the analysis of the mechanism of injury is the most important element of the scene size-up and possibly of the entire assessment. However, forming an index of suspicion for individual abdominal injuries is very difficult because the signs and symptoms are, for the most part, limited and nonspecific. In fact, more than 30 percent of patients with serious abdominal injury may present with no specific signs or symptoms of abdominal injury whatsoever. Additionally, other less life-threatening but more painful injuries may overshadow signs and symptoms of the patient's abdominal injury. Also, those signs and symptoms that are present may become less specific in nature with time and the progressive nature of peritonitis. Last, the patient's reporting of his condition may be unreliable due to the effects of alcohol or drug ingestion, head injury, or shock.

For the patient who has sustained abdominal injury, the analysis of the mechanism of injury is the most important element of the scene size-up and possibly of the entire assessment.

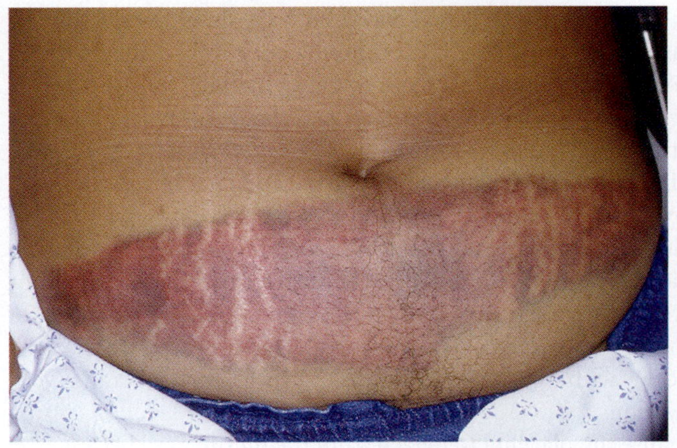

■ **Figure 26-7** Use the mechanism of injury to identify where signs of injury might be found—for example, contusions resulting from compression by a seat belt. *(© Mark C. Ide)*

If the patient has suffered blunt trauma, identify the strength and direction of the forces and where on the body they were delivered. Focus your observation and palpation on that site during the primary and rapid secondary assessments and place your highest suspicion of injury there. Begin to develop a list of possible organs injured (the index of suspicion) and the immediate and delayed effects they will have on the patient's condition. In serious blunt trauma or deep penetrating trauma, expect internal and uncontrolled hemorrhage.

If the patient was involved in an auto crash, identify whether seat belts were used and if they were used properly (Figure 26-7 ■). Remember that improper placement (above the iliac crests) may increase the likelihood of abdominal compression (and lumbar spine) injury. Lack of seat belt use increases the incidence and severity of all types of injuries, including abdominal injury. Examine the vehicle interior for signs of impact like the deformity of a bent steering wheel, a deflated air bag, or a structural intrusion into the passenger compartment. Frontal impact is most likely to compress the abdomen, injuring the liver and spleen and possibly rupturing distended hollow organs like the stomach and bladder. Right-side impact frequently induces liver, ascending colon, and pelvic injury, while left-side impact induces splenic, descending colon, and pelvic injuries. Pedestrians, and especially children, are likely to sustain lower abdominal injury, especially if the vehicle impacts the patient's midsection. It is important to determine the velocity of impact and the distance the patient was thrown. Motorcyclists and, to a lesser degree, bicyclists are likely to sustain abdominal injury as they are propelled forward while the handlebars restrain the pelvis and lower abdomen. In assaults and other isolated impacts, be observant for left flank impact and splenic or renal damage and right-side impact causing renal or hepatic (liver) injury. If the impact involves the superior abdomen, suspect liver, stomach, spleen, and pancreatic injury, while impact to the middle or lower abdomen will likely damage the small bowel, kidneys, and bladder.

With a patient who has experienced penetrating trauma, determine the nature of the offending agent. If it is a knife, arrow, or impaled object, determine the probable angle and depth of insertion (Figure 26-8 ■). Do not move or remove the impaled object.

With gunshot wounds, determine whether the weapon was a hand gun, shotgun, or rifle; the distance from the gun to the victim; and the gun's caliber. Also determine the number of shots fired, if possible, and the angle from which the gun was fired. Be prepared to examine the flanks, the buttocks, and the back for any sign of additional or exit wounds. Attempt to estimate the amount of blood lost at the scene and communicate this, with the other information previously listed, to the emergency department physician.

The internal damage done by a bullet does not correlate well to the appearance of the entrance or exit wound.

Gunshot wounds provide a challenge to assessment. The damage done does not correlate well to the appearance of the entrance or exit wound. It is more related to the bullet's kinetic energy (velocity and mass) as it enters the body and to its energy exchange characteristics as it travels into and through tissue. Low-velocity bullets cause little damage beyond the bullet's actual path. However, these projectiles are easily deflected from their paths by contact with clothing, bone, or, in some cases, soft tissue. They also carry pieces of clothing and other debris into the body and do not tend to pass through the body.

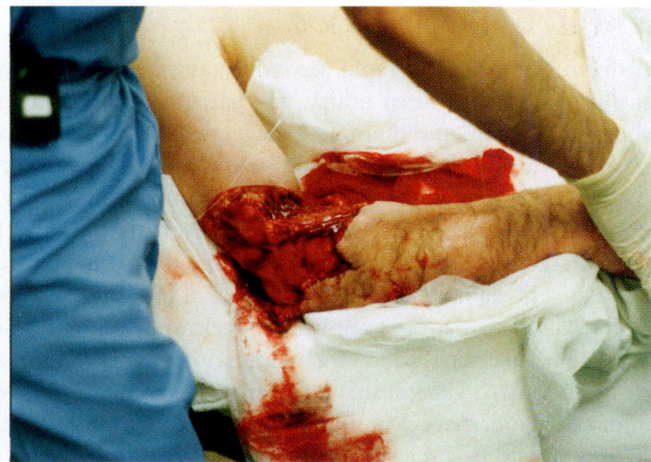

■ **Figure 26-8** Analyze the mechanism of a penetrating trauma in an attempt to determine the probable angle and depth of the wound. (*© Mark C. Ide*)

High-velocity weapons and the wounds they cause were once seen only in the military setting, but now more powerful hand guns are causing similar wounds and internal injuries in the civilian world. Their projectiles cause injury well beyond the bullet's path and injure tissue as the projectile creates a cavity and compresses and stretches neighboring tissue (cavitation). The wounding process also draws debris into the wound, where the damaged and devitalized (without circulation) tissue forms a good medium for bacterial growth. The wounding process may create secondary projectiles as the bullet hits bone, breaks it apart, and then drives the fragments into adjacent tissue. The high-velocity bullet may also fragment and transmit its injuring potential to several pathways.

With either significant blunt or any penetrating trauma to the abdomen, suspect serious and continuing internal hemorrhage. Be especially watchful of the patient during your assessment and initiate shock care at the first signs and symptoms of hypoperfusion. These signs and symptoms include diminishing level of consciousness or orientation, increasing anxiety or restlessness, thirst, increasing pulse rate, decreasing pulse pressure, and increasing capillary refill time.

With significant blunt or penetrating trauma, suspect serious and continuing internal hemorrhage.

Information you gather at the scene is invaluable to the attending emergency department physician. That information, however, will be unavailable unless you document it carefully and report it upon your arrival at the hospital. Doing this is essential to assuring that the patient receives the best care in both the prehospital and in-hospital settings.

PRIMARY ASSESSMENT

As you begin the primary assessment, carefully note your patient's level of consciousness and orientation as well as any indication that he may be affected by alcohol, drugs, head injury, or shock. These agents and conditions reduce the reliability of your patient's reporting of the signs and symptoms of abdominal injury. Any decrease in the level of orientation or consciousness should alert you to the need to maintain a higher index of suspicion for abdominal injury and to perform more careful initial and rapid trauma assessments. The patient may also complain of dizziness or lightheadedness when moving from a supine to a seated or standing position. (Do not ask the patient to move: however, he may have moved on his own before your arrival.) Any of these signs and symptoms should lead you to suspect hypovolemia, possibly from an abdominal injury. Use your initial evaluation as a baseline against which to trend any changes in the patient's level of consciousness or orientation.

As you evaluate airway, breathing, and circulation, be observant for any associated signs and symptoms of hypovolemia, especially if they occur early in your care or are out of proportion with the obvious or expected injuries. Note any rapid shallow respirations, diminished pulse pressure, rapid pulse rate, slow capillary refill time, or thirst. Limited chest movement may be due to the pain of peritonitis or blood irritating the diaphragm. Shallow respirations may be due to abdominal contents in the thorax from a ruptured diaphragm. Be prepared to protect the airway because abdominal trauma patients are likely to vomit.

RAPID SECONDARY ASSESSMENT

Perform the usual full rapid secondary assessment, but if you have developed a high index of suspicion for abdominal injury, pay particular attention to that region. Carefully examine the abdomen for evidence of injury as suggested by the mechanism of injury or by signs or symptoms observed during the primary assessment. When you suspect that the patient has received blunt trauma, look carefully over the entire abdominal surface for the slight reddening of erythema or minor abrasions associated with superficial soft-tissue injury. Remember that any trauma must pass through the exterior of the abdomen before it can do damage within.

Quickly examine the anterior surface of the abdomen and then flanks, then carefully and gently log roll the patient to examine the back, looking for any signs of injury, erythema, ecchymosis, contusions, or open wounds, including eviscerations and impaled objects (Figure 26-9 ■). Also look at the abdomen's general shape and any signs of distention. Visualize the inguinal area for signs of injury or hemorrhage. Jeans may contain hemorrhage without any indication of the accumulation so they should be cut away or removed to assess this region when injury is suspected. Remember that the abdominal cavity can contain a very large volume of blood (on the order of 1.5 liters) before it becomes noticeably distended. In obese patients the volume of blood loss may be even greater before distention is visible. Also be aware that the signs and symptoms of hemoperitoneum or retroperitoneal hemorrhage are minimal.

The abdomen may contain up to 1.5 liters of blood before distention becomes noticeable.

Visualize and palpate the pelvis for signs of injury or instability. Apply gentle pressure directed posteriorly, then medially, on the iliac crests, then place pressure downward on the symphysis pubis. If you note any crepitus or instability, suspect pelvic fracture and both injury to the organs of the lower abdomen and severe internal hemorrhage. If you already suspect pelvic injury, do not test or apply any pressure and be very careful during movement to the ambulance and transport to the hospital. Any manipulation of the fracture site may restart or increase hemorrhage.

Question the patient about pain or discomfort in each quadrant, then palpate the quadrants individually, leaving any quadrant with anticipated injury or patient complaint of pain to last. If you palpate an injured quadrant first, the pain may lead the patient to guard during any remaining palpation. Feel for any spasm or guarding as you palpate, then note any patient report of pain when you quickly release the pressure of your palpation (rebound tenderness). If you palpate an abdomen that is board hard, expect injury to the pancreas, duodenum, or stomach, especially if the time since the injury has been short.

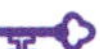

Abnormal pulsations in the abdomen suggest arterial injury.

Auscultation for bowel sounds is not recommended during assessment of the abdominal trauma patient.

Also note any unusual pulsations in the abdomen. You may visualize some pulsing in the thin, young, healthy, athletic patient, but most patients will not have any visible or palpable pulses in the abdomen. Abnormal pulsation suggests arterial injury. Injuries to the thorax or pelvis also suggest abdominal injury, especially if there are lower rib fractures or the pelvic ring is unstable. Auscultation is not recommended during assessment of the abdominal trauma patient. It takes a great deal of time to adequately listen for bowel sounds, and their presence or absence neither confirm nor rule out possible injury.

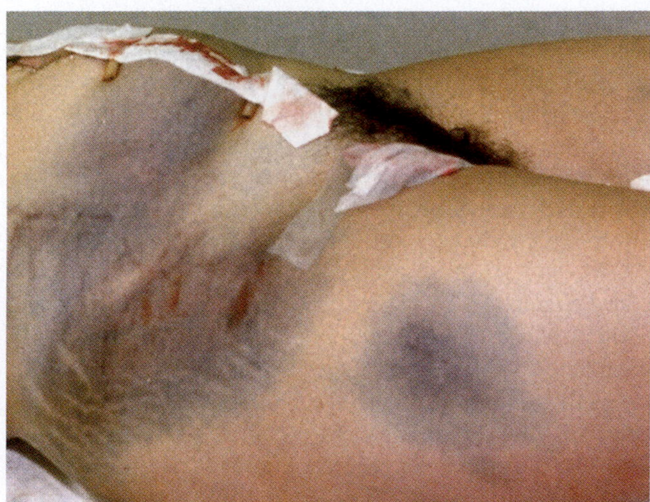

■ **Figure 26-9** Examine the abdomen for signs of injury.

When evaluating the patient with penetrating trauma to the abdomen, look carefully at the entrance wound, and note its appearance, size, and depth. Point-blank discharge of a gun against tissue will introduce the barrel exhaust into the wound created by the bullet. You may notice powder debris and the crackling of subcutaneous emphysema. Look for contamination and any signs of serious blood loss. Then examine the patient for an exit wound. Exit wounds may look more "blown out" in nature and are generally larger and more serious in appearance than entrance wounds. Count the number of entry and exit wounds and note whether they are paired or if an inequality suggests that some projectiles did not exit. The wounds from a projectile may be very small and difficult to see, while still carrying the potential to cause lethal injury. (It is not advisable to note entrance and exit wounds on the patient care report, as it is often difficult to distinguish between the two and there are legal ramifications to mis-identifying wounds.) Anticipate the injuries that occurred as the object or bullet sped into and through the body, but remember that it is not uncommon for a bullet to alter its path. Be suspicious of any projectile wound in the proximal extremities because the projectile may travel along the limb and into the body's interior. Also keep in mind that a bullet wound to the thorax may then deflect and penetrate the abdomen, or vice versa.

Do not identify entrance and exit wounds in your written reports, as they may confound the crime investigation.

While performing the rapid secondary assessment, carefully question the patient about the characteristics of any pain he feels and ask specifically about any abdominal sensations or other symptoms. Serious injury may result while the patient feels limited pain or injury sensation, especially when other more painful injuries elsewhere might be distracting them. The evaluation of abdominal pain from the patient's complaint may, however, be subjective as patients often vary in their response to pain. In the male, retroperitoneal pain may be referred to the testicular region. Thirst may be one of the few symptoms of abdominal injury as significant hemorrhage draws down the body's blood volume. Be sure to record any symptoms in the patient's own words and ensure that these comments and your findings are documented on the prehospital care report and reported to the attending physician.

When investigating the rest of the patient history, give special consideration to the last oral intake. The bladder, bowel, and stomach are much more likely to rupture if full and distended. Ask about when the patient last ate or drank and how much he consumed. Relate the intake to the type of impact received, especially blunt trauma to the trunk. Conclude the rapid secondary assessment by gathering a set of baseline vital signs.

At the end of the rapid secondary assessment, reevaluate the patient's priority for transport. The potential for an abdominal injury must factor into this determination. Remember that serious internal hemorrhage from blunt or penetrating trauma frequently occurs with few overt signs and symptoms. Any patient with a history of significant blunt or any penetrating trauma to the torso is a candidate for rapid transport to the trauma center. Always err on the side of providing more patient care and early transport rather than underestimating the seriousness of trauma to the abdomen.

Any patient with a history of significant blunt or any penetrating trauma to the torso is a candidate for rapid transport to the trauma center.

Special Assessment Considerations with Pregnant Patients

If the patient you are treating is pregnant, pay special attention to the abdomen and the possibility of injury. Remember that the maternal blood volume is increased by up to 45 percent in the third trimester and blood loss can exceed 30 percent before the normal signs and symptoms of hypovolemia reveal themselves. Watch for the earliest signs of shock. Ensure that the uterus does not compress the vena cava by placing the noticeably pregnant mother in the left lateral recumbent position. If spinal injury is also suspected, immobilize her firmly to the spine board and, when placed on the stretcher, rotate her onto her left side. Carefully evaluate the maternal vital signs and remember that the fetus is likely to experience distress before the mother shows any signs of hypotension or hypoperfusion.

Place the late pregnancy patient on her left side to prevent compression of the inferior vena cava.

Trauma to the abdomen in late pregnancy may cause several specific uterine injuries and requires careful assessment. The normal uterus will be firm and round to palpation. It will be palpable above the iliac crests after the first 12 weeks of pregnancy and progress upward in the abdominal cavity until it reaches the costal border at about 32 weeks. Your palpation may result in tenderness and muscular contractions of the uterus, which are normal secondary to uterine contusions. These contractions will often be self-limiting; however, any tenderness, pain, or contractions should raise your suspicions of abruptio placentae. The mother may complain of cramping, generally related to palpable uterine contractions and, in some cases, experience vaginal hemorrhage. Abruptio placentae represents a serious risk to the fetus and mother and is a true emergency requiring rapid transport.

Palpation of the uterus that reveals an asymmetrical uterus or permits you to recognize the irregular features of the fetus suggests uterine rupture. This condition may also present with uterine contractions, but the fundus of the uterus is not palpable and the mass does not harden with the contractions.

If uterine rupture or abruptio placentae are suspected or if you suspect any serious injury to the abdomen of the pregnant patient, ask for the mother's Rh status and report it to the emergency department. Alert the emergency department well before your arrival if you are transporting a pregnant mother who was injured by trauma. This allows department personnel to prepare for the special monitoring necessary for both the mother and fetus.

REASSESSMENT

The reassessment is an essential part of the continuing care process for the patient with possible abdominal injury. During it, you will look for the signs of progressing abdominal injury or continuing hemorrhage. Perform it every 5 minutes in patients with any significant suggestion of abdominal injury. Often the progressive nature of peritonitis leads to greater and greater patient complaints or may make abdominal signs and symptoms more evident as you care for and reduce the pain of other injuries. The signs of ongoing hemorrhage are equally progressive and may not clearly present until well into your patient care.

Pay close attention to the signs of hidden hemorrhage during ongoing assessments of the patient with potential abdominal injury. Watch the blood pressure, pulse rate, capillary refill time, and the patient's appearance and level of consciousness and orientation. A decrease in the difference between the systolic and diastolic blood pressures (the pulse pressure) suggests the body is compensating for shock. An increasing pulse rate (especially if the strength of the pulse is diminishing) and an increasing capillary refill time both suggest hypovolemic compensation. Also observe for the skin becoming cool, clammy, cyanotic, or ashen, and watch for pulse oximetry readings that become more erratic. A change in either the level of consciousness or, more subtly, a lowering of the patient's orientation suggests the brain is being hypoperfused. These findings all indicate the body is employing increasing levels of shock compensation. If you cannot account for a continuing blood loss elsewhere, suspect internal and continuing abdominal hemorrhage. Subtle changes may be the only apparent signs of gradually worsening shock.

Another sign of continuing blood loss from an abdominal hemorrhage is aggressive fluid resuscitation that appears ineffective.

Another sign of continuing blood loss from an abdominal hemorrhage is aggressive fluid resuscitation that appears ineffective. Note your patient's response to fluid resuscitation. If his vital signs do not improve and all external hemorrhage is controlled, suspect continuing internal hemorrhage.

MANAGEMENT OF THE ABDOMINAL INJURY PATIENT

Content Review

Management of the Abdominal Injury Patient

- Position the patient properly.
- Ensure oxygenation and ventilation.
- Control external bleeding.
- Be prepared for aggressive fluid resuscitation.

Management of the patient with abdominal injuries is supportive, with the major emphasis on bringing the patient to surgery as quickly as possible. Prehospital care centers on rapid packaging and transport and fluid resuscitation, as needed. Specific care steps for the abdominal injury patient include proper positioning, general shock care, fluid resuscitation, and care for specific injuries (open wounds and eviscerations).

The patient with minor or severe abdominal pain should be positioned for comfort (unless the positioning is contraindicated by suspicion of spinal injury). Flex the patient's knees to relax the abdominal muscles. If the injuries permit, place the patient in the left lateral recumbent position to maintain knee flexure and the relaxed state of the abdominal muscles, and facilitate the clearing of emesis from the airway.

Ensure good ventilation and consider early administration of high-flow, high-concentration oxygen for the abdominal injury patient. The pain associated with peritonitis or diaphragmatic irritation may reduce respiratory excursion, adding to the potential for early shock development in these patients.

Control any moderate or serious external hemorrhage with direct pressure and bandaging. Minor bleeding may be controlled during transport if at all.

When a serious mechanism of injury is found and the patient does not present with the signs and symptoms of shock, act in anticipation of it. Be prepared to administer repeated fluid boluses if any signs of shock develop and the systolic blood pressure drops below 80 mmHg. Monitor the pulse rate and blood pressure. If the pulse does not slow and the pulse pressure does not rise, consider administering additional fluid boluses. Use this access if the patient's blood pressure begins to drop below 80 mmHg. Do not delay transport to initiate any IV access. Start the IV access en route to the hospital if necessary. Prehospital infusion is usually limited to 3,000 mL of fluid. Titrate your administration rate to maintain a systolic blood pressure of 80 mmHg and ensure that you do not exceed this volume of fluid during field care and transport.

When a serious mechanism of injury is found and the patient does not present with the signs and symptoms of shock, act in anticipation of it.

As you should with all serious trauma patients, communicate frequently with the abdominal injury patient to reduce anxiety and provide emotional support. Also watch for any changes in the patient's description of the pain or injury's character or intensity. Be wary of patient hypothermia, especially when providing fluid resuscitation. Provide ample blankets, keep the patient compartment of the vehicle warm, take patient complaints of being cold seriously, and warm infusion fluids when possible. Hypothermia is a special consideration with pediatric patients because they have a disproportionately large body surface area to body volume and will rapidly lose heat to the environment.

Cover any exposed abdominal organs with a dressing moistened with sterile saline (Procedure 26–1). Be careful to keep the region clean and do not replace any exposed organs. Cover the wet dressing with a sterile occlusive dressing like clear plastic wrap to keep the site as clean as possible and yet retain the moisture. If the transport is lengthy, check the dressing from time to time and remoisten as necessary.

Another wound that deserves special attention is the impaled object. Do all that you can to keep the object from moving and do not remove it from the victim. Any motion causes further injury, disrupts the clotting mechanisms, and continues the hemorrhage. Removal may withdraw the object from a blood vessel, thereby permitting increased internal and uncontrollable hemorrhage. Pad around the object with bulky trauma dressings and wrap around the trunk with soft, self-adherent roller bandaging to secure it firmly. Apply direct pressure around the object if hemorrhage is anything but minor. If the object is too long to accommodate during transport or it is affixed to an immovable object, attempt to cut it. Use a saw, cutter, or torch, but be very careful to ensure that vibration, jarring, and heat are not transmitted to the patient.

Stabilize impaled objects to prevent further injury and reduce associated hemorrhage.

Carefully observe and care for penetrating wounds that may traverse both the abdominal and thoracic cavities. If the wound is large and may have penetrated the diaphragm or otherwise entered the thoracic cavity, seal the wound with an occlusive dressing taped on three sides to permit the release of the buildup of air pressure that occurs in a tension pneumothorax. Be especially watchful of respiratory excursion and effort.

In some systems, the PASG may be used for the patient with abdominal injury and the early signs of shock. However, it should not be used if there is concurrent penetrating trauma to the chest. The PASG applies circumferential pressure to the abdominal cavity, thereby raising intraabdominal pressure and reducing the rate of intraabdominal hemorrhage. Its use is generally contraindicated (inflate the leg sections only) in females in late pregnancy, abdominal evisceration patients, or patients with impaled objects. If the patient with an evisceration experiences a blood pressure below 50 mmHg, consider inflating the abdominal section of the garment as the risks associated with injury to the exposed bowel are less than those of profound hypotension. Incrementally inflate the PASG to maintain blood pressure and pulse rate, not to return them to preinjury levels.

Inflate the PASG in increments to maintain blood pressure and pulse, not to return them to preinjury levels.

MANAGEMENT OF THE PREGNANT PATIENT

Special care is offered to the pregnant patient because of the anatomical and physiological changes induced by pregnancy. Place the late-term mother, when possible, in the left lateral recumbent position. This assures that the weight of the uterus does not compress the vena cava, reduce blood return to the heart, and cause hypotension. It also facilitates airway care. Administer high-flow, high-concentration oxygen early in your care because the mother's respiratory reserve volume is diminished, because the work necessary for her to move air is greater because of the increased

Procedure 26-1 Eviscertion Care

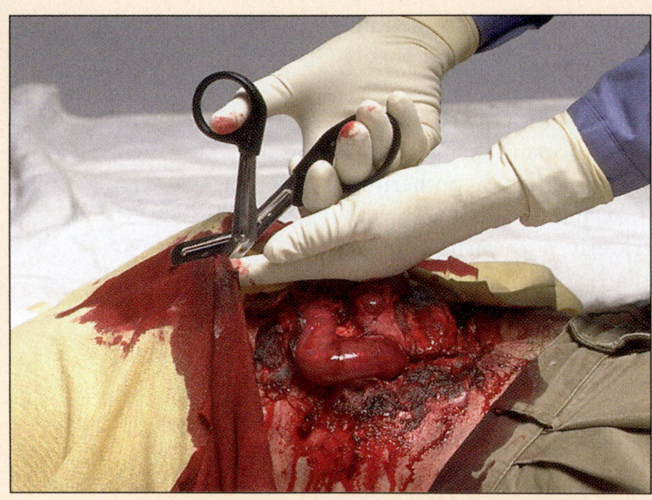

26-1a Remove clothing from around the abdominal wound.

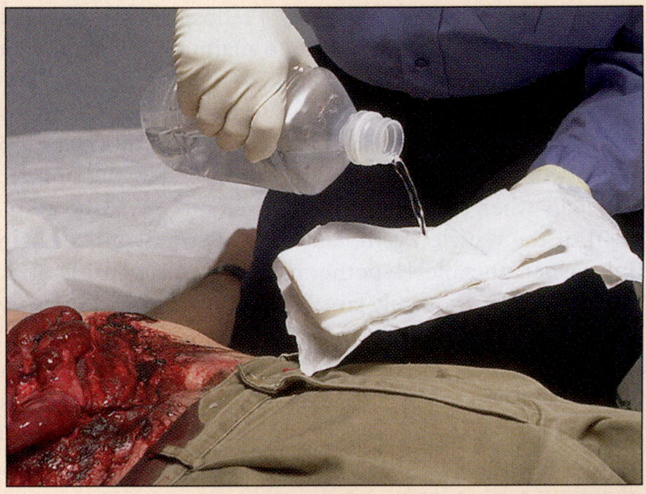

26-1b Cover the wound with a sterile dressing soaked with sterile normal saline.

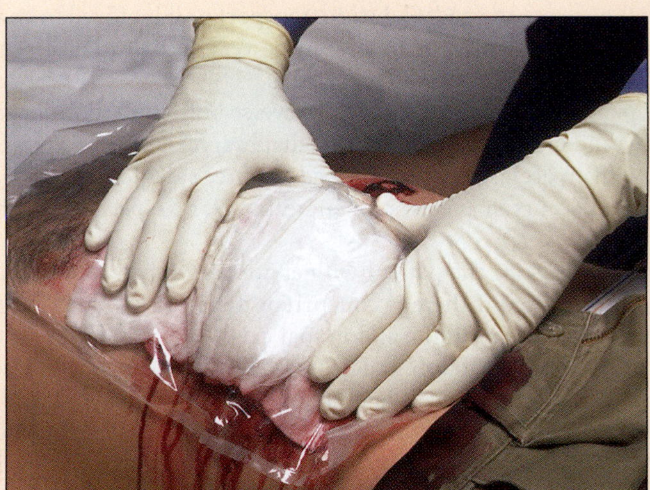

26-1c Cover the moistened dressing with a sterile occlusive dressing to prevent evaporative drying.

intra-abdominal pressure, and because the fetus is especially susceptible to hypoxia. If necessary, employ intermittent positive pressure ventilation early in your care. Also consider aggressive airway care. The pregnant mother is prone to vomiting and aspiration. If she has a significantly reduced level of consciousness, consider rapid-sequence intubation.

Maintain a high index of suspicion for internal hemorrhage since the increased blood volume of the third-trimester mother may permit an increased blood loss before the signs and symptoms of hypovolemia become evident. The fetus may be at risk early in the blood loss, well before the mother displays any signs. Initiate IV therapy early, but remember that pregnancy induces a relative anemia and that aggressive fluid resuscitation may further dilute the erythrocyte concentrations and lead to ineffective circulation.

Summary

Blunt or penetrating abdominal trauma can result in serious organ damage and life-threatening hemorrhage. Concurrently, the signs of injury are limited, non-specific, and do not reflect the seriousness of abdominal pathology. It is thus very important for your assessment to carefully determine the mechanism of injury and the region of the abdomen it affects. This information must be communicated to the emergency department to ensure that its personnel acknowledge the significance of your firsthand knowledge of the mechanism of injury.

Care for significant abdominal injury is provided by rapid transport to the trauma center. Most significant abdominal injury results in serious internal bleeding or organ injury that can neither be cared for nor stabilized in the prehospital setting. Further, the definitive care for the patient with serious abdominal injury is provided via surgery. The patient must be transported to a facility capable of providing immediate surgical intervention when needed. This is a trauma center. Prehospital care is supportive of the airway and breathing, and preventive for shock.

The pregnant patient with abdominal injury deserves special attention because her vascular volume is increased and she will likely not show the signs of shock until the fetus is at risk. Careful observation while preparing for rapid transport to the trauma center is in order. If any of the slightest signs of hypoperfusion is noted, initiate fluid resuscitation.

Review Questions

1. Unlike other major body containers, the abdomen is bound by ____________ rather than skeletal structures.
   a. cartilage
   b. muscle
   c. skin
   d. mucous membranes
2. Blunt trauma to the abdomen causes injury through all of the following mechanisms *except:*
   a. deceleration.
   b. torque.
   c. compression.
   d. shear.

3. Hollow organs like the stomach, bowel, bladder, and pregnant uterus may __________ with compression from blunt forces.
   a. rupture
   b. contract
   c. expand
   d. invert
4. Penetrating trauma most frequently involves the __________ and small bowel.
   a. liver
   b. spleen
   c. kidneys
   d. aorta
5. A protrusion of organs from a wound is called an:
   a. extravasation.
   b. evisceration.
   c. ecchymosis.
   d. exsanguination.
6. Inflammation of the lining of the anterior abdomen, caused by bacterial or chemical irritation, is called:
   a. traumatic bowel.
   b. appendicitis.
   c. gastric convulsion.
   d. peritonitis.
7. __________ is the number one killer of pregnant females.
   a. Hypertension
   b. Toxemia
   c. Trauma
   d. Sepsis
8. Significant blunt or penetrating trauma to the abdomen may cause internal hemorrhage and shock. First signs and symptoms of shock include all of the following *except:*
   a. lethargy.
   b. diminishing level of consciousness.
   c. decreasing pulse pressure.
   d. increasing capillary refill time.
9. Palpation of an injured abdominal quadrant is most likely to:
   a. reveal the mechanism of injury.
   b. aggravate existing injuries.
   c. help determine which organs are injured.
   d. cause guarding.
10. It is very important to ensure early fluid resuscitation of the potentially hypotensive pregnant mother. This statement is true because it may take a maternal blood loss of between __________ percent before changes in maternal blood pressure or heart rate are evident.
    a. 10 and 15
    b. 20 and 25
    c. 30 and 35
    d. 40 and 45

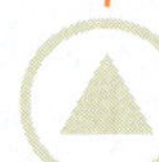

See Answers to Review Questions at the back of this book.

Division 4

Medical Emergencies

Chapter

27

Pulmonology

Objectives

After reading this chapter, you should be able to:

1. Discuss the epidemiology of pulmonary diseases and pulmonary conditions. (p. 1081)
2. Identify and describe the function of the structures located in the upper and lower airway. (see Chapter 3)
3. Discuss the physiology of ventilation and respiration. (pp. 1081–1084; also see Chapter 3)
4. Identify common pathological events that affect the pulmonary system. (pp. 1084–1086)
5. Compare various airway and ventilation techniques used in the management of pulmonary diseases. (pp. 1098–1118)
6. Review the use of equipment utilized during the physical examination of patients with complaints associated with respiratory diseases and conditions. (pp. 1091–1092, 1093–1098)
7. Identify the epidemiology, anatomy, physiology, pathophysiology, assessment findings, and management (including prehospital medications) for the following respiratory diseases and conditions:
   - A. Adult respiratory distress syndrome (pp. 1100–1101)
   - B. Bronchial asthma (pp. 1101–1102, 1105–1108)
   - C. Chronic bronchitis (pp. 1101–1102, 1104–1105)
   - D. Emphysema (pp. 1101–1104)
   - E. Pneumonia (pp. 1109–1110)
   - F. Pulmonary edema (pp. 1100–1101)
   - G. Pulmonary thromboembolism (pp. 1114–1116)
   - H. Neoplasms of the lung (pp. 1112–1113)
   - I. Upper respiratory infections (pp. 1108–1109)
   - J. Spontaneous pneumothorax (p. 1116)
   - K. Hyperventilation syndrome (pp. 1116–1117)
8. Given several preprogrammed patients with nontraumatic pulmonary problems, provide the appropriate assessment, prehospital care, and transport. (pp. 1081–1118)

Key Terms

adult respiratory distress syndrome (ARDS), p. 1100
apnea, p. 1084
asphyxia, p. 1088
bradypnea, p. 1093
COPD, p. 1081
cor pulmonale, p. 1102
crepitus, p. 1090
cyanosis, p. 1088
diaphoresis, p. 1088
diffusion, p. 1082
dyspnea, p. 1089
flail chest, p. 1084
hemoglobin, p. 1082
hemoptysis, p. 1089
hemothorax, p. 1084
hypoxia, p. 1086
nasal flaring, p. 1088
orthopnea, p. 1089
pallor, p. 1088
paroxysmal nocturnal dyspnea, p. 1089
perfusion, p. 1082
pleuritic, p. 1110
pneumothorax, p. 1084
polycythemia, p. 1103
positive end-expiratory pressure (PEEP), p. 1101
respiration, p. 1084
spontaneous pneumothorax, p. 1116
subcutaneous emphysema, p. 1090
tachycardia, p. 1089
tachypnea, p. 1093
tactile fremitus, p. 1091
tracheal deviation, p. 1091
tracheal tugging, p. 1088
ventilation, p. 1082

INTRODUCTION

According to one U.S. study, respiratory complaints accounted for over 28 percent of all EMS calls. More than 200,000 people die each year as a result of respiratory emergencies. Several factors increase the risk of developing respiratory disease. *Intrinsic risk factors* are those within or influenced by the patient. The most important of these is genetic predisposition. For example, bronchial asthma, **COPD,** and lung cancer are more common in those who have family members with these diseases.

The most important intrinsic factor in the development of respiratory disorders is genetic predisposition. The most important extrinsic factor is smoking.

COPD *a disease characterized by a decreased ability of the lungs to perform the function of ventilation.*

Certain respiratory conditions are increased in patients with underlying cardiac or circulatory problems. Cardiac conditions that result in ineffective pumping of blood tend to cause pulmonary edema. Cardiac and circulatory diseases may allow blood to pool in the large veins of the pelvis and lower extremities, causing pulmonary emboli. Stress may increase the severity of any respiratory complaint and can precipitate acute episodes of asthma or COPD.

Extrinsic risk factors are those that are external to the patient. The most important of these is cigarette smoking. There is a strong link between cigarette smoking and the development of pulmonary diseases such as lung carcinoma and COPD. Also, diseases such as pneumonia and pulmonary emboli are more likely in patients who smoke. Finally, cigarette smoking has been implicated as a risk factor in the development of cardiac disease. In any case, underlying lung damage caused by cigarette smoking worsens virtually all lung disorders.

Another key extrinsic risk factor is environmental pollutants. The prevalence of COPD is markedly increased in areas with high environmental pollutants, as are the number and severity of acute attacks of asthma and COPD.

This chapter explores the pathophysiology of respiratory disease and how to integrate this knowledge with your assessment findings to develop a field impression and manage the patient with respiratory problems.

PHYSIOLOGICAL PROCESSES

The major function of the respiratory system is to exchange gases with the environment. Oxygen is taken in while carbon dioxide is eliminated, a process known as gas exchange.

Oxygen is vital to our bodies, allowing us to generate the energy that drives our many body functions. Oxygen from the atmosphere diffuses into the bloodstream through the lungs. Oxygen is then available for use in cellular metabolism by the body's 100 trillion cells. Waste products, including carbon dioxide, produced by cellular metabolism, must be eliminated from the body. In the lungs, carbon dioxide is exchanged for oxygen and the carbon dioxide is excreted from the lungs.

Three important processes allow gas exchange to occur:

★ Ventilation
★ Diffusion
★ Perfusion

Content Review

Processes of Gas Exchange

- Ventilation
- Diffusion
- Perfusion

Ventilation

ventilation *the mechanical process of moving air in and out of the lungs.*

Ventilation is the mechanical process of moving air in and out of the lungs. For ventilation to occur, several body structures must be intact, including the chest wall, nerve pathways, diaphragm, pleural cavity, and brainstem.

Ventilation is divided into two phases: inspiration and expiration. During inspiration, air is drawn into the lungs. During expiration, air leaves the lungs. These phases of ventilation depend on changes in the volume of the thoracic cavity, as discussed in Chapter 3, "Anatomy and Physiology."

Diffusion

diffusion *the movement of molecules through a membrane from an area of greater concentration to an area of lesser concentration.*

Diffusion is the process by which gases move between the alveoli and the pulmonary capillaries. Remember that gases tend to flow from areas in which there is a high concentration of gas into an area of low concentration. The normal concentration of oxygen in the alveoli is 104 mmHg as opposed to a concentration of 40 mmHg in the pulmonary arterial circulation. Therefore, oxygen will move from the oxygen-rich alveoli into the oxygen-poor capillaries in response to the gradient that exists in the concentration of gases. As the red blood cells move through the pulmonary capillaries, they become enriched with oxygen. Less oxygen will pass into the bloodstream as the gradient between alveolar and capillary oxygen concentration decreases.

Similarly, carbon dioxide passes out of the blood in response to a gradient that exists between the concentration of carbon dioxide in the blood in the pulmonary capillaries (45 mmHg) and in the alveoli (40 mmHg). By the time blood leaves the pulmonary capillaries, it has a dissolved concentration of oxygen of 104 mmHg and a carbon dioxide concentration of 40 mmHg.

The respiratory membrane, which normally measures 0.5 to 1.0 micrometer in thickness, must remain intact for gas exchange to occur. Any disorder that damages the alveoli or allows them to collapse will impede oxygen from entering the body and will reduce carbon dioxide elimination. Changes in the respiratory membrane or any increase in the interstitial space will also impede the process of diffusion. For example, fluid accumulation in the interstitial space as the result of pulmonary edema or pneumonia will prevent proper diffusion of gases. Finally, the endothelial lining of the capillaries must be intact for exchange of oxygen and carbon dioxide to occur. Diseases that produce thickening of the endothelial lining will also interfere with the process of diffusion.

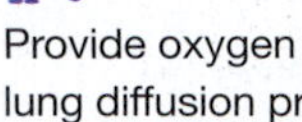

Provide oxygen to a patient with a lung diffusion problem to increase the concentration gradient that drives oxygen into the capillaries. When fluid accumulation or inflammation is present, consider administering diuretics or anti-inflammatory drugs.

There are certain measures that you can take to address problems with lung diffusion. Providing the patient with high concentrations of oxygen is one simple step that can be utilized. Remember that the concentration gradient provides the driving force in moving oxygen into the capillaries. Therefore, the larger the difference between the concentration of oxygen in the alveoli and the capillaries, the greater the diffusion of oxygen into the bloodstream. Similarly, when fluid accumulation or inflammation is the underlying cause of the thickening of the interstitial space within the alveoli, medications such as diuretic agents or anti-inflammatory drugs (corticosteroids, antibiotics) are given to reduce fluid and inflammation.

Perfusion

perfusion *the circulation of blood through the capillaries.*

One additional process that occurs in the lungs is **perfusion.** Lung perfusion is the circulation of blood through the lungs or, more specifically, the pulmonary capillaries. Lung perfusion is dependent on three conditions:

- Adequate blood volume
- Intact pulmonary capillaries
- Efficient pumping of blood by the heart

hemoglobin *the transport protein that carries oxygen in the blood.*

For perfusion to proceed effectively, there must be an adequate volume of blood in the bloodstream. Equally important is the concentration of **hemoglobin,** which is the transport protein that carries oxygen in the blood. Remember that oxygen is transported in the bloodstream in one of two ways: bound to hemoglobin or dissolved in the plasma. Under normal conditions, less than 2 percent of all oxygen is transported while dissolved in plasma (as measured by the PO_2), whereas more than 98 percent is carried by hemoglobin.

Hemoglobin has some unique properties. It is made up of four iron-containing heme molecules and a protein-containing globin portion. Oxygen molecules bind to the heme portion of the

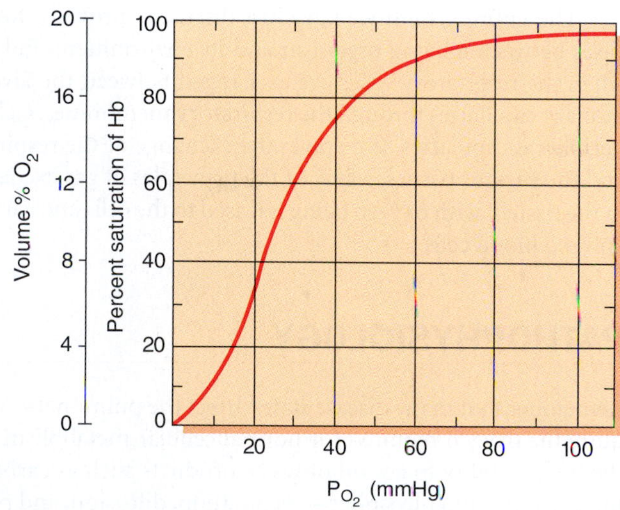

■ **Figure 27-1** Oxygen dissociation curve.

hemoglobin molecule. As oxygen binds to hemoglobin, its structure changes so that it more readily binds additional oxygen molecules. Similarly, as fully oxygen-bound hemoglobin begins to release oxygen, it more readily sheds additional oxygen. The relationship is described by the *oxygen dissociation curve* (Figure 27-1 ■). You can see that with between 10 and 50 mmHg, there is a marked increase in the saturation of hemoglobin. However, as the PO_2 increases above 70 mmHg, there is only a small change in the saturation of hemoglobin which is already near 100 percent.

Changes in the body temperature, the blood pH, and the PCO_2 can alter the oxygen dissociation curve. Within the tissues, as hemoglobin becomes bound with carbon dioxide, it loses its affinity for oxygen. As a result, more oxygen is released and is thus available to cells for metabolism (called the Bohr effect).

Carbon dioxide is transported from the cells to the lungs in one of three ways:

★ As bicarbonate ion
★ Bound to the globin portion of the hemoglobin molecule
★ Dissolved in plasma (measured as PCO_2)

The greatest portion of CO_2 produced in cells during metabolism is converted into bicarbonate ion. As the CO_2 is released into the capillaries, it enters the red blood cell where an enzyme (carbonic anhydrase) combines carbon dioxide with water to form two ions, hydrogen (H^+) and bicarbonate (HCO_3^-). Bicarbonate is then released from the red blood cell and transported in plasma. In the lungs, the reverse process takes place, producing water and carbon dioxide. The carbon dioxide then diffuses into the alveoli where it is eliminated during exhalation.

The carbon dioxide that is bound to hemoglobin is released in the lung because of the lower concentration of this gas in the alveoli. Additionally, as the heme portion of the hemoglobin molecule becomes saturated with oxygen, more carbon dioxide is released (called the Haldane effect). Finally, the approximately 10 percent of carbon dioxide that is dissolved in the plasma flows into the alveoli due to the gradient that exists between the concentration of gases (PCO_2 of 45 mmHg in pulmonary artery versus 40 mmHg in the alveoli).

For perfusion to take place, in addition to having adequate blood volume, the pulmonary capillaries must be able to transport blood through all portions of the lung tissue. These vessels must be open and not occluded, or blocked. For example, a pulmonary embolism will occlude the pulmonary artery in which it lodges, making that artery unavailable for perfusion of the portion of the lung it usually supplies with blood. Finally, the heart must pump efficiently in order to push blood effectively through the pulmonary capillaries to perfuse the lung tissues.

To maintain perfusion, you must ensure that the patient has an adequate circulating blood volume. In addition, take the necessary steps to improve the pumping action of the heart. For example, in patients with acute pulmonary edema the use of diuretic agents reduces the blood return (preload) to an ineffectively pumping heart and improves cardiac efficiency.

To maintain perfusion, ensure that the patient has an adequate circulating blood volume. Also, take all necessary steps to improve the pumping action of the heart.

respiration *the exchange of gases between a living organism and its environment.*

The entire system we have just discussed provides for **respiration,** which is the exchange of gases between a living organism and its environment. Pulmonary respiration occurs in the lungs when the respiratory gases are exchanged between the alveoli and the red blood cells in the pulmonary capillaries through the respiratory membranes. Cellular respiration, however, occurs in the peripheral capillaries. It involves the exchange of the respiratory gases between the red blood cells and the various tissues. Many of the principles of gas exchange that occur in the lungs are reversed in the tissues, with oxygen being released to the cells and carbon dioxide accumulating in the plasma and red blood cells.

PATHOPHYSIOLOGY

Your understanding of the normal processes of ventilation, diffusion, and perfusion will aid in understanding specific disease processes and direct you toward appropriate corrective actions.

Remember that many disease states affect the pulmonary system and interfere with its ability to acquire the oxygen required for normal cellular metabolism. Additionally, respiratory diseases limit the body's ability to get rid of waste products such as carbon dioxide. Your understanding of normal anatomy and physiology—ventilation, diffusion, and perfusion—will aid in understanding the mechanism of each disease process and will direct you toward the appropriate corrective actions. Ultimately, any disease process that impairs the pulmonary system will result in a derangement in ventilation, diffusion, perfusion, or a combination of these processes.

DISRUPTION IN VENTILATION

Diseases that affect ventilation will result in obstruction of the normal conducting pathways of the upper or lower respiratory tract, impairment of the normal function of the chest wall, or abnormalities involving the nervous system's control of ventilation.

Upper and Lower Respiratory Tracts

Disease states that affect the upper respiratory tract will result in obstruction of air flow to the lower structures. Upper airway trauma, for example, produces both significant hemorrhage and swelling. Infections of the upper airway structures, including epiglottitis, soft-tissue infections of the neck, tonsillitis, and abscess formation within the pharynx (peritonsillar abscess and retropharyngeal abscess), can obstruct air flow. Similarly, lower airway obstruction may be produced by trauma, foreign body aspiration, mucus accumulation (as in asthmatics), smooth muscle constriction (in asthma and COPD), and airway edema produced by infection or burns.

pneumothorax *a collection of air in the pleural space, causing a loss of the negative pressure that binds the lung to the chest wall. In an* open pneumothorax, *air enters the pleural space through an injury to the chest wall. In a* closed pneumothorax, *air enters the pleural space through an opening in the pleura that covers the lung. A* tension pneumothorax *develops when air in the pleural space cannot escape, causing a buildup of pressure and collapse of the lung.*

hemothorax *a collection of blood in the pleural space.*

flail chest *one or more ribs fractured in two or more places, creating an unattached rib segment.*

apnea *absence of breathing.*

Chest Wall and Diaphragm

As you read earlier, the chest wall and diaphragm are mechanical components that are essential for normal ventilation. Traumatic injuries to these areas will disrupt the normal mechanics causing loss of negative pressure within the pleural space. This occurs in patients with **pneumothorax,** including open pneumothorax, tension pneumothorax, or **hemothorax.** Infectious processes such as empyema (pus accumulation in the pleural space) or inflammatory conditions produce similar effects. Chest wall injuries including rib fractures or **flail chest** and diaphragmatic rupture limit the patient's ability to expand the thoracic cavity. Certain neuromuscular diseases, such as muscular dystrophy, multiple sclerosis, or amyotrophic lateral sclerosis (ALS or Lou Gehrig's disease), impair muscular function so as to limit the ability to generate a negative pressure within the chest cavity.

Nervous System

Any disease process that impairs the nervous system's regulation of breathing may also alter ventilation. Central nervous system depressants such as alcohol, benzodiazepines, or barbiturates, alone or in combination, can alter the brain's response to important signals such as rising PCO_2. Similarly, stroke, diseases, or injuries that involve the respiratory centers within the central nervous system can change the normal ventilatory pattern. In fact, certain abnormal respiratory patterns are produced by specific brain injury (Figure 27-2 ■):

- *Cheyne-Stokes respirations* are a ventilatory pattern with progressively increasing tidal volume, followed by a declining volume, separated by periods of **apnea** at the end of

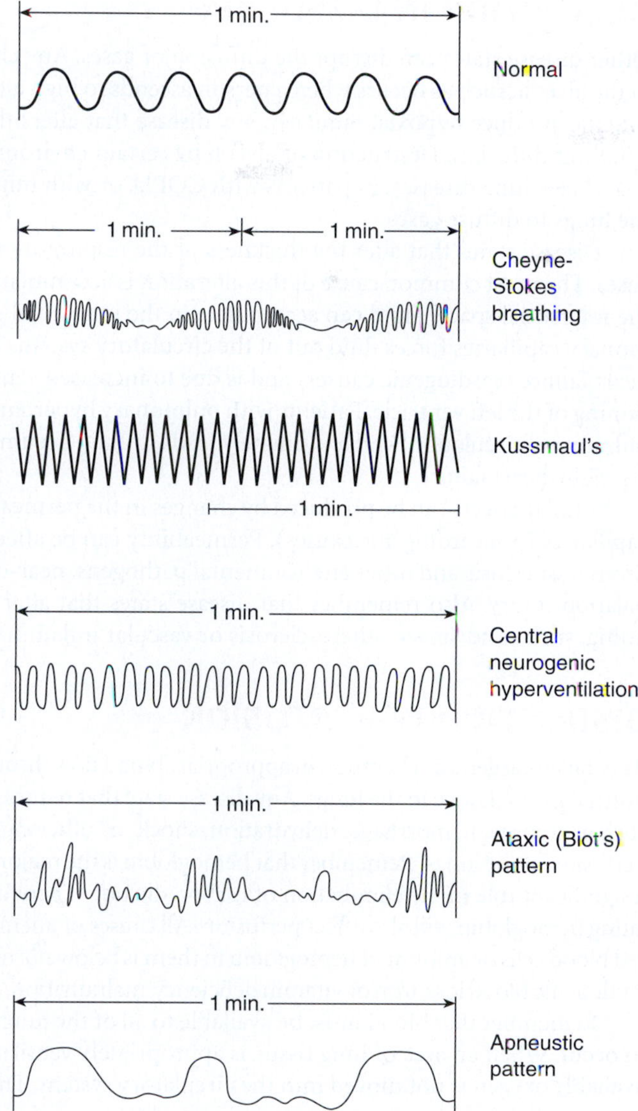

■ Figure 27-2 Abnormal respiratory patterns.

expiration. This pattern is typically seen in older patients with terminal illness or brain injury.

- ★ *Kussmaul's respirations* are deep, rapid breaths that result as a corrective measure against conditions such as diabetic ketoacidosis that produce metabolic acidosis.
- ★ *Central neurogenic hyperventilation* also produces deep, rapid respirations that are caused by strokes or injury to the brainstem. In this case, there is loss of normal regulation of ventilatory controls and respiratory alkalosis is often seen.
- ★ *Ataxic (Biot's) respirations* are characterized by repeated episodes of gasping ventilations separated by periods of apnea. This pattern is seen in patients with increased intracranial pressure.
- ★ *Apneustic respiration* is characterized by long, deep breaths that are stopped during the inspiratory phase and separated by periods of apnea. This pattern is a result of stroke or severe central nervous system disease.

Also remember that damage to the major peripheral nerves that supply the diaphragm and intercostal muscles, the phrenic nerve, and intercostal nerves will also affect normal ventilatory mechanics. Traumatic disruption of the phrenic nerve during chest surgery, with penetrating trauma, or by neoplastic (cancerous, tumorous) invasion of the nerve can paralyze the diaphragm on the side of involvement.

DISRUPTION IN DIFFUSION

hypoxia *state in which insufficient oxygen is available to meet the oxygen requirements of the cells.*

Other disease states can disrupt the diffusion of gases. Any change in the concentration of oxygen in the alveoli, such as occurs when a person ascends to high altitudes, can limit the diffusion of oxygen and produce **hypoxia.** Similarly, any disease that alters the structure or patency of the alveoli will limit diffusion. Destruction of alveoli by certain environmental pathogens such as asbestos or coal (black lung disease), in patients with COPD, or with inhalation injury reduces the capacity of the lungs to diffuse gases.

Disease states that alter the thickness of the respiratory membrane will limit the diffusion of gases. The most common cause of this alteration is accumulation of fluid and inflammatory cells in the interstitial space. Fluid can accumulate in the interstitial space if high pressure within the pulmonary capillaries forces fluid out of the circulatory system. This is seen in patients with left-sided heart failure (cardiogenic causes) and is due to increased venous pressure as a result of poor functioning of the left ventricle. Patients with pulmonary hypertension have high resting pressures in the pulmonary circulation which ultimately leads to fluid accumulation in the interstitial space, causing right-heart failure.

Similar effects can be produced by changes in the permeability (or leakiness) of the pulmonary capillaries (noncardiogenic causes). Permeability can be affected by adult respiratory distress syndrome, asbestosis and other environmental pathogens, near-drowning, prolonged hypoxia, and inhalation injury. Also remember that disease states that alter the pulmonary capillary endothelial lining, such as advanced atherosclerosis or vascular inflammatory states, can affect diffusion.

DISRUPTION IN PERFUSION

As detailed earlier, any alteration in appropriate blood flow through the pulmonary capillaries will limit normal gas exchange in the lungs. Any disease state that reduces the normal circulating blood volume, such as trauma, hemorrhage, dehydration, shock, or other causes of hypovolemia, will limit normal perfusion of the lungs. Remember that hemoglobin is the major transport protein for oxygen and plays a significant role in the elimination of carbon dioxide. Therefore, any reduction in the normal circulating hemoglobin will also affect perfusion. All causes of anemia, a condition in which the number of red blood cells or amount of hemoglobin in them is below normal, must be considered. Such causes include acute blood loss, iron or vitamin deficiency, malnutrition, and anemia from chronic disease states.

Remember that blood must be available to all of the lung segments for maximum gas exchange to occur. When an area of lung tissue is appropriately ventilated but no capillary perfusion occurs, available oxygen is not moved into the circulatory system. This is referred to as a *pulmonary shunting.* In patients with pulmonary embolism, a blockage of a division of the pulmonary artery by a clot prevents perfusion of the lung segments supplied by that branch of the artery. As a result, there may be significant shunt with return of unoxygenated blood to the pulmonary venous circulation.

ASSESSMENT OF THE RESPIRATORY SYSTEM

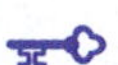

If the patient's complaints suggest respiratory system involvement, direct the focused history and physical examination to this aspect.

Assessment of the respiratory system is a vital aspect of prehospital care. You must quickly assess the airway and ventilation status during the initial assessment. If the patient's complaints suggest that the respiratory system is involved in the patient's problem, the focused history and physical examination should be directed to this aspect of the assessment.

SCENE SIZE-UP

When you approach the scene, consider: (1) Is the scene safe? and (2) Are there visual clues to the patient's medical complaint?

When you approach the scene, you should consider two major questions: (1) Is the scene safe to approach the patient? and (2) Are there visual clues that might provide information regarding the patient's medical complaint?

Remember that there are several hazards that may result in respiratory complaints by the patient that are also potentially dangerous for emergency care providers. Certain gases and toxic products that are causing respiratory complaints from your patient may also present a significant risk to you. Carbon monoxide, for example, is a colorless and odorless gas that may be present in quantities large enough to overcome unsuspecting emergency care personnel. Other toxins from incomplete combustion produced in fires or industrial processes pose a similar risk. Recent incidents involving chemical agents such as sarin gas or biologic agents like anthrax highlight the need for emergency care providers to be aware of hazards to themselves as well as to their patient.

You should also be aware that there are certain rescue environments in which the concentration of available oxygen is significantly reduced. This would include areas such as grain silos, enclosed storage containers, or any enclosed space in which there is an active fire. You must take the appropriate precautions before entering such environments, including the use of your own supplemental oxygen supply.

In any situation where you believe there is a hazard to you as a care provider, make sure that the scene is appropriately secured before you enter. If specific protective items such as hazardous materials suits, self-contained breathing apparatus, or supplemental oxygen are needed, make sure they are available before you attempt to care for your patient. Similarly, if other personnel such as fire suppression units or hazmat teams are required, contact dispatch and have them available on scene before putting yourself at risk.

Once it is safe to enter the scene, look for clues that will provide information regarding the patient's complaints. Do you see evidence of cigarette packs or ashtrays to suggest that the patient or family members are smokers? Look for any home nebulizer machines or supplemental oxygen tanks that may suggest a patient with underlying COPD or asthma. If the patient is a small child, look for small items lying around the house that could suggest potential ingested foreign bodies. Using your eyes, ears, and nose can lead you to several important clues that are useful as you begin your assessment of the patient.

PRIMARY ASSESSMENT

General Impression

Take the following considerations and steps to help form your initial impression of the patient's respiratory status:

★ *Position.* Consider the patient's position. Patients with respiratory diseases tend to tolerate an upright posture better than lying flat. Indications of severe respiratory distress include a patient who is sitting upright with feet dangling over the side of the bed. In the most severe cases, the patient will assume the "tripod" position in which he leans forward and supports his weight with the arms extended (Figure 27-3 ■).

Content Review

General Impression of Respiratory Status

- Position
- Color
- Mental status
- Ability to speak
- Respiratory effort

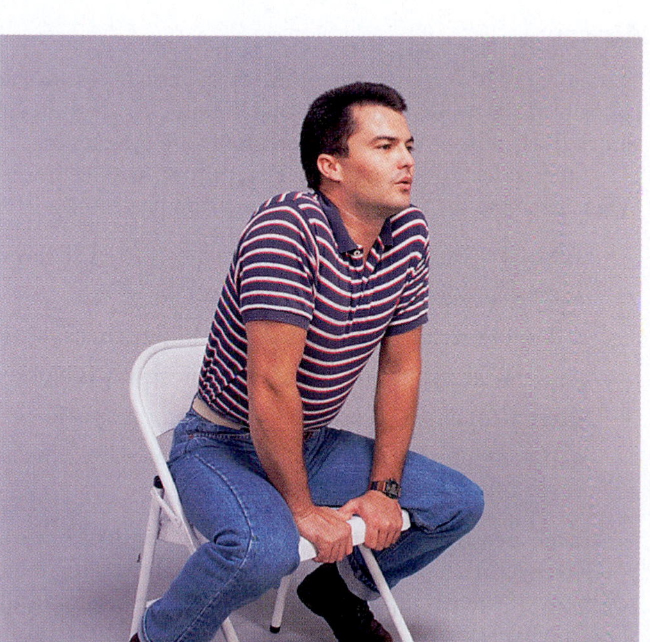

■ Figure 27-3 Tripod position.

pallor *paleness.*

diaphoresis *sweatiness.*

cyanosis *bluish discoloration of the skin due to an increase in reduced hemoglobin in the blood. The condition is directly related to poor ventilation.*

- *Color.* Patients with severe respiratory distress display **pallor** and **diaphoresis.** **Cyanosis** is a late finding and may be absent even with significant hypoxia. Peripheral cyanosis (bluish discoloration involving only the distal extremities) is not a specific finding and is also found in patients with poor circulation. Peripheral cyanosis reflects the slowing of blood flow and increased extraction of oxygen from red blood cells. Central cyanosis (involving the lips, tongue, and truncal skin) is a more ominous finding seen in hypoxia.
- *Mental status.* Briefly assess the patient's mental status. The hypoxic patient will become restless and agitated. Confusion is seen with both hypoxia (deficiency of oxygen) and hypercarbia (excess of carbon dioxide). When respiratory failure is imminent, the patient will appear severely lethargic and somnolent. The eyelids will begin to droop and the head will bob with each respiratory effort.
- *Ability to speak.* Assess the patient's ability to speak in full, coherent sentences. Determine the ease with which the patient can discuss symptoms. Patients with respiratory distress will be able to speak only one to two words before they need to pause to catch their breath. Rambling, incoherent speech indicates fear, anxiety, or hypoxia.
- *Respiratory effort.* As described, normal ventilation is an active process. However, the use of accessory muscles in the neck (scalenes and sternocleidomastoids) and visible contractions of the intercostal muscles indicate significant breathing effort.

As you form your general impression, also make specific note of any of the following signs of respiratory distress:

nasal flaring *excessive widening of the nares with respiration.*

- **Nasal flaring**
- Intercostal muscle retraction
- Use of the accessory respiratory muscles
- Cyanosis
- Pursed lips
- **Tracheal tugging**

tracheal tugging *retraction of the tissues of the neck due to airway obstruction or dyspnea.*

Your initial assessment of the patient is directed at identification of any life-threatening conditions resulting from compromise of airway, breathing, or circulation (the ABCs). Because this chapter concerns the respiratory system, we will focus here on assessment of airway and breathing.

Airway

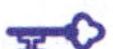

Any significant abnormality in the respiratory tract must be viewed as potentially life threatening.

Remember that oxygen is one of the most basic necessities for life, and the respiratory system is responsible for supplying it to the body tissues. As a result, any significant abnormality in the respiratory tract must be viewed as potentially life threatening.

After quickly forming your general impression, immediately focus on the patient's airway. When assessing the airway, keep these principles in mind:

asphyxia *a decrease in the amount of oxygen and an increase in the amount of carbon dioxide as a result of some interference with respiration.*

- Noisy breathing nearly always means partial airway obstruction.
- Obstructed breathing is not always noisy.
- The brain can survive only a few minutes in **asphyxia.**
- Artificial respiration is useless if the airway is blocked.
- A patent airway is useless if the patient is apneic.
- If you note airway obstruction, do not waste time looking for help or equipment. Act immediately.

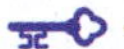

If the airway is compromised, quickly institute basic airway management techniques. Once you have secured a patent airway, ensure that the patient has adequate ventilation.

If the airway is compromised, quickly institute basic airway management techniques. Once you have secured a patent airway, ensure that the patient has adequate ventilation. Your initial assessment of the respiratory system should be brief and directed. A more detailed examination should be conducted once you have been able to establish that an immediate threat to life does not exist.

Breathing

The following signs should suggest a possible life-threatening respiratory problem in adults. They are listed in order from most ominous to least severe:

- ★ Alterations in mental status
- ★ Severe central cyanosis
- ★ Absent breath sounds
- ★ Audible stridor
- ★ One-to-two-word **dyspnea** (need to breathe between every word or two)
- ★ **Tachycardia** ≥ 130 beats per minute
- ★ Pallor and diaphoresis
- ★ Presence of intercostal and sternocleidomastoid retractions
- ★ Use of accessory muscles

dyspnea *difficult or labored breathing; a sensation of "shortness of breath."*

tachycardia *rapid heart rate.*

If any of these signs are present, direct your efforts toward immediate resuscitation and transport of the patient to a medical facility.

SECONDARY ASSESSMENT

History

The history and physical exam should be directed at problem areas as determined by the patient's chief complaint or primary problem. Patients with respiratory diseases will often present with a complaint of "shortness of breath" (dyspnea). Obtain a SAMPLE history. If the chief complaint suggests respiratory disease, ask the OPQRST–ASPN questions, including the following questions about the current symptoms. The answers to these or similar questions will provide you with a pertinent patient history:

If a patient complains of dyspnea, obtain a SAMPLE history. If the chief complaint suggests respiratory disease, ask the OPQRST–ASPN questions about current symptoms.

How long has the dyspnea been present?

Was the onset gradual or abrupt?

Is the dyspnea better or worse by position? Is there associated **orthopnea** or **paroxysmal nocturnal dyspnea?**

Has the patient been coughing? If so, is the cough productive?

What is the character and color of the sputum?

Is there any **hemoptysis** (coughing up of blood)?

Is there any chest pain associated with the dyspnea?

If so, what is the location of the pain?

Was the onset of pain sudden or slow?

What was the duration of the pain?

Does the pain radiate to any area?

Does the pain increase with respiration?

Are there associated symptoms of fever or chills?

What is the patient's past medical history?

Does the patient have obstructive sleep apnea?

Has the patient experienced wheezing?

Is the patient or close family member a smoker?

orthopnea *dyspnea while lying supine.*

paroxysmal nocturnal dyspnea *short attacks of dyspnea that occur at night and interrupt sleep.*

hemoptysis *expectoration of blood from the respiratory tree.*

It is also important to ask the patient if he has ever experienced similar symptoms in the past. Patients with chronic medical conditions such as COPD or asthma can usually relate the severity of their current presenting complaints to other episodes that they have experienced. Question the patient or family about prior hospitalizations for respiratory disease. In particular, you should try to determine whether the patient required care in the intensive care unit (ICU) for breathing problems. Ask if the patient has ever required endotracheal intubation and ventilatory support. Consider patients who have been previously intubated to be potentially seriously ill and approach them with great caution.

Similarly, it is important to ask the patient if he already has a known respiratory disease. The most common reason for a call to emergency care personnel is a worsening of an already present respiratory disease. This is typical for patients with COPD, asthma, or lung cancer. If you are not familiar with the patient's diagnosis (for example, alpha-1 antitrypsin deficiency), try to determine if the disease is affecting the process of ventilation, diffusion, or perfusion.

Continue history taking by determining: What current medications is the patient taking? (Pay particular attention to oxygen therapy, oral bronchodilators, corticosteroids, and antibiotics.) Does the patient have any allergies?

A good history of medication use is essential and may provide useful clues to the diagnosis. If time permits, gather the patient's current medications and transport them with the patient. This is a great benefit to the emergency department personnel who will be evaluating the patient. Pay particular attention to any medications that suggest pulmonary disease. These would include inhaled or oral sympathomimetics such as albuterol and related agents that are used to treat diseases such as COPD or asthma. Also ask about steroid preparations, which are used in these conditions. Other common medications used by patients with COPD or asthma include cromolyn sodium, methylxanthines like theophylline, and antibiotic agents.

Ask if the patient has a home nebulizer unit and how frequently it is used. Inquire about the use of a continuous positive airway pressure (CPAP) device (or similar device) for obstructive sleep apnea. Also ask about drugs used for cardiac conditions since cardiac patients often present with dyspnea. Nitrates, calcium channel blockers, diuretic agents, digoxin, and antidysrhythmic agents are all commonly used by patients with cardiac disease.

Finally, inquire about medication allergies. This information is important because it helps to avoid administering agents to which the patient is allergic. It is also possible that a specific medication may be the cause of an allergic reaction that has resulted in upper airway edema and respiratory complaints.

Content Review

Physical Exam of Respiratory System

- Head
- Neck
- Chest
  - Inspection
  - Palpation
  - Percussion
  - Auscultation
- Extremities

Physical Examination

First address the patient's head and neck. Look at the lips. Pursed lips indicate significant respiratory distress. This is the patient's way of maintaining positive pressure during expiration and preventing alveolar collapse. Also examine the nose, mouth, and throat for any signs of swelling or infection that might be causing upper airway obstruction.

Occasionally, the patient may produce sputum, which can suggest an underlying cause of the patient's complaints. An increase in the amount of sputum produced suggests infection of the lungs or bronchial passages (bronchitis). Thick green or brown sputum is characteristic of these infections. However, thin yellow or pale-gray sputum is more typical of inflammation or an allergic cause. Pink, frothy sputum is a sign of severe pulmonary edema. Truly bloody sputum (hemoptysis) may be seen with cancer, tuberculosis, and bronchial infection.

Assess the neck for signs of swelling or infection. Remember to look at the jugular veins for evidence of distention (Figure 27-4 ■). This occurs when the right side of the heart is not pumping blood effectively, causing a "backup" in the venous circulation. Such findings are often accompanied by left-sided heart failure and pulmonary edema.

Physical examination of the respiratory system should follow the standard steps of patient assessment: *inspection, palpation, percussion,* and *auscultation.*

- ★ *Inspection.* Inspection should include an examination of the anterior-posterior dimensions and general shape of the chest. An increased anterior-posterior diameter is suggestive of COPD. Inspect the chest for symmetrical movement. Any asymmetry may be suggestive of trauma. A paradoxical movement (moving in a fashion opposite to that expected) is suggestive of flail chest. Note any chest scars, lesions, wounds, or deformities.
- ★ *Palpation.* Palpate the chest, both front and back, for abnormalities. Note any tenderness, **crepitus,** or **subcutaneous emphysema.** Palpate the anterior chest first,

crepitus *crackling sounds.*

subcutaneous emphysema *presence of air in the subcutaneous tissue.*

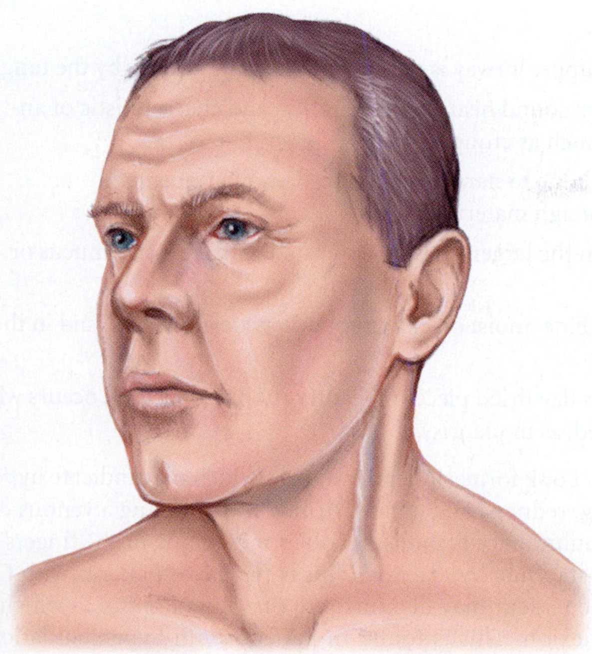

■ **Figure 27-4** Jugular vein distention.

then the posterior. Inspect your gloved hands for blood each time you remove them from behind the patient's chest. In some instances, it may be appropriate to evaluate **tactile fremitus,** the vibration felt in the chest during speaking. When evaluating tactile fremitus, compare one side of the chest with the other. Simultaneously, palpate the trachea for **tracheal deviation,** which is suggestive of a tension pneumothorax.

tactile fremitus *vibratory tremors felt through the chest by palpation.*

tracheal deviation *any position of the trachea other than midline.*

★ *Percussion.* If indicated, quickly percuss the chest. Limit percussion to suspected cases of pneumothorax and pulmonary edema. A hollow sound on percussion is often indicative of pneumothorax or emphysema. In contrast, a dull sound is indicative of pulmonary edema, hemothorax, or pneumonia. Remember, however, that percussion may be of little value in the noisy environment typical of most emergency scenes.

★ *Auscultation.* Auscultate the chest. Begin by listening to the patient without a stethoscope and from a distance. Note any loud stridor, wheezing, or cough. If possible, the patient should be in the sitting position and the chest auscultated in a symmetrical pattern. If the patient cannot sit up, auscultate the anterior and lateral parts of the chest. Each area should be auscultated for one respiratory cycle.

Normal breath sounds heard during auscultation can be characterized according to the following descriptions:

Normal Breath Sounds

★ Bronchial (or tubular)
  - Loud, high-pitched breath sounds heard over the trachea
  - Expiratory phase lasts longer than inspiratory phase

★ Bronchovesicular
  - Softer, medium-pitched breath sounds heard over the mainstem bronchi (below clavicles or between scapulae)
  - Expiratory phase and inspiratory phase equal

★ Vesicular
  - Soft, low-pitched breath sounds heard in the lung periphery

While the patient breathes in and out deeply with the mouth open, note any abnormal breath sounds and their location. Many terms are used to describe abnormal breath sounds. The following list includes some of the more common terms.

Abnormal Breath Sounds

- ★ *Snoring.* Occurs when the upper airway is partially obstructed, usually by the tongue.
- ★ *Stridor.* Harsh, high-pitched sound heard on inspiration and characteristic of an upper airway obstruction such as croup.
- ★ *Wheezing.* Whistling sound due to narrowing of the airways by edema, bronchoconstriction, or foreign materials.
- ★ *Rhonchi.* Rattling sounds in the larger airways associated with excessive mucus or other material.
- ★ *Crackles (also called rales).* Fine, moist crackling sounds associated with fluid in the smaller airways.
- ★ *Pleural friction rub.* Sounds like dried pieces of leather rubbing together; occurs when the pleura become inflamed, as in pleurisy.

Also examine the extremities. Look for peripheral cyanosis, which may indicate hypoxia. Examine the extremities for swelling, redness, and a hard, firm cord indicating a venous clot. This may suggest a possible cause for pulmonary embolism. Look for clubbing of the fingers (Figures 27-5a and b ■), suggesting long-standing hypoxemia. This is typical of patients with COPD or cyanotic heart disease. Finally, the patient may demonstrate *carpopedal spasm* in which the fingers and toes are contracted in flexion. This is found in patients with hyperventilation and is caused by transient shifts in the blood calcium concentration due to changes in the serum CO_2 and pH levels.

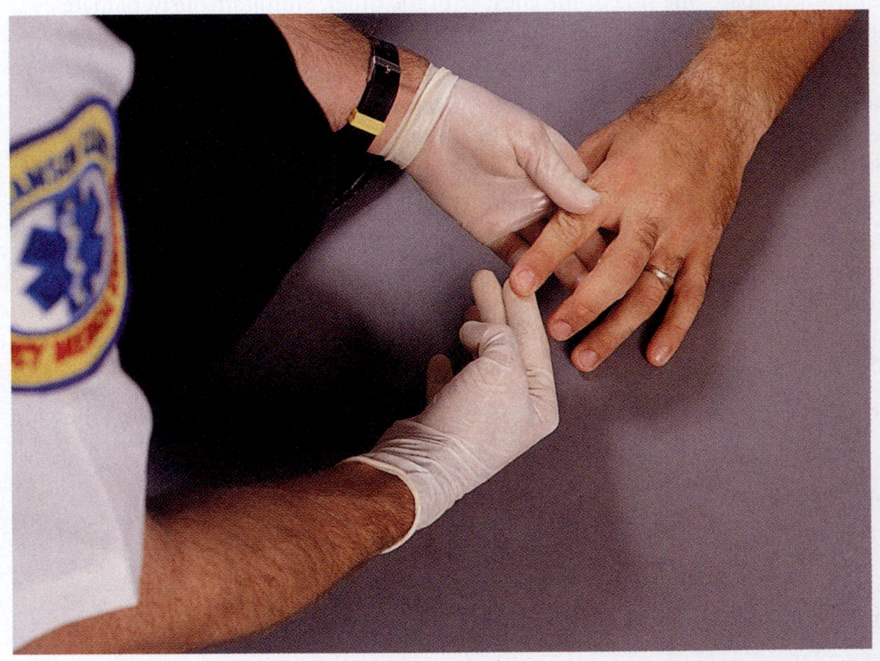

■ **Figure 27-5** (a) Inspect for finger clubbing. Any clubbing may indicate chronic respiratory or cardiac disease. (b) Characteristics of finger clubbing include large fingertips and a loss of the normal angle at the nail bed.

Vital Signs

The patient's vital signs may also provide information regarding the severity of the respiratory complaints. In general, tachycardia (rapid heart rate) is a very nonspecific finding, seen with fear, anxiety, and fever. In patients with respiratory complaints, however, tachycardia may also indicate hypoxia. Remember that the patient may have recently used sympathomimetic drugs such as albuterol, which will accelerate the heart rate. These same drugs will elevate the patient's blood pressure as well. During your assessment of the blood pressure, a patient will occasionally exhibit *pulsus paradoxus,* a drop in the systolic blood pressure of 10 mmHg or more with each respiratory cycle. Pulsus paradoxus is associated with COPD and cardiac tamponade. As a rule, however, you should not take the time to look for pulsus paradoxus.

A change in a patient's respiratory rate may be one of the earliest indicators of respiratory disease. The patient's respiratory rate can be influenced by several factors, including respiratory difficulty, fear, anxiety, fever, and underlying metabolic disease. Assume that an elevated respiratory rate in a patient with dyspnea is caused by hypoxia. Although fluctuations in the respiratory rate are common, a persistently *slow* rate indicates impending respiratory arrest.

Assume that an elevated respiratory rate in a patient with dyspnea is caused by hypoxia. A persistently slow rate indicates impending respiratory arrest.

Continually reassess the patient's respiratory rate during the time that you are caring for the patient. Trends in the respiratory rate (for example, an increasing rate) can give you an overall assessment of the effectiveness of any intervention you have made. Also assess the patient's respiratory pattern. The normal respiratory pattern (eupnea) is steady, even breaths occurring 12 to 20 times per minute with an expiratory phase that lasts between three to four times the inspiratory phase. **Tachypnea** describes a respiratory pattern with a rate that exceeds 20 breaths per minute. **Bradypnea** describes a respiratory pattern with a rate slower than 12 breaths per minute. Look also for any abnormal respiratory patterns (e.g., Cheyne-Stokes, Kussmaul's, or other) as discussed earlier in the chapter.

tachypnea *rapid respiration.*

bradypnea *slow respiration.*

Constantly reassess the patient's respiratory rate and pattern.

Diagnostic Testing

Three diagnostic measurements are of value in assessing the patient's respiratory status: *pulse oximetry, peak flow,* and *capnography.*

Content Review

Prehospital Diagnostic Tests

- Pulse oximetry
- Peak flow
- Capnography

Pulse Oximetry Pulse oximetry offers a rapid and accurate means for assessing oxygen saturation. The pulse oximeter can be quickly applied to a finger or earlobe. The pulse rate and oxygen saturation can be continuously recorded (Figure 27-6 ■).

Pulse oximeter probes contain two light-emitting diodes (LEDs). One diode emits light in the red (660 nm) range and the other emits light in the infrared (940 nm) range. Photodetectors on the opposite side of the probe detect the two wavelengths of light that penetrate the tissues. Deoxyhemoglobin absorbs more red light than does oxyhemoglobin; oxyhemoglobin absorbs more infrared light

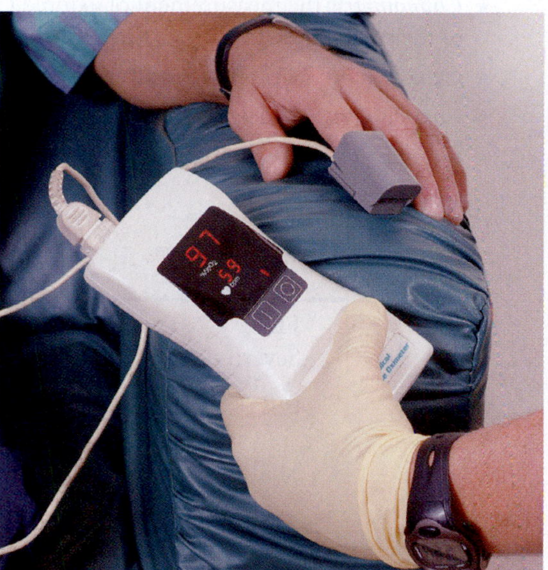

■ Figure 27-6 Sensing unit for pulse oximetry. This device transmits light through a vascular bed, such as in the finger, and can determine the oxygen saturation of red blood cells. To use the pulse oximeter, it is only necessary to turn the device on and attach the sensor to a finger. The desired graphic mode on the oximeter should be selected. The oxygen saturation and pulse rate can be continuously monitored.

■ Figure 27-7 Wright spirometer for determining peak expiratory flow rate (PEFR).

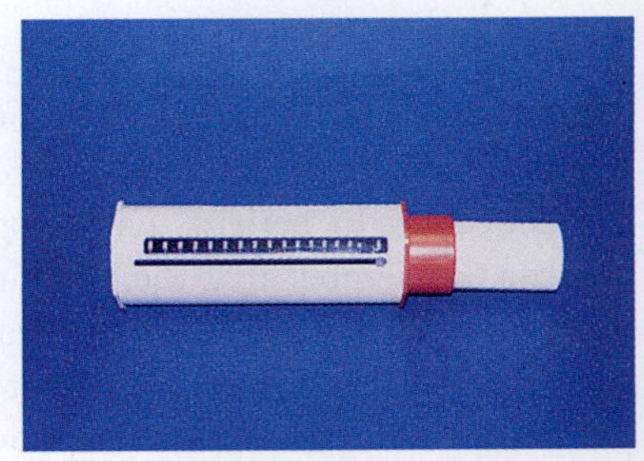

than red light. The ratio of the two types of absorbed light is calculated by the oximeter and compared against standardized values. The concentration of oxyhemoglobin (and thus oxygen saturation) is displayed as a percentage called the hemoglobin oxygen saturation. The oxygen saturation measurement obtained through pulse oximetry is abbreviated as SpO_2. Oxygen saturations obtained through blood gas analysis in hospitals are abbreviated SaO_2. Normally, the SpO_2 and SaO_2 are the same. Older pulse oximeters were prone to give abnormal or inconsistent readings in patients with peripheral vasoconstriction (as in sepsis or hypothermia). They may also be inaccurate under conditions in which an abnormal substance such as carbon monoxide binds to hemoglobin, since the instrument measures the saturation of hemoglobin without indicating what substance has saturated it. Fortunately, second-generation pulse oximeters have technology (filters, signal processors) that minimizes these effects, making them more accurate and much less sensitive to extraneous factors.

Peak Flow Handheld devices are available for use in determining the patient's peak expiratory flow rate (PEFR). The normal expected peak flow rate is based on the patient's sex, age, and height. Remember that the measurement of the peak expiratory flow rate is somewhat effort dependent; you must have a cooperative patient who understands the use of the device to get an accurate reading.

The PEFR is obtained using a Wright spirometer (Figure 27-7 ■), which is inexpensive and easy to use. Place the disposable mouthpiece into the meter. First have the patient take in the deepest possible inspiration. Then encourage the patient to seal his lips around the device and forcibly exhale. The peak rate of exhaled gas is recorded in liters per minute. This should be repeated twice, with the highest reading recorded as the patient's PEFR (Table 27–1).

Capnography As discussed in Chapter 8, "Airway Management and Ventilation," capnography has become a commonly used diagnostic tool for prehospital care. End-tidal carbon dioxide ($ETCO_2$) monitoring is a noninvasive method of measuring the levels of carbon dioxide (CO_2) in the exhaled breath.

The following terms have been applied to capnography:

- *Capnometry:* the measurement of expired CO_2 (It typically provides a numeric display of the partial pressure of CO_2 [in torr or mmHg] or the percentage of CO_2 present.)
- *Capnography:* a graphic recording or display of the capnometry reading over time
- *Capnograph:* a device that measures expired CO_2 levels
- *Capnogram:* the visual representation of the expired CO_2 waveform

Table 27–1 Spirometry and Peak Flow Values for Adults

FEV_1 Severity	FEV_1 (Liters)	FVC (%)	Peak Flow (Liters/Min)
Normal	4.0–6.0 L	80–90%	550–650 (Male) 400–500 (Female)
Mild	3.0 L	70%	300–400
Moderate	1.6 L	50%	200–300
Severe	0.6 L	40%	100

★ *End-tidal CO_2 ($ETCO_2$):* the measurement of the CO_2 concentration at the end of expiration (maximum CO_2)

★ *$PETCO_2$:* the partial pressure of end-tidal CO_2 in a mixed gas solution

★ *$PaCO_2$:* the partial pressure of CO_2 in the arterial blood

CO_2, a normal end product of metabolism, is transported by the venous system to the right side of the heart. It is then pumped from the right ventricle to the pulmonary artery and eventually enters the pulmonary capillaries. There it diffuses into the alveoli and is removed from the body through exhalation. When circulation is normal, $ETCO_2$ levels change with ventilation and are a reliable estimate of the partial pressure of carbon dioxide in the arterial system ($PaCO_2$). Normal $ETCO_2$ is 1–2 mm less than the partial pressure of carbon dioxide ($PaCO_2$), or approximately 5 percent. A normal partial pressure of end-tidal CO_2 ($PETCO_2$) is approximately 38 mmHg (0.05×760 mmHg = 38 mmHg). ($ETCO_2$ is normally expressed as a percentage, while $PETCO_2$, a partial pressure, is expressed in mmHg.) When perfusion decreases, as in shock or cardiac arrest, $ETCO_2$ levels reflect pulmonary blood flow and cardiac output, not ventilation.

Decreased $ETCO_2$ levels can be found in shock, cardiac arrest, pulmonary embolism, bronchospasm, and with incomplete airway obstruction (such as mucous plugging). Increased $ETCO_2$ levels are found with hypoventilation, respiratory depression, and hyperthermia (Table 27–2).

Table 27–2 Basic Rules of Capnography

Symptom	Possible Cause
Sudden drop of $ETCO_2$ to zero	• Esophageal intubation • Ventilator disconnection or defect in ventilator • Defect in CO_2 analyzer
Sudden decrease of $ETCO_2$ (not to zero)	• Leak in ventilator system; obstruction • Partial disconnect in ventilator circuit • Partial airway obstruction (secretions)
Exponential decrease of $ETCO_2$	• Pulmonary embolism • Cardiac arrest • Hypotension (sudden) • Severe hyperventilation
Change in CO_2 baseline	• Calibration error • Water droplet in analyzer • Mechanical failure (ventilator)
Sudden increase in $ETCO_2$	• Accessing an area of lung previously obstructed • Release of tourniquet • Sudden increase in blood pressure
Gradual lowering of $ETCO_2$	• Hypovolemia • Decreasing cardiac output • Decreasing body temperature; hypothermia; drop in metabolism
Gradual increase in $ETCO_2$	• Rising body temperature • Hypoventilation • CO_2 absorption • Partial airway obstruction (foreign body); reactive airway disease

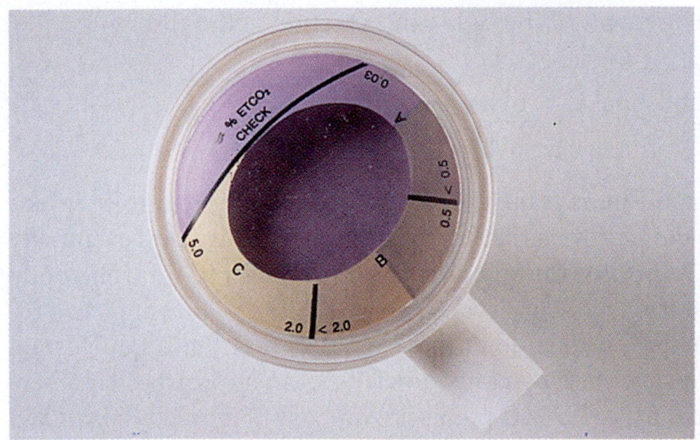

■ **Figure 27-8** Colorimetric end-tidal CO_2 detector. *(© Scott Metcalfe)*

Capnometry provides a noninvasive measure of $ETCO_2$ levels, thus providing medical personnel with information about the status of systemic metabolism, circulation, and ventilation. The use of capnography has become commonplace in the operating room, emergency department, and prehospital setting.

When first introduced into prehospital care, $ETCO_2$ monitoring was used exclusively to verify proper endotracheal tube placement in the trachea. The presence of adequate CO_2 levels following intubation confirms the tube is in the trachea through the presence of exhaled CO_2. CO_2 is detected by using either a colorimetric or an infrared device.

Colorimetric Devices The colorimetric device is a disposable $ETCO_2$ detector that contains pH-sensitive, chemically impregnated paper encased within a plastic chamber (Figure 27-8 ■). It is placed in the airway circuit between the patient and the ventilation device. When the paper is exposed to CO_2, hydrogen ions (H^+) are generated, causing a color change in the paper. The color change is reversible and changes breath to breath. A color scale on the device estimates the $ETCO_2$ level. Colorimetric devices cannot detect hypercarbia or hypocarbia (increased or decreased CO_2 levels). If gastric contents or acidic drugs (e.g., endotracheal epinephrine) contact the paper in the device, subsequent readings may be unreliable.

Electronic Devices Electronic $ETCO_2$ detectors use an infrared technique to detect CO_2 in the exhaled breath (Figure 27-9 ■). A heated element in the sensor generates infrared radiation. The CO_2 molecules absorb infrared light at a very specific wavelength and can thus be measured. Electronic $ETCO_2$ detectors may be either qualitative (i.e., they simply detect the presence of CO_2) or quantitative (i.e., they determine how much CO_2 is present). Quantitative devices are now routinely used in prehospital care. Most can provide a digital waveform (capnogram) that reflects the entire respiratory cycle (Figure 27-10 ■).

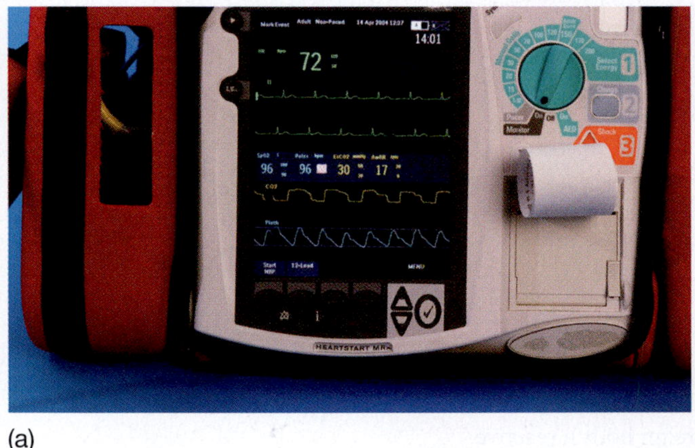

(a)

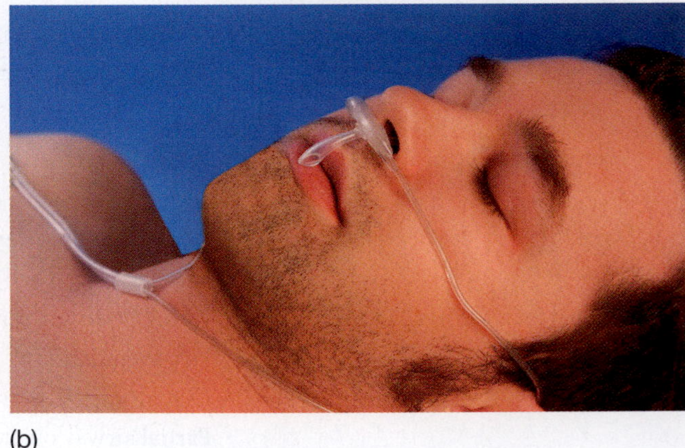

(b)

■ **Figure 27-9** (a) Electronic end-tidal CO_2 detector. (b) Electronic end-tidal CO_2 detector on a patient. *(© Scott Metcalfe)*

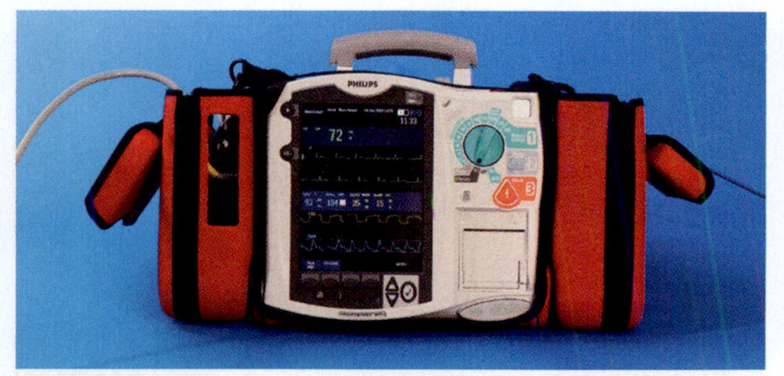

■ **Figure 27-10** Most quantitative electronic $ETCO_2$ detectors can provide a digital waveform (capnogram) that reflects the entire respiratory cycle. *(© Scott Metcalfe)*

Capnogram The capnogram reflects CO_2 concentrations over time. It is typically divided into four phases (Figure 27-11 ■).

★ *Phase I* (AB in Figure 27-11) is the respiratory baseline. It is flat when no CO_2 is present and corresponds to the late phase of inspiration and the early part of expiration (in which dead-space gases without CO_2 are released).

★ *Phase II* (BC in Figure 27-11) is the respiratory upstroke. This reflects the appearance of CO_2 in the alveoli.

★ *Phase III* (CD in Figure 27-11) is the respiratory plateau. It reflects the air flow through uniformly ventilated alveoli with a nearly constant CO_2 level. The highest level of the plateau (point D in Figure 27-11) is called the $ETCO_2$ and is recorded as such by the capnometer.

★ *Phase IV* (DE in Figure 27-11) is the inspiratory phase. It is a sudden downstroke and ultimately returns to the baseline during inspiration. The respiratory pause restarts the cycle (EA in Figure 27-11).

Clinical Applications Initially, as noted earlier, $ETCO_2$ detection was used only to determine proper endotracheal tube placement. Typically, a qualitative $ETCO_2$ device was applied to the airway circuit following intubation. If $ETCO_2$ levels were detected, then proper tube placement was verified. However, it is difficult to continuously monitor the airway with a quantitative device. Now, continuous waveform capnography is available and allows continuous monitoring of airway placement and ventilation for intubated patients. Continuous waveform capnography also has utility in monitoring nonintubated patients. By following trends in the capnogram, prehospital personnel can continuously monitor the patient's condition, detect trends, and document the response to medications.

$ETCO_2$ detection is also useful in CPR. During cardiac arrest, CO_2 levels fall abruptly following the onset of cardiac arrest. They begin to rise with the onset of effective CPR and return to near-normal levels with a return of spontaneous circulation. During effective CPR, $ETCO_2$ levels have been found to correlate well with cardiac output, coronary perfusion pressure, and even with the effectiveness of CPR compressions.

Continuous waveform capnography is rapidly becoming a standard of care in EMS (Figure 27-12 ■). Misplaced endotracheal tubes represent a significant area of liability in EMS and the

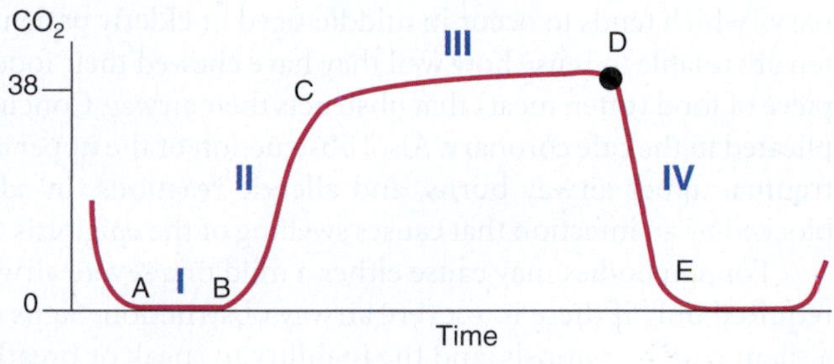

■ **Figure 27-11** Normal capnogram. AB = *Phase I:* late inspiration, early expiration (no CO_2). BC = *Phase II:* appearance of CO_2 in exhaled gas. CD = *Phase III:* plateau (constant CO_2). D = highest point ($ETCO_2$). DE = *Phase IV:* rapid descent during inspiration. EA = respiratory pause.

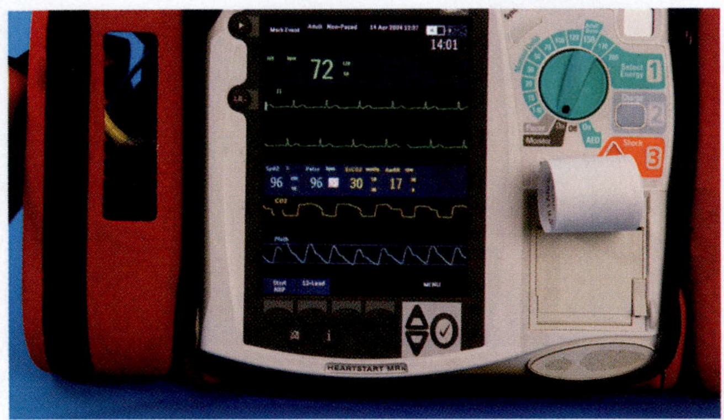

■ Figure 27-12 Continuous waveform capnography. (© Scott Metcalfe)

documentation provided by this technology can provide irrefutable evidence of proper endotracheal tube placement.

MANAGEMENT OF RESPIRATORY DISORDERS

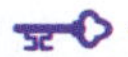

Principles of management for respiratory disorders include (1) give first priority to the airway, and (2) always provide oxygen to patients with respiratory distress or the possibility of hypoxia, including patients with COPD.

The following sections will address the pathophysiology, assessment, and management of the more common respiratory disorders encountered in prehospital care. The discussion begins with a look at general principles that can and should be applied to all respiratory emergencies.

In cases of acute respiratory insufficiency, the following principles should guide your actions in the prehospital setting:

★ The airway always has first priority. In trauma victims who may have associated cervical spine injuries, protect and maintain the airway without extending the neck.

★ Any patient with respiratory distress should receive oxygen.

★ Any patient whose illness or injury suggests the possibility of hypoxia should receive oxygen.

★ If there is a question whether oxygen should be given, as in COPD, administer it. *Oxygen should never be withheld from a patient suspected of suffering hypoxia.*

Keep these precautions in mind as you read through the descriptions of pathophysiology, assessment, and management of respiratory disorders frequently encountered in the field.

SPECIFIC RESPIRATORY DISEASES

UPPER AIRWAY OBSTRUCTION

Content Review

Common Causes of Airway Obstruction

- Tongue
- Foreign matter
- Trauma
- Burns
- Allergic reaction
- Infection

The most common cause of upper airway obstruction is the relaxed tongue. In an unconscious patient in the supine position, the tongue can fall into the back of the throat and obstruct the upper airway. Additionally, the upper airway can become obstructed by such common materials as food, dentures, or other foreign bodies. A typical example of upper airway obstruction is the "cafe coronary," which tends to occur in middle-aged or elderly patients who wear dentures. These people often are unable to sense how well they have chewed their food. Thus, they accidentally inhale a large piece of food (often meat) that obstructs their airway. Concurrent alcohol consumption is often implicated in the cafe coronary. Also, obstruction of the upper airway can be the result of facial or neck trauma, upper airway burns, and allergic reactions. In addition, the upper airway can become blocked by an infection that causes swelling of the epiglottis (epiglottitis) or subglottic area (croup).

Foreign bodies may cause either a mild or a severe airway obstruction. Intervention is usually required only if there is a severe airway obstruction. Signs of a severe airway obstruction include a silent cough, cyanosis, and the inability to speak or breathe. If the patient is conscious ask, "Are you choking?" If the victim indicates yes (by nodding the head) without speaking, you should assume the obstruction is severe.

Assessment

Assessment of the patient with an upper airway obstruction varies, depending on the cause of the obstruction and the history of the event. The unresponsive patient should be evaluated for snoring respirations, possibly indicating tongue or denture obstruction. If confronted by a patient suffering a cafe coronary, determine whether the victim can speak. Speech indicates that, at present, the obstruction is incomplete. If the victim is unresponsive and has been eating, strongly suspect a food bolus lodged in the trachea. If a burn is present or suspected, assume laryngeal edema until proven otherwise.

Patients who may be having an allergic reaction to food or medications will often report an itching sensation in the palate followed by a "lump" in the throat. The situation may progress to hoarseness, inspiratory stridor, and complete obstruction. Pay particular attention to the presence of urticaria (hives). Intercostal muscle retraction and use of the strap muscles of the neck for breathing suggest attempts to ventilate against a partially closed airway.

Capnography can be useful in identifying upper airway obstruction. Generally, depending on the degree of upper airway obstruction, you will see a steady increase in $ETCO_2$ levels.

Management

Management of the obstructed airway is based on the nature of the obstruction. Blockage by the tongue can be corrected by opening the airway, using the head-tilt/chin-lift, the jaw-thrust, or the modified jaw-thrust maneuver. The airway can be maintained by employing either a nasopharyngeal or oropharyngeal airway. If possible, remove obstructing foreign bodies using the following basic airway maneuvers:

Conscious Adult In an adult patient (or child >1 year of age) who is conscious:

1. Determine if there is a complete obstruction or poor air exchange. Ask the patient: "Are you choking?" "Can you speak?" If the patient can speak, he should be asked to produce a forceful cough to expel the foreign body.
2. If the patient has a severe obstruction or poor air exchange, provide rapid abdominal thrusts until the obstruction is relieved. If abdominal thrusts are ineffective (or if the patient is obese), attempt chest thrusts. Also, if the patient is pregnant, omit the abdominal thrusts and proceed straight to the chest thrusts. Often, more than one technique is required. These should be applied in rapid sequence until the obstruction is relieved.

Unconscious Adult If the patient is unconscious or loses consciousness:

1. Use the head-tilt/chin-lift, or the jaw-thrust without head extension in an attempt to open the airway.
2. Begin CPR.
3. Every time you open the airway to begin ventilations, look for and remove any foreign objects seen in the oropharynx.
4. If the obstruction persists and ventilation cannot be provided, visualize the airway with the laryngoscope. If you can see the foreign body, grasp it with the Magill forceps and remove. After it is removed, begin ventilation and administer supplemental oxygen.

In cases of airway obstruction caused by laryngeal edema (e.g., anaphylactic reactions, angioedema), establish the airway by the head-tilt/chin-lift, the jaw-thrust, or the jaw-thrust without head extension. Then administer supplemental oxygen. Attempt bag-valve-mask ventilation. Often, air can be forced past the obstruction and the patient adequately ventilated using this technique. Next, start an IV with a crystalloid solution and administer subcutaneous epinephrine. Then administer diphenhydramine (Benadryl). Transtracheal ventilation may be required if the patient does not respond to the treatments described.

See Chapter 42, "Pediatrics," for pediatric techniques.

NONCARDIOGENIC PULMONARY EDEMA/ ADULT RESPIRATORY DISTRESS SYNDROME

adult respiratory distress syndrome (ARDS) *form of pulmonary edema that is caused by fluid accumulation in the interstitial space within the lungs.*

Adult respiratory distress syndrome (ARDS) is a form of pulmonary edema that is caused by fluid accumulation in the interstitial space within the lungs. Patients with *cardiogenic* pulmonary edema have a poorly functioning left ventricle. This leads to increases in hydrostatic pressure and fluid accumulation in the interstitial space. In patients with ARDS, however, fluid accumulation occurs as the result of increased vascular permeability and decreased fluid removal from the lung tissue. This occurs in response to a wide variety of lung insults including:

- ★ Sepsis, particularly with gram-negative organisms
- ★ Aspiration
- ★ Pneumonia or other respiratory infections
- ★ Pulmonary injury
- ★ Burns
- ★ Inhalation injury
- ★ Oxygen toxicity
- ★ Drugs such as aspirin or opiates
- ★ High altitude
- ★ Hypothermia
- ★ Near-drowning
- ★ Head injury
- ★ Emboli from blood clot, fat, or amniotic fluid
- ★ Tumor destruction
- ★ Pancreatitis
- ★ Procedures such as cardiopulmonary bypass or hemodialysis
- ★ Other insults such as hypoxia, hypotension, or cardiac arrest

The mortality in patients who develop ARDS is quite high, approaching 70 percent. While many patients die as the result of respiratory failure, many succumb to failure of several organ systems, including the liver and kidneys.

Pathophysiology

ARDS is a disorder of lung diffusion that results from increased fluid in the interstitial space. Each of the underlying conditions cited previously results in the inability to maintain a proper fluid balance in the interstitial space. Severe hypotension, significant hypoxemia as the result of cardiac arrest, drowning, seizure activity or hypoventilation, high altitude exposure, environmental toxins, and endotoxins released in septic shock all can cause disruption of the alveolar-capillary membrane. Increases in pulmonary capillary permeability, destruction of the capillary lining, and increases in osmotic forces act to draw fluid into the interstitial space and contribute to interstitial edema. This increases the thickness of the respiratory membrane and limits diffusion of oxygen. In advanced cases, fluid also accumulates in the alveoli, causing loss of surfactant, collapse of the alveolar sacs, and impaired gas exchange. This results in a significant amount of pulmonary shunting with unoxygenated blood returning to the circulation. The result is significant hypoxia.

Assessment

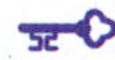

With ARDS, symptoms are related to the underlying cause.

Specific clinical symptoms are related to the underlying cause of ARDS. For example, patients who develop ARDS as the result of sepsis will have symptoms related to their underlying infection. Determine if there is a history of prolonged hypoxia, head or chest trauma, inhalation of gases, or ascent to a high altitude without prior acclimation, all of which can suggest an underlying cause for the respiratory complaints.

Patients with ARDS experience a gradual decline in their respiratory status. In rare cases, a seemingly healthy patient has a sudden onset of respiratory failure and hypoxia. Such a presentation is characteristic of patients with high altitude pulmonary edema (HAPE).

Dyspnea, confusion, and agitation are often found in patients with noncardiogenic pulmonary edema. Patients may also report fatigue and reduced exercise ability. Symptoms such as orthopnea, paroxysmal nocturnal dyspnea, or sputum production are not commonly reported but may be seen.

The prominent physical findings are generally those associated with the underlying lung insult. Tachypnea and tachycardia are often found in association with ARDS. Crackles (rales) are audible in both lungs. Wheezing may also be heard if there is any element of bronchospasm. Severe tachypnea, central cyanosis, and signs of imminent respiratory failure are seen in severe cases. Pulse oximetry will demonstrate low oxygen saturations in those patients with advanced disease. In those patients requiring ventilatory support, a decreased lung compliance will be noted. (It will require more operator force to deliver an adequate lung volume.)

Management

Specific management of the patient's underlying medical condition is the hallmark of treatment for this disorder. Treatment of gram-negative sepsis with appropriate antibiotics, removal of the patient from any inciting toxin, or rapid descent to a lower altitude in patients with HAPE are the most important therapies for this condition. The patient will usually tolerate an upright position with the legs dangling off the cart.

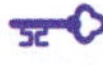

Management of the patient's underlying medical condition is the hallmark of treatment for ARDS.

Since the hypoxia seen in ARDS is the result of diffusion defects, oxygen supplementation is essential for all patients with this condition. Establish intravenous access, but provide fluids only if hypovolemia exists. Establish cardiac monitoring. Suctioning of lung secretions is often required to maintain airway patency.

Oxygen supplementation is essential for all ARDS patients.

Use positive-pressure ventilation to support any ARDS patient who demonstrates signs of respiratory failure. Use bag-valve-mask ventilation for initial respiratory support while preparing a CPAP device. Use of CPAP can often avoid the need for endotracheal intubation and mechanical ventilation. **Positive end-expiratory pressure (PEEP)**, via CPAP, is often required to maintain patency of the alveoli and adequate oxygenation. Diuretics and nitrates, which are used in patients with cardiogenic pulmonary edema, are usually not helpful in patients with ARDS. Your medical director may occasionally order corticosteroids for patients with ARDS/noncardiogenic pulmonary edema. Corticosteroids are thought to stabilize the alveolar-capillary membrane, although clinical studies have not demonstrated any benefit to their use.

positive end-expiratory pressure (PEEP) *a method of holding the alveoli open by increasing expiratory pressure. Some bag-valve units used in EMS have PEEP attachments. EMS personnel also sometimes transport patients who are on ventilators with PEEP attachments.*

Maintain cardiac monitoring and pulse oximetry throughout transport of the patient. Transport patients to a facility capable of advanced hemodynamic monitoring (including Swan-Ganz catheter) and mechanical ventilation support.

OBSTRUCTIVE LUNG DISEASE

Obstructive lung disease is widespread in our society. The most common obstructive lung diseases encountered in prehospital care are asthma, emphysema, and chronic bronchitis (the last two are often discussed together as chronic obstructive pulmonary disease, or COPD). Asthma afflicts 4 to 5 percent of the U.S. population and COPD is found in 25 percent of all adults. Chronic bronchitis alone affects one in five adult males. Patients with COPD have a 50 percent mortality within 10 years of the diagnosis.

Content Review

Obstructive Lung Diseases

- Emphysema
- Chronic bronchitis
- Asthma

Although asthma may have a genetic predisposition, COPD is known to be directly caused by cigarette smoking and environmental toxins. Other factors have been shown to precipitate symptoms in patients who already have obstructive airway disease. Intrinsic factors include stress, upper respiratory infections, and exercise. Extrinsic factors include tobacco smoke, drugs, occupational hazards (chemical fumes, dust, and others), and allergens such as foods, animal danders, dusts, and molds.

Obstructive lung diseases all have abnormal ventilation as a common feature. This abnormal ventilation is a result of obstruction that occurs primarily in the bronchioles. Several changes occur within these air conduits. Bronchospasm (sustained smooth muscle contraction) occurs, which may be reversed by beta-adrenergic receptor stimulation. Agents such as terbutaline, albuterol, levalbuterol, and epinephrine are used to accomplish this stimulation. Increased mucus production by goblet cells that line the respiratory tree also contribute to obstruction. This effect may be worsened by the fact that in many patients, the cilia are destroyed, resulting in poor clearance of excess mucus. Finally, inflammation of the bronchial passages results in the accumulation of fluid and inflammatory cells. Depending on the underlying cause, some elements of bronchial obstruction are reversible, whereas others are not. Ipratropium (Atrovent), a parasympathetic blocker, may aid in drying of bronchial secretions and in reversing bronchospasm.

During inspiration, the bronchioles will naturally dilate, allowing air to be drawn into the alveoli. As the patient begins to exhale, the bronchioles constrict. When this natural constriction occurs—in addition to the underlying bronchospasm, increased mucus production, and inflammation that exist in patients with obstructive airway disease—the result is significant air trapping distal to the obstruction. This is one of the hallmarks of obstructive lung disease. This section will discuss each of these disease processes—emphysema, chronic bronchitis, and asthma—detailing the pathophysiology, assessment, and treatment.

EMPHYSEMA

Emphysema results from destruction of the alveolar walls distal to the terminal bronchioles. It is more common in men than in women. The major factor contributing to emphysema in our society is cigarette smoking. Significant exposure to environmental toxins is another contributing factor.

Pathophysiology

Continued exposure to noxious substances, such as cigarette smoke, results in the gradual destruction of the walls of the alveoli. This process decreases the alveolar membrane surface area, thus lessening the area available for gas exchange. The progressive loss of the respiratory membrane results in an increased ratio of air to lung tissue. The result is diffusion defects. Additionally, the number of pulmonary capillaries in the lung is decreased, thus increasing resistance to pulmonary blood flow. This condition ultimately causes pulmonary hypertension, which in turn may lead to right-heart failure, **cor pulmonale,** and death (Figure 27-13 ■).

cor pulmonale *hypertrophy of the right ventricle resulting from disorders of the lung.*

Emphysema also causes weakening of the walls of the small bronchioles. When the walls of the alveoli and small bronchioles are destroyed, the lungs lose their capacity to recoil and air becomes trapped in the lungs. Thus, residual volume increases while vital capacity remains relatively normal. The destroyed lung tissue (called *blebs*) results in alveolar collapse. To counteract this effect, patients

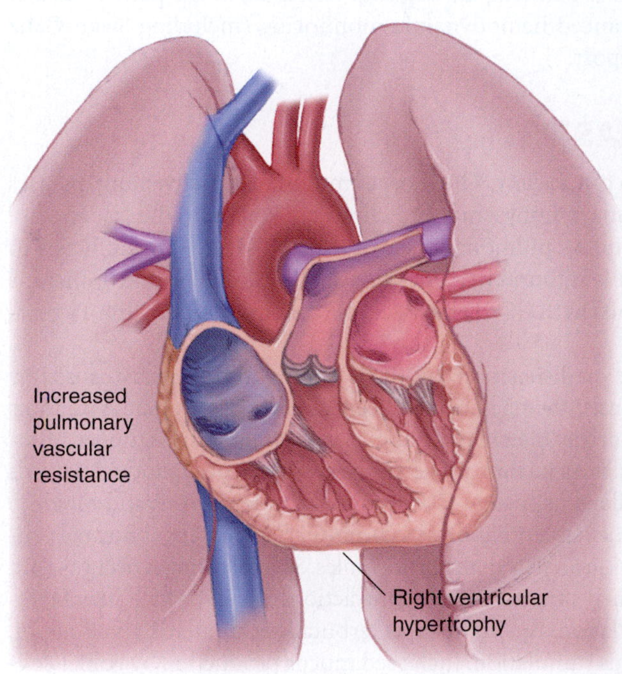

■ Figure 27-13 Chronic obstructive pulmonary disease of long standing can cause pulmonary hypertension, which in turn may lead to cor pulmonale.

tend to breathe through pursed lips. This creates continued positive pressure similar to PEEP and prevents alveolar collapse.

As the disease progresses, the PaO_2 further decreases, which may lead to increased red blood cell production and **polycythemia** (an excess of red blood cells resulting in an abnormally high hematocrit). The $PaCO_2$ also increases and becomes chronically elevated, forcing the body to depend on hypoxic drive to control respirations. Finally, remember that emphysema is characterized by irreversible airway obstruction.

polycythemia *an excess of red blood cells.*

Patients with emphysema are more susceptible to acute respiratory infections, such as pneumonia, and to cardiac dysrhythmias. Chronic emphysema patients ultimately become dependent on bronchodilators, corticosteroids, and, in the final stages, supplemental oxygen.

Assessment

The patient with emphysema may report a history of recent weight loss, increased dyspnea on exertion, and progressive limitation of physical activity. Unlike chronic bronchitis, discussed in subsequent sections, emphysema is rarely associated with a cough, except in the morning. Question the patient about cigarette and tobacco usage. This is generally reported in pack/years. Ask the number of cigarette packs (20 cigarettes/pack) smoked per day and the number of years the patient has smoked. Multiply the number of packs smoked per day by the number of years. For example, a man who has smoked 2 packs per day for 15 years would have a 30 pack/year smoking history. Medical problems related to smoking, such as emphysema, chronic bronchitis, and lung cancer, usually begin after a patient surpasses a 20 pack/year history, although this can vary significantly.

Emphysema is rarely associated with a cough except in the morning.

Physical exam of the emphysema patient usually reveals a barrel chest evidenced by an increase in the anterior/posterior chest diameter. You may also note decreased chest excursion with a prolonged expiratory phase and a rapid resting respiratory rate. Patients with emphysema are often thin since they must use a significant amount of their caloric intake for respiration. They tend to be pink in color due to polycythemia (excess of red blood cells) and are referred to as "pink puffers." Emphysema patients often have hypertrophy of the accessory respiratory muscles (Figure 27-14 ■).

Emphysema patients usually have a barrel chest, are often thin, and have a pink color ("pink puffers").

The patient will often involuntarily purse his lips to create continuous positive airway pressure. Clubbing of the fingers is common. Breath sounds are usually diminished. Wheezes and rhonchi

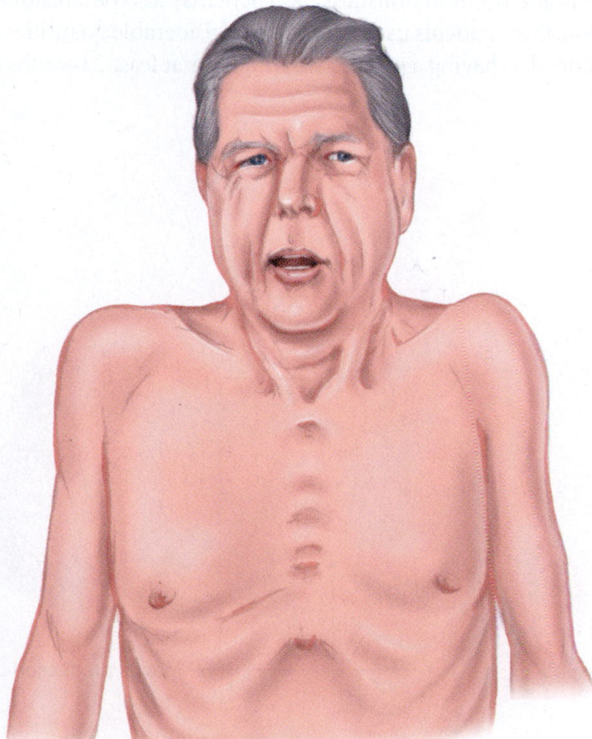

■ **Figure 27-14** Typical appearance of patient with emphysema. There are well-developed accessory muscles and suprasternal retraction.

may or may not be present, depending on the amount of obstruction to air flow. The patient may exhibit signs of right-heart failure as evidenced by jugular vein distention, peripheral edema, and hepatic congestion. Signs of severe respiratory impairment in all patients with obstructive lung disease include confusion, agitation, somnolence, one-to-two-word dyspnea, and use of accessory muscles to assist ventilation.

Management

Although emphysema differs in the disease process from chronic bronchitis, the two respiratory disorders share several of the same symptoms and pathophysiology. As a result, you will treat the two disorders in a similar manner. The discussion of management of emphysema will be taken up with chronic bronchitis in the following section.

CHRONIC BRONCHITIS

Chronic bronchitis results from an increase in the number of the goblet (mucus-secreting) cells in the respiratory tree (Figure 27-15 ■). It is characterized by the production of a large quantity of sputum. This often occurs after prolonged exposure to cigarette smoke.

Pathophysiology

Unlike emphysema, in chronic bronchitis the alveoli are not severely affected and diffusion remains normal. Gas exchange is decreased because of the lowered alveolar ventilation, which ultimately results in hypoxia and hypercarbia. Hypoxia may increase red blood cell production, which in turn leads to polycythemia (as occurs in emphysema). Increased $PaCO_2$ levels may lead to irritability, somnolence, decreased intellectual abilities, headaches, and personality changes. Physiologically, an increased $PaCO_2$ causes pulmonary vasoconstriction, resulting in pulmonary hypertension and, eventually, cor pulmonale. Unlike emphysema, the vital capacity is decreased, while the residual volume is normal or decreased.

Assessment

Chronic bronchitis is usually associated with a productive cough and copious sputum production.

The patient with chronic bronchitis often will have a history of heavy cigarette smoking, but the disease may also occur in nonsmokers. There may also be a history of frequent respiratory infections. In addition, these patients usually produce considerable quantities of sputum daily. Clinically, the patient is described as having a productive cough for at least 2 months per year for 2 or more consecutive years.

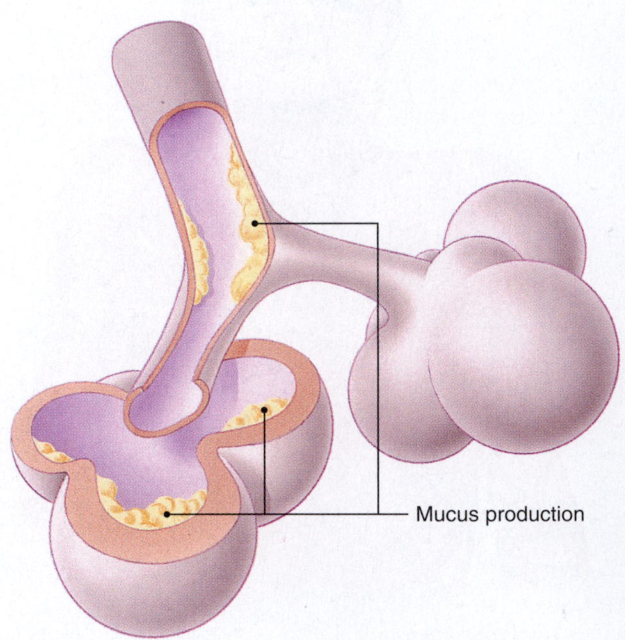

■ **Figure 27-15** Chronic mucus production and plugging of the airways occur in chronic bronchitis.

Patients with chronic bronchitis tend to be overweight and can be cyanotic. Because of this, they are often referred to as "blue bloaters." This can be contrasted with the "pink puffer" image of emphysema patients just described. Auscultation of the thorax often will reveal rhonchi due to occlusion of the larger airways with mucus plugs. The patient may also exhibit signs and symptoms of right-heart failure such as jugular vein distention, ankle edema, and hepatic congestion.

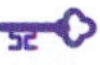

Chronic bronchitis patients tend to be overweight and are often cyanotic ("blue bloaters").

Management

The primary goals in the emergency management of the patient with either emphysema or chronic bronchitis are to relieve hypoxia and reverse any bronchoconstriction that may be present. However, many of these patients are dependent on hypoxic respiratory drive. As a result, the supplemental administration of oxygen may decrease respiratory drive and inhibit ventilation. You must continually monitor the patient and be prepared to assist ventilations if signs of respiratory depression develop.

The first step in treating a patient suffering an exacerbation of emphysema or chronic bronchitis is to establish an airway. Then place the patient in a seated or semiseated position to assist the accessory respiratory muscles. Apply a pulse oximeter and determine the blood oxygen saturation (SpO_2). Administer supplemental oxygen at a low flow rate while maintaining an oxygen saturation above 90 percent. A nasal cannula can often be used, but you must constantly monitor the respiratory rate and depth as well as oxygen saturation. Alternatively, you may use a Venturi mask at a low concentration (24 to 35 percent). If hypoxia or respiratory failure is evident, then increase the concentration of delivered oxygen. Be prepared to support the ventilation with bag-valve-mask assistance. CPAP may prove beneficial in COPD and can, in some instances, prevent the need for endotracheal intubation. It is best to keep PEEP pressures <10 cm/H_2O to avoid possible barotraumas. Regardless, intubation may be required if CPAP fails and respiratory failure is imminent.

Establish an intravenous line with lactated Ringer's or normal saline at a "to keep open" rate. More aggressive fluid administration is suggested if there are signs of dehydration present. This may also aid in loosening thick mucus secretions. Then, if ordered by medical direction, administer a bronchodilator medication, such as albuterol, levalbuterol, metaproterenol, or ipratropium bromide, through a small-volume nebulizer. Consider the addition of ipratropium bromide (Atrovent) during the initial nebulizer treatment. Corticosteroids are also commonly used in the early management of patients with COPD.

Content Review

Emphysema and Chronic Bronchitis: Management Goals

- Relieve hypoxia
- Reverse bronchoconstriction

Administer oxygen to the COPD patient who needs it to relieve hypoxia. Since this may decrease the respiratory drive in the COPD patient, monitor the patient and be prepared to assist ventilations, if necessary.

ASTHMA

Asthma is a common respiratory illness that affects many persons. Although deaths from other respiratory diseases are steadily declining, deaths from asthma have significantly increased during the last decade. Most of the increased asthma deaths have occurred in patients aged 45 years or older. In addition, the death rate for black asthmatics has been twice as high as for their white counterparts. Approximately 50 percent of patients who die from asthma do so before reaching the hospital. Thus, EMS personnel are frequently called on to treat patients suffering an asthma attack. Prompt recognition followed by appropriate treatment can significantly improve the patient's condition and enhance his chance of survival.

Pathophysiology

Asthma is a chronic inflammatory disorder of the airways. In susceptible individuals, this inflammation causes symptoms usually associated with widespread but variable air flow obstruction. In addition to air flow obstruction, the airway becomes hyperresponsive. The air flow obstruction and hyperresponsiveness are often reversible with treatment. These conditions may also reverse spontaneously.

Asthma may be induced by one of many different factors. These factors, commonly referred to as "triggers" or "inducers," vary from one individual to the next. In allergic individuals, environmental allergens are a major cause of inflammation. These may occur both indoors and outdoors. In addition to allergens, asthma may be triggered by cold air, exercise, foods, irritants, stress, and certain medications. Often, a specific trigger cannot be identified. Extrinsic triggers tend predominantly to affect children, whereas intrinsic factors trigger asthma in adults.

Within minutes of exposure to the offending trigger, a two-phase reaction occurs. The first phase of the reaction is characterized by the release of chemical mediators such as histamine. These mediators cause contraction of the bronchial smooth muscle and leakage of fluid from peribronchial capillaries.

This results in both bronchoconstriction and bronchial edema. These two factors can significantly decrease expiratory air flow causing the typical "asthma attack."

Often, the asthma attack will resolve spontaneously in 1–2 hours or may be aborted by the use of inhaled bronchodilator medications such as albuterol. However, within 6–8 hours after exposure to the trigger, a second reaction occurs. This late phase is characterized by inflammation of the bronchioles as cells of the immune system (eosinophils, neutrophils, and lymphocytes) invade the mucosa of the respiratory tract. This leads to additional edema and swelling of the bronchioles and a further decrease in expiratory air flow.

The second phase reaction will not typically respond to inhaled beta-agonist drugs such as metaproterenol or albuterol. Instead, anti-inflammatory agents such as corticosteroids are often required. It is important to point out that the severe inflammatory changes seen in an acute asthma attack do not develop over a few hours or even a few days. The inflammation will often begin several days or several weeks before the onset of the actual asthma attack.

Assessment

Content Review

Asthma: Common Presenting Signs

- Dyspnea
- Wheezing
- Cough

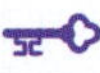

Note that some asthmatics do not wheeze; rather, they present with a frequent, persistent cough.

Begin the initial prehospital assessment of the asthmatic by considering immediate threats to the airway, breathing, or circulation. Then turn your attention to the secondary assessment.

The most common presenting symptoms of asthma are dyspnea, wheezing, and cough. Wheezing results from turbulent air flow through the inflamed and narrowed bronchioles. Many asthmatics will have a persistent cough. This is primarily due to hyperresponsiveness of the airway. It is important to point out that some asthmatics do not wheeze. Instead, their initial presentation may be a frequent and persistent cough. As asthma severity increases, the patient may exhibit hyperinflation of the chest due to trapping of air in the alveoli. In addition, tachypnea (rapid respiration) will occur. The patient may start to use accessory muscles to aid respiration.

Symptoms of a severe asthma attack include one-to-two-word dyspnea (the inability to complete a phrase or sentence without having to stop to breathe), pulsus paradoxus (a drop of systolic blood pressure of 10 mmHg or more with inspiration), tachycardia, and decreased oxygen saturation on pulse oximetry. As hypoxia develops the patient may become agitated and anxious.

When conducting the secondary assessment, start by obtaining a brief patient history. Most asthmatics will report that they suffer from asthma. In addition, the patient's home medications may help confirm a history of asthma. Common asthma medications include inhaled beta-agonists (albuterol, levalbuterol, metaproterenol), inhaled corticosteroids (betamethasone, beclomethasone), inhaled cromolyn sodium, and inhaled anticholinergics (ipratropium bromide). Often the patient will be taking oral bronchodilators such as theophylline or may be taking oral corticosteroids (prednisone).

Determine when symptoms started and what the patient has taken in an attempt to abort the attack. Also, find out whether the patient is allergic to any medications. Question the patient about hospitalizations for asthma. If the patient has been hospitalized, ask whether the patient has ever required intubation and mechanical ventilation. A prior history of intubation and mechanical ventilation should heighten your index of suspicion. Similarly, an asthmatic who is on continuous corticosteroid therapy is also a high-risk patient.

After you obtain the pertinent history, perform a brief physical examination. Place particular emphasis on the chest and neck. Examination of the chest should begin with inspection. Note any increase in the diameter of the chest that may indicate air trapping. Also, note the use of accessory muscles, including retraction of the intercostal muscles or use of the strap muscles of the neck. Following inspection, palpate the chest, noting any deformity, crepitus, or asymmetry. Next, auscultate the posterior chest. Note any abnormal breath sounds such as wheezing or rhonchi. Listen to the symmetry of breath sounds. Unilateral wheezing may indicate an aspirated foreign body or a pneumothorax.

Obtain accurate vital signs. One of the most important vital signs is the respiratory rate. An increase in the respiratory rate is one of the earliest symptoms of a respiratory problem. Many EMS personnel inaccurately measure the respiratory rate. The easiest method is to simply place your fingers on the patient's radial artery as if you were measuring the pulse rate. This will make the patient think you are obtaining the pulse rate, and he will not alter his breathing pattern. Measure the respiratory rate for at least 30 seconds. At the same time, note any alterations in the respiratory pattern. Pulse oximetry is an excellent adjunct to respiratory assessment. It will pro-

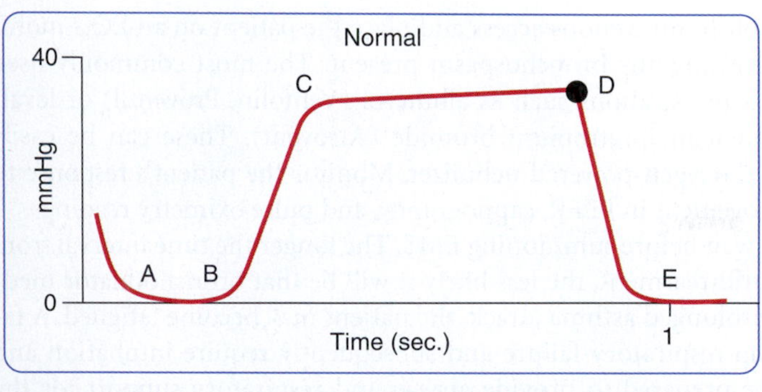

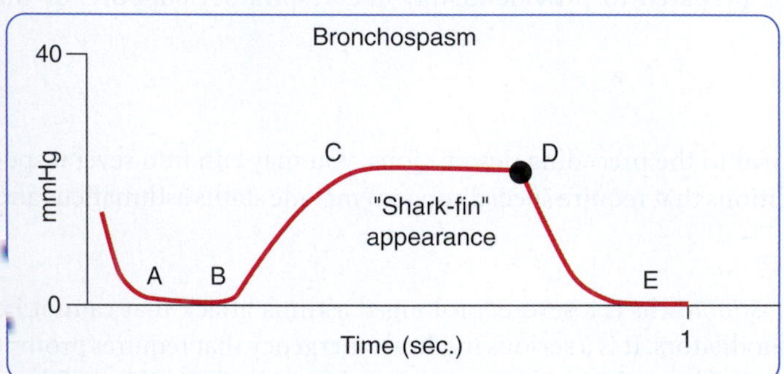

■ Figure 27-16
Comparison of normal and asthmatic capnogram waveforms.

vice you with data regarding the oxygen saturation status (SpO_2) as well as an audible measure of the pulse rate.

EMS systems should be able to measure the peak expiratory flow rate (PEFR). The PEFR is a reliable indicator of air flow. If possible, measure peak flow rates to determine the severity of an asthma attack and the degree of response to treatment. The more severe the asthma attack, the lower will be the PEFR.

Continuous waveform capnography can assist in identifying asthma (and other types of lung disease) and can also help determine the severity of air flow obstruction. Patients with an acute asthma exacerbation will often exhibit a "shark fin" configuration on their capnogram (Figure 27-16 ■). This results from slower emptying of the alveoli, which causes an increase in the slope of the ascending phase and the alveolar plateau. During an acute asthma exacerbation, patients tend to hyperventilate in order to maintain adequate oxygenation. This causes a fall in the $ETCO_2$ level (usually < 35 mmHg). As the exacerbation progresses untreated, the patient will begin to tire and the $ETCO_2$ will rise back to the normal range (35–45 mmHg). If effective treatment is not provided or the patient fails to respond to treatment, the $ETCO_2$ levels will continue to rise to dangerous levels (> 50 mmHg) (Table 27–3). Thus, considering both the shark fin configuration and the $ETCO_2$ level, it is possible to detect asthma and estimate the severity of an asthma patient's exacerbation.

Management

Treatment of asthma is designed to correct hypoxia, reverse any bronchospasm, and treat the inflammatory changes associated with the disease. Administer oxygen at a high flow rate and high

Table 27–3 Phases of Acute Asthma Exacerbation

Phase	Clinical Assessment	$ETCO_2$ Levels (mmHg)
Mild	Hyperventilating	< 35
Moderate	Tiring	35–50
Severe	Tired	> 50

Review

Content

Asthma: Management Goals

- Correct hypoxia
- Reverse bronchospasm
- Reduce inflammation

concentration (100 percent). Establish intravenous access and place the patient on an ECG monitor. Direct initial treatment at reversing any bronchospasm present. The most commonly used drugs are the inhaled beta-agonist preparations such as albuterol (Ventolin, Proventil) or levalbuterol (Xopenex) in conjunction with ipratropium bromide (Atrovent). These can be easily administered with a small-volume, oxygen-powered nebulizer. Monitor the patient's response to these medications by noting improvement in PEFR, capnography, and pulse oximetry readings.

Many asthmatic patients will wait before summoning EMS. The longer the time interval from the onset of the asthma attack until treatment, the less likely it will be that bronchodilator medications will work. Often, after a prolonged asthma attack, the patient may become fatigued. A fatigued patient can quickly develop respiratory failure and subsequently require intubation and mechanical ventilation. Always be prepared to provide airway and respiratory support for the asthmatic.

Special Cases

While most cases of asthma conform to the preceding descriptions, you may run into several special cases in the field. Asthma conditions that require special concern include status asthmaticus and asthmatic attacks in children.

Status Asthmaticus *Status asthmaticus* is a severe, prolonged asthma attack that cannot be broken by repeated doses of bronchodilators. It is a serious medical emergency that requires prompt recognition, treatment, and transport. The patient suffering status asthmaticus frequently will have a greatly distended chest from continued air trapping. Breath sounds, and often wheezing, may be absent. The patient is usually exhausted, severely acidotic, and dehydrated. The management of status asthmaticus is basically the same as for asthma. *Recognize that respiratory arrest is imminent and be prepared for endotracheal intubation.* Transport immediately and continue aggressive treatment en route.

Asthma in Children Asthma in children is common. The pathophysiology and treatment are essentially the same as in adults, with altered medication dosages. Several additional medications are used in the treatment of childhood asthma. (Asthma in children is discussed in greater detail in Chapter 42, "Pediatrics.")

UPPER RESPIRATORY INFECTION

Infections involving the upper airway and respiratory tract are among the most common infections for which patients seek medical attention. Although these conditions are rarely life threatening, upper respiratory infections (URIs) can make many existing pulmonary diseases worse or lead to direct pulmonary infection. The best defense against the spread of upper respiratory infection is common practices such as good hand washing and covering the mouth during coughing and sneezing. Attention to such details is important when caring for patients with underlying pulmonary disease or those who are immunosuppressed (HIV infection, cancer) because URIs are more severe in these populations. Because of the prevalence of such infections, complete protection is impossible.

Pathophysiology

Remember that the upper airway begins at the nose and mouth, passes through the pharynx, and ends at the larynx. Other related structures are the paranasal sinuses and the eustachian tubes that connect the pharynx and the middle ear. In addition, several collections of lymphoid tissue found in the pharynx (palatine, pharyngeal, and lingual tonsils) produce antibodies and provide immune protection.

The vast majority of URIs are caused by viruses. A variety of bacteria may also produce infection of the upper respiratory tract. The most significant is group A streptococcus, which is the causative organism in "strep throat" and accounts for up to 30 percent of URIs. This bacteria is also implicated in sinusitis and middle ear infections. Up to 50 percent of patients who have pharyngitis (inflammation of the pharynx) are not found to have a viral or bacterial cause. Fortunately, most URIs are self-limiting illnesses that resolve after several days of symptoms.

Table 27–4	Locations and Signs and Symptoms of Upper Respiratory Infections		
Structure	**Infection**	**Symptoms**	**Signs**
Nose	Rhinitis	Runny nose, congestion, sneezing	Rhinorrhea
Pharynx	Pharyngitis	Sore throat, pain on swallowing	Erythematous pharynx, tonsil enlargement, pus on tonsils, cervical lymph node enlargement
Middle Ear	Otitis media	Ear pain, decreased hearing	Red, bulging eardrum, pus behind eardrum, lymph node enlargement in front of or behind ear
Larynx	Laryngitis	Sore throat, hoarseness, pain on speaking	Red pharynx, hoarse quality to voice, cervical lymph node enlargement
Epiglottis	Epiglottitis	Sore throat, drooling, ill appearing	Upright position, drooling, ill appearing
Sinuses	Sinusitis	Headache, congestion	Tenderness over the sinuses, worsening of pain with leaning forward, yellow nasal discharge

Assessment

The major symptoms of URI are determined by the portion of the upper respiratory tract that is predominantly affected (Table 27–4). Patients with URIs will often have accompanying symptoms such as fever, chills, myalgias (muscle pains), and fatigue.

Remember that any child with suspected epiglottitis (see Chapter 42, "Pediatrics") should be supported in a position of comfort. Do not attempt examination of the throat as this may produce severe laryngospasm. Adults do occasionally also develop epiglottitis, but this is generally a more benign condition.

Support the child with suspected epiglottitis in a position of comfort. Do not attempt examination of the throat, which may produce severe laryngospasm.

Management

In most cases, the diagnosis and treatment of upper respiratory conditions is based on the history and physical findings. Patients with pharyngitis are often diagnosed by obtaining a throat culture that confirms the presence of a bacterial cause of symptoms. A rapid test is also available. In patients with sinusitis and otitis media, treatment is based on a presumed bacterial cause.

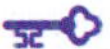

In URI, as with other medical conditions, focus attention on the patient's airway and ventilation. Give supplemental oxygen to any patient with underlying pulmonary disease.

As with other medical conditions, focus your attention on the patient's airway and ventilation. Generally, no intervention is required except in children with epiglottitis and in some complicated upper respiratory infections where a collection of pus may occlude the airway. Give oxygen supplementation to any patient who has underlying pulmonary disease.

Most upper respiratory infections are treated symptomatically. Acetaminophen or ibuprofen is prescribed for fever, headache, and myalgias. Encourage patients to drink plenty of fluids. Saltwater gargles may be used for throat discomfort. Decongestants and antihistamines may be used to reduce mucous secretion. Encourage patients being treated with antibiotics for bacterial causes of URI to continue these agents.

In some patients with asthma or COPD, a URI may produce a worsening of their underlying medical condition. Use inhaled bronchodilators and corticosteroid agents according to local protocols or on advice of medical direction. Transport patients with underlying medical conditions to a health care facility capable of continued evaluation and management of the underlying condition. Continue appropriate monitoring with pulse oximetry and ECG during transport.

PNEUMONIA

Pneumonia is an infection of the lungs and a common medical problem, especially in the aged and those infected with the human immunodeficiency virus (HIV). In fact, pneumonia is one of the leading causes of death in both groups of patients and is the fifth-leading overall cause of death in the United States.

Patients with HIV infection and those on immune suppressive therapy (cancer patients) are at high risk of developing pneumonia. In addition, the very young and very old are at higher risk of acquiring pneumonia because of ineffective protective mechanisms. Other risk factors include a history of alcoholism, cigarette smoking, and exposure to cold temperatures.

Pathophysiology

Pneumonia is a collection of related respiratory diseases caused when a variety of infectious agents invade the lungs. Mucus production and the action of respiratory tract cilia play a role in protecting the body against bacterial invasion. When considering which patients are at risk, the unifying concept is that there is a defect in mucus production, ciliary action, or both.

Bacterial and viral pneumonias are the most frequent, although fungal and other forms of pneumonia exist. More unusual forms of pneumonia are seen in those patients who are currently or recently have been hospitalized where they are exposed to a more unusual variety of microorganisms. This is referred to as hospital-acquired pneumonia. (Cases that develop in the out-of-hospital setting are described as community-acquired pneumonia.)

The infection begins in one part of the lung and often spreads to nearby alveoli. The infection may ultimately involve the entire lung. As the disease progresses, fluid and inflammatory cells collect in the alveoli, and alveolar collapse may occur. Pneumonia is primarily a ventilation disorder. Occasionally, the infection will extend beyond the lungs into the bloodstream and to more distant sites in the body. This systemic spread may lead to septic shock.

Assessment

pleuritic *sharp or tearing, as a description of pain.*

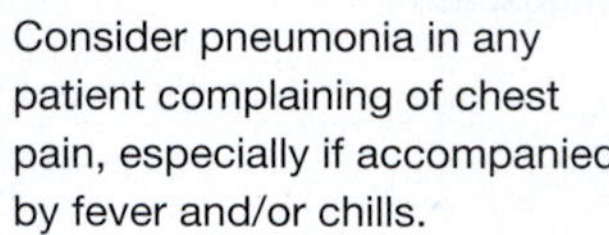

Consider pneumonia in any patient complaining of chest pain, especially if accompanied by fever and/or chills.

A patient with pneumonia will generally appear ill. He may report a recent history of fever and chills. These chills are commonly described as "bed shaking." There is usually a generalized weakness and malaise. The patient will tend to complain of a deep, productive cough and may expel yellow to brown sputum, often streaked with blood. Many cases involve associated **pleuritic** chest pain. Therefore, pneumonia should be considered in any patient who presents complaining of chest pain, especially if accompanied by fever and/or chills. In pneumonia involving the lower lobes of the lungs, a patient may complain of nothing more than upper abdominal pain.

Physical examination will commonly reveal fever, tachypnea, tachycardia, and a cough. Respiratory distress may be present. Auscultation of the chest usually demonstrates crackles (rales) in the involved lung segment, although wheezes or rhonchi may be heard. There usually is decreased air movement in the areas filled with infection. Percussion of the chest may reveal dullness over these areas. *Egophony* (a change in the spoken "E" sound to an "A" sound on auscultation) may also be noted.

In the forms of pneumonia involving viral, fungal, and rare bacterial causes, the typical symptoms as described are not seen. Instead, these patients may report a nonproductive cough with less prominent lung findings. Systemic symptoms such as headache, malaise, fatigue, muscle aches, sore throat, and abdominal complaints including nausea, vomiting, and diarrhea are more prominent. Fever and chills are not as impressive as in bacterial pneumonia.

Management

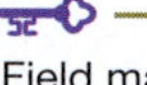

Field management of suspected pneumonia is purely supportive. Place the patient in a position of comfort and administer high-flow, high-concentration oxygen.

Pneumonia is generally diagnosed on the basis of physical examination, X-ray findings, and laboratory cultures. Therefore, diagnosis in the field is unlikely. The primary treatment is antibiotics to which the causative organism is susceptible. In the field, however, antibiotics are not indicated and treatment is purely supportive.

Place the patient in a comfortable position, and administer high-flow, high-concentration oxygen. Use pulse oximetry to assess the patient's oxygen requirements. In severe cases, ventilatory assistance is needed and endotracheal intubation may be required. Establish intravenous access and base fluid resuscitation on the patient's hydration status. Administering fluids for dehydration is appropriate, but overhydration can also worsen the respiratory condition. Medical direction may sometimes order a breathing treatment with a beta-agonist, particularly if wheezing is present. Because patients with pneumonia often have some bronchospasm, these drugs will afford the patient some symptomatic relief. Give antipyretic agents such as acetaminophen or ibuprofen to reduce a high fever. Also, a cool, moistened wash cloth may soothe the patient.

Remember to be extremely careful when caring for patients over age 65 with suspected pneumonia. These patients have high mortality and complication rates. Transport them to a facility capable of handling the significant complications associated with the disease for this population.

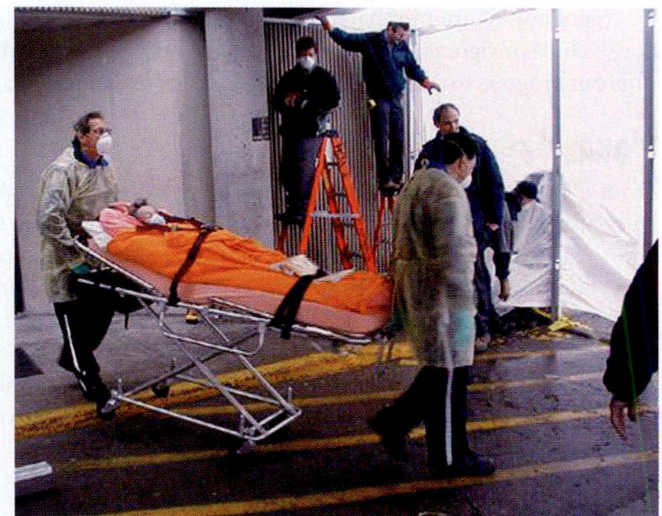

■ **Figure 27-17** Health care personnel donned protective clothing and installed plastic sheeting to help isolate infected patients during the Toronto SARS epidemic. *(© Brian Schwartz, MD)*

SEVERE ACUTE RESPIRATORY SYNDROME (SARS)

Severe acute respiratory syndrome (SARS) is a viral respiratory illness that first appeared in southern China in November 2002. It became a global threat in March 2003 by spreading internationally via Hong Kong. Ultimately, 8,098 people worldwide were affected with SARS during that outbreak. Of these, 774 died. SARS entered Canada and several other countries and spread rapidly. Toronto, Ontario, was particularly affected. In fact, SARS placed a significant stress on the Toronto EMS system. Four paramedics contracted the disease, and more than 400 paramedics were placed on "working quarantine." The four paramedics who contracted SARS reportedly did so before mandatory PPE measures were undertaken (Figure 27-17 ■). SARS appears to be an ongoing threat because of the highly infectious nature of the illness.

Pathophysiology

The virus that causes SARS, which was previously unrecognized, is called SARS-associated coronavirus (SARS-CoV). Coronaviruses play a major role in upper respiratory infections and the common cold. Preliminary studies indicated that SARS-CoV may survive in the environment for several days. Other infectious agents may play a role in SARS as well.

SARS is spread by close person-to-person contact. SARS-CoV is transmitted by respiratory droplets produced when an infected person coughs or sneezes. Disease transmission occurs when these droplets are deposited on the mucous membranes of the mouth, nose, and eyes of persons who are nearby. SARS-CoV can also be contracted by touching a surface or object contaminated by infectious droplets.

The incubation period (time from exposure until onset of symptoms) is generally 2–7 days, although some cases have had an incubation period of as long as 10–14 days. A person with SARS is considered to be contagious as long as he has symptoms. Furthermore, there have been no reported cases of disease transmission before the source patient develops symptoms. Persons with documented SARS should be quarantined to their home for at least 10 days after the fever has abated and symptoms have cleared.

Assessment

If a SARS outbreak has been identified, all personnel should use appropriate PPE on every call or as directed by local health authorities. If, in a non-SARS epidemic area, a case is encountered that has SARS-like symptoms, all involved should immediately don appropriate PPE.

As for any patient with a respiratory illness, first address signs of severe respiratory distress. Look for altered mental status, one-to-two-word speech dyspnea, cough, cyanosis, and hypoxia as documented by pulse oximetry. Patients with underlying respiratory disease (asthma, emphysema, chronic bronchitis) and those with chronic illnesses are at increased risk of SARS-related problems.

Signs and symptoms that have been associated with SARS include sore throat, rhinorrhea (runny nose), chills or rigors (sudden paroxysmal chills), myalgias (muscle aches), headache, and diarrhea. This can progress to cough, sputum production, respiratory distress, and eventual respiratory failure.

Management

From a management standpoint, any patient suspected of SARS should be treated as any patient with suspected pneumonia or other respiratory illness. Place the patient in a comfortable position and administer high-flow, high-concentration oxygen. Use pulse oximetry to assess the patient's oxygenation requirements. In severe cases, ventilatory assistance may be needed and endotracheal intubation may be required. Establish intravenous access, and base fluid administration on the patient's hydration status. If the patient is wheezing, consider the administration of a nebulized bronchodilator. If SARS is suspected, notify the receiving hospital of your suspicions so that they can take appropriate measures for isolation of the patient and protection of health care workers.

LUNG CANCER

Lung cancer (neoplasm) is the leading cause of cancer-related death in the United States in both men and women. Most patients with lung cancer are between the ages of 55 and 65 years. There is a high mortality rate for patients with lung cancer after only 1 year with the disease.

There are currently four major types of lung cancer based on the predominant cell type. Twenty percent of cases involve only the lung tissue. Another 35 percent involve spread to the lymphatic system, and 45 percent have distant metastases (cancer cells spreading to other tissues). In those cases where there is lung tissue invasion, the primary problem is disruption of diffusion. In some larger cancers, there may also be alterations in ventilation by obstruction of the conducting bronchioles.

Cigarette smoking has long been known to be a risk factor for development of lung cancer. Environmental exposure to asbestos, hydrocarbons, radiation, and fumes from metal production have also been identified as risk factors. Finally, home exposure to radon has been implicated in the development of lung cancer. Preventive strategies include educating teenagers about the dangers of cigarette smoking and encouraging current smokers to quit. Implementing environmental safety standards that reduce the risk of exposure to such substances as asbestos will also reduce the risk of lung cancer. Finally, cancer screening of populations at risk is encouraged.

Pathophysiology

Although cancers that start elsewhere in the body can spread to the lungs, the vast majority of lung cancers are caused by carcinogens (cancer-producing substances) from cigarette smoking. A small portion of lung cancers are caused by inhalation of occupational agents such as asbestos and arsenic. These substances irritate and adversely affect the various tissues of the lung, ultimately leading to the development of abnormal (cancerous) cells.

There are four major types of lung cancers depending on the type of lung tissue involved. The most common type of lung cancer is referred to as *adenocarcinoma.* This cancer arises from glandular-type (i.e., mucus-producing) cells found in the lungs and bronchioles. The next most frequently encountered type of lung cancer is *small cell carcinoma* (also called "oat cell" carcinoma). Small cell carcinoma arises from bronchial tissues. The third type of lung cancer is referred to as *epidermoid carcinoma.* Finally, *large cell carcinoma* is the fourth major type of lung cancer. Like small cell carcinoma, epidermoid and large cell carcinomas typically arise from the bronchial tissues. Lung cancers generally have a bad prognosis with most patients dying within a year of the diagnosis.

Assessment

In lung cancer, as with other respiratory diseases, your first priority is to address signs of respiratory distress.

As with other respiratory diseases, your first priority is to address signs of severe respiratory distress. Look for altered mental status, one-to-two-word dyspnea, cyanosis, hemoptysis, and hypoxia as documented by pulse oximeter. Severe uncontrolled hemoptysis can be a particularly life-threatening presentation.

Patients with lung cancer will present with a variety of complaints, depending on whether they are related to direct lung involvement, invasion of local structures, or metastatic spread. Patients with localized disease will present with cough, dyspnea, hoarseness, vague chest pain, and hemoptysis. Fever, chills, and pleuritic chest pain are seen in patients who develop pneumonia. Symptoms related to local invasion include pain on swallowing (dysphagia), weakness or numbness in the arm, and shoulder pain. Metastatic symptoms are related to the area of spread and include headache, seizures, bone pain, abdominal pain, nausea, and malaise.

Many patients with lung cancer will have coexisting COPD from years of tobacco smoking.

Physical findings are nonspecific. Patients with advanced disease have profound weight loss and cachexia (general physical wasting and malnutrition). Crackles (rales), rhonchi, wheezes, and diminished breath sounds may be heard in the affected lung. Venous distention in the arms and neck may be present if there is occlusion of the superior vena cava (called *superior vena cava syndrome*).

Management

Content Review

Lung Cancer: Management Goals

- Administer oxygen
- Support ventilation
- Be aware of any DNR order
- Provide emotional support

Administer supplemental oxygen as needed based on the clinical status and pulse oximetry measurement. Support the patient's ventilation as needed and intubate as necessary. Be attentive, however, for any Do Not Resuscitate order or other advance directive, such as a living will, and follow your local protocol regarding these legal instruments. Consult medical direction if questions arise.

Initiate an IV of 0.9 percent normal saline and provide fluids if signs of dehydration are present. Follow your local protocol regarding the access of permanent indwelling catheters that many cancer patients have in place.

Prehospital drug therapy consists of bronchodilator agents and corticosteroids when signs of obstructive lung disease are present. Continue any prescribed antibiotics. Transport the patient and monitor mental status, vital signs, and oxygen status, as appropriate. Be prepared to provide emotional support for both the patient and family during transport.

TOXIC INHALATION

Inhalation of toxic substances into the respiratory tract can cause pain, inflammation, or destruction of pulmonary tissues. Significant inhalations can affect the ability of the alveoli to exchange oxygen, thus resulting in hypoxemia.

Pathophysiology

The possibility of inhalation of products toxic to the respiratory system should be considered in any dyspneic patient. Causes of toxic inhalation include superheated air, toxic products of combustion, chemical irritants, and inhalation of steam. Each of these agents can result in upper airway obstruction due to edema and laryngospasm. In such cases, bronchospasm and lower airway edema may additionally appear. In severe inhalations, disruption of the alveolar-capillary membranes may result in life-threatening pulmonary edema.

Assessment

When assessing the patient with possible toxic inhalation, determine the nature of the inhalant or combusted material.

When assessing the patient with possible toxic inhalation exposure, determine the nature of the inhalant or the combusted material. Several products can result in the formation of corrosive acids or alkalis that irritate and damage the airway. These include ammonia (ammonium hydroxide), nitrogen oxide (nitric acid), sulfur dioxide (sulfurous acid), sulfur trioxide (sulfuric acid), and chlorine (hydrochloric acid).

Content Review

Toxic Inhalation: Management Sequence

- Ensure safety of rescue personnel
- Remove patient from toxic environment
- Maintain an open airway
- Provide humidified, high-flow, high-concentration oxygen

It is also crucial to determine the duration of the exposure, whether the patient was in an enclosed area at the time of the exposure, or if he experienced a loss of consciousness. Loss of consciousness may cause the airway to become vulnerable as a result of the loss of airway protective mechanisms.

During physical examination, pay particular attention to the face, mouth, and throat. Note any burns or particulate matter. Next, auscultate the chest for the presence of any wheezes or crackles (rales). Wheezing may indicate bronchospasm, while crackles may suggest pulmonary edema.

Management

After ensuring the safety of rescue personnel, remove the patient from the hazardous environment. Next, establish and maintain an open airway. Remember that the airway is often irritable and attempts at endotracheal intubation may result in laryngospasm, completely obstructing the airway. Laryngeal edema, as evidenced by hoarseness, brassy cough, and stridor, is ominous and may require prompt endotracheal intubation. Administer humidified oxygen at a high flow rate and high concentration. As a precaution, start an IV of a crystalloid solution to provide rapid venous access. Transport promptly.

CARBON MONOXIDE INHALATION

Carbon monoxide is an odorless, tasteless, colorless gas produced from the incomplete burning of fossil fuels and other carbon-containing compounds. Carbon monoxide can be encountered in industrial sites, such as mines and factories. It is present in the environment in various concentrations primarily because of automotive exhaust emissions. Most poisonings occur from automobile emissions and home-heating devices used in poorly ventilated areas. Carbon monoxide is often used in suicide attempts. In addition, it is a particular hazard for firefighters and rescue personnel.

Pathophysiology

Carbon monoxide exposure is potentially life threatening because it easily binds to the hemoglobin molecule. It has an affinity for hemoglobin 200–250 times that of oxygen. Once bound, receptor sites on the hemoglobin can no longer transport oxygen to the peripheral tissues. Hemoglobin with carbon monoxide bound is referred to as **carboxyhemoglobin**. The result is hypoxia at the cellular level and, ultimately, metabolic acidosis. Additionally, carbon monoxide binds to iron-containing enzymes and proteins (myoglobin) within the cells, leading to worsening cellular acidosis.

carboxyhemoglobin *hemoglobin with carbon monoxide bound.*

Assessment

With carbon monoxide poisoning, determine the source of exposure, its length, and the location.

When confronted by a patient suffering possible carbon monoxide poisoning, determine the source of exposure, its length, and the location. Less time is required to develop a significant exposure in a closed space compared to one in an area that is fairly well ventilated.

Signs and symptoms of carbon monoxide poisoning include headache, nausea and vomiting, confusion, agitation, loss of coordination, chest pain, loss of consciousness, and even seizures. On physical examination, the skin may be cyanotic or it may be bright cherry red (a very late finding). There may be other signs of hypoxia such as peripheral cyanosis or confusion. Noninvasive carboxyhemoglobin levels can now be measured in the prehospital setting through CO-oximetry. A CO-oximeter is similar to a pulse oximeter, but uses eight different wavelengths of light instead of two. It can detect carboxyhemoglobin, methemoglobin (on certain models), oxyhemoglobin, and deoxyhemogobin. Carboxyhemoglobin levels (SpCO) are reported in percentage of carboxyhemoglobin present. Normally, carboxyhemoglobin levels are less than 1% in nonsmokers and 3% in smokers.

Content Review

Carbon Monoxide Inhalation: Management Sequence

- Ensure safety of rescue personnel
- Remove patient from exposure site
- Maintain an open airway
- Provide high-flow, high-concentration oxygen

Management

On detection of carbon monoxide poisoning, first ensure the safety of rescue personnel, then remove the patient from the site of exposure. Ensure and maintain the airway. Administer supplemental oxygen at the highest possible concentration. If the patient is breathing spontaneously, apply a *tight-fitting* nonrebreather mask. If respiratory depression is noted, assist respirations. If shock is present, treat. Prompt transport is essential.

Hyperbaric oxygen therapy may be used in the treatment of severe carbon monoxide poisoning. Many EMS systems have protocols established whereby patients suffering carbon monoxide poisoning are transported to hospitals with hyperbaric oxygen therapy facilities. Hyperbaric oxygen increases the PaO_2, thus promoting increased oxygen uptake and displacement of the carbon monoxide from the hemoglobin.

PULMONARY EMBOLISM

A pulmonary embolism is a blood clot (thrombus) or some other particle that lodges in a pulmonary artery, effectively blocking blood flow through that vessel. This condition is potentially life threatening because it can significantly decrease pulmonary blood flow, thus leading to hypoxemia (inadequate levels of oxygen in the blood). Pulmonary thromboembolism accounts for 50,000 deaths annually in the United States. In fact, one in five cases of sudden death are caused by pulmonary emboli. The great majority of patients with pulmonary emboli survive; only one in ten cases of documented pulmonary emboli result in death.

The incidence of pulmonary emboli is increased in certain populations. Any condition that results in immobility of the extremities can increase the risk of thromboembolism. Such conditions include recent surgery, long-bone fractures (with immobilization in casts or splints), bedridden condition, or prolonged immobilization as with long-distance travel. Venous pooling that occurs during pregnancy can also lead to pulmonary emboli. Certain disease states increase the likelihood of blood clot formation. These include cancer, infections, thrombophlebitis, atrial fibrillation, and sickle cell anemia. Also, the incidence of thromboembolic disease is increased in patients taking oral birth control pills, particularly among smokers.

Pathophysiology

Sources of pulmonary emboli include air embolism, such as can occur during the placement of a central line; fat embolism, which can occur following a fracture; amniotic fluid embolism; and blood clots. It is also possible for a foreign body (such as part of a venous catheter) to become dislodged in the venous circulation. The vast majority of cases, however, are caused by blood clots that develop in the deep venous system of the lower extremities.

As a rule, a significant amount of blood passes through the veins of the lower extremity. During normal use of our legs, muscular contractions propel the blood through the venous system with the aid of valves that are present in the lower extremity veins. This action prevents blood from flowing backward through the venous system. When there is infection, venous injury, or any other condition that leads to pooling of blood in the deep veins of the lower extremity, clot formation occurs. If a portion of the clot becomes dislodged, it will pass through the right side of the heart and become lodged in the pulmonary vasculature.

When a pulmonary embolism occurs, the blockage of blood flow through the affected artery causes the right heart to pump against increased resistance. This results in an increase in pulmonary capillary pressure. The area of the lung supplied by the occluded pulmonary vessel can no longer effectively function in gas exchange since it receives no effective blood supply. The major derangement in patients with pulmonary emboli is a perfusion disorder. The involved lung segment is still ventilated, producing a ventilation-perfusion mismatch.

Assessment

Signs and symptoms of a patient suffering a pulmonary embolism will vary, depending on the size and location of the obstruction. The patient suffering acute pulmonary embolism may report a sudden onset of severe unexplained dyspnea, which may or may not be associated with pleuritic chest pain. The patient may also report a cough which is usually not productive but may occasionally produce blood (hemoptysis). There may be a recent history of immobilization such as hip fracture, surgery, or debilitating illness.

The patient with acute pulmonary embolism may have a sudden onset of severe unexplained dyspnea, with or without pleuritic chest pain.

The physical examination may reveal labored breathing, tachypnea, and tachycardia. In massive pulmonary emboli, there may be signs of right-heart failure such as jugular venous distention and, in some cases, falling blood pressure. In many cases, auscultation of the chest may reveal no significant lung findings, although rare crackles and wheezing may be noted. Occasionally, a pleural friction rub (leathery sound heard with inspiration) may be heard.

Always examine the extremities. In up to 50 percent of cases, findings suggestive of deep venous thrombosis will be evident. These include a warm, swollen extremity with a thick cord palpated along the medial thigh and pain on palpation or when extending the calf.

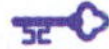

With suspected pulmonary embolism, always examine the extremities. In up to 50 percent of cases, findings suggestive of deep venous thrombosis will be evident.

In extreme cases, the patient may present with extreme confusion as the result of hypoxia, severe cyanosis, profound hypotension, and even cardiac arrest. Physical examination may reveal petechiae (small hemorrhagic spots) on the arms and chest wall in these cases.

Management

As with all respiratory conditions, your first priorities are the airway, breathing, and circulation. Remember that a large pulmonary embolism may lead to cardiac arrest. Perform CPR if needed.

If you suspect a patient is suffering a pulmonary embolism, establish and maintain an airway. Assist ventilations as required. Administer supplemental oxygen at the highest possible concentration. Endotracheal intubation may be required.

With pulmonary embolism, as with all respiratory conditions, your first priorities are the airway, breathing, and circulation. Remember that a large pulmonary embolism may lead to cardiac arrest. Be prepared to perform CPR, if needed.

Pulmonary embolism has a high complication rate and significant mortality. Carefully monitor vital signs and cardiac rhythm. Transport to a facility with the capability of caring for the critical needs of the patient.

Establish an IV of lactated Ringer's or normal saline at a "to keep open" rate. The diagnosis of pulmonary embolism is often difficult and requires a high index of suspicion. Remember that patients with suspected pulmonary embolism may require a significant amount of care. This disorder has a high complication rate and a significant mortality. Carefully monitor the patient's vital signs and cardiac rhythm. Quickly transport the patient to a facility with the capabilities to care for the critical needs of the patient. Treatment in the hospital setting may include the use of various medications such as fibrinolytic agents and blood thinners like heparin.

SPONTANEOUS PNEUMOTHORAX

spontaneous pneumothorax *a pneumothorax (collection of air in the pleural space) that occurs spontaneously, in the absence of blunt or penetrating trauma.*

A **spontaneous pneumothorax** is defined as a pneumothorax that occurs in the absence of blunt or penetrating trauma. Spontaneous pneumothorax is a common clinical condition, with 18 cases occurring for every 100,000 population. There is also a high recurrence rate. Fifty percent of patients will have a recurrent episode within 2 years.

There is a 5:1 ratio of male to female patients with spontaneous pneumothorax. Other risk factors include a tall, thin stature and a history of cigarette smoking. This disorder tends to develop in patients between the ages of 20 and 40 years. Patients with COPD have a higher incidence of spontaneous pneumothorax, presumably because of the presence of thinned lung tissue (blebs) that may rupture.

Pathophysiology

The primary derangement is one of ventilation as the negative pressure that normally exists in the pleural space is lost. This prevents proper expansion of the lung in concert with the chest wall. A pneumothorax occupying 15 to 20 percent of the chest cavity is generally well tolerated by the patient unless there is significant underlying lung disease.

Assessment

The patient with a spontaneous pneumothorax will have a sudden onset of pleuritic chest or shoulder pain, often precipitated by coughing or lifting.

The patient with a spontaneous pneumothorax presents with a sudden onset of sharp, pleuritic chest or shoulder pain. Often, the symptoms are precipitated by coughing or lifting. Dyspnea is commonly reported. The degree of symptoms is not strictly related to the size of the pneumothorax.

The physical examination is usually not impressive. Decreased breath sounds on the involved side may be difficult to note. They may be best heard at the lung apex. Even more subtle is hyperresonance to percussion of the chest. Occasionally, the patient may have subcutaneous emphysema, which may be palpated as a crackling under the skin overlying the chest. Tachypnea, diaphoresis, and pallor are also seen. Cyanosis is rarely found.

Management

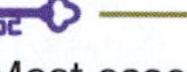

Most cases of spontaneous pneumothorax require only supplemental oxygen.

Use the patient's symptoms and pulse oximetry readings as guides to therapy. For most cases of spontaneous pneumothorax, supplemental oxygen is all that is required. Ventilatory support and endotracheal intubation are rarely required.

Be careful when ventilating a patient with suspected spontaneous pneumothorax. Too much pressure may result in a tension pneumothorax.

Be careful when managing patients with a spontaneous pneumothorax who require positive-pressure ventilation by mask or endotracheal tube. They are at risk for the development of a *tension pneumothorax.* You may note that the patient will become physically difficult to ventilate. Hypoxia, cyanosis, and hypotension may also develop. In addition to the usual signs of a pneumothorax, the patient will develop jugular vein distention and deviation of the trachea away from the pneumothorax. Needle decompression of a tension pneumothorax may be required.

Other management measures should include placing the patient in a position of comfort. Reserve intravenous access and electrocardiographic monitoring for patients with significant symptoms or severe underlying respiratory disease. Carefully monitor such patients during transport.

HYPERVENTILATION SYNDROME

Hyperventilation syndrome is characterized by rapid breathing, chest pains, numbness, and other symptoms usually associated with anxiety or a situational reaction. However, as shown in Table 27–5,

Table 27–5 Causes of Hyperventilation Syndrome	
Acidosis	Interstitial pneumonitis, fibrosis, edema
Beta-adrenergic agonists	Metabolic disorders
Bronchial asthma	Methylxanthine derivatives
Cardiovascular disorders	Neurologic disorders
Central nervous system infection or tumors	Pain
Congestive heart failure	Pneumonia
Drugs	Pregnancy
Fever, sepsis	Progesterone
Hepatic failure	Psychogenic or anxiety hypertension
High altitude	Pulmonary disease
Hypotension	Pulmonary emboli, vascular disease
Hypoxia	Salicylate

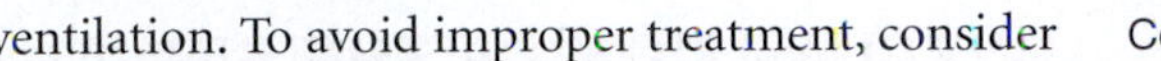

many serious medical problems can cause hyperventilation. To avoid improper treatment, consider hyperventilation to be indicative of a serious medical problem until proven otherwise.

Consider hyperventilation indicative of a serious medical problem until proven otherwise.

Pathophysiology

Hyperventilation syndrome frequently occurs in anxious patients. The patient often senses that he cannot "catch his breath." The patient will then begin to breathe rapidly. Hyperventilation in a purely anxious patient results in the excess elimination of CO_2, causing a respiratory alkalosis. This increases the amount of bound calcium, producing a relative hypocalcemia. This results in cramping of the muscles of the feet and hands, which is called *carpopedal spasm.*

Assessment

With a hyperventilating patient, you may elicit a history of fatigue, nervousness, dizziness, dyspnea, chest pain, and numbness and tingling around the mouth, hands, and feet. The physical examination will reveal an anxious patient with tachypnea and tachycardia. As noted, spasm of the fingers and feet may also be present. If the patient has a history of seizure disorder, the hyperventilation episode may precipitate a seizure. Other symptoms are related to the underlying cause of the hyperventilation syndrome.

Management

The primary treatment for hyperventilation syndrome is reassurance. Instruct the patient to voluntarily reduce his respiratory rate and depth of breathing. Mechanisms that will assist in increasing the PCO_2, such as breath holding or breathing into a paper bag, are discouraged in prehospital care. Hyperventilating patients require oxygen. Allowing them to rebreathe into a paper bag can be deadly. Many EMS systems permit paramedics to use rebreathing techniques only on physician order. It is important to exclude other medical causes before determining that a patient is hyperventilating. Check the oxygen saturation by applying a pulse oximeter. Do not withhold oxygen.

The primary treatment for hyperventilation is reassurance. Instruct the patient to reduce his respiratory rate and depth.

The hyperventilating patient can often present a dilemma for prehospital personnel. Although anxiety is the most common cause of hyperventilation, other more serious diseases can present in exactly the same manner. For example, pulmonary embolism or acute myocardial infarction can exhibit symptoms similar to hyperventilation syndrome.

CENTRAL NERVOUS SYSTEM DYSFUNCTION

Except in the case of drug overdose or massive stroke, central nervous system dysfunction is rarely the cause of respiratory emergencies.

Central nervous system dysfunction, with the exception of drug overdose and massive stroke, is a relatively rare cause of respiratory emergencies. However, always consider the possibility of central nervous system dysfunction in any dyspneic patient.

Pathophysiology

Central nervous system dysfunction can be a causative factor in respiratory depression and arrest. Causes include head trauma, stroke, brain tumors, and various drugs. Several medications, such as narcotics and barbiturates, make the respiratory centers in the brain less responsive to increases in $PaCO_2$. These agents also depress areas of the brain responsible for initiating respirations.

Assessment

The assessment of patients with central nervous system dysfunction should follow the same approach as for any respiratory emergency. However, you should be alert for nonrespiratory system problems such as CNS trauma or drug ingestion. Be careful to note any variation in the respiratory pattern, which can be an indication of central nervous system dysfunction.

Management

With suspected central nervous system dysfunction, establish and maintain an open airway. If respiratory depression is noted or respirations are absent, initiate mechanical ventilation with supplemental oxygen and establish an IV of normal saline at a "to keep open" rate.

If central nervous system dysfunction is suspected, establish and maintain an open airway. If respiratory depression is noted or if respirations are absent, initiate mechanical ventilation. Administer supplemental oxygen, and establish an IV of normal saline at a "to keep open" rate. Direct specific therapy at the underlying problem, if it is known.

DYSFUNCTION OF THE SPINAL CORD, NERVES, OR RESPIRATORY MUSCLES

Several disease processes can affect the spinal cord, nerves, and/or respiratory muscles. Dysfunction of these structures can lead to hypoventilation and progressive hypoxemia.

Pathophysiology

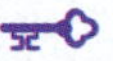

Disorders that affect the spinal cord, nerves, or respiratory muscles and can interfere with respiratory function include spinal cord trauma, polio, ALS, myasthenia gravis, and tumors that impinge on the spinal cord.

Numerous disorders can interfere with respiratory function. These include spinal cord trauma, polio, amyotrophic lateral sclerosis (ALS or Lou Gehrig's disease), and myasthenia gravis. Viral infections, in certain cases, can cause dysfunction of the nervous system. An example of this is *Guillain-Barré syndrome (GBS)*. In GBS, the myelin-covering of the nerve is damaged resulting in relative loss of nerve impulse conduction. This affects virtually every peripheral nerve. Approximately 30 percent of patients with GBS will require ventilatory assistance, as the nerves that stimulate respiration are impaired.

Certain tumors can impinge on the spinal cord, depressing respiratory function. These disorders result in an inability of the respiratory muscles to contract normally, thus causing hypoventilation. Tidal volume and minute volume are decreased. You should also be aware that patients with these disorders do not have the ability to generate an adequate cough reflex and as a result are at risk of developing pneumonia.

Assessment

Patients with possible dysfunction of the spinal cord, nerves, or respiratory muscles may have a history of trauma that is not readily apparent. Always question the patient about injuries or falls. If there is any doubt about a possible injury, act accordingly and immobilize the cervical spine. Also, inquire about signs or symptoms that may suggest a problem with the peripheral nerves. These include such findings as numbness, pain, or sensory dysfunction. The assessment of patients with possible dysfunction of the spinal cord, nerves, or respiratory muscles should follow the same approach as for any respiratory emergency. However, be alert for subtle findings that may indicate a problem with the peripheral nervous system. Always be ready to protect the airway and support ventilation if the patient has symptoms of possible airway obstruction or respiratory failure.

Management

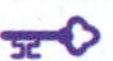

Management of spinal cord and respiratory muscle dysfunction is purely supportive.

Management of spinal cord and respiratory muscle dysfunction is purely supportive. Establish an airway and provide ventilatory support. If myasthenia gravis is present and if transport time is long, the physician may request the administration of one of several agents effective in treating such patients.

Summary

Respiratory emergencies are commonly encountered in prehospital care. It is important to recognize that all respiratory disorders may produce derangements in ventilation, perfusion, or diffusion. Recognition and treatment must be prompt. Understanding the underlying cause of the respiratory disorder can guide therapy. The primary treatment is to correct hypoxia. Necessary steps include establishing and maintaining the airway, assisting ventilations as required, and administering supplemental oxygen. Appropriate pharmacological agents may be subsequently ordered by medical direction.

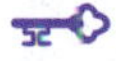

No matter the underlying cause of respiratory dysfunction, the primary treatment is to establish and maintain the airway, administer oxygen, and assist ventilations as required.

Review Questions

1. ___________ risk factors are those that are influenced by or are from within the patient.
   a. Intrinsic
   b. Inherent
   c. Extrinsic
   d. Generic
2. The oxygen dissociation curve can be altered by changes in the:
   a. PCO_2.
   b. blood pH.
   c. body temperature.
   d. all of the above
3. Cellular respiration occurs in the peripheral:
   a. veins.
   b. arteries.
   c. capillaries.
   d. arterioles.
4. ______________________ is (are) characterized by long, deep breaths that are stopped during the inspiratory phase and separated by periods of apnea; this pattern is a result of stroke or severe central nervous system disease.
   a. Kussmaul's respirations
   b. Apneustic respirations
   c. Ataxic (Biot's) respirations
   d. Central neurogenic hyperventilation
5. Common medications used by patients with COPD include all of the following except:
   a. chlorpropamide.
   b. theophylline.
   c. cromolyn sodium.
   d. antibiotic agents.
6. A whistling sound due to narrowing of the airways by edema, bronchoconstriction, or foreign materials describes:
   a. stridor.
   b. snoring.
   c. rhonchi.
   d. wheezing.
7. The preferred abbreviation to describe oxygen saturation measurement is:
   a. O_2.
   b. SpO_2.
   c. PaO_2.
   d. SaO_2.

8. ____________ is a graphic recording or display of the capnometry reading over time.
   a. Capnogram
   b. Capnograph
   c. Capnography
   d. Capnometry
9. __________ describes an excess of red blood cells resulting in an abnormally high hematocrit.
   a. Anemia
   b. Hypoxemia
   c. Polycythemia
   d. Thrombocytopenia
10. The paramedic should measure ____________ to determine the severity of an asthma attack and the degree of response to treatment.
   a. CO_2
   b. PCO_2
   c. PEFR
   d. $ETCO_2$

See Answers to Review Questions at the back of this book.

Chapter 28

Cardiology

Objectives

Part 1: Cardiovascular Anatomy and Physiology, ECG Monitoring, and Dysrhythmia Analysis (begins on p. 1127)

After reading Part 1 of this chapter, you should be able to:

1. Describe the incidence, morbidity, and mortality of cardiovascular disease. (p. 1126)
2. Discuss prevention strategies that may reduce the morbidity and mortality of cardiovascular disease. (p. 1126)
3. Identify the risk factors most predisposing to coronary artery disease. (p. 1126)
4. Describe the anatomy of the heart, including the position in the thoracic cavity, layers of the heart, chambers of the heart, and location and function of cardiac valves. (pp. 1127–1128; also see Chapter 3)
5. Identify the major structures of the vascular system, the factors affecting venous return, the components of cardiac output, and the phases of the cardiac cycle. (pp. 1128–1130; also see Chapter 3)
6. Define preload, afterload, and left ventricular end-diastolic pressure and relate each to the pathophysiology of heart failure. (see Chapter 3)
7. Identify the arterial blood supply to any given area of the myocardium. (p. 1128; also see Chapter 3)
8. Compare and contrast the coronary arterial distribution to the major portions of the cardiac conduction system. (p. 1128; also see Chapter 3)
9. Identify the structure and course of all divisions and subdivisions of the cardiac conduction system. (pp. 1129–1130; also see Chapter 3)
10. Identify and describe how the heart's pacemaking control, rate, and rhythm are determined. (p. 1130; also see Chapter 3)
11. Explain the physiological basis of conduction delay in the AV node. (see Chapter 3)
12. Define the functional properties of cardiac muscle. (see Chapter 3)
13. Define the events comprising electrical potential. (see Chapter 3)
14. List the most important ions involved in myocardial action potential and their primary function in this process. (see Chapter 3)
15. Describe the events involved in the steps from excitation to contraction of cardiac muscle fibers. (p. 1130; also see Chapter 3)
16. Describe the clinical significance of Starling's law. (see Chapter 3)

17. Identify the structures of the autonomic nervous system and their effect on heart rate, rhythm, and contractility. (see Chapter 3)
18. Define and give examples of positive and negative inotropism, chronotropism, and dromotropism. (see Chapter 3)
19. Discuss the pathophysiology of cardiac disease and injury. (pp. 1142–1185)
20. Explain the purpose of ECG monitoring and its limitations. (p. 1130)
21. Correlate the electrophysiological and hemodynamic events occurring throughout the entire cardiac cycle with the various ECG waveforms, segments, and intervals. (pp. 1134–1141)
22. Identify how heart rates, durations, and amplitudes may be determined from ECG recordings. (pp. 1134–1141)
23. Relate the cardiac surfaces or areas represented by the ECG leads. (pp. 1131–1132, 1140)
24. Differentiate among the primary mechanisms responsible for producing cardiac dysrhythmias. (pp. 1140, 1142–1185)
25. Describe a systematic approach to the analysis and interpretation of cardiac dysrhythmias. (pp. 1141–1185)
26. Describe the dysrhythmias originating in the sinus node, the AV junction, the atria, and the ventricles. (pp. 1144–1185)
27. Describe the process and pitfalls of differentiating wide QRS complex tachycardias. (pp. 1174–1176)
28. Describe the conditions of pulseless electrical activity. (pp. 1182–1183)
29. Describe the phenomena of reentry, aberration, and accessory pathways. (pp. 1143–1144, 1153, 1184–1185)
30. Identify the ECG changes characteristically produced by electrolyte imbalances and specify their clinical implications. (p. 1185)
31. Identify patient situations where ECG rhythm analysis is indicated. (pp. 1142–1185)
32. Recognize the ECG changes that may reflect evidence of myocardial ischemia and injury and their limitations. (p. 1140)
33. Correlate abnormal ECG findings with clinical interpretation. (pp. 1142–1185)
34. Identify the major mechanical, pharmacological, and electrical therapeutic objectives in the treatment of the patient with any dysrhythmia. (pp. 1142–1185)
35. Describe artifacts that may cause confusion when evaluating the ECG of a patient with a pacemaker. (pp. 1131, 1179, 1181–1182)
36. List the possible complications of pacing. (pp. 1181–1182)
37. List the causes and implications of pacemaker failure. (pp. 1181–1182)
38. Identify additional hazards that interfere with artificial pacemaker function. (pp. 1181–1182)
39. Recognize the complications of artificial pacemakers as evidenced on an ECG. (pp. 1181–1182)

Part 2: Assessment and Management of the Cardiovascular Patient (begins on p. 1186)

After reading Part 2 of this chapter, you should be able to:

1. Identify and describe the components of the focused history as it relates to the patient with cardiovascular compromise. (pp. 1187–1191)
2. Identify and describe the details of inspection, auscultation, and palpation specific to the cardiovascular system. (pp. 1191–1194)
3. Identify and define the heart sounds and relate them to hemodynamic events in the cardiac cycle. (pp. 1192–1193)
4. Describe the differences between normal and abnormal heart sounds. (pp. 1192–1193)

5. Define pulse deficit, pulsus paradoxus, and pulsus alternans. (pp. 1194, 1222)
6. Identify the normal characteristics of the point of maximum impulse (PMI). (p. 1193)
7. Based on field impressions, identify the need for rapid intervention for the patient in cardiovascular compromise. (pp. 1186–1194)
8. Describe the incidence, morbidity, and mortality associated with myocardial conduction defects. (p. 1216)
9. Identify the clinical indications, components, and the function of transcutaneous and permanent artificial cardiac pacing. (pp. 1179, 1181–1182, 1206, 1207–1208)
10. Explain what each setting and indicator on a transcutaneous pacing system represents and how the settings may be adjusted. (pp. 1207–1208)
11. Describe the techniques of applying a transcutaneous pacing system. (pp. 1206, 1207)
12. Describe the characteristics of an implanted pacemaking system. (pp. 1179, 1181–1182)
13. Describe the epidemiology, morbidity, mortality, and pathophysiology of angina pectoris. (pp. 1211–1212)
14. Describe the assessment and management of a patient with angina pectoris. (pp. 1213–1214)
15. Identify what is meant by the OPQRST of chest pain assessment. (pp. 1187–1188)
16. List other clinical conditions that may mimic signs and symptoms of coronary artery disease and angina pectoris. (p. 1212)
17. Identify the ECG findings in patients with angina pectoris. (p. 1213)
18. Based on the pathophysiology and clinical evaluation of the patient with chest pain, list the anticipated clinical problems according to their life-threatening potential. (p. 1212)
19. Describe the epidemiology, morbidity, mortality, and pathophysiology of myocardial infarction. (pp. 1214–1215)
20. List the mechanisms by which a myocardial infarction may be produced from traumatic and nontraumatic events. (p. 1214)
21. Identify the primary hemodynamic changes produced in myocardial infarction. (pp. 1214–1215)
22. List and describe the assessment parameters to be evaluated in a patient with a suspected myocardial infarction. (pp. 1215–1216)
23. Identify the anticipated clinical presentation of a patient with a suspected acute myocardial infarction. (pp. 1215–1216)
24. Differentiate the characteristics of the pain/discomfort occurring in angina pectoris and acute myocardial infarction. (p. 1215)
25. Identify the ECG changes characteristically seen during evolution of an acute myocardial infarction. (p. 1216)
26. Identify the most common complications of an acute myocardial infarction. (pp. 1214–1216)
27. List the characteristics of a patient eligible for fibrinolytic therapy. (pp. 1218–1220)
28. Describe the “window of opportunity” as it pertains to reperfusion of a myocardial injury or infarction. (p. 1218)
29. Based on the pathophysiology and clinical evaluation of the patient with a suspected acute myocardial infarction, list the anticipated clinical problems according to their life-threatening potential. (pp. 1214–1220)
30. Specify the measures that may be taken to prevent or minimize complications in the patient suspected of myocardial infarction. (pp. 1216–1220)
31. Describe the most commonly used cardiac drugs in terms of therapeutic effect and dosages, routes of administration, side effects, and toxic effects. (pp. 1199, 1200, 1218; also see Chapter 6)

32. Describe the epidemiology, morbidity, mortality, and physiology associated with heart failure. (pp. 1220–1221)
33. Identify the factors that may precipitate or aggravate heart failure. (pp. 1220–1221)
34. Define acute pulmonary edema and describe its relationship to left ventricular failure. (pp. 1220–1221)
35. Differentiate between early and late signs and symptoms of left ventricular failure and those of right ventricular failure. (pp. 1220–1221)
36. Define and explain the clinical significance of paroxysmal nocturnal dyspnea, pulmonary edema, and dependent edema. (pp. 1221–1222)
37. List the interventions prescribed for the patient in acute congestive heart failure. (pp. 1223–1224)
38. Describe the most commonly used pharmacological agents in the management of congestive heart failure in terms of therapeutic effect, dosages, routes of administration, side effects, and toxic effects. (pp. 1999, 1200, 1223; also see Chapter 6)
39. Define and describe the incidence, mortality, morbidity, pathophysiology, assessment, and management of the following cardiac related problems:
    - ★ Cardiac tamponade (pp. 1224–1225)
    - ★ Hypertensive emergency (pp. 1225–1226)
    - ★ Cardiogenic shock (pp. 1226–1229)
    - ★ Cardiac arrest (pp. 1229–1233)
40. Identify the limiting factor of pericardial anatomy that determines intrapericardiac pressure. (p. 1224)
41. Describe how to determine if pulsus paradoxus, pulsus alternans, or electrical alternans is present. (pp. 1222, 1224)
42. Explain the essential pathophysiological defect of hypertension in terms of Starling's law of the heart. (pp. 1221, 1226)
43. Rank the clinical problems of patients in hypertensive emergencies according to their sense of urgency. (pp. 1225–1226)
44. Identify the drugs of choice for hypertensive emergencies, cardiogenic shock, and cardiac arrest, including their indications, contraindications, side effects, route of administration, and dosages. (pp. 1999, 1200, 1226, 1227–1229, 1230; also see Chapter 6)
45. Describe the major systemic effects of reduced tissue perfusion caused by cardiogenic shock. (pp. 1226–1227)
46. Explain the primary mechanisms by which the heart may compensate for a diminished cardiac output and describe their efficiency in cardiogenic shock. (pp. 1226–1227)
47. Identify the clinical criteria and progressive stages of cardiogenic shock. (pp. 1226–1227)
48. Describe the dysrhythmias seen in cardiac arrest. (p. 1229)
49. Explain how to confirm asystole using the 3-lead ECG. (p. 1229)
50. Define the terms *defibrillation* and *synchronized cardioversion*. (pp. 1199, 1204)
51. Specify the methods of supporting the patient with a suspected ineffective implanted defibrillation device. (p. 1201)
52. Describe resuscitation and identify circumstances and situations where resuscitation efforts would not be initiated. (pp. 1229–1233)
53. Identify communication and documentation protocols with medical direction and law enforcement used for termination of resuscitation efforts. (pp. 1232–1233)
54. Describe the incidence, morbidity, mortality, pathophysiology, assessment, and management of vascular disorders including occlusive disease, phlebitis, aortic aneurysm, and peripheral artery occlusion. (pp. 1233–1237)

55. Identify the clinical significance of claudication and presence of arterial bruits in a patient with peripheral vascular disorders. (pp. 1233–1237)

56. Describe the clinical significance of unequal arterial blood pressure readings in the arms. (p. 1236)

57. Recognize and describe the signs and symptoms of dissecting thoracic or abdominal aneurysm. (pp. 1233–1234)

58. Differentiate between signs and symptoms of cardiac tamponade, hypertensive emergencies, cardiogenic shock, and cardiac arrest. (pp. 1224–1229)

59. Utilize the results of the patient history, assessment findings, and ECG analysis to differentiate between, and provide treatment for, patients with the following conditions (pp. 1186–1237):
   - ★ Cardiovascular disease
   - ★ Chest pain
   - ★ In need of a pacemaker
   - ★ Angina pectoris
   - ★ A suspected myocardial infarction
   - ★ Heart failure
   - ★ Cardiac tamponade
   - ★ A hypertensive emergency
   - ★ Cardiogenic shock
   - ★ Cardiac arrest

60. Based on the pathophysiology and clinical evaluation of the patient with chest pain, characterize the clinical problems according to their life-threatening potential. (p. 1212)

61. Given several preprogrammed patients with cardiac complaints, provide the appropriate assessment, treatment, and transport. (pp. 1186–1237)

Key Terms

aberrant conduction, p. 1184
absolute refractory period, p. 1140
acute arterial occlusion, p. 1235
acute coronary syndrome (ACS), p. 1211
acute pulmonary embolism, p. 1234
aneurysm, p. 1233
angina pectoris, p. 1212
arrhythmia, p. 1143
arteriosclerosis, p. 1233
artifact, p. 1131
atherosclerosis, p. 1233
augmented limb leads, p. 1132
bipolar limb leads, p. 1131
bradycardia, p. 1141
bruit, p. 1155
bundle branch block, p. 1184
bundle of Kent, p. 1185
cardiac arrest, p. 1229
cardiac tamponade, p. 1224
cardiogenic shock, p. 1226
cardiovascular disease (CVD), p. 1126
claudication, p. 1233
compensatory pause, p. 1166
congestive heart failure (CHF), p. 1221
coronary heart disease (CHD), p. 1126
corrected QT (QTc), p. 1140
coupling interval, p. 1173
cystic medial necrosis, p. 1234
deep venous thrombosis, p. 1235
defibrillation, p. 1199
dissecting aortic aneurysm, p. 1234
downtime, p. 1229
dysrhythmia, p. 1143
ectopic beat, p. 1143
ectopic focus, p. 1143
Einthoven's triangle, p. 1132
electrocardiogram (ECG), p. 1131
heart failure, p. 1221
hypertensive emergency, p. 1225
hypertensive encephalopathy, p. 1225
interpolated beat, p. 1172
myocardial infarction (MI), p. 1214
noncompensatory pause, p. 1152
non-ST-elevation myocardial infarction (NSTEMI), p. 1214
normal sinus rhythm, p. 1142
paroxysmal nocturnal dyspnea (PND), p. 1222
peripheral arterial atherosclerotic disease, p. 1235
precordial (chest) leads, p. 1132
Prinzmetal's angina, p. 1212
prolonged QT interval, p. 1140
pulmonary embolism (PE), p. 1221
QT interval, p. 1140
refractory period, p. 1140
relative refractory period, p. 1140
resuscitation, p. 1229

return of spontaneous circulation (ROSC), p. 1230
rhythm strip, p. 1130
ST-elevation myocardial infarction (STEMI), p. 1214
subendocardial infarction, p. 1214
sudden death, p. 1229
survival, p. 1230
synchronized cardioversion, p. 1204
tachycardia, p. 1141
total downtime, p. 1229
transmural infarction, p. 1214
unipolar limb leads, p. 1132
varicose veins, p. 1235
vasculitis, p. 1235

INTRODUCTION

cardiovascular disease (CVD) *disease affecting the heart, peripheral blood vessels, or both.*

coronary heart disease (CHD) *a type of CVD; the single largest killer of Americans.*

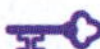

More than 60 million Americans have some form of cardiovascular disease.

According to current estimates, more than 60 million Americans have some form of **cardiovascular disease (CVD). Coronary heart disease (CHD)**, a type of CVD, is the single largest killer of Americans. Each year, on average, 466,000 people die of CHD. Approximately 225,000 of them, a little less than half, die before ever reaching the hospital. Another way of looking at the impact of coronary heart disease is this: one American will suffer a nonfatal heart attack every 29 seconds. About once every minute, an American will die from CHD. These deaths are usually sudden and often due to lethal cardiac rhythm disturbances that result in cardiac arrest.

Sudden death from CHD is often preventable. To decrease the chances of sudden death, the patient must recognize the signs and symptoms early and seek health care. Then, the health care system must provide definitive care promptly, usually within the first hour after the onset of symptoms.

Public education about CHD has focused on two strategies. The first is to educate the public about the risk factors for the development of CHD. This program encourages patients to modify their lifestyle to minimize these risk factors. The following factors have been *proven* to increase the risk of cardiovascular disease:

- ★ Smoking
- ★ Older age
- ★ Family history of cardiac disease
- ★ Hypertension (high blood pressure)
- ★ Hypercholesterolemia (excessive cholesterol in the blood)
- ★ Carbohydrate intolerance (diabetes mellitus)
- ★ Cocaine use
- ★ Male gender
- ★ Lack of exercise

Factors that are *thought* to increase the risk of coronary heart disease include:

- ★ Diet
- ★ Obesity
- ★ Oral contraceptives (birth control pills)
- ★ Sedentary lifestyle
- ★ Type A personality (competitive, aggressive, hostile)
- ★ Psychosocial tensions (stress)

The second component of public education is to teach recognition of the signs and symptoms of heart attack. Patients can only benefit from medical intervention if they recognize the signs and symptoms and promptly access the health care system. Patients are encouraged to access the EMS system early. As a paramedic, you will treat patients who already have developed the manifestations of cardiac disease. This will be an opportunity for you to further serve your patients by teaching preventive strategies, including early recognition of symptoms, education, and alteration of lifestyle.

This chapter discusses the advanced prehospital care of cardiovascular emergencies. First, we will review the pertinent anatomy and physiology, and then we will use that knowledge to discuss assessing, recognizing, and treating cardiovascular disorders.

Part 1: Cardiovascular Anatomy and Physiology, ECG Monitoring, and Dysrhythmia Analysis

REVIEW OF CARDIOVASCULAR ANATOMY AND PHYSIOLOGY

Cardiac anatomy and physiology were discussed in detail in Chapter 3, "Anatomy and Physiology." The following is a brief review of that information.

CARDIOVASCULAR ANATOMY

The heart is located in the center of the chest in the *mediastinum.* It is a muscular organ, consisting of three tissue layers: *endocardium* (the innermost layer that lines the chambers), *myocardium* (the middle layer with its unique ability to generate and conduct electrical impulses, causing the heart to contract), and *pericardium* (the protective sac surrounding the heart).

The heart (Figure 28-1 ■) contains four chambers—two superior, the *atria*, and two inferior, the *ventricles.* Valves control the flow of blood through the heart: the *mitral valve* between the left atrium and ventricle; the *tricuspid valve* between the right atrium and ventricle; the *aortic valve*

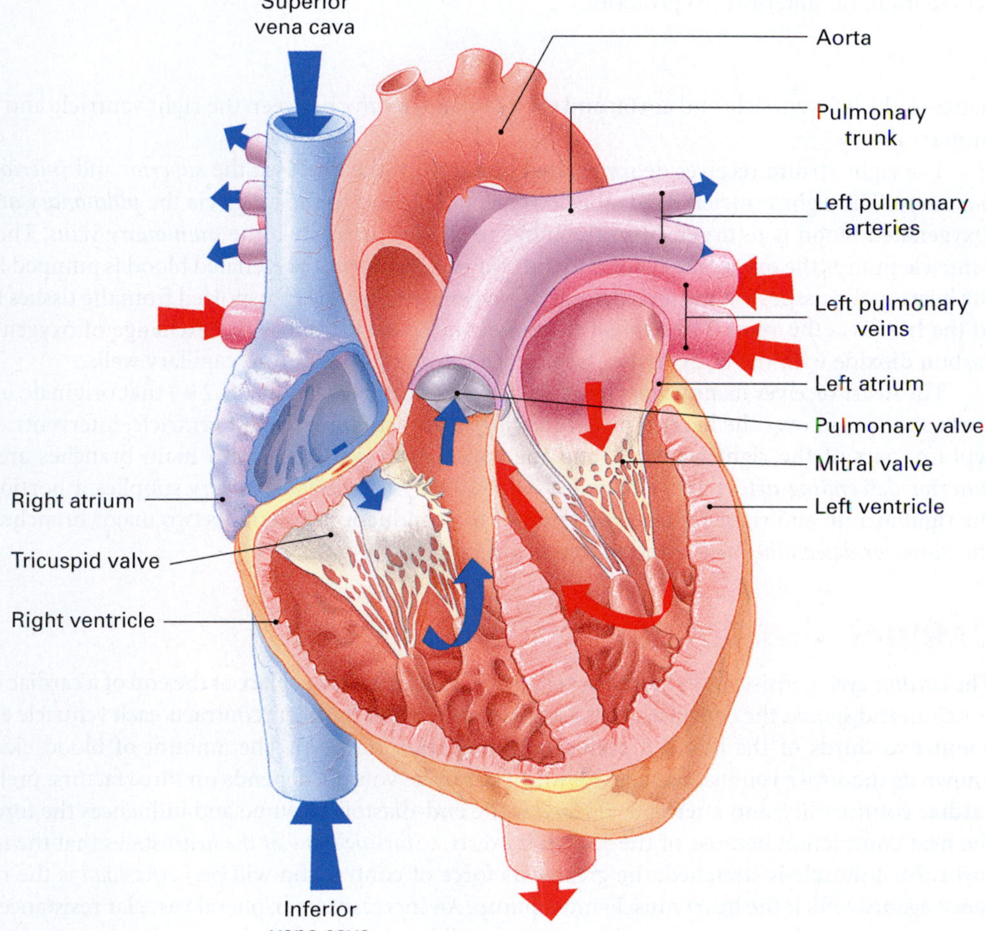

■ Figure 28-1 Blood flow through the heart.

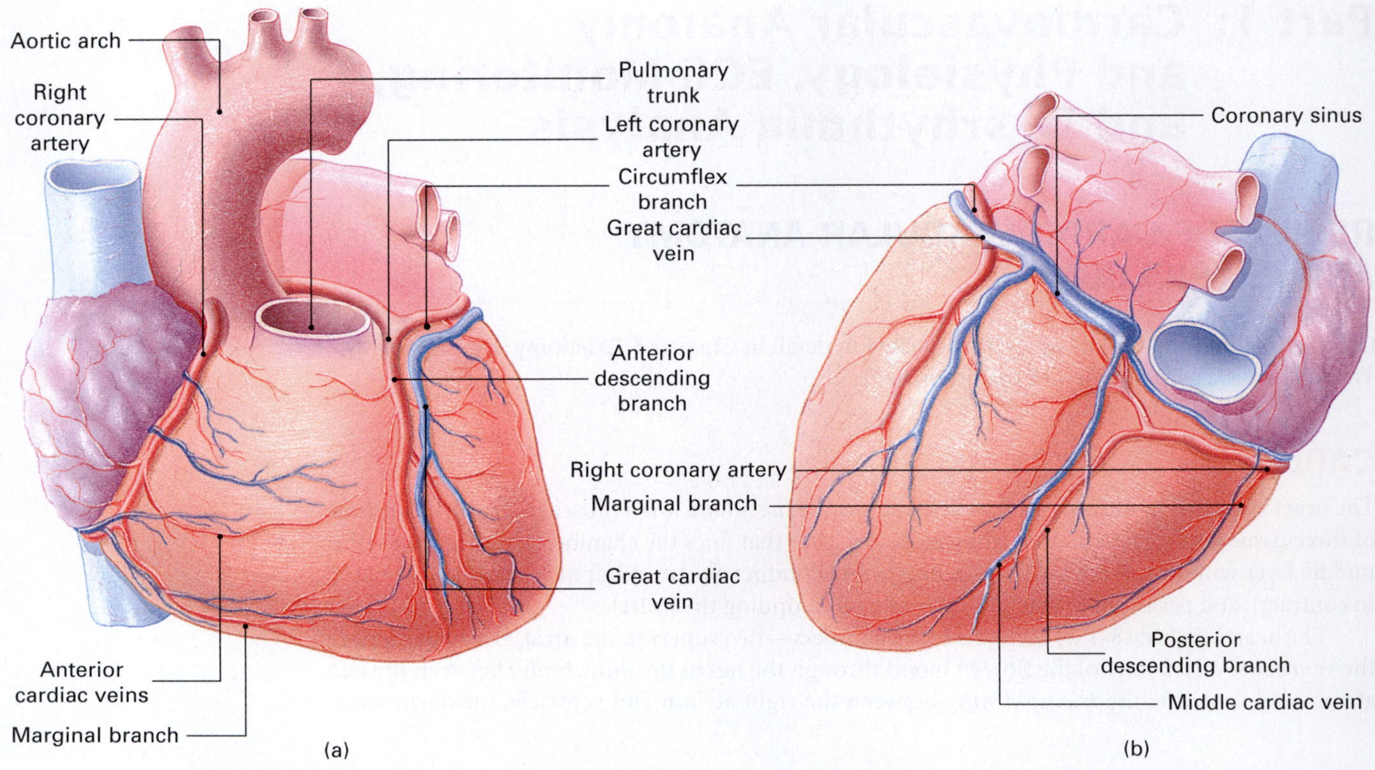

Figure 28-2 The coronary circulation: (a) anterior; (b) posterior.

between the left ventricle and aorta; and the *pulmonary valve* between the right ventricle and pulmonary artery.

The right atrium receives deoxygenated blood from the body via the *superior* and *inferior venae cavae.* The right ventricle sends the deoxygenated blood to the lungs via the *pulmonary artery.* Oxygenated blood is returned from the lungs to the *left atrium* via the *pulmonary veins.* The left ventricle pumps the oxygenated blood to the body via the *aorta.* Oxygenated blood is pumped from the heart to the tissues via the *arteries,* and deoxygenated blood is transported from the tissues back to the heart via the *veins.* The *capillaries* connect arteries and veins. The exchange of oxygen and carbon dioxide with the body tissues takes place through the very thin capillary walls.

The heart receives its nutrients from the *coronary arteries* (Figure 28-2 ■) that originate in the aorta and spread over the heart. The *left coronary artery* supplies the left ventricle, interventricular septum, part of the right ventricle, and the conduction system. Its two main branches are the *anterior descending artery* and *circumflex artery.* The *right coronary artery* supplies a portion of the right atrium and right ventricle and part of the conduction system. Its two major branches are the *posterior descending artery* and *marginal artery.*

CARDIAC PHYSIOLOGY

The *cardiac cycle* consists of *diastole,* the relaxation phase that takes place at the end of a cardiac contraction, and *systole,* the contraction phase. Normally, when the heart contracts each ventricle ejects about two-thirds of the blood it contains (the *ejection fraction*). The amount of blood ejected, known as the *stroke volume,* averages 70 mL. The stroke volume depends on three factors: preload, cardiac contractility, and afterload. *Preload* is the end-diastolic volume and influences the force of the next contraction because of the stretch it exerts. (*Starling's law of the heart* states that the more myocardial muscle is stretched, the greater its force of contraction will be.) *Afterload* is the resistance against which the heart muscle must pump. An increase in peripheral vascular resistance will decrease stroke volume; a decrease in resistance will increase stroke volume.

Cardiac output is calculated as stroke volume times heart rate. Since the normal heart rate is 60–100 beats per minute and the average stroke volume is 70 mL, the average cardiac output is about 5 liters (5,000 milliliters) per minute (70 mL × 70 bpm = 4,900 mL/min).

Heart function is regulated by the sympathetic and parasympathetic nervous components of the autonomic nervous system, working in opposition to one another to maintain a balance. During stress, the sympathetic system dominates to raise the heart rate and increase contractile force. During sleep, the parasympathetic system dominates to decrease heart rate and contractile force. The terms *chronotropy* (referring to heart rate), *inotropy* (referring to contractile strength), and *dromotropy* (referring to rate of nervous impulse conduction) describe autonomic control of the heart.

Cardiac function depends heavily on electrolyte balances. Electrolytes that affect cardiac function include sodium (Na^+), calcium (Ca^{++}), potassium (K^+), chloride (Cl^-), and magnesium (Mg^{++}). Sodium plays a major role in depolarizing the myocardium. Calcium takes part in myocardial depolarization and myocardial contraction. Potassium influences repolarization. Research is ongoing into the roles of magnesium and chloride.

ELECTROPHYSIOLOGY

Within the cardiac muscle fibers are special structures called *intercalated discs.* These discs connect cardiac muscle fibers and conduct electrical impulses quickly from one muscle fiber to the next. Thus, when one cell becomes excited, the action potential spreads rapidly across the entire group of cells, resulting in a coordinated contraction. This functional unit is a *syncytium.* The heart has two syncytia—the *atrial syncytium* and the *ventricular syncytium.* The atrial syncytium contracts from superior to inferior, so that the atria express blood to the ventricles. The ventricular syncytium contracts from inferior to superior, expelling blood from the ventricles into the aorta and pulmonary arteries. An impulse can be conducted from the atria to the ventricles only through the *atrioventricular (AV) bundle.*

Cardiac muscle functions according to an "all-or-none" principle. That is, if a single muscle fiber becomes *depolarized,* the action potential will spread through the whole syncytium. Stimulating a single atrial fiber will thus completely depolarize the atria, and stimulating a single ventricular fiber will completely depolarize the ventricles.

Cardiac Depolarization

Normally, an ionic difference exists on the two sides of a cell membrane. The cell's sodium-potassium pump expels sodium (Na^+) from the cell, leaving the inside of the cell more negatively charged than the outside. This difference is called the *resting potential.* When the myocardial cell is stimulated, the membrane changes to allow positively charged sodium ions to rush into the cell, giving the inside of the cell a greater positive charge than the outside. This change of membrane polarity is the *action potential.* After the influx of sodium, a slower influx of calcium ions (Ca^{++}) increases the positive charge inside the cell.

This change from the resting potential (when the inside of the cell is more negatively charged) to a relatively more positive charge inside the cell is called *cardiac depolarization.* Once depolarization occurs in a muscle fiber, it is transmitted throughout the entire syncytium, via the intercalated discs, until the entire muscle mass is depolarized. Contraction of the muscle follows depolarization. The cell membrane remains permeable to sodium for only a fraction of a second. Thereafter, sodium influx stops and potassium escapes from inside the cell. This returns the charge inside the cell to normal (negative). In addition, sodium is actively pumped outside the cell, allowing the cell to *repolarize* and return to its normal resting state.

Understanding the process of cardiac depolarization is critical to understanding and interpreting electrocardiograms (ECGs).

The Cardiac Conductive System

The cardiac conductive system stimulates the ventricles to depolarize in the proper direction. It initiates an impulse, spreads it through the atria, transmits it to the apex of the heart, and then stimulates the ventricles to depolarize from inferior to superior. The conduction system relies on specialized conductive fibers that transmit the depolarization potential through the heart very quickly.

■ Figure 28-3 The cardiac conductive system.

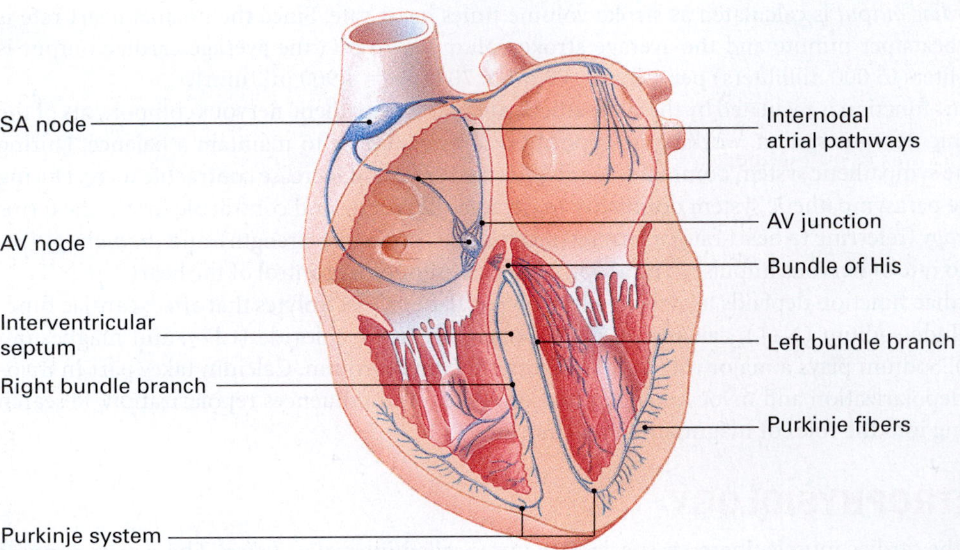

To accomplish their task, the cardiac conductive cells have:

★ *Excitability.* The cells can respond to an electrical stimulus.

★ *Conductivity.* The cells can propagate the electrical impulse from cell to cell.

★ *Automaticity.* Each conductive cell can depolarize without any outside impulse (called self-excitation). Generally, the cell with the fastest rate of discharge becomes the heart's pacemaker. Usually, this is the sinoatrial (SA) node; however, if one pacemaker cell fails to discharge, then the cell with the next fastest rate becomes the pacemaker.

★ *Contractility.* The cells have the ability to contract.

Internodal atrial pathways connect the SA node to the AV node (Figure 28-3 ■). These internodal pathways conduct the depolarization impulse to the atrial muscle mass and through the atria to the AV junction. The AV junction (the "gatekeeper") slows the impulse and allows the ventricles time to fill. Then, the impulse passes through the AV junction into the AV node and on to the AV fibers, which conduct the impulse from the atria to the ventricles. In the ventricles the AV fibers form the *bundle of His.*

The bundle of His subsequently divides into the right and left bundle branches. The *right bundle branch* delivers the impulse to the apex of the right ventricle. From there the *Purkinje system* spreads it across the myocardium. The *left bundle branch* divides into *anterior and posterior fascicles* that also ultimately terminate in the Purkinje system. At the same time that the impulse is transmitted to the right ventricle, the Purkinje system spreads it across the mass of the myocardium. Repolarization predominantly occurs in the opposite direction.

Each conductive system component has an intrinsic rate of self-excitation (SA node 60–100 bpm; AV node 40–60 bpm; Purkinje system 15–40 bpm).

ELECTROCARDIOGRAPHIC MONITORING

rhythm strip *electrocardiogram printout.*

One of your most important skills as a paramedic will be obtaining and interpreting ECG rhythm strips.

One of your most important skills as a paramedic will be obtaining and interpreting electrocardiographic (ECG) **rhythm strips.** Your patient's subsequent treatment will be based on rapid, accurate interpretation of these strips. At first, rhythm strips may seem difficult to read, for only through classroom instruction and repeated practice can you master their interpretation. Nor will every rhythm strip you encounter be a "textbook" example; you must be comfortable with all possible variants. With practice and a systematic approach, however, you will soon be skilled in their interpretation. This section presents basic information about ECG monitoring, as well as recognizing and interpreting dysrhythmias.

THE ELECTROCARDIOGRAM

The **electrocardiogram** (ECG) is a graphic record of the heart's electrical activity. However, it tells you nothing about the heart's pumping ability, which you must evaluate by pulse and blood pressure.

electrocardiogram (ECG) *the graphic recording of the heart's electrical activity. It may be displayed either on paper or on an oscilloscope.*

The electrocardiogram was invented by the Dutch physiologist Dr. Willem Einthoven in 1903. The device was first described in Dutch and referred to as an *elektrokardiograaf,* and thus the abbreviation *EKG* was applied. The abbreviation *EKG* is often interchanged with the English abbreviation *ECG.* Interestingly, Einthoven chose the letters *P, Q, R, S,* and *T* to describe points along the ECG waveform simply because they were in the middle of the alphabet and would not be confused with mathematic variables and similar commonly used letters.

Electrodes on the skin can detect the total electrical activity within the heart at any given time. The electrical impulses on the skin surface have a very low voltage. The ECG machine amplifies these impulses and records them over time on ECG graph paper or a monitor. *Positive impulses* appear as *upward* deflections on the paper, *negative impulses* as *downward* deflections. The absence of any electrical impulse produces an *isoelectric line,* which is flat.

Artifacts are deflections on the ECG produced by factors other than the heart's electrical activity. Common causes of artifacts include:

artifact *deflection on the ECG produced by factors other than the heart's electrical activity.*

- ★ Muscle tremors
- ★ Shivering
- ★ Patient movement
- ★ Loose electrodes
- ★ 60 hertz interference
- ★ Machine malfunction

It is important for ECGs to be free of artifacts. When an artifact is present, you must first try to eliminate it before recording the ECG. Loose electrodes should be replaced. Occasionally, patients may be quite diaphoretic, thus preventing the electrodes from adhering well to the skin. In these cases, you may need to wipe the skin and apply tincture of Benzoin before applying the electrode.

ECG Leads

Review

Content

ECG Leads

- Bipolar (limb)
- Augmented (unipolar)
- Precordial (chest)

You can obtain many views of the heart's electrical activity by monitoring the voltage change through *electrodes* placed at various places on the body surface. Each pair of electrodes is a *lead.* In the hospital, 12 leads are normally used. As a rule, most EMS systems use only 3 leads in the field. In fact, a single lead is adequate for detecting life-threatening dysrhythmias. With the advent of fibrinolytic therapy and computer interpretation, however, 12-lead ECGs are becoming more common in the field, especially in rural EMS systems.

The three types of ECG leads are bipolar, augmented, and precordial. **Bipolar limb leads,** the kind most frequently used, have one positive electrode and one negative electrode. Any electrical impulse moving toward the positive electrode will cause a positive (upward) deflection on the ECG paper. Any electrical impulse moving toward the negative electrode will cause a negative (downward) deflection. The absence of a positive or negative deflection means either that there is no electrical impulse or that the impulse is moving perpendicular to the lead. Leads I, II, and III, commonly called *limb leads,* are bipolar. They are the most frequently used leads in the field. Table 28–1 lists their placement sites.

bipolar limb leads *electrocardiogram leads applied to the arms and legs that contain two electrodes of opposite (positive and negative) polarity; leads I, II, and III.*

Table 28–1 Bipolar Lead Placement Sites

Lead	Positive Electrode	Negative Electrode
I	Left arm	Right arm
II	Left leg	Right arm
III	Left leg	Left arm

■ Figure 28-4 Einthoven's triangle as formed by leads I, II, and III.

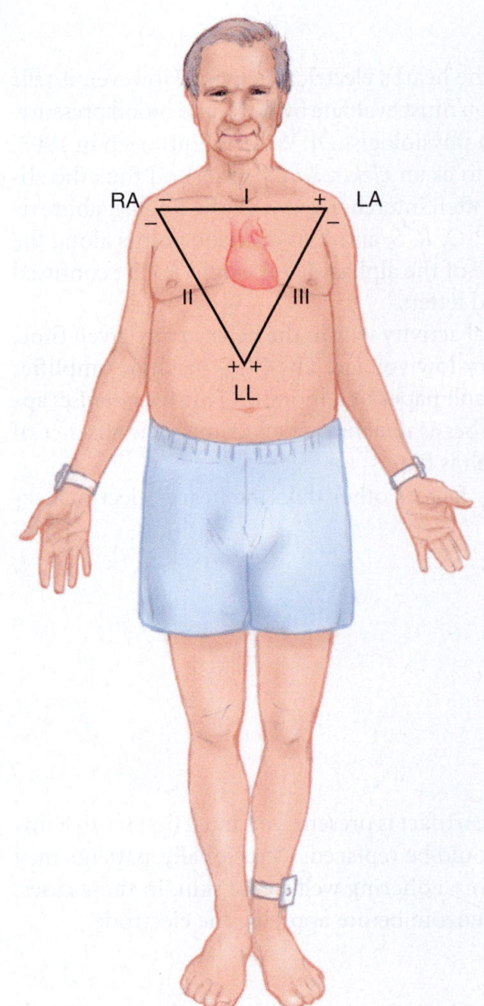

Einthoven's triangle *the triangle around the heart formed by the bipolar limb leads.*

augmented limb leads *another term for unipolar limb leads (see the following definition), reflecting the fact that the ground lead is disconnected, which increases the amplitude of deflection on the ECG tracing.*

unipolar limb leads *electrocardiogram leads applied to the arms and legs, consisting of one polarized (positive) electrode and a nonpolarized reference point that is created by the ECG machine combining two additional electrodes; also called augmented limb leads; leads aVR, aVL, and aVF.*

precordial (chest) leads *electrocardiogram leads applied to the chest in a pattern that permits a view of the horizontal plane of the heart; leads V_1, V_2, V_3, V_4, V_5, and V_6.*

These three bipolar leads form **Einthoven's triangle**, named after the inventor of the ECG machine (Figure 28-4 ■). The direction from the negative to the positive electrode is the lead's *axis.* Each lead shows a different axis of the heart. Lead I, at the top of Einthoven's triangle, has an axis of 0°. Lead II forms the right side of the triangle and has an axis of 60°. Lead III forms the left side of the triangle and has an axis of 120°.

The bipolar leads provide only three views of the heart. **Augmented limb leads**, or **unipolar limb leads**, provide additional views that are sometimes useful. Although these leads evaluate different axes than the bipolar leads, they utilize the same electrodes. They do this by electronically combining the negative electrodes of two of the bipolar leads to obtain an axis. These augmented leads are designated aVR, aVL, and aVF. The letter *a* indicates that the lead is augmented. The letter *V* identifies it as a unipolar lead. The *R, L,* and *F* identify the extremity on which the lead is placed (R = right arm, L = left arm, and F = left foot).

In addition, six **precordial (chest) leads** can be placed across the surface of the chest to measure electrical cardiac activity on a horizontal axis. These leads help in viewing the left ventricle and septum. They are designated V_1 through V_6, with the letter *V* identifying them as unipolar leads.

Routine ECG Monitoring

Whether in the ambulance, emergency department, or coronary care unit, routine ECG monitoring generally uses only one lead. The most common monitoring leads are either lead II or the *modified chest lead 1* (MCL_1). Of these, lead II is used more frequently because most of the heart's electrical current flows toward its positive axis. This gives the best view of the ECG waves and best depicts the conduction system's activity. MCL_1 is a special monitoring lead that some systems use selectively to help determine the origin of abnormal complexes such as premature beats. To avoid confusion, we will use lead II as the monitor lead throughout this text.

Lead II gives the best view of the ECG waves and best depicts the conduction system's activity.

Einthoven's triangle offers a basis for placing the leads. Usually you should place the electrodes on the chest wall instead of the extremities. This helps to reduce artifacts from arm movement. (If you use the arms, place the lead as high as possible on the extremity to decrease movement.) Make certain the skin is clean and free of hair before you place the electrodes on the chest wall. For lead II, the positive electrode is usually placed at the apex of the heart on the chest wall (or on the left leg), the negative electrode below the right clavicle (or on the right arm). The third electrode, the ground, is placed somewhere on the left, upper chest wall (or on the left arm).

A single monitoring lead can provide considerable information, including:

★ Rate of the heartbeat
★ Regularity of the heartbeat
★ Time it takes to conduct the impulse through the various parts of the heart

A single lead cannot provide the following information:

★ Presence or location of an infarct
★ Axis deviation or chamber enlargement
★ Right-to-left differences in conduction or impulse formation
★ Quality or presence of pumping action

ECG Graph Paper

ECG graph paper is standardized to allow comparative analysis of ECG patterns. The paper moves across the stylus at a standard speed of 25 mm/sec (Figure 28-5 ■). The *amplitude* of the ECG *deflection* is also standardized. When properly calibrated, the ECG stylus should deflect two large boxes when one millivolt (1 mV) is present. Most machines have calibration buttons, and a calibration curve should be placed at the beginning of the first ECG strip. Many machines do this automatically when they are first turned on.

The ECG graph is divided into a grid of light and heavy lines. The light lines are 1 mm apart, and the heavy lines are 5 mm apart. The heavy lines thus enclose large squares, each containing 25 of the smaller squares formed by the lighter lines (Figure 28-6 ■). The following relationships apply to the horizontal axis:

1 small box = 0.04 sec

1 large box = 0.20 sec (0.04 sec × 5 = 0.20 sec)

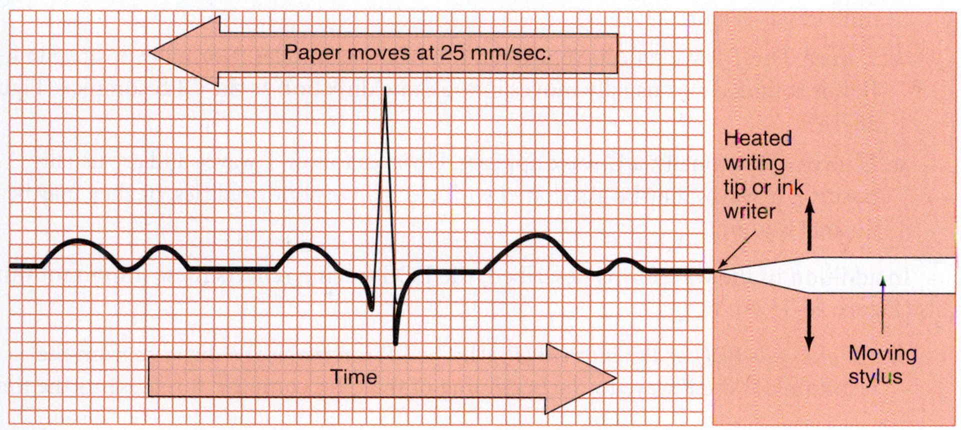

■ Figure 28-5 Recording of the ECG.

■ Figure 28-6 The ECG paper and markings.

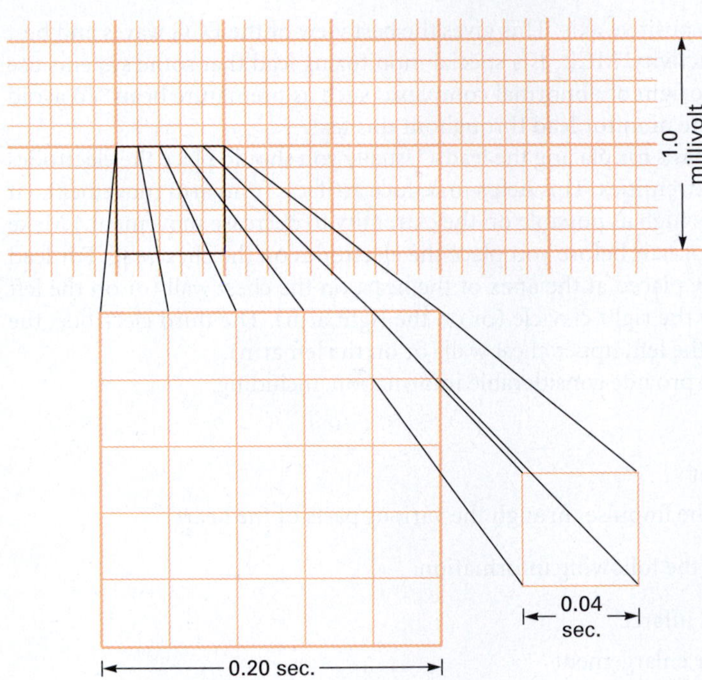

These increments measure the duration of the ECG complexes and time intervals. The vertical axis reflects the voltage amplitude in millivolts (mV). Two large boxes equal 1 mV.

In addition to the grid, ECG paper has time interval markings at the top. These marks are placed at 3-second intervals. Each 3-second interval contains 15 large boxes (0.2 sec × 15 boxes = 3.0 sec). The time markings measure heart rate.

RELATIONSHIP OF THE ECG TO ELECTRICAL EVENTS IN THE HEART

Content Review

ECG Components

- P wave
- QRS complex
- T wave
- U wave

The ECG tracing's components reflect electrical changes in the heart (Figure 28-7 ■):

- ★ *P wave.* The first component of the ECG, the P wave corresponds to atrial depolarization. On lead II, it is a positive, rounded wave before the QRS complex (Figures 28-8 ■ to 28-12 ■).
- ★ *QRS complex.* The QRS complex reflects ventricular depolarization. The *Q wave* is the first negative deflection after the P wave; the *R wave* is the first positive deflection after the P wave; and the *S wave* is the first negative deflection after the R wave. Not all three waves are always present, and the shape of the QRS complex can vary among individuals (Figure 28-13 ■).
- ★ *T wave.* The T wave reflects repolarization of the ventricles. Normally positive in lead II, it is rounded and usually moves in the same direction as the QRS complex (Figure 28-14 ■).
- ★ *U wave.* Occasionally, a U wave appears. U waves follow T waves and are usually positive. U waves may be associated with electrolyte abnormalities, or they may be a normal finding.

Content Review

ECG Time Intervals

- PR interval
- QRS interval
- ST segment

In addition to the waveforms described, the ECG tracing reflects these important time intervals (Figure 28-15 ■):

- ★ *PR interval (PRI) or PQ interval (PQI).* The PR interval is the distance from the beginning of the P wave to the beginning of the QRS complex. It represents the time

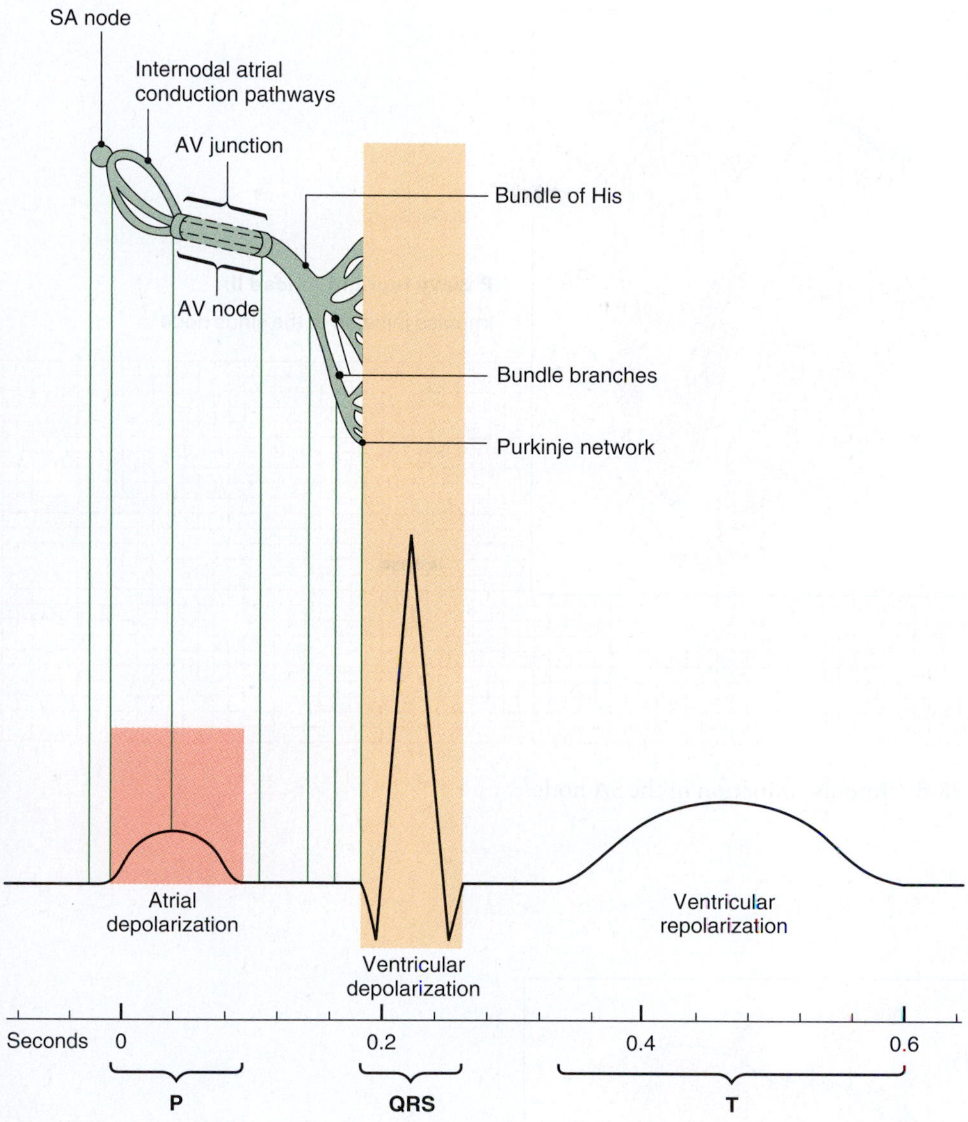

SA node
Internodal atrial conduction pathways
AV junction
Bundle of His
AV node
Bundle branches
Purkinje network
Atrial depolarization
Ventricular depolarization
Ventricular repolarization
Seconds 0 0.2 0.4 0.6
P QRS T

Figure 28-7 Relationship of the ECG to electrical activities in the heart.

the impulse takes to travel from the atria to the ventricles. Occasionally, the R wave is absent, in which case this interval is called the PQ interval. The terms *PR interval* and *PQ interval* may be used interchangeably.

- ★ *QRS interval.* The QRS interval is the distance from the first deflection of the QRS complex to the last. It represents the time necessary for ventricular depolarization.
- ★ *ST segment.* The ST segment is the distance from the S wave to the beginning of the T wave. Usually it is an isoelectric line; however, it may be elevated or depressed in certain disease states such as ischemia.

A normal PR interval is 0.12–0.20 second. A short PRI lasts less than 0.12 second; a prolonged PRI lasts longer than 0.20 second. A prolonged PRI indicates a delay in the AV node. A normal QRS complex lasts between 0.04 and 0.12 second. A value of less than 0.12 second means that the ventricles depolarized in a normal length of time.

Content Review

Normal Interval Durations

- PR 0.12–0.20 sec
- QRS 0.04–0.12 sec
- QT 0.33–0.42 sec

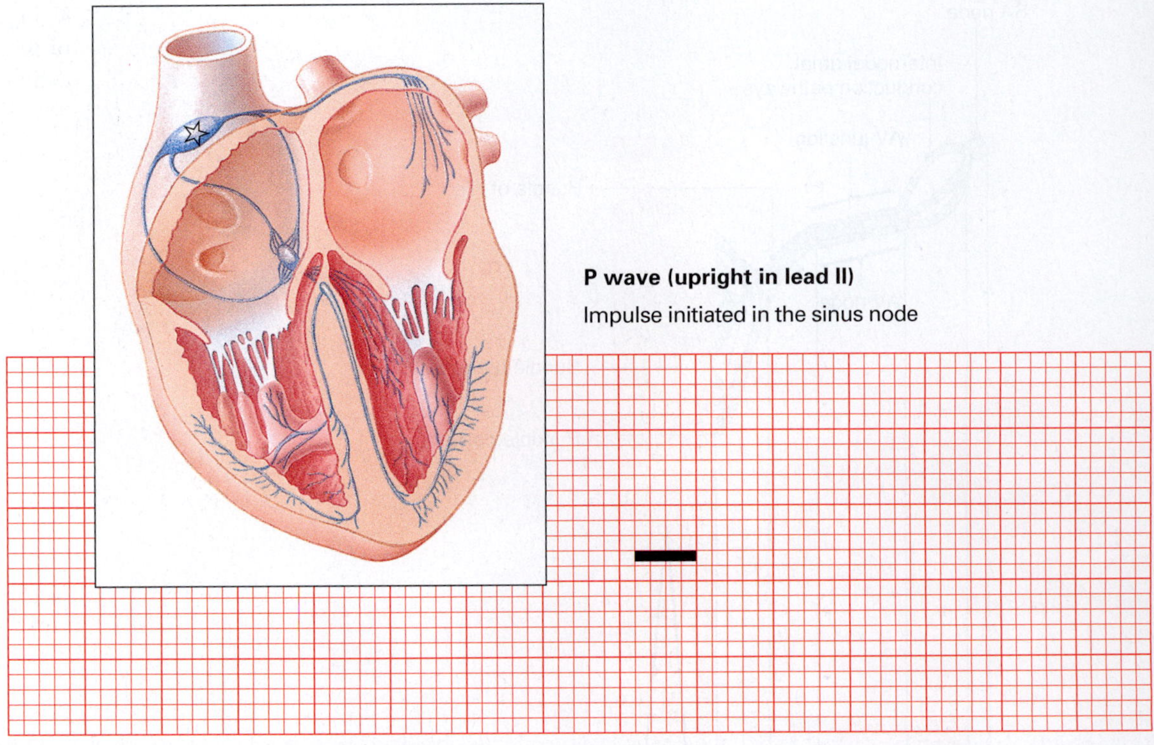

■ **Figure 28-8** Impulse initiation in the SA node.

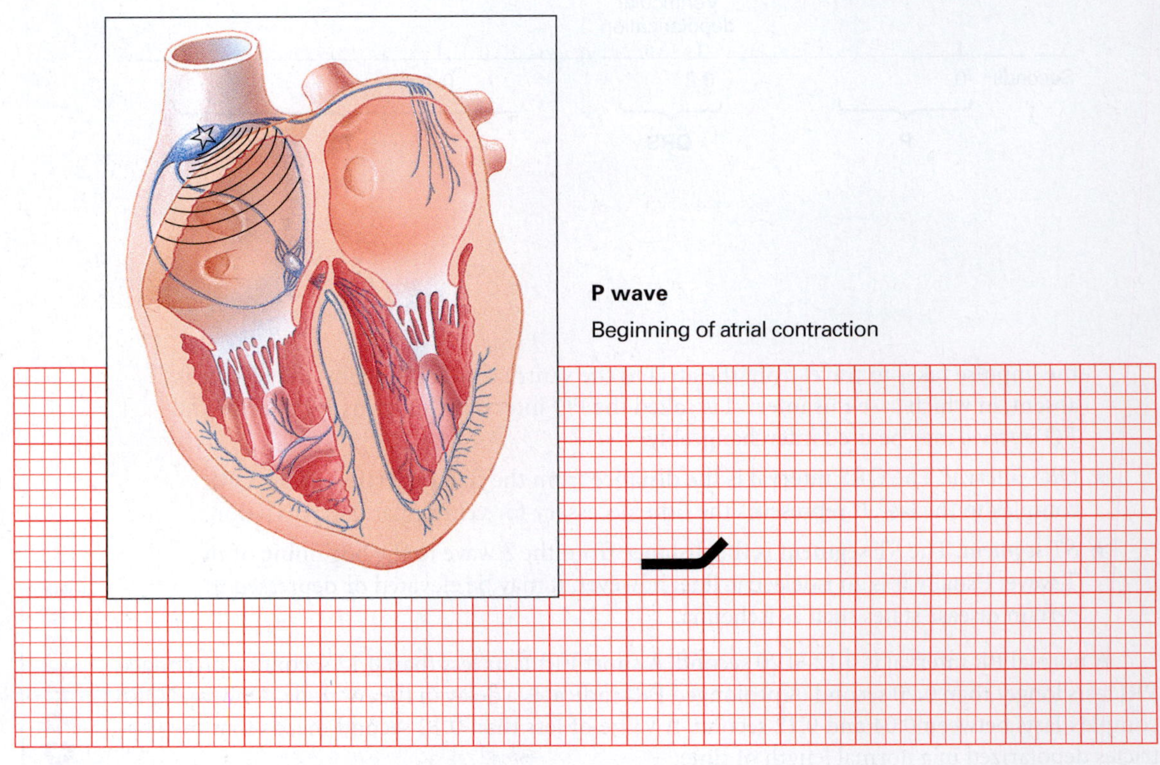

■ **Figure 28-9** Beginning of atrial contraction.

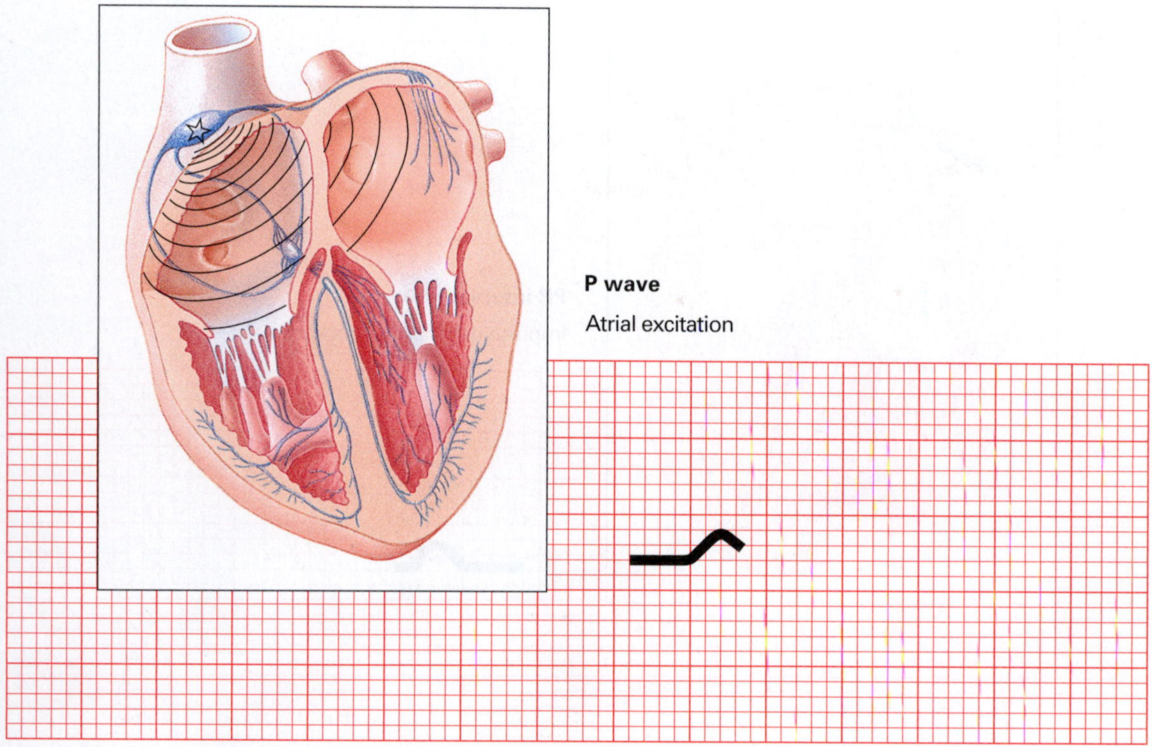

■ **Figure 28-10** Atrial excitation.

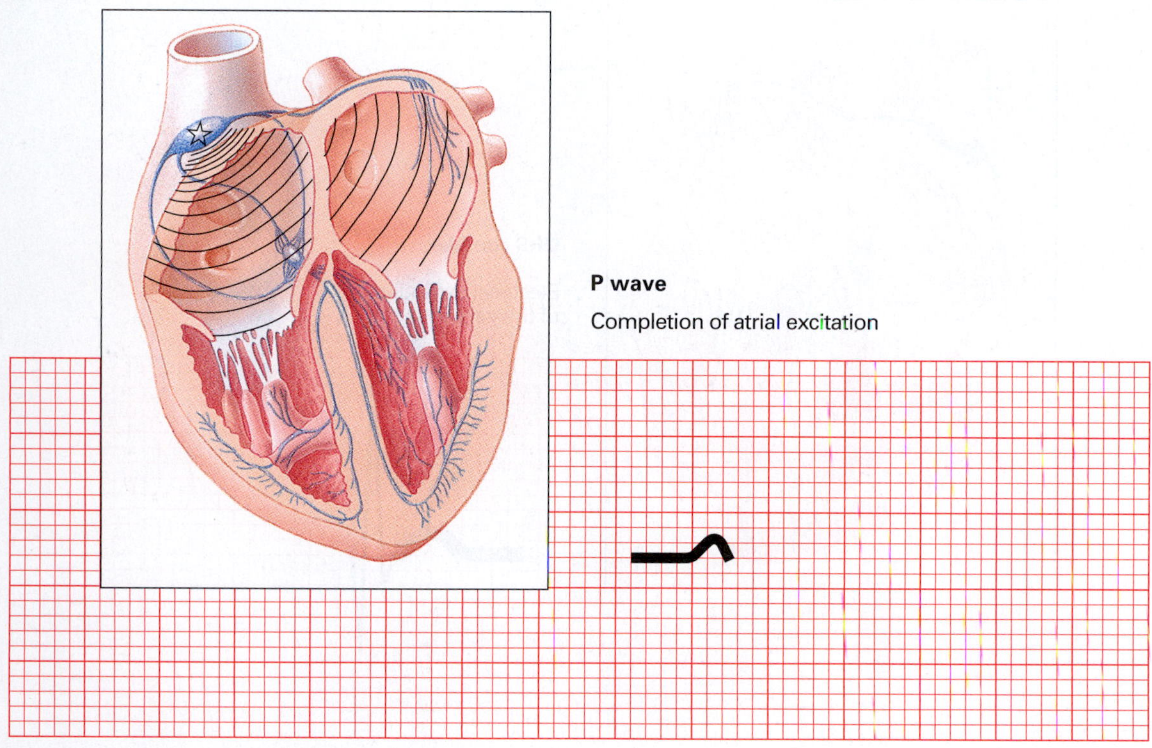

■ **Figure 28-11** Completion of atrial excitation.

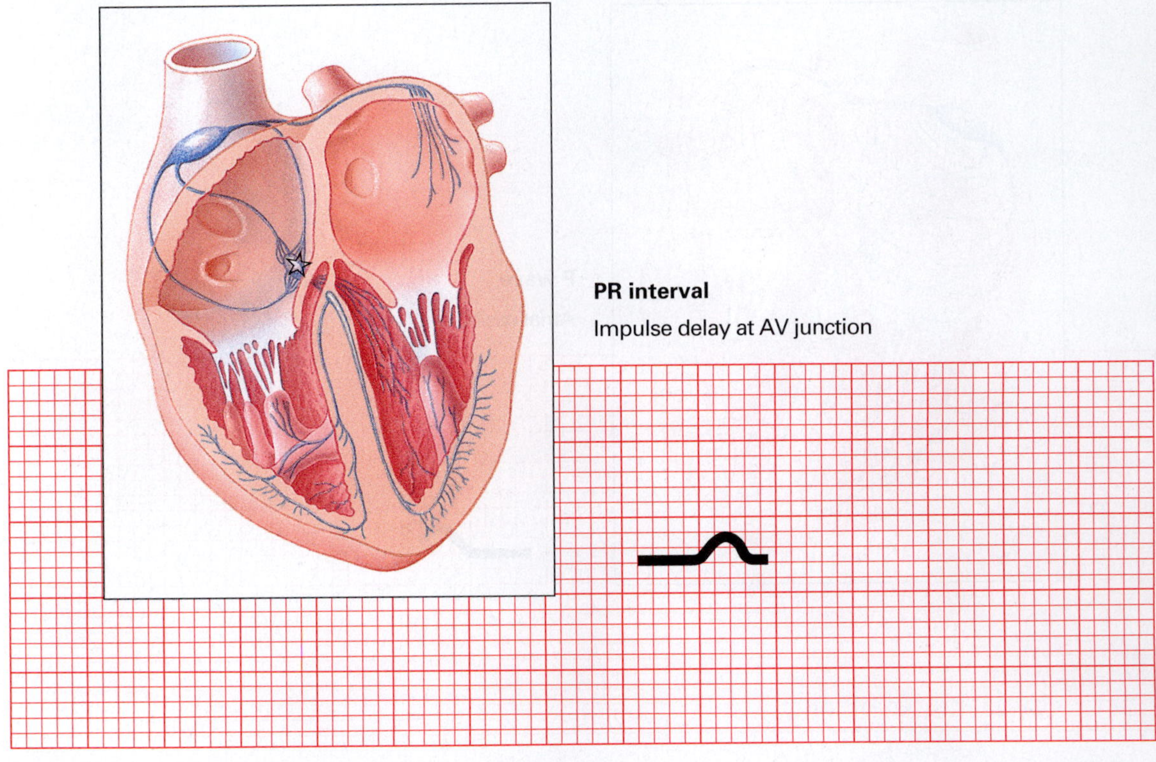

Figure 28-12 Impulse delay at the AV junction.

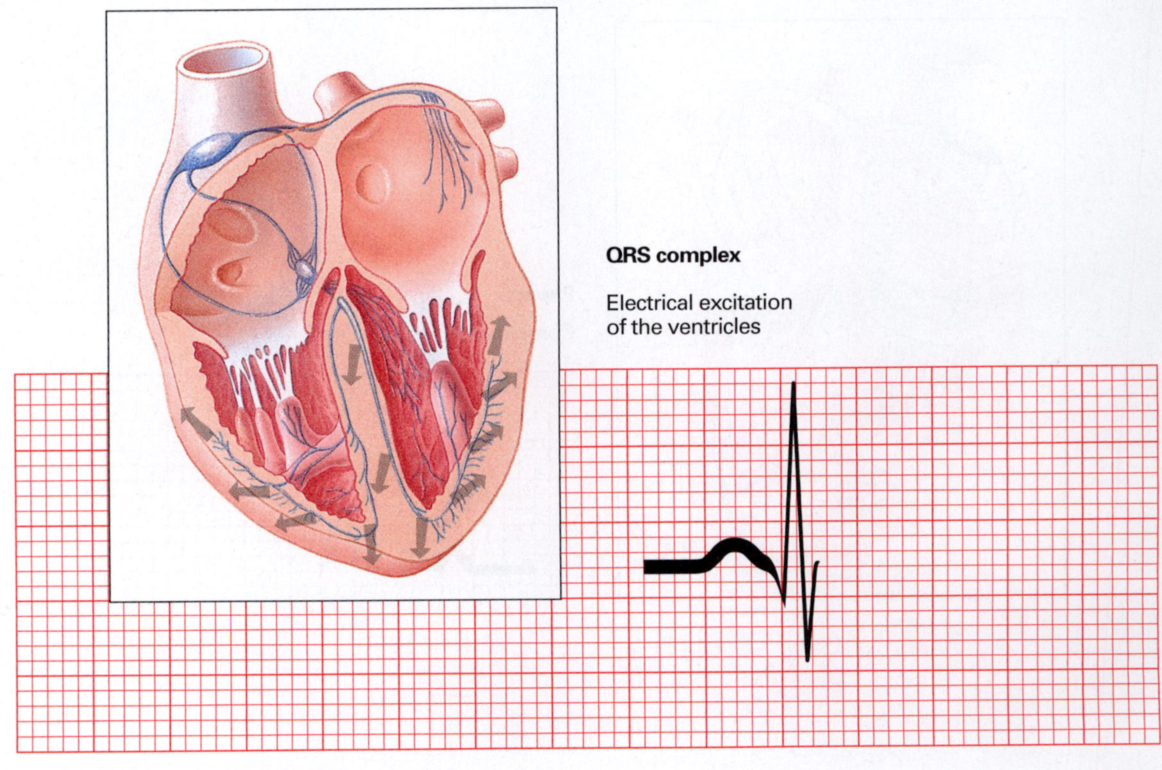

Figure 28-13 Electrical excitation of the ventricles.

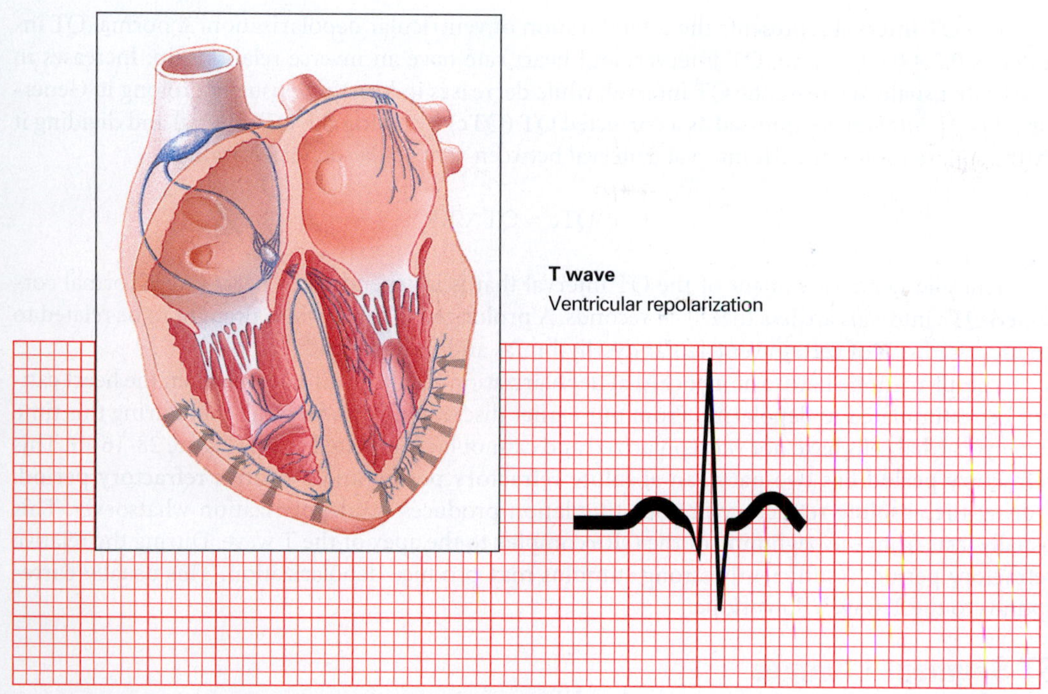

■ **Figure 28-14** Ventricular repolarization.

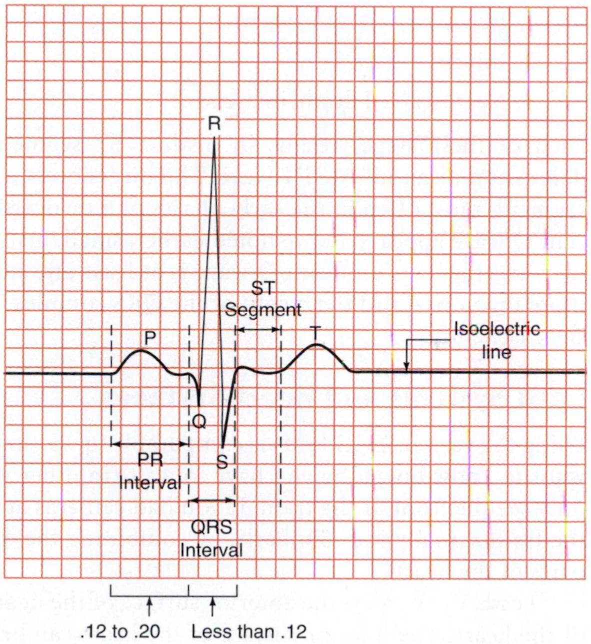

■ **Figure 28-15** The ECG.

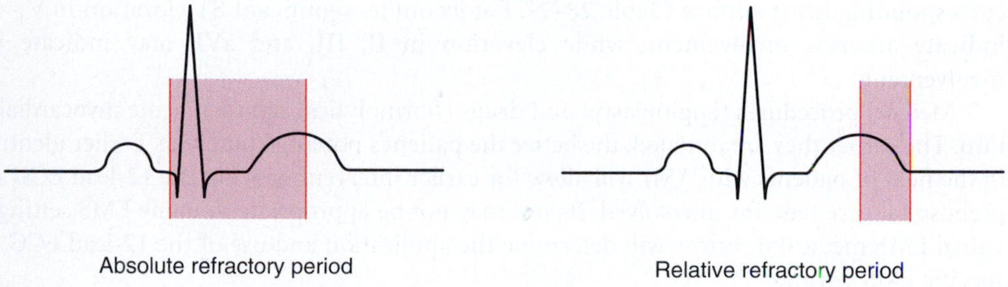

■ **Figure 28-16** Refractory periods of the cardiac cycle.

QT interval *period from the beginning of the QRS to the end of the T wave.*

corrected QT (QTc) *QT interval divided by the square root of the RR interval.*

prolonged QT interval *QT interval greater than 0.44 second.*

refractory period *the period of time when myocardial cells have not yet completely repolarized and cannot be stimulated again.*

absolute refractory period *the period of the cardiac cycle when stimulation will not produce any depolarization whatsoever.*

relative refractory period *the period of the cardiac cycle when a sufficiently strong stimulus may produce depolarization.*

The **QT interval** represents the total duration of ventricular depolarization. A normal QT interval is 0.33–0.42 second. QT intervals and heart rate have an inverse relationship: Increases in heart rate usually decrease the QT interval, while decreases in heart rate usually prolong it. Generally, the QT interval is expressed as a **corrected QT (QTc)** by taking the QT interval and dividing it by the square root of the RR interval (interval between ventricular depolarizations):

$$\text{QTc} = \text{QT}\ \sqrt{\text{RR}}$$

This allows an assessment of the QT interval that is independent of heart rate. Normal corrected QTc intervals are less than 0.44 seconds. A **prolonged QT interval** is thought to be related to an increased risk of certain ventricular dysrhythmias and sudden death.

The all-or-none nature of myocardial depolarization results in an interval when the heart cannot be restimulated to depolarize. From our earlier discussion you will recall that during this time the myocardial cells have not yet repolarized and cannot be stimulated again (Figure 28-16 ■). This **refractory period** has two parts, an **absolute refractory period** and a **relative refractory period.** During the absolute refractory period stimulation produces no depolarization whatsoever. This usually lasts from the beginning of the QRS complex to the apex of the T wave. During the relative refractory period, a sufficiently strong stimulus may produce depolarization. This usually corresponds to the T wave's downslope.

ST Segment Changes

The ST segment is usually an isoelectric line. Myocardial infarctions, which are caused by lack of blood flow to a part of the heart, produce changes in this line. The affected area is then electrically dead and cannot conduct electrical impulses. Myocardial infarctions usually follow this sequence:

1. Ischemia (lack of oxygen)
2. Injury
3. Necrosis (cell death, infarction)

Each of these stages results in distinct ST segment changes. Ischemia causes ST segment depression or an inverted T wave. The inversion is usually symmetrical. Injury elevates the ST segment, most often in the early phases of a myocardial infarction. As the tissue dies, a significant Q wave appears. As we noted earlier, small, insignificant Q waves may show up in normal ECG tracings. A significant Q wave is at least one small square wide, lasting 0.04 second, or is more than one-third the height of the QRS complex. Q waves may also indicate extensive transient ischemia.

Lead Systems and Heart Surfaces

Using the various ECG leads is comparable to waiting for a train at a railroad crossing. You will want to know how long you have to wait (in other words, how long is the train), but you can only see the front of the train. If you had cameras at other viewpoints, you could see how long the train actually was. Similarly, by combining the different ECG leads you can view different parts of the heart.

Leads V_1–V_4 view the anterior surface of the heart. Leads I and aVL view the lateral surface of the heart. The inferior surface of the heart can be visualized in leads II, III, and aVF. These leads can show ischemia, injury, and necrotic changes and can provide information about the corresponding heart surface (Table 28–2). For example, significant ST elevation in V_1–V_4 may indicate anterior involvement, while elevation in II, III, and aVF may indicate inferior involvement.

Earlier identification in the field of patients with AMI will allow for earlier intervention.

Medical procedures (angioplasty) and drugs (fibrinolytics) can treat acute myocardial infarction. The earlier they are initiated, the better the patient's potential outcome. Earlier identification in the field of patients with AMI will allow for earlier interventions, but the 12-lead ECG's role in prehospital care remains unresolved. Its use may not be appropriate in many EMS settings. Individual EMS medical directors will determine the application and use of the 12-lead ECG in their specific EMS settings.

Table 28–2 Overview of ECG Lead Groupings

Leads	Portion of the Heart Examined
I and aVL	The left side of the heart in a vertical plane
II, III, and aVF	The inferior (diaphragmatic) side of the heart
aVR	The right side of the heart in a vertical plane
V_1 and V_2	The right ventricle
V_3 and V_4	The intraventricular septum and the anterior wall of the left ventricle
V_5 and V_6	The anterior and lateral walls of the left ventricle

INTERPRETATION OF RHYTHM STRIPS

The key to interpreting rhythm strips is to approach each strip logically and systematically. Attempts to nonanalytically "eyeball" the strip often lead to incorrect interpretations. Your approach to rhythm strip interpretation should include the following basic criteria:

The key to interpreting rhythm strips is to approach each strip logically and systematically.

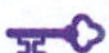

Use ECG calipers to measure ECG tracings to ensure accuracy and to avoid misinterpretation.

- ★ Always be consistent and analytical.
- ★ Memorize the rules for each dysrhythmia.
- ★ Analyze a given rhythm strip according to a specific format.
- ★ Compare your analysis to the rules for each dysrhythmia.
- ★ Identify the dysrhythmia by its similarity to established rules.

The health care profession uses several standard formats for ECG analysis. We will use the following five-step procedure. Analyze the:

1. Rate.
2. Rhythm.
3. P waves.
4. PR interval.
5. QRS complex.

Analyzing Rate

The first step in ECG strip interpretation is to analyze the heart rate. Usually this means the ventricular rate; however, if the atrial and ventricular rates differ, you must calculate both. The normal heart rate is 60–100 beats per minute. A heart rate greater than 100 beats per minute is a **tachycardia.** A heart rate less than 60 beats per minute is a **bradycardia.** You can use any of the following methods to calculate the rate:

tachycardia *a heart rate greater than 100 beats per minute.*

bradycardia *a heart rate less than 60 beats per minute.*

- ★ *Six-second method.* Count the number of complexes in a 6-second interval. Mark off a 6-second interval by noting two 3-second marks at the top of the ECG paper. Then multiply the number of complexes within the 6-second strip by 10.
- ★ *Heart rate calculator rulers.* Commercially available heart rate calculator rulers allow you to determine heart rates rapidly. Always use them according to the accompanying directions, since variations occur among different manufacturers. Also learn a manual method so you can still calculate rates if you forget your ruler.
- ★ *RR interval.* The RR interval is related directly to heart rate. The RR interval method is accurate only if the heart rhythm is regular. You can calculate it in the following ways:
  - Measure the duration between R waves in seconds. Divide this number into 60, giving the heart rate per minute.

Example: *60 ÷ 0.65 second = 92 (heart rate)*

  - Count the number of large squares within an RR interval, and divide the number of squares into 300.

Example: *300 ÷ 3.5 large boxes = 86 (heart rate)*

- Count the number of small squares within an RR interval, and divide the number of squares into 1,500.

Example: *1,500 ÷ 29 small boxes = 52 (heart rate)*

- ★ *Triplicate method.* Another method, also useful only with regular rhythms, is to locate an R wave that falls on a dark line bordering a large box on the graph paper. Then assign numbers corresponding to the heart rate to the next six dark lines to the right. The order is: 300, 150, 100, 75, 60, and 50. The number corresponding to the dark line closest to the peak of the next R wave is a rough estimate of the heart rate.

Pick one of these methods and become comfortable with it. Use it to determine the rate on all strips that you analyze.

Analyzing Rhythm

The next step is to analyze the rhythm. First, measure the RR interval across the strip. Normally, the RR rhythm is fairly regular. Some minimal variation, associated with respirations, should be expected. If the rhythm is irregular, note whether it fits one of the following patterns:

- ★ Occasionally irregular (only one or two RR intervals on the strip are irregular)
- ★ Regularly irregular (patterned irregularity or group beating)
- ★ Irregularly irregular (no relationship among RR intervals)

Analyzing P Waves

The P waves reflect atrial depolarization. Normally, the atria depolarize away from the SA node and toward the ventricles. In lead II, this appears as a positive, rounded P wave. When analyzing the P waves, ask yourself the following questions:

- ★ Are P waves present?
- ★ Are the P waves regular?
- ★ Is there one P wave for each QRS complex?
- ★ Are the P waves upright or inverted (compared to the QRS complex)?
- ★ Do all the P waves look alike?

Analyzing the PR Interval

The PR interval represents the time needed for atrial depolarization and conduction of the impulse up to the AV node. Remember, the normal PR interval is 0.12–0.20 sec (three to five small boxes). Any deviation is an abnormal finding. The PR interval should be consistent across the strip.

Analyzing the QRS Complex

The QRS complex represents ventricular depolarization. When evaluating the QRS complex, ask yourself the following questions:

- ★ Do all of the QRS complexes look alike?
- ★ What is the QRS duration?

Remember, the QRS duration is usually 0.04–0.12 sec. Anything longer than 0.12 sec (three small boxes) is abnormal.

DYSRHYTHMIAS

normal sinus rhythm *the normal heart rhythm.*

On a normal ECG, the heart rate is between 60 and 100 beats per minute. The rhythm is regular (both PP and RR). The P waves are normal in shape, upright, and appear only before each QRS complex. The PR interval lasts 0.12–0.20 sec and is constant. The QRS complex has a normal morphology, and its duration is less than 0.12 sec. All of these factors indicate a **normal sinus rhythm**

Parenteral penicillin injections are the most common cause of fatal anaphylactic reactions. Insect stings are the second most frequent cause of fatal anaphylactic reactions. Insects in the order *Hymenoptera* are the most frequent offending insects. There are three families in this order: fire ants (*Formicoidea*); wasps, yellow jackets, and hornets (*Vespidae*); and the honey bees (*Apoidea*). All produce a unique venom, although there are similar components in each. Honey bees often will leave their stinger embedded in the victim following a sting.

Following exposure to a particular allergen, large quantities of IgE antibodies are released. These antibodies attach to the membranes of **basophils** and **mast cells**—specialized cells of the immune system which contain chemicals that assist in the immune response. When the allergen binds to IgE attached to the basophils and mast cells, these cells release histamine, heparin, and other substances into the surrounding tissues. Histamine and other substances are stored in *granules* found within the basophils and mast cells. In fact, because of this feature, basophils and mast cells are often called *granulocytes*. The process of releasing these substances from the cells is called *degranulation*. This release results in what people call an *allergic reaction* which can be very mild or very severe.

basophil *type of white blood cell that participates in allergic responses.*

mast cell *specialized cell of the immune system which contains chemicals that assist in the immune response.*

The principal chemical mediator of an allergic reaction is histamine. **Histamine** is a potent substance that causes bronchoconstriction, increased intestinal motility, vasodilation, and increased vascular permeability. Increased vascular permeability causes the leakage of fluid from the circulatory system into the surrounding tissues. A common manifestation of severe allergic reactions and anaphylaxis is angioneurotic edema. **Angioneurotic edema,** also called *angioedema,* is marked edema of the skin and usually involves the head, neck, face, and upper airway. Histamine acts by activating specialized histamine receptors present throughout the body.

histamine *a product of mast cells and basophils that causes vasodilation, capillary permeability, bronchoconstriction, and contraction of the gut.*

There are two classes of histamine receptors. H_1 receptors, when stimulated, cause bronchoconstriction and contraction of the intestines. H_2 receptors cause peripheral vasodilation and secretion of gastric acids. The goal of histamine release is to minimize the body's exposure to the antigen. Bronchoconstriction decreases the possibility of the antigen entering through the respiratory tract. Increased gastric acid production helps destroy an ingested antigen. Increased intestinal motility serves to move the antigen quickly through the gastrointestinal system with minimal absorption of the antigen into the body. Vasodilation and capillary permeability help remove the allergen from the circulation where it has the potential to do the most harm.

angioneurotic edema *marked edema of the skin that usually involves the head, neck, face, and upper airway; a common manifestation of severe allergic reactions and anaphylaxis.*

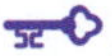

There are four types of allergic reactions:
Type I—Immediate (e.g., anaphylaxis)
Type II—Cytotoxic (e.g., transfusion reaction)
Type III—Immune complex (e.g., lupus erythematosis)
Type IV—Delayed (e.g., poison ivy/oak)

ANAPHYLAXIS

Anaphylaxis usually occurs when a specific allergen is injected directly into the circulation. This is the reason anaphylaxis is more common following injections of drugs and diagnostic agents and following bee stings. When the allergen enters the circulation, it is distributed widely throughout the body. The allergen interacts with both basophils and mast cells, resulting in the massive dumping of histamine and other substances associated with anaphylaxis. The principal body systems affected by anaphylaxis are the cardiovascular, respiratory, and gastrointestinal systems, and the skin. Histamine causes widespread peripheral vasodilation as well as increased permeability of the capillaries. Increased capillary permeability results in marked loss of plasma from the circulation. People sustaining anaphylaxis can actually die from circulatory shock.

Also released from the basophils and mast cells is a substance called **slow-reacting substance of anaphylaxis (SRS-A)**. This causes spasm of the bronchial smooth muscle, resulting in an asthma-like attack and occasionally asphyxia. SRS-A potentiates the effects of histamine, especially on the respiratory system.

slow-reacting substance of anaphylaxis (SRS-A) *substance released from basophils and mast cells that causes spasm of the bronchiole smooth muscle, resulting in an asthma-like attack and occasionally asphyxia.*

ASSESSMENT FINDINGS IN ANAPHYLAXIS

The signs and symptoms of anaphylaxis begin within 30–60 seconds following exposure to the offending allergen. In a small percentage of patients the onset of signs and symptoms may be delayed over an hour. The signs and symptoms of anaphylaxis can vary significantly. The severity of the reaction is often related to the speed of onset. Reactions that develop very quickly tend to be much more severe.

A rapid and focused assessment is crucial to the early detection and treatment of anaphylaxis. Patients suffering an anaphylactic reaction often have a sense of impending doom. This sense of impending doom is often followed by development of additional signs and symptoms.

If the patient's condition permits, a brief history should be gathered, including previous allergen exposures and reactions. If possible, try to determine how quickly symptoms started and how severe they were.

Next, quickly evaluate the patient's level of consciousness. Upper airway problems, including laryngeal edema, may result in the patient being unable to speak. As the emergency progresses, the patient will become restless. As cardiovascular collapse continues, the patient will exhibit a decreased level of consciousness. If untreated, this may continue to unresponsiveness.

As noted earlier, a common manifestation of anaphylaxis is angioneurotic edema, involving the face and neck. Laryngeal edema is also a frequent complication and can threaten the airway. Initially, laryngeal edema will cause a hoarse voice. As the edema worsens, the patient may develop stridor. Finally, this all may lead to complete airway obstruction from either massive laryngeal edema, laryngospasm, or pharyngeal edema, or a combination of any of these.

The respiratory system is significantly involved in an anaphylactic reaction. Initially, the patient will become tachypneic. Later, as lower airway edema and bronchospasm develop, respirations will become labored as evidenced by retractions, accessory muscle usage, and prolonged expirations. Wheezing, resulting from bronchospasm and edema of the smaller airways, is a common manifestation and may be so pronounced that it can be heard without the aid of a stethoscope. Ultimately, anaphylaxis can result in markedly diminished lung sounds, which reflect decreased air movement and hypoventilation.

urticaria *the raised areas, or wheals, that occur on the skin, associated with vasodilation due to histamine release; commonly called "hives."*

The skin is typically involved early in severe allergic reactions and anaphylaxis. Generally, a fine red rash will appear diffusely on the body. As histamine is released, fluid will diffuse from leaky capillaries, resulting in urticaria. **Urticaria,** also called "hives," is a wheal and flare reaction characterized by red, raised bumps which may appear and disappear across the body (Figure 31-1 ■). As cardiovascular collapse and dyspnea progresses, the patient will become diaphoretic. This may, if untreated, progress to cyanosis and pallor.

The effect of histamine on the gastrointestinal system is pronounced. Initially, the patient may note a rumbling sensation in the abdomen as gastrointestinal motility increases. On physical examination, this may be evident as hyperactive bowel sounds. Later, nausea, vomiting, and diarrhea develop as the body tries to rid itself of the offending allergen.

The vital signs will vary depending on the severity and stage of the severe allergic or anaphylactic reaction. Initially there will be an increase in both the heart and respiratory rate. As airway edema and dyspnea occurs, the respiratory rate can fall—an ominous finding. The blood pressure will fall when significant capillary leakage and peripheral vasodilation occurs. This will often result in a reflex tachycardia as the body attempts to compensate for the fall in blood pressure. Very late in anaphylaxis the heart rate will fall. This too should be considered a very ominous sign.

State-of-the-art advanced prehospital care of anaphylaxis includes use of all available monitoring devices. These include the cardiac monitor, the pulse oximeter, and, if the patient is intu-

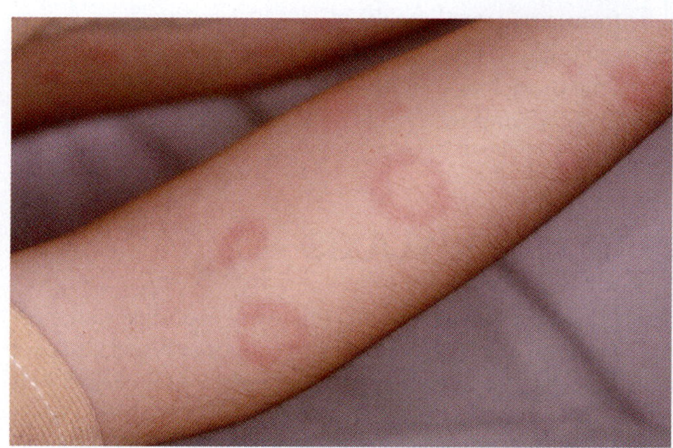

■ **Figure 31-1** Hives are red, itchy blotches, sometimes raised, that often accompany an allergic reaction.

bated, an end-tidal carbon dioxide detector. As anaphylaxis progresses, the end-tidal carbon dioxide level may climb due to the development of both respiratory and metabolic acidosis, which results in increased carbon dioxide elimination.

MANAGEMENT OF ANAPHYLAXIS

When responding to a patient with an anaphylactic reaction, first ensure that the scene is safe to approach. The presence of chemicals or patrolling bees can pose a risk to EMS personnel as well as to the patient and bystanders. If the patient is still in contact with the agent causing the reaction, he should be moved a safe distance away. Honey bees often leave their stinger behind during a sting. If present, the stinger should be removed by scraping the skin with a fingernail or scalpel blade.

Always consider the possibility of trauma in anaphylaxis. If there is any suspicion of coincidental trauma, stabilize the cervical spine. It is not uncommon for people to fall or otherwise injure themselves as they try to escape from wasps and bees. Signs and symptoms of trauma may be masked by those of anaphylaxis.

PROTECT THE AIRWAY

Position the patient and protect the airway. Administer oxygen via a nonrebreather mask. If the patient is hypoventilating or apneic, initiate ventilatory assistance. If an airway problem is detected, first apply basic airway maneuvers such as head positioning or the modified jaw-thrust maneuver. Use oropharyngeal and nasopharyngeal airways with caution as they can cause laryngospasm. If the patient is having severe airway problems, consider early endotracheal intubation to prevent complete occlusion of the airway. It is important to remember that the glottic opening may be smaller than expected due to laryngeal edema. Also, the larynx will be irritable, and any manipulation of the airway may lead to laryngospasm. Ideally, the most experienced member of the crew should perform endotracheal intubation, as only one attempt may be possible. Have available equipment for placement of a surgical airway, such as a needle cricothyrotomy, in case it is needed.

Establish an IV as soon as possible with a crystalloid solution such as lactated Ringer's or normal saline. Remember that patients suffering anaphylaxis are volume depleted due to histamine-mediated third spacing of fluid. If the patient is hypotensive, administer fluids wide open. If time allows, place a second IV line.

ADMINISTER MEDICATIONS

The primary treatment for anaphylaxis is pharmacological. If the necessary drugs cannot be administered in the field, then the patient should be transported to the emergency department immediately. Emergency medications used in the treatment of anaphylaxis include oxygen, epinephrine, antihistamines, corticosteroids, and vasopressors. Occasionally, inhaled beta-agonists, such as albuterol, may be required.

Oxygen Oxygen is always the first drug to administer to a patient with an anaphylactic reaction. Administer high-concentration oxygen with a nonrebreather mask or similar device. If mechanical ventilation is required, attach supplemental oxygen to ensure as high an oxygen delivery as possible.

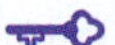

Epinephrine is the primary drug for management of anaphylaxis.

Epinephrine The primary drug for use in treatment of severe allergic reactions and anaphylaxis is epinephrine. Epinephrine is a sympathetic agonist. It causes an increase in heart rate, an increase in the strength of the cardiac contractile force, and peripheral vasoconstriction. It can also reverse some of the bronchospasm associated with anaphylaxis. Epinephrine also reverses much of the capillary permeability caused by histamine. It acts within minutes of administration. In severe anaphylaxis, characterized by hypotension and/or severe airway obstruction, administer epinephrine

1:10,000 intravenously. Epinephrine 1:10,000 contains 1 mg of epinephrine in 10 mL of solvent. The standard adult dose is 0.3–0.5 mg; child dose is 0.01 mg/kg. The effects of intravenous epinephrine wear off in 3–5 minutes, so repeat boluses may be required. In severe cases of sustained anaphylaxis, medical direction may order the preparation and administration of an epinephrine drip.

Antihistamines Antihistamines are second-line agents in the treatment of anaphylaxis. They should only be given following the administration of epinephrine. Antihistamines block the effects of histamine by blocking histamine receptors. They do not displace histamine from the receptors; they only block additional histamine from binding. They also help reduce histamine release from mast cells and basophils. Most antihistamines are nonselective and block both H_1 and H_2 receptors. Others are more selective for either H_1 or H_2 receptors.

Diphenhydramine (Benadryl) is probably the most frequently used antihistamine in the treatment of allergic reactions and anaphylaxis. It is nonselective and acts on both H_1 and H_2 receptors. The standard dose of diphenhydramine is 25–50 mg intravenously or intramuscularly. It should be administered slowly when given intravenously. The pediatric dose of diphenhydramine is 1–2 mg/kg of body weight. Other nonselective antihistamines frequently used are hydroxyzine (Atarax, Vistaril) and promethazine (Phenergan). Hydroxyzine is a potent antihistamine, but it can only be administered intramuscularly. Promethazine can be administered intravenously or intramuscularly, but does not appear to be as potent as diphenhydramine.

Selective histamine blockers are primarily H_2 blockers used to treat ulcer disease. Blockage of the H_2 receptors decreases gastric acid secretion. However, H_2 receptors are also present in the peripheral blood vessels. Administration of H_2 blockers conceivably will reverse some of the vasodilation associated with anaphylaxis. The two most frequently used H_2 blockers are cimetadine (Tagamet) and ranitidine (Zantac). Typically, 300 mg of cimetadine or 50 mg of ranitidine are administered by slow IV push (over 3–5 minutes). (Some recent studies have questioned the effectiveness of H_2 blockers in the treatment of allergic reactions.) Also, these agents are more expensive than the nonselective antihistamines.

Corticosteroids Corticosteroids are important in the treatment and prevention of anaphylaxis. Although they are of little benefit in the initial stages of treatment they help suppress the inflammatory response associated with these emergencies. Commonly used corticosteroids include methylprednisolone (Solu-Medrol), hydrocortisone (Solu-Cortef), and dexamethasone (Decadron).

Vasopressors Severe and prolonged anaphylactic reactions may require the use of potent vasopressors to support blood pressure. Use these medications in conjunction with first-line therapy and adequate fluid resuscitation. Commonly used agents include dopamine, norepinephrine, and epinephrine. These medications are prepared as infusions and are continuously administered to support blood pressure and cardiac output.

Beta-agonists Many patients with severe allergic reactions and anaphylaxis will develop bronchospasm, laryngeal edema, or both. In these cases, an inhaled beta-agonist can be useful. The most frequently used beta-agonist in prehospital care is albuterol (Ventolin, Proventil). Although usually used in the treatment of asthma, these agents will help reverse some of the bronchospasm and laryngeal edema associated with anaphylaxis. Give the adult patient 0.5 mL of albuterol in 3 mL of normal saline via a handheld nebulizer. Children should receive 0.2–0.5 mL of albuterol based on their weight. Other beta-agonists, such as metaproterenol (Alupent) and levalbuterol (Xopenex), may be used instead of albuterol.

Other Agents Other drugs occasionally used in the treatment of anaphylaxis include aminophylline and cromolyn sodium. Certain medications have been identified as potentially beneficial for anaphylaxis. These include vasopressin, atropine, and glucagon. There is some evidence that vasopressin may benefit hypotensive patients while atropine may benefit those with bradycardia; glucagon should be considered in those who are unresponsive to epinephrine—especially those receiving beta blockers.

OFFER PSYCHOLOGICAL SUPPORT

A severe allergic or anaphylactic reaction is a harrowing experience for the patient. Although it is essential to work fast, prehospital crews should provide the patient emotional support and explain the treatment regimen. Caution patients about the potential side effects of administered medications. For example, epinephrine will often cause a rapid heart rate, anxiety, and tremulousness. Likewise, the antihistamines may cause a dry mouth, thirst, and sedation. Careful explanation and emotional support will help allay patient anxiety and apprehension.

ASSESSMENT FINDINGS IN ALLERGIC REACTION

Many patients you will be called to treat will be suffering from forms of allergic reaction less severe than anaphylaxis. An allergic reaction, as contrasted with an anaphylactic reaction, will have a more gradual onset with milder signs and symptoms and the patient will have a normal mental status (Table 31–2).

MANAGEMENT OF ALLERGIC REACTION

Common manifestations of mild (nonanaphylactic) allergic reactions include itching, rash, and urticaria. Patients with simple itching and nonurticarial rashes may be treated with antihistamines alone. In addition to antihistamines, epinephrine is often necessary for the treatment of urticaria.

Any patient suffering an allergic reaction who exhibits dyspnea or wheezing should receive supplemental oxygen. This should be followed by subcutaneous epinephrine 1:1,000. Lesser allergic reactions that are not accompanied by hypotension or airway problems can be adequately treated with epinephrine 1:1,000 administered subcutaneously (Figure 31-2 ■). Epinephrine 1:1,000 contains 1 mg of epinephrine in 1 mL of solvent. When administered into the subcutaneous tissue, the drug is absorbed more slowly and the effect prolonged. The subcutaneous dose is the same as the intravenous dose (0.3–0.5 mg). The subcutaneous route should not be used in severe anaphylaxis. Many physicians prefer to give epinephrine 1:1,000 intramuscularly, because this has a faster rate of onset although it has a shorter duration of action.

Table 31–2 Signs and Symptoms of Allergic and Anaphylactic Reactions

Mild Allergic Reaction	Severe Allergic Reaction or Anaphylaxis
Onset: Gradual	*Onset:* Sudden (30–60 seconds but can be more than an hour after exposure)
Skin/vascular system: Mild flushing, edema rash, or hives	*Skin/vascular system:* Severe flushing, rash, or hives; angioneurotic to the face and neck
Respiration: Mild bronchoconstriction	*Respiration:* Severe bronchoconstriction (wheezing), laryngospasm (stridor), breathing difficulty
GI system: Mild cramps, diarrhea	*GI system:* Severe cramps, abdominal rumbling, diarrhea, vomiting
Vital signs: Normal to slightly abnormal	*Vital signs:* Increased pulse early, may fall in late/severe case; increased respiratory rate early, falling respiratory rate late; falling blood pressure late
Mental status: Normal	*Mental status:* Anxiety, sense of impending doom, may decrease to confusion and to unconsciousness
	Other clues: Symptoms occur shortly after exposure to parenteral penicillin, *Hymenoptera* sting (fire ant, wasp, yellow jacket, hornet, bee), or ingestion of foods to which patient is allergic such as nuts or shellfish
	Ominous signs: Respiratory distress, signs of shock, falling respiratory rate, falling pulse rate, falling blood pressure

Note: Not all signs and symptoms will be present in every case.

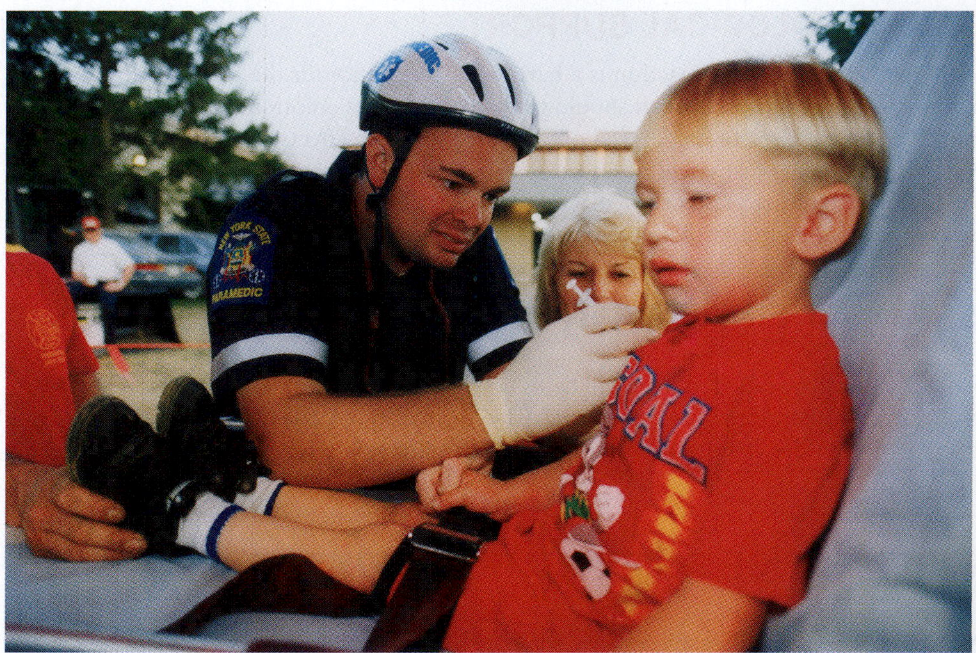

■ **Figure 31-2** Epinephrine being administered to a pediatric patient. *(© Craig Jackson/In the Dark Photography)*

Summary

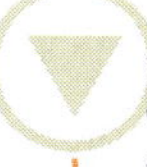

Fortunately, severe allergies and anaphylaxis are uncommon. However, when they do occur, they can progress quickly and result in death in minutes. The central physiological action in anaphylaxis is the massive release of histamine and other mediators. Histamine causes bronchospasm, airway edema, peripheral vasodilation, and increased capillary permeability. The prehospital treatment of anaphylaxis is intended to reverse the effects of these agents.

The primary, and most important, drug used in the treatment of anaphylaxis is epinephrine. Epinephrine helps reverse the effects of histamine. It also supports the blood pressure and reverses detrimental capillary leakage. Following the administration of epinephrine, potent antihistamines should be used to block the adverse effects of the massive histamine release. Inhaled beta-agonists are useful in cases of severe bronchospasm and airway involvement. Intravenous fluid replacement is crucial in preventing hypovolemia and hypotension.

The key to successful prehospital management of anaphylaxis is prompt recognition and treatment.

Review Questions

1. The ___________ system is a complicated body system responsible for combating infection.
   a. immune
   b. nervous
   c. respiratory
   d. cardiovascular
2. Innate immunity is also called:
   a. acquired immunity.
   b. natural immunity.
   c. naturally acquired immunity.
   d. induced active immunity.

3. The initial exposure of an individual to an antigen is referred to as:
   a. allergy.
   b. sensitization.
   c. hypersensitivity.
   d. active immunity.
4. ___________ ___________ are the second most frequent cause of fatal anaphylactic reactions.
   a. Insect stings
   b. Inhaled substances
   c. Ingested substances
   d. Injected penicillin
5. A type of white blood cell that participates in allergic responses is a(n):
   a. histamine.
   b. antibody.
   c. basophil.
   d. erythrocyte.
6. People sustaining anaphylaxis can die from ___________ shock.
   a. septic
   b. neurogenic
   c. respiratory
   d. circulatory
7. ___________ is the primary drug for the management of anaphylaxis.
   a. Oxygen
   b. Dexamethasone
   c. Albuterol
   d. Epinephrine
8. Commonly used vasopressor agents include:
   a. dopamine.
   b. epinephrine.
   c. norepinephrine.
   d. all of the above

See Answers to Review Questions at the back of this book.

Chapter

32 Gastroenterology

Objectives

After reading this chapter, you should be able to:

1. Describe the incidence, morbidity, and mortality of gastrointestinal emergencies. (p. 1307)
2. Identify the risk factors most predisposing to gastrointestinal emergencies. (p. 1307)
3. Discuss the anatomy and physiology of the gastrointestinal system. (see Chapter 3)
4. Discuss the pathophysiology of abdominal inflammation and its relationship to acute pain. (pp. 1307–1308)
5. Define somatic, visceral, and referred pain as they relate to gastroenterology. (p. 1308)
6. Differentiate between hemorrhagic and nonhemorrhagic abdominal pain. (p. 1310)
7. Discuss the signs and symptoms and differentiate between local, general, and peritoneal inflammation relative to acute abdominal pain. (p. 1308)
8. Describe the questioning technique and specific questions when gathering a focused history in a patient with abdominal pain. (pp. 1309–1310)
9. Describe the technique for performing a comprehensive physical examination on a patient complaining of abdominal pain. (p. 1310)
10. Discuss the pathophysiology, assessment findings, and management of the following gastroenterological problems:
    - ★ Upper gastrointestinal bleeding (pp. 1311–1312)
    - ★ Lower gastrointestinal bleeding (pp. 1317–1318)
    - ★ Acute gastroenteritis (pp. 1314–1315)
    - ★ Colitis (p. 1318)
    - ★ Gastroenteritis (pp. 1314–1315)
    - ★ Diverticulitis (pp. 1319–1320)
    - ★ Appendicitis (pp. 1322–1323)
    - ★ Ulcer disease (pp. 1315–1317)
    - ★ Bowel obstruction (pp. 1320–1322)

★ Crohn's disease (pp. 1318–1319)
★ Pancreatitis (p. 1324)
★ Esophageal varices (pp. 1313–1314)
★ Hemorrhoids (p. 1320)
★ Cholecystitis (pp. 1323–1324)
★ Acute hepatitis (pp. 1324–1325)

11. Differentiate between gastrointestinal emergencies based on assessment findings. (pp. 1308–1310)
12. Given several preprogrammed patients with abdominal pain and symptoms, provide the appropriate assessment, treatment, and transport. (pp. 1307–1325)

Key Terms

acute gastroenteritis, p. 1314
adhesion, p. 1320
appendicitis, p. 1322
bowel obstruction, p. 1320
chronic gastroenteritis, p. 1315
cirrhosis, p. 1313
colic, p. 1318
Crohn's disease, p. 1318
Cullen's sign, p. 1310
diverticula, p. 1319
diverticulitis, p. 1319
diverticulosis, p. 1319
esophageal varix, p. 1313
Grey Turner's sign, p. 1310
hematemesis, p. 1312
hematochezia, p. 1314
hemorrhoid, p. 1320
hernia, p. 1320
infarction, p. 1320
intussusception, p. 1320
ligament of Treitz, p. 1311
lower gastrointestinal bleeding, p. 1317
Mallory-Weiss tear, p. 1311
McBurney's point, p. 1322
melena, p. 1312
Murphy's sign, p. 1324
pancolitis, p. 1318
peptic ulcer, p. 1315
peritonitis, p. 1308
portal, p. 1313
proctitis, p. 1318
referred pain, p. 1308
Sengstaken-Blakemore tube, p. 1312
somatic pain, p. 1308
upper gastrointestinal bleeding, p. 1311
visceral pain, p. 1308
volvulus, p. 1320
Zollinger-Ellison syndrome, p. 1316

INTRODUCTION

Gastrointestinal emergencies account for over 500,000 emergency visits and hospitalizations every year, or approximately 5 percent of all visits to the emergency department. Of that number, more than 300,000 are due to gastrointestinal bleeding. These figures will probably increase as more and more people treat themselves with over-the-counter medications and delay seeing a physician until their symptoms become severe. Perhaps more important, the numbers will rise as the general population ages. In the last few years the number of patients over 60 years of age included in these statistics has risen from approximately 3 percent to more than 45 percent.

Content Review

Gastrointestinal Disease Risk Factors

- Excessive alcohol consumption
- Excessive smoking
- Increased stress
- Ingestion of caustic substances
- Poor bowel habits

GENERAL PATHOPHYSIOLOGY, ASSESSMENT, AND TREATMENT

Gastrointestinal (GI) emergencies usually result from an underlying pathologic process that can be predicted by evaluating numerous risk factors. These risk factors are commonly known to physicians; most are self-induced by patients. They include excessive alcohol consumption, excessive smoking, increased stress, ingestion of caustic substances, and poor bowel habits. The wide variety of risk factors and potential causes requires the emergency care provider to complete a thorough secondary assessment before making a field diagnosis, along with assessing the seriousness of the emergency and the need for any prevention strategy to minimize organ damage.

Gastrointestinal illnesses require the emergency care provider to complete a thorough assessment before making a field diagnosis.

Content Review

Types of Gastrointestinal Pain

- Visceral
- Somatic
- Referred

visceral pain *dull, poorly localized pain that originates in the walls of hollow organs.*

Pain from hollow organs tends to be vague and nondescript, whereas pain from solid organs tends to be localized.

peritonitis *inflammation of the peritoneum, which lines the abdominal cavity.*

somatic pain *sharp, localized pain that originates in walls of the body such as skeletal muscles.*

referred pain *pain that originates in a region other than where it is felt.*

GENERAL PATHOPHYSIOLOGY

Pain is the hallmark of the acute abdominal emergency. The three main classifications of abdominal pain are visceral, somatic, and referred. **Visceral pain** originates in the walls of hollow organs such as the gallbladder or appendix, in the capsules of solid organs such as the kidney or liver, or in the visceral peritoneum. Three separate mechanisms can produce this pain—inflammation, distention (being stretched out or inflated), and ischemia (inadequate blood flow). Because these processes progress at varying rates, they likewise can cause varying intensities, characteristics, and locations of pain.

Inflammation, distention, and ischemia all transmit a pain signal from visceral afferent neural fibers back to the spinal column. Because the nerves enter the spinal column at various levels, visceral pain usually is not localized to any one specific area. Instead, it is often described as very vague or poorly localized, dull, or crampy. The body most often responds to this vague pain with sympathetic stimulation that causes nausea and vomiting, diaphoresis, and tachycardia.

Organs that consist of hollow viscera, for example, the gallbladder (cholecystitis) and the small and large intestines, can frequently cause visceral pain. Many hollow organs first cause visceral pain when they become distended and then cause a different, more specific type of pain (somatic pain, described next) when they rupture or tear. For example, appendicitis initially presents with vague periumbilical abdominal pain that is classified as visceral. If the appendix ruptures it can spill its contents into the peritoneal cavity, causing bacterial **peritonitis** and generating somatic pain. Various microbes associated with pelvic inflammatory diseases can also cause bacterial peritonitis.

Somatic pain, as contrasted to visceral pain, is a sharp type of pain that travels along definite neural routes (determined by the dermatomes, or tissue blocks, present during embryonic development) to the spinal column. Because these routes are clearly defined, the pain can be localized to a particular region or area. As previously noted, bacterial and chemical irritations of the abdomen commonly cause somatic pain. Bacterial irritation can originate from a perforated or ruptured appendix or gallbladder. Chemical irritation of the abdomen can result from leakage of acidic juices from a perforated ulcer or from an inflamed pancreas. Whether the cause is bacterial or chemical, the resulting peritonitis can lead to sepsis and even death. The degree of pain is initially proportional to the spread of the irritant through the abdominal cavity. Somatic pain allows the examiner to locate the specific area of irritation, providing valuable information.

The third type of pain, referred pain, is not a true pain-producing mechanism. As its name implies, **referred pain** originates in a region other than where it is felt. Many neural pathways from various organs pass through or over regions where the organ was formed during embryonic development. For example, the afferent neural pathways that originate in the diaphragm enter the spinal column at the cervical enlargement at the fourth cervical vertebra. Therefore, patients who have an inflammation or injury of the diaphragm often feel pain in their necks or shoulders. One of the most significant hemorrhagic emergencies, the dissecting abdominal aortic artery, produces referred pain felt between the shoulder blades. Some common nonhemorrhagic emergencies are associated with referred-pain patterns, too. Appendicitis often presents with periumbilical pain, whereas pneumonia can cause pain below the lower margin of the rib cage.

GENERAL ASSESSMENT

Your assessment of a patient who complains of abdominal discomfort or whom you suspect of having an abdominal pathology is similar to a trauma assessment with an expanded history. Do not approach the patient until you and your partner have determined the scene to be free and clear of any apparent dangers. Always take appropriate Standard Precautions, including gloves, eyewear, mask, and disposable body gown, to prevent contamination. As you approach the patient, survey the scene for potential evidence of your patient's problem. Medication bottles, alcohol containers, ashtrays, and buckets with emesis or sputum, for instance, can provide valuable information.

Scene Size-Up and Primary Assessment

As you approach, look for mechanisms of injury to help determine whether the call is medical or trauma. If you suspect trauma, always immobilize the cervical spine as you assess the adequacy of the patient's airway and his level of responsiveness. In the vast majority of medical patients you can check responsiveness and airway patency by asking the patient his name and chief complaint (why he called the ambulance today) and noting the answers. You can further evaluate the rate, depth, and quality of the patient's respirations fairly rapidly and without great difficulty. As you evaluate the respiratory functions, quickly palpate a pulse and check skin color, temperature, and circulation, including signs of bleeding and capillary refill. If you discover a life-threatening condition during the primary assessment, treat it and then rapidly continue the assessment to identify any other life threats.

History and Physical Exam

Once you have completed the primary assessment and dealt with any life threats, conduct the secondary assessment. Your ability to obtain a history from the patient will depend on his level of responsiveness. In some cases, you may detect deterioration of the patient's mental status over time as you take the history.

History An accurate and thorough history can provide invaluable information. After you conduct the SAMPLE history (*s*ymptoms, *a*llergies, *m*edications, *p*ast medical history, *l*ast oral intake, and *e*vents), you can take a more thorough, focused history, exploring the chief complaint, the history of the present illness, the past medical history, and the current health status. The history of the present illness and the past medical history will be especially helpful in sorting the multitude of signs and symptoms and piecing together a clear picture of the underlying pathophysiology.

The history of the present illness and the past medical history will be especially helpful in piecing together a clear picture of the underlying gastrointestinal pathophysiology.

History of the Present Illness Your OPQRST–ASPN history for gastrointestinal patients should address the following specific concerns:

- ★ *Onset.* When did the pain first start? Was the onset sudden or gradual? Sudden onsets of abdominal pain are generally caused by perforations of abdominal organs or capsules. Gradual onset of pain usually is associated with the blockage of hollow organs.
- ★ *Provocation/palliation.* What makes the pain worse? What makes the pain better? If the pain lessens when the patient draws his legs up to his chest or lies on his side, it usually indicates peritoneal inflammation, which is often of GI origin. If walking relieves the pain, the cause may be in the GI or urinary systems—perhaps an obstruction of the gallbladder or a stone caught in the renal pelvis or ureter.
- ★ *Quality.* How would you describe the pain: dull, sharp, constant, intermittent? Localized, tearing pain is usually associated with the rupture of an organ. Dull, steadily increasing pain may indicate a bowel obstruction. Sharp pain, particularly in the flank, may indicate a kidney stone.
- ★ *Region/radiation.* Does the pain travel to any other part of your body? Radiated pain, or pain that seems to change location, is common because it involves the same neural routes as referred pain. Pain referred to the shoulder or neck is usually associated with an irritation of the diaphragm, such as happens with cholecystitis.
- ★ *Severity.* On a scale of 1 to 10, with 10 representing the worst pain possible, how would you rate the pain you are feeling now? The severity of pain usually worsens as the pathology (ischemia, inflammation, or stretching) of the organ advances.
- ★ *Time.* When did the pain first start? Estimation of the pain's time of onset is important to determine its possible causes. Any abdominal pain lasting over 6 hours is considered a surgical emergency and needs to be evaluated in the emergency department.
- ★ *Associated symptoms.* Have you experienced any associated nausea and/or vomiting with the discomfort? If yes, try to determine the content, color, and smell of the vomitus. Ask if the vomitus contained any bright red blood, "coffee grounds," or clots. Determining if your patient has an active gastrointestinal bleed is imperative.

  Have you experienced any changes in bowel habits—constipation or diarrhea—associated with this discomfort/pain? Question the patient further to determine if there have been any changes in feces such as a tarry, foul-smelling stool. Changes in bowel morphology, color, or smell can be the only indication of such conditions as a lower GI hemorrhage, gastritis, or bleeding diverticula.

Have you had an associated loss of appetite or weight loss? Patients who have an acute abdomen usually have an associated loss of appetite.

★ *Pertinent negatives.* The absence of symptoms associated with GI function or the presence of symptoms related to urinary function may mean the problem originates in the urinary system. Pain in the lowest part of the abdomen, the pelvis, can be due to problems in the reproductive system. Last, remember that an inferior myocardial infarction (MI) can irritate the diaphragm and generate its referred-pain pattern. Be sure to check for cardiovascular history when this pain pattern (pain in shoulder and/or neck area) is present.

Keep in mind the information that your SAMPLE history provides about your patient's last oral intake. It can help you to differentiate the possible causes of your patient's pain if the problem is in the GI system.

Not all abdominal emergencies result in abdominal pain. Some may cause chest pain. This, typically, is referred pain. Common gastrointestinal emergencies that can cause chest pain include gastroesophageal reflux, gastric ulcers, duodenal ulcers, and, in some cases, gallbladder disease. When confronted by a patient with chest pain, always consider the gastrointestinal system as a possible cause.

Past Medical History Have you ever experienced this same type of pain or discomfort before? If the patient answers yes, then investigate whether he saw a physician for the problem and how it was diagnosed. Commonly, patients have been treated for the complaint in the past and the pain is a flare-up of an old problem.

Usually patients with severe abdominal pathology lie as still as possible, often in the fetal position.

Physical Examination While you are conducting the history you can also begin the physical examination. Your patient's general appearance and posture strongly suggest his apparent state of health and the severity of his complaint. Usually patients with severe abdominal pathology lie as still as possible, often in the fetal position. They do not writhe around on the floor or cry out, because doing so increases the pain. You also should continually monitor the patient's level of consciousness for any subtle changes that indicate early signs of shock.

Take a complete set of vital signs to establish a baseline for further evaluation and treatment. These include pulse, respiratory rate, blood pressure, and pulse oximetry. You can also ascertain additional important information such as body temperature.

Distention of the abdomen may be an ominous sign.

Cullen's sign *ecchymosis in the periumbilical area.*

Grey Turner's sign *ecchymosis in the flank.*

Visually inspect the abdomen before palpating it, auscultating it, or moving the patient. Remove the patient's clothing as necessary to freely visualize the entire abdomen. Distention of the abdomen may be an ominous sign. It can be caused by a buildup of free air due to an obstruction of the bowel. If the distention is caused by hemorrhage, the patient has lost a large amount of his circulating volume, for the abdomen can hold from 4–6 L of fluid before any noticeable change in abdominal girth occurs. Other signs of fluid loss include periumbilical ecchymosis (**Cullen's sign**) and ecchymosis in the flank (**Grey Turner's sign**).

If you auscultate the abdomen, you must do so before palpating it.

Auscultating the abdomen usually provides little helpful information because bowel sounds are heard throughout this area. If you auscultate the abdomen, you must do so before palpating it. Listen for at least 2 minutes in each quadrant, beginning with the quadrant farthest from the affected area and auscultating the affected area last. Like auscultation, percussion requires a quiet environment and an experienced clinician. It too provides little or no useful information and, therefore, is not routinely performed in the field.

Palpating the abdomen can give you a plethora of information.

Palpating the abdomen, however, can give you a plethora of information. It can define the area of pain and identify the associated organs. Before palpating, ask the patient to point to where he is experiencing the most discomfort. Then work in reverse order, palpating that area last. Palpate the abdomen with a gentle pressure, feeling for muscle tension or its absence, as well as for masses, pulsations, and tenderness beneath the muscle. If you identify a pulsating mass, stop palpating at once; the increase in pressure may cause the affected blood vessel or organ to rupture.

GENERAL TREATMENT

Your highest priority when treating a patient with abdominal pain is to secure and maintain his airway, breathing, and circulation.

Once you have completed the primary assessment and the secondary assessment, you can address treatment and transport. Your highest priority when treating a patient with abdominal pain is to secure and maintain his airway, breathing, and circulation. Be prepared to suction the airway of vomitus and blood. High-flow, high-concentration oxygen and aggressive airway management may be indicated, depending on your patient's status. Monitor circulation by placing the patient on a cardiac monitor and frequently assessing his blood pressure. Measurement of the hematocrit will give an indirect measure of blood loss.

Establish a large-bore IV line in patients who complain of abdominal discomfort for use if emergency blood transfusion becomes necessary. You can use the IV for pharmacological intervention or to replace volume lost to hemorrhage or dehydration. In general, the need to avoid masking any abdominal pain for further evaluation will limit your pharmacological interventions to palliative agents such as antiemetics. Place the patient in a comfortable position and provide emotional reassurance based on your field assessment, any conversation with hospital staff or family, and knowledge of estimated transport time. Keep your voice and actions quiet and collected. Calm, as well as anxiety, are transmitted easily to patients and family. How you transport the patient will depend on his physiological status. Normally, gentle but rapid transport is sufficient. Remember that persistent abdominal pain lasting longer than 6 hours is classified as a surgical emergency and always requires transport. In all cases, be sure to maintain monitoring of mental status and vital signs and to give nothing by mouth. Bring vomitus to the emergency department for evaluation.

Persistent abdominal pain lasting longer than 6 hours always requires transport.

SPECIFIC ILLNESSES

The gastrointestinal (GI) tract is essentially one long tube divided structurally and functionally into different parts. Three other organs, the liver, gallbladder, and pancreas, are intimately associated with it, as is the small structure called the vermiform appendix, which protrudes from the first portion of the large intestine. Collectively, these organs are called the GI, or digestive, system. The GI system converts food into nutrient molecules that individual cells can use, and it excretes solid wastes from the body.

Content Review

The Gastrointestinal System

- GI tract
- Liver
- Gallbladder
- Pancreas
- Appendix

UPPER GASTROINTESTINAL DISEASES

For convenience, clinicians often divide the GI tract broadly into the upper and lower GI tracts. The upper GI tract consists of the mouth, esophagus, stomach, and duodenum, the latter being the first part of the small intestine. Physical digestion of food and some chemical digestion take place here. As food passes through the lower GI tract, consisting of the remainder of the small intestine and the large intestine, nutrients are absorbed into the blood and solid wastes are formed and excreted.

Content Review

The Upper GI Tract

- Mouth
- Esophagus
- Stomach
- Duodenum

Upper GI Bleeding

Upper gastrointestinal bleeding can be defined as bleeding within the gastrointestinal tract proximal to the **ligament of Treitz,** which supports the duodenojejunal junction, the point where the first two sections of the small intestine (the duodenum and the jejunum) meet.

upper gastrointestinal bleeding *bleeding within the gastrointestinal tract proximal to the ligament of Treitz.*

ligament of Treitz *ligament that supports the duodenojejunal junction.*

Upper gastrointestinal bleeds account for more than 300,000 hospitalizations per year. The mortality rate has remained fairly steady at approximately 10 percent over the past years. Many factors contribute to this high mortality. First, the number of patients who treat their symptoms with home remedies and over-the-counter medications is increasing rapidly. Many of these patients come under medical care only when their disease has caused significant damage, such as large-scale hemorrhage from an ulcerated lesion. Second, the overall age of the population is increasing. The infirmities of age and its greater likelihood of coexisting illnesses, such as hypertension, atherosclerosis, diabetes, and substance abuse (including abuse of medications), make this older population more vulnerable to the effects of upper gastrointestinal bleeds. The mortality rate is highest in those over 60 years of age. One prevention strategy for the field is to check for such coexisting problems, especially in elderly patients, and to treat accordingly. In particular, look at the history and physical for evidence of tobacco or alcohol use, or both.

The six major identifiable causes of upper GI hemorrhage, in descending order of frequency, are peptic ulcer disease, gastritis, variceal rupture, **Mallory-Weiss tear** (esophageal laceration, usually secondary to vomiting), esophagitis, and duodenitis. Peptic ulcer disease accounts for approximately 50 percent of upper GI bleeds, with gastritis accounting for an additional 25 percent.

Mallory-Weiss tear *esophageal laceration, usually secondary to vomiting.*

Content Review

Major Causes of Upper GI Hemorrhage

- Peptic ulcer disease
- Gastritis
- Varix rupture
- Mallory-Weiss tear
- Esophagitis
- Duodenitis

If an ulcer erodes through the gastric mucosa, if the esophagus tears, or if varices rupture, an acute, life-threatening, and difficult-to-control hemorrhage can result.

hematemesis *bloody vomitus.*

melena *dark, tarry, foul-smelling stool indicating the presence of partially digested blood.*

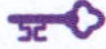

The key to managing an acute hemorrhage is to recognize its subtle indicators early and treat the condition before it worsens.

Sengstaken-Blakemore tube *three-lumen tube used in treating esophageal bleeding.*

Overall, irritation or erosion of the gastric lining of the stomach causes more than 75 percent of upper GI bleeds. Most cases of upper GI bleeding are chronic irritations or inflammations that cause minimal discomfort and minor hemorrhage. Physicians can manage these conditions on an outpatient basis; however, if a peptic ulcer erodes through the gastric mucosa, if the esophagus is lacerated in Mallory-Weiss syndrome, or if varices (often secondary to alcoholic liver damage) rupture, an acute-onset, life-threatening, and difficult-to-control hemorrhage can result.

Upper GI bleeds may be obvious, or they may present quite subtly. Most often patients will complain of some type of abdominal discomfort ranging from a vague burning sensation to an upset stomach, gas pain, or tearing pain in the upper quadrants. Because blood severely irritates the GI system, most cases present with nausea and vomiting. If the bleeding is in the upper GI tract, the patient may experience **hematemesis** (bloody vomitus), or, if it passes through the lower GI tract, **melena.** The partially digested blood will turn the stool black and tarry. For melena to be recognizable, approximately 150 cc of blood must drain into the GI tract and remain there for 5 to 8 hours. Blood in emesis may be bright red (new, fresh blood) or look like coffee grounds (old, partially digested blood).

Upper GI bleeding may be light or it may be brisk and life threatening. Patients who suffer a rupture of an esophageal varix or a tear or disruption in the esophageal or gastric lining may vomit copious amounts of blood. These hemorrhages can cause the classic signs and symptoms of shock, including alteration in mental status, tachycardia, peripheral vasoconstriction, diaphoresis (sweating that produces pale, cool, clammy skin), and hemodynamic instability. Besides shock, the vomitus itself can compromise the airway, resulting in impaired respirations, aspiration, and ultimately respiratory arrest.

A frequently employed clinical indicator is the tilt test, which indicates if the patient has orthostatic hypotension (a 10-mmHg change in blood pressure or a 20-bpm change in heart rate when the patient rises from supine to standing). Hypotension suggests a decreased circulating volume. The human body can compensate for a circulating volume deficit of approximately 15 percent before clinical indicators such as the tilt test show positive results. Thus, those patients whose systolic blood pressure drops 10 mmHg or whose heart rate increases 20 bpm or more need aggressive fluid resuscitation.

When evaluating the patient and his laboratory values, remember that the hematocrit might be within normal ranges when the patient is in the early phase of an acute hemorrhage. The key prevention strategy is to identify subtle indicators and treat the condition before it worsens. More general complaints include malaise, weakness, syncopal (fainting) and near-syncopal (light-headed) spells, tachycardia, and indigestion.

Your patient's general appearance may be the best indicator of his condition's severity. Because the hemorrhage is internal and histories are often misleading, you must perform a thorough physical examination. The patient may present doubled over in pain or lying very still. The latter is usually an ominous sign that any movement causes extreme pain. If you place the patient supine, be alert to the possibility of vomitus compromising the airway. Patients with a history of GI problems may have scars from past surgeries.

Examination in cases of suspected hemorrhage may be very helpful. Abdominal inspection may show symmetric distention or bulging in one region of the abdomen. Ecchymosis may be present if much blood has been lost into the abdominal cavity. If auscultation is subsequently performed, bowel sounds may be absent if the bleeding is severe or they may be hyperactive if the bleeding is minimal.

Prehospital treatment of an upper gastrointestinal bleed centers on maintaining a patent airway, oxygenation, and circulatory status. Place the patient in the left lateral recumbent or high semi-Fowler's position to prevent aspiration. To maximize the remaining hemoglobin molecules' carrying capability, administer high-flow, high-concentration oxygen via a nonrebreather mask to all patients with a suspected gastrointestinal bleed.

Establish two large-bore (14–16 gauge) IVs in any patient whom you suspect of having a gastrointestinal bleed. Start one with blood tubing for possible transfusion and one with volume-replacement 0.9 percent NaCl. Base fluid resuscitation on the patient's condition and response to the treatment. In general you can administer a 20 cc/kg fluid bolus to begin treating hemorrhagic hypovolemia.

Once the patient reaches the emergency department, treatment may include gastric decompression and lavage with a nasogastric tube, further fluid/blood resuscitation, endoscopy, **Sengstaken-Blakemore tube** placement, antacid and histamine antagonist administration, or immediate surgery.

Esophageal Varices

An **esophageal varix** is a swollen vein of the esophagus. Often these varices rupture and hemorrhage. When they do, the mortality rate is over 35 percent.

The cause of esophageal varices usually is an increase in **portal** pressure (portal hypertension). The blood flows from the abdominal organs, through the portal vein, and into the liver, where nutrients are absorbed into liver tissue and numerous compounds are detoxified and returned to the blood. From the liver, blood courses directly into the inferior vena cava through the hepatic veins. Blood flow through the liver ordinarily encounters little, if any, resistance. Damage to that organ, however, can impede circulation, causing blood to back up into the left gastric vein and, from there, into the esophageal veins. The dramatically higher pressure in these normally low-pressure pathways causes the esophageal veins to dilate and emerge from their sheaths (to evaginate, or "outpocket"). These small evaginations are called esophageal varices (Figures 32-1a and b ■). As they become engorged, the varices continue to dilate outward under extreme pressure until they rupture, causing massive hemorrhage. They may also erode through the submucosal layer and directly into the esophagus.

The primary causes of esophageal varices are the consumption of alcohol and the ingestion of caustic substances. Alcoholic liver cirrhosis accounts for two-thirds of cases of esophageal varices. Over time, alcohol consumption can cause a degenerative process known as **cirrhosis** of the liver. Cirrhosis results in fatty deposits and fibrosis in the liver parenchymal tissue, thus obstructing portal blood flow. Consequently, esophageal varices are common in the United States and the Western Hemisphere in general, where the alcohol consumption rate is high. In fact, cirrhosis is one of the leading causes of death in the Western Hemisphere. Caustic substances such as battery acid or drain cleaners can erode the esophagus from the inside out, causing hemorrhage of a vessel. Caustic ingestion, along with variceal formation due to viral hepatitis and erosive esophagitis, accounts for the remaining one-third of cases of esophageal varices.

Patients suffering from leaking or ruptured esophageal varices often present initially with painless bleeding and signs of hemodynamic instability. They may complain of hematemesis with bright red blood, dysphagia (difficulty swallowing), and a burning or tearing sensation as the varices continue to bleed, irritating the lining of the esophagus. The hematemesis can be forceful and copious if the hemorrhage is large. Clotting time increases because the high portal pressure backs up blood into the spleen, destroying platelets. The patient may exhibit the classic signs of shock, including an increased pulse, increased respirations, and cool, clammy, diaphoretic skin, possibly associated with an altered level of consciousness and hypotension.

Content Review

Upper GI Diseases

- Esophageal varices
- Acute gastroenteritis
- Chronic gastroenteritis
- Peptic ulcers

esophageal varix *swollen vein of the esophagus.*

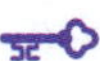

When varices rupture and hemorrhage, the mortality rate is over 35 percent.

portal *pertaining to the flow of blood into the liver.*

cirrhosis *degenerative disease of the liver.*

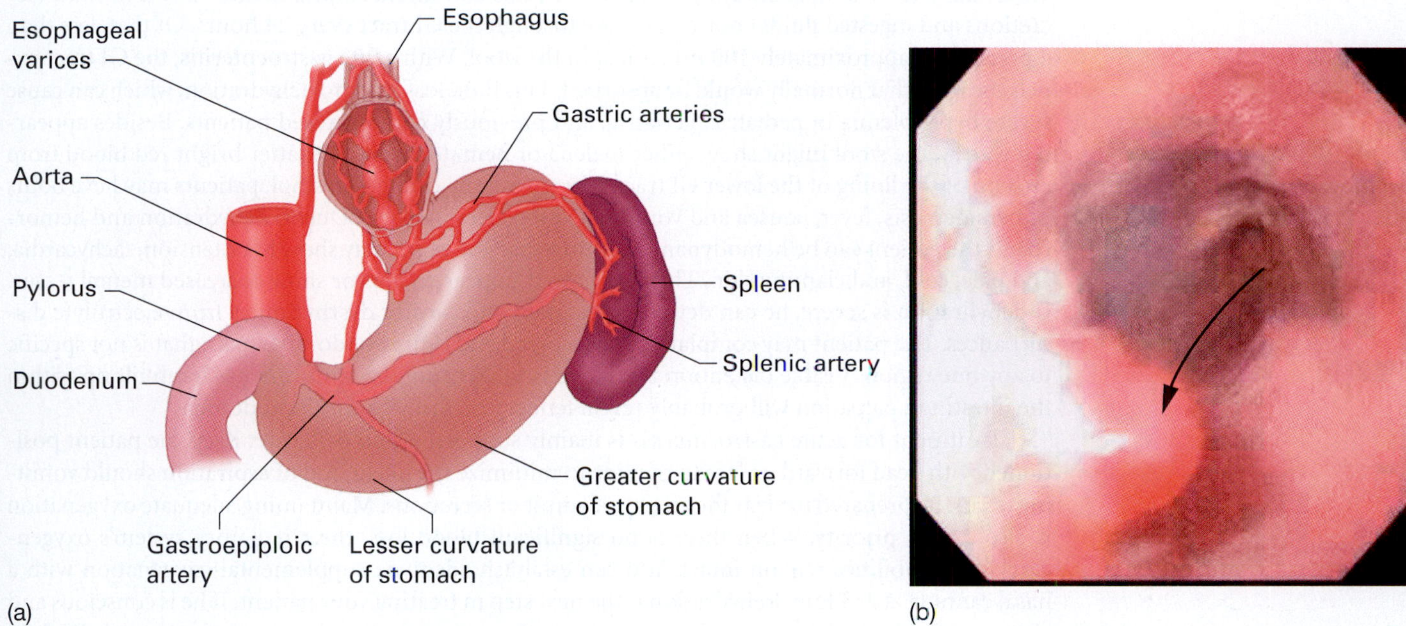

■ **Figure 32-1** Esophageal varices occur when the esophageal veins dilate and emerge from their sheaths.

Because paramedics cannot tamponade the bleeding in the prehospital setting, your care should focus on aggressive airway management, intravenous fluid resuscitation, and rapid transport to the emergency department. Airway management is a top priority. You may need to suction emesis frequently and diligently from the airway. Orotracheal intubation also may be needed to maintain airway patency. To maximize oxygenation, administer high-flow, high-concentration oxygen via a nonrebreather mask. If the patient shows signs and symptoms of shock, place him in the shock position and begin fluid resuscitation. If the patient continues to hemorrhage, management in the emergency department might include the use of a Sengstaken-Blakemore tube to tamponade the bleeding, endoscopic cauterization, or sclerotherapy (injection of a thrombus-forming drug into the vein itself).

Prehospital placement of nasogastric tubes should be avoided in cases of suspected esophageal varices.

Acute Gastroenteritis

acute gastroenteritis *sudden onset of inflammation of the stomach and intestines.*

Acute gastroenteritis is defined as inflammation of the stomach and intestines with associated sudden onset of vomiting and/or diarrhea. It affects from 3 to 5 million people yearly worldwide and affects approximately 20 percent of all hospitalized patients. The pathologic inflammation causes hemorrhage and erosion of the mucosal and submucosal layers of the gastrointestinal tract. This inflammation and erosion can in turn damage the villi inside the intestine, which absorb water and nutrients. The water that healthy villi normally would absorb now moves through the bowel at an increased rate. Dehydration secondary to diarrhea is a common cause of death in developing nations but is seen far less frequently in the United States. Adequate volume replacement is your major prehospital prevention strategy to minimize the likelihood of hypovolemia, or even possible hypovolemic shock.

Individuals who abuse alcohol and tobacco are at high risk for gastritis (inflammation of the stomach) and gastroenteritis (inflammation of the stomach and intestines). A wide variety of chemical agents and incidents can lead to acute gastritis. One of the most common is the use of nonsteroidal anti-inflammatory drugs such as aspirin, which break down the mucosal surfaces of the stomach and GI tract. Other causes include excessive alcohol intake and tobacco use; alcohol and nicotine have the same irritating effect on the mucosa as nonsteroidal anti-inflammatory drugs. Stress, chemotherapeutic agents, and the ingestion of acidic or alkalotic agents can also cause acute gastroenteritis. Both systemic infection (salmonellosis) and infection from ingested pathogens (staphylococcus) can cause infectious acute gastroenteritis.

As the name implies, the onset of acute gastroenteritis is rapid and usually severe. The swift movement of fluid through the gastrointestinal tract causes multiple problems. First, and most obvious, diarrhea is almost always associated with this condition. Approximately 7–9 L of fluid (secretions and ingested fluids) normally move through the GI tract every 24 hours. Of that, less than 2 percent, or approximately 100 mL, is lost in the stool. With acute gastroenteritis, the GI tract expels the fluid that normally would be absorbed. This fluid loss leads to dehydration, which can cause severe hypovolemia in pediatric, geriatric, and previously compromised patients. Besides appearing watery, the stool might show either melena or **hematochezia,** the latter bright red blood from erosion of the lining of the lower GI tract. Along with the changes in stool, patients may have bouts of hematemesis, fever, nausea and vomiting, and general malaise. Due to dehydration and hemorrhage, the patient can be hemodynamically unstable; the exam may show hypotension, tachycardia, and pale, cool, and clammy skin. The patient may appear restless or show decreased mental status. If dehydration is severe, he can develop chest pain and cardiac dysrhythmias from electrolyte disturbances. The patient may complain of widespread and diffuse abdominal pain that is not specific to any one region. Visible distention is relatively unlikely unless significant gas has built up within the intestines; palpation will probably reveal tenderness throughout the abdomen.

hematochezia *bright red blood in the stool.*

Treatment for acute gastroenteritis is mainly supportive and palliative. Keep the patient positioned with head forward or face to the side to minimize the likelihood of aspiration should vomiting occur. Be prepared to clear the airway of vomit or secretions. Maintaining adequate oxygenation is also a high priority. When there is no significant blood loss, the circulatory system's oxygen-carrying capabilities remain intact. You can establish adequate supplemental oxygenation with a nasal cannula at 2–4 lpm. Rehydration is the next step in treating your patient. If he is conscious and alert, oral fluid rehydration may be appropriate. The easiest and quickest route, however, is IV fluid administration. In the prehospital setting, the fluid of choice is either 0.9 percent NaCl or lactated

Ringer's solution to replace the patient's circulating volume. In-hospital treatment will switch the fluid to D_5/LR or D_5/NS to replace electrolytes. Pharmacological treatment can involve antiemetics such as prochlorperazine (Compazine) or promethazine (Phenergan). Additional replacement of electrolytes such as potassium may be needed. Offer emotional support during transport. Exercise extreme caution and use Standard Precautions throughout patient contact to prevent any spread of infectious disease.

Chronic Gastroenteritis

Chronic gastroenteritis is inflammation of gastrointestinal mucosa marked by long-term mucosal changes or permanent mucosal damage. Unlike acute gastroenteritis, chronic gastroenteritis is due primarily to microbial infection. The most prevalent pathogen in the United States is the *Helicobacter pylori* bacillus. Other bacteria that can cause chronic gastroenteritis include *Escherichia coli, Klebsiella pneumoniae, Enterobacter, Campylobacter jejuni, Vibrio cholerae, Shigella,* and *Salmonella.* Many of these bacteria can be found as part of normal enteric flora, and effective vaccination against pathogenic strains has not been possible. *Shigella* and *Salmonella* are not part of the normal spectrum of intestinal flora. Viral pathogens include the Norwalk virus and rotavirus. Among the parasitic causes are the protozoa *Giardia lamblia, Cryptosporidium parvum,* and *Cyclosporidium cayetenis.*

chronic gastroenteritis *non-acute inflammation of the gastrointestinal mucosa.*

Most cases of gastroenteritis are viral. Patients with bacterial gastroenteritis tend to be considerably more ill than those with viral gastroenteritis.

All of these microbes and their associated gastric disorders are far more common in underdeveloped countries. They are transmitted via the fecal–oral route or through infected food or water. Fecal–oral transmission can occur when people practice poor personal hygiene or food-handling techniques. Local water supplies can become contaminated during natural disasters that disrupt normal water distribution and sewage treatment practices. In such instances, people from outside the endemic area may be more vulnerable to infection than is the local population. *Cyclosporidium* infection reportedly can be contracted by swimming in contaminated water.

Gastroenteritis patients commonly present with nausea and vomiting, fever, diarrhea, abdominal pain, cramping, anorexia (loss of appetite), lethargy, and in severe cases, shock. Usually the intensity of signs and symptoms reflects the degree of microbial contamination. However infection with *H. pylori,* the most common infectious gastroenteritis in the United States, often presents with common signs such as heartburn, abdominal pain, and, on endoscopic examination, gastric ulcers.

Helicobacter pylori is associated with gastric and duodenal ulcers.

When in contaminated conditions, be sure to decontaminate the drinking water or use a different water source; when in doubt about the reliability of the water, drink only beverages that have been brisk boiled or disinfected. Make sure proper sanitation and preparation of foods is maintained. Hand washing and Standard Precautions will protect most EMS providers and prevent transmitting the organism further. To avoid transmitting the disease to patients, health care providers should not work when they are ill.

Prehospital treatment involves protecting yourself and the patient from further contamination, monitoring the ABCs, and transport. Medical treatment of infectious gastroenteritis will require identification of the offending organism. Some of the causative microorganisms are sensitive to antibiotics, but for most the patient will be supported while the disease takes its natural path.

Peptic Ulcers

Peptic ulcers are erosions caused by gastric acid (Figure 32-2a ■). They can occur anywhere in the gastrointestinal tract; terminology is based on the portion of the GI tract affected. Duodenal ulcers (Figure 32-2b ■) most frequently occur in the proximal portion of the duodenum; gastric ulcers occur exclusively in the stomach. Overall, peptic ulcers occur in males four times more frequently than in females, and duodenal ulcers occur from two to three times more frequently than do gastric ulcers. Current statistics place the number of peptic ulcers at 4 to 5 million, with approximately 500,000 new cases diagnosed yearly. Those patients who are more likely to have gastric ulcers are over 50 years old and work in jobs requiring physical activity. Their pain usually increases after eating or with a full stomach and they usually have no pain at night. Duodenal ulcers are more common in patients from 25 to 50 years old who are executives or leaders under high stress. There is also some familial tendency toward duodenal ulcer, suggesting genetic predisposition. Patients with duodenal ulcers commonly have pain at night or whenever their stomach is empty. Thus, it is important in taking the focused history to get family history and a reliable estimate of the patient's last oral intake. Measurement of hematocrit may substantiate any suspicions of chronic or acute hemorrhage.

peptic ulcer *erosion caused by gastric acid.*

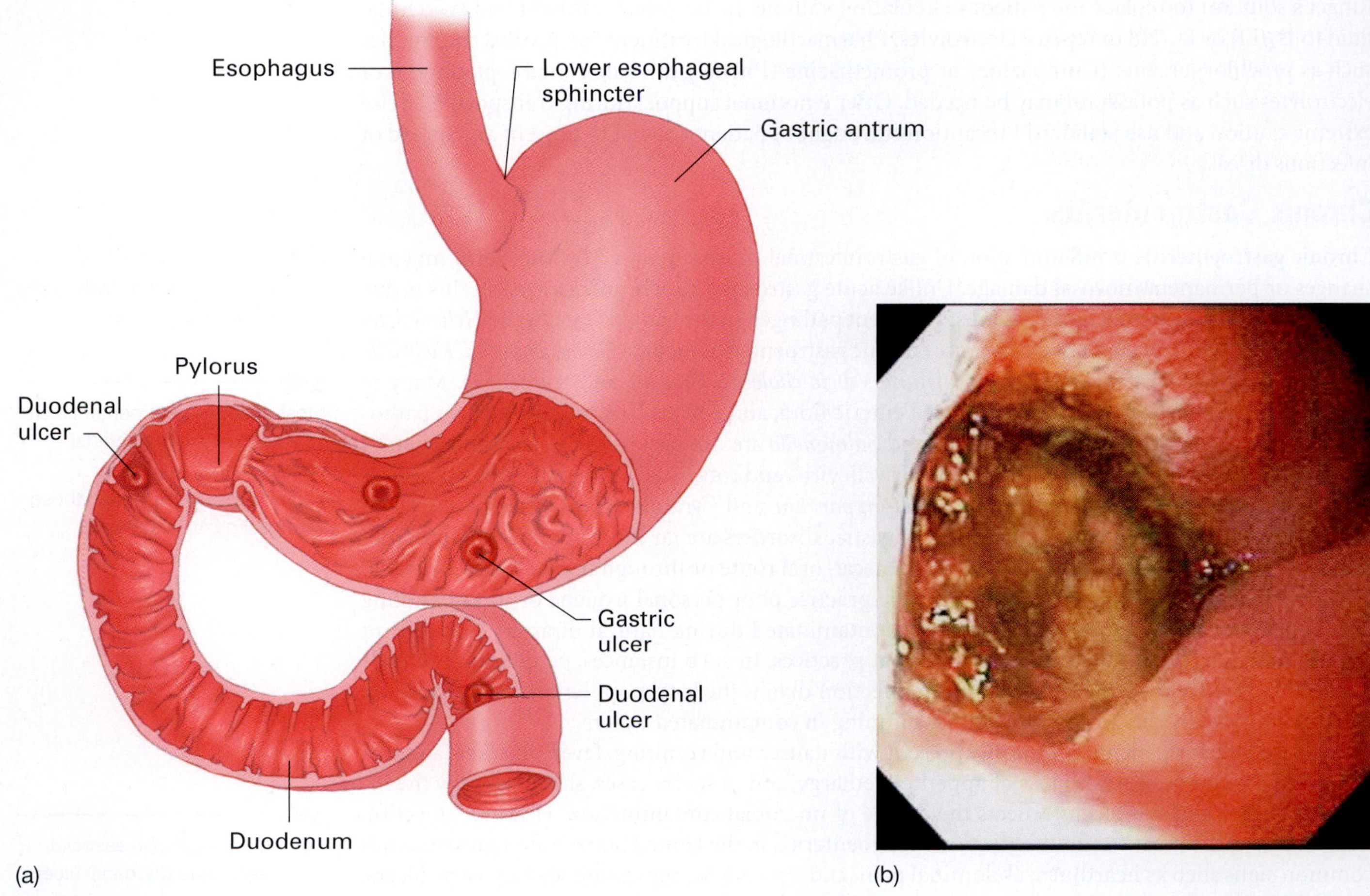

■ **Figure 32-2** Peptic ulcer.

Nonsteroidal anti-inflammatory medications (aspirin, Motrin, Advil, Naprosyn), acid-stimulating products (alcohol, nicotine), or *Helicobacter pylori* bacteria are the most common causes of peptic ulcers. To help break down food boluses, the stomach secretes hydrochloric acid. One enzyme that controls this secretion is pepsinogen. The hydrochloric acid helps to convert pepsinogen into its active form, pepsin. Between them, the pepsin and the hydrochloric acid can make the digestive enzymes very irritating to the GI tract's mucosal lining. Ordinarily, mucous gland secretions protect the stomach's mucosal barrier from these irritants, but when nonsteroidal anti-inflammatory medications, acid stimulators, or *H. pylori* damage the barrier, the mucosa is exposed to the highly acidic fluid, and peptic ulcers result. Prostaglandin, an important locally acting hormone, decreases the stimulation for blood flow through the gastric mucosa, thus allowing its further destruction. Treatment strategies in the prehospital setting focus on antacid treatment and support of any complications such as hemorrhage.

The recent discovery that *Helicobacter pylori* bacteria appear in over 80 percent of gastric and duodenal ulcers has enabled physicians to treat the disease by eliminating its cause with antacids and antibiotics, rather than merely treating its symptoms. Definitive treatment includes tamponade of any bleed, possibly by surgical resection, and antibiotic therapy along with histamine blockers and antacids. If medical therapy fails and the problem persists, it may require surgical resection of the vagus nerve (vagotomy) to reduce the stimulation for acid secretion.

Zollinger-Ellison syndrome *condition that causes the stomach to secrete excessive amounts of hydrochloric acid and pepsin.*

A blocked pancreatic duct can also contribute to duodenal ulcers. As chyme passes through the pyloric sphincter from the stomach into the duodenum, the pancreas secretes an alkalotic solution laden with bicarbonate ions that neutralize the acidic hydrogen ions in the chyme. If the pancreatic duct is blocked, however, the acidic chyme can cause ulcerations throughout the intestine. One other cause of duodenal ulcers is **Zollinger-Ellison syndrome,** in which an acid-secreting tumor provokes the ulcerations.

Findings on clinical examination of a patient with peptic ulcer can vary. Chronic ulcers can cause a slow bleed with resulting anemia. Visual inspection of the abdomen is usually helpful only if significant hemorrhage has occurred, in which case the same signs of ecchymosis and distention are found as in other causes of upper GI bleeding. On palpation, pain may be localized or diffuse. These patients often have relief of pain after eating or coating their GI tract with a liquid such as milk.

Acute, severe pain is probably due to a rupture of the ulcer into the peritoneal cavity causing hemorrhage. Depending on the ulcer's location, the patient may have hematemesis or may have melena-colored stool. Bouts of nausea and vomiting due to the irritation of the mucosa are common. If the ulcer has eroded through a highly vascular area, massive hemorrhage can occur. Along with the signs of hemorrhage on visual inspection, these patients will appear very ill and have signs of hemodynamic instability such as pale, cool, and clammy skin; tachycardia; decreased blood pressure; and, possibly, altered mental status. Most patients will lie still to decrease the pain. They may have surgical scars from previous ulcer repair. Bowel sounds will usually be absent.

Treatment for peptic ulcers depends on the severity of the patient's pain. Those who have abdominal pain or hemodynamic instability may require comfortable positioning and psychological support; high-flow, high-concentration oxygen; IV access for fluid resuscitation and pharmacological administration; and rapid transport. Common medications to reduce the mucosal irritation include histamine blockers such as Zantac and Pepcid and antacids such as Carafate.

LOWER GASTROINTESTINAL DISEASES

The lower GI tract consists of the jejunum and ileum of the small intestine and the entire large intestine, the rectum, and the anus. As digestive fluid moves through the small intestine (approximately 6 meters long), nutrients are absorbed into the blood. Water is absorbed and solid wastes form in the large intestine, also called the large bowel or colon, which is roughly 1.5 meters long.

Content Review

Lower GI Tract

- Jejunum
- Ileum
- Large intestine
- Rectum
- Anus

Lower GI Bleeding

Lower gastrointestinal bleeding occurs in the GI tract distal to the ligament of Treitz. Lower GI hemorrhages most frequently occur in conjunction with chronic disorders and anatomic changes associated with advanced age. The most common cause is diverticulosis, which is most prevalent in elderly people. Other causes are colon lesions (cancer or benign polyps), rectal lesions (hemorrhoids, anal fissures, anal fistulas), and inflammatory bowel disorders such as ulcerative colitis and Crohn's disease. These chronic disorders and diverticulosis rarely result in a massive hemorrhage such as that which can occur in the esophagus or stomach.

lower gastrointestinal bleeding *bleeding in the gastrointestinal tract distal to the ligament of Treitz.*

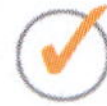

Content Review

Major Causes of Lower GI Hemorrhage

- Diverticulosis
- Colon lesions
- Rectal lesions
- Inflammatory bowel disorder

Your assessment of patients with suspected lower GI bleeds will be identical to your assessment of those with suspected upper GI bleeds. After you complete your primary assessment and treat all life-threatening conditions, you can conduct your secondary assessment. First, ask the patient whether this is a new complaint or a chronic problem. If a chronic problem, check the abdomen visually for scars from previous surgery. Frequent complaints with lower GI bleeding include cramping pain that may be described as similar to a muscle cramp or to gas pain, nausea and vomiting, and changes in stool. Melenic stool usually indicates a slow GI bleed. If the stool contains bright red blood, the hemorrhage either is very large (thus passing through the intestines before melenic change can occur) or has occurred in the distal colon. In the latter case, hemorrhoids or rectal fissures are possible causes. The abdominal exam will show findings similar to those for a bleeding peptic ulcer. If the abdomen has the distention or ecchymosis characteristic of significant hemorrhage, check for signs of early shock such as pale, cool, and clammy skin; tachycardia; decreased blood pressure; and, possibly, altered mental status. Because most patients with lower GI bleeds have not lost significant amounts of blood, they will present with hemodynamic stability, including warm dry skin, on physical exam.

Lower gastrointestinal bleeding is usually chronic and rarely results in exsanguinating hemorrhage.

How you manage the patient with a lower GI bleed will depend on his physiological status. Watch his airway and oxygenation status closely. If hypoventilation or inadequate respirations develop, administer high-flow, high-concentration oxygen via a nonrebreather mask or positive-pressure ventilation. Establish IV access and fluid resuscitation based on your patient's hemodynamic status. If you find a drop in hematocrit along with other signs of significant blood loss, be especially sure that one IV line is of sufficiently large bore for emergency transfusion. Place him in a comfortable position, offer psychological support, and transport him for further examination. If hemodynamic instability develops during transport, consider use of the pneumatic antishock garment (PASG) if directed in local protocols.

Review

Content

Lower GI Diseases

- Ulcerative colitis
- Crohn's disease
- Diverticulitis
- Hemorrhoids
- Bowel obstruction

Ulcerative Colitis

Ulcerative colitis is classified as an idiopathic inflammatory bowel disorder (IBD), that is, one of unknown origin. The inflammatory (ulcerative) process creates a continuous length of chronic ulcers in the mucosal layer of the colon; extension of the ulcers into the submucosal layer is uncommon. As ulcers heal, granular tissue replaces the ulcerations, thickening the mucosa. Approximately 75 percent of all ulcerative colitis involves the rectum or rectosigmoid portion of the large intestine. The inflammatory process usually starts in the rectum and then extends proximally into the colon, sometimes affecting the entire large intestine. If it spreads throughout the entire colon it is called **pancolitis;** if limited to the rectum, it is called **proctitis.**

pancolitis *ulcerative colitis spread throughout the entire colon.*

proctitis *ulcerative colitis limited to the rectum.*

Though ulcerative colitis is relatively unusual in Africa or Asia, its occurrence in the Western Hemisphere is increasing rapidly. In the United States, more than 10,000 new cases are diagnosed each year. It most frequently strikes people between the ages of 20 and 40 years. While researchers have not found a specific pathogen or cause of ulcerative colitis, they have determined many different contributing factors—psychological, allergic, toxic, environmental, immunological, and infectious. Current research has found that the release of cytokines can cause an overwhelming inflammatory response in the submucosa much like the release of histamines during anaphylaxis.

Acute ulcerative colitis is difficult to differentiate from other causes of lower GI bleeding. Because of its insidious presentation, diagnosing, tracking, and treating ulcerative colitis may require hematocrit and hemoglobin results, guaiac analyses of the stool, and endoscopic examinations. The severity of ulcerative colitis's signs and symptoms is usually related directly to the extent and severity of current inflammation in the colon. In patients with mild signs and symptoms, the disease often is isolated in one distal segment of the GI tract. Severe presentations, however normally involve the entire colon.

Typically, ulcerative colitis presents as a recurrent disorder with occasional bloody diarrhea or stool that contains mucus. Accompanying the stool abnormalities are **colicky** abdominal pain (cramping), nausea and vomiting, and, occasionally, fever (suggesting infection) or weight loss (suggesting severe or longer term colonic dysfunction). The cramping is usually limited to the lower quadrants, depending on the extent of colonic involvement, and it occurs when hypertrophic muscles lying beneath the submucosa prevent the colon from stretching in response to pressure from its contents. These patients will typically appear restless due to abdominal discomfort but will not show signs of hemodynamic instability (that is, skin will be warm and dry rather than cool and clammy).

colic *acute pain associated with cramping or spasms in the abdominal organs.*

Patients with ulcerative colitis are at increased risk of developing colon cancer.

More severe cases may present with bloody diarrhea and intense colicky abdominal pain, electrolyte derangements due to fluid loss through the colon, ischemic damage to the colon itself, or, eventually, perforation of the bowel. Often these patients present with signs and symptoms of hypovolemic shock such as pale, cool, clammy skin; hypotension; and tachycardia. Such patients with advanced disease and ongoing hemorrhage may have distention or ecchymosis on the skin and may show guarding of the lower quadrants during the physical examination. Significant hemorrhage is common in patients with ulcerative colitis.

Your management of the patient with ulcerative colitis will depend on his physiological status. If he presents with signs and symptoms of hypovolemic shock, administer high-flow, high-concentration oxygen and circulatory support including intravenous access and fluid resuscitation. If your patient has bouts of nausea and vomiting, you must diligently manage his airway to prevent aspiration of vomitus. Additional management may include antiemetics and antispasmodic medications. Transport any patient who presents with lower GI bleeding or colicky pain to the emergency department for diagnostic evaluation.

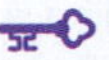

Transport any patient who presents with lower GI bleeding or colicky pain to the emergency department for diagnostic evaluation.

Crohn's Disease

Crohn's disease, along with ulcerative colitis, is the other idiopathic inflammatory bowel disorder in humans. It is more common in the Western Hemisphere, with from 20,000 to 30,000 new cases reported annually in the United States. This disease, which strongly tends to run in families, is most prevalent among white females, those under frequent stress, and in the Jewish population.

Crohn's disease *idiopathic inflammatory bowel disorder associated with the small intestine.*

Unlike ulcerative colitis, which affects the large intestine, Crohn's disease can occur anywhere from the mouth to the rectum. Between 35 and 45 percent of less severe cases involve the small intestine only; approximately 40 percent involve the colon itself. Severe cases of Crohn's disease may involve any portion of the GI tract, causing a variety of problems ranging from diarrhea to intestinal and perianal abscesses and fistulas (the latter, abnormal passages connecting two internal organs or different lengths of intestine). Complete intestinal obstruction, a surgical emergency, can also occur. Significant lower GI bleeding, however, is rare with Crohn's disease.

As the pathologic inflammation begins, it damages the innermost layer of tissue, the mucosa. Granulomas then form and further break down the mucosal and submucosal layers. The affected section of intestinal wall eventually becomes rubbery and nondistendable due to hypertrophy and fibrosis of the muscles underlying the submucosa. The patchwork-quilt formation of granulomas, fibrosis, and hypertrophy also decreases the intestine's internal diameter, resulting in fissures (incomplete tears) in the mucosa and possibly deeper into the submucosa as food boluses pass through. If a tear extends into the blood vessels in the submucosal layer, small bleeds result. The same pathologic pattern of ulceration and scarring can lead to creation of fistulas, most commonly between lengths of small intestine, or to obstruction of the small bowel. Increased suppressor T lymphocyte activity suggests an immune-mediated role in the inflammatory process.

Crohn's patients' clinical presentations can vary drastically as the disease progresses, and prehospital diagnosis is difficult or next to impossible. Common signs and symptoms include GI bleeding, recent weight loss, intermittent abdominal cramping/pain, nausea and vomiting, diarrhea, and fever. Onset of a flare-up in disease activity is usually rapid, often requiring a visit to the emergency department or physician's office. Abdominal pain cannot be localized to any specific quadrant since the disease can affect any portion of the small intestine and often affects more than one. The physical exam is also nonspecific and nonlocalized, with diffuse tenderness the most commonly found sign. Absence of bowel sounds in a patient with Crohn's disease strongly suggests intestinal obstruction, a surgical emergency.

Prehospital diagnosis of Crohn's disease is next to impossible because the patient's clinical presentations can vary drastically as the disease progresses.

Because the vast majority of patients with Crohn's disease are hemodynamically stable, prehospital treatment is largely palliative. Your management depends on the patient's physiological status. If he has bouts of nausea and vomiting you must diligently manage the airway to prevent aspiration of vomitus. Additional management may include antiemetics and antispasmodic medications. Particularly if he presents with signs and symptoms of obstruction or significant hemorrhage, administer high-flow, high-concentration oxygen and circulatory support including intravenous access and fluid resuscitation. As always, calmly and quietly inform the patient of all measures taken and offer psychological support en route to the emergency facility.

Diverticulitis

Diverticulitis is a relatively common complication of diverticulosis. **Diverticulosis** is a condition characterized by the presence in the intestine of **diverticula,** small outpouchings of mucosal and submucosal tissue that push through the outermost layer of the intestine, the muscle. Colonic diverticula are far more common in developed countries such as the United States and increase markedly in prevalence with increased age. They are present in more than half of patients over 60 years of age. Diverticulitis is an inflammation of diverticula secondary to infection. Unlike diverticulosis, it is symptomatic; patients will complain of lower left-sided pain (because most diverticula are in the sigmoid colon); exam and testing will show fever and an increased white blood cell count.

diverticulitis *inflammation of diverticula.*

diverticulosis *presence of diverticula, with or without associated bleeding.*

diverticula *small outpouchings in the mucosal lining of the intestinal tract.*

The pathogenesis of an acquired diverticulum is twofold. First, stool passes sluggishly through the colon, a condition associated with the relatively low-fiber diets common in developed countries. The colon responds with muscle spasms that increase bulk movement by raising the pressure on the contents inside the colon and pushing the fecal material forward. Second, the outermost layer of colon tissue is made up of fibrous bands of muscle wrapped around one another. Among them are muscles called the teniae coli. Nerves and blood vessels enter the colon through small openings within the teniae coli. These openings become weakened with age, and the increased pressure of muscle spasms can cause the inner layers of tissue, the mucosa and submucosa, to herniate through the openings, forming diverticula.

These diverticula commonly trap small amounts of fecal material, including sunflower seeds, popcorn fragments, okra seeds, sesame seeds, and others. The entrapped feces may allow bacteria other than the normal flora to grow and cause an infection. The problem is compounded when the diverticula become inflamed, causing diverticulitis. Complications secondary to diverticulitis include possible hemorrhage or larger perforations of the colon wall through which the infected fecal contents can spill into the peritoneal cavity and cause peritonitis.

The most common presentation of diverticulitis is colicky pain—usually on the lower left side—associated with a low-grade fever, nausea and vomiting, and tenderness upon palpation.

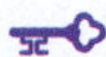

The presence of diverticuli in the colon is common in the elderly. Some patients with diverticuli will develop bleeding, while others will develop an infection (diverticulitis).

The most common presentation of diverticulitis is colicky pain associated with a low-grade fever, nausea and vomiting, and tenderness upon palpation. The pain is usually localized to the lower left side because the sigmoid colon is involved in 95 percent of reported cases. Thus, diverticulitis is often called left-sided appendicitis. If the diverticula begin to bleed significantly, the usual signs and symptoms associated with severe lower GI bleeding may be present: cool, clammy skin; tachycardia; and diaphoresis. Bleeding diverticula can also result in bright red and bloody feces (hematochezia) because of their close proximity to the rectum. Patients may additionally complain of the perception that they cannot empty their rectums, even after defecation.

Prehospital treatment for diverticulitis is mainly supportive. Measures to counter hypovolemic shock will only be needed when significant hemorrhage has occurred. Monitor the patient's airway and oxygenation and provide supplemental oxygen if needed. Establish intravenous access and begin fluid resuscitation if the patient is hemodynamically unstable. Antiemetics (Phenergan or Vistaril) may comfort the patient. Treatment in the hospital includes antibiotic therapy, endoscopy, and radiological tests to locate the diverticula. Long-term treatment includes implementing a high-fiber diet to stimulate daily bowel movements.

Hemorrhoids

hemorrhoid *small mass of swollen veins in the anus or rectum.*

Hemorrhoids are small masses of swollen veins that occur in the anus (external) or rectum (internal). They frequently develop during the fourth decade of life. Most hemmorhoids are idiopathic (of unknown cause), although they can result from pregnancy or portal hypertension. External hemorrhoids often result from lifting a heavy object. Other causes of hemorrhoids include straining at defecation and a diet low in fiber. Overall, hemorrhoids are common, particularly in persons over the age of 50 years. Their morbidity is low in most cases; one marked exception is in alcoholic patients with cirrhosis of the liver.

Rarely do hemorrhoids cause a massive hemorrhage.

Internal hemorrhoids most often involve the inferior hemorrhoidal plexus and vasculature. They commonly bleed during the process of defecation due to straining and then thrombose into a closed state again. External hemorrhoids result from thrombosis of a vein, often following lifting or straining, causing bright red bleeding with a bowel movement. The increased venous pressure sometimes causes the vessels to erode and bleed spontaneously, which increases the risk of infection. Rarely do hemorrhoids cause a significant hemorrhage.

Patients with hemorrhoids commonly call for emergency care because of bright red bleeding and pain on defecation. Physical assessment usually reveals a hemodynamically stable patient with relatively normal appearance (warm, dry skin, perhaps with slight tachycardia consistent with anxiety) who bleed with defecation. Visual examination of the stool may reveal gross bleeding. Treatment for hemorrhoids depends on the patient's condition. Most frequently, emotional reassurance and transport are all that is needed; however, you should remain alert to the possibility that the bleeding could be from a lower GI bleed, potentially resulting in uncontrolled hemorrhage. Either significant hemorrhage or bleeding hemorrhoids in an alcoholic patient warrant closer monitoring and transport for immediate follow-up.

bowel obstruction *blockage of the hollow space within the intestines.*

hernia *protrusion of an organ through its protective sheath.*

intussusception *condition that occurs when part of an intestine slips into the part just distal to itself.*

adhesion *union of normally separate tissue surfaces by a fibrous band of new tissue.*

volvulus *twisting of the intestine on itself.*

infarction *area of dead tissue caused by lack of blood.*

Bowel Obstruction

Bowel obstructions are blockages of the hollow space, or lumen, within the small and large intestines. Obstructions can be either partial or complete. An obstructed bowel segment can be catastrophic if not rapidly diagnosed and treated. Of this malady's varied causes, **hernias, intussusception, adhesions,** and **volvulus** are the four most frequent, accounting for over 70 percent of all reported cases (Figure 32-3 ■). Other common causes are foreign bodies, gallstones, tumors, adhesions from previous abdominal surgery, and bowel **infarction.** The most common location for obstructions is the small intestine, due to its smaller diameter and greater length, flexibility, and mobility.

An obstructed bowel segment can be catastrophic if not rapidly diagnosed and treated.

The obstruction may be chronic, as with tumor growth or adhesion progression, or its onset may be sudden and acute, as with obstruction by a foreign body. Chronic obstruction usually re-

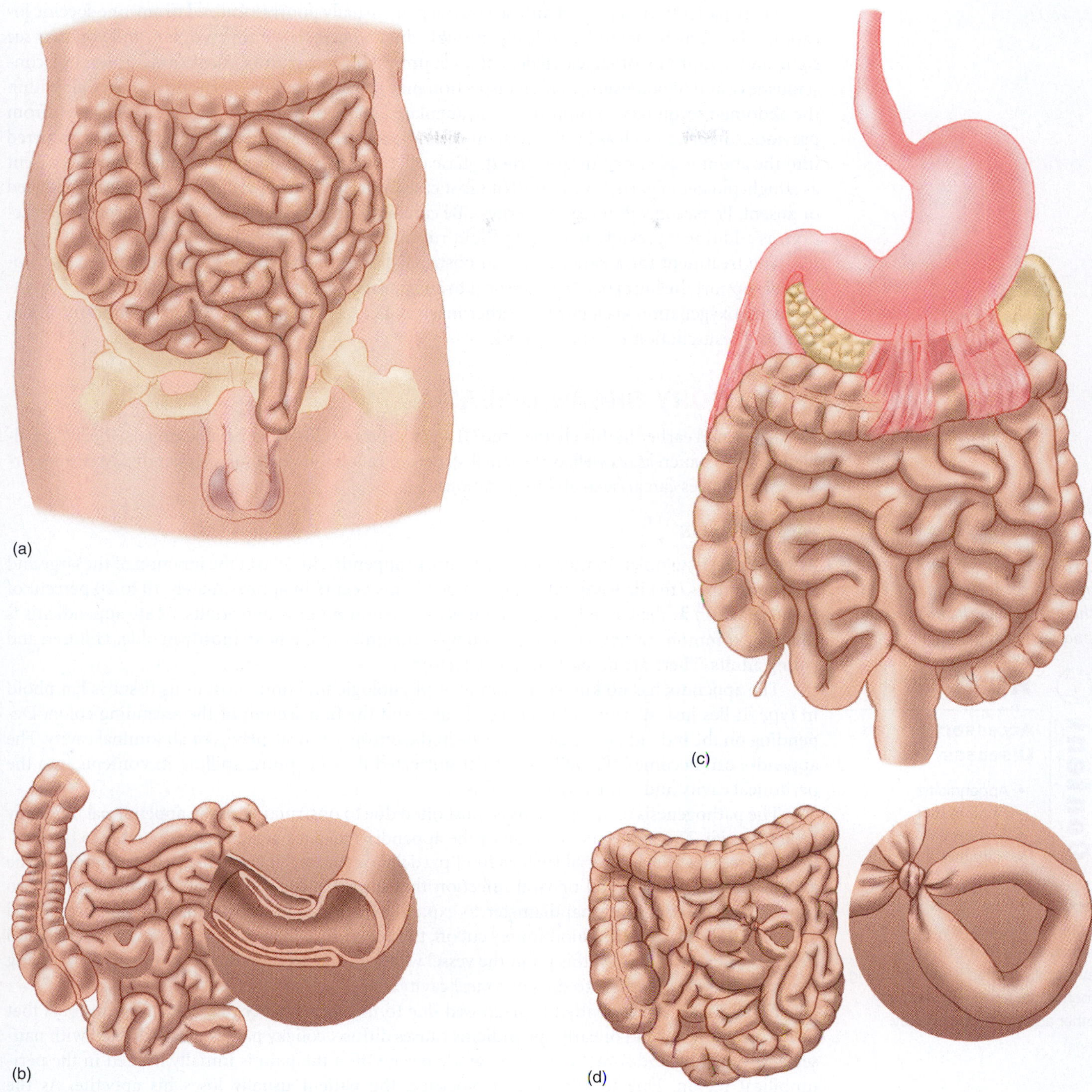

■ **Figure 32-3** The most common causes of bowel obstruction: (a) hernia, (b) intussusception, (c) adhesion, (d) volvulus.

sults in a decreased appetite, fever, malaise, nausea and vomiting, weight loss, or, if rupture occurs, peritonitis. Acute-onset pain may follow ingestion of a foreign body. Pain might also be due to a strangulated hernia, one that has rotated through the muscle wall of the abdomen such that blood flow is suddenly cut off (the herniated tissue has been "strangulated") and ischemia, or even infarction, of tissue occurs. Patients with bowel obstruction will frequently vomit, with the vomitus often containing a significant amount of bile. Severe bowel obstructions may result in the patient's vomiting material that looks and smells like feces. All of these findings suggest a bowel obstruction.

These patients present with diffuse visceral pain, usually poorly localized to any one specific location. They may be hemodynamically unstable due to necrosis within an organ, and you may see signs and symptoms of shock (pale, cool, clammy skin; tachycardia; alterations in level of consciousness; and hypotension). Visual inspection may reveal distention, peritonitis, or free air within the abdomen secondary to rupture of a strangulated segment of intestine. Look for scars left from previous surgery, as well as for the ecchymosis indicating that significant hemorrhage has occurred into the abdominal cavity. In the earliest phase of acute obstruction, bowel sounds may be present as a high-pitched obstruction sound. In most cases, however, bowel sounds will be greatly reduced or absent. Palpation will reveal tenderness. Be careful to palpate very lightly if you suspect obstruction, as additional pressure may bring about rupture of the obstructed segment.

The treatment for a patient with an obstructed bowel is based on physiological and psychological support during expedited transport to an appropriate facility. Measures include airway management, oxygenation via a nonrebreather mask at 15 lpm, position of comfort or shock position, and fluid resuscitation to prevent shock.

ACCESSORY ORGAN DISEASES

As you learned earlier in this chapter, the GI tract has three closely associated organs, the liver, gallbladder, and pancreas, as well as the small structure called the vermiform appendix. Accessory organ emergencies can arise in all four locations.

Appendicitis

appendicitis *inflammation of the vermiform appendix at the juncture of the large and small intestines.*

Review

Content

Accessory Organ Diseases

- Appendicitis
- Cholecystitis
- Pancreatitis
- Hepatitis

Appendicitis is evaluated in the emergency department and eventually treated in the operating room more frequently than any other abdominal emergency.

Appendicitis is an inflammation of the vermiform appendix, located at the junction of the large and small intestines (the ileocecal junction). Appendicitis occurs in approximately 10 to 20 percent of the population in the United States, and it is most common in young adults. Acute appendicitis is the most common surgical emergency you will encounter in the field, mostly in older children and young adults. There are no particular risk factors.

The appendix has no known anatomic or physiologic function; most of its tissue is lymphoid in type. It lies just inferior to the ileocecal valve and the first section of the ascending colon. Depending on the individual patient, it may be in the retroperitoneal, pelvic, or abdominal cavity. The appendix can become inflamed, and if left untreated it can rupture, spilling its contents into the peritoneal cavity and setting up peritonitis.

The pathogenesis of appendicitis is most often due to obstruction of the appendiceal lumen by fecal material. The shape and location of the appendix make it particularly vulnerable to obstruction by feces or other material such as food particles or tumor. This inflames the lymphoid tissue and often leads to bacterial or viral infection that ulcerates the mucosa. The inflammation also causes the appendix's internal diameter to expand, which can block the appendicular artery and cause thrombosis. With its blood supply cut off, the appendix becomes ischemic, and infarction and necrosis of tissue follow. At this point the vessel walls often weaken to the point of rupture, spilling the appendiceal contents into the peritoneal cavity.

McBurney's point *common site of pain from appendicitis, 1 to 2 inches above the anterior iliac crest in a direct line with the umbilicus.*

Appendicitis is frequently misdiagnosed due to the wide variety of signs and symptoms that can accompany it. Mild or early appendicitis causes diffuse, colicky pain often associated with nausea and vomiting and sometimes a low-grade fever. Often the pain is initially located in the periumbilical region. Due to appendiceal blockage, the patient usually loses his appetite. As the appendix continues to dilate, the pain will localize in the right lower quadrant. A common site of pain is **McBurney's point,** 1 to 2 inches above the anterior iliac crest along a direct line from the anterior crest to the umbilicus (Figure 32-4 ■). Once the appendix ruptures the pain becomes diffuse due to development of peritonitis.

Physical assessment will find a patient who appears to be in discomfort. The abdominal exam will reveal tenderness or guarding around the umbilicus or right lower quadrant. Do not repeatedly palpate for rebound tenderness. The pressure that this procedure exerts can cause an inflamed appendix to rupture.

Prehospital care for appendicitis includes placing the patient in a position of comfort, giving psychological support, diligently managing his airway to prevent aspiration, establishing intravenous access, and transporting him. In most cases the appendix will not have ruptured, and the

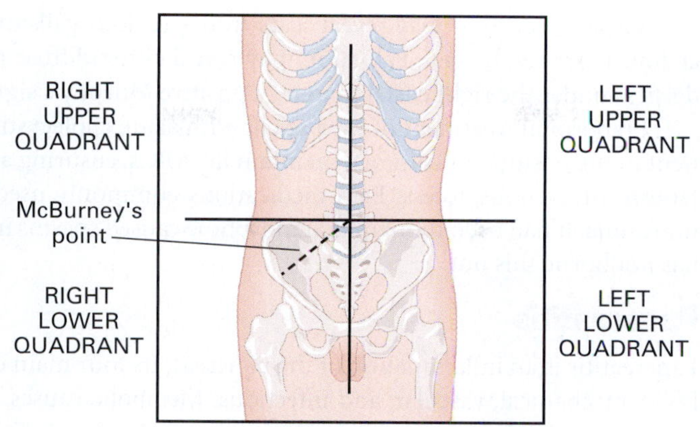

■ **Figure 32-4** McBurney's point is a common site of pain in appendicitis.

patient will remain hemodynamically stable. Monitor as you would for bowel obstruction, and treat any complications such as tachycardia or other signs of shock as they arise.

Cholecystitis

Cholecystitis is an inflammation of the gallbladder. Cholelithiasis (the formation of gallstones), which causes 90 percent of cholecystitis cases, occurs in approximately 15 percent of the adult population in the United States, with over 1 million new cases diagnosed annually. There are two types of gallstones, cholesterol based and bilirubin based. Cholesterol-based stones are far more common and are associated with a specific risk profile: obese, middle-aged women with more than one biological child.

Definitive treatment of acute cholecystitis includes antibiotic therapy, laparoscopic surgery, lithotripsy (ultrasound treatment to break up the stones), and surgery if the other, less invasive therapies fail. With the advent of laparoscopic surgery, mortality has fallen to less than 1 percent, with an overall morbidity of approximately 6 percent.

Cholecystitis caused by gallstones can be chronic or acute. The liver produces bile, the primary vehicle for removing cholesterol from the body. The bile travels down the common bile duct to empty into the small intestine at the sphincter of Oddi. The sphincter of Oddi opens when chyme exits the stomach through the pyloric sphincter. When the sphincter of Oddi closes, the flow of bile backs up into the gallbladder via the cystic duct. The bile remains in the gallbladder until the sphincter of Oddi opens again.

The bile can become supersaturated and calculi—stonelike masses based on bilirubin, cholesterol, or both—form. These calculi travel down the cystic duct, frequently lodging in the common bile duct. When they obstruct the flow of bile, gallbladder inflammation and irritation result. The bile salts subsequently attack the mucosal membrane lining the gallbladder, leaving the underlying epithelial tissue without protection. Prostaglandins are also released, further irritating the epithelial wall. As irritation continues, the inflammation grows, increasing intraluminal pressure and ultimately reducing blood flow to the epithelium.

Other causes of cholecystitis include acalculus cholecystitis (cholecystitis without associated stones) and chronic inflammation caused by bacterial infection. Acalculus cholecystitis usually results from burns, sepsis, diabetes, and multiple organ failure. Chronic cholecystitis resulting from a bacterial infection (*Escherichia coli* and enterococci) presents with an inflammatory process similar to cholelithiasis.

An inflamed gallbladder usually causes an acute attack of upper right quadrant abdominal pain. The inflammation can cause an irritation of the diaphragm with referred pain in the right shoulder. If the gallstones are lodged in the cystic duct, the pain may be colicky, due to expansion and contraction of the duct. Often the pain occurs after a meal that is high in fat content because of the secondary release of bile from the gallbladder. The right subcostal region may be tender because of abdominal muscle spasms. Patients may experience extreme pain as the epithelium in the gallbladder erodes away. Sympathetic stimulation because of the pain may cause pale, cool, clammy skin. If peritonitis occurs, the skin may be warm due to increased blood flow to the inflamed peritoneum. Nausea and vomiting are common, due to cystic duct spasm.

Gallbladder pain is located in the right upper quadrant or epigastrium and is colicky in nature. The problem tends to recur unless surgery is performed.

Visual inspection may reveal scars from previous gallstone surgeries, but distention and ecchymosis are rarely seen. Palpation may reveal either diffuse right-sided tenderness or point tenderness under the right costal margin, a positive **Murphy's sign.**

Murphy's sign *pain caused when an inflamed gallbladder is palpated by pressing under the right costal margin.*

Prehospital treatment of the patient with acute cholecystitis is mainly palliative. Place the patient in the position of comfort; maintain his ABCs, ensuring adequate oxygenation; and finally establish intravenous access. Pain medications commonly used include fentanyl (Sublimaze) and morphine. It had been thought that morphine caused spasms in the sphincter of Oddi, but research has not borne this out.

Pancreatitis

Acute pancreatitis is most often due to alcohol abuse or gallstones.

Content Review

Causes of Acute Pancreatitis

- Alcohol abuse
- Gallstones
- Elevated serum lipids (cholesterol and triglycerides)
- Drug induced

Pancreatitis is an inflammation of the pancreas. Its four main categories, based on cause, are metabolic, mechanical, vascular, and infectious. Metabolic causes, specifically alcoholism, account for approximately 80 percent of all cases; consequently, pancreatitis is widespread in the United States, due to the high incidence of alcoholism. Mechanical obstructions caused by gallstones or elevated serum lipids account for another 9 percent. Vascular injuries caused by thromboembolisms or shock, along with infectious diseases, account for the remaining 11 percent. Overall mortality in acute pancreatitis is relatively high, approximately 30–40 percent, mainly due to accompanying sepsis and shock, which lead to multisystem organ failure. In acute pancreatitis, the rate of serious morbidity and mortality has been found to be 14 percent in patients with fewer than three positive findings. The mortality rate exceeded 95 percent when there were three or more positive findings.

The vast bulk of the pancreas's tissue is arranged in glandular structures called *acini* (singular, *acinus*). These cells produce digestive enzymes that empty into the duodenum at the ampulla of Vater, near the junction with the stomach. The other function of the pancreas is endocrine: A small amount of tissue located in isolated islets of tissue secretes the hormones insulin and glucagon. Frequently, gallstones leaving the common bile duct become lodged at the ampulla of Vater and obstruct the pancreatic duct. These obstructions back up pancreatic digestive enzymes into the pancreatic duct and the pancreas itself. The digestive enzymes inflame the pancreas and cause edema, which reduces blood flow, as in the pathogenesis of acute appendicitis. In turn, the decreased blood flow causes ischemia and, finally, acinar destruction. This is often called acute pancreatitis based on rapidity of onset.

Content Review

Pancreatitis (Mild) Signs and Symptoms

- Epigastric pain
- Abdominal distention
- Nausea/vomiting
- Elevated amylase and lipase

Acinar tissue destruction causes a second form of pancreatitis, chronic pancreatitis. Acinar tissue destruction commonly occurs due to chronic alcohol intake, drug toxicity, ischemia, or infectious diseases. Alcohol ingestion results in the deposit of platelet plugs in the acinar tissue. The plugs disrupt enzyme flow from the pancreas. When digestive juices back up into the pancreas from the ampulla of Vater, the digestive enzymes can become activated and begin to digest the pancreas itself. Morphologically this autodigestion appears as lesions and fatty tissue changes on the pancreas.

Content Review

Pancreatitis (Severe) Signs and Symptoms

- Refractory hypotensive shock
- Blood loss
- Respiratory failure

As tissue digestion continues, the lesion can erode and begin to hemorrhage. This acute exacerbation of pancreatitis causes intense abdominal pain. Its intensity reflects the number of lesions affected or the degree of acinar tissue death. The pain can be localized to the left upper quadrant or may radiate to the back or the epigastric region. Most patients experience nausea followed by uncontrolled vomiting and retching that can further aggravate the hemorrhage. Visual inspection may reveal previous surgical scars for lesion removal; ecchymosis and swelling of the left upper quadrant may also be present due to hemorrhage or significant organ edema. The patient will appear acutely ill with diaphoresis, tachycardia, and possible hypotension if massive hemorrhaging is involved.

Prehospital treatment is supportive and aimed at maintaining the ABCs by providing high-flow, high-concentration oxygen and establishing intravenous access. Fluid resuscitation with crystalloid may be warranted if the patient appears hemodynamically unstable. Definitive treatment involves gastric intubation and suctioning for emesis control, diagnostic peritoneal lavage, antibiotic therapy, fluid resuscitation, and surgery to remove the blockage.

Hepatitis

Hepatitis involves any injury to hepatocytes (liver cells) associated with an inflammation or infection. Due to its wide range of potential causes, hepatitis has a high mortality rate. Five viruses—hepatitis types A, B, C, D, and E—are the disease's most common causes, resulting in five different kinds of hepatitis that together account for 60–70 percent of all cases. Alcoholic hepatitis, which arises from alcoholic cirrhosis, rather than an infectious agent, is responsible for another 20–30 percent. Trauma and other diseases account for the remaining 10 percent. Factors that increase the risk of contracting hepatitis include, to name a few, crowded and unsanitary living conditions, poor personal hygiene that invites oral–fecal transmission, exposure to bloodborne pathogens, and chronic alcohol intake. (Specific risk factors are associated with the different types of hepatitis—A, B, C, D, and E.)

The liver is in the upper right abdominal quadrant. A highly vascular organ, it filters and detoxifies blood returning from the abdomen and certain abdominal organs. Its other important functions include synthesizing fatty acids, converting glucose to glycogen, and helping to remove toxic products such as ammonia from the body. Any of the viral pathogens, alcoholic exposure, or trauma can injure the hepatocytes, causing inflammation and, possibly, chronic liver disease. Whatever its cause the results are usually similar. The changes in the liver include enlargement and hypertrophy, fatty changes, loss of architecture, and appearance of lesions and spontaneous hemorrhages. The symptoms' severity can range from mild to complete liver failure and death.

Of the five types of viral hepatitis, hepatitis A (HAV) is probably the best known. Commonly referred to as infectious hepatitis, HAV spreads by the oral–fecal route. The disease is self-limiting, usually lasting between 2 and 8 weeks. It rarely causes severe hepatic injury and, thus, has a very low mortality rate. Hepatitis B (HBV), known as "serum hepatitis," is transmitted as a bloodborne pathogen that can stay active in bodily fluids outside the body for days. With well over 310 million carriers worldwide, HBV is an epidemic. Its effects may be only minimal, but they can also range to severe liver ischemia and necrosis. Hepatitis C (HCV) is caused by the pathogen most commonly responsible for spreading hepatitis through blood transfusions. Hepatitis C is marked by chronic and often debilitating damage to the liver. Hepatitis D (HDV) is a less common disorder because its pathogen is dormant until activated by HBV. Hepatitis E (HEV) is a waterborne infection that has caused epidemics in Africa, Mexico, and other third-world nations. Its mortality rate for pregnant women is high.

With well over 310 million carriers worldwide, HBV is an epidemic.

Be wary of HIV, but fear hepatitis B and C. Do not forget to use personal protective equipment (PPE) and Standard Precautions.

Patients with hepatitis commonly present with symptoms relative to the severity of their disease. Usually they complain of upper right quadrant abdominal tenderness, not relieved by antacids, food, or positioning. They may lose their appetite and become anorexic, usually losing weight. The decrease in bile production changes their stool to a clay color, and increased bilirubin retention causes jaundice, a yellow coloring of the skin, and scleral icterus, a yellowing of the white of the eyes. Other symptoms include severe nausea and vomiting, general malaise, photophobia, pharyngitis, and coughing.

Physical examination will reveal a sick patient, possibly with a jaundiced appearance. Depending on the patient's severity, his positioning can range from standing up and walking around to lying in a fetal position with his knees drawn to his chest. Pain may present in the right upper quadrant or the right shoulder (referred from diaphragmatic irritation). Fever may be secondary to infection or to tissue necrosis. Inspection may yield nonspecific findings. Palpation may reveal an enlarged liver. Skin color and temperature can range from warm and dry (due to the infection) to cool, clammy, and diaphoretic if a hepatic lesion has ruptured and begun to bleed.

Prehospital treatment is mainly palliative. Secure the ABCs and establish intravenous access for fluid resuscitation or antiemetic administration. You must carefully consider any pharmacological administration because the liver breaks down many active drug metabolites. Definitive treatment involves antiviral and anti-inflammatory medications and symptomatic treatment.

If you suspect hepatitis, you must consider carefully any pharmacological administration because the liver breaks down many active drug metabolites.

Several large fire departments on the eastern seaboard of the United States have experienced increased rates of hepatitis C in their personnel. So always take precautions and work closely with your department infection control officer.

Summary

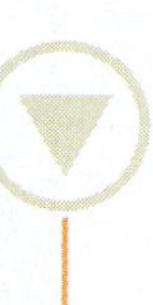

Abdominal pain can originate from a wide variety of causes, either from the abdominal organs or from areas outside of the abdominal cavity. The prehospital management priorities for the abdominal patient are to establish and maintain his airway, breathing, and circulation. The differential diagnosis can include a multitude of causes that usually cannot be identified without laboratory and radiographic analysis. Airway management is of paramount importance, since patients frequently

The key to successful treatment of gastrointestinal ailments is prompt recognition, treatment, and rapid transport to the hospital.

suffer from severe bouts of nausea and vomiting. Be prepared to turn the patient onto his side if necessary to clear large amounts of vomitus from the airway. Oxygenation usually can be adequately stabilized by placing the patient on high-flow, high-concentration oxygen via a nonrebreather mask. Fluid loss, hemorrhage, or sepsis may compromise the circulatory status. Initiate fluid resuscitation for the hemodynamically unstable patient in the field, but never delay transport. Patients who have abdominal pain lasting over 6 hours should always be evaluated by a physician.

Review Questions

1. ___________ is the hallmark of the acute abdominal emergency.
   a. Pain
   b. Fever
   c. Nausea
   d. Vomiting
2. ___________ pain is a sharp type of pain that travels along definite neural routes to the spinal column.
   a. Tearing
   b. Somatic
   c. Referred
   d. Visceral
3. The abdomen can hold from ___________ of fluid before any noticeable change in abdominal girth occurs.
   a. 4 to 6 pints
   b. 6 to 10 pints
   c. 6 to 10 liters
   d. 4 to 6 liters
4. Persistent abdominal pain lasting longer than ___________ hours is classified as a surgical emergency and always requires transport.
   a. 2
   b. 4
   c. 6
   d. 5
5. The paramedic should administer a ___________ cc/kg fluid bolus to begin treating hemorrhagic hypovolemia.
   a. 20
   b. 40
   c. 60
   d. 80
6. The most common cause of lower GI hemorrhages is:
   a. benign polyps.
   b. Crohn's disease.
   c. diverticulosis.
   d. ulcerative colitis.
7. Acute ___________ is the most common surgical emergency the paramedic will encounter in the field, mostly in older children and young adults.
   a. gastritis
   b. appendicitis
   c. cholecystitis
   d. diverticulitis

8. An inflamed gallbladder usually causes an acute attack of __________ quadrant abdominal pain.
   a. upper left
   b. lower left
   c. upper right
   d. lower right
9. Liver cells are called:
   a. hepatocytes.
   b. leukocytes.
   c. lymphocytes.
   d. phagocytes.
10. Hepatitis __________ is a waterborne infection that has caused epidemics in Africa, Mexico, and other third-world nations.
   a. A
   b. C
   c. D
   d. E

See Answers to Review Questions at the back of this book.

Chapter 33

Urology and Nephrology

Objectives

After reading this chapter, you should be able to:

1. Describe the incidence, morbidity, mortality, and risk factors predisposing to urologic and nephrologic emergencies. (pp. 1329–1330, 1335, 1338–1339, 1343–1344, 1345–1346)
2. Discuss the anatomy and physiology of the organs and structures related to the urinary system. (see Chapter 3)
3. Define referred pain and visceral pain as they relate to urology. (p. 1331)
4. Describe the questioning technique and specific questions the paramedic should use when gathering a focused history in a patient with abdominal pain. (pp. 1332–1333)
5. Describe the technique for performing a comprehensive physical examination of a patient complaining of abdominal pain. (pp. 1333–1334)
6. Define acute renal failure. (p. 1335)
7. Discuss the pathophysiology of acute renal failure. (pp. 1335–1337)
8. Recognize the signs and symptoms related to acute renal failure. (pp. 1337–1338)
9. Describe the management of acute renal failure. (p. 1338)
10. Integrate pathophysiological principles and assessment findings to formulate a field impression and implement a treatment plan for the patient with acute renal failure. (pp. 1335–1338)
11. Define chronic renal failure. (pp. 1338–1339)
12. Discuss the pathophysiology of chronic renal failure. (pp. 1339–1340)
13. Recognize the signs and symptoms related to chronic renal failure. (pp. 1340–1341)
14. Describe the management of chronic renal failure. (pp. 1341–1343)
15. Integrate pathophysiological principles and assessment findings to formulate a field impression and implement a treatment plan for the patient with chronic renal failure. (pp. 1339–1343)
16. Define renal dialysis. (pp. 1342–1343)
17. Discuss the common complications of renal dialysis. (pp. 1342–1343)

18. Define renal calculi. (pp. 1343–1344)
19. Discuss the pathophysiology of renal calculi. (p. 1344)
20. Recognize the signs and symptoms related to renal calculi. (p. 1345)
21. Describe the management of renal calculi. (p. 1345)
22. Integrate pathophysiological principles and assessment findings to formulate a field impression and implement a treatment plan for the patient with renal calculi. (pp. 1343–1345)
23. Define urinary tract infection. (pp. 1345–1346)
24. Discuss the pathophysiology of urinary tract infection. (pp. 1346–1347)
25. Recognize the signs and symptoms related to urinary tract infection. (p. 1347)
26. Describe the management of a urinary tract infection. (p. 1347)
27. Integrate pathophysiological principles and assessment findings to formulate a field impression and implement a treatment plan for the patient with a urinary tract infection. (pp. 1345–1347)
28. Apply epidemiology to develop prevention strategies for urologic and nephrologic emergencies. (p. 1330)
29. Integrate pathophysiological principles to the assessment of a patient with abdominal pain. (pp. 1331–1334)
30. Synthesize assessment findings and patient history information to accurately differentiate between pain of a urologic or nephrologic emergency and that of another origin. (pp. 1331–1334)
31. Develop, execute, and evaluate a treatment plan based on the field impression made in the assessment. (pp. 1329–1347)

Key Terms

acute renal failure (ARF), p. 1335
acute tubular necrosis, p. 1337
anuria, p. 1335
benign prostatic hypertrophy, p. 1330
chronic renal failure (CRF), p. 1338
community-acquired infection, p. 1346
cystitis, p. 1346
dialysate, p. 1342
end-stage renal failure, p. 1338
genitourinary system, p. 1330
glucose intolerance, p. 1339
hemodialysis, p. 1342
interstitial nephritis, p. 1337
intrarenal abscess, p. 1346
isosthenuria, p. 1339
microangiopathy, p. 1336
nephrology, p. 1330
nosocomial infection, p. 1346
oliguria, p. 1335
perinephric abscess, p. 1346
peritoneal dialysis, p. 1343
post-renal acute renal failure, p. 1337
prerenal acute renal failure, p. 1336
priapism, p. 1345
prostatitis, p. 1346
pyelonephritis, p. 1346
reduced nephron mass, p. 1339
reduced renal mass, p. 1339
renal, p. 1330
renal acute renal failure, p. 1336
renal calculi, p. 1343
renal dialysis, p. 1342
urea, p. 1330
uremia, p. 1339
urethritis, p. 1346
urinary stasis, p. 1346
urinary system, p. 1329
urinary tract infection (UTI), p. 1345
urine, p. 1330
urology, p. 1330

INTRODUCTION

The **urinary system** performs a number of vital functions. It maintains blood volume and the proper balance of water, electrolytes, and pH (acid–base balance). It ensures that key substances such as glucose remain in the bloodstream, yet it also removes a variety of toxic wastes from the blood. It plays a major role in arterial blood pressure regulation. In addition, the urinary system controls development of red blood cells, or erythrocytes.

urinary system *the group of organs that produces urine, maintaining fluid and electrolyte balance for the body.*

urine *the fluid made by the kidney and eliminated from the body.*

urea *waste derived from ammonia produced through protein metabolism.*

genitourinary system *the male organ system that includes reproductive and urinary structures.*

nephrology *the medical specialty dealing with the kidneys.*

urology *the surgical specialty dealing with the urinary/genitourinary system.*

renal *pertaining to the kidneys.*

benign prostatic hypertrophy *a noncancerous enlargement of the prostate associated with aging.*

The body eliminates water and other substances removed from blood in the form of the fluid **urine.** The kidneys' regulation of water and other important substances in blood is an example of homeostasis, the body's ability to maintain an appropriate internal environment despite changing conditions. Metabolism, the intracellular processes that generate the energy and materials necessary for cell growth and repair, also creates many waste products. For example, significant amounts of ammonia form in the liver when amino acids are broken down in gluconeogenesis, a process that produces glucose between meals. Ammonia is highly toxic to body cells, particularly brain cells. Liver cells convert the ammonia into **urea,** a less toxic compound. The kidneys remove urea efficiently from the blood and pass it into the urine. Moreover, the urinary system eliminates many foreign chemicals such as drug metabolites.

The urinary system in women is physically distinct from the reproductive system. They share no structures. (Chapters 39 and 40 discuss medical emergencies related to the female reproductive system.) In contrast, the urinary system in men shares some structures with the reproductive system. For instance, both urine and the male reproductive fluid are eliminated from the body through the opening at the tip of the penis. Consequently, the term **genitourinary system** is often used with men. The urinary and reproductive systems' proximity in women and their shared structures in men are due to the common embryonic origin of their tissues.

The most significant medical disorders involving the urinary system affect the kidneys and kidney function. **Nephrology** (from the Greek *nephros,* kidney) is the medical specialty devoted to kidney disorders. **Urology** is the surgical specialty devoted to care of the entire urinary system in women and the genitourinary system in men. We will use nephrology and nephrologic (or the preferred adjective, **renal,** from the Latin *renes,* kidneys) to refer to conditions primarily affecting the kidneys. We will use urology and urologic to refer to conditions that significantly affect other parts of the urinary or genitourinary systems.

Renal and urologic disorders are common, affecting about 20 million Americans. Many disorders are very serious. More than 50,000 Americans die annually from kidney disease. More than 250,000 Americans suffer from the most severe form of long-term kidney failure, end-stage renal failure. They require either dialysis, a process that artificially performs the most important kidney functions, or kidney transplantation, implantation of a kidney from another person, to survive. The leading causes of end-stage renal failure are poorly controlled diabetes mellitus (both Type I and Type II) and uncontrolled or inadequately controlled hypertension.

Among acute, or sudden-onset, disorders, renal calculi, or kidney stones, are very common. More than 500,000 Americans are treated for kidney stones each year. Infections are also common, and they may have different causes in women and men. A woman complaining of burning pain on urination probably has an infection in the urinary system. Men with the same chief complaint may have an infection that arose in the urinary system or as a sexually transmitted disease. Noncancerous enlargement of the prostate gland, or **benign prostatic hypertrophy,** affects about 60 percent of men by age 50 and about 80 percent by age 80. If prostatic hypertrophy obstructs urine flow, a medical emergency involving sharp pain and inability to urinate results.

All of these conditions, as well as others described later, are sufficiently common that you will see them in the field. In any case where existing kidney function may be jeopardized, prehospital care includes preventive strategies, or steps to minimize the likelihood of any further loss of function. Our discussion of assessment and management will cover these procedures.

Content Review

Mechanisms of Nontraumatic Urologic Disorders

- Inflammatory or immune-mediated disease
- Infectious disease
- Physical obstruction
- Hemorrhage

GENERAL MECHANISMS OF NONTRAUMATIC TISSUE PROBLEMS

Both traumatic and nontraumatic problems can affect the urinary system, particularly the kidneys. The kidneys' retroperitoneal location protects them relatively well against injury. Nontraumatic renal and urologic disorders result from four general mechanisms: inflammatory or immune-mediated disease, infectious disease, physical obstruction, or hemorrhage. Traumatic renal and urologic disorders are discussed in Chapter 26. We will discuss nontraumatic disorders later in this chapter.

GENERAL PATHOPHYSIOLOGY, ASSESSMENT, AND MANAGEMENT

Because of many gastrointestinal and urologic emergencies' similar presentation, you may have difficulty determining the source of an abdominal problem when pain is the sole complaint.

As you learned in Chapter 32, "Gastroenterology," abdominal emergencies are common. Because of the similar presentations of gastrointestinal (GI) and urologic emergencies, you may have difficulty determining the source of an abdominal problem when pain is the sole complaint. You can often find clues to the eventual diagnosis when you take a focused history and perform the focused physical exam. Before reading further, you may want to review the discussion of GI pathophysiology, assessment, and management in Chapter 32, "Gastroenterology."

PATHOPHYSIOLOGIC BASIS OF PAIN

The nerve fibers that carry pain messages to the brain are triggered by different stimuli. Some are triggered when damage to the epithelial lining of an organ exposes the underlying tissue layer, where the nerve endings are located. Others respond to stretching forces generated when an organ is inflamed or enlarged by internal hemorrhage or obstruction.

Causes of Pain

Bacterial infection damages the epithelial tissue that lines structures such as the urethra and urinary bladder. This damage causes pain that often worsens when urine flows over the affected tissue during urination. Bacteria normally found on the skin can cause infections in women. In men, the same symptom, pain on voiding, is often due to a sexually transmitted disease such as gonorrhea. Distention of a ureter by a renal calculus (kidney stone) causes a sharp pain that may ease or worsen when the stone shifts position inside the ureter.

Types of Pain

The most common types of pain in urologic emergencies are visceral and referred. *Visceral pain* usually arises in hollow structures such as the ureters, urinary bladder, and urethra, or the vas deferens or epididymis in males. Its chief characteristic, an aching or crampy pain felt deep within the body and poorly localized, is due to the relatively low number of nerve fibers in the involved structures. Visceral pain can also be the initial presentation of urinary tract infection or of renal calculi. *Referred pain* is felt in a location other than its site of origin. This occurs when afferent nerve fibers carrying the pain message merge with other pain-carrying fibers at the junction with the spinal cord. If that junction has far more nerve fibers from one or more other locations than from the site of origin, the brain may perceive the pain as coming from those locations rather than the affected one. Pyelonephritis, inflammation associated with kidney infection, is not only associated with pain in the flank, the skin surface closest to the kidney, but sometimes with pain in the neck or shoulder. The referred pain originates in diaphragmatic irritation due to kidney inflammation, but the brain perceives the pain as coming from the area of the neck or shoulder.

ASSESSMENT AND MANAGEMENT

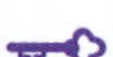

Do not try to pinpoint the cause of abdominal pain in the field.

The assessment steps are the same for all abdominal emergencies. Do not try to pinpoint the cause of abdominal pain in the field; diagnosis is often difficult even in the hospital setting. However, you do need to do an assessment to detect and manage life-threatening conditions such as shock and to provide historical and physical information that will be helpful in the hospital.

Scene Size-Up

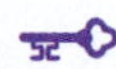

Blood always calls for personal protective equipment and proper sample handling on your part.

During scene size-up, look for evidence of a traumatic versus medical cause and for signs of a life-threatening situation, perhaps an observer performing CPR or the presence of blood. Remember to employ personal protective equipment and proper handling.

Primary Assessment

Primary assessment of the patient concentrates on the ABCs of airway, breathing, and circulation, as well as on patient disability (for example, signs of agitation and confused mental state). If the patient is conscious and responsive, ask for the chief complaint.

During the secondary assessment, your job is to gather the historical and physical evidence that can be used in the hospital and to make sure the patient is supported before and during transport.

Secondary Assessment

Information about Pain. When the chief complaint is pain or involves pain, initial questions should elicit information about the timing, character, and associated symptoms of the pain. The OPQRST–ASPN template is useful for beginning your questions.

- ★ *Onset.* When did the pain start, and what were you doing at the time? Visceral pain often arises gradually, with the patient first aware of vague discomfort and only later aware of pain.
- ★ *Provocation/palliation.* What makes the pain worse or better? Increased pain on urination, particularly in light of a fever or history of fever, suggests urinary/genitourinary tract infection. Pain associated with the inability to urinate, particularly in elderly men, points toward urethral obstruction due to prostatic enlargement. Improvement with knees drawn up to the chest points toward peritonitis, whereas improvement with walking may indicate a kidney stone that moved into a less painful position.
- ★ *Quality.* What is the pain like? Visceral pain is frequently described as dull or crampy; because many urinary-system structures are hollow, visceral pain is common in these emergencies. Vague discomfort followed by a change to sharp pain localized in the flank, for instance, may indicate ureteral obstruction due to a kidney stone that has moved.
- ★ *Region/radiation.* Where is the pain located, or do you feel pain in several places? Does the pain seem to move from one part of your body to another? Listen for patterns of referred pain such as pain in the lower back and the neck or shoulder, as well as changes in perception of pain on movement of a limb or whole body. In postpubertal women, be sure to ask for menstrual history, particularly if menstrual-like cramps are described or blood is present in the perineal area. (For more on gynecologic and obstetrical emergencies, see Chapters 39 and 40.)
- ★ *Severity.* Where is the pain on a scale of 1 to 10? Has the intensity changed over time, and if so, how? Sudden changes to sharp pain, particularly when associated with decreased responsiveness and early signs of shock, may indicate rupture of an internal organ such as the appendix in appendicitis or the fallopian tube in an ectopic pregnancy. Most urologic problems will not show this pattern of abrupt and significant shift in severity and type of pain.
- ★ *Time.* How long ago did the pain start? Is it constant or does it come and go? Remember that any case of abdominal pain lasting about 6 hours or longer is considered a surgical emergency until proven otherwise, and the patient should be transported to an appropriate facility. Pelvic visceral pain of long duration and unchanging intensity, particularly if associated with signs suggesting urinary tract origin such as fever and increased pain on urination, suggests a medical case rather than a surgical one, but you still may need to transport the patient to the hospital. When confronted with an acute abdomen (sudden onset of severe abdominal pain), always err on the side of considering it a potential surgical emergency.
- ★ *Previous history of similar event.* Some urologic emergencies such as renal calculus and infection may recur. This makes it especially important to elicit any history of a similar event, the diagnosis at the time, and the treatment given. Because increased risk for renal calculi is genetic in some cases, listen for a history of family members similarly affected.

- ★ *Nausea/vomiting.* As you learned in Chapter 32, "Gastroenterology" severe pain is often associated with autonomic nervous system discharge producing the signs of nausea, possibly with vomiting, along with profuse sweating, clammy skin, and rapid heart rate. Remember that such a presentation does not necessarily indicate that the problem is in the GI system. For instance, the severe pain of a kidney stone can cause this presentation.
- ★ *Changes in bowel habits and stool.* Frequent stools, especially if they are diarrheal or contain signs of blood (either melena or hematochezia), suggest a problem in the GI system. Recent constipation may not be relevant except in the context of physical findings.
- ★ *Weight loss.* Significant weight loss over a very short period (hours or days) almost always reflects water loss, and signs of dehydration will be evident. Longer term weight loss may suggest chronic illness or GI dysfunction. Be sure to ask about conditions including diabetes, cardiovascular disease, and cancer, as well as medications and medication changes.
- ★ *Last oral intake.* The timing and content of the last meal may indicate an acute, progressive problem (a normal appetite, normal meal) or exacerbation of a long-standing one (poor appetite, small meal). Ask explicitly about fluid intake, because patients may not consider beverages to be food. The timing of the last oral intake is also important if the patient will be undergoing general anesthesia for a surgical procedure.
- ★ *Chest pain.* Chest pain, particularly left sided, does not necessarily indicate a myocardial infarction (MI). Assess whether the pain pattern suggests angina (for example, chest pain associated with radiation to jaw and left arm). Also remember that patients with long-standing or severe diabetes may not show the typical pain pattern of an MI due to diabetic neuropathy (nerve damage), but signs of ischemia may appear on an ECG.

Focused Physical Examination

The focused examination includes forming an overall impression as well as examining the abdomen. Remember that you will not be able to diagnose most cases of abdominal pain in the field. Your job is to gather the historical and physical evidence that can be used in the hospital and to make sure the patient is supported before and during transport.

Appearance In general, any person with significant pain, particularly pain of some duration, will appear uncomfortable. A patient may show discomfort by rigidly maintaining the position of least pain or by constantly pacing if walking helps ease the pain.

Posture Lying with knees drawn to the chest suggests peritonitis, which is often of GI origin. Relief with walking suggests visceral pain; kidney stones may shift position during walking, easing the sharp pain. Check visually if the patient who is walking is upright or favoring one side. Someone who looks feverish and walks hunched up, leaning to one side, and complaining of back pain may have a pyelonephritis (kidney infection).

Level of Consciousness In the absence of fever, acute-onset decreases in responsiveness often suggest hemorrhage and evolution of hypovolemic shock. Hemorrhage is far more often tied to GI or reproductive (namely, obstetric) emergencies than to urinary system problems. You may see a decreased level of consciousness in sick patients who are undergoing dialysis, the artificial technique that replaces some vital kidney functions, including maintenance of electrolyte balance and removal of wastes. Try to determine if the change in responsiveness is acute or chronic, which may suggest a new problem or an aggravation of preexistent problems.

Apparent State of Health Patients with chronic illness, whether or not it originates in the urinary system, often look ill even without an acute problem. Extreme thinness, pale skin or mucous membranes, or the presence of home health equipment such as a bedside toilet, dialysis machine, or an oxygen tank all suggest chronic problems. In significant emergency states, the patient will usually not be tidy and neatly dressed. If he is, this may suggest that the emergency occurred suddenly, as with a hemorrhage or painful passage of a stone.

Skin Color Pale, dry, cool skin and mucous membranes may suggest chronic anemia such as that found in persons with chronic renal failure. Pale clammy skin suggests severe pain or shock, whereas flushed, dry skin may accompany fever.

Examination of the Abdomen The four components of the abdominal exam are inspection, auscultation, percussion, and palpation.

Always inspect the abdomen first. Note any ecchymotic discoloration or distention, as well as any surgical or traumatic scars. Most nephrologic and urologic emergencies will not show acute abnormalities on exam, whereas a number of GI emergencies will. Auscultation rarely produces a positive finding because bowel sounds are almost always present. Absence of bowel sounds, however, is important and suggests a GI emergency such as bowel obstruction.

Percussion and palpation may be more useful in the field. Percussion of the abdomen or other involved areas may produce clues to the origin of a urologic problem. Pain induced by percussion of the flanks, especially when accompanied by fever, strongly suggests pyelonephritis, or kidney infection. Pain on percussion just above the pelvic rim of the abdomen, especially when accompanied by fever and an increased urge to void, suggests cystitis, bladder infection. Constant, sharp pain increased by percussion of the affected flank may indicate where a kidney stone has lodged in a ureter.

Pain on percussion of the costovertebral angle (CVA—where the last rib meets the lumbar vertebrae) is known as Lloyd's sign and is indicative of pyelonephritis (infection of the kidney and renal pelvis).

In postpubescent girls and women, abdominal palpation may reveal pregnancy if you feel the firm, muscular mass of the gravid uterus above the pelvic rim. A ruptured ectopic pregnancy is possible when palpation increases pain in the lower quadrant, particularly when accompanied by evidence of hemorrhage or early shock. A vaginal exam is rarely indicated in the field; however, you should check for blood or other discharge at the urethral or vaginal openings. In all cases, ask the patient for the date of her last menstrual period.

Palpation of the lower abdomen may help diagnose acute urinary obstruction in older men due to prostatic enlargement. If enough urine has been retained, you will feel a large (up to roughly the size of a 2-liter bottle), painful, fluctuant mass above the pelvic rim of the abdomen. This represents the distended bladder. The male abdominal exam should also include inspection of the penis and scrotum. Purulent discharge from the penis may indicate a sexually transmitted disease (STD). Palpation of the scrotum may detect a testicular mass (remember that testicular cancer is far more common in younger men—the opposite of the age risk for prostatic cancer). Palpable nontesticular masses may be painful (infectious epididymitis) or nonpainful (varicocele, a noninfectious swelling of the epididymis). Ask relevant questions, such as whether swelling has been present for some time (as occurs with a varicocele) or is of recent onset (epididymitis).

Assessment Tools A hematocrit may detect significant or chronic bleeding. If blood is present in underwear or on the perineum itself, consider obtaining a small amount of material from the rectum, penile opening, or opening of the vagina to be checked for visible blood or occult bleeding. The latter may help to localize the affected system.

Vital Signs Temperature is important because fever suggests an infectious process. If you found high blood pressure, increased heart rate, or both during the ABC assessment, put those findings into context with other impressions from the exam. For instance, both heart rate and blood pressure commonly increase in someone with severe pain. However, it is also important to find out the patient's usual readings, if either he or a bystander can tell you. Uncontrolled chronic hypertension is one of the two most common causes of nephron damage and chronic renal failure (with the other cause being diabetes mellitus).

Management and Treatment Plans

Management of the patient with abdominal pain includes general and case-specific elements.

Airway, Breathing, Circulation Field management always starts with the ABCs—airway, breathing, and circulation. Be sure to maintain an open airway and use high-flow, high-concentration oxygen by mask. Be prepared for vomiting in any patient with severe pain, whether or not it is likely of genitourinary origin. Circulatory support is also vital, especially when there is any indication of hemorrhage, dehydration, or shock or the patient appears to have any compromise of renal function. Monitor blood pressure closely, and monitor cardiac status with ECG per local protocol or discussion with medical direction.

Pharmacological Interventions Consider placing a large-bore IV line for volume replacement or drug administration. Where possible, use a needle of sufficiently large bore for any emergency blood transfusion. In almost all cases involving abdominal pain, the question of analgesics, pain-relieving medications, will arise. The positive aspects of analgesic use are that the patient is more comfortable during transport and that pain- or stress-induced tachycardia, hypertension, or both may be abated. However, analgesics may mask the problem's signs and symptoms, making it difficult to accurately gauge progression of the pathologic process. Use analgesics as sparingly as possible; local protocol or discussion with medical direction may be advisable.

In cases of abdominal pain, use analgesics as sparingly as possible.

Nonpharmacological Interventions Remember that patients with an acute abdominal problem are possible surgical cases. Thus, nothing should be given by mouth. Administer fluid or medication only by IV or IM routes. Monitor vital signs closely and look for any change in level of consciousness. Be sure the patient is in a position of relative comfort, but also ensure that the position minimizes risk of aspiration if vomiting occurs.

Transport Considerations Each patient with abdominal pain of greater than 6 hours is considered a surgical emergency until hospital evaluation proves otherwise. Rapidly yet gently transport all such patients. During transportation, talk quietly to the patient, both to calm him and to keep him informed of time until arrival or other pertinent matters. All of your actions, both with the patient and any family or friends in the ambulance, should reflect caring and competence.

Content Review

Patients Most at Risk for Significant Kidney Problems

- Older patients
- Patients with diabetes
- Patients with chronic hypertension
- Patients with more than one risk factor

RENAL AND UROLOGIC EMERGENCIES

You must know how to respond properly and quickly to each major type of urinary or genitourinary emergency. Prevention strategies, procedures that minimize further loss of any existing kidney function, are vital. Most of this discussion focuses on renal emergencies, those affecting the kidneys. The leading causes of kidney failure are diabetes mellitus (both types) and uncontrolled or inadequately controlled hypertension. Add to that profile the fact that nephron number decreases with age, and you have the general profiles of patients most at risk for significant problems affecting kidney function: older patients, those with diabetes or chronic hypertension, or those with more than one risk factor.

We will discuss three renal emergencies—acute renal failure, chronic renal failure, and renal calculi (kidney stones). We will also discuss one urologic disorder, urinary tract infection, which can affect any or all parts of the urinary/genitourinary system.

Content Review

Most Common Renal Emergencies

- Acute renal failure
- Chronic renal failure
- Renal calculi

ACUTE RENAL FAILURE

Acute renal failure (ARF) is a sudden (often over a period of days) drop in urine output to less than 400–500 mL per day, a condition called **oliguria.** Output may literally fall to zero, a condition called **anuria.** ARF is not uncommon among severely ill, hospitalized patients. It is less common in the field. Noting ARF in the prehospital setting is vital because the condition may be reversible, dependent on the cause and extent of damage associated with the disorder. Overall mortality is roughly 50 percent, in part because the condition usually appears in significantly injured or ill persons.

acute renal failure (ARF) *the sudden-onset of severely decreased urine production.*

oliguria *decreased urine elimination to 400–500 mL or less per day.*

Pathophysiology

The three types of ARF are prerenal, renal, and post-renal. The distinct initial pathophysiology of each type determines both the severity of ARF and the likelihood for reversal and preserving renal

anuria *no elimination of urine.*

Content Review

Types of ARF

- Prerenal
- Renal
- Post-renal

function. The common point among the three types is their clinical presentation: sudden-onset oliguria or anuria. You may wish to reread the summary of kidney physiology before reading about the pathophysiology for each type of ARF.

prerenal acute renal failure *ARF due to decreased blood perfusion of kidneys.*

Prerenal ARF **Prerenal acute renal failure** begins with dysfunction before the level of the kidney; that is, with insufficient blood supply to the kidneys, or hypoperfusion. Prerenal ARF not only accounts for the highest proportion of ARF cases—40 to 80 percent—but also is often reversible through restoration of proper perfusion. These factors make it extremely important to know conditions associated with increased risk of renal hypoperfusion and to treat the patient quickly and properly. Problems that can trigger prerenal ARF include some common field conditions: hemorrhage, heart failure (MI or CHF), sepsis, and shock (Table 33–1). These triggers decrease renal blood supply through a drop in blood volume, blood pressure, or both. In addition, any anomaly directly affecting blood flow into the kidneys (such as thrombosis of a renal artery or vein) can trigger prerenal ARF through an increase in renal vascular resistance. When renal vascular resistance becomes higher in the renal vessels than in systemic vessels, blood is effectively shunted away from the kidneys.

Normally, the kidneys receive about 20 to 25 percent of cardiac output. This high level of perfusion is essential to sustaining a glomerular filtration rate sufficient to maintain blood volume and composition and to clear wastes such as urea and creatinine from the bloodstream. As the filtration rate drops, less urine forms, and the bloodstream retains water, electrolytes, and wastes such as urea and creatinine. Because the retained electrolytes include H^+ and K^+, metabolic acidosis and hyperkalemia may appear.

If hypoperfusion is prolonged or worsens in degree, two things happen. First, GFR decreases still further, and less filtrate means still less urine formation. Second, the nephron tubular cells become ischemic and active reabsorption and secretion decrease or cease. All of these metabolic effects of decreased nephron function further stress the body, particularly the cardiovascular system, and increase the likelihood that tubular ischemia will advance toward tubular cell death. At this point, the process is renal ARF, not prerenal.

renal acute renal failure *ARF due to pathology within the kidney tissue itself.*

microangiopathy *a disease affecting the smallest blood vessels.*

Renal ARF In **renal acute renal failure,** the pathologic process is within the kidney tissue, or renal parenchyma, itself. Three different processes cause renal ARF. The first is injury to small blood vessels (or **microangiopathy**) or glomerular capillaries; the second is injury to tubular cells; the third is inflammation or infection in the interstitial tissue surrounding nephrons (Table 33–1).

Microangiopathy and glomerular injury both result in obstruction of these minute vessels that are a vital part of the blood vessel-tubule structure of the nephron; consequently, nephron function is lost. Microangiopathy and glomerular injury are often immune mediated and may be associated with systemic immune-mediated diseases such as diabetes mellitus Type I and systemic lupus erythematosus. In these cases, ARF involves both preexistent and ongoing (that is, chronic and acute) nephron destruction.

Table 33–1 Causes of Prerenal, Renal, and Post-renal Acute Renal Failure (ARF)

Prerenal ARF	Renal ARF	Post-renal ARF
Hypovolemia (hemorrhage, dehydration, burns)	Small vessel/glomerular damage (vasculitis—often immune-mediated, acute glomerulonephritis, malignant hypertension)	Abrupt obstruction of both ureters (secondary to large stones, blood clots, tumor)
Cardiac failure (myocardial infarction, congestive heart failure, valvular disease)	Tubular cell damage (acute tubular necrosis—either ischemic or secondary to toxins)	Abrupt obstruction of the bladder neck (secondary to benign prostatic hypertrophy, stones, tumor, clots)
Cardiovascular collapse (shock, sepsis)	Interstitial damage (acute pyelonephritis, acute allergic interstitial reactions)	Abrupt obstruction of the urethra (secondary to inflammation, infection, stones, foreign body)
Renal vascular anomalies (renal artery stenosis, thrombosis, embolism of renal vein)		

Note: ARF secondary to transplant rejection is considered an immune-mediated form of renal ARF.

Tubular cell death, or **acute tubular necrosis,** can follow prerenal ARF or can develop directly due to toxin deposition. Along with heavy metals and miscellaneous inorganic and organic compounds, a number of medications (including some antibiotics and cisplatin, an anticancer agent) can cause acute tubular necrosis.

acute tubular necrosis *a particular syndrome characterized by the sudden death of tubular cells.*

Interstitial nephritis, a chronic inflammatory process also commonly due to toxic compounds including drugs (antibiotics, nonsteroidal anti-inflammatory drugs, diuretics), can also result in renal ARF.

interstitial nephritis *an inflammation within the tissue surrounding the nephrons.*

Post-renal ARF

The third form of ARF, **post-renal acute renal failure,** originates in a structure distal to the kidney—the ureters, bladder, or urethra. In its earliest phase (before urine has backed up into the kidneys, shutting down further urine formation), post-renal ARF is reversible simply by removing the obstruction that is preventing elimination of urine. Urinary tract obstruction causes fewer than 5 percent of ARF cases, but like prerenal ARF, it is important to identify because the odds of reversal are good. If obstruction is not cleared, renal ARF may develop secondary to nephron and interstitial injury caused by renovascular obstruction.

post-renal acute renal failure *ARF due to obstruction distal to the kidney.*

Because both ureters must be blocked simultaneously for post-renal ARF to develop (assuming two kidneys are present), it is probably the least likely cause of the cases you will see. Far more common will be obstruction of the bladder neck or of the urethra.

Regardless of probable cause, treat ARF aggressively in the field so the patient will have the best chance for recovery.

Assessment

The focused history will often provide clues to the severity and duration of ARF. For instance, if the patient complains of inability to void for a number of hours associated with a feeling of painful bladder fullness, the cause may simply be acute obstruction at the bladder neck or urethra. In contrast, a patient with poor mentation may be unable to give a coherent history, and a family member will tell you that the patient has felt increasingly ill for several days and has not urinated at all within the past 12 hours or so. Questions likely to provide useful information include the following:

- ★ *When was the decrease or absence of urine first noticed, and has there been any observed change in output since the problem was first noted?* What was the patient's previous output? The last question may be useful because patients with chronic renal failure due to inadequate renal function can develop ARF as a complication.
- ★ *Has the patient noted development of edema (swelling) in the face, hands, feet, or torso? How about feelings of heart palpitations or irregular rhythm?* Has a family member or friend noticed decreased mental function, lethargy, or overt coma? If the patient continued to consume fluids after ARF developed, retention of water and Na^+ can lead to visible edema in a relatively short time. Retention of K^+ can lead to hyperkalemia, a condition that can be lethal, especially in a person with previously compromised heart function. Increasingly poor mentation can be a sign of metabolic acidosis.

The focused physical examination may be helpful in assessing the degree of ARF present, the antecedent condition, and any immediate threats to life. Impaired mentation or clear decreases in consciousness in a person with previously good mental function suggest severe ARF and a potential threat to life. In a patient without evidence of shock, cardiovascular findings may include hypertension due to fluid retention, tachycardia, and ECG evidence of hyperkalemia (Figure 33-1 ■). If shock triggered the ARF or has developed more recently, profound hypotension may be present, accompanied by tachycardia and hyperkalemia.

Impaired mentation or clear decreases in consciousness in a person with previously good mental function suggest severe ARF and a potential threat to life.

General visual inspection will usually show pale, cool, moist skin; if shock is not present, these findings may still represent homeostatic shunting of blood to the internal organs, including the kidneys. Look for edema in the face, hands, and feet (Figure 33-2 ■). Examination of the abdomen will reveal very different findings dependent on the cause of ARF. As with any abdominal complaint, look for scars, ecchymosis, and distention. If the abdomen is distended, note whether the swelling is symmetric. Palpate for pulsing masses, which may indicate an abdominal aortic aneurysm. Auscultation is rarely helpful in renal and urological emergencies, and bowel sounds may be muffled if

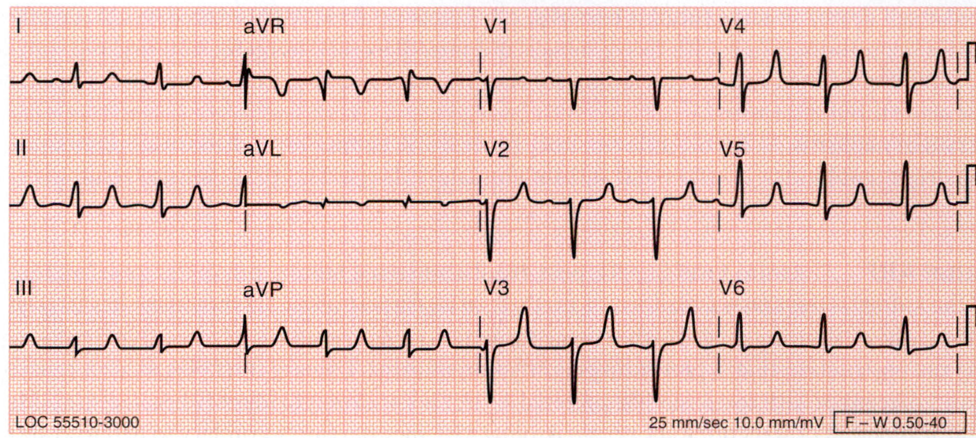

■ **Figure 33-1** ECG with signs of hyperkalemia.

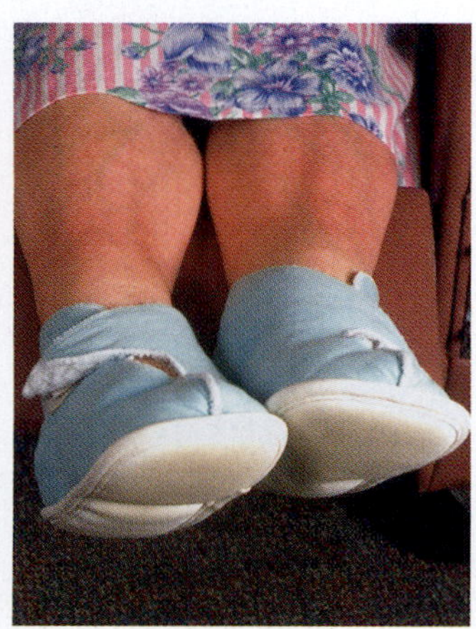

■ **Figure 33-2** Edema of the feet consistent with fluid retention in acute renal failure.

ascites (fluid within the abdomen) is present. Percussion and palpation findings will depend on the trigger condition.

A hematocrit may be useful if either acute hemorrhage or chronic anemia is suspected (the latter common in patients with cancer or chronic renal failure). Urinalysis can offer useful information very quickly. Proteinuria and glycosuria (urinary protein and glucose, respectively) suggest renal dysfunction. In some infections, notably pyelonephritis, the urine may contain so many white blood cells that they form a visible sediment in the specimen.

Renal function is clinically evaluated by laboratory analysis of the blood. Two frequently used indicators of renal function are the blood urea nitrogen (BUN) level and the serum creatinine. An elevation in either of these two values points toward renal insufficiency or failure. Usually, the ratio of BUN to creatinine (BUN/creatinine ratio) should be less than 20. A BUN/creatinine ratio greater than 20 indicates prerenal or post-renal problems, while a BUN/creatinine ratio of less than 20 indicates a renal problem.

Management

Because ARF can lead to life-threatening metabolic derangements, monitoring and supporting the ABCs is vital.

Because ARF can lead to life-threatening metabolic derangements, monitoring and supporting the ABCs is vital. Use high-flow, high-concentration oxygen to maximize breathing efficiency; couple this with circulatory supports such as positioning with head down and legs up to assist blood flow to the brain and internal organs and IV fluid resuscitation (bolus followed by drip) if hypovolemia is present. Patients who undergo peritoneal dialysis may benefit from fluid lavage of the abdomen; consult with medical direction to see if this is an option. Monitor ECG readings closely and adjust supports per local protocol or discussion with medical direction.

The chief prevention strategies are protecting fluid volume and cardiovascular function, as indicated by some of the steps previously noted, and eliminating or reducing exposure to any nephrotoxic agents or medications. If you are unsure whether an antibiotic, analgesic, or other drug is nephrotoxic and you are not in a position to check, discontinue the medication until the patient is at the appropriate care facility.

During transportation, be sure to talk quietly to the patient, both to calm him and to keep him informed of time until arrival or other pertinent matters. As always, your actions should reflect caring competence. Even if the patient is confused or comatose, you should still address him respectfully as you perform procedures and avoid saying anything you do not want him to hear.

CHRONIC RENAL FAILURE

chronic renal failure (CRF) *permanently inadequate renal function due to nephron loss.*

end-stage renal failure *an extreme failure of kidney function due to nephron loss.*

Chronic renal failure (CRF) is inadequate kidney function due to permanent loss of nephrons. Usually, at least 70 percent of the nephrons (healthy norm, 1 million per kidney) must be lost before significant clinical problems develop and the diagnosis is made. Metabolic instability does not occur until about 80 percent or more of nephrons are destroyed. When this point of dysfunction is reached, an individual is said to have developed **end-stage renal failure,** and must have either dialysis or a kidney transplant to survive. Anuria is not necessarily present in either CRF or end-stage renal failure.

Together, diabetes mellitus and hypertension cause more than half of all cases of end-stage renal failure. The death toll from CRF is high: More than 250,000 Americans have end-stage renal failure, and more than 50,000 die yearly from kidney disease. Roughly 30,000 new cases of CRF are diagnosed each year. The number of donor kidneys available in recent years has been sufficient for only about one third of the persons on the waiting list to receive a kidney.

Pathophysiology

The three pathologic processes that initiate the nephron damage of CRF are the same as those underlying renal ARF: microangiopathy or glomerular capillary injury, tubular cell injury, and inflammation or infection in interstitial tissue (Table 33–2). Although the cause of initial nephron destruction is different for each of the three pathological processes, the same cycle of ongoing nephron damage becomes established: Functional nephrons adapt by increasing glomerular filtration primarily (through decreased vascular resistance in glomerular vessels and hypertrophy of capillary vessels) and by increasing tubular reabsorption and secretion secondarily (through cellular hypertrophy and functional adaptation of tubular cells). After a time, the compensatory changes damage these nephrons, leading to their destruction and initiating adaptive changes in additional, functional nephrons. Most of the damage seems to affect the glomeruli. Under the microscope, surviving nephrons often show dilated, abnormal glomeruli, and nonfunctional nephrons have heavily scarred glomeruli or no visible glomeruli, only sclerotic tissue.

This characteristic loss of nephrons, or **reduced nephron mass,** is also visible at the level of gross anatomy as shrunken, scarred kidneys, or **reduced renal mass.** Physiologically, each of the kidney's four major functions is highly disturbed or absent, depending on the degree of renal failure:

reduced nephron mass *the decrease in number of functional nephrons that causes chronic renal failure.*

reduced renal mass *the decrease in kidney size associated with chronic renal failure.*

isosthenuria *the inability to concentrate or dilute urine relative to the osmolarity of blood.*

- ★ *Maintenance of blood volume with proper balance of water, electrolytes, and pH.* In CRF, active transport in the tubules decreases significantly or ceases. Filtrate simply passes through the tubules, leading to characteristic **isosthenuria,** the inability to concentrate or dilute urine. As overall GFR falls over time, retention of Na^+ and water increases, causing a high-volume stress on the cardiovascular system. Retention of K^+ can lead to dangerous hyperkalemia, and retention of H^+ can lead to equally dangerous metabolic acidosis. Hypocalcemia is also common. It results from several causes, including renal retention of phosphate ions (with higher levels of serum phosphate facilitating Ca^{++} absorption into bone) and lack of renal production of vitamin D.
- ★ *Retention of key compounds such as glucose with excretion of wastes such as urea.* Glucose and other substances that normally are actively reabsorbed are also lost in urine as filtrate flows passively through the nephron. Any hypoglycemic effect is overshadowed, however, by the significant hyperglycemic effect (**glucose intolerance**) in most patients due to cellular resistance to insulin. The wastes urea and creatinine accumulate in blood almost in direct proportion to the number of nephrons lost. In fact, the general syndrome of signs and symptoms caused by severe CRF is termed **uremia,** for this characteristic buildup of blood urea.

glucose intolerance *the body cells' inability to take up glucose from the bloodstream.*

uremia *the syndrome of signs and symptoms associated with chronic renal failure.*

Table 33–2 Causes of Chronic Renal Failure

Type of Tissue Injury	Examples
Microangiopathy, glomerular injury	Systemic hypertension, diabetes mellitus, atherosclerosis, glomerulonephritis, systemic lupus erythematosus
Tubular cell injury	Nephrotoxins including analgesics and heavy metals, stones, obstruction at bladder neck or urethra
Interstitial injury	Infections including pyelonephritis, tuberculosis

Note: Congenital disorders resulting in CRF include polycystic disease and renal hypoplasia.

★ *Control of arterial blood pressure.* The renin-angiotensin loop is disrupted; even small amounts of renin can lead to severe hypertension. Hypertension may also develop due to retention of Na^+ and water. Cardiac decompensation, with hypotension and tachycardia, can develop suddenly, especially if cardiac function has been independently impaired.

★ *Regulation of erythrocyte development.* Because erythropoietin is no longer produced in normal quantities (or at all, in some end-stage patients), chronic anemia develops. Anemia is another cardiac stressor, and it can contribute to cardiac failure.

Always be alert for shock or other major physiologic instability when dealing with CRF or end-stage disease, even when the patient initially appears stable.

Assessment

During the focused history and physical exam, you will probably find many characteristics of uremia in patients with CRF and end-stage disease. Table 33–3 lists some of these signs and symptoms, which affect nearly every organ system. Many of the listed problems can precipitate shock or other major physiologic instability; this is one reason you must always be alert when dealing with patients

Table 33–3 Common Elements of Uremic Syndrome

System	Pathophysiology	Clinical Sign/Symptom
Fluid/Electrolyte	$Water/Na^+$ retention	Edema, arterial hypertension[1]
	K^+ retention	Hyperkalemia[1]
	H^+ retention	Metabolic acidosis
	HPO_4 retention	Hyperphosphatemia/hypocalcemia[1]
Cardiovascular/Pulmonary	Fluid volume overload	Ascites, pulmonary edema
	Arterial hypertension	Congestive heart failure, accelerated atherosclerosis
	Dysfunctional fat metabolism; retention urea, other wastes	Pericarditis
Neuromuscular		
Central Nervous System	Retention urea, other wastes	Headache, sleep disorders, impaired mentation, lethargy, coma, seizures
Skeletal Muscle	Retention urea, other wastes; hypocalcemia	Muscular irritability and cramps, muscle twitching
Gastrointestinal (GI)	Retention urea, other wastes	Anorexia, nausea, vomiting
	Impaired hemostasis	Peptic ulcer, GI bleeding
Endocrine-Metabolic	Low vitamin D, other factors	Osteodystrophy
	Cellular resistance to insulin	Glucose intolerance
	Mechanisms unclear	Poor growth and development, delayed sexual maturation[2]
Dermatologic	Chronic anemia	Pallor skin, mucous membranes
	Retention urea, pigments	Jaundice, uremic frost
	Clotting disorders	Ecchymoses, easy bleeding
	Secondary hyperparathyroidism	Pruritus, scratches
Hematologic	Lack of renal erythropoietin	Chronic anemia
	Impaired platelet function and prothrombin consumption	Impaired hemostasis, with easy bleeding, bruising; splenomegaly
Immunologic	Lymphopenia, general leukopenia	Vulnerability to infection

[1]Although relatively uncommon, fluctuations to the other extreme (example, hypokalemia) may occur if oral intake is poor over prolonged period or during or after dialysis treatment.

[2]Primarily seen in children, adolescents, young adults.

with CRF or end-stage disease, even when they initially appear stable. In addition, this list is by no means exhaustive. Kidney failure affects almost every organ and major function in the body.

The focused history will typically show GI symptoms such as anorexia and nausea, sometimes with vomiting. The patient's mentation as he speaks is an important clue to CNS impairment. Signs may be as subtle as anxiety or mood swings or as immediately serious as seizures or coma.

Your general impression before the focused physical exam is likely to note marked abnormalities. Skin will typically be pale, moist, and cool. Scratches and ecchymoses are common skin changes associated with CRF. Mucous membranes may also be very pale, dependent on the degree of anemia. Jaundice may be present, dependent on the degree of retention of urea and other pigmented metabolic wastes. A skin condition called uremic frost appears when excessive amounts of urea are eliminated through sweat. As the sweat dries, a white "frosty" dust of urea may appear on the skin.

The major organ systems often show significant abnormalities on direct examination (Table 33–3). Because of the failure of vital urinary system functions, cardiovascular stress can be enormous. Either hypertension or hypotension may occur, dependent on the degree of fluid retention (retention detectable as peripheral edema or pulmonary edema) and the level of cardiac function; tachycardia is common with both presentations. ECG findings may include a dysrhythmia secondary to hyperkalemia. Metabolic acidosis, when present, compounds the effects of hyperkalemia. Pericarditis is also common, and a rub may be heard on chest auscultation. Neuromuscular abnormalities, in addition to impaired mentation, include muscle cramps and "restless legs syndrome," as well as muscle twitching or tonic-clonic or other forms of seizure.

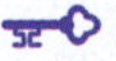

In CRF emergencies, the challenge is to separate chronic findings from those of recent onset or those aggravated by the emergency that led to your call.

Your abdominal exam will reveal many abnormalities. The challenge is to begin separating (by exam and history) chronic findings from those of recent onset or aggravated by the emergency that led to your call. For instance, you know that ecchymoses on the abdomen or flank may suggest acute hemorrhage. You may find a patient with ecchymoses scattered over the body surface. Look for evidence of new abdominal ecchymoses versus older bruises or a clear history of recent onset as signs of a current problem. Be sure to note abdominal contour, including the presence of symmetric distention or localized bulges, scars, and ecchymoses, before the exam and to clearly document the pre-exam appearance. Findings on auscultation, percussion, and palpation will depend on the presenting problem.

The hematocrit and urinalysis generally have less value in CRF than in ARF. A hematocrit is useful only if you know the patient's baseline value, and recent changes in the amount of urinary output may be more significant than the content. The exceptions are blood (red blood cells) in urine, which is always a significant finding on dipstick analysis, and visible amounts of white blood cells, which suggest significant infection.

Management

Immediate Management As with ARF, CRF can lead to life-threatening complications, so monitoring and supporting the ABCs is vital. Use high-flow, high-concentration oxygen to maximize breathing efficiency. Couple this with circulatory supports such as positioning with the head down and the legs up to support blood flow to the brain and internal organs. Consider a small IV bolus for fluid resuscitation if hypovolemia is evident. Indications for fluid lavage (in peritoneal dialysis patients) are the same as those for patients with ARF. Monitor the ECG readings closely and adjust supports according to your local protocol or discussion with medical direction.

The chief prevention strategies are regulation of fluid volume and cardiovascular function and major electrolyte disturbances (for example, use of a vasopressor in hypotension and administration of bicarbonate for partial correction of acidosis, respectively) and elimination or reduction of exposure to any nephrotoxic agents or medications. Although uncommon, severe swings in electrolyte levels may occur during and after dialysis, so be cautious about replacement measures in the field in these patients. Err on the side of conservative treatment except for clearly life-threatening complications. If you are unsure whether a drug is nephrotoxic and you are not in a position to check, discontinue it until the patient is at the emergency department.

In CRF, err on the side of conservative treatment except for clearly life-threatening complications.

Expedite transportation to an appropriate facility in the same manner appropriate for patients with ARF. Be sure to talk quietly to the patient, both to calm him and to keep him informed of the time until arrival or other pertinent matters. If the patient is confused, ask short orientation questions periodically to assess lucidity and level of consciousness.

renal dialysis *artificial replacement of some critical kidney functions.*

Content Review

Types of Dialysis

- Hemodialysis
- Peritoneal dialysis

dialysate *the solution used in dialysis that is hypoosmolar to many of the wastes and key electrolytes in blood.*

hemodialysis *a dialysis procedure relying on vascular access to the blood and on an artificial membrane.*

Long-Term Management Renal dialysis, the artificial replacement of some of the kidney's most critical functions, is a fact of life for most patients with CRF and end-stage disease. Although dialysis is necessary for survival, it is not without risk. One risk that you have already learned about is the possibility of physiologically destabilizing shifts in blood volume, blood composition, and arterial blood pressure.

Dialysis was first developed about 30 years ago. Since then, two different technologies, hemodialysis and peritoneal dialysis, have been refined. Both rely on the same physiologic principles: osmosis and equalization of osmolarity across a semipermeable membrane such as that of the renal nephron. (You may wish to reread the explanation of osmosis in this chapter's physiology section before reading further.) In dialysis, the patient's blood flows past a semipermeable membrane that has a special cleansing fluid on the other side that is hypoosmolar to blood for a number of impurities (such as urea, creatinine) and critical substances (such as Na^+, K^+, H^+). As the blood flows over the membrane, these substances in blood move into the hypoosmolar solution, called the **dialysate,** and their concentrations in blood are thus reduced. The effect of dialysis is to temporarily lessen or eliminate volume overload and toxically high blood concentrations of electrolytes, urea, and other substances.

In **hemodialysis** (*hemo*=blood, *dia*=across, *lysis*=separation), the patient's blood is passed through a machine that contains an artificial membrane and the dialysate solution. Vascular access is required to achieve the necessary blood flow of 300 to 400 mL/minute. Often, a superficial, internal fistula is created surgically by anastamosing an artery and vein in the lower forearm. If the required healthy artery and vein are not available, surgeons can insert a special vascular graft made of artificial material between an artery and vein (Figure 33-3 ■). If creating such a fistula is not possible, an indwelling catheter may need to be placed in the internal jugular vein. Because hemodialysis can be performed in settings including outpatient clinics and at home, you may see patients both between and during hemodialysis sessions. The three most common complications relate to vascular access. Two of the three complications are bleeding from the needle puncture site and local infection. The third is the narrowing or closing of the internal fistula. Under normal flow conditions, the internal fistula will have a palpable thrill (vibration), or bruit, due to the relatively high-volume turbulent flow from artery into vein. If the fistula narrows significantly or closes, however, this vibration is lost. The leading complications that require hospitalization are thrombosis, infection, and aneurysm development. They are particularly common in patients with grafts of artificial material.

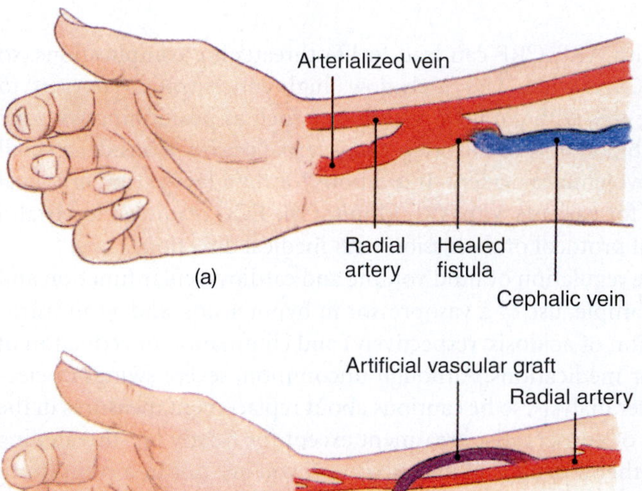

■ **Figure 33-3** Vascular access for hemodialysis: (a) arteriovenous fistula; (b) artificial graft between artery and vein.

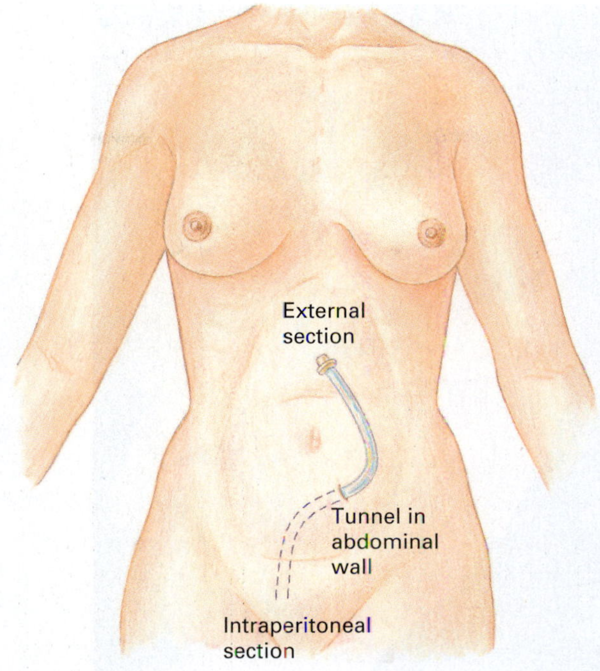

■ **Figure 33-4** Peritoneal dialysis.

Peritoneal dialysis uses the peritoneal membrane within the patient's abdomen as the semipermeable dialysis membrane, and dialysate solution is introduced and removed from the abdominal cavity via an indwelling catheter (Figure 33-4 ■). This simpler technique, which used to be significantly less effective than hemodialysis, has been improved greatly in recent years. Currently, many patients practice either chronic peritoneal lavage (intermittent cycles in which dialysate is introduced, allowed to remain for an extended period, and then removed) or continuous peritoneal lavage (in which dialysate is introduced via a closed system that allows the patient to remain ambulatory during dialysis). Peritoneal dialysis avoids some of the risk of fluid and electrolyte shifts seen during hemodialysis, but its success requires additional physical characteristics (such as healthy vasculature around the peritoneum). The most common complication is infection in the catheter, the abdominal tunnel containing the catheter, or the peritoneum itself. The incidence of peritonitis is about one episode per year, so you may find its signs in these patients.

peritoneal dialysis *a dialysis procedure relying on the peritoneal membrane as the semipermeable membrane.*

Both forms of dialysis have complications not related to vascular access in common. They include hypotension, shortness of breath, chest pain, and neurologic abnormalities ranging from headache to seizure or coma. If the patient is hypotensive, check for dehydration, hemorrhage, or infection. Shortness of breath and chest pain may reflect cardiac dysrhythmias (often secondary to hyperkalemia) or may be without identifiable cause. Be aware that these patients, many of whom have cardiac compromise, are at higher risk for ischemia or MI during these periods. Neurologic abnormalities may occur before, during, or after treatment. In most cases they represent neurotoxicity of accumulated blood urea; in some cases rapid removal of urea from blood causes an osmotic diuresis from brain tissue with a resulting increase in intracranial pressure. Benzodiazepines may be useful in patients who develop seizures.

RENAL CALCULI

Kidney stones, or **renal calculi** (singular, *calculus*), represent crystal aggregation in the kidney's collecting system (Figure 33-5 ■). This condition is also called nephrolithiasis (from Greek *lithos*, stone). Kidney stones affect about 500,000 persons each year. Brief hospitalization is common due to the severity of pain as a stone travels from the renal pelvis, through the ureter, to the bladder, and is eliminated in urine. If necessary, additional inpatient treatment may include shockwave lithotripsy, a procedure that uses sound waves to break large stones into smaller ones. Overall morbidity and mortality are low, however, unless a complication such as hemorrhage or urinary tract

renal calculi *kidney stones.*

Kidney stones occur more frequently in summer and fall.

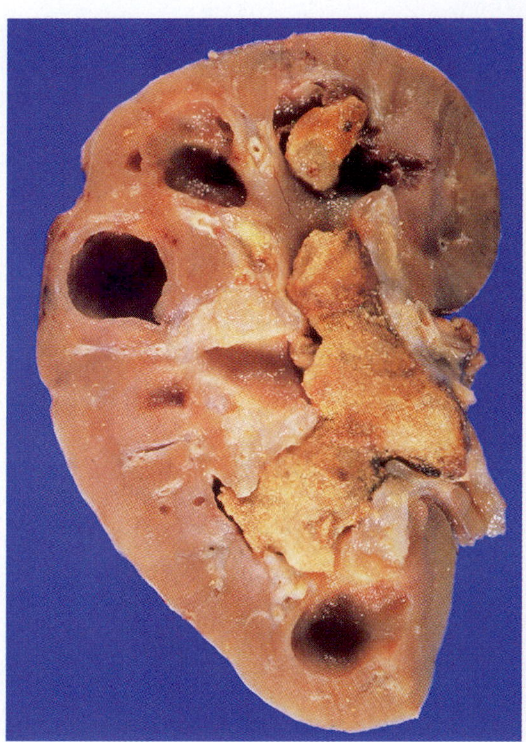

■ **Figure 33-5** Sectioned kidney with kidney stones. *(© SIU/Photo Researchers, Inc.)*

obstruction results. Stones form more commonly in men than women, although the ratio varies for types of stones with different compositions. Certain stones also occur in familial patterns, suggesting hereditary factors. Another risk factor for calculus formation is immobilization due to surgery or injury, with the latter including immobilization secondary to paraplegia or other paralysis syndromes that involve the absence of motor impulses, sensation, or both. Last, the use of certain medications, including anesthetics, opiates, and psychotropic drugs, increases the risk for stones.

Pathophysiology

Stones may form in metabolic disorders such as gout and primary hyperparathyroidism, which produce excessive amounts of uric acid and calcium, respectively. More often, they occur when the general balance between water conservation and dissolution of relatively insoluble substances such as mineral ions and uric acid is lost and excessive amounts of the insolubles aggregate into stones. The problem boils down to "too much insoluble stuff" and urine "too concentrated," a situation that may more likely arise with change in diet, climate, or physical activity.

Stones consisting of calcium salts (namely, calcium oxalate and calcium phosphate) are by far the most common. These compounds are found in 75 to 85 percent of all stones. Calcium stones are from two to three times more common in men than in women, and the average age at onset is between 20 and 30 years. Their formation frequently runs in families, and anyone who has had a calcium stone is at fairly high risk to form another within 2 to 3 years.

Struvite stones (chemically denoted $MgNH_4PO_4$) are also common, representing about 10 to 15 percent of all stones. The pathophysiology of struvite stones differs from that of calcium stones. Their formation is associated with chronic urinary tract infection (UTI) or frequent bladder catheterization. The association with bacterial UTI makes struvite stones much more common in women than in men. These stones can grow to fill the renal pelvis, producing a characteristic "staghorn" appearance on X-rays.

Far less common are stones made of uric acid or cystine. Uric acid stones form more often in men than in women and tend to occur in families; about half of all patients with uric acid stones have gout. Cystine stones are the least common. They are associated with excess levels of cystine in filtrate and are probably due at least in part to hereditary factors, as they often run in families.

Assessment

The focused history almost always centers on pain. (Kidney stones are generally conceded to be among the most painful of human medical conditions.) Typically, the patient first notes discomfort as a vague, visceral pain in one flank. Within 30 to 60 minutes it progresses to an extremely sharp pain that may remain in the flank or migrate downward and anteriorly toward the groin. Migrating pain indicates that the stone has passed into the lowest third of the ureter. Stones that lodge in the lowest part of the ureter, within the bladder wall, often cause characteristic bladder symptoms such as frequency during the day or during the night (nocturia), urgency, and painful urination. Because these latter three symptoms far more frequently suggest bladder infection, making the probable diagnosis may be difficult, particularly in women. Visible hematuria is not uncommon in urine specimens taken during passage of a stone. Fever, however, is not typical unless infection is present. When kidney stones are suspected, be sure to get the patient's personal medical history and family history, because both will often provide useful information.

When kidney stones are suspected, be sure to get the patient's personal medical history and family history.

The physical exam will almost always reveal someone who is very uncomfortable. The patient may be agitated or physically restless; walking sometimes reduces the pain. Vital signs will vary with level of discomfort, with highest blood pressure and heart rate associated with greatest pain. Skin will typically be pale, cool, and clammy. Abdominal examination may be difficult, depending on the patient's ability to remain still. First inspect the abdomen for contour and symmetry. Auscultation and percussion are generally useful only in ruling out GI conditions. Palpation results will vary and may depend, in part, on whether pain is so great that muscle guarding is present, making palpation of underlying structures impossible.

Many male patients with kidney stones present with testicular pain on the affected side.

Management

As always, management begins with the ABCs. Positioning should center on comfort, but be prepared for vomiting due to the severe pain, especially if the patient's last meal was within several hours. Consider analgesia en route to the hospital, according to your local protocol and your perception of the patient's condition. Use narcotics cautiously if a GI condition is at all possible or if mentation is impaired. If the pain is in the initial, intermittent, colicky phase, consider coaching pain management through breathing techniques similar to those used for women in labor. An IV line is useful for volume replacement or drug administration. The usual prevention strategy, if kidney function is adequate, is IV fluid to promote urine formation and movement through the system. Transport is the same as that for other abdominal conditions; that is, position of comfort and supportive care.

Parenteral narcotic analgesics or ketorolac (Toradol) should be considered for the patient with renal colic.

PRIAPISM

Priapism is a painful and prolonged erection of the penis. Priapism affects only the *corpora cavernosa.* The *corpora spongiosum* remains flaccid. Although in many instances the cause is unclear, priapism has been associated with certain disease processes. The most common cause of nontraumatic priapism is sickle cell disease, in which sickling of erythrocytes prevents normal venous drainage of the penis. Other causes of priapism include leukemia, multiple myeloma, tumors, spinal cord injury, spinal anesthesia, carbon monoxide poisoning, malaria, and black widow spider bites. Priapism has also been associated with use of the following drugs: psychotropic omeprazole, hydroxyzine, prazosin, calcium channel blockers, anticoagulants, cocaine, marijuana, ethanol, and MDMA (ecstasy). Some of the erectile dysfunction drugs, especially vardenafil (Levitra), have been associated with priapism.

priapism *a painful, prolonged erection of the penis.*

A priapism is a medical emergency and requires prompt intervention by a urologist to prevent permanent damage and penile dysfunction.

URINARY TRACT INFECTION

Urinary tract infection (UTI) affects the urethra, bladder, or kidney, as well as the prostate gland in men. UTIs are extremely common, accounting for over 6 million office visits yearly. Almost all UTIs start with pathogenic colonization of the bladder by bacteria that enter through the urethra. Thus,

urinary tract infection (UTI) *an infection, usually bacterial, at any site in the urinary tract.*

females in general are at higher risk because of their relatively short urethra. Other groups at risk for UTI are paraplegic patients or patients with nerve disruption to the bladder, including some diabetic persons. Any condition that promotes **urinary stasis** (incomplete urination with urine remaining in the bladder that may serve as nutrition for pathogens) places a person at higher risk. Pregnant women often have urinary stasis due to pressure from the gravid uterus. People with neurological impairment (some patients with spina bifida or with diabetic neuropathy, for example) also tend to have urinary stasis, which predisposes them to infection. The use of instrumentation in patients who require bladder catheterization places them at even higher risk of UTIs.

urinary stasis *a condition in which the bladder empties incompletely during urination.*

Morbidities such as scarring, abscesses, or eventual development of CRF are most likely in persons with anatomic abnormalities of the urinary system or chronic calculi (the latter acting as a focus for continuing infection and inflammation), those who are immunocompromised, or those who have renal disease due to diabetes mellitus or another condition.

Pathophysiology

UTIs are generally divided into those of the lower urinary tract, namely, urethritis (urethra), cystitis (bladder), and prostatitis (prostate gland), and those of the upper urinary tract, pyelonephritis (kidney).

Lower UTIs are far more common than upper UTIs, for two reasons. First, seeding of infection via the bloodstream is rare. Second, asymptomatic bacterial colonization of the urethra, especially in females, is very common, and can predispose a person to infection by other, pathogenic bacteria.

In females, infection may begin when gram-negative bacteria normally found in the bowel (that is, the enteric flora) colonize the urethra and bladder. Symptomatic **urethritis,** inflammation secondary to urethral infection, is very uncommon. More often you will see joint symptomatic infection of the urethra and bladder (urethritis and **cystitis,** respectively). Sexually active females are at higher risk, which may be attributed to use of contraceptive devices or agents, to the introduction of enteric flora during intercourse, or both. Recently, homosexually active men who engage in anal sex have also been found to be at higher risk for bacterial cystitis, possibly due to introduction of enteric bacterial flora during intercourse. In any case, sexually active persons who suffer from urinary stasis are at even higher risk for infection. Persons who urinate after intercourse might lower their risk because voiding eliminates some bacteria. The pathophysiology for persons using bladder catheterization probably differs only in that pathogenic bacteria are introduced directly into the bladder via the catheter. In general, the likelihood that active cystitis will develop, that antibiotic treatment will clear such infections, and that reinfection will occur are all determined by the interplay of the pathogen's virulence, the size of its colony, its sensitivity to antibiotic treatment, and the strength of the host's local and systemic immune functions.

urethritis *an infection and inflammation of the urethra.*

cystitis *an infection and inflammation of the urinary bladder.*

Prostatitis, inflammation of the prostate gland, in our context denotes inflammation secondary to bacterial infection, as well as any general inflammatory condition. Men with acute bacterial prostatitis, the closest parallel to acute cystitis in women, also tend to show evidence of joint urethritis, and the same bowel flora tend to be involved. The major difference between acute bacterial prostatitis and acute cystitis is the much lower incidence of prostatitis among men who do not require bladder catheterization.

prostatitis *infection and inflammation of the prostate gland.*

Upper UTIs usually evolve from infection that spreads upward into the kidney. **Pyelonephritis** is an infectious inflammation of the renal parenchyma: nephrons, interstitial tissue, or both. Acute pyelonephritis is 10 times more common in women than in men. Its incidence is highest in pregnancy and during periods of sexual activity, reflecting the epidemiology of lower UTIs. If the infection of pyelonephritis persists, intrarenal or perinephric abscesses may occur, but these complications are uncommon. **Intrarenal abscesses** form within the renal parenchyma. If they rupture and spill their contents into the adjacent fatty tissue, **perinephric abscesses** may result. From 20 to 60 percent of patients who develop perinephric abscesses have a clear predisposing factor such as renal calculi, anatomic abnormalities of the kidney, history of urologic surgery or injury, or diabetic renal disease.

pyelonephritis *an infection and inflammation of the kidney.*

intrarenal abscess *a pocket of infection within kidney tissue.*

perinephric abscess *a pocket of infection in the layer of fat surrounding the kidney.*

Urinary tract infections may be community acquired or nosocomial. Among **community-acquired infections,** gram-negative enteric bacteria predominate. In fact, *E. coli* accounts for roughly 80 percent of infections in persons without the complicating factors of bladder catheterization, renal calculi, or anatomic abnormalities. In **nosocomial infections,** cases acquired in an inpatient setting or related to catheterization, *Proteus, Klebsiella,* and *Pseudomonas* are commonly

community-acquired infection *an infection occurring in a nonhospitalized patient who is not undergoing regular medical procedures, including the use of instruments such as catheters.*

nosocomial infection *an infection acquired in a medical setting.*

identified. Less common, but still important, are sexually transmitted pathogens (among women and men) such as *Chlamydia* and *N. gonorrhoeae.* Fungi such as *Candida* are rarely seen except in catheterized or immunocompromised patients or patients with diabetes mellitus.

Assessment

The focused history of lower UTI typically centers on three symptoms: painful urination, frequent urge to urinate, and difficulty in beginning and continuing to void. Pain often begins as visceral discomfort that progresses to severe, burning pain, particularly during and just after urination. The evolution of pain corresponds roughly to the degree of epithelial damage caused by the pathogen. In both men and women, pain is often localized to the pelvis and perceived as in the bladder (in women) or bladder and prostate (in men). The patient may complain of a strong or foul odor in the urine. Many women will give a history of similar episodes, which may or may not have been diagnosed or treated. Patients with pyelonephritis are more likely to feel generally ill or feverish. They typically complain of constant, moderately severe or severe pain in a flank or lower back (just under the rib cage). Pain may be referred to the shoulder or neck. The triad of urgency, pain, and difficulty may or may not be present or included in the past history.

On physical exam, patients with UTI appear restless and uncomfortable. Typically, patients with pyelonephritis appear more ill and are far more likely to have a fever. Skin will often be pale, cool, and moist (in lower UTI) or warm and dry (in febrile upper UTI). Vital signs will vary with the degree of illness and pain, but in an otherwise healthy individual they should not be far from the norms. Inspect and auscultate the abdomen to document findings, but neither procedure is likely to be very useful, as visible appearance and bowel sounds are usually within normal limits. Percussion and palpation will probably reveal painful tenderness over the pubis in lower UTI and at the flank in upper UTI. Lloyd's sign, tenderness to percussion of the lower back at the costovertebral angle (CVA), indicates pyelonephritis.

The patient with acute pyelonephritis will usually appear quite ill. The patient with cystitis, however, will be uncomfortable but will not appear toxic.

Management

UTI management should center on the ABCs and circulatory support. If pain is severe, help the patient to a comfortable position, but consider the risk of aspiration during vomiting. Analgesics should be considered as with renal calculi; they will probably be needed only for severely painful cases of pyelonephritis. Consider nonpharmacological pain management with breathing and relaxation techniques. The best prevention technique is hydration to increase blood flow through the kidneys and to produce a more dilute urine. In many cases, this is better accomplished by IV administration, which eliminates the risk of vomiting and satisfies the guidelines for possible surgical cases. Expedite transport to an appropriate facility.

Summary

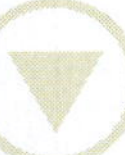

The urinary system (1) maintains blood volume and the proper balance of water, electrolytes, and pH; (2) enables the blood to retain key substances such as glucose and removes a variety of toxic wastes from the blood; (3) plays a major role in regulation of arterial blood pressure; and (4) controls maturation of red blood cells. Kidney nephrons produce urine. Homeostasis through urine production is responsible for the first two functions and assists in the third, regulating blood pressure, by producing renin, the enzyme through which blood pressure is controlled. Other kidney cells produce erythropoietin, the hormone that stimulates red blood cell maturation.

Renal and urologic emergencies typically present as an acute abdomen. The most common are acute renal failure (ARF), chronic renal failure (CRF, with the subset of end-stage renal disease), and renal calculi. Both ARF and CRF may present with life-threatening complications and impaired function of other systems. Be prepared for apparently stable patients to acutely develop destabilizing complications (often, cardiovascular). Urinary tract infections (UTIs) are divided into those of the lower urinary tract (urethra, bladder, and prostate in men) and those of the upper urinary tract (kidney). Both types of infection can present with considerable pain, but pyelonephritis is the more serious, with fever likely and complications including abscesses possible.

Because renal function is often lowered in the elderly and in persons with hypertension or diabetes, consider it potentially impaired in all of these patients. The best prevention strategies are to minimize the likelihood of prerenal failure by protecting blood volume and blood pressure and to investigate possible post-renal urinary tract obstruction.

Review Questions

1. ________ is the surgical specialty devoted to care of the entire urinary system in women and the genitourinary system in men.
   a. Urology
   b. Neurology
   c. Nephrology
   d. Renology
2. The general profiles of patients most at risk for significant problems affecting kidney function include:
   a. older patients.
   b. those with more than one risk factor.
   c. patients with diabetes or chronic hypertension.
   d. all of the above
3. A drop in urine output to 400–500 mL per day or less describes a condition called:
   a. anuria.
   b. oliguria.
   c. dysuria.
   d. polyuria.
4. "A chronic inflammatory process commonly due to toxic compounds, including drugs, can result in renal ARF" describes:
   a. cystitis.
   b. post-renal ARF.
   c. interstitial nephritis.
   d. chronic renal failure.
5. Relative to hemodialysis, the leading complications that require hospitalization are:
   a. infection.
   b. thrombosis.
   c. aneurysm development.
   d. all of the above
6. Kidney stones most commonly consist of:
   a. cystine.
   b. struvite.
   c. uric acid.
   d. calcium salts.
7. ________ is an infectious inflammation of the renal parenchyma: nephrons, interstitial tissue, or both.
   a. Cystitis
   b. Urethritis
   c. Pyelonephritis
   d. Prostatitis
8. Types of ARF include:
   a. renal.
   b. prerenal.
   c. post-renal.
   d. all of the above

See Answers to Review Questions at the back of this book.

Chapter 34

Toxicology and Substance Abuse

Objectives

After reading this chapter, you should be able to:

1. Describe the incidence, morbidity, and mortality of toxic and drug abuse emergencies. (p. 1351)
2. Identify the risk factors most predisposing to toxic emergencies. (p. 1351)
3. Discuss the anatomy and physiology of the organs and structures related to toxic emergencies. (pp. 1352–1353)
4. Describe the routes of entry of toxic substances into the body. (pp. 1352–1353)
5. Discuss the role of poison control centers in the United States. (p. 1351)
6. Discuss the pathophysiology, assessment findings, need for rapid intervention and transport, and management of toxic emergencies. (pp. 1350–1386)
7. List the most common poisonings, pathophysiology, assessment findings, and management of poisoning by ingestion, inhalation, absorption, injection, and overdose. (pp. 1352–1386)
8. Define the following terms:
   - **A.** Substance or drug abuse (p. 1380)
   - **B.** Substance or drug dependence (p. 1380)
   - **C.** Tolerance (p. 1380)
   - **D.** Withdrawal (p. 1380)
   - **E.** Addiction (p. 1380)
9. List the most commonly abused drugs (both by chemical name and by street names). (pp. 1381, 1382–1383)
10. Describe the pathophysiology, assessment findings, and management of commonly used drugs. (pp. 1380–1386)
11. List the clinical uses, street names, pharmacology, assessment findings, and management for patients who have taken the following drugs or been exposed to the following substances:
    - **A.** Cocaine (pp. 1361, 1381, 1382)
    - **B.** Marijuana and cannabis compounds (p. 1383)

C. Amphetamines and amphetamine-like drugs (pp. 1381, 1383)
D. Barbiturates (pp. 1381, 1382)
E. Sedative-hypnotics (p. 1383)
F. Cyanide (pp. 1359, 1362)
G. Narcotics/opiates (pp. 1361, 1381, 1382)
H. Cardiac medications (p. 1363)
I. Caustics (pp. 1363–1364)
J. Common household substances (pp. 1363–1364)
K. Drugs abused for sexual purposes/sexual gratification (p. 1381)
L. Carbon monoxide (pp. 1359, 1361, 1362–1363)
M. Alcohols (pp. 1361, 1381, 1382, 1383–1386)
N. Hydrocarbons (p. 1365)
O. Psychiatric medications (pp. 1365–1367)
P. Newer antidepressants and serotonin syndromes (pp. 1366–1367)
Q. Lithium (p. 1367)
R. MAO inhibitors (p. 1366)
S. Nonprescription pain medications: (1) nonsteroidal antiinflammatory agents; (2) salicylates; (3) acetaminophen (pp. 1368–1369)
T. Theophylline (p. 1369)
U. Metals (pp. 1361, 1369–1370)
V. Plants and mushrooms (pp. 1371–1372)

12. Discuss common causative agents or offending organisms, pharmacology, assessment findings, and management for a patient with food poisoning, a bite, or a sting. (pp. 1370–1371, 1373–1380)
13. Given several scenarios of poisoning or overdose, provide the appropriate assessment, treatment, and transport. (pp. 1350–1386)

Key Terms

acid, p. 1363
activated charcoal, p. 1354
addiction, p. 1380
alkali, p. 1363
antidote, p. 1355
decontamination, p. 1354
delirium tremens (DTs), p. 1386
drug overdose, p. 1380
enterotoxin, p. 1370
exotoxin, p. 1370
gastric lavage, p. 1354
ingestion, p. 1352
inhalation, p. 1352
injection, p. 1353
organophosphates, p. 1352
substance abuse, p. 1380
surface absorption, p. 1352
therapeutic index, p. 1365
tolerance, p. 1380
toxicology, p. 1350
toxidrome, p. 1359
toxin, p. 1350
whole bowel irrigation, p. 1355
withdrawal, p. 1380

INTRODUCTION

toxicology *study of the detection, chemistry, pharmacological actions, and antidotes of toxic substances.*

toxin *any chemical (drug, poison, or other) that causes adverse effects on an organism that is exposed to it.*

Toxicology is the study of **toxins** (drugs and poisons) and their antidotes, as well as their effects on living organisms. Toxicological emergencies result from the ingestion, inhalation, surface absorption, or injection of toxic substances that then exert their adverse effects on the body's tissues and metabolic mechanisms. Theoretically all toxicological emergencies can be classified as poisoning. However, in this discussion, the term *poisoning* will be used to describe exposure to nonpharmacological substances. The term *overdose* will be used to describe exposure to pharmacological substances, whether the overdose is accidental or intentional. Substance abuse, although technically a form of poisoning, will be addressed separately.

In this chapter we will discuss various aspects of toxicological emergencies as they apply to prehospital care. We will establish general treatment guidelines for each type of toxic exposure, then address the specific issues surrounding some of the more common substances involved. Because the field of toxicology is rapidly changing, it is virtually impossible for a paramedic to remain up-to-date on treatment guidelines for each type of toxic exposure. Specific treatment should be supervised by medical direction in association with a poison control center. This plan ensures that the patient receives the most current level of care available.

EPIDEMIOLOGY

Over the years, the occurrence of toxicological emergencies has continued to increase in number and severity. The following figures reveal the high potential for toxic substance involvement on an EMS call:

- ★ The American Association of Poison Control Centers estimates more than 4 million poisonings occur annually.
- ★ Ten percent of all emergency department visits and EMS responses involve toxic exposures.
- ★ Seventy percent of accidental poisonings occur in children under the age of 6 years.
- ★ A child who has experienced an accidental ingestion has a 25 percent chance of another, similar ingestion within 1 year.
- ★ Eighty percent of all attempted suicides involve a drug overdose.

Although more than half of all poisonings occur in children ages 1–5, they are generally accidental and relatively mild, accounting for only 10 percent of hospital admissions for poisoning and only 5 percent of the fatalities. EMS personnel must be aware that more serious poisonings, especially in children older than 5 years, may represent intentional poisoning by parents or caretakers. Unfortunately, poisoning due to drug experimentation and suicide attempts are also becoming a common consideration in older children.

Adult poisonings and overdoses, although less frequent, account for 90 percent of hospital admissions for toxic substance exposure. They also account for 95 percent of the fatalities in this category. Most adult poisonings and overdoses are intentional. Intentional poisonings and overdoses can be due to illicit drug use, alcohol abuse, attempted suicide, and "suicidal gesturing" in which the patient is making a cry for help but may miscalculate and take a type or amount of toxin that does actually cause injury. More rarely, intentional poisoning can result from attempted homicide or chemical warfare. Accidental poisonings are increasingly caused by exposure to chemicals and toxins on the farm or in the industrial workplace. More often they are the result of idiosyncratic (individual hypersensitivity) reactions or dosage errors when taking prescribed medications, but these usually do not require medical attention.

POISON CONTROL CENTERS

Poison control centers have been set up across the United States and Canada to assist in the treatment of poison victims and to provide information on new products and new treatment recommendations. They are usually based in major medical centers and teaching hospitals and serve a large population. Almost all poison control centers now have computer systems to rapidly access information.

Poison control centers are usually staffed by physicians, toxicologists, pharmacists, nurses, or paramedics with special training in toxicology. These experts provide information to callers 24 hours a day, 7 days a week. They update information regularly and offer the most current treatment guidelines.

Memorize the number of the nearest poison control center and access it routinely. There are several advantages to this. First, the poison control center can help you immediately determine potential toxicity based on the type of agent, amount and time of exposure, and physical condition of the patient. Second, the most current, definitive treatment can sometimes be started in the field. The poison control center also can notify the receiving hospital of current treatment and recommendations even before arrival of the patient.

Memorize the number of the nearest poison control center and access it routinely for information regarding a poisoning or overdose.

Review

Content

Routes of Toxic Exposure

- Ingestion
- Inhalation
- Surface absorption
- Injection

It is important to remember that toxic substances have both immediate and delayed effects.

ingestion *entry of a substance into the body through the gastrointestinal tract.*

inhalation *entry of a substance into the body through the respiratory tract.*

surface absorption *entry of a substance into the body directly through the skin or mucous membrane.*

organophosphates *phosphorus-containing organic chemicals.*

ROUTES OF TOXIC EXPOSURE

In order to have a destructive effect, poisons must gain entrance into the body. The four portals of entry are *ingestion, inhalation, surface absorption,* and *injection.* It is important to note that, regardless of the portal of entry, toxic substances have both immediate and delayed effects.

INGESTION

Ingestion is the most common route of entry for toxic exposure. Frequently ingested poisons include:

- ★ Household products
- ★ Petroleum-based agents (gasoline, paint)
- ★ Cleaning agents (alkalis and soaps)
- ★ Cosmetics
- ★ Drugs (prescription, nonprescription, illicit)
- ★ Plants
- ★ Foods

Immediate toxic effects of ingestion of corrosive substances, such as strong acids or alkalis, can involve burns to the lips, tongue, throat, and esophagus. Delayed effects result from absorption of the poison from the gastrointestinal tract. Most absorption occurs in the small intestine, with only a small amount being absorbed from the stomach. Some poisons may remain in the stomach for up to several hours, because the intake of a large bolus of poison can retard absorption. Aspirin ingestion is a classic example of this. When a patient ingests a large number of aspirin tablets, the tablets can bind together to form a large bolus that is difficult to remove or break down.

INHALATION

Inhalation of a poison results in rapid absorption of the toxic agent through the alveolar-capillary membrane in the lungs. Inhaled toxins can irritate pulmonary passages, causing extensive edema and destroying tissue. When these toxins are absorbed, wider systemic effects can occur. Causative agents can appear as gases, vapors, fumes, or aerosols. Common inhaled poisons include:

- ★ Toxic gases
- ★ Carbon monoxide
- ★ Ammonia
- ★ Chlorine
- ★ Freon
- ★ Toxic vapors, fumes, or aerosols
- ★ Carbon tetrachloride
- ★ Methyl chloride
- ★ Tear gas
- ★ Mustard gas
- ★ Nitrous oxide

SURFACE ABSORPTION

Surface absorption is the entry of a toxic substance through the skin or mucous membranes. This most frequently occurs from contact with poisonous plants such as poison ivy, poison sumac, and poison oak. Many toxic chemicals may also be absorbed through the skin. **Organophosphates,** often used as pesticides, are easily absorbed through dermal contact.

INJECTION

Injection of a toxic agent under the skin, into muscle, or into a blood vessel results in both immediate and delayed effects. The immediate reaction is usually localized to the site of the injection and appears as red, irritated, edematous skin. An allergic or anaphylactic reaction can also appear (see Chapter 31, "Allergies and Anaphylaxis"). Later, as the toxin is distributed throughout the body by the circulatory system, delayed systemic reactions can occur.

injection *entry of a substance into the body through a break in the skin.*

Other than intentional injection of illicit drugs, most poisonings by injection result from the bites and stings of insects and animals. Most insects that can sting and bite belong to the class *Hymenoptera*, which includes honeybees, hornets, yellow jackets, wasps, and fire ants. Only the females in this group can sting. In addition, spiders, ticks, and other arachnids, such as scorpions, are notorious for causing poisonings by injection. Higher animals that bite and sting include snakes and certain marine animals. Marine animals with venomous stings include jellyfish (especially the Portuguese man-of-war), stingrays, anemones, coral, hydras, and certain spiny fish.

GENERAL PRINCIPLES OF TOXICOLOGIC ASSESSMENT AND MANAGEMENT

Although specific protocols for managing toxicological emergencies may vary, certain basic principles apply to most situations. Keep in mind the importance of recognizing the poisoning promptly. Have a high index of suspicion if circumstances suggest involvement of a toxin in the emergency.

Review Content

Standard Toxicological Emergency Procedures

- Recognize a poisoning promptly (have a high index of suspicion).
- Assess the patient thoroughly to identify the toxin and measures required to control it.
- Initiate standard treatment procedures for all toxicological emergencies:
  - — Protect rescuer safety
  - — Remove patient from toxic environment
  - — Support ABCs
  - — Decontaminate patient
  - — Administer antidote if one exists

SCENE SIZE-UP

Always begin assessment with a thorough evaluation of the scene. Take note of where you are and who is around you. Be alert for any potential danger to you, the rescuer. Remember, despite your natural urge to immediately assess and treat the patient, if you are incapacitated you will not be able to help anyone and you will become a patient yourself. In toxicological emergencies there are specific hazards to keep in mind:

- ★ Patients who are suicidal may have the potential for violence. They are often intoxicated, may act irrationally, and will not always be cooperative or happy to see you. Therefore, look for signs of overdose such as empty pill bottles and used needles or other drug paraphernalia. Never put your hand blindly into a patient's pocket as it may contain used needles.
- ★ Chemical spills and hazardous material emergencies can quickly incapacitate any individuals who are nearby. Make sure you have the proper clothing and equipment needed for the particular emergency. Distribute this gear to rescuers who have been trained in their use.

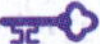

Rescuer safety takes particular priority during scene size-up for a toxicological emergency.

PRIMARY ASSESSMENT

After the scene size-up, perform the standard primary assessment. Form a general impression and quickly assess mental status. Assessment of the ABCs is critical in toxicological emergencies because airway and respiratory compromise are common complications. This can be due to direct airway injury, pulmonary injury, profuse secretions, or decreased respiratory effort secondary to altered mental status. After assessing the ABCs, set a transport priority for the patient.

SECONDARY ASSESSMENT AND REASSESSMENT

For responsive patients, start by obtaining a history. It is important to find out not only what toxin the patient was exposed to but when the exposure took place, since toxic effects develop over time. Then proceed to a focused physical exam with full vital signs. With unresponsive patients, start with a rapid head-to-toe exam. Be alert for signs of trauma inconsistent with the suspected intoxication.

It is important to find out not only what toxin the patient was exposed to but when the exposure took place, since toxic effects develop over time.

Then proceed to obtain a history from relatives or other bystanders. Relay this information to the local poison control center. The center will advise you on the most current protocol for treatment. Be aware of your local policy, which will outline whether you can initiate this protocol or whether you must first contact on-line medical direction. Never delay supportive measures or immediate transport to the hospital based on a delay in contacting or obtaining information from the poison control center.

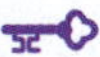

Never delay supportive measures or immediate transport based on a delay in contacting the poison control center.

A detailed physical exam can be performed en route if time and the patient's condition permit. Reassessment is essential for these patients. Poisoned patients can deteriorate suddenly and quickly. Repeat the primary assessment and vitals and reevaluate every 5 minutes for critical/unstable patients and every 15 minutes for stable patients.

TREATMENT

Decontamination

Once you have initiated supportive treatment (airway control, breathing assistance, and IV fluids), proceed to a mode of treatment that is specific to toxicological emergencies: decontamination. **Decontamination** is the process of minimizing toxicity by reducing the amount of toxin absorbed into the body. There are three steps to decontamination:

decontamination *the process of minimizing toxicity by reducing the amount of toxin absorbed into the body.*

Content Review

Principles of Decontamination

- Reduce intake
- Reduce absorption
- Enhance elimination

1. *Reduce intake of toxin.* This means that you must remove a person from an environment where he is inhaling toxic fumes, or you must properly remove a stinger and sac from someone stung by a bee. A classic example involves a person who has had organophosphates spilled on him. The patient's clothes must be removed and the skin cleaned with soap and water to reduce absorption of the toxins.
2. *Reduce absorption of toxin once in the body.* This usually applies to ingested toxins, which wait in the stomach and intestines while the body absorbs them into the bloodstream.

   In the past, syrup of ipecac was used to induce vomiting in order to empty the stomach. *Use of syrup of ipecac is no longer recommended except in rare cases.* These include the following:

   - ★ There is no contraindication to the use of ipecac syrup; and
   - ★ There is a significant risk of serious toxicity in the victim; and
   - ★ There is no alternative therapy available or effective to decrease gastrointestinal absorption (e.g., activated charcoal); and
   - ★ There will be a delay greater than 1 hour before the patient will arrive at the emergency department and ipecac syrup can be administered within 30–90 minutes of the ingestion; and
   - ★ Ipecac syrup administration will not adversely affect more definitive treatment that might be provided at a hospital.

   Gastric lavage ("pumping the stomach") has also been found to be of limited use. This process involves passing a tube into the stomach and repeatedly filling and emptying the stomach with water or saline in hopes of removing the ingested poison. Most studies have shown that gastric lavage removes almost no poisons from the stomach unless it is initiated within 1 hour of the ingestion. Possible complications, such as aspiration or perforation, make this procedure a risk without much benefit. Except in limited situations with ingestions of highly toxic substances that do not bind to charcoal and for which there is no antidote, gastric lavage has become an uncommon decontamination procedure.

   gastric lavage *removing an ingested poison by repeatedly filling and emptying the stomach with water or saline via a gastric tube; also known as "pumping the stomach."*

   The most effective and widely used method of reducing absorption of toxins is **activated charcoal.** Because of its extremely large surface area, it can adsorb, or bind, molecules from the offending toxin and prevent their absorption into the bloodstream.

   activated charcoal *a powder, usually premixed with water, that will adsorb (bind) some poisons and help prevent them from being absorbed by the body.*

3. *Enhance elimination of toxin.* Cathartics, such as sorbitol (often mixed with activated charcoal), increase gastric motility, thereby shortening the amount of time toxins stay in the gastrointestinal tract to be absorbed. Cathartics must be used cautiously, since there is controversy regarding their effectiveness. Cathartics should not be used in pediatric patients because of the potential to cause severe electrolyte derangements.

Table 34–1 Antidotes for Toxicological Emergencies

Toxin	Antidote	Adult Dosage (Pediatric Dosage)
Acetaminophen	N-Acetylcysteine	Initial: 140 mg/kg
Arsenic	*see* Mercury, Arsenic, Gold	
Atropine	Physostigmine	Initial: 0.5–2 mg IV
Benzodiazepines	Flumazenil	Initial: 0.2 mg q 1 min to total of 1–3 mg
Carbon monoxide	Oxygen	
Cyanide	Amyl nitrite	Inhale crushed pearl for 30 seconds, then oxygen for 30 seconds
	then sodium nitrite	10 mL of 3 percent sol'n over 3 min IV (Pediatric: 0.33 mL/kg)
	then sodium thiosulfate	50 mL of 25 percent sol'n over 10 min IV (Pediatric: 1.65 mL/kg)
Ethylene glycol	Fomepizole (or as methyl alcohol)	Initial: 15 mg/kg IV
Gold	*see* Mercury, Arsenic, Gold	
Iron	Defroxamine	Initial: 10–15 mg/kg/hr IV
Lead	Edetate calcium disodium	1 amp/250 mL $D_{50}W$ over 1 hr
	or Dimercaptosuccinic acid (DMSA)	250 mg PO
Mercury, Arsenic, Gold	BAL (British anti-Lewisite)	5 mg/kg IM
	DMSA	250 mg PO
Methyl alcohol	Ethyl alcohol +/− dialysis	1 mL/kg of 100 percent ethanol IV
Nitrates	Methylene blue	0.2 mL/kg of 1 percent sol'n IV over 5 min
Opiates	Naloxone	0.4–2.0 mg IV
Organophosphates	Atropine	Initial: 2–5 mg IV
	Pralidoxime (Protopam)	Initial: 1 g IV

Whole bowel irrigation is another method of enhancing elimination. Using a gastric tube, polyethylene glycol electrolyte solution is administered continuously at 1–2 L/hr until the rectal effluent is clear or objects recovered. This technique seems effective with few complications and is therefore gaining popularity. Its availability, however, is limited to a few centers.

whole bowel irrigation *administration of polyethylene glycol continuously at 1–2 L/hr through a nasogastric tube until the effluent is clear or objects are recovered.*

Antidotes

Finally, if indicated, the appropriate antidote should be administered. An **antidote** is a substance that will neutralize a specific toxin or counteract its effect on the body. There are not many antidotes (Table 34–1), and they will rarely be 100 percent effective. Most poisonings will not require the administration of an antidote.

antidote *a substance that will neutralize a specific toxin or counteract its effect on the body.*

The specific actions you take when dealing with toxicological emergencies will be dictated by consultation with medical direction, by protocols obtained from the poison control center, and by your local policy and procedures on initiating these protocols.

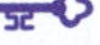

Specific actions in a toxicological emergency will be dictated by consultation with medical direction, protocols from the poison control center, and local policy on initiating these protocols.

SUICIDAL PATIENTS AND PROTECTIVE CUSTODY

Before leaving a suicidal patient who claims to have been "just kidding," consider the legal ramifications. You may be charged later with patient abandonment. At the same time, be aware of protective custody laws in your state. Always involve law enforcement personnel in these cases and involve them early. Only law enforcement personnel can place a patient in protective custody and ultimately consent to treatment.

Involve law enforcement early in any possible suicide case.

INGESTED TOXINS

Poisoning by ingestion is the most common route of poisoning you will encounter in prehospital care. It is essential to initiate the following principles of assessment and treatment promptly.

Assessment

It takes time for an ingested toxin to make its way from the gastrointestinal system into the circulatory system. Therefore, you need to find out not only what was ingested but when it was ingested. Following are some general guidelines for managing patients who have ingested toxins as well as information about specific substances.

History Begin your history by trying to find out the type of toxin ingested, the quantity of the toxin, the time elapsed since ingestion, and whether the patient took any alcohol or other potentiating substance. Also ask the patient about drug habituation or abuse and underlying medical illnesses and allergies. Remember that in cases of poisoning, inaccuracies creep into nearly half the histories because of drug-induced confusion, patient misinformation, or deliberate patient attempts at deception.

In cases of poisoning, histories are often unreliable because of drug-induced confusion, patient misinformation, or deliberate deception.

The following questions will help you to develop a relevant history:

- ★ What did you ingest? (Obtain pill containers and any remaining contents, samples of the ingested substance, or samples of vomitus. Bring them with the patient to the emergency department.)
- ★ When did you ingest the substance? (Time is critical for decisions regarding lab tests and the use of gastric lavage and/or antidotes.)
- ★ How much did you ingest?
- ★ Did you drink any alcohol?
- ★ Have you attempted to treat yourself (including inducing vomiting)?
- ★ Have you been under psychiatric care? If so, why? (Answers may indicate a potential for suicide.)
- ★ What is your weight?

Physical Examination Because the history can be unreliable, the physical examination is extremely important. It has two purposes: (1) to provide physical evidence of intoxication and (2) to find any underlying illnesses that may account for the patient's symptoms or that may affect the outcome of the poisoning. As you complete the primary assessment and rapid physical exam, pay attention to the following patient features:

- ★ *Skin.* Is there evidence of cyanosis, pallor, wasting, or needle marks? Flushing of the skin may indicate poisoning with an anticholinergic substance. Staining of the skin may occur from chronic exposure to mercuric chloride, bromine, or similar chemicals.
- ★ *Eyes.* Constriction or dilation of the pupils can occur with various types of poisons (e.g., marijuana, methamphetamines, narcotics). Ask about impaired vision, blurring of vision, or coloration of vision.
- ★ *Mouth.* Look for signs of caustic ingestion, presence of the gag reflex, the amount of salivation, any breath odor, or the presence of vomitus.
- ★ *Chest.* Breath sounds may reveal evidence of aspiration, atelectasis, or excessive pulmonary secretions.
- ★ *Circulation.* Cardiac examination may give clues as to the type of toxin ingested. For example, the presence of tachydysrhythmias (e.g., from methamphetamine) or bradydysrhythmias (e.g., from organophosphates) may suggest specific toxins.
- ★ *Abdomen.* Abdominal pain may result from poisoning by salicylates, methyl alcohol, caustics, or botulism toxin.

You can frequently expect to encounter patients who have ingested more than one toxin. This may be the result of a suicide attempt or of experimentation with illicit drugs. Such multiple ingestions present a diagnostic and therapeutic dilemma. Signs and symptoms may be inconsistent with a single diagnosis, and attempted treatment may produce unexpected results. A common example of this is the "speedball" (heroin mixed with cocaine). If the narcotic overdose is treated, the rescuer is often presented with a patient who is now in a cocaine-induced catecholamine crisis (tachycardia, hypertension, seizures). In such cases, or if you cannot identify what the patient has ingested, consult medical direction and/or the poison control center according to your local protocols.

Management

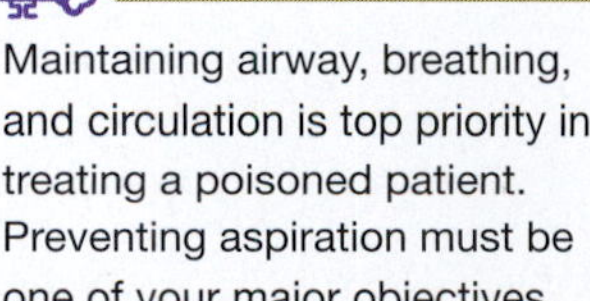
Maintaining airway, breathing, and circulation is top priority in treating a poisoned patient. Preventing aspiration must be one of your major objectives.

Prevent Aspiration As previously discussed, initiation of supportive measures (maintaining airway, breathing, and circulation) is top priority in the treatment of the poisoned patient. Aspiration is a frequent complication of poisoning, resulting from an altered level of consciousness and a decreased gag reflex. Preventing aspiration must be one of your major objectives. If insertion of an endotracheal tube is necessary, nasotracheal intubation is preferred in patients who have a gag reflex.

Poisoning is a situation where rapid-sequence intubation (RSI) may be required (see Chapter 8, "Airway Management and Ventilation"). It is not uncommon to encounter a patient with altered mental status who is vomiting. The prevention of aspiration is a primary concern, but attempts at endotracheal intubation fail because the patient will "clamp down" his teeth. In these situations, it is often prudent to use RSI to quickly control and maintain the airway. This is far superior to waiting for the patient to deteriorate to the point where an endotracheal tube can be placed without the aid of neuromuscular blockers. Remember, most poisoning patients will have compromised respiration or circulation, so routinely give high-flow, high-concentration oxygen.

Administer Fluids and Drugs Once you have ensured the ABCs, establish intravenous access. An IV of lactated Ringer's or normal saline at a to-keep-open rate is recommended for all potentially dangerous ingestions. In addition to volume replacement with a crystalloid solution, conduct cardiac monitoring and repeat assessments, including frequent monitoring of vital signs.

Many EMS systems still utilize an empiric therapeutic regimen for comatose patients consisting of $D_{50}W$, naloxone (Narcan), and thiamine (vitamin B_1). This so-called coma cocktail should not be used. Instead, treatment should be guided by objective patient information obtained on scene. If immediate determination of blood glucose levels is available (glucometer and chemstrips), withhold the administration of $D_{50}W$ until determination of hypoglycemia is made. If indicated, use 25–50 g of $D_{50}W$ IV push. If narcotic intoxication is suspected (respiratory depression or pinpoint pupils), give 1–2 mg of naloxone IV push. Naloxone reverses the effects of narcotic intoxication. If chronic alcoholism is suspected, consider administration of 100 mg of thiamine IV to address possible encephalopathy. Do not give these medications empirically!

Follow these supportive measures with the decontamination procedures outlined earlier. Often, decontamination is performed in the emergency department rather than on scene or during transport. This also applies to the use of most antidotes. There are exceptions, of course, and each case needs to be treated individually. Consult the poison control center and medical direction according to local protocols.

Do Not Induce Vomiting As mentioned earlier, induction of vomiting is no longer an accepted routine intervention for patients who have ingested toxins. It is still important to contact the poison control center about this, since, in rare cases of pediatric ingestion, induction of vomiting may play some role. However, for the overwhelming majority of cases, inducement of vomiting is not required and may even be contraindicated.

INHALED TOXINS

Toxic inhalations can be self-induced or the result of accidental exposure from such sources as house fires or industrial accidents. Commonly abused inhaled toxins include paint (and other hydrocarbons), Freon, propellants, glue, amyl nitrite, butyl nitrite, and nitrous oxide. The general guidelines for assessment and management of toxicological emergencies apply to inhaled toxins, but the following provides some specifics.

Assessment

Inhaled toxic substances produce signs and symptoms primarily in the respiratory system. These symptoms are particularly severe in patients who have inhaled chemicals and propellants concentrated in paper or plastic bags. Patients who inhale paint or propellants are often referred to as "huffers." Look for the presence of paint on the upper or lower lip. "Huffers," who report it to be more potent, often prefer gold paint. The presence of paint on the upper or lower lips should alert you to the possibility of inhalant abuse. The sniffing of paint, propellants, or hydrocarbons has become an epidemic problem in many developing countries. This is particularly true in the lower socioeconomic groups, most notably the legions of street children in Latin and South America. "Huffing" can lead to serious, irreversible brain damage. As the toxins are inhaled, oxygen is gradually displaced from the respiratory system, producing a relative hypoxia. Signs and symptoms of aerosol inhalation include:

- ★ *Central nervous system:* dizziness, headache, confusion, seizures, hallucinations, coma
- ★ *Respiratory:* tachypnea, cough, hoarseness, stridor, dyspnea, retractions, wheezing, chest pain or tightness, crackles, or rhonchi
- ★ *Cardiac:* dysrhythmias

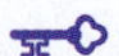

Your first priority in any inhalation emergency is personal safety, then removal of the patient from the toxic environment.

Management

Your first priority in the case of toxin inhalation is to remove the patient from the source as soon as it is safe to do so. Then follow these guidelines:

- ★ Safely remove the patient from the poisonous environment. In doing so, take the following essential precautions:
  - Wear protective clothing.
  - Use appropriate respiratory protection.
  - Remove the patient's contaminated clothing.
- ★ Perform the primary assessment, history, and physical exam.
- ★ Initiate supportive measures.
- ★ Contact the poison control center and medical direction according to your local protocols.

SURFACE-ABSORBED TOXINS

Many poisons, including organophosphates, cyanide, and other toxins, can be absorbed through the skin and mucous membranes.

Assessment and Management

Signs and symptoms of absorbed poisons can vary depending on the toxin involved. See the discussion of specific toxins in the sections that follow. When you suspect absorption of a toxin (especially cyanide or organophosphates), take the following steps:

Your first priority in any surface-absorbed poisoning emergency is personal safety, then removal of the patient from the toxic environment.

- ★ Safely remove the patient from the poisonous environment. It is essential that you follow these guidelines:
  - Wear protective clothing.
  - Use appropriate respiratory protection.
  - Remove the patient's contaminated clothing.
  - Perform the primary assessment, history, and physical exam.

- Initiate supportive measures.
- Contact the poison control center and medical direction according to your local protocols.

SPECIFIC TOXINS

To recognize and implement the proper procedure in a given poisoning, you must be familiar with the signs and symptoms that a particular toxin will trigger. Often, you may not be able to identify the exact toxin a patient has been exposed to, but usually a group of toxins will have similar manifestations and effects and will require similar interventions. Similar toxins with similar signs and symptoms are organized into **toxidromes** (toxic syndromes), which make remembering the details of their effects much simpler. Study the toxidromes listed in Table 34–2.

toxidrome *a toxic syndrome; a group of typical signs and symptoms consistently associated with exposure to a particular type of toxin.*

The following sections address specific toxins commonly encountered. While the standard toxicological emergency procedures, discussed earlier, apply to all of these toxins, pay close attention to variations in treatment. Variations include specific procedures you must perform in a particular case or a poisoning in which an antidote is available or immediately necessary. Management of injected toxins, drug overdose, and substance abuse will be covered later in the chapter.

CYANIDE

Cyanide can enter the body by a variety of routes. It is present in many commercial and household items that can be either ingested or absorbed—rodenticides, silver polish, and fruit pits and seeds (apricots, cherries, pears, and so on). It also can be inhaled, especially in fires that release cyanide from products containing nitrogen. A roomful of burning plastics, silks, or synthetic carpeting can also be a roomful of cyanide-filled smoke. Cyanide also forms in patients on long-term sodium nitroprusside therapy. Suicidal patients have been known to take cyanide salt. Regardless of the entry route, cyanide is an extremely fast-acting toxin. Once cyanide enters the body, it acts as a *cellular asphyxiant.* It inflicts its damage by inhibiting an enzyme vital to cellular use of oxygen.

Signs and Symptoms

Signs and symptoms of cyanide poisoning include:

- ★ Burning sensation in the mouth and throat
- ★ Headache, confusion, combative behavior
- ★ Hypertension and tachycardia followed by hypotension and further dysrhythmias
- ★ Seizures and coma
- ★ Pulmonary edema

Management

First safely remove the patient from the source of exposure. To prevent inhalation, always wear breathing equipment when entering the scene of a fire. Initiate supportive measures immediately. Follow this with the cyanide antidote kit (Figure 34-1 ■). This kit contains amyl nitrite ampules, a sodium nitrite, and a sodium thiosulfate solution. Adding nitrites to blood converts some hemoglobin to *methemoglobin,* which allows cyanide to bind to it. Thiosulfate then binds with the cyanide to form thiocyanate, a nontoxic substance readily excreted renally. Because cyanide is rapidly toxic, you must administer the cyanide antidote kit without delay. If your unit carries this kit, familiarize yourself with its contents and use.

CARBON MONOXIDE

Carbon monoxide (CO) is an odorless, tasteless gas that is often the by-product of incomplete combustion. Because of its chemical structure, it has more than 200 times the affinity of oxygen to bind with the red blood cell's hemoglobin (producing carboxyhemoglobin). Once this molecule has

Table 34–2 Toxic Syndromes

Toxidromes	Toxin			Signs and Symptoms
Anticholinergic	Belladonna alkaloids: Atropine (hyoscyamine)			Dry skin and mucous membranes
	Belladonna alkaloid mixtures: belladonna leaf, fluid extract, tincture			Thirst
	Homatropine			Dysphagia
	Methscopolamine			Vision blurred for near objects
	Methylatropine nitrate			Fixed dilated pupils
	Plants: *Atropa belladonna, Datura stramonium, Hyoscyamus niger, Amanita muscaria* or *pantherina*			Tachycardia
				Sometimes hypertension
	Scopolamine (I-hyoscine)			Rash, like scarlet fever
	Synthetic anticholinergics			Hyperthermia, flushing
	Adiphenine	Isopropamide	Pipenzolate	Urinary urgency and retention
	Anisotropine	Mepenzolate	Piperiodolate	Lethargy
	Cyclopentolate	Methantheline	Poldine	Confusion to restlessness, excitement
	Dicyclomine	Methixene	Propantheline	Delirium, hallucinations
	Diphemanil	Oxyphenonium	Thiphenamil	Ataxia
	Eucatropine	Oxyphencyclimine	Tridihexethyl	Seizures
	Glycopyrrolate	Pentapiperide	Tropicamide	Respiratory failure
	Hexocyclium			Cardiovascular collapse
	Incidental anticholinergics			
	Antihistamines	Benactyzine	Phenothiazines	
	Tricyclic antidepressants			
Acetylcholinesterase inhibition	Organophosphates			Sweating, constricted pupils, lacrimation, excessive salivation, wheezing, cramps, vomiting, diarrhea, tenesmus, bradycardia *or* tachycardia, hypotension *or* hypertension, blurred vision, urinary incontinence
	TEPP	Methylparathion		
	OMPA	Malathion		
	Dipterex	Systox		Striated muscle: cramps, weakness, twitching, paralysis, respiratory failure, cyanosis, arrest
	Chlorthion	EPN		
	Di-Syston	Diazinon		
	Co-ral	Guthion		Sympathetic ganglia: tachycardia, elevated blood pressure
	Phosdrin	Trithion		
	Parathion			CNS effects: anxiety, restlessness, ataxia, seizures, insomnia, coma, absent reflexes, Cheyne-Stokes respirations, respiratory and circulation depression
Cholinergic	Acetylcholine	Betel nut	Methacholine	Sweating, constricted pupils, lacrimation, excessive salivation, wheezing, cramps, vomiting, diarrhea, tenesmus, bradycardia *or* tachycardia, hypotension *or* hypertension, blurred vision, urinary incontinence
	Area catechu	Bethanechol	Muscarine	
	Carbachol	Pilocarpine		
	Clitocybe dealbata	*Pilocarpus species*		
Extrapyramidal	Acetophenazine	Mesoridazine	Thioridazine	Parkinsonian
	Butaperazine	Perphenazine	Thiothixene	Dysphagia, eye muscle spasm, rigidity, tremor, neck spasm, shrieking, jaw spasm, laryngospasm
	Carphenazine	Piperacetaxine	Trifluoperazine	
	Chlorpromazine	Promazine	Triflupromazine	
	Haloperidol			

Hemoglobinopathies	Carbon monoxide Methemoglobin			Headache, nausea, vomiting, dizziness, dyspnea, seizures, coma, death Cutaneous blisters, gastroenteritis Epidemic occurrence with carbon monoxide Cyanosis, chocolate blood with nonfunctional hemoglobin
Metal fume fever	Fumes of oxides of: Brass Cadmium Copper Zinc	Iron Magnesium Mercury	Nickel Titanium Tungsten	Chills, fever, nausea, vomiting, muscular pain, throat dryness, headache, fatigue, weakness, leukocytosis, respiratory disease
Narcotic	Alphaprodine Anileridine Codeine Cyclazocine Dextromethorphan Dextromoramide Diacetylmorphine Dihydrocodeine Dihydrocodeinone Dipipanone Diphenoxylate (Lomotil)	Ethylmorphine Ethoheptazine (meperidene metabolite) Fentanyl Heroin Hydromorphone Levorphanol Meperidine Methadone Metopon Morphine	Normeperidene Opium Oxycodone Oxymorphone Pentazocine Phenazocine Piminodine Propoxyphene Racemorphan	CNS depression Pinpoint pupils Slowed respirations Hypotension Response to naloxone Pupils may be dilated and excitement may predominate Normeperidine: tremor, CNS excitation, seizures
Sympathomimetic	Aminophylline Amphetamines Caffeine *Catha edulus* (Khat) Cocaehylene Cocaine Dopamine	Ephedrine Epinephrine Fenfluramine Levarterenol Metaraminol Methamphetamine Methcathinone	Methylphenidate (Ritalin) Pemoline Phencyclidine Phenmetrazine Phentermine	CNS excitation, seizures Hypertension Hypotension with caffeine Tachycardia
Withdrawal	Alcohol Barbiturates Benzodiazepines Chloral hydrate	Cocaine Ethchlorvynol Glutethimide Meprobamate	Methaqualone Methyprylon Opioids Paraldehyde	Diarrhea, large pupils, piloerection, hypertension, tachycardia, insomnia, lacrimation, muscle cramps, restlessness, yawning, hallucinations Depression with cocaine

Adapted from Done, A.K. *Poisoning—A Systematic Approach for the Emergency Department Physician.* Presented Aug. 6–9, 1979, at Snowmass Village, CO, Symposium sponsored by Rocky Mountain Poison Center. Used by permission.

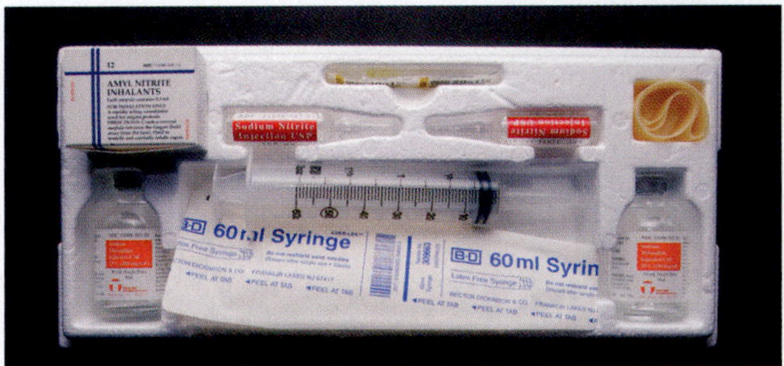

■ **Figure 34-1** Cyanide antidote kit. *(© Jeff Forster)*

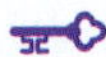

Pulse oximetry may give a falsely elevated reading in CO poisoning and should be used with extreme caution.

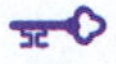

Devices are now available to measure CO levels in the prehospital setting.

bound with hemoglobin, it is very resistant to removal and causes an effective hypoxia. Because of the variability of the signs and symptoms, people usually ignore CO poisoning until toxic levels occur. Common circumstances for CO poisoning include improperly vented heating systems or the use of a small barbecue to heat a house or camper. Symptoms of early poisoning are similar to those of the flu. Be alert for CO poisoning in multiple patients living together in a poorly heated and vented space who have "flulike" symptoms.

Signs and Symptoms

Signs and symptoms of CO poisoning include:

- Headache
- Nausea, vomiting
- Confusion or other altered mental status
- Tachypnea

Management

Because of the difficulty in removing CO from hemoglobin, definitive treatment is often performed in a hyperbaric chamber (Figure 34-2 ■). In this specially designed environment, oxygen under several atmospheres of pressure surrounds the body. This increases oxygenation of available hemoglobin. In field settings, take the following supportive steps:

- Ensure safety of rescue personnel.
- Remove the patient from the contaminated area.

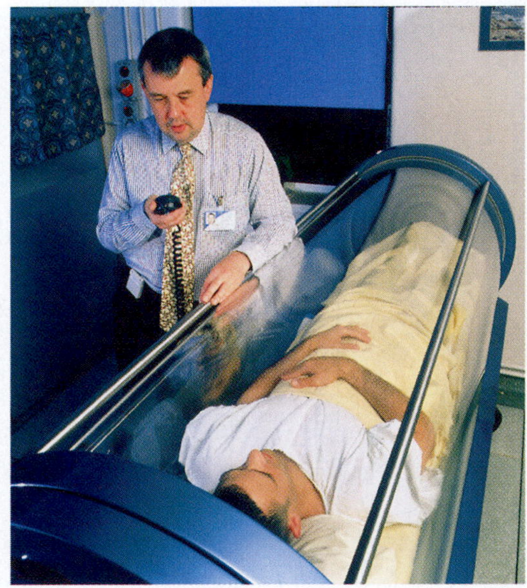

■ **Figure 34-2** Hyperbaric chamber. *(© James Kingholmes/Science Photo Library/Photo Researchers, Inc.)*

- ★ Begin immediate ventilation of the area.
- ★ Initiate supportive measures. High-flow, high-concentration oxygen by nonrebreather is critical in this setting.

CARDIAC MEDICATIONS

The list of cardiac medications grows almost daily. Many classes of these drugs exist, including antidysrythmics, beta-blockers, calcium channel blockers, glycosides, and ACE inhibitors. Generally these medications regulate heart function by decreasing heart rate, suppressing automaticity, and/or reducing vascular tone. Overdoses of these drugs can be intentional but are more often due to errors in dosage.

Signs and Symptoms

In overdose quantities, signs and symptoms of cardiac medication poisoning include:

- ★ Nausea and vomiting
- ★ Headache, dizziness, confusion
- ★ Profound hypotension
- ★ Cardiac dysrhythmias (usually bradycardia)
- ★ Heart conduction blocks
- ★ Bronchospasm and pulmonary edema (especially beta-blockers)

Management

Initiate standard toxicological emergency assessment and treatment immediately. Be aware that severe bradycardia may not respond well to atropine; therefore, you may need to use an external pacing device. Some cardiac medications do have antidotes that may help with severe adverse effects. These include calcium for calcium channel blockers, glucagon for beta-blockers, and digoxin-specific Fab (Digibind) for digoxin. Contact medical direction before giving these antidotes.

CAUSTIC SUBSTANCES

Caustic substances are either **acids** or **alkalis** (bases) that are found in both the home and the industrial workplace. Approximately 12,000 exposures occur annually with 150 major complications or deaths. Strong caustics can produce severe burns at the site of contact and, if ingested, cause tissue destruction at the lips, mouth, esophagus, and other areas of the gastrointestinal tract.

acid *a substance that liberates hydrogen ions (H^+) when in solution.*

alkali *a substance that liberates hydroxyl ions (OH^-) when in solution; a strong base.*

Strong *acids* have a pH less than 2. They are found in plumbing liquids such as drain openers and bathroom cleaners. Contact with strong acids usually produces immediate and severe pain. This is a result of tissue coagulation and necrosis. Often this type of contact injury will produce *eschar* at the burn site, which will act like a shield and prevent further penetration or damage to deeper tissues. If ingested, acids will cause local burns to the mouth and throat. Because of the rapid transit through the esophagus, the esophagus is not usually damaged. More likely, the stomach lining will be injured. Immediate or delayed hemorrhage can occur and may be associated with perforation. Pain is severe and usually due to direct injury and spasm from irritation. Absorption of acids into the vascular system will occur quite readily, causing a significant acidemia, which will need to be managed along with the direct local effects.

Strong *alkaline* agents typically have a pH greater than 12.5. They can be in solid or liquid form (such as in Drano or Liquid Plumber) and are routinely found around the house. These agents cause injury by inducing liquefaction necrosis. Pain is often delayed, which allows for longer tissue contact and deeper tissue injury before the exposure is even recognized. Solid alkaline agents can stick to the oropharynx or esophagus. This can cause perforation, bleeding, and inflammation of central chest structures. Liquid alkalis are more likely to injure the stomach because they pass quickly through the esophagus. Within 2–3 days of exposure, complete loss of the protective mucosal tissue can occur, followed by either gradual healing and recovery or further bleeding, necrosis, and stricture formation.

Signs and Symptoms

Signs and symptoms of caustic injury include:

- ★ Facial burns
- ★ Pain in the lips, tongue, throat, or gums
- ★ Drooling, trouble swallowing
- ★ Hoarseness, stridor, or shortness of breath
- ★ Shock from bleeding, vomiting

Management

Assessment and intervention must be aggressive and rapid to minimize morbidity and mortality. Take precautions to prevent injury to rescuers. Initiate standard toxicological emergency assessment and treatment, but pay particular attention to establishing an airway. Injury to the oropharynx and larynx may make airway control and ventilation difficult and may even require cricothyrotomy. Since caustics will not adsorb to activated charcoal, there is no indication to administer it. In the past, rescuers often gave water or milk to dilute any ingested caustics but there is controversy as to whether this is beneficial. Rapid transport to the emergency department is essential.

HYDROFLUORIC ACID

Hydrofluoric acid is used to clean glass in lab settings and for etching glass in art.

Hydrofluoric (HF) acid deserves special attention because it is extremely toxic and can be lethal despite the appearance of only moderate burns on skin contact. HF acid penetrates deeply into tissues and is inactivated only when it comes in contact with *cations* such as calcium. Calcium fluoride is formed by this inactivation and settles in the tissue as a salt. The removal of calcium from cells causes a total disruption of cell functioning and can even cause bone destruction as calcium is leached out of the bones. Death has been reported from exposure of < 2.5 percent body surface area to a highly concentrated solution.

Signs and Symptoms

Signs and symptoms of HF acid exposure include:

- ★ Burning at site of contact
- ★ Trouble breathing
- ★ Confusion
- ★ Palpitations
- ★ Muscle cramps

Management

Management includes:

- ★ Ensure the safety of rescue personnel.
- ★ Initiate supportive measures.
- ★ Remove exposed clothing.
- ★ Irrigate the affected area with water thoroughly.
- ★ Immerse the affected limb in iced water with magnesium sulfate, calcium salts, or benzethonium chloride.
- ★ Transport immediately for definitive care.

ALCOHOL

See the section on Alcohol Abuse later in this chapter.

HYDROCARBONS

Hydrocarbons are organic compounds of mostly carbon and hydrogen. They include such common recognizable names as kerosene, naphtha, turpentine, mineral oil, chloroform, toluene, and benzene. These chemicals are found in common household products such as lighter fluid, paint, glue, lubricants, solvents, and aerosol propellants. Toxicity from hydrocarbons can occur through any route, including ingestion, inhalation, or surface absorption.

Signs and Symptoms

Signs and symptoms of hydrocarbon poisoning will vary with the type and route of exposure but may include:

- ★ Burns due to local contact
- ★ Wheezing, dyspnea, hypoxia, and pneumonitis from aspiration/inhalation
- ★ Headache, dizziness, slurred speech, ataxia (irregular and difficult-to-control movements), and obtundation (dulled reflexes)
- ★ Foot and wrist drop with numbness and tingling
- ★ Cardiac dysrhythmias

Management

Recent studies have shown that very few poisonings with hydrocarbons are serious, and less than 1 percent require physician intervention. If you know the exact chemical that the patient has been exposed to and the patient is asymptomatic, medical direction may suggest that the patient can be left at home. However, a few hydrocarbon poisonings can be very serious. Any patient who is symptomatic, does not know what he has taken, or who has taken a hydrocarbon that requires gastrointestinal decontamination (halogenated or aromatic hydrocarbons) must be treated using standard toxicological emergency procedures. Since charcoal will not bind hydrocarbons, this may be one of the few cases in which gastric lavage can be useful.

TRICYCLIC ANTIDEPRESSANTS

Tricyclic antidepressants were once commonly used to treat depression. Close monitoring was required because these medications have a narrow **therapeutic index,** meaning that a relatively small increase in dose can quickly lead to toxic effects. The very nature of their use, treating depression, presents a dilemma because the patients most seriously in need of treatment may also be the most likely to attempt to take an overdose. Deaths due to antidepressant overdose have dropped significantly in recent years since the development and rapid acceptance of safer agents unrelated to tricyclics. However, tricyclic antidepressants are still used for various clinical problems such as chronic pain or migraine prophylaxis and may still be responsible for more deaths due to intentional overdose than any other medication. Common agents include amitriptyline (Elavil), amoxapine, clomipramine, doxepin, imipramine, and nortriptyline.

therapeutic index *the maximum tolerated dose divided by the minimum curative dose of a drug; the range between curative and toxic dosages; also called* therapeutic window.

Signs and Symptoms

Signs and symptoms of tricyclic antidepressant toxicity include:

- ★ Dry mouth
- ★ Blurred vision
- ★ Urinary retention
- ★ Constipation

Late into an overdose, more severe toxicity may produce:

- ★ Confusion, hallucinations
- ★ Hyperthermia
- ★ Respiratory depression

- Seizures
- Tachycardia and hypotension
- Cardiac dysrhythmias (heart block, wide QRS, *torsades de pointes*)

Management

Toxicity from tricyclic antidepressants requires immediate initiation of standard toxicological emergency procedures. Cardiac monitoring is critical since dysrhythmias are the most common cause of death. If you suspect a mixed overdose with benzodiazepines, do *not* use Flumazenil, since it may precipitate seizures. If significant cardiac toxicity occurs, sodium bicarbonate can be used as an additional therapy. Contact medical direction as necessary.

If you suspect a mixed overdose with benzodiazepines, do NOT use Flumazenil, since it may precipitate seizures.

MAO INHIBITORS

Monoamine oxidase inhibitors (MAOIs) have been used, although rarely, to treat depression. Recently they have been used, on a limited basis, to treat obsessive-compulsive disorders. They are relatively unpopular because of a narrow therapeutic index, multiple-drug interactions, serious interactions with foods containing *tyramine* (for example, red wine and cheese), and high morbidity and mortality when taken in overdose. These drugs inhibit the breakdown of neurotransmitters such as norepinephrine and dopamine while increasing the availability of the components needed to make even more neurotransmitters. When taken in overdose, MAOIs can be extremely dangerous, although symptoms may not appear for up to 6 hours.

Signs and Symptoms

Signs and symptoms of MAOI overdose include:

- Headache, agitation, restlessness, tremor
- Nausea
- Palpitations
- Tachycardia
- Severe hypertension
- Hyperthermia
- Eventually bradycardia, hypotension, coma, and death occur

New MAOIs have recently entered the marketplace. These next-generation drugs are reversible, less toxic, and do not have the same reactions with food as the older MAOIs. Data are not yet available on the outcome of patients overdosing with these newer agents.

Management

No antidote exists for MAOI overdose because the inhibition is not reversible except with newer drugs. Therefore, institute standard toxicological emergency procedures as soon as possible. If necessary, give symptomatic support for seizures and hyperthermia using benzodiazepines. If vasopressors are needed, use norepinephrine.

NEWER ANTIDEPRESSANTS

In recent years, several new agents have been developed to treat depression. Because of their high safety profile in therapeutic and overdose amounts, these drugs have been widely accepted and have virtually replaced tricyclic antidepressants.

Recently introduced drugs include trazodone (Desyrel), bupropion (Wellbutrin), and the large group of popular *selective serotonin reuptake inhibitors*, or SSRIs (Prozac, Luvox, Paxil, Zoloft). SSRIs prevent the reuptake of serotonin in the brain, theoretically making it more available for brain functions. The true mechanism by which these drugs treat depression is unclear.

Signs and Symptoms

When these drugs are taken in overdose, usually the signs and symptoms are mild. Occasionally trazodone and bupropion will cause CNS depression and seizures, but deaths are rare and have only been reported in mixed overdoses with multiple ingestions. More commonly, signs and symptoms of overdose with the newer antidepressant agents include:

★ Drowsiness
★ Tremor
★ Nausea and vomiting
★ Sinus tachycardia

SSRIs are now also associated with *serotonin syndrome.* This syndrome is caused by increased serotonin levels and is often triggered by increasing the dose of SSRI or adding a second drug such as Demerol, codeine, dextromethorphan (cough syrup), or other antidepressants. Signs and symptoms of serotonin syndrome include:

★ Agitation, anxiety, confusion, insomnia
★ Headache, drowsiness, coma
★ Nausea, salivation, diarrhea, abdominal cramps
★ Cutaneous piloerection, flushed skin
★ Hyperthermia, tachycardia
★ Rigidity, shivering, incoordination, myoclonic jerks

Management

Overdose with these new antidepressants is not as life threatening as with previous agents unless other drugs or alcohol are taken simultaneously. Consequently, treat overdoses with the standard toxicological emergency procedures. Also have the patient discontinue all serotonergic drugs and implement supportive measures. Benzodiazepines or beta-blockers occasionally are used to improve patient comfort, but these are rarely given in the field.

LITHIUM

In the treatment of bipolar (manic-depressive) disorder, no other drug has been proven to be more effective than lithium. It is unclear how lithium exerts its therapeutic effect. However, like tricyclic antidepressants, lithium has a narrow therapeutic index which results in toxicity during normal use and in overdose situations.

Signs and Symptoms

Signs and symptoms of lithium toxicity include:

★ Thirst, dry mouth
★ Tremor, muscle twitching, increased reflexes
★ Confusion, stupor, seizures, coma
★ Nausea, vomiting, diarrhea
★ Bradycardia, dysrhythmias

Management

Treat lithium overdose with mostly supportive measures. Use the standard toxicological emergency procedures, but remember that activated charcoal will not bind lithium and need not be given. Alkalinizing the urine with sodium bicarbonate and osmotic diuresis using mannitol may increase elimination of lithium, but severe toxic cases require hemodialysis.

SALICYLATES

Salicylates are some of the more common drugs taken in overdose, largely due to the fact that they are readily available over the counter. The most recognizable forms are aspirin, oil of wintergreen, and some prescription combination medications.

Aspirin in large doses can cause serious consequences. About 300 mg/kg is required to cause toxicity. In such amounts, salicylates inhibit normal energy production and acid buffering in the body. This results in a metabolic acidosis, which further injures other organ systems.

Signs and Symptoms

Signs and symptoms of salicylate overdose include:

- ★ Rapid respirations
- ★ Hyperthermia
- ★ Confusion, lethargy, coma
- ★ Cardiac failure, dysrhythmias
- ★ Abdominal pain, vomiting
- ★ Pulmonary edema, ARDS (adult respiratory distress syndrome)

Chronic overdose symptoms are somewhat less severe and do not tend to include abdominal complaints. It is difficult to distinguish chronic overdose from very early acute overdose or early overdose that has progressed past the abdominal irritation stage.

Management

In all cases, salicylate poisoning should be treated using standard toxicological emergency procedures. Activated charcoal definitely reduces drug absorption and should be used. If possible, find out the time of ingestion, since blood levels measured at the right time can indicate the expected degree of injury. Most symptomatic patients will require generous IV fluids and may need urine alkalinization with sodium bicarbonate. Severe cases may require dialysis.

ACETAMINOPHEN

Due to its few side effects in normal dosages, acetaminophen (e.g., paracetamol, Tylenol) is one of the most common drugs in use today. It is used to treat fever and/or pain and is a common ingredient in hundreds of over-the-counter preparations. It also can be obtained by prescription in combination with various other drugs.

In large doses, however, acetaminophen can be a very dangerous pharmaceutical. A dose of 150 mg/kg is considered toxic and may result in death due to injury to the liver. A highly reactive byproduct of acetaminophen metabolism is responsible for most adverse effects, but this is usually avoided by the body's detoxification system. When large amounts of acetaminophen enter the system, the detoxification system is overwhelmed and gradually depleted, leaving the toxic metabolite in the circulation to cause hepatic necrosis.

Signs and Symptoms

Signs and symptoms of acetaminophen toxicity appear in four stages:

Stage 1	½ hour to 24 hours	Nausea, vomiting, weakness, fatigue
Stage 2	24–48 hours	Abdominal pain, decreased urine, elevated liver enzymes
Stage 3	72–96 hours	Liver function disruption
Stage 4	4–14 days	Gradual recovery or progressive liver failure

Management

Treat acetaminophen overdose with standard toxicological emergency procedures. Find out the time of ingestion since blood levels taken at the right time can predict the potential for injury. An antidote called N-acetylcysteine (NAC, Mucomyst) is available and highly effective. However, NAC is usually administered based on clinical and laboratory studies and is rarely given in the prehospital setting.

OTHER NONPRESCRIPTION PAIN MEDICATIONS

Nonsteroidal anti-inflammatory drugs (NSAIDs) are another group of medications that are readily available and are often overdosed. Common examples include naproxen sodium, indomethacin, ibuprofen, and ketorolac (Toradol).

Signs and Symptoms

The presentation of toxicity caused by NSAIDs varies greatly but can include:

- ★ Headache
- ★ Ringing in the ears (tinnitus)
- ★ Nausea, vomiting, abdominal pain
- ★ Swelling of the extremities
- ★ Mild drowsiness
- ★ Dyspnea, wheezing, pulmonary edema
- ★ Rash, itching

Management

There is no specific antidote for NSAID toxicity. Use general overdose procedures, including supportive care, as soon as possible and transport to the emergency department for observation and any necessary symptomatic treatment.

THEOPHYLLINE

Theophylline, which belongs to a group of medications called xanthines, is usually used for patients with asthma or COPD because of its moderate bronchodilation and mild anti-inflammatory effects. Like other drugs with a narrow therapeutic index and high toxicity, theophylline has become less popular recently and therefore is not implicated in as many overdose injuries as in the past.

Signs and Symptoms

Symptoms of theophylline toxicity include:

- ★ Agitation
- ★ Tremors
- ★ Seizures
- ★ Cardiac dysrhythmias
- ★ Nausea and vomiting

Management

Theophylline can cause significant morbidity and mortality. In overdose situations, it is essential that you institute toxicological emergency procedures immediately. In fact, theophylline is on the small list of drugs that have significant *enterohepatic circulation.* This means that multiple doses of activated charcoal over time will continuously remove more and more of the drug from the body. Treat any dysrhythmias according to ACLS procedures.

METALS

With the exception of iron, overdose of heavy metals is a rare occurrence. Other possible involved metals include lead, arsenic, and mercury. All metals affect numerous enzyme systems within the body and therefore present with a variety of symptoms. Some also have direct local effects when ingested and when accumulated in various organs.

Iron

The body only requires small amounts of iron on a daily basis to maintain a sufficient store for enzyme and hemoglobin production. Excess amounts are easily obtained from nonprescription supplements and multivitamins. Children have a tendency to accidentally overdose on iron by taking too many candy-flavored chewable vitamins containing iron. To determine the amount of iron ingested, calculate the amount of elemental iron present in the type of pill ingested. Symptoms occur when more than 20 mg/kg of elemental iron are ingested.

Signs and Symptoms Excess iron will cause gastrointestinal injury and possible shock from hemorrhage, especially if it forms *concretions* (lumps of iron formed when tablets fuse together after being swallowed). Patients with significant iron ingestions will often have visible tablets or concretions in the stomach or small intestine on X-ray. Other signs and symptoms of iron ingestion include:

- Vomiting (often hematemesis), diarrhea
- Abdominal pain, shock
- Liver failure
- Metabolic acidosis with tachypnea
- Eventual bowel scarring and possible obstruction

Management It is essential to initiate standard toxicological emergency procedures immediately. Since iron tends to inhibit gastrointestinal motility, pills sit longer in the stomach and may possibly be easier to remove through gastric lavage. Because activated charcoal will not bind iron (or any metals), it should not be used. Deferoxamine, a chelating agent, may be used in iron overdose as an antidote since it binds to iron so that less is moved into cells and tissues to cause damage.

Lead and Mercury

Both lead and mercury are heavy metals found in varying amounts in the environment. Lead was often used in glazes and paints before the toxic potential of such exposure became apparent. Mercury is a contaminant from industrial processing but is also found in thermometers and temperature-control switches in most homes. Chronic and acute exposures are possible with both metals.

Signs and Symptoms Signs and symptoms of heavy metal toxicity include:

- Headache, irritability, confusion, coma
- Memory disturbance
- Tremor, weakness, agitation
- Abdominal pain

Management Chronic poisoning can cause permanent neurological injury, which makes it imperative that the proper agencies monitor heavy metal levels in the environment of a patient who has presented with toxicity. Learn to recognize the signs of heavy metal toxicity and institute standard toxicology emergency procedures as needed. Activated charcoal will not bind heavy metals, but various chelating agents (DMSA, BAL, CDE) are available and may be used in definitive management in the hospital.

CONTAMINATED FOOD

Food poisoning is caused by a spectrum of different factors. For example, bacteria, viruses, and toxic chemicals notoriously produce varying levels of gastrointestinal distress. The patient may present with nausea, vomiting, diarrhea, and diffuse abdominal pain.

exotoxin *a soluble poisonous substance secreted during growth of a bacterium.*

enterotoxin *an exotoxin that produces gastrointestinal symptoms and diseases such as food poisoning.*

Bacterial food poisonings range in severity. Bacterial **exotoxins** (secreted by bacteria) or **enterotoxins** (exotoxins associated with gastrointestinal diseases, including food poisoning) cause the adverse GI complaints noted previously. Food contaminated with other bacteria such as *Shigella*, *Salmonella*, or *E. coli* can produce even more severe gastrointestinal reactions, often leading to electrolyte imbalance and hypovolemia. *Clostridium botulinum*, the world's most toxic poison, presents as severe respiratory distress or arrest. The incubation of this toxin can range from 4 hours to 8 days. Fortunately, botulism rarely occurs, except in cases of improper food storage methods such as canning.

A variety of seafood poisonings are a result of specific toxins found in dinoflagellate-contaminated shellfish such as clams, mussels, oysters, and scallops and can produce a syndrome referred to as *paralytic shellfish poisoning*. This condition can lead to respiratory arrest in addition to standard gastrointestinal symptoms.

Increased fish consumption by North Americans has also increased the number of cases of poisonings from toxins found in many commonly eaten fish. *Ciguatera (bony fish) poisoning* most frequently turns up in fish caught in the Pacific Ocean or along the tropical reefs of Florida and the West Indies. Ciguatera normally takes 2–6 hours to incubate and may produce myalgia and paresthesia. *Scombroid (histamine) poisoning* results from bacterial contamination of mackerel, tuna, bonitos, and albacore. Both types of poisoning cause the common gastrointestinal symptoms. Scombroid poisoning will present with an immediate facial flushing as histamines cause vasodilation.

Signs and Symptoms

As mentioned, signs and symptoms of food poisoning may include:

- ★ Nausea, vomiting, diarrhea, abdominal pain
- ★ Facial flushing, respiratory distress (with some seafood poisonings)

Management

Except for botulism, food poisoning is rarely life threatening. Treatment, therefore, is largely supportive. In suspected cases of food poisoning, contact poison control and medical direction, and take the following steps:

- ★ Perform the necessary assessment.
- ★ Collect samples of the suspected contaminated food source.
- ★ Perform the following management actions:
  - Establish and maintain the airway.
  - Administer high-flow, high-concentration oxygen.
  - Intubate and assist ventilations, if appropriate.
  - Establish venous access.
- ★ Consider the administration of antihistamines (especially in seafood poisonings) and antiemetics.

POISONOUS PLANTS AND MUSHROOMS

Plants, trees, and mushrooms contribute heavily to the number of accidental toxic ingestions. While the vast majority of plants are nontoxic, many of the popular decorative houseplants can present a danger to children, who frequently ingest nonfood items. Most poison control centers distribute pamphlets that identify toxic household plants. (These pamphlets will help "poison proof" the home.)

It is impossible to cover all the toxic plants and mushrooms. Few rescuers are trained as botanists, and they find it difficult to identify the offending material. Mushrooms are particularly difficult to identify from small pieces. Additionally, most people recognize mushrooms and other plants by common names rather than by the nomenclature of scientific species. A general approach is to obtain a sample of the plant, if possible. Try to find a full leaf, stem, and any flowers.

Since many ornamental plants contain irritating chemicals or crystals, examine the patient's mouth and throat for redness, blistering, or edema. Identify other abnormal signs during the focused physical exam.

Mushroom poisonings generally fall into two categories: people seeking edible mushrooms and accidental ingestions by children. Fortunately, few of the many mushroom species possess extremely dangerous toxins. Toxic mushrooms fall into seven classes. *Amanita* and *Galerina* belong to

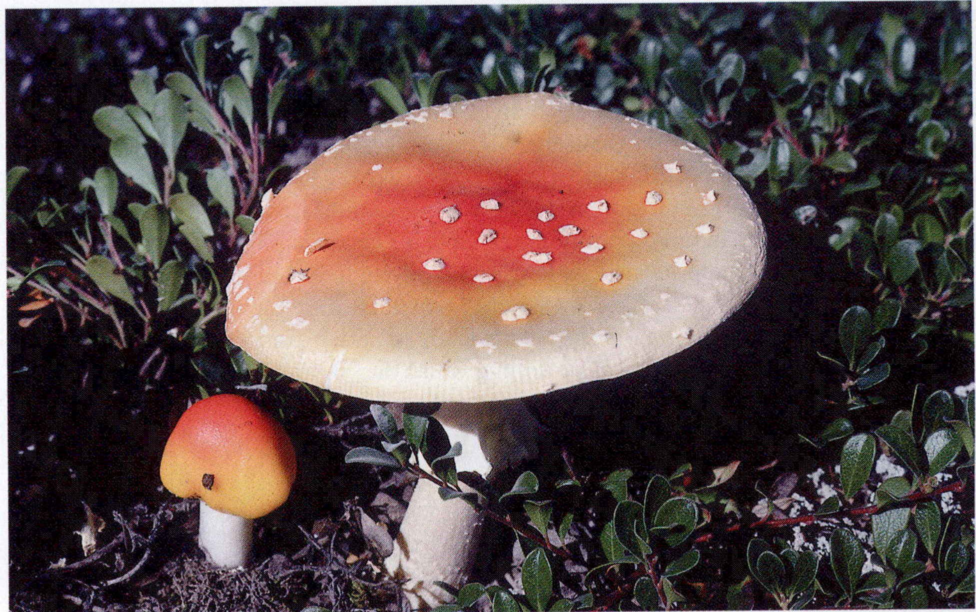

■ Figure 34-3 Poisonous mushrooms from Amanita and Galerina class. *(© Leonard Lee Rue III/Photo Researchers, Inc.)*

the deadly *cyclopeptide* group (Figure 34-3 ■). (*Amanita* accounts for over 90 percent of all deaths.) These mushrooms produce a poison that is extremely toxic to the liver, with a mortality rate of about 50 percent.

Signs and Symptoms

Signs and symptoms of poisonous plant ingestion include:

- ★ Excessive salivation, lacrimation (secretion of tears), diaphoresis
- ★ Abdominal cramps, nausea, vomiting, diarrhea
- ★ Decreasing levels of consciousness, eventually progressing to coma

Management

For guidance on the treatment of plant poisonings, call the poison control center. If contact cannot be made, use the procedures outlined under treatment of food poisoning earlier.

INJECTED TOXINS

Although we generally think of intentional or accidental drug overdoses as sources of injected poisons, the most common source for these poisonings is the animal kingdom. Bites and stings from a variety of insects, reptiles, and animals are among the most common injuries sustained by humans. Further injury can result from bacterial contamination or from a reaction produced by an injected substance.

GENERAL PRINCIPLES OF MANAGEMENT

In the case of a bite or sting, remember to protect rescue personnel. The offending organism may still be around.

The general principles of field management for bites and stings include:

- ★ Protect rescue personnel—the offending organism may still be around.
- ★ Remove the patient from danger of repeated injection, especially in the case of yellow jackets, wasps, or hornets.
- ★ If possible, identify the insect, reptile, or animal that caused the injury and bring it to the emergency department along with the patient (if it can be done safely).
- ★ Perform an initial assessment and rapid physical exam.
- ★ Prevent or delay further absorption of the poison.

- ★ Initiate supportive measures as indicated.
- ★ Watch for anaphylactic reaction (see Chapter 5, "Life-Span Development").
- ★ Transport the patient as rapidly as possible.
- ★ Contact the poison control center and medical direction according to your local protocols.

INSECT BITES AND STINGS

Insect Stings

Many people die from allergic reactions to the stings from an order of insects known as *Hymenoptera.* As mentioned earlier, *Hymenoptera* includes wasps, bees, hornets, and ants. Only the common honeybee leaves a stinger. Wasps, yellow jackets, hornets, and fire ants sting repeatedly until removal from contact.

In most cases of insect bite, local treatment is all that is necessary. Unless an allergic reaction occurs, most patients will tolerate the isolated *Hymenoptera* sting.

Signs and Symptoms Signs and symptoms include:

- ★ Localized pain
- ★ Redness
- ★ Swelling
- ★ Skin wheal

Idiosyncratic reactions to the toxin may occur, resulting in a progressing localized swelling and edema. This is not an allergic reaction, however, if it responds well to an antihistamine such as diphenhydramine hydrochloride. The major problem resulting from a *Hymenoptera* sting is an allergic reaction or anaphylaxis. Signs and symptoms of allergic reaction include the following:

- ★ Localized pain, redness, swelling, and a skin wheal
- ★ Itching or flushing of the skin, rash
- ★ Tachycardia, hypotension, bronchospasm, or laryngeal edema
- ★ Facial edema, uvular swelling

Management For *Hymenoptera* stings, take the following supportive measures:

- ★ Wash the area.
- ★ Gently remove the stinger, if present, by scraping without squeezing the venom sac.
- ★ Apply cool compresses to the injection site.
- ★ Observe for and treat allergic reactions and/or anaphylaxis (see Chapter 31, "Allergies and Anaphylaxis").

Africanized Honeybees In the past decade, Africanized honeybees (AHBs), also referred to as "Africanized bees" or "killer bees," have begun invading North America primarily through south Texas. The bees have spread across the southwestern United States and into California.

Africanized bees acquired the name "killer bees" because they will viciously attack people and animals who unwittingly stray into their territory, often resulting in serious injury or death. Only a minimal disturbance is all that is necessary to cause an AHB attack. Although all honeybees respond to threats to their colonies, AHBs respond more quickly and in much greater numbers than do European honeybees.

AHBs pose a particular risk for firefighters and EMS personnel. Heavy turnout gear can provide good protection as long as a properly fitting bee veil is used. Hazardous material suits can also be used. AHBs can be immobilized and killed with wetting agents (surfactants) including commercial dishwashing soaps.

■ Figure 34-4 Brown recluse spider.

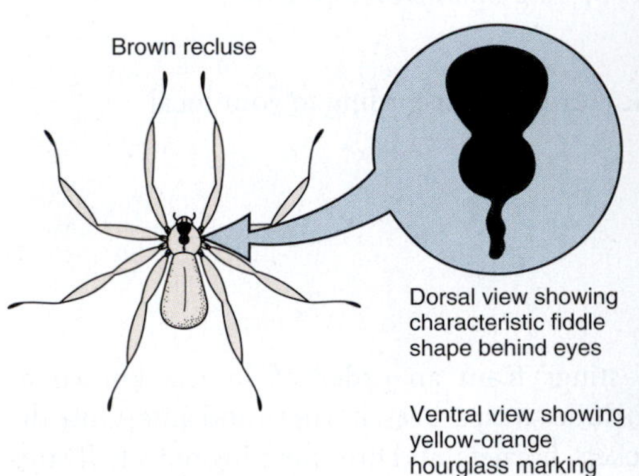

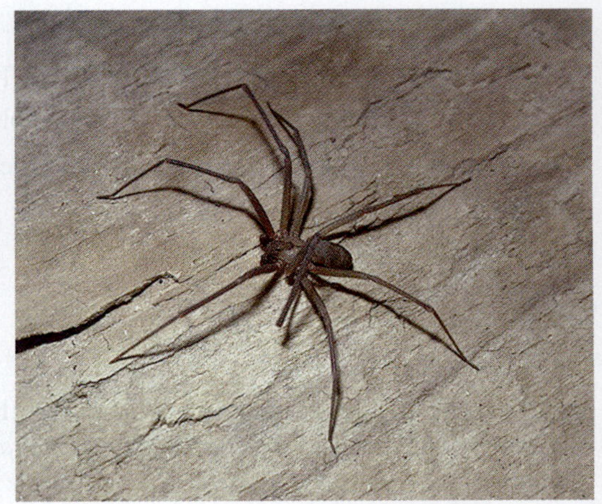

Brown Recluse Spider Bites

The brown recluse spider lives in the southern and midwestern states. It is found in large numbers in Tennessee, Arkansas, Oklahoma, and Texas. It has also been reported in Hawaii and California.

The brown recluse is about 15 mm in length. It generally lives in dark, dry locations and can often be found in and around the house. There is a characteristic violin-shaped marking on the back, giving the spider its nickname, "fiddleback spider" (Figure 34-4 ■). Another identifying feature is the presence of six eyes (three pairs in a semicircle), instead of the eight eyes common to most spiders.

Signs and Symptoms Brown recluse spider bites are usually painless. Not uncommonly, bites occur at night while the patient sleeps. Most victims are unaware they have been bitten until the local reaction starts. Initially a small erythematous macule surrounded by a white ring forms at the site (Figure 34-5 ■). This usually appears within a few minutes of the bite. Over the next 8 hours localized pain, redness, and swelling develop. Tissue necrosis at the site occurs over days to weeks (Figure 34-6 ■). Other symptoms include chills, fever, nausea and vomiting, joint pain, and, in severe situations, bleeding disorders (disseminated intravascular coagulation).

Management Treatment is mostly supportive. Since there is no antivenin, the emergency department treatment consists of antihistamines to reduce systemic reactions and possible surgical excision of necrotic tissue.

Black Widow Spider Bites

Black widow spiders live in all parts of the continental United States. They are usually found in woodpiles or brush. The female spider is responsible for bites and can be easily identified by the characteristic orange hourglass marking on her black abdomen (Figure 34-7 ■). The venom of the legendary black widow is very potent, causing excessive neurotransmitter release at the synaptic junctions.

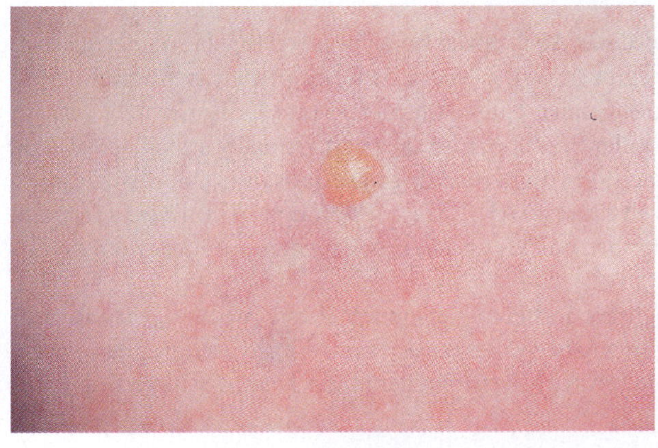

■ Figure 34-5 Brown recluse spider bite 24 hours after bite. Note the bleb and surrounding white halo. *(Scott and White Hospital and Clinic)*

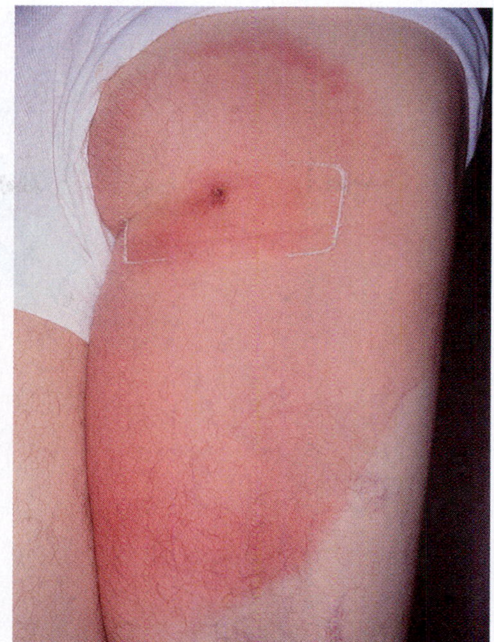

■ **Figure 34-6** Brown recluse spider bite 4 days after the bite. Note the spread of erythema and early necrosis. *(Scott and White Hospital and Clinic)*

Signs and Symptoms Signs and symptoms of black widow spider bites start as immediate localized pain, redness, and swelling. Progressive muscle spasms of all large muscle groups can occur and are usually associated with severe pain. Other systemic symptoms include nausea, vomiting, sweating, seizures, paralysis, and decreased level of consciousness.

Management Prehospital treatment is mostly supportive. It is important to reassure the patient. IV muscle relaxants may be necessary for severe spasms. With physician order you may use diazepam (2.5–10 mg IV) or calcium gluconate (0.1–0.2/kg of 10 percent solution IV). Note that calcium chloride is not effective and should not be used. Since hypertensive crisis is possible, monitor blood pressure carefully. Antivenin is available, so transfer the patient to the emergency department as soon as possible.

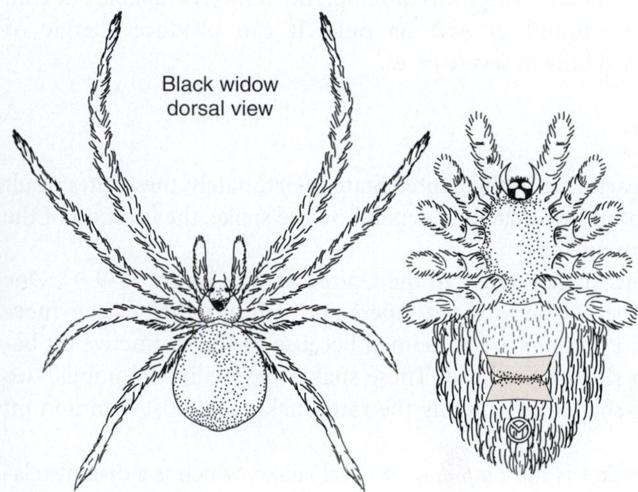

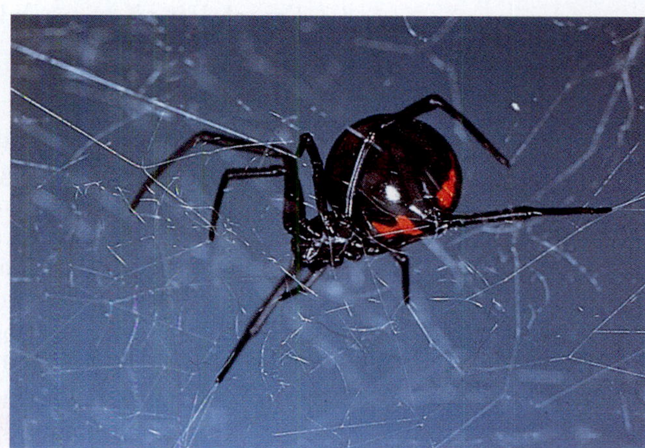

■ **Figure 34-7** Black widow spider.

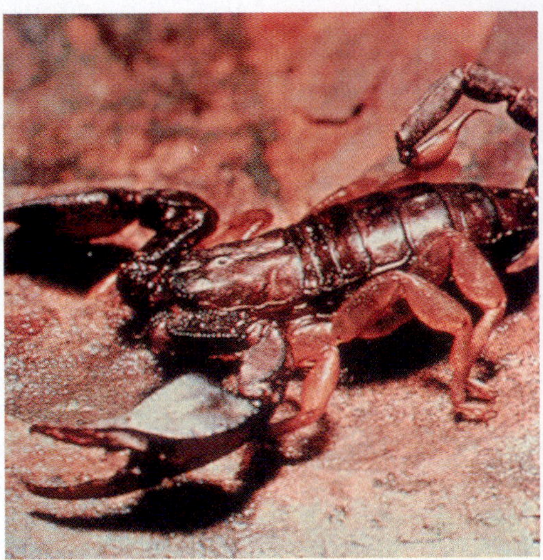

■ **Figure 34-8** Scorpion.

Scorpion Stings

There are many species of scorpion in the United States (Figure 34-8 ■). All can sting, causing localized pain, but only one, the bark scorpion, has caused fatalities. These arthropods live mostly in Arizona and adjacent areas of California, Nevada, New Mexico, and Texas. There have been no deaths in Arizona from scorpion stings since 1970.

Scorpions move mostly at night, hiding in the day under debris and buildings. The venom they inject is stored in a bulb at the end of the tail. If provoked the scorpion will sting with its tail, injecting only a small amount of poison.

Signs and Symptoms The bark scorpion's venom acts on the nervous system, producing a burning and tingling effect without much evidence of injury initially. Gradually this progresses to numbness. Systemic effects are more pronounced with slurred speech, restlessness (hyperactivity in 80 percent of children), muscle twitching, salivation, abdominal cramping, nausea and vomiting, and seizures.

Management Begin treatment by reassuring the patient. Apply a constricting band above the wound site no tighter than a watchband to occlude lymphatic flow only. Avoid the use of analgesics, which may increase toxicity and potentiate the venom's effect on airway control. Transport the patient to the emergency department if systemic symptoms develop. Antivenin is available but is an unlicensed goat-serum-derived product found in Arizona only. It can produce allergic or anaphylactic reactions and should be used only in severe cases.

SNAKEBITES

There are several thousand snakebites each year in the United States. Fortunately, these bites result in very few deaths. The signs and symptoms of snakebite depend on the snake, the location of the bite, and the type and amount of venom injected.

There are two families of poisonous snakes native to the United States (Figure 34-9 ■). One family (*Crotalidae*) includes the pit vipers. Common pit vipers are cottonmouths (water moccasins), rattlesnakes, and copperheads. Pit vipers are so named because of the distinctive pit between the eye and the nostril on each side of the head. These snakes have elliptical pupils, two well-developed fangs, and a triangular-shaped head. Only the rattlesnake, the most common pit viper, has rattles on the end of its tail.

The second family of poisonous snakes is the *Elapidae,* or coral snake, which is a distant relative of the cobra. Several varieties of coral snakes are found in the United States, primarily in the

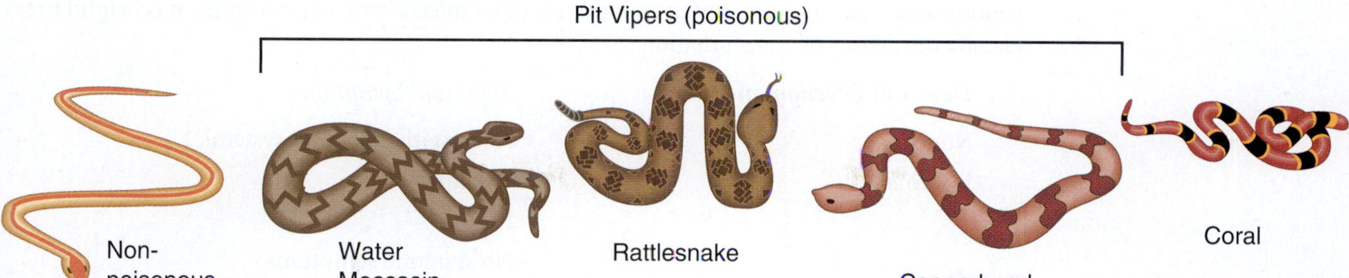

■ Figure 34-9 Venomous snakes in the United States.

southwest. Because it is a small snake and has small fangs, the coral snake cannot readily attach itself to a large surface, such as an arm or leg. The coral snake has round eyes, a narrow head, and no pit. It has characteristic yellow-banded red and black rings around its body. Several nonpoisonous snakes, such as the king snake, mimic this coloration pattern. Keep in mind a helpful mnemonic: "red touch yellow, kill a fellow; red touch black, venom lack." This rhyme indicates the distinctive pattern of the coral snake—a pattern that signals danger.

Pit-Viper Bites

Pit-viper venom contains hydrolytic enzymes that are capable of destroying proteins and most other tissue components. These enzymes may produce destruction of red blood cells and other tissue components and may affect the body's blood clotting system within the blood vessels. This will produce infarction and tissue necrosis, especially at the site of the bite.

A severe pit-viper bite can result in death from shock within 30 minutes. However, most deaths from pit-viper bites occur from 6 to 30 hours after the bite, with 90 percent occurring within the first 48 hours.

Signs and Symptoms Signs and symptoms of pit-viper bite include:

- Fang marks (often little more than a scratch mark or abrasion)
- Swelling and pain at the wound site
- Continued oozing at the wound site
- Weakness, dizziness, or faintness
- Sweating and/or chills
- Thirst
- Nausea and vomiting
- Diarrhea
- Tachycardia and hypotension
- Bloody urine and gastrointestinal hemorrhage (late)
- Ecchymosis
- Necrosis
- Shallow respirations progressing to respiratory failure
- Numbness and tingling around face and head (classic)

Management In treating a person who has been bitten by a pit viper, the primary goal is to slow absorption of the venom. Remember, about 25 percent of all rattlesnake bites are "dry" and no venom is injected. The amount of venom a pit viper injects varies significantly. It is helpful to try to classify the degree of envenomation:

Degree of Envenomation	*Signs and Symptoms*
None	None (either local or systemic)
Minimal	Swelling Pain No systemic symptoms
Moderate	Progressive swelling Mild systemic symptoms – paresthesias – nausea and vomiting – unusual tastes – mild hypotension – mild tachycardia – tachypnea
Severe	Swelling (spreading rapidly) Severe pain Systemic symptoms – altered mental status – nausea and vomiting – hypotension (systolic <80) – severe tachycardia – severe respiratory distress Blood oozes freely from puncture wounds

Antivenin is available for the various common pit vipers found in the United States. However, antivenin should only be considered for severe cases where there is marked envenomation as evidenced by severe systemic symptoms. In some cases, people become more ill from the antivenin than they do from the snakebite itself. Routine emergency treatment of pit-viper bites includes the following steps:

- ★ Keep the patient supine.
- ★ Immobilize the limb with a splint.
- ★ Maintain the extremity in a neutral position. Do not apply constricting bands.

Initiate supportive care using the following guidelines:

- ★ Apply high-flow, high-concentration oxygen.
- ★ Start IV with crystalloid fluid.
- ★ Transport the patient to the emergency department for management, which may include the administration of antivenin.
- ★ DO NOT apply ice, cold pack, or Freon spray to the wound.
- ★ DO NOT apply an arterial tourniquet.
- ★ DO NOT apply electrical stimulation from any device in an attempt to retard or reverse venom spread.

Coral Snake Bites

The venom of the coral snake contains some of the enzymes found in pit-viper venom. However, because of the presence of neurotoxin, coral snake venom primarily affects nervous tissue. The classic, severe coral snake bite will result in respiratory and skeletal muscle paralysis.

Signs and Symptoms After the bite of a coral snake, there may be no local manifestations or even any systemic effects for as long as 12–24 hours. Signs and symptoms of a coral snake bite include:

- ★ Localized numbness, weakness, and drowsiness
- ★ Ataxia
- ★ Slurred speech and excessive salivation
- ★ Paralysis of the tongue and larynx (produces difficulty breathing and swallowing)
- ★ Drooping of eyelids, double vision, dilated pupils
- ★ Abdominal pain
- ★ Nausea and vomiting
- ★ Loss of consciousness
- ★ Seizures
- ★ Respiratory failure
- ★ Hypotension

Management Treatment in cases of suspected coral snake bites includes the following steps:

- ★ Wash the wound with copious amounts of water.
- ★ Apply a compression bandage and keep the extremity at the level of the heart.
- ★ Immobilize the limb with a splint.
- ★ Start an IV using crystalloid fluid.
- ★ Transport the patient to the emergency department for administration of antivenin.
- ★ DO NOT apply ice, cold pack, or Freon sprays to the wound.
- ★ DO NOT incise the wound.
- ★ DO NOT apply electrical stimulation from any device in an attempt to retard or reverse venom spread.

MARINE ANIMAL INJECTION

Although most dangerous marine life prefer warm, tropical waters, some can be found in more northern waters. With the large number of people who flock to beaches and coastal recreation areas every year, the number of injuries from marine life has increased moderately. The most common encounters occur while the person is walking on the beach but can also happen while wading in shallow waters or scuba diving in deeper waters. Injection of toxins from marine life can result from stings of jellyfish and corals or from punctures by the bony spines of animals such as sea urchins and stingrays (Figure 34-10 ■). All venoms of marine animals contain substances that produce pain out of proportion to the size of the injury. These poisonous toxins are unstable and heat sensitive. Heat will relieve pain and inactivate the venom.

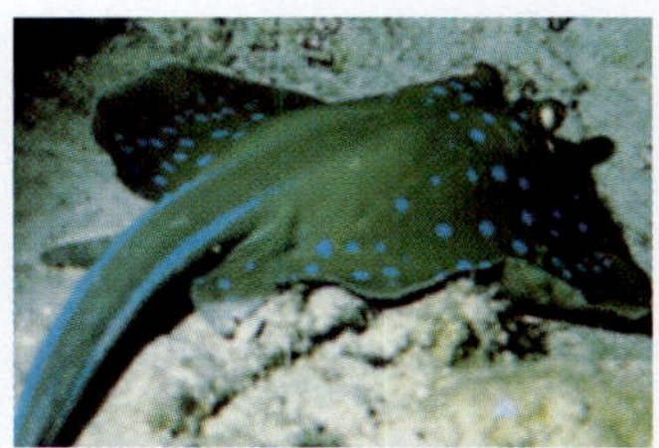

■ **Figure 34-10** Stingray.

Both freshwater and saltwater contain considerable bacterial and viral pollution. Therefore, secondary infection is always a possibility in injuries from marine animals. Particularly severe and life-threatening infections can be inflicted by a number of organisms. In all cases of marine-acquired infections, *Vibrio* species must be considered.

Signs and Symptoms Signs and symptoms of marine animal injection include:

- ★ Intense local pain and swelling
- ★ Weakness
- ★ Nausea and vomiting
- ★ Dyspnea
- ★ Tachycardia
- ★ Hypotension or shock (severe cases)

Management In suspected cases of marine animal injection, take the following steps:

- ★ Establish and maintain the airway.
- ★ Apply a constricting band between the wound and the heart no tighter than a watchband to occlude lymphatic flow only.
- ★ Apply heat or hot water (110°–113°F).
- ★ Inactivate or remove any stingers.

SUBSTANCE ABUSE AND OVERDOSE

substance abuse *use of a pharmacological substance for purposes other than medically defined reasons.*

addiction *compulsive and overwhelming dependence on a drug; an addiction may be physiological dependence, a psychological dependence, or both.*

tolerance *the need to progressively increase the dose of a drug to reproduce the effect originally achieved by smaller doses.*

withdrawal *referring to alcohol or drug withdrawal in which the patient's body reacts severely when deprived of the abused substance.*

Substance abuse, the use of a pharmacological substance for purposes other than medically defined reasons, is a very serious problem in our nation. Drugs are abused because they stimulate a feeling of euphoria in the abuser. Eventually, abusers begin to crave the feeling the drug gives them and therefore develop a *dependence* on the drug, also called **addiction.** An addiction exists when a person repeatedly uses and feels an overwhelming need to obtain and continue using a particular drug. Becoming accustomed to the use of the drug is called *habituation. Physiological dependence* is the resulting condition if removal of the drug causes adverse physical reactions. There can also be *psychological dependence,* in which use of the drug is required to prevent or relieve tension or emotional stress. With continued use, **tolerance** develops, which means that the abuser must use increasingly larger doses to get the same effect.

Attempts to stop the drug can trigger a psychological or physical reaction known as **withdrawal.** Withdrawal reactions can be quite unpleasant and severe. In some cases (especially with alcohol), withdrawal can be severe enough to cause death. These reactions further strengthen the victim's dependence on the drug. At this point the abuser may begin to withdraw from regular activities. He may have conflicts with family, friends, and coworkers as his personality and priorities change. Often the abuser will be involved in criminal activities to support the habit. The abuser has formed an addiction at the point when the substance abuse begins to affect some part of his life. This includes affecting the abuser's health, work, or relationships. Also, the abuser begins to act in a manner so as to seek out the drug he abuses.

The National Institute on Drug Abuse performed a survey to estimate national use and exposure to illicit drugs. The results were astounding:

- ★ 28 million Americans used illicit drugs at least once.
- ★ 14.5 million Americans use illicit drugs regularly.
- ★ 20 million Americans have tried cocaine.
- ★ 860,000 Americans use cocaine weekly.
- ★ 11.6 million Americans use marijuana regularly.
- ★ 770,000 Americans use hallucinogens such as PCP or LSD regularly.
- ★ 2.5 million Americans have used heroin.

The use of illicit drugs has fluctuated in recent years. Most recently, heroin has regained popularity, especially among middle- to upper-class teenagers and young adults. Beyond hurting themselves, substance abusers are 18 times more likely to be involved in criminal activities. These include violent crimes as well as theft to support drug habits. (The Secretary of Health and Human Services has estimated that cocaine is a $65 billion per year industry.)

drug overdose *poisoning from a pharmacological substance in excess of that usually prescribed or that the body can tolerate.*

In general terms, **drug overdose** refers to poisoning from a pharmacological substance, either legal or illegal. This can occur by accident, miscalculation, changes in the strength of a drug, suicide, polydrug use, or recreational drug usage. Many overdose emergencies seen in the field occur in the habitual drug abuser. It is most difficult to obtain a good history in these cases. However, if the paramedic is familiar with street-drug slang, a more accurate history may be obtained. It is imperative that the paramedic maintain a nonjudgmental attitude in these cases, even though this may be difficult.

The presentation of the drug overdose will vary based on the substance used. Management should be the same as for any ingested, inhaled, or injected poison. Poison control should be contacted for additional direction.

DRUGS OF ABUSE

Drugs Commonly Abused

Drugs of abuse are both common and dangerous. These drugs all have various signs and symptoms and require supportive treatment and general toxicological emergency management. Refer to Table 34–3 for further details on what you may find on assessment and the interventions required.

Remember these specific guidelines for patients who have taken the following drugs:

- ★ *Alcohol.* May require thiamine and $D_{50}W$ for hypoglycemia.
- ★ *Cocaine.* Benzodiazepines (diazepam) may be needed for sedation and to treat seizures. Beta-blockers are absolutely contraindicated because unopposed alpha receptor stimulation can cause cardiac ischemia, hypertension, and hyperthermia.
- ★ *Narcotics/opiates.* Naloxone is effective in reversing respiratory depression and sedation, but be careful, since it may trigger a withdrawal reaction in chronic opiate abusers.
- ★ *Amphetamines.* Use benzodiazepines (diazepam) for seizures and in combination with haloperidol for hyperactivity.
- ★ *Hallucinogens.* Use benzodiazepines for seizures and in combination with haloperidol for hyperactivity.
- ★ *Benzodiazepines.* Use flumazenil to counteract adverse effects. Be careful not to trigger a withdrawal syndrome with seizures.
- ★ *Barbiturates.* Forced diuresis and alkalinization of the urine improve elimination of barbiturates from the body.

Drugs Used for Sexual Purposes

There are a number of drugs that deserve mention as a separate category. These drugs are used to stimulate and enhance the sexual experience, but without medically approved indications for such use. *Ecstasy,* also called *MDMA,* is one such drug. Ecstasy is a modified form of methamphetamines and has similar, although milder effects. It is very popular in today's university and nightclub environments.

Use of Ecstasy initially causes anxiety, nausea, tachycardia, and elevated blood pressure, followed by relaxation, euphoria, and feelings of enhanced emotional insight. No definitive data exist as to whether the experience of sexual intercourse is improved. Studies show that prolonged use may cause brain damage. Some deaths from MDMA ingestion have been reported. These cases present with confusion, agitation, tremor, high temperature, and diarrhea. No specific treatment exists. Standard supportive measures should be initiated.

Rohypnol (flunitrazepam) is another drug abused for sexual purposes. Illegal in the United States, it is commonly called the "date rape drug," because it can be slipped secretly into a woman's drink. This drug is a strong benzodiazepine like diazepam, lorazepam, and midazolam. The resulting sedation and amnesia allows the perpetrator to rape the victim. Treatment is the same as for any benzodiazepine, but consequences of the sexual assault require attention as well.

ALCOHOL ABUSE

Alcohol is the most common substance of abuse in the United States and most of the world. Almost 75 percent of Americans have at least one drink per year. The average American consumes 2.5 gallons of pure ethanol every year. Alcohol has been linked to 5 percent of deaths in the United States. Alcoholism costs over $100 billion per year due to lost work time and medical costs to treat complications and injuries. Alcoholism progresses in much the same way as drug dependence, discussed earlier.

PHYSIOLOGICAL EFFECTS

Alcohol (ethyl alcohol, or ethanol) depresses the central nervous system, potentially to the point of stupor, coma, and death. In patients with severe liver disease, metabolism of alcohol may become

Table 34–3 Common Drugs of Abuse

Drug	Signs and Symptoms	Routes	Prehospital Management
Alcohol	CNS depression	Oral	ABCs
Beer	Slurred speech		Respiratory support
Whiskey	Disordered thought		Oxygenate
Gin	Impaired judgment		Establish IV access
Vodka	Diuresis		Administer 100 mg thiamine IV
Wine	Stumbling gait		ECG monitor
Tequila	Stupor		Check glucose level
	Coma		Administer $D_{50}W$, if hypoglycemic
Barbiturates	Lethargy	Oral	ABCs
Thiopental	Emotional lability	IV	Respiratory support
Phenobarbital	Incoordination		Oxygenate
Primidone	Slurred speech		Establish IV access
	Nystagmus		ECG monitor
	Coma		Contact Poison Control—may order bicarbonate
	Hypotension		
	Respiratory depression		
Cocaine	Euphoria	Snorting	ABCs
Crack	Hyperactivity	Injection	Respiratory support
Rock	Dilated pupils	Smoking (freebasing)	Oxygenate
	Psychosis		ECG monitor
	Twitching		Establish IV access
	Anxiety		Treat life-threatening dysrhythmias
	Hypertension		Seizure precautions: diazepam 5–10 mg
	Tachycardia		
	Dysrhythmias		
	Seizures		
	Chest pain		
Narcotics	CNS depression	Oral	ABCs
Heroin	Constricted pupils	Injection	Respiratory support
Codeine	Respiratory depression		Oxygenate
Meperidine	Hypotension		Establish IV access
Morphine	Bradycardia		Administer 1–2 mg naloxone IV or endotracheally as ordered by medical direction until respirations improve.*
Hydromorphone	Pulmonary edema		
Pentazocine	Coma		Larger than average doses (2–5 mg) have been used in the management of Darvon overdose and alcoholic coma
Darvon	Death		
Darvocet			
Methadone			ECG monitor

*With the advent of the opiate antagonist naloxone, narcotic overdosage became easier to manage. It is possible to titrate this effective medication to increase respirations to normal levels without fully awakening the patient. In the case of narcotics addicts, this prevents hostile and confrontational episodes.

Table 34–3 Common Drugs of Abuse

Drug	Signs and Symptoms	Routes	Prehospital Management
Marijuana	Euphoria	Smoked	ABCs
Grass	Dry mouth	Oral	Reassure the patient
Weed	Dilated pupils		Speak in a quiet voice
Hashish	Altered sensation		ECG monitor if indicated
Amphetamines	Exhilaration	Oral	ABCs
Benzedrine	Hyperactivity	Injection	Oxygenate
Dexedrine	Dilated pupils		ECG monitor
Ritalin	Hypertension		Establish IV access
"Speed"	Psychosis		Treat life-threatening dysrhythmias
	Tremors		Seizure precautions: diazepam 5–10 mg
	Seizures		
Hallucinogens	Psychosis	Oral	ABCs
LSD	Nausea	Smoked	Reassure the patient
STP	Dilated pupils		"Talk down" the "high" patient
Mescaline	Rambling speech		Protect the patient from injury
Psilocybin	Headache		Provide a dark, quiet environment
PCP**	Dizziness		Speak in a soft, quiet voice
	Suggestibility		Seizure precautions: diazepam 5–10 mg
	Distortion of sensory perceptions		
	Hallucinations		
Sedatives	Altered mental status	Oral	ABCs
Seconal	Hypotension		Respiratory support
Valium	Slurred speech		Oxygenate
Librium	Respiratory depression		Establish IV access
Xanax	Shock		ECG monitor
Halcion	Bradycardia		Medical direction may order naloxone
Restoril	Seizures		
Dalmane			
Phenobarbital			
*Benzodiazepines****	Altered mental status	Oral	ABCs
Valium	Slurred speech		Respiratory support
Librium	Dysrhythmias		Oxygenate
Xanax	Coma		Activated charcoal as ordered by medical direction
Halcion			Establish IV access
Restoril			ECG monitor
Dalmane			Contact poison control
Centrax			
Ativan			
Serax			

**While PCP was originally an animal tranquilizer, it manifests hallucinogenic properties when used by humans. In addition to bizarre delusions, it can cause violent and dangerous outbursts of aggressive behavior. The rescuer is advised to remain safe when attempting to treat this type of overdose. PCP patients have been known to have almost superhuman strength and high pain tolerance.

***Deaths due to pure benzodiazepine are rare. Minor toxicity ranges are 500–1,500 mg. A benzodiazepine antagonist (Romazicon) is available (IV dosage 1–10 mg or infusion 0.5 mg/hr). It may cause seizures in a benzodiazepine dependent patient.

impaired, which increases the course and severity of intoxication. At low doses, alcohol has excitatory and stimulating effects, thus depressing inhibitions. At higher doses alcohol's depressive effect is more obvious. Alcohol abuse and dependence is called *alcoholism.* It is a major problem, contributing to highway traffic fatalities, drownings, burns, trauma, and drug overdoses.

Alcohol is completely absorbed from the stomach and intestinal tract in approximately 30 to 120 minutes after ingestion. Once absorbed, alcohol is distributed to all body tissues and fluids, with concentrations of alcohol in the brain rapidly approaching the alcohol level in the blood.

Some alcoholics will drink methanol (wood alcohol) or ethylene glycol (a component of antifreeze) if ethanol is unavailable. Ingestion of these chemicals can cause blindness or death.

In addition, alcohol causes a peripheral vasodilator effect on the cardiovascular system, resulting in flushing and a feeling of warmth. In cold conditions, alcohol's dilation of the blood vessels results in an increased loss of body heat. The diuretic effect seen when large amounts of alcohol are ingested is due to the inhibition of *vasopressin,* which is the hormone responsible for the conservation of body fluids. Without vasopressin, an increase in urine flow occurs. The "dry mouth syndrome" experienced after alcohol consumption may be the result of alcohol-induced cellular dehydration.

In addition, methanol will also cause visual disturbances, abdominal pain, and nausea and vomiting even at low doses. In fact, death has been reported after ingestion of only 15 mL of a 40 percent solution. Occasionally patients will complain of headache or dizziness and may even present with seizures and obtundation. Ethylene glycol ingestion has similar symptoms, but the CNS effects such as hallucinations, coma, and seizures are more pronounced in the early stages.

GENERAL ALCOHOLIC PROFILE

Most alcoholics are not unkempt street people but are functional people at all levels of society who are able to mask their addiction.

The classic alcoholic portrayed in movies is an unkempt, continually intoxicated street person who is completely nonfunctional. Although alcoholics of this type exist, it would be a grave error to consider this the typical picture of someone dependent on alcohol. More commonly, alcoholism is characterized by impaired control over drinking, preoccupation with the drug ethanol, use of ethanol despite adverse consequences, and distortions in thinking, such as denial. This is the definition used by the National Council on Alcoholism and Drug Dependence. Obviously, this definition applies to many people, including many functional people at all levels of society who have masked their addiction well. Take note of these warning signs, which may indicate alcohol abuse:

- Drinks early in the day
- Prone to drink alone and secretly
- Periodic binges (may last for several days)
- Partial or total loss of memory ("blackouts") during period of drinking
- Unexplained history of gastrointestinal problems (especially bleeding)
- "Green tongue syndrome" (using chlorophyll-containing substances to disguise the odor of alcohol on the breath)
- Cigarette burns on clothing
- Chronically flushed face and palms
- Tremulousness
- Odor of alcohol on breath under inappropriate conditions

CONSEQUENCES OF CHRONIC ALCOHOL INGESTION

Alcohol has many deleterious effects on the body. Chronic abuse can be devastating, affecting every organ system as shown in Figure 34-11 ■. Some of the more common effects include:

- Poor nutrition
- Alcohol hepatitis

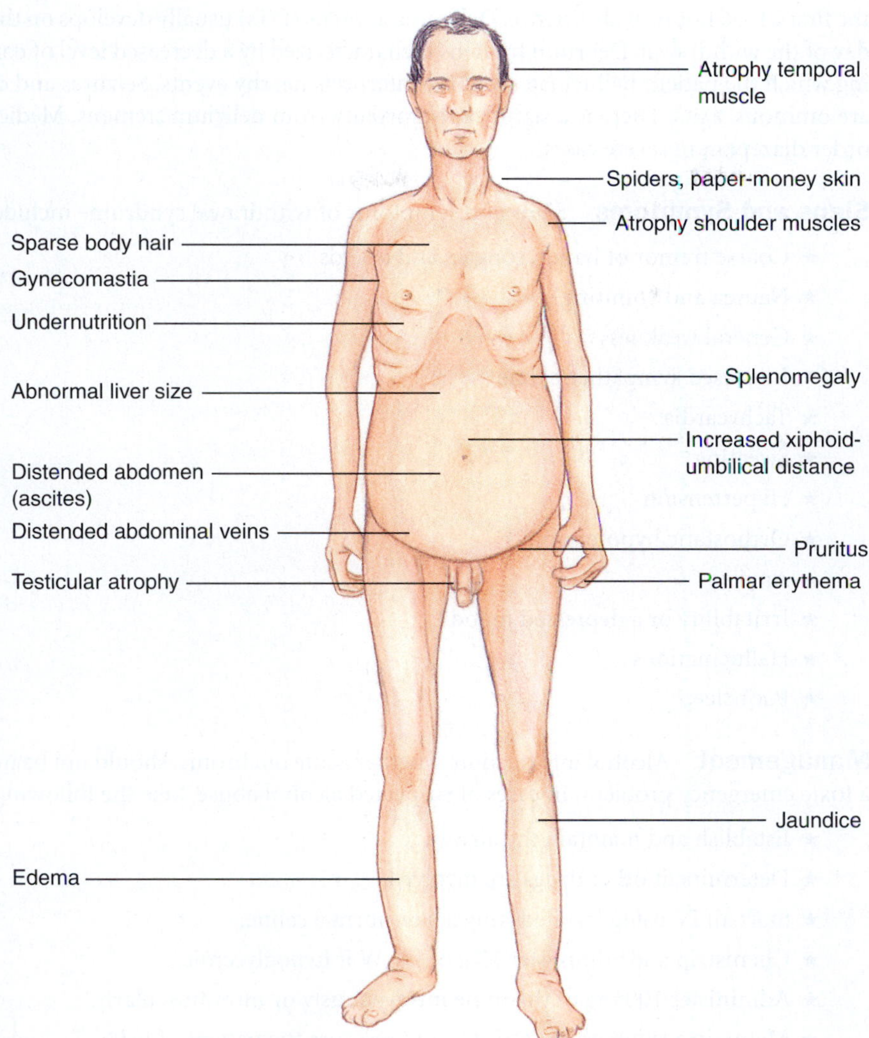

■ Figure 34-11 The chronic alcoholic.

★ Liver cirrhosis with subsequent esophageal varices
★ Loss of sensation in hands and feet
★ Loss of cerebellar function (balance and coordination)
★ Pancreatitis
★ Upper gastrointestinal hemorrhage (often fatal)
★ Hypoglycemia
★ Subdural hematoma (due to falls)
★ Rib and extremity fractures (due to falls)

Keep in mind that conditions such as subdural hematomas, sepsis, and other life-threatening disease processes may mimic the signs and symptoms of alcohol intoxication. For example, diabetic ketoacidosis produces a breath odor that can easily be confused with the odor of alcohol.

Conditions such as subdural hematomas, sepsis, and other diseases may mimic signs and symptoms of alcohol intoxication. For example, ketoacidosis produces an odor similar to alcohol on the breath.

Withdrawal Syndrome

The alcoholic may suffer a withdrawal reaction from either abrupt discontinuation of ingestion after prolonged use or from a rapid fall in blood alcohol level after acute intoxication. Alcohol withdrawal can be potentially fatal. Withdrawal symptoms can occur several hours after sudden abstinence and can last up to 5 to 7 days. Seizures (sometimes called "rum fits") may occur within

delirium tremens (DTs) *disorder found in habitual and excessive users of alcoholic beverages after cessation of drinking for 48–72 hours. Patients experience visual, tactile, and auditory disturbances. Death may result in severe cases.*

the first 24–36 hours of abstinence. **Delirium tremens (DTs)** usually develops on the second or third day of the withdrawal. Delirium tremens is characterized by a decreased level of consciousness during which the patient hallucinates and misinterprets nearby events. Seizures and delirium tremens are ominous signs. There is a significant mortality from delirium tremens. Medical direction may order diazepam in severe cases.

Signs and Symptoms Signs and symptoms of withdrawal syndrome include:

- ★ Coarse tremor of hands, tongue, and eyelids
- ★ Nausea and vomiting
- ★ General weakness
- ★ Increased sympathetic tone
- ★ Tachycardia
- ★ Sweating
- ★ Hypertension
- ★ Orthostatic hypotension
- ★ Anxiety
- ★ Irritability or a depressed mood
- ★ Hallucinations
- ★ Poor sleep

Do not underestimate alcohol intoxication as a toxic emergency.

Management Alcohol intoxication, whether acute or chronic, should not be underestimated as a toxic emergency problem. In cases of suspected alcohol abuse, take the following steps:

- ★ Establish and maintain the airway.
- ★ Determine if other drugs are involved.
- ★ Start an IV using lactated Ringer's or normal saline.
- ★ Chemstrip and administer 25 g of $D_{50}W$ if hypoglycemic.
- ★ Administer 100 mg of thiamine intravenously or intramuscularly.
- ★ Maintain a sympathetic attitude and reassure the patient of help.
- ★ Transport to the emergency department for further care.

Summary

Clearly, there is much to remember when dealing with toxicological emergencies. To effectively manage these situations you must focus on three things:

- ★ *Recognize the poisoning promptly.* In other words, you must have a high index of suspicion when circumstances suggest a toxin may be involved.
- ★ *Be thorough in your initial assessment and evaluation of the patient.* This will facilitate your efforts to identify the toxin and the measures needed to control the situation.
- ★ *Initiate the standard treatment procedures required for all toxicological emergencies.* Beyond the usual concern for rescuer safety and rapid implementation of ABCs and supportive measures, consider the methods needed to minimize any further exposure to the toxin, decontaminate the patient from the toxins already involved, and finally administer any useful antidote if one exists for the particular toxin.

If you remember these three steps, you will be equipped to handle most toxicological emergencies promptly and efficiently.

Review Questions

1. The American Association of Poison Control Centers estimates more than ___________ poisonings occur annually.
   a. 2 million
   b. 4 million
   c. 2 thousand
   d. 8 thousand
2. ___________ is the most common route of entry for toxic exposure.
   a. Injection
   b. Inhalation
   c. Ingestion
   d. Surface absorption
3. Common inhaled poisons include:
   a. Freon.
   b. chlorine.
   c. ammonia.
   d. all of the above.
4. The most effective and widely used method of reducing absorption of toxins is:
   a. gastric lavage.
   b. activated charcoal.
   c. syrup of ipecac.
   d. whole bowel irrigation.
5. Amitriptyline, amoxapine, clomipramine, doxepin, imipramine, and nortriptyline are common agents called:
   a. hydrocarbons.
   b. antiemetics.
   c. tricyclic antidepressants.
   d. calcium channel blockers.
6. In the treatment of bipolar disorder, no other drug has been proven to be more effective than:
   a. lithium.
   b. codeine.
   c. valium.
   d. dextromethorphan.
7. The most common pit viper is the:
   a. copperhead.
   b. rattlesnake.
   c. water moccasin.
   d. coral snake.
8. Because of the presence of neurotoxin, coral snake venom primarily affects ___________ tissue.
   a. cardiac
   b. nervous
   c. muscle
   d. skeletal
9. ___________ is(are) the most common substance of abuse in the United States and most of the world.
   a. Cocaine
   b. Alcohol
   c. Amphetamines
   d. Narcotics/opiates

10. In cases of poisoning, patient histories are often unreliable because of:
    a. deliberate deception.
    b. patient misinformation.
    c. drug-induced confusion.
    d. all of the above.

See Answers to Review Questions at the back of this book.

Chapter 35

Hematology

Objectives

After reading this chapter, you should be able to:

1. Identify the anatomy and physiology of the hematopoietic system. (see Chapter 3)
2. Discuss the following: (see Chapter 3)
   - ★ Plasma
   - ★ Red blood cells (erythrocytes)
   - ★ Hemoglobin
   - ★ Hematocrit
   - ★ White blood cells (leukocytes)
   - ★ Platelets, clotting, and fibrinolysis
   - ★ Hemostasis
3. Identify the following: (see Chapter 4)
   - ★ Inflammatory process
   - ★ Cellular and humoral immunity
   - ★ Alterations in immunological response
4. Identify blood groups. (pp. 1390–1391)
5. List erythrocyte disorders. (pp. 1397–1399)
6. List leukocyte disorders. (pp. 1399–1401)
7. List platelet and clotting disorders. (pp. 1401–1402)
8. Describe how acquired factor deficiencies may occur. (pp. 1401–1402)
9. Identify the components of the physical assessment as they relate to the hematology system. (pp. 1392–1396)
10. Describe the pathology and clinical manifestations and prognosis associated with:
    - ★ Anemia (pp. 1397–1398)
    - ★ Leukemia (p. 1400)
    - ★ Lymphomas (pp. 1400–1401)
    - ★ Polycythemia (p. 1399)
    - ★ Disseminated intravascular coagulopathy (p. 1402)
    - ★ Hemophilia (pp. 1401–1402)
    - ★ Sickle cell disease (pp. 1398–1399)
    - ★ Multiple myeloma (pp. 1402–1403)
11. Given several preprogrammed patients with hematological problems, provide the appropriate assessment, management, and transport. (pp. 1390–1403)

Key Terms

anemia, p. 1397
antigen, p. 1390
disseminated intravascular coagulation (DIC), p. 1402
hematology, p. 1390
hemophilia, p. 1401
leukemia, p. 1400
leukocytosis, p. 1399
leukopenia, p. 1399
lymphoma, p. 1400
multiple myeloma, p. 1402
neutropenia, p. 1399
polycythemia, p. 1397
sickle cell anemia, p. 1398
thrombocytopenia, p. 1401
thrombocytosis, p. 1401
von Willebrand's disease, p. 1402

INTRODUCTION

hematology *the study of blood and the blood-forming organs.*

Hematology is the study of the blood and the blood-forming organs. It exemplifies the way that multiple organ systems interact to maintain homeostasis, the normal balance of body functions. Hematological disorders are common and include red blood cell disorders, white blood cell disorders, platelet disorders, and coagulation problems. Although these disorders are common, they rarely are the primary cause of a medical emergency. They usually accompany other ongoing disease processes. Some hematological diseases are genetic in origin. Hemophilia A is a classic example. It is a sex-linked disease that causes abnormally low levels of an essential blood clotting protein (Factor VIII). It affects approximately 1–2 persons per 10,000 in the United States. Some hematological diseases are more common in certain ethnic groups. For example, among the population as a whole, sickle cell anemia is relatively uncommon. However, among African Americans specifically, 8 percent of the population has the sickle cell trait. In addition to their primary effects, hematological disorders may predispose patients to infection and intolerance to exercise, hypoxia, acidosis, and blood loss.

Patients with hematological problems often complain of signs and symptoms that do not point directly to a specific disease process. Careful examination and history taking may be necessary to further clarify the diagnosis. Often, however, laboratory findings will be needed to confirm the diagnosis. Thus, the final diagnosis of patients for whom you provide prehospital care is often not immediately apparent. You must use your assessment skills to recognize and treat injuries, pain, and instabilities, while formulating a field impression that enables you to anticipate further complications and thus enhance patient outcome and survivability. Because of this, it is essential that you have a good understanding of the basic pathophysiological processes of your patients' disease, including hematological disorders.

BLOOD PRODUCTS AND BLOOD TYPING

A blood transfusion is the transplantation of blood or a component of blood from one person to another. It is accomplished by IV infusion (Figure 35-1 ■). Various types of transfusions are given for various purposes (Table 35–1).

antigen *protein on the surface of a donor's red blood cells that the patient's body recognizes as "not self."*

In the 1800s when patients received blood from others, some had a reaction that led to multiple organ failure and death. Karl Landsteiner discovered the reason for this was reaction **antigens,** proteins on the surface of the donor's red blood cells that the patient's body recognized as "not self." Following transfusion, antibodies in the patient's own blood attacked the foreign antigens present in the transfused blood. Landsteiner named the antigens A and B and the opposing antibodies anti-A and anti-B. Someone with A antigen on his red blood cells would have anti-B antibodies. His blood type would be A. Someone with B antigens on the red blood cell surface would have anti-A antibodies; his type would be B. Some people's red blood cells have both antigens on their surface but neither antibody. Their blood type is AB. Others have neither antigen but both antibodies; their blood type is O (for zero antigens, but pronounced "Oh"). Blood type is an inherited trait. Approximately 45 percent of the U.S. population has type O, 39 percent type A, 11 percent type B, and 5 percent type AB.

Content Review

Blood Types

- A
- B
- AB
- O

Since only the antibodies recognize and attack foreign tissue, a person with no antibodies (type AB) can receive any blood type in an emergency, and the body will not attack the cells. So a person with type AB blood is called a *universal recipient.* Conversely, blood with no antigens to any other blood group type (type O) would not trigger a reaction, as the recipient's blood recognizes nothing "foreign." So people with type O blood are called *universal donors.*

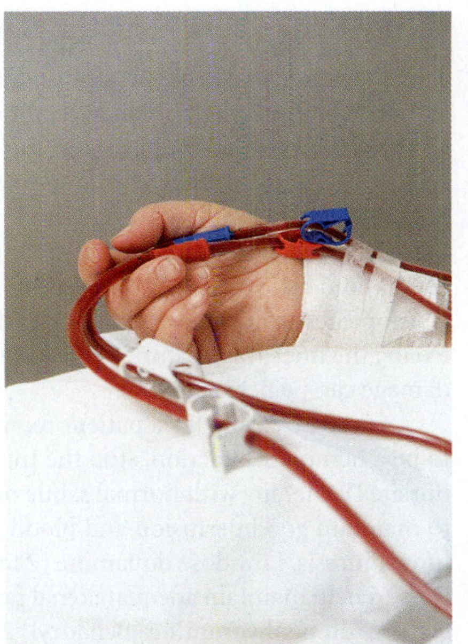

■ **Figure 35-1** Blood transfusion. *(© Gaillard/Jerrican/Photo Researchers, Inc.)*

Crossmatching blood involves checking samples from both donor and recipient to ensure the greatest compatibility. If a donor's blood does not clump together, or agglutinate, when mixed with the recipient's blood, they are compatible. Reliance on the universal donor and recipient concept is useful only in an emergency, when there is no time to check samples.

Blood transfusion is not as simple as that, however. Approximately 40 years after the discovery of A and B antigens, Landsteiner and A. S. Weiner observed another antigen present on red blood cells. Research leading to this antigen's discovery used rhesus monkey blood, so the antigen was called the Rh factor. If a person has the Rh factor, he is Rh positive; if not, he is Rh negative.

As many as 500 other lesser antigens have since been identified but they usually do not cause the severe hemolytic reaction seen in the patients sensitized to the Rh factor. *Erythroblastosis fetalis,* more commonly called hemolytic disease of the newborn, can lead to a fatal hemolytic reaction in neonates. In this disease, the mother who is Rh– is sensitized by previous exposure to the Rh antigen during a previous pregnancy with an Rh+ child or from a previous blood transfusion. Therefore, if she subsequently becomes pregnant with an Rh+ child, the mother produces antibodies that attack the fetus's red blood cells, leading to a severe and often fatal hemolytic reaction. Fortunately, the incidence of hemolytic disease of newborns has been declining due to the administration of Rh immune globulin (RhoGAM) to mothers. This inhibits formation of anti-Rh antibodies. Additionally, transfusions in *utero* or fetal exchange transfusions immediately after birth can diminish or eliminate the likelihood of infant death.

Table 35–1 Types of Transfusions

Type of Transfusion	Contents	Use
Whole blood	All cells, platelets, clotting factors, and plasma	Replace blood loss from hemorrhage
Packed red blood cells (PRBCs)	Red blood cells and some plasma	Replace red blood cells in anemic patients
Platelets	Thrombocytes and some plasma	Replace platelets in a patient with thrombocytopenia
Fresh frozen plasma (FFP)	Plasma, a combination of fluids, clotting factors, and proteins	Replace volume in a burn patient or in hypovolemia secondary to low oncotic pressure
Clotting factors	Specific clotting factors needed for coagulation	Replace factors missing due to inadequate production as in hemophilia

TRANSFUSION REACTIONS

There are many types of transfusion reactions. One, hemolytic transfusion reaction, occurs when a donor's and recipient's blood are not compatible. Antigens on the donor's red blood cells trigger a response from the antibodies in the recipient's blood. The antibodies attach to the red blood cells, which are then *hemolyzed,* or taken up by the fixed macrophages of the spleen's reticuloendothelial system.

Signs and symptoms of a hemolytic transfusion reaction may include facial flushing, hyperventilation, tachycardia, and a sense of dread. Hives may appear on the skin, and the patient may develop chest pain, wheezing, fever, chills, and cyanosis. Flank pain may occur as small clots begin to clog the microvasculature of the kidneys, which can lead to kidney failure requiring dialysis. The damage can be permanent.

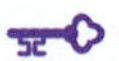

If a patient receiving a blood transfusion develops what you believe to be a hemolytic reaction, stop the transfusion immediately.

If you are caring for a patient receiving a blood transfusion and he develops what you believe to be a hemolytic reaction, stop the transfusion immediately. Change all associated IV tubing and initiate IV therapy with normal saline or lactated Ringer's solution. Administer a bolus as necessary to maintain good perfusion and blood pressure. Furosemide (Lasix) is often administered to promote diuresis. Low dose dopamine (2 to 5 mcg/kg/minute) should be considered along with the IV fluid to help maintain adequate renal perfusion. If you observe evidence of an allergic reaction, you can give diphenhydramine (Benadryl) 25 to 50 mg IV to help with some of the histamine-mediated effects such as itching or hives. In extreme cases of anaphylactic reaction, you may need to administer IV epinephrine if the patient is hypotensive or demonstrates severe bronchospasm.

The most common transfusion reaction is the febrile nonhemolytic reaction. It is caused by sensitization to antigens on the white blood cells, platelets, or plasma proteins. Signs and symptoms include headache, fever, and chills. As with any other transfusion reaction, always stop the transfusion before attempting to treat it. After stopping the blood product, change all tubing, and initiate normal saline IV. Patients are often given diphenhydramine (Benadryl) and an antipyretic (ibuprofen, acetaminophen) for the fever. No further treatment may be necessary, as this reaction rarely progresses to more serious complications. However, close observation is required to exclude development of a hemolytic reaction. In the event of any transfusion reaction, return all blood bags, tubing, and filters to the blood bank for analysis. Medical direction may order you to take blood and urine samples.

Because blood transfusion adds fluid to the system, a patient may experience signs and symptoms of circulatory overload. In fact, signs and symptoms are the same as those for left ventricular failure and may include pulmonary edema, dyspnea, and chest pain. Hypotension is not usually a problem, and you may treat the patient successfully by slowing the heart rate and administering diuretics.

GENERAL ASSESSMENT AND MANAGEMENT

In general, patients with disorders of the hematopoietic system may present with a variety of complaints and physical findings. Patients with infection, white blood cell abnormalities (immunocompromised and prone to infection), or transfusion reactions may present with febrile symptoms. Subsequently, these patients may develop hemodynamic instability as infection progresses to sepsis or as the transfusion reaction leads to a hemolytic reaction, renal failure, and disseminated intravascular coagulation (DIC). Acute hemodynamic compromise can also be found in patients with anemia secondary to acute blood loss, coagulation defects, or autoimmune disease. These disease processes may not be easily differentiated in the field and often require significant laboratory testing to confirm the diagnosis. In most cases, however, if you obtain a careful history, you will have a good working diagnosis.

Most hematopoietic disorders are chronic conditions that present with acute exacerbation when the patient is exposed to an additional stress such as infection or trauma. Treatment of patients with disorders of the hematopoietic system, in most cases, is supportive. Some patients may have hemodynamic instability from blood or fluid loss. These patients may require intravenous fluids to support end-organ perfusion and prevent shock. In addition, they should receive oxygen therapy to prevent hypoxia from poor perfusion and diminished oxygen-carrying capacity of the blood. It is important to recognize the need for rapid transport in patients with hemodynamic instability who may require transfusion or other definitive care measures. Always contact medical direction for questions or problems.

SCENE SIZE-UP

Assessment of the patient with a possible hematopoietic abnormality begins the same as for any other patient. Perform a scene size-up and use Standard Precautions. During your approach, form a general impression of the patient. Is the patient a trauma or medical patient? In how much distress is the patient?

PRIMARY ASSESSMENT

Complete a primary assessment for life threats. Determine responsiveness and assess the airway, breathing, and circulation. Alterations in the hematopoietic system may present as life-threatening bleeds or overwhelming infections with septic shock. Do not spend time obtaining a complete set of vital signs during the primary assessment. Check the ABCs and quickly determine your priority for transport. Critical or unstable patients should be considered candidates for expeditious transport.

SECONDARY ASSESSMENT

Next, complete a secondary assessment. Use your general impression to choose a format for a responsive or unresponsive medical patient or trauma patient with significant or nonsignificant mechanism of injury. Each format follows a sequence of history gathering and examination designed to meet the needs of that particular patient. Trauma patients and unresponsive medical patients often present life-threatening problems that are noted in your primary assessment.

SAMPLE History

For a responsive medical patient, obtain a SAMPLE history and perform a physical exam. Obtain a set of vital signs and place the pulse oximeter. Keep in mind that an anemic patient will have increased heart and respiratory rates as his body attempts to compensate for less oxygen reaching the tissues. Ask for the chief complaint—why did the patient call for assistance? What signs or symptoms (SAMPLE) accompanied or preceded the complaint? Pay attention to generalized complaints such as fatigue, lethargy, malaise, apprehension, or confusion. These may indicate inadequate oxygen delivery to the tissues. Have there been any unusual skin changes such as coloring or bruising? Does the patient complain of itching? Inquire about lymph node enlargement (swollen glands), sore throat, or pain on swallowing. These may indicate infection.

Any change in the blood's ability to deliver oxygen to the body will appear in the cardiovascular and respiratory systems. Note dyspnea, palpitations, and dizziness with changes in the patient's position. Patients with hematological problems may suffer syncope. Did the patient have a syncopal episode or is he just weak? Syncope can be due to several factors but is often related to a sudden change in position in a patient who has a marked anemia. Bleeding abnormalities may be disguised as gastrointestinal upset. Ask about overt bleeding with vomiting or diarrhea, but do not overlook complaints of nausea or anorexia, vomiting of "coffee ground" material, or having black tarry or cranberry, sticky, odoriferous stools. Many patients will notice bleeding of the gums when they brush their teeth. This can, on occasion, be hard to control. Atraumatic bleeding of the gums almost always points to an underlying hematologic abnormality. Ask about changes in urination, hematuria (blood in the urine), and alterations in the usual menstrual pattern in females. Keep in mind that hematological disorders are often diagnosed when the patient seeks assistance for another medical condition.

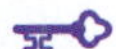

Keep in mind that hematological disorders are often diagnosed when the patient seeks assistance for another medical condition.

Determine any allergies (SAMPLE). Be sure to ask about use of prescription or over-the-counter medications (SAMPLE). Make note of the patient's medication, dose, and the condition for which he takes the medication. Also, if time allows, note the dosing schedule of the medications. Ask about compliance. Does the patient take medication as prescribed? When was the last dose taken? Medications that may indicate an alteration in the hematologic system, or that might make the patient more susceptible to an alteration in the system, include pain relievers, antibiotics, anticoagulants, hormones, and medications for heart disease, arthritis, and seizures.

When asking about past medical history (SAMPLE), make note of surgeries such as a splenectomy, heart-valve replacement, or placement of long-term venous-access devices. Ask about bloodborne infections such as HIV or hepatitis B or C. Make note of liver or bone marrow disease or cancers. Include questions about family history such as hemophilia, sickle cell disease, cancer, or death at an early age that was not trauma related. Inquire also about social habits such as smoking, alcohol consumption, IV drug use, or long-term exposure to chemicals or radiation.

If you find a significant history, ask about the last episode of an incident or last use of a medication. Remember to include the usual questions about last oral intake (SAMPLE). Also, inquire about any unusual events (SAMPLE) that preceded the onset of the complaint such as the start of a new medication, recent transfusion, fall, or injury.

Physical Exam

When performing the physical exam, evaluate each system methodically as you would in any other patient. If the history suggests a hematopoietic problem, look for potential pathology during the physical exam that may confirm your working diagnosis and be a clue to developing complications.

- ★ *Nervous system.* Always evaluate the nervous system in any patient with a suspected hematological problem. First, note the patient's level of consciousness using the AVPU system. Be alert for other nervous system disorders. Many patients with hematological problems will complain of being "weak and dizzy." Try to clarify this further. Is the patient fatigued, weak all over, or does he have focal weakness? Is he dizzy or is he suffering true vertigo? Both can be associated with hematological problems such as anemia. Ask if the patient has any numbness or motor deficits. Pernicious anemia can cause sensory deficits that are often unilateral. Try to determine whether the patient had a syncopal episode. What were the patient's condition and position immediately prior to the syncopal episode? Many of the hematological diseases, especially the autoimmune diseases, will affect the eye. Always examine the eyes for abnormalities. Question the patient about any visual disturbances or visual loss. In addition to the autoimmune diseases, sickle cell anemia is notorious for causing eye problems.
- ★ *Skin.* Note the patient's skin color (Figure 35-2 ■). Jaundice (yellow skin) may indicate liver disease or hemolysis of red blood cells, while a florid (reddish) appearance is often associated with polycythemia. Patients with anemia typically exhibit pallor. Observe for petechiae (tiny red dots in the skin), purpura (large purplish blotches related to multiple hemorrhages into the skin), and bruising. Inquire about pruritus (itching). Patients with hematological disorders often develop pruritus. Some hematological problems, such as sickle cell anemia, cause the destruction of red blood cells. This results in hemoglobin's spilling into the circulatory system. Macrophages then break down the hemoglobin. The iron is removed and transported to the bones or liver. The porphyrin portion of the hemoglobin is subsequently converted into bilirubin, which is taken up by the liver. An excess of bilirubin, either from liver disease or from the breakdown of hemoglobin associated with the hemolytic anemias, can cause pruritis. Often, patients will develop itching over a bruise. As the hemoglobin breaks down within the bruise, the localized accumulation of bilirubin causes the itching. This is most common 1 to 2 weeks after the bruise occurs. When examining the skin, be alert for any evidence of prolonged bleeding. The patient may have several bandages over relatively minor wounds where he could not stop the bleeding.
- ★ *Lymphatic.* The lymphatic system is affected early in hematopoietic diseases, especially those of the immune system. During your physical exam, pay particular attention to the lymph nodes. Palpate the lymph nodes of the neck, clavicle, axilla, and groin. Note any enlargement. Compare sides. Splenomegaly (an enlarged spleen) is also often present, but this can be hard to examine in the field.
- ★ *Gastrointestinal.* The gastrointestinal effects of hematological problems can be quite varied. Epistaxis (nosebleed) is common. The nasal mucosa is quite vascular as it warms and humidifies the inhaled air. A slight crack in the nasal mucosa can result in brisk bleeding. This is a particular problem in people with blood clotting abnormalities, as stopping the bleeding is very difficult for them. These patients may

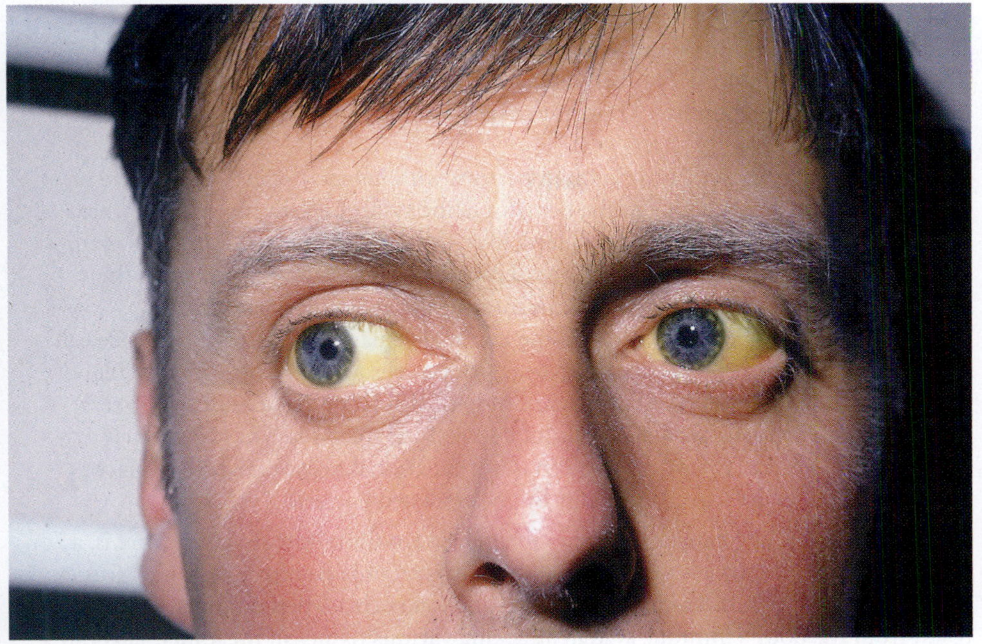

(A)

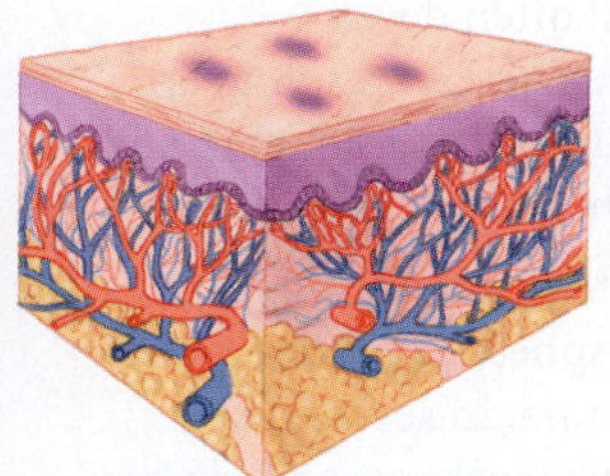

Petechiae – Reddish-purple spots, diameter less than 0.5 cm

(B)

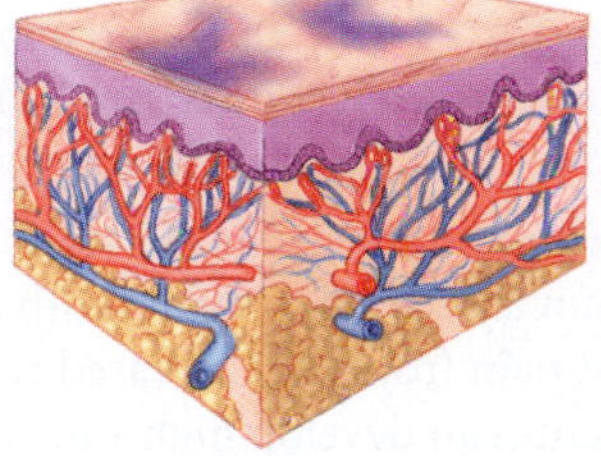

Purpura – Reddish-purple blotches, diameter more than 0.5 cm

(C)

■ **Figure 35-2** Abnormal skin colors: (A)jaundice, (B)petechiae, (C)purpura. *(John Callan/Shout Picture Library)*

swallow a great deal of blood and may become nauseated. Also, blood acts as a cathartic (laxative). Patients who swallow even moderate amounts of blood will often report loose bowel movements. These are often dark (melena). Blood present in emesis may be bright red or appear like coffee grounds.

Bleeding of the gums is one of the earliest findings of hematological problems. Patients with blood clotting abnormalities and low platelet levels will often develop atraumatic bleeding of the gums. Any patient with bleeding gums requires a detailed investigation for a possible hematological disorder. Gingivitis (infection of the gums) can be due to poor hygiene, disease, or both. However, chronic gingivitis should cause increased suspicion of a hematological disorder, especially involving the immune system. Also, gingivitis increases a patient's risk of developing sepsis. Slight trauma, such as brushing the teeth, can cause the bacteria to enter the circulatory system, resulting in generalized sepsis. Always note the presence of gingivitis when examining for bleeding gums. Ulcerations of the gums and oral mucosa are typically due to viral diseases. These infections are more common in immunosuppressed patients. Thrush (yeast infection in the mouth) in adults is almost always associated with AIDS. (Thrush in children is common and not a reason for concern.)

Bleeding gums are often associated with a decreased platelet count.

An oral yeast infection in an adult is commonly associated with AIDS.

The liver plays a major role in manufacturing many of the substances required for blood clotting. Liver disease can slow blood clotting. This is most evident in a prolonged prothrombin (PT) time. Also, as the liver fails, the bilirubin level will increase, resulting in jaundice. Thus, any patient with jaundice should be evaluated for liver disease.

Abdominal pain is not uncommon in persons with hematological disease. Two of the major organs associated with the hematopoeitic system, the liver and spleen, are in the abdomen. Problems with the spleen, liver, or both can lead to abdominal pain. Splenomegaly is common in hematological problems, as the spleen is active in the removal of abnormal or aged red cells. In some of the anemias, especially the hemolytic anemias, the spleen can become markedly enlarged. Patients with sickle cell anemia will often develop splenic infarcts as sickled cells accumulate and block blood supply to parts of the spleen. By the time children with sickle cell disease are 5 years of age, they are virtually asplenic (without a spleen), as the disease has completely infarcted their spleen. Because the spleen is not functional, these patients are placed at increased risk of infection, especially by encapsulated bacteria.

- ★ *Musculoskeletal.* Many hematopoietic problems are autoimmune in nature. That is, a problem develops in which the immune system has trouble determining which tissues are self and which are nonself. Autoimmune diseases such as rheumatoid arthritis result from the body's immune system attacking various tissues in the joints. This can cause arthralgia (pain and swelling of the joints). Autoimmune diseases tend to affect more than one joint, whereas infectious processes tend to affect only a single joint. Patients with blood clotting disorders such as hemophilia will often develop hemarthrosis (bleeding into a joint) with only minor trauma. This can result in an extremely swollen, discolored, and painful joint. Always inquire about joint pain and examine the major joints in any patient suspected of having hematopoietic disease.

Be alert for high-output heart failure in patients with severe anemia.

- ★ *Cardiorespiratory.* The effects of hematopoietic problems on the cardiorespiratory system are varied. Patients with anemia will often develop dyspnea, tachycardia, and chest pain from the increased cardiac work caused by the anemia. In severe cases, patients can develop high-output heart failure, where the heart works excessively hard to compensate for a profound anemia. If untreated, heart failure and pulmonary edema can result. Patients with bleeding disorders may report expectorating blood with coughing. This can be due to small tears in the respiratory mucosa from the coughing. Normally, these heal quickly. Patients with bleeding disorders, however, will continue to bleed, resulting in potential airway obstruction and, in severe cases, shock. Always auscultate for breath sounds. Note crackles or rhonchi indicative of heart problems or infection.

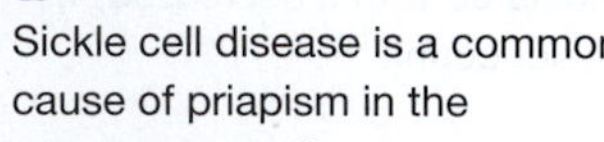

Sickle cell disease is a common cause of priapism in the emergency setting.

- ★ *Genitourinary.* The genitourinary effects of hematopoietic problems are typically due to bleeding disorders or infection. Bleeding disorders can cause hematuria (blood in the urine) and blood in the scrotal sac in males. A woman who still has her uterus may develop menorrhagia (heavy menstrual bleeding) or frank vaginal bleeding (dysfunctional uterine bleeding). Immunocompromised patients are at increased risk for developing genitourinary infections. These can range from recurrent urinary tract infections to severe sexually transmitted diseases. Sickle cell anemia, especially in the later stages, can cause priapism. This is a prolonged, painful erection due to obstruction of the blood vessels that drain the penis and allow for detumescence. Sickle cell disease is the most common cause of priapism in the emergency setting. All of these require additional evaluation in the emergency department. Detailed evaluation of the genitourinary system is not appropriate for field settings.

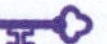

Pay close attention to the airway and ventilation status of patients experiencing any alteration in the hematopoietic system.

GENERAL MANAGEMENT OF HEMATOPOIETIC EMERGENCIES

Pay close attention to the airway and ventilation status of patients experiencing any alteration in the hematopoietic system. Place the patient on high-flow, high-concentration supplemental oxygen and monitor breathing for difficulty or fatigue. Be ready to assist ventilations with a bag-valve-mask.

Assess the circulatory system. Consider fluid volume replacement, but remember that crystalloid solutions cannot carry oxygen. Too much fluid can "dilute" the blood and reduce its capacity per unit volume to carry oxygen. Be alert for dysrhythmias and treat accordingly. Based on your assessment and evaluation, create the optimum environment for the blood to perform its tasks of oxygen delivery and waste product removal. Creating such an environment may include giving the patient aspirin to inhibit platelet aggregation or ventilating the patient to compensate for acidosis and to allow oxygen to unload from hemoglobin at the tissues.

Transport the patient to the appropriate facility, provide comfort measures including analgesia, and provide psychological support to both the patient and his family.

MANAGING SPECIFIC PATIENT PROBLEMS

The rest of this chapter will detail the more common hematopoietic diseases that you might encounter in prehospital care. Again, it is important to remember that many hematological problems occur in conjunction with other illnesses. For example, someone with a cancer or significant renal disease quite commonly will have a coexisting anemia. In the following sections we will first examine diseases of the red blood cells. These are the most common hematological problems encountered. Second, we will look at the white blood cell diseases. These include the leukemias, lymphomas, and similar illnesses. Finally, we will present diseases of the platelets and blood coagulation disorders.

Remember that many hematological problems occur in conjunction with other illnesses.

DISEASES OF THE RED BLOOD CELLS

Red blood cell diseases result in too many red blood cells, too few red blood cells, or improperly functioning red blood cells. An excess of red blood cells is called **polycythemia.** Although uncommon, several conditions can cause polycythemia. An inadequate number of red blood cells or inadequate hemoglobin within the red blood cells is called **anemia.** Anemia is common, and several types are frequently encountered. Finally, red blood cell function can be impaired. Most commonly, this is due to problems with either hemoglobin structure and function or with the red blood cell membrane. Problems with red blood cell function include the thalassemias and sickle cell anemia.

polycythemia *an excess of red blood cells.*

anemia *an inadequate number of red blood cells or inadequate hemoglobin within the red blood cells.*

Content Review

Diseases of the Red Blood Cells

- Anemia
- Sickle cell disease
- Polycythemia

Anemias

The most common diseases of the red blood cells are the anemias. Anemia is typically classified as a hematocrit of less than 37 percent in women or less than 40 percent in men. Most patients with anemia will remain asymptomatic until the hematocrit drops below 30 percent. The decreased hematocrit in anemia is due to a reduction in the number of red blood cells or in the amount or quality of hemoglobin in the red blood cells. Anemia is actually a sign of an underlying disease process that is either destroying red blood cells and hemoglobin or decreasing the production of red blood cells and hemoglobin. Blood loss, either acute or chronic, also can cause anemia. Anemia can be a self-limited disease or it can be a lifelong illness requiring periodic transfusions. Anemias that result from the destruction of red blood cells are called hemolytic anemias. These can be hereditary or acquired. Examples of hereditary hemolytic anemias include sickle cell anemia, thalassemia, and glucose-6-phosphate dehydrogenase deficiency (G6PD). Acquired hemolytic anemias can result from immune system disorders, drug effects, or environmental effects. Anemias caused by inadequate red blood cell production include such problems as iron deficiency anemia, pernicious anemia, and anemia of chronic disease. Table 35–2 shows the numerous types of anemia, all of which must be confirmed by laboratory diagnosis.

Anemia is a sign, not a disease process in itself. Since the red blood cells' primary purpose is to transport oxygen, anemia results in hypoxia. The signs and symptoms of anemia vary, depending on the rapidity of its onset and on the patient's age and underlying general health. A mild anemia may not exhibit signs or symptoms until the body is stressed, as during exercise. Then a mild dyspnea, fatigue, palpitations, and syncope may be present. Chronic anemias may present signs or symptoms of pica (the craving of unusual substances such as clay or ice), headache, dizziness, ringing in the ears, irritability or difficulty concentrating, pallor, and tachycardia. Angina pectoris can be an important indicator.

Table 35–2 Types of Anemia

Cause	Type	Pathophysiology
Inadequate production of red blood cells	Aplastic	Failure to produce red blood cells
	Iron deficiency	Iron is primary component of hemoglobin
	Pernicious	Vitamin B_{12} is necessary for correct red blood cell division during its development
	Sickle cell	Genetic alteration causes production of a hemoglobin that changes shape of red blood cell to a *C*, or sickle, in low oxygen states
Increased red blood cell destruction	Hemolytic	Body destroys red blood cells at greater rate than production; red blood cell parts interfere with blood flow
Blood cell loss or dilution	Chronic disease	Hemorrhage leads to cell loss while excessive fluid leads to a dilution of red blood cell concentration

If anemia develops rapidly, the body does not have time to compensate for the change. Signs and symptoms of shock may be present, including postural hypotension and decreased cardiac output, resulting in a shunting of blood away from the periphery to the heart, lungs, and brain. Compensatory mechanisms can cause diaphoresis, pallor, cool skin, anxiety, thirst, and air hunger. If the anemia's onset is slower, the body can adjust to oxygen's reduced availability with a right shift of the oxyhemoglobin dissociation curve and an increase in plasma volume.

Prehospital treatment of anemia is primarily symptomatic. Direct your attention at maximizing oxygenation, stemming blood loss, and transporting to a medical facility for treatment of the cause. Start volume replacement if there is evidence of dehydration.

Sickle Cell Disease

sickle cell anemia *an inherited disorder of red blood cell production, so named because the red blood cells become sickle-shaped when oxygen levels are low.*

Sickle cell anemia, often termed "sickle cell disease," is a disorder of red blood cell production. Normal hemoglobin is very flexible, and the red blood cell can pass easily through the tiny capillaries. Sickle hemoglobin has an abnormal chemical sequence that gives red blood cells a *C*, or sickle, shape when oxygen levels are low (Figure 35-3 ■). Patients with sickle cell disease will have a chronic anemia that results from destruction of abnormal red blood cells (hemolytic anemia). The average life span of sickled red blood cells is 10 to 20 days compared to 120 days for normal red blood cells. In addition, sickled red blood cells increase the blood's viscosity, leading to sludging and obstruction of the capillaries and small blood vessels. Blockage of blood flow to various tissues and organs is common and usually occurs following a period of stress. This process, called a vasoocclusive crisis, is characteristic of sickle cell anemia. Because of the vasoocclusive crisis, tissues and organs are eventually damaged. Adult sickle cell patients often have multiple organ problems, including cardiopulmonary disease, renal disease, and neurological disorders.

Sickle cell disease is inherited. It primarily affects African Americans although other ethnic groups can be affected. These include Puerto Ricans and people of Spanish, French, Italian, Greek, and Turkish heritage. If both parents carry a gene for sickle cell anemia, the chances are 1 in 4 that the child will have normal hemoglobin. The chances are 2 in 4 that he will have both normal hemoglobin and sickle hemoglobin, which is referred to as *sickle cell trait.* The chances are 1 in 4 that he will have only sickle hemoglobin (no normal hemoglobin). This condition is referred to as *sickle cell disease.*

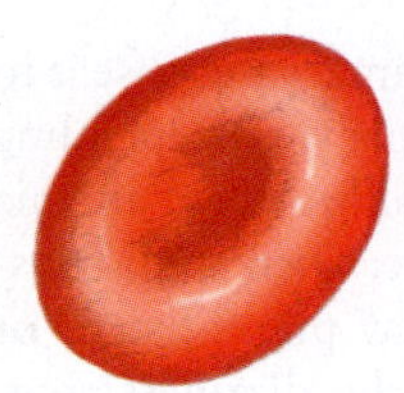

■ Figure 35-3 A normal red blood cell contrasted with a sickle cell.

Patients with sickle cell disease will develop three types of problems. *Vasoocclusive crises* cause musculoskeletal pain, abdominal pain, priapisms, pulmonary problems, renal crises (renal infarctions), and central nervous system crises (cerebral infarctions). In addition, they will develop *hematological crises* that consist of a fall in the hemoglobin level, sequestration of red blood cells in the spleen, and problems with bone marrow function. In severe cases, the bone marrow can shut down, causing an aplastic crisis. These are usually self-limited. Finally, sickle cell patients often develop *infectious crises.* They are functionally immunosuppressed, and the loss of splenic function makes them particularly vulnerable to encapsulated bacteria. Infections become common and are often the cause of death in sickle cell anemia.

Content Review

Sickle Cell Crises

- Vasoocclusive
- Hematological
- Infectious

Prehospital care for patients in sickle cell crisis is primarily supportive. Begin high-flow, high-concentration oxygen to saturate as much hemoglobin as possible. Initiate IV therapy with an isotonic crystalloid solution. These patients are often dehydrated and hydration will sometimes help with the vasoocclusive process. Venous access is sometimes difficult in older patients with sickle cell disease due to the large number of IV starts they have required in their lifetime. Placing a central line is occasionally necessary. Vasoocclusive crises can be extremely painful. Start analgesic therapy in the field, if possible. Often these patients will require large amounts of narcotics for pain control. Always consult medical direction if there is a question regarding management. Transport is indicated.

Polycythemia

Polycythemia is an abnormally high hematocrit. It is due to excess production of red blood cells. Polycythemia is a relatively rare disorder and typically occurs in patients 50 years of age or older. It can occur secondarily to dehydration. The increased red blood cell load increases the patient's risk of thrombosis. Most deaths from polycythemia are due to thrombosis.

Polycythemia's signs and symptoms vary. The principal finding is a hematocrit of 50 percent or greater. The patient will usually have an increased number of white blood cells and platelets. However, the large number of red blood cells may cause a platelet dysfunction. This can result in bleeding abnormalities such as epistaxis, spontaneous bruising, and gastrointestinal bleeding. Patients with polycythemia may complain of headache, dizziness, blurred vision, itching, and gastrointestinal disease. Severe cases can result in congestive heart failure.

The prehospital treatment of polycythemia is supportive. Ensure that the airway and breathing are adequate. Administer supplemental oxygen as required. Initiate an IV with an isotonic crystalloid solution. The principal treatment is phlebotomy, which removes excess red blood cells.

DISEASES OF THE WHITE BLOOD CELLS

The white blood cells are the body's principal defense system. Problems with white blood cells typically result from too few white blood cells (**leukopenia**), too many white blood cells (**leukocytosis**), or improper white blood cell function. The neutrophil is the main blood component protecting against a bacterial or fungal infection. A reduction in the number of neutrophils (**neutropenia**) predisposes the patient to bacterial and fungal infections.

leukopenia *too few white blood cells.*

leukocytosis *too many white blood cells.*

neutropenia *a reduction in the number of neutrophils.*

Leukopenia/Neutropenia

The status of the white blood cells is easily determined by obtaining a complete blood count. A normal white blood cell count ranges from 5,000 to 9,000 per cubic millimeter of blood. A decrease in the number of white blood cells indicates a problem with white blood cell production in the marrow or destruction of white blood cells. Because bacterial infections pose a major risk to humans, an absolute neutrophil count is a better indicator of the immune system's status. The prehospital treatment of leukopenia/neutropenia is supportive. Pay special attention to preventing infection in the patient, as his immune system is overstressed or may be functioning inadequately.

Content Review

Diseases of the White Blood Cells

- Leukopenia/neutropenia
- Leukocytosis
- Leukemia
- Lymphoma

Leukocytosis

Leukocytosis is an increase in the number of circulating white blood cells. This occurs when the body is exposed to an infectious agent or is particularly stressed. Following exposure, the immune system is stimulated and the marrow and spleen start releasing white blood cells to help the body fight infection. A white blood cell count between 10,800 and 23,000 per cubic millimeter of blood is characteristic of a bacterial infection. During periods of stress, immature neutrophils may be released into the circulation. These differ from mature neutrophils in that they have a segmented nucleus. These cells are referred to as "bands" or "segs." An increase in the number of bands is indicative of a significant bacterial infection. Causes of leukocytosis include bacterial infection, rheumatoid arthritis, DKA, leukemia, pain, and exercise. Viral infections tend to have little effect on the white blood cell count or, in some cases, actually cause a decrease in the white blood cell count. A white blood cell count greater than 30,000 per cubic millimeter is called a *leukemoid reaction.* A white blood cell count this high indicates a problem with excess white blood cell production. Any patient with a significantly elevated white blood cell count should be evaluated for possible leukemia.

Leukemia

leukemia *a cancer of the hematopoietic cells.*

Leukemias are cancers of hematopoietic cells. Precursors of white blood cells in the bone marrow begin to replicate abnormally. The cells proliferate initially in the bone marrow and then spread to the peripheral blood. Leukemias affect approximately 13 in 100,000 persons. They are classified by the type of cell or cells involved. The most common types of leukemia are:

- ★ Acute lymphocytic leukemia (ALL)
- ★ Acute myelogenous leukemia (AML)
- ★ Chronic lymphocytic leukemia (CLL)
- ★ Chronic myelogenous leukemia (CML)
- ★ Hairy cell leukemia

Discussion of the pathology of the various leukemias is not within the scope of this text. ALL is primarily a disease of children and young adults. CML occurs in both children and adults. AML, CLL, and hairy cell leukemia tend to occur in the sixth and seventh decades of life. Medicine has made significant advances in the treatment of leukemia. Treatments such as chemotherapy, radiation therapy, and bone marrow transplantation have resulted in cures of certain types of leukemias. The treatment of pediatric leukemia is one of the great successes of modern medicine. More than 50 percent of pediatric patients with ALL live a normal life with the disease in remission or cured. Infections are a common complication of leukemia, primarily due to the low number of circulating neutrophils. Deaths from leukemias are typically secondary to infection or bleeding.

The signs and symptoms of leukemia vary. Most patients will have a moderate to severe anemia as the cancerous cell production overwhelms the bone marrow. Thrombocytopenia (an abnormal decrease in platelets) is common for the same reason. Many leukemia patients will present with bleeding, usually due to the thrombocytopenia. With the initial presentation, leukemia patients will appear acutely ill. They will be febrile and weak, usually due to a secondary infection. Various lymph nodes may be enlarged. Patients often have a history of weight loss and anorexia. In addition, liver and spleen enlargement are typical, resulting in a sensation of abdominal fullness or abdominal pain. The sternum may be tender, secondary to the increased bone marrow activity. Fatigue is a common complaint.

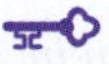

Employ proper isolation techniques for leukemia patients, who are at increased risk of developing infection.

The prehospital treatment of the patient with leukemia is primarily supportive. Place the patient in a position of comfort. Administer supplemental oxygen via a nonrebreather mask. Initiate an IV with an isotonic crystalloid solution such as lactated Ringer's or normal saline. Consider a fluid bolus if the patient is dehydrated. If the patient is having pain secondary to the leukemia, consider administration of an analgesic. Remember, leukemia patients are at increased risk of developing infection. Employ proper isolation techniques.

Lymphomas

lymphoma *a cancer of the lymphatic system.*

Lymphomas are cancers of the lymphatic system. Malignant lymphoma is typically classified as follows:

- ★ Hodgkin's lymphoma
- ★ Non-Hodgkin's lymphoma

Malignant lymphoma is classified by the cell type involved, which indicates the stem cell from which the malignancy arises. In the United States, each year approximately 40,000 persons are diagnosed with non-Hodgkin's lymphoma, and 7,500 are diagnosed with Hodgkin's lymphoma. The long-term survival rate is much better with Hodgkin's lymphoma. In fact, many patients with Hodgkin's lymphoma who have been treated with radiation, chemotherapy, or both are considered cured.

The most common presenting sign of non-Hodgkin's lymphoma is painless swelling of the lymph nodes. The majority of patients with Hodgkin's lymphoma typically have no related symptoms. Patients with lymphoma may report fever, night sweats, anorexia, weight loss, fatigue, and pruritis. Treat patients with lymphomas symptomatically. Place the patient in a position of comfort. Administer supplemental oxygen via a nonrebreather mask. Initiate an IV with an isotonic crystalloid solution such as lactated Ringer's or normal saline. Consider a fluid bolus if the patient is dehydrated. If the patient is having pain secondary to the lymphoma, consider administration of an analgesic. As with leukemia patients, lymphoma patients are at increased risk of developing infection. Employ proper isolation techniques.

Lymphoma patients are at increased risk of developing infection. Use proper isolation techniques.

DISEASES OF THE PLATELETS/ BLOOD CLOTTING ABNORMALITIES

Content Review

Platelet Abnormalities

- Thrombocytosis
- Thrombocytopenia
- Hemophilia
- von Willebrand's disease

Various disorders can affect the platelets or the body's blood clotting system. Some of these are hereditary, while others may be acquired. Examples of platelet abnormalities include thrombocytosis (increased platelets) and thrombocytopenia (reduced platelets). Various disorders can affect the coagulation system, including hemophilia A and hemophilia B (Christmas disease).

Thrombocytosis

thrombocytosis *an abnormal increase in the number of platelets.*

Thrombocytosis is an increase in the number of platelets, usually due to increased platelet production (essential thrombocytosis). It is also seen in polycythemia vera where both red blood cells and platelets are increased. Thrombocytosis often complicates chronic myelogenous leukemia. Thrombocytosis can be secondary to other disorders such as malignant diseases, hemolytic anemias, acute hemorrhage, and autoinflammatory diseases. Most patients with thrombocytosis are asymptomatic. Prehospital treatment is supportive.

Thrombocytopenia

thrombocytopenia *an abnormal decrease in the number of platelets.*

Thrombocytopenia is an abnormal decrease in the number of platelets. It is due to decreased platelet production, sequestration of platelets in the spleen, destruction of platelets, or any combination of the three. Many drugs can induce thrombocytopenia. *Acute idiopathic thrombocytopenia purpura (ITP)* results from destruction of platelets by the immune system. It is most commonly seen in children following a viral infection. ITP is characterized by easy bruising, bleeding, and a falling platelet count. Chronic ITP usually occurs in adult women and is often associated with autoimmune disease. Prehospital treatment is supportive.

Hemophilia

hemophilia *a blood disorder in which one of the proteins necessary for blood clotting is missing or defective.*

Hemophilia is a blood disorder in which one of the proteins necessary for blood clotting is missing or defective. A deficiency of factor VIII is called hemophilia A. A deficiency of factor IX is known as hemophilia B (Christmas disease). Hemophilia A is the most common inherited disorder of hemostasis. The severity of the disease is directly related to the amount of circulating factor VIII available. Patients are classified as mild, moderate, or severe, based on the amount of circulating factor VIII. Hemophilia B is more rare, but also more severe, than hemophilia A.

When a person with hemophilia is injured, the bleeding will take longer to stop because the body cannot form stable fibrin clots. Simple trauma such as nosebleeds or tooth extractions can lead to prolonged, occasionally life-threatening bleeds. In extensive trauma such as pelvic fractures, blood loss can be overwhelming. A common problem with hemophilia is hemarthrosis (bleeding into the joint space). This can result from even the most minor trauma. Eventually, repeated bleeding episodes will lead to permanent joint damage.

Hemophilia is a sex-linked, inherited bleeding disorder. The gene with the defective information is carried on the X chromosome. Females have two X chromosomes, one from their mother and one from their father. If one chromosome has the defective gene and the other does not, the disease is not expressed. Females who have one X chromosome containing the defective gene are referred to as carriers. Males, however, have an X chromosome from their mother and a Y chromosome from their father. If that X chromosome carries the defective gene, males will express the disease. Hemophilia A affects approximately 1 in 10,000 males. A female, however, can inherit hemophilia only if she receives two X chromosomes that express the disease. That is, she must be the offspring of a carrier mother and a father with hemophilia.

The signs and symptoms of hemophilia include numerous bruises, deep muscle bleeding characterized as pain or a "pulled muscle," and the joint bleeding called hemarthrosis. Most patients will be aware of their diagnosis and will tell you. Some may wear Medic Alert bracelets or similar devices.

Hemophiliacs can be treated in the hospital with infusions of factor VIII. In addition to factor VIII, some hemophiliacs will require blood transfusions due to bleeding from trauma. Unfortunately, before blood and blood products were routinely tested, transfusions infected many hemophiliacs with the human immunodeficiency virus, hepatitis B, and/or hepatitis C.

Prehospital treatment of the patient with hemophilia should be comprehensive. The normal hemostatic mechanisms of vasoconstriction and platelet aggregation will still occur, but the platelet plug will not be stable, due to the deficiency of factor VIII. Thus, you should be attentive to prolonged bleeding or possible rebleeds. The hemophiliac is at risk of both. Administer supplemental oxygen via a nonrebreather mask and initiate IV therapy with an isotonic crystalloid such as normal saline. Be careful to help prevent additional trauma, which can result in further hemorrhage. If the patient sustained a joint injury with resultant hemarthrosis, splinting the extremity will sometimes help control pain. Occasionally, analgesics will be required.

If your patient has hemophilia, be especially careful to help prevent additional trauma, which can result in further hemorrhage.

von Willebrand's Disease

von Willebrand's disease *condition in which the vWF component of factor VIII is deficient.*

Factor VIII actually consists of several components. One of these components is factor VIII:vWF, also called von Willebrand's factor. In **von Willebrand's disease,** this component of factor VIII is deficient. It is produced by the endothelial cells and is necessary for normal platelet adhesion. Thus, in addition to the clotting problem, platelet function is abnormal in patients with von Willebrand's disease. While the disease is inherited, it is not sex linked, equally affecting both females and males. A sign of this disease is excessive bleeding, primarily after surgery or injury. It is not associated with the deep muscle or joint bleeding of hemophilia, nor is it usually as serious, although nosebleeds, excessive menstruation, and gastrointestinal bleeds can occur. Prehospital treatment is supportive. Aspirin is generally contraindicated as it further inhibits platelet aggregation, thus exacerbating the disease. Definitive treatment is the administration of von Willebrand factor.

OTHER HEMATOPOIETIC DISORDERS

Disseminated Intravascular Coagulation

disseminated intravascular coagulation (DIC) *a disorder of coagulation caused by systemic activation of the coagulation cascade.*

Disseminated intravascular coagulation (DIC), also called consumption coagulopathy, is a disorder of coagulation caused by systemic activation of the coagulation cascade. Normally, inhibitory mechanisms localize coagulation to the affected area. A combination of protein inhibitors, rapid blood flow, and absorption of the fibrin clot restricts circulating free thrombin to the site of coagulation. In DIC, circulating thrombin cleaves fibrinogen to form fibrin clots throughout the circulation. This can cause widespread thrombosis and, occasionally, end-organ ischemia. Bleeding is the most frequent sign of DIC and is due to the reduced fibrinogen level, consumption of coagulation factors, and thrombocytopenia. DIC most commonly results from sepsis, hypotension, obstetric complications, severe tissue injury, brain injury, cancer, and major hemolytic transfusion reactions. The disease is quite grave. Its signs include oozing blood at venipuncture and wound sites. The patient may exhibit a purpuric rash, often over the chest and abdomen. Minute hemorrhages may be noted just under the skin. Prehospital care is symptomatic. The DIC patient may be hemodynamically unstable and may require IV fluids. Definitive treatment includes the administration of fresh frozen plasma and platelets.

Multiple Myeloma

multiple myeloma *a cancerous disorder of plasma cells.*

Multiple myeloma is a cancerous disorder of plasma cells. Plasma cells are a type of B cell responsible for producing immunoglobulins (antibodies). The disease is rarely found in persons under the age of 40. Approximately 14,000 new cases are diagnosed each year. Usually, multiple myeloma begins with a change or mutation in a plasma cell in the bone marrow. These cancerous plasma cells crowd out healthy cells and lead to a reduction in blood cell production. The patient then becomes anemic and prone to infection.

The first sign of multiple myeloma often is pain in the back or ribs. The diseased marrow weakens the bones and *pathological fractures* (those occurring with minimal or no trauma) may occur. The resulting anemia leads to fatigue, and reduced platelet production places the patient at risk for bleeding. Laboratory evaluation will reveal an elevation in the level of a circulating antibody or part of an antibody (light chain) due to the proliferation of plasma cells. Despite this, the patient is at increased risk of infection, as the plasma cells do not secrete specific antibodies in response to infection. In addition, the calcium level is often elevated due to bone destruction. This can lead to renal failure.

Treatment of multiple myeloma includes chemotherapy, radiation, and bone marrow transplants. Prehospital care is supportive. Establish an IV of isotonic crystalloid solution. Consider a fluid bolus if there are symptoms of dehydration. Multiple myeloma can be very painful due to the proliferation of the plasma cells and destruction of the marrow. Consider analgesics if pain is severe. A pathological fracture in a patient with multiple myeloma is very painful, and you should start analgesic therapy if so indicated.

Summary

Hematology is the study of the blood and blood-forming organs. Hematological disorders include red blood cell disorders, white blood cell disorders, platelet disorders, and coagulation problems. Problems can also be caused when the body has an immunological response to antigens present on red blood cells from a foreign donor. Although hematological disorders are common, they are seldom the primary reason for an emergency call. Rather, they are likely to accompany another ongoing disease process.

The signs and symptoms that accompany hematological problems seldom point directly to the underlying disease. Generally, lab findings are necessary to clarify the diagnosis. However, an understanding of hematological pathophysiology is important to understanding the disease process your patient may be undergoing and to helping you to form a field impression and make appropriate decisions about emergency care.

Review Questions

1. A person with type ___________ blood is called a universal recipient.
   a. O
   b. A
   c. AB
   d. B
2. Because blood transfusion adds fluid to the system, a patient may experience signs and symptoms of ___________, such as pulmonary edema, dyspnea, and chest pain.
   a. aplastic anemia
   b. acute hemophilia
   c. cellular polycythemia
   d. circulatory overload
3. ___________ is typically classified as a hematocrit of less than 37 percent in women or less than 40 percent in men.
   a. Anemia
   b. Leukemia
   c. Polycythemia
   d. Thrombocytopenia

4. Many leukemia patients will present with bleeding, usually due to:
   a. anemia.
   b. infection.
   c. hypoxemia.
   d. thrombocytopenia.
5. A cancer of the lymphatic system is known as:
   a. lymphoma.
   b. leukopenia.
   c. leukemia.
   d. myeloma.
6. Hemophilia is a blood disorder in which one of the proteins necessary for __________ is missing or defective.
   a. clotting
   b. metabolism
   c. diffusion
   d. phagocytosis
7. von Willebrand's disease is:
   a. inherited.
   b. sex-linked.
   c. more common in men.
   d. all of the above
8. __________ is the most frequent sign of DIC and is due to the reduced fibrinogen level, consumption of coagulation factors, and thrombocytopenia.
   a. Fever
   b. Bleeding
   c. Purpuric rash
   d. Oozing blood at wound sites

See Answers to Review Questions at the back of this book.

Chapter 36

Environmental Emergencies

Objectives

After reading this chapter, you should be able to:

1. Define "environmental emergency." (p. 1407)
2. Describe the incidence, morbidity, and mortality associated with environmental emergencies. (p. 1423)
3. Identify risk factors most predisposing to environmental emergencies. (p. 1407)
4. Identify environmental factors that may cause illness or exacerbate a preexisting illness or complicate treatment or transport decisions. (p. 1407)
5. Define "homeostasis" and relate the concept to environmental influences. (p.1407)
6. Identify normal, critically high, and critically low body temperatures. (pp. 1408–1410)
7. Describe several methods of temperature monitoring. (p. 1409)
8. Describe human thermal regulation, including system components, substances used, and wastes generated. (pp. 1407–1411, 1416)
9. List the common forms of heat and cold disorders. (pp. 1411–1423)
10. List the common predisposing factors and preventive measures associated with heat and cold disorders. (pp. 1411–1412, 1416–1417)
11. Define heat illness, hypothermia, frostbite, near-drowning, decompression illness, and altitude illness. (pp. 1411, 1416, 1422, 1423, 1428, 1433)
12. Describe the pathophysiology, signs and symptoms, and predisposing factors, preventive actions, and treatment for heat cramps, heat exhaustion, heatstroke, and fever. (pp. 1411–1416)
13. Describe the contribution of dehydration to the development of heat disorders. (p. 1415)
14. Describe the differences between classical and exertional heatstroke. (p. 1414)
15. Identify the fundamental thermoregulatory difference between fever and heatstroke. (p. 1415)
16. Discuss the role of fluid therapy in the treatment of heat disorders. (pp. 1412, 1413, 1414)
17. Describe the pathophysiology, predisposing factors, signs, symptoms, and management of the following:
    - ★ hypothermia (pp. 1416–1422)
    - ★ superficial and deep frostbite (pp. 1422–1423)

- ★ near-drowning (pp. 1423–1426)
- ★ decompression illness (pp. 1428, 1429–1431)
- ★ diving emergency (pp. 1427–1433)
- ★ altitude illness (pp. 1433–1436)

18. Identify differences between mild, severe, chronic, and acute hypothermia. (p. 1417)
19. Discuss the impact of severe hypothermia on standard BCLS and ACLS algorithms and transport considerations. (pp. 1419–1422)
20. Differentiate between freshwater and saltwater immersion as they relate to near-drowning. (p. 1424)
21. Discuss the incidence of "wet" versus "dry" drownings and the differences in their management. (p. 1424)
22. Discuss the complications and protective role of hypothermia in the context of near-drowning. (pp. 1423, 1424)
23. Define self-contained underwater breathing apparatus (scuba). (p. 1426)
24. Describe the laws of gases and relate them to diving emergencies and altitude illness. (pp. 1426–1427)
25. Differentiate between the various diving emergencies. (pp. 1427–1428)
26. Identify the various conditions that may result from pulmonary overpressure accidents. (pp. 1428, 1431)
27. Describe the function of the Divers Alert Network (DAN) and how its members may aid in the management of diving-related illnesses. (p. 1433)
28. Describe the specific function and benefit of hyperbaric oxygen therapy for the management of diving accidents. (pp. 1429–1430)
29. Define acute mountain sickness (AMS), high altitude pulmonary edema (HAPE), and high altitude cerebral edema (HACE). (pp. 1434–1436)
30. Discuss the symptomatic variations presented in progressive altitude illnesses. (pp. 1434–1436)
31. Discuss the pharmacology appropriate for the treatment of altitude illnesses. (pp. 1435–1436)
32. Given several preprogrammed simulated environmental emergency patients, provide the appropriate assessment, management, and transportation. (pp. 1407–1436)

Key Terms

acclimatization, p. 1412
arterial gas embolism (AGE), p. 1428
autonomic neuropathy, p. 1411
barotrauma, p. 1428
basal metabolic rate (BMR), p. 1410
conduction, p. 1408
convection, p. 1408
core temperature, p. 1408
decompression illness, p. 1428
deep frostbite, p. 1422
drowning, p. 1423
environmental emergency, p. 1407
evaporation, p. 1408
exertional metabolic rate, p. 1410
frostbite, p. 1422
heat cramps, p. 1412
heat exhaustion, p. 1413
heat illness, p. 1411
heatstroke, p. 1413
homeostasis, p. 1407
hyperbaric oxygen chamber, p. 1429
hyperthermia, p. 1411
hypothalamus, p. 1409
hypothermia, p. 1416
J wave, p. 1419
mammalian diving reflex, p. 1424
near-drowning, p. 1423
negative feedback, p. 1409
nitrogen narcosis, p. 1428
pneumomediastinum, p. 1428
pneumothorax, p. 1428
pulmonary overpressure, p. 1428
pyrexia, p. 1415
pyrogen, p. 1415
radiation, p. 1408
recompression, p. 1429
respiration, p. 1408
scuba, p. 1426
superficial frostbite, p. 1422
surfactant, p. 1424
thermal gradient, p. 1408
thermogenesis, p. 1408
thermoregulation, p. 1408
trench foot, p. 1423

INTRODUCTION

The *environment* can be defined as all of the surrounding external factors that affect the development and functioning of a living organism. Human beings obviously depend on the environment for life, but they also must be protected from its extremes. When factors such as temperature, weather, terrain, and atmospheric pressure act on the body, they can create stresses for which the body is unable to compensate. A medical condition caused or exacerbated by such environmental factors is known as an **environmental emergency.**

environmental emergency *a medical condition caused or exacerbated by the weather, terrain, atmospheric pressure, or other local factors.*

Environmental emergencies include a variety of conditions such as heatstroke, hypothermia, drowning or near-drowning, altitude sickness, and diving accidents or barotraumas. Such emergencies often call for special rescue resources.

Although environmental emergencies can affect anyone, several risk factors predispose certain individuals to developing environmental illnesses. These factors include:

- Age—especially very young children and older adults, who do not tolerate environmental extremes very well
- Poor general health
- Fatigue
- Predisposing medical conditions
- Certain medications—either prescription or over-the-counter

Environmental factors must also be considered when determining the risk for environmental emergencies. For example, climate in a particular place may vary greatly from moment to moment. Areas where change in temperature can be drastic over the course of the day may catch unwary individuals off guard. For example, desert areas can have temperatures of 105°F during the day but drop below freezing at night, placing unprepared travelers in a difficult situation. Temperatures in parts of southern Alberta can change drastically when the Chinook winds kick up. Other considerations include the current season, local weather patterns, atmospheric pressures (high altitude or underwater), and the type of terrain, which can cause injury or hinder rescue efforts.

As a paramedic, you will frequently be called on to treat medical emergencies related to environmental conditions. It is critical that you understand the particular conditions that prevail in your region. If you live in a mountain area, near large caves, in an area with swift moving water, or in a resort area where diving is prominent, you need to be familiar with the specialized rescue resources these situations may require and the particular environmental emergencies they may cause. Understanding their causes and underlying pathophysiologies can help you recognize these emergencies promptly and manage them effectively.

Although many environmental factors can result in medical emergencies, this chapter will focus primarily on problems related to temperature extremes, drowning or near-drowning, diving emergencies, and high altitude illness.

For the human body to function properly, it must interact with the environment to obtain oxygen, nutrients, and other necessities, but it must also avoid being damaged by extreme external environmental conditions. The process of maintaining constant suitable conditions within the body is called **homeostasis.** Various body systems respond in an effort to maintain the correct core and peripheral temperature, oxygen level, and energy supply to maintain life.

homeostasis *the natural tendency of the body to maintain a steady and normal internal environment.*

The following sections address how the body attempts to maintain these normal settings and what happens when certain environmental conditions exceed the ability of the body to compensate.

PATHOPHYSIOLOGY OF HEAT AND COLD DISORDERS

MECHANISMS OF HEAT GAIN AND LOSS

The body gains and loses heat in two ways, from within the body itself and by contact with the external environment.

thermal gradient *the difference in temperature between the environment and the body.*

The body receives heat from, or loses it to, the environment via the thermal gradient. The **thermal gradient** is the difference in temperature between the environment (the ambient temperature) and the body. The ambient temperature is usually different from body temperature. If the environment is warmer than the body, heat flows from the environment to the body. If the body is warmer than the environment, heat flows from the body to the environment. Other environmental factors, including wind and relative humidity (the percentage of water vapor in the air), also affect heat gain and loss.

The mechanisms by which heat is generated within the body and by which heat is gained or lost to the environment are discussed in more detail in the following sections.

THERMOGENESIS (HEAT GENERATION)

The amount of heat in the body continually fluctuates as a result of the heat generated or gained and the heat lost. The body gains heat from both external and internal sources. In addition to the heat the body absorbs from the environment, the body also generates heat through energy-producing chemical reactions (metabolism).

thermogenesis *the production of heat, especially within the body.*

The creation of heat is called **thermogenesis.** There are several types of thermogenesis. One is *work-induced thermogenesis* that results from exercise. Our muscles need to create heat because warm muscles work more effectively than cold ones. One way muscles can produce heat is by shivering. Another type, *thermoregulatory thermogenesis,* is controlled by the endocrine system. The hormones norepinephrine and epinephrine can cause an immediate increase in the rate of cellular metabolism, which in turn increases heat production. The last type, metabolic thermogenesis, or *diet-induced thermogenesis,* is caused by the processing of food and nutrients. When a meal is eaten, digested, absorbed, and metabolized, heat is produced as a by-product of these activities.

THERMOLYSIS (HEAT LOSS)

The heat generated by the body is constantly lost to the environment. This occurs because the body is usually warmer than the surrounding environment. The transfer of heat into the environment occurs through the following mechanisms (Figure 36-1 ■):

conduction *moving electrons, ions, heat, or sound waves through a conductor or conducting medium.*

convection *transfer of heat via currents in liquids or gases.*

radiation *transfer of energy through space or matter.*

evaporation *change from liquid to a gaseous state.*

respiration *the exchange of gases between a living organism and its environment.*

- ★ **Conduction.** Direct contact of the body's surface to another, cooler object causes the body to lose heat by conduction. Heat flows from higher temperature matter to lower temperature matter.
- ★ **Convection.** Heat loss to air currents passing over the body. Heat, however, must first be conducted to the air before being carried away by convection currents.
- ★ **Radiation.** An unclothed person will lose approximately 60 percent of total body heat by radiation at normal room temperature. This heat loss is in the form of infrared rays. All objects not at absolute zero temperature will radiate heat into the atmosphere.
- ★ **Evaporation.** The change of a liquid to vapor. Evaporative heat loss occurs as water evaporates from the skin. Additionally, a great deal of heat loss occurs through evaporation of fluids in the lungs. Water evaporates from the skin and lungs at approximately 600 mL/day.
- ★ **Respiration.** Combines the mechanisms of convection, radiation, and evaporation. It accounts for a large proportion of the body's heat loss. Heat is transferred from the lungs to inspired air by convection and radiation. Evaporation in the lungs humidifies the inspired air (adds water vapor to it). During expiration this warm, humidified air is released into the environment, creating heat loss.

thermoregulation *the maintenance or regulation of a particular temperature of the body.*

core temperature *the body temperature of the deep tissues, which usually does not vary more than a degree or so from its normal 37°C (98.6°F).*

THERMOREGULATION

Thermoregulation is the maintenance or regulation of temperature. The body temperature of the deep tissues, commonly called the **core temperature,** usually does not vary more than a degree or so from its normal 98.6°F (37°C). A naked person can be exposed to an external environment ranging anywhere from 55°F to 144°F and still maintain a fairly constant internal body temperature.

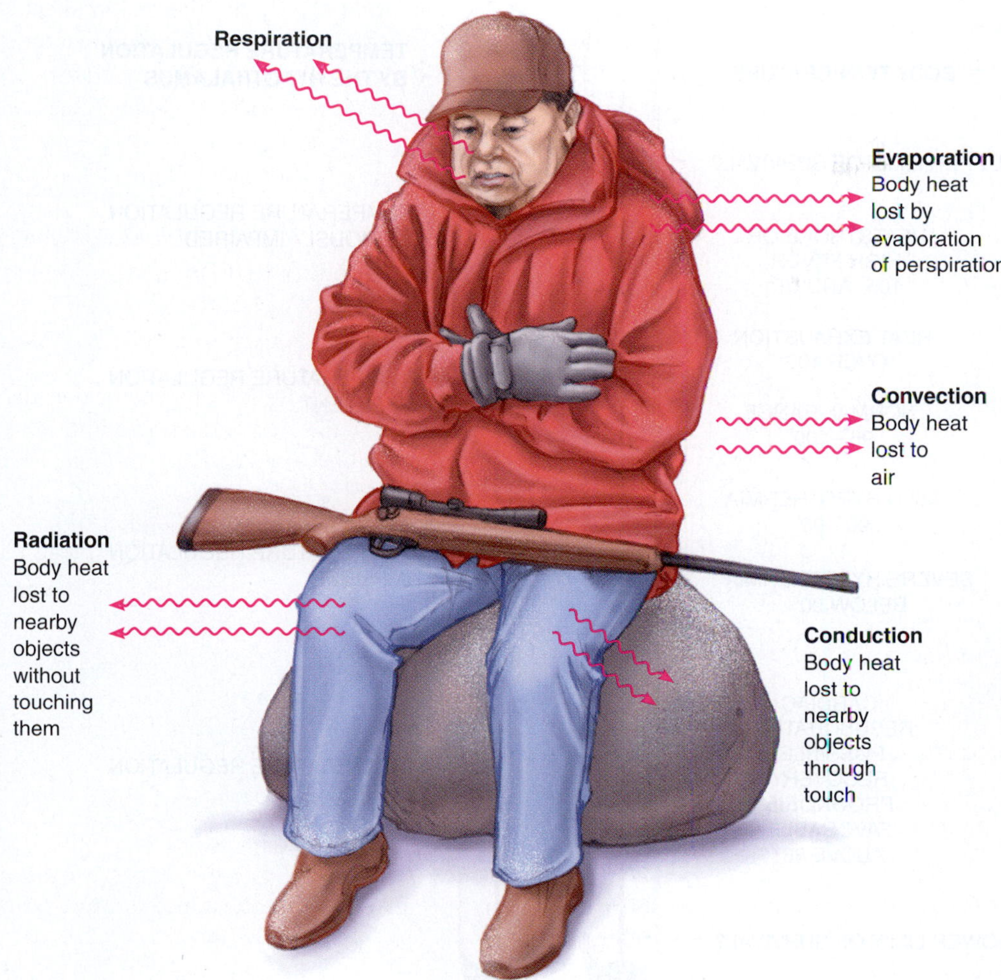

■ **Figure 36-1** Heat loss by the body.

Content Review

Comparative Body Temperatures

Celsius	*Fahrenheit*
40.6°	105°
37.8°	100°
37°	98.6°
35°	95°
32°	89.6°
30°	86°
20°	68°

This characteristic of warm-blooded animals is called *steady-state metabolism.* The various biochemical reactions occurring within the cell are most efficient when the body temperature is within this narrow temperature range.

Evaluation of peripheral body temperature can be measured by touch or by taking the temperature by oral or axillary means. Core body temperatures can be measured using tympanic or rectal thermometers.

The body maintains a balance between the production and loss of heat almost entirely through the nervous system and negative feedback mechanisms. The **hypothalamus,** located at the base of the brain, is responsible for temperature regulation. It functions as a thermostat, controlling temperature through the release of neurosecretions (secretions produced by nerve cells). When the hypothalamus senses an increased body temperature, it shuts off the mechanisms designed to create heat, for example, shivering. When it senses a decrease in body temperature, the hypothalamus shuts off mechanisms designed to cool the body, for example, sweating. Because the action involved requires stopping, or negating, a process, it is called a **negative feedback** system.

When the heat-regulating function of the hypothalamus is disrupted, the result can be an abnormally high or low body temperature. At the extremes, such abnormal temperatures can result in death (Figure 36-2 ■).

hypothalamus *portion of the diencephalon producing neurosecretions important in the control of certain metabolic activities, including body temperature regulation.*

negative feedback *homeostatic mechanism in which a change in a variable (here, core temperature) ultimately inhibits the process that led to the shift.*

Content Review

Mechanisms of Heat Dissipation

- Sweating
- Vasodilation

Mechanisms of Heat Conservation

- Shivering
- Vasoconstriction

Thermoreceptors

Although the hypothalamus plays a key role in body temperature regulation, temperature receptors in other parts of the body also help to moderate temperatures. There are thermoreceptors in the skin and certain mucous membranes (peripheral thermoreceptors) as well as in certain deep tissues of the

■ **Figure 36-2** Temperature regulation by the hypothalamus.

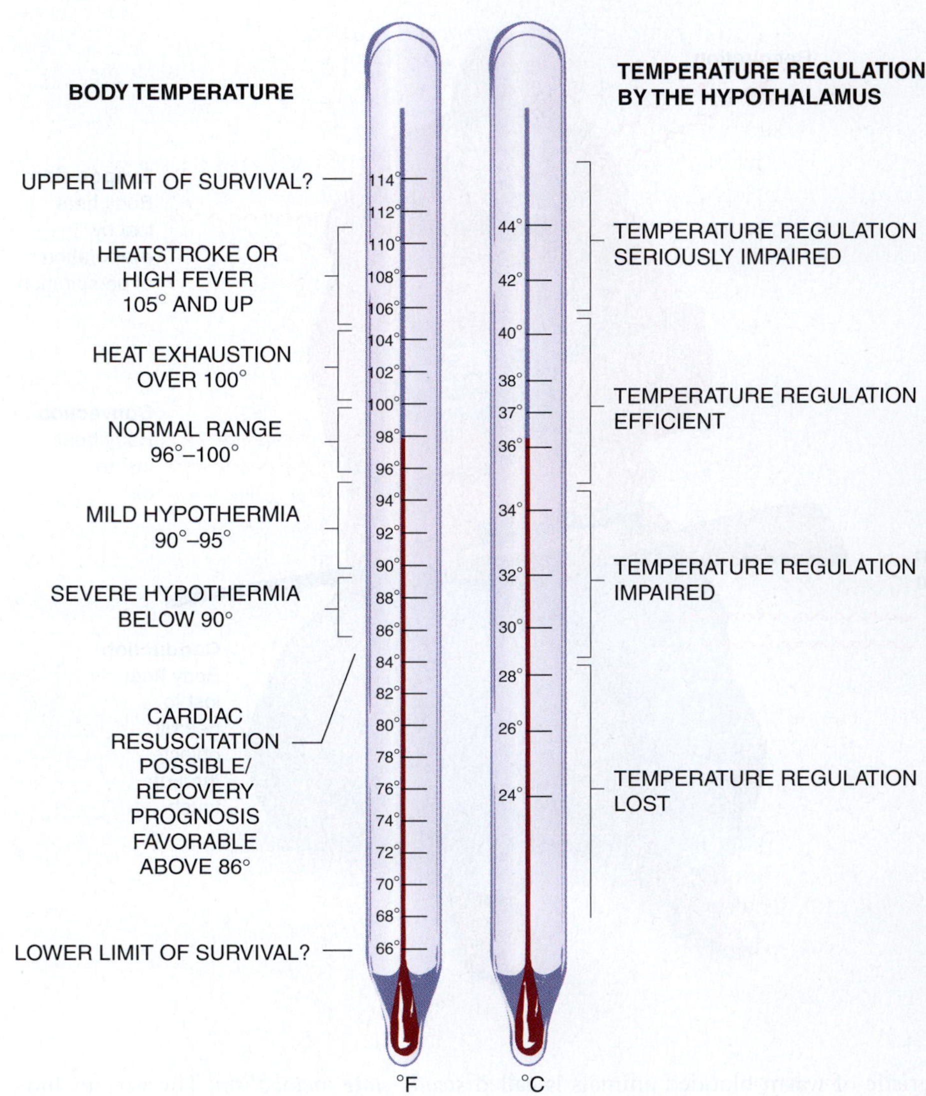

body (central thermoreceptors). The skin has both cold and warm receptors. Because cold receptors outnumber warm receptors, peripheral detection of temperature consists mainly of detecting cold rather than warmth. Deep body temperature receptors lie mostly in the spinal cord, abdominal viscera, and in or around the great veins. These receptors are exposed to the body's core temperature rather than the peripheral temperature. They also respond mainly to cold rather than warmth. Both peripheral and central thermoreceptors act to prevent lowering of the body temperature.

basal metabolic rate (BMR) *rate at which the body consumes energy just to maintain stability; the basic metabolic rate (measured by the rate of oxygen consumption) of an awake, relaxed person 12 to 14 hours after eating and at a comfortable temperature.*

exertional metabolic rate *rate at which the body consumes energy during activity. It is faster than the basal metabolic rate.*

Metabolic Rate

The **basal metabolic rate** (BMR) is the metabolism that occurs when the body is completely at rest. It is the rate at which the body consumes energy just to maintain itself—the rate of metabolism that maintains brain function, circulation, and cell stability. Any additional activity that the body performs demands energy consumption beyond that supported by the basal rate, metabolizing more nutrients and releasing more calories (units of heat). The rate of metabolism that supports this additional activity is called an **exertional metabolic rate.**

The body continually adjusts the metabolic rate to maintain the temperature of the core (where the crucial structures like the heart and brain are located). The body also achieves temperature maintenance by dilating some blood vessels and constricting others so that the blood carries the excess heat from the core to the periphery where it is close to the skin. This allows heat to dissipate through the skin into the environment.

Conversely, when the environment is too cold, *counter-current heat exchange* is used to shunt warm blood away from the superficial veins near the skin and back into the deep veins near the core to keep vital structures warm. Another body response that counters a cold environment is shivering, a physical activity that increases metabolism and generates heat.

It is important to note that these various mechanisms can create a difference between the core body temperature and the peripheral body temperature. Core temperature is the crucial measurement since, as noted, the core is where the major organs are located. Therefore, it is important in any heat-related or cold-related emergency to obtain a core temperature reading such as from the rectum. Oral and axillary temperatures may provide convenient approximations in some situations but may lead to incorrect interventions if relied on for treatment of the patient with an environmental illness.

HEAT DISORDERS

Disruption of the body's normal thermoregulatory mechanisms can produce a number of heat illnesses, such as hyperthermia and fever. **Heat illness** is increased *core body temperature (CBT)* due to inadequate thermolysis.

heat illness *increased core body temperature due to inadequate thermolysis.*

HYPERTHERMIA

Hyperthermia is a state of unusually high body temperature, specifically the core body temperature. Hyperthermia is usually caused by heat transfer from the external environment for which the body cannot compensate. Occasionally it is caused by excessive generation of heat within the body.

Review

Content

Heat Disorders

- Hyperthermia
- Heat cramps
- Heat exhaustion
- Heatstroke

hyperthermia *unusually high core body temperature.*

As the body attempts to eliminate this excessive heat, you will see the general signs of thermolysis (heat loss). These signs are caused by the body's two chief methods of heat dissipation, sweating (which leads to evaporative heat loss) and vasodilation (which allows the blood to carry heat to the periphery for dissipation through the skin). These include:

- ★ Diaphoresis (sweating)
- ★ Increased skin temperature
- ★ Flushing

As heat illness progresses, you will also note signs of thermolytic inadequacy (the failure of the body's thermoregulatory mechanisms to compensate adequately):

- ★ Altered mentation
- ★ Altered level of consciousness

Hyperthermia can manifest as heat cramps, heat exhaustion, or heatstroke, which will be discussed in the following sections.

PREDISPOSING FACTORS

Age, general health, and medications are predisposing factors in hyperthermia. Factors that may contribute to a susceptibility to hyperthermia include:

- ★ *Age of the patient.* Pediatric and geriatric populations can tolerate less variation in temperature and their heat-regulating mechanisms are not as responsive as those of young adult and adult populations.
- ★ *Health of the patient.* Diabetics can become hyperthermic more easily because they develop **autonomic neuropathy.** This condition damages the autonomic nervous system, which may interfere with thermoregulatory input and with vasodilation and perspiration, which normally dissipate heat.
- ★ *Medications.* Various medications can affect body temperature in the following ways:
  - *Diuretics* predispose to dehydration, which worsens hyperthermia.

autonomic neuropathy *condition that damages the autonomic nervous system, which usually senses changes in core temperature and controls vasodilation and perspiration to dissipate heat.*

- *Beta-blockers* interfere with vasodilation and reduce the capacity to increase heart rate in response to volume loss and may also interfere with thermoregulatory input.
- *Psychotropics and antihistamines,* such as antipsychotics and phenothiazines, interfere with central thermoregulation.

acclimatization *the reversible changes in body structure and function by which the body becomes adjusted to a change in environment.*

★ *Level of acclimatization.* **Acclimatization** is the process of becoming adjusted to a change in environment. In response to an environmental change, reversible changes in body structure and function take place that help to maintain homeostasis.

★ *Length of exposure*

★ *Intensity of exposure*

★ *Environmental factors* such as humidity and wind.

PREVENTIVE MEASURES

Ideally, prevention of heat disorders is preferable to treating an illness already in progress. Measures to prevent hyperthermia include the following:

★ Maintain adequate fluid intake, remembering that thirst is an inadequate indicator of dehydration.

★ Allow time for gradual acclimatization to being out in the heat. Acclimatization results in more perspiration with lower salt concentration and increases body-fluid volume.

★ Limit exposure to hot environments.

SPECIFIC HEAT DISORDERS

Inevitably, you will be required to respond to heat-related emergencies: heat cramps, heat exhaustion, or heatstroke. Heat cramps and heat exhaustion result from dehydration and depletion of sodium and other electrolytes. Heatstroke, a far more serious and potentially life-threatening condition, results from the failure of the body's thermoregulatory mechanisms.

Signs and symptoms and emergency care procedures for heat cramps, heat exhaustion, and heatstroke are discussed in the following sections.

Heat (Muscle) Cramps

heat cramps *acute painful spasms of the voluntary muscles following strenuous activity in a hot environment without adequate fluid or salt intake.*

Heat cramps are muscle cramps caused by overexertion and dehydration in the presence of high atmospheric temperatures. Sweating occurs as sodium (salt) is transported to the skin. Because "water follows sodium," water is deposited on the skin surface where evaporation occurs, aiding in the cooling process. Since sweating involves not only the loss of water but also the loss of electrolytes (such as sodium), intermittent cramping of skeletal muscles may occur. Heat cramps are painful but are not considered to be an actual heat illness.

Signs and Symptoms The patient with heat cramps will present with cramps in the fingers, arms, legs, or abdominal muscles. He will generally be mentally alert with a feeling of weakness. He may feel dizzy or faint. Vital signs will be stable. Body temperature may be normal or slightly elevated. The skin is likely to be moist and warm.

Treatment Treatment of the patient with heat cramps is usually easily accomplished:

1. *Remove the patient from the environment.* Place the patient in a cool environment such as a shaded area or the air-conditioned back of the ambulance.

In the case of severe cramps:

2. *Administer an oral saline solution* (approximately 4 teaspoons of salt to a gallon of water) or a sports drink. Do NOT administer salt tablets, which are not absorbed as readily and may cause stomach irritation and ulceration or hypernatremia. *If the patient is unable to take fluids orally, an IV of normal saline may be needed.*

Some EMS systems recommend massaging the painful muscles. Application of moist towels to the patient's forehead and over the cramped muscles may also be helpful.

Heat Exhaustion

Heat exhaustion, which is considered to be a mild heat illness, is an acute reaction to heat exposure. It is the most common heat-related illness seen by prehospital personnel. An individual performing work in a hot environment will lose 1 to 2 liters of water an hour. Each liter lost contains 20 to 50 milliequivalents of sodium. The resulting loss of water and sodium, combined with general vasodilation, leads to a decreased circulating blood volume, venous pooling, and reduced cardiac output.

heat exhaustion *a mild heat illness; an acute reaction to heat exposure.*

Dehydration and sodium loss due to sweating account for the presenting symptoms. However, these signs and symptoms are not exclusive to heat exhaustion. Instead, they mimic those of an individual suffering from fluid and sodium loss from any of a number of other causes. A history of exposure to high environmental temperatures is needed to obtain an accurate assessment.

If not treated, heat exhaustion may progress to heatstroke.

Signs and Symptoms Signs and symptoms that you may encounter include increased body temperature (over 100°F or 37.8°C), skin that is cool and clammy with heavy perspiration, breathing that is rapid and shallow, and a weak pulse. There may be signs of active thermolysis such as diarrhea and muscle cramps. The patient will feel weak and, in some cases, may lose consciousness. There may be central nervous system (CNS) symptoms such as headache, anxiety, paresthesia, and impaired judgment or even psychosis.

Treatment Prehospital management of the patient with heat exhaustion is aimed at immediate cooling and fluid replacement. Steps include:

1. *Remove the patient from the environment.* Place the patient in a cool environment such as a shaded area or the air-conditioned ambulance.
2. *Place the patient in a supine position.*
3. *Administer an oral saline solution* (approximately 4 teaspoons of salt to a gallon of water) or a sports drink. Do NOT administer salt tablets, which are not absorbed as readily and may cause stomach irritation and ulceration or hypernatremia. *If the patient is unable to take fluids orally, an IV of normal saline may be needed.*
4. *Remove some clothing and fan the patient.* Remove enough clothing to cool the patient without chilling him. Fanning increases evaporation and cooling. Again, be careful not to cool the patient to the point of chilling. If the patient begins to shiver, stop fanning and perhaps cover the patient lightly.
5. *Treat for shock, if shock is suspected.* However, be careful not to cover the patient to the point of overheating him.

Symptoms should resolve with fluids, rest, and supine posturing with knees elevated. If they do not, consider that the symptoms may be due to an increased core body temperature, which is predictive of impending heatstroke and should be treated aggressively, as outlined in the following section.

Heatstroke

Heatstroke is a true environmental emergency that occurs when the body's hypothalamic temperature regulation is lost, causing uncompensated hyperthermia. This in turn causes cell death and damage to the brain, liver, and kidneys. There is no arbitrary core temperature at which heatstroke begins. However, heatstroke is generally characterized by a body temperature of at least 105°F (40.6°C), central nervous system disturbances, and usually the cessation of sweating.

heatstroke *acute, dangerous reaction to heat exposure, characterized by a body temperature usually above 105°F (40.6°C) and central nervous system disturbances. The body usually ceases to perspire.*

Signs and Symptoms Sweating is thought to stop due to destruction of the sweat glands or when sensory overload causes them to temporarily dysfunction. However, the patient's skin may be either dry or covered with sweat that is still present on the skin from earlier exertion. In either case, the skin will be hot.

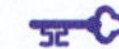

Heatstroke is a true environmental emergency.

The patient may present with the following signs and symptoms:

- ★ Cessation of sweating
- ★ Hot skin that is dry or moist
- ★ Very high core temperature
- ★ Deep respirations that become shallow, rapid at first but may later slow
- ★ Rapid, full pulse, may slow later
- ★ Hypotension with low or absent diastolic reading
- ★ Confusion or disorientation or unconsciousness
- ★ Possible seizures

Classic heatstroke commonly presents in those with chronic illnesses, with the increased core body temperature due to deficient thermoregulatory function. Predisposing conditions include age, diabetes, and other medical conditions. In this type of heatstroke hot, red, dry skin is common.

Exertional heatstroke commonly presents in those who are in good general health, with the increased core body temperature due to overwhelming heat stress. There is excessive ambient temperature as well as excessive exertion with prolonged exposure and poor acclimatization. In this type of heatstroke you will find that, although sweating has ceased and the skin is hot, moisture from prior sweating may still be present.

If the patient develops heatstroke due to exertion, he may go into severe metabolic acidosis caused by lactic acid accumulation. Hyperkalemia (excessive potassium in blood) may also develop because of the release of potassium from injured muscle cells, renal failure, or metabolic acidosis.

The heatstroke patient should be cooled immediately and given fluids.

Treatment Prehospital management of the heatstroke patient is aimed at immediate cooling and replacement of fluids. Steps include:

1. *Remove the patient from the environment.* This first step is essential. If you do not remove the patient from the hot environment, any other measures will be only minimally useful. Move the patient to a cool environment, such as the air-conditioned ambulance.
2. *Initiate rapid active cooling.* Body temperature must be lowered to 102°F (39°C). A target of 102°F (39°C) is used to avoid an overshoot. This can be accomplished en route to the hospital. Remove the patient's clothing and cover the patient with sheets soaked in tepid water. Fanning and misting may also be used if necessary. Refrain from overcooling, as this may cause reflex hypothermia (low body temperature). This results in shivering, which can raise the core temperature again. Tepid water is used because ice packs and cold-water immersion may affect peripheral thermoreceptors, producing reflex vasoconstriction and shivering.
3. *Administer oxygen.* Administer high-flow, high-concentration oxygen by nonrebreather mask. If respirations are shallow, assist with a bag-valve-mask unit supplied with 100 percent oxygen. Utilize pulse oximetry, if available.
4. *Administer fluid therapy if the patient is alert and able to swallow.*
   - —*Oral fluids.* In many cases oral fluid therapy will be all that is needed. Some salt additive is beneficial, but salt tablets should be avoided as they may cause gastrointestinal irritation and ulceration or hypernatremia. There is a very limited need for other electrolytes in oral rehydration.
   - —*Intravenous fluids.* Begin 1 to 2 IVs, using normal saline. Initially infuse them wide open.
5. *Monitor the ECG.* Cardiac dysrhythmias may occur at any time. ST segment depression, nonspecific T wave changes with occasional PVCs, and supraventricular tachycardias are common.
6. *Avoid vasopressors and anticholinergic drugs.* These agents may potentiate heatstroke by inhibiting sweating. They can also produce a hypermetabolic state in the presence of high environmental temperatures and relatively high humidity.

7. *Monitor body temperature.* EMS systems operating in extremely warm climates should carry some device to record the body temperature, whether a simple rectal thermometer or a sophisticated electronic device. Simple glass thermometers generally do not measure above 106°F (41°C) or below 95°F (35°C). This may become significant during long transport when it is essential to detect changes in the patient's condition.

ROLE OF DEHYDRATION IN HEAT DISORDERS

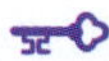

Dehydration often goes hand-in-hand with heat disorders.

Dehydration often goes hand-in-hand with heat disorders because it inhibits vasodilation and therefore thermolysis. Dehydration leads to orthostatic hypotension (increased pulse and decreased blood pressure on rising from a supine position) and the following symptoms which may occur along with the signs and symptoms of heatstroke:

- ★ Nausea, vomiting, and abdominal distress
- ★ Vision disturbances
- ★ Decreased urine output
- ★ Poor skin turgor
- ★ Signs of hypovolemic shock

Thirst is a poor indication of the degree of dehydration present.

When these signs and symptoms are present, rehydration of the patient is critical. Oral fluids may be administered if the patient is alert and not nauseated. Administration of IV fluids may be necessary, especially if the patient has an altered mental status or is nauseated. It is not uncommon for the adult patient with moderate-to-severe dehydration to require 2 to 3 liters of IV fluids (occasionally more!).

FEVER (PYREXIA)

A fever (**pyrexia**) is the elevation of the body temperature above the normal temperature for that person. (An individual person's normal temperature may be 1 or 2 degrees above or below 98.6°F or 37°C.) The body develops a fever when pathogens enter and cause infection, which in turn stimulates the production of pyrogens.

pyrexia *fever, or above-normal body temperature.*

Pyrogens are any substances that cause fever, such as viruses and bacteria or substances produced within the body in response to infection or inflammation. They reset the hypothalamic thermostat to a higher level. Metabolism is increased, which produces the elevation of temperature. The increased body temperature fights infection by making the body a less hospitable environment for the invading organism. The hypothalamic thermostat will reset to normal when pyrogen production stops or when pathogens end their attack on the body.

pyrogen *any substance causing a fever, such as viruses and bacteria or substances produced within the body in response to infection or inflammation.*

Fever is sometimes difficult to differentiate from heatstroke, and neurological symptoms may present with either, but there is usually a history of infection or illness with a fever. While the heatstroke patient usually has a history of exertion and exposure to high ambient temperatures, this is not always the case. In some cases, heatstroke can be caused by impaired functioning of the hypothalamus without exertion or exposure to ambient heat. Treat for heatstroke if you are unsure which it is.

When unsure if the problem is heatstroke or fever, treat for heatstroke.

Although fever may be beneficial, it can be disconcerting to the parents of children with fever. In addition, fever can be uncomfortable for the patient. If the patient is uncomfortable, measures should be taken to treat the fever. Also, if a child has a history of febrile seizures, the fever should be treated. Parents will often have their febrile children wrapped in several layers of clothing or blankets because the child is "cold." These should be removed, leaving only the diaper or underclothes, exposing the child to the ambient air. This will allow a controlled cooling.

Do not use sponge baths to cool febrile children.

Sponge baths and cool-water immersion should not be used. These cause a rapid drop in the body core temperature and result in shivering. This again elevates the core temperature, which complicates the process. Several medications are good antipyretics (that is, they lower body temperature in fever). These include acetaminophen (Tylenol) and ibuprofen (Motrin). Many EMS systems will utilize an antipyretic in the treatment of fever, particularly in pediatric patients. Liquid acetaminophen and ibuprofen are easy to administer and effective. Acetaminophen is also available in a

Consider administering an antipyretic, primarily for patient comfort. This is especially important in services with long transportation times.

suppository form for patients with active vomiting. These antipyretics are typically dosed based on the patient's weight:

- ★ *Acetaminophen.* 15 mg/kg for pediatric patients; adult dose is typically 650 mg.
- ★ *Ibuprofen.* 10 mg/kg for pediatric patients; adult dose is typically 600–800 mg.

These liquid medications should be dosed with syringes as teaspoons are inaccurate measuring devices. EMS services with prolonged transport times should consider the use of antipyretics for patient comfort as well as for the prevention of febrile seizures.

Content Review

Cold Disorders

- Hypothermia
- Frostbite
- Trench foot

COLD DISORDERS

Disruption of the body's normal thermoregulation may produce cold-related disorders such as hypothermia, frostbite, and trench foot.

HYPOTHERMIA

hypothermia *state of low body temperature, particularly low core body temperature.*

Hypothermia is a state of low body temperature, specifically low core temperature. When the core temperature of the body drops below 95°F (35°C), an individual is considered to be hypothermic. Hypothermia can be attributed to inadequate thermogenesis, excessive cold stress, or a combination of both.

MECHANISMS OF HEAT CONSERVATION AND LOSS

Exposure to cold normally triggers compensatory mechanisms designed to conserve and generate heat to maintain a normal body temperature. One such mechanism is piloerection (hair standing on end, "goose bumps") to impede air flow across the skin. Shivering and increased muscle tone occur, resulting in increased metabolism. There is peripheral vasoconstriction with an increase in cardiac output and respiratory rate. When these mechanisms can no longer adequately compensate for heat lost from the body surface, the body temperature falls. As the body temperature falls, so do the metabolic rate and cardiac output.

As discussed, major mechanisms of body heat loss are conduction, convection, radiation, evaporation, and respiration. Heat loss can be increased by the removal of clothing (decreased insulation, increased radiation), the wetting of clothing by rain or snow (increased conduction and evaporation), air movement around the body (increased convection), or contact with a cold surface or cold-water immersion (increased conduction).

PREDISPOSING FACTORS

Several factors can contribute to the risk of developing hypothermia. They also contribute to the severity of damage if cold injury occurs. Risk factors that increase the danger of developing hypothermia include:

- ★ *Age of the patient.* Pediatric or geriatric patients cannot tolerate cold environments and have less responsive heat-generating mechanisms to combat cold exposure. Elderly persons often become hypothermic in environments that seem only mildly cool to others.
- ★ *Health of the patient.* Hypothyroidism suppresses metabolism, preventing patients from responding appropriately to cold stress. Malnutrition, hypoglycemia, Parkinson's disease, fatigue, and other medical conditions can interfere with the body's ability to combat cold exposure.
- ★ *Medications.* Some drugs interfere with proper heat-generating mechanisms. These include narcotics, alcohol, phenothiazines, barbiturates, antiseizure medications, antihistamines and other allergy medications, antipsychotics, sedatives, antidepressants, and various pain medications such as aspirin, acetaminophen, and NSAIDs.

★ *Prolonged or intense exposure.* The length and severity of cold exposure have a direct effect on morbidity and mortality.

★ *Coexisting weather conditions.* High humidity, brisk winds, or accompanying rain can all magnify the effect of cold exposure on the human body by accelerating the loss of heat from skin surfaces.

PREVENTIVE MEASURES

Certain precautions can decrease the risk of morbidity related to cold injury:

★ Dress warmly.

★ Get plenty of rest to maximize the ability of heat-generating mechanisms to replenish energy supplies.

★ Eat appropriately and at regular intervals to support metabolism.

★ Limit exposure to cold environments.

DEGREES OF HYPOTHERMIA

Hypothermia can be classified as mild or severe, as follows:

★ *Mild.* A core temperature greater than 90°F (32°C) with signs and symptoms of hypothermia.

★ *Severe.* A core temperature less than 90°F (32°C) with signs and symptoms of hypothermia

Initially some patients may exhibit *compensated* hypothermia. In this case signs and symptoms of hypothermia will be present but with a normal core body temperature, temporarily maintained by thermogenesis. As energy stores from the liver and muscle glycogen are exhausted, the core body temperature will drop.

The onset of symptoms may be *acute,* as occurs when a person suddenly falls through ice into a frigid lake. *Subacute* exposure can occur in situations such as when mountain climbers are trapped in a snowy, cold environment. Finally, *chronic* exposure to cold is a growing problem in our inner cities where homeless people endure frequent and prolonged cold stress without shelter.

In some cases cold exposure is the primary cause of hypothermia, but in others, hypothermia may develop secondary to other problems, such as medical problems. For example, hypothyroidism depresses the body's heat-producing mechanisms. Brain tumors or head trauma can depress the hypothalamic temperature control center, causing hypothermia. Other conditions such as myocardial infarction, diabetes, hypoglycemia, drugs, poor nutrition, sepsis, or old age can also contribute to metabolic and circulatory disorders that predispose to hypothermia. Any patient thought to have hypothermia, but with no history of exposure to a cold environment, should be assessed for any predisposing factors. Evaluate the patient for level of consciousness, cool skin, and shivering. Also, evaluate the rectal temperature. A rectal temperature of less than 95°F (35°C) indicates hypothermia. Key findings at different degrees of hypothermia are summarized in Table 36–1.

Patients who experience body temperatures above 86°F (30°C) will usually have a favorable prognosis. Those with temperatures below 86°F (30°C) show a significant increase in mortality rate. Remember that most thermometers used in medicine do not register below 95°F (35°C). EMS systems in colder areas should carry special thermometers for recording subnormal temperature readings as there is no reliable correlation between signs and symptoms and actual core body temperature.

Services operating in colder environments should carry specialized hypothermia thermometers for cold exposure victims.

ASSESSMENT AND MANAGEMENT OF HYPOTHERMIA

Signs and Symptoms

Signs and symptoms of hypothermia are summarized in Table 36–2. Patients experiencing mild hypothermia (core temperature >90°F or 32°C) will generally exhibit shivering. The patient may be

Table 36–1 Key Findings at Different Degrees of Hypothermia

C°	F°	Clinical Findings
37.6	99.6	Normal rectal temperature
37	98.6	Normal oral temperature
36	96.8	Metabolic rate increased
35	95	Maximum shivering seen Impaired judgment
34	93.2	Amnesia Slurred speech
33	91.4	Severe clouding of consciousness/apathy Uncoordinated movement
32	89.6	Most shivering ceases Pupils dilate
31	87.8	Blood pressure may no longer be obtainable
30	86	Atrial fibrillation/other dysrhythmias develop Pulse and cardiac output decreased by 33 percent
29	84.2	Progressive decrease in pulse and breathing Progressive decrease in level of consciousness
28	82.4	Pulse and oxygen consumption decreased by 50 percent Severe slowing of respiration Increased muscle rigidity Loss of consciousness High risk of ventricular fibrillation
27	80.6	Loss of reflexes and voluntary movement Patients appear clinically dead
26	78.8	No reflexes or response to painful stimuli
25	77	Cerebral blood flow decreased by 66 percent
24	75.2	Marked hypotension
22	71.6	Maximum risk for ventricular fibrillation
19	66.2	Flat electroencephalogram (EEG)
18	64.4	Asystole
16	60.8	Lowest reported adult survival from accidental exposure
15.2	59.2	Lowest reported infant survival from accidental exposure
10	50	Oxygen consumption 8 percent of normal
9	48.2	Lowest reported survivor from therapeutic exposure

Table 36–2 Hypothermia: Signs and Symptoms

Mild	Severe
Lethargy	No shivering
Shivering	Dysrhythmias, asystole
Lack of coordination	Loss of voluntary muscle control
Pale, cold, dry skin	Hypotension
Early rise in blood pressure, heart, and respiratory rates	Undetectable pulse and respirations

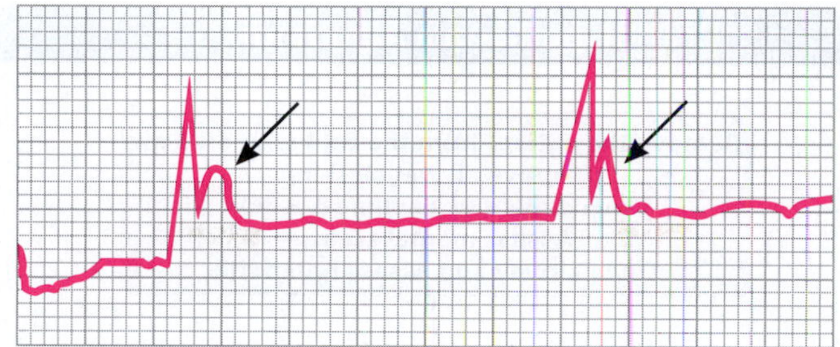

■ **Figure 36-3** ECG tracing showing J wave following the QRS complex as seen in hypothermia.

lethargic and somewhat dulled mentally. (In some cases, however, the patient may be fully oriented.) Muscles may be stiff and uncoordinated, causing the patient to walk with a stumbling, staggering gait.

Patients experiencing severe hypothermia (core temperature <90°F or 32°C) may be disoriented and confused. As their temperatures continue to fall, they will proceed into stupor and complete coma. Shivering will usually stop, and physical activity will become uncoordinated. Muscles may be stiff and rigid. Continuous cardiac monitoring is indicated for anyone experiencing hypothermia. The ECG will frequently show pathognomonic (indicative of a disease) **J waves,** also called Osborn waves, associated with the QRS complexes (Figure 36-3 ■), but these are not useful diagnostically. Atrial fibrillation is the most common presenting dysrhythmia seen in hypothermia. As the body cools, however, the myocardium becomes progressively more irritable and may develop a variety of dysrhythmias. In severe hypothermia, bradycardia is inevitable.

J wave *ECG deflection found at the junction of the QRS complex and the ST segment. It is associated with hypothermia and seen at core temperatures below 32°C, most commonly in leads II and V_6; also called an* Osborn wave.

Ventricular fibrillation becomes more probable as the body's core temperature falls below 86°F (30°C). The severely hypothermic patient requires assessment of pulse and respirations for at least 30 seconds every 1 to 2 minutes.

Treatment

All victims of hypothermia should have the following care (Figure 36-4 ■):

1. *Remove wet garments.*
2. *Protect against further heat loss and wind chill.* Use *passive external warming* methods such as application of blankets, insulating materials, and moisture barriers.
3. *Maintain the patient in a horizontal position.*
4. *Avoid rough handling,* which can trigger dysrhythmias.
5. *Monitor the core temperature.*
6. *Monitor the cardiac rhythm.*

Rewarming is not the mirror image of the cooling process.

Active Rewarming Victims of mild hypothermia may also be rewarmed, using *active external methods.* This includes the use of warmed blankets and/or heat packs placed over areas of high heat transfer with the core: the base of the neck, the axilla, and the groin. Be sure to insulate between the heat packs and the skin to prevent burning. Intravenous fluid heaters (i.e., Hot I.V.) can be used to warm the IV fluid to 95° to 100°F (35° to 38°C). Warmed IV fluids are helpful in treating mild-to-moderate hypothermia. Heat guns and lights may also be used, but this will most likely take place in the emergency department. Warm water immersion in water between 102° and 104°F (38.9° to 40.0°C) may be used but can induce rewarming shock (see the following section), so this method also has little application in an out-of-hospital setting.

Active rewarming of the severely hypothermic patient is best carried out in the hospital using a prearranged protocol. Most patients who die during rewarming die from ventricular fibrillation, the risk of which is related to both the depth and the duration of hypothermia. Rough handling of the hypothermic patient may also induce ventricular fibrillation. Active rewarming should not be attempted in the field unless travel to the emergency department will take more than 15 minutes.

If such is the case, active internal rewarming methods may also be used, including the use of warmed (102° to 104°F or 38.9° to 40.0°C) humidified oxygen, and administration of warmed IV fluids

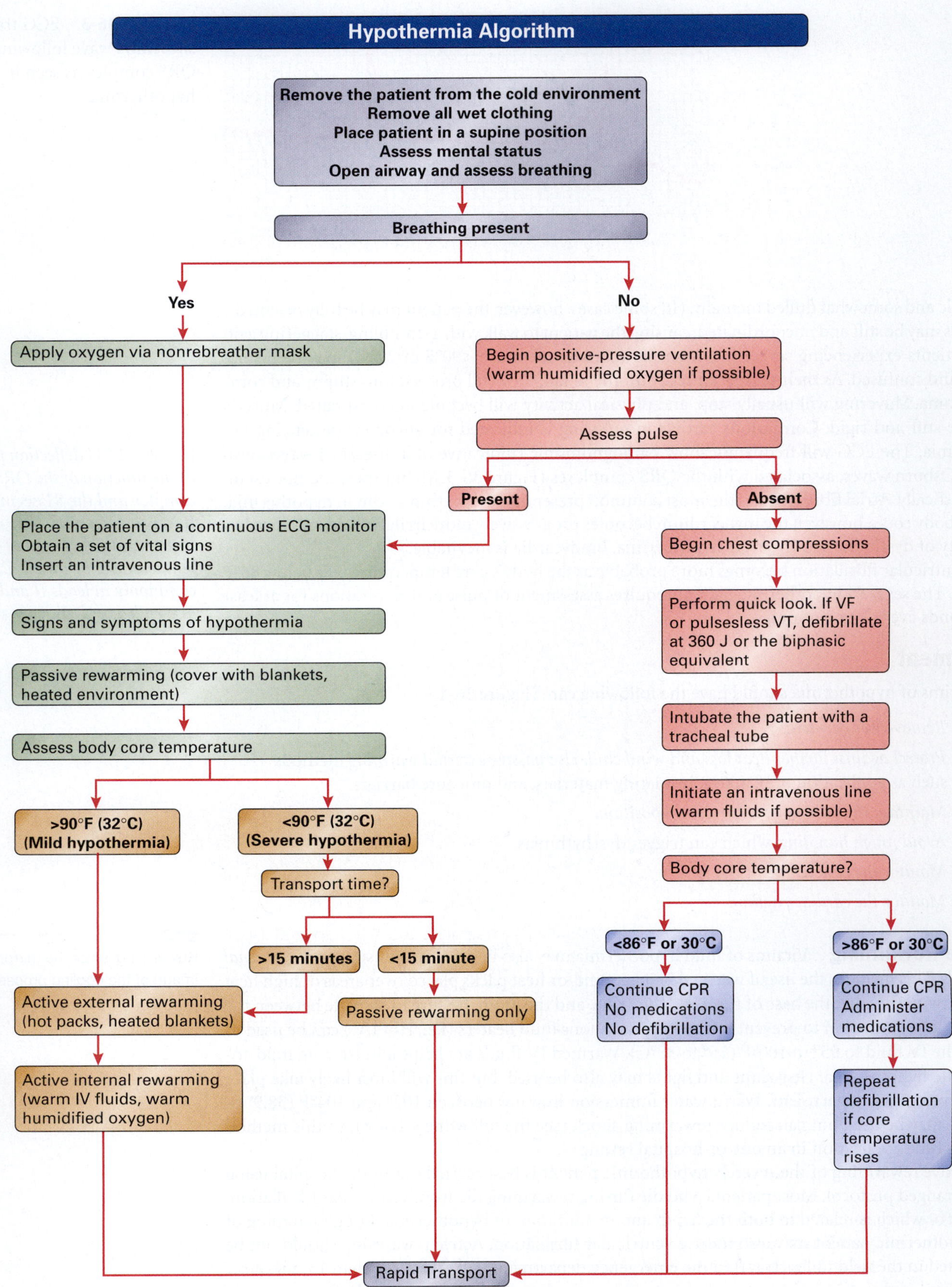

■ **Figure 36-4** Algorithm for treatment of hypothermia.

(also warmed to 102° to 104°F or 38° to 40°C). This is crucial to prevent further heat loss, but actual heat transferred is minimal, so there is limited contribution to the rewarming effort.

Rewarming Shock While application of warmed blankets is a safe and effective means of rewarming the hypothermic patient, application of external heat, as with heat packs, is usually not recommended in the prehospital setting. For effective rewarming, more heat transference is generally required than is possible with prehospital methods. Additionally, application of external heat may result in *rewarming shock* by causing reflex peripheral vasodilation. This reflex vasodilation causes the return of cool blood and acids from the extremities to the core. This may cause a paradoxical "afterdrop" core temperature decrease and further worsen core hypothermia. This, in turn, may cause the blood pressure to fall, especially when there is also volume depletion.

If active rewarming is necessary in the prehospital setting (for example, when transport is delayed), administration of warmed IV fluids during rewarming can prevent the onset of rewarming shock.

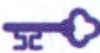

Active rewarming of the severely hypothermic patient should be deferred until the patient is at the hospital unless transport time is long and rewarming is ordered by medical direction.

Cold Diuresis Volume depletion can occur as a result of *cold diuresis.* Core vasoconstriction causes increased blood volume and blood pressure, so the kidneys remove excess fluid to reduce the pressure, thus causing diuresis. A warmed IV volume expander (e.g., normal saline) should be used both to prevent rewarming shock and to replace fluid lost from cold diuresis.

The conscious patient who is able to manage his airway may be given warmed, sweetened fluids. Alcohol and caffeine should be avoided.

Resuscitation

There are certain resuscitation considerations when handling cardiac arrest victims with core temperatures below 86°F (30°C).

Basic Cardiac Life Support BLS providers should start cardiopulmonary resuscitation (CPR) immediately, although pulse and respirations may need to be checked for longer periods to detect minimal cardiopulmonary efforts. Use normal chest compression and ventilation rates and ventilate with warmed, humidified oxygen. If an AED is available and ventricular fibrillation is detected, a single shock may be given. Further shocks should be avoided until after rewarming to above 86°F. CPR, rewarming, and rapid transport should immediately follow the defibrillation attempt.

Advanced Cardiac Life Support Since there is no increased risk of inducing ventricular fibrillation from orotracheal or nasotracheal intubation, ALS providers may intubate the patient and ventilate with warmed, humidified oxygen. Drug metabolism is reduced, however, so administered medications such as epinephrine, lidocaine, and procainamide may accumulate to toxic levels if used repeatedly in the severely hypothermic victim. In addition, administered drugs may remain in the peripheral circulation. When the patient is rewarmed and perfusion resumes, large, toxic boluses of these medications may be delivered to the central circulation and target tissues. Lidocaine and procainamide may also paradoxically lower the fibrillatory threshold in a hypothermic heart and increase resistance to defibrillation. Bretylium and magnesium sulfate, however, may be effective even in hypothermic hearts.

The American Heart Association recommends that, if the patient fails to respond to initial defibrillation attempts or initial drug therapy, subsequent defibrillations or boluses of medication should be avoided until the core temperature is about 86°F (30°C). This is because it is generally impossible to electrically defibrillate a heart that is colder than 86°F. Active core rewarming techniques are the primary modality in hypothermia victims who are either in cardiac arrest or unconscious with a slow heart rate.

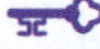

If the hypothermic cardiac arrest patient fails to respond to initial defibrillation attempts or drug therapy, avoid subsequent defibrillations or medication until the core temperature is about 86°F (30°C). It is generally impossible to defibrillate a heart that is colder than 86°F.

Techniques that may be used include the administration of heated, humidified oxygen and warmed intravenous fluids, preferably normal saline, infused centrally at rates of 150 to 200 mL/hour to avoid overhydration. Peritoneal lavage with warmed potassium-free fluid administered 2 L at a time may be used, as may extracorporeal blood warming with partial cardiac bypass. Obviously some of these techniques may only be carried out in a hospital setting.

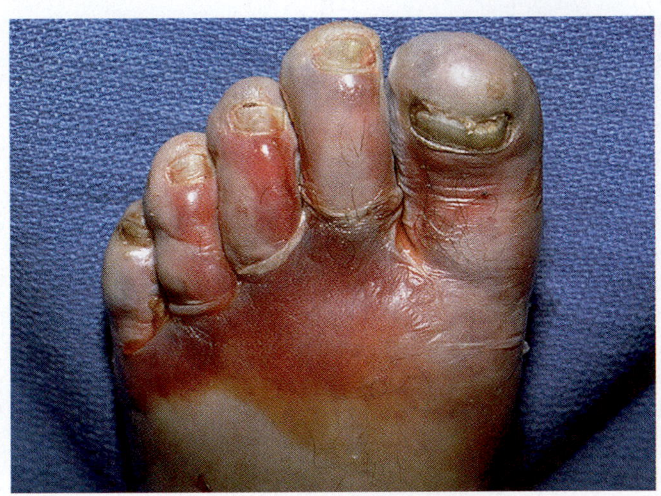

■ **Figure 36-5** Frostbite.

Transportation

When transporting a hypothermic patient, remember that gentle transportation is necessary due to myocardial irritability and that the patient should be kept level or slightly inclined with head down. Contact the receiving hospital for general rewarming options. When determining your destination, consider the availability of cardiac bypass rewarming.

FROSTBITE

frostbite *environmentally induced freezing of body tissues causing destruction of cells.*

Frostbite is environmentally induced freezing of body tissues (Figure 36-5 ■). As the tissues freeze, ice crystals form within and water is drawn out of the cells into the extracellular space. These ice crystals expand, causing the destruction of cells. During this process, intracellular electrolyte concentrations increase, further destroying cells. Damage to blood vessels from ice crystal formation causes loss of vascular integrity, resulting in tissue swelling and loss of distal nutritional flow.

Superficial and Deep Frostbite

superficial frostbite *freezing involving only epidermal tissues resulting in redness followed by blanching and diminished sensation; also called* frostnip.

deep frostbite *freezing involving epidermal and subcutaneous tissues resulting in a white appearance, hard (frozen) feeling on palpation, and loss of sensation.*

Generally, there are two types of frostbite: superficial and deep. **Superficial frostbite** (frostnip) exhibits some freezing of epidermal tissue, resulting in initial redness, followed by blanching. There will also be diminished sensation. **Deep frostbite** affects the epidermal and subcutaneous layers. There is a white appearance and the area feels hard (frozen) to palpation. There is also loss of sensation in deep frostbite.

Frostbite mainly occurs in the extremities and in areas of the head and face exposed to the environment. Subfreezing temperatures are required for frostbite to occur, although they are not necessary to produce hypothermia. Many patients who have frostbite will also have hypothermia.

There can be tremendous variation in how an individual can present with frostbite. For example, some patients feel little pain at onset. Others will report severe pain. A certain degree of compliance may be felt beneath the frozen layer in superficial frostbite, but in deep frostbite, the frozen part will be hard and noncompliant.

Treatment

Do not thaw frozen flesh if there is any possibility of refreezing. Do not massage the frozen area or rub it with snow.

In treating frostbite, take the following recommended steps:

- Do not thaw the affected area if there is any possibility of refreezing.
- Do not massage the frozen area or rub with snow. Rubbing the affected area may cause ice crystals within the tissues to damage the already injured tissues more seriously.
- Administer analgesia prior to thawing.

- ★ Transport to the hospital for rewarming by immersion. If transport will be delayed, thaw the frozen part by immersion in a 102–104°F (39°–40°C) water bath. Water temperature will fall rapidly, requiring additions of warm water throughout the process.
- ★ Cover the thawed part with loosely applied dry, sterile dressings.
- ★ Elevate and immobilize the thawed part.
- ★ Do not puncture or drain blisters.
- ★ Do not rewarm frozen feet if they are required for walking out of a hazardous situation.

TRENCH FOOT

Trench foot (immersion foot) is similar to frostbite, but it occurs at temperatures above freezing. It is rarely seen in the civilian population. It received its name in World War I, when troops confined to trenches with standing cold water developed progressive symptoms over days. Symptoms are similar to frostbite, but there may be pain. Blisters may form on spontaneous rewarming.

trench foot *a painful foot disorder resembling frostbite and resulting from exposure to cold and wet, which can eventually result in tissue sloughing or gangrene; also called* immersion foot.

Treatment

Treatment of trench foot requires early recognition of developing symptoms and immediate steps to warm, dry, aerate, and elevate the feet. Measures to prevent trench foot are most effective, such as avoiding prolonged exposure to standing water, changing wet socks frequently, and never sleeping in wet boots or socks.

NEAR-DROWNING AND DROWNING

Drowning is asphyxiation resulting from submersion in liquid. The term *drowning* can be differentiated from the term *near-drowning. Drowning* means that death occurred within 24 hours of submersion, whereas **near-drowning** indicates that death either did not occur or occurred more than 24 hours after submersion.

drowning *asphyxiation resulting from submersion in liquid with death occurring within 24 hours of submersion.*

near-drowning *an incident of potentially fatal submersion in liquid which did not result in death or in which death occurred more than 24 hours after submersion.*

It is estimated that, in the United States, approximately 4,500 persons die annually due to drowning. Many more sustain serious injury due to near-drowning. This makes drowning the third most common cause of accidental death in the United States. Approximately 40 percent of these deaths are in children under 5 years of age. There is a second peak incidence in teenagers and a final third peak in the elderly as a result of accidental bathtub drownings. Approximately 85 percent of near-drowning victims are male, and two-thirds of these do not know how to swim. Most commonly, these situations are due to freshwater submersion, especially in swimming pools. Unfortunately, alcohol use by the victim or the supervising adult is frequently associated with this type of accident.

It is important to note that other emergency conditions are often associated with near-drowning. If the cause of the submersion is unknown, consider the possibility of trauma and treat the patient accordingly.

Frequently the submersion occurs in cold water, causing hypothermia. Hypothermia slows the body's metabolic processes, thereby decreasing the need for oxygen. This can have a protective effect on organs and tissues which become hypoxic (low in oxygen) in submersion situations. However, it is important to treat the hypoxia first, once you have initiated rescue.

PATHOPHYSIOLOGY OF DROWNING AND NEAR-DROWNING

As a paramedic, you need to understand the sequence of events in drowning or near-drowning. Following submersion, if the victim is conscious, he will undergo a period of complete apnea for up to 3 minutes. This apnea is an involuntary reflex as the victim strives to keep his head above water. During this time, blood is shunted to the heart and brain because of the mammalian diving reflex, which is described later in this chapter.

When the victim is apneic, the $PaCO_2$ in the blood rises to greater than 50 mmHg. Meanwhile, the PaO_2 of the blood falls below 50 mmHg. The stimulus from the hypoxia ultimately overrides the sedative effects of the hypercarbia, resulting in central nervous system stimulation.

Dry versus Wet Drowning

Until unconscious, the victim experiences a great deal of panic. During this stage the victim makes violent inspiratory and swallowing efforts. At this point, copious amounts of water enter the mouth, posterior oropharynx, and stomach, stimulating severe laryngospasm (airway obstruction due to aspirated water) and bronchospasm. In approximately 10 percent of drowning victims, and in a much greater percentage of near-drowning victims, this laryngospasm prevents the influx of water into the lungs. If a significant amount of water does not enter the lungs, it is referred to as a *dry drowning.* Conversely, if a laryngospasm does not occur, and a significant quantity of water does enter the lungs, it is referred to as a *wet drowning.*

The laryngospasm further aggravates the hypoxia, with coma ultimately ensuing. Persistent anoxia (absence of oxygen) results in a deeper coma. Following unconsciousness, reflex swallowing continues, resulting in gastric distention and increased risk of vomiting and aspiration. If untreated, hypotension, bradycardia, and death result in a short period.

Drowning and near-drowning are primarily due to asphyxia from airway obstruction in the lung secondary to the aspirated water or the laryngospasm. If, in a near-drowning episode, this process does not end in death, any fluid that has entered the lungs may cause lower airway disease.

Freshwater versus Saltwater Drowning

Although the physiology of freshwater and saltwater drownings differ, there is no difference in the end result or in prehospital management.

You should expect different physiological reactions in cases of freshwater and saltwater drownings or near-drownings. However, these mechanistic differences make no difference in the end metabolic result or in the prehospital management.

Freshwater Drowning In freshwater drowning or near-drowning, the large surface area of the alveoli and small airways allow a massive amount of hypotonic water to diffuse across the alveolar/capillary membrane and into the vascular space. This results in hemodilution, an expansion in blood plasma volume and relative reduction in red blood cell concentration. *Hemodilution* produces a thickening of the alveolar walls with inflammatory cells, hemorrhagic pneumonitis (bleeding lung inflammation), and destruction of surfactant.

surfactant *a compound secreted by cells in the lungs that regulates the surface tension of the fluid that lines the alveoli, which is important in keeping the alveoli open for gas exchange.*

Surfactant is a substance in the alveoli responsible for keeping the alveoli open. In drowning, some surfactant is lost when the capillaries of the alveoli are damaged. Plasma proteins then leak back into the alveoli, resulting in the accumulation of fluid in the small airways. This in turn leads to multiple areas of atelectasis—areas of alveolar collapse. Atelectasis causes shunting, which is the return of unoxygenated blood from the damaged alveoli to the bloodstream. In other words, blood is traveling through the lungs without being oxygenated. The result is hypoxemia (inadequate oxygenation of the blood) (Figure 36-6 ■).

Saltwater Drowning In saltwater drowning or near-drowning, the hypertonic nature of seawater, which is three to four times more hypertonic than plasma, draws water from the bloodstream into the alveoli (Figure 36-6). This produces pulmonary edema, leading to profound shunting. The result is failure of oxygenation, producing hypoxemia. Additionally, respiratory and metabolic acidosis develop due to the retention of CO_2 and developing anaerobic (without-oxygen) metabolism.

Factors Affecting Survival

A number of factors have an impact on drowning and near-drowning survival rates. These include the cleanliness of the water, the length of time submerged, and the age and general health of the victim. Children have a longer survival time and a greater probability of a successful resuscitation. Even more significant is the water temperature. The concept of developing brain death after 4 to 6 minutes without oxygen is not applicable in cases of near-drowning in cold water. Some patients in cold water (below 68°F) can be resuscitated after 30 minutes or more in cardiac arrest. However, persons under water 60 minutes or longer usually cannot be resuscitated.

mammalian diving reflex *a complex cardiovascular reflex, resulting from submersion of the face and nose in water, that constricts blood flow everywhere except to the brain.*

A possible contribution to survival may be the **mammalian diving reflex.** When a person dives into cold water, he reacts to the submersion of the face. Breathing is inhibited, the heart rate be-

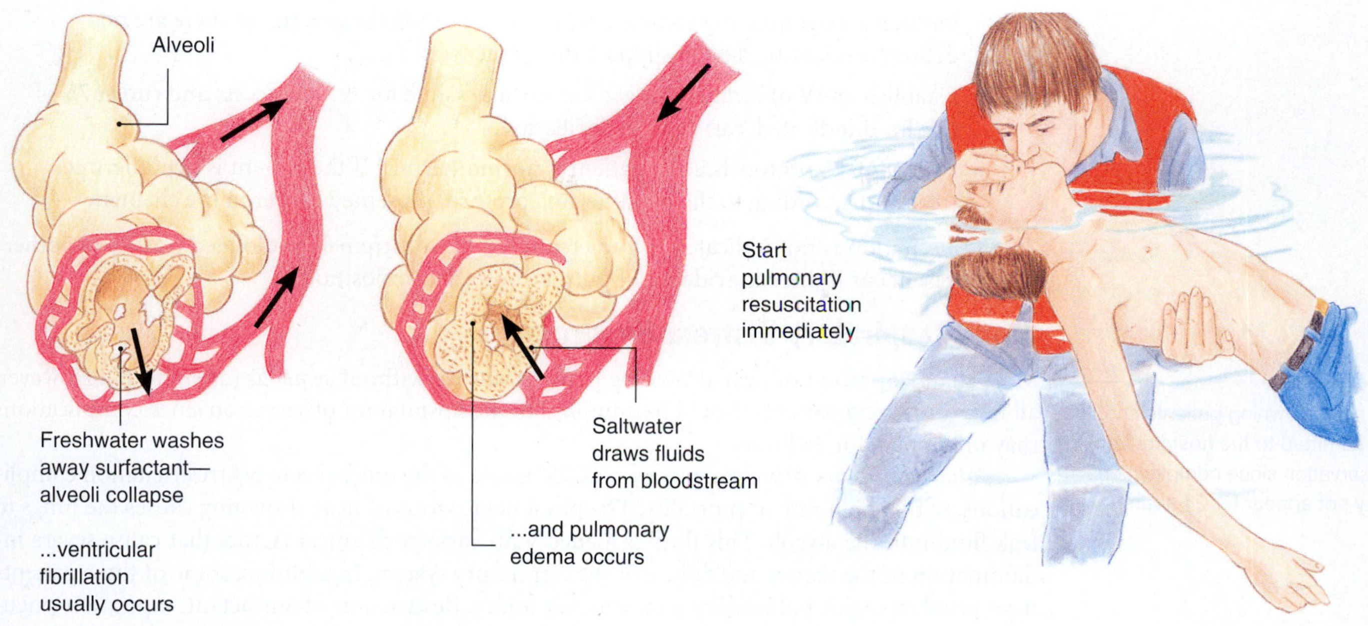

■ **Figure 36-6** Pathophysiological effects of drowning.

comes bradycardic, and vasoconstriction develops in tissues relatively resistant to asphyxia. Meanwhile, cerebral and cardiac blood flow is maintained. In this way, oxygen is sent and used only where it is immediately needed to sustain life. The colder the water, the more oxygen is diverted to the heart and brain. A common saying in emergency medicine states: "The cold-water drowning victim is not dead until he is warm and dead." In other words, a person who has been submerged in cold water may only seem to be dead, but due to the continued supply of oxygen to the heart and brain may indeed still be alive.

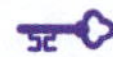

The cold-water drowning victim is not dead until he is warm and dead.

TREATMENT FOR NEAR-DROWNING

Since freshwater and saltwater near-drownings both involve factors that disrupt normal pulmonary function, initial field treatment must be directed toward correcting the profound hypoxia. Take the following steps:

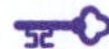

Never attempt to rescue a drowning victim unless you have been trained and have the necessary safety equipment.

- ★ Remove the patient from the water as soon as possible. This should be done by a trained rescue swimmer.
- ★ Initiate ventilation while the patient is still in the water. Rescue personnel should wear protective clothing if water temperature is less than 70°F. In addition, attach a safety line to the rescue swimmer. In fast water, it is essential to use personnel specifically trained for this type of rescue.
- ★ Suspect head and neck injury if the patient experienced a fall or was diving. Rapidly place the victim on a long backboard and remove him from the water. Use C-spine precautions throughout care.
- ★ Protect the patient from heat loss. Avoid laying the patient on a cold surface. Remove wet clothing and cover the body to the extent possible.
- ★ Examine the patient for airway patency, breathing, and pulse. If indicated, begin CPR and defibrillation.
- ★ Manage the airway using proper suctioning and airway adjuncts.
- ★ Administer oxygen at a 100 percent concentration.
- ★ Use respiratory rewarming, if available, and if transport time is longer than 15 minutes. (In the past, prophylactic abdominal thrusts were used to clear the airway,

but there are conflicting recommendations regarding the practice as there are no definitive scientific data to support this maneuver.)

- ★ Establish an IV of lactated Ringer's or normal saline for venous access and run at 75 mL/hr. If indicated, carry out defibrillation.
- ★ Follow ACLS protocols if the patient is normothermic. If the patient is hypothermic, treat him according to the hypothermia protocol presented earlier in the chapter.

Resuscitation is not indicated if immersion has been extremely prolonged (unless hypothermia is present) or if there is evidence of putrefaction (decomposition).

Adult Respiratory Distress Syndrome

All near-drowning patients should be admitted to the hospital for observation since complications may not appear for 24 hours.

More than 90 percent of near-drowning patients survive without *sequelae* (aftereffects). However, all near-drowning patients should be admitted to the hospital for observation since complications may not appear for 24 hours.

Adult respiratory distress syndrome (ARDS) is one of the more severe postresuscitation complications, with a high rate of mortality. The physiologic stress of near-drowning causes the lungs to leak fluid into the alveoli. This fluid is loaded with various chemical factors that cause severe inflammation of the tissues and failure of the respiratory system. In addition, some of these patients have problems with pulmonary parenchymal injury, destruction of surfactant, aspiration pneumonitis, or pneumothorax. A number require an extended hospital stay due to renal failure, hypoxia, hypercarbia, and mixed metabolic and respiratory acidosis. The effects of cerebral hypoxia occasionally require treatment throughout hospitalization and beyond.

DIVING EMERGENCIES

scuba *acronym for self-contained underwater breathing apparatus, portable apparatus that contains compressed air which allows the diver to breathe underwater.*

Scuba diving has become an extremely popular recreational sport. Divers wear portable equipment containing compressed air, which allows the diver to breathe underwater. Although scuba diving accidents are fairly uncommon, inexperienced divers have a higher rate of injury. Scuba diving emergencies can occur on the surface, in 3 feet of water, or at any depth. The more serious emergencies usually occur following a dive. To better assess and care for diving injuries, it is important to understand a few principles of pressure.

THE EFFECTS OF AIR PRESSURE ON GASES

Content Review

Boyle's Law

The volume of a gas is inversely proportional to its pressure if the temperature is kept constant.

Dalton's Law

The total pressure of a mixture of gases is equal to the sum of the partial pressures of the individual gases.

Henry's Law

The amount of gas dissolved in a given volume of fluid is proportional to the pressure of the gas above it.

Water is an incompressible liquid. Fresh water has a density, or weight per unit of volume, of 62.4 pounds per cubic foot. Saltwater has a density of 64 pounds per cubic foot. This density can be equated to pressure, which is defined as the weight or force acting on a unit area. Thus, a cubic foot of freshwater exerts a pressure ("weight") of 62.4 pounds over an area of 1 square foot. This measurement is typically stated in pounds per square inch (psi).

Humans at sea level live in an atmosphere of air, which is a mixture of gases. These gases weigh and exert a pressure of 14.7 pounds per square inch (760 mmHg). This pressure, however, may vary within the environment. For example, ascending to an altitude of 1 mile will decrease the atmospheric pressure by 17 percent to approximately 12.2 pounds.

To understand how air pressure affects diving accidents, we look at three physical laws: Boyle's law, Dalton's law, and Henry's law.

Boyle's Law

Boyle's law states that the volume of a gas is inversely proportional to its pressure if the temperature is kept constant. As you increase pressure, the gas is compressed into a smaller space. For example, doubling the pressure of a gas mixture will decrease its volume by one-half. The pressure of air at sea level is 14.7 lb/in.^{2} or 760 mmHg. This pressure is called 1 "atmosphere absolute" or 1 "ata." Two ata occur at a depth of 33 feet of water, 3 ata occur at a depth of 66 feet of water, and so on. Therefore, 1 L of air at the surface is compressed to 500 mL at 33 feet. At 66 feet, 1 L of air would be compressed to 250 mL.

Dalton's Law

Dalton's law states that the total pressure of a mixture of gases is equal to the sum of the partial pressures of the individual gases. The air we breathe is a mixture of nitrogen (about 78 percent), oxygen (about 21 percent), and carbon dioxide plus traces of argon, helium, and other rare gases (about 1 percent). Since the pressure of air at sea level is 760 mmHg, the pressure of nitrogen is about 593 mmHg, the pressure of oxygen is about 160 mmHg, and the pressure of carbon dioxide is somewhat less than 4 mmHg—each gas exerting its proportion of the total pressure of the mixture.

At different altitudes above sea level or depths below sea level, the pressure of air will change (less at higher altitudes, more at greater depths), but the component gases will still account for the same proportion of whatever the total pressure is at that level: nitrogen 78 percent, oxygen 21 percent, and carbon dioxide less than 1 percent.

Henry's Law

Henry's law states that the amount of gas dissolved in a given volume of fluid is proportional to the pressure of the gas above it. When we descend below sea level, and the pressure bearing down on us increases, the gases that make up the air we breathe tend to dissolve in the liquids (mainly blood plasma) and tissues of the body.

Let us compare what happens to the two chief components of the air we breathe—oxygen and nitrogen—when a person descends to greater and greater depths below sea level. Much of the oxygen is used up in the normal metabolism of the cells, leaving only a small amount to be dissolved in the blood and tissues. Nitrogen, however, is an inert gas and, as such, is not used by the body. Therefore, a far greater quantity of nitrogen is available to dissolve in the blood and tissues as a person descends below sea level. In brief, at depths below sea level, oxygen metabolizes but nitrogen dissolves.

When the person ascends toward sea level again, the gases that are dissolved in the blood and tissues, being under less and less pressure, come out of the blood and tissues and, if the ascent is too rapid, form bubbles. To understand this phenomenon, compare the human body to a bottled carbonated soft drink—that is, a liquid in which carbon dioxide gas is dissolved. The gas is kept dissolved in the liquid by the cap on the bottle and a high-pressure gas under the cap, on top of the liquid. When the cap is removed and the pressure is released, the gas bubbles out of the liquid, causing a fizz that will sometimes rise completely out of the bottle.

In the following sections, we will discuss how the phenomena of gases and pressure can cause serious problems for divers.

PATHOPHYSIOLOGY OF DIVING EMERGENCIES

As noted, gases are dissolved in the diver's blood and tissues under pressure. As the diver goes deeper into the water, pressure increases, causing more gas to dissolve in the blood (Henry's law). According to Boyle's law, these gases will have a smaller volume due to the increased ambient pressure. During *controlled* ascent, with decreasing pressure, dissolved gases come out of the blood and tissues slowly, escaping gradually through respiration.

If ascent is *too rapid*, however, the dissolved gases, mostly nitrogen, come out of solution and expand quickly, forming bubbles in the blood, brain, spinal cord, skin, inner ear, muscles, and joints. Once bubbles of nitrogen have formed in various tissues, it is difficult for the body to remove them. The ascending diver who comes to the surface too rapidly, not adhering to safety measures, is at risk of becoming a veritable living bottle of soda.

CLASSIFICATION OF DIVING INJURIES

Scuba diving injuries are due to barotrauma, pulmonary overpressure, arterial gas embolism, decompression illness, cold, panic, or a combination of these. Accidents generally occur at one of the following four stages of a dive:

- ★ On the surface
- ★ During descent

- ★ On the bottom
- ★ During ascent

Injuries on the Surface

Surface injuries can involve any of several factors. One such factor can be entanglement of lines or entanglement in kelp fields while swimming to the area of the dive. Divers in these situations may panic, become fatigued, even drown. Another factor may be cold water that produces shivering and blackout. Boats in the area are another potential source of injury to the diver. To prevent such accidents, divers will usually mark the area of their dive with a flag. Maritime rules require boat operators to stay clear of a flagged area.

barotrauma *injuries caused by changes in pressure. Barotrauma that occurs from increasing pressure during a diving descent is commonly called "the squeeze."*

nitrogen narcosis *a state of stupor that develops during deep dives due to nitrogen's effect on cerebral function; also called "raptures of the deep."*

decompression illness *development of nitrogen bubbles within the tissues due to a rapid reduction of air pressure when a diver returns to the surface; also called "the bends."*

pulmonary overpressure *expansion of air held in the lungs during ascent. If not exhaled, the expanded air may cause injury to the lungs and surrounding structures.*

arterial gas embolism (AGE) *an air bubble, or air embolism, that enters the circulatory system from a damaged lung.*

pneumomediastinum *the presence of air in the mediastinum.*

pneumothorax *a collection of air in the pleural space. Air may enter the pleural space through an injury to the chest wall or through an injury to the lungs. In a tension pneumothorax, pressure builds because there is no way for the air to escape, causing lung collapse.*

Injuries during Descent

Barotrauma means injuries caused by changes in pressure. Barotrauma during descent is commonly called "the squeeze." It can occur if the diver cannot equilibrate the pressure between the nasopharynx and the middle ear through the eustachian tube. The diver can experience middle ear pain, ringing in the ears, dizziness, and hearing loss. In severe cases, rupture of the eardrum can occur. A diver who has an upper respiratory infection, and who therefore cannot clear the middle ear through the eustachian tube, should not dive. A similar lack of equilibration can occur in the sinuses, producing severe frontal headaches or pain beneath the eye in the maxillary sinuses.

Injuries on the Bottom

Major diving emergencies while at the bottom of the dive often involve **nitrogen narcosis** (a state of stupor), commonly called "raptures of the deep." This is due to nitrogen's effect on cerebral function. The diver may appear to be intoxicated and may take unnecessary risks. Other emergencies occur when a diver runs low on or out of air. The diver who panics will exacerbate this situation by consuming even more oxygen and producing even more carbon dioxide.

Injuries during Ascent

Serious and life-threatening emergencies, many involving barotrauma, can occur during the ascent. For example, as during descent, an ascending diver may be unable to equilibrate inner ear and nasopharyngeal pressure.

Dives below 33 feet may require staged ascent to prevent **decompression illness,** also called "the bends." This condition develops in divers subjected to rapid reduction of air pressure while ascending to the surface following exposure to compressed air, with formation of nitrogen bubbles causing severe pain, especially in the abdomen and the joints.

The most serious barotrauma that occurs during ascent is injury to the lung from **pulmonary overpressure.** This can occur with a deep dive, or it can occur with a dive of as little as 3 feet below the surface. The injury results from the diver holding his breath during the ascent. As the diver ascends, the air in the lung, which has been compressed, expands. If it is not exhaled, the alveoli may rupture. If this occurs, the result will be structural damage to the lung and, possibly, **arterial gas embolism (AGE),** an air bubble, or air embolism, that enters the circulatory system from the damaged lung. Another result may be **pneumomediastinum,** the release of gas (air) through the visceral pleura into the mediastinum and pericardial sac around the heart as well as into the tissues of the neck. **Pneumothorax** is possible if the alveoli rupture into the pleural cavity. Air embolism can occur if the air ruptures into the pulmonary veins or arteries and returns to the left atrium and finally into the left ventricle and out into the systemic circulation.

GENERAL ASSESSMENT OF DIVING EMERGENCIES

In the early assessment of diving accidents, all symptoms of air embolism and decompression illness are considered together. Early assessment and treatment of a diving injury is of more importance than trying to distinguish the exact problem. One of your most important tasks in a diving-related injury is elicitation of a diving history or profile. Several essential factors to consider are as follows:

- ★ Time at which the signs and symptoms occurred
- ★ Type of breathing apparatus utilized
- ★ Type of hypothermia protective garment worn
- ★ Parameters of the dive:
  - Depth of dive(s)
  - Number of dives
  - Duration of dive(s)
- ★ Aircraft travel following a dive (in a pressurized cabin)
- ★ Rate of ascent
- ★ Associated panic forcing rapid ascent
- ★ Experience of the diver, for example, student, inexperienced, or "pro"
- ★ Properly functioning depth gauge
- ★ Previous medical diseases
- ★ Old injuries
- ★ Previous episodes of decompression illness
- ★ Use of medications
- ★ Use of alcohol

From a quick assessment of the patient's diving profile, you can rapidly determine if the diver is a likely candidate for a pressure disorder.

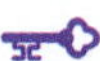

In a diving emergency, consider all symptoms of air embolism and decompression illness together. Early assessment and treatment are more important than identifying the exact problem.

PRESSURE DISORDERS

Injuries caused by pressure, as noted earlier, are known as *barotrauma*. In the case of diving accidents, most barotrauma results from a pressure imbalance between the external environment and gases within the body. The following sections describe some of the most common forms of barotrauma involved in diving accidents.

Decompression Illness

Decompression illness develops in divers subjected to rapid reduction of air pressure after ascending to the surface following exposure to compressed air. A number of general and individual factors can contribute to the development of decompression illness, or the bends (Table 36–3). Decompression illness results as nitrogen bubbles come out of solution in the blood and tissues, causing increased pressure in various body structures and occluding circulation in the small blood vessels. This occurs in joints, tendons, the spinal cord, skin, brain, and inner ear. Symptoms develop when a diver rapidly ascends after being exposed to a depth of 33 feet or more for a time sufficient to allow the body's tissues to be saturated with nitrogen.

Signs and Symptoms The principal signs and symptoms of decompression illnesses are joint and abdominal pain, fatigue, paresthesias, and CNS disturbances. The nitrogen bubbles produced by rapid decompression are thought to produce obstruction of blood flow and lead to local ischemia, subjecting tissues to anoxic stress. In some cases, this stress may lead to tissue damage.

Treatment Patients with decompression illness usually seek medical treatment within 12 hours of ascent from a dive. Some patients may not seek treatment for as long as 24 hours after the last dive. It is generally safe to assume that signs or symptoms developing more than 36 hours after a dive cannot reasonably be attributed to decompression illness.

Decompression illness may require urgent definitive care through **recompression.** This can be accomplished by placing the patient in a **hyperbaric oxygen chamber** (Figure 36-7 ■). There the

recompression *resubmission of a person to a greater pressure so that gradual decompression can be achieved; often used in the treatment of diving emergencies.*

hyperbaric oxygen chamber *recompression chamber used to treat patients suffering from barotrauma.*

Table 36-3 Factors Related to the Development of Decompression Illness

General Factors	Individual Factors
Cold water dives	Age—older individuals
Diving in rough water	Obesity
Strenuous diving conditions	Fatigue—lack of sleep prior to dive
History of previous decompression dive incident	Alcohol—consumption before or after dive
Overstaying time at given dive depth	History of medical problems
Dive at 80 feet or greater	
Rapid ascent—panic, inexperience, unfamiliarity with equipment	
Heavy exercise before or after dive to the point of muscle soreness	
Flying after diving (24 hour wait is recommended)	
Driving to high altitude after dive	

Recompression in a hyperbaric oxygen chamber may be required for the patient suspected of suffering decompression illness or an air embolism.

patient is subjected to oxygen under greater-than-atmospheric pressure to force the nitrogen in the body to redissolve, and then is gradually decompressed to allow the nitrogen to escape without forming bubbles. However, prompt stabilization at the nearest emergency department should be accomplished before transportation to a recompression chamber.

Early oxygen therapy may substantially reduce symptoms of decompression illness. Divers who are administered high-flow, high-concentration oxygen have a considerably better treatment outcome. The following list outlines some of the steps in the prehospital management of decompression illnesses:

- ★ Assess the ABCs.
- ★ Administer CPR, if required.
- ★ Administer oxygen at 100 percent concentration with a nonrebreather mask. An unconscious diver should be intubated.

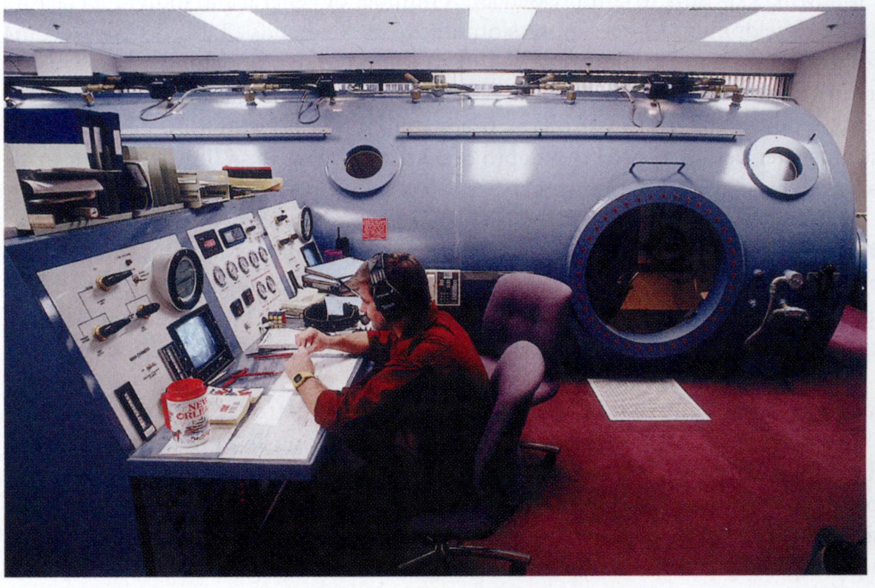

■ **Figure 36-7** Hyperbaric oxygen chamber used in the treatment of decompression illness. *(© Gregory G. Dimijian/Photo Researchers, Inc.)*

- ★ Keep the patient in the supine position.
- ★ Protect the patient from excessive heat, cold, wetness, or noxious fumes.
- ★ Give the conscious, alert patient nonalcoholic liquids such as fruit juices or oral balanced salt solutions.
- ★ Evaluate and stabilize the patient at the nearest emergency department prior to transport to a recompression chamber. Begin IV fluid replacement with electrolyte solutions for unconscious or seriously injured patients. You may use lactated Ringer's or normal saline. Do not use 5 percent dextrose in water.
- ★ If there is evidence of CNS involvement, administer dexamethasone, heparin, or Valium as ordered by medical direction.
- ★ If air evacuation is used, do not expose the patient to decreased barometric pressure. Cabin pressure must be maintained at sea level; otherwise the patient must fly at the lowest possible safe altitude.
- ★ Send the patient's diving equipment with the patient for examination. If that is impossible, arrange for local examination and gas analysis.

Pulmonary Overpressure Accidents

Lung overinflation due to rapid ascent is the common cause of a number of emergencies, particularly at shallow depths of less than 6 feet. Air can become trapped in the lungs by mucous plugs, bronchospasm, or simple breath holding. With rapid ascent, ambient pressure drops quickly, causing the trapped air to expand. Air expansion can rupture the alveolar membranes. This can result in hemorrhage, reduced oxygen and carbon dioxide transport, and capillary and alveolar inflammation. Air can also escape from the lung into other nearby tissues and cause pneumothorax and tension pneumothorax, subcutaneous emphysema, or pneumomediastinum.

Signs and Symptoms Divers with this type of condition will complain of substernal chest pain. Respiratory distress and diminished breath sounds are common findings on examination.

Treatment Treatment for this condition is the same as for pneumothorax caused by any other mechanism (see Chapter 27, "Pulmonology"). Rest and supplemental oxygen are important but hyperbaric oxygen is not usually necessary.

Arterial Gas Embolism

As described, a pressure buildup in the lung can damage and rupture alveoli. This can allow air in the form of a large bubble to escape into the circulation. This air embolism, or arterial gas embolism (AGE), can travel to the left atrium and ventricle of the heart and out into various parts of the body where it may lodge and obstruct blood flow, causing ischemia and possibly infarct. Such obstruction of blood flow can have devastating effects triggered by cardiac, pulmonary, and cerebral compromise.

Signs and Symptoms Signs and symptoms of air embolism include onset within 2 to 10 minutes of ascent; a rapid and dramatic onset of sharp, tearing pain; and other symptoms related to the organ system affected by blocked blood flow. The most common presentation mimics a stroke with confusion, vertigo, visual disturbances, and loss of consciousness. Although rare, you may also encounter paralysis on one side of the body (hemiplegia), as well as cardiac and pulmonary collapse. If any person using scuba equipment presents with neurologic deficits during or immediately after ascent, an air embolism should be suspected. As death or serious disability can result, prompt medical treatment is crucial.

Treatment Management of air embolism includes the following steps:

- ★ Assess ABCs.
- ★ Administer oxygen by nonrebreather mask at 100 percent.
- ★ Place the patient in a supine position.

- ★ Monitor vital signs frequently.
- ★ Administer IV fluids at a TKO rate.
- ★ Administer a corticosteroid agent, if ordered by medical direction.
- ★ Transport to a recompression chamber as rapidly as possible. If air transport is utilized, it is very important to use a pressurized aircraft or to fly at a low altitude.

Pneumomediastinum

As noted earlier, a pneumomediastinum is the release of gas (air) through the visceral pleura into the mediastinum and pericardial sac around the heart. It can result from a pulmonary overpressure accident during rapid ascent from a dive.

Signs and Symptoms Signs and symptoms of a pneumomediastinum include substernal chest pain, irregular pulse, abnormal heart sounds, reduced blood pressure and narrow pulse pressure, and a change in voice. There may or may not be evidence of cyanosis.

Treatment The field management of pneumomediastinum includes:

- ★ Administer high-flow, high-concentration oxygen via nonrebreather mask.
- ★ Start an IV of lactated Ringer's or normal saline per medical direction.
- ★ Transport to the emergency department.

Treatment generally ranges from observation to recompression for relief of acute symptoms. The patient should be observed for 24 hours for any other signs of lung overpressure. He should not be recompressed unless air embolism or decompression illness is also present.

Nitrogen Narcosis

Nitrogen narcosis develops during deep dives and contributes to major diving emergencies while the diver is at the bottom. With an elevated partial pressure, more nitrogen dissolves in the bloodstream. With higher concentrations of nitrogen in the body, including the brain, the result is intoxication and altered levels of consciousness similar to the effects of alcohol or narcotic use. Between 70 and 100 feet these effects become apparent in most divers, but at 200 feet most divers become so impaired that they cannot do any useful work. At 300 to 350 feet unconsciousness occurs. The main concern with nitrogen narcosis is the same as with any person who is intoxicated while in a situation requiring alertness and common sense. Impaired judgment during a deep dive can cause accidents and unnecessary risk taking.

Signs and Symptoms Signs and symptoms include altered levels of consciousness and impaired judgment.

Treatment Treatment simply requires return to a shallow depth since this condition is self-resolving on ascent. To avoid this problem altogether in deep dives, oxygen mixed with helium is used, since helium does not have the anesthetic effect of nitrogen.

OTHER DIVING-RELATED ILLNESSES

There are less frequent problems that can occur as a result of scuba diving. For example, oxygen toxicity caused by prolonged exposure to high partial pressures of oxygen can cause lung damage or even convulsions. Hyperventilation due to excitement or panic may lead to a decreased level of consciousness or muscle cramps and spasm. This will impair the diver's ability to function properly, possibly leading to injury. Inadequate breathing or faulty equipment may lead to increased CO_2 levels, or *hypercapnia*. This also may cause unconsciousness. Finally, poorly prepared air tanks may be contaminated with other gases, which can increase the risk of hypoxia, narcosis, and accidental injury.

DIVERS ALERT NETWORK

Clearly, scuba diving has a unique set of potential problems. With the popularity of this activity rising so dramatically, it is important for EMS personnel in popular diving areas to become familiar with recognition and treatment of these problems. If assistance is needed, the Divers Alert Network (DAN) operates a nonprofit consultation and referral service in affiliation with Duke University Medical Center. In an emergency, contact (919) 684-8111. For nonemergency situations call (919) 684-2948.

HIGH ALTITUDE ILLNESS

In contrast to illnesses related to diving and high atmospheric pressure, high altitude illnesses are caused by a decrease in ambient pressure. Essentially, high altitude is a low-oxygen environment. As noted in the discussion of Dalton's law, oxygen concentration in the atmosphere remains constant at 21 percent. Therefore, as you go higher and barometric pressure decreases, the partial pressure of oxygen also decreases (is 21 percent of a lower total pressure). Oxygen becomes less available, triggering a number of related illnesses as well as aggravating preexisting conditions such as angina, congestive heart failure, chronic obstructive pulmonary disease, and hypertension.

Even in healthy individuals, ascent to high altitude, especially if it is very rapid, can cause illness. It is difficult to predict who will be affected and to what degree. The only predictor is the hypoxic ventilatory response.

High altitude illnesses start to become manifest at altitudes greater than 8,000 ft.

Every year millions of visitors to mountains expose themselves to altitudes greater than 2,400 m (8,000 ft), the altitude at which high altitude illnesses start to become manifest. For reference purposes, Denver, Colorado, is at 1,610 m where there is 17 percent less oxygen than at sea level. Aspen at 2,438 m has 26 percent less oxygen, and at the top of Mount Everest (8,848 m or 29,028 ft) there is 66 percent less oxygen than at sea level. At *high altitude* (4,900 to 11,500 ft) the hypoxic environment causes decreased exercise performance, although without major disruption of normal oxygen transport in the body. However, if ascent is very rapid, altitude illness will commonly occur at 8,000 ft and beyond. *Very high altitude* (11,500 to 18,000 ft) will result in extreme hypoxia during exercise or sleep. It is important to ascend to these altitudes slowly, thereby allowing for acclimatization to the environment. *Extreme altitude* beyond 18,000 ft will cause severe illness in almost everyone.

Some of the signs and symptoms of altitude illness are malaise, anorexia, headache, sleep disturbances, and respiratory distress that increases with exertion.

PREVENTION

Acclimatization, exertion, sleep, diet, and medication are key considerations in preventing or limiting high altitude medical emergencies. A description of each follows.

Gradual Ascent

To avoid developing high altitude medical problems, it is important to allow a period of acclimatization. Slow, gradual ascent over days to weeks gives the body a chance to adjust to the hypoxic state caused by high altitudes. A person who would normally become short of breath, dizzy, and confused by a rapid drop in oxygen can function quite well if the oxygen level is decreased to the same level gradually over a long period of time. Acclimatization occurs through several mechanisms. They are:

- *Ventilatory changes.* The *hypoxic ventilatory response (HVR)* is triggered by decreased oxygen. When oxygen is decreased, ventilation increases. This hyperventilation causes a decrease in CO_2, but the kidneys compensate by eliminating more bicarbonate from the body. In essence, the body resets its normal ventilation and operating level of CO_2. The process takes 4 to 7 days at a given altitude.
- *Cardiovascular changes.* The heart rate increases at high altitude, allowing more oxygen to be delivered to the tissues. In addition, peripheral veins constrict, increasing the central blood volume. In response, the central receptors, which sense blood volume, induce a diuresis, which causes concentration of the blood.

Unfortunately, pulmonary circulation also constricts in a hypoxic environment. This causes or exacerbates preexisting hypertension and predisposes to developing high altitude pulmonary edema.

★ *Blood changes.* Within 2 hours of ascent to high altitude the body begins making more red blood cells to carry oxygen. Over time, this mechanism will significantly compensate for the hypoxic environment. It is this mechanism that fostered the idea of "blood-doping" during athletic competition, especially at high altitudes. Athletes donate their own blood long in advance of a competition at high altitude. This allows them time to rebuild their red blood cells. Just before the competition they receive a transfusion of their own blood to increase their oxygen-carrying capacity. This practice is frowned on by most athletic governing bodies.

Limited Exertion

Clearly, one of the easiest ways to avoid some effects of high altitude is to limit the amount of exertion. By limiting the body's need for oxygen, the effect of oxygen deprivation will be minimized.

Sleeping Altitude

Sleep is often disrupted by high altitude. Hypoxia causes abnormal breathing patterns and frequent awakenings in the middle of the night. Descending to a lower altitude for sleep improves rest and allows the body to recover from hypoxia. This practice will, however, interfere with the process of acclimatization.

High Carbohydrate Diet

Carbohydrates are converted by the body into glucose and are rapidly released into the bloodstream, providing quick energy. The theory that this is helpful in acclimatizing to high altitude is controversial.

Medications

Two medications will limit or prevent the development of medical conditions related to high altitude. They are:

★ *Acetazolamide.* Acetazolamide (Diamox) acts as a diuretic. It forces bicarbonate out of the body, which greatly enhances the process of acclimatization as discussed earlier. The hypoxic ventilatory response reaches a new set point more quickly. This improves ventilation and oxygen transport with less alkalosis. In addition, the periodic breathing that occurs at high altitude is resolved, thereby preventing sudden drops in oxygen.

★ *Nifedipine.* Nifedipine (Procardia, Adalat) is a medication used to treat high blood pressure. It causes blood vessels to dilate, preventing the increase in pulmonary pressure that often causes pulmonary edema.

Other treatments are currently under evaluation. Phenytoin (Dilantin), for example, is being studied because of its membrane stabilization effects. Steroids are commonly used but their efficacy is still controversial.

TYPES OF HIGH ALTITUDE ILLNESS

A variety of symptoms occur when the average person ascends rapidly to high altitude. These may range from fatigue and decreased exercise tolerance to headache, sleep disturbance, and respiratory distress. The following section will deal with some of the specific syndromes that will occur.

Acute Mountain Sickness

Acute mountain sickness (AMS) usually manifests in an unacclimatized person who ascends rapidly to an altitude of 2,000 m (6,600 ft) or greater.

Signs and Symptoms The mild form of acute mountain sickness presents with the following symptoms:

- ★ Lightheadedness
- ★ Breathlessness
- ★ Weakness
- ★ Headache
- ★ Nausea and vomiting

These symptoms can develop from 6 to 24 hours after ascent. More severe cases can develop especially if the person continues to ascend to higher altitudes. These symptoms include:

- ★ Weakness (requiring assistance to eat and dress)
- ★ Severe vomiting
- ★ Decreased urine output
- ★ Shortness of breath
- ★ Altered level of consciousness

Mild AMS is self-limiting and will often improve within 1 to 2 days if no further ascent occurs.

Treatment Treatment of AMS consists of halting ascent, possibly lowering altitude, and using acetazolamide (Diamox) and antinauseants such as prochlorperazine (Compazine) as necessary. It is not usually necessary to descend to sea level. Supplemental oxygen will relieve symptoms but is usually used only in severe cases. In severe cases oxygen, if available, will help. In addition, immediate descent is the definitive treatment. For very severe cases, hyperbaric oxygen may be necessary.

Definitive treatment of all high altitude illnesses is descent to a lower altitude. Administration of supplemental oxygen is also important.

High Altitude Pulmonary Edema (HAPE)

High altitude pulmonary edema (HAPE) develops as a result of increased pulmonary pressure and hypertension caused by changes in blood flow at high altitude. Children are most susceptible, and men are more susceptible than women.

Signs and Symptoms Initially symptoms include dry cough, mild shortness of breath on exertion, and slight crackles in the lungs. As the condition progresses, so will the symptoms. Dyspnea can become quite severe and cause cyanosis. Coughing may be productive of frothy sputum, and weakness may progress to coma and death.

Treatment In the early stages, HAPE is completely and easily reversible with descent and the administration of oxygen. It is therefore critical to recognize the illness early and initiate appropriate treatment. If immediate descent is not possible, supplemental oxygen can completely reverse HAPE but requires 36 to 72 hours. Such a supply of oxygen is rarely available to mountain climbers. In this situation the portable hyperbaric bag can be very useful. This is a sealed bag that can be inflated to 2 psi, which simulates a descent of approximately 5,000 feet. Acetazolamide can be used to decrease symptoms. Medications such as morphine, nifedipine (Procardia), and furosemide (Lasix) have been used with some success, but they carry complications such as hypotension and dehydration and should be used with caution.

High Altitude Cerebral Edema

The exact cause of high altitude cerebral edema (HACE) is not known. It usually manifests as progressive neurological deterioration in a patient with AMS or HAPE. The increased fluid in the brain tissue causes a rise in intracranial pressure.

Signs and Symptoms The symptoms of high altitude cerebral edema include:

- ★ Altered mental status
- ★ Ataxia (poor coordination)

★ Decreased level of consciousness

★ Coma

Headache, nausea, and vomiting are less common. Occasionally actual focal neurological changes may occur.

Treatment As in all altitude illnesses, definitive treatment is descent to lower altitude. Oxygen and steroids may also help to improve recovery. If descent is not possible, the use of oxygen with steroids and a hyperbaric bag may be sufficient, although often unavailable. If coma develops, it may persist for days after descent to sea level but usually resolves, although sometimes leaving residual disability.

Summary

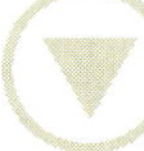

Our environment provides us with all that we need to survive and prosper. The extremes of our environment, however, can have significant impact on human metabolism. Our bodies will, of course, compensate for these extremes, but sometimes it is not enough. Sometimes the heat gain or loss is too much. Sometimes the pressure change is too much. As a result, medical illnesses and emergencies arise. These can range from abnormal core body temperatures to decompensation, shock, and even death.

Basic knowledge of common environmental, recreational, and exposure emergencies is necessary in order for you to administer prompt and proper treatment in the prehospital setting. It is not easy to remember this type of information since these problems are not usually encountered on a daily basis. Remember the general principles involved. Remove the environmental influence causing the problem. Support the patient's own attempt to compensate. Finally, select a definitive care location and transport the patient as rapidly as possible.

In every case, remember that you must maintain your own safety. There are too many cases in which paramedics have lost their lives as a result of attempting a rescue for which they were not properly trained. Rapid action is always necessary when performing an environmental rescue; however, common sense must prevail.

Review Questions

1. The type of thermogenesis that results from exercise is:
   a. metabolic.
   b. diet induced.
   c. work induced.
   d. thermoregulatory.
2. Through the mechanism called evaporation, water evaporates from the skin and lungs at approximately ___________ mL/day.
   a. 200
   b. 400
   c. 600
   d. 800
3. It is important in any heat-related or cold-related emergency to obtain a core temperature reading such as from the:
   a. ear.
   b. mouth.
   c. rectum.
   d. axillary.

4. Factors that may contribute to a susceptibility to hyperthermia include:
   a. medications.
   b. age of the patient.
   c. health of the patient.
   d. all of the above
5. Treatment of the patient with heat cramps includes all of the following except:
   a. administer salt tablets.
   b. administer an oral saline solution.
   c. place the patient in a cool environment.
   d. if the patient is unable to take fluids orally, consider an IV of normal saline.
6. When the core temperature of the body drops below ___________ an individual is considered to be hypothermic.
   a. 95°F
   b. 96°F
   c. 97°F
   d. 98°F
7. ___________ is the most common presenting dysrhythmia seen in hypothermia.
   a. Atrial flutter
   b. Sinus bradycardia
   c. Atrial fibrillation
   d. Ventricular fibrillation
8. The third most common cause of accidental death in the United States is:
   a. stroke.
   b. trauma.
   c. drowning.
   d. heart disease.
9. The return of unoxygenated blood from the damaged alveoli to the bloodstream is called:
   a. shunting.
   b. pneumonitis.
   c. atelectasis.
   d. hemodilution.
10. All near-drowning patients should be admitted to the hospital for observation since complications may not appear for ___________ hours.
    a. 10
    b. 16
    c. 20
    d. 24
11. ___________ law states that the volume of a gas is inversely proportional to its pressure if the temperature is kept constant.
    a. Henry's
    b. Boyle's
    c. Dalton's
    d. Starling's
12. ___________ is the condition that develops in divers subjected to rapid reduction of air pressure while ascending to the surface following exposure to compressed air, with formation of nitrogen bubbles causing severe pain, especially in the abdomen and the joints.
    a. Nitrogen narcosis
    b. Arterial gas embolism
    c. Decompression illness
    d. Pulmonary overpressure

13. ___________ develops as a result of increased pulmonary pressure and hypertension caused by changes in blood flow at high altitude.
    a. AMS
    b. HACE
    c. HAPE
    d. AGE
14. If any person using scuba equipment presents with neurologic deficits during or immediately after ascent, ___________ should be suspected.
    a. nitrogen narcosis
    b. air embolism
    c. decompression illness
    d. pulmonary overpressure
15. If ascent is very rapid, altitude illness will commonly occur at ___________ and beyond.
    a. 1,200 m (4,000 ft)
    b. 2,400 m (8,000 ft)
    c. 3,600 m (12,000 ft)
    d. 4,800 m (16,000 ft)

See Answers to Review Questions at the back of this book.

Chapter 37

Infectious Disease

Objectives

After reading this chapter, you should be able to:

1. Describe the specific anatomy and physiology pertinent to infectious and communicable diseases. (pp. 1443–1446; also see Chapter 4)
2. Define specific terminology identified with infectious/communicable diseases. (pp. 1441–1482)
3. Discuss public health principles relevant to infectious/communicable diseases. (pp. 1441–1442)
4. Identify public health agencies involved in the prevention and management of disease outbreaks. (p. 1442)
5. List and describe the steps of an infectious process. (pp. 1446–1449)
6. Discuss the risks associated with infection. (pp. 1441, 1446–1449)
7. List and describe the stages of infectious diseases. (pp. 1446–1449)
8. List and describe infectious agents, including bacteria, viruses, fungi, protozoans, and helminths (worms). (pp. 1443–1446)
9. Describe characteristics of the immune system. (see Chapters 4 and 31)
10. Describe the processes of the immune system defenses, including humoral and cell-mediated immunity. (see Chapters 4 and 31)
11. In specific diseases, identify and discuss the issues of personal isolation. (pp. 1449–1484)
12. Describe and discuss the rationale for the various types of personal protection equipment. (pp. 1449–1453)
13. Discuss what constitutes a significant exposure to an infectious agent. (pp. 1453–1454)
14. Describe the assessment of a patient suspected of, or identified as having, an infectious/communicable disease. (pp. 1454–1455)
15. Discuss the proper disposal of contaminated supplies such as sharps, gauze, sponges, and tourniquets. (pp. 1451–1452)
16. Discuss disinfection of patient care equipment and areas where patient care occurred. (pp. 1452–1453)

17. Discuss the seroconversion rate after direct significant HIV exposure. (pp. 1448–1449)

18. Discuss the causative agent, body systems affected and potential secondary complications, routes of transmission, susceptibility and resistance, signs and symptoms, patient management and protective measures, and immunization for each of the following:

- ★ HIV (pp. 1447, 1451, 1456–1458)
- ★ Hepatitis A (pp. 1447, 1459)
- ★ Hepatitis B (pp. 1447, 1459–1460)
- ★ Hepatitis C (pp. 1447, 1460)
- ★ Hepatitis D (p. 1460)
- ★ Hepatitis E (p. 1460)
- ★ Hepatitis G (pp. 1460–1461)
- ★ Tuberculosis (pp. 1461–1463)
- ★ Meningococcal meningitis (pp. 1466–1468)
- ★ Pneumonia (pp. 1447, 1463–1464)
- ★ Tetanus (pp. 1476–1477)
- ★ Rabies (pp. 1475–1476)
- ★ Hantavirus (p. 1473)
- ★ Chickenpox (pp. 1465–1466)
- ★ Mumps (pp. 1447, 1469)
- ★ Rubella (p. 1470)
- ★ Measles (pp. 1447, 1469–1470)
- ★ Pertussis (whooping cough) (pp. 1470–1471)
- ★ Influenza (pp. 1447, 1468–1469)
- ★ Mononucleosis (p. 1471)
- ★ Herpes simplex 1 and 2 (pp. 1447, 1471–1472, 1480)
- ★ Syphilis (pp. 1447, 1478–1479)
- ★ Gonorrhea (pp. 1447, 1478)
- ★ Chlamydia (p. 1480)
- ★ Scabies (p. 1482)
- ★ Lice (pp. 1481–1482)
- ★ Lyme disease (pp. 1447, 1477–1478)
- ★ Gastroenteritis (pp. 1473–1474)

19. Discuss other infectious agents known to cause meningitis including streptococcus pneumonia, haemophilus influenza type B, and various varieties of viruses. (pp. 1466–1468)

20. Identify common pediatric viral diseases. (pp. 1465–1466, 1469–1471, 1472)

21. Discuss the characteristics of and organisms associated with febrile and afebrile diseases including bronchiolitis, bronchitis, laryngitis, croup, epiglottitis, and the common cold. (pp. 1468–1473)

22. Articulate the pathophysiological principles of an infectious process given a case study of a patient with an infectious/communicable disease. (pp. 1441–1484)

23. Given several preprogrammed infectious disease patients, provide the appropriate Standard Precautions, assessment, management, and transport. (pp. 1441–1484)

Key Terms

airborne, p. 1447
antibody, p. 1448
antigen, p. 1448
bacteria, p. 1443
bactericidal, p. 1444
bacteriostatic, p. 1444
bloodborne, p. 1447
Brudzinski's sign, p. 1467
chancroid, p. 1481
chlamydia, p. 1480
communicable, p. 1448
communicable period, p. 1448
contamination, p. 1448
croup, p. 1472
decontaminate, p. 1452
disease period, p. 1449
disinfect, p. 1452
encephalitis, p. 1475
endotoxin, p. 1444
epiglottitis, p. 1472
exotoxin, p. 1444
fecal–oral route, p. 1447
food poisoning, p. 1474
fungi, p. 1445
gastroenteritis, p. 1473
gonorrhea, p. 1478
Gram stain, p. 1444
hantavirus, p. 1473
hepatitis, p. 1458
herpes simplex virus, p. 1471
hookworms, p. 1446
human immunodeficiency virus (HIV), p. 1456
impetigo, p. 1481
incubation period, p. 1448
index case, p. 1442
infection, p. 1448
infectious disease, p. 1441
infestation, p. 1481
influenza, p. 1468
Kernig's sign, p. 1467
latent period, p. 1448
lice, p. 1481
Lyme disease, p. 1477
mask, p. 1462
measles, p. 1469
meningitis, p. 1466
mononucleosis, p. 1471
mumps, p. 1469
normal flora, p. 1443
nosocomial, p. 1482
obligate intracellular parasite, p. 1444
opportunistic pathogen, p. 1443
parasites, p. 1446
pathogen, p. 1443
pertussis, p. 1470
pharyngitis, p. 1472
pinworms, p. 1446
pneumonia, p. 1463
PPD, p. 1450
prions, p. 1445
protozoa, p. 1445
rabies, p. 1475
reservoir, p. 1446
resistance, p. 1448
respirator, p. 1462
respiratory syncytial virus (RSV), p. 1470
rubella (German measles), p. 1470
Ryan White Act, p. 1453
scabies, p. 1482
seroconversion, p. 1448
severe acute respiratory syndrome (SARS), p. 1464
sexually transmitted disease (STD), p. 1478
sinusitis, p. 1472
sterilize, p. 1453
syphilis, p. 1478
tetanus, p. 1476
trichinosis, p. 1446
trichomoniasis, p. 1480
tuberculosis (TB), p. 1461
varicella, p. 1465
virulence, p. 1448
viruses, p. 1444
window phase, p. 1448

INTRODUCTION

Infectious diseases are illnesses caused by infestation of the body by biological organisms such as bacteria, viruses, fungi, protozoans, and helminths (worms). Most infectious disease states are not life threatening and the patient recovers completely. Some types of infection, however, such as human immunodeficiency virus (HIV), hepatitis B virus (HBV), and acute bacterial meningitis, are particularly dangerous and may result in death or permanent disability.

infectious disease *illness caused by infestation of the body by biological organisms.*

All health care professionals must maintain a strong working knowledge of public health principles and infectious diseases. This is especially true for paramedics, who are often the first to encounter patients with communicable diseases. Early recognition and management of these patients may make a difference in how the patient is treated and may also ensure that care providers take necessary precautions to prevent the spread of the disease to others.

This chapter discusses infectious diseases, including the types of disease-causing organisms, functions of the immune system, and general pathophysiology of infectious diseases. It emphasizes the specific diseases, discussing those that you may encounter during interhospital transports or out-of-hospital care, especially those that you are most likely to encounter in the field.

PUBLIC HEALTH PRINCIPLES

When dealing with infectious diseases, you must consider the impact of the disease process on the community as well as on the infected patient. An infectious agent is a "hazardous material" that can affect large numbers of people.

Epidemiologists, health professionals who study how infectious diseases affect populations, attempt to describe and predict how diseases move from individuals to populations. Through various clinically based studies and statistical techniques, they try to determine how effectively an infectious agent can travel through a population. Using the population of infected individuals as a standard, they attempt to predict those individuals in the larger population who may be most at risk for contracting the infectious agent. Recognizing that risk may be predictable, and not just random, is important. The characteristics of the host, the infectious agent, and the environment may yield clues as to how the infectious agent is transmitted and reveal individuals or populations susceptible to infection.

How a population is identified is important. It may be defined by such parameters as geographic boundary, workplace, school, correctional institution, age group, income level, or ethnic group. All of the characteristics of a certain population are known as its demographics. The population's tendency to expand, decline, or move is important as well. Besides stimulating social and economic progress, the movement of people and animals within and among other societies also provides a vehicle for infectious agents.

index case *the individual who first introduced an infectious agent to a population.*

To track the progress of infection within a population, epidemiologists work backward through the chain of infection to determine the **index case,** that individual who first introduced the infectious agent to the population. From the index case, they then retrace the chain forward to verify their reconstruction of the infection's pattern.

To gauge a disease's potential impact on the community, paramedics must evaluate the host (patient), what they believe to be the infectious agent, and the environment. Based on that assessment, they may use more aggressive personal protective equipment. They must also consider the patient, those in the patient's immediate environment, and those in the environment where the patient is being transported all to be at risk for infection. On a more personal level, paramedics must appreciate that they and their families could also be at risk.

PUBLIC HEALTH AGENCIES

Local agencies are the first line of defense in disease surveillance and outbreak.

Local agencies are the first line of defense in disease surveillance and outbreak. Municipal, city, and county agencies, including fire departments, ambulance services, and health departments, must cooperate to monitor and report the incidence and prevalence of disease.

At the state level, a designated agency (health department or board of health, for instance) generally monitors infectious diseases. These agencies may set policies requiring vaccinations and regulate or implement control programs in vector and animal control, food preparation, water, sewer, and other sanitation control programs. State and local laws sometimes require these agencies to meet or exceed federal guidelines and recommendations.

A number of federal agencies are involved in tracking the morbidity and mortality of infectious diseases. The U.S. Department of Health and Human Services (DHHS) Centers for Disease Control and Prevention (CDC) in Atlanta, Georgia, is the most visible federal agency. The CDC monitors national disease data and freely disseminates this information to all health care providers. It sends personnel nationally and internationally to assist with studying, characterizing, and managing serious disease outbreaks. The CDC is also involved in researching infectious diseases. The National Institute for Occupational Safety and Health (NIOSH), also under the aegis of DHHS, works with the U.S. Department of Labor's Occupational Safety and Health Administration (OSHA) in setting standards and guidelines for workplace and worker controls to prevent infectious diseases in the workplace. This level of federal government involvement would not be possible without the leadership of the U.S. Congress in establishing national health policies and in drafting the federal budget.

Other organizations and governmental agencies that might serve as resources to your organization include the Federal Emergency Management Agency (FEMA), the National Fire Protection Association (NFPA), the United States Fire Protection Administration (USFPA), and the International Association of Firefighters (IAFF). These groups develop helpful blueprints for incorporating OSHA, NIOSH, and other standards and guidelines into daily operations.

MICROORGANISMS

The vast majority of disease-causing organisms are microscopic (visible only under a microscope). These microorganisms surround us. They are on our skin and in the air we breathe, and they colonize virtually every orifice of our bodies. Some can even live in the highly acidic environment of our stomachs, which destroys other disease-producing microorganisms or deactivates their toxic products. Microorganisms that reside in our bodies without ordinarily causing disease are part of the *host defenses* known as **normal flora.** Normal flora help keep us disease free by creating environmental conditions that are not conducive to disease-producing microorganisms, or **pathogens.** Competition between colonies of normal flora and pathogens also discourages the survival of pathogens. Common bacterial pathogens include *Staphylococci, Streptococci,* and *Enterobacteriaceae.* Certain viruses, rickettsiae, fungi, and protozoans are also pathogenic.

normal flora *organisms that live inside our bodies without ordinarily causing disease.*

pathogen *organism capable of causing disease.*

opportunistic pathogen *ordinarily nonharmful bacterium that causes disease only under unusual circumstances.*

Opportunistic pathogens are ordinarily nonharmful bacteria that cause disease only under unusual circumstances. Most opportunistic pathogens are normal flora. Patients who have a weakened immune system or who are under unusual stress become susceptible to diseases caused by opportunistic organisms. For example, the fungus *Pneumocystis carinii* is usually harmless but can cause a deadly form of pneumonia in patients with HIV. The fungus overwhelms the weakened immune system and begins to reproduce rapidly in the lungs. Left untreated, *P. carinii* pneumonia may be fatal. Organ transplant recipients are also at increased risk for infectious diseases because they must take immunosuppressant medications to prevent organ rejection. A more common (and less harmful) opportunistic infection is thrush (oral candidiasis), often seen in patients who take broad-spectrum antibiotics. As the antibiotic kills normal bacterial flora in the mouth, the fungus *Candida albicans* grows almost uninhibited on the tongue and in the pharynx, producing a white coating on the mucosa.

BACTERIA

Bacteria are microscopic single-celled organisms that range in length from 1 to 20 micrometers (Figure 37-1 ■). These living cells are classified as *prokaryotes* because they do not have a distinct nuclear membrane and possess only one chromosome in the cytoplasm. Bacteria reproduce independently, but they require a host to supply food and a supportive environment. Some common diseases caused by pathogenic bacteria include sinusitis, otitis media, bacterial pneumonia, pharyngitis (strep throat), tuberculosis, and most urinary tract infections.

bacteria *microscopic single-celled organisms that range in length from 1 to 20 micrometers.*

Most bacteria are easily identifiable with stains or by their appearance under a microscope. Similar colorfastness indicates similarities in cell wall structure and other anatomic features. The

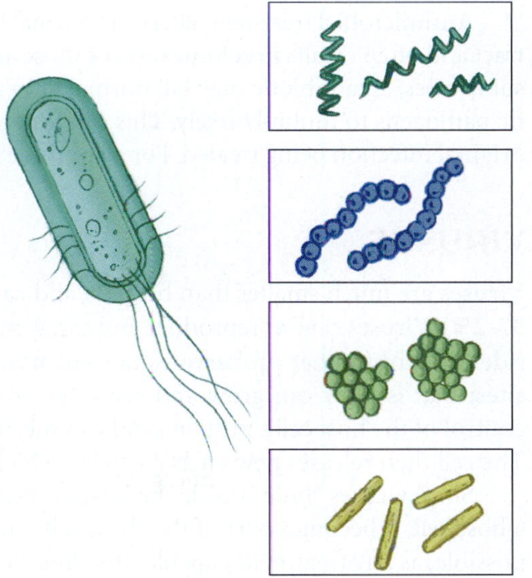

■ **Figure 37-1** Bacteria are single-celled organisms that range in length from 1 to 20 micrometers.

Gram stain *method of differentiating types of bacteria according to their reaction to a chemical stain process.*

Review

Content

Types of Bacteria

- Spheres (cocci)
- Rods
- Spirals

Gram stain is the most common method of differentiating bacteria. Bacteria that this process turns purple are known as gram-positive bacteria; those it turns red are gram-negative. Because of the similarities in their cell walls, bacteria that stain alike may respond to similar treatments.

Bacteria are further categorized into groups based on their general appearance: Cocci, or spheres (staphylococcus, streptococcus), are round; rods (*Enterobacter* sp., *E. coli*) are elongated; and spirals (spirochetes, vibrio) are coiled. *Enterobacter* sp. and *E. coli* are gram-negative rods. *Staphylococci* and *Streptococci* are gram-positive cocci. Regardless of how bacteria stain or appear under a microscope, it is the specific tissues and organs which are infected that chiefly determine the patient's signs and symptoms.

exotoxin *toxic waste products released by living bacteria.*

endotoxin *toxic products released when bacteria die and decompose.*

Pathogenic bacteria may harm their human hosts in a number of ways. Heavy colonization may result in direct damage to tissues as the bacteria feed. Bacteria may also cause indirect damage by releasing toxic chemicals that can have localized or systemic effects. The two general categories of toxins are exotoxins and endotoxins. This classification is no longer based primarily on where they originate, as their names imply, but by their chemical structures. **Exotoxins** are poisonous proteins shed by bacteria during bacterial growth. They stimulate the immune system to form antibodies to these proteins, and they may also be deactivated by chemicals, light, or heat. Exotoxins are more toxic than endotoxins. The infectious agent of toxic shock syndrome, *S. aureus*, releases an exotoxin, as does anthrax, which can be delivered as a biological weapon of mass destruction.

Endotoxins consist of proteins, polysaccharides (large sugar molecules), and lipids. The immune system cannot form antibodies specific to a particular endotoxin unless both the protein and polysaccharide portions are present. Endotoxins come from the bacterial cell wall and are released when the bacterial cell is destroyed. They are more stable in heat than exotoxins. Only gram-negative bacteria make endotoxins. The skin lesions of meningococcemia and the signs of shock that sometimes accompany it are due to large amounts of endotoxin released by the infectious agent, *N. meningitidis*.

bactericidal *capable of killing bacteria.*

bacteriostatic *capable of inhibiting bacterial growth or reproduction.*

Most bacterial infections respond to treatment with antibiotics that are either **bactericidal** (kill bacteria) or **bacteriostatic** (inhibit bacterial growth or reproduction). Antibiotics are prescribed based on bacterial sensitivity; different antibiotics are required to treat different bacteria. Their administration usually decreases bacterial presence and reduces symptoms. Some types of bacterial infections respond quickly to antibiotics; others take longer. In recent years, a number of bacterial strains have developed resistance to antibiotic therapy, making treatment more difficult. The more a type of bacterium is exposed to an antibiotic, the greater the likelihood of its developing resistance. The overuse of antibiotics in both medical and veterinary settings has contributed to this serious problem. Resistant forms of tuberculosis (mycobacterium) are of particular concern. Antibiotics may now be ineffective against this disease, and its mortality rate is high. The willingness of some physicians to prescribe the newest antibiotics for relatively minor infections and the widespread addition of antibiotics to animal feed have only added to the problem.

Antimicrobial treatment alters the normal flora of the skin, mouth, mucosa, and gastrointestinal tract and often results in colonization of those areas by new microorganisms that resist antibiotics. In some cases, an antibiotic may kill normal flora and allow more virulent and dangerous opportunistic pathogens to multiply freely. This can lead to a secondary infection that is more severe than the original infection being treated. For all of these reasons, antibiotics should be prescribed cautiously.

VIRUSES

viruses *disease-causing organisms that can be seen only with an electron microscope.*

obligate intracellular parasite *organism that can grow and reproduce only within a host cell.*

Viruses are much smaller than bacteria and can be seen only with an electron microscope (Figure 37-2 ■). Viruses cannot reproduce and carry on metabolism by themselves. Therefore, they are considered to be neither prokaryotes nor eukaryotes. Instead, viruses are **obligate intracellular parasites;** that is, they can grow and reproduce only within a host cell. Once inside, the virus takes control of the host cell's protein synthesis mechanism and directs it to begin reproducing the virus. The cell then releases new virus particles, which infect nearby cells.

Since viruses "hide" inside the host's cells, they resist antibiotic treatment. Once a virus enters a host cell, it becomes part of that host cell, making selective eradication of the virus virtually impossible, as any treatment capable of killing the virus will generally kill the host cell as well. This is the major obstacle facing researchers as they work to find cures for HIV and other viruses.

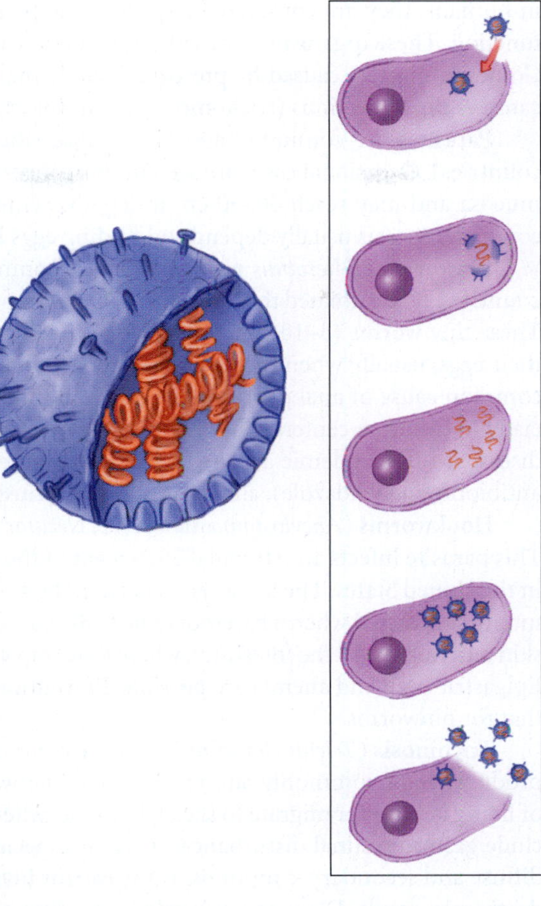

Figure 37-2 Viruses are much smaller than bacteria and can be seen only with an electron microscope. They grow and reproduce only within a host cell.

Approximately 400 types of viruses have been identified. One frequently encountered viral disorder, the common cold, is caused by a number of different viruses (nearly 200) that all produce similar symptoms. Fortunately, most viral diseases are mild and self-limiting. They run their course until the patient's immune system eventually fights them off. A host is generally susceptible to any particular virus only once. Once a person's immune system develops active immunity against a particular type of virus, it becomes attuned to similar attacking viruses and will destroy them.

OTHER MICROORGANISMS

Prions are a new classification of disease-producing agents that microbiologists used to refer to as "slow viruses." They are neither prokaryotes nor eukaryotes but particles of protein, folded in such a way that proteases (enzymes that break down proteins) cannot act on them. These protein particles accumulate in nervous system and brain tissue, destroying them and giving them a spongy appearance on gross examination. Prions are known to cause progressive, untreatable dementia in kuru, Creutzfeldt-Jakob disease, mad cow disease, and fatal familial insomnia. Although EMS providers will rarely respond to patients with diseases caused by prions, a general discussion of infectious agents must acknowledge their existence.

prions *particles of protein, folded in such a way that protease enzymes cannot act on them.*

Fungi are plantlike microorganisms, most of which are not pathogenic. Yeasts, molds, and mushrooms are types of fungi. Some fungi have a capsule around the cell wall that provides additional protection against phagocytes. While fungi compose a large part of the body's normal flora, they may become pathogenic in patients with compromised immune function, such as those with HIV. Fungi may also lead to disease states in patients taking broad-spectrum antibiotics. As the antibiotics kill off bacteria, the fungi are able to grow uninhibited. Fungi are a common cause of vaginal infections and often cause pneumonia in patients with weakened immune systems.

fungi *plantlike microorganisms; singular: fungus.*

Protozoa are single-celled parasitic organisms with flexible membranes and the ability to move. Most protozoa live in the soil and ingest decaying organic matter. Although rarely a cause of disease

protozoa *single-celled parasitic organisms with flexible membranes and the ability to move.*

in humans, they are considered opportunistic pathogens in patients with compromised immune function. These organisms may enter the body by the fecal–oral route or through a mosquito bite. Common diseases caused by protozoa include malaria and forms of gastroenteritis. Protozoa also cause vaginal infections (trichomoniasis) in women with normal immune function.

parasites *organisms that live in or on another organism.*

Parasites are common causes of disease where sanitation is poor (generally in developing countries). Occasional cases are seen in this country. Roundworms (ascarides) live in the intestinal mucosa and may reach 30–50 cm in length. Symptoms include abdominal cramping, fever, and cough. Diagnosis usually depends on finding eggs in the patient's stool.

pinworms *parasites that are 3 to 10 mm long and live in the distal colon.*

Pinworms (*Enterobius vermicularis*) are common in the United States and in other civilized countries. It is estimated that 20 percent of children living in temperate climates harbor this disease. These tiny worms (3–10 mm long) live in the distal colon and crawl onto the anal mucosa to lay their eggs, usually when the host is asleep. Although the disease may remain asymptomatic, it is a common cause of anal pruritus (itching) and infection and is easily spread among children, especially in childcare centers. Children may carry the disease home and infect their entire family. This disease is often endemic among institutionalized children. Treatment involves a single dose of an antibiotic (mebendazole); all family members must be treated simultaneously to avoid reinfection.

hookworms *parasites that attach to the host's intestinal lining.*

Hookworms (*Ancylostoma duodenale, Necator americanus*) are found in warm, moist climates. This parasite infects an estimated 25 percent of the world's population, although it is relatively rare in the United States. The larvae are passed in the stool of infected animals. The disease is most commonly contracted when a barefoot child walks in a contaminated area. The larvae enter through the skin and migrate to the intestines, where they grip and irritate the intestinal wall and feed on blood. Epigastric pain and anemia are possible. Prevention involves wearing shoes; treatment is similar to that for pinworms.

trichinosis *disease resulting from an infestation of* Trichinella spiralis.

Trichinosis (*Trichinella spiralis*) may be contracted by eating raw or inadequately cooked pork products, most commonly sausage. Females burrow into the intestinal wall and produce thousands of living larvae that migrate to skeletal muscle, where each forms a cyst and remains. Symptoms include gastrointestinal disturbances, edema (especially of the eyelids), fever, and a variety of other diffuse and secondary symptoms. If the worms invade the heart, lungs, or brain in large numbers, death may result. Diagnosis is made by finding encysted worms during examination of muscle biopsy. Mebendazole is the antibiotic of choice.

Other types of worms such as tapeworms and flukes are rarely encountered in the United States.

CONTRACTION, TRANSMISSION, AND STAGES OF DISEASE

As a paramedic you must understand the relationship between the pathophysiology and the assessment and management of patients with infections or diseases resulting from infections. This knowledge will prepare you for leadership in recognizing infectious diseases and curbing their transmission.

The interactions of host, infectious agent, and environment are the elements of disease transmission. Studying each of these factors individually and then looking for relationships among them often reveals how an infectious agent has been effectively transmitted. Infectious agents exist in all types of **reservoirs**—animals, humans, insects, and the environment. While inhabiting animal or insect reservoirs, they do not cause disease. Their presence at any time in a given environment is affected by their life cycle, by the presence of stressors that may force them outside of their normal reservoirs, and by the climate. The initiation of therapy can sometimes disrupt the life cycle of the infectious agent and may eradicate the infection. When a host and infectious agent come together at the right time and under the right conditions, disease transmission takes place.

reservoir *any living creature or environment (water, soil, and so on) that can harbor an infectious agent.*

Infectious agents may invade hosts through one of two basic mechanisms. The more common is direct transmission from person to person through a cough, sneeze, kiss, or sexual contact. The other mechanism, indirect transmission, can spread organisms in a number of ways. Infected persons often shed organisms into the environment. These organisms come to rest on doorknobs, handrails, computer keyboards, and so on. Other people who contact those surfaces are at risk for contracting the disease. Similarly, microorganisms may be transmitted via food products, water, or even through the soil.

Bloodborne diseases are transmitted by contact with the blood or body fluids of an infected person. They include AIDS, hepatitis B, C, and D, and syphilis. The risk of transmission of bloodborne diseases increases if a patient has open wounds, active bleeding, or increased secretions. Assume that every patient has an infectious bloodborne disease and take precautions to avoid contact with blood and other body fluids.

Some infectious diseases may be transmitted through the air on droplets expelled during a productive cough or sneeze. They include tuberculosis, meningitis, mumps, measles, rubella, and chickenpox (varicella). Other, more common diseases such as the common cold, influenza, and respiratory syncytial virus (RSV) may also be transmitted by the **airborne** route.

Some infectious diseases are transmitted orally (primarily by eating) or by the **fecal–oral route,** in which enteric microorganisms (normally found in the GI system and the feces) are transmitted between potential hosts, as in shaking hands or other social customs, and then having the recipient somehow introduce the infectious agent into his mouth by scratching or eating with his hands. Fecal–oral diseases are prevalent in third-world countries or in areas with unsanitary conditions. Hepatitis A and E and other viruses can be transmitted by this route. Foodborne illnesses include food poisoning, certain parasitic infections, and trichinosis.

The risk of infection is considered *theoretical* if transmission is acknowledged to be possible but has not actually been reported. It is considered *measurable* if factors in the infectious agent's transmission and their associated risks have been identified or deduced from reported data. Generally, the risk of disease transmission rises if a patient has open wounds, increased secretions, active coughing, or any ongoing invasive treatment where exposure to an infectious body fluid is likely (Table 37–1). In the prehospital setting, the unpredictable environment and behavior of patients increase the risk of exposure. For example, a patient with a closed head injury and multiple lacerations may be combative, thereby contaminating EMS personnel with blood or other body fluids. Broken windshield glass contaminated with blood may easily penetrate examination gloves and skin. Patients who are violent and aggressive may deliberately bite, scratch, or spit at rescuers. Many EMS patient care activities occur in a closed, poorly ventilated environment such as the back of an ambulance. Thus, you must have available, and routinely use, protective clothing and other barrier devices, as indicated.

bloodborne *transmitted by contact with blood or body fluids.*

airborne *transmitted through the air by droplets or particles.*

fecal–oral route *transmission of organisms picked up from the gastrointestinal tract (e.g., feces) into the mouth.*

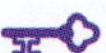

Generally, the risk of disease transmission rises if a patient has open wounds, increased secretions, active coughing, or any ongoing invasive treatment where exposure to an infectious body fluid is likely.

Content Review

Factors Affecting Disease Transmission

- Mode of entry
- Virulence
- Number of organisms transmitted
- Host resistance

Table 37–1 Modes of Transmission of Infectious Diseases

Disease	Bloodborne	Airborne	Sexual	Indirect	Opportunist	Oral–Fecal
Hepatitis A						✓
Hepatitis B	✓					
Hepatitis C	✓					
HIV	✓		✓			
Influenza		✓	✓	✓		
Syphilis			✓			
Gonorrhea			✓			
Measles		✓				
Mumps		✓				
Strep throat		✓			✓	
Herpes virus	✓		✓	✓		
Food poisoning		✓		✓		✓
Lyme disease	✓					
Pneumonia		✓			✓	

communicable *capable of being transmitted to another host.*

contamination *presence of an agent only on the surface of the host without penetrating it.*

infection *presence of an agent within the host, without necessarily causing disease.*

virulence *an organism's strength or ability to infect or overcome the body's defenses.*

resistance *a host's ability to fight off infection.*

latent period *time when a host cannot transmit an infectious agent to someone else.*

communicable period *time when a host can transmit an infectious agent to someone else.*

incubation period *time between a host's exposure to infectious agent and the appearance of symptoms.*

antigen *surface protein on most viruses and bacteria that identifies them as self or non-self.*

antibody *protein that is produced in response to and that attacks a disease antigen.*

seroconversion *creation of antibodies after exposure to a disease.*

window phase *time between exposure to a disease and seroconversion.*

Not all exposures to microorganisms from body fluids or infected patients will result in transmission of those agents. Nor are all infectious agents and diseases **communicable** (capable of being transmitted to another host). Communicability depends on several factors. Exposure to an infectious agent may just result in **contamination,** in which the agent exists only on the surface of the host without penetrating it. Penetration of the host implies that **infection** has occurred, but infection should never be equated with disease. Factors that affect the likelihood that an exposed individual will become infected and then actually develop disease include:

- ★ *Correct mode of entry.* Certain external barriers in hosts, particularly the skin, make it impossible for infectious agents to establish themselves. Mucous membranes, however, often present an effective point of entry.
- ★ *Virulence.* **Virulence** is an organism's strength or ability to infect or overcome the body's defenses. Some organisms, such as the hepatitis B virus (HBV), are highly virulent and can remain infectious on a surface for weeks. Others, such as HIV and syphilis, die when exposed to air and light. Some bacteria (Clostridium) may remain dormant in the soil for months and be capable of causing disease if contracted. Infection generally occurs either when a highly virulent microorganism interacts with a normal, intact host or when a less virulent microorganism enters a host with impaired defenses (immunosuppression).
- ★ *Number of organisms transmitted (dose).* For most diseases, a minimum number of organisms must enter the host to cause infection. As a rule, the higher the number, the greater the likelihood of contracting the disease.
- ★ *Host resistance.* **Resistance** is the host's ability to fight off infection. Several factors affect the host's resistance. They include general health and fitness, genetic predisposition or resistance to infection, nutrition status, recent exposure to stressors, hygiene, and the presence of underlying disease processes. Persons with decreased immune function are at significantly increased risk for contracting infectious diseases. Cigarette smokers and those regularly exposed to secondhand cigarette smoke are also at increased risk due to damage to mucus-producing cells.
- ★ *Other host factors.* The tendency of the host to travel or be in contact with other potential hosts, the age and socioeconomic status of the host, and the characteristics of other hosts within the population of which the infected host is a member all affect the likelihood of contracting disease.

PHASES OF THE INFECTIOUS PROCESS

Disease progression varies greatly, depending on the infectious agent and the host. Conditions can manifest themselves in various ways. Once infected with an infectious agent, the host goes through a **latent period** when he cannot transmit the agent to someone else. Following the latent period is a **communicable period** when the host may exhibit signs of clinical disease and can transmit the infectious agent to another host.

The appearance of symptoms often lags after exposure to an infectious disease. The time between exposure and presentation, known as the **incubation period,** may range from a few days, as in the common cold, to months or years, as in AIDS or hepatitis. Thus, prehospital personnel must be notified if any patient for whom they provide care subsequently develops a life-threatening infectious disease.

Most viruses and bacteria have surface proteins, or **antigens,** that stimulate the body to produce **antibodies.** These antibodies react to or unite with the antigens. The antibodies' presence in the blood indicates exposure to the particular disease that they fight. Although testing for the presence of a specific disease antigen is difficult, laboratory tests can often spot antibodies that are specific for the disease or antigen. For example, they detect the human immunodeficiency virus (HIV) through the presence of antibodies specific to HIV. When a person develops antibodies after exposure to a disease, his previously negative test will be positive and **seroconversion** has occurred. The time between exposure to disease and seroconversion is referred to as the **window phase.** A person in the window phase may test negative even though he is infected. From the standpoint of the immune system response, the window phase is the period when antigen is present but antibody production has not reached detectable levels. The **disease period** is the duration from the onset of signs and symptoms of disease until the resolution of symptoms or death. Keep in mind that the resolution of symptoms does not necessarily imply that the infectious agent has been eradicated.

disease period *the duration from the onset of signs and symptoms of disease until the resolution of symptoms or death.*

INFECTION CONTROL IN PREHOSPITAL CARE

To supplement the body's natural defenses against disease, EMS providers must protect themselves from infectious exposures.

The body protects itself from disease in many ways. At the basic level, skin defends against invading pathogens. Turbulent air flow through the airway and nasal hair assist in capturing foreign bodies. Mucus can trap and kill foreign materials. Coughing and sneezing expel foreign materials. Further, as you learned in Chapter 4 on pathophysiology, the body has a very sophisiticated immune system. The complement and lymphatic systems also assist in fighting infection through inflammatory responses and filtering of body fluids.

To supplement the body's natural defenses against disease, EMS providers must protect themselves from infectious exposures (Figure 37-3 ■). The four phases of infection control in prehospital care include preparation for response, response, patient contact, and recovery.

Content Review

Phases of Prehospital Infection Control

- Preparation for response
- Response
- Patient contact
- Recovery

PREPARATION FOR RESPONSE

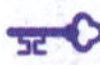

Infection control begins long before an emergency call.

Infection control begins long before an emergency call. To ensure proper protection, the EMS agency should implement the following procedures:

- ★ Establish and maintain written standard operating procedures (SOPs) for infection control, and monitor employee compliance.

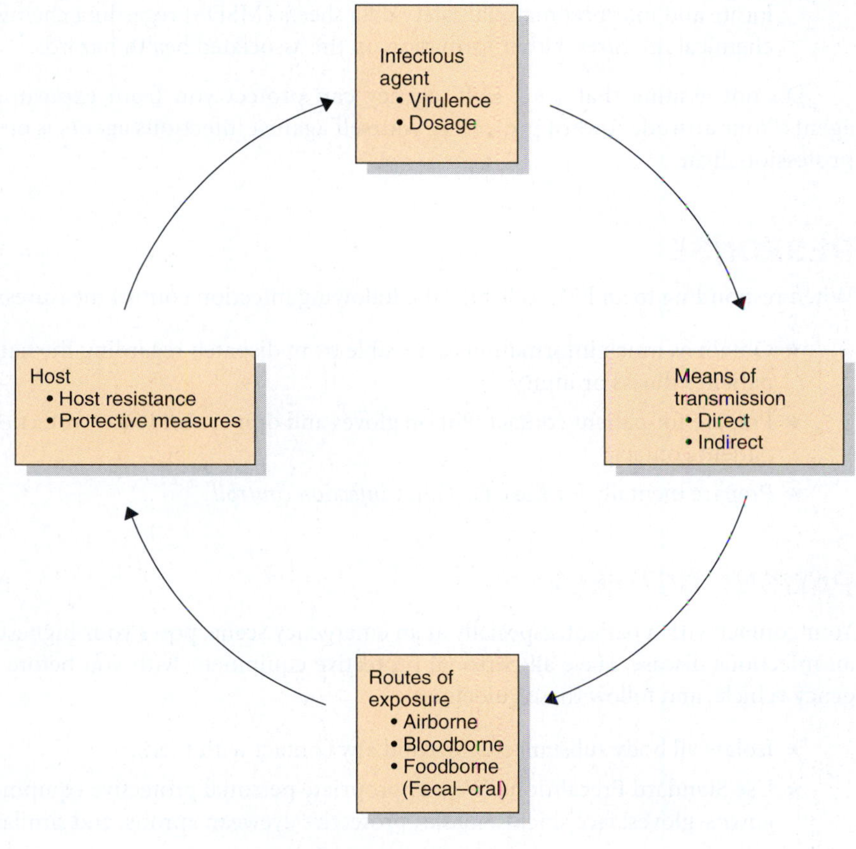

■ **Figure 37-3** Interruption of infectious disease transmission is a role of prehospital personnel.

- ★ Prepare an infection control plan that includes a schedule of when and how to implement OSHA, NIOSH, and CDC pathogen standards and guidelines.
- ★ Provide adequate original and ongoing infection control training to all personnel, including engineering and work practice controls.
- ★ Ensure that all employees are provided with personal protective equipment (PPE) and that it is fitted appropriately, checked regularly, maintained properly, and can be located easily.
- ★ Ensure that all EMS personnel treat and bandage all personal wounds (e.g., open sores, cuts, or skin breaks) before any emergency response.
- ★ Use disposable supplies and equipment when possible. The risk of transmitting disease is generally much lower than when reusing items, even though they have been cleaned or disinfected.
- ★ Ensure that all EMS personnel have access to the facilities and supplies needed to maintain a high level of personal hygiene.
- ★ Do not allow EMS personnel to deliver patient care if they exhibit signs or symptoms of an infectious disease.
- ★ Monitor all EMS personnel for compliance with vaccinations and appropriate diagnostic tests (e.g., **PPD,** antibody titers).
- ★ Appoint a designated infectious disease control officer (IDCO) to serve as a contact person for personnel exposed to an infectious disease and monitor the infection control program.
- ★ Identify specific job classifications and work processes in which the possibility of exposure exists.
- ★ Provide hazmat (hazardous materials) education for employees, including how to locate and interpret material safety data sheets (MSDS) regarding chemicals or chemical mixtures with information on the associated health hazards.

PPD *purified protein derivative, the substance used in a test for tuberculosis.*

Do not assume that your EMS agency can protect you from exposure to all infectious agents. Your attitude toward protecting yourself against infectious agents is one measure of your professionalism.

RESPONSE

When responding to an EMS call, take the following infection control measures:

- ★ Obtain as much information as possible from dispatch regarding the nature of the patient's illness or injury.
- ★ Prepare for patient contact. Put on gloves and don eye and face protection before patient contact.
- ★ Prepare mentally for the call. Think *infection control!*

PATIENT CONTACT

Your contact with a patient, especially at an emergency scene, poses your highest risk for acquiring an infectious disease.

Your contact with a patient, especially at an emergency scene, poses your highest risk for acquiring an infectious disease. Have all personal protective equipment with you before leaving the emergency vehicle, and follow these guidelines:

- ★ Isolate all body substances and avoid any contact with them.
- ★ Use Standard Precautions. Wear appropriate personal protective equipment such as gowns, gloves, face shields, masks, protective eyewear, aprons, and similar items.
- ★ Allow only necessary personnel to make patient contact. Limit the risk to as few people as possible, thus minimizing exposure.

- ★ Use airway adjuncts such as a pocket mask or bag-valve-mask unit to minimize exposure. Disposable items are preferable.
- ★ Properly dispose of biohazardous waste.
- ★ Use extreme caution with sharp instruments. Utilize retractable IV needles and needleless injection systems when possible. Never bend, recap, or remove contaminated needles. Dispose of all contaminated sharps in properly labeled puncture-resistant containers.
- ★ Never smoke, eat, or drink in the patient compartment of the ambulance. Each service should have strict guidelines regarding the presence of food and drink in the driver compartment during down times. Strictly adhere to OSHA guidelines.
- ★ Do not apply cosmetics or lip balm or handle contact lenses when a likelihood of exposure exists.

Table 37–2 details specific measures for protection against HIV and HBV infections.

RECOVERY

Infection control does not end when you deliver the patient to the emergency department. Decontaminating the ambulance and equipment is essential. Take the following steps at the completion of each response:

Infection control does not end when you deliver the patient to the emergency department.

- ★ Wash hands immediately after patient contact. Ample data substantiate that *effective, vigorous* hand washing is superior to some disinfectants. On scene, you can wipe your hands with a waterless hand-cleansing solution. However, this provides for only partial cleansing because it cannot grossly remove the particles to which microorganisms adhere. Only soap and water can do that. On returning to quarters, or at the earliest opportunity, thoroughly wash your hands with soap and warm water, paying attention to the webs between fingers. Overlooking this important habit may result in the inadvertent contamination of personal clothing or anything else that you contact. Such oversight can result in transmitting the disease to family and friends.

Table 37–2 Guidelines for Prevention of Transmission of HIV and HBV to Prehospital Personnel

Task or Activity	Disposable Gloves	Gown	Mask	Protective Eyewear
Bleeding control with active bleeding	Yes	Yes	Yes	Yes
Bleeding control with minimal bleeding	Yes	No	No	No
Emergency childbirth	Yes	Yes	Yes	Yes
Blood drawing	Yes	No	No	No
IV insertion	Yes	No	No	No
Endotracheal intubation	Yes	No	Yes	Yes
EOA insertion	Yes	No	Yes	Yes
Oral/nasal suctioning; manually clearing airway	Yes	Yes	Yes	Yes
Handling/cleaning instruments with possible contamination	Yes	Yes	Yes	Yes
Measuring blood pressure	Yes	No	No	No
Giving an injection	Yes	No	No	No
Measuring temperature	Yes	No	No	No
Rescuing from a building fire	Yes	No	No	No
Cleaning back of ambulance after a medical call	Yes	No	No	No

■ Figure 37-4 Bag all linen, and label it infectious.

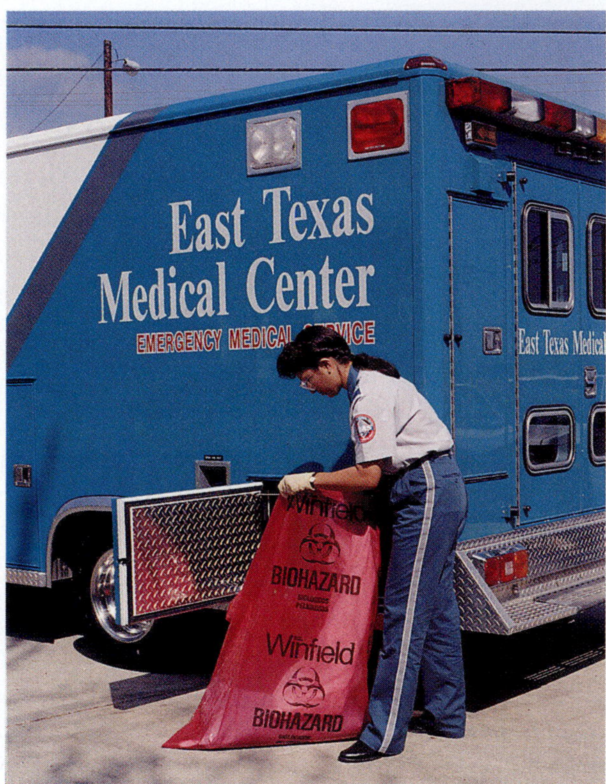

★ If you sustain a wound and are exposed to the body fluids of others, vigorously wash the wound with soap and warm water immediately, *before* contacting your employer or IDCO.

★ Dispose of all biohazardous wastes in accordance with local laws and regulations.

★ Place potentially infectious wastes in leakproof biohazard bags. Bag any soiled linen and label for laundry personnel (Figure 37-4 ■).

★ Decontaminate all contaminated clothing and reusable equipment.

★ Handle uniforms in accordance with the agency's standard procedures for personal protective equipment.

Decontamination Methods and Procedures

decontaminate *to destroy or remove pathogens.*

Decontaminate infected equipment according to local protocol and SOPs established by the EMS agency. Perform decontamination in a designated area that is properly marked and secured. The room should have a suitable ventilation system and adequate drainage. Be sure to wear gloves, gowns, boots, protective eyewear, and a face mask. To begin decontamination, remove surface dirt and debris with soap and water. Then disinfect and, if required, sterilize all items. The four levels of decontamination are low-level disinfection, intermediate-level disinfection, high-level disinfection, and sterilization.

Content Review

Decontamination Levels

- Low-level disinfection
- Intermediate-level disinfection
- High-level disinfection
- Sterilization

Low-Level Disinfection Low-level **disinfection** destroys most bacteria and some viruses and fungi. It does not destroy *Mycobacterium tuberculosis* or bacterial spores. Use low-level disinfection for routine housekeeping and cleaning, as well as for removing visible body fluids. All EPA-registered disinfectants are suitable for low-level disinfection.

disinfect *to destroy certain forms of microorganisms, but not all.*

Intermediate-Level Disinfection Intermediate-level disinfection destroys *Mycobacterium tuberculosis* and most viruses and fungi. It does not, however, destroy bacterial spores. Use it for all equipment that has come into contact with intact skin such as stethoscopes, splints, and blood pressure cuffs. A 1:10 to 1:100 dilution of water and chlorine bleach is acceptable for intermediate-level disinfection. Hard-surface germicides and EPA-registered disinfectants/chemical germicides are also effective.

High-Level Disinfection High-level disinfection destroys all forms of microorganisms except certain bacterial spores. High-level disinfection is required for all reusable devices that have come into contact with mucous membranes, including laryngoscopes, Magill forceps, and airway adjuncts. For high-level disinfection, immerse objects in an EPA-approved chemical-sterilizing agent for 10 to 45 seconds (depending on the manufacturer's instructions). Alternatively, immerse the device in hot water (176° to 212°F) for 30 minutes.

Sterilization **Sterilization** destroys all microorganisms and is required for all contaminated invasive instruments. An autoclave that uses pressurized steam or ethylene-oxide gas effectively sterilizes equipment. These methods, however, are rarely available outside of a hospital setting. Alternatively, prolonged immersion (6 to 10 hours, depending on the manufacturer's instructions) in an EPA-approved chemical-sterilizing agent is usually adequate. When possible, use disposable instruments for invasive procedures.

sterilize *to destroy all microorganisms.*

INFECTIOUS DISEASE EXPOSURES

Infectious disease exposures occur during all hours of a work shift. Since you may not always be able to contact an agency administrator, you need a working knowledge of your agency's standard operating procedures as well as the laws and regulations applicable to exposures. The following recommendations will help to ensure that exposure management will protect you, other emergency responders and health care professionals, the agency, and the confidentiality of patient information.

Reporting an Infectious Disease Exposure

Immediately report exposures of EMS personnel to the designated IDCO, according to local protocol. Report all exposures to blood, blood products, or any potentially infectious material, regardless of their perceived severity. This will permit immediate medical follow-up, including counseling for the EMS provider and identification of the infectious agent. It also enables the IDCO to evaluate the circumstances of the exposure and implement changes to prevent future exposures, if needed. Finally, it facilitates follow-up testing if the source individual consents.

Report all exposures to blood, blood products, or any potentially infectious material, regardless of their perceived severity.

The Ryan White Act

The **Ryan White Act** is a federal law that outlines the rights and responsibilities of agencies and health care workers when an infectious disease exposure occurs. Under its provisions, the exposed employee has the right to ask the source patient's infection status, but neither the agency nor the employee can force the source individual to be tested. Employers must also tell their employees what to do if an exposure occurs.

Federal law further mandates that each agency designate an IDCO to whom exposures are reported. This officer coordinates implementation of the exposure control plan and follows local reporting requirements.

Ryan White Act *federal law that outlines the rights and responsibilities of agencies and health care workers when an infectious disease exposure occurs.*

Postexposure

Employers are required to provide a medical evaluation and treatment for any paramedic or other EMS provider exposed to an infectious disease. The nature of the exposure is assessed based on the route, dose, and nature of the infectious agent. As part of the medical evaluation, employees are entitled to receive counseling about alternatives for treatment, the risks of treatment, signs, symptoms, the possibility of developing disease, and preventing further spread of the potential infection. This includes the available medications, their potential side effects, and their contraindications. Treatment must be in line with current U.S. Public Health Service recommendations.

After a paramedic is exposed to an infectious disease, he has the option to submit a blood sample for baseline testing. If the employee does not consent to having his blood screened for specific diseases, the blood samples are normally maintained for 90 days in the event that he changes his mind.

The IDCO or other health care professional who specializes in occupational infectious diseases should counsel the exposed employee and obtain informed consent for postexposure prophylaxis (PEP) based on CDC guidelines. All records related to employee counseling and PEP are forwarded to the IDCO. Vaccines may be made available to the employee if deemed appropriate by an occupational medicine physician.

Confidentiality

The IDCO will maintain records of all exposures as required by law. All of these exposure records (like any medical records) are confidential. They must not be released to anyone without express written permission from the employee.

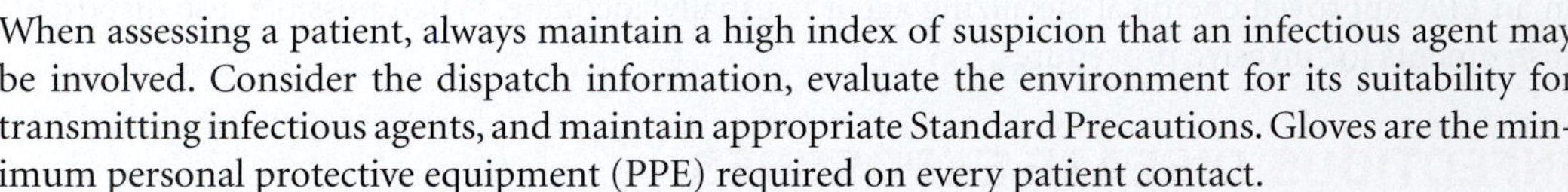

ASSESSMENT OF THE PATIENT WITH INFECTIOUS DISEASE

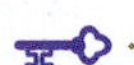

Approach every scene with a high index of suspicion that a patient may have an infectious disease.

When assessing a patient, always maintain a high index of suspicion that an infectious agent may be involved. Consider the dispatch information, evaluate the environment for its suitability for transmitting infectious agents, and maintain appropriate Standard Precautions. Gloves are the minimum personal protective equipment (PPE) required on every patient contact.

When approaching a patient with a possible infectious disease, look for general indicators of infection such as unusual skin signs, fever, weakness, profuse sweating, malaise, anorexia, and unexplained worsening of existing disease states. If an infection is localized, signs of inflammation may include redness, swelling, tenderness to palpation, capillary streaking, and warmth in the affected area. A rash or other diagnostic skin signs may make identifying an infectious disease much easier.

PAST MEDICAL HISTORY

The patient's past medical history (PMH) may provide valuable clues to his illness. Patients who have AIDS or are taking immunosuppressant medications such as steroids are particularly susceptible to infection. COPD patients, patients with autoimmune diseases, and transplant recipients frequently take steroids and immunosuppressants. Persons with diabetes and other endocrine disorders are also more likely to get infections due to additional stressors on their immune systems. Other conditions that increase the risk for developing infectious diseases include alcoholism, malnutrition, IV drug abuse, malignancy (cancer), and splenectomy (removal of the spleen), as well as artificial heart valves (aortic or mitral) or joints (hip or knee). Any significant increase in emotional stress may also increase a person's risk of significant illness, including infectious diseases.

A patient with a PMH of numerous untreated throat infections who suddenly develops a heart murmur, fever, and malaise may have rheumatic fever, a streptococcal infection that can affect the heart. Such patients are often found in medically underserved areas where access to primary care is difficult or nonexistent. Patients with cancer are at increased risk for acquiring numerous opportunistic infectious diseases. A recently transmitted sexual disease may precede systemic infection. Recent unfinished antibiotic treatment may lead to the proliferation of drug-resistant infectious agents, causing recurrent, persistent bacterial infections or development of other opportunistic infections.

In addition to determining past or current illnesses or diseases, thoroughly investigate the patient's chief complaint and any history of the present illness including:

- When did signs and symptoms begin?
- Is fever present? How has the temperature changed over time?
- Has the patient taken any aspirin, acetaminophen, or other medications?
- Does the patient have any neck pain or stiffness when his head is moved, especially during flexion (nuchal rigidity)?
- Has the patient had any difficulty swallowing?
- Has the patient had any previous symptoms or illnesses similar to this one?

THE PHYSICAL EXAMINATION

Physical examination of the patient whom you suspect of having an infectious disease follows the standard format for assessing a medical patient. Determine the patient's level of consciousness and vital signs early on. Increased temperature commonly indicates infection. Significant increases in pulse may occur due to the infection and as a result of elevated body temperature. As a consequence, metabolic needs will increase. The patient will require more oxygen and more nutrients to maintain normal physiologic function. This may be a serious problem for elderly, very young, or debilitated patients with concurrent illnesses that limit their cardiovascular and respiratory reserve.

Every EMS unit should have the capability of measuring and monitoring body temperature (e.g., a tympanic thermometer).

Hypotension in the patient with an infectious disease may result from dehydration, vasodilation, or both, as in septic shock. In rare cases, infections of the heart muscle (endocarditis) may result in decreased cardiac output (cardiogenic shock). In any case, assess the cause of hypotension and treat it promptly. If the lungs are clear, the judicious use of fluids may be beneficial; if fluid status is not a problem, vasopressors such as dopamine may be necessary.

Dehydration is a common consequence of infectious diseases. Increased body temperature is often accompanied by increased respiratory rate and concomitant fluid loss, of which the patient is often unaware (insensible fluid loss). Vomiting or diarrhea can quickly cause life-threatening dehydration, especially in pediatric patients who have large body surface areas relative to their volume. Electrolyte imbalances often occur with fluid loss. Advances in technology that may soon make the prehospital evaluation of electrolytes cost effective may be indicated in the setting of significant dehydration. Clinically significant dehydration will usually cause tachycardia and hypotension, but be vigilant for more subtle signs that include thirst, poor skin turgor, and a shrunken and furrowed tongue. A history of decreased fluid intake, fever, vomiting, and/or diarrhea should trigger a thorough assessment of fluid status. While performing a physical exam similar to that for any patient with a medical emergency, assess the following:

- Skin for temperature, hydration, color, or rash
- Sclera for icterus
- Reaction to neck flexion (Is nuchal rigidity [neck stiffness] present?)
- Lymph nodes for swelling or tenderness (lymphadenopathy)
- Breath sounds (for adventitious sounds and evidence of consolidation)
- Hepatomegaly (enlargement of the liver)
- Purulent (pus-filled) lesions

SELECTED INFECTIOUS DISEASES

The following section profiles infectious diseases that either may be encountered in the prehospital setting or are commonly known by emergency health care practitioners. The first major category includes diseases of immediate concern to EMS. General profiles of other diseases follow. You should be familiar with the terminology of these profiles, realize which diseases you will more commonly encounter in your patients. Always employ Standard Precautions.

Content Review

Diseases of Immediate Concern to EMS Providers

- HIV
- Hepatitis
- Tuberculosis
- Pneumonia
- SARS
- Chickenpox
- Meningitis

DISEASES OF IMMEDIATE CONCERN TO EMS PROVIDERS

The diseases of immediate concern to EMS providers include HIV, hepatitis, tuberculosis, pneumonia, chickenpox, and bacterial meningitis. They are infectious diseases that have gained notoriety, pose a high risk for communicability and debilitating disease, or are relevant to direct patient care. While most attention focuses on reducing transmission from patient to health care worker, the profiles also consider reverse transmission, because responsible health care workers protect both themselves and their patients. The inclusion of chickenpox may surprise some EMS personnel, but the disease is highly communicable and poses a serious occupational risk for unvaccinated or previously unexposed health care workers.

Human Immunodeficiency Virus

human immunodeficiency virus (HIV) *organism responsible for acquired immunodeficiency syndrome (AIDS).*

The **human immunodeficiency virus** (HIV) is the most discussed and feared infectious agent of the modern era, especially of the last two decades. The clinical condition that it causes, acquired immunodeficiency syndrome (AIDS), is not a disease *per se,* but a collection of signs and symptoms that share common anatomical, physiological, and biochemical derangements in the immune system. Like other viruses, HIV utilizes the host cell's reproductive apparatus to copy itself. HIV is a retrovirus; that is, it normally carries its genetic material in RNA (instead of DNA) and utilizes an enzyme called *reverse transcriptase* (hence the designation "*retro*virus") to use RNA to synthesize DNA. This is the reverse of the usual process of transcription of DNA into RNA. The action of reverse transcriptase enables genetic material from a retrovirus to become permanently incorporated into the DNA of an infected cell. Two types of HIV have been identified, HIV-1 and HIV-2. Most research targets the HIV-1 variant, which has proven much more pathogenic than HIV-2.

The emergence of HIV and AIDS, more than any other infectious process, has increased emergency and health care workers' awareness of the dangers of infectious disease. The worldwide research and educational activities resulting from concern about HIV and AIDS are effective models for teaching health care workers and lay persons about how other infectious diseases are transmitted and for providing personal and community action plans to prevent the spread of infectious agents. Although it is a worldwide epidemic, with an especially high mortality rate in sub-Saharan Africa, AIDS poses a significantly lower *occupational* risk to health care workers in developed countries than other infectious agents.

Pathogenesis In recent years, we have learned about the dynamics of HIV infection and the development of AIDS. It was first assumed that the virus caused a cellular immune system response and then remained in a dormant phase. The humoral response was known to produce antibodies within 1 to 3 months after infection, with clinical disease developing in from 1 to 10 years. For unexplained reasons, the virus would become active, and the worsening clinical signs were attributed to an increasing viral population. The extent of immune cell activity during the incubation phase, reported to be from months to 10 years, was not immediately understood.

Research in the mid-1980s and early 1990s determined that HIV specifically targets T lymphocytes with the CD4 marker, a surface molecule that attaches the virus to the cell, and as a result a better understanding of the cellular immune response and CD4 markers emerged. A reasonably reliable correlation between disease progression and the decrease in CD4 T lymphocyte count was developed. Physicians could predict the development of specific clinical events as the CD4 count decreased. For example, *P. carinii* pneumonia (PCP), an opportunistic AIDS infection, frequently develops when CD4 counts drop to a certain level. The CD4 count thus became a guide to treatment. Its usefulness, however, was limited because it only reflected the immune system's destruction.

Recent advances in molecular biology and more reliable and cost-effective assays of proteins and other biochemical molecules have revealed a tremendous increase in virus production immediately after infection and have shown that the immune system increases its activity to counter it. Eventually the number of immune system cells (T lymphocytes) offsets the viral load, reflected by the HIV RNA. This equilibrium, or set point, may take years to establish. Even during the dynamic phase when the equilibrium has not yet been set, measurement of viral load is still the best available indicator of response to therapy and long-term clinical outcome.

Risk to the General Public HIV is transmitted through contact with blood, blood products, and body fluids. The virus has been noted in blood, semen, vaginal secretions, and breast milk. Although not yet reported, tears, amniotic fluid, urine, saliva, and bronchial secretions may theoretically transmit the disease.

The virus can enter the body through breaks in the skin, mucous membranes, the eyes, or by placental transmission. Reports of the transmission rate from mother to infant range from 13 to 30 percent. The virus is most commonly contracted through sexual contact or sharing contaminated needles. Before the initiation of stringent controls in screening donor blood and blood products, hemophiliacs and individuals needing frequent blood transfusions were at increased risk. Other groups initially identified at high risk included IV drug abusers and homosexual or bisexual males. The morbidity of heterosexual transmission of HIV has been steadily increasing, with vaginal and anal sex the primary concerns. The risk of oral sex has not been quantified but is believed to be low. Vector transmission by mosquitoes has been postulated but not yet reported. Coexisting sexually transmitted disease, especially with ulceration, appears to increase the risk of infection in sexual transmission. Ethnicity and gender are not established risk factors, and the period of maximum infectiousness cannot be effectively determined. No recovery from AIDS has ever been reported, although postexposure prophylaxis has been demonstrated to decrease the severity of disease and delay mortality.

Risk to Health Care Workers Although contact with contaminated blood or body secretions potentially places health care workers at risk, infection from HIV-positive patients has been exceedingly rare, with an estimated probability of from 0.2 to 0.44 percent after exposure to virus-containing blood. Accidental needle-stick injuries are the most frequent source of infection in health care workers.

The risk for effective transmission of HIV to health care workers initially depends on whether the exposure to HIV was percutaneous, mucosal, or cutaneous (to intact skin). Within each of these categories, the risk depends on fluid type. Blood is the most dangerous, followed by fluids that may or may not contain blood: semen, vaginal secretions, and cerebrospinal, synovial, pleural, peritoneal, pericardial, and amniotic fluid. Urine and saliva, unlikely to contain blood, pose a very low risk. Source patients (those possibly infecting health care workers) who are HIV positive or die within 2 months after the health care worker's exposure, are considered to increase the risk. The highest risk exposure involves a large volume of blood, high antibody titer against a retrovirus in the source patient, deep percutaneous injury, or actual intramuscular injection.

Clinical Presentation The Centers for Disease Control first established the case definition of what constituted AIDS in 1982. Since then, it has expanded the definition of the syndrome to include other diseases such as extrapulmonary and pulmonary tuberculosis, recurrent pneumonia, wasting syndrome, HIV dementia, and sensory neuropathy. The AIDS patient may first develop a mononucleosis-like syndrome with nonspecific signs and symptoms such as fatigue, fever, sore throat, lymphadenopathy (lymph node disease), splenomegaly (enlarged spleen), rash, and diarrhea. Since not all of those signs are present, the situation may seem so trivial that the patient does not seek health care. Many patients develop purplish skin lesions known as Kaposi sarcoma. Kaposi sarcoma is a cancerous lesion that was quite rare until HIV appeared. As the disease progresses, many patients develop life-threatening opportunistic infections such as *P. carinii* pneumonia. Secondary infections caused by *M. tuberculosis* may also be present. As AIDS progresses, it involves the central nervous system; dementia, psychosis, encephalopathy, and peripheral neurological disorders may develop.

Postexposure Prophylaxis There is no cure or vaccine for AIDS. After an exposure to a confirmed HIV-positive source patient, the health care worker should immediately seek evaluation and possible initiation of treatment by an occupational medicine or infectious disease physician. The basic regimen includes zidovudine (Retrovir, ZDV, AZT) and lamivudine (Epivir, 3TC). These two medications are available as a combination preparation called Combivir. Current CDC recommendations establish two hours as the optimum time within which to start occupational postexposure prophylaxis therapy. This is because early, aggressive treatment may decrease the viral load and alter the set point. Counseling by the IDCO or a trained occupational infectious disease specialist must supplement the postexposure evaluation as part of the agency's exposure control plan. EMS personnel should not attempt to determine their own risk and need for postexposure prophylaxis. Health care workers have significantly underestimated their own risk and need for medical intervention regarding other infections, and the element of denial in HIV increases that tendency.

Summary of HIV HIV-positive patients generally do not present in life-threatening situations to EMS; however, they pose substantial psychosocial challenges. Despite changes in societal attitudes and increased tolerance of differences, HIV-positive individuals are often marginalized and shunned. Their subsequent feeling of social isolation is often worsened by depression. In spite of this, these patients are usually forthcoming about their infection status when dealing with health care workers. Although a paramedic generally has little to offer in terms of treatment, it is vitally important that care be compassionate, understanding, and nonjudgmental. Take appropriate precautions to prevent disease transmission, but if you truly understand the risk as it applies to you as a health care worker, it should be no barrier to your providing professional and emotionally supportive care, including a caring touch. In the EMS environment, physical isolation of the HIV-positive patient is unjustified.

Standard Precautions The CDC, OSHA, and NIOSH recommend Standard Precautions for health care workers at increased risk for exposure to HIV and other bloodborne pathogens. Since reliably determining which patients have bloodborne infections is impossible, the following precautions are recommended for all patients:

- ★ All health care workers should routinely use appropriate barrier precautions to prevent exposure of the skin and mucous membranes to any contact with blood, or other body fluids, from any patient. Wear disposable gloves when touching blood and body fluids, mucous membranes, or broken skin; handling items or surfaces soiled with blood or body fluids; and performing venipuncture or other vascular access procedures. Change and discard gloves after contact with each patient. To prevent exposure of the mucous membranes of the mouth, nose, and eyes, wear masks and protective eyewear or protective face shields during procedures likely to aerosolize blood or other body fluids. If a glove is torn or a needle stick occurs, remove the glove and replace it as soon as possible. Discard the needle or instrument and obtain another. Wear gowns or aprons during any procedure likely to generate splashes of bloods or other body fluids.
- ★ Wash your hands (including the webs between your fingers) and other skin surfaces thoroughly with soap and warm water after removal of gloves and especially after contamination with blood or other body fluids.
- ★ Take precautions to prevent injuries caused by needles, scalpels, or other sharp instruments or devices when performing procedures, cleaning instruments, or disposing of instruments. To prevent needle-stick injuries, needles should not be recapped, purposely bent, broken by hand, removed from disposable syringes, or otherwise manipulated by hand. Position puncture-resistant containers as close as possible to work areas and place disposable syringes and needles, scalpel blades, and other sharp items in them for disposal.
- ★ Although saliva has not been directly implicated in HIV transmission, use mouthpieces with one-way valves or filters, bag-valve-mask devices, and other ventilation devices to avoid mouth-to-mouth contact. Place these resuscitation items where the need for resuscitation is predictable.
- ★ Do not put gloved hands close to your mouth, and avoid wiping your face with your forearms or the backs of your gloved hands. Use clean towels to deal with perspiration.
- ★ If you have exudative or weeping skin lesions, refrain from direct patient care and from handling patient care equipment until the condition resolves.
- ★ Pregnant health care workers are not believed to be at greater risk of HIV infection than health care workers who are not pregnant. If a health care worker develops HIV infection during pregnancy, however, the infant is at risk for transplacental transmission. Therefore, pregnant health care workers should be especially familiar with, and strictly adhere to, precautions to minimize the risk of HIV transmission.
- ★ Disinfection of diagnostic or therapeutic equipment and supplies is mandatory.

Hepatitis

hepatitis *inflammation of the liver characterized by diffuse or patchy tissue necrosis.*

Hepatitis is an inflammation of the liver caused by viruses, bacteria, fungi, parasites, excessive alcohol consumption, or medications. Viruses are by far the most common cause of hepatitis. The clinical signs and symptoms of hepatitis secondary to viral infection are the same regardless of the type of virus. Initially they include headache, fever, weakness, joint pain, anorexia, nausea and vomiting, and, in some cases, right upper quadrant abdominal pain. As disease progresses, the patient may become jaundiced, with fever often resolving at the onset of jaundice. This stage is sometimes marked by a darkened urine and the development of clay-colored stools. The various types of hepatitis are transmitted in specific ways. Hepatitis A, B, C, D, E, and G represent the greatest potential for communicable disease. Paramedics who practice Standard Precautions against bloodborne and fecal–oral transmission will drastically reduce their risk of contracting hepatitis through occupational exposure.

Hepatitis A Hepatitis A (infectious or viral hepatitis) is transmitted by the fecal–oral route. The causative agent, hepatitis A virus, is usually found in the stool of infected persons, who may not exercise suitable personal hygiene. After these individuals handle food or contact another individual by something as casual as shaking hands, the virus can then be transmitted via contaminated hands, food, water, ice, and eating utensils. Furthermore, the virus can exist on unwashed hands for as long as 4 hours. Many hepatitis A infections are asymptomatic. They do not present with obvious signs like jaundice and are recognizable only by liver function studies. This is especially true of children, who represent most cases of infection and often transmit the virus to others by close social contact. Sexual contact can also spread the virus. Transmission by needle-stick injury is unlikely and has not been reported.

Diaper changing, especially in childcare centers with an infected child, is known to increase risk. Travelers to areas with poor sanitary conditions are also at risk. Two inactivated hepatitis A vaccines (Havrix and Vaqta) provide effective active immunization. Health care workers serving on disaster medical teams to Africa, the Middle East, Central and South America, and Asia should be immunized. Immunization is not generally recommended for health care workers in the United States but may be advised in some areas where hepatitis A prevalence is unusually high. Passive pre-exposure immunization with immune globulin (gamma globulin) is therefore falling out of favor, but immunization may be used after exposure in selected incidents.

The hepatitis A virus's incubation period averages from 3 to 5 weeks, with the greatest probability of transmission in the latter half of that period. Afflicted individuals are most infectious during the first week of symptoms. The disease follows a mild course, is rarely serious, and lasts from 2 to 6 weeks.

Hepatitis B The hepatitis B (serum hepatitis) virus is transmitted through direct contact with contaminated body fluids (blood, semen, vaginal fluids, and saliva) and therefore represents a substantial risk to EMS providers. Hepatitis B is much more contagious than HIV. The potential for transmitting hepatitis B following exposure to infected blood ranges from 1.9 to 40 percent and by needle stick from 5 to 35 percent. The incidence of antibodies in hepatitis B in health care workers has been reported to be two to four times greater than in the community at large. Health care workers infected by hepatitis B can develop acute hepatitis, cirrhosis, and liver cancer. From 5 to 10 percent of infected health care workers may become asymptomatic chronic carriers and pose an infection risk to family and other intimate contacts. The effectiveness of the three series of immunizations has been reported to be close to 90 percent in adults and higher in children, but low rates of health care worker compliance with immunization are distressingly common. No clearly identifiable populations are at risk except for those individuals who are exposed to high-risk body fluids in the course of their employment.

In the general populace, sexual transmission of hepatitis B is common. Transmission has also been known to occur with transfusion, dialysis, needle and syringe sharing in IV drug use, tattooing, acupuncture, and communally used razors and toothbrushes. The virus is stable on surfaces with dried, visible blood for more than 7 days. Infection of toddlers from household contacts with family member carriers has been reported. Transmission by insect vectors or the fecal–oral route has not been reported.

Serum markers that reflect amounts of antigen or antibody from surface or core molecules of the virus reliably reflect active infection, communicability, the window phase of infection, and peak virus replication levels. A detailed discussion of the clinical significance of these markers and how they guide therapy is beyond the scope of this text.

With as much as is known about hepatitis B's disease process and its consequences, combined with the fact that effective vaccines exist, the number of health care workers who have not been immunized or are unaware of their immune status is alarming. Two vaccines, Recombivax HB and Engerix B, which are both products of genetic recombinant technology, are available. They are reported to be as effective as the previously available Heptavax, derived from blood plasma, without the risk of HIV transmission or other viral infection. The immunization regimen is a series of three intramuscular injections.

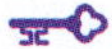
All EMS workers should receive the hepatitis B vaccination series.

Following the initial dose, booster doses are administered at 1 and 6 months. After the immunization regimen, antibody assays are obtained to confirm active immunity.

The target antibody titer is 10 milli-international units per mL (10 mIU/mL), with a recommendation to draw for antibody titer from 4 to 6 weeks after the series is completed. An additional booster may be necessary if the individual does not develop adequate antibody levels. The duration of protection is thought to be 5 years, perhaps longer. The vaccine is safe in pregnancy. Its side effects include local redness, occasional low grade fever, rash, nausea, joint pain, or mild fatigue.

Hepatitis B's incubation period lasts from 8 to 24 weeks. Joint pain and rash are more common with hepatitis B infection than with other types of hepatitis, but 60 to 80 percent of hepatitis B infections are asymptomatic.

Hepatitis C The prevalence of hepatitis C (HCV) in the United States is believed to be 1.8 percent in the adult population and from 2.7 to 10 percent in health care workers. The virus is transmitted primarily by IV drug abuse and sexual contact. Sexual contact, however, does not appear to transmit hepatitis C as effectively as it does hepatitis B. After 1989, effective blood donor screening for hepatitis C practically eliminated the risk of transfusion-associated infection. Fecal–oral transmission and household contact have not been reported as factors in transmission, and no specific groups have been identified to be at greater risk for hepatitis C infection.

Hepatitis C is a chronic condition in about 85 percent of infected people. Because of its chronic nature and its ability to cause active disease years later, it poses a great international public health problem. Antibodies can be produced against hepatitis C and provide the laboratory method for determining infection. However, the antibodies are not effective in eliminating the virus, and their presence does not indicate immunity. The ineffectiveness of antibodies is attributed to the virus's high mutation rate. Consequently, the cellular immune response, which results in the immune system's killing infected cells, is very aggressive and is believed, ironically, to cause most of the associated liver injury.

Hepatitis C infection, formerly called non-A, non-B hepatitis, often causes liver fibrosis, which progresses over decades to cirrhosis and is estimated to develop in about 20 percent of infected individuals. This progression is known to be accelerated in persons older than 50 at the time of initial infection, in those consuming more than 50 g of alcohol per day, and in men. Cirrhosis has also been known to occur in those who have not consumed alcohol and can worsen to end-stage liver disease with jaundice, ascites, and esophageal varices.

No effective vaccination for hepatitis C exists. Treatment with alpha interferon has had limited success, with about 15 to 20 percent of patients responding positively, as defined by the liver enzymes' return to normal levels. Another drug, ribavirin (an antiviral), administered orally, is known to potentiate interferon's immune system effects, and researchers are now focusing their efforts on improving the results of combination therapy with ribavirin and alpha interferon.

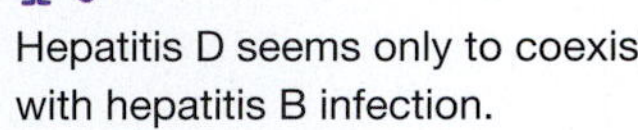

Hepatitis D seems only to coexist with hepatitis B infection.

Hepatitis D The hepatitis D virus (HDV), formerly called delta hepatitis, depends on a surface antigen of the hepatitis B virus (HBV) to produce its structural protein shell. Thus, HDV infection seems to exist only with a coexisting HBV infection. Immunization against HBV therefore confers immunity to HDV. When a patient who has HBV infection with liver disease develops an overlying HDV infection, mortality rates are very high.

Parenteral HDV transmission occurs similarly to HBV in western Europe and North America. Fortunately, cases in health care workers are extremely rare. Frequent epidemics of nonparenteral transmission occur in central Africa, the Middle East, and the Mediterranean countries. HDV's incubation period has not been determined.

Hepatitis E Hepatitis E (HEV) is transmitted like hepatitis A virus (HAV), through the fecal–oral route, and seems to be associated with contaminated drinking water more commonly than HAV. It occurs primarily in young adults, with highest rates in pregnant women. First described in India, outbreaks have occurred in Russia, Nepal, Southeast Asia, the Middle East, Pakistan, and China. Only six cases were reported in the United States from 1989 to 1992, most likely because of more sanitary sources of drinking water.

Hepatitis G Hepatitis G virus is a newly identified virus. It was found after people who had a blood transfusion developed post-transfusion hepatitis that could not be identified as any known virus. Infection with the hepatitis G virus can lead to persistent infection in 15 to 30 percent of adults. The long-term outcomes of the infection are not yet known. People with hepatitis A, B, or C can be co- or super-infected with hepatitis G. There is no vaccine available for hepatitis G.

Tuberculosis

Tuberculosis (TB) is the most common preventable adult infectious disease in the world. TB is caused by bacteria known collectively as the *Mycobacterium tuberculosis* complex, which includes *M. tuberculosis, M. bovis,* and *M. africanum.* Other bacteria in the *Mycobacterium* family can cause tuberculosis, particularly in immunocompromised patients. These other types of *Mycobacterium* are referred to as atypicals. It primarily affects the respiratory system, including a highly contagious form in the larynx. Untreated or undertreated, it may spread to other organ systems, causing extrapulmonary TB and other complications. The disease appeared about 7,000 years ago and peaked in the eighteenth century. The number of new cases in the United States has increased steadily since 1985, in large part because of TB in AIDS patients and in recently arrived immigrants from countries where the disease is prevalent.

tuberculosis (TB) *disease caused by a bacterium known as* Mycobacterium tuberculosis *that primarily affects the respiratory system.*

TB is the most common preventable adult infectious disease in the world. Its incidence in the United States has been rising since 1985.

The development of multiple drug-resistant tuberculosis (MDR-TB) has been known since the late 1940s. Drug resistance occurs when drug-resistant bacteria outgrow drug-susceptible bacteria. These bacteria acquire resistance either because of patient noncompliance with therapy or inadequate treatment regimens. Drug resistance occurs early in therapy, especially when only one drug is used. For this reason, most current CDC recommendations for the initiation of therapy in the United States involve several options for treatment, each calling for multiple medications, including isoniazid (INH), rifampin, pyrazinamide, ethambutol, and streptomycin, among others.

M. tuberculosis is most commonly transmitted through airborne respiratory droplets but may also be contracted by direct inoculation through mucous membranes and broken skin or by drinking contaminated milk. Animal reservoirs for the bacteria include cattle, swine, badgers, and primates. Coughing and other expiratory actions (sneezing, speaking, singing) create bacteria-containing droplets from 5 to 10 microns in size, which susceptible individuals inhale into the alveoli.

The risk of transmitting tuberculosis is not as high as the risk of measles. Although the average case infects only about a third of his close contacts, prolonged exposure to a person with active TB is always listed as a risk factor. Communicability varies from case to case. Although a single occupational exposure to a patient with active TB is highly unlikely to transmit the disease to a paramedic, Standard Precautions against TB should still be employed.

Skin Testing The commonly used purified protein derivative (PPD) skin test effectively identifies candidates for prophylactic drug therapy (to prevent active TB) in large groups of health care workers. It has limited value in guiding individual therapy in those with active TB because a positive PPD indicates previous infection but does not distinguish active from dormant disease. Another health care worker experienced in interpreting the results should read the skin test, rather than the worker tested, because health care workers are known to underinterpret positive results. In addition, the skin test must be interpreted on the basis of the disease's prevalence in the community. A negative test does not rule out active disease, particularly in immunosuppressed individuals or in those who were infected so recently that their immune systems have not yet had time to mount the cellular mediated response that causes a positive PPD.

EMS workers should receive TB screening on an annual basis.

Most EMS agencies require skin testing at least annually. This may be sufficient, but again, decisions about the frequency of testing should be based on the disease's prevalence in the community. For individuals who have not been previously skin tested or who have no documentation of a negative PPD in the last 12 months, two-step testing may be reasonable. In these individuals, an initial negative test may be due to weak reactivity to the PPD. A second skin test is administered from 1 to 3 weeks later. A positive reaction to the second test probably represents a boosted reaction, which means that the individual has been previously infected, and should be evaluated for possible prophylaxis. If the second test is negative, that individual is classified as uninfected. A positive reaction to any subsequent test would represent a new infection by *M. tuberculosis.*

Pathogenesis TB's incubation period is 4 to 12 weeks. In most people with subclinical infections, immediate disease (primary TB) does not develop because of a cell-mediated immune response. Development of disease normally occurs 6 to 12 months after infection. Susceptibility to primary infection is increased in persons who are malnourished and those persons whose immune systems are suppressed, such as the elderly, HIV patients, and people taking immunosuppressant drugs. Children less than 3 years of age are at risk because of underdeveloped immune systems, with older children identified at lowest risk. As expected, the aged are at high risk, and the reactivation of latent infections in this age group implies that the immune system has difficulty dealing with the complex nature of the *M. tuberculosis* infection. Once the bacteria enter the lungs, alveolar macrophages attack them and attempt to "wall them off" (forming granulomas) in a localized immune response. For this reason, most TB infections do not produce disease. Healed sites leave lesions of calcified areas known as Ghon foci. When Ghon foci combine with lymph nodes, they form a Ghon complex, which creates small, sharply defined shadows on a chest X-ray.

If the macrophages cannot destroy them, the bacteria lie dormant within the macrophages and are then distributed to other sites within the body. They remain dormant until some event, usually a depression of the immune system, triggers their reactivation into secondary TB. The sites of reactivation are greatest in areas of the lung with the highest oxygen tension, the apices or upper lobes. Reactivation in extrapulmonary sites such as lymph nodes, pleura, and pericardium are much more common in HIV-infected persons. In AIDS patients, the disease may spread to the thoracic and lumbar spine, destroying intervertebral disks and adjacent vertebral bodies. TB is also known to lead to subacute meningitis and granulomas in the brain.

Clinical Presentation The signs and symptoms of active TB can be very nonspecific and can be manifestations of other clinical conditions. However, a typical list would include chills, fever, fatigue, productive or nonproductive chronic cough, and weight loss. Many patients report night sweats, leaving their bed linens drenched with perspiration. Hemoptysis (expectorating blood) is very suggestive of active TB. Reactivation of dormant TB manifests as signs and symptoms specific to the organ systems involved.

EMS Response Your acceptance of responsibility for protecting yourself from *M. tuberculosis* is the most important step in preventing disease transmission. A proactive, high-index-of-suspicion-driven response is essential. The factors that increase a paramedic's risk of transmission are close and sometimes prolonged contact with the patient. Care and transport are provided in a very small, often ineffectively ventilated space, and the patient may effect various expiratory actions while in contact with EMS personnel. Placing a mask over the patient, when it does not create undue anxiety or dyspnea, effectively decreases the number of expectorated droplet nuclei. Also, nebulized medications may be administered more safely with a nebulization mask. Use appropriate respiratory precautions while performing CPR and intubation.

You should don a protective respirator on contact with a patient you suspect may have TB. Your knowledge of the prevalence of TB and the most susceptible populations in your jurisdiction should reinforce your index of suspicion. The most current NIOSH/OSHA standards for protecting health care workers from TB call for N95 **respirators,** which are designed to prevent contaminated air from reaching the health care workers wearing them (Figure 37-5a ■). High-efficiency particulate aspirator (HEPA) respirators (Figure 37-5b ■) are no longer required in TB, but EMS agencies may opt to continue their use. They are more expensive, bulky, and sometimes difficult to breathe through.

respirator *an apparatus worn that cleanses or qualifies the air.*

mask *a device for protecting the face.*

Masks, as opposed to respirators, work primarily as barriers against larger particles and are not certified to prevent contaminated air from reaching the paramedic. However, they effectively prevent the transmission of many airborne pathogens, especially when both provider and patient wear them. They also provide a more comfortable and cost-effective alternative to the routine use of respirators. The extensive terminology and guidelines relative to the design, construction, and classification of various respirators is beyond the scope of this text. EMS agencies and their IDCOs are responsible for educating their personnel in the proper use and application of respirators and for ensuring proper fit and easy access. According to the NIOSH classification, N series respirators provide protection against non-oil-based aerosols, including the droplet nuclei from TB patients. These N-type respirators must filter 95 percent of particles that are no larger than 0.3 microns in diameter, hence the designation N95. This is a very safe standard since the diameter of TB aerosol droplets ranges from 5 to 10 microns. Health care workers' noncompliance causes most respirator failures.

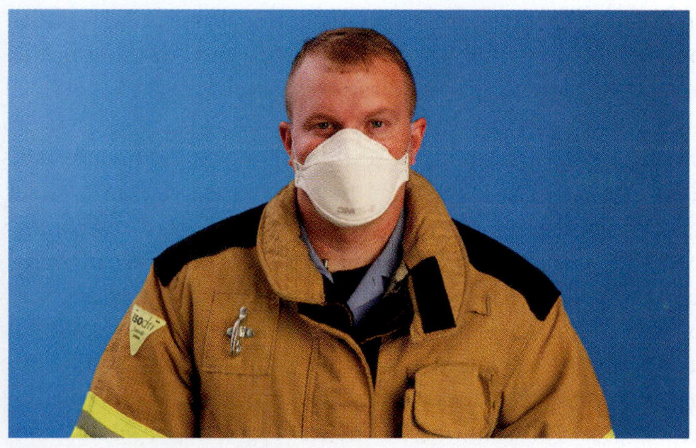

■ **Figure 37-5a** NIOSH/OSHA standards call for N95 respirators when caring for patients with tuberculosis. *(© Scott Metcalfe)*

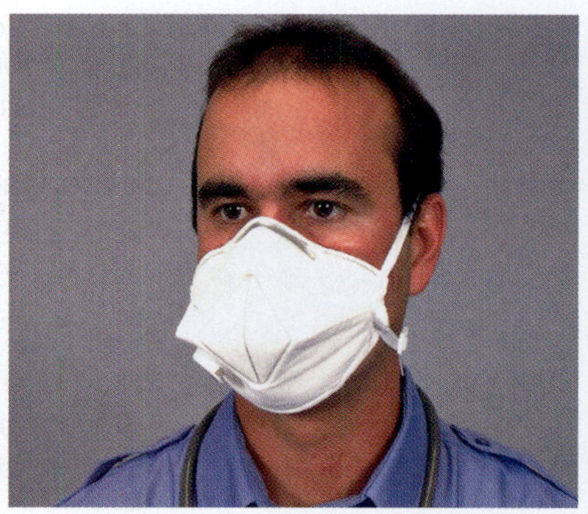

■ **Figure 37-5b** EMS agencies may opt to use high efficiency particulate aspirator (HEPA) respirators in TB.

Ventilation systems currently being marketed in selected ambulances claim to effectively recycle and filter enough air to ensure the expulsion of infected droplet nuclei. Such ventilation systems should include HEPA filtration in addition to recycling the patient compartment air volume according to OSHA standards. Do not open patient compartment windows to increase ventilation and dilute the concentration of droplet nuclei. The moving ambulance may create a Bernoulli effect that draws engine exhaust, including carbon monoxide, into the patient compartment.

Postexposure Identification and Management Early identification of exposure and drug prophylaxis, if deemed necessary, are the keys to effectively preventing active TB in health care workers. An occupational medicine physician should assess TB skin test results and determine the appropriateness of chest X-rays, sputum cultures, and a myriad of other diagnostic procedures to confirm infection or the presence of frank disease. The polymerase chain reaction (PCR) test, which eliminates the need to wait for cultures and provides a diagnosis in 6 hours, may soon become the gold standard for identifying the presence of *M. tuberculosis.*

Pneumonia

Patients with difficulty breathing often confront paramedics with the enigma of differentiating pneumonia from mild exacerbations of congestive heart failure (CHF) and its more severe form, acute pulmonary edema. The mistaken assumption that a patient has CHF may lead to aggressive treatment that reduces the patient's respiratory drive, dries protective mucous secretions, and contributes to hypotension.

pneumonia *acute infection of the lung, including alveolar spaces and interstitial tissue.*

Pneumonia, an acute lung inflammation, is not a single disease but a family of diseases that result from respiratory infection by viruses, bacteria, or fungi. The infectious agent most often associated with pneumonia, and against which the pneumococcal vaccine is targeted, is *Streptococcus pneumoniae,* gram-positive spheres found in pairs or chains. Other microorganisms known to cause pneumonia are *Mycoplasma pneumoniae* (primary atypical pneumonia), *H. influenzae, Klebsiella pneumoniae, M. catarrhalis, Legionella, S. aureus* in nosocomial infections, and *P. carinii.* These agents are also known to cause meningitis, ear infections, and pharyngitis. In addition to droplet nuclei, the infectious agents are also spread by direct contact and through linens soiled with respiratory secretions.

Those at highest risk for pneumonia are the immunocompromised, patients with sickle cell disease, transplanted organs, cardiovascular disease, diabetes mellitus, kidney disease, multiple myeloma, lymphoma, Hodgkin's disease, those without functioning spleens, and the elderly, particularly those in common residential situations. Low-birth-weight neonates and malnourished infants are very susceptible. In otherwise healthy individuals, susceptibility is increased by a previous respiratory infection like influenza, exposure to inhaled toxins, chronic lung disease, and aspiration (postalcohol ingestion, near-drowning, ingested toxins, or gastric distention from BVM ventilation). When patients contract infectious agents of pneumonia outside of a hospital or other health care institution, they are referred to as cases of community-acquired pneumonia.

History and Assessment Always consider the possibility of community-acquired pneumonia. In geriatric communities where residents live in their own home but may share common social facilities, ask if neighbors recently have been diagnosed with pneumonia or other respiratory infections. Signs and symptoms in previously healthy individuals include an acute onset of chills, high-grade fever, dyspnea, pleuritic chest pain worsened by deep inspiration, and cough, which may be productive with phlegm of various colors. The absence of fever does not rule out pneumonia. Breath sounds may include adventitious lung sounds (crackles, wheezes) and signs of consolidation. When purulent fluids accumulate in many lobes of the lung because of inflammation, alveoli collapse and their acoustic properties change to those of solid tissue, hence the name *consolidation.* Consolidation causes the expiratory sounds in the peripheral lung fields to develop the same duration as inspiration and to be just as loud. Assessment with pulse oximetry may be useful. In geriatric patients, the only presenting sign may be an altered mental status; fever is often absent, and headache, aches and pain, nausea, diarrhea, and nonproductive cough, if present, do not allow you to rule out pneumonia. In children, fever, tachypnea, and retractions are ominous signs but are not specific to pneumonia; this triad of signs, however, reliably indicates respiratory distress secondary to an infectious process in pediatric patients.

Patient Management and PPE Management of the pneumonia patient aims at supporting adequate ventilation and oxygenation, with supplemental oxygen often providing relief. Always consider TB a possibility in any patient with pneumonia and place a mask either on yourself or on your patient.

Immunization and Postexposure Management An effective vaccination exists against most serotypes of *S. pneumoniae* known to cause disease. It is highly recommended for children 2 years and younger, for adults over 65, and for those without spleens. Routine vaccination of EMS workers is not necessary. In health care settings, health care workers who routinely treat elderly, immunocompromised, or other at-risk patients may be required to be immunized because they pose the risk of patient transmission. Because EMS workers are predominantly healthy, exposure to a single patient with pneumonia generally will not result in infection or disease. A number of antimicrobial agents are effective against the infectious agents known to cause pneumonia. However, multidrug-resistant strains have been reported.

Severe Acute Respiratory Syndrome

severe acute respiratory syndrome (SARS) *a highly infectious viral respiratory illness that first appeared in southern China in 2002.*

As noted in Chapter 27, "Pulmonology," **severe acute respiratory syndrome** (**SARS**) is a viral respiratory illness that first appeared in southern China in 2002 and became a global threat in 2003 by spreading internationally. In that outbreak, 8,098 people worldwide were affected, and 774 died. Toronto, Ontario, was particularly affected, placing a significant stress on the Toronto EMS system. Four paramedics contracted the disease, reportedly before mandatory PPE measures were undertaken (Figure 37-6 ■). SARS is considered to be an ongoing threat because of its highly infectious nature.

Pathophysiology The virus that causes SARS, unrecognized before its 2002 appearance, is called SARS-associated coronavirus (SARS-CoV). Coronaviruses play a major role in upper respiratory infections and the common cold. SARS-CoV apparently may survive in the environment for several days and is spread by close person-to-person contact via respiratory droplets when an infected person coughs or sneezes. SARS-CoV can also be contracted by touching a contaminated object.

The incubation period is generally 2 to 7 days but in some cases has been as long as 10 to 14 days. A person with SARS is considered to be contagious as long as he has symptoms. There have been no reported cases of disease transmission before the source patient develops symptoms. Persons with documented SARS should be quarantined to their home for at least 10 days after the fever has abated and symptoms cleared.

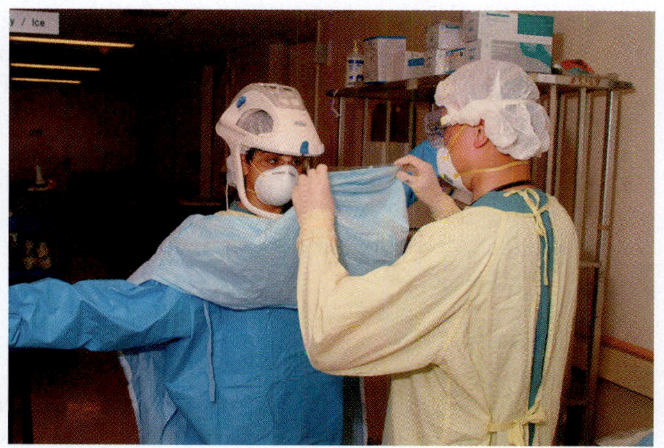

■ **Figure 37-6** During the Toronto SARS outbreak, health care workers donned mandated PPE. *(© Brian Schwartz, MD)*

Assessment If a SARS outbreak has been identified, all personnel should use appropriate PPE on every call or as directed by local health authorities. If a case is encountered in a non-SARS-epidemic area that has SARS-like symptoms, all involved should immediately don appropriate PPE.

As with any respiratory illness, first address signs of severe respiratory distress: altered mental status, one-to-two-word speech dyspnea, cough, cyanosis, and hypoxia. Patients with underlying respiratory disease (asthma, emphysema, chronic bronchitis) and those with chronic illnesses are at increased risk.

Signs and symptoms associated with SARS include sore throat, rhinorrhea (runny nose), chills, rigors (sudden paroxysmal chills), myalgias (muscle aches), headache, and diarrhea. This can progress to cough, sputum production, respiratory distress, and eventual respiratory failure.

Management Any patient suspected of having SARS should be treated like any patient with suspected pneumonia or other respiratory illness. Place the patient in a comfortable position and administer high-flow, high-concentration oxygen. Use pulse oximetry to assess the patient's oxygenation requirements. Provide ventilatory assistance and endotracheal intubation if required. Establish IV access and administer fluids if the patient is dehydrated. If the patient is wheezing, consider administering a nebulized bronchodilator. Notify the receiving hospital if you suspect SARS so that they can take appropriate protective measures.

Chickenpox

Chickenpox is caused by the varicella zoster virus (VZV). The varicella zoster virus is in the herpes virus family. Although chickenpox (**varicella**) in pediatrics is considered a self-limited disease that rarely causes severe complications, it is much more lethal in adults. It results in fewer than 100 deaths per year in the United States, but while adults represent only 2 percent of the morbidity, they account for 50 percent of the mortality. Thus, health care workers who have not been immunized against VZV or been exposed to it as children must increase their awareness of this infection and its consequences. It is estimated that 10 percent of adults have not contracted VZV during childhood. VZV is also the infectious agent of shingles (herpes zoster), a painful condition that causes skin lesions along the course of peripheral nerves and dermatome bands. Approximately 15 percent of patients with chickenpox will eventually develop shingles.

varicella *viral disease characterized by a rash of fluid-filled vesicles that rupture, forming small ulcers that eventually scab; commonly called* chickenpox.

Clinical Presentation Chickenpox usually occurs in clusters during winter and spring and presents with respiratory symptoms, malaise, and low-grade fever, followed by a rash that starts on the face and trunk and progresses to the rest of the body, including mucous membranes. The rash may be the first sign of illness, and infected persons may have anywhere from a few to 500 lesions. It is more profuse on the trunk, with less distribution to the extremities and scalp. The fluid-filled vesicles that form the rash soon rupture, forming small ulcers that eventually scab over within 1 week, at which point the patient is no longer contagious. Transmission occurs through inhalation of airborne droplets and direct contact with weeping lesions and tainted linen. The incubation period is from 10 to 21 days.

In adults, varicella's most common complication is a VZV pneumonia. A large percentage of adult deaths from VZV occur in immunocompromised patients. The most alarming aspect of adult epidemiology, however, is a significant death rate in previously healthy patients. Therefore, it is important for unexposed or unvaccinated paramedics to be immunized.

Assessing Immunity Most people develop immunity for life after recovery from childhood chickenpox infections. Thus, a history of chickenpox is considered adequate evidence of immunity. An available blood test can determine immunity in those who are unsure about their history or who have not had chickenpox.

Immunization A chickenpox vaccine, Varivax, has been licensed in the United States since 1995, and the Advisory Committee on Immunization Practices (ACIP) of CDC now recommends that all states require children entering childcare facilities and elementary school to be vaccinated or have some other evidence of immunity. Such evidence would include a primary care provider's diagnosis of chickenpox, a reliable history of the disease, or blood test confirming immunity. Vaccination is also routinely recommended for all susceptible health care workers. ACIP has also strengthened its recommendations for all other susceptible persons 13 years old or younger to include any adolescents living in the same household with younger children.

The vaccine is administered as one subcutaneous dose in children under age 12 and as two doses in susceptible adolescents and adults. Among vaccinated people 13 years or older, 78 percent developed protective antibodies, with 99 percent seroconverting after the second dose. Health care workers who receive the vaccination should have their antibody level checked 6 weeks after the second vaccination.

Patients with active TB, malignant conditions, or those being treated with immunosuppressants should not receive varicella vaccine. Its use in those taking steroids depends on a variety of factors beyond the scope of this discussion. Few adverse effects have been reported through CDC's Vaccine Adverse Events Reporting System (VAERS). The most frequent was rash, with some cases of herpes zoster. No incidents of chickenpox have been reported. Although a few serious adverse effects were reported, no cause-and-effect relationship was clearly established with the vaccination. The vaccine manufacturer discourages taking aspirin within 6 weeks after receiving the vaccination.

EMS transport of a patient with chickenpox should be followed by extensive decontamination of the ambulance and any equipment used.

EMS Response and Postexposure Observe Standard Precautions and place masks on patients. If a patient only has chickenpox, he should remain at home until the lesions are crusted and dry. If a susceptible paramedic is exposed to chickenpox, postexposure vaccination may be warranted. Recent data indicate that if used within 3 days, and possibly up to 5 days, Varivax may be effective in preventing chickenpox or lessening its severity. Varicella-zoster immune globulin (VZIG) is an alternative postexposure prophylaxis. Unlike Varivax, it provides passive immunity, and the most current recommendation for its use is in immunocompromised patients. The use of acyclovir, which inhibits replication of the virus, within 24 hours of the onset of rash may decrease the disease's severity in adults and adolescents.

Meningitis

meningitis *inflammation of the meninges, usually caused by an infection.*

Meningitis is an inflammation of the meninges (the membranes protecting the brain and spinal cord) and cerebrospinal fluid, caused by bacterial and viral infections. Meningococcal meningitis (spinal meningitis), caused by *Neisseria meningitidis,* is the disease variant of greatest concern to EMS responders.

Other agents are, or have been, known to cause meningitis. *Streptococcus pneumoniae,* the primary infectious agent of concern in pneumonia, is the second most common cause of pneumonia in adults and the most common cause of otitis media in children. Vaccines have proven very effective, especially in children. *Haemophilus influenzae* type B, a gram-negative rod, was once the leading cause of meningitis in children age 6 months to 3 years. However, with the implementation of effective childhood vaccination against *H. influenzae* since 1981, *N. meningitidis* has become the bacterium most commonly implicated in serious meningitis cases. Viruses and other microorganisms are known to cause meningitis, with similar disease profiles. Enteroviruses are implicated in 90 percent of patients with viral (aseptic) meningitis. In healthy individuals, viral meningitis is a self-limited disease that lasts about 7 to 10 days.

Transmission Factors *N. meningitidis* asymptomatically colonizes the upper respiratory tract of healthy individuals and is then transmitted by respiratory droplets. Up to 35 percent of the general population may be infected with the bacterium, which is prevented from gaining access to the CSF by the epithelial lining of the pharynx. Almost every human has probably been a carrier at some point in his life. Conversion from carrier to clinical disease is rare in developed countries and occurs in clusters in developing nations. The disease appears to peak in midwinter months with low temperature and humidity. This has been validated by observations of epidemic seasonal variations in the "meningitis belt" of sub-Saharan Africa. Epidemiologists have hypothesized that this pattern may represent a herd immunity, in which host resistance factors may be more a function of the population's general immunity than of the immunity of individuals within that population. One theory that could explain the phenomenon of herd immunity holds that another species within the genus *Neisseria* may be "mistaken" for *N. meningitidis* (a cross-reaction), resulting in effective antibody production against the pathogen. Meningococcal meningitis occurs more commonly in some areas of the United States, and the world, for reasons not yet understood. Other factors that have been implicated in transmission of *N. meningitidis* include contacting oral secretions of the index case (kissing, sharing food or drink), crowding, close contact, smoking, and lower socioeconomic status. For the EMS responder, contact with secretions during mouth-to-mask ventilation, intubation, or suctioning would increase the probability of transmission.

Clinical Presentation The incubation period most commonly ranges from 2 to 4 days but may last as long as 10 days. As with most bacterial infections, signs and symptoms develop rapidly within a few hours or 1 to 2 days of exposure and include fever, chills, headache, nuchal rigidity with flexion, arthralgia, lethargy, malaise, altered mental status, vomiting, and seizures. An upper respiratory or ear infection may precede the disease. A characteristic rash may appear and develop into hemorrhagic spots, or petechiae. Roughly 10 percent of patients may develop septic shock. Acute adrenal insufficiency, disseminated intravascular coagulation (DIC), and coma are other consequences. Death can ensue in 6 to 8 hours.

Newborns and infants may seem slow or inactive, vomit, appear irritable, or feed poorly. Fever in newborns should be evaluated with a high index of suspicion for meningococcemia. Rarely, bulging of an open anterior fontanel is seen. In older children, assessment techniques that stretch the inflamed meninges and cause pain may reveal positive Brudzinski's and Kernig's signs. **Brudzinski's sign** is a physical exam finding suggestive of meningitis. Due to irritation of the meninges, flexion of the neck causes flexion of the hips and knees. To test for Brudzinski's sign, have the patient lie supine without a pillow. Flex the neck while observing the hips and knees. Flexion of the hips or knees when the neck is flexed is considered a positive Brudzinski's sign. **Kernig's sign** is likewise suggestive of meningitis. To elicit Kernig's sign, have the patient sit or lie and flex the hips. With the hips flexed, attempt to extend (straighten) the knee. Inability to fully extend the knee is due to meningeal irritation and is considered a positive Kernig's sign. Maternal antibodies protect newborns from meningitis and other infections until up to 6 months of age (slightly longer in breast-fed children). Infants from 6 months to 2 years are especially susceptible to meningitis because they no longer have circulating maternal antibodies and their immune systems are immature and incompetent.

Brudzinski's sign *physical exam finding in which flexion of the neck causes flexion of the hips and knees.*

Kernig's sign *inability to fully extend the knees with hips flexed.*

Immunization *N. meningitidis* has several serotypes (A, B, C, X, Y, Z, 29-E, W-135), with B and C causing most disease outbreaks in the United States. The A serotype is the most common cause of epidemics in Africa and Asia. An effective vaccine has been developed against the A, C, Y, and W-135 serotypes. Attempts to develop one against the B serotype have so far resulted in weak immune responses. The meningococcal vaccine is not presently recommended for routine immunization of health care workers. Travelers to endemic areas and children younger than 2 years who are asplenic (without a spleen) or have a certain deficiency in their complement system are candidates for vaccination.

EMS Response and Postexposure Observing Standard Precautions and using masks on yourself and/or your patients with suspected meningococcal meningitis will adequately protect you against all the infectious agents of meningitis. Postexposure prophylaxis with rifampin, ciprofloxacin

(Cipro), or ceftriaxone (Rocephin) is the primary means of preventing meningococcal disease. Prophylaxis should be started within 24 hours after exposure because the rate of effective transmission in close contacts (EMS responders) with the index-case patient has been estimated to be 500 to 800 times that of the general population. Initiation of chemoprophylaxis 14 days or more after the onset of illness in the index case is of limited or no value. All postexposure medications are easily complied with and have few side effects.

Review

Content

Other Job-Related Airborne Diseases

- Influenza and the common cold
- Measles
- Mumps
- Rubella
- Respiratory syncytial virus
- Pertussis

Other Job-Related Airborne Diseases

Influenza and colds, rubella, measles, mumps, and respiratory syncytial virus (RSV) are viral infections that may be contracted in the EMS environment. Pertussis, a highly contagious bacterial disease, also poses a risk. These diseases are transmitted by direct inhalation of infected droplets or through exposed mucosal surfaces. Handling contaminated surfaces or objects and subsequently introducing the virus by scratching, wiping, or other activities with unwashed hands (autoinoculation) is another route of transmission. Masks and ventilation are recommended for measles. Precautions against autoinoculation with RSV infections, influenza, and colds include masks, more practically placed on patients, and possibly gloves, gowns, and goggles. Avoid touching your face and areas of broken skin while in contact with the patient. Effective, vigorous hand washing with soap and warm water after patient contact is the most important personal precaution against disease transmission.

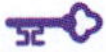

Effective, vigorous hand washing with soap and warm water after patient contact is the most important personal precaution against disease transmission.

influenza *disease caused by a group of viruses.*

Influenza and the Common Cold **Influenza** is caused by viruses designated types A, B, and C. Within these types are various subtypes that mutate so often that they are identified on the basis of where they were isolated, the culture number, and year of isolation—for instance, A/Japan/305/57. Two glycoproteins, hemagglutinin and neuraminidase, on the outer membrane of an influenza virus determine its virulence. The letters H and N, which denote these two glycoproteins, are often seen in parentheses along with a number, as in A (H1N1). This method of classification helps epidemiologists to more specifically identify a flu virus, since it is based on the immune responses to hemagglutinin and neuraminidase.

Influenza is a leading cause of respiratory disease worldwide, and various strains cause epidemics, mainly during the winter months. It is easily transmittable in crowded spaces such as public transportation vehicles, and can be spread by direct contact. The virus can persist on environmental surfaces for hours, especially in low humidity and cold temperatures. Thus, it has a high potential for transmission by autoinoculation. It is much more serious than the common cold and has caused worldwide epidemics with high mortality rates. The last great epidemic was in 1918, and CDC and the World Health Organization (WHO) closely monitor worldwide disease outbreaks.

Influenza is characterized by the sudden onset of fever, chills, malaise, muscle aches, nasal discharge, and cough. The disease is more serious in the very young, the very old, and those with underlying disease. Its incubation period is from 1 to 3 days. Fever generally lasts 3 to 5 days. Signs include mild sore throat, nonproductive cough, and nasal discharge. The cough may be severe and of long duration. Secondary infections may occur as the virus damages respiratory epithelial cells, thereby decreasing resistance to other, primarily bacterial, disorders. Severe cases may result in pneumonia, hemorrhagic bronchitis, and death. The uncomplicated disease usually lasts 2 to 7 days and full recovery is the norm.

Management is primarily supportive. Fever may increase body temperature to as high as 105°F. Begin cooling measures for patients with temperatures of 104°F or greater. Increased body temperature may lead to significant insensible fluid loss and dehydration. Determine hydration status early and begin fluid replacement if indicated.

Everyone is susceptible to influenza. Although infection confers resistance after recovery, the influenza viruses mutate so rapidly that protection is effective only against the particular strain or variant from which the person has just recovered. An immunization is available and is recommended for the elderly, those who live or work in correctional institutions, and military recruits. Patients should be immunized between early September and mid-November for maximum effectiveness. The CDC recommends vaccination for EMS personnel to reduce transmission of influenza to patients and to decrease worker absenteeism. EMS responders who are diabetics, especially those requiring frequent medical follow-up, are strongly urged to be immunized. Three antiviral drugs, amantadine (Symmetrel), oseltamivir (Tamiflu), and rimantadine (Flumadine), are available for the prevention and treatment of influenza; however, they only work against the type A influenza virus. They are as effective as vaccines when used preventively, and they shorten the illness's duration when used as a treatment. A new agent, zanamavir (Relenza), which is effective against type B, was recently released. However, its use is limited because only 35 percent of influenza cases are type B and because it must be delivered by aerosol nebulizer.

The common cold, or viral rhinitis, is caused by the rhinoviruses, of which there are more than 100 serotypes. Its incidence in the United States rises in fall, winter, and spring, is highest in children younger than 5 years, and declines in older adults, displaced by more serious diseases. Transmission is by direct contact, airborne droplets, or, more importantly, by hands and linen soiled with discharges from infected individuals. The incubation period ranges from 12 hours to 5 days and averages 48 hours. The disease's course is mild, often without fever and generally without muscle aching. Aside from severity, it is often difficult to differentiate from influenza. Mortality has not been reported, but a cold may lead to more serious complications such as otitis media and sinusitis.

Measles Measles (rubeola, hard measles), a systemic disease caused by the measles virus of the genus *Morbilli,* is highly communicable. It is most common in children but may affect older persons who have not had it. Immunity following disease is usually lifelong. Maternal antibodies protect neonates for about 4 to 5 months after birth.

measles *highly contagious, acute viral disease characterized by a reddish rash that appears on the fourth or fifth day of illness.*

Measles is transmitted by inhalation of infective droplets and direct contact. The incubation period ranges from 7 to 14 days, averaging 10 days. The infected person presents prodromally like a severe cold, with fever, conjunctivitis, swelling of the eyelids, photophobia, malaise, cough, and nasopharyngeal congestion. The fever increases, rising to as high as 104° to 106°F, when the rash reaches its maximum. A day or two before the rash develops, Koplik's spots (bluish-white specks with a red halo approximately 1 mm in diameter) appear on the oral mucosa. The red, bumpy (maculopapular) rash normally lasts about 6 days and spreads from head to feet by the third day. At that point, it appears to thicken on the head and shoulders and then disappear in the same direction as its progression.

Measles is so highly communicable that the slightest contact with an active case may infect a susceptible person. Infectivity is greatest before the prodrome and subsides about 4 days after the rash appears or as it fades. Everyone should be immunized. Immunization is 99 percent effective in children, for whom vaccination is mandatory since there is no specific treatment. Unimmunized or previously unexposed paramedics should mask their measles patients and be vigilant about handling linens and touching their face during and after the call. Postexposure hand washing is critical.

In otherwise healthy children or adults, uncomplicated measles has a low mortality rate. Potential complications include bacterial pneumonia, eye damage, and myocarditis. The most life-threatening sequela is encephalitis in children and adolescents that causes gradual decreases in mental capacity and muscle coordination.

Mumps The **mumps** virus, a member of the genus *Paramyxovirus,* is transmitted through respiratory droplets and direct contact with the saliva of infected patients. It is characterized by painful enlargement of the salivary glands. Most cases occur in the 5- to 15-year age group. After a 12 to 25-day incubation period, mumps presents as a feverish cold that is soon followed by swelling and stiffening of the parotid salivary gland in front of the ear. The condition is often found bilaterally. The patient may also experience earache and difficulty chewing and swallowing. In most cases, the submaxillary and sublingual glands are very tender to palpation. Most cases resolve spontaneously within 1 week without intervention.

mumps *acute viral disease characterized by painful enlargement of the salivary glands.*

Mumps occurs in epidemics, with danger of transmission beginning 1 week before the infected person feels sick and lasting about 2 weeks. Lifelong immunity is generally conferred after infection, even in the absence of disease (subclinical infection).

Mumps is generally benign and self-limiting; however, complications may occur. In postpubescent patients, inflammation of the testicles (orchitis), breasts (mastitis), or ovaries (oophoritis) may occur, but is of short duration and of no serious consequence. Meningoencephalitis is fairly common but resolves without residual neurological sequelae.

A mumps live-virus vaccine is available and should be administered with measles and rubella vaccines to all children over 1 year of age. Mumps is not easily transmitted, and with Standard

Precautions the risk of contracting the disease is minimal. For the benefit of their patients, EMS workers should not work without an established mumps/measles/rubella (MMR) immunity.

rubella (German measles) *systemic viral disease characterized by a fine pink rash that appears on the face, trunk, and extremities and fades quickly.*

Rubella Rubella (German measles) is a systemic viral disease caused by the rubella virus, of the genus *Rubivirus,* transmitted by inhalation of infective droplets. Generally milder than measles, it is characterized by sore throat and low-grade fever, accompanied by a fine pink rash on the face, trunk, and extremities that lasts about 3 days. The incubation period is 12 to 19 days, with natural infection conferring lifelong immunity, as does immunization. Transfer of maternal antibodies does not confer lifelong immunity but does protect the neonate. There is no specific treatment for rubella. More serious complications that occur in measles do not occur in rubella, but young females sometimes develop a short course of arthritis.

Rubella is devastating to a developing fetus. Mothers infected during the first trimester are at risk for abnormal fetal development, with offspring often developing congenital rubella syndrome and shedding large quantities of virus in their secretions. An infant acquiring this infection *in utero* (in the uterus) is likely to be developmentally delayed and suffer eye inflammation, deafness, and congenital heart defects. All females, therefore, should be immunized against rubella before becoming pregnant.

Vaccines for measles, mumps, and rubella are commonly combined in an MMR vaccination, which can be given safely with the varicella vaccine. Immunization is 98 to 99 percent effective but is not recommended for pregnant women because of a theoretical possibility of birth defects. Health care workers have been identified as the source in numerous outbreaks. For this reason, and for their own protection, all EMS providers should be required to receive the MMR vaccination before they are allowed to work. Immunizations, along with placing a mask on the patient, are an effective method of preventing these diseases.

Paramedics should not be allowed to work until they have received the MMR vaccination.

respiratory syncytial virus (RSV) *common cause of pneumonia and bronchiolitis in children.*

Respiratory Syncytial Virus Respiratory syncytial virus (RSV) is a common cause of pneumonia and bronchiolitis in infants and young children. In this age group, RSV may be fatal. In older children and adults RSV is less common, and its symptoms are generally milder. RSV is often associated with outbreaks of lower respiratory infections from November to April. If a patient with pneumonia or bronchitis simultaneously contracts this virus, the disease becomes more severe. RSV commonly begins as an upper respiratory infection, and is often misdiagnosed as a simple cold. Children with RSV infection will initially develop a runny nose and nasal congestion. Later, this will spread to lower airway involvement evidenced by wheezing, tachypnea, and signs of respiratory distress. It is a common infection that can be diagnosed by a rapid assay using nasal washings. In winter months, wheezing in children under 1 year of age should be presumed to be due to RSV until proven otherwise. High-risk children (those with congenital heart conditions, prematurity, or cancers, for instance) can be treated with the antiviral agent ribavirin (Virazole). However, this treatment is quite expensive and poses a significant risk to unborn babies of pregnant health care workers. Postexposure prophylaxis with Respi-Gam (RSV immune globulin) is also an option.

pertussis *disease characterized by severe, violent coughing; whooping cough.*

Content Review

Phases of Pertussis

- Catarrhal
- Paroxysmal
- Convalescent

Pertussis The word *pertussis* means "violent cough." **Pertussis** (whooping cough) is caused by the bacterium *Bordetella pertussis,* affecting the oropharynx in three clinical phases after an incubation period of from 6 to 20 days. The *catarrhal phase,* characterized by symptoms similar to those of the common cold, lasts from 1 to 2 weeks. The *paroxysmal phase,* during which the fever subsides, can last a month or longer. The patient develops a mild cough that quickly becomes severe and violent. Rapid consecutive coughs are followed by a deep, high-pitched inspiration. (This characteristic "whoop" often is not present in infants and adults.) The cough often produces large amounts of thick mucus, and vomiting may also occur. Sustained coughing may lead to increased intracranial pressure and intracerebral hemorrhage. Continually high intrapulmonary pressure and vigorous chest movement may cause pneumothorax. During the *convalescent phase* the frequency and severity of coughing attacks decrease, and the patient is not contagious.

The widespread vaccination of children in a combination diphtheria-tetanus-pertussis (DTP) vaccine caused a dramatic decrease in the incidence of pertussis until the early 1980s. Over the past 20 years, however, its incidence has steadily grown, with the greatest increase in persons aged 5 years or older. This has occurred in spite of unprecedented pertussis vaccination coverage. One factor in the increase may be a waning effectiveness of the vaccine among adolescents and adults vaccinated during childhood. Although disease is likely to confer immunity against pertussis, the duration of that immunity is unknown. Previously immunized and exposed adolescents and adults therefore may be at risk of infection. Thus, booster doses are recommended.

For patients with pertussis, EMS is most likely to be requested during the paroxysmal phase, when the primary treatment will be calming and oxygenating the patient. Anticipate the needs to intubate patients with respiratory failure and to perform chest decompression for those whose coughing paroxysms might have caused a pneumothorax. During the response, remember that pertussis is highly contagious. Fortunately, the communicable period is thought to be greatest before the paroxysmal phase. Transmission occurs via respiratory secretions or in an aerosolized form. Mask the patient and observe Standard Precautions, including postexposure hand washing.

Everyone is susceptible to *B. pertussis* infection. Routine immunization of EMS workers against pertussis is not yet recommended. Evaluation of pertussis vaccination is ongoing, however, and considering the unknown duration of immunity with past immunization or exposure, adolescent and adult immunization may be recommended in the future. Erythromycin is known to decrease the period of communicability, but can reduce symptoms only if administered before the onset of violent coughing.

Viral Diseases Transmitted by Contact

Review

Content

Viral Diseases Transmitted by Contact

- Mononucleosis
- Herpes simplex virus type 1

Mononucleosis and herpes simplex type 1 infections pose little risk to EMS providers who observe Standard Precautions and wash their hands after patient contact. Since these diseases cause relatively minor symptoms, patients may not even be aware of their infection status. The public is highly aware of these two diseases, however, so as health care providers, paramedics should be familiar with them.

mononucleosis *acute disease caused by the Epstein-Barr virus.*

Mononucleosis **Mononucleosis** is caused by the Epstein-Barr virus (EBV). It affects the oropharynx, tonsils, and the reticuloendothelial system (the phagocytes). A 4- to 6-week incubation period precedes the development of symptoms, which characteristically begin with fatigue. Fever, severe sore throat, oral discharges, and enlarged, tender lymph nodes generally follow several days to weeks later. Splenomegaly (enlargement of the spleen) is present in approximately one-half of patients. The disease is common; over 95 percent of the general population has antibodies to the virus. One-half of all children will have contracted it before the age of 5 years. Infection by EBV generally confers immunity for life.

Mononucleosis is most commonly transmitted through oropharyngeal contact involving the exchange of saliva between an uninfected person and one who has the disease but who is asymptomatic. Kissing is implicated in adolescents and adults, and transmission from caregivers to young children is common. Blood transfusions can be a mode of transmission, but with few cases of disease attributed to it. Active disease is most common in those between 15 and 25 years of age. The risk of contracting the disease without close facial contact is minimal. Symptoms generally dissipate within a few weeks, but full recuperation may take several months. There is no specific treatment for mononucleosis, and immunization is unavailable. Corticosteroids are occasionally administered to help minimize tonsillar swelling. Nonsteroidal anti-inflammatory drugs (NSAIDs) may provide symptomatic relief.

herpes simplex virus *organism that causes infections characterized by fluid-filled vesicles, usually in the oral cavity or on the genitals.*

Herpes Simplex Virus Type 1 There are two types of **herpes simplex virus,** herpes simplex virus type 1 (HSV-1) and herpes simplex virus type 2 (HSV-2). HSV-2 will be discussed in the section on sexually transmitted diseases. HSV-1 is transmitted in the saliva of carriers and commonly infects the oropharynx, face, lips, skin, fingers, and toes. Everyone is susceptible. Infections of health care workers' hands and fingers can result in herpetic whitlow, weeping inflammations at the distal fingers and toes. The incubation period following exposure ranges from 2 to 12 days. In the oral cavity, fluid-filled vesicles develop into cold sores or fever blisters that soon deteriorate into small ulcers. Fever, malaise, and dehydration may accompany these primary lesions, which usually disappear in 2 to 3 weeks. They may recur spontaneously, especially following periods of stress or other illness. Recurrent HSV labialis (lip lesions) may cause problems for many years in some adults.

Although primarily recognized for causing skin and mucous membrane disorders, HSV-1 can cause meningoencephalitis in newborns and aseptic meningitis in adults. A high index of suspicion for HSV-1 in these situations may result in timely treatment with antiviral agents such as acyclovir, which is somewhat effective against HSV-1.

Standard Precautions, primarily gloves, are absolutely essential, especially if an intimate contact or family member of the EMS worker is afflicted. Breaks in the skin place everyone at greater risk, and may not be visible to the naked eye. Treatment with acyclovir (Zovirax) provides relief when used topically or orally. Immunization is not available.

Review

Content

Other Infectious Respiratory Conditions

- Epiglottitis
- Croup
- Pharyngitis
- Sinusitis
- Hantavirus

OTHER INFECTIOUS CONDITIONS OF THE RESPIRATORY SYSTEM

The majority of profiles in this section discuss pathological conditions of the airway caused by a variety of infectious agents. They are not diseases, per se. Chapter 42, "Pediatrics," discusses croup and epiglottitis in greater detail. Hantavirus is included here, although its sites of pathology extend beyond the airways.

Epiglottitis

epiglottitis *infection and inflammation of the epiglottis.*

Epiglottitis is an inflammation of the epiglottis and may also involve the areas just above and below it. In children it is a true emergency, usually caused by *H. influenzae*, with an abrupt onset over several hours and without any immediate history of upper respiratory disease. Patients present with one or more of the "four Ds": dysphonia, drooling, dysphagia, or distress. Epiglottitis can also occur in teenagers and adults. In the older age groups, stridor, sore throat, fever, and drooling usually develop over days, not hours. Due to natural immunity from initial infection, epiglottitis is not known to reoccur in any age group. Increased immunization against *H. influenzae* has reduced the incidence of epiglottitis caused by this bacterium. However, *S. pneumoniae* and *S. aureus* have been implicated as causative agents of epiglottitis.

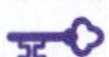

Epiglottitis is a bacterial infection that affects the glottis and the tissue above the glottis, while croup is a viral infection that affects the tissues below the glottis.

Croup

croup *viral illness characterized by inspiratory and expiratory stridor and a seal-barklike cough.*

Croup (laryngotracheobronchitis) is a common cause of acute upper airway obstruction in children. A viral illness characterized by inspiratory and expiratory stridor and a "seal-bark" cough, it is most common in children under the age of 3 years. Although generally not life threatening, croup may create panic in parents and children alike. Viruses implicated in croup include the parainfluenza viruses, rhinoviruses, and RSV. Croup is often preceded by an upper respiratory infection. The child commonly awakens during the night with acute respiratory distress, tachypnea, and retractions. Seasonal outbreaks of this disease are common. Total airway obstruction is rare.

Pharyngitis

pharyngitis *infection of the pharynx and tonsils.*

Pharyngitis is a common infection of the pharynx and tonsils. It may be caused by a virus or bacteria and is characterized by a sudden onset of sore throat and fever. The tonsils and palate become red and swollen, and the cervical lymph nodes enlarge. Headache, neck pain, nausea, and vomiting may also be present. Most cases occur in late winter and early spring. Although this disease may occur in any age group, most cases are seen in 5- to 11-year-olds.

Group A streptococcus (strep throat) causes a particularly serious pharyngitis that, if left untreated, in certain cases, can progress to rheumatic fever. There are several subtypes of group A streptococcus. One strain causes rheumatic fever. Another strain is responsible for scarlet fever (scarletina). Patients infected with this bacterium may present with a scarlet-colored rash. Because strep throat is very contagious, wear a mask when assessing and managing these patients. Although laboratory tests can easily determine which cases of pharyngitis are caused by strep, it is virtually impossible to tell clinically. Assume that all cases of pharyngitis are serious and contagious until proven otherwise. Antibiotics (penicillin, amoxicillin, erythromycin, azithromycin) effectively treat strep throat.

Sinusitis

sinusitis *inflammation of the paranasal sinuses.*

Sinusitis is an inflammation of the paranasal (ethmoid, frontal, maxillary, or sphenoid) sinuses. It occurs when mucus and pus cannot drain and become trapped in the sinus. Sinusitis is usually preceded by a viral upper respiratory infection or exposure to allergens, either of which may cause nasal congestion and blocked sinus passages. Postnasal drip may develop and nasal drainage may be blood tinged and purulent. As fluids collect in the sinus, a sensation of pressure or fullness generally develops. If left untreated, the condition may become painful, and the infection can cause an abscess or spread into the cranium and attack the brain. Discomfort often worsens when the patient bends forward or when pressure is applied over the affected sinus. Sinusitis is occasionally a causative factor of meningitis. Management includes antibiotics, decongestants, and supportive care. Apply a heat pack directly over the affected sinus to help relieve pain and facilitate drainage.

Hantavirus

hantavirus *family of viruses that are carried by the deer mouse and transmitted by ticks and other arthropods.*

Hantavirus is a family of viruses carried by rodents such as the deer mouse. Other known carriers are the rice and cotton rats in the southeastern United States and the white-footed mouse of the northeastern states. The common house mouse is not known to carry the virus. Most cases of hantavirus infection have occurred in the southwestern United States, particularly the Four Corners region. Transmission is primarily by inhalation of aerosols created by stirring up the dried urine, saliva, and fecal droppings of these rodents. Contamination of food and autoinoculation after handling objects tainted by rodent droppings may also cause transmission. Direct bites are possible routes, but are thought to be rare. Person-to-person transmission is not possible.

The virus causes hantavirus pulmonary syndrome (HPS), to which anyone is susceptible. The initial symptoms are fatigue, fever, and muscle aches, especially of large muscle groups. Headaches, nausea, vomiting, diarrhea, and abdominal pain are also common. Earache, sore throat, and rash are uncommon. Approximately 4 to 10 days later, symptoms of pulmonary edema occur. Patients with fatal infections appear to have severe myocardial depression, which can progress to sinus bradycardia and subsequent electromechanical dissociation, ventricular tachycardia, or fibrillation. Hemodynamic compromise occurs a median of 5 days after symptoms' onset—usually dramatically within the first day of hospitalization. The only specific treatment is intensive supportive care, and no immunization is available.

EMS responders who find themselves in dusty, unoccupied buildings for extended times should wear face masks to prevent inhaling aerosolized rodent droppings.

GI SYSTEM INFECTIONS

Content Review

GI System Infections

- Gastroenteritis
- Food poisoning

You may on occasion respond to scenes with single or multiple cases of foodborne illness. Although you cannot determine the causative agent outside of the hospital, you must have a basic knowledge of the infectious process and guidelines for assessment, management, and safe handling of these patients. Many EMS personnel are being recruited and volunteering for domestic and international disaster medical teams. In these situations, when the sanitation infrastructure (water treatment and distribution, sewer, animal control, and so forth) is disrupted, GI system infections increase significantly.

Gastroenteritis

gastroenteritis *generalized disorder involving nausea, vomiting, gastrointestinal cramping or discomfort, and diarrhea.*

Gastroenteritis is a gastrointestinal disorder manifested by nausea, vomiting, gastrointestinal cramping or discomfort, anorexia, and diarrhea. In more advanced cases, which are rare, it can cause lassitude and shock. It is a common disease that many of us in developed countries have experienced. The reference to "stomach flu" in these situations is incorrect, since an influenza of the GI system has not yet been identified. What this distressing and uncomfortable condition usually represents, at least in developed countries, is a viral gastroenteritis. The causative agents may be viruses (Norwalk virus, rotavirus, and others), bacteria (*E. coli, K. pneumoniae, C. jejuni, E. aerogenes, V. cholerae, Shigella,* and *Salmonella*), and parasites (*G. lamblia, C. parvum, C. cayetensis*). Gastroenteritis is highly contagious via the fecal–oral route, including the ingestion of contaminated food and water. It is especially contagious during natural disasters in epidemic proportions. International travelers into endemic areas are very susceptible, while native populations are generally resistant.

In otherwise healthy persons, gastroenteritis is generally self-limiting and benign; however, in the very young, the very old, or those with preexisting disease, it can be serious and often fatal. Prolonged vomiting and/or diarrhea may result in dehydration and electrolyte disturbances. Patients generally experience painful and severe abdominal cramping, and some develop hypovolemic shock. Always consider dehydration in any patient who presents with signs of gastroenteritis. If a patient has vomited many times or is actively vomiting, has multiple medical problems, is debilitated, or is at risk by virtue of age and general health, start an IV with isotonic saline. Pay careful attention to hydration status. If the patient is in shock, the management objectives are no different than for hemorrhagic shock. If the patient is not in shock, the judicious use of fluids is warranted. A good rule of thumb is to replace fluids at approximately the rate they are lost. The World Health Organization and other international disaster response agencies have found oral rehydration very effective in treating fluid loss, even with cholera. Do not feel compelled to pour in IV fluids. If prolonged vomiting or retching is present, administer an antiemetic such as droperidol (Inapsine), prochlorperazine (Compazine), or promethazine (Phenergan). Remember that vehicle movements often aggravate symptoms and increase the probability of vomiting.

With isolated cases of gastroenteritis, compliance with Standard Precautions and postexposure hand washing are critical to avoiding infection. In times of disaster, EMS responders must be more focused on environmental health and sanitation issues: preparing food, identifying clean sources of water, using mosquito netting while sleeping, and general sanitation. Eat hot foods only and drink hot beverages that have been brisk boiled. Be careful to avoid personal habits that facilitate fecal–oral transmission. Prevention is important because even though antimicrobials may be available to treat isolated cases, resources for treating gastroenteritis during disasters or in developing countries may be limited. In those situations, many people receive symptomatic treatment.

Food Poisoning

food poisoning *nonspecific term often applied to gastroenteritis that occurs suddenly and that is caused by the ingestion of food containing preformed toxins.*

Food poisoning is a nonspecific term often applied to gastroenteritis. Food poisoning occurs suddenly and is caused by eating. Diarrhea, vomiting, and gastrointestinal discomfort characterize its more benign presentation. Most cases are caused by bacteria and their toxic products. In the majority of cases, only the GI system is affected, but other systems may be affected in some cases, as with botulism or *Escherichia coli* O157:H7, causing debilitating illness or death. *Clostridium botulinum* produces a very potent neurotoxin that causes flaccid paralysis by blocking the release of acetylcholine at motor end plates and preganglionic autonomic synapses.

E. coli O157:H7, transmitted by the ingestion of uncooked or undercooked ground beef, often causes severe bloody diarrhea and abdominal cramps; sometimes the infection causes nonbloody diarrhea or no symptoms. Drinking unpasteurized milk and swimming in or drinking sewage-contaminated water can also cause infection. Little or no fever is usually present, and the illness resolves in 5 to 10 days. In some persons, particularly children under 5 years of age and the elderly, the infection can cause a complication called hemolytic uremic syndrome, in which the red blood cells are destroyed and the kidneys fail. About 2 to 7 percent of infections lead to this complication. In the United States, hemolytic uremic syndrome is the principal cause of acute kidney failure in children, and *E. coli* O157:H7 causes most cases of hemolytic uremic syndrome.

Other bacteria implicated in food poisoning include *Campylobacter, Salmonella, Shigella,* and *Vibrio cholerae.* Microorganisms may be transmitted in other meats that are insufficiently cooked. *Salmonella* is commonly transmitted through incompletely cooked poultry. It may also be spread through contaminated cookware and utensils used in preparation of poultry. Hepatitis A and Norwalk virus are known to have been ingested in undercooked seafood. Bacterial gastrointestinal infections tend to be much more severe than viral gastrointestinal infections. With bacterial infections, the patient will appear more toxic. There is often a history of bloody, foul-smelling diarrhea (especially with shigellosis). The presence of leukocytes in a fecal smear is suggestive of bacterial disease. Ultimately, stool cultures are required to confirm a bacterial cause of gastroenteritis.

Initiate standard advanced life support (ALS) protocols, including assessment of airway and ventilatory status, oxygenation, initiation of an IV, and cardiac monitoring. Fluid resuscitation with isotonic crystalloids is often required. It is not uncommon for an adult with severe gastroenteritis to require 2 to 3 liters of fluid. In patients with significant vomiting or diarrhea, also consider antiemetics. Constant reassessment of ventilatory status is essential since the neurotoxin in *C. botulinum* ingestion may cause respiratory arrest. Observing Standard Precautions should protect against foodborne transmission of infectious agents. No immunization against these agents or their toxins exists.

Prevention efforts are the primary means of reducing foodborne illness. Advances in technology may provide better alternatives for food supply surveillance, an aspect of foodborne disease prevention that could be improved. Lawrence Berkeley National Laboratory has developed plastic strips that turn from blue to red in the presence of toxic strains of *E. coli*. This technology's basis could become a prototype for other simple reagent strips that can detect foodborne pathogens.

NERVOUS SYSTEM INFECTIONS

Review

Content

Nervous System Infections

- Encephalitis
- Rabies
- Tetanus
- Lyme disease

Encephalitis, rabies, tetanus, and Lyme disease all have significant effects on the nervous system. These infectious conditions or diseases do not necessarily pose occupational risks to EMS providers. They are well-known to the general public, however, and are often associated with recreational activities in which EMS responders participate.

Encephalitis

encephalitis *acute infection of the brain, usually caused by a virus.*

Encephalitis is an inflammation caused by infection of the brain and its structures, usually by viruses such as equine viruses, arboviruses, the rubella virus, or the mumps virus. These viral infections usually result in one of the following:

1. They cause no pathology until they are transported to cerebral neurons, which they invade, and then replicate (the rabies and arthropod-borne viruses, for instance).
2. They first injure nonnervous tissues and then, rarely, invade the cerebral neurons (for example, herpes simplex 1 and varicella-zoster virus).

Bacteria, fungi, or parasites may also cause encephalitis, but the viruses are the predominant infectious agents.

The clinical presentation of encephalitis is similar to that of meningitis since they often coexist. Signs and symptoms include decreased level of consciousness, fever, headache, drowsiness, coma, tremors, and a stiff neck and back. Seizures may occur in patients of any age but are most common in infants. Characteristic neurological signs include uncoordinated and involuntary movements; weakness of the arms, legs, or other portions of the body; or unusual sensitivity of the skin to various types of stimuli.

Treatment is difficult, even when the virus is known. Despite the severity of illness, many patients suffer no long-term neurological deficits; however, as many as 50 percent of children younger than 1 year may suffer irreversible brain damage after contracting eastern or western equine encephalitis, diseases of horses and mules transmitted to humans by mosquitoes.

Rabies

rabies *viral disorder that affects the nervous system.*

Rabies is transmitted by the rabies virus, a member of the Rhabdovirus family and *Lyssavirus* genus, which affects the nervous system. It exists in two epidemiological forms: *urban*, propagated chiefly through unimmunized domestic dogs and cats, and *sylvatic*, propagated by skunks, foxes, raccoons, mongooses, coyotes, wolves, and bats. Humans are especially susceptible when bitten by infected animals. The virus is transmitted in the saliva of infected mammals by bites, an opening in the skin, or direct contact with a mucous membrane. It passes along motor and sensory fibers to the spinal ganglia corresponding to the site of invasion, and then to the brain, creating an *encephalomyelitis* that is almost always fatal. Although rare, transmission is also known to occur by inhalation of aerosolized virus, through nasal nerve fibers and mucosa, along the olfactory nerve, and then to the brain. Mammals are highly susceptible to infection. Transmission is known to be affected by the severity of the wound, abundance of the nerve supply close to the wound, the distance to the CNS, the amount and strain of virus, protective clothing, and other undetermined factors. The highly variable incubation period is usually from 3 to 8 weeks but can be as short as 9 days (rare) or as long as 10 years. It is believed to be dependent on the bite site, with bites to the head and neck generally followed by shorter incubation periods.

Rabies is characterized by a nonspecific *prodrome* (symptoms that precede the appearance of a disease) of malaise, headache, fever, chills, sore throat, myalgias, anorexia, nausea, vomiting, and diarrhea. The prodrome typically lasts from 1 to 4 days. The next phase, the *encephalitic phase,* begins with periods of excessive motor activity, excitation, and agitation. This is soon followed by confusion, hallucinations, combativeness, bizarre aberrations of thought, muscle twitches and tetany, and seizures. Soon, focal paralysis appears. When left untreated, it can cause death within 2 to 6 days. Attempts to drink water may produce laryngospasm, causing the characteristic profuse drooling commonly known as hydrophobia (fear of water).

Rabies in the United States has become more prevalent in the wild. From 1980 to 1999, 58 of the rabies cases diagnosed in the United States have been attributed to bat variants. It is not surprising, then, that the CDC has identified wildlife as the most important potential source of infection for humans and domestic animals in this country. In Africa, Asia, and Latin America, dogs remain the major source. Human rabies is rare in the United States, but each year 16,000 to 39,000 people receive postexposure prophylaxis. This is not a matter of paranoia. The CDC estimates that up to one-third of persons who have contracted rabies cannot accurately relate a history of having been bitten by an animal. Thus, epidemiologists now believe that the inhalation route, once thought to be theoretical, may be more common than previously believed. Human-to-human transmission of rabies is not known to occur; however, paramedics should take Standard Precautions to protect themselves from contact with infectious saliva. The use of masks in environments where a patient has been exposed may be prudent, judging from the recent epidemiological evidence in the United States with bats.

When caring for a bite patient, first inspect the site of the wound for bite pattern and the presence of saliva. Then rinse the wound with copious amounts of normal saline to remove saliva and blood. Do not bandage or dress the wound, but allow it to drain freely during transport. Irrigation en route from a 10- or 15-drop/mL IV administration set may be beneficial. If the patient refuses transport to the emergency department, inform him of the consequences of the bite and the importance of medical follow-up. If time and circumstances permit, ensure that the suspect animal has been secured and contained for transport to the hospital or animal control shelter for subsequent postmortem examination of cerebral tissue.

If you are bitten or exposed to an animal you believe is rabid, take the following measures:

1. Vigorously wash the wound with soap and warm water.
2. Debride and irrigate the wound, and allow it to drain freely on the way to the emergency department.
3. Discuss postexposure prophylaxis with the physician. Consultation with public health officials may be necessary. Unless you have an actual bite from an animal whose behavior is consistent with rabies infection, exposure is a medical urgency, not emergency.
4. Consider the need for tetanus and other antibiotic therapy as the attending physician deems appropriate.

Several alternatives now exist for rabies immunization. Individuals who should be immunized include animal care workers and shelter personnel, and those who work outdoors and have frequent contact with wild animals known to transmit rabies.

Tetanus

tetanus *acute bacterial infection of the central nervous system.*

Tetanus is an acute bacterial infection of the central nervous system. It presents with musculoskeletal signs and symptoms caused by tetanospasmin, an exotoxin of the *Clostridium tetani* bacillus. *C. tetani* is present as extremely durable spores in the soil, street dust, and feces and is in the same genus as *C. perfringens,* the causative organism of gas gangrene. Since *Clostridium* species favor an anaerobic environment, the bacteria are particularly suited to colonizing dead or necrotic tissue. Infection has been contracted through wounds considered too minor to warrant medical attention and through burns. Although puncture wounds are classically associated with *C. tetani* infection, deep lacerations can also be suitable environments. Transmission can even occur by injection of contaminated drugs and surgical procedures, leading to the conclusion that *C. tetani* spores are found everywhere. The incubation period is variable (usually from 3 to 21 days, sometimes from 1 day to several months) and depends on the wound's severity and location. Generally, a shorter incubation period leads to a more severe illness. The mortality rate increases in direct proportion to age. The general population is susceptible, but incidence is highest in agricultural areas where unimmunized people are in frequent contact with animal feces. The disease is rare in the United States, with fewer than 100 cases reported each year.

Localized tetanus symptoms include rigidity of muscles in close proximity to the injury site. Subsequent generalized symptoms may include pain and stiffness in the jaw muscles and may progress to cause muscle spasm and rigidity of the entire body. Respiratory arrest may result. In children, abdominal rigidity may be the first sign. Rigidity occurs after the toxin is taken up at the myoneural junction and transported to the CNS. The toxin then acts on inhibitory neurons, which normally suppress unnecessary efferent impulses and muscle movements. The reduction in inhibitory action results in the muscles' receiving more nervous impulses and tetany. Sometimes a sardonic grin, *risus sardonicus,* accompanies the lock jaw and conjures memories of the Cheshire Cat in *Alice in Wonderland.*

EMS responders will rarely encounter this disease, much less recognize its signs and symptoms, until they are advanced to the point of tetany. A possible EMS scenario would be the transfer of a patient from a rural community hospital to an urban medical center for intensive care. Standard Precautions should provide adequate protection. Masks probably are not necessary unless the infectious agent is unknown. Respiratory arrest is a possibility, so you should consider wearing masks while performing endotracheal intubation. If you incur a wound in the course of treating a patient, wash the wound thoroughly or, if warranted, have it inspected and debrided in the emergency department. Wounds that are cared for within 6 hours pose a lower risk for growth of anaerobic microorganisms. Consideration should be given to postexposure prophylaxis with tetanus immune globulin (TIG), diphtheria-tetanus toxoid (Td), or diphtheria-tetanus-pertussis (DTP).

Immunizations, which generally begin in childhood as DTP vaccinations, include boosters before entering elementary school and every 10 years thereafter. A booster administered every 10 years is believed to confer effective active immunity. Previous documented infection is not known to confer lifelong immunity.

Lyme Disease

Lyme disease is a recurrent inflammatory disorder accompanied by skin lesions, polyarthritis, and involvement of the heart and nervous system. Caused by the tick-borne spirochete *Borrelia burgdorferi,* similar in shape to the causative organism of syphilis, it is the most commonly reported vector-borne disease in the United States. The tick that carries Lyme disease is common in the Northeast, the Upper Midwest, and along the Pacific Coast. Deer and mice are both reservoirs of the tick, and the disease is common in people living and recreating near wooded areas with high deer populations. Most infections occur in spring and summer, when tick exposure is most likely. Everyone is susceptible, and natural infection does not appear to confer immunity. The incubation period ranges from 3 to 21 days.

Lyme disease *recurrent inflammatory disorder caused by a tick-borne spirochete.*

Lyme disease progresses in three stages:

★ *Early localized stage.* A painless, flat, red lesion appears at the bite site. In some patients, a ringlike rash, *erythema migrans (EM),* develops and spreads outward. The outer border remains bright red, with the center becoming clear, blue, or even necrotic. The rash—often called a "bull's eye" rash—usually disappears in time, whether treated or not. At this stage, patients also may complain of headache, malaise, and muscle aches. Although uncommon, the patient's neck may be stiff.

★ *Early disseminated stage.* The spirochete spreads to the skin, nervous system, heart, and joints. More EM lesions develop. CNS sequelae include meningitis, seventh-cranial-nerve Bell's palsy, and peripheral neuropathy. Cardiac abnormalities include conduction defects and myopathy. Arthritis and myalgia are common months after infection. Approximately 8 percent of patients will have some cardiac involvement. The most common manifestations are varying degrees of atrioventricular block (first degree, Wenckebach, and complete heart block). Less commonly, myocarditis and left ventricular dysfunction are seen. Cardiac involvement typically lasts only a few weeks, but can recur.

★ *Late stage (persistent infection).* The late stage can occur months or years after the initial exposure. Although the incidence of cardiac problems is lower, it involves the same neurological complications as second stage, plus encephalopathy with cognitive deficits, depression, and sleep disorders. Monoarthritis of large joints and more than one joint concurrently (polyarthritis) is common.

Content Review

Stages of Lyme Disease

- Early localized
- Early disseminated
- Late

Development of erythema migrans, the bull's eye rash, usually 3 to 30 days after tick exposure, is presumptive for the diagnosis.

The EMS response to Lyme disease will probably be to treat its clinical consequences, especially those of the disseminated and late stages. ALS treatment is directed toward those consequences, not the infection. Adhere to Standard Precautions. After responding to calls in heavily wooded areas infested by ticks, always check both your and the patient's clothing, shoes, socks, and body for ticks. Spray the ambulance compartment with an insecticide effective against arthropods. Available antibiotic therapies are effective for the stages of the disease progression. Protection against Lyme disease (LYMErix) is now available as a series of three vaccinations, with the second dose given at 1 month and the third at 12 months. It is recommended for persons aged 15 to 70 years whose activities result in frequent exposure to tick habitats, and for selected travelers to endemic areas where exposure to tick habitats is anticipated.

Review

Content

Sexually Transmitted Diseases

- Gonorrhea
- Syphilis
- Genital warts
- Herpes simplex type 2
- Chlamydia
- Trichomoniasis
- Chancroid

SEXUALLY TRANSMITTED DISEASES

sexually transmitted disease (STD) *illness most commonly transmitted through sexual contact.*

Infectious diseases transmitted through sexual contact are known as **sexually transmitted diseases,** or **STDs.** They represent some of the most prevalent communicable diseases. A variety of bacterial (gonorrhea, syphilis, chancroid, chlamydia), viral (HIV, herpes), and parasitic (*Pediculosis, Trichomonas*) infections are spread by this route. Other illnesses that are generally not considered STDs, including hepatitis A, B, C, D, salmonella, and shigella, may also be transmitted through sexual contact. STDs affect the genital organs, often resulting in pathology to reproductive structures. Although EMS responders do not treat these diseases, other emergency health care personnel commonly know the information in the following profiles. Your knowledge of these diseases will put you on a "level playing field" with those other health care workers and bolster your credibility. When you treat or transport patients with STDs, observe Standard Precautions, avoid contact with lesions and exudates, and wash your hands vigorously after exposure.

Gonorrhea

gonorrhea *sexually transmitted disease caused by a gram-negative bacterium.*

Gonorrhea, caused by *Neisseria gonorrhoeae,* a gram-negative bacterium, is one of the most commonly diagnosed communicable diseases in the United States. More than 1 million cases are treated annually. Everyone is susceptible to infection, and although antibodies develop after exposure and confer immunity, they do so only for the specific serotype that caused the infection. Thus, persons contracting gonorrhea would not be immune to penicillinase-producing *N. gonorrhoeae* (PPNG), a strain of *N. gonorrhoeae* known by military personnel during the Vietnam War as black clap. Most commonly seen in males in their early 20s, gonorrhea is transmitted by direct contact with exudates of mucous membranes, primarily from direct sexual contact. In men, the disease presents as painful urination and a purulent urethral discharge. Untreated, it can lead to epididymitis, prostatitis, and urethral strictures. The majority of women contracting the disease have no pain and minimal discharge. In some cases, symptoms include urinary frequency, vaginal discharge, fever, and abdominal pain. Pelvic inflammatory disease (PID) often results after menstruation when bacteria spread from the cervix to the upper genital tract. Affected females are at increased risk for sterility, ectopic pregnancy, abscesses within reproductive structures, and peritonitis.

Gonorrhea may occasionally become systemic, causing sepsis or meningitis. Septic arthritis may result, presenting with fever, pain, swelling, and limited range of motion in one or two joints, sometimes leading to progressive deterioration. In the United States, single dosing is often effective in treating localized gonorrhea (genitourinary only). Treating systemic gonorrhea often involves additional treatment. When gonorrhea infection coexists with chlamydial infections (as is estimated to occur in about 50 percent of gonorrhea patients), two-drug therapy is routinely advised. No immunization is available.

Syphilis

syphilis *bloodborne sexually transmitted disease caused by the spirochete* Treponema pallidum.

Syphilis, a disease caused by the spirochete *Treponema pallidum,* is transmitted by direct contact with exudates from other syphilitic lesions of skin and mucous membranes, semen, blood, saliva, and vaginal discharges. It is therefore most commonly contracted through sexual intercourse but also may be transmitted by kissing or close contact with an open lesion. An estimated 30 percent of exposures result in infection. In congenital syphilis, infants contract the disease before birth from an infected mother. Everyone is susceptible to infection. Although the risk of transmission by blood transfusion or needle-stick injury is low, health care workers have been infected after physical examination involving manual contact with a lesion. A gradual immunity does develop after infection, but aggressive antimicrobial therapy may interfere with this natural antibody formation, especially during the primary and secondary stages.

Review

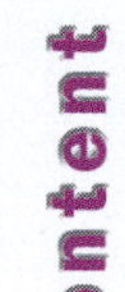

Stages of Syphilis

- Primary
- Secondary
- Latent
- Tertiary

Syphilis is characterized by lesions that may involve virtually any organ or tissue. It usually has cutaneous manifestations with frequent relapses, and it may remain latent for years. The incubation period is 3 weeks. Syphilis may occur in four stages, depending on how early and aggressively treatment is initiated:

★ *Primary syphilis (first stage)* presents as a painless lesion, or chancre. In heterosexual men, the chancre is usually on the penis. In homosexual men, the chancre is often found on the anal canal, rectum, tongue, lips, or other point of entry. The chancre typically occurs 3 to 6 weeks after exposure. Nontender enlargement of regional lymph nodes may also occur.

★ *Secondary syphilis (second stage),* or the bacteremic stage, begins 5 to 6 weeks after the chancre has healed. It is characterized by a maculopapular skin rash (small, red, flat lesions) on the palms and soles, condyloma latum (painless, wartlike lesions on warm, moist skin areas that are very infectious), and cutaneous infection in areas of hair growth causing loss of hair and/or eyebrows. These skin signs last for about 6 weeks. CNS disease (syphilitic meningitis) and arthritis may occur, as can infections of the eyes and kidneys.

★ *Latent syphilis (third stage),* a period when symptoms improve or disappear completely, may last from months to many years. Twenty-five percent of cases may relapse with secondary stage symptoms; however, relapses usually do not occur after 4 years. Thirty-three percent of cases will progress to tertiary syphilis, and the rest will remain asymptomatic.

★ *Tertiary syphilis (fourth stage)* is the stage of syphilis that justifies its reputation as a "great imitator." Lesions with sharp borders, called gummas, may appear on skin and bones, causing a deep, gnawing pain. Cardiovascular syphilis may appear, usually 10 years after the primary infection, resulting in aortic aneurysms that antibiotic therapy does not reverse. Neurosyphilis is diagnosed when there are neurological signs in seropositive patients. Meningitis may result, with possible spinal cord disease causing loss of reflexes, and reduced sensation of pain and temperature. The spirochetes can also invade the cerebral vessels, causing a stroke. A progressive dementia can also occur during this stage.

EMS responders may treat a variety of clinical complications of syphilis, often without being aware of infection as the primary etiology. ALS is directed toward treating the clinical presentation, which may include seizures, an acute onset of dementia, signs of a stroke, aortic aneurysm, or acute myocardial infarction. Avoid frequent contact with lesions on any part of the patient's body, and pay attention to hand washing technique after patient contact since *T. pallidum* is easily killed by heat, soap, and water.

For presumptive screening after exposure, rapid plasmin reagin (RPR) and venereal disease research lab (VDRL) tests are available. Because RPR or VDRL have fairly high rates of false-positive reactions, more specific tests should always follow. Treatment of primary syphilis is benzathine penicillin, with erythromycin and doxycycline (Vibramycin) as alternatives for patients allergic to penicillin. No immunization is available.

Genital Warts

Genital warts (condyloma acuminatum) are caused by the human papillomavirus (HPV), a DNA virus. To date, research has identified 70 HPV types, with most known to cause specific clinical manifestations. Some of the types known to cause genital warts are associated with cervical cancer. Genital warts are contagious and easily spread. In males, they generally appear as cauliflowerlike, fleshy growths on the penis, anus, and mucosa of the anal canal. In females, they usually appear on the labial surfaces. Genital warts are sometimes difficult to distinguish from the condyloma latum seen in the secondary stage of syphilis. HPV has been implicated as a causative factor of cervical cancer in females.

Herpes Simplex Virus Type 2

HSV-2 causes 70 to 90 percent of all genital herpes cases. Transmission is usually by sexual contact. Everyone is susceptible, but adolescents and young adults are most commonly afflicted. Neonates are often infected during passage through the birth canal. The prevalence of HSV-2 antibody, which does not confer immunity, is greater in lower socioeconomic groups and persons with multiple sex partners. The disease presents as vesicular lesions on the penis, anus, rectum, and mouth of the male depending on sexual activity. Females are sometimes asymptomatic, but can display lesions of the vagina, vulva, perineum, rectum, mouth, and cervix. Recurrent infections in females are often found on the vulva, buttocks, legs, and the perineum. Patients may present with fever and enlarged lymph nodes during the initial infection. Lesions may last up to several weeks before eventually crusting over and healing. The most serious consequence of HSV-2 infection is that painful lesions may recur periodically during the patient's lifetime, significantly diminishing quality of life. Recent evidence suggests that symptomatic treatment with the antiviral agent acyclovir orally, intravenously, or topically may decrease the incidence of recurrences and lessen the severity of their symptoms. Other treatment alternatives include CO_2 laser removal, cryotherapy (freezing and removal) with liquid nitrogen, electrical cauterization, and interferon. Immunization is not currently available.

Chlamydia

chlamydia *group of intracellular parasites that cause sexually transmitted diseases.*

Chlamydia is a genus of intracellular parasites most like gram-negative bacteria. Once thought to be viruses, the chlamydiae are now known to have an inner and outer membrane, to contain both DNA and RNA, and to be susceptible to numerous antibiotics. However, they lack peptidoglycan, a net of polysaccharides found in all true bacterial walls.

From the standpoint of STDs, *Chlamydia trachomatis* is the most clinically significant species, affecting the genital area, eyes, and respiratory system. Everyone is susceptible, and up to 25 percent of men may be carriers. *C. trachomatis* is responsible for roughly 50 percent of all cases of nongonococcal urethritis (NGU) in men, with dysuria and penile discharge common. It is transmitted by sexual activity and by hand-to-hand transfer of eye secretions, causing conjunctivitis. Internationally, this is the leading cause of preventable blindness. Because children are the major reservoir and the common use of infected linen can transmit chlamydia, childcare centers and school workers should exercise caution in handling blankets, sheets, and towels.

The symptoms are similar to gonorrhea's but less severe, often making the clinical differentiation difficult. In addition, the progression of disease in women is identical, with both causing a mucopurulent discharge that often accompanies cervicitis. Some women may have retrograde infections of the reproductive tract, causing pelvic inflammatory disease. Sterility may result. Newborns may be infected during passage through an infected birth canal, resulting in infant pneumonia or blindness.

No immunization is available, but *C. trachomatis* infection responds to a variety of antimicrobial agents such as tetracycline, doxycycline (Vibramycin), erythromycin (PCE), and orally administered azithromycin (Zithromax). Natural infection is not known to confer immunity.

Another species of Chlamydia, *C. pneumoniae,* has been found in atherosclerotic lesions of patients who have died of myocardial infarction. This has led to speculation about the relationship between *C. pneumoniae* infection and atherosclerosis as an inflammatory process.

Trichomoniasis

trichomoniasis *sexually transmitted disease caused by the protozoan* Trichomonas vaginalis.

Trichomonas vaginalis, a protozoan parasite, is a common cause of vaginitis. In women, the symptoms of **trichomoniasis** include a greenish-yellow vaginal discharge, irritation of the perineum and thighs, and dysuria. This disease is frequently present with gonorrhea. Men are generally asymptomatic carriers of the disease. When present, symptoms include dysuria, urethral discharge, and discomfort in the perineum. The infection is currently treated with metronidazole (Flagyl).

Chancroid

Chancroid is a highly contagious ulcer caused by *Haemophilus ducreyi,* a gram-negative bacterium. It is more frequently diagnosed in men, particularly those who have sex with prostitutes. Uncircumcised men are at higher risk. It is spread by direct contact, mostly sexual, with open lesions and pus. Autoinoculation has occurred in infected persons. Its incubation period is typically 3 to 5 days but may be as long as 14 days.

chancroid *highly contagious sexually transmitted ulcer.*

The disease begins with a painful, inflamed pustule or ulcer that may appear on the penis, anus, urethra, or vulva. It spreads easily to other sites such as breasts, fingers, and thighs. Lymph nodes may become swollen and tender, and fever may be present. Chancroid ulcer is linked with increased risk of HIV infection. Chancroid lesions in children beyond the neonatal period should alert EMS responders to the possibility of reportable child sexual abuse.

Health care workers have contracted the disease by contacting patients' ulcers. Immunization is not available, and infection does not appear to confer immunity. Several effective antimicrobials (for example, erythromycin) are available.

DISEASES OF THE SKIN

EMS responders' interactions with patients or the general public may expose them to contagious skin infections such as impetigo or the ectoparasites lice and scabies. Because the public frequently attempts to consult paramedics about general topics in personal and community health, your knowledge of ectoparasites may enable you to provide education and customer service. As always, use Standard Precautions and effective postexposure hand washing.

Content Review

Diseases of the Skin

- Impetigo
- Lice
- Scabies

Impetigo

Impetigo is a very contagious infection of the skin caused by staphylococci or streptococci. The disease begins as a single vesicle that ruptures and forms a thick, honey-colored crust with a yellowish-red center. Lesions most commonly occur on the extremities and joints. Although few patients call an ambulance for this condition, it often appears on patients who seek EMS for other reasons. EMS responders who develop impetigo should not report for work until cleared by their physician. It is easily transmitted by direct skin-to-skin contact, so Standard Precautions should provide ample protection.

impetigo *infection of the skin caused by staphylococci or streptococci.*

Lice

Lice (pediculosis) is a parasitic **infestation** of the skin of the scalp, trunk, or pubic area. Lice infest hosts rather than infect them because they do not break the skin. The three different varieties of infestations are *Pediculus humanus var. capitis* (head lice), *Pediculus humanus var. corporis* (body lice), and *Pthirus pubis* (pubic lice, or crabs). Historically, head lice have been involved in outbreaks of typhus, trench fever in World War I, and relapsing fever. Head and body lice appear similar, both being 3 to 4 mm long. Head lice are transmitted by sharing of combs or hats and are fairly common among young school-age children regardless of socioeconomic status. Outbreaks in childcare centers and schools are common. Head lice are easily diagnosed by the presence of small, white, oval-shaped eggs (nits) attached to the hair shafts. Nits can be seen with the naked eye but are more easily found with a magnifying glass. Lice themselves are rarely seen. They tend to leave febrile hosts, so high environmental temperatures and crowding favor transmission. Lice have a three-stage life cycle of eggs, nymphs, and adults. Eggs hatch in 7 to 10 days but cannot hatch below 72°F. The nymph stage lasts about 7 to 13 days, again depending on temperature, with a total egg-to-egg cycle of 3 weeks.

lice *parasitic infestation of the skin of the scalp, trunk, or pubic area.*

infestation *presence of parasites that do not break the host's skin.*

Anyone can be infested, and repeated infestations may cause an allergic response. Infestation often occurs on eyebrows and eyelashes, hair, mustaches, and beards. Symptoms are generally limited to severe itching. Body lice often infest clothing along seams close to skin surfaces and attach to the skin only to feed. They can be vectors of bacteria. Red macules, papules, and urticaria commonly appear on the shoulders, buttocks, and abdomen. Pubic lice infest through sexual contact by attaching to hair in the genital and anal regions but can also infest facial hair.

Any EMS responder exposed to a patient with lice may be treated with one of several nonprescription agents. Pyrethrin preparations such as RID are commonly used, but require two applications

1 week apart because they do not kill eggs. Permethrin agents such as Nix or Elimite theoretically require only a single application because they kill adults and eggs. Lindane 1 percent shampoo (Kwell) may be used, but it is available only by prescription and is more toxic than the other treatments. Eliminating the eggs by combing the hair is essential. Nits are more easily removed (nit picking) after soaking combs in a white vinegar solution or using a commercial preparation such as the Step 2 Nit Removal System. Separately bagging linen in an occupational setting is unnecessary. At home, however, isolating infested linen and clothing is advisable to avoid exposing uninfested laundry for extended periods. Lice are not known to jump great distances like fleas, so spraying the ambulance's interior close to the cot and the area by the patient's head with an insecticide, preferably one containing permethrin, should be sufficient after a call. Clean and wipe all sprayed areas to remove insecticide residues.

Scabies

scabies *skin disease caused by mite infestation and characterized by intense itching.*

Scabies is caused by infestation of a mite (*Sarcoptes scabiei*) that is barely visible without magnification. Exposure to the mite is through close personal contact, from hand holding to sexual relations. The mite can remain viable on clothing or in bedding for up to 48 hours.

On attaching to a new host, the female tunnels into the skin within 2.5 minutes and lays up to three eggs a day along the "burrow" in the epidermis. The larvae hatch shortly thereafter, leading to a full-grown adult 10 to 20 days later. The adults remain near hair follicles and forage for nourishment with their jaws and the claws of their forelegs.

The primary symptom is intense itching (hence the name "7-year itch"), usually at night. It generally occurs from 2 to 6 weeks after infestation. The irritation results from sensitization to the mite and its droppings. Inflammatory lesions appear as fine, wavy, dark lines, usually not more than 1 cm long. In males they most commonly occur on the webs of the fingers, wrists, elbows, armpits, belt line, thighs, and external genitalia. In females, they most often involve the areolae and nipples, abdomen, and lower portions of the buttocks. In infants, the head, neck, palms, and soles are frequently involved. Older children exhibit patterns similar to adults. Complications are generally due to infections of lesions that are broken by scratching.

Although everyone is susceptible to infection, immunocompromised patients sometimes develop Norwegian scabies, a more severe form of scabies. Persons with previous exposure appear to have fewer mites on subsequent exposures and develop symptoms much sooner (in from 1 to 4 days), suggesting an amnestic (remembered) immune system response. Outbreaks of scabies resistant to lindane (Kwell) have been reported in several nursing homes across the country.

Scabies remains communicable until all mites and eggs are destroyed. Because of the long incubation period, all household members and/or close contacts of infested EMS responders should be treated simultaneously. Although some experts recommend that clothing and uniforms worn within 2 days of treatment, along with towels and bed linen, should be washed in hot water or dry cleaned, this necessity is questionable for most infestations. It is essential, however, for articles contacting patients with Norwegian scabies. Bag and remove all linens from the ambulance immediately after you deliver the patient. To prevent spread of the mite, clean the stretcher and patient compartment as recommended for lice. Remove and decontaminate any clothing that may have contacted the patient.

The scabicides of choice are permethrin cream (Elimite) or lindane (Kwell), which is applied to the skin from the neck down, left on for 8 to 14 hours, and then washed off. This should be repeated within 1 week. If permethrin is ineffective, 10 percent crotamiton (Eurax) and ivermectin (Stromectol) are also available.

NOSOCOMIAL INFECTIONS

nosocomial *acquired while in the hospital.*

Hospitalized patients, especially those with compromised immune function, often acquire new infectious diseases. Especially virulent strains of microorganisms may cause these **nosocomial** (hospital-acquired) diseases. Bacteria that resist antibiotics are of particular concern. Recently, vancomycin-resistant enterococcus (VRE) and methicillin-resistant *Staphylococcus aureus* (MRSA) have become especially alarming. Both of these organisms can cause severe host damage, and both are difficult to treat. They rapidly colonize patients in whom broad-spectrum antibiotics have eliminated normal flora. Hospitalized patients may also contract resistant strains of tuberculosis that spread easily from patient to patient if protective clothing and hand washing precautions are not strictly observed.

PREVENTING DISEASE TRANSMISSION

Preventing or limiting exposure to infectious or communicable diseases cannot be overemphasized. While some infectious diseases are relatively minor with no long-term effects, others can be very serious and even life threatening. As a paramedic, you must be extremely vigilant during patient contact and take every step possible to ensure your health and safety. Personal accountability is important. Do not go to work if you:

As a paramedic, you must be extremely vigilant during your patient contact to take every step possible to ensure your health and safety.

- Have diarrhea.
- Have a draining wound or any type of wet lesions. Allow them to dry and crust over before returning to work.
- Are jaundiced.
- Have mononucleosis.
- Have been exposed to lice or scabies and have not yet been treated.
- Have strep throat and have not been taking antibiotics for at least 24 hours.
- Have a cold.

Keep the following immunizations current: MMR, hepatitis A (if deemed appropriate in your jurisdiction), hepatitis B, DPT, polio, chickenpox, influenza (seasonal), and rabies (if appropriate).

Always approach the scene cautiously with a high index of suspicion. On arrival, control the scene to decrease the likelihood of body fluid exposure for everyone present. Observe Standard Precautions. Always wear gloves. If there is the remotest possibility of splashing or aerosolization of body fluids, wear protective eyewear or a mask with face shield. If large volumes of blood or other fluids may result from the response, don a gown. When contacting a patient who has or may have active TB, wear the appropriate N95 respirator.

Patients who have coughs, fever, headache, general weakness, recent weight loss, or nuchal rigidity or are taking certain medications may raise your awareness of the potential for contracting an infectious agent. With experience, you will develop your intuition and associate certain symptoms with infectious patients you have treated. Bolster your experience by increasing your knowledge, particularly your clinical acumen in recognizing the immunocompromised patient.

After a call, wash your hands first. Decontaminate and disinfect your equipment and the interior of the ambulance. Using commercially available disinfectants that certify bactericidal activity against *M. tuberculosis* should provide ample disinfection of those infectious agents that pose your greatest occupational risk. Remember that HIV is a fragile virus that any vigorous application of soap and water will kill. Utilize high-level disinfection on airway equipment. If the patient or the situation surrounding the response presents the possibility of lice, scabies, or ticks, spray the gurney and interior of the ambulance with the appropriate insecticide and wipe or mop up any residue. Ensure that linen will not be taken home. If practical, do not wear uniforms home. To discourage that practice, some EMS agencies consider uniforms as PPE. Report any infectious exposure to the IDCO, human resources director, or appropriate designated official.

The topics mandated by OSHA/NIOSH for compliance with published standards and guidelines (that is, bloodborne pathogens and TB) reflect the paramedic's minimum needed knowledge of infectious diseases. Proactive EMS agencies offer their personnel continuing education in infectious diseases that have high incidence or prevalence in the communities they serve. Continuing education sessions should include identification of causative agents, modes of transmission, epidemiological patterns within the community, signs and symptoms, methods to avoid infection, and special postexposure considerations, including postexposure prophylaxis, if appropriate.

To maintain a perspective on personal risk, always consider the interaction of three major factors: infectious agent, host, and environment. Are you aware of the infectious agent's virulence? Do you have some idea of the dose of the organism involved? For example, was a large volume of body fluid involved? How healthy are you? Do you have any chronic medical conditions or take any medications that would classify you as immunocompromised? What was the nature of the exposure? Is it significantly high? The probability of risk is sometimes just a measure of exposure. Not all infectious diseases are communicable. If they are communicable, they may not necessarily pose a high probability of developing disease. The risk and potential for HIV transmission to health care workers may be high, but the probability of transmission, which averages approximately 0.3 percent, is very low.

As you are promoted within your organization, your first additional responsibility may be as a preceptor for a new paramedic or student. You therefore assume responsibility for his well-being. Are you familiar with your local protocols and procedures for reporting and recording an exposure? Can you adequately document the circumstances surrounding the exposure to facilitate review by the IDCO, physician, or agency administrator? If you cannot, what kind of a role model are you for that new employee or student?

Paramedics cannot allow their personal prejudices to interfere with providing optimum care for their patients. Patients should not be treated differently because they have an infectious disease that might reflect on their ethnicity, culture, sexual preference, or social status. You should not avoid certain procedures because you find a disease process or its consequences personally repulsive. It is sometimes helpful to think about doing things *for* patients, as opposed to doing things *to* them.

Summary

Over the past 30 years, medical science has made tremendous progress in diagnosing and treating infectious diseases. New vaccines and antibiotics are continually being developed. Advances in laboratory technology, notably the polymerase chain reaction (PCR), have made the presence and identification of microorganisms easier, quicker, and more accurate. Despite these tremendous advances, many infectious diseases cannot be effectively treated. Specific treatments for most viral diseases remain elusive, and each year countless people die from AIDS, hepatitis, pneumonia, sexually transmitted diseases, and other infectious diseases.

EMS can have a significant impact on the incidence of infectious disease if providers remain knowledgeable, are leaders in public education, and are consistently alert in protecting themselves and their patients. The title of the International Association of Fire Fighters (IAFF) hepatitis B curriculum, *The Silent War,* provides a metaphor for the dilemma of infectious diseases in EMS: EMS personnel deal with few infectious disease emergencies; however, when we do respond to such emergencies, we often are unaware of the disease's presence until after the call. Standard Precautions, often written for clinical and research facilities with more predictable hazards and risks, are increased to body substance isolation (BSI) for emergency health care providers because of the uncertainties of our profession. Constant vigilance and personal accountability are the keys to reducing those risks.

All body fluids are possibly infectious. Standard Precautions should be followed at all times.

Review Questions

1. All of the characteristics of a certain population are known as its:
   a. boundary.
   b. workplace.
   c. parameters.
   d. demographics.
2. The ___________ monitors national disease data and freely disseminates this information to all health care providers.
   a. AHA
   b. CDC
   c. OSHA
   d. HHHS

3. The infectious agent of toxic shock syndrome, *S. aureus,* releases a/an ___________, as does anthrax, which can be delivered as a biological weapon of mass destruction.
   a. protein
   b. exotoxin
   c. endotoxin
   d. polysaccharide
4. ___________ are single-celled parasitic organisms with flexible membranes and the ability to move.
   a. Fungi
   b. Pinworms
   c. Protozoa
   d. Parasites
5. Factors that affect the likelihood that an exposed individual will become infected and then actually develop disease include:
   a. virulence.
   b. correct mode of entry.
   c. number of organisms.
   d. all of the above
6. The time between exposure to and presentation of an infection, which may range from a few days to months or years, is known as the:
   a. latent period.
   b. incubation period.
   c. communicable period.
   d. window phase.
7. The presence of HIV has been noted in all of these fluids except:
   a. semen.
   b. blood or body fluids.
   c. saliva.
   d. vaginal secretions.
8. The hepatitis ___________ virus is transmitted through direct contact with contaminated body fluids (blood, semen, vaginal fluids, and saliva) and therefore represents a substantial risk to EMS providers.
   a. A
   b. B
   c. C
   d. E
9. ___________ is the most common preventable adult infectious disease in the world.
   a. TB
   b. AIDS
   c. Pneumonia
   d. Hepatitis B
10. ___________ is a viral illness that is characterized by inspiratory and expiratory stridor and a seal-barklike cough, and is most common in children under the age of 3 years.
    a. Sinusitis
    b. Pharyngitis
    c. Epiglottitis
    d. Laryngotracheobronchitis

See Answers to Review Questions at the back of this book.

Chapter

38

Psychiatric and Behavioral Disorders

Objectives

After reading this chapter, you should be able to:

1. Define behavior and distinguish among normal behavior, abnormal behavior, and the behavioral emergency. (pp. 1487–1488)
2. Discuss the prevalence of behavioral and psychiatric disorders. (pp. 1487–1488)
3. Discuss the pathophysiology of behavioral and psychiatric disorders. (pp. 1488–1489)
4. Discuss the factors that may alter the behavioral or emotional status of an ill or injured individual. (pp. 1488–1489)
5. Describe the medical legal considerations for management of emotionally disturbed patients. (p. 1504)
6. Describe the overt behaviors associated with behavioral and psychiatric disorders. (pp. 1492–1502)
7. Define the following terms:
   - ★ Affect (p. 1490)
   - ★ Anger (p. 1495)
   - ★ Anxiety (p. 1494)
   - ★ Confusion (p. 1490)
   - ★ Depression (p. 1495)
   - ★ Fear (p. 1490)
   - ★ Mental status (p. 1490)
   - ★ Open-ended question (p. 1490)
   - ★ Posture (p. 1489)
8. Describe verbal techniques useful in managing the emotionally disturbed patient. (pp. 1490–1491)
9. List the appropriate measures to ensure the safety of the paramedic, the patient, and others. (pp. 1489, 1504)
10. Describe the circumstances when relatives, bystanders, and others should be removed from the scene. (p. 1490)

11. Describe techniques to systematically gather information from the disturbed patient. (pp. 1490–1491, 1503–1504)
12. Identify techniques for physical assessment in a patient with behavioral problems. (pp. 1489–1491, 1502–1507)
13. List situations in which you are expected to transport a patient forcibly and against his will. (p. 1504)
14. Describe restraint methods necessary in managing the emotionally disturbed patient. (pp. 1504–1507)
15. List the risk factors and behaviors that indicate a patient is at risk for suicide. (p. 1501)
16. Use the assessment and patient history to differentiate among the various behavioral and psychiatric disorders. (pp. 1489–1502)
17. Given several preprogrammed behavioral emergency patients, provide the appropriate scene size-up, primary assessment, secondary assessment, and detailed assessment, then provide the appropriate care and patient transport. (pp. 1487–1507)

Key Terms

affint, p. 1490

INTRODUCTION

A significant difference between behavioral and psychiatric conditions and other types of medical emergencies is that most of your assessment and care will depend on your people skills. You can evaluate a bradycardia with a cardiac monitor and treat it with atropine or a pacing unit. You evaluate the psychiatric patient, however, by observing his behavior, by gathering information from his family and bystanders, and by interviewing him. Your care, which includes support, calming reassurance, and occasionally restraint, requires interpersonal skills more than diagnostic equipment.

BEHAVIORAL EMERGENCIES

Behavior is a person's observable conduct and activity. A **behavioral emergency** is a situation in which a patient's behavior becomes so unusual, bizarre, threatening, or dangerous that it alarms the patient or another person such as a family member or bystander and requires the intervention of emergency service and/or mental health personnel.

Notice that the definition of behavioral emergency does not use the word *abnormal*. The differentiation between normal and abnormal is largely subjective. What is normal varies based on

behavior *a person's observable conduct and activity.*

behavioral emergency *situation in which a patient's behavior becomes so unusual that it alarms the patient or another person and requires intervention.*

culture, ethnic group, socioeconomic class, and personal interpretation and opinion. What one person considers normal, another might consider highly abnormal. Generally, however, normal behavior can be defined as behavior that is readily acceptable in a society.

Indications of a behavioral or psychological condition include actions that:

- ★ Interfere with core life functions (eating, sleeping, ability to maintain housing, interpersonal or sexual relations)
- ★ Pose a threat to the life or well-being of the patient or others
- ★ Significantly deviate from society's expectations or norms

PATHOPHYSIOLOGY OF PSYCHIATRIC DISORDERS

Most patients who suffer from disorders such as anxiety, depression, eating disorders, or mild personality disorders function normally on a daily basis, going unnoticed in society.

Experts estimate that up to 20 percent of the population has some type of mental health problem and that as many as one person in seven will actually require treatment for an emotional disturbance. These problems may be severely disabling and require inpatient care, or the patient may quietly tolerate them with no outward symptoms. That all people with psychiatric conditions exhibit bizarre or unusual behavior is a misconception. The small percentage of patients with psychiatric disorders who publicly exhibit bizarre behavior tend to create this misconception among lay people. In reality, most patients who suffer from disorders such as anxiety, depression, eating disorders, or mild personality disorders function normally on a daily basis, going unnoticed in society. Nonetheless, behavioral and psychiatric disorders incapacitate more people than all other health problems combined. Most patients with mental illness are cared for in outpatient settings such as public mental health centers. Only those with severe psychiatric illnesses remain institutionalized. Because of this, EMS providers are increasingly being called to care for patients with behavioral complaints. A common reason for EMS intervention in psychiatric illness is patients' failure to take their psychiatric medications. When mental health patients such as schizophrenics begin to deteriorate and develop bizarre behavior, more often than not they have not been adhering to their psychiatric medication regimen.

Content Review

General Causes of Behavioral Emergencies

- Biological (organic)
- Psychosocial (personal)
- Social (situational)

Another common misconception is that all mental patients are unstable and dangerous and that their conditions are incurable. This is simply not true. Research in psychiatry, like other areas in medicine, has made great strides in determining causes and treatments for many psychiatric conditions. Suffering from a mental disorder is not reason for embarrassment or shame, although society often stigmatizes these patients unfairly. The general causes of behavioral emergencies are biological (or organic), psychosocial, and sociocultural. Each of these three possible causes should guide your questioning during the patient interview. Keep in mind, however, that a patient's condition may result from more than one pathological process.

BIOLOGICAL

biological/organic *related to disease processes or structural changes.*

For many years, medical practitioners have used the terms **biological** and **organic** interchangeably when discussing certain types of psychiatric disorders whose causes are physical rather than purely psychological. They result from disease processes such as infections and tumors or from structural changes in the brain such as those brought on by the abuse of alcohol or drugs (including over-the-counter and prescription medications). It could be argued, however, that even purely psychological conditions originate in the brain and for that very reason are organic. Indeed, many psychiatric conditions do originate from alterations in brain chemistry.

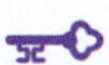

Never assume a patient with an altered mental status or unusual behavior is suffering from a purely psychological condition or disease until you have completely ruled out medical conditions and substance abuse.

Behavioral emergencies frequently involve biological conditions. Never assume a patient with an altered mental status or unusual behavior is suffering from a purely psychological condition or disease until you have completely ruled out medical conditions and substance abuse.

PSYCHOSOCIAL

psychosocial *related to a patient's personality style, dynamics of unresolved conflict, or crisis management methods.*

Psychosocial (personal) conditions are related to a patient's personality style, dynamics of unresolved conflict, or crisis management methods. These disorders are not attributable to substance abuse or medical conditions.

Environment plays a large part in psychosocial development. Traumatic childhood incidents may affect a person throughout life. Parents or other persons in positions of authority can have a tremendous impact on a child's development. Dysfunctional families, abusive parents, alcohol or drug abuse by parents, or neglect can cause behavioral problems from childhood through adulthood. Such conditions, in addition to—or in combination with—genetic predisposition and brain chemistry, form the basis for psychosocial conditions.

SOCIOCULTURAL

Sociocultural (situational) causes of behavioral disorders are related to the patient's actions and interactions within society and to factors such as socioeconomic status, social habits, social skills, and values. These problems are usually attributable to events that change the patient's social space (relationships, support systems), social isolation, or otherwise have an impact on socialization.

sociocultural *related to the patient's actions and interactions within society.*

Some events in the lives of children and adults that may cause a profound psychological change are rape, assault, witnessing the victimization of another, death of a loved one, and acts of violence such as war or riots. Events that occur over time may also have an impact on the individual. These include the loss of a job, economic problems such as poverty, and ongoing prejudice or discrimination. Sometimes simply doing anything outside the norms of society can lead to stress and psychological changes.

ASSESSMENT OF BEHAVIORAL EMERGENCY PATIENTS

The assessment and care of behavioral emergency patients is similar to that for other medical conditions. The order of assessment (scene size-up, primary assessment, secondary assessment) remains unchanged. Potential medical conditions that mimic behavioral emergencies require you to perform a thorough medical assessment.

Among the differences between your assessment and care of a patient with a medical condition and one with a behavioral emergency is that, as already noted, you actually begin your care at the same time you begin your assessment by developing a rapport with the patient. Interpersonal skills are important for all patients, but perhaps never more than for one who is experiencing a behavioral emergency. Additionally, the secondary assessment for a behavioral emergency includes a mental status examination.

SCENE SIZE-UP

As with any call, determining scene safety is of the utmost importance. Approach the scene carefully. If a patient is experiencing a behavioral emergency that is significant enough to warrant EMS, it is most likely significant enough to have law enforcement authorities respond. Most patients experiencing behavioral emergencies or crises will not attack you; however, those who are behaving unusually, experiencing hallucinations or delusions, or are under the effect of a substance may become violent. Approach every patient cautiously to protect yourself and your crew from injury (Figure 38-1 ■).

Approach every patient cautiously to protect yourself and your crew from injury.

The scene size-up also includes making observations that relate to patient care. Look for evidence of substance use or abuse, for therapeutic medications that may indicate an underlying medical condition (or abuse of that medication), and for signs of violence or destruction of property. Examine the general environmental condition and, when possible, observe the patient from a distance to note any visible behavior patterns or violent behavior.

PRIMARY ASSESSMENT

Because many behavioral emergencies are caused by or are concurrent with medical conditions, you should be acutely suspicious of life-threatening emergencies. As with any other injury or condition, assess the ABCs and intervene when necessary. Continue to observe the patient for any clues to his underlying condition. Be cautious of any overt behavior such as **posture** or hand gestures. Note any

posture *position, attitude, or bearing of the body.*

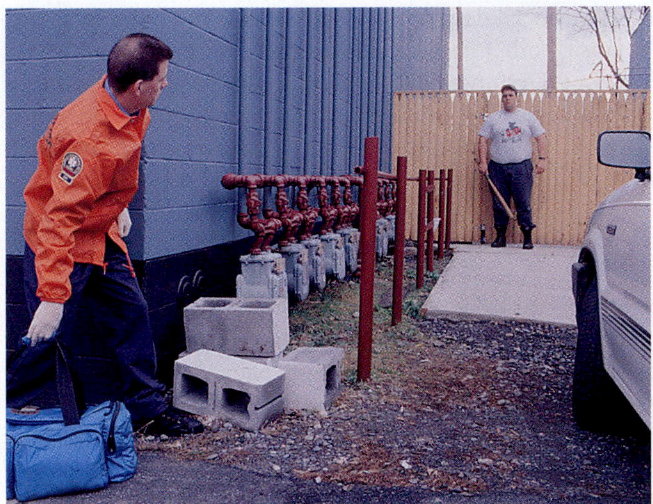

■ Figure 38-1 Approach every patient cautiously. If you determine a potential for violence, request police assistance.

fear *feeling of alarm and discontentment in the expectation of danger.*

confusion *state of being unclear or unable to make a decision easily.*

mental status *the state of the patient's cerebral functioning.*

affect *visible indicators of mood.*

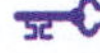

Stay alert for signs of aggression.

emotional response such as rage, **fear,** anxiety, **confusion,** or anger. Early in the evaluation, try to determine the patient's **mental status,** the state of his cerebral functioning. Continue assessing mental status throughout the patient encounter by evaluating his awareness, orientation, cognitive abilities, and **affect** (visible indicators of mood).

Control the scene as soon as possible. Remove anyone who agitates the patient or adds confusion to the scene. Generally, a limited number of people around the patient is best. At times, performing an effective assessment and care may necessitate totally clearing a room or moving the patient to a quiet area. Finally, observe the patient's affect in greater detail. To avoid being grabbed or struck by the patient, stay alert for signs of aggression.

SECONDARY ASSESSMENT

Your examination of a patient experiencing a behavioral emergency is largely conversational. This makes your interpersonal technique very important. Just as starting an IV with poor technique most likely will not establish a patent IV line, interviewing with poor interpersonal skills most likely will not obtain significant information. Remove the patient from the crisis area and limit interruptions. Focus your questioning and assessment on the immediate problem and follow these guidelines:

- ★ *Listen.* Ask open-ended questions (those that require more than a yes-or-no response). These will encourage your patient to respond in detail and share important information. Listen to the answer. Pay attention. No one likes being ignored. When you need information from a patient, listen.
- ★ *Spend time.* Rushing the patient's answers, cutting him off, or appearing hurried will cause him to "shut down" and stop answering questions.
- ★ *Be assured.* Communicate self-confidence, honesty, and professionalism.
- ★ *Do not threaten.* Avoid rapid or sudden movements or questions that the patient might interpret as threats. Approach him slowly and confidently.
- ★ *Do not fear silence.* Silence can be appropriate. Encourage the patient to tell his story, but do not be forceful or antagonizing.
- ★ *Place yourself at the patient's level.* Standing over the patient may be intimidating. Unless you are intentionally attempting to gain a position of authority, crouch, kneel, or sit near the patient. Do not position yourself where you cannot respond appropriately to danger or attack.
- ★ *Keep a safe and proper distance.* The surest way to make a behavioral emergency patient violent is to invade his "personal space" (Figure 38-2 ■). This is an area within

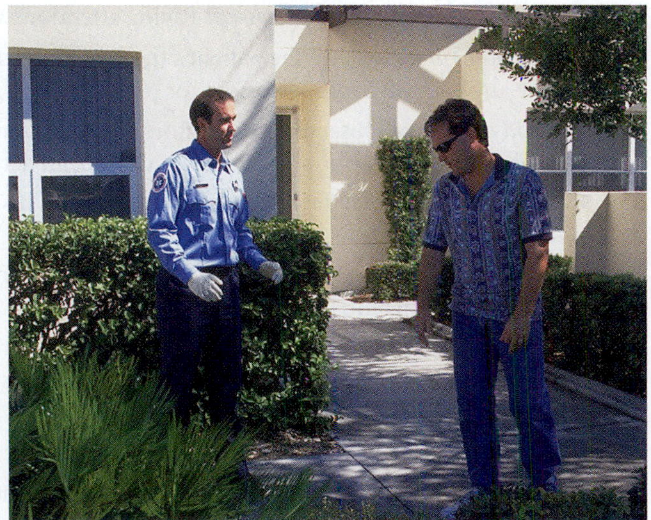

■ Figure 38-2 Avoid invading the patient's personal space, the area within about 3 feet of the patient.

an approximately 3-foot radius around every person; encroaching on it causes anxiety. If appropriate, however, you may touch the patient's shoulder or use another consoling touch when he allows.

★ *Appear comfortable.* Do not appear uncomfortable—even if you are. Talking to patients about suicide, self-mutilation, or other psychological conditions is difficult. If the patient sees that you are uncomfortable, however, he is unlikely to open up to you. Would you expect a patient to tell you his reasons for attempting suicide when you appear uncomfortable even saying the word? To help, use terms the patient has used. If he says he wanted to "end it all," begin with that. Caregivers sometimes hesitate to use the word *suicide* because it might give the patient ideas of suicide. If you are there to care for a suicidal or potentially suicidal patient, however, he has already had those thoughts.

★ *Avoid appearing judgmental.* Patients who are experiencing behavioral emergencies may feel strong emotions toward their caregivers. The patient should believe that you are interested in his condition and welfare. Be supportive and empathetic, and avoid judgments, pity, anger, or any other emotions that may damage your relationship with the patient.

★ *Never lie to the patient.* Honesty is the best policy. Do not reinforce false beliefs or hallucinations or mislead the patient in any way.

MENTAL STATUS EXAMINATION

As part of the secondary assessment for behavioral emergencies, do not overlook any physical or medical complaint. In addition to the medical evaluation, which is covered in depth throughout this and the other volumes of this program, your examination of the patient with psychiatric or behavioral disorders should include a psychological evaluation, also known as a **mental status examination (MSE)**. The components of the MSE include:

mental status examination (MSE) *a structured exam designed to quickly evaluate a patient's level of mental functioning.*

★ *General appearance.* The patient's appearance can provide important information. Observe hygiene, clothing, and overall appearance.

★ *Behavioral observations.* Observe verbal or nonverbal behavior, strange or threatening appearance, or facial expressions. Note tone of voice, rate, volume, and quality.

★ *Orientation.* Does the patient know who he is and who others are? Is he oriented to current events? Can he concentrate on simple questions and answer them?

★ *Memory.* Is the patient's memory intact for recent and long-term events?

- *Sensorium.* Is the patient focused? Paying attention? What is his level of awareness?
- *Perceptual processes.* Are the patient's thought patterns ordered? Does he appear to have any hallucinations, delusions, or phobias?
- *Mood and affect.* Observe for indicators of the patient's mood. Is it appropriate? What is his prevailing emotion? Depression, elation, anxiety, or agitation? Other?
- *Intelligence.* Evaluate the patient's speech. What is his level of vocabulary? His ability to formulate an idea?
- *Thought processes.* What is the patient's apparent form of thought? Are his thoughts logical and coherent?
- *Insight.* Does the patient have insight into his own problem? Does he recognize that a problem exists? Does he deny or blame others for his problem?
- *Judgment.* Does the patient base his life decisions on sound, reasonable judgments? Does he approach problems thoughtfully, carefully, and rationally?
- *Psychomotor.* Does the patient exhibit an unusual posture or is he making unusual movements? Patients with hallucinations may react to them. For example, a patient who believes he is covered with insects may be picking at his skin to remove the "bugs."

PSYCHIATRIC MEDICATIONS

Many patients who suffer from psychiatric or behavioral disorders are under the care of a mental health professional and may be taking prescription medications. During the interview and history-taking process, determine whether the patient is taking medications and, if so, what type. The patient's use of such medications can provide clues to his underlying condition. Additionally, if a patient is not taking a medication as directed, his condition may deteriorate. Some schizophrenic patients may receive periodic injections of extremely long-acting antipsychotics (for example, haloperidol deconoate) because of poor compliance. They will often carry an identification card or may report that they "go to the clinic every 3 weeks for a shot." Types of psychiatric medications are discussed in Chapter 6, "General Principles of Pharmacology."

SPECIFIC PSYCHIATRIC DISORDERS

Almost all psychiatric disorders have two diagnostic elements: symptoms of the disease or disorder and indications that the disease or disorder has impaired major life functions resulting in loss of relationships, a job, or housing or in another significant social problem. To define specific conditions, mental health professionals use the *Diagnostic and Statistical Manual of Mental Disorders,* Fourth Edition (*DSM-IV*). Published by the American Psychiatric Association (APA), the *DSM-IV* details diagnostic criteria for all currently defined psychiatric disorders, which are grouped according to the patient's signs and symptoms. The recognized types of behavioral and psychiatric disorders include:

- Cognitive disorders
- Schizophrenia
- Anxiety disorders
- Mood disorders
- Substance-related disorders
- Somatoform disorders
- Factitious disorders
- Dissociative disorders
- Eating disorders
- Personality disorders
- Impulse control disorders

The following summaries of these illnesses' major criteria do not imply that you should diagnose behavioral disorders. Even for skilled psychologists and psychiatrists, diagnosis is complicated by the considerable overlap in symptoms from one disease to another. A patient may actually fit into several categories. You should use the information here only as a guide to better understand the science of psychiatry and the criteria applied to patients with behavioral emergencies. Knowledge of these terms and conditions will also allow you to communicate better with psychiatric care providers.

COGNITIVE DISORDERS

Review

Content

Cognitive Disorders

- Delirium
- Dementia

Psychiatric disorders with organic causes such as brain injury or disease are known as cognitive disorders. This family of disorders includes conditions caused by metabolic disease, infections, neoplasm, endocrine disease, degenerative neurological disease, and cardiovascular disease. They might also be caused by physical or chemical injuries due to trauma, drug abuse, or reactions to prescribed drugs. The specific brain pathology will differ based on the type of disease. Two types of cognitive disorders are delirium and dementia.

Delirium

Delirium is characterized by a relatively rapid onset of widespread disorganized thought. These patients suffer from inattention, memory impairment, disorientation, and a general clouding of consciousness. In some cases, individuals may experience vivid visual hallucinations. Delirium is characterized by a fairly acute onset (hours or days) and may be reversible. Delirium may be due to a medical condition, substance intoxication, substance withdrawal, or multiple etiologies. Confusion is a hallmark of delirium.

delirium *condition characterized by relatively rapid onset of widespread disorganized thought.*

Dementia

Dementia may be due to several medical problems. Included among the more common causes of dementia are Alzheimer's disease (both early and late onset), vascular problems, AIDS, head trauma, Parkinson's disease, and substance abuse. Regardless of its cause, dementia involves memory impairment, cognitive disturbance, and pervasive impairment of abstract thinking and judgment. Unlike delirium, dementia usually develops over months and, in many cases, is irreversible.

dementia *condition involving gradual development of memory impairment and cognitive disturbance.*

Dementia involves cognitive deficits manifested by both memory impairment (diminished ability to learn new information or to recall previously learned information) and one or more of the following cognitive disturbances:

- ★ *Aphasia.* Impaired ability to communicate verbally.
- ★ *Apraxia.* Impaired ability to carry out motor activities despite intact sensory function.
- ★ *Agnosia.* Failure to recognize objects or stimuli despite intact sensory function.
- ★ *Disturbance in executive functioning.* Impaired ability to plan, organize, or sequence.

These conditions must significantly impair social or occupational functioning and represent a significant decline from a previous level of functioning. Your approach to patients with either of these conditions should be supportive. Assess and manage any medical complaints or conditions and transport to an appropriate medical facility.

SCHIZOPHRENIA

Schizophrenia is a common mental health problem, affecting an estimated 1 percent of the U.S. population. Its hallmark is a significant change in behavior and a loss of contact with reality. Signs and symptoms often include hallucinations, delusions, and depression. The schizophrenic patient may live in his "own world" and be preoccupied with inner fantasies. Although several biological and psychosocial theories attempt to explain the condition and its manifestations, its definitive cause is unknown.

schizophrenia *common disorder involving significant change in behavior often including hallucinations, delusions, and depression.*

The symptoms of schizophrenia include:

- ★ **Delusions.** Fixed, false beliefs that are not widely held within the context of the individual's cultural or religious group.
- ★ **Hallucinations.** Sensory perceptions with no basis in reality—often auditory ("hearing voices").

delusions *fixed, false beliefs not widely held within the individual's cultural or religious group.*

hallucinations *sensory perceptions with no basis in reality.*

★ *Disorganized speech.* Frequent derailment or incoherence.
★ **Catatonia.** Grossly disorganized behavior.
★ **Flat affect.** Negative symptoms.

catatonia *condition characterized by immobility and stupor, often a sign of schizophrenia.*

flat affect *appearance of being disinterested, often lacking facial expression.*

A diagnosis of schizophrenia requires that two or more symptoms must each be present for a significant portion of each month over the course of 6 months. The symptoms must cause a social or occupational dysfunction (decline in social relations or work from the predisease state). Most schizophrenics are diagnosed in early adulthood.

The *DSM-IV* defines several major types of schizophrenia:

★ *Paranoid.* The patient is preoccupied with a feeling of persecution and may suffer delusions or auditory hallucinations.
★ *Disorganized.* The patient often displays disorganized behavior, dress, or speech.
★ *Catatonic.* The patient exhibits catatonic rigidity, immobility, stupor, or peculiar voluntary movements. Catatonic schizophrenia is exceedingly rare.
★ *Undifferentiated.* The patient does not readily fit into one of the previous categories.

Content Review

Major Types of Schizophrenia

– Paranoid
– Disorganized
– Catatonic
– Undifferentiated

Your approach to the schizophrenic patient should be supportive and nonjudgmental. Do not reinforce the patient's hallucinations, but understand that he considers them real. Speak openly and honestly with him. Be encouraging yet realistic. Remain alert for aggressive behavior, and restrain the patient if he becomes violent or presents a danger to you, to himself, or to others.

ANXIETY AND RELATED DISORDERS

anxiety disorder *condition characterized by dominating apprehension and fear.*

anxiety *state of uneasiness, discomfort, apprehension, and restlessness.*

panic attack *extreme period of anxiety resulting in great emotional distress.*

The group of illnesses known as **anxiety disorders** is characterized by dominating apprehension and fear. These disorders affect approximately 2 to 4 percent of the population. Broadly defined, **anxiety** is a state of uneasiness, discomfort, apprehension, and restlessness. More specifically, anxiety disorders fall into three categories: panic disorder, phobia, and post-traumatic stress syndrome.

Panic Attack The *DSM-IV* does not list **panic attacks** in themselves as a disease. Characterized by recurrent, extreme periods of anxiety resulting in great emotional distress, they are symptoms of disease and are included among the criteria for other disorders (panic disorder, agoraphobia). Panic attacks differ from generalized feelings of anxiety in their acute nature. They are usually unprovoked, peaking within 10 minutes of their onset and dissipating in less than 1 hour.

Content Review

Anxiety-Related Disorders

- Panic attack
- Phobia
- Posttraumatic stress syndrome

The presentation of panic and anxiety may resemble a cardiac or respiratory condition. This presents a dilemma for EMS personnel. Ruling out those conditions is difficult in the prehospital setting; psychiatrists usually diagnose anxiety or panic disorders by excluding known medical conditions. Keys to identifying panic or anxiety in the field are the patient's having a history of the condition and being outside the expected age range for certain cardiac or respiratory illnesses. This, of course, is not to say that young people cannot have myocardial infarction. Many symptoms of panic resemble those of hyperventilation, and some do appear to be correlated, such as the paresthesia from panic being due largely to hyperventilation.

The diagnostic criteria for a panic attack require a discrete period of intense fear or discomfort, during which four or more of the following symptoms develop abruptly and reach a peak within 10 minutes:

★ Palpitations, pounding heart, or accelerated heart rate
★ Sweating
★ Trembling or shaking
★ Sensations of shortness of breath or smothering
★ Feeling of choking
★ Chest pain or discomfort
★ Nausea or abdominal distress
★ Feeling dizzy, unsteady, lightheaded, or faint

★ Derealization (feelings of unreality) or depersonalization (being detached from oneself)

★ Fear of losing control or going crazy

★ Fear of dying

★ Paresthesia (numbness or tingling sensations)

★ Chills or hot flashes

Management for anxiety disorders is generally simple and supportive. Show empathy. Assess any medical complaints and manage them appropriately. If the patient experiences hyperventilation, calm and reassure him in order to decrease his respiratory rate to normal. Patients with severe or incapacitating symptoms may benefit from the administration of a sedative. Benzodiazepines, such as diazepam (Valium) and lorazepam (Ativan), can be administered in the prehospital setting. In addition, antihistamines, such as hydroxyzine (Vistaril) and diphenhydramine (Benadryl), have sedative effects and are useful in treating patients with significant anxiety. Consult medical direction in accordance with local protocol and transport to an appropriate medical facility.

Phobias All people have some source of fear or anxiety that they consciously avoid. When this fear becomes excessive and interferes with functioning, it is a **phobia.** A phobia, generally considered an intense, irrational fear, may be due to animals, the sight of blood (or injection or injury), situational factors (elevators, enclosed spaces), or environmental conditions (heights or water). Exposure to the situation or item will induce anxiety or a panic attack. Some patients experience extreme phobias that prevent or limit their normal daily activities. For example, a patient suffering from agoraphobia (fear of crowds) may confine himself to his home and avoid ever venturing outdoors. In most patients, however, the phobia is less severe; the patient realizes that his fear is unreasonable, and the anxiety dissipates.

phobia *excessive fear that interferes with functioning.*

Management for a patient with a phobia is supportive. Understand that the patient's fear is very real. Do not force him to do anything that he opposes. Manage any underlying problems and transport for evaluation.

Post-traumatic Stress Syndrome EMS providers often are particularly interested in **post-traumatic stress syndrome** because their responsibilities may make them susceptible to it. Originally recognized on the battlefields of war, post-traumatic stress syndrome is a reaction to an extreme, usually life-threatening stressor such as a natural disaster, victimization (rape, for instance), or other emotionally taxing situation. It is characterized by a desire to avoid similar situations, recurrent intrusive thoughts, depression, sleep disturbances, nightmares, and persistent symptoms of increased arousal. The patient may feel guilty for having survived the incident, and substance abuse may frequently complicate his condition.

post-traumatic stress syndrome *reaction to an extreme stressor.*

Treat any post-traumatic stress syndrome patient with respect, empathy, and support, and transport him to an appropriate facility for evaluation.

MOOD DISORDERS

The *DSM-IV* defines mood as "a pervasive and sustained emotion that colors a person's perception of the world." Common examples of mood alterations include depression, elation, **anger,** and anxiety. The main **mood disorders** are depression and bipolar disorder.

anger *hostility or rage to compensate for an underlying feeling of anxiety.*

mood disorder *pervasive and sustained emotion that colors a person's perception of the world.*

depression *profound sadness or feeling of melancholy.*

Depression **Depression** is characterized by a profound sadness or feeling of melancholy. It is common in everyday life and is to be expected following the breakup of a relationship or the loss of a loved one. Most of us have experienced some sort of depression, at least in its mildest form. It is one of the most prevalent psychiatric conditions, affecting from 10 to 15 percent of the population. When depression becomes prolonged or severe, however, it is diagnosed as a *major depressive episode.*

The symptoms of major depressive disorder include:

★ Depressed mood most of the day, nearly every day, as indicated by subjective report or observation by others

Content Review

Mood Disorders

- Depression
- Bipolar disorder

- ★ Markedly diminished interest in pleasure in all, or almost all, activities most of the day nearly every day
- ★ Significant weight loss (without dieting) or weight gain—a 5 percent change in body weight is considered significant
- ★ Insomnia or hypersomnia nearly every day
- ★ Psychomotor agitation or retardation every day (observable by others, not just the subjective feeling of the patient)
- ★ Feelings of worthlessness or excessive inappropriate guilt (may be delusional) nearly every day
- ★ Diminished ability to think or concentrate, or indecisiveness nearly every day
- ★ Recurrent thoughts of death (not just fear of dying), recurrent suicidal ideation without a specific plan, or a suicide attempt or a specific plan for committing suicide (Depression greatly increases the risk of suicide.)

The diagnostic criteria for major depressive disorder require that five or more of the symptoms have been present during the same 2-week period and represent a change from previous functioning; at least one of the symptoms must be either a depressed mood or loss of interest in pleasure. The condition must cause clinically significant distress or impairment in social, occupational, or other important functions. Further, it must not meet the criteria for a mixed episode (mixtures of mania and depression); it must not be due to the direct physiological effects of a substance such as drug abuse or a medication, or to a general medical condition such as hypothyroidism; finally, it must not be better accounted for by **bereavement.** The acronym *In SAD CAGES* provides a screening mnemonic for major depression.

bereavement *death of a loved one.*

- ★ *In*terest
- ★ *S*leep
- ★ *A*ppetite
- ★ *D*epressed mood
- ★ *C*oncentration
- ★ *A*ctivity
- ★ *G*uilt
- ★ *E*nergy
- ★ *S*uicide

Depression may occur as an isolated condition, but it is often accompanied by other disorders such as substance abuse, anxiety disorders, and schizophrenia. Depression can also affect a patient without meeting all of the identified clinical criteria. It can affect different people in different ways and is often atypical. Bereavement is one of the situations in which depression is expected. If the depression lasts longer than 2 months or is accompanied by suicidal ideation or marked functional impairment, it could be classified as a major depressive episode. Depression is more prevalent in females and is spread evenly throughout the life span.

bipolar disorder *condition characterized by one or more manic episodes, with or without periods of depression.*

manic *characterized by excessive excitement or activity (mania).*

Bipolar Disorder **Bipolar disorder** is characterized by one or more **manic** episodes (periods of elation), with or without subsequent or alternating periods of depression. In the past, the term *manic-depressive* was used to describe this condition. Bipolar disorder is not particularly common, affecting approximately less than 1 percent of the population.

Manic-depressive episodes are not the "Jekyll and Hyde" transformations that television and the movies often portray. However, they often begin suddenly and escalate rapidly over a few days. In contrast to major depressive disorders, bipolar disorders usually develop in adolescence or early adulthood and occur as often in males as in females. Some patients with major depressive episodes will eventually develop a bipolar disorder and experience manic episodes. Commonly patients have several depressive episodes before having a manic episode.

The diagnostic criteria for a manic episode require a distinct period of abnormally and persistently elevated, expansive, or irritable mood lasting for at least 1 week (or for any duration when hospitalization is necessary). Three or more (four or more if the mood is only irritable) of the following symptoms must have been present to a certain degree and must have persisted during that time:

- ★ Inflated self-esteem or grandiosity
- ★ Decreased need for sleep
- ★ More talkative than usual or pressure to keep talking
- ★ Flight of ideas or subjective experience that thoughts are racing
- ★ Distractibility
- ★ Increase in goal-directed activity (socially, at work or school, or sexually) or psychomotor agitation
- ★ Excessive involvement in pleasurable activities that have a high potential for painful consequences (buying sprees, sexual indiscretions, foolish business investments)
- ★ Delusional thoughts (grandiose ideas or unrealistic plans)

The symptoms must not meet the criteria for a mixed episode. The mood disturbance must be severe enough to markedly impair occupational or social functioning, to require hospitalizing the patient to prevent harm to himself or others, or present with psychotic features. As with depression, the symptoms must not be due to the direct physiological effects of a substance or a general medical condition. Patients with bipolar illness are often prescribed lithium (Lithobid, Eskalith) for treatment.

Management of these patients includes maintaining a calm, protective environment. Avoid confronting the manic patient. Never leave a depressed or suicidal patient alone. Assess and manage any other coexisting medical problems, and transport to an appropriate medical facility. Bipolar patients in an extreme manic phase may be overtly psychotic. In these cases, medication with an antipsychotic medication such as haloperidol may be indicated. Always contact medical direction for treatment options.

Many patients with bipolar disorder are treated with lithium. Lithium has a very narrow therapeutic index, making lithium toxicity a significant complicating factor.

SUBSTANCE-RELATED DISORDERS

Substance abuse is a common disorder. Any patient exhibiting symptoms of a psychiatric or behavioral disorder should be screened for substance use and/or abuse. Substance abuse patients may present as being depressed, psychotic, or delirious, and their signs and symptoms may mimic those of many behavioral disorders. The *DSM-IV* lists substance abuse as a psychiatric disorder; you should consider it a serious condition. Any mood-altering chemical has the potential for abuse. Alcohol is a common part of our culture, but can be abused. The user of a substance may be intoxicated from the effects of the chemical or may be ill from addiction or withdrawal of the chemical. Intoxication, in and of itself, may cause behavioral problems.

Repetitive use of a mood-altering chemical may lead to dependence or addiction. Dependence on a substance is characterized by repeated use of the substance. Dependence may be either psychological, physical, or both. Psychological dependence is a compelling desire to use the substance, inability to reduce or stop use, and repeated efforts to quit. Physical dependence is characterized by the need for increased amounts of the chemical to obtain the desired effect. Also, the presence of withdrawal symptoms when the substance is reduced or stopped is characteristic of physical dependence. All drugs have the potential to cause psychological dependence; many have the potential to cause physical dependence as well.

somatoform disorder *condition characterized by physical symptoms that have no apparent physiological cause and are attributable to psychological factors.*

SOMATOFORM DISORDERS

Somatoform disorders are characterized by physical symptoms that have no apparent physiological cause. They are believed to be attributable to psychological factors. People who suffer from somatoform disorders believe their symptoms are serious and real. The major types of somatoform disorder are:

- ★ *Somatization disorder.* The patient is preoccupied with physical symptoms.
- ★ *Conversion disorder.* The patient sustains a loss of function, usually involving the nervous system (for instance, blindness or paralysis), unexplained by any medical illness.

Content Review

Somatoform Disorders

- Somatization disorder
- Conversion disorder
- Hypochondriasis
- Body dysmorphic disorder
- Pain disorder

★ *Hypochondriasis.* Exaggerated interpretation of physical symptoms as a serious illness.

★ *Body dysmorphic disorder.* A person believes he has a defect in physical appearance.

★ *Pain disorder.* The patient suffers from pain, usually severe, that is unexplained by a physical ailment.

Somatoform disorders are often difficult to identify and diagnose. They can mimic and be confused with various bona fide physical conditions. Never attribute physical symptoms to a behavioral disorder until medical conditions have been ruled out.

FACTITIOUS DISORDERS

factitious disorder *condition in which the patient feigns illness in order to assume the sick role.*

dissociative disorder *condition in which the individual avoids stress by separating from his core personality.*

Review

Content

Dissociative Disorders

- Psychogenic amnesia
- Fugue state
- Multiple personality disorder
- Depersonalization

Factitious disorders are sometimes confused with somatoform disorders. They are characterized by the following three criteria:

★ An intentional production of physical or psychological signs or symptoms is present.

★ Motivation for the behavior is to assume the "sick role."

★ External incentives for the behavior (e.g., economic gain, avoiding work, avoiding police) are absent.

While patients suffering from factitious disorders essentially feign their illnesses, that does not preclude the possibility of true physical or psychological symptoms. The disorder is apparently more common in males than in females. In severe cases, patients will go to great length to obtain medical or psychological treatment. Patients with factitious disorders often will voluntarily produce symptoms and will present with a very plausible history. They often have an extensive knowledge of medical terminology and can be very demanding and disruptive. In severe cases (Munchausen syndrome), patients will undergo multiple surgical operations and other painful procedures.

DISSOCIATIVE DISORDERS

Like somatoform disorders, **dissociative disorders** are attempts to avoid stressful situations while still gratifying needs. In a manner, they permit the person to deny personal responsibility for unacceptable behavior. The individual avoids stress by *dissociating* from his core personality. These behavior patterns can be complex but are quite rare. The disorders include the following.

psychogenic amnesia *failure to recall, as opposed to inability to recall.*

fugue state *condition in which an amnesiac patient physically flees.*

multiple personality disorder *manifestation of two or more complete systems of personality.*

depersonalization *feeling detached from oneself.*

Psychogenic Amnesia

While amnesia is a partial or total *inability* to recall or identify past events, **psychogenic amnesia** is a *failure* to recall. The "forgotten" material is present but "hidden" beneath the level of consciousness.

Fugue State

An amnesic individual may withdraw even further by retreating in what is known as a **fugue state.** A patient in a fugue state actually flees as a defense mechanism and may travel hundreds of miles from home.

Multiple Personality Disorder

In **multiple personality disorder** the patient reacts to an identifiable stress by manifesting two or more complete systems of personality. While such disorders have received a great deal of attention in television, film, and novels, they are actually quite rare.

Depersonalization

Depersonalization is a relatively more frequent dissociative disorder that occurs predominantly in young adults. Patients experience a loss of the sense of one's self. Such individuals suddenly feel "different"—that they are someone else or that their body has taken on a different form. The disorder is often precipitated by acute stress.

Review

Content

Eating Disorders

- Anorexia nervosa
- Bulimia nervosa

EATING DISORDERS

The two classifications of eating disorders are anorexia nervosa and bulimia nervosa. Both generally occur between adolescence and the age of 25. The condition afflicts women more than men at a rate of 20:1.

Anorexia Nervosa Anorexia is the loss of appetite. **Anorexia nervosa** is a disorder marked by excessive fasting. Individuals with this disorder have an intense fear of obesity and often complain of being fat even though their body weight is low. They suffer from weight loss (25 percent of body weight or more), refusal to maintain body weight, and often a cessation of menstruation from severe malnutrition.

anorexia nervosa *psychological disorder characterized by voluntary refusal to eat.*

Bulimia Nervosa Recurrent episodes of seemingly uncontrollable binge eating with compensatory self-induced vomiting or diarrhea, excessive exercise, or dieting and with a full awareness of the behavior's abnormality characterize **bulimia nervosa.** Individuals often display personality traits of perfectionism, low self-esteem, and social withdrawal.

bulimia nervosa *recurrent episodes of binge eating.*

The weight loss and body changes experienced by anorexic and bulimic patients can lead to serious physical problems. Starvation and attempts to purge can have drastic consequences such as anemia, dehydration, vitamin deficiencies, hypoglycemia, and cardiovascular problems. In addition to psychological support, prehospital care is likely to include treatment for dehydration and physical problems. Both disorders have a high potential morbidity and mortality.

PERSONALITY DISORDERS

Most adults' personalities are attuned to social demands. Some individuals, however, often seem ill equipped to function adequately in society. These people might be suffering from a **personality disorder.** Stemming largely from immature and distorted personality development, these personality, or character, disorders result in persistently maladaptive ways of perceiving, thinking, and relating to the world.

personality disorder *condition that results in persistently maladaptive behavior.*

The broad category of personality disorder includes problems that vary greatly in form and severity. Although others might describe them as "eccentric" or "troublesome," some patients with personality disorders function adequately. In extreme cases, patients act out against or attempt to manipulate society.

Personality Disorder Clusters

The *DSM-IV* groups similar personality disorders into three broad types: cluster A, cluster B, and cluster C.

Cluster A Individuals in cluster A often act odd or eccentric. Their unusual behavior can take drastically different forms. This cluster includes the following:

- ★ *Paranoid personality disorder.* Pattern of distrust and suspiciousness.
- ★ *Schizoid personality disorder.* Pattern of detachment from social relationships.
- ★ *Schizotypal personality disorder.* Pattern of acute discomfort in close relationships, cognitive distortions, and eccentric behavior.

Cluster B Individuals in cluster B often appear dramatic, emotional, or fearful. This cluster includes the following:

- ★ *Antisocial personality disorder.* Pattern of disregard for the rights of others.
- ★ *Borderline personality disorder.* Pattern of instability in interpersonal relationships, self-image, and impulsivity.
- ★ *Histrionic personality disorder.* Pattern of excessive emotions and attention seeking.
- ★ *Narcissistic personality disorder.* Pattern of grandiosity, need for admiration, and lack of empathy.

Cluster C Individuals in cluster C often appear anxious or fearful. This cluster includes the following:

- ★ *Avoidant personality disorder.* Pattern of social inhibition, feelings of inadequacy, and hypersensitivity to criticism.

Content Review

Personality Disorder Clusters

- Cluster A personality disorders
  - –Paranoid
  - –Schizoid
  - –Schizotypal
- Cluster B personality disorders
  - –Antisocial
  - –Borderline
  - –Histrionic
  - –Narcissistic
- Cluster C personality disorders
  - –Avoidant
  - –Dependent
  - –Obsessive-compulsive

★ *Dependent personality disorder.* Pattern of submissive and clinging behavior related to an excessive need to be cared for.

★ *Obsessive-compulsive disorder.* Pattern of preoccupation with orderliness, perfectionism, and control.

Diagnosing a personality disorder requires evaluating the individual's long-term functioning and behavior. In many cases, the individual suffers from multiple disorders. A complete interview, history, and assessment will assist you in determining your approach. Your prehospital care will vary based on the patient's chief complaint and overall presentation.

IMPULSE CONTROL DISORDERS

impulse control disorder *condition characterized by the patient's failure to control recurrent impulses.*

Related to the personality disorders are the **impulse control disorders.** Recurrent impulses and the patient's failure to control them characterize these disorders. Examples of impulse control disorders include:

★ *Kleptomania.* A recurrent failure to resist impulses to steal objects not for immediate use or for their monetary value.

★ *Pyromania.* A recurrent failure to resist impulses to set fires.

★ *Pathological gambling.* A chronic and progressive preoccupation with gambling and the urge to gamble.

★ *Trichotillomania.* A recurrent impulse to pull out one's own hair.

★ *Intermittent explosive disorder.* Recurrent and paroxysmal episodes of significant loss of control of aggressive responses.

Disorders of impulse control may be harmful to the patient and others. Prior to committing the act the patient will have an increasing sense of tension. After the act, he will either have pleasure gratification or release.

SUICIDE

Suicide, simply stated, is when a person intentionally takes his own life. Suicide is alarmingly common. It is the ninth leading cause of death overall, and it is the third leading cause in the 15- to 24-year age group. Suicide rates have risen dramatically in the younger age groups and have also increased significantly in the elderly population. Women attempt suicide more than men, but men—especially those over 55 years of age—are more likely to succeed. Statistically, suicide successes and methods vary widely by race, sex, and culture. The most common methods of suicide are:

1. Bullet wound (60 percent)
2. Poisoning (18 percent)
3. Strangulation (15 percent)
4. Cutting (1 percent)
5. Other, or unspecified (6 percent)

Assessing Potentially Suicidal Patients

Document observations at the scene of an attempted suicide, especially any detailed suicide plans, suicide notes, and statements by the patient and bystanders.

In cases of attempted suicide, many focus on whether the patient really wanted to kill himself. Indeed this question will be at the heart of the patient's future psychiatric care, and information from the paramedic will be crucial to making that determination. However, never lose sight of patient care while probing the psychological nature of attempted suicide.

Perform an appropriate secondary assessment concurrently with providing sound psychological care. Mental health professionals are rarely on the scene. It is up to you to document observations at the scene, especially any detailed suicide plans, any suicide notes, and any statements of the patient and bystanders. This information may not be available after the event when the patient receives psychiatric screening at the hospital. Such care and observations at the scene, combined with detailed documentation, are critical to the patient's long-term psychological care.

Risk Factors for Suicide

The risk factors for suicide are numerous. When assessing a patient who has indicated suicidal intentions, screen for any of these risk factors:

- ★ Previous attempts (Eighty percent of persons who successfully commit suicide have made a previous attempt.)
- ★ Depression (Suicide is 500 times more common among patients who are severely depressed than those who are not.)
- ★ Age (Incidence is high between the ages of 15 and 24 years and over the age of 40.)
- ★ Alcohol or drug abuse
- ★ Divorced or widowed (The rate is five times higher than among other groups.)
- ★ Giving away personal belongings, especially cherished possessions
- ★ Living alone or in increased isolation
- ★ The presence of **psychosis** with depression (for example, suicidal or destructive thoughts or hallucinations about killing or death)
- ★ Homosexuality (especially homosexuals who are depressed, aging, alcoholic, or HIV infected)
- ★ Major separation trauma (mate, loved one, job, money)
- ★ Major physical stresses (surgery, childbirth, sleep deprivation)
- ★ Loss of independence (disabling illness)
- ★ Lack of goals and plans for the future
- ★ Suicide of same-sexed parent
- ★ Expression of a plan for committing suicide
- ★ Possession of the mechanism for suicide (gun, pills, rope)

psychosis *extreme response to stress characterized by impaired ability to deal with reality.*

Patients who have attempted suicide must be evaluated in a hospital or psychiatric facility. Many people assume that "they were just looking for attention." Applied to the wrong patient, that conjecture may contribute to his death.

AGE-RELATED CONDITIONS

Some behavioral disorders are particularly common among patients at the ends of the age spectrum—the young and the elderly. Your awareness of age-related conditions will help you to assess and interact with these patients.

Crisis in the Geriatric Patient

Common physical problems among the elderly include dementia, chronic illness, and diminished eyesight and hearing. The elderly also experience depression that is often mistaken for dementia. When confronted with an elderly person in a crisis, take the following steps:

- ★ Assess the patient's ability to communicate.
- ★ Provide continual reassurance.
- ★ Compensate for the patient's loss of sight and hearing with reassuring physical contact.
- ★ Treat the patient with respect. Call the patient by name and title, such as "Mrs. Jones." Avoid such terms as "dear," "honey," and "babe."
- ★ Avoid administering medication.
- ★ Describe what you are going to do before you do it.
- ★ Take your time. Do not convey the impression that you are in a hurry.
- ★ Allow family members and friends to remain with the patient, if possible.

CRISIS IN THE PEDIATRIC PATIENT

Behavioral emergencies are not limited to adults. Children also have behavioral crises. While the child's developmental stage will affect his behavior, these general guidelines will assist you when confronting an emotionally distraught or disruptive child:

- ★ Avoid separating a young child from his parent.
- ★ Attempt to prevent the child from seeing things that will increase his distress.
- ★ Make all explanations brief and simple, and repeat them often.
- ★ Be calm and speak slowly.
- ★ Identify yourself by giving both your name and your function.
- ★ Be truthful with the child. Telling the truth will develop trust.
- ★ Encourage the child to help with his care.
- ★ Reassure the child by carrying out all interventions gently.
- ★ Do not discourage the child from crying or showing emotion.
- ★ If you must be separated from the child, introduce the person who will assume responsibility for his care.
- ★ Allow the child to keep a favorite blanket or toy.
- ★ Do not leave the child alone, even for a short period.

Always be mindful of every young or elderly patient's uniqueness. Treat him equally and fairly, as you would any other patient.

MANAGEMENT OF BEHAVIORAL EMERGENCIES

Patients who are experiencing behavioral emergencies require both medical and psychological care. In general, take the following measures when you treat a patient who is experiencing a behavioral emergency:

1. Ensure scene safety and use Standard Precautions.
2. Provide a supportive and calm environment.
3. Treat any existing medical conditions.
4. Do not allow the suicidal patient to be alone.
5. Do not confront or argue with the patient.
6. Provide realistic reassurance.
7. Respond to the patient in a direct, simple manner.
8. Transport to an appropriate receiving facility.

Remember to treat the whole patient. Never overlook any serious, or potentially serious, medical complaints while focusing on the psychiatric assessment.

MEDICAL

Patients who are experiencing apparent behavioral emergencies often have concurrent medical conditions—some of which may be responsible for the behavioral problem. Current literature indicates that medical conditions and/or substance abuse cause a much higher proportion of behavioral emergencies than previously believed. Medical care may include treatment for overdose, lacerations, toxic inhalation, hypoxia, or metabolic conditions. Many patients with chronic psychiatric conditions take medications for their illnesses; when abused, those medications have extremely toxic side effects. (Refer to Chapter 6, "General Principles of Pharmacology.") Additionally these patients often live in conditions ranging from substandard housing to the street. This existence may predispose them to other medical problems such as exposure, infections, and untreated illnesses.

Never overlook any serious, or potentially serious, medical complaints while focusing on the psychiatric assessment.

PSYCHOLOGICAL

Patients who present with an apparent behavioral emergency also require psychological care. The time you spend developing a rapport with the patient—before, during, and after assessment—is actually a part of the care you provide. In effect, when you begin an assessment you are also beginning your care, and you will continue to perform psychological assessment and care concurrently with medical assessment and care. Be calm and reassuring while you interview your patient.

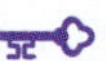

The time you spend developing a rapport with the behavioral emergency patient—before, during, and after assessment—is actually a part of the care you provide.

Since much of your care will be aimed at the psychological problem, you should steer your conversation and actions in that direction. Visualize your patients on a continuum ranging from agitated and out of control to introverted and depressed (Figure 38-3 ■). As a paramedic, you will need to defuse the agitated patient and attempt to communicate with the withdrawn patient. These situations especially will require the interviewing skills you learned earlier in this chapter.

As you approach the patient, introduce yourself and state that you want to help, since this might not be intuitively clear to a person with distorted perceptions. As you begin to converse, note how the patient reacts to you. Generally, if he responds appropriately to your actions, you should continue what you are doing. If the patient becomes more agitated or further withdrawn, rethink. Perhaps you are getting too close, talking too fast, or addressing difficult topics too early. Be sure your exit path is not blocked.

Your approach to these patients requires excellent people skills—especially listening and observing. If you do not use these skills, or if you rush or seem disinterested, your care will likely fail. Therapeutic communication, as this interaction has been called, is an art. "Talking down" the behavioral emergency patient requires effort and skill. Some patients, however, will not react favorably even to the best people skills. Extremely withdrawn patients or those with severe psychotic symptoms may never fully respond during the time you spend with them out of the hospital. These patients still deserve quality care and compassion, even when they are uncommunicative or restrained.

Talking down the behavioral emergency patient is an art that requires effort and skill.

Just as we must observe the patient, the patient observes us. Patients may actually be able to "read" us as accurately (or more accurately) than we read them. Perform your assessment and care confidently and competently. If patients sense uneasiness or indecision, they are more likely to act out. Never play along with a patient's hallucinations or delusions. It may seem to be the easiest route, but ultimately it may be harmful. Often the patient will recognize that you are patronizing

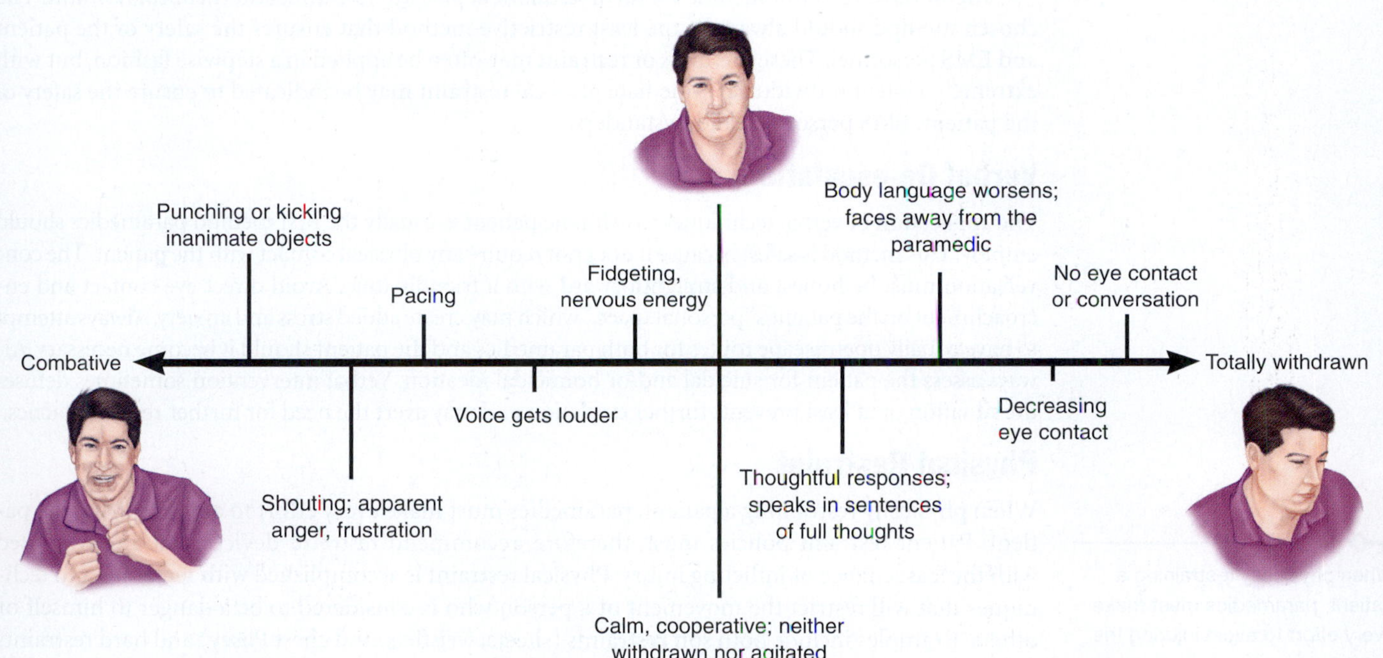

■ **Figure 38-3** Continuum of patient responses during behavioral emergency. Whether dealing with an agitated or withdrawn patient, you will use your interpersonal skills to bring him to the calm, cooperative state in the middle of the continuum.

him. Or the patient may talk of hallucinations or appear delusional, but not fully believe what he says. If you play along, you will lose credibility.

VIOLENT PATIENTS AND RESTRAINT

Providing medical care in the prehospital environment often places paramedics in harm's way. Agitation or confusion can result from a variety of medical or traumatic conditions. Additionally, various psychiatric and behavioral disorders can result in violent patients who pose a risk to paramedics, to themselves, and to others.

The restraint of violent patients at an emergency scene is a controversial aspect of modern EMS. In fact, because of several deaths related to patient restraint in the prehospital environment, the practice has come under increasing scrutiny. As a result, in 2002 the National Association of EMS Physicians (NAEMSP) adopted a position paper titled "Patient Restraint in Emergency Medical Services Systems." The purpose of this document was to provide guidelines that will help to minimize the possibility of injury to patients and EMS personnel.

It is important to remember that many medical and trauma conditions can result in agitation and combativeness.

It is important to remember that many medical and trauma conditions can result in agitation and combativeness. Because of this, paramedics must be knowledgeable about these conditions and their appropriate treatment. All EMS systems should have protocols in place for the restraint and management of agitated and combative patients.

METHODS OF RESTRAINT

The safety of EMS personnel is always a paramount concern.

If a patient is known to be violent, EMS personnel should ensure that law enforcement personnel secure the scene before EMS enters. However, this is not always possible, and paramedics should always be alert for unexpectedly agitated patients or those with escalating emotions. The safety of EMS personnel is paramount, and it is appropriate for paramedics to withdraw from a violent situation until after law enforcement or other additional resources arrive.

Paramedics should anticipate the potential for exposure to blood and body fluids during patient restraint. Restraint procedures can expose EMS providers to blood, saliva, urine, or feces. Based on the situation, appropriate barrier protection should be worn during patient restraint.

Methods of restraint include *verbal de-escalation, physical restraint,* and *chemical restraint.* The chosen method should always be the least restrictive method that ensures the safety of the patient and EMS personnel. These methods of restraint may often be applied in a stepwise fashion, but with extremely violent individuals immediate physical restraint may be indicated to ensure the safety of the patient, EMS personnel, and bystanders.

Verbal De-escalation

The application of verbal techniques to calm the patient is usually the first method paramedics should employ. This method is safest because it does not require any physical contact with the patient. The conversation must be honest and straightforward with a friendly tone. Avoid direct eye contact and encroachment on the patient's "personal space," which may create added stress and anxiety. Always attempt to have equally open escape routes for both paramedics and the patient should it become necessary. Always assess the patient for suicidal and/or homicidal ideation. Verbal intervention sometimes defuses the situation or at least prevents further escalation and may avert the need for further restraint tactics.

Physical Restraint

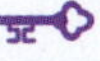

When physically restraining a patient, paramedics must make every effort to avoid injuring the patient.

When physically restraining a patient, paramedics must make every effort to avoid injuring the patient. Patient restraint policies must, therefore, recommend restraint devices that are associated with the least chance of inflicting injury. Physical restraint is accomplished with materials and techniques that will restrict the movement of a person who is considered to be a danger to himself or others. Examples include both soft restraints (sheets, wristlets, and chest Posey) and hard restraints (plastic ties, handcuffs, and leathers).

In general, EMS personnel should avoid using hard restraints. If an EMS system chooses to use hard restraints, all personnel should be trained to proficiency in their use, and the patient's extremities should be evaluated frequently for injury or possible neurovascular compromise.

Ideally, a minimum of five people should be present to safely apply physical restraint to a violent patient, which allows for control of the head and each limb. This requirement may be difficult for some EMS systems to accomplish because of limits on the number of available personnel. At a minimum, however, four rescuers should work together to accomplish restraint (Procedure 38–1). Before beginning physical restraint, there should be a plan and a team leader who will direct the restraining process.

Four-point restraints (restraining both arms and both legs) are preferred over two-point restraints. It is often helpful to tether the hips, thighs, and chest. Tethering the thighs just above the knees is often more effective in preventing kicking than restraint of the ankles.

Contrary to the methods recommended in the U.S. DOT National Standard Curriculum for EMT-Paramedics, patients should *not* be transported while restrained in a prone position. Restraint in a prone position has been associated with **positional asphyxia.** In addition, nothing should be placed over the face, head, or neck of the patient. A surgical mask placed loosely on the patient may prevent spitting. A hard cervical collar may limit the mobility of the patient's neck and may decrease the range of head motion necessary for the patient to attempt to bite.

positional asphyxia *death from positioning that prevents sufficient intake of oxygen.*

While gaining initial control of the patient, it may be acceptable to restrain him in a prone position *temporarily*—or to sandwich the patient with mattresses or backboards *temporarily*—but *personnel must be extremely vigilant for respiratory compromise.* Gaining initial control of the patient in the prone position limits the patient's visual awareness of the environment and decreases the range of motion of the extremities. As soon as the team has control of the patient's movement, however, the team must work to move the patient into a supine four-point restrained position.

A patient should *never* be hobbled or "hog tied" with the arms and legs tied together behind the back. During transport, a patient should *never* be restrained to a stretcher in the prone position or sandwiched between backboards or mattresses.

Once the patient has been restrained, he should never be left unattended. If a patient vomits, it will be necessary to immediately position him and possibly to suction him to protect the airway. Also, paramedics should perform and document frequent neurovascular assessments of the restrained extremities to ensure adequate circulation. A patient who has undergone physical restraint should not be allowed to continue to struggle against the restraints (see "Chemical Restraint"). Struggling against restraints may lead to severe acidosis and fatal dysrhythmia. In general, for the safety of the patient and EMS personnel, physical restraints applied in the field should not be removed until the patient is reevaluated on arrival at the receiving hospital.

A restrained patient should never be transported in a prone position.

A patient should never be hobbled or "hog tied" with the arms and legs tied together behind the back.

Weapons used by law enforcement officers, including but not limited to pepper spray, mace defensive spray, stun guns, air tasers, stun batons, and telescoping steel batons, are *not* appropriate choices for patient restraint by EMS. They can exacerbate the patient's agitation and increase the risk of injury or death. While appropriately trained law enforcement officers may use these weapons, their use should be excluded from routine EMS protocols.

Chemical Restraint

Chemical restraint is defined as the administration of specific pharmacological agents to decrease agitation and increase the cooperation of patients who require medical care and transportation. EMS systems may use a variety of agents for chemical restraint of the agitated or combative patient. The goal is to subdue the patient's excessive agitation and his struggle against physical restraints. Ideally, this pharmacological sedation will change the patient's behavior without reaching the point of amnesia or altering the patient's level of consciousness.

Law enforcement weapons must never be used as a part of EMS patient restraint.

Butyrophenones (haloperidol, droperidol) and/or benzodiazepines (diazepam, midazolam, lorazepam) are the medications most commonly used for chemical restraint in emergency departments and in prehospital care. Other historical but less advisable medications include the barbiturates (pentothal), opioids (morphine), and phenothiazines (chlorpromazine).

Chemical restraint protocols often include a butyrophenone, a benzodiazepine, or a combination of both. Diazepam (Valium), lorazepam (Ativan), and midazolam (Versed) are the benzodiazepines that are most commonly used for patient restraint. Droperidol (Inapsine) and haloperidol (Haldol) are the butyrophenones that are commonly used. All five of these medications can be given intramuscularly or intravenously.

While several limited prehospital studies support the effectiveness of droperidol in decreasing the agitation of combative patients in the prehospital setting, the FDA has issued a warning of possible dysrhythmias associated with droperidol administration. Droperidol has been associated with

Procedure 38–1 Restraining a Patient

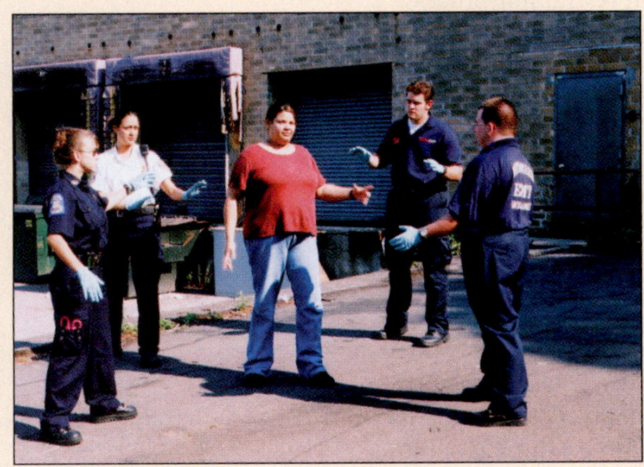

38-1a Plan your approach to the patient.

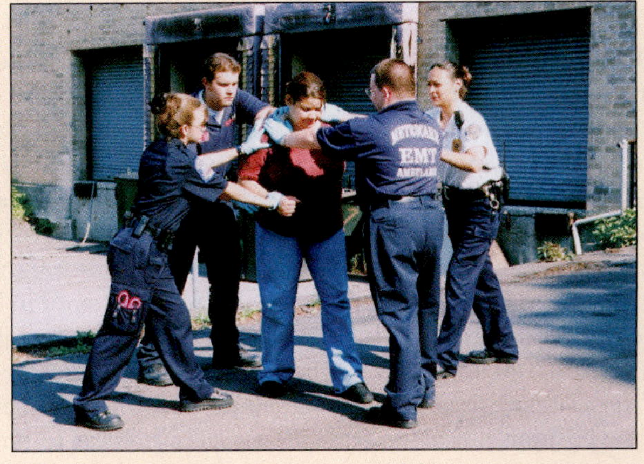

38-1b Assign one rescuer to each limb.

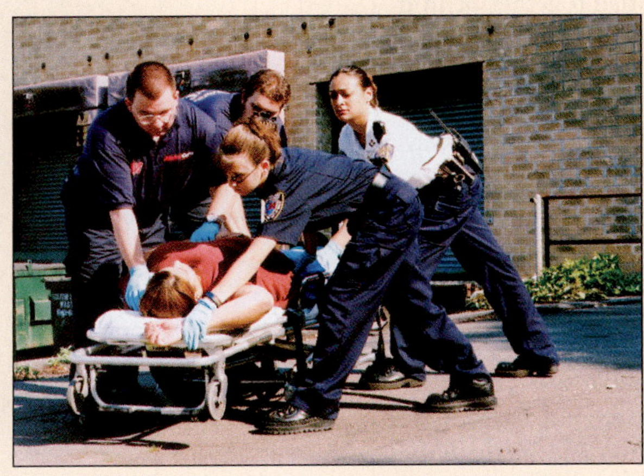

38-1c Place the patient supine on the stretcher.

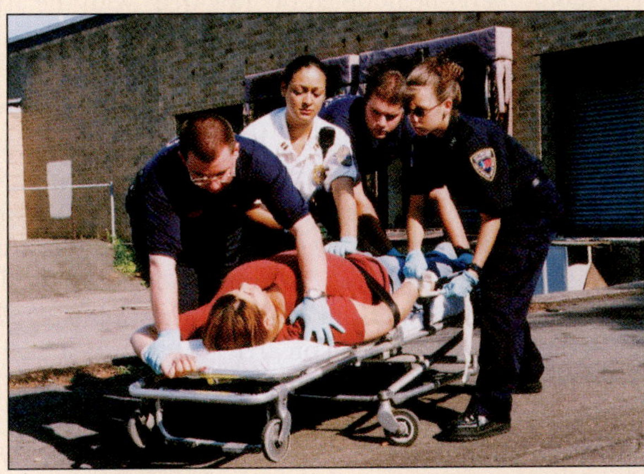

38-1d Use soft restraints to secure the patient to the stretcher.

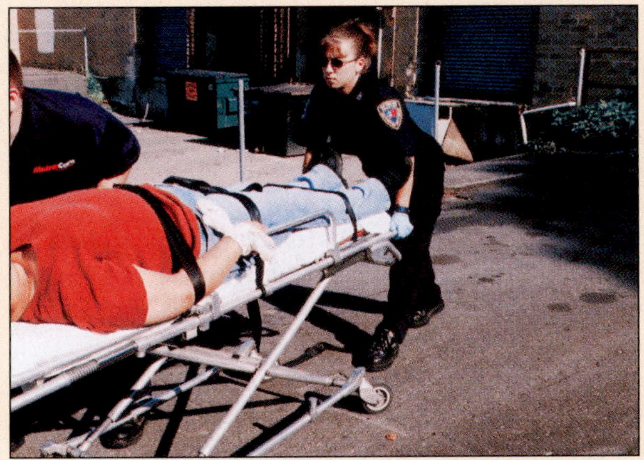

38-1e Assess distal circulation and continually monitor the airway and breathing.

Note: A fifth rescuer, if available, can control the patient's head—taking special care, however, not to be bitten.

(Photos © Craig Jackson/In the Dark Photography)

problems in patients who have a prolonged QT interval on their ECG. Because of this, many experts recommend obtaining a 12-lead ECG on patients prior to administering droperidol. This is not always practical in agitated or combative patients and this makes droperidol a less desirable agent for chemical restraint. Haloperidol and the benzodiazepines have been shown to be effective in the emergency department setting, and they are probably also effective in the prehospital environment.

Neuromuscular-blocking medications that are used with endotracheal intubation are never indicated to paralyze a patient solely for the purpose of restraining violent behavior. Only patients who have coexisting medical conditions—for example, severe head injury or respiratory failure—may benefit from paralysis and intubation. In all cases, the decision to paralyze a patient should be based on medical indications beyond violent or combative behavior.

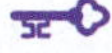

Neuromuscular-blocking medications with endotracheal intubation are never indicated to paralyze a patient solely for the purpose of restraining violent behavior.

When considering the use of chemical restraint, paramedics must weigh the risks of the patient struggling while physically restrained against the side-effect profile of the medications being considered for sedation of the agitated patient. At present, there is no consensus on the best medication or dosage for chemical restraint, and these decisions are best deferred to the individual EMS system and its medical director.

Summary

Calls involving psychiatric and behavioral emergencies will challenge your skills as a paramedic. Differentiating physiological and psychological conditions will try your diagnostic skills, and developing the interview abilities that form the basis of psychiatric assessment and care will test your people skills. Ultimately, you will be called on to help patients in a time of great need—the time of crisis. Once you determine that the patient is experiencing a purely behavioral emergency your compassion and communication skills rather than medications and procedures will benefit him most.

Emergency medical services providers routinely encounter patients who are violent or combative as a result of behavioral illness or a medical condition or trauma. Verbal, physical, and chemical restraint techniques provide effective ways of restraining patients who are a threat to themselves or others or who require medical assessment and treatment for a condition associated with combative or agitated behavior. Life-threatening adverse events have occurred in restrained individuals, but adherence to the principles of restraint presented in this chapter will minimize the occurrence of such adverse events. EMS personnel and their medical directors should ensure that their systems are prepared to treat violent or combative patients responsibly by providing appropriate training, policies, and protocols to deal with these situations.

Situations involving crisis can drain your emotions. Observing a suicide or attempted suicide or struggling with or restraining a patient can take its toll. Take care of yourself before, during, and after these calls.

Review Questions

1. ___________ is defined as a person's observable conduct and activity.
   a. Affect
   b. Conduct
   c. Behavior
   d. Personality
2. The general cause(s) of behavioral emergencies are:
   a. social.
   b. biological.
   c. psychosocial.
   d. all of the above

3. __________ causes of behavioral disorders are related to the patient's actions and interactions within society.
   a. Organic
   b. Personal
   c. Sociocultural
   d. Psychosocial
4. Visible indicators of mood describe a person's:
   a. fear.
   b. affect.
   c. posture.
   d. behavior.
5. The area within an approximately 3-foot radius around every person, which when encroached upon causes anxiety, is the:
   a. comfort zone.
   b. safety zone.
   c. personal space.
   d. private space.
6. Observing hygiene, clothing, and overall appearance describes which component of the MSE?
   a. orientation
   b. general appearance
   c. perceptual processes
   d. thought processes
7. Published by the American Psychiatric Association (APA), the __________ details diagnostic criteria for all currently defined psychiatric disorders, which are grouped according to the patient's signs and symptoms.
   a. *PDR*
   b. *CDC*
   c. *DSM-V*
   d. *DSM-IV*
8. Psychiatric disorders with organic causes such as brain injury or disease are known as __________ disorders.
   a. mood
   b. cognitive
   c. anxiety
   d. dissociative
9. Failure to recognize objects or stimuli despite intact sensory function describes:
   a. agnosia.
   b. aphasia.
   c. apraxia.
   d. dysphagia.
10. Feeling detached from oneself defines:
    a. fugue state.
    b. psychogenic amnesia.
    c. depersonalization.
    d. multiple personality disorder.

See Answers to Review Questions at the back of this book.

Gynecology

Objectives

After reading this chapter, you should be able to:

1. Review the anatomic structures and physiology of the female reproductive system. (see Chapter 3)
2. Identify the normal events of the menstrual cycle. (see Chapter 3)
3. Describe how to assess a patient with a gynecological complaint. (pp. 1510–1511)
4. Explain how to recognize a gynecological emergency. (pp. 1510–1511)
5. Describe the general care for any patient experiencing a gynecological emergency. (pp. 1512, 1514, 1515)
6. Describe the pathophysiology, assessment, and management of the following gynecological emergencies:
   - ★ Pelvic inflammatory disease (pp. 1512–1513)
   - ★ Ruptured ovarian cyst (p. 1513)
   - ★ Cystitis (p. 1513)
   - ★ Mittelschmerz (p. 1513)
   - ★ Endometritis (p. 1513)
   - ★ Endometriosis (pp. 1513–1514)
   - ★ Ectopic pregnancy (p. 1514)
   - ★ Vaginal hemorrhage (p. 1514)
7. Describe the assessment, care, and emotional support of the sexual assault patient. (pp. 1515–1516)
8. Given several preprogrammed gynecological patients, provide the appropriate assessment, management, and transportation. (pp. 1510–1516)

Key Terms

cystitis, p. 1513
dysmenorrhea, p. 1510
dyspareunia, p. 1510
dysuria, p. 1513
ectopic pregnancy, p. 1514
endometriosis, p. 1513
endometritis, p. 1513
gynecology, p. 1510
menorrhagia, p. 1514
miscarriage, p. 1513
mittelschmerz, p. 1513
obstetrics, p. 1510
pelvic inflammatory disease (PID), p. 1512

INTRODUCTION

gynecology *the branch of medicine that deals with the health maintenance and the diseases of women, primarily of the reproductive organs.*

obstetrics *the branch of medicine that deals with the care of women throughout pregnancy.*

Gynecology, derived from the Greek word *gynaik,* meaning "woman," is the branch of medicine that deals with the health maintenance and the diseases of women, primarily of their reproductive organs. **Obstetrics** is the branch of medicine that deals with the care of women throughout pregnancy. This chapter focuses on the assessment and care of nonpregnant patients with problems of the reproductive system. The assessment and care of the obstetrical patient is the subject of the next chapter.

ASSESSMENT OF THE GYNECOLOGICAL PATIENT

Content Review

Most Common Emergency Gynecological Complaints

- Abdominal pain
- Vaginal bleeding

Beyond labor and delivery, the most common emergency complaints of women in the childbearing years are abdominal pain and vaginal bleeding. Abdominal pain is often due to problems of the reproductive organs. In addition to the usual history and physical assessment activities, you will need to ask specific questions pertinent to reproductive function and dysfunction. However, do not allow yourself to get distracted from getting complete past medical histories including chronic medical problems, medications, and allergies.

You may feel uncomfortable asking a patient about her reproductive history, but remember that you are a health care professional who is trying to obtain pertinent information in order to provide the best possible care for your patient. If you conduct yourself in this manner, it should not be uncomfortable for you or your patient. Assess your patient's emotional state. If she is reluctant to discuss her complaint in detail, respect her wishes and transport her to the emergency department where a more thorough assessment can be done.

HISTORY

dysmenorrhea *painful menstruation.*

dyspareunia *painful sexual intercourse.*

Use the SAMPLE approach for obtaining additional information about the history of the present illness. If the chief complaint is pain, then use the mnemonic OPQRST–ASPN to gather more information. Is the patient's pain abdominal or in the pelvic region? Is it localized in a specific quadrant of the pelvis? Is she having her menstrual period? If so, how does the pain she is having now compare with how she usually feels? Some women have severe discomfort, called **dysmenorrhea** during their menstrual periods. Others may experience **dyspareunia,** painful sexual intercourse. Does walking or defecation aggravate her pain? What, if anything, alleviates her pain? Does positioning herself on her back or side with her knees bent relieve her discomfort?

You need to determine if there are any associated signs or symptoms that will be helpful in determining what is wrong with your patient. For instance, does your patient report a fever or chills? Is she reporting signs of gastrointestinal problems such as nausea, vomiting, diarrhea, or constipation? Is she complaining of urinary problems such as frequency, painful urination, or "colicky" urinary cramping? Does she report a vaginal discharge or bleeding? If so, obtain information about the color, amount, frequency, or odors associated with either vaginal bleeding or discharge. If she reports vaginal bleeding, how does the amount compare with the volume of her usual menstrual period? Does she report dizziness with changes in position (orthostatic hypotension), syncope, or diaphoresis?

You will need to obtain specific information about your patient's obstetric history. Has she ever been pregnant? *Gravida* (G) is the term used to describe the number of times a woman has been pregnant, including this one if she is pregnant. How many of those pregnancies ended in the delivery of a viable infant? *Para* or *parity* (P) refers to the number of deliveries. *Abortion* (A or AB) refers to any pregnancy that ends before 20 weeks of gestation, regardless of cause. You may see this information recorded in shorthand, for example, G_3 P_2 ($T_2P_0A_1L_2$). *T* refers to pregnancies that went to term. *P* refers to premature deliveries. *A* refers to abortions (therapeutic or miscarriage). *L* refers to live births. These terms refer to the number of pregnancies and deliveries, not the number of infants delivered, so even twins or triplets counts only as one pregnancy and one delivery.

You will also need to obtain a gynecological history. Question the patient about previous ectopic pregnancies, infections, cesarean sections, pelvic surgeries such as tubal ligation, abortions (either elective or therapeutic), and dilation and curettage (D&C) procedures. Also ask the patient about any prior history of trauma to the reproductive tract. It is often helpful to find out whether the patient, if sexually active, has had pain or bleeding during or after sexual intercourse.

In the female patient of child-bearing age, always document the LMP.

It is important to document the date of the patient's last menstrual period, commonly abbreviated LMP (or LNMP for "last normal menstrual period"). Ask whether the period was of a normal length and whether the flow was heavier or lighter than usual. An easy way for women to estimate menstrual flow is by the number of pads or tampons used. She can easily compare this number to her routine usage. It is also important to inquire how regular the patient's periods tend to be. Ask her what form of birth control, if any, she uses. Also, find out if she uses it regularly. Direct questions such as "Could you be pregnant?" are generally unlikely to get an accurate response. Indirect questioning is often more helpful in determining the likelihood of pregnancy, such as "When did your last menstrual period start?" If you suspect pregnancy, inquire about other signs, including a late or missed period, breast tenderness, bloating, urinary frequency, or nausea and vomiting. Until proven otherwise, you should assume that any missed or late period is due to pregnancy even though your patient may deny it.

Any patient of reproductive age who still has her uterus should be considered to be pregnant until proven otherwise.

Contraception, or the prevention of pregnancy, takes many forms. Remember that many contraceptives are medications, so ask about their use. With the exception of oral contraceptives ("the pill") and intrauterine devices (IUDs), side effects caused by contraceptives are relatively rare. Oral contraceptives have been associated with hypertension, rare incidents of stroke and heart attack, and possibly pulmonary embolism. IUDs can cause perforation of the uterus, uterine infection, or irregular uterine bleeding. This is especially true for IUDs that have remained in place longer than the time recommended by the manufacturer, which rarely exceeds 2 years.

PHYSICAL EXAM

Physical examination of the gynecological patient is limited in the field. More than at any other time, the patient's comfort level should guide your actions. Respect your patient's modesty and maintain her privacy. This may mean that you need to exclude parents from the room when assessing adolescent patients or that you need to exclude spouses of married patients. Recognizing that most people are not comfortable discussing matters related to sexuality or reproductive organs, take your cues from the patient. Maintain a professional demeanor. Explain all procedures thoroughly so that your patient can understand them prior to initiating any care. Some women may feel more comfortable if they can be cared for by a female paramedic.

As always, the level of consciousness is the best indicator of your patient's status. Assess your patient's general appearance, paying particular attention to the color of her skin and mucous membranes. Cyanosis and pallor may indicate shock or a gas-exchange problem, while a flushed appearance is more indicative of fever.

Remember that vital signs are useful clues to the nature of your patient's problem. Pain and fever tend to cause an increase in pulse and respiratory rates along with a slight increase in blood pressure. Significant bleeding will cause increased pulse and respiratory rates as well as narrowing pulse pressures (the difference between systolic and diastolic pressures). Perform a tilt test to assess for orthostatic changes in her vital signs (a decrease in blood pressure and an increase in pulse rate when the patient rises from a supine or seated position), which again points to significant blood loss.

Assess your patient for evidence of vaginal bleeding or discharge. If possible, estimate blood loss. The use of more than two sanitary pads per hour is considered significant bleeding. If serious bleeding is reported or evident, it may be necessary to inspect the patient's perineum. Document the color and character of the discharge, as well as the amount, and the presence or absence of clots. *Do not perform an internal vaginal exam in the field.*

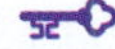

Do not perform an internal vaginal exam in the field.

Pay particular attention to the abdominal examination. Auscultate the abdomen and note whether bowel sounds are absent or hyperactive. Gently palpate the abdomen. Document and report any masses, distention, guarding, localized tenderness, or rebound tenderness. In thin patients, a palpable mass in the lower abdomen may be an intrauterine pregnancy. At 3 months, the uterus is barely palpable above the symphysis pubis. At 4 months, the uterus is palpable midway between the umbilicus and the symphysis pubis. At 5 months (approximately 20 weeks), the uterus is palpable at the level of the umbilicus.

MANAGEMENT OF GYNECOLOGICAL EMERGENCIES

General management of gynecological emergencies is focused on supportive care.

In general, the management of the patient experiencing a gynecological emergency is focused on supportive care. Rely on your primary assessment to guide your decision making about the need for oxygen therapy or intravenous access. If your patient's status warrants it, administer oxygen or assist ventilation as necessary. As a rule, intravenous access and fluid replacement is usually not indicated. However, if your patient has excessive bleeding or demonstrates signs of shock, then establish at least one large-bore IV and administer normal saline at a rate indicated by the patient's presentation. You may also want to initiate cardiac monitoring if your patient is unstable.

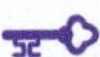

Do not pack dressings in the vagina.

Continue to monitor and evaluate serious bleeding. *Do not pack dressings in the vagina.* Discourage the use of tampons to absorb blood flow. If your patient is bleeding heavily, count and document the number of sanitary pads used. If your patient demonstrates signs of impending shock, you may elect to place her in the Trendelenburg position (head lower than feet). The use of a pneumatic anti-shock garment in this situation should be governed by your local protocol. If shock is not a consideration, then position your patient for comfort in the left lateral recumbent position or supine with her knees bent, as this decreases tension on the peritoneum. Analgesics (pain-control medications) are not usually given in the field for gynecological complaints because these drugs tend to mask signs and symptoms of a deteriorating condition and make assessment and diagnosis difficult.

Since it is not appropriate to perform an internal vaginal exam in the field, most patients with gynecological complaints will be transported to be evaluated by a physician. Some problems may require surgical intervention, so you should consider emergency transport to the appropriate facility based on your local protocols.

Psychological support is particularly important when caring for patients with gynecological complaints. Keep calm. Maintain your patient's modesty and privacy. Remember that this is likely to be a very stressful situation for your patient, and she will appreciate your gentle, considerate care.

SPECIFIC GYNECOLOGICAL EMERGENCIES

Gynecological emergencies can be generally divided into two categories—medical and traumatic.

MEDICAL GYNECOLOGICAL EMERGENCIES

Gynecological emergencies of a medical nature are often hard to diagnose in the field. The most common symptoms of a medical gynecological emergency are abdominal pain and/or vaginal bleeding.

Gynecological Abdominal Pain

pelvic inflammatory disease (PID) *an acute infection of the reproductive organs that can be caused by a bacteria, virus, or fungus.*

Pelvic Inflammatory Disease Probably the most common cause of nontraumatic abdominal pain is **pelvic inflammatory disease (PID),** an infection of the female reproductive tract that can be caused by a bacterium, virus, or fungus. The organs most commonly involved are the uterus, fallopian tubes, and ovaries. Occasionally the adjoining structures, such as the peritoneum and intestines, become involved. PID is the most common cause of abdominal pain in women in the childbearing years, occurring in 1 percent of that population. The highest rate of infection occurs in sexually active women ages 15 to 24. The most common causes of PID are gonorrhea (*Neisseria gonorrhoeae*) or chlamydia (*Chlamydia trachomatis*), although rarely streptococcus or staphylococcus bacteria may cause it. Commonly, gonorrhea or chlamydia progresses undetected in a female until frank PID develops.

PID is a major risk factor for pelvic adhesions.

Predisposing factors include multiple sexual partners, prior history of PID, recent gynecological procedure, or an IUD. Postinfection damage to the fallopian tubes is a common cause for infertility. PID may be either acute or chronic. If it is allowed to progress untreated, sepsis may develop. Additionally, PID may cause adhesions, in which the pelvic organs "stick together." Adhesions are a common cause of chronic pelvic pain and increase the frequency of infertility and ectopic pregnancies.

While it is possible for a patient with pelvic inflammatory disease to be asymptomatic, most patients with PID complain of abdominal pain. It is often diffuse and located in the lower abdomen.

It may be moderate to severe, which occasionally makes it difficult to distinguish it from appendicitis. Pain may intensify either before or after the menstrual period. It may also worsen during sexual intercourse, as movement of the cervix tends to cause increased discomfort. Patients with PID tend to walk with a shuffling gait, since walking often intensifies their pain. In severe cases, fever, chills, nausea, vomiting, or even sepsis may accompany PID. Occasionally, patients have a foul-smelling vaginal discharge, often yellow in color, as well as irregular menses. It is common also to have midcycle bleeding.

Generally, on physical examination, the patient with PID appears acutely ill or toxic. The blood pressure is normal, although the pulse rate may be slightly increased. Fever may or may not be present. Palpation of the lower abdomen generally elicits moderate to severe pain. Occasionally, in severe cases, the abdomen will be tense with obvious rebound tenderness. Such cases may be impossible to distinguish from appendicitis in the prehospital setting.

The primary treatment for PID is antibiotics, often administered intravenously over an extended period. Once the causative organism is determined, the sexual partner may also require treatment. In the field, the primary goal is to make the patient as comfortable as possible. Place the patient on the ambulance stretcher in the position in which she is most comfortable. She may wish to draw her knees up toward her chest, as this decreases tension on the peritoneum. *Do not perform a vaginal examination.* If your patient has signs of sepsis, administer oxygen and establish intravenous access.

Ruptured Ovarian Cyst *Cysts* are fluid-filled pockets. When they develop in the ovary, they can rupture and be a source of abdominal pain. When an egg is released from the ovary, a cyst, known as a corpus luteum cyst, is often left in its place. Occasionally, cysts develop independent of ovulation. When the cysts rupture, a small amount of blood is spilled into the abdomen. Because blood irritates the peritoneum, it can cause abdominal pain and rebound tenderness. Ovarian cysts may be found during a routine pelvic examination. However, in the field setting, your patient is likely to complain of moderate to severe unilateral abdominal pain, which may radiate to her back. She may also report a history of dyspareunia, irregular bleeding, or a delayed menstrual period. It is not uncommon for patients to rupture ovarian cysts during intercourse or physical activity. This often results in immediate, severe abdominal pain causing the patient to immediately stop intercourse or other physical activity. Ruptured ovarian cysts may be associated with vaginal bleeding.

Cystitis Urinary bladder infection, or **cystitis,** is a common cause of abdominal pain. Bacteria usually enter the urinary tract via the urethra, ascending into the bladder and ureters. The bladder lies anterior to the reproductive organs and, when inflamed, causes pain, generally immediately above the symphysis pubis. If untreated, the infection can progress to the kidneys. In addition to abdominal pain, your patient may report urinary frequency, pain or burning with urination (**dysuria**), and a low-grade fever. Occasionally the urine may be blood tinged.

cystitis *infection of the urinary bladder.*

dysuria *painful urination often associated with cystitis.*

Mittelschmerz Occasionally, ovulation is accompanied by midcycle abdominal pain known as **mittelschmerz.** It is thought that the pain is related to peritoneal irritation due to follicle rupture or bleeding at the time of ovulation. The unilateral lower quadrant pain is usually self-limited and may be accompanied by midcycle spotting. While some women may report a low-grade fever, it should be noted that body temperature normally increases at the time of ovulation and remains elevated until the day prior to the onset of the menstrual period. Treatment is symptomatic.

mittelschmerz *abdominal pain associated with ovulation.*

Endometritis An infection of the uterine lining called **endometritis** is an occasional complication of **miscarriage,** childbirth, or gynecological procedures such as dilatation and curettage (D&C). Commonly reported signs and symptoms include mild to severe lower abdominal pain; a bloody, foul-smelling discharge; and fever (101° to 104°F). The onset of symptoms is usually 48 to 72 hours after the gynecological procedure or miscarriage. These infections often mimic the presentation of PID and can be quite serious if not quickly treated with the appropriate antibiotics. Complications of endometritis may include sterility, sepsis, or even death.

endometritis *infection of the endometrium.*

miscarriage *commonly used term to describe a pregnancy which ends before 20 weeks' gestation; may also be called spontaneous abortion.*

Endometriosis **Endometriosis** is a condition in which endometrial tissue is found outside of the uterus. Most commonly it is found in the abdomen and pelvis, although it has been found

endometriosis *condition in which endometrial tissue grows outside of the uterus.*

virtually everywhere in the body, including the central nervous system and lungs. Regardless of its site, the tissue responds to the hormonal changes associated with the menstrual cycle and thus bleeds in a cyclic manner. This bleeding causes inflammation, scarring of adjacent tissues, and the subsequent development of adhesions, particularly in the pelvic cavity.

Endometriosis is usually seen in women between the ages of 30 to 40 and is rarely seen in postmenopausal women. The exact cause is unknown. The most common symptom is dull, cramping pelvic pain that is usually related to menstruation. Dyspareunia and abnormal uterine bleeding are also commonly reported. Painful bowel movements have also been reported when the endometrial tissue has invaded the gastrointestinal tract. It is not uncommon for endometriosis to be diagnosed when the patient is being evaluated for infertility. Definitive treatment may include medical management with hormones, analgesics, and anti-inflammatory drugs, and/or surgery to remove the excessive endometrial tissue or adhesions from other organs.

ectopic pregnancy *the implantation of a developing fetus outside of the uterus, often in a fallopian tube.*

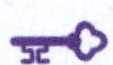

Ectopic pregnancy is a life-threatening condition.

Ectopic Pregnancy An **ectopic pregnancy** is the implantation of a fetus outside of the uterus. The most common site is within the fallopian tubes. This is a surgical emergency, because the tube can rupture, triggering a massive hemorrhage. Patients with ectopic pregnancy often have severe unilateral abdominal pain which may radiate to the shoulder on the affected side, a late or missed menstrual period, and, occasionally, vaginal bleeding. Additional discussion of ectopic pregnancy is presented in the next chapter.

Content Review

Treatment for Abdominal Pain

- Make the patient comfortable.
- Transport the patient.

Management of Gynecological Abdominal Pain

Any woman with significant abdominal pain should be treated and transported to the hospital for evaluation. Administer oxygen and establish intravenous access, if indicated. Refer to the earlier section on management of gynecological emergencies for additional information.

Nontraumatic Vaginal Bleeding

menorrhagia *excessive menstrual flow.*

The most common cause of nontraumatic vaginal bleeding is spontaneous abortion (miscarriage).

Nontraumatic vaginal bleeding is rarely seen in the field unless it is severe. Refer to the earlier section in this chapter on completing a patient history. You should not presume that vaginal bleeding is due to normal menstruation. Occasionally a woman will experience **menorrhagia,** or excessive menstrual flow, but it is rarely the cause for a 911 call. Hemorrhage, regardless of cause, is always potentially life threatening, so be alert for signs of impending shock.

The most common cause of nontraumatic vaginal bleeding is a spontaneous abortion (miscarriage). If it has been more than 60 days since your patient's LMP, you should assume that this is the cause. Vaginal bleeding due to miscarriage is often associated with cramping abdominal pain and the passage of clots and tissue. The loss of a pregnancy, even at a very early phase, is a significant emotional event for your patient, so your kind and considerate care is important. Spontaneous abortion and other causes of bleeding in the obstetric patient will be discussed further in the next chapter. Other potential causes of vaginal bleeding include cancerous lesions, PID, or the onset of labor.

Content Review

Treatment for Vaginal Bleeding

- Absorb blood flow, but do not pack the vagina.
- Transport the patient.
- Initiate oxygen therapy and IV access based on the patient's condition.

Management of Nontraumatic Vaginal Bleeding

Your field management of patients suffering nontraumatic vaginal bleeding will depend on the severity of the situation and your assessment of the patient's status. Absorb the blood flow. *Do not pack the vagina.* If your patient is passing clots or tissue, save these for evaluation by a physician. Transport your patient in a position of comfort. The initiation of oxygen therapy and intravenous access should be guided by the patient's condition.

TRAUMATIC GYNECOLOGICAL EMERGENCIES

Most cases of vaginal bleeding result from obstetrical problems or are related to the menstrual period. However, trauma to the vagina and perineum can also cause bleeding and abdominal pain.

Causes of Gynecological Trauma

The incidence of genital trauma is increasing, with vaginal injury occurring far more commonly than male genital injury. Gynecological trauma may occur at any age. Blunt trauma occurs more frequently than penetrating trauma. Straddle injury (such as may occur with riding a bicycle) is the most common form of blunt trauma. Vaginal injuries are most often lacerations due to sexual assault. Other causes of gynecological trauma include blunt force to the lower abdomen due to assault or seatbelt injuries, direct blows to the perineal area, foreign bodies inserted into the vagina, self-attempts at abortion, and lacerations following childbirth.

Management of Gynecological Trauma

Injuries to the external genitalia should be managed by direct pressure over the laceration or a chemical cold pack applied to a hematoma. In most cases of vaginal bleeding, the source is not readily apparent. If bleeding is severe or your patient demonstrates signs of shock, establish IV access to maintain intravascular volume and monitor vital signs closely. Blunt force may cause organ rupture leading to the development of peritonitis or sepsis. *Never* pack the vagina with any material or dressing, regardless of the severity of the bleeding. Expedite transport to the emergency department since surgical intervention is often required.

Sexual Assault

Sexual assault continues to represent the most rapidly growing violent crime in America. Over 700,000 women are sexually assaulted annually. Unfortunately, it is estimated that more than 60 percent of all sexual assaults are never reported to authorities. Male victims represent 5 percent of reported sexual assaults. Sexual abuse of children is reported even less frequently. It is estimated that the incidence of sexual abuse in children ranges from 50,000 to 350,000/year. There is no "typical victim" of sexual assault. Nobody, from small children to aged adults, is immune.

Most victims of sexual assault know their assailants. Friends, acquaintances, intimates, and family members commit the vast majority (80 percent) of sexual assaults against women. Acquaintance rape is particularly common among adolescent victims. Sexual assault is a crime of violence, not passion, that is motivated by aggression and a need to control, humiliate, or inflict pain. There are very few predictors of who is capable of committing sexual assault, as age, economic status, and ethnic origins vary widely. Common behavioral characteristics found among rapists include poor impulse control, the need to achieve sexual satisfaction within the context of violence, and immaturity.

The definition of sexual assault varies from state to state. The common element of any definition is sexual contact without consent. Generally, rape is defined as penetration of the vagina or rectum of an unwilling female or the rectum in an unwilling male. In most states, penetration must occur for an act to be classified as rape. Sexual assault also includes oral-genital sex. Regardless of the legal definition, sexual assault is a crime of violence with serious physical and psychological implications.

Assessment The victim of sexual assault is a unique patient with unique needs. Your patient needs emergency medical treatment and psychological support. Your patient also needs to have legal evidence gathered. *Your* objectivity is essential, as your attitude may affect long-term psychological recovery. As a rule, victims of sexual abuse *should not* be questioned about the incident in the field. Do not ask questions about specific details of the assault. It is not important, from the standpoint of prehospital care, to determine whether penetration took place. Do not inquire about the patient's sexual practices. Confine your questions to the physical injuries the patient received. Even well-intentioned questions may lead to guilt feelings in the patient.

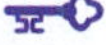

Do not ask about specific details of a sexual assault.

The psychological response of sexual assault victims is widely variable. The victim of sexual assault may be withdrawn or hysterical. Some use denial, anger, or fear as defense mechanisms. Approach the patient calmly and professionally. Allay the patient's fear and anxiety. Respond to the patient's feelings but be aware of your own. If the patient is incompletely dressed, a cover should be offered. Respect the patient's modesty. Explain all procedures and obtain the patient's permission before beginning them. Avoid touching the patient other than to take vital signs or examine other physical injuries. *Do not* examine the genitalia unless there is life-threatening hemorrhage.

Do not examine the external genitalia of a sexual assault victim unless there is a life-threatening hemorrhage.

Management In most situations, psychological and emotional support is the most important help you can offer. Maintain a nonjudgmental attitude and assure the patient of confidentiality. If the patient is female, allow her to be cared for by a female EMT or paramedic (if available). If the patient desires, have a female accompany her to the hospital (Figure 39-1 ■). Provide a safe environment, such as the back of a well-lit ambulance. Respond to the patient's feelings and respect the patient's wishes. Unless your patient is unconscious, do not touch the patient unless given

Psychological and emotional support are the most important elements of care for the sexual assault victim.

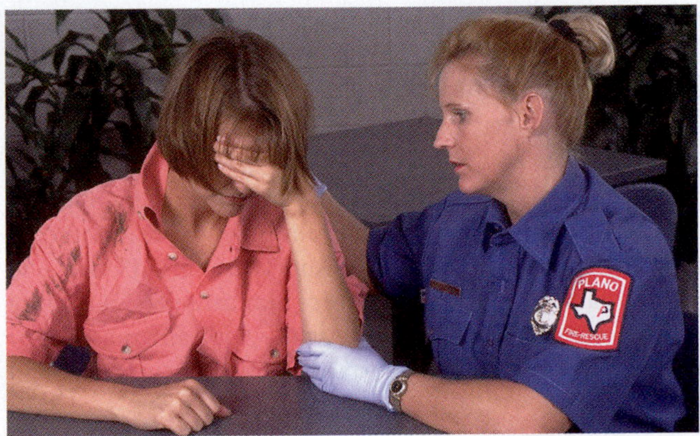

■ **Figure 39-1** If possible, have a female EMT or paramedic accompany the sexual assault victim to the hospital.

permission. Even when your patient appears to have an altered level of consciousness, explain what's going to be done before initiating any treatment.

Preservation of physical evidence is important. When the patient arrives at the hospital, a physician or sexual assault nurse examiner will complete a sexual assault examination to gather physical evidence. To protect this evidence, it is important that you adhere to the following guidelines:

- ★ Consider the patient a crime scene and protect that scene.
- ★ Handle clothing as little as possible, if at all.
- ★ If you must remove clothing, separately bag each item.
- ★ Do not cut through any tears or holes in the clothing.
- ★ Place bloody articles in brown paper bags.
- ★ Do not examine the perineal area.
- ★ If the assault took place within the hour or the patient is bleeding, put an absorbent underpad (e.g., Chux) under the patient's hips to collect that evidence.
- ★ If you cover the patient with a sheet or blanket, turn that over to the hospital as evidence.
- ★ Do not allow patients to change their clothes, bathe, or douche (if female) before the medical examination.
- ★ Do not allow patients to comb their hair, brush their teeth, or clean their fingernails.
- ★ Do not clean wounds, if at all possible.
- ★ If you must initiate care on scene, avoid disruption of the crime scene.

Documentation When completing your patient care report, keep the following documentation guidelines in mind:

- ★ State patient remarks accurately.
- ★ Objectively state your observations of the patient's physical condition, environment, or torn clothing.
- ★ Document any evidence (e.g., clothing, sheets) turned over to the hospital staff and the name of the individual to whom you gave it.
- ★ Do NOT include your opinions as to whether rape occurred.

Summary

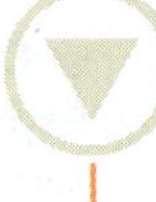

Most gynecological emergency patients have either abdominal pain or vaginal bleeding. The patient with abdominal pain should be made comfortable and transported to the emergency department. The management of vaginal bleeding depends on the severity. Minor bleeding should be simply monitored. Severe bleeding should be treated with IV fluids, if indicated.

In the case of sexual assault, first determine if any life-threatening physical injuries exist. Second, respect the patient's wishes and offer emotional support. Third, in treating victims of sexual assault, make every effort to preserve physical evidence. As with any type of emergency care, the primary concern is the patient.

Review Questions

1. Painful menstruation is known as:
   a. dysmenorrhea.
   b. dyspareunia.
   c. dysuria.
   d. menorrhagia.
2. In the female patient of childbearing age, it is important to document the LMP. LMP stands for:
   a. late menstrual period.
   b. last menstrual period.
   c. latent menstrual period.
   d. longest menstrual period.
3. ___________ is thought to be the most common cause of nontraumatic abdominal pain.
   a. Endometriosis
   b. Ectopic pregnancy
   c. Ruptured ovarian cyst
   d. Pelvic inflammatory disease
4. Abdominal pain associated with ovulation is called:
   a. dysuria.
   b. endometritis.
   c. mittelschmerz.
   d. endometriosis.
5. A condition in which endometrial tissue is found outside of the uterus is:
   a. endometritis.
   b. endometriosis.
   c. ectopic pregnancy.
   d. pelvic inflammatory disease.
6. The most common cause of nontraumatic vaginal bleeding is:
   a. pelvic inflammatory disease.
   b. the onset of labor.
   c. spontaneous abortion.
   d. cancerous lesions.
7. ___________ is a life-threatening condition.
   a. Menorrhagia
   b. Endometritis
   c. Endometriosis
   d. Ectopic pregnancy
8. In the case of sexual assault, the paramedic should:
   a. determine if any life-threatening physical injuries exist.
   b. respect the patient's wishes and offer emotional support.
   c. make every effort to preserve physical evidence.
   d. do all of the above.

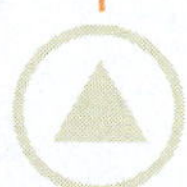

See Answers to Review Questions at the back of this book.

Chapter

40

Obstetrics

Objectives

After reading this chapter, you should be able to:

1. Describe the anatomic structures and physiology of the reproductive system during pregnancy. (pp. 1519–1522)
2. Identify the normal events of pregnancy. (pp. 1522–1525)
3. Describe how to assess an obstetrical patient. (pp. 1525–1527)
4. Identify the stages of labor and the paramedic's role in each stage. (pp. 1537–1539)
5. Differentiate between normal and abnormal delivery. (pp. 1544–1549)
6. Identify and describe complications associated with pregnancy and delivery. (pp. 1527–1537, 1549–1550)
7. Identify predelivery emergencies. (pp. 1527–1537)
8. State indications of an imminent delivery. (pp. 1538–1539)
9. Identify the contents of an obstetrical kit and explain the use of each item. (pp. 1539–1542)
10. Differentiate the management of a patient with predelivery emergencies from a normal delivery. (p. 1527)
11. State the steps in the predelivery preparation of the mother. (pp. 1538–1539)
12. Establish the relationship between Standard Precautions and childbirth. (p. 1539)
13. State the steps to assist in the delivery of a newborn. (pp. 1539–1542)
14. Describe how to care for the newborn. (pp. 1542–1544)
15. Describe how and when to cut the umbilical cord. (p. 1542)
16. Discuss the steps in the delivery of the placenta. (pp. 1541, 1542)
17. Describe the management of the mother postdelivery. (pp. 1542, 1549–1550)
18. Summarize neonatal resuscitation procedures. (pp. 1543–1544)
19. Describe the procedures for handling abnormal deliveries, complications of pregnancy, and maternal complications of labor. (pp. 1527–1537, 1544–1550)
20. Describe special considerations when meconium is present in amniotic fluid or during delivery. (p. 1549)
21. Describe special considerations of a premature baby. (pp. 1536–1537)
22. Given several simulated delivery situations, provide the appropriate assessment, management, and transport for the mother and child. (pp. 1519–1550)

Key Terms

abortion, p. 1528
afterbirth, p. 1519
amniotic fluid, p. 1521
amniotic sac, p. 1521
crowning, p. 1527
effacement, p. 1536
estimated date of confinement (EDC), p. 1522
labor, p. 1537
neonate, p. 1542
ovulation, p. 1519
placenta, p. 1519
puerperium, p. 1537
tocolysis, p. 1537
umbilical cord, p. 1520

INTRODUCTION

Pregnancy, childbirth, and the potential complications of each are the focus of this chapter. Pregnancy is a normal, natural process of life that results from ovulation and fertilization. Complications of pregnancy are uncommon, but when they do occur, you must be prepared to recognize them quickly and manage them. Childbirth occurs daily, usually requiring only the most basic assistance. This chapter will prepare you to assess and care for the female patient throughout her pregnancy and the delivery of her child.

THE PRENATAL PERIOD

The *prenatal period* (literally "prebirth period") is the time from conception until delivery of the fetus. During this period, fetal development takes place. In addition, significant physiological changes occur in the mother.

ANATOMY AND PHYSIOLOGY OF THE OBSTETRIC PATIENT

As you learned in the previous chapter, the first 2 weeks of the menstrual cycle are dominated by the hormone estrogen, which causes the endometrium (the inner lining of the uterus) to thicken and become engorged with blood. In response to a surge of luteinizing hormone (LH) and follicle-stimulating hormone (FSH), **ovulation,** or release of an egg (ovum) from the ovary, takes place. The egg travels down the fallopian tube to the uterus. If the egg has been fertilized, it becomes implanted in the uterus and pregnancy begins. If the egg has not been fertilized, menstruation (discharge of blood, mucus, and cellular debris from the endometrium) takes place 14 days after ovulation. (The time from ovulation to menstruation is always exactly 14 days. However, the time from menstruation to the next ovulation may vary by several days from the average of 14 days, which is why it can be difficult for couples to find the optimum time of the month to conceive, or to avoid conceiving, a baby.)

ovulation *the release of an egg from the ovary.*

If the woman has had intercourse within 24 to 48 hours before ovulation, fertilization may occur. The male's seminal fluid carrying numerous spermatozoa, or male sex cells, enters the vagina and uterus and travels toward the fallopian tubes. Fertilization, which usually takes place in the distal third of the fallopian tube, occurs when a male spermatozoan fuses with the female ovum (Figure 40-1 ■). After fertilization, the ovum begins cellular division immediately, which continues as it moves through the fallopian tube to the uterus. The ovum then becomes a *blastocyst* (a hollow ball of cells). The blastocyst normally implants in the thickened uterine lining, which has been prepared for implantation by the hormone progesterone, where the fetus and placenta subsequently develop.

Approximately 3 weeks after fertilization, the placenta develops on the uterine wall at the site where the blastocyst attached (Figure 40-2 ■). The **placenta,** known as the "organ of pregnancy," is a temporary, blood-rich structure that serves as the lifeline for the developing fetus. It transfers heat while exchanging oxygen and carbon dioxide; delivering nutrients such as glucose, potassium, sodium, and chloride; and carrying away wastes such as urea, uric acid, and creatinine. The placenta also serves as an endocrine gland throughout pregnancy, secreting hormones necessary for fetal survival as well as the estrogen and progesterone required to maintain the pregnancy. Additionally, the placenta serves as a protective barrier against harmful substances. (However, some drugs such as narcotics, steroids, and some antibiotics are able to cross the placental membrane from the mother to the fetus.) When expelled from the uterus following birth of the child, the placenta and accompanying membranes are called the **afterbirth.**

placenta *the organ that serves as a lifeline for the developing fetus. The placenta is attached to the wall of the uterus and the umbilical cord.*

afterbirth *the placenta and accompanying membranes that are expelled from the uterus after the birth of a child.*

Figure 40-1 Fertilization and implantation of the ovum.

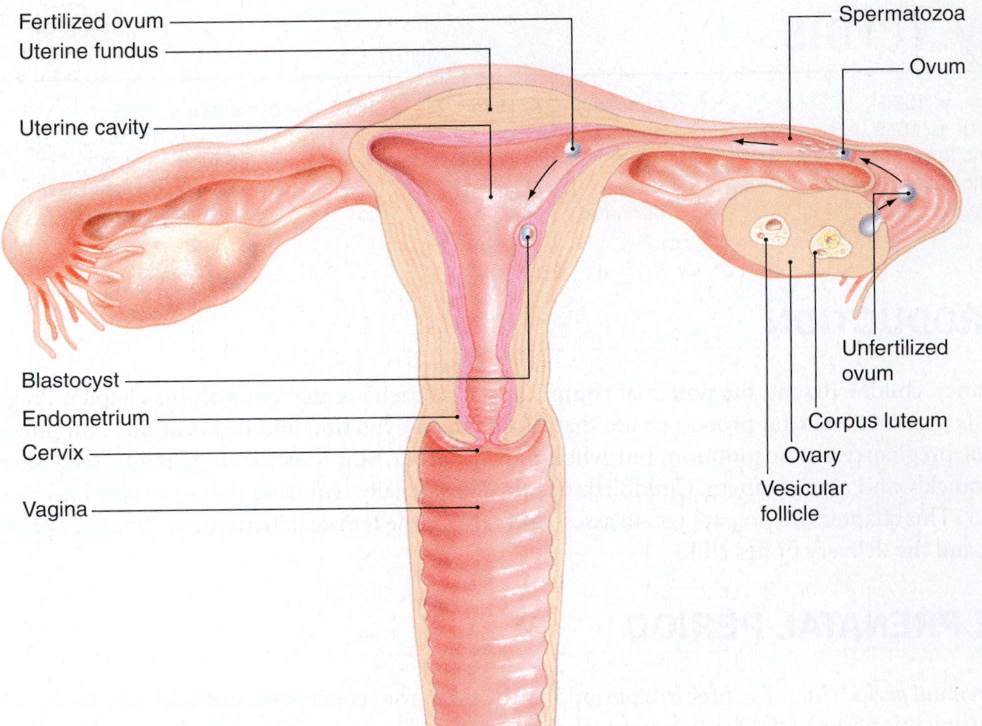

umbilical cord *structure containing two arteries and one vein that connects the placenta and the fetus.*

The placenta is connected to the fetus by the **umbilical cord,** a flexible, ropelike structure approximately 2 feet in length and 0.75 inch in diameter. Normally, the umbilical cord contains two arteries and one vein. The umbilical vein transports oxygenated blood to the fetus, while the umbilical arteries return relatively deoxygenated blood to the placenta.

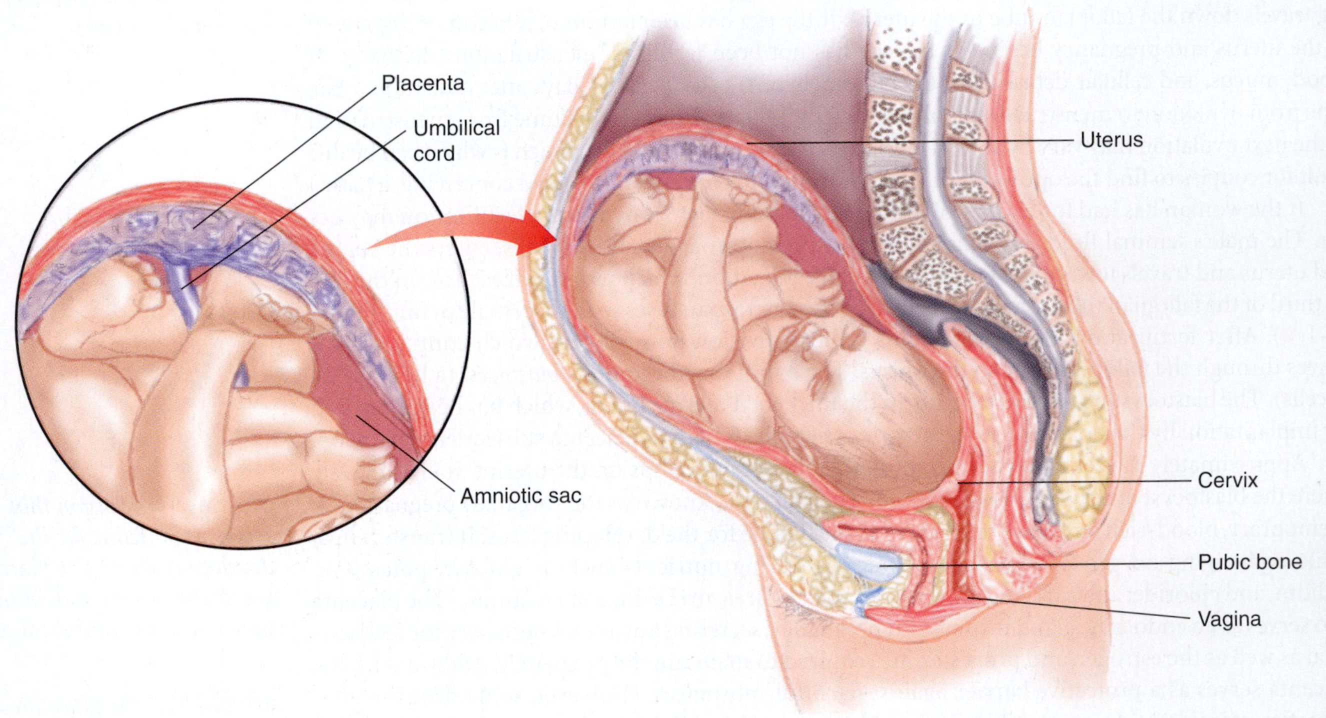

Figure 40-2 Anatomy of the placenta.

The fetus develops within the **amniotic sac,** sometimes called the "bag of waters" (BOW). This thin-walled membranous covering holds the **amniotic fluid** that surrounds and protects the fetus during intrauterine development. The amniotic fluid increases in volume throughout the course of the pregnancy. After the 20th week of gestation, the volume varies from 500 to 1,000 cc. The presence of amniotic fluid allows for fetal movement within the uterus and serves to cushion and protect the fetus from trauma. The volume changes constantly as amniotic fluid moves back and forth across the placental membrane. During the latter part of the pregnancy, the fetus contributes to the volume by secretions from the lungs and urination. Although it may rupture earlier, the amniotic sac usually breaks during labor, and the amniotic fluid or "water" flows out of the vagina. This is called *rupture of the membranes (ROM)*. It is what has happened when the pregnant woman says, "My water has broken."

amniotic sac *the membranes that surround and protect the developing fetus throughout the period of intrauterine development.*

amniotic fluid *clear, watery fluid that surrounds and protects the developing fetus.*

Physiologic Changes of Pregnancy

The physiologic changes associated with pregnancy are due to an altered hormonal state, the mechanical effects of the enlarging uterus and its significant vascularity, and the increasing metabolic demands on the maternal system. It is important for you to understand the physiologic changes associated with pregnancy so that you can better assess your pregnant patients.

Reproductive System It is understandable that the most significant pregnancy-related changes occur in the uterus. In its nonpregnant state, the uterus is a small pear-shaped organ weighing about 60 g (2 oz) with a capacity of approximately 10 cc. By the end of pregnancy, its weight has increased to 1,000 g (slightly more than 2 pounds) while its capacity is now approximately 5,000 mL (Figure 40-3 ■). Another notable change is that during pregnancy the vascular system of the uterus contains about one-sixth (16 percent) of the mother's total blood volume.

Other changes include the formation of a mucous plug in the cervix that protects the developing fetus and helps to prevent infection. This plug will be expelled when cervical dilatation begins prior to delivery. Estrogen causes the vaginal mucosa to thicken, vaginal secretions to increase, and the connective tissue to loosen to allow for delivery. The breasts enlarge and become more nodular as the mammary glands increase in number and size in preparation for lactation.

Respiratory System As maternal oxygen demands increase, progesterone causes a decrease in airway resistance. This results in a 20 percent increase in oxygen consumption and a 40 percent

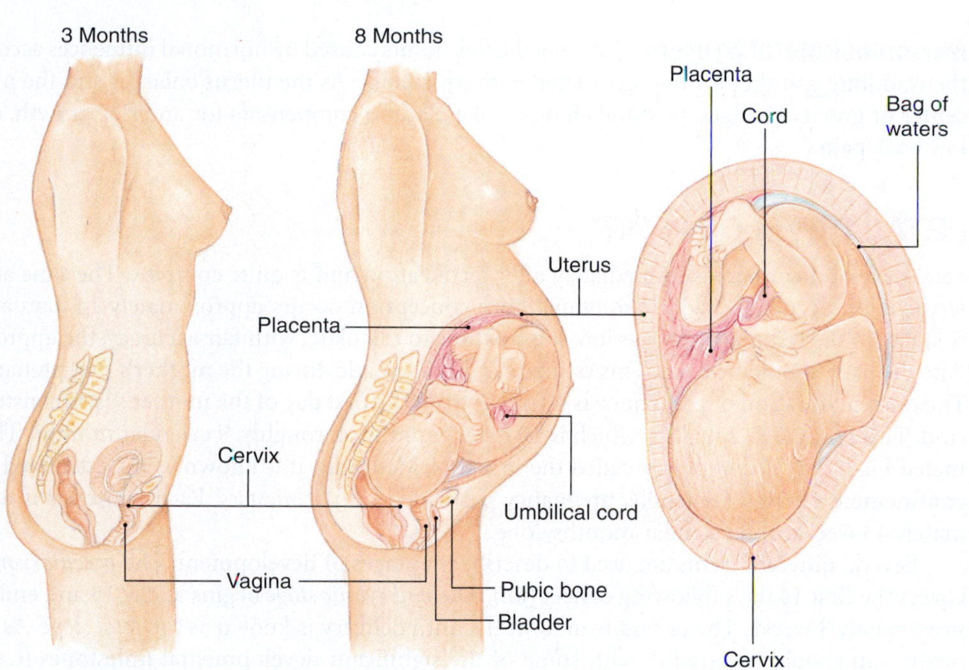

■ **Figure 40-3** Uterine changes associated with pregnancy.

increase in tidal volume. There is only a slight increase in respiratory rate. The diaphragm is pushed up by the enlarging uterus, resulting in flaring of the rib margins to maintain intrathoracic volume.

Cardiovascular System Various changes take place in the cardiovascular system during pregnancy. Cardiac output increases throughout pregnancy, peaking at 6 to 7 liters/minute by the time the fetus is fully developed. The maternal blood volume increases by 45 percent and, although both red blood cells and plasma increase, there is slightly more plasma, resulting in a relative anemia. To combat this anemia, pregnant women receive supplemental iron to increase the oxygen-carrying capacity of their red blood cells. Due to the increase in blood volume, the pregnant female may suffer a blood loss of 30 to 35 percent without a significant change in vital signs. The maternal heart rate increases by 10 to 15 bpm. Blood pressure decreases slightly during the first two trimesters, then rises to near nonpregnant levels during the third trimester.

Supine hypotensive syndrome occurs when the gravid uterus compresses the inferior vena cava when the mother lies in a supine position, causing decreased venous return to the right atrium, which lowers blood pressure. Current research suggests that the abdominal aorta may also be compressed. The enlarging uterus also may press on the pelvic and femoral vessels, causing impaired venous return from the legs and venous stasis. This may lead to the development of varicose veins, dependent edema, and postural hypotension. Some patients are predisposed to this problem because of an overall decrease in circulating blood volume or because of anemia. Assessment and management of supine hypotensive syndrome will be discussed later in this chapter.

Gastrointestinal System Nausea and vomiting are common in the first trimester as a result of hormone levels and changed carbohydrate needs. Peristalsis is slowed, so delayed gastric emptying is likely and bloating or constipation is common. As the uterus enlarges, abdominal organs are compressed, and the resulting compartmentalization of abdominal organs makes assessment difficult.

Urinary System Renal blood flow increases during pregnancy. The glomerular filtration rate increases by nearly 50 percent in the second trimester and remains elevated throughout the remainder of the pregnancy. As a result, the renal tubular absorption also increases. Occasionally glucosuria (large amounts of sugar in the urine) may result from the kidney's inability to reabsorb all of the glucose being filtered. Glucosuria may be normal or may indicate the development of gestational diabetes. The urinary bladder gets displaced anteriorly and superiorly increasing the potential for rupture. As a result, urinary frequency is common, particularly in the first and third trimesters.

Musculoskeletal System Loosened pelvic joints caused by hormonal influences account for the waddling gait that is often associated with pregnancy. As the uterus enlarges and the mother's center of gravity changes, postural changes take place to compensate for anterior growth, causing low back pain.

FETAL DEVELOPMENT

Fetal development begins immediately after fertilization and is quite complex. The time at which fertilization occurs is called *conception.* Since conception occurs approximately 14 days after the first day of the last menstrual period, it is possible to calculate, with fair accuracy, the approximate date the baby should be born. This estimate is usually made during the mother's first prenatal visit. The normal duration of pregnancy is 40 weeks from the first day of the mother's last menstrual period. This is equal to 280 days, which is 10 lunar months or, roughly, 9 calendar months. This estimated birth date is commonly called the *due date.* Medically, it is known as the **estimated date of confinement** (**EDC**). Generally, pregnancy is divided into *trimesters.* Each trimester is approximately 13 weeks, or 3 calendar months, long.

estimated date of confinement (EDC) *the approximate day the infant will be born. This date is usually set at 40 weeks after the date of the mother's last menstrual period (LMP).*

Several different terms are used to describe the stages of development. The *preembryonic stage* covers the first 14 days following conception. The *embryonic stage* begins at day 15 and ends at approximately 8 weeks. The period from 8 weeks until delivery is known as the *fetal stage.* As a paramedic you should be familiar with some of the significant developmental milestones that occur

Table 40–1	Significant Fetal Developmental Milestones
	Preembryonic Stage
2 weeks	Rapid cellular multiplication and differentiation
	Embryonic Stage
4 weeks	Fetal heart begins to beat
8 weeks	All body systems and external structures are formed Size: approximately 3 centimeters (1.2 inches)
	Fetal Stage
8–12 weeks	Fetal heart tones audible with Doppler Kidneys begin to produce urine Size: 8 centimeters (3.2 inches), weight about 1.6 ounces Fetus most vulnerable to toxins
16 weeks	Sex can be determined visually Fetus swallows amniotic fluid and produces meconium Looks like a baby, although thin
20 weeks	Fetal heart tones audible with stethoscope Mother able to feel fetal movement Baby develops schedule of sucking, kicking, and sleeping Hair, eyebrows, and eyelashes present Size: 19 centimeters (8 inches), weight approximately 16 ounces
24 weeks	Increased activity Begins respiratory movement Size: 28 centimeters (11.2 inches), weight 1 pound 10 ounces
28 weeks	Surfactant necessary for lung function is formed Eyes begin to open and close Weighs 2 to 3 pounds
32 weeks	Bones are fully developed but soft and flexible Subcutaneous fat being deposited Fingernails and toenails present
38–40 weeks	Considered to be full-term Baby fills uterine cavity Baby receives maternal antibodies

during these three periods (Table 40–1). During normal fetal development, the sex of the infant can usually be determined by 16 weeks' gestation. By the 20th week, *fetal heart tones (FHTs)* can be detected by stethoscope. The mother also has generally felt fetal movement. By 24 weeks, the baby may be able to survive if born prematurely. Fetuses born after 28 weeks have an excellent chance of survival. By the 38th week the baby is considered *term,* or fully developed.

Most of the fetus's organ systems develop during the first trimester. Therefore, this is when the fetus is most vulnerable to the development of birth defects.

FETAL CIRCULATION

The fetus receives its oxygen and nutrients from its mother through the placenta. Thus, while in the uterus, the fetus does not need to use its respiratory system or its gastrointestinal tract. Because of this, the fetal circulation shunts blood around the lungs and gastrointestinal tract.

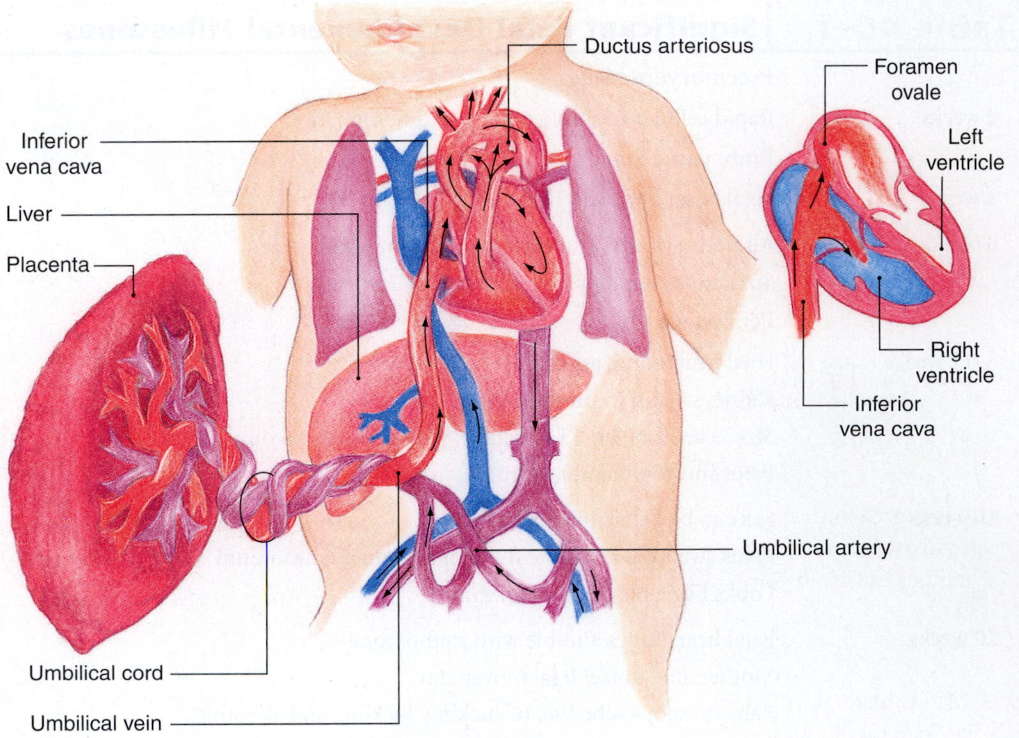

■ **Figure 40-4** The maternal-fetal circulation.

The infant receives its blood from the placenta by means of the umbilical vein (Figure 40-4 ■). The umbilical vein connects directly to the inferior vena cava by a specialized structure called the *ductus venosus.* Blood then travels through the inferior vena cava to the heart. The blood enters the right atrium and passes through the tricuspid valve into the right ventricle. It then exits the right ventricle, through the pulmonic valve, into the pulmonary artery. The fetus's heart has a hole between the right and left atria, termed the *foramen ovale,* which allows mixing of the oxygenated blood in the right atrium with that leaving the left ventricle bound for the aorta.

At this time, the blood is still oxygenated. Once in the pulmonary artery, the blood enters the *ductus arteriosus,* which connects the pulmonary artery with the aorta. The ductus arteriosus causes blood to bypass the uninflated lungs. Once in the aorta, blood flow is basically the same as in extrauterine life. Deoxygenated blood containing waste products exits the fetus, after passage through the liver, via the umbilical arteries.

The fetal circulation changes immediately at birth. As soon as the baby takes its first breath, the lungs inflate, greatly decreasing pulmonary vascular resistance to blood flow. Also, the ductus arteriosus closes, diverting blood to the lungs. In addition, the ductus venosus closes, stopping blood flow from the placenta. The foramen ovale also closes as a result of pressure changes in the heart, which stops blood flow from the right to left atrium.

Obstetric Terminology

The field of obstetrics has its own unique terminology. You should be familiar with this terminology, since patient documentation and communications with other health care workers and physicians often require it.

Antepartum	The time interval prior to delivery of the fetus
Postpartum	The time interval after delivery of the fetus
Prenatal	The time interval prior to birth, synonymous with antepartum
Natal	Relating to birth or the date of birth
*Gravidity**	The number of times a woman has been pregnant
*Parity**	Number of pregnancies carried to full term
Primigravida	A woman who is pregnant for the first time

Primipara	A woman who has given birth to her first child
Multigravida	A woman who has been pregnant more than once
Nulligravida	A woman who has not been pregnant
Multipara	A woman who has delivered more than one baby
Nullipara	A woman who has yet to deliver her first child
Grand multiparity	A woman who has delivered at least seven babies
Gestation	Period of time for intrauterine fetal development

*The gravidity and parity of a woman is expressed in the following "shorthand": G_4 P_2. "G" refers to the gravidity, and "P" refers to the parity. The woman in this example would have had four pregnancies and two births.

GENERAL ASSESSMENT OF THE OBSTETRIC PATIENT

PRIMARY ASSESSMENT

The initial approach to the obstetrical patient should be the same as for the nonobstetrical patient, with special attention paid to the developing fetus. Complete the primary assessment quickly and then obtain essential obstetric information.

HISTORY

The SAMPLE history will allow you to gain specific information about the mother's situation as well as her pertinent medical history.

General Information

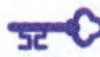

Obtain information about the pregnancy. Ask about gravidity, parity, length of gestation, and EDC. Ask about past gynecological or obstetrical complications and prenatal care. Determine current medications and any drug allergies.

You will want to obtain information about the pregnancy, such as the mother's gravidity and parity, the length of gestation, and the estimated date of confinement (EDC), if known. In addition, you should determine whether the patient has had any cesarean sections or any gynecological or obstetrical complications in the past. It is also important to ascertain whether the patient has had any prenatal care. Determine what type of health care professional (physician or nurse midwife) is providing her care and when she was last evaluated. Ask the patient whether a sonogram examination was done. A sonogram reveals the age of the fetus, the presence of more than one fetus, abnormal presentations, and certain birth defects. A general overview of the patient's current state of health is important. Pay particular attention to current medications and drug and/or medication allergies.

Preexisting or Aggravated Medical Conditions

Pregnancy can aggravate preexisting medical conditions such as diabetes, heart disease, hypertension, seizure disorders, and neuromuscular disorders, and may trigger new ones. (However, a remission of neurological disorder symptoms during pregnancy is not unusual.)

Pregnancy aggravates many preexisting medical conditions and may trigger new ones.

Diabetes Previously diagnosed diabetes can become unstable during pregnancy due to altered insulin requirements. Diabetics are at increased risk of developing preeclampsia and hypertension (discussed later in this chapter). Pregnancy may also accelerate the progression of vascular disease complications of diabetes. It is not uncommon for pregnant diabetics to have problems with fluctuating blood sugar levels, causing hypoglycemic or hyperglycemic episodes. Also, many patients develop diabetes during pregnancy *(gestational diabetes)*. Pregnant diabetics cannot be managed with oral hypoglycemic agents because these drugs tend to cross the placenta and affect the fetus. Therefore, all pregnant diabetics are placed on insulin, if their blood sugar levels cannot be controlled by diet alone. It has been shown that maintaining careful control of the mother's blood sugar between 70 and 120 mg/dL reduces risks to mother and fetus.

Diabetes also affects the infant. Infants of diabetic mothers, especially those with poorly controlled blood sugar levels, tend to be large. This complicates delivery. Such infants also may have trouble maintaining body temperature after birth and may be subject to hypoglycemia. Babies born to diabetic mothers are also at increased risk of congenital anomalies (birth defects).

Heart Disease During pregnancy, cardiac output increases up to 30 percent. Patients who have serious preexisting heart disease may develop congestive heart failure in pregnancy. When confronted by a pregnant patient in obvious or suspected heart failure, inquire about preexisting heart disease or murmurs. It is important to be aware, however, that most patients develop a quiet systolic flow murmur during pregnancy. This is caused by increased cardiac output and is rarely a source of concern.

Hypertension Hypertension is also aggravated by pregnancy. Generally, blood pressure is lower in pregnancy than in the nonpregnant state. However, women who were borderline hypertensive before becoming pregnant may become dangerously hypertensive when pregnant. Also, many common blood pressure medications cannot be used during pregnancy. In addition, preeclampsia (discussed later in this chapter) may contribute to maternal hypertension. Persistent hypertension may adversely affect the placenta, thus compromising the fetus as well as placing the mother at increased risk for stroke, seizure, or renal failure.

Seizure Disorders Most women with a history of seizure disorders controlled by medication have uneventful pregnancies and deliver healthy babies. However, women who have poorly controlled seizure disorders are likely to have increased seizure activity during pregnancy. Medications to control seizures are commonly administered throughout the pregnancy.

Neuromuscular Disorders Disabilities associated with neuromuscular disorders, such as multiple sclerosis, may be aggravated by pregnancy. However, it is more common that pregnant women enjoy remission of symptoms during pregnancy and a slight increase in relapse rate during the postpartum period. The strength of uterine contractions is not diminished in these patients. Also, their subjective sensation of pain is often less than seen in other patients.

When the patient complains of pain, determine onset, character, and especially the regularity of occurrence.

Pain

If the patient is in pain, try to determine when the pain started and whether its onset was sudden or slow. Also, attempt to define the character of the pain—its duration, location, and radiation, if any. It is especially important to determine whether the pain is occurring on a regular basis.

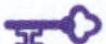

If there is vaginal bleeding, determine events prior to its start. Assess the amount by the number of sanitary pads used and save any clots or passed tissue.

Vaginal Bleeding

The presence of vaginal bleeding or spotting is a major concern in an obstetrical patient. Ask about events immediately prior to the start of bleeding. You also need to gain information about the color, amount, and duration. To assess the amount of bleeding, count the number of sanitary pads used. If your patient is passing clots or tissue, save this material for evaluation. In addition, question the patient about the presence of other vaginal discharges, as well as the color, amount, and duration.

For a patient in labor, determine if she feels the need to push or move her bowels or if her membranes have ruptured (her "water broke")—which are all signs of possible imminent delivery.

Active Labor

When confronted with a patient in active labor, assess whether the mother feels the need to push or has the urge to move her bowels. Determine whether the patient thinks her membranes have ruptured. Patients often sense this as a dribbling of water or, in some cases, a true gush of water.

PHYSICAL EXAMINATION

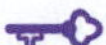

Always protect the patient's modesty.

Physical examination of the obstetric patient is essentially the same as for any emergency patient. However, you should be particularly careful to protect the patient's modesty as well as to maintain her dignity and privacy.

When examining a pregnant patient, first estimate the date of the pregnancy by measuring the *fundal height*. The fundal height is the distance from the symphysis pubis to the top of the uterine fundus. Each centimeter of fundal height roughly corresponds to a week of gestation. For example, a woman with a fundal height of 24 centimeters has a gestational age of approximately 24 weeks. If the fundus is just palpable above the symphysis pubis, the pregnancy is about 12 to 16 weeks' gestation. When the uterine fundus reaches the umbilicus, the pregnancy is about 20 weeks. As pregnancy reaches term, the fundus is palpable near the xiphoid process. If fetal movement is felt when the abdomen is palpated, the pregnancy is at least 20 weeks. Fetal heart tones can be heard by stethoscope at approximately 18 to 20 weeks. The normal fetal heart rate ranges from 140 to 160 beats per minute.

Generally, vital signs in the pregnant patient should be taken with the patient lying on her left side. As noted earlier, as pregnancy progresses, the uterus increases in size. Ultimately, when the patient is supine, the weight of the uterus compresses the inferior vena cava, severely compromising venous blood return from the lower extremities. Turning the patient to her left side alleviates this problem. Occasionally, it may be helpful to perform orthostatic vital signs. First, obtain the blood pressure and pulse rate after the patient has rested for 5 minutes in the left lateral recumbent position. Then repeat the vital signs with the patient sitting up or standing. A drop in the blood pressure level of 15 mmHg or more, or an increase in the pulse rate of 20 beats per minute or more, is considered significant and should be reported and documented. When performing this maneuver, it is always important to be alert for syncope. This procedure should *not* be performed if the patient is in obvious shock.

You may need to examine the genitals to evaluate any vaginal discharge, the progression of labor, or the presence of a *prolapsed cord,* an umbilical cord that comes out of the uterus ahead of the fetus. This can be accomplished simply by looking at the perineum. If, during the physical examination, the patient reports that she feels the need to push, or if she feels as though she must move her bowels, examine her for crowning. **Crowning** is the bulging of the fetal head past the opening of the vagina during a contraction. Crowning is an indication of impending delivery. Examine for crowning only during a contraction. *Do not perform an internal vaginal examination in the field.*

crowning *the bulging of the fetal head past the opening of the vagina during a contraction. Crowning is an indication of impending delivery.*

GENERAL MANAGEMENT OF THE OBSTETRIC PATIENT

The first consideration for managing emergencies in obstetric patients is to remember that you are in fact caring for two patients, the mother and the fetus. Fetal well-being is dependent on maternal well-being. Also keep in mind that your calm, professional demeanor and caring attitude will go a long way in reducing the emotional stress during any obstetric emergency. Remember to protect your patient's privacy and maintain her modesty.

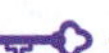

Do not perform an internal vaginal examination in the field.

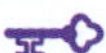

Always remember that you are caring for two patients, the mother and the fetus.

The physiologic priorities for obstetric emergencies are identical to those for any other emergency situation. Focus your efforts on maintaining the airway, breathing, and circulation. Administer high-flow, high-concentration oxygen as needed based on the patient's condition. Initiate intravenous access by using a large-bore catheter in a large vein and consider fluid resuscitation based on your local protocols. If your patient is bleeding or showing signs of shock, establish two IV lines. Cardiac monitoring is also appropriate. Place your patient in a position of comfort, but remember that left lateral recumbent is preferred after the 24th week.

Focus on airway, breathing, and circulation. Monitor for shock. As needed, administer oxygen, initiate IV access, consider fluid resuscitation, and monitor the heart. Place the patient in a position of comfort. The left lateral recumbent position is preferred after the 24th week.

If pain is the primary complaint, administer analgesics such as morphine. However, analgesics should be used with caution since they can alter your ability to assess a deteriorating condition as well as other changes in patient status and may negatively affect the fetus. Nitrous oxide is the preferred analgesic in pregnancy, but narcotics are acceptable.

When transport is indicated, transport immediately to a hospital that is capable of managing emergency obstetric and neonatal care. Report the situation to the receiving hospital prior to your arrival, as emergency department personnel may want to summon obstetrics department staff to assist with patient care.

COMPLICATIONS OF PREGNANCY

Pregnancy is a normal process. However, women who are pregnant are not immune from injury or other health problems. There may also be complications associated with the pregnancy itself.

TRAUMA

Paramedics frequently receive calls to help a pregnant woman who has been in a motor vehicle accident or who has sustained a fall. In pregnancy, syncope occurs frequently. The syncope of pregnancy often results from compression of the inferior vena cava, as described earlier, or from normal changes in the cardiovascular system associated with pregnancy. Also, the weight of the gravid uterus alters the patient's balance, making her more susceptible to falls.

Pregnant victims of major trauma are more susceptible to life-threatening injury than are nonpregnant victims because of the increased vascularity of the gravid uterus. Trauma is the most frequent, nonobstetric cause of death in pregnant women. Some form of trauma, usually a motor vehicle crash or a fall but sometimes physical abuse, occurs in 6 to 7 percent of all pregnancies. Since the primary cause for fetal mortality is maternal mortality, the pregnant trauma patient presents a unique challenge. The later in the pregnancy, the larger the uterus and the greater the likelihood of injury. All patients at 20 weeks' (or more) gestation with a history of direct or indirect injury should be transported for evaluation by a physician.

Transport all trauma patients at 20 weeks' or more gestation. Anticipate the development of shock.

Paramedics should *anticipate* the development of shock based on the mechanism of injury rather than waiting for overt signs and symptoms. Due to the cardiovascular changes of pregnancy, overt signs of shock are late and inconsistent. Trauma significant enough to cause maternal shock is associated with a 70 to 80 percent fetal mortality. In the face of acute blood loss, significant vasoconstriction will occur in response to catecholamine release, resulting in maintenance of a normotensive state for the mother. However, this causes significant uterine hypoperfusion (20 to 30 percent decrease in cardiac output) and fetal bradycardia.

Generally, the amniotic fluid cushions the fetus from blunt trauma fairly well. However, in direct abdominal trauma, the pregnant patient may suffer premature separation of the placenta from the uterine wall, premature labor, abortion, uterine rupture, and possibly fetal death. The presence of vaginal bleeding or a tender abdomen in a pregnant patient should increase your suspicion of serious injury. Fetal death may result from death of the mother, separation of the placenta from the uterine wall, maternal shock, uterine rupture, or fetal head injury. Any pregnant patient who has suffered trauma should be immediately transported to the emergency department and evaluated by a physician. Trauma management essentials include the following:

- ★ Apply a C-collar to provide cervical stabilization and immobilize on a long backboard.
- ★ Administer high-flow, high-concentration oxygen.
- ★ Initiate two large-bore IVs for crystalloid administration per protocol.
- ★ Transport tilted to the left to minimize supine hypotension.
- ★ Reassess frequently.
- ★ Monitor the fetus.

Any pregnant patient with abdominal pain should be evaluated by a physician.

MEDICAL CONDITIONS

The pregnant patient is subject to all of the medical problems that occur in the nonpregnant state. Abdominal pain, a common complaint, is often caused by the stretching of the ligaments that support the uterus. However, appendicitis and cholecystitis can also occur. Pregnant women are at increased risk of developing gallstones as a result of hormonal influences that delay emptying of the gallbladder. In pregnancy, the abdominal organs are displaced because of the increased mass of the gravid uterus in the abdomen, which makes assessment more difficult. The pregnant patient with appendicitis may complain of right upper quadrant pain or even back pain. The symptoms of acute cholecystitis may also differ from those in nonpregnant patients. Any pregnant patient with abdominal pain should be evaluated by a physician.

Content Review

Causes of Bleeding during Pregnancy

- Abortion
- Ectopic pregnancy
- Placenta previa
- Abruptio placentae

abortion *termination of pregnancy before the 20th week of gestation. The term refers to both miscarriage and induced abortion. Commonly, abortion is used for elective termination of pregnancy and miscarriage for the loss of a fetus by natural means. A miscarriage is sometimes called a "spontaneous abortion."*

BLEEDING IN PREGNANCY

Vaginal bleeding may occur at any time during pregnancy. Bleeding is usually due to abortion, ectopic pregnancy, placenta previa, or abruptio placentae. Generally, the exact etiology of vaginal bleeding during pregnancy cannot be determined in the field. Refer to the earlier discussion in this chapter and your own local protocols for management of obstetric emergencies. Vaginal bleeding is associated with potential fetal loss. Keep in mind that this is an emotional and stressful situation for your patient, so a professional, caring demeanor is imperative.

Abortion

Abortion, the expulsion of the fetus prior to 20 weeks' gestation, is the most common cause of bleeding in the first and second trimesters of pregnancy. The terms *abortion* and *miscarriage* can be used interchangeably. Generally, the lay public think of abortion as termination of pregnancy at maternal request and of miscarriage as an accident of nature. Medically, the term *abortion* applies to both kinds of fetal loss. Spontaneous abortion, the naturally occurring termination of pregnancy that is often called miscarriage, is most commonly seen between 12 and 14 weeks of gestation. It is estimated that 10 to 20 percent of all pregnancies end in spontaneous abortion. If the pregnancy has not yet been confirmed, the mother often assumes she is merely having a period with unusually heavy flow.

About half of all abortions are due to fetal chromosomal anomalies. Other causes include maternal reproductive system abnormalities, maternal use of drugs, placental defects, or maternal infections. Although many people believe that trauma and psychological stress can cause abortion, research does not support that belief.

Assessment The patient experiencing an abortion is likely to report cramping abdominal pain and a backache. She is also likely to report vaginal bleeding, which is often accompanied by the passage of clots and tissue. If the abortion was not recent, then frank signs and symptoms of infection may be present. In addition to your routine emergency assessments, assess for orthostatic vital sign changes and ascertain the amount of vaginal bleeding.

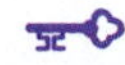

Signs and symptoms of an abortion include cramping abdominal pain, backache, and vaginal bleeding, often accompanied by passage of clots and tissue.

Management Place the patient who is experiencing an abortion in a position of comfort. Treat for shock with oxygen therapy and IV access for fluid resuscitation. As mentioned earlier, any tissue or large clots should be retained and given to emergency department personnel. If the abortion occurs during the late first trimester or later, a fetus may be passed. Often, the placenta does not detach, and the fetus is suspended by the umbilical cord. In such a case, place the umbilical clamps from the OB kit on the cord and cut it. Carefully wrap the fetus in linen or other suitable material and transport it to the hospital with the mother.

An abortion is generally a very sad occurrence. Provide emotional support to the parents. This can be a devastating psychological experience for the mother, so avoid saying trite but inaccurate phrases meant to provide comfort. Inappropriate remarks include "You can always get pregnant again" or "This is nature's way of dealing with a defective fetus." Parents who wish to view the fetus should be allowed to do so.

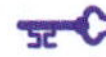

Treat the patient suffering an abortion as you would any patient at risk for hypovolemic shock. Provide emotional support to the parents.

Classifications of Abortion

Since you will be interacting with other health care professionals, be familiar with the variety of terms used to describe the classifications of abortion.

Complete abortion	An abortion in which all of the uterine contents including the fetus and placenta have been expelled.
Incomplete abortion	An abortion in which some, but not all, fetal tissue has been passed. Incomplete abortions are associated with a high incidence of infection.
Threatened abortion	A potential abortion characterized by unexplained vaginal bleeding during the first half of pregnancy in which the cervix is slightly open and the fetus remains in the uterus and is still alive. In some cases of threatened abortion, the fetus still can be saved.
Inevitable abortion	A potential abortion, characterized by vaginal bleeding accompanied by severe abdominal cramping and cervical dilatation, in which the fetus has not yet passed from the uterus, but the fetus cannot be saved.
Spontaneous abortion	Naturally occurring expulsion of the fetus prior to viability, generally as a result of chromosomal abnormalities. Most spontaneous abortions occur before week 12 of pregnancy. Many occur within 2 weeks after conception and are mistaken for menstrual periods. Commonly called a *miscarriage.*
Elective abortion	An abortion in which the termination of pregnancy is desired and requested by the mother. Elective abortions during the first and second

	trimesters of pregnancy have been legal in the United States since 1973. Most elective abortions are performed during the first trimester. Some clinics perform second-trimester abortions. Second-trimester abortions have a higher complication rate than first-trimester abortions. Third-trimester elective abortions are generally illegal in this country.
Criminal abortion	Intentional termination of a pregnancy under any condition not allowed by law. It is usually the attempt to destroy a fetus by a person who is not licensed or permitted to do so. Criminal abortions often are attempted by amateurs and they are rarely performed in aseptic surroundings.
Therapeutic abortion	Termination of a pregnancy deemed necessary by a physician, usually to protect maternal health and well-being.
Missed abortion	An abortion in which fetal death occurs but the fetus is not expelled. This poses a potential threat to the life of the mother if the fetus is retained beyond 6 weeks.
Habitual abortion	Spontaneous abortions that occur in three or more consecutive pregnancies.

Ectopic Pregnancy

As you learned earlier, the fertilized egg normally is implanted in the endometrial lining of the uterine wall. The term *ectopic pregnancy* refers to the abnormal implantation of the fertilized egg outside of the uterus. Approximately 95 percent are implanted in the fallopian tube. Occasionally (< 1 percent), the egg is implanted in the abdominal cavity. Current research indicates that the incidence of ectopic pregnancy is 1 in 44 live births. Improved diagnostic technology is credited with an increased incidence, as most are detected between the 2nd and 12th week. Ectopic pregnancy accounts for approximately 10 percent of maternal mortality.

Predisposing factors in the development of ectopic pregnancy include scarring of the fallopian tubes due to pelvic inflammatory disease (PID), a previous ectopic pregnancy, or previous pelvic or tubal surgery, such as a tubal ligation. Other factors include endometriosis or use of an intrauterine device (IUD) for birth control.

Assessment Ectopic pregnancy most often presents as abdominal pain, which starts out as diffuse tenderness and then localizes as a sharp pain in the lower abdominal quadrant on the affected side. This pain is due to rupture of the fallopian tube when the fetus outgrows the available space. The woman often reports that she missed a period or that her LMP occurred 4 to 6 weeks ago, but with decreased menstrual flow that was brownish in color and of shorter duration than usual. As the intraabdominal bleeding continues, the abdomen becomes rigid and the pain intensifies and is often referred to the shoulder on the affected side. The pain is often accompanied by syncope, vaginal bleeding, and shock.

Assume that any female of childbearing age with lower abdominal pain is experiencing an ectopic pregnancy.

Assume that any female of childbearing age with lower abdominal pain is experiencing an ectopic pregnancy.

Management Ectopic pregnancy poses a significant life threat to the mother. Transport this patient immediately, since surgery is often required to resolve the situation. Interim care measures should include oxygen therapy and IV access for fluid resuscitation. Trendelenburg position or the use of a pneumatic anti-shock garment may be indicated by your local protocols.

Ectopic pregnancy is life-threatening. Transport the patient immediately.

Placenta Previa

Third-trimester bleeding should be attributed to either placenta previa or abruptio placentae until proven otherwise. Placenta previa usually presents with painless bleeding. Abruptio placentae usually presents with sharp pain, with or without bleeding.

Placenta previa occurs as a result of abnormal implantation of the placenta on the lower half of the uterine wall, resulting in partial or complete coverage of the cervical opening (Figure 40-5 ■). Vaginal bleeding, which may initially be intermittent, occurs after the 7th month of the pregnancy as the lower uterus begins to contract and dilate in preparation for the onset of labor. This process pulls the placenta away from the uterine wall, causing bright red vaginal bleeding. Placenta previa occurs in about 1 in 250 live births. It is classified as complete, partial, or marginal, depending on whether the placenta covers all or part of the cervical opening or is merely in close proximity to the opening.

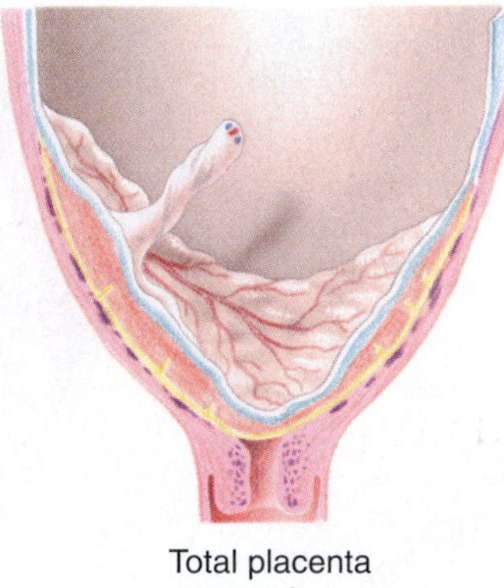

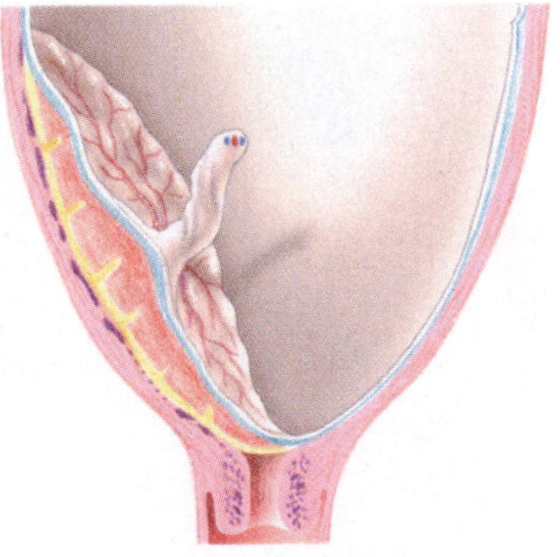

■ **Figure 40-5** Placenta previa (abnormal implantation).

Although the exact cause of placenta previa is unknown, certain predisposing factors are commonly seen. These factors include a previous history of placenta previa, multiparity, or increased maternal age. Other factors include the presence of uterine scars from cesarean sections, a large placenta, or defective development of blood vessels in the uterine wall.

Assessment The patient with placenta previa is usually a multigravida in her third trimester of pregnancy. She may have a history of prior placenta previa or of bleeding early in the current pregnancy. She may report a recent episode of sexual intercourse or vaginal examination just before vaginal bleeding began, or she may not bleed until the onset of labor. The onset of painless bright red vaginal bleeding, which may occur as spotting or recurrent hemorrhage, is the hallmark of placenta previa. In fact, any painless bleeding in pregnancy is considered placenta previa until proven otherwise. The bleeding may or may not be associated with uterine contractions. The uterus is usually soft, and the fetus may be in an unusual presentation. *Vaginal examination should never be attempted, as an examining finger can puncture the placenta, causing fatal hemorrhage.*

Never attempt vaginal examination since an examining finger can puncture the placenta and cause fatal hemorrhage.

The presence of placenta previa may already have been diagnosed with an ultrasound during prenatal care, in which case the mother is anticipating the onset of symptoms. The prognosis for the fetus is dependent on the extent of the previa. Obviously, in profuse hemorrhage the fetus is at risk of severe hypoxia and the viability of the placenta is compromised. You should perform your assessment and physical exam as discussed earlier in this chapter.

Management If the placenta previa was previously diagnosed, your patient may already have been managed by placing her on bed rest. Because of the potential for profuse hemorrhage, you should treat for shock. Administer oxygen and initiate intravenous access. Additionally, continue to monitor the maternal vital signs and FHTs. Since the definitive treatment is delivery of the fetus by cesarean section, it is imperative to transport the patient to a hospital with obstetric surgical capability.

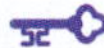

Because of the potential for profuse hemorrhage, always treat the patient with suspected placenta previa for shock. Transport immediately since definitive treatment is delivery by cesarean section.

Abruptio Placentae

Abruptio placentae, or the premature separation (abruption) of a normally implanted placenta from the uterine wall, poses a potential life threat for both mother and fetus (Figure 40-6 ■). The incidence of abruptio placentae is 1 in 120 live births. It is associated with 20 to 30 percent fetal mortality, which rises to 100 percent in cases where the majority of the placenta has separated. Maternal mortality is relatively uncommon, although it rises markedly if shock is inadequately treated. Abruptio placentae is classified as marginal (or partial), central (severe), or complete, as explained next.

Although the cause of abruptio placentae is unknown, predisposing factors include multiparity, maternal hypertension, trauma, cocaine use, increasing maternal age, and history of abruption in previous pregnancy.

Signs and symptoms of abruptio placentae vary. With a marginal abruption, there will be bleeding but no pain. With a central abruption, there will be sharp, tearing pain and a stiff, boardlike abdomen. Complete abruption will result in massive hemorrhage.

Assessment The presenting signs and symptoms of abruptio placentae vary depending on the extent and character of the abruption. Partial abruptions can be marginal or central. Marginal abruptio is characterized by vaginal bleeding but no increase in pain. In central abruptio, the

■ Figure 40-6 Abruptio placentae (premature separation).

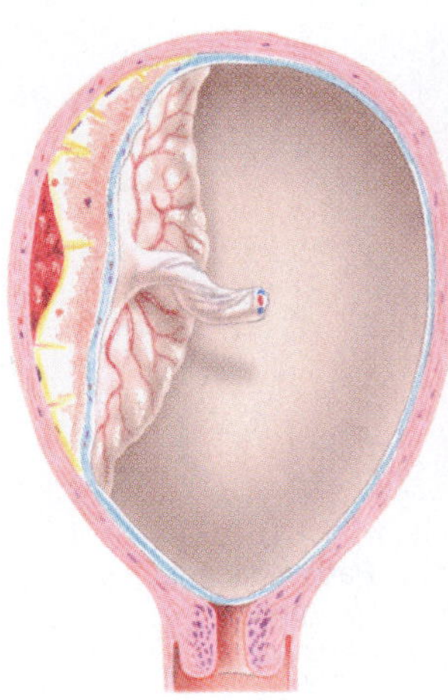

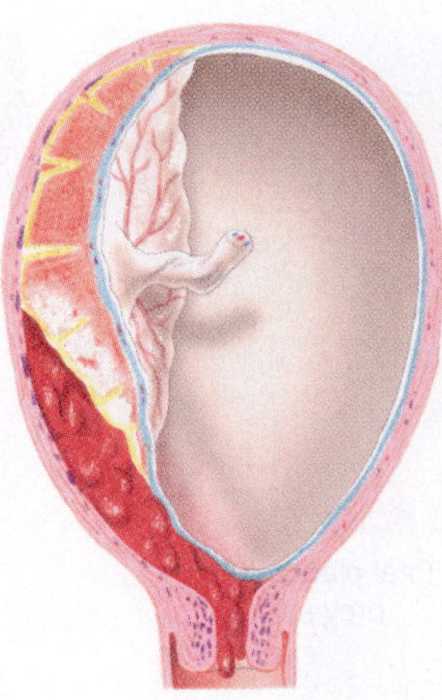

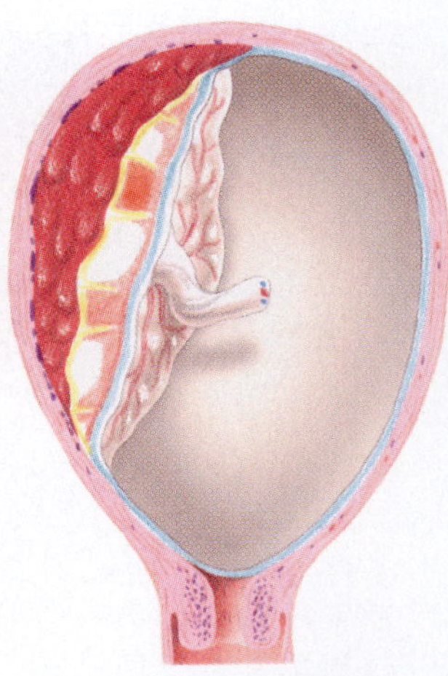

placenta separates centrally and the bleeding is trapped between the placenta and the uterine wall, or "concealed," so there is no vaginal bleeding. However, there is a sudden sharp, tearing pain and development of a stiff, boardlike abdomen. In complete abruptio placentae there is massive vaginal bleeding and profound maternal hypotension. If the patient is in labor at the time of the abruptio, separation of the placenta from the uterine wall will progress rapidly, with fetal distress versus fetal demise dependent on percentage of separation.

Abruptio placentae is a life-threatening emergency. Treat for shock, including fluid resuscitation, and transport immediately in the left lateral recumbent position.

Management Abruptio placentae is a life-threatening obstetrical emergency. Immediate intervention to maintain maternal oxygenation and perfusion is imperative. Immediately place two large-bore intravenous lines and begin fluid resuscitation. Position your patient in the left lateral recumbent position. Transport immediately to a hospital with available surgical obstetric and high-risk neonatal care.

Content Review

Medical Complications of Pregnancy

- Hypertensive disorders of pregnancy
- Supine hypotensive syndrome
- Gestational diabetes

MEDICAL COMPLICATIONS OF PREGNANCY

As discussed earlier, pregnancy can exacerbate preexisting medical conditions such as diabetes, heart disease, hypertension, and seizure or neuromuscular disorder.

Hypertensive Disorders of Pregnancy

The American College of Obstetricians and Gynecologists has identified four classifications of *hypertensive disorders of pregnancy* (formerly called "toxemia of pregnancy"). They include the following:

★ ***Preeclampsia and eclampsia***

Hypertensive disorders of pregnancy (HDP), which include preeclampsia and eclampsia, occur in approximately 5 percent of all pregnancies. Preeclampsia is the most common hypertensive disorder seen in pregnancy. There is a higher incidence among primigravidas, particularly if they are teenagers or over the age of 35. Others at increased risk are diabetics, women with a history of preeclampsia, and those who are carrying multiple fetuses.

Preeclampsia is a progressive disorder that is usually categorized as mild or severe. Seizures (or coma) develop in its most severe form, known as eclampsia. Preeclampsia is defined as an increase in systolic blood pressure by 30 mmHg and/or a diastolic increase of 15 mmHg over baseline on at least two occasions at least 6 hours apart. Remember that maternal blood pressure normally drops during pregnancy, so a woman may be hypertensive at 120/80 if her baseline in early pregnancy was 90/66. If there is no baseline blood pressure available then a reading ≥ 140/90 is considered to be hypertensive.

Preeclampsia is most commonly seen in the last 10 weeks of gestation, during labor, or in the first 48 hours postpartum. The exact cause of preeclampsia is unknown. It is thought to be caused by abnormal vasospasm, which results in increased maternal blood pressure and other associated symptoms. Additionally, the vasospasm causes decreased placental perfusion, contributing to fetal growth retardation and chronic fetal hypoxia.

Mild preeclampsia is characterized by hypertension, edema, and protein in the urine. Severe preeclampsia progresses rapidly with maternal blood pressures reaching 160/110 or higher, while the edema becomes generalized and the amount of protein in the urine increases significantly. Other commonly seen signs and symptoms in the severe state include headache, visual disturbances, hyperactive reflexes, and the development of pulmonary edema, along with a dramatic decrease in urine output.

Patients who are preeclamptic have intravascular volume depletion, since a great deal of their body fluid is in the third space. Those who develop severe preeclampsia and eclampsia are at increased risk for cerebral hemorrhage, pulmonary embolism, abruptio placentae, disseminated intravascular coagulopathy (DIC), and the development of renal failure.

Eclampsia, the most serious manifestation of the hypertensive disorders of pregnancy, is characterized by generalized tonic-clonic (major motor) seizure activity. Eclampsia is often preceded by visual disturbances, such as flashing lights or spots before the eyes. Also, the development of epigastric pain or pain in the right upper abdominal quadrant often indicates impending seizure. Eclampsia can often be distinguished from epilepsy by the history and physical appearance of the patient. Patients who become eclamptic are usually grossly edematous and have markedly elevated blood pressure, while epileptics usually have a prior history of seizures and are usually taking anticonvulsant medications. If eclampsia develops, death of the mother and fetus frequently results. The risk of fetal mortality increases by 10 percent with each maternal seizure.

★ ***Chronic hypertension***

Hypertension is considered chronic when the blood pressure is ≥ 140/90 before pregnancy or prior to the 20th week of gestation, or if it persists for more than 42 days postpartum. As a general rule, if the diastolic pressure exceeds 80 mmHg during the second trimester, chronic hypertension is likely. The cause of chronic hypertension is unknown. The goal of management is to prevent the development of preeclampsia.

★ ***Chronic hypertension superimposed with preeclampsia***

It is not uncommon for the chronic hypertensive who develops preeclampsia to progress rapidly to eclampsia even prior to the 30th week of gestation. The same diagnostic criteria for preeclampsia are used (systolic blood pressure increases > 30 mmHg over baseline, edema, and protein in the urine).

★ ***Transient hypertension***

Transient hypertension is defined as a temporary rise in blood pressure which occurs during labor or early in postpartum and which normalizes within 10 days.

Assessment Obtaining an accurate history is extremely important when you suspect one of the hypertensive disorders of pregnancy (HDP). Question the patient about excessive weight gain, headaches, visual problems, epigastric or right upper quadrant abdominal pain, apprehension, or seizures. On physical exam, patients with HDP or preeclampsia are usually markedly edematous. They are often pale and apprehensive. The reflexes are hyperactive. The blood pressure, which is usually elevated, should be taken after the patient has rested for 5 minutes in the left lateral recumbent position.

With suspected hypertensive disorder, it is critical to obtain an accurate history, including information about weight gain, headaches, visual problems, epigastric or right upper quadrant abdominal pain, apprehension, or seizures.

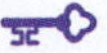

Preeclampsia and eclampsia are life threatening. Keep the patient calm. Dim the lights. Place the patient in the left lateral recumbent position and transport quickly without lights or siren. Administer magnesium sulfate to control seizures if they occur. Medical direction may request administration of antihypertensive or sedative drugs.

Management Definitive treatment of the hypertensive disorders of pregnancy is delivery of the fetus. However, in the field, use the following management tactics to prevent dangerously high blood pressures or seizure activity.

★ ***Hypertension***

Closely monitor the patient who is pregnant and has elevated blood pressure without edema or other signs of preeclampsia. Record the fetal heart tones and the mother's blood pressure level.

★ ***Preeclampsia***

The patient who is hypertensive and shows other signs and symptoms of preeclampsia, such as edema, headaches, and visual disturbances, should be treated quickly. Keep the patient calm and dim the lights. Place the patient in the left lateral recumbent position and quickly carry out the primary assessment. Begin an IV of normal saline. Transport the patient rapidly, without lights or siren. If the blood pressure is dangerously high (diastolic > 110), medical direction may request the administration of hydralazine (Apresoline) or similar antihypertensives that are safe for use in pregnancy. If the transport time is long, the administration of magnesium sulfate may also be ordered.

★ ***Eclampsia***

If the patient has already suffered a seizure or a seizure appears to be imminent, then, in addition to the previous measures, administer oxygen and manage the airway appropriately. Administer a bolus dose of magnesium sulfate (2 to 5 g diluted in 50 to 100 mL slow IV push) to control the seizures. If you are unable to control the seizures with magnesium sulfate, consider diazepam (Valium) or some other sedative. It is important to keep calcium gluconate available for use as an antidote to magnesium sulfate. Also monitor your patient closely for signs (vaginal bleeding or abdominal rigidity) of abruptio placentae or developing pulmonary edema. Transport immediately to a hospital with surgical obstetric and neonatal care availability.

Supine-Hypotensive Syndrome

Supine-hypotensive syndrome usually occurs in the third trimester of pregnancy. Also known as vena caval syndrome, supine hypotensive syndrome occurs when the gravid uterus compresses the inferior vena cava when the mother lies in a supine position (Figure 40-7 ■).

Assessment Supine-hypotensive syndrome usually occurs in a patient late in her pregnancy who has been supine for a period of time. The patient may complain of dizziness, which results from the decrease in venous return to the right atrium and consequent lowering of the patient's blood pressure. Question the patient about prior episodes of a similar nature and about any recent hemorrhage or fluid loss. Direct the physical examination at determining whether the patient is volume depleted.

Treat supine-hypotensive syndrome by placing the patient in the left lateral recumbent position or elevating her right hip. Monitor fetal heart tones and maternal vital signs. If volume depletion is evident, initiate an IV of normal saline.

Management If there are no indications of volume depletion, such as decreased skin turgor or thirst, place the patient in the left lateral recumbent position or elevate her right hip. Monitor the fetal heart tones and maternal vital signs frequently. If there is clinical evidence of volume depletion, administer oxygen and start an IV of normal saline. Check for orthostatic changes (a decrease in blood pressure and increase in heart rate when rising from the supine position) and place electrodes for cardiac monitoring. Transport the patient promptly in the left lateral recumbent position.

Gestational Diabetes

Diabetes mellitus occurs in approximately 4 percent of all pregnancies. Hormonal influences cause an increase in insulin production as well as an increased tissue response to insulin during the first 20 weeks of gestation. However, during the last 20 weeks placental hormones cause an increased resistance to insulin and a decreased glucose tolerance. This causes catabolism (the "breaking down" phase

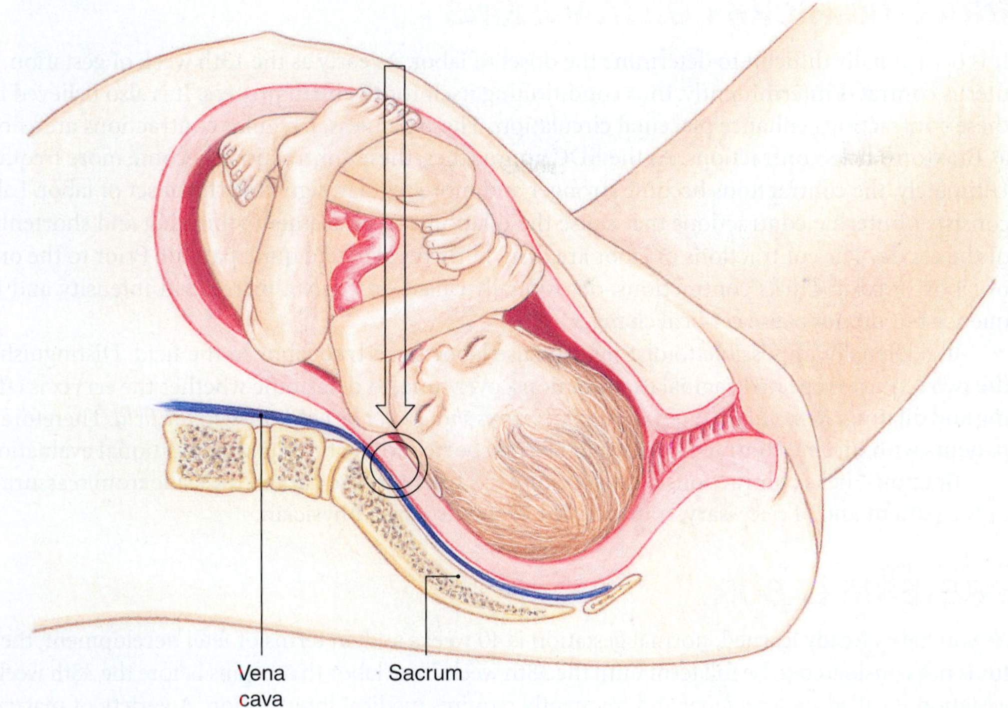

■ **Figure 40-7** The supine-hypotensive syndrome results from compression of the inferior vena cava by the gravid uterus.

of metabolism) between meals and during the night. At these times, ketones may be present in the urine because fats are metabolized more rapidly. Further, maternal glucose stores are used up, as they are the sole source of glucose to meet the energy needs of the growing fetus. This is known as the *diabetogenic* (diabetes-causing) *effect of pregnancy.* Gestational diabetes usually subsides after pregnancy.

Routine prenatal care includes screening to detect diabetes throughout the pregnancy. Women who are considered to be at high risk for developing gestational diabetes are given a glucose tolerance test at their first prenatal visit. High risk is associated with maternal age (over 35), obesity, hypertension, family history of diabetes, and history of prior stillbirth.

Management of gestational diabetes requires good prenatal care. The mother will be instructed on diabetic management and the importance of balancing diet and exercise as well as how to monitor her glucose levels and administer insulin. Fetal development will be monitored on an ongoing basis throughout the pregnancy.

Assessment When you encounter a pregnant patient with an altered mental status, consider hypoglycemia as a likely cause. Remember that the clinical signs and symptoms of hypoglycemia are many and varied. An abnormal mental status is the most important. Physical signs may include diaphoresis and tachycardia. If the blood sugar falls to a critically low level, she may sustain a hypoglycemic seizure or become comatose, which poses a potential life threat to the mother and fetus. Obtaining an accurate history of associated signs and symptoms, such as nausea, vomiting, abdominal pain, increased urination, or a recent infection, will allow you to ascertain whether diabetic ketoacidosis might be the cause of your patient's altered mental status. Determine the blood glucose level in addition to obtaining baseline vital signs and FHTs.

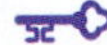

Consider hypoglycemia when encountering a pregnant patient with altered mental status.

Management If the blood glucose level is noted to be less than 60 mg/dL, draw a tube of blood and start an IV of normal saline. Next, administer 50 to 100 mL (25 to 50 g) of 50 percent dextrose intravenously. If the patient is conscious and able to swallow, complete glucose administration with orange juice, sugared soft drinks, or commercially available glucose pastes.

If the blood glucose level is in excess of 200 mg/dL, draw a red-top tube (or the tube specified by local protocols) of blood and then establish IV access to administer 1 to 2 L of 0.9 percent sodium chloride per protocol. If transport time is lengthy, medical direction may request intravenous or subcutaneous administration of regular insulin.

If blood glucose is below 60 mg/dL, draw a red-top tube of blood, start an IV of normal saline, and administer 25 grams of 50 percent dextrose. If blood glucose is above 200 mg/dL, draw a red-top tube of blood and administer 1 to 2 liters of normal saline by IV per protocol.

BRAXTON-HICKS CONTRACTIONS

It is occasionally difficult to determine the onset of labor. As early as the 13th week of gestation, the uterus contracts intermittently, thus conditioning itself for the birth process. It is also believed that these contractions enhance placental circulation. These painless, irregular contractions are known as Braxton-Hicks contractions. As the EDC approaches, these contractions become more frequent. Ultimately, the contractions become stronger and more regular, signaling the onset of labor. Labor consists of uterine contractions that cause the dilation and **effacement** (thinning and shortening) of the cervix. The contractions of labor are firm, fairly regular, and quite painful. Prior to the onset of labor Braxton-Hicks contractions, occasionally called *false labor,* increase in intensity and frequency but do not cause cervical changes.

effacement *the thinning and shortening of the cervix during labor.*

It is virtually impossible to distinguish false labor from true labor in the field. Distinguishing the two requires repeated vaginal examinations, over time, to determine whether the cervix is effacing and dilating. *Remember: Internal vaginal exams should not be performed in the field.* Therefore, all patients with uterine contractions should be transported to the hospital for additional evaluation.

Braxton-Hicks contractions do not require treatment by the paramedic aside from reassurance of the patient and, if necessary, transport for evaluation by a physician.

PRETERM LABOR

As you have already learned, normal gestation is 40 weeks and, in terms of fetal development, the fetus is not considered to be full term until the 38th week. True labor that begins before the 38th week of gestation is called *preterm labor* and frequently requires medical intervention. A variety of maternal, fetal, or placental factors may cause this potentially life-threatening situation for the mother and fetus:

- ★ Maternal factors
  - Cardiovascular disease
  - Renal disease
  - Hypertensive disorders of pregnancy (HDP)
  - Diabetes
  - Abdominal surgery during gestation
  - Uterine and cervical abnormalities
  - Maternal infection
  - Trauma, particularly blows to the abdomen
  - Contributory factors: history of preterm birth, smoking, and cocaine abuse
- ★ Placental factors
  - Placenta previa
  - Abruptio placentae
- ★ Fetal factors
  - Multiple gestation
  - Excessive amniotic fluid
  - Fetal infection

In many cases, physicians attempt to stop preterm labor to give the fetus additional time to develop in the uterus. Prematurity is the primary neonatal health problem in the nation and occurs in 7 to 10 percent of all live births. All of the preterm infant's organ systems are immature to some degree, but lung development is of greatest concern. Although technological advances in the care of preterm infants have improved the prognosis dramatically, the consequences of a preterm birth can last a lifetime.

Assessment When confronted by a patient with uterine contractions, first determine the approximate gestational age of the fetus. If it is less than 38 weeks, then suspect preterm labor. If gestational age is greater than 38 weeks, treat the patient as a term patient, as described later in this chapter.

After determining gestational age, obtain a brief obstetrical history. Then question the mother about the urge to push or the need to move her bowels or urinate. Also ask if her membranes have ruptured. Any sensation of fluid leakage or "gushing" from the vagina should be interpreted as ruptured membranes until proven otherwise. Next, palpate the contractions by placing your hand on the patient's abdomen. Note the intensity and length of the contractions, as well as the interval between contractions.

Commonly reported signs and symptoms of preterm labor include contractions that occur every 10 minutes or less, low abdominal cramping that is similar to menstrual cramps, or a sensation of pelvic pressure. Other complaints such as low backache, changes in vaginal discharge, and abdominal cramping with or without diarrhea may also be reported. Rupture of the membranes is confirmatory for preterm labor.

Management Preterm labor, especially if quite early in the pregnancy, should be stopped if possible. The process of stopping labor, or **tocolysis,** is frequently practiced in obstetrics. However, it is infrequently done in the field.

tocolysis *the process of stopping labor.*

There are three general approaches to tocolysis. The first is to sedate the patient, often with narcotics or barbiturates, thus allowing her to rest. Often, after a period of rest, the contractions stop on their own. The second approach is to administer a fluid bolus intravenously. The administration of approximately 1 liter of fluid intravenously increases the intravascular fluid volume, thus inhibiting ADH secretion from the posterior pituitary. Since oxytocin and ADH are secreted from the same area of the pituitary gland, the inhibition of ADH secretion also inhibits oxytocin release, often causing cessation of uterine contractions. Ultimately, if the previous methods fail, magnesium sulfate or a beta-agonist, such as terbutaline or ritodrine, may be administered to stop labor by inhibiting uterine smooth muscle contraction. Current research in tocolysis includes the administration of calcium channel blockers, such as nifedipine, and prostaglandin inhibitors, such as indomethacin. You may also find that a patient with preterm labor has been given corticosteroids to accelerate fetal lung maturity.

As a rule, tocolysis in the field is limited to sedation and hydration, especially if transport time is long. Paramedics may, however, transport a patient from one medical facility to another with beta-agonist administration underway. You should therefore be familiar with its use. Commonly associated side effects include being jittery, tachycardia usually described by the patient as palpitations, and occasionally abdominal pain. You will, of course, want to transport your patient to the nearest facility that has neonatal intensive care capabilities. Careful and frequent monitoring of maternal vital signs and FHTs is imperative during tocolysis.

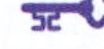

The patient with suspected preterm labor should be transported immediately.

THE PUERPERIUM

The **puerperium** is the time period surrounding birth of the fetus. Childbirth generally occurs in a hospital or similar facility with appropriate equipment. Occasionally, prehospital personnel may be called on to attend a delivery in the field. Therefore, you should be familiar with the birth process and some of the complications that may be associated with it.

puerperium *the time period surrounding the birth of the fetus.*

LABOR

Childbirth, or the delivery of the fetus, is the culmination of pregnancy. The process by which delivery occurs is called **labor,** the physiologic and mechanical process in which the baby, placenta, and amniotic sac are expelled through the birth canal. The duration of labor is widely variable.

labor *the time and processes that occur during childbirth; the physiologic and mechanical process in which the baby, placenta, and amniotic sac are expelled through the birth canal.*

Prior to the onset of true labor, the head of the fetus descends into the bony pelvis area. The frequency and intensity of the Braxton-Hicks contractions increase in preparation for true labor. Increased vaginal secretions and softening of the cervix occur. Bloody show, pink-tinged secretions, is generally considered a sign of imminent labor as the mucous plug is expelled from the cervix. Labor then usually begins within 24 to 48 hours. Many people also consider the rupture of the membranes as a sign of impending labor. If labor does not begin spontaneously within 12 to 24 hours after rupture, labor will likely require induction because of the risk of infection.

Pressure exerted by the fetus on the cervix causes changes that lead to the subsequent expulsion of the fetus. Muscular uterine contractions increase in frequency, strength, and duration. You can assess the frequency and duration of contractions by placing one hand on the fundus of the uterus. Time contractions from the beginning of one contraction until the beginning of the next. It is important to note whether the uterus relaxes completely between contractions. It is also desirable to monitor fetal heart tones during and between contractions. Occasional fetal bradycardia occurs during contractions, but the heart rate should increase to a normal rate (120 to 160) after the contraction ends. Failure of the heart rate to return to normal between contractions is a sign of fetal distress.

Labor is generally divided into three stages:

Review

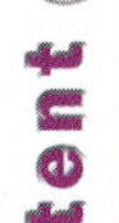
Content

Stages of Labor

- Stage one: dilatation
- Stage two: expulsion
- Stage three: placental

★ ***Stage One (Dilatation Stage)***

The first stage of labor begins with the onset of true labor contractions and ends with the complete dilatation and effacement of the cervix. Early in pregnancy the cervix is quite thick and long, but after complete *effacement* it is short and paper thin. Effacement usually begins several days before active labor ensues. *Dilatation* is the progressive stretching of the cervical opening. The cervix dilates from its closed position to 10 centimeters, which is considered complete dilation. This stage lasts approximately 8 to 10 hours for the woman in her first labor, the nullipara, and about 5 to 7 hours in the woman who has given birth previously, the multipara. Early in this stage the contractions are usually mild, lasting for 15 to 20 seconds with a frequency of 10 to 20 minutes. As labor progresses, the contractions increase in intensity and occur approximately every 2 to 3 minutes with a duration of 60 seconds.

★ ***Stage Two (Expulsion Stage)***

The second stage of labor begins with the complete dilatation of the cervix and ends with the delivery of the fetus. In the nullipara, this stage lasts 50 to 60 minutes, while it takes about half that amount of time for the multipara. The contractions are very strong, occurring every 2 minutes and lasting for 60 to 75 seconds. Often, the patient feels pain in her lower back as the fetus descends into the pelvis. The urge to push or "bear down" usually begins in the second stage. The membranes usually rupture at this time, if they have not ruptured previously. Crowning during contractions is evident as the delivery of the fetus nears. Crowning occurs when the head (or other presenting part of the fetus) is visible at the vaginal opening during a contraction and is the definitive sign that birth is imminent. The most common presentation is for the infant to be delivered headfirst, face down (vertex position).

★ ***Stage Three (Placental Stage)***

The third and final stage of labor begins immediately after the birth of the infant and ends with the delivery of the placenta. The placenta generally delivers within 5 to 20 minutes. There is no need to delay transport to wait for its delivery. Classic signs of placental separation include a gush of blood from the vagina; a change in size, shape, or consistency of the uterus; lengthening of the umbilical cord protruding from the vagina; and the mother's report that she has the urge to push.

MANAGEMENT OF A PATIENT IN LABOR

Transport the patient in labor unless delivery is imminent. Maternal urge to push or the presence of crowning indicates imminent delivery. Delivery at the scene or in the ambulance will be necessary.

Probably one of the most important decisions you must make with a patient in labor is whether to attempt to deliver the infant at the scene or to transport the patient to the hospital. It is generally preferable to transport the mother unless delivery is imminent. There are several factors to take into consideration when making this decision. They include the patient's number of previous pregnancies, the length of labor during the previous pregnancies, the frequency of contractions, the maternal urge to push, and the presence of crowning. Some women have rapid labors and may be completely dilated in a short period of time. Also, as mentioned, multiparas generally have shorter labors than nulliparas. The maternal urge to push or the presence of crowning indicates that delivery is imminent. In such cases, the infant should be delivered at the scene or in the ambulance.

Traditionally, a woman who had previously delivered by a cesarean section was advised to deliver all subsequent infants by cesarean sections. However, current thinking encourages women to attempt vaginal birth after cesarean (VBAC). If your patient has had prenatal care during this pregnancy she has probably already discussed this with her health care provider. The only absolute contraindication for VBAC is a classic vertical uterine incision. However, most cesarean sections done today are done using a low transverse uterine incision. (Note that a horizontal skin incision does not assure that the uterine incision is horizontal.) A labor patient who is opting for VBAC requires no more special care than any other labor patient does.

However, certain factors should prompt immediate transport, despite the threat of delivery. These include prolonged rupture of membranes (> 24 hours), since prolonged time between rupture and delivery often leads to fetal infection; abnormal presentation, such as breech or transverse; prolapsed cord; or fetal distress, as evidenced by fetal bradycardia or meconium staining (the presence of meconium, the first fetal stools, in the amniotic fluid). The presence of multiple fetuses may also contribute to your decision to transport. You will read more about these conditions later in this chapter.

FIELD DELIVERY

If delivery is imminent, you can assist the mother to deliver the baby in the field (Procedure 40–1 and Figures 40-8 ■ through 40-16 ■). Equipment and facilities must be quickly prepared. Set up a delivery area. This should be out of public view, such as in a bedroom or the back of the ambulance. Administer oxygen to the mother via nasal cannula or nonrebreather mask. If time permits, establish intravenous access and administer normal saline at a keep-open rate. Place the patient on her back with knees and hips flexed and buttocks slightly elevated. It should be noted that this position is easier on you than the mother. She may prefer to squat or lie in a semi-Fowler's position with her knees and hips flexed. Either of these positions enables gravity to facilitate the delivery. If time permits, drape the mother with toweling from the OB kit. Place one towel under the buttocks, another below the vaginal opening, and another across the lower abdomen.

Remember: Childbirth is a normal event. Your primary job will be to assist the mother in the delivery of the child.

Until delivery, the fetal heart rate should be monitored frequently. A drop in the fetal heart rate to less than 90 beats per minute indicates fetal distress and requires immediate transport with the mother in the left lateral recumbent position. Coach the mother to breathe deeply between contractions and to push with contractions. If the baby does not deliver after 20 minutes of contractions every 2 to 3 minutes, *transport immediately.*

Prepare the OB equipment and don sterile gloves, gown, and face shield or goggles. If time permits, wash your hands and forearms prior to gloving. As the head crowns, control it with gentle pressure. Providing support to the head and perineum decreases the likelihood of vaginal and perineal tearing and decreases the potential for rapid expulsion of the baby's skull through the birth canal which may cause intracranial injury. Support the head as it emerges from the vagina and begins to turn. If it is still enclosed in the amniotic sac, tear the sac open to permit escape of the amniotic fluid and enable the baby to breathe.

Gently slide your finger along the head and neck to ensure that the umbilical cord is not wrapped around the baby's neck. If it is, try to gently slip it over the shoulder and head. If this cannot be done and it is so wrapped tightly as to inhibit labor, carefully place two umbilical cord clamps approximately 2 inches apart and cut the cord between the clamps. As soon as the infant's head is clear of the vagina, instruct the mother to stop pushing. While supporting the head, suction the baby's mouth, then nose, using a bulb syringe. If meconium-stained fluid is noted, suction the mouth, nares, and pharynx with mechanical suction to prevent aspiration. Then tell the mother to resume pushing, while you support the infant's head as it rotates.

Gently guide the baby's head downward to allow delivery of the upper shoulder. Do not pull! Gently guide the baby's body upward to allow delivery of the lower shoulder. Once the head and shoulders have been delivered, the rest of the body will follow rapidly. Be prepared to support the infant's body as it emerges. Remember to keep the baby at the level of the vagina to prevent over- or

Procedure 40–1 **Normal Delivery**

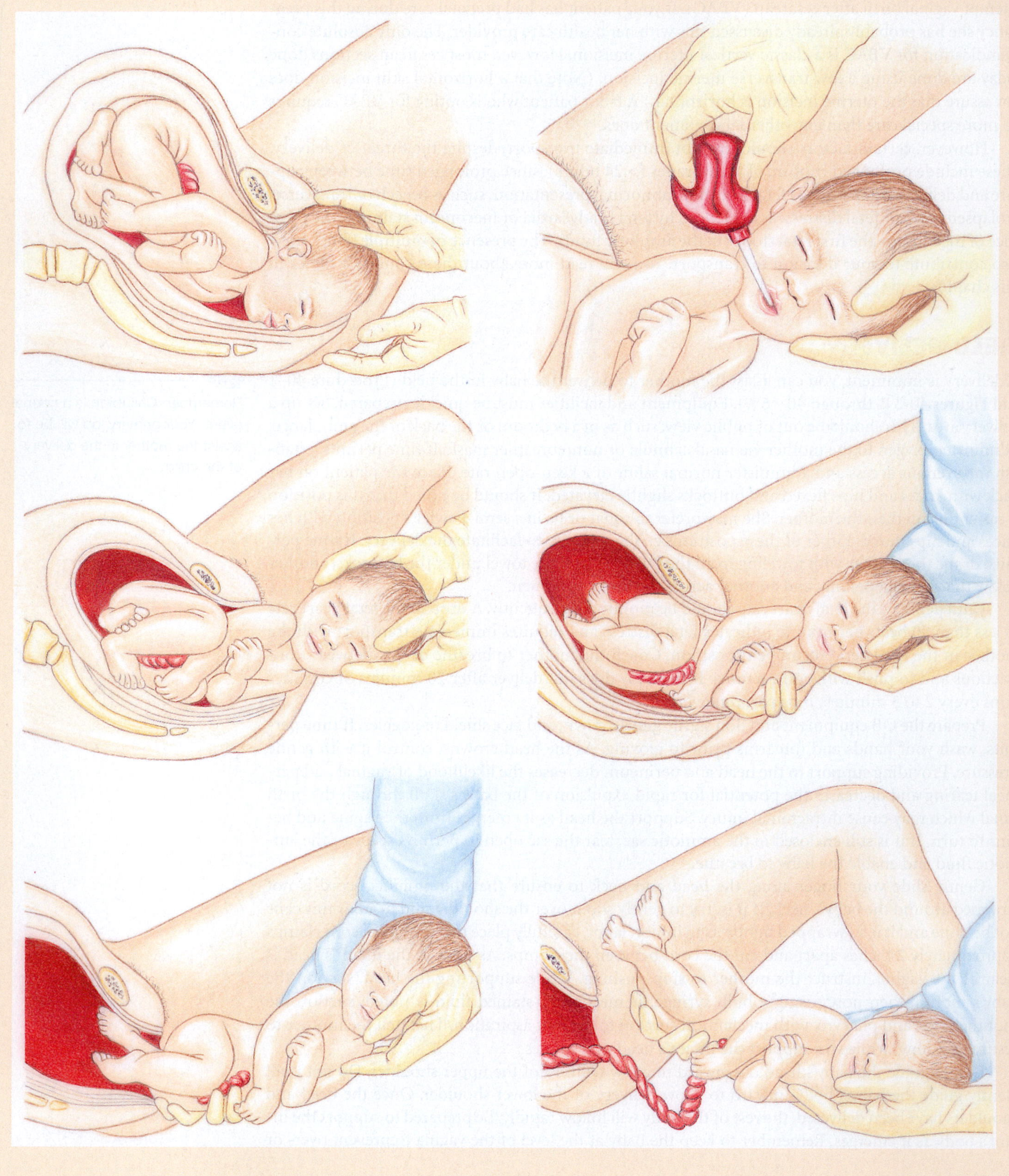

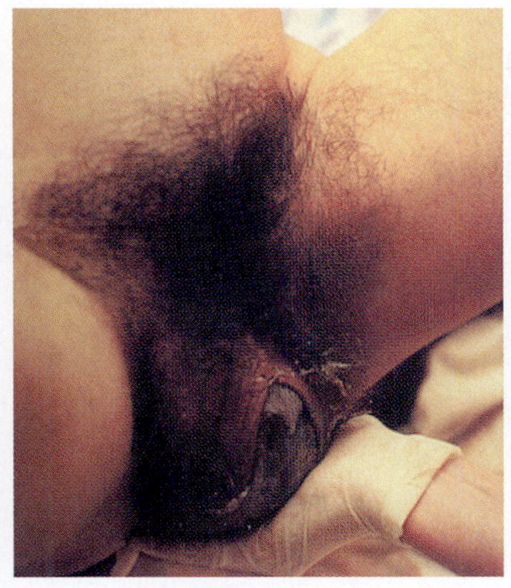

■ Figure 40-8 Crowning.

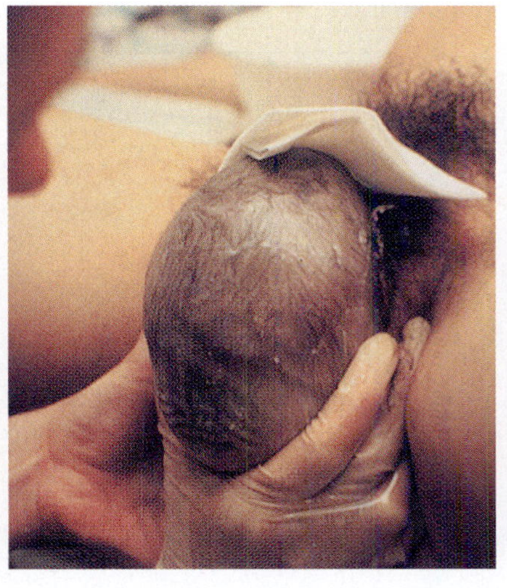

■ Figure 40-9 Delivery of the head.

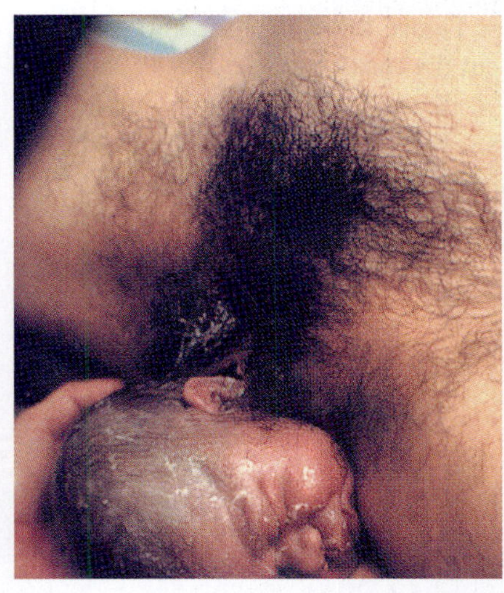

■ Figure 40-10 External rotation of the head.

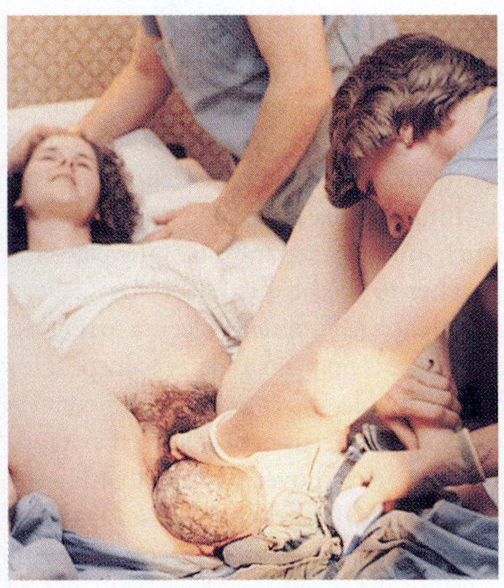

■ Figure 40-11 As soon as possible, suction the mouth, then the nose.

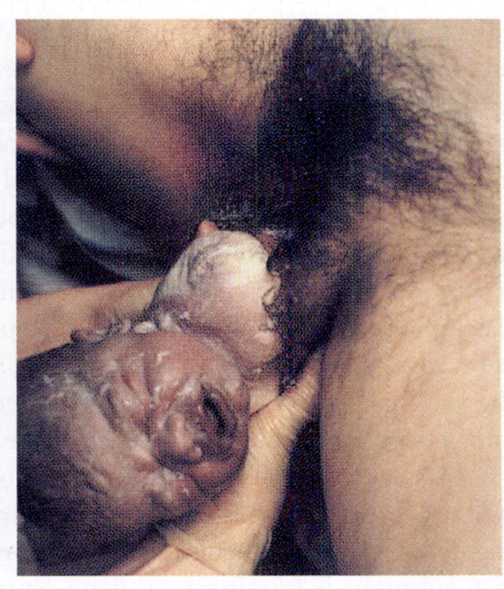

■ Figure 40-12 Delivery of the anterior shoulder.

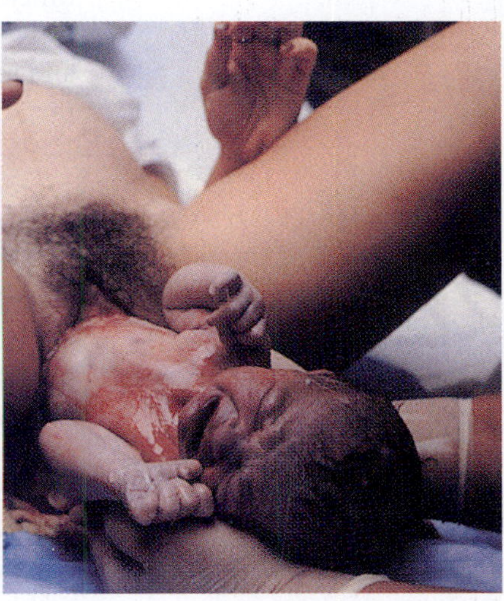

■ Figure 40-13 Complete delivery of the infant.

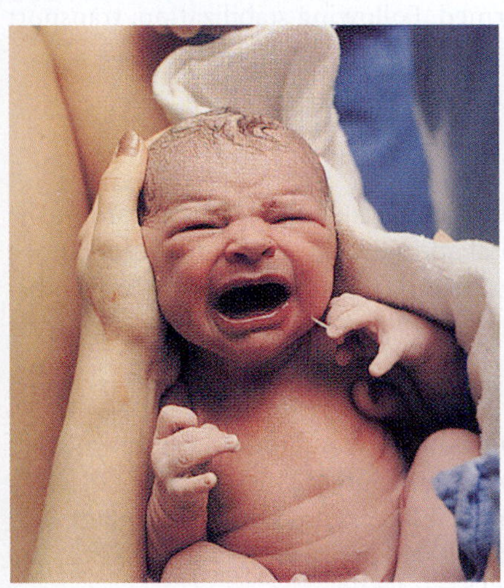

■ Figure 40-14 Dry the infant.

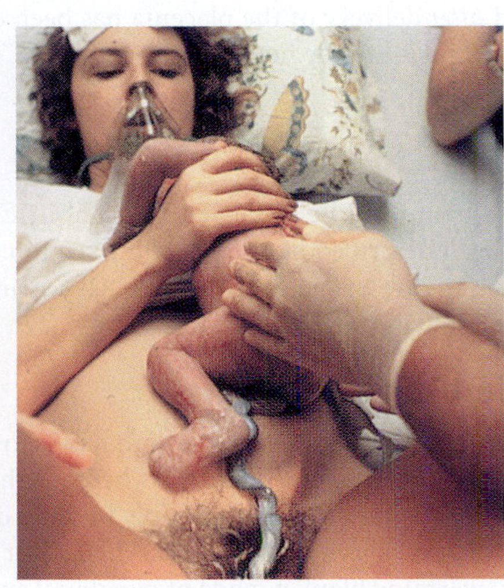

■ Figure 40-15 Place the infant on the mother's stomach.

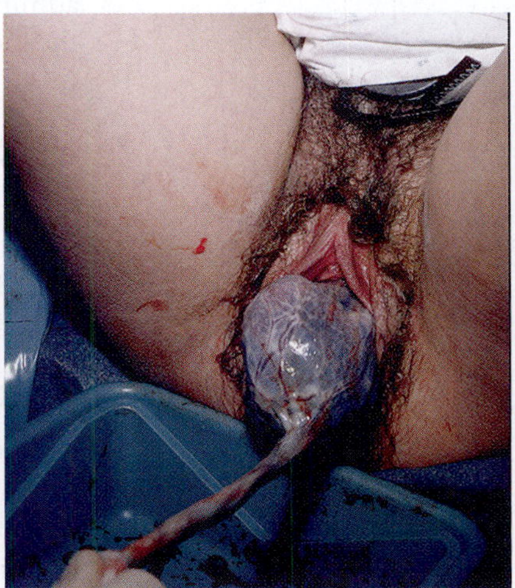

■ Figure 40-16 Deliver the placenta and save it for transport with the mother and infant.

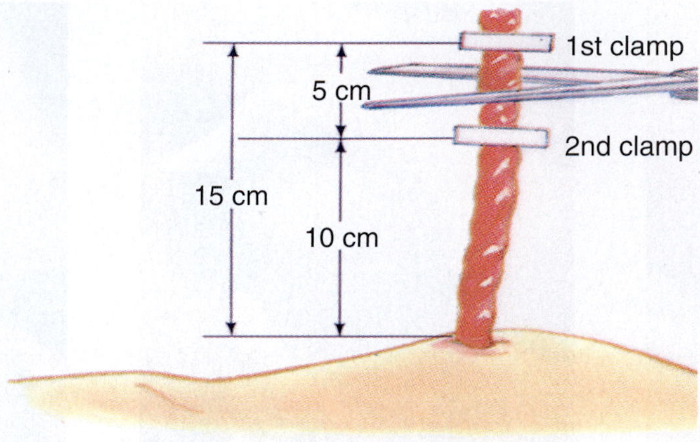

■ **Figure 40-17** Clamp and cut the cord.

undertransfusion of blood from the cord. Never "milk" the cord. Clamp and cut the cord as follows (Figure 40-17 ■). Supporting the baby's body, place the first umbilical clamp approximately 10 centimeters from the baby. Place the second clamp approximately 5 centimeters above the first. Then carefully cut the umbilical cord between the clamps. Wipe the baby's face clean of blood and mucus and repeat suctioning of the mouth and nose until the airway is clear. Dry the infant thoroughly and then cover with warm, dry blankets or towels, and position on his side. Record the time of birth.

Usual maternal blood loss with delivery is 1 pint (about 500 cc). Following delivery, if the uterus is contracting normally, the fundus should be at the level of the umbilicus and have the size and consistency of a grapefruit. After birth, the mother's vagina should continue to ooze blood. Do not pull on the umbilical cord. Eventually, the cord will appear to lengthen, which indicates separation of the placenta. The placenta should be delivered and transported with the mother to the hospital. If it does deliver, place it in a plastic biohazard bag and bring it to the hospital for evaluation. Retained placenta may cause maternal hemorrhage or become a source of infection. However, there is no need to delay transport for delivery of the placenta. At this time, massage the uterine fundus by placing one hand immediately above the symphysis pubis and the other on the uterine fundus. Cup the uterus between the two hands and support it. Massage until the uterus assumes a woody hardness. Avoid overmassage. Putting the baby to the mother's breast also stimulates uterine contractions, which will further decrease bleeding.

Following delivery, inspect the mother's perineum for tears. If any tears are present, apply direct pressure. Continuously monitor vital signs. Note the presence of continued hemorrhage and report it to medical direction. In some systems, paramedics may administer oxytocin (Pitocin) to facilitate uterine contraction in the control of postpartum hemorrhage. Oxytocin should only be administered *after* delivery of the placenta has been confirmed. Following stabilization, transport the mother and infant to the hospital.

NEONATAL CARE

neonate *newborn infant.*

Care of the **neonate** will be discussed in detail in Chapter 41, "Neonatology." Initial care of the neonate has been described in the preceding section. Several additional important considerations regarding routine care of the neonate, APGAR scoring, and neonatal resuscitation are briefly discussed in the following sections.

Routine Care of the Neonate

Support the infant's head and torso, using both hands. Maintain warmth, repeat suctioning of the mouth and nose as needed, and assess using APGAR scoring.

Newborns are slippery and will require both hands to support the head and torso. Position yourself so that you can work close to the surface where you have placed the infant.

Maintain warmth! Cold infants rapidly become distressed infants. Quickly dry the infant with towels, discarding each as it becomes wet. Then cover the infant with a dry receiving blanket or use a commercial warming blanket made of a material such as Thinsulate™.

Repeat suctioning of the mouth and nose as needed until the infant's airway is clear. Generally, suctioning and drying the baby will stimulate respirations, crying, and activity. This should cause

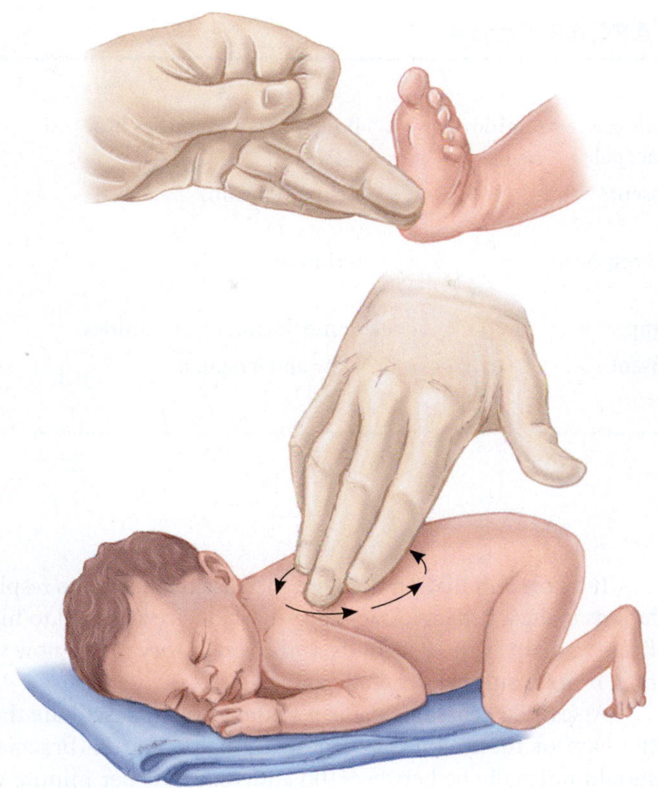

■ **Figure 40-18** Stimulate the infant as required.

the infant to "pink up." (Do not be alarmed if the extremities remain dusky. This is known as *acrocyanosis* and is very common in the first hours of life.) If this is not effective, you may try flicking your finger against the soles of the feet or rubbing gently in a circular motion in the middle of the back (Figure 40-18 ■).

Assess the neonate as soon as possible after birth. The normal neonatal respiratory rate should average 30 to 60 breaths per minute while the heart rate should be 100 to 180 beats per minute. If resuscitation is not indicated, assign APGAR scores. Do not, however, delay resuscitative efforts and transport in order to complete APGAR scoring.

APGAR Scoring

Named for Dr. Virginia Apgar, who developed the assessment tool, the APGAR scoring system is a means of evaluating the status of a newborn's vital functions at 1 minute and 5 minutes after delivery. There are five parameters and each is given a score from a low value of 0 to a normal value of 2. APGAR is an acronym for the names of the five parameters, which are *a*ppearance (skin color), *p*ulse rate, *g*rimace (irritability), *a*ctivity (muscle tone), and *r*espiratory effort (Table 40–2).

The majority of infants are healthy and active and have total scores between 7 and 10, requiring only routine care. Infants scoring between 4 and 6 are moderately depressed and require oxygen and stimulation to breathe. Infants scoring 0 to 3 are severely depressed and require immediate ventilatory and circulatory assistance. By repeating the score at 1 and 5 minutes, it is possible to determine whether intervention has caused a change in infant status.

Neonatal Resuscitation

It is estimated that approximately 6 percent of all neonates born in a hospital require resuscitation. It is likely that this percentage is higher for out-of-hospital deliveries, although the exact numbers are not available. Factors that contribute to the need for resuscitation include prematurity, pregnancy and delivery complications, maternal health problems, or inadequate prenatal care.

Table 40–2 The APGAR Score

Element	0	1	2	Score
Appearance (Skin color)	Body and extremities blue, pale	Body pink, extremities blue	Completely pink	
Pulse rate	Absent	Below 100/min	100/min or above	
Grimace (Irritability)	No response	Grimace	Cough, sneeze, cry	
Activity (Muscle tone)	Limp	Some flexion of extremities	Active motion	
Respiratory effort	Absent	Slow and irregular	Strong cry	
			Total Score =	

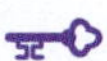

If the infant's respirations are below 30 per minute and tactile stimulation does not increase the rate to a normal range, immediately assist ventilations using a pediatric bag-valve-mask with high-flow, high-concentration oxygen. If the heart rate is below 60 and does not respond to ventilations, initiate chest compressions. Transport to a facility with neonatal intensive care capabilities.

If tactile stimulation does not increase the neonate's respiratory rate, immediately assist ventilations using a pediatric bag-valve-mask device attached to high-flow, high-concentration oxygen. Reassess after 15 to 30 seconds. If the respiratory rate is now within normal limits, assess the heart rate. If not, continue ventilations.

Assess the heart rate using a stethoscope to auscultate the apical pulse, by feeling the pulse at the base of the umbilical cord, or by palpating the brachial or femoral artery. The heart rate should normally be between 100 and 180 beats per minute with a range of 140 to 160 beats per minute being optimal. If the pulse is 100 or greater with spontaneous respirations, continue assessment. If less than 100, continue positive-pressure ventilations. If less than 60 and not responding to ventilations, initiate chest compressions. Continue to reassess respiratory status and heart rate frequently.

Make every effort to expedite transport to a facility capable of providing neonatal intensive care while you continue resuscitative efforts. If you have a long transport time, it may be necessary to initiate vascular access in order to administer medications or fluid resuscitation. The most logical (and easiest) access is the umbilical vein. If this is not feasible, consider peripheral veins or an intraosseous access. While many medications (epinephrine, atropine, lidocaine, and naloxone) can be administered via the endotracheal route, this route is not suitable for fluid resuscitation. During transport, continue to maintain warmth while supporting ventilations, oxygenation, and circulation. Refer to Chapter 41, "Neonatology," for more information on neonatal resuscitation.

Content Review

Abnormal Deliveries

- Breech presentation
- Prolapsed cord
- Limb presentation
- Occiput posterior

ABNORMAL DELIVERY SITUATIONS

Breech Presentation

Most infants present head first and face down, which is called the vertex position. Breech presentation is the term used to describe the situation in which either the buttocks or both feet present first. This occurs in approximately 4 percent of all live births. In such presentations, there is an increased risk for delivery trauma to the mother, as well as an increased potential for cord prolapse, cord compression, or anoxic insult for the infant. Although the cause is unknown, breech presentations are most commonly associated with preterm birth, placenta previa, multiple gestation, and uterine and fetal anomalies.

Management Because cesarean section is often required, delivery of the breech presentation is best accomplished at the hospital. However, if field delivery is unavoidable, the following maneuvers are recommended. First, position the mother with her buttocks at the edge of a firm bed. Ask her to hold her legs in a flexed position. She will often require assistance in doing this. As the infant delivers, do not pull on the infant's legs. Simply support them. Allow the entire body to be delivered with contractions while you merely continue to support the infant's body (Figure 40-19 ■).

As the head passes the pubis, apply gentle upward traction until the mouth appears over the perineum. If the head does not deliver, and the baby begins to breathe spontaneously with its face pressed against the vaginal wall, place a gloved hand in the vagina with the palm toward the infant's face. Form a "V" with the index and middle fingers on either side of the infant's nose, and push the vaginal wall away from the infant's face to allow unrestricted respiration (Figure 40-20 ■). If necessary, continue during transport.

Alternatively, you may find that the shoulders, not the head, are the most difficult part to deliver. In that case, allow the body to deliver to the level of the umbilicus. Support the infant's body in your palm while gently extracting approximately 4 to 6 inches of umbilical cord. Be very careful that you do not compress the cord during this extraction. Gently rotate the infant's body so that the shoulders are now in an anterior-posterior position. Apply gentle traction to the body until the axilla become visible. Guide the infant's body upward to deliver the posterior shoulder. Then, guide the neonate downward to facilitate delivery of the anterior shoulder. Now gently ease the head through the birth canal. Continue your care of the mother and infant as you would with a normal delivery.

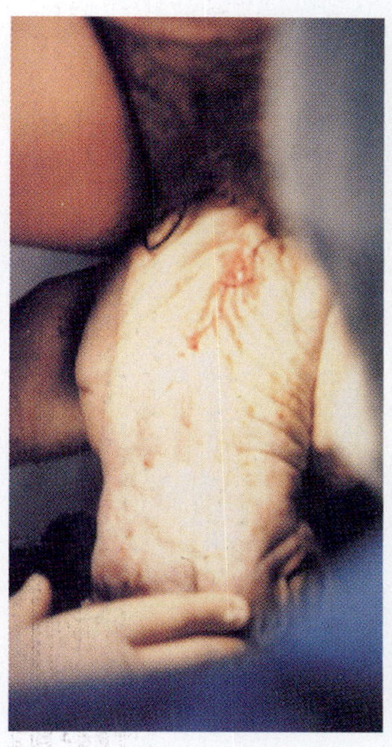

■ Figure 40-19 Breech delivery.

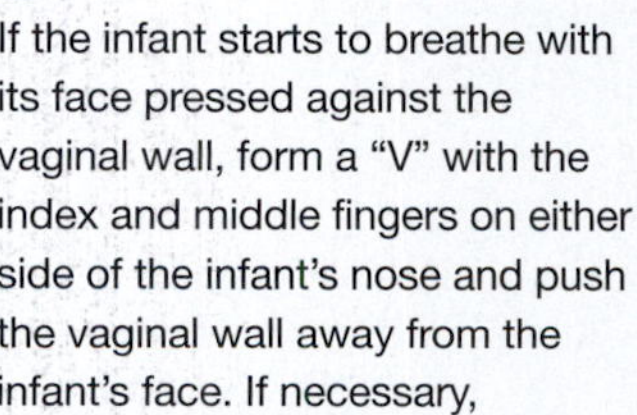

If the infant starts to breathe with its face pressed against the vaginal wall, form a "V" with the index and middle fingers on either side of the infant's nose and push the vaginal wall away from the infant's face. If necessary, continue during transport.

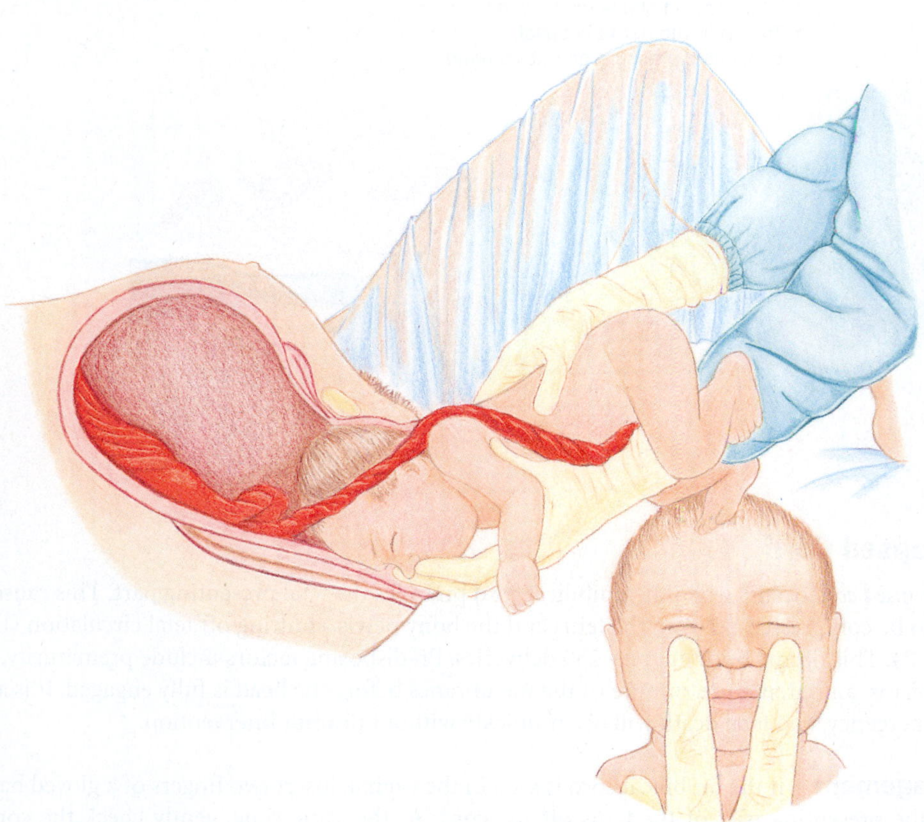

■ Figure 40-20 Placement of the fingers to maintain the airway in a breech birth.

■ Figure 40-21 Prolapsed cord.

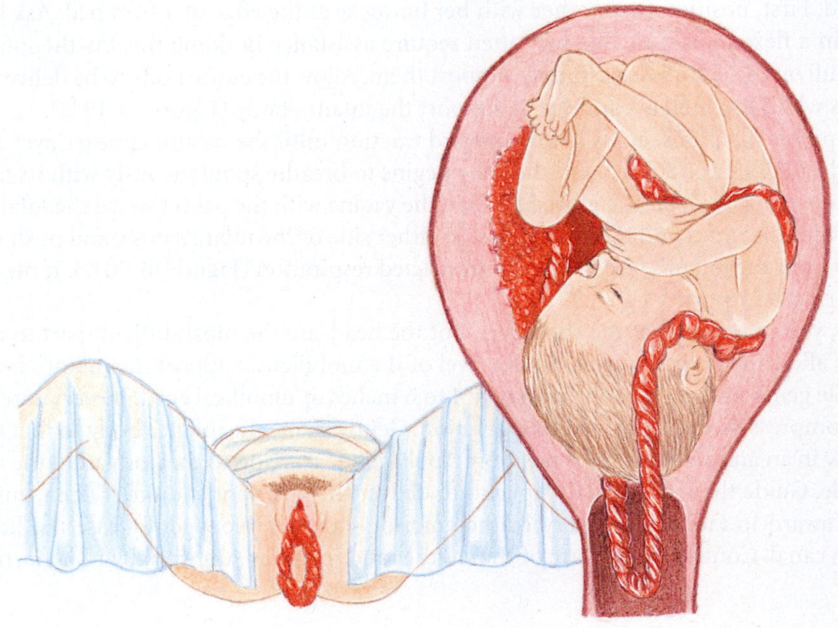

Prolapsed Cord

A *prolapsed cord* occurs when the umbilical cord precedes the fetal presenting part. This causes the cord to be compressed between the fetus and the bony pelvis, shutting off fetal circulation (Figure 40-21 ■). This occurs once in every 250 deliveries. Predisposing factors include prematurity, multiple births, and premature rupture of the membranes before the head is fully engaged. It is a serious emergency, and fetal death will occur quickly without prompt intervention.

If the umbilical cord is seen in the vagina, insert two gloved fingers to raise the fetus off the cord. Place the mother in the Trendelenburg or knee-chest position, administer oxygen, and transport immediately. Do not attempt delivery.

Management If the umbilical cord is seen in the vagina, insert two fingers of a gloved hand to raise the presenting part of the fetus off the cord. At the same time, gently check the cord for pulsations, but take great care to ensure that you do not compress the cord. Place the mother in a Trendelenburg or knee-chest position (Figure 40-22 ■). Administer high-flow, high-concentration oxygen to the mother and transport her immediately, with the fingers continuing to hold the

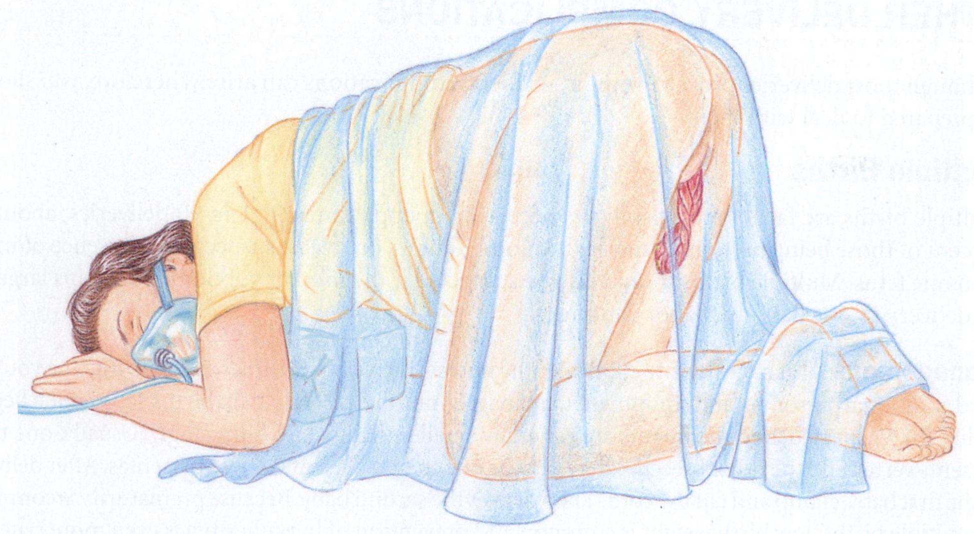

■ Figure 40-22 Patient positioning for prolapsed cord.

presenting part off the umbilical cord. If assistance is available, apply a dressing moistened with sterile saline to the exposed cord. *Do not attempt delivery! Do not pull on the cord! Do not attempt to push the cord back into the vagina!*

Limb Presentation

Sometimes, if the baby is in a transverse lie across the uterus, an arm or leg is the presenting part protruding from the vagina. This is seen in less than 1 percent of births and is more commonly associated with preterm birth and multiple gestation.

Management When examination of the perineum reveals a single arm or leg protruding from the birth canal, a cesarean section is necessary. Under no circumstance should you attempt a field delivery. Do not touch the extremity, as to do so may stimulate the infant to gasp, risking inhalation and aspiration of amniotic fluid. *Do not pull on the extremity or attempt to push it back into the vagina!*

Assist the mother into a knee-chest position as is also done when there is a prolapsed cord and administer oxygen via nonrebreather mask. Provide reassurance to the mother. Transport immediately (still in the knee-chest position) for emergency cesarean section.

With limb presentation, place the mother in the knee-chest position, administer oxygen, and transport immediately. Do not attempt delivery.

Other Abnormal Presentations

Other abnormal presentations can complicate delivery. One of the most common is the *occiput posterior position.* Normally, as the infant descends into the pelvis, its face is turned posteriorly. This is important, as extension of the head assists delivery. However, if the infant descends facing forward, or occiput posterior, its passage through the pelvis is delayed. This presentation occurs most frequently in primigravidas. In multigravidas it usually resolves spontaneously.

The presenting part may also be the face or brow, rather than the crown of the head. Occasionally, during these presentations, the face or brow can be seen high in the pelvis during a contraction. Usually, vaginal delivery is impossible in these cases.

As described earlier for a limb presentation, the fetus can lie transversely in the uterus. In such a case, the fetus cannot enter the pelvis for delivery. If the membranes rupture, the umbilical cord can prolapse, or an arm or leg can enter the vagina. Vaginal delivery is impossible.

When an abnormal presentation or position of the fetus makes normal delivery impossible, reassure the mother, administer oxygen, and transport immediately. Do not attempt field delivery in these circumstances.

Management Early recognition of an abnormal presentation is important. If one is suspected, the mother should be reassured, placed on oxygen, and transported immediately, since forceps or cesarean delivery is often required.

Content Review

Other Delivery Complications

- Multiple births
- Cephalopelvic disproportion
- Precipitous delivery
- Shoulder dystocia
- Meconium staining

OTHER DELIVERY COMPLICATIONS

Although most deliveries proceed without incident, complications can arise. Therefore, you should be prepared to deal with them.

Multiple Births

Multiple births are fairly rare, with twins occurring in approximately 1 in 90 deliveries, about 40 percent of those being preterm. Usually, the mother knows or at least suspects the presence of more than one fetus. Multiple births should also be suspected if the mother's abdomen remains large after delivery of one baby and labor continues.

Management Manage this situation with the normal delivery guidelines, recognizing that you will need additional personnel and equipment to manage a multiple birth. In twin births, labor often begins earlier than expected, and the infants are generally smaller than babies born singly. Usually, one twin presents vertex and the other breech. There may be one shared placenta or two placentas. After delivery of the first baby, clamp and cut the cord. Then deliver the second baby. Because prematurity is common in multiple births, low birth weight is common and prevention of hypothermia is even more crucial.

Cephalopelvic Disproportion

Cephalopelvic disproportion occurs when the infant's head is too big to pass through the maternal pelvis easily. This may be caused by an oversized fetus. Large fetuses are associated with diabetes, multiparity, or postmaturity. Fetal abnormalities such as hydrocephalus, conjoined twins, or fetal tumors may make vaginal delivery impossible. Women of short stature or women with contracted pelvises are at increased risk for this problem. If cephalopelvic disproportion is not recognized and managed appropriately, fetal demise or uterine rupture may occur.

Cephalopelvic disproportion tends to develop most frequently in the primigravida. There may be strong contractions for an extended period of time. On physical examination, the fetus may feel large. Also, labor generally does not progress. The fetus may be in distress, as evidenced by fetal bradycardia or meconium staining.

Management The usual management of cephalopelvic disproportion is cesarean section. Administer oxygen to the mother and establish intravenous access. Transport should be immediate and rapid.

Precipitous Delivery

A *precipitous delivery* is a delivery that occurs after less than 3 hours of labor. This type of delivery occurs most frequently in the grand multipara and is associated with a higher-than-normal incidence of fetal trauma, tearing of the umbilical cord, or maternal lacerations.

Management The best way to handle precipitous delivery is to be prepared. Do not turn your attention from the mother. Be ready for a rapid delivery, and attempt to control the infant's head. Once delivered, the baby may have some difficulty with temperature regulation and must be kept warm.

Shoulder Dystocia

A *shoulder dystocia* occurs when the infant's shoulders are larger than its head. This occurs most frequently with diabetic and obese mothers and in post-term pregnancies. In shoulder dystocia, labor progresses normally and the head is delivered routinely. However, immediately after the head is delivered, it retracts back into the perineum because the shoulders are trapped between the symphysis pubis and the sacrum ("turtle sign").

Management If a shoulder dystocia occurs, *do not pull on the infant's head.* Administer oxygen to the mother and have her drop her buttocks off the end of the bed. Then flex her thighs upward to facilitate delivery and apply firm pressure with an open hand immediately above the symphysis pubis. If delivery does not occur, transport the patient immediately.

Meconium Staining

Meconium staining occurs when the fetus passes feces into the amniotic fluid. Between 10 and 30 percent of all deliveries have meconium-stained fluid. It is always indicative of a fetal hypoxic incident. Hypoxia causes an increase in fetal peristalsis along with relaxation of the anal sphincter, causing meconium to pass into the amniotic fluid. In addition to the stress that caused the incident, there is a risk of aspiration of the meconium-stained fluid.

Meconium staining is often associated with prolonged labor but may be seen in term, post-term, and low-birth-weight infants. The incident may occur a few days prior to delivery or during labor. Some meconium staining is virtually always associated with breech deliveries as a result of vagal stimulation, which occurs as a result of the pressure of the contracting uterus on the fetus's head.

Evidence of meconium staining is readily observable. Normally the amniotic fluid is clear or possibly light straw colored. When meconium is present, the color varies from a light yellowish-green to light green or, worst case, dark green, which is sometimes described as "pea soup." As a rule, the thicker and darker the color, the higher the risk of fetal morbidity.

If meconium is thick, visualize the infant's glottis and suction the hypopharynx and trachea using a clean endotracheal tube each time until all meconium has been cleared from the airway.

Management As noted earlier, once the head of the newborn is out of the birth canal you should suction the mouth and nose on the perineum. If the meconium is thin and light colored no further treatment is required, and you should continue with the delivery and routine care. However, if the meconium is thick, visualize the glottis and suction the hypopharynx and trachea using a clean endotracheal tube each time until you have cleared all of the meconium from the newborn's airway. Failure to do so will cause the meconium to be pushed farther into the airway and down into the lungs during the delivery process.

MATERNAL COMPLICATIONS OF LABOR AND DELIVERY

Content Review

Maternal Complications

- Postpartum hemorrhage
- Uterine rupture
- Uterine inversion
- Pulmonary embolism

Several maternal problems can arise during and after delivery. These include postpartum hemorrhage, uterine rupture, uterine inversion, and pulmonary embolism.

Postpartum Hemorrhage

Postpartum hemorrhage is the loss of more than 500 cc of blood immediately following delivery. It occurs in approximately 5 percent of deliveries. The most common cause of postpartum hemorrhage is *uterine atony,* or lack of uterine muscle tone. This tends to occur most frequently in the multigravida and is most common following multiple births or births of large infants. Uterine atony also occurs after precipitous deliveries and prolonged labors. In addition to uterine atony, postpartum hemorrhage can be caused by placenta previa, abruptio placentae, retained placental parts, clotting disorders in the mother, or vaginal and cervical tears. Occasionally, the uterus fails to return to its normal size during the postpartum period, and postpartum hemorrhage occurs long after the birth, potentially as much as 2 weeks postpartum.

Assessment of the patient with postpartum hemorrhage should focus on the history and the predisposing factors as described. You must rely heavily on the clinical appearance of the patient and her vital signs. Often, the uterus will feel boggy and soft on physical examination. Vaginal bleeding is usually obvious as a steady, free flow of blood. Counting the number of sanitary pads used is a good way to monitor the bleeding. When postpartum bleeding takes place in the hospital setting the pads are often weighed, since 500 cc of blood weighs approximately 1 pound. You should also examine the perineum for evidence of traumatic injury, which may be the source of the bleeding.

When there is a loss of more than 500 cc of blood immediately following delivery, administer oxygen and begin fundal massage. Establish two large-bore IVs of normal saline. Treat for shock as necessary. Follow local protocols regarding application of anti-shock trousers.

Management When confronted by a patient with postpartum hemorrhage, complete the primary assessment immediately. Administer oxygen and begin fundal massage. Establish at least one, preferably two, large-bore IVs of normal saline. If shock is evident, apply anti-shock trousers according to your local protocols. Never attempt to force delivery of the placenta or pack the vagina with dressings. In severe cases, medical direction may request the administration of oxytocin (Pitocin). The usual dose is 10 to 20 USP units (20 mg) oxytocin in 1 L of normal saline to run at 125 cc/hr titrated to response. If IV access cannot be obtained, an alternative therapy is to administer 10 USP units intramuscularly.

Uterine Rupture

Uterine rupture is the actual tearing, or rupture, of the uterus. It usually occurs with the onset of labor. However, it can also occur before labor as a result of blunt abdominal trauma. During labor, it often results from prolonged uterine contractions or a surgically scarred uterus, such as occurs from previous cesarean sections, especially in those with the classic vertical incision. It can also occur following a prolonged or obstructed labor, as in the case of cephalopelvic disproportion or in conjunction with abnormal presentations. Although it is a rare occurrence, it carries with it an extremely high maternal and fetal mortality rate.

The patient with uterine rupture will complain of excruciating abdominal pain and will often be in shock. Uterine rupture is virtually always associated with the cessation of labor contractions. If the rupture is complete, the pain usually subsides. On physical examination, there is often profound shock without evidence of external hemorrhage, although it is sometimes associated with vaginal bleeding. Fetal heart tones are absent. The abdomen is often tender and rigid and may exhibit rebound tenderness. It is often possible to palpate the uterus as a separate hard mass found next to the fetus.

Management Management is the same as for any patient in shock. Administer oxygen at high flow and high concentration. Next, establish two large-bore IVs with normal saline and begin fluid resuscitation. Monitor vital signs and fetal heart tones continuously. Transport the patient rapidly. If the fetus is still viable, the definitive treatment is cesarean section with subsequent repair or removal of the uterus.

Uterine Inversion

Uterine inversion is a rare emergency occurring only once in every 2,500 live births. It occurs when the uterus turns inside out after delivery and extends through the cervix. When uterine inversion occurs, the supporting ligaments and blood vessels supplying blood to the uterus are torn, usually causing profound shock. The average blood loss associated with uterine inversion ranges from 800 to 1,800 cc. Uterine inversion usually results from pulling on the umbilical cord while awaiting delivery of the placenta or from attempts to express the placenta when the uterus is relaxed.

In the rare occurrence of uterine inversion, begin fluid resuscitation, then make one attempt to replace the uterus. If this fails, cover the uterus with towels moistened with saline and transport immediately.

Management If uterine inversion occurs, you must act quickly. First, place the patient in a supine position and begin oxygen administration. *Do not* attempt to detach the placenta or pull on the cord. Initiate two large-bore IVs of normal saline and begin fluid resuscitation. Make one attempt to replace the uterus, using the following technique. With the palm of the hand, push the fundus of the inverted uterus toward the vagina. If this single attempt is unsuccessful, cover the uterus with towels moistened with saline and transport the patient immediately.

Pulmonary Embolism

Pulmonary embolism is the presence of a blood clot in the pulmonary vascular system (see Chapter 27, "Pulmonology"). It can occur after pregnancy, usually as a result of venous thromboembolism. It is one of the most common causes of maternal death and appears to occur more frequently following cesarean section than vaginal delivery. Pulmonary embolism may occur at any time during pregnancy. There is usually a sudden onset of severe dyspnea accompanied by sharp chest pain. Some patients also report a sense of impending doom. On physical examination, the patient may show tachycardia, tachypnea, jugular vein distention, and, in severe cases, hypotension.

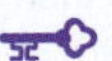

Pulmonary embolism usually presents with sudden severe dyspnea and sharp chest pain. Administer high-flow, high-concentration oxygen and support ventilations as needed. Establish an IV of normal saline. Transport immediately, monitoring the heart, vital signs, and oxygen saturation.

Management Management of pulmonary embolism consists of administration of high-flow, high-concentration oxygen and ventilatory support as needed. Also establish an IV of normal saline at a keep-open rate. Initiate cardiac monitoring and carefully monitor the patient's vital signs and oxygen saturation while transporting her immediately.

Summary

Childbirth is a normal process and obstetrical emergencies are fairly uncommon. However, all pregnant patients are at risk for developing complications, and it is impossible to predict which ones will actually occur. It is therefore important to recognize these complications and act accordingly. Keep in mind that you are caring for two patients; as long as you remember the priorities of patient care, the situation should go smoothly. Relax and enjoy the opportunity to help bring a new life into the world.

Review Questions

1. The first 2 weeks of the menstrual cycle are dominated by the hormone ___________, which causes the endometrium to thicken and become engorged with blood.
   a. pitocin
   b. estrogen
   c. epinephrine
   d. progesterone
2. During normal fetal development, the sex of the infant can usually be determined by ___________ weeks' gestation.
   a. 10
   b. 12
   c. 14
   d. 16
3. A woman who has given birth to her first child is termed:
   a. multipara.
   b. primipara.
   c. primigravida.
   d. multigravida.
4. Generally, vital signs in the pregnant patient should be taken with the patient:
   a. sitting upright.
   b. lying on her right side.
   c. lying on her left side.
   d. lying flat on her back.
5. ___________ is the preferred analgesic in pregnancy.
   a. Codeine
   b. Demerol
   c. Nitrous oxide
   d. Morphine sulfate
6. Intentional termination of a pregnancy under any condition not allowed by law is termed:
   a. missed abortion.
   b. elective abortion.
   c. criminal abortion.
   d. therapeutic abortion.
7. ___________ occurs as a result of abnormal implantation of the placenta on the lower half of the uterine wall, resulting in partial or complete coverage of the cervical opening.
   a. Placenta previa
   b. Ectopic pregnancy
   c. Abruptio placentae
   d. Incomplete abortion

8. An abortion in which fetal death occurs but the fetus is not expelled is termed:
   a. missed abortion.
   b. criminal abortion.
   c. habitual abortion.
   d. incomplete abortion.
9. The ___________ stage of labor begins with the complete dilatation of the cervix and ends with the delivery of the fetus.
   a. first
   b. third
   c. second
   d. dilatation
10. Infants scoring ___________ on the APGAR scoring system are moderately depressed and require oxygen and stimulation to breathe.
    a. 7 to 10
    b. 0 to 3
    c. 6 to 9
    d. 4 to 6

See Answers to Review Questions at the back of this book.

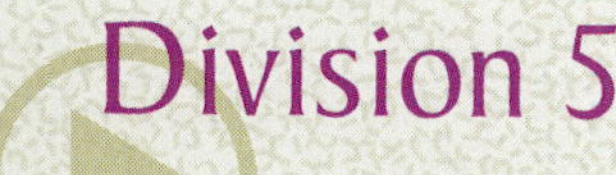

Division 5

Special Considerations/ Operations

Chapter

41

Neonatology

Objectives

After reading this chapter, you should be able to:

1. Define newborn and neonate. (p. 1555)
2. Identify important antepartum factors that can affect childbirth. (p. 1556)
3. Identify important intrapartum factors that can determine high-risk newborn patients. (p. 1556)
4. Identify the factors that lead to premature birth and low-birth-weight newborns. (pp. 1556, 1573, 1576–1577)
5. Distinguish between primary and secondary apnea. (p. 1557)
6. Discuss pulmonary perfusion and asphyxia. (p. 1557)
7. Identify the primary signs utilized for evaluating a newborn during resuscitation. (pp. 1559–1560)
8. Identify the appropriate use of the APGAR scale. (pp. 1559–1560)
9. Calculate the APGAR score given various newborn situations. (pp. 1559–1560; see also Chapter 40)
10. Formulate an appropriate treatment plan for providing initial care to a newborn. (pp. 1560–1563)
11. Describe the indications, equipment needed, application, and evaluation of the following management techniques for the newborn in distress:
    - ★ Blow-by oxygen (pp. 1565, 1567)
    - ★ Ventilatory assistance (pp. 1565, 1567–1568)
    - ★ Endotracheal intubation (pp. 1564, 1566–1567, 1568)
    - ★ Orogastric tube (p. 1570)
    - ★ Chest compressions (pp. 1570, 1571)
    - ★ Vascular access (pp. 1570, 1571)
12. Discuss the routes of medication administration for a newborn. (pp. 1570, 1571, 1572)
13. Discuss the signs of hypovolemia in a newborn. (p. 1578)
14. Discuss the initial steps in resuscitation of a newborn. (pp. 1564–1573)
15. Discuss the effects of maternal narcotic usage on the newborn. (p. 1573)

16. Determine the appropriate treatment for the newborn with narcotic depression. (p. 1573)
17. Discuss appropriate transport guidelines for a newborn. (p. 1573)
18. Determine appropriate receiving facilities for low- and high-risk newborns. (p. 1573)
19. Describe the epidemiology, including the incidence, morbidity/mortality, risk factors and prevention strategies, pathophysiology, assessment findings, and management for the following neonatal problems:
    - ★ Meconium aspiration (pp. 1574–1575)
    - ★ Apnea (p. 1575)
    - ★ Diaphragmatic hernia (pp. 1575–1576)
    - ★ Bradycardia (p. 1576)
    - ★ Prematurity (pp. 1576–1577)
    - ★ Respiratory distress/cyanosis (pp. 1577–1578)
    - ★ Seizures (pp. 1578–1579)
    - ★ Fever (p. 1579)
    - ★ Hypothermia (pp. 1579–1580)
    - ★ Hypoglycemia (p. 1580)
    - ★ Vomiting (pp. 1580–1581)
    - ★ Diarrhea (p. 1581)
    - ★ Common birth injuries (pp. 1581–1582)
    - ★ Cardiac arrest (p. 1582)
    - ★ Post-arrest management (p. 1582)
20. Given several neonatal emergencies, provide the appropriate procedures for assessment, management, and transport. (pp. 1555–1582)

Key Terms

acrocyanosis, p. 1579
antepartum, p. 1556
APGAR scoring, p. 1559
birth injury, p. 1581
choanal atresia, p. 1559
cleft lip, p. 1559
cleft palate, p. 1559
DeLee suction trap, p. 1560
diaphragmatic hernia, p. 1559
ductus arteriosus, p. 1557
extrauterine, p. 1557
glottic function, p. 1569
herniation, p. 1575
hyperbilirubinemia, p. 1563
intrapartum, p. 1556
isolette, p. 1573
meconium, p. 1560
meningomyelocele, p. 1559
nasogastric tube, p. 1570
neonatal abstinence syndrome (NAS), p. 1581
neonate, p. 1555
newborn, p. 1555
omphalocele, p. 1559
orogastric tube, p. 1570
PEEP, p. 1569
persistent fetal circulation, p. 1557
phototherapy, p. 1581
Pierre Robin syndrome, p. 1559
polycythemia, p. 1563
thyrotoxicosis, p. 1581
vagal response, p. 1564

INTRODUCTION

Babies pass through stages of physical and emotional development. This chapter concerns itself with babies 1 month old and under. Babies less than 1 month old are called **neonates.** Recently born neonates—those in the first few hours of their lives—may also be called **newborns** or *newly born infants* (Figure 41-1 ■).

neonate *an infant from the time of birth to 1 month of age.*

newborn *a baby in the first few hours of its life; also called a* newly born infant.

After an unscheduled delivery in the field, you have two patients to manage—the mother and the baby. You can review information on care of the mother in Chapter 40, "Obstetrics." The present chapter will describe the initial care of newborns, focusing on the special needs of distressed and premature newborns.

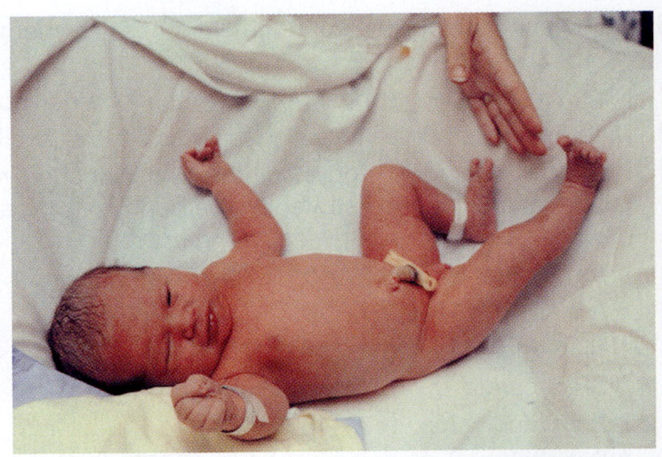

■ **Figure 41-1** Term newborn.

GENERAL PATHOPHYSIOLOGY, ASSESSMENT, AND MANAGEMENT

The care of newborns follows the same priorities as for all patients. You should complete the primary assessment first. Correct any problems detected during the primary assessment before proceeding to the next step. The vast majority of newborns require no resuscitation beyond suctioning the airway, mild stimulation, and maintenance of body temperature. However, for newborns who require additional care, your quick actions can make the difference between life and death.

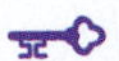

For newborns that require additional care, your quick actions can make the difference between life and death.

EPIDEMIOLOGY

Approximately 6 percent of field deliveries require life support procedures. The incidence of complications increases as the birth weight decreases. About 80 percent of newborns weighing less than 1,500 grams (3 pounds, 5 ounces) at birth require resuscitation. Determine if a newborn is at risk by considering the **antepartum** and **intrapartum** factors that may indicate complications at the time of delivery (Table 41–1).

antepartum *before the onset of labor.*

intrapartum *occurring during childbirth.*

Your success in resuscitating at-risk infants increases with training, ongoing practice, and proper stocking of equipment on board the ambulance. Make sure your ambulance carries a basic OB kit and resuscitation equipment for newborns of various sizes. (See the list in the "Resuscitation" section later in this chapter.)

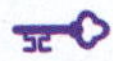

Your success in treating at-risk newborns increases with training, ongoing practice, and proper stocking of equipment on board the ambulance.

Plan transport in advance. Know the types of facilities available in your locality and local protocols governing use of these facilities. A nearby neonatal intensive care unit (NICU) makes the best choice for at-risk newborns. However, if you must transport to a distant NICU, determine whether it might be in the best interests of the infant to transport him to the nearest facility for stabilization. Follow local protocols and consult medical direction as needed.

Table 41–1 Risk Factors Indicating Possible Complications in Newborns

Antepartum Factors	Intrapartum Factors
Multiple gestation	Premature labor
Inadequate prenatal care	Meconium-stained amniotic fluid
Mother's age (<16 or >35)	Rupture of membranes more than 24 hours prior to delivery
History of perinatal morbidity or mortality	Use of narcotics within 4 hours of delivery
Post-term gestation	Abnormal presentation
Drugs/medications	Prolonged labor or precipitous delivery
Toxemia, hypertension, diabetes	Prolapsed cord or bleeding

PATHOPHYSIOLOGY

On birth, dramatic changes occur within the newborn to prepare it for **extrauterine** life. The respiratory system, which is essentially nonfunctional when the fetus is in the uterus, must suddenly initiate and maintain respirations. While in the uterus, fetal lung fluid fills the fetal lungs. The capillaries and arterioles of the lungs are closed. Most blood pumped by the heart bypasses the nonfunctional respiratory system by flowing through the **ductus arteriosus.**

On birth, dramatic changes take place within the newborn to prepare it for extrauterine life.

extrauterine *outside the uterus.*

ductus arteriosus *channel between the main pulmonary artery and the aorta of the fetus.*

Approximately one-third of fetal lung fluid is removed through compression of the chest during vaginal delivery. Under normal conditions, the newborn takes its first breath within the first few seconds after delivery. The timing of the first breath is unrelated to the cutting of the umbilical cord. Factors that stimulate the baby's first breath include:

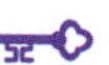

The time of a newborn's first breath is unrelated to the cutting of the umbilical cord.

- ★ Mild acidosis
- ★ Initiation of stretch reflexes in the lungs
- ★ Hypoxia
- ★ Hypothermia

With the first breaths, the lungs rapidly fill with air, which displaces the remaining fetal fluid. The pulmonary arterioles and capillaries open, decreasing pulmonary vascular resistance. At this point, the resistance to blood flow in the lungs is now less than the resistance of the ductus arteriosus. Because of this pressure difference, blood flow is diverted from the ductus arteriosus to the lungs, where it picks up oxygen for transport to the peripheral tissues (Figure 41-2 ■).

Soon, there is no need for the ductus arteriosus, and it eventually closes and becomes the *ligamentum arteriosum.* However, if hypoxia or severe acidosis occurs, the pulmonary vascular bed may constrict again and the ductus may reopen. This will retrigger fetal circulation with its attendant shunting and ongoing hypoxia. (This condition is called **persistent fetal circulation.**) To help the newborn make its transition to extrauterine life, it is very important for the paramedic to facilitate its first few breaths and to prevent ongoing hypoxia and acidosis.

persistent fetal circulation *condition in which blood continues to bypass the fetal respiratory system, resulting in ongoing hypoxia.*

Remain alert at all times to signs of respiratory distress. Infants are susceptible to hypoxemia, which can lead to permanent brain damage. After initial hypoxia, the infant rapidly gasps for breath. If the asphyxia continues, respiratory movements cease altogether, the heart rate begins to fall, and neuromuscular tone gradually diminishes. The infant then enters a period of apnea known as *primary apnea.* In most cases, simple stimulation and exposure to oxygen will reverse bradycardia and assist in the development of pulmonary perfusion.

With ongoing asphyxia, however, the infant will enter a period known as *secondary apnea.* During secondary apnea, the infant takes several last deep gasping respirations. The heart rate, blood pressure, and oxygen saturation in the blood continue to fall. The infant becomes unresponsive to stimulation and will not spontaneously resume respiration on its own. Death will occur unless you promptly initiate resuscitation. For this reason, always assume that apnea in the newborn is secondary apnea and rapidly treat it with ventilatory assistance with oxygen and, when appropriate, chest compressions.

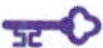

Always assume that apnea in the newborn is secondary apnea and rapidly treat it with ventilatory assistance.

Congenital Anomalies

Approximately 2 percent of infants are born with some sort of congenital problem. Congenital problems typically arise from a problem in fetal development. Most fetal development occurs during the first trimester of pregnancy. It is during this time that the developing fetus is most sensitive to environmental factors and substances that can affect normal development.

There are many types of congenital anomalies. These may affect a single organ or structure or may affect many organs or structures. Congenital anomalies are the leading cause of death in infants, causing approximately one quarter of infant deaths. Several recognized patterns, called *syndromes,* occur. It is not within the scope of this text to discuss all of the various congenital anomalies. However, a few of the congenital anomalies may make resuscitation of the neonate more difficult. Among the congenital anomalies encountered, congenital heart defects are the most common. The cause of these is largely unknown. Congenital heart defects are often classified by whether or not they increase pulmonary blood flow, decrease pulmonary blood flow, or obstruct blood flow.

Newborns may have congenital anomalies that make resuscitation more difficult.

Some congenital heart problems result in increased pulmonary blood flow. These include cases where the *ductus arteriosus* fails to close, a condition referred to as *patent ductus arteriosus* (also called a *persistent ductus arteriosus*). Also, septal defects (a hole in the wall between the atria or the

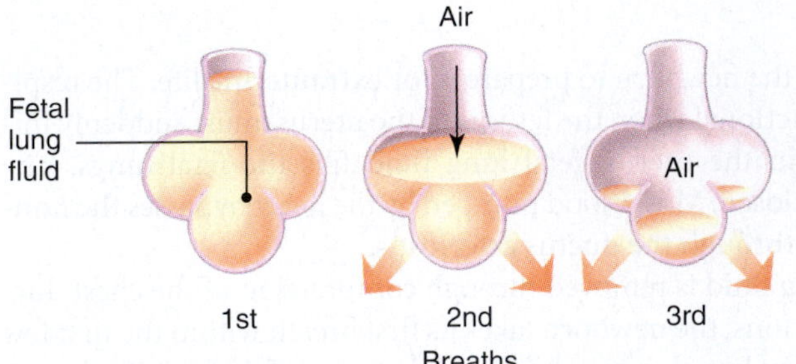

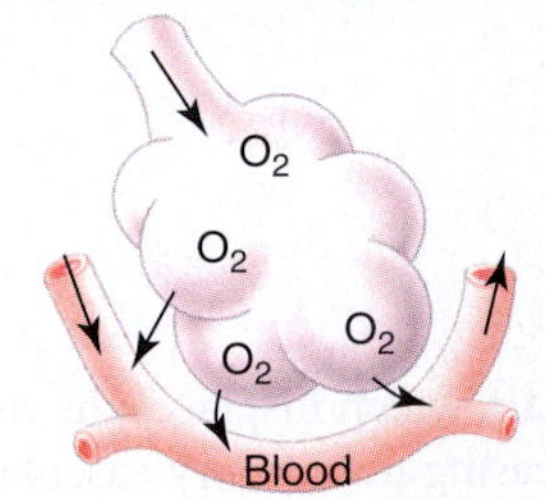

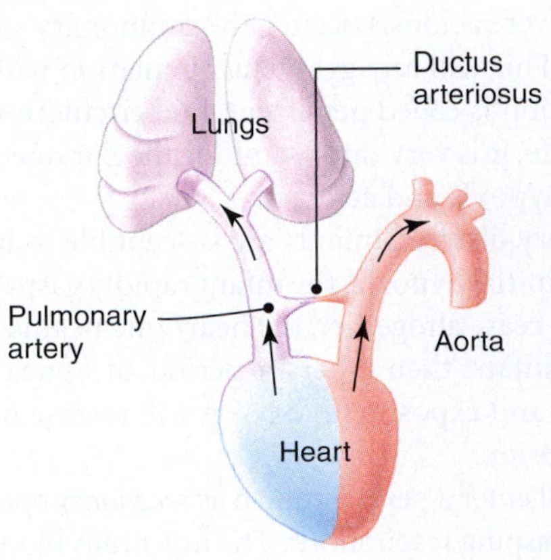

■ **Figure 41-2**
Hemodynamic changes in the newborn at birth.

ventricles) can result in increased pulmonary blood flow. With *atrial septal defect,* there is a hole between the atria that allows the comixing of blood. With a *ventricular septal defect,* there is a hole between the two ventricles that allows comixing of blood. The increase in pulmonary blood flow that results from either type of septal defect can lead to congestive heart failure.

Other congenital cardiac anomalies can lead to decreased pulmonary blood flow, which decreases the ability of the lungs to oxygenate the blood. These defects include *tetralogy of Fallot,* which is a combination of four congenital conditions. In addition, a condition called *transposition of the great vessels* can occur whereby the normal outflow tracts of the right and left ventricles are switched.

Finally, some congenital cardiac anomalies can result in obstruction of blood flow. Causes of blood flow obstruction include coarctation of the aorta, aortic or mitral stenosis/atresia, and hypoplastic left heart syndrome. With *coarctation of the aorta,* there is a narrowing in the arch of the aorta that obstructs blood flow. Problems with either the mitral or the aortic valve can cause blood flow obstruction, a condition called *mitral stenosis* or *aortic stenosis.* With *hypoplastic left heart syndrome,* the left side of the heart is underdeveloped, a condition that is usually fatal by 1 month of age if untreated.

There are some noncardiac congenital anomalies of note. For example, some children may be born with a defect in the diaphragm that allows some of the abdominal contents to enter the chest through the defect. This abnormality is referred to as a **diaphragmatic hernia.** If you suspect a diaphragmatic hernia, do not treat the infant with bag-valve-mask ventilation. If there is a diaphragmatic hernia, bag-valve-mask or other positive-pressure ventilation will cause stomach distention, which will cause the stomach to protrude into the chest cavity, thus decreasing ventilatory capacity. Instead, immediately intubate the infant. Diaphragmatic hernia will be discussed in more detail later in this chapter.

diaphragmatic hernia *protrusion of abdominal contents into the thoracic cavity through an opening in the diaphragm.*

Some infants are born with a defect in the spinal cord. In some cases, the spinal cord and associated structures may be exposed. This abnormality is called a **meningomyelocele.** Infants born with a meningomyelocele should not be placed on the back. Instead, place them on the stomach or side and conduct resuscitation in this position, if possible. Cover the spinal defect with sterile gauze pads soaked in warm sterile saline and inserted in a plastic covering.

meningomyelocele *herniation of the spinal cord and membranes through a defect in the spinal column.*

A newborn may exhibit a defect in the area of the umbilicus. In some cases, the abdominal contents will fill this defect, resulting in an **omphalocele.** If you encounter a newborn with an omphalocele, cover the defect with an occlusive plastic covering to decrease water and heat loss.

omphalocele *congenital hernia of the umbilicus.*

Because newborns are obligate nose breathers, **choanal atresia** can cause upper airway obstruction and respiratory distress. Choanal atresia is the most common birth defect involving the nose and is due to the presence of a bony or membranous septum between the nasal cavity and the pharynx. Suspect this condition if you are unable to pass a catheter through either nare into the oropharynx. An oral airway will usually bypass the obstruction.

choanal atresia *congenital closure of the passage between the nose and pharynx by a bony or membranous structure.*

A fairly common congenital anomaly is cleft lip and cleft palate. During fetal development, the lip and palate come together in the middle forming the oral cavity. Failure of the palate to completely close during fetal development can result in a defect known as **cleft palate.** Cleft palate may also be associated with failure of the upper lip to close. This condition, referred to as **cleft lip,** can make it difficult to obtain an adequate seal for effective mask ventilation. If a child with a cleft lip or cleft palate will require more than brief mechanical ventilation, you should place an endotracheal tube.

cleft palate *congenital fissure in the roof of the mouth, forming a passageway between oral and nasal cavities.*

cleft lip *congenital vertical fissure in the upper lip.*

Pierre Robin syndrome is a congenital condition characterized by a small jaw and large tongue in conjunction with a cleft palate. In this condition, the tongue is likely to obstruct the upper airway. A nasal or oral airway usually bypasses the obstruction. If the obstruction cannot be bypassed with a simple airway, then intubation will be necessary, although it can be very difficult to carry out on newborns with this condition.

Pierre Robin syndrome *unusually small jaw, combined with a cleft palate, downward displacement of the tongue, and an absent gag reflex.*

ASSESSMENT

Assess the newborn immediately after birth. (Ideally, if two paramedics are available, one paramedic attends the mother while the other attends the newborn.) Make a mental note of the time of birth and then quickly obtain vital signs. Remember that newborns are slippery and will require both hands to support the head and torso. Position yourself so that you can work close to the surface where you have placed the infant.

APGAR scoring *a numerical system of rating the condition of a newborn. It evaluates the newborn's heart rate, respiratory rate, muscle tone, reflex irritability, and color.*

The newborn's respiratory rate should average 40 to 60 breaths per minute. If respirations are not adequate or if the newborn is gasping, immediately start positive-pressure ventilation.

Expect a normal heart rate of 150 to 180 beats per minute at birth, slowing to 130 to 140 beats per minute thereafter. A pulse rate of less than 100 beats per minute indicates distress and requires emergency intervention.

Evaluate the skin color as well. Some cyanosis of the extremities is common immediately after birth. However, cyanosis of the central part of the body is abnormal, as is persistent peripheral cyanosis. In such cases, administer 100 percent oxygen until the cause is determined or the condition is corrected.

Content Review

APGAR

- Appearance
- Pulse rate
- Grimace
- Activity
- Respiratory effort

The APGAR Score

As discussed in Chapter 40, "Obstetrics," assign the newborn an **APGAR score** as soon as possible, (see Table 40–2 in Chapter 40). Ideally, try to do this at 1 and 5 minutes after birth. However, if the newborn is not breathing, DO NOT withhold resuscitation in order to determine the APGAR score.

If a newborn is not breathing, DO NOT withhold resuscitation in order to determine the APGAR score.

Table 41–2	Guidelines for Tracheal Tube Sizes and Depth of Insertion in the Newborn		
Tube Size, mm ID	**Depth of Insertion from Upper Lip, cm**	**Weight, g**	**Gestation, wk**
2.5	6.5–7	<1,000	<28
3.0	7–8	1,000–2,000	28–34
3.5	8–9	2,000–3,000	34–38
3.5–4.0	>9	>3,000	>38

American Heart Association: *2000 Handbook of Cardiovascular Care for Healthcare Providers* © 2000, American Heart Association.

The APGAR scoring system helps distinguish between newborns who need only routine care and those who need greater assistance. The system also predicts long-term survival.

A score of 0, 1, or 2 is given for each of the previous parameters. The minimum total score is 0 and the maximum is 10. A score of 7 to 10 indicates an active and vigorous newborn who requires only routine care. A score of 4 to 6 indicates a moderately distressed newborn who requires oxygenation and stimulation. Severely distressed newborns, those with APGAR scores of less than 4, require immediate resuscitation.

Severely distressed newborns, those with APGAR scores of less than 4, require immediate resuscitation.

TREATMENT

Treatment starts prior to delivery. Begin care by preparing the environment and assembling the equipment needed for delivery and immediate care of the newborn. The primary care of a newborn follows the same priorities as for all patients. Complete the primary assessment first. Correct any problems detected during the primary assessment before proceeding to the next step. The vast majority of term newborns—approximately 80 percent—require no resuscitation beyond suctioning of the airway, mild stimulation, and maintenance of body temperature by drying and warming with blankets.

Airway management is one of the most critical steps in caring for the newborn.

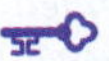

Always suction the mouth first so that there is nothing for the infant to aspirate if he gasps when the nose is suctioned.

Establishing the Airway

Airway management is one of the most critical steps in caring for the newborn. During delivery, fluid is forced out of the baby's lungs, into the oropharynx, and out through the nose and mouth. Fluid drainage occurs independently of gravity. As soon as you deliver the newborn's head, suction the mouth and then the nose, using a bulb suction. Always suction the mouth first so that there is nothing for the infant to aspirate if he gasps when the nose is suctioned.

DeLee suction trap *a suction device that contains a suction trap connected to a suction catheter. The negative pressure that powers it can come either from the mouth of the operator or, preferably, from an external vacuum source.*

meconium *dark green material found in the intestine of the full-term newborn. It can be expelled from the intestine into the amniotic fluid during periods of fetal distress.*

Immediately following delivery, maintain the newborn at the same level as the mother's vagina, with the head approximately 15 degrees below the torso. This facilitates the drainage of secretions and helps to prevent aspiration. If there appears to be a large amount of secretions, attach a **DeLee suction trap** to a suction source. As previously explained, suction the mouth first and then the nose (Figure 41-3a ■). Repeat these steps until the airway is clear. If you detect **meconium,** do not suction the infant if he is vigorous, but if he is not vigorous, prepare intubation equipment and a meconium aspirator (Figure 41-3b ■). (Meconium staining will be discussed in more detail in several later sections of this chapter.)

Drying and suctioning produce enough stimulation to initiate respirations in most newborns. If the newborn does not immediately cry, stimulate it by flicking the soles of its feet or gently rubbing its back (Figure 41-4 ■). DO NOT spank or vigorously rub a newborn baby.

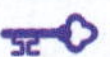

If the newborn does not cry immediately, stimulate it by gently rubbing its back or flicking the soles of its feet. DO NOT spank or vigorously rub a newborn baby.

Preventing Heat Loss

Heat loss can be a life-threatening condition in newborns. Cold infants quickly become distressed infants. Heat loss occurs through evaporation, convection, conduction, and radiation. Most heat loss in newborns results from evaporation, since the newborn comes into the world wet, and the

When head is delivered

As soon as the baby's head is delivered (prior to delivery of the shoulders) *the mouth, oropharynx, and hypopharynx should be thoroughly suctioned,* using a 10-Fr. DeLee suction catheter or other flexible suction catheter. Any catheter used should be no smaller than a 10 Fr.

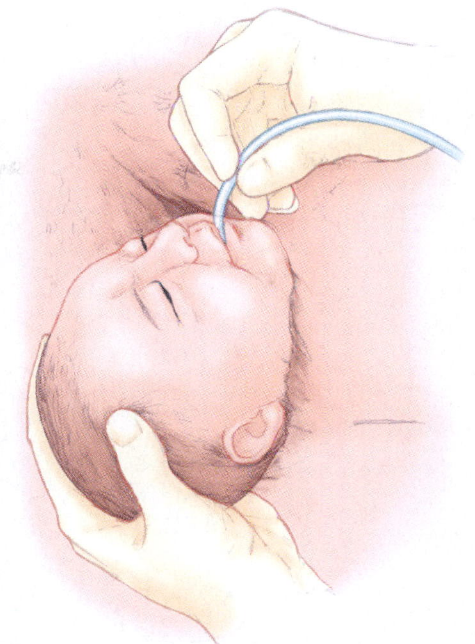

■ Figure 41-3a Suctioning of the mouth using flexible suction catheter.

Following delivery

After delivery of the infant, if a great deal of meconium is present, the trachea should be intubated and any residual meconium removed from the lower airway.

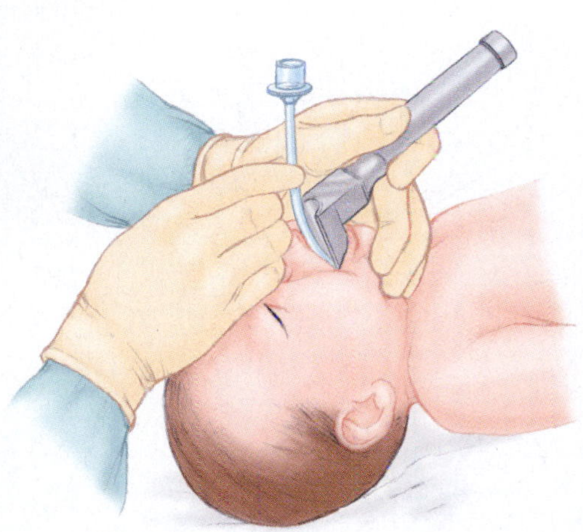

■ Figure 41-3b Intubation for removal of residual meconium.

amniotic fluid quickly evaporates. Immediately after birth, the newborn's core temperature can drop 1°C (1.8°F) or more from its birth temperature of 38°C (100.4°F).

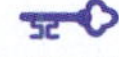

Cold infants quickly become distressed infants.

Loss of heat can also occur through convection, depending on the temperature of the room and the movement of the air around the newborn. The newborn can lose additional heat through contact with surrounding surfaces (convection) or by radiating heat to colder objects nearby.

To prevent heat loss, take these steps:

- ★ Dry the newborn immediately to prevent evaporative cooling (Figure 41-5 ■).
- ★ Maintain the ambient temperature—the temperature in the delivery room or ambulance—at a *minimum* of 23 to 24°C (74° to 76°F).
- ★ Close all windows and doors.
- ★ Discard the towel used to dry the newborn and swaddle the infant in a warm, dry receiving blanket or other suitable material. Cover the head.
- ★ In colder areas, place well-insulated water bottles or rubber gloves filled with warm water (40°C or 104°F) around the newborn to help maintain a warm body temperature. To avoid burns, do not place these items against the skin. Be sure the newborn is wrapped in a blanket and place the water bottle or rubber glove against the blanket.

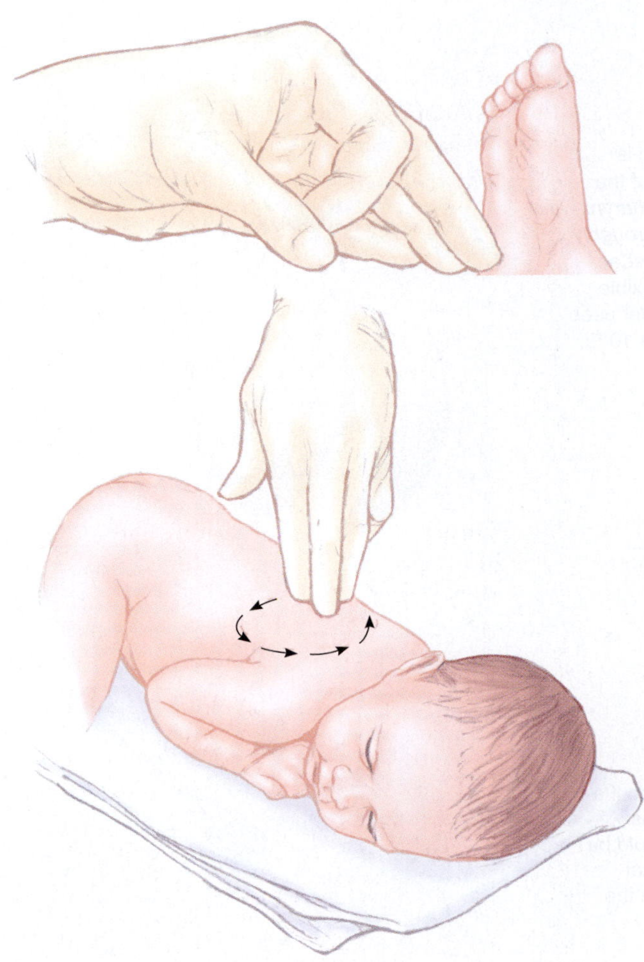

■ **Figure 41-4** Stimulate the newborn as required.

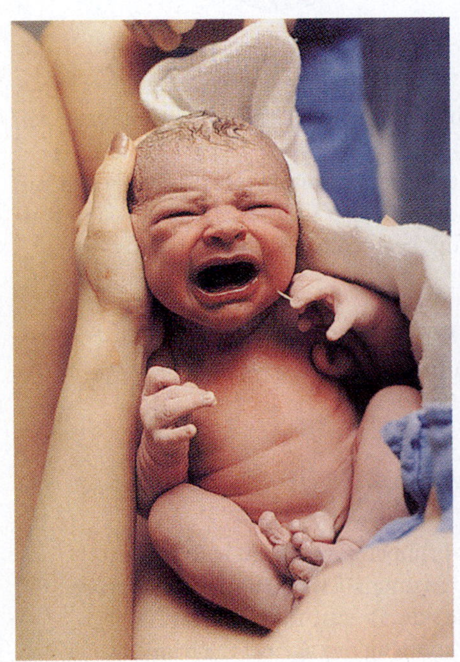

■ **Figure 41-5** Dry the infant to prevent loss of evaporative heat.

Cutting the Umbilical Cord

After you have stabilized the newborn's airway and minimized heat loss, clamp and cut the umbilical cord. You can prevent over- and undertransfusion of blood by maintaining the baby at the same level as the mother's vagina, as previously described. Do not "milk" or strip the umbilical cord, since this increases blood viscosity, or **polycythemia.** Polycythemia can cause cardiopulmonary problems. It can also contribute to excessive red blood cell destruction, which may in turn lead to **hyperbilirubinemia**—an increased level of bilirubin in the blood that causes jaundice.

Apply the umbilical clamps within 30 to 45 seconds after birth. Place the first clamp approximately 10 cm (4 inches) from the newborn. Place the second clamp about 5 cm (2 inches) farther away than the first. Then cut the cord between the two clamps (see Figure 40-17 in Chapter 40, "Obstetrics"). After the cord is cut, inspect it periodically to make sure there is no additional bleeding.

Do not "milk" or strip the umbilical cord.

polycythemia *an excess of red blood cells. In a newborn, the condition may reflect hypovolemia or prolonged intrauterine hypoxia.*

hyperbilirubinemia *an excessive amount of bilirubin—the orange-colored pigment associated with bile—in the blood. In newborns, the condition appears as jaundice. Precipitating factors include maternal Rh or ABO incompatibility, neonatal sepsis, anoxia, hypoglycemia, and congenital liver or gastrointestinal defects.*

THE DISTRESSED NEWBORN

The distressed newborn can be either full term or premature. (See the "Prematurity" section later in this chapter.) The presence of fetal meconium at birth indicates that fetal distress has occurred at some point during pregnancy. If the newborn is simply meconium stained, then distress may have occurred at a remote time. If you see *particulate* meconium, however, distress may have occurred recently and the newborn should be managed accordingly.

Aspiration of meconium can cause significant respiratory problems and should be prevented. When you spot meconium during delivery, do not induce respiratory effort until you have removed the meconium from the trachea by suctioning under direct visualization with the laryngoscope. (More will be said about this topic in the "Meconium-Stained Amniotic Fluid" section later.) Be sure to report the presence of meconium to the medical direction physician.

The most common problems experienced by newborns during the first minutes of life involve the airway. For this reason, resuscitation usually consists of ventilation and oxygenation. Except in special situations, the use of IV fluids, drugs, or cardiac equipment is usually not indicated. (See "Inverted Pyramid for Resuscitation" later.) The most important procedures include suctioning, drying, and stimulating the distressed newborn.

Of the vital signs, fetal heart rate is the most important indicator of neonatal distress. The newborn has a relatively fixed stroke volume. Thus, cardiac output depends more on heart rate than on stroke volume. Bradycardia, as caused by hypoxia, results in decreased cardiac output and, ultimately, poor perfusion. A pulse rate of less than 60 beats per minute in a distressed newborn should be treated with chest compressions. In distressed newborns, monitor the heart rate manually. Do not depend on external electronic monitors.

Of the vital signs, fetal heart rate is the most important indicator of neonatal distress.

RESUSCITATION

The vast majority of newborns do not require resuscitation beyond stimulation, maintenance of the airway, and maintenance of body temperature. Unfortunately, it is difficult to predict which newborns ultimately will require resuscitation. Each EMS unit, therefore, should carry a neonatal resuscitation kit that contains the following items:

- ★ Neonatal bag-valve-mask unit
- ★ Bulb syringe
- ★ DeLee suction trap
- ★ Meconium aspirator
- ★ Laryngoscope with size 0 and 1 blades (usually Miller)
- ★ Uncuffed endotracheal tubes (2.5, 3.0, 3.5, 4.0) with appropriate suction catheters
- ★ Endotracheal tube stylet
- ★ Tape or device to secure endotracheal tube
- ★ Umbilical catheter and 10-mL syringe

- ★ Three-way stopcock
- ★ 20-mL syringe and 8-French (Fr.) feeding tube for gastric suction
- ★ Glucometer
- ★ Assorted syringes and needles
- ★ Towels (sterile)
- ★ Medications:
  - – Epinephrine 1:10,000 and 1:1,000
  - – Neonatal naloxone (Narcan)
  - – Volume expander (lactated Ringer's solution or saline)
  - – Sodium bicarbonate (10 mEq in 10 mL)

INVERTED PYRAMID FOR RESUSCITATION

Resuscitation of the newborn follows an inverted pyramid (Figure 41-6 ■). As this pyramid indicates, most distressed newborns respond to relatively simple maneuvers. Few require CPR or advanced life support measures.

The following are steps for the initial care of the newborn. Also see the resuscitation steps illustrated in Procedure 41–1 and listed in Figure 41-7 ■.

Step 1: Drying, Warming, Positioning, Suctioning, and Tactile Stimulation

Resuscitation begins with drying, warming, positioning, suctioning, and stimulating the newborn. Immediately on delivery, minimize heat loss by drying the newborn. Next, place the newborn in a warm, dry blanket. Make sure the environment is warm and free of drafts.

After you have dried the newborn, place the infant on its back with its head slightly below its body and its neck slightly extended (Figure 41-8 ■). This facilitates drainage of secretions and fluids from the lungs. Place a small blanket, folded to a 2-cm (3/4-inch) thickness, under the newborn's shoulders to help maintain this position.

vagal response *stimulation of the vagus nerve causing a parasympathetic response.*

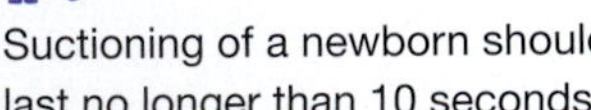

Suctioning of a newborn should last no longer than 10 seconds.

Next, suction the newborn again, using a bulb syringe or DeLee suction trap. Deep suctioning can cause a **vagal response,** resulting in bradycardia. Because of this, suctioning should last no longer than 10 seconds. If meconium is present, avoid stimulating the infant and visualize the airway with a laryngoscope. Suction the meconium, preferably with a DeLee suction trap. If there is a great deal of meconium, place an appropriately sized endotracheal tube (Table 41–2) and suction the meconium directly through the tube. Remove the tube and discard. Do not use the same tube

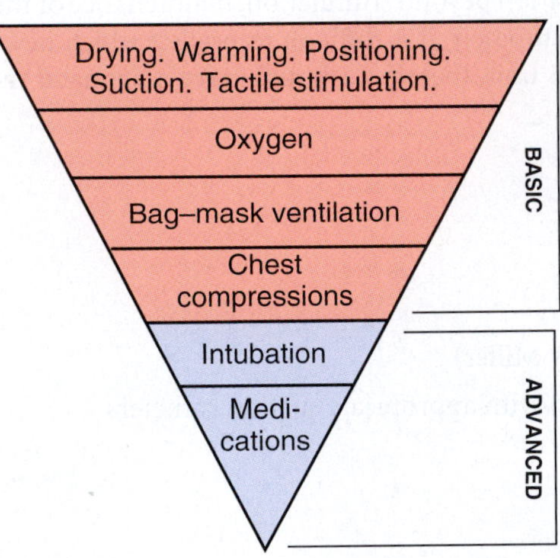

■ Figure 41-6 The inverted pyramid of neonatal resuscitation showing approximate relative frequencies of neonatal care and resuscitative efforts. Note that a majority of infants respond to the simple measures noted at the top, wide part of the pyramid.

Procedure 41–1 Resuscitation of the Distressed Newborn

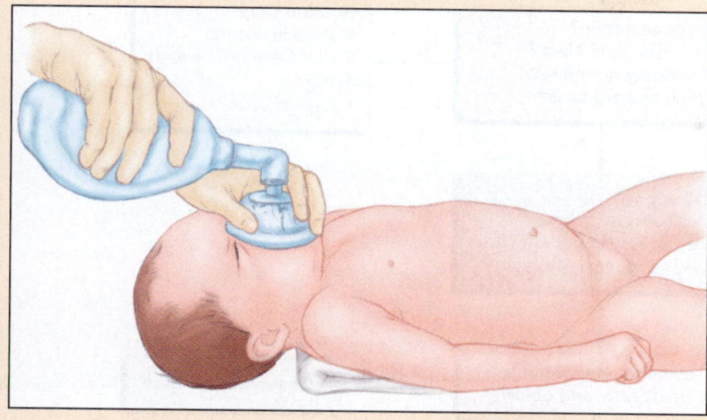

41-1a Ventilate with 100 percent oxygen for 15 to 30 seconds.

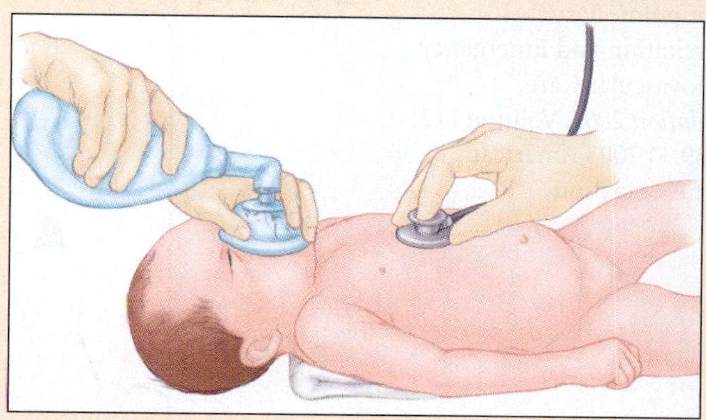

41-1b Evaluate heart rate.

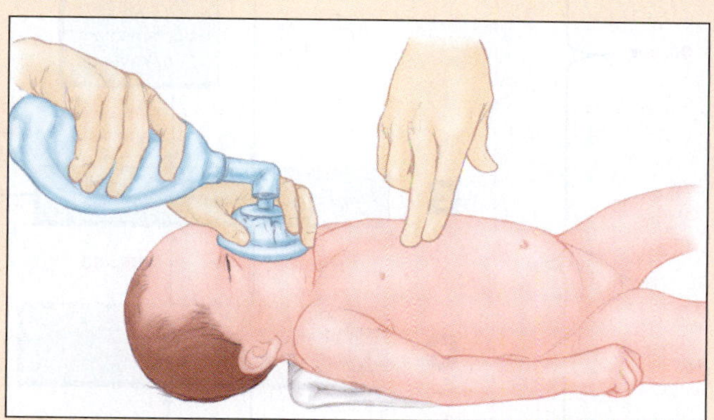

41-1c Initiate chest compressions if heart rate is less than 60.

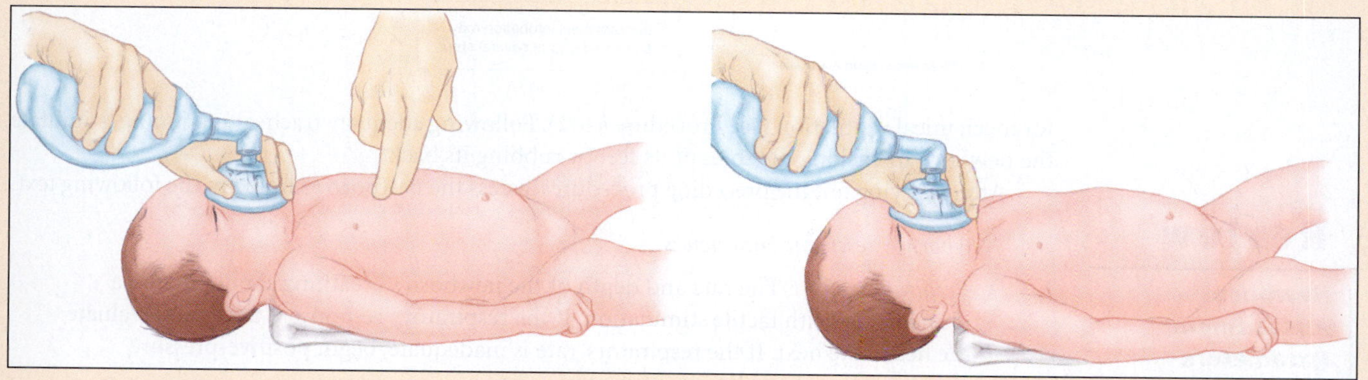

41-1d Evaluate heart rate: *Below 60*—Continue chest compressions, *60 or above*—Discontinue chest compressions.

■ Figure 41-7 Neonatal flow algorithm. Reproduced with permission from "2005 American Heart Association Guidelines for Cardiopulmonary Resuscitation and Emergency Cardiovascular Care," *Circulation 2005*, Volume 112, IV-189. © 2005 American Heart Association.

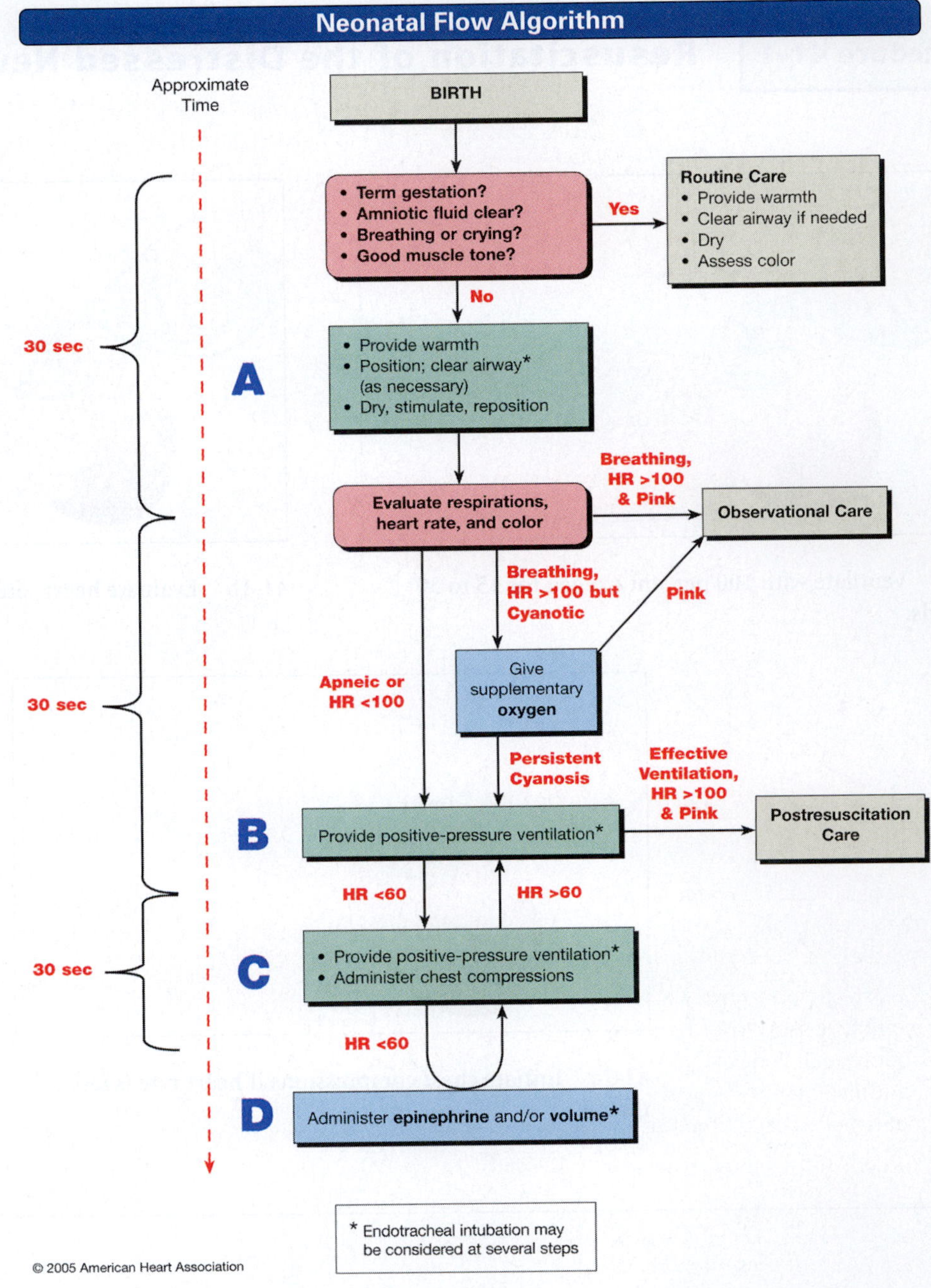

for mechanical ventilation (see Procedure 41–2). Following adequate tracheal suctioning, stimulate the newborn by flicking the soles of its feet or rubbing its back.

After carrying out the preceding procedures, assess the newborn as noted in the following text.

Content Review

Newborn Assessment Parameters

- Respiratory effort
- Heart rate
- Color
- APGAR score

Newborn Assessment Parameters

★ *Respiratory effort.* The rate and depth of the newborn's breathing should increase immediately with tactile stimulation. If the respiratory response is adequate, evaluate the heart rate next. If the respiratory rate is inadequate, begin positive-pressure ventilation (see Step 3).

★ *Heart rate.* As noted earlier, heart rate is critical in the newborn. Check the heart rate by listening to the apical area of the heart with a stethoscope, feeling the pulse by lightly grasping the umbilical cord, or feeling either the brachial or femoral pulse. If

CORRECT

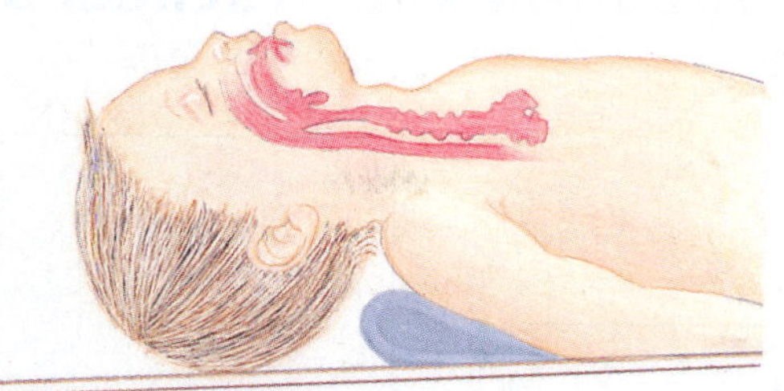

Neck slightly extended

Care should be taken to prevent hyperextension or underextension of the neck since either may decrease air entry.

INCORRECT

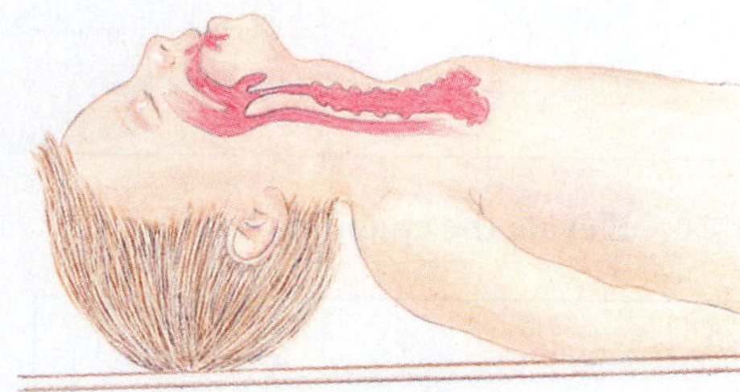

Neck hyperextended

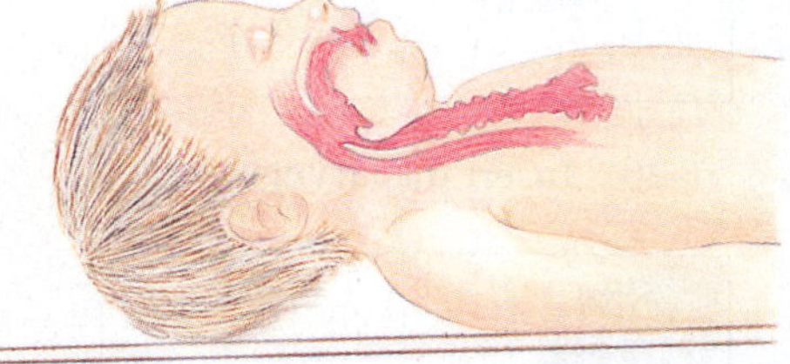

Neck underextended

■ Figure 41-8 Positioning the newborn to open the airway.

the heart rate is greater than 100 and spontaneous respirations are present, continue the assessment. If the heart rate is less than 100, immediately begin positive-pressure ventilation (see Step 3).

- ★ *Color.* A newborn may be cyanotic despite a heart rate greater than 100 and spontaneous respirations. If you note central cyanosis, or cyanosis of the chest and abdomen, in a newborn with adequate ventilation and a pulse rate greater than 100, administer supplemental oxygen (see Step 2). Newborns with peripheral cyanosis do not usually need supplemental oxygen UNLESS the cyanosis is prolonged.
- ★ *APGAR score.* Unless resuscitation is required, obtain 1- and 5-minute APGAR scores.

Content Review

Normal Newborn Vital Signs

- Respirations 30 to 60
- Heart rate 100 to 180
- Blood pressure 60 to 90 systolic
- Temperature 36.7° to 37.8°C (98° to 100°F)

Step 2: Supplemental Oxygen

If central cyanosis is present or the adequacy of ventilation is uncertain, administer supplemental oxygen by blowing oxygen across the newborn's face (Figure 41-9 ■). If possible, the oxygen should be warmed and humidified. Continue oxygen administration until the newborn's color has improved. Although oxygen toxicity is a concern, this condition usually results from prolonged usage over several days. Administration of blow-by oxygen in the prehospital setting will not cause problems. NEVER DEPRIVE A NEWBORN OF OXYGEN IN THE PREHOSPITAL SETTING FOR FEAR OF OXYGEN TOXICITY.

Never deprive a newborn of oxygen in the prehospital setting for fear of oxygen toxicity.

Step 3: Ventilation

Begin positive-pressure ventilation if *any* of the following conditions is present:

- ★ Heart rate less than 100 beats per minute
- ★ Apnea
- ★ Persistence of central cyanosis after administration of supplemental oxygen

Procedure 41-2

Endotracheal Intubation and Tracheal Suctioning in the Newborn

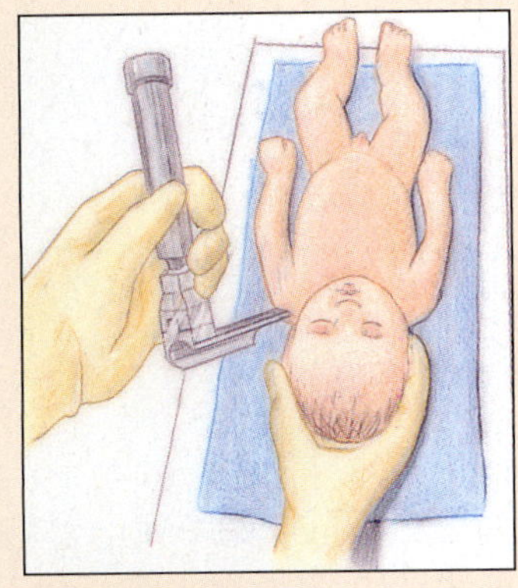

41-2a Position the infant.

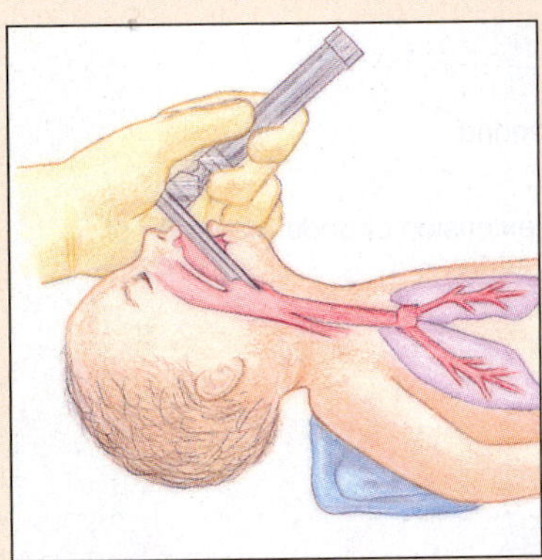

41-2b Insert the laryngoscope.

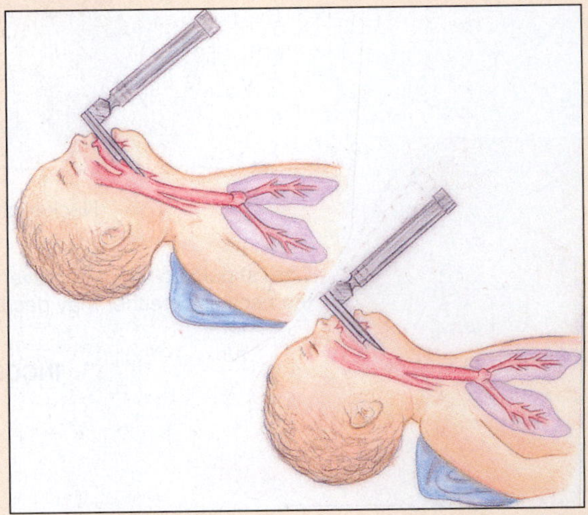

41-2c Elevate the epiglottis by lifting.

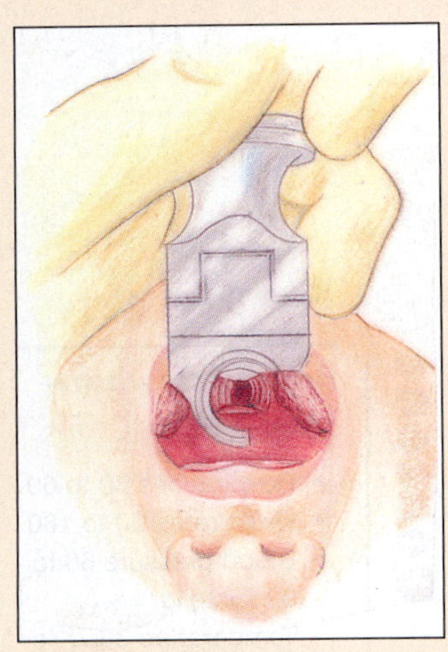

41-2d Visualize the cords.

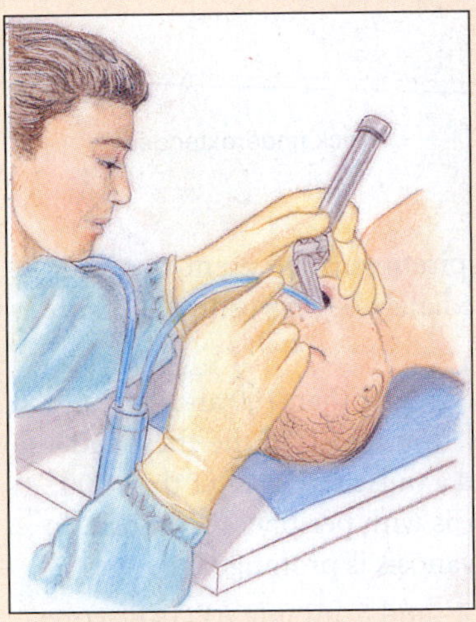

41-2e Suction any meconium present.

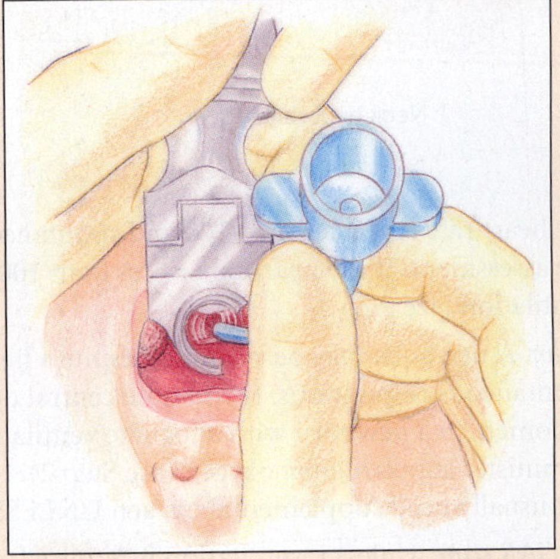

41-2f Insert a fresh tube for ventilation.

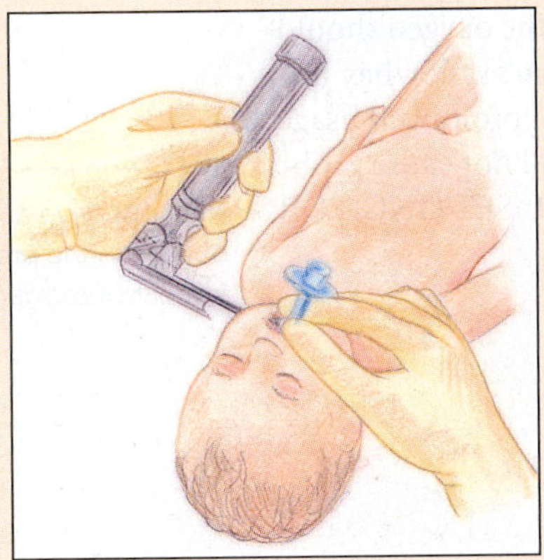

41-2g Remove the laryngoscope.

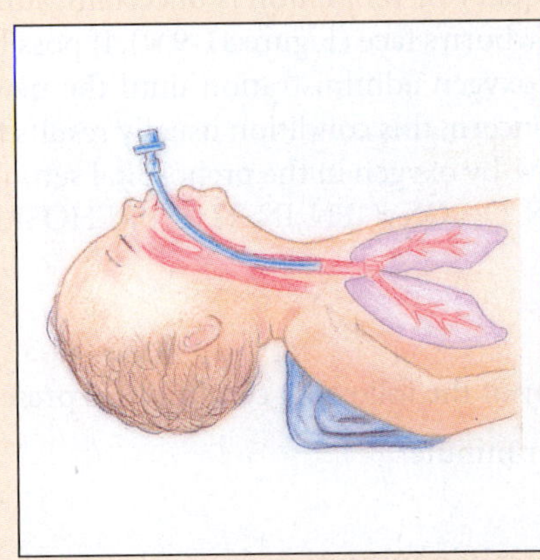

41-2h Check proper tube placement.

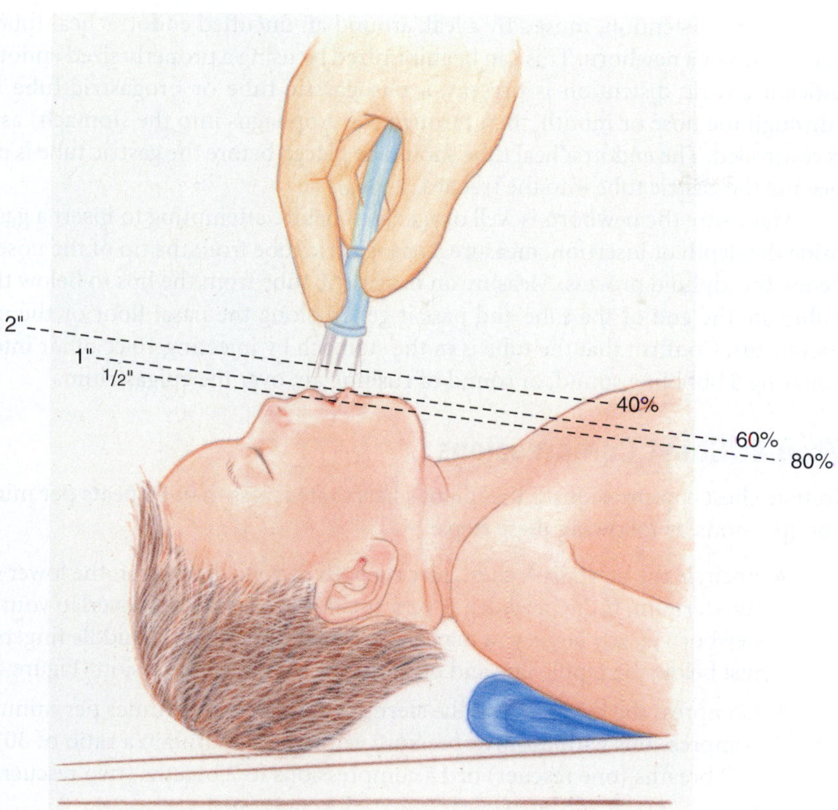

■ **Figure 41-9** Guidelines for estimating oxygen concentration. Based in oxygen flow rate of 5 liters per minute.

A ventilatory rate of 40 to 60 breaths per minute is usually adequate. A bag-valve-mask unit is the device of choice. A self-inflating bag of an appropriate size (450 mL is optimal) should be used. Many self-inflating bags have a pressure-limiting pop-off valve that is preset at 30 to 45 cm H_2O. However, since the initial pressures required to ventilate a newborn may be as high as 60 cm H_2O, you may have to depress the pop-off valve to deactivate it and ensure adequate ventilation. If prolonged ventilation is required, you may have to disable the pop-off valve.

Face masks in various sizes must be available. The most effective ones are designed to fit the contours of the newborn's face and have a low dead space volume (less than 5 mL). When a mask is correctly sized and positioned, it covers the newborn's nose and mouth, but not the eyes.

Endotracheal intubation of a newborn should be carried out in the following situations:

- ★ The bag-valve-mask unit does not work.
- ★ Tracheal suctioning is required (such as in cases of thick meconium).
- ★ Prolonged ventilation will be required.
- ★ A diaphragmatic hernia is suspected.
- ★ Inadequate respiratory effort is found.

Because of the narrowness of the neonatal airway at the level of the cricoid cartilage, always use an *uncuffed* endotracheal tube. (Review Table 41–2 regarding tube size.) After inserting the tube, ensure proper placement by noting symmetrical chest wall motion and equal breath sounds. (Review Procedure 41–2.)

Intubation has several effects in the newborn. First, it bypasses **glottic function.** Second, it eliminates PEEP—the physiologic positive end-expiratory pressure created during normal coughing and crying. To maintain adequate functional residual capacity, a PEEP of 2 to 4 cm/H_2O should be provided when mechanical ventilation is initiated by adding a magnetic-disk PEEP valve to the bag-valve outlet.

When resuscitating a distressed nenonate, avoid large-volume ventilations as these may damage the infant's lungs. Avoid hyperventilation.

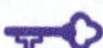

It is reasonable to begin neonatal ventilations with an oxygen concentration less than 100 percent or to start with no supplemental oxygen. If there is no appreciable improvement in 90 seconds, supplemental oxygen should be added.

glottic function *opening and closing of the glottic space.*

PEEP *positive end-expiratory pressure.*

nasogastric tube/orogastric tube *a tube that runs through the nose or mouth and esophagus into the stomach, used for administering liquid nutrients or medications or for removing air or liquids from the stomach.*

Gastric distention, caused by a leak around an uncuffed endotracheal tube, may compromise ventilation of a newborn. This can be minimized by using a properly sized endotracheal tube. If significant gastric distention is present, a **nasogastric tube** or **orogastric tube** should be inserted (through the nose or mouth, then through the esophagus into the stomach) as soon as the airway is controlled. The endotracheal tube should be placed before the gastric tube is placed to avoid misplacing the gastric tube into the trachea.

Make sure the newborn is well oxygenated before attempting to insert a gastric tube. To determine the depth of insertion, measure a nasogastric tube from the tip of the nose, around the ear, to below the xiphoid process. Measure an orogastric tube from the lips to below the xiphoid process. Lubricate the end of the tube and pass it gently along the nasal floor or the mouth and into the esophagus. Confirm that the tube is in the stomach by injecting 10 cc of air into the tube and auscultating a bubbling sound, or sound of rushing air, over the epigastrium.

Step 4: Chest Compressions

With neonatal CPR, *push hard* (⅓ to ½ the antero-posterior diameter of the chest), *push fast* (100 compressions per minute), *release the chest completely* to allow full recoil, and *minimize interruptions* in chest compressions.

Initiate chest compressions if the infant's heart rate is less than 60 beats per minute. Perform chest compressions by following these steps:

- ★ Encircle the newborn's chest, placing both of your thumbs on the lower one-third of the sternum. If the newborn is very small, you may need to overlap your thumbs. If the newborn is very large, you may need to place the ring and middle fingers of one hand just below the nipple line and perform two-finger compression (Figure 41-10 ■).
- ★ Compress the lower half of the sternum at a rate of 100 times per minute. Accompany compressions with positive-pressure ventilation. Maintain a ratio of 30 compressions to 2 breaths (one rescuer) or 15 compressions to 2 breaths (two rescuers).
- ★ Reassess heart rate, respiration, and color every 30 seconds. Coordinate with compressions and ventilations.
- ★ Discontinue compressions if the spontaneous heart rate exceeds 60.

Step 5: Medications and Fluids

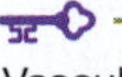

Vascular access for the administration of fluids and drugs can most readily be managed by using the umbilical vein.

Most cardiopulmonary arrests in newborns result from hypoxia. Because of this, initial therapy consists of ventilation and oxygenation. However, when these measures fail, fluid and medications should be administered. They may also be necessary in cases of persistent bradycardia, hypovolemia, respiratory depression secondary to narcotics, and metabolic acidosis.

Vascular access for the administration of fluids and drugs can most readily be managed by using the umbilical vein. The umbilical cord contains three vessels—two arteries and one vein. The vein is larger than the arteries and has a thinner wall (Figure 41-11 ■). To establish venous access, follow these procedures:

- ★ Trim the umbilical cord with a scalpel blade to 1 cm above the abdomen. Be sure to save enough of the umbilical cord stump in case neonatal personnel have to place additional lines.
- ★ Insert a 5-Fr. umbilical catheter into the umbilical vein. Connect the catheter to a three-way stopcock and fill it with saline.
- ★ Insert the catheter until the tip is just below the skin and you note the free flow of blood. (If the catheter is inserted too far, it may become wedged against the liver, and it will not function.)
- ★ After the catheter is in place, secure it with umbilical tape.

If an umbilical vein catheter cannot be placed, some medications can be given via the endotracheal tube. They include lidocaine, epinephrine, atropine, and naloxone. Other options for vascular access are peripheral vein cannulation and intraosseous cannulation. Table 41–3 lists recommended

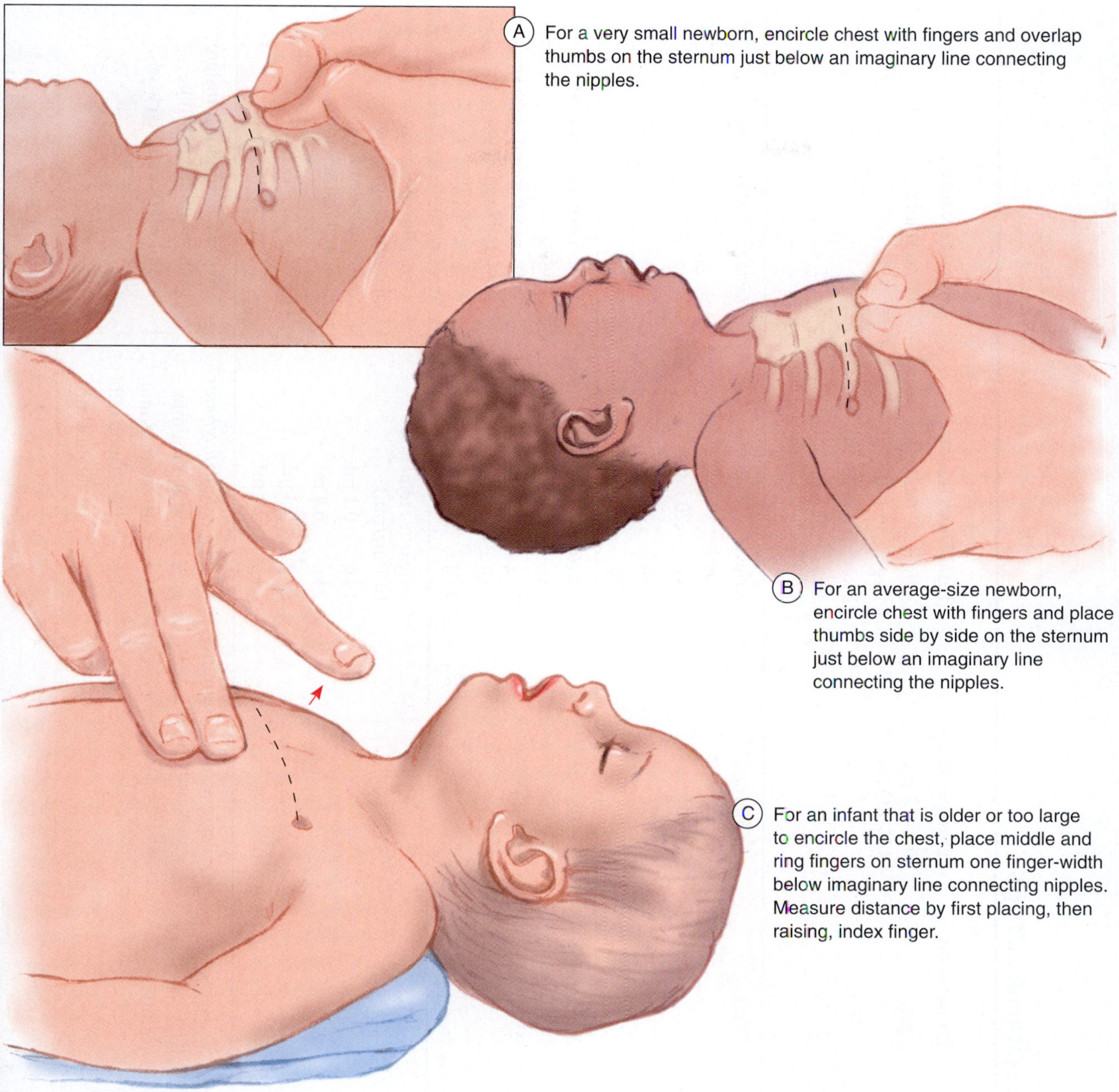

A For a very small newborn, encircle chest with fingers and overlap thumbs on the sternum just below an imaginary line connecting the nipples.
B For an average-size newborn, encircle chest with fingers and place thumbs side by side on the sternum just below an imaginary line connecting the nipples.
C For an infant that is older or too large to encircle the chest, place middle and ring fingers on sternum one finger-width below imaginary line connecting nipples. Measure distance by first placing, then raising, index finger.

■ **Figure 41-10** Position fingers for chest compressions according to the size of the infant.

Umbilical cord
Umbilical vein
Umbilical arteries

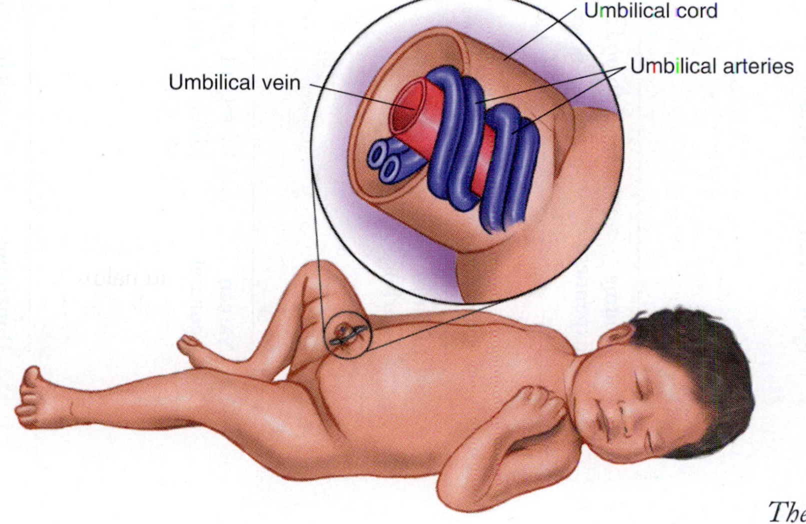

■ **Figure 41-11** The umbilical cord contains two arteries and one vein. The umbilical vein can be accessed for vascular administration of fluids and drugs. The vein is larger than the arteries and has a thinner wall.

Table 41–3 Neonatal Resuscitation Drugs

Medication	Concentration to Administer	Preparation	Dosage/Route*	Total Dose/Infant	Rate/Precautions
Epinephrine	1:10,000	1 mL	0.1–0.3 mL/kg I.V., I.O., or I.T.	*weight . . . total mLs* 1 kg 0.1–0.3 mL 2 kg 0.2–0.6 mL 3 kg 0.3–0.9 mL 4 kg 0.4–1.2 mL	Give rapidly.
Volume Expanders	Whole blood 5% Albumin normal saline Lactated Ringer's	40 mL	10 mL/kg I.V.	*weight . . . total mls* 1 kg 10 mL 2 kg 20 mL 3 kg 30 mL 4 kg 40 mL	Give over 5–10 min.
Sodium Bicarbonate	0.5 mEq/mL	20 mL or two 10-mL prefilled syringes	2 mEq/kg I.V.	*weight . . . total dose . . . mLs* 1 kg 2 mEq 4 mL 2 kg 4 mEq 8 mL 3 kg 6 mEq 12 mL 4 kg 8 mEq 16 mL	Give slowly, over at least 2 min. Give only if infant is being effectively ventilated.
Narcan Neonatal	1.0 mg/mL or 0.4 mg/mL (dilute 1.0 mg in 9 mL of saline)	2 mL	0.1 mg/kg I.V., I.M., S.Q., I.O., or I.T.	*weight . . . total mLs* (0.1 mg/mL) 1 kg 0.1 mL 2 kg 0.2 mL 3 kg 0.3 mL 4 kg 0.4 mL	Generally speaking, naloxone is no longer recommended for neonatal resuscitation.
Dopamine	$\frac{6 \times \text{weight (kg)} \times \text{desired dose (mcg/kg/min)}}{\text{desired fluid (mL/hr)}} =$	mg of dopamine per 100 mL of solution	Begin at 5 mcg/kg/min (may increase to 20 mcg/kg/min if necessary) I.V.	*weight . . . total mcg/min* 1 kg 5–20 mcg/min 2 kg 10–40 mcg/min 3 kg 15–60 mcg/min 4 kg 20–80 mcg/min	Give as continuous infusion using an infusion pump. Monitor HR and BP closely. Seek consultation.

From *Textbook of Neonatal Resuscitation* © 2001, American Heart Association.

*I.M. = Intramuscular, I.T. = Intratracheal, I.V. = Intravenous, S.Q. = Subcutaneous

medications and doses for the newborn. Fluid therapy should consist of 10 mL/kg of saline or lactated Ringer's solution given by syringe as a slow IV push.

MATERNAL NARCOTIC USE

Maternal abuse of narcotics—either illegal or prescribed—can complicate field deliveries. Maternal narcotic use has been shown to produce low-birth-weight infants. Such infants may demonstrate withdrawal symptoms—tremors, startles, and decreased alertness. They also face a serious risk of respiratory depression at birth.

Naloxone (Narcan), which is extremely safe even at high doses, is the treatment of choice for respiratory depression secondary to maternal narcotic use *within 4 hours of delivery.* Ventilatory support must be provided prior to administration of naloxone. Because the duration of the narcotics ingested by the mother prior to delivery may exceed that of the naloxone, repeat administration as necessary. Keep in mind, however, that the naloxone may induce a withdrawal reaction in an infant born to a *narcotic-addicted* mother. Medical direction may advise that naloxone NOT be administered if the mother is drug addicted, advising that prolonged ventilatory support be provided instead.

Keep in mind that naloxone may induce a withdrawal reaction with an infant born to a narcotic-addicted mother.

The dosage of naloxone is 0.1 mg/kg. The initial dose may be repeated every 2 to 3 minutes as needed. Naloxone may be given by intravenous, intraosseous, endotracheal, subcutaneous, or intramuscular routes.

As with other newborns, continue all resuscitative measures until the newborn is resuscitated or until the emergency staff assumes care.

NEONATAL TRANSPORT

Healthy newborns should be allowed to begin the bonding process with the mother as soon as possible (Figure 41-12 ■). Distressed newborns, however, must be positioned on their side to prevent aspiration and rapidly transported.

In addition to field deliveries, paramedics are frequently called on to transport a high-risk newborn from a facility where stabilization has occurred to a neonatal intensive care unit (NICU). The trip may be across the street or across the state. Usually, a pediatric nurse, respiratory therapist, and, often, a physician accompany the newborn. During transport, a paramedic crew will help maintain a newborn's body temperature, control oxygen administration, and maintain ventilatory support. Often, a transport **isolette** with its own heat, light, and oxygen source is available. In such cases, intravenous medications are usually infused through the umbilical vein. The umbilical artery is catheterized as well.

isolette *also known as an* incubator; *a clear plastic-enclosed bassinet used to keep prematurely born infants warm. The temperature of an isolette can be adjusted regardless of the room temperature. Some isolettes also provide humidity control.*

If a self-contained isolette is not available for transport, it is important to keep the ambulance warm. Wrap the newborn in several blankets, keep the head covered, and place hot-water bottles containing water heated to no more than 40°C (104°F) near, but not touching, the newborn. Do not use chemical packs to keep the newborn warm. These can generate excessive heat and may burn the infant.

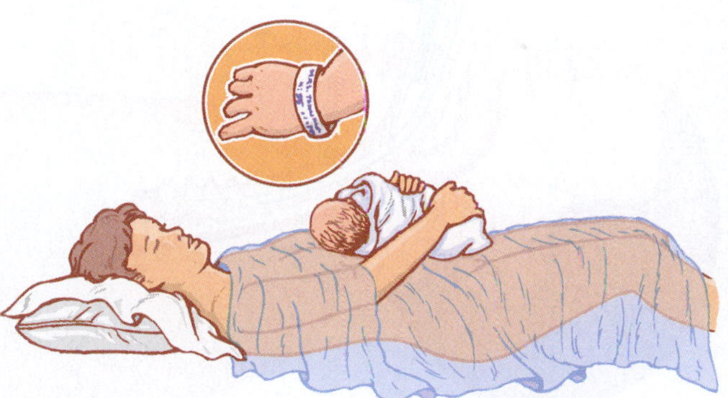

■ Figure 41-12 A healthy newborn can be placed on the mother's abdomen. Write the mother's last name and time of delivery on a tape and place it around the infant's wrist. (Do not allow adhesive to contact the infant's skin.)

SPECIFIC NEONATAL SITUATIONS

Rapid assessment and treatment of a distressed newborn is the key to the infant's survival. The following information will help you to formulate treatment plans for specific emergencies involving newborns. Remember that, unless otherwise directed, you will need to transport these infants to a facility that is able to handle high-risk neonates. A reference card should be available in the ambulance and in the dispatch office that tracks the availability of neonatal unit beds. When possible, keep the parents advised of what is happening and the reason for any treatments being given to the infant. However, do not discuss "chances of survival" with the family or caregivers.

Do not discuss "chances of survival" with a newborn's family or caregivers.

MECONIUM-STAINED AMNIOTIC FLUID

Meconium-stained amniotic fluid occurs in approximately 10 to 15 percent of deliveries, mostly in post-term or in small-for-gestational-age (SGA) newborns. The mortality rate for meconium-stained infants is considerably higher than the mortality rate for non-meconium-stained infants, and meconium aspiration accounts for a significant proportion of neonatal deaths.

Fetal distress and hypoxia can cause the passage of meconium into the amniotic fluid. Meconium is a dark green substance found in the digestive tract of full-term newborns. It arises from secretions of the various digestive glands and amniotic fluid. Either *in utero* or, more often, with the first breath, thick meconium is aspirated into the lungs, resulting in small-airway obstruction and aspiration pneumonia. This may produce respiratory distress within the first hours, or even minutes, of life as evidenced by tachypnea, retraction, grunting, and cyanosis in severely affected newborns.

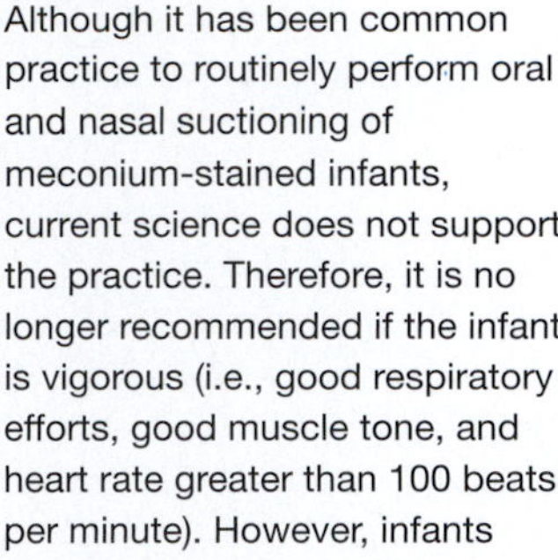

Although it has been common practice to routinely perform oral and nasal suctioning of meconium-stained infants, current science does not support the practice. Therefore, it is no longer recommended if the infant is vigorous (i.e., good respiratory efforts, good muscle tone, and heart rate greater than 100 beats per minute). However, infants who are not vigorous should receive endotracheal suctioning.

The partial obstruction of some airways may lead to pneumothorax. A pneumothorax may occur in an infant, cause no distress, and require no active treatment. If, however, the infant has significant respiratory distress, then the pneumothorax must be evacuated. If tension pneumothorax has occurred, needle decompression may be required.

An infant born through thin meconium may not require treatment, but depressed infants born through thick, particulate (pea-soup) meconium-stained fluid should be intubated immediately, prior to the first ventilation (Figure 41-13 ■). Aspiration of meconium by a newborn can result in either partial or complete airway obstruction. Complete airway obstruction causes atelectasis (collapsed or airless lungs). In addition, some aspects of fetal blood flow resume a right-to-left shunt of blood across the foramen ovale (the opening between the atria of the fetal heart). This results from increased pulmonary pressures. Incomplete obstruction can act as a ball-valve in the smaller airways, thus preventing exhalation. Also, the newborn is at increased risk of developing a pneumothorax.

Before stimulating the infant to breathe, apply suction with a meconium aspirator attached to an endotracheal tube. Connect to suction at 100 cm/H_2O or less to remove meconium from the airway. Withdraw the endotracheal tube as suction is applied.

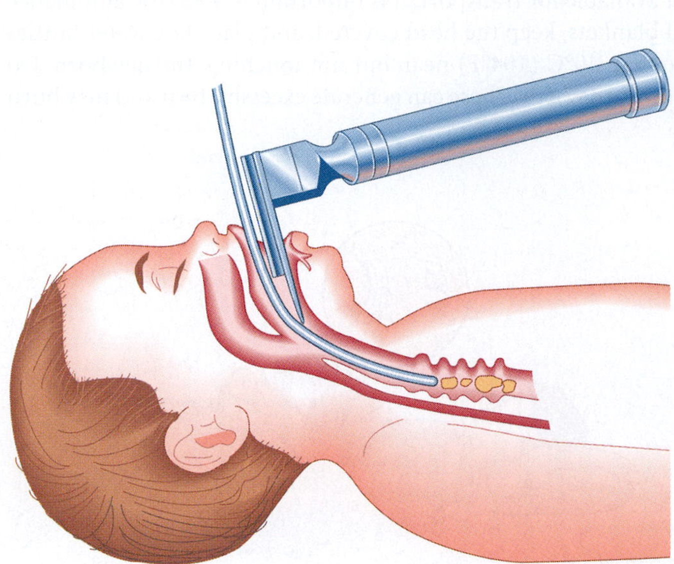

■ **Figure 41-13** Intubate the infant born through particulate, thick meconium immediately—prior to the first ventilation.

Repeat intubation with a clean ET tube and suction until the meconium clears, usually not more than two times. Once the airway is clear and the infant is able to breathe on its own, ventilate with 100 percent oxygen. If the infant is found to be hypotensive, consider a fluid challenge. Remember to warm the infant to prevent hypothermia. The parents will probably question the treatment being performed on the infant. Explain what you are doing and why, without discussing chances of survival. Stress the need for rapid transport to a facility able to handle high-risk infants.

APNEA

Apnea is a common finding in preterm infants, infants weighing less than 1,500 grams (3 pounds, 5 ounces), infants exposed to drugs, or infants born after prolonged or difficult labor and delivery. Typically, the infant fails to breathe spontaneously after stimulation, or the infant experiences respiratory pauses of greater than 20 seconds.

Although apnea is usually due to hypoxia or hypothermia, there may be other causative factors. These include:

- ★ Narcotic or central nervous depressants
- ★ Weakness of the respiratory muscles
- ★ Septicemia
- ★ Metabolic disorders
- ★ Central nervous system disorders

Begin management of apnea with tactile stimulation. Flick the soles of the infant's feet or gently rub his back. If necessary, ventilate using a bag-valve-mask unit with the pop-off valve disabled, as explained earlier. If the infant still does not breathe on its own, or if it has a heart rate of less than 60 with adequate ventilation and chest compressions, perform tracheal intubation with direct visualization. Gain circulatory access, and monitor the heart rate continuously. If the apnea is due to narcotics administered within the previous 4 hours, consider naloxone. As noted earlier, however, the use of narcotic antagonists is generally contraindicated if the mother is a drug abuser.

Early and aggressive treatment of apnea usually results in a good outcome. Throughout treatment, keep the infant warm to prevent hypothermia. Also explain procedures to parents and the need for rapid transport.

Content Review

Causes of Apnea in Newborns

- Hypoxia
- Hypothermia
- Narcotics
- Respiratory muscle weakness
- Septicemia
- Metabolic disorder
- Central nervous system disorder

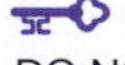

DO NOT utilize narcotic antagonists if the mother is a drug abuser.

DIAPHRAGMATIC HERNIA

Diaphragmatic hernias rarely occur. They are seen in approximately 1 out of every 2,200 live births. When they do appear, the **herniation** takes place most often in the posterolateral segments of the diaphragm, and most commonly (90 percent) on the left side. The defect is caused by the failure of the pleuroperitoneal canal (foramen of Bochdalek) to close completely. The survival rate for infants who require mechanical ventilation in the first 18 to 24 hours is approximately 50 percent. However, if there is no respiratory distress in the first 24 hours of life, the survival rate approaches 100 percent.

herniation *protrusion or projection of an organ or part of an organ through the wall of the cavity that normally contains it.*

Protrusion of abdominal viscera through the hernia into the thoracic cavity occurs in varying degrees. In severe cases, the stomach and a large part of the intestines and the spleen, liver, and kidneys displace the lungs and heart to the opposite side. The lung on the affected side is compressed, causing diminished total lung volume. In at least one-third of patients, pulmonary hypertension is present. With a patent ductus arteriosus, severe right-to-left shunting may occur, further aggravating tissue hypoxia.

Assessment findings may include:

- ★ Little to severe distress present from birth
- ★ Dyspnea and cyanosis unresponsive to ventilations
- ★ Small, flat (scaphoid) abdomen
- ★ Bowel sounds in the chest
- ★ Heart sounds displaced to the right

■ Figure 41-14 If a diaphragmatic hernia is suspected, position the infant with its head and thorax higher than the abdomen and feet to facilitate downward displacement of abdominal organs.

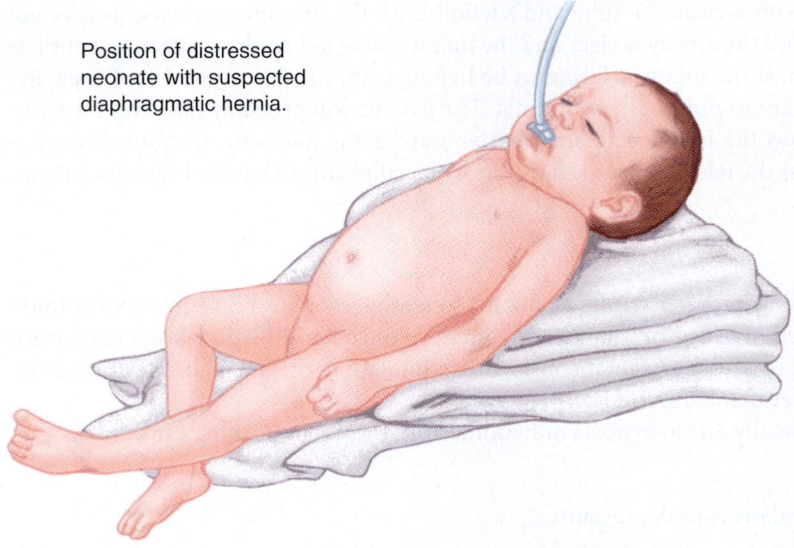

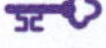

If you suspect a diaphragmatic hernia, DO NOT use bag-valve-mask ventilation, which can worsen the condition by causing gastric distention.

As soon as you suspect a diaphragmatic hernia, position the infant with its head and thorax higher than the abdomen and feet (Figure 41-14 ■). This will help facilitate the downward displacement of the abdominal organs. Place a nasogastric or orogastric tube and apply low, intermittent suctioning. This will decrease the entrapment of air and fluid within the herniated viscera and will reduce the degree of ventilatory compromise. DO NOT use bag-valve-mask ventilation, which can worsen this condition by causing gastric distention. If necessary, cautiously administer positive-pressure ventilation through an endotracheal tube.

This condition usually requires surgical repair. Explain the possible need for surgery to parents, assuring them that their newborn child will be transported quickly to the facility best able to handle this procedure.

BRADYCARDIA

Bradycardia in the newborn is most commonly caused by hypoxia. However, it may also be due to several other factors, including increased intracranial pressure, hypothyroidism, or acidosis.

Resist the temptation to treat bradycardia in a newborn with pharmacological measures alone.

In cases of hypoxia, the infant experiences minimal risk if the hypoxia is corrected quickly. In providing treatment, follow the procedures in the inverted pyramid, as discussed earlier. Check for secretions in the airway, check tongue and soft-tissue positioning, and check for possible foreign body obstruction. Resist the inclination to treat the bradycardia with pharmacological measures alone. Atropine should not be used. Although epinephrine may be necessary, in all likelihood you will be able to correct the problem with suctioning, positioning, administration of oxygen (blow-by or bag-valve mask), or tracheal intubation. Throughout treatment, keep the newborn warm and transport to the nearest facility.

PREMATURITY

A premature newborn is an infant born prior to 37 weeks of gestation or with weight ranging from 0.6 to 2.2 kg (1 pound, 5 ounces to 4 pounds, 13 ounces). Healthy premature infants weighing more than 1,700 grams (3 pounds, 12 ounces) have a survivability and outcome approximately equal to that of full-term infants. The mortality rate decreases weekly as the gestational age surpasses the age of fetal viability. With the technology currently available, fetal viability is considered to be 23 to 24 weeks of gestation.

Premature newborns are at greater risk of respiratory suppression, head or brain injury caused by hypoxemia, changes in blood pressure, intraventricular hemorrhage, and fluctuations in serum osmolarity. They are also more susceptible to hypothermia than full-term newborns. Reasons premature newborns lose heat more readily include the following:

- ★ The premature newborn has a relatively large body surface area and comparatively small weight.

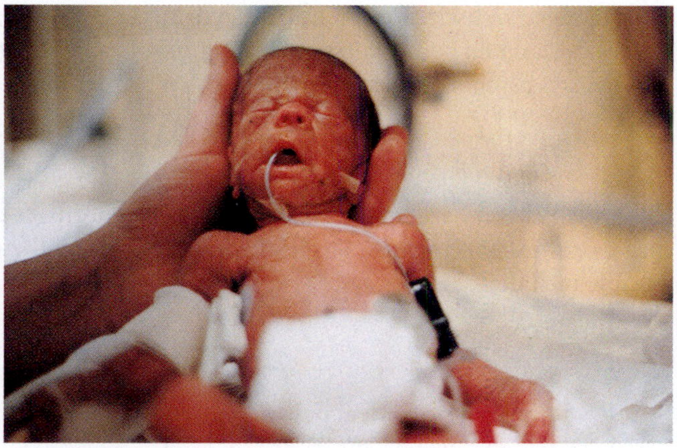

■ Figure 41-15 The premature newborn.

★ The premature newborn has not sufficiently developed the various control mechanisms needed to regulate body temperature.

★ The premature newborn has smaller subcutaneous stores of insulating fat.

★ Newborns cannot shiver and must maintain body temperature through other mechanisms.

The degree of immaturity determines the physical characteristics of a premature newborn (Figure 41-15 ■). Premature newborns often appear to have a larger head relative to body size. They may have large trunks and short extremities, transparent skin, and few wrinkles.

Prematurity should not be a factor in short-term treatment. Resuscitation should be attempted if there is any sign of life, and the measures of resuscitation should be the same as those for newborns of normal weight and maturity. Maintain a patent airway and avoid potential aspiration of gastric contents. Medical direction may advise administration of epinephrine. Throughout treatment, maintain the newborn's body temperature and transport to a facility with special services for low-birth-weight newborns.

Prematurity should not be a factor in short-term treatment. Resuscitation should be attempted if there is any sign of life.

RESPIRATORY DISTRESS/CYANOSIS

Prematurity is the single most common factor causing respiratory distress and cyanosis in the newborn. The problem occurs most frequently in infants weighing less than 1,200 grams (2 pounds, 10 ounces) and at less than 30 weeks of gestation. Premature infants have an immature central respiratory control center and are easily affected by environmental or metabolic changes. Multiple gestations or prenatal maternal complications may also increase the risk of respiratory distress and cyanosis.

The severely ill newborn with respiratory distress and cyanosis presents a difficult diagnostic challenge. Contributing factors include lung or heart disease, central nervous system disorders, meconium aspiration, metabolic problems, obstruction of the nasal passages, shock and sepsis, diaphragmatic hernia, and more. Assessment findings include:

★ Tachypnea

★ Paradoxical breathing

★ Intercostal retractions

★ Nasal flaring

★ Expiratory grunt

Follow the inverted pyramid of treatment (Figure 41-6), paying particular attention to airway and ventilation. Suction as needed and provide high-flow, high-concentration oxygen. Ventilate, as needed, with a bag-valve-mask unit. If prolonged ventilation will be required, consider placing an endotracheal tube. Perform chest compressions, if indicated. Sodium bicarbonate may be helpful for prolonged resuscitation. Consider dextrose ($D_{10}W$ or $D_{25}W$) solution if the newborn is hypoglycemic. Maintain body temperature and transport. Be sure to keep the parents informed and provide needed psychological support.

HYPOVOLEMIA

Hypovolemia is the leading cause of shock in newborns. It may result from dehydration, hemorrhage, or third-spacing of fluids. Dehydration is by far the most common cause. Signs of hypovolemia include:

- ★ Pale color
- ★ Cool skin
- ★ Diminished peripheral pulses
- ★ Delayed capillary refill, despite normal ambient temperature
- ★ Mental status changes
- ★ Diminished urination (oliguria)

When you observe these signs, administer a fluid bolus and assess the infant's response. If signs of shock continue, administer a second bolus. Additional boluses should be infused as indicated by repeated assessments. A hypovolemic infant may often need 40 to 60 mL/kg of fluid during the first hour of resuscitation.

Fluid bolus resuscitation consists of 10 mL/kg of an isotonic crystalloid solution, such as Ringer's lactate or normal saline. Administer the bolus over 5 to 10 minutes as soon as intravascular or intraosseous access is obtained. Do not use solutions containing dextrose, because they can produce hypokalemia or worsen ischemic brain injury.

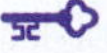

In treating hypovolemia in a newborn, do not use solutions containing dextrose, as they can produce hypokalemia or worsen ischemic brain injury.

SEIZURES

Although seizures occur in a very small percentage of all newborns, they usually indicate a serious underlying abnormality and represent a medical emergency. Prolonged and frequent multiple seizures may result in metabolic changes and cardiopulmonary difficulties.

Neonatal seizures differ from seizures in a child or an adult, because generalized tonic-clonic convulsions normally do not occur during the first month of life. Seizures in neonates include these types:

- ★ *Subtle seizures.* These seizures consist of chewing motions, excessive salivation, blinking, sucking, swimming movements of the arms, pedaling movements of the legs, apnea, and changes in color.
- ★ *Tonic seizures.* These seizures are characterized by rigid posturing of the extremities and trunk. They are sometimes associated with fixed deviation of the eyes. They occur more commonly in premature infants, especially those with an intraventricular hemorrhage.
- ★ *Focal clonic seizures.* These seizures consist of rhythmic twitching of muscle groups, particularly the extremities and face. They may occur in both full-term and premature infants.
- ★ *Multifocal seizures.* These seizures are similar to focal clonic seizures, except that multiple muscle groups are involved. Clonic activity randomly migrates. These seizures occur primarily in full-term newborns.
- ★ *Myoclonic seizures.* These seizures involve brief focal or generalized jerks of the extremities or parts of the body that tend to involve distal muscle groups. They may occur singly or in a series of repetitive jerks.

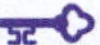

Always check the glucose level in a neonate with seizures.

Causes of neonatal seizures include sepsis, fever, hypoglycemia, hypoxic-ischemic encephalopathy, metabolic disturbances, meningitis, developmental abnormalities, or drug withdrawal. Assessment findings include a decreased level of consciousness and seizure activities such as those just described. Treatment focuses on airway management and oxygen saturation. With medical direction, consider administration of an anticonvulsant. You might also administer a benzodiazepine (usually lorazepam) for status epilepticus or dextrose ($D_{10}W$ or $D_{25}W$) for hypoglycemia. As with all distressed newborns, maintain body temperature and transport rapidly.

FEVER

Average normal temperature in a newborn is 37.5°C (99.5°F). A rectal temperature of 38.0°C (100.4°F) or higher is considered fever. Neonates do not develop fever as readily as older children. Thus, any fever in a neonate requires extensive evaluation because it may be caused by life-threatening conditions such as pneumonia, sepsis, or meningitis. Fever may be the only sign of meningitis in a neonate. Because of their immature development, they do not develop the classic symptoms such as a stiff neck. Thus, any neonate with a fever should be considered to have meningitis until proven otherwise.

Any neonate with a fever should be considered to have meningitis until proven otherwise.

In assessing a neonate with fever, remember that infants have a limited ability to control their body temperature. As a result, fever can be a serious problem. Assessment findings will probably include the following:

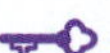

In assessing a neonate with fever, remember that infants have a limited ability to control their body temperature. As a result, fever can be a serious condition.

- ★ Mental status changes (irritability/somnolence)
- ★ Decreased feeding
- ★ Skin warm to the touch
- ★ Rashes or *petechiae* (small, purplish, hemorrhagic spots on the skin)

Term infants may produce beads of sweat on their brow but not on the rest of their body. Premature infants will have no visible sweat at all.

Treatment of a neonate with fever will, for the most part, be limited to ensuring a patent airway and adequate ventilation. Do not use cold packs, which may drop the temperature too quickly and may also cause seizures. If the newborn becomes bradycardic, provide chest compressions. In the prehospital setting, administration of an antipyretic agent to a neonate is of questionable benefit and should be avoided. Select the appropriate treatment facility and explain the need for transport to the parents or caregivers.

HYPOTHERMIA

As previously noted, hypothermia presents a common and life-threatening condition for newborns. Adults sometimes fail to realize that a newborn may die because of exposure to temperatures that adults find comfortable. The increased surface-to-volume relationship in newborns makes them extremely sensitive to environmental temperatures, especially right after delivery when they are wet. As a result, it is important to control the four methods of heat loss: evaporation, conduction, convection, and radiation.

In treating hypothermia—a body temperature below 35°C (95°F)—keep in mind that it can also be an indicator of sepsis in the newborn. Regardless of the cause, the increased metabolic demands created by hypothermia can produce a variety of related conditions including metabolic acidosis, pulmonary hypertension, and hypoxemia.

In assessing a hypothermic newborn, remember that they do not shiver. Instead, expect these findings:

- ★ Pale color
- ★ Skin cool to the touch, particularly in the extremities
- ★ Acrocyanosis
- ★ Respiratory distress
- ★ Possible apnea
- ★ Bradycardia
- ★ Central cyanosis
- ★ Initial irritability
- ★ Lethargy in later stages

acrocyanosis *cyanosis of the extremities.*

Management focuses on ensuring adequate ventilations and oxygenation. Chest compressions may be performed, if necessary. With medical direction, you might administer warm fluids through an IV fluid heater. Do not microwave fluids, because great variations in fluid temperature can result. Dextrose ($D_{10}W$ or $D_{25}W$) may also be given if the newborn is hypoglycemic. Above all, the newborn must be kept warm. Set the ambulance temperature at 24° to 26°C (75.2° to 78.8°F). Also remember to warm your hands before touching the newborn. Select the appropriate receiving facility and transport rapidly.

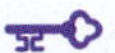

Remember to warm your hands before touching a neonate.

HYPOGLYCEMIA

Newborns are the only age group that can develop severe hypoglycemia and not have diabetes mellitus. Hypoglycemia may be due to inadequate glucose intake or increased glucose utilization. Stress and other factors can also cause the blood sugar to fall, sometimes to a critical level.

Hypoglycemia is more common in premature or small-for-gestational-age (SGA) infants, the smaller twin, and newborns of a diabetic mother, because these infants often have decreased glycogen stores. Hypoglycemia can also develop due to increased glucose utilization. Causes include respiratory illnesses, hypothermia, toxemia, CNS hemorrhage, asphyxia, meningitis, and sepsis. In an older infant, hypoglycemia may be due to an inadequate glucose intake or increased utilization of glucose. Infants receiving glucose infusions can develop hypoglycemia if the infusion is suddenly stopped.

Infants with hypoglycemia may be asymptomatic or they may exhibit symptoms such as apnea, color changes, respiratory distress, lethargy, seizures, acidosis, and poor myocardial contractility.

Persistent hypoglycemia can have catastrophic effects on the brain. The normal newborn's glycogen stores are sufficient to meet glucose requirements for only 8 to 12 hours. This time frame is diminished in infants with decreased glycogen stores or the presence of other problems where glucose utilization increases. As a result, you should determine the blood glucose level on all sick infants. A blood glucose screening test of less than 45 mg/dL indicates hypoglycemia.

Because hypoglycemia can have a catastrophic effect on a neonate's brain, you should determine the blood glucose on all sick infants.

In response to hypoglycemia, the newborn's body will release counterregulatory hormones such as glucagon, epinephrine, cortisol, and growth hormone. These hormones help raise the blood glucose level by mobilizing glucose stores. In fact, this hormone response may cause transient symptoms of hyperglycemia that can last for several hours. However, when the infant's glucose stores are depleted, the glucose level will again fall.

In assessing hypoglycemic newborns, expect these findings:

- Twitching or seizures
- Limpness
- Lethargy
- Eye-rolling
- High-pitched cry
- Apnea
- Irregular respirations
- Possible cyanosis

Treatment begins with management of the airway and ventilations. Ensure adequate oxygenation. Perform chest compressions, if indicated. With medical direction, administer dextrose ($D_{10}W$ or $D_{25}W$). Maintain a normal body temperature in the newborn and transport to the appropriate facility.

VOMITING

Vomiting in a neonate may result from a variety of causes and rarely presents as an isolated symptom. Vomiting (a forceful ejection of stomach contents) is uncommon during the first weeks of life and may be confused with regurgitation (a simple backflow of stomach contents into the mouth, or "spitting up"). Vomiting in the neonate usually occurs because of an anatomical abnormality such as a tracheoesophageal fistula or upper gastrointestinal obstruction. More often, it may be a symptom of some disease such as increased intracranial pressure or an infection. Vomitus containing dark blood often signals a life-threatening illness. Keep in mind, however, that vomiting of mucus—which may occasionally be blood streaked—in the first few hours after birth is not uncommon.

Assessment findings may include a distended stomach, signs of infection, increased intracranial pressure, or drug withdrawal. Because vomitus can be aspirated, management considerations focus on ensuring a patent airway. If you detect respiratory difficulties or obstruction of the airway, suction or clear vomitus from the airway and ensure adequate oxygenation. Fluid administration may be needed to prevent dehydration. Also remember that, as with older patients, vagal stimulation may cause bradycardia in the neonate.

After you have protected the airway, place the infant on its side and transport to an appropriate facility. As with all other situations involving distressed neonates, advise parents or caregivers of the steps taken and why.

DIARRHEA

Diarrhea in a neonate can cause severe dehydration and electrolyte imbalances. Although diarrhea may be harder to assess in neonates than in other patients, consider five to six stools per day as normal, especially in breast-fed infants.

Causes of diarrhea in a neonate include:

★ Bacterial or viral infection
★ Gastroenteritis
★ Lactose intolerance
★ **Phototherapy**
★ **Neonatal abstinence syndrome** (NAS)
★ **Thyrotoxicosis**
★ Cystic fibrosis

In treating neonates with diarrhea, remember to take appropriate Standard Precautions, just as you would do in any situation involving body fluids. Expect to find loose stools, decreased urinary output, and other signs of dehydration such as prolonged capillary refill time, cool extremities, and listlessness or lethargy. It is often difficult for the parents to estimate the number of stools. In such cases, it might be better to inquire about the number of diapers the baby is using.

Management consists of maintenance of airway and ventilations, adequate oxygenation, and chest compressions, if indicated. With medical direction, you might also consider fluid therapy. Explain all treatments to parents or caregivers, and transport the neonate to a facility able to handle high-risk infants.

phototherapy *exposure to sunlight or artificial light for therapeutic purposes. In newborns, light is used to treat hyperbilirubinemia or jaundice.*

neonatal abstinence syndrome (NAS) *a generalized disorder presenting a clinical picture of CNS hyperirritability, gastrointestinal dysfunction, respiratory distress, and vague autonomic symptoms. It may be due to intrauterine exposure to heroin, methadone, or other less potent opiates. Nonopiate central nervous system depressants may also cause NAS.*

thyrotoxicosis *toxic condition characterized by tachycardia, nervous symptoms, and rapid metabolism due to hyperactivity of the thyroid gland.*

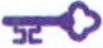

In treating a neonate with diarrhea, remember to take appropriate Standard Precautions.

COMMON BIRTH INJURIES

A **birth injury** occurs in an estimated 2 to 7 of every 1,000 live births in the United States. About 5 to 8 of every 100,000 infants die of birth trauma and 25 of every 100,000 die of anoxic injuries. Such injuries account for 2 to 3 percent of infant deaths. Risk factors for birth injury include:

★ Prematurity
★ Postmaturity
★ Cephalopelvic disproportion
★ Prolonged labor
★ Breech presentation
★ Explosive delivery
★ Diabetic mother

Birth injuries take various forms. Cranial injuries may include molding of the head and overriding of the parietal bones, erythema (reddening of the skin), abrasions, ecchymosis (black-and-blue

birth injury *avoidable and unavoidable mechanical and anoxic trauma incurred by the newborn during labor and delivery.*

discoloration) and subcutaneous fat necrosis, subconjunctival and retinal hemorrhage, subperiosteal hemorrhage, and fracture of the skull. Intracranial hemorrhage may result from trauma or asphyxia. Often the infant will develop a large scalp hematoma during the birth process. This injury, called *caput succedaneum,* will usually resolve over a week's time. Damage to the spine and spinal cord may occur as a result of strong traction exerted when the spine is hyperextended or there is a lateral pull. Other birth injuries include peripheral nerve injury, injury to the liver, rupture of the spleen, adrenal hemorrhage, fractures of the clavicle or extremities, and, of course, hypoxia-ischemia.

Assessment findings may include:

- ★ Diffuse, sometimes ecchymotic, edematous swelling of soft tissues around the scalp
- ★ Paralysis below the level of the spinal cord injury
- ★ Paralysis of the upper arm with or without paralysis of the forearm
- ★ Diaphragmatic paralysis
- ★ Movement on only one side of the face when crying
- ★ Inability to move the arm freely on the side of the fractured clavicle
- ★ Lack of spontaneous movement of the affected extremity
- ★ Hypoxia
- ★ Shock

Management of a newborn or newborn with birth injuries usually centers on protection of the airway, provision of adequate ventilation and oxygen, and, if needed, chest compressions. With medical direction, you may administer medications or take other nonpharmacological steps to support the specific injury. Newborns with birth injuries usually require treatment at specialized facilities. As in the management of other neonatal emergencies, provide professional and compassionate communication to parents or caregivers.

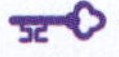

In treating distressed neonates with birth injuries or other critical conditions, provide professional and compassionate communication to the parents or caregivers.

CARDIAC RESUSCITATION, POSTRESUSCITATION, AND STABILIZATION

The incidence of neonatal cardiac arrest is related primarily to hypoxia. As previously explained, the outcome will be poor unless you immediately initiate appropriate interventions. As you might expect, cases involving cardiac arrest have an increased chance of brain and organ damage. Risk factors for cardiac arrest in newborns include:

- ★ Bradycardia
- ★ Intrauterine asphyxia
- ★ Prematurity
- ★ Drugs administered to or taken by the mother
- ★ Congenital neuromuscular diseases
- ★ Congenital malformations
- ★ Intrapartum hypoxemia

Content Review

Causes of Neonatal Cardiac Arrest

- Primary or secondary apnea
- Bradycardia
- Persistent fetal circulation
- Pulmonary hypertension

Cardiac arrest can be caused by primary or secondary apnea, bradycardia, persistent fetal circulation, or pulmonary hypertension. Assessment findings may include peripheral cyanosis, inadequate respiratory effort, and ineffective or absent heart rate.

In managing neonatal cardiac arrest, follow the inverted pyramid for resuscitation (Figure 41-6). Administer drugs or fluids according to medical direction. Maintain normal body temperature while you transport the distressed newborn to the appropriate facility. This situation will require delicate handling of the parents or caregivers. Explain what is being done for the infant, without discussing the possibilities of survival.

Summary

After a woman gives birth, you must care for two patients—the mother and her newborn child. The newborn has several special needs, the most important of which are protection of the airway and support of ventilations. The newborn must be kept warm at all times. If assessment reveals a distressed newborn, you should initiate ventilatory support, stimulation, and, if required, CPR. If possible, newborns should be transported to a facility with an NICU. Maintain communications with family members or caregivers, explaining all procedures performed on the newborn.

Review Questions

1. About 80 percent of newborns weighing less than ___________ grams at birth require resuscitation.
   a. 1,500
   b. 2,000
   c. 2,500
   d. 2,800
2. Factors that stimulate the baby's first breath include all of the following *except:*
   a. hypoxia.
   b. hyperthermia.
   c. mild acidosis.
   d. initiation of stretch reflexes in the lungs.
3. Most fetal development occurs during the ___________ trimester of pregnancy.
   a. last
   b. third
   c. first
   d. second
4. The newborn's respiratory rate should average ___________ breaths per minute and the heart rate should fall within the range of ___________ beats per minute.
   a. 20 to 30, 90 to 110
   b. 25 to 35, 100 to 110
   c. 30 to 40, 110 to 120
   d. 40 to 60, 130 to 140
5. The maximum APGAR score is:
   a. 6.
   b. 7.
   c. 8.
   d. 10.
6. Most heat loss in newborns results from:
   a. radiation.
   b. convection.
   c. conduction.
   d. evaporation.
7. In a newborn, ___________ refers to an excess of red blood cells and may reflect hypovolemia or prolonged intrauterine hypoxia.
   a. choanal atresia
   b. polycythemia
   c. omphalocele
   d. Pierre Robin syndrome

8. When caring for a newborn, suctioning should last no longer than __________ seconds.
   a. 5
   b. 10
   c. 15
   d. 20
9. In the newborn, vascular access for the administration of fluids and drugs can most readily be managed by using the __________ vein.
   a. cephalic
   b. brachial
   c. umbilical
   d. saphenous
10. A premature newborn is an infant born prior to __________ weeks of gestation or with weight ranging from 0.6 to 2.2 kg.
    a. 40
    b. 39
    c. 38
    d. 37

See Answers to Review Questions at the back of this book.

Chapter 42

Pediatrics

Objectives

After reading this chapter, you should be able to:

1. Discuss the paramedic's role in the reduction of infant and childhood morbidity and mortality from acute illness and injury. (pp. 1587–1589)
2. Identify methods/mechanisms that prevent injuries to infants and children. (pp. 1588–1589)
3. Describe Emergency Medical Services for Children (EMSC) and how it can affect patient outcome. (p. 1588)
4. Identify the common family responses to acute illness and injury of an infant or child. (p. 1590)
5. Describe techniques for successful interaction with families of acutely ill or injured infants and children. (p. 1590)
6. Identify key anatomical, physiological, growth, and developmental characteristics of infants and children and their implications. (pp. 1590–1593)
7. Outline differences in adult and childhood anatomy, physiology, and "normal" age-group-related vital signs. (pp. 1593–1597)
8. Describe techniques for successful assessment and treatment of infants and children. (pp. 1597–1623)
9. Discuss the appropriate equipment used to obtain pediatric vital signs. (p. 1605)
10. Determine appropriate airway adjuncts, ventilation devices, and endotracheal intubation equipment; their proper use; and complications of use for infants and children. (pp. 1606–1617)
11. List the indications and methods of gastric decompression for infants and children. (pp. 1617–1619)
12. Define pediatric respiratory distress, failure, and arrest. (pp. 1624–1626)
13. Differentiate between upper airway obstruction and lower airway disease. (pp. 1626–1632)
14. Describe the general approach to the treatment of children with respiratory distress, failure, or arrest from upper airway obstruction or lower airway disease. (pp. 1626–1632)

15. Discuss the common causes and relative severity of hypoperfusion in infants and children. (pp. 1632–1636)
16. Identify the major classifications of pediatric cardiac rhythms. (pp. 1637–1640)
17. Discuss the primary etiologies of cardiopulmonary arrest in infants and children. (pp. 1624–1625, 1632)
18. Discuss age-appropriate sites, equipment, techniques, and complications of vascular access for infants and children. (pp. 1619–1620)
19. Describe the primary etiologies of altered level of consciousness in infants and children. (pp. 1623–1648, 1653–1654, 1663)
20. Identify common lethal mechanisms of injury in infants and children. (pp. 1649–1651)
21. Discuss anatomical features of children that predispose or protect them from certain injuries. (pp. 1654–1655)
22. Describe aspects of infant and child airway management that are affected by potential cervical spine injury. (pp. 1651–1653)
23. Identify infant and child trauma patients who require spinal immobilization. (pp. 1621, 1623)
24. Discuss fluid management and shock treatment for infant and child trauma patients. (pp. 1632–1636, 1653)
25. Determine when pain management and sedation are appropriate for infants and children. (p. 1653)
26. Define child abuse, child neglect, and sudden infant death syndrome (SIDS). (pp. 1656–1661)
27. Discuss the parent/caregiver responses to the death of an infant or child. (p. 1657)
28. Define children with special health care needs and technology-assisted children. (pp. 1661–1664)
29. Discuss basic cardiac life support (CPR) guidelines for infants and children. (pp. 1599–1602, 1606–1611)
30. Integrate advanced life support skills with basic cardiac life support for infants and children. (pp. 1611–1621, 1637–1640)
31. Discuss the indications, dosage, route of administration, and special considerations for medication administration in infants and children. (pp. 1620–1622)
32. Discuss appropriate transport guidelines for low- and high-risk infants and children. (p. 1623)
33. Describe the epidemiology, including the incidence, morbidity/mortality, risk factors, prevention strategies, pathophysiology, assessment, and treatment of infants and children with:
    - ★ Respiratory distress/failure (pp. 1624–1632)
    - ★ Hypoperfusion (pp. 1632–1636)
    - ★ Cardiac dysrhythmias (pp. 1637–1640)
    - ★ Neurologic emergencies (pp. 1640, 1642–1643)
    - ★ Trauma (pp. 1648–1651)
    - ★ Abuse and neglect (pp. 1657–1661)
    - ★ Special health-care needs, including technology-assisted children (pp. 1661–1664)
    - ★ SIDS (pp. 1656–1657)
34. Given several preprogrammed simulated pediatric patients, provide the appropriate assessment, treatment, and transport. (pp. 1587–1664)

Key Terms

asthma, p. 1630
bacterial tracheitis, p. 1629
bend fractures, p. 1655
bronchiolitis, p. 1631
buckle fractures, p. 1655
cardiogenic shock, p. 1634
central IV line, p. 1662
congenital, p. 1636
croup, p. 1626
diabetic ketoacidosis, p. 1645
distributive shock, p. 1634
Emergency Medical Services for Children (EMSC), p. 1588
epiglottitis, p. 1627
febrile seizures, p. 1642
foreign body airway obstruction (FBAO), p. 1591
greenstick fractures, p. 1655
growth plate, p. 1596
hyperglycemia, p. 1645
hypoglycemia, p. 1644
hypovolemic shock, p. 1634
JumpSTART Pediatric MCI Triage Tool, p. 1664
noncardiogenic shock, p. 1634
shunt, p. 1663
status asthmaticus, p. 1630
status epilepticus, p. 1642
stoma, p. 1661
sudden infant death syndrome (SIDS), p. 1656
tracheostomy, p. 1661

INTRODUCTION

The ill or injured child presents special concerns for prehospital personnel. Current research indicates that more than 20,000 pediatric deaths occur each year in the United States. The leading causes of death are age specific. They include motor vehicle collisions, burns, drownings, suicides, and homicides. These alarming facts become even more troublesome when experts theorize that many of them could have been prevented by early intervention. Tragedies involving children—neonates to adolescents—account for some of the most stressful incidents that you will encounter in EMS practice.

Treatment of pediatric patients presents a number of challenges for the paramedic. Children, especially young ones, often cannot describe what is bothering them or what has happened to them. In addition to the child patient, you must deal with the parents or caregivers. Finally, a child's size often makes routine procedures more difficult. Keep in mind that children are not simply small adults. They have special considerations and needs. This chapter will present the topic of pediatric emergencies as it applies to advanced prehospital care.

Content Review

Top Causes of Pediatric Deaths

- Motor vehicle accidents
- Burns
- Drownings
- Suicides
- Homicides

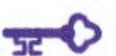

Tragedies involving children account for some of the most stressful incidents that you will encounter in EMS practice.

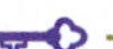

Children are not simply small adults.

ROLE OF PARAMEDICS IN PEDIATRIC CARE

When considering the reduction of pediatric morbidity and mortality, your role as a paramedic centers around two key concepts. First, you must realize that pediatric injuries have become a major health concern. Second, you should remember that children are at a higher risk of injury than adults and that they are more likely to be adversely affected by the injuries that they suffer.

Numerous factors account for the high pediatric injury rates. Some factors, such as geography and weather, cannot be altered. However, other factors, particularly dangers within the home and community, can be eliminated or minimized. As health care professionals, we must all get involved in identifying and implementing methods and mechanisms that prevent injuries to infants and children. Those of us who deliver prehospital care must do more than simply enter the picture after an injury has taken place.

In addition to treating pediatric injuries, paramedics are often responsible for treating the ill child. There are many aspects of disease and disease processes that are unique to children. It is important that the paramedic be familiar with these, because early intervention is often the key to reduced morbidity and mortality.

CONTINUING EDUCATION AND TRAINING

Your role in improving the health care offered to pediatric patients begins with your own training. Because you will encounter pediatric patients less frequently than adult patients, you have a professional

Because you will encounter pediatric patients less frequently than adult patients, you have a professional responsibility to maintain and improve on your pediatric knowledge, particularly your clinical skills.

responsibility to maintain and improve on your pediatric knowledge, particularly your clinical skills. Continuing education programs include:

- ★ Pediatric Advanced Life Support (PALS)
- ★ Pediatric Education for Paramedic Professionals (PEPP)
- ★ Advanced Pediatric Life Support (APLS)
- ★ Prehospital Pediatric Care (PPC)

In addition to these programs, you can also attend regional conferences and seminars designed to increase your knowledge of pediatric care. These are often conducted by regional children's hospitals. You can further enhance your clinical skills by spending time in pediatric emergency departments, pediatric hospitals, or pediatric departments in local hospitals. You might also visit the offices of pediatricians or talk with pediatric nurse practitioners—advanced-practice registered nurses who provide primary health care to children.

For self-study, you can choose among many excellent pediatric textbooks that are currently available or read articles on pediatric care in the various EMS journals. Many good pediatric educational sites are available on the Internet. A particularly useful source of information is the Center for Pediatric Medicine (CPEM), established in 1985 at the New York University Medical Center and Bellevue Hospital. This federally funded center promotes education, research, and development of systems aimed at improving emergency medical services for children in the United States. CPEM has made available the *Teaching Resource for Instructors in Prehospital Pediatrics* (TRIPP), a progressive and comprehensive resource for instructors of prehospital providers. This resource contains a thorough review of prehospital pediatric emergencies.

IMPROVED HEALTH CARE AND INJURY PREVENTION

Emergency Medical Services for Children (EMSC) *federally funded program aimed at improving the health of pediatric patients who suffer from life-threatening illnesses and injuries.*

Funding for CPEM comes largely from a program known as the **Emergency Medical Services for Children (EMSC).** This federally funded program falls under the management of the Maternal and Child Health Bureau, an agency of the U.S. Department of Health and Human Services. The EMSC was formed for the express purpose of improving the health of pediatric patients who suffer potentially life-threatening illnesses or injuries. This nationally coordinated effort has identified a number of pediatric health care concerns, including:

- ★ Community education
- ★ Data collection
- ★ Quality improvement
- ★ Injury prevention
- ★ Access
- ★ Prehospital care
- ★ Emergency care
- ★ Definitive care
- ★ Finance
- ★ Rehabilitation
- ★ A systems approach to pediatric care
- ★ Ongoing health care from birth to young adulthood

As a paramedic, you can take part in this national effort by actively participating in programs that promote injury prevention. Let's face it—as prehospital care providers, we see the consequences of pediatric trauma all too often. You can help reduce the rate of injury by taking advantage of opportunities to share "teaching points" in your daily life, both personally and professionally. Take part in, or offer to organize, school or community programs in injury prevention or health care. Engage student interest in the EMS profession by volunteering to speak at "career days," emphasizing those aspects of your job that relate to young people. Use nonurgent ambulance calls as a chance to educate family members or caregivers on the importance of "childproofing" a home or neighborhood. Work with appropriate agencies in initiating or conducting safety inspections, block watches, and more.

There has been an increased effort to identify the severity and nature of prehospital pediatric emergencies. Many regions now have both pediatric and trauma registries. These, in addition to standard epidemiological research conducted by local health departments, are dependent on quality prehospital documentation. If your area is participating in a registry program or research study, be sure to obtain and record all required data. Information gained from these registries will help identify the need for more or specialized resources.

GENERAL APPROACH TO PEDIATRIC EMERGENCIES

The approach to the pediatric patient varies with the age of the patient and with the problem being treated. Foremost in approaching any pediatric emergency is consideration of the patient's emotional and physiological development. Care also involves the family members or caregivers responsible for the child. They will demand information, express fears, and, ultimately, give or refuse consent for treatment and/or transport.

COMMUNICATION AND PSYCHOLOGICAL SUPPORT

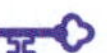

Treatment of an infant, child, or teenager begins with communication and psychological support.

Treatment of an infant, child, or teenager begins with communication and psychological support. Interaction with pediatric patients and related adults continues throughout assessment and management. When obtaining the medical history of the pediatric patient, you should gather information as quickly and as accurately as possible. The parents and caregivers are often the primary source of information, especially in the case of infants. However, as children become older, they can also be a good source of information. Older children, for example, can often give accurate descriptions of symptoms or other details. Treat pediatric patients with respect, allowing them to express opinions and ask questions. Your listening skills will play an important role in alleviating the fears of child patients. You can even communicate a calm and caring attitude to infants, who respond to touch and voice just like any other human being.

Responding to Patient Needs

As previously mentioned, a child's response to an emergency will vary, depending on the age and emotional maturity of the child. The child's most common response to illness or injury is fear. Common fears of children include:

- ★ Fear of being separated from the parents or caregivers
- ★ Fear of being removed from a family place, such as home, and never returning
- ★ Fear of being hurt
- ★ Fear of being mutilated or disfigured
- ★ Fear of the unknown

These fears may be intensified if the child detects fear or anxiety from the parents or caregivers. The general chaos and panic that often surround pediatric emergency situations may further distress the child.

Remember that children have the right to know what is being done to them. Be as honest as possible.

Remember that children have the right to know what is being done to them. You should be as honest as possible with them. If a procedure such as an IV needle stick will hurt, tell them so—but tell them immediately before performing a procedure. Do not say that a procedure will be painful and then take 5 minutes to prepare the equipment, allowing time for the child's anticipation of pain to build.

Always use language that is appropriate for the age of the child. Medical and anatomical terms that we routinely use may be completely foreign to children. Telling a child that you are going to "apply a cervical collar" means nothing. Instead, tell the child: "I'm going to put this collar around your neck to keep it from moving." "Try to hold your head still." "Tell me if it is too tight." This will involve children in their own care and reduce their feelings of helplessness.

Responding to Parents or Caregivers

As you might expect, the reaction of parents or caregivers to a pediatric emergency will vary. Initial reactions might include shock, grief, denial, anger, guilt, fear, or complete loss of control. Their behavior may change during the course of the emergency. Communication is the key. Preferably only one paramedic will speak with adults at the scene. This will reduce the chance of providing conflicting information and allow a second paramedic to focus on the child. If parents or caregivers sense your confidence and professionalism, they will regain control and trust your suggestions for care. As with the child, most parents and caregivers feel overwhelmed by fear. They often express their fears in questions such as the following:

"Is my child going to die?"

"Did my child suffer brain damage?"

"Is my child going to be all right?"

"What are you doing to my child?"

"Will my child be able to walk?"

It may be difficult to answer these questions in the prehospital setting. However, the following actions may help allay parents' fears:

- ★ Tell them your name and qualifications.
- ★ Acknowledge their fears and concerns.
- ★ Reassure them that it is all right to feel the way they do.
- ★ Redirect their energies toward helping you care for the child.
- ★ Remain calm and appear in control of the emergency.
- ★ Keep the parents or caregivers informed as to what you are doing.
- ★ Don't "talk down" to them.
- ★ Assure them that everything possible is being done for their child.

If conditions permit, you should allow one of the parents or caregivers to remain with the child at all times. Some family members may be extremely emotional in emergency situations. The child will react more positively to a family member who appears calm and reassuring. If a parent or caregiver is "out of control," have another person take him away from the immediate area to settle down. Maintain a reasonable level of suspicion if a child shows a pattern of injuries, some old and some new. In such cases, the parent or caregiver may try to cover up what may be an abusive situation. They may also try to block examination and treatment. (Potential abuse or neglect will be discussed in more detail later in this chapter.)

GROWTH AND DEVELOPMENT

Children progress through developmental stages on their way to adulthood. You should tailor your approach to the developmental level of your pediatric patient.

Newborns (First Hours after Birth)

Although the terms *newborn* and *neonate* are often used interchangeably, *newborn* refers to a baby in the first hours of extrauterine life. The term *neonate* describes infants from birth to 1 month of age. The method most frequently used to assess newborns is the *APGAR scoring system,* which was described in Chapter 40, "Obstetrics." Resuscitation of the newborn generally follows the inverted pyramid described in Chapter 41, "Neonatology," and the guidelines established in the Neonatal Advanced Life Support (NALS) curriculum.

Neonates (Ages Birth to 1 Month)

The neonate, as just noted and as described in Chapter 41, is an infant up to 1 month of age. This is a major stage of development. Soon after birth, the neonate typically loses up to 10 percent of its birth weight as it adjusts to extrauterine life. This lost weight, however, is ordinarily recovered within 10 days. Gestational age affects early growth. Children born at term (40 weeks) should follow accepted developmental guidelines. Infants born prematurely will not be as developed, either neurologically or physically, as their term counterparts.

The neonatal stage of development centers on reflexes. The neonate's personality also begins to form. The infant is close to the mother and may stare at faces and smile. The mother, and occasionally the father, can comfort and quiet the child. Common illnesses in this age group include jaundice, vomiting, and respiratory distress. Serious illnesses, such as meningitis, are difficult to distinguish from minor illnesses in neonates. Often, fever is the only sign, although the majority of neonates with fever have minor illnesses (96 to 97 percent). The few that are seriously ill can be easily missed. For this reason, any fever in a neonate requires extensive evaluation.

The approach to this age group should include several factors. First, the neonate should always be kept warm. Observe skin color, tone, and respiratory activity. The absence of tears when crying may indicate dehydration. The lungs should be auscultated early during the exam, while the infant is quiet. You might find it helpful to have the neonate suck on a pacifier during the examination. Allowing the neonate to remain in a parent's or caregiver's lap may help keep the child calm. Obviously, the history must be obtained from the parents or caregivers. However, it is also important to observe the neonate.

Infants (Ages 1 to 5 Months)

Infants should have doubled their birth weight by 5 to 6 months of age. They should be able to follow the movements of others with their eyes. Muscle control develops in a cephalocaudal progression. This means, literally, that development of muscular control begins at the head (cephalo) and moves toward the tail (caudal). Muscular control also spreads from the trunk toward the extremities during this period. The infant's personality at this stage still centers closely on the parents or caregivers. The history must be obtained from these individuals, with close attention to possible illnesses and accidents, including sudden infant death syndrome (SIDS), vomiting, dehydration, meningitis, child abuse, and household accidents.

Concentrate on keeping these patients warm and comfortable. Allow the infant to remain in the parent's or caregiver's lap. A pacifier or bottle may help keep the baby quiet during the exam.

Infants (Ages 6 to 12 Months)

Infants in this age group may stand or even walk with assistance. They are quite active and enjoy exploring the world with their mouths. In this stage of development, the risk of **foreign body airway obstruction** (FBAO) becomes a serious concern.

foreign body airway obstruction (FBAO) *blockage or obstruction of the airway by an object that impairs respiration; in the case of pediatric patients, tongues, abundant secretions, and deciduous (baby) teeth are more likely to block airways.*

Infants 6 months and older have more fully formed personalities and express themselves more readily. They have considerable anxiety toward strangers. They don't like lying on their backs. Children in this age group tend to cling to the primary caregiver, though other family members "will do" in many cases. Common illnesses and accidents include febrile seizures, vomiting, diarrhea, dehydration, bronchiolitis, motor vehicle collisions, croup, child abuse, poisonings, falls, airway obstructions, bronchitis, and meningitis.

These children should be examined while sitting in the lap of the parent or caregiver (Figure 42-1 ■). The exam should progress in a toe-to-head order, since starting at the face may upset the child. If time and conditions permit, allow the child to become familiar with you before beginning the examination.

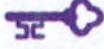

Examine infants and toddlers in a toe-to-head order.

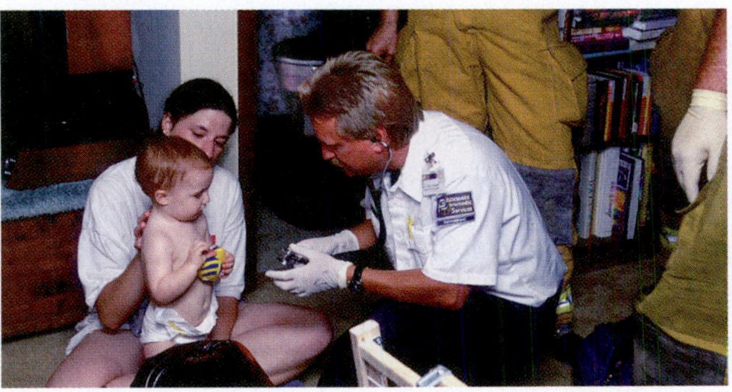

■ **Figure 42-1** Infants and young children should be allowed to remain in their mother's arms. *(© Jeff Forster)*

Toddlers (Ages 1 to 3 Years)

Great strides occur in gross motor development during this stage. Children tend to run underneath or stand on almost everything. They seem to always be on the move. As they grow older, toddlers become braver and more curious or stubborn. They begin to stray away from the parents or caregivers more frequently. Yet these remain the only people who can comfort them quickly, and most children will cling to a parent or caregiver if frightened.

At ages 1 to 3 years, language development begins. Often children can understand better than they can speak. Therefore, the majority of the medical history will still come from the parents or caregivers. Remember, however, that you can ask toddlers simple and specific questions.

Accidents of all types are the leading cause of injury deaths in pediatric patients ages 1 to 15 years. Common accidents in this age group include motor vehicle collisions, homicides, burn injuries, drownings, and pedestrian collisions. Common illnesses and injuries in the toddler age group include vomiting, diarrhea, febrile seizures, poisonings, falls, child abuse, croup, and meningitis. Keep in mind that FBAO is still a high risk for toddlers.

Be cautious when treating toddlers. Approach toddlers slowly and try to gain their confidence. Conduct the exam in a toe-to-head order. The child may be difficult to examine and may resist being touched. Speak quietly and use only simple words. Avoid asking questions that allow the child to say "no." If the situation permits, allow toddlers to hold transitional objects such as a favorite blanket or toy. Be sure to tell the child if something will hurt. If at all possible, avoid procedures on the dominant arm/hand, which the child will try to pull away.

Preschoolers (Ages 3 to 5 Years)

Children in this age group show a tremendous increase in fine and gross motor development. Language skills increase greatly. Children in this age group know how to talk. However, if frightened, they often refuse to speak, especially to strangers. They often have vivid imaginations and may see monsters as part of their world. Preschoolers may have tempers and will express them. During this stage of development, children fear mutilation and may feel threatened by treatment. Avoid frightening or misleading comments.

Preschoolers often run to a particular parent or caregiver, depending on the occasion. They stick up for the people they love and are openly affectionate. They still seek support and comfort from within the home.

When evaluating children in this age group, question the child first, keeping in mind that imagination may interfere with the facts. The child often has a distorted sense of time, and thus you must rely on the parents or caregivers to fill in the gaps. Common illnesses and accidents in this age group include croup, asthma, poisonings, motor vehicle collisions, burns, child abuse, ingestion of foreign bodies, drownings, epiglottitis, febrile seizures, and meningitis.

Do not trick or lie to the child, and always explain what you are going to do.

Treatment of preschoolers requires tact. Avoid baby talk. If time and situation permit, give the child simple health care choices. Often the use of a doll or stuffed animal will assist in the examination. Allow the child to hold a piece of equipment, such as a stethoscope, and to use it. Let the child sit on your lap. Start the examination with the chest and evaluate the head last. Avoid misleading comments. Do not trick or lie to the child, and always explain what you are going to do.

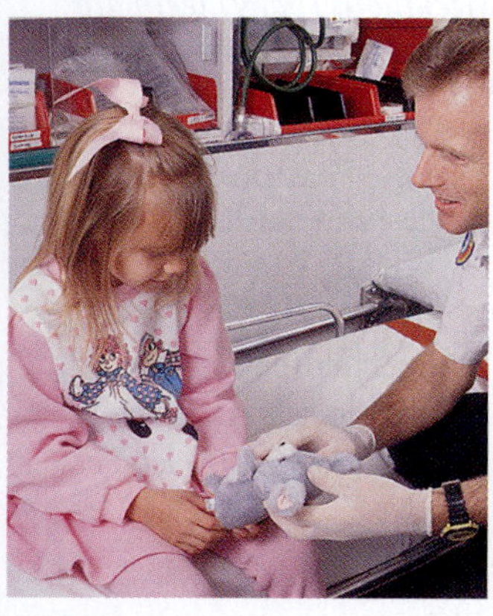

Figure 42-2 A small toy may calm a child in the 6 to 10 year age range.

School-Age Children (Ages 6 to 12 Years)

Children in this age group are active and carefree. Growth spurts sometimes lead to clumsiness. The personality continues to develop. School-age children are protective and proud of their parents or caregivers and seek their attention. They value peers, but also need home support.

When examining school-age children, give them the responsibility of providing the history. However, remember that children may be reluctant to provide information if they sustained an injury while doing something forbidden. The parents or caregivers can fill in the pertinent details. When assessing children in this age group, it is important to respect their modesty. Be honest and tell the child what is wrong. A small toy may help to calm the child (Figure 42-2). Common illnesses and injuries for this age group include drownings, auto collisions, bicycle accidents, falls, fractures, sports injuries, child abuse, and burns.

Adolescents (Ages 13 to 18 Years)

Adolescence covers the period from the end of childhood to the start of adulthood (age 18). It begins with puberty, roughly age 13 for male children and age 11 for female children. (For this reason, adolescence is often defined as including ages 11 to 18, rather than 13 to 18.) Puberty is highly child specific and can begin at various ages. A female child, for example, may experience her first menstrual period as early as age 7 or 8.

Adolescents vary significantly in their development. Those over age 15 are physically nearer to adults in terms of their vital signs but emotionally may still be children. Regardless of physical maturity, remember that teenagers as a group are "body conscious." They worry about their physical image more than any other pediatric age group. You should tactfully address their stated concerns about body integrity or disfigurement. The slightest possibility of a lasting scar may be a tremendous issue to the adolescent patient.

Although patients in this age group are not yet legally adults, most consider themselves to be grown up. They take offense at the use of the word *child.* They have a strong desire to be liked by their peers and to be included. Relationships with parents and caregivers may at times be strained as the adolescent demands greater independence. They value the opinions of other adolescents, especially members of the opposite sex. Generally, these patients make good historians. Do not be surprised, however, if their perception of events differs from that of their parents or caregivers.

Common illnesses and injuries in this age group include mononucleosis, asthma, motor vehicle collisions, sports injuries, drug and alcohol problems, suicide, depression, and sexual abuse. Remember that pregnancy is also possible in female adolescents. When assessing teenagers, remember that vital signs will approach those of adults. In gathering a history, be factual and address the patient's questions. It may be wise to interview the patient away from the parents or caregivers. Listen to what the teenager is saying, as well as what he is *not* saying. If you suspect substance abuse or endangerment of the patient or others, approach the subject with tact and compassion. If you must perform a detailed physical exam, respect the teenager's sense of privacy. If the patient exhibits modesty or bodily shame, have a paramedic of the same sex as the teenager conduct the examination, if possible. Regardless of the situation, provide psychological support and reassurance.

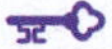

It may be wise to interview the adolescent patient away from the parents or caregivers.

ANATOMY AND PHYSIOLOGY

The differences between the anatomy and physiology of infants and children and that of adults form the basis for the differences in the emergency medical care offered to the two groups (Table 42–1). As previously mentioned, children are not simply small adults. They possess bodies well suited to growth. As a rule, they have healthier organs, a greater ability to compensate for most illnesses, and softer, more flexible tissues. Because you will probably have infrequent contact with pediatric patients, you need to regularly review the physical characteristics that distinguish them from the adult patients that you encounter more often.

Head

The pediatric patient's head is proportionately larger than an adult's and the occipital region is significantly larger. In comparison to their head size, most pediatric patients have small faces and flat noses, which makes it difficult to obtain a good face-mask seal.

With infants, pay special attention to the fontanelles—areas of the skull that have not yet fused. The fontanelles allow for compression of the head during childbirth and for rapid growth of the brain during early life. The posterior fontanelle generally closes by 4 months of age. The anterior fontanelle diminishes after 6 months of age and usually closes between 9 and 18 months.

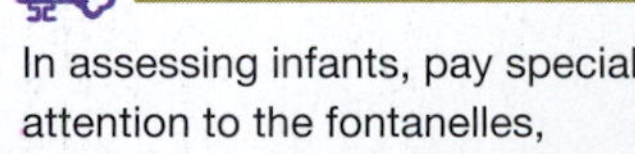

In assessing infants, pay special attention to the fontanelles, especially the anterior fontanelle.

During assessment, always inspect the anterior fontanelle. Normally, it should be level with the surface of the skull or slightly sunken. It also may pulsate. With increased intracranial pressure, as with meningitis or head trauma, the fontanelle may become tight and bulging and pulsations may diminish or disappear. In the presence of dehydration, the anterior fontanelle often falls below the level of the skull and appears sunken.

Table 42–1 Anatomical and Physiological Characteristics of Infants and Children

Differences in Infants and Children as Compared to Adults	Potential Effects That May Impact Assessment and Care
Tongue proportionately larger	More likely to block airway
Smaller airway structures	More easily blocked
Abundant secretions	Can block the airway
Deciduous (baby) teeth	Easily dislodged; can block the airway
Flat nose and face	Difficult to obtain good face mask seal
Head heavier relative to body and less-developed neck structures and muscles	Head may be propelled more forcefully than body producing a higher incidence of head injury in trauma
Fontanelle and open sutures (soft spots) palpable on top of young infant's head	Bulging fontanelle can be a sign of increased intracranial pressure (but may be normal if infant is crying); shrunken fontanelle may indicate dehydration
Thinner, softer brain tissue	Susceptible to serious brain injury
Head larger in proportion to body	Tips forward when supine; possible flexion of neck, which makes neutral alignment of airway difficult
Shorter, narrower, more elastic (flexible) trachea	Can close off trachea with hyperextension of neck
Short neck	Difficult to stabilize or immobilize
Abdominal breathers	Difficult to evaluate breathing
Faster respiratory rate	Muscles easily fatigue, causing respiratory distress
Newborns breathe primarily through the nose (obligate nose breathers)	May not automatically open mouth to breathe if nose is blocked; airway more easily blocked
Larger body surface relative to body mass	Prone to hypothermia
Softer bones	More flexible, less easily fractured; traumatic forces may be transmitted to internal organs, causing injury without fracturing the ribs; lungs easily damaged with trauma
Spleen and liver more exposed	Organ injury likely with significant force to abdomen

The heavy head relative to body size places an infant or child at risk of blunt head trauma. In accidents, the head may be propelled more forcefully than the body, resulting in a higher incidence of brain injury. Head size also affects the airway positioning techniques you should use in treating pediatric patients. In general, follow these guidelines:

- ★ In treating seriously injured patients less than 3 years of age, place a thin layer of padding under their back to obtain a neutral position. This will prevent the head from tipping forward when supine, causing flexion of the neck (Figure 42-3 ■).
- ★ In treating medically ill children over 3 years of age, place a folded sheet or towel under the occiput to obtain a sniffing position (neck flexed slightly forward, head extended slightly backward to align pharynx and trachea).

Airway

In managing the airway of an infant or child, keep in mind these anatomical and physiological considerations:

- ★ Pediatric patients have narrower airways than adults at all levels and these are more easily blocked by secretions or obstructions.
- ★ Infants are obligate nose breathers. If their noses are blocked by secretions, for example, they may not automatically "know" to open their mouths to breathe.
- ★ The tongue takes up more space proportionately in a child's mouth than in an adult's and can more easily obstruct breathing in an unconscious patient.

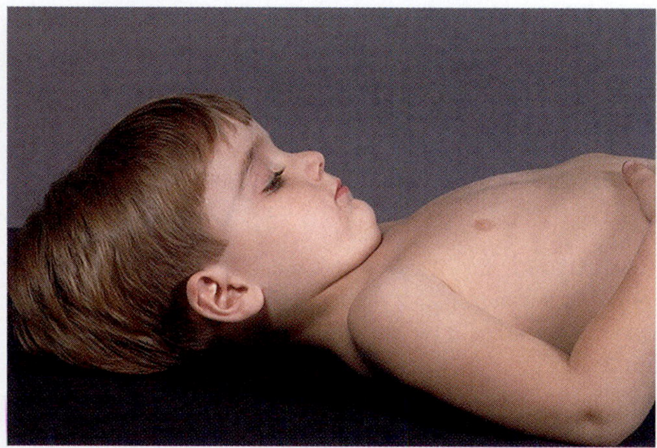

■ Figure 42-3a In the supine position, an infant's or child's larger head tips forward, causing airway obstruction.

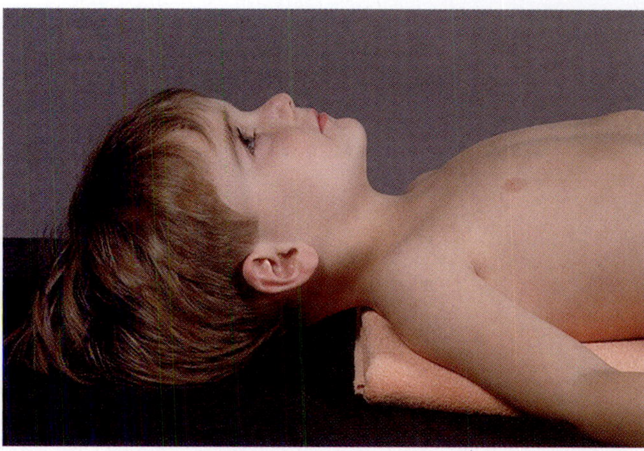

■ Figure 42-3b Placing padding under the patient's back and shoulders will bring the airway to a neutral or slightly extended position.

- ★ The trachea is softer and more flexible in a child than in an adult and can collapse if the neck and head are hyperextended.
- ★ A child's larynx is more superior (C-3 to C-4) than an adult's and extends into the pharynx.
- ★ In young children, the cricoid ring is the narrowest part of the airway.
- ★ Infants have an omega-shaped (horseshoe-shaped) epiglottis that extends at a 45-degree angle into the airway. Because epiglottic folds in pediatric patients have softer cartilage than in adults, they can be more floppy, especially in infants.

Take these anatomical and physiological differences into account by following these general procedures: Always keep the nares clear in infants less than 6 months of age. Do not overextend the neck, which may collapse the trachea. Open the airway gently to avoid soft-tissue injury. Because any device placed in the infant's or child's airway further narrows the passage's diameter and may result in localized swelling, consider use of an oral or a nasal airway only after other manual maneuvers have failed to keep the airway open. (More information on pediatric airway management will be provided later in this chapter.)

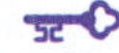

Consider use of an oral or nasal airway in a pediatric patient only after other manual maneuvers have failed to keep the airway open.

Chest and Lungs

In evaluating the chest and lungs of an infant or child, remember that tissues and muscles are more immature than in adults. Chest muscles tire easily, and lung tissues are more fragile. The soft, pliable ribs offer less protection to organs. Expect the ribs to be positioned horizontally and the mediastinum to be more mobile.

Take into account the following anatomical and physiological considerations when assessing the chest and lungs of a pediatric patient:

- ★ Infants and children are diaphragmatic breathers.
- ★ Pediatric patients, especially young infants, are prone to gastric distention.
- ★ Although rib fractures occur less frequently in children, they are not uncommon in cases of child abuse.
- ★ Because of the softness of a child's ribs, greater energy can be transmitted to underlying organs following trauma. As a result, significant internal injury can be present without external signs.
- ★ Pulmonary contusions are more common in pediatric patients who have been subjected to major trauma.
- ★ An infant's or child's lungs are more prone than an adult's to pneumothorax following barotrauma.

- ★ The mediastinum of a child or infant will shift more with tension pneumothorax than in an adult.
- ★ Thin chest walls in infants and children allow for easily transmitted breath sounds. This may result in perception of breath sounds from elsewhere in the chest, which may cause you to miss a pneumothorax or misplaced intubation.

Abdomen

Note that the liver and spleen, both very vascular organs, are proportionately larger in the pediatric patient than in the adult patient. Abdominal organs lie closer together. Because of the immature abdominal muscles in an infant or child, expect to find more frequent damage to the liver and spleen and more multiple organ injuries than in an adult.

Extremities

Until pediatric patients reach adolescence, they have softer and more porous bones than adults. Therefore, you should treat "sprains" and "strains" as fractures and immobilize them accordingly.

During early stages of development, injuries to the **growth plate** may also disrupt bone growth. Keep this in mind when inserting an intraosseous needle, which could mistakenly pierce the plate. (Intraosseous infusion will be discussed later in this chapter.)

growth plate *the area just below the head of a long bone in which growth in bone length occurs; the epiphyseal plate.*

During the early stages of development, injuries to the growth plate by an intraosseous needle may disrupt bone growth.

Skin and Body Surface Area (BSA)

The pediatric patient's skin and body surface area (BSA) have three distinguishing features. First, the skin of an infant or child is thinner than that of an adult. Second, infants and children generally have less subcutaneous fat. Finally, they have a larger BSA-to-weight ratio.

As a result of these features, children risk greater injury from extremes in temperature or thermal exposure. They lose fluids and heat more quickly than adults and have a greater likelihood of dehydration and hypothermia. They also burn more easily and deeply than adults, explaining why burns account for one of the leading causes of death among pediatric trauma patients.

Respiratory System

Although infants and children have a tidal volume proportionately similar to that of adolescents and adults, they require double the metabolic oxygen. They also have proportionately smaller oxygen reserves. The combination of increased oxygen requirements and decreased oxygen reserves makes infants and children especially susceptible to hypoxia.

Cardiovascular System

Infants and children increase their cardiac output by increasing their heart rate. They have a very limited capacity to increase their stroke volume.

Cardiac output is rate dependent in infants and small children. They possess vigorous, but limited, cardiovascular reserves. Although infants and children have a circulating blood volume proportionately larger than that of adults, their absolute blood volume is smaller. As a result, they can maintain blood pressure longer than an adult but still be at risk of shock (hypoperfusion). In assessing a pediatric patient for shock, keep in mind the following points:

- ★ A smaller absolute volume of fluid/blood loss is needed to cause shock in infants and children.
- ★ A larger proportional volume of fluid/blood loss is needed to cause shock in these same patients.
- ★ As with all categories of patients, hypotension is a late sign of shock. In pediatric patients, it is an ominous sign of imminent cardiopulmonary arrest.
- ★ A child may be in shock despite a normal blood pressure.
- ★ Shock assessment in children and infants is based on clinical signs of tissue perfusion. (See the later discussion of circulation assessment.)
- ★ Suspect shock if tachycardia is present.
- ★ Monitor the pediatric patient carefully for the development of hypotension.

Once again, remember that children are not small adults. Bleeding that would not be dangerous in an adult may be a serious and life-threatening condition in an infant or child. Shock can develop in the small child who has a laceration to the scalp (with its many blood vessels) or in the 3-year-old who loses as little as a cup of blood. (Management of shock in pediatric patients will be discussed in detail later in the chapter.)

Bleeding that would not be dangerous in an adult may be life threatening in an infant or child.

Nervous System

The nervous system develops continually throughout childhood. Even so, the neural tissue remains more fragile than in adults. The skull and spinal column, which are softer and more pliable than in adults, offer less protection of the brain and spinal cord. Therefore, greater force can be transmitted to a child's neural tissue with more devastating consequences. These injuries can occur without injury to the skull or to the spinal column. (Treatment of head and neck trauma will be discussed later in the chapter.)

Metabolic Differences

You may have noticed the repeated emphasis on the need to keep neonatal and pediatric patients warm during treatment and transport. The emphasis on warming techniques is based on the following metabolic considerations:

★ Infants and children have a limited store of glycogen and glucose.

★ Pediatric patients are prone to hypothermia because of their greater BSA-to-weight ratio.

★ Significant volume loss can result from vomiting and diarrhea.

★ Newborns and neonates lack the ability to shiver.

To prevent heat loss, always cover the patient's head and maintain adequate temperature controls in the ambulance. Ensure that the ambulance is always stocked with an adequate supply of blankets and, if you live in a cold area, hot water bottles.

GENERAL APPROACH TO PEDIATRIC ASSESSMENT

Priorities in the management of the pediatric patient, as with all patients, are established on a threat-to-life basis. If life-threatening problems are not present, you will complete each of the general steps discussed in the following sections.

BASIC CONSIDERATIONS

Many of the components of the primary patient assessment can be done during a visual examination of the scene. (This is sometimes called the "assessment from the doorway," during which you quickly note signs of an ill child such as lethargy.) When possible, involve the parent or caregiver in efforts to calm or comfort the child. Depending on the situation, you may decide to allow the parent or caregiver to remain with the child during treatment and transport. As previously mentioned, the developmental stage of the patient and the coping skills of the parents or guardians will be key factors in making this decision.

When interacting with parents or other responsible adults, keep in mind the communication techniques suggested earlier. Pay attention to the way in which parents or caregivers interact with the child. Are the interactions appropriate to the emergency? Are family members concerned? Are they angry? Are they overly emotional or entirely indifferent?

From the time of dispatch, you will continually acquire information relative to the patient's condition. As with all patients, personal safety must be your first priority. In treating pediatric patients, follow the same guidelines in approaching the scene as you would with any other patient. Observe for potentially hazardous situations and make sure you use Standard Precautions. Remember that infants and young children are at especially high risk of an infectious process.

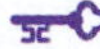

Remember to use Standard Precautions when treating infants and children.

SCENE SIZE-UP

On arrival, conduct a quick scene size-up. Dispatch information received en route, as well as your own observations, can provide critical indicators of scene safety. Be aware of the increased anxiety and stress in any situation involving an infant or child. Try to set aside thoughts of your own children and adopt the professional, systematic approach to assessment necessary for scene safety and effective patient management. If you find yourself getting angry or upset, temporarily turn over care to another paramedic until you compose yourself.

As you survey the scene, look for clues to the mechanism of injury (MOI) or the nature of the illness (NOI). These clues will help guide your assessment and determine appropriate interventions. Note the presence of dangerous substances (for example, medicine bottles, household chemicals, or poisonous plants) that the child may have ingested. Spot environmental hazards such as unprotected stairwells, kerosene heaters, and so on. Identify possible causes of trauma, especially in motor vehicle collisions. Remain alert for evidence of child abuse, particularly in cases in which the injury and history do not coincide. As already mentioned, pay attention to the way parents or caregivers respond to the child and the way the child responds to them.

Keep the child in mind while conducting your scene size-up. Pace your approach to give the child time to adjust to your presence. Speak in a soft voice, using simple words. As soon as you reach the child, position yourself at eye level with the patient and make every effort to win his trust. If the child bonds more readily with one member of the team than another, allow that person to remain with the child and, if possible, to conduct most of the physical exam.

PRIMARY ASSESSMENT

The patient's condition determines the course of your primary assessment. An active and alert child will allow for a more comfortable approach, with more time spent on communication with the child and appropriate adults. A critically ill or injured child, however, may require quick intervention and rapid transport. Your choice of action depends on your general impression of the patient.

General Impression

The major points in forming your general impression are outlined in an assessment tool called the *pediatric assessment triangle.* Many experts recommend this assessment tool as a way of quickly evaluating the level of severity and the need for immediate intervention. It is a rapid "eyes-open, hands-on" approach that allows you to detect a life-threatening situation without the use of a stethoscope, blood pressure cuff, pulse oximeter, or other medical device. The triangle's three components are:

- ★ *Appearance.* Focuses on the child's mental status and muscle tone.
- ★ *Breathing.* Directs attention to respiratory rate and respiratory effort.
- ★ *Circulation.* Uses skin signs and color as well as capillary refill as indicators of the patient's circulatory status.

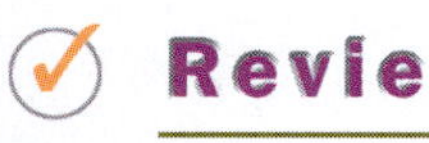

Content Review

Pediatric Assessment Triangle

- Appearance
- Breathing
- Circulation

Vital Functions

After quickly applying the pediatric assessment triangle to form a general impression, you will evaluate vital functions—mental status (level of consciousness) and the ABCs—as they apply to infants and children. Although assessment steps are basically the same as for adults, certain modifications must be made to collect accurate data.

Level of Consciousness Employ the AVPU method (*a*lert, responds to *v*erbal stimuli, responds to *p*ainful stimuli, *u*nresponsive) to evaluate the pediatric patient's level of consciousness. Adjust the techniques for the child's age. With an infant, you may need to shout to elicit a response (perhaps crying) to verbal stimulus. An infant should withdraw from a noxious stimulus. *Never shake an infant or child.*

Never shake an infant or child.

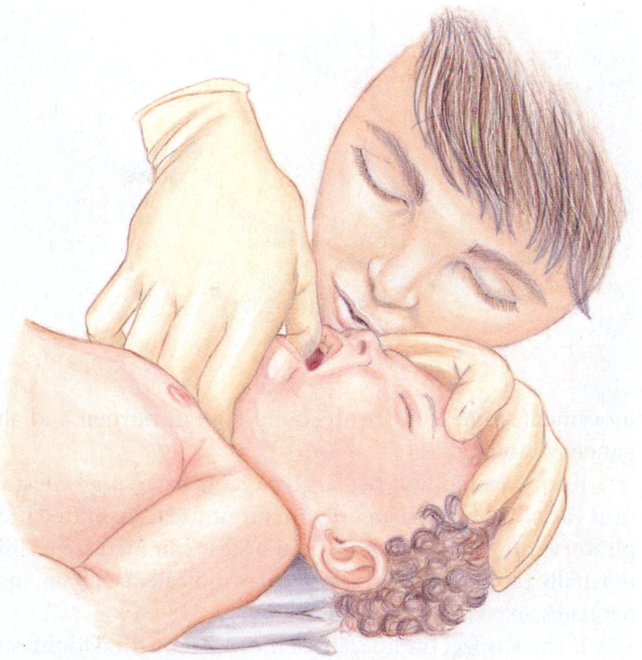

■ Figure 42-4 Opening the airway in a child.

Never shake an infant or child.

Airway Assess the airway using the techniques shown in Figures 42-4 ■ through 42-7 ■. If at any point the patient shows little or no movement of air, intervene immediately. Keep this fact in mind: *Airway and respiratory problems are the most common cause of cardiac arrest in infants and young children.*

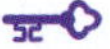

Airway and respiratory problems are the most common cause of cardiac arrest in infants and young children.

As you inspect the airway, ask yourself the following questions:

- ★ Is the airway patent?
- ★ Is the airway maintainable with head positioning, suctioning, or airway adjuncts?
- ★ Is the airway *not* maintainable? If so, what action is required? (Airway management techniques will be discussed later in this chapter.)

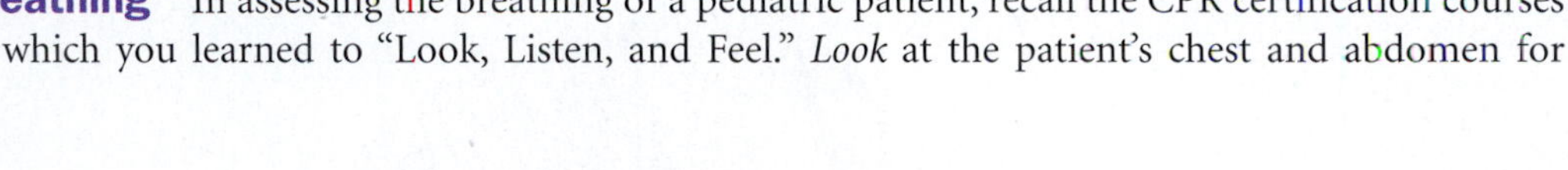

Breathing In assessing the breathing of a pediatric patient, recall the CPR certification courses in which you learned to "Look, Listen, and Feel." *Look* at the patient's chest and abdomen for

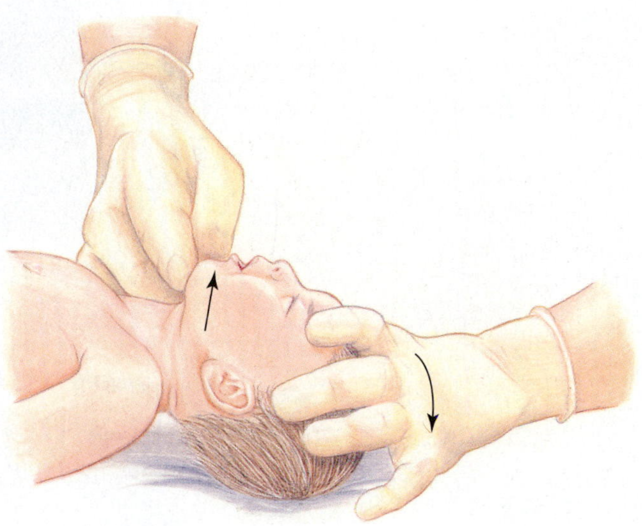

■ Figure 42-5 Head-tilt/chin-lift method.

■ Figure 42-6 Jaw-thrust method.

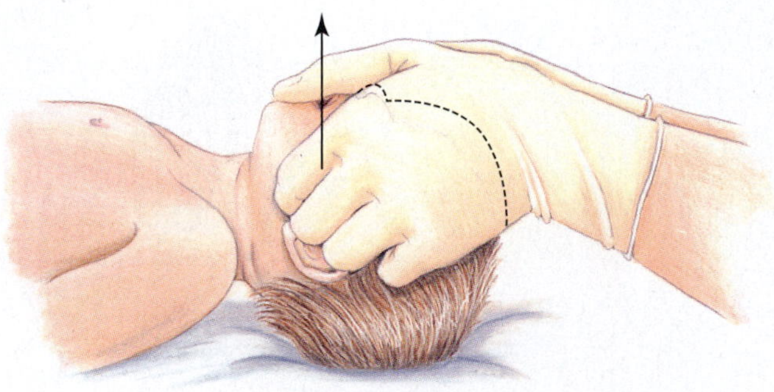

movement. *Listen* for breath sounds—both normal and abnormal. *Feel* for air movement at the patient's mouth.

Keep in mind that pediatric patients have small chests. For this reason, place the stethoscope near each of the axillae in order to minimize transmitted breath sounds. When considering the respiratory rate, remember that pain or fear can increase a child's respiratory rate. Tachypnea, an abnormally rapid rate of breathing, may indicate fear, pain, inadequate oxygenation, or, in the case of neonates, exposure to cold.

If you suspect trauma, check the infant or child for life-threatening chest injuries. Keep in mind that even a minor injury to the chest can interfere with a child's breathing efforts. A chest injury can also interfere with your effort to provide adequate oxygenation or ventilation.

Your goal is to identify any evidence of compromised breathing. Evaluation of breathing includes assessment of the following conditions:

★ *Respiratory rate.* Tachypnea is often the first manifestation of respiratory distress in infants. Regardless of the cause, an infant breathing at a rapid rate will eventually tire. Keep in mind that a decreasing respiratory rate may be a result of tiring and is not necessarily a sign of improvement. A slow respiratory rate in an acutely ill infant or child is an ominous sign. (Normal respiratory rates are listed in Table 42–2.) In short, be alert for a respiratory rate that is *either* abnormally fast *or* abnormally slow.

★ *Respiratory effort.* The quality of air entry can be assessed by observing for chest rise, breath sounds, stridor, or wheezing. An increased respiratory effort in the infant or

■ Figure 42-7 Assessing breathing.

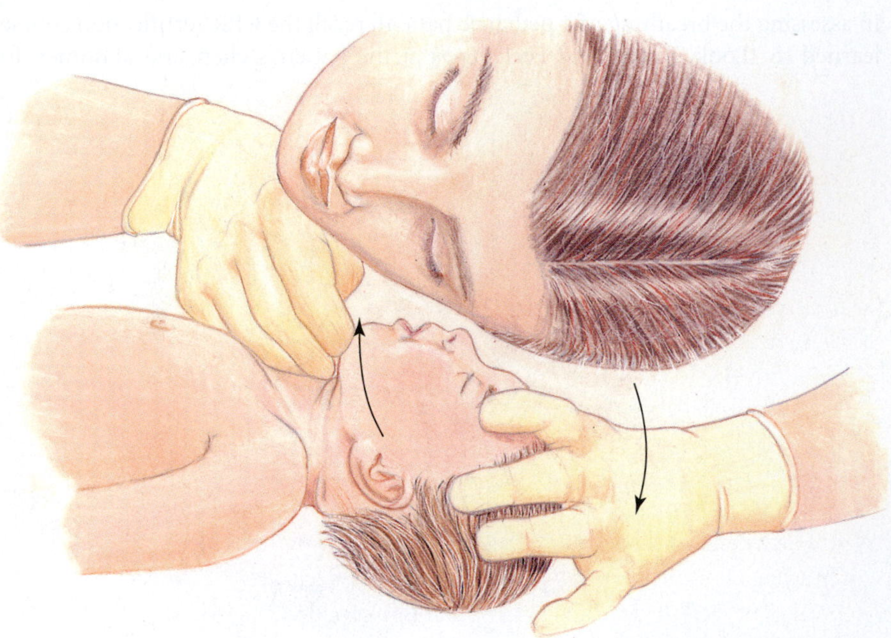

Table 42–2 Normal Vital Signs: Infants and Children*

Normal Pulse Rates (Beats per Minute, at Rest)		
Newborn	100 to 180	
Infant (0 to 5 months)	100 to 160	
Infant (6 to 12 months)	100 to 160	
Toddler (1 to 3 years)	80 to 110	
Preschooler (3 to 5 years)	70 to 110	
School Age (6 to 10 years)	65 to 110	
Early Adolescence (11 to 14 years)	60 to 90	
Normal Respiration Rates (Breaths per Minute, at Rest)		
Newborn	30 to 60	
Infant (0 to 5 months)	30 to 60	
Infant (6 to 12 months)	30 to 60	
Toddler (1 to 3 years)	24 to 40	
Preschooler (3 to 5 years)	22 to 34	
School Age (6 to 10 years)	18 to 30	
Early Adolescence (11 to 14 years)	12 to 26	
Normal Blood Pressure Ranges (mmHg, at Rest)		
	Systolic	**Diastolic**
	Approx. 90 plus 2 × age	Approx. ⅔ systolic
Preschooler (3 to 5 years)	average 98 (78 to 116)	average 65
School age (6 to 10 years)	average 105 (80 to 122)	average 69
Early Adolescence (11 to 14 years)	average 114 (88 to 140)	average 76

* Adolescents ages 15 to 18 approach the vital signs of adults.

Note: A high pulse in an infant or child is not as great a concern as a low pulse. A low pulse may indicate imminent cardiac arrest. Blood pressure is usually not taken in a child under 3 years of age. In cases of blood loss or shock, a child's blood pressure will remain within normal limits until near the end, then fall swiftly.

child is also evidenced by nasal flaring and the use of accessory respiratory muscles. (Signs of respiratory effort are listed in Table 42–3.)

★ *Color.* Cyanosis is a fairly late sign of respiratory failure and is most frequently seen in the mucous membranes of the mouth and the nail beds. Cyanosis of the extremities alone is more likely due to circulatory failure (shock) than to respiratory failure.

Circulation As mentioned earlier, you should assess a pediatric patient's circulation by first checking the child's color. Keep in mind that the pediatric patient tends to become hypothermic; therefore, you should check the capillary refill time in an area of central circulation, such as the sternum or forehead. (Note that capillary refill time, as discussed later in this chapter, is considered reliable as a sign of perfusion primarily in children less than 6 years of age.) In general, evaluate the following conditions when assessing circulation during the primary assessment:

★ *Heart rate.* As previously mentioned, infants develop sinus tachycardia in response to stress. Thus, any tachycardia in an infant or child requires further evaluation to determine the cause. Bradycardia in a distressed infant or child may indicate hypoxia and is an ominous sign of potential cardiac arrest. (Normal heart rates are listed in Table 42–2.)

★ *Peripheral circulation.* The presence of peripheral pulses is a good indicator of the adequacy of end-organ perfusion. Loss of central pulses is an ominous sign.

Table 42–3	Signs of Increased Respiratory Effort
Retraction	Visible sinking of the skin and soft tissues of the chest around and below the ribs and above the collarbone
Nasal flaring	Widening of the nostrils; seen primarily on inspiration
Head bobbing	Observed when the head lifts and tilts back as the child inhales and then moves forward as the child exhales
Grunting	Sound heard when an infant attempts to keep the alveoli open by building back pressure during expiration
Wheezing	Passage of air over mucous secretions in bronchi; heard more commonly on expiration; a low- or high-pitched sound
Gurgling	Coarse, abnormal bubbling sound heard in the airway during inspiration or expiration; may indicate an open chest wound
Stridor	Abnormal, musical, high-pitched sound, more commonly heard on inspiration

- ★ *End-organ perfusion.* End-organ perfusion is most evident in the skin, kidneys, and brain. Decreased perfusion of the skin is an early sign of shock. A capillary refill time of greater than 2 seconds is indicative of low cardiac output. Impairment of brain perfusion is usually evidenced by a change in mental status. The child may become confused or lethargic. Seizures may occur. Failure of the child to recognize the parents' faces is often an ominous sign. Urine output directly relates to kidney perfusion. Normal urine output is 1 to 2 mL/kg/hr. Urine flow of less than 1 mL/kg/hr is an indicator of poor renal perfusion.

Remember that evaluation of mental status and ABCs during the primary assessment is rapid and not detailed, because it is aimed at discovering and correcting immediate life threats. More thorough measurements will be performed during the secondary assessment.

Anticipating Cardiopulmonary Arrest

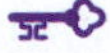

At each stage of evaluating vital functions, ask yourself "Does this child have pulmonary or circulatory failure that may lead to cardiopulmonary arrest?"

Your primary assessment and the repeated assessments that follow help you to recognize and prevent cardiopulmonary arrest. At each stage of evaluating vital functions, ask yourself this question: *"Does this child have pulmonary or circulatory failure that may lead to cardiopulmonary arrest?"* Early recognition of the physiologically unstable child is one of the main goals of pediatric advanced life support (PALS). Conditions that place a pediatric patient at risk of cardiopulmonary arrest include:

- ★ Respiratory rate greater than 60
- ★ Heart rate greater than 180 or less than 80 (under 5 years)
- ★ Heart rate greater than 180 or less than 60 (over 5 years)
- ★ Respiratory distress
- ★ Trauma
- ★ Burns
- ★ Cyanosis
- ★ Altered level of consciousness
- ★ Seizures
- ★ Fever with petechiae (small purple spots resulting from skin hemorrhages)

Evaluate the patient for these conditions throughout assessment and transport. Cardiopulmonary arrest in infants and children is usually not a sudden event. Instead, it is the end result of progressive deterioration in respiratory and cardiac function. Therefore, you need to determine whether the patient's condition is deteriorating or improving. Any decompensation or change in the patient's status will prompt you to perform basic or advanced life support measures, as appropriate.

Table 42–4 Glasgow Coma Scale Modifications for Infants

Category	Response	Score
Verbal	Happy, coos, babbles, or cries spontaneously	5
	Irritable crying, but consolable	4
	Cries to pain, weak cry	3
	Moans to pain	2
	None	1
Motor	Spontaneous movement	6
	Withdraws to touch	5
	Withdraws to pain	4
	Abnormal flexion	3
	Abnormal extension	2
	None	1
Eye opening (same as adult)	Spontaneous	4
	To speech	3
	To pain	2
	None	1

Source: Adapted from James, H. E. "Neurologic Evaluation and Support in the Child with Acute Brain Insult." *Pediatric Annals, 15* (1) (1986): 17.

Transport Priority

Based on your primary assessment, you will assign the patient one of the following transport priorities:

- ★ *Urgent.* Proceed with the rapid secondary assessment, if trauma is suspected, then transport immediately with further assessment and treatment performed en route.
- ★ *Nonurgent.* Complete the secondary assessment at the scene, then transport.

To help determine transport priority, some EMS systems use a trauma score that is modified for pediatric patients, which includes the elements of the Glasgow Coma Scale, also modified for pediatric patients (Table 42–4). These scores can help predict patient outcome and help in the decision on whether rapid transport to a trauma center is required. If used in your EMS system, your medical director and/or system protocols will determine what numerical score mandates rapid transport.

Transitional Phase

The way in which the pediatric patient is transferred to EMS care depends entirely on the seriousness of the patient's condition. A transitional phase is intended for the conscious, nonacutely ill child. This phase of assessment allows the infant or child to become familiar with you and the equipment that you will be using. When dealing with the unconscious or acutely ill patient, however, you will skip this phase and proceed directly to the treatment and transport phases of assessment. In essence, you assign the patient an "urgent" status.

SECONDARY ASSESSMENT

After you have prioritized patient care at the end of the primary assessment, you will obtain a history and perform a physical exam. If the patient has a medical illness, the history will precede the physical exam. If the patient is suffering from trauma, the physical exam will take precedence. If partners are working together, the history and physical exam may be performed simultaneously.

History

When a patient is identified as a priority patient, then the focused history will occur en route to the hospital, after essential treatments or interventions for life-threatening conditions have been performed.

To obtain a history for a pediatric patient, you will probably need to involve a family member or caregiver. Remember, however, that school-age children and adolescents like to take part in their own care. As previously mentioned, you can elicit valuable information from even very young patients. As a general precaution, question older adolescent patients in private, especially about issues such as sexual activity, pregnancy, or illicit drug and alcohol use. If you question adolescents about these subjects in the presence of an adult, they will probably be more reticent for fear of later repercussions.

As with any patient, you will use the history to uncover additional pertinent injuries or medical conditions. The history should center on the chief complaint and past medical history.

To evaluate the nature of the chief complaint, determine each of the following:

- ★ Nature of the illness/injury
- ★ Length of time the patient has been sick/injured
- ★ Presence of fever
- ★ Effects of the illness/injury on patient behavior
- ★ Bowel/urine habits
- ★ Presence of vomiting/diarrhea
- ★ Frequency of urination

The past medical history identifies chronic illnesses, use of medications, and allergies. Be sure to inquire whether the infant or child is currently under a doctor's care. If so, obtain the name of the physician and present it at the receiving hospital. In the case of trauma patients, reconsider the mechanism of injury and the results of your on-scene physical examination (which, as noted earlier, will precede the history in the case of trauma).

Physical Exam

Focused Exam Carry out the physical exam after all life-threatening conditions have been identified and addressed. If there is a significant mechanism of injury or if the patient is unresponsive, perform a complete rapid trauma assessment or rapid medical assessment. Use the toe-to-head approach with the younger child (or begin with the chest and examine the head last) and the head-to-toe approach in the older child. If the injury is minor or if the ill patient is responsive, perform a physical exam that is focused on the affected areas and systems.

Perform the physical exam as described in Chapter 11, "Physical Exam Techniques." Depending on the particular situation, some or all of the following assessment techniques may be appropriate to include in the exam:

- ★ *Pupils.* Inspect the patient's pupils for equality and reaction to light.
- ★ *Capillary refill.* As noted earlier, this technique is valuable for pediatric patients less than 6 years of age. Blanch the nail bed, base of the thumb, or sole of one of the feet. Remember that normal capillary refill is 2 seconds or less. Recall that this technique is less reliable in cold environments.
- ★ *Hydration.* Note skin turgor, presence of tears and saliva and, with infants, the condition of the fontanelles.
- ★ *Pulse oximetry.* Use this mechanical device on moderately injured or ill infants and children. Readings will give you immediate information regarding peripheral oxygen saturation and allow you to follow trends in the patient's pulse rate and oxygenation status. Keep in mind, however, that hypothermia or shock can affect readings.

Content Review

Elements of the Glasgow Coma Scale

- Verbal responses
- Motor functions
- Eye movements

Glasgow Coma Scale In cases of trauma, you may need to apply the Glasgow Coma Scale (GCS), a scoring system for monitoring the neurologic status of patients with possible head injuries. The GCS assigns scores based on verbal responses, motor functions, and eye movements.

In using the Glasgow Coma Scale with pediatric patients, you will have to make certain modifications. The younger the patient, the more adjustments you will need to make. Verbal responses, for example, will not be possible for neonates and infants. However, motor function may be assessed in very young children by observing voluntary movement. Infants under 4 months of age should have a grasp reflex when an object is placed on the palmar surface of their hand. The grasp should be immediate. Children over 3 years of age will follow directions, when encouraged. Sensory function can be observed by the withdrawal reaction from "tickling" the patient. (Review Table 42–4 for a modified GCS for pediatric patients.)

In using the Glasgow Coma Scale with pediatric patients, you will have to make certain modifications. The younger the patient, the more adjustments you will need to make.

After you score the GCS for the patient, prioritize the patient according to severity. Guidelines are:

- ★ *Mild.* GCS 13 to 15.
- ★ *Moderate.* GCS 9 to 12.
- ★ *Severe.* GCS less than or equal to 8.

Vital Signs Remember that poorly taken vital signs are of less value than no vital signs at all. The following guidelines will help you obtain accurate pediatric readings. (Review Table 42–2 for normal pediatric vital signs.)

Remember that poorly taken vital signs are of less value than no vital signs at all.

- ★ Take vital signs with the patient in as close to a resting state as possible. If necessary, allow the child to calm down before attempting vital signs. Vital signs in the field should include pulse, respiration, blood pressure, and temperature.
- ★ Obtain blood pressure with an appropriate-sized cuff. The cuff should be two-thirds the width of the upper arm. Note that the pulse pressure (the difference between the systolic and diastolic blood pressure) narrows as shock develops. *Note that hypotension is a late and often sudden sign of cardiovascular decompensation.* Even mild hypotension should be taken seriously and treated quickly and vigorously, since cardiopulmonary arrest is probably imminent.
- ★ Feel for peripheral, brachial, or femoral pulses. There is often a significant variation in pulse rate in children due to varied respirations. Therefore, it is important to monitor the pulse for at least 30 seconds, with 1 full minute being preferable.
- ★ It is generally not possible to weigh the child. However, if medications are required, make a good estimate of the child's weight. Often the parents or caregivers can provide a fairly reliable weight from a recent visit to the doctor.
- ★ Observe respiratory rate before beginning the examination. After the examination is started, the child will often begin to cry. It will then be impossible to determine respiratory rate. For an estimate of the upper limit of respiratory rate, subtract the child's age from 40. It is also important to identify respiratory pattern, as well as retractions, nasal flaring, or paradoxical chest movement.
- ★ Measure temperature early in the patient encounter and repeat toward the end. IV fluid and exposure to the environment can cause a drop in core temperature.
- ★ Continue to observe the child for level of consciousness. The level of consciousness and activity during treatment may vary widely.

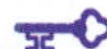

Even mild hypotension should be taken seriously in infants and young children.

Noninvasive Monitoring Modern noninvasive monitoring devices all have their application in pediatric emergency care (Figure 42-8 ■). These may include the pulse oximeter, automated blood pressure devices, self-registering thermometers, and ECGs. To promote the goal of early recognition of cardiopulmonary arrest, every seriously ill or injured child should receive continuous pulse oximetry. This will provide you with essential information regarding the patient's heart rate and peripheral O_2 saturation. It will also help you to monitor the effects of any medications administered. An ECG and automated blood pressure/pulse monitor should also be considered. However, these devices may frighten the child. Before applying any monitoring device, explain what you are going to do. Demonstrate the display or lights. If the monitoring device makes noise, allow the child to hear the noise before you apply it. Reassure the child that the device will not hurt him.

Every seriously ill or injured child should receive continuous ECG monitoring.

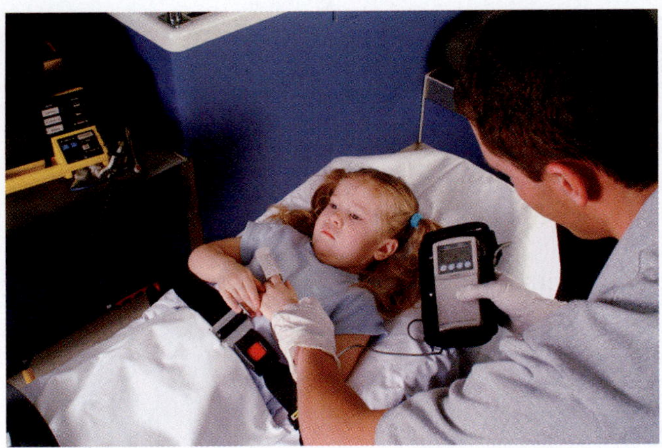

■ Figure 42-8 If available, noninvasive monitoring, including pulse oximetry and temperature measurement, should be used in prehospital pediatric care. *(© Ken Kerr)*

REASSESSMENT

Because a pediatric patient's condition can rapidly change for the better or the worse, it is necessary to repeat relevant portions of the assessment. You should continually monitor the patient's respiratory effort, skin color, mental status, temperature, and pulse oximetry. Retake vital signs and compare them with baseline vitals. In general, reassess stable patients every 15 minutes, critical patients every 5 minutes.

GENERAL MANAGEMENT OF PEDIATRIC PATIENTS

The same ABCs that guide the management of adult patients apply to pediatric patients: Your top priorities in treating an infant or child are airway, breathing, and circulation. However, because of the special anatomical and physiological considerations that influence the management of pediatric patients, you need to practice these skills on an ongoing and regular basis.

BASIC AIRWAY MANAGEMENT

In treating the pediatric patient, basic life support (BLS) should be applied according to current standards and protocols. BLS should include maintenance of the airway, artificial ventilation, and, if required, chest compressions. (See Table 42–5.) As with all patients, your priority is to ensure an open airway. The following modifications of BLS airway skills will ensure that you take into account the clinical implications of the pediatric airway.

Manual Positioning

Allow the pediatric patient to assume a position of comfort, if possible. When placing the patient in a supine position, avoid hyperextension of the neck. As previously mentioned, infants and small children risk collapsed tracheas from hyperextension of the neck. For trauma patients less than 3 years old, place support under the torso. For supine medical patients 3 years old and older, provide occipital elevation.

Foreign Body Airway Obstruction (FBAO)

Before administering treatment, determine if an airway obstruction is mild or severe. Infants or children with a mild airway obstruction will have a cough, hoarse voice or cry, stridor, or some other evidence that at least some air is passing through the airway. If the obstruction is mild, avoid any maneuvers that will turn it into a severe obstruction. Instead, place the patient in a position of comfort and transport immediately.

In the case of severe airway obstruction, take one of the following age-specific maneuvers:

- ★ *Children.* For children older than 1 year of age, perform a series of abdominal thrusts until the item is expelled or the patient becomes unresponsive.
- ★ *Infants.* For an infant, deliver a series of five back blows followed by five chest thrusts. Inspect the infant's mouth on completion of each series.

Table 42–5 Summary of BLS Maneuvers in Infants and Children

Target of Maneuver	Infant (< 1 year)	Child (1 to puberty)
Airway		
Open airway	Head-tilt/chin-lift (unless trauma present) Jaw-thrust	Head-tilt/chin-lift (unless trauma present) Jaw-thrust
Clear foreign body obstruction	Back blows/chest thrusts	Abdominal thrusts
Breathing		
Initial	2 breaths that make the chest rise	2 breaths that make the chest rise
Subsequent	1 breath every 3 seconds (12–20/minute)	1 breath every 3 seconds (12–20 minutes)
Circulation		
Pulse check	Brachial/femoral	Carotid
Compression area	Lower third of sternum	Lower third of sternum
Compression width	Two or three fingers	Heel of 1 hand
Depth	Approximately ⅓ to ½ anteroposterior diameter of chest	Approximately ⅓ to ½ anteroposterior diameter of chest
Rate	At least 100/minute	100/minute
Compression-ventilation ratio	30:2 (1 rescuer); 15:2 (2 rescuers)	30:2 (1 rescuer); 15:2 (2 rescuers)

As you recall from the basic CPR courses, never check a pediatric patient's mouth with blind finger sweeps.

Never use blind finger sweeps in a pediatric patient.

Suctioning

Apply suctioning when you detect heavy secretions in the nose or mouth of a pediatric patient, especially if the patient has a diminished level of consciousness. You can use a bulb syringe, flexible suction catheter, or rigid-tip suction catheter, depending on the patient's age or size (Figure 42-9 ■). Make sure that flexible catheters are correctly sized (Table 42–6).

Although pediatric suctioning techniques differ very little from adult suctioning techniques, keep the following modifications in mind:

- ★ Decrease suction pressure to less than 100 mmHg in infants.
- ★ Avoid excessive suctioning time (suction less than 10 seconds) in order to decrease the possibility of hypoxia.

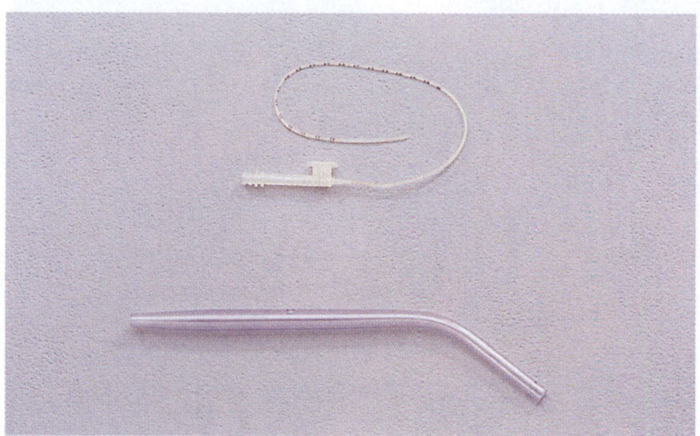

■ **Figure 42-9** Pediatric-size suction catheters. Top: Soft suction catheter. Bottom: Rigid or hard suction catheter.

Table 42-6	Suction Catheter Sizes for Infants and Children
Age	**Suction Catheter Size (French)**
Up to 1 year	8
2 to 6 years	10
7 to 15 years	12
16 years	12 to 14

- ★ Avoid stimulation of the vagus nerve, which may produce bradycardia. As a general rule, suction no deeper than you can see and for no more than 10 seconds per attempt.
- ★ Frequently check the patient's pulse. If bradycardia occurs, stop suctioning immediately and oxygenate.

Oxygenation

Adequate oxygenation is the hallmark of pediatric patient management.

Adequate oxygenation is the hallmark of pediatric patient management. Methods of oxygen delivery include "blow-by" techniques (especially for neonates) and pediatric-sized nonrebreather masks. Although nonrebreather masks provide the highest concentration of supplemental oxygen, children may resist their use. Try to overcome their fear by demonstrating the use of the mask on yourself (Figure 42-10 ■). Better yet, enlist the support of a parent or caregiver, and ask them to demonstrate the mask. As an alternative, you might place the mask over the face of a stuffed animal.

If the child refuses to accept the nonrebreather mask, resort to high-flow, high-concentration blow-by oxygen. Some units place oxygen tubing through the bottom of a colorful paper cup and use it to deliver the blow-by supplemental oxygen. Children often find a familiar object less frightening than complicated medical equipment.

Airway Adjuncts

Use airway adjuncts in pediatric patients only if prolonged artificial ventilations are required.

As a general rule, use airway adjuncts in pediatric patients only if prolonged artificial ventilations are required. There are two reasons for this. First, infants and children often improve quickly through the administration of 100 percent oxygen. Second, airway adjuncts may create greater complications in children than in adults. Pediatric patients risk soft-tissue damage, vomiting, and stimulation of the vagus nerve.

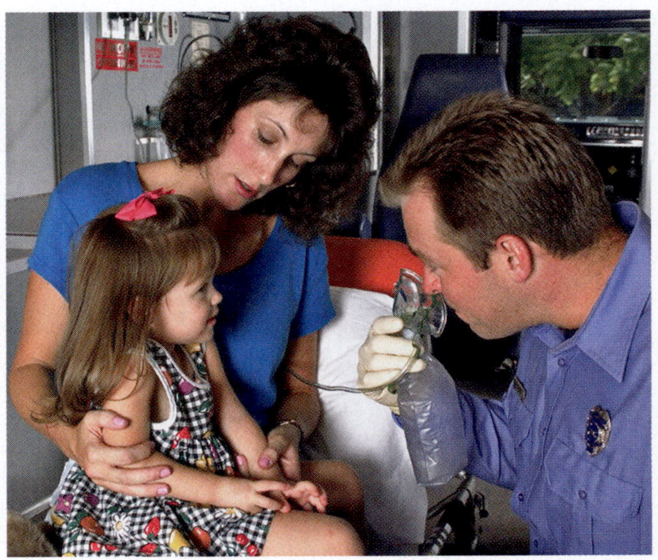

■ Figure 42-10 To overcome the child's fear of the nonrebreather mask, try it on yourself or have the parent try it on before attempting to place it on the child.

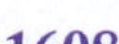

Table 42–7 Equipment Guidelines According to Age and Weight

Equipment	Premie (1 to 2.5 kg)	Neonate (2.5 to 4.0 kg)	6 Months (7.0 kg)	1 to 2 Years (10 to 12 kg)	5 Years (16 to 18 kg)	5 to 10 Years (24 to 30 kg)
	Age (50th Percentile Weight)					
Airway	Infant	Infant (small)	Small	Small	Medium	Medium large
Oral	(00)	(0)	(1)	(2)	(3)	(4.5)
Breathing						
Self-inflating bag	Infant	Infant	Child	Child	Child	Child/adult
O_2 *ventilation mask*	Premature	Newborn	Infant/child	Child	Child	Small adult
Endotracheal tube	2.5 to 3.0 (uncuffed)	3.0 to 3.5 (uncuffed)	3.5 to 4.0	4.0 to 4.5	5.0 to 5.5	5.5 to 6.5
Laryngoscope blade	0 (straight)	1 (straight)	1 (straight)	1 to 2 (straight)	2 (straight or curved)	2 to 3 (straight or curved)
Suction/stylet (F)	6 to 8/6	8/6	8 to 10/6	10/6	14/14	14/14
Circulation						
BP cuff	Newborn	Newborn	Infant	Child	Child	Child/adult
Venous access						
Angiocath	22 to 24	22 to 24	22 to 24	20 to 22	18 to 20	16 to 20
Butterfly needle	25	23 to 25	23 to 25	23	20 to 23	18 to 21
Intracath	—	—	19	19	16	14
Arm board	6″	6″	6″ to 8″	8″	8″ to 15″	15″
Orogastric tube (F)	5	5 to 8	8	10	10 to 12	14 to 18
Chest tube (F)	10 to 14	12 to 18	14 to 20	14 to 24	20 to 32	28 to 38

Oropharyngeal Airways Oropharyngeal airways should be used only in pediatric patients who lack a gag reflex. (Patients with a gag reflex risk vomiting and bradycardia.) Size the airway by measuring from the corner of the mouth to the front of the earlobe. Remember, oropharyngeal airways that are too small can obstruct breathing; ones that are too large can both block the airway and cause trauma. (For general sizing suggestions, see Table 42–7.)

In placing an oropharyngeal airway, use a tongue blade to depress the tongue and jaw (Figure 42-11 ■). If you detect a gag reflex, continue to maintain an open airway with a manual maneuver (jaw-thrust or head-tilt/chin-lift) and consider the use of a nasal airway. Remember that with a pediatric patient, the oral airway is inserted with the tip pointing toward the tongue and pharynx.

Nasopharyngeal Airways Use nasopharyngeal airways for those children who possess a gag reflex and who require prolonged artificial ventilations. *DO NOT* use them on any child with midface or head trauma. You might mistakenly pass the airway through a fracture into the sinuses or the brain.

DO NOT use nasal airways on a child with midface or head trauma.

Size a nasal airway in the same fashion as for adult patients. (Use the outside diameter of the patient's little finger as a measure.) Although nasopharyngeal airways come in a variety of sizes, they

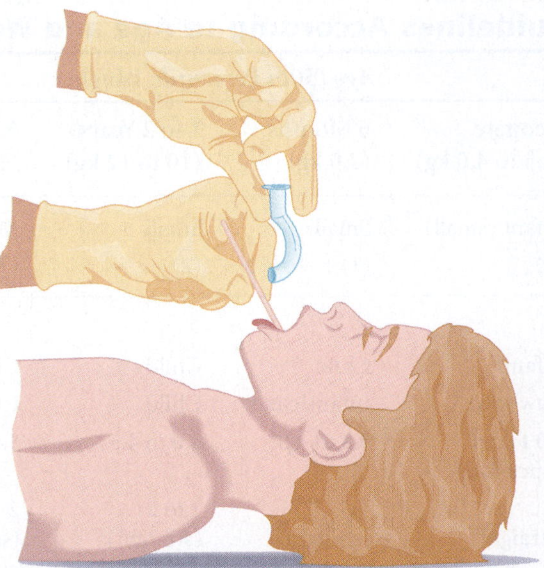

■ **Figure 42-11** Inserting an oropharyngeal airway in a child with the use of a tongue blade.

are not readily available for infants less than 1 year old. Equipment required for insertion of a nasal airway includes:

- ★ Appropriately sized soft, flexible latex tubing
- ★ Water-based lubricant

When inserting the nasal airway, follow the same basic method as you would in an adult patient. It is important to remember that younger children often have enlarged adenoids (lymphatic tissues in the nasopharynx), which can be easily traumatized when inserting a nasopharyngeal airway. Because of this, always use care when inserting a nasopharyngeal airway in a younger child. If resistance is met, do not force the airway because significant bleeding can result.

Ventilation

Adequate tidal volume and ventilatory rate provide more than just a high oxygen saturation for your patient. Ventilation is a two-way physiological street: Maintenance of appropriate oxygen levels results in appropriate carbon dioxide levels as well. However, you will achieve neither of these clinically important events without tailoring the ventilatory device and technique to your pediatric patient. Important points to remember include the following:

- ★ Avoid excessive bag pressure and volume. Ventilate at an age-appropriate rate, using only enough ventilation to make the chest rise.
- ★ Use a properly sized mask to ensure a good fit. In general, the mask should fit on the bridge of the nose and the cleft of the chin (Figure 42-12 ■).
- ★ Obtain a chest rise with each breath.
- ★ Allow adequate time for full chest recoil and exhalation.
- ★ Assess bag-valve-mask (BVM) ventilation. (Provide 100 percent oxygen by using a reservoir attached to the BVM.)
- ★ Remember that flow-restricted, oxygen-powered ventilation devices are contraindicated in pediatric resuscitation.
- ★ Do not use BVMs with pop-off valves unless they can be readily occluded, if necessary. (Ventilatory pressures required during pediatric CPR may exceed the limit of the pop-off valve.)

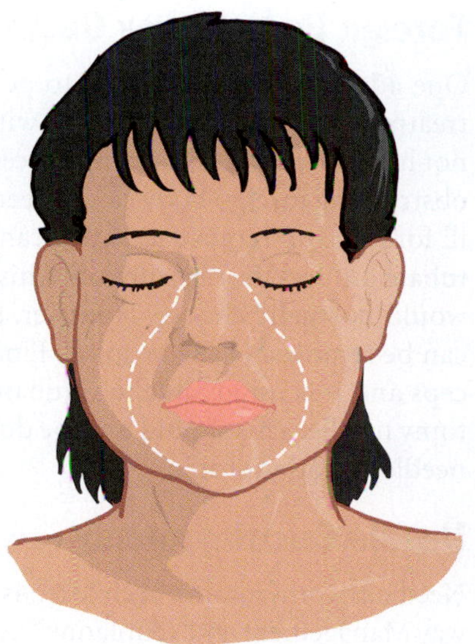

■ Figure 42-12 In placing a mask on a child, it should fit on the bridge of the nose and the cleft of the chin.

★ Apply cricoid pressure through application of the Sellick maneuver to minimize gastric inflation and passive regurgitation (Figure 42-13 ■).

★ Ensure correct positioning to avoid hyperextension of the neck.

ADVANCED AIRWAY AND VENTILATORY MANAGEMENT

As a paramedic, you will be expected to master the advanced life support (ALS) procedures that make you a leader in the EMS system. Your clinical skills will help save the lives of pediatric patients whose respiratory systems have failed so severely that BLS measures are insufficient. When signs of impending cardiopulmonary arrest have been identified (as discussed earlier), you may be called on to implement the following pediatric advanced life support (PALS) techniques, either in your own unit or in a transfer of care from a BLS unit. The success of these techniques requires knowledge of the procedures that set pediatric skills apart from the ALS skills used on adults. (Review the advanced airway skills for adults discussed in Chapter 8, "Airway Management and Ventilation.")

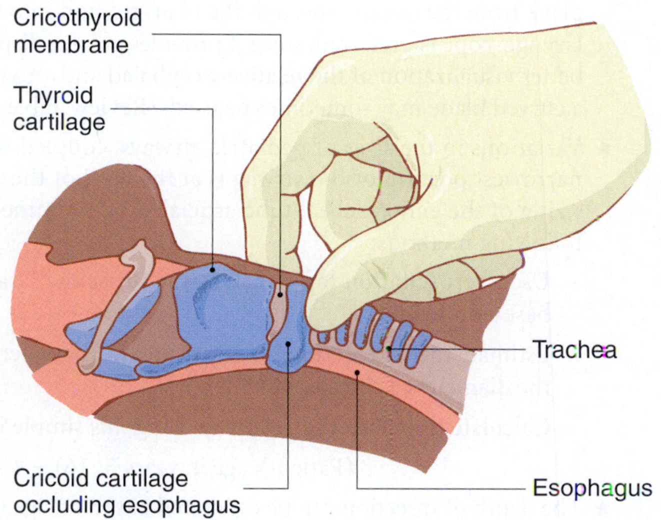

■ Figure 42-13 In the Sellick maneuver, pressure is placed on the cricoid cartilage, compressing the esophagus. This reduces regurgitation and helps bring the vocal cords into view, which is useful if intubation is to be performed.

Foreign Body Airway Obstruction

One advantage of being able to perform endotracheal intubation is that it gives you another treatment modality for children with foreign body airway obstructions. If a child's airway cannot be cleared by basic airway procedures, visualize the airway with the laryngoscope. Often, the obstructing foreign body can be seen. Once it is visualized, grasp the foreign body with the Magill forceps and remove it. If you cannot remove the foreign body with Magill forceps, try to intubate around the obstruction. This often requires using an endotracheal tube smaller than you would normally choose. However, this will provide an adequate airway until the foreign body can be removed at the hospital. Finally, if the foreign body cannot be removed with Magill forceps and it is impossible to intubate around it, then you should consider placing a cricothyrotomy needle. This should only be done as a last resort. Be sure to follow local protocols regarding needle cricothyrotomy.

Needle Cricothyrotomy

Needle cricothyrotomy in children is the same as for adult patients (as discussed in Chapter 8, "Airway Management and Ventilation"). It is important to remember that the anatomical landmarks are smaller and more difficult to identify. For years it was taught that needle cricothyrotomy was contraindicated in children less than 1 year of age. However, current thinking is that the possible benefit (life) exceeds the risks (bleeding, local tissue damage). Remember, the only indication for cricothyrotomy is failure to obtain an airway by any other method.

The only indication for cricothyrotomy is failure to obtain an airway by any other method.

Endotracheal Intubation

Endotracheal intubation allows direct visualization of the lower airway through the trachea, bypassing the entire upper airway. It is the most effective method of controlling a patient's airway, whether it be an adult or a child. However, endotracheal intubation is not without complications. It is an invasive technique with little room for error. A tube that is mistakenly sized or misplaced, especially in an apneic patient, can quickly lead to hypoxia and death.

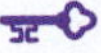

Remember: An endotracheal tube that is mistakenly sized or misplaced, especially in the apneic patient, can quickly lead to hypoxia and death.

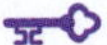

Alternative airways (EOA, PtL, ETC) cannot be used in children. A properly sized laryngeal mask airway (LMA) can be used in the pediatric patient. However, you should remember that LMAs do not protect the airway from aspiration.

Anatomical and Physiological Concerns Although endotracheal intubation of a child and an adult follow the same basic procedures, the special features of the pediatric airway complicate placement of any orotracheal tube. In fact, variations in the airway size of children preclude the use of certain airways, including esophageal obturator airways (EOA), pharyngotracheal lumen airways (PtL), and Esophageal Tracheal CombiTubes (ETC). Properly sized laryngeal mask airways (LMAs) may be used in children but do not protect the airway from aspiration. In using an endotracheal tube, keep in mind these points:

- ★ In infants and small children, it is often more difficult to create a single clear visual plane from the mouth, through the pharynx, and into the glottis. A straight-blade laryngoscope is preferred, since it provides greater displacement of the tongue and better visualization of the relatively cephalad and anterior glottis. For larger children, a curved blade may sometimes be used. (Review Table 42–7.)
- ★ Variations in the sizes of pediatric airways, coupled with the fact that the narrowest portion of the airway is at the level of the cricoid ring, make proper sizing of the endotracheal tube crucial. To determine correct size, apply any of the following methods:
  - – Use a resuscitation tape, such as the Broselow™ tape, to estimate tube size based on height.
  - – Estimate the correct tube size by using the diameter of the patient's little finger or the diameter of the nasal opening.
  - – Calculate the correct tube size by using this simple numerical formula:

$$(\text{Patient's age in years} + 16) \div 4 = \text{Tube size}$$

- ★ The depth of insertion can be estimated based on age (Table 42–8). However, the best method of determining depth is direct visualization. Due to the distance between the

National Center for Injury Prevention and Control states arrest rates for homicide, rape, robbery, and aggravated assault are consistently higher for ages 15 to 34 than for all other age groups.

Approximately one in six victims of violent crimes requires medical attention, often by the emergency medical services. Many victims fail to report the violence to the police. As a result, the EMS may be a victim's only contact with professionals who can intervene to prevent further harm.

EMS providers find it almost impossible to predict exactly when and where a violent incident will occur. Nearly all calls that a paramedic handles on a given day will progress without any threat of danger. In fact, you have a higher risk of being injured by oncoming traffic than by a violent act. Even so, you cannot let down your "crime scene awareness." Otherwise, you risk becoming a victim or hostage of a violent situation. Your most important safety tactic is an ability to identify potentially violent situations as soon as possible. Also be aware of local issues that hold a potential for violence, such as the presence of street gangs or a known area of drug activity.

Equally as important, familiarize yourself with standard operating procedures (SOPs) for handling violent situations and/or the specialized resources that you can call on for backup. Find out, for example, whether your unit has access to a **tactical emergency medical service** (TEMS), which is a unit that provides on-site medical support to law enforcement. If so, know how and when to access it. Above all else, remain alert to the signs of danger from the start of a call to the time you return your ambulance to service.

tactical emergency medical services (TEMS) *a specially trained unit that provides on-site medical support to law enforcement.*

APPROACH TO THE SCENE

Your safety strategy begins with dispatch. Emergency medical dispatchers try to keep callers on the line to obtain as much information as possible, remaining alert to background noises such as fighting or intoxicated persons, so they can warn incoming units of these dangers. Modern computer-aided dispatch programs provide instant information on previous calls at a location and display "caution indicators" to notify dispatchers when a location has a history of violence.

Your safety strategy begins as soon as you are dispatched on a call.

Even in the age of computers, however, some of your best information can still come from your own experience and that of other crews. Your memory of previous calls can serve as an important indicator of trouble. For example, if a bar or club has a reputation for fights and you are summoned there, you will already have a high suspicion of danger before you arrive.

POSSIBLE SCENARIOS

There are three possible scenarios for violence during a call. The dispatcher may advise you of a potentially violent scene en route to the call and you will be alert to danger from the start. In other cases, you may not spot danger until you arrive on the scene and begin your size-up and approach. In yet a third scenario, you may not face danger until the start of patient care or transport.

Advised of Danger En Route

When the dispatcher reports possible danger, do not approach the scene until it has been secured by law enforcement. Remember that lights and siren can draw a crowd and/or alert the perpetrator of a crime, so use them cautiously or not at all. Never follow police units to the scene; doing so might place you at the center of violence. If you arrive first, keep the ambulance out of sight so that the rig does not attract the attention of bystanders or parties involved in the incident. While you wait for police to secure the scene, set up a Staging Area.

Never follow police units to the scene. To do so might place you at the center of violence.

Management of the incident requires interagency cooperation. Communicate with the police—you are in this together. Be sure you understand any differences in dispatch terminology. For example, what is a code 1 emergency for police units may be a code 3 emergency for EMS units. Work with police to determine if and when you should approach the scene.

Keep in mind that violence can occur or resume even with the police present. Furthermore, depending on your uniform colors and the use of badges, people might mistake you for the police, especially if you exit from a vehicle with flashing lights and siren. They might expect you to intervene in a violent situation, or they might direct aggression toward you as an authority figure. If the scene cannot be made safe, retreat immediately (Figure 48-31 ■).

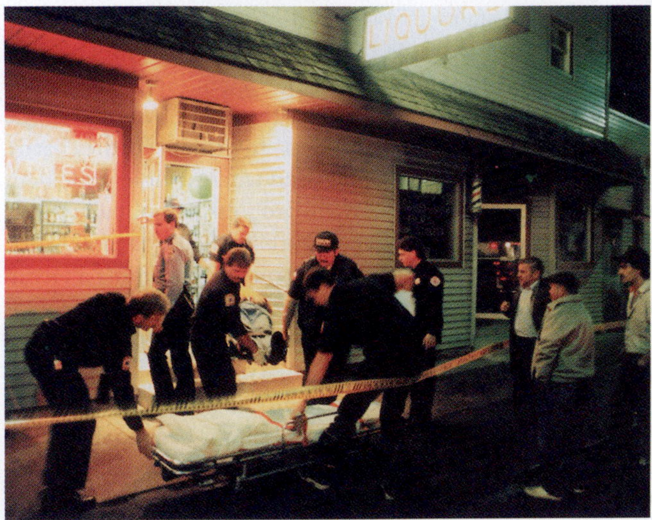

■ **Figure 48-31** Never approach the scene until you are advised that the scene is secure. Remember, even if a scene has been declared secure, violence may still erupt. *(© Craig Jackson/In the Dark Photography)*

Observing Danger on Arrival

Even if dispatch has not alerted you to danger, you must still keep this possibility in mind once you arrive. One of the main purposes of the scene size-up is to search for any possible hazards such as downed power lines or hazmats. As you look for these, observe for other signs of trouble such as crowds gathering on the street, an unusual silence, or a darkened residence. Obviously, you will adopt a different approach for a confirmed medical emergency than for an "unknown problem, caller hang-up." Even so, do not exit the vehicle until you have ruled out all immediate hazards.

If you have any doubts about a call, park away from the scene. If you must park in view of the location, take an unconventional approach to the door (Figure 48-32 ■). People will expect you to use the sidewalk, so approach from the side, the lawn, or flush against the house. Avoid getting between a residence and the lighted ambulance so you do not "backlight" yourself. Hold your flashlight to the side rather than in front of you (Figure 48-33 ■). Assailants often fire at the light.

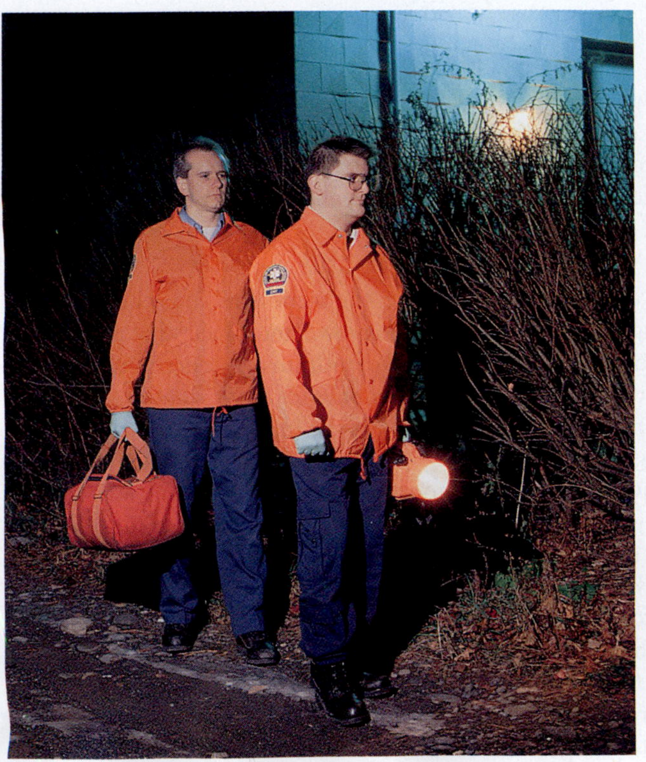

■ **Figure 48-32** Approach potentially unstable scenes single file along an unconventional path.

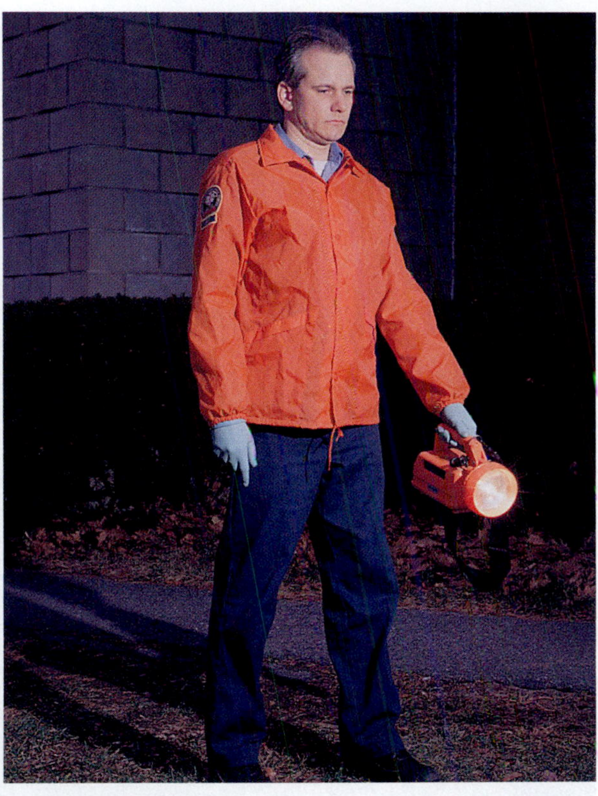

■ Figure 48-33 Hold a flashlight to the side of your body, not in front of it. Armed assailants usually aim at the light.

Before announcing your presence, observe for signs of danger. If you can, look into windows for evidence of fighting, weapons, or the use of alcohol or drugs. Gradually make your way to the doorknob side of the door or the side opposite the hinges (Figure 48-34 ■). Listen for any signs of danger such as loud noises, items breaking, incoherent speech, or the lack of any sounds at all.

If you spot danger at any time during your approach, immediately stop and reevaluate the situation. Decide whether it is in the interest of your own safety to continue or to retreat until law enforcement officials can be summoned. Rather than risk becoming injured or killed, err on the side of safety.

Rather than risk becoming injured or killed, err on the side of safety.

Eruption of Danger during Care or Transport

Remain alert throughout a call, especially in areas with a history of violence. You may enter the scene and spot weapons or drugs. Additional combative people may arrive on scene. The patient or bystanders may become agitated or threatening. Even if treatment has begun, you must place your own safety first. You now have two tactical options: (1) quickly package the patient and leave the scene with the patient or (2) retreat without the patient.

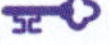

In most cases, you can legally leave a patient behind when there is a documented danger.

Your choice of action depends on the level of danger. Abandonment is always a concern. However, in most cases, you can legally leave a patient behind when there is a documented danger. As discussed later, keep accurate records of incidents involving violence. If you must defend yourself, use the minimum amount of force necessary. Immediately summon police and retreat as needed.

Regardless of the situation, always have a way out. Failure to plan will eventually get you into trouble. Make sure SOPs include an escape plan. Then adhere to this plan so you do not become a victim of violence yourself.

Content Review

Potentially Dangerous Scenes

- Highway encounters
- Violent street incidents
- Murders, assaults, robberies
- Dangerous crowds
- Street gangs
- Drug-related crimes
- Clandestine drug labs
- Domestic violence

SPECIFIC DANGEROUS SCENES

Most prehospital services were developed to meet the needs of individual patients in controlled situations. However, in recent years, EMS personnel trained for this limited role have been pressed increasingly into service in potentially hazardous situations. The following are some of the known dangers that you may face "on the street." (Tactical safety strategies are discussed later.)

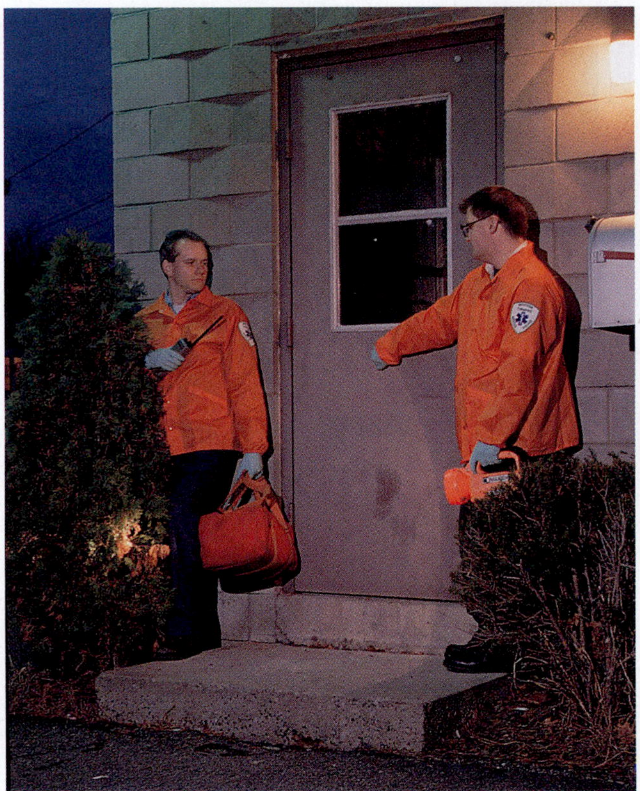

Figure 48-34 Stand to the side of the door when knocking. Do not stand directly in front of a door or window, making yourself an unwitting target.

HIGHWAY ENCOUNTERS

The preceding examples of known dangers have focused largely on residences. However, EMS units frequently report to roadside calls involving motor vehicle collisions, disabled vehicles, or sick and/or unresponsive people inside a car, for example, "man slumped over wheel" calls. Dangers of highway operations and the steps that you should take to protect yourself were discussed earlier in the chapter. However, highway operations also hold the risk of violence from occupants who may be fleeing felons, intoxicated or drugged, fleeing from the police, or in possession of weapons. Some potential warning signs of danger include:

- ★ Violent or abusive behavior
- ★ An altered mental state
- ★ Grabbing or hiding items inside the vehicle
- ★ Arguing or fighting among passengers
- ★ Lack of activity where activity is expected
- ★ Physical signs of alcohol or drug abuse (e.g., liquor bottles, beer cans, or syringes)
- ★ Open or unlatched trunks (a potential hiding spot for people or weapons)
- ★ Differing stories told by occupants

To make a safe approach to a vehicle at a roadside emergency, follow these steps:

- ★ Park the ambulance in a position that provides safety from traffic.
- ★ Notify dispatch of the situation, location, the vehicle make and model, and the state and number of the license plate.
- ★ Use a one-person approach. The driver should remain in the ambulance, which is elevated and provides greater visibility.
- ★ The driver should remain prepared to radio for immediate help and to back or drive away rapidly once the other medic returns.

- ★ At nighttime, use the ambulance lights to illuminate the vehicle. However, do not walk between the ambulance and the other vehicle. You will be backlighted, forming an easy target.
- ★ Because police approach vehicles from the driver's side, you should approach from the passenger's side—an unexpected route.
- ★ Use the A, B, and C door posts for cover.
- ★ Observe the rear seat. Do not move forward of the C post unless you are sure there are no threats in the rear seat or foot wells.
- ★ Retreat to the ambulance (or another strategic position of cover) at the first sign of danger.
- ★ Make sure you have mapped out your intended retreat and escape with the ambulance driver.

VIOLENT STREET INCIDENTS

The following are some of the dangerous street situations that you may face at some point in your EMS career.

Murder, Assault, and Robbery

Violent acts take place at residences, schools, and commercial establishments. However, according to the U.S. Department of Justice, the most common location is on the streets. In order of occurrence, the most frequent crimes are simple assaults, aggravated assaults, rapes and sexual assaults, robberies, and homicides. In one-quarter of violent crimes, offenders used or threatened the use of a weapon. Homicides are most commonly committed with handguns, but knives, blunt objects, and other types of guns or weapons may also be used. About one in five violent victimizations involves the use of alcohol.

Although motives vary, there has been a recent rise in **hate crimes**—crimes committed against a person solely on the basis of the individual's actual or perceived race, color, national origin, ethnicity, gender, disability, or sexual orientation. A number of states or communities have passed legislation on the management of hate crimes, including the steps to be taken on scene. Determine whether these laws exist in your area, and establish protocols that your agency should follow. Crew assignments, for example, should be well thought out in advance of the response to a hate crime. You should also know the specific type of information that must be documented for later use by the courts.

hate crimes *crimes committed against a person wholly on the basis of the individual's actual or perceived race, color, national origin, ethnicity, gender, disability, or sexual orientation.*

Crew assignments should be well thought out in advance of the response to a hate crime.

In responding to the scene of any violent crime, keep these points in mind:

- ★ Dangerous weapons may have been used in the crime.
- ★ Perpetrators may still be on-scene or could return to the scene.
- ★ Patients may sometimes exhibit violence toward EMS, particularly if they risk criminal penalties as a result of the original incident.

Dangerous Crowds and Bystanders

Crowds can quickly become large and volatile, especially in the case of a hate crime. Violence can be directed against anyone or anything in the path of an angry crowd. Your status as an EMS provider does not give you immunity. Whenever a crowd is present, look for these warning signs:

- ★ Shouts or increasingly loud voices
- ★ Pushing or shoving
- ★ Hostilities toward anyone on scene, including the perpetrator of a crime, the victim, and police
- ★ Rapid increase in the crowd size
- ★ Inability of law enforcement officials to control bystanders

Constantly monitor the crowd and retreat if necessary. If possible, take the patient with you. Rapid transport may require limited or tactical assessment at the scene with more in-depth assessment done inside the safety of the ambulance. Be sure to document reasons for the quick assessment and transport.

Street Gangs

Street gangs can be found in big cities, suburban towns, and lately in rural America. In fact, some organized gangs have purposely branched out into smaller towns in an effort to escape surveillance and expand their illicit businesses. Gangs account for a disproportionate amount of youth violence. Gang activity is associated with high levels of delinquency, illegal drug use, physical violence, and weapons possession. Young people from all demographic backgrounds report some knowledge of gangs or gang activity.

Some of the largest and best known gangs include the Crips, Bloods, Almighty Latin King Nation (Latin Kings), Hell's Angels, Outlaws, Pagans, MS-13, and Banditos. Local variations can be found throughout the country. In some places, gangs have used firebombs, Molotov cocktails, and, on a limited basis, hand grenades as weapons of revenge and intimidation. Links have been drawn between street gangs and the sale of drugs, which finances gang activities.

Commonly observed gang characteristics include the following:

★ *Appearance.* Gang members frequently wear unique clothing specific to the group. Because the clothing is often a particular color or hue, it is referred to as the gang's "colors." Wearing a color, even a bandana, can signify gang membership. Within the gang, members sometimes wear different articles to signify rank.

★ *Graffiti.* Gangs have territories, or "turfs." Members often mark their turf with graffiti of the gang's logo, and also use it to warn away intruders, brag about crimes, insult rival gangs, or taunt police.

★ *Tattoos.* Many gang members wear tattoos or other body markings to identify their gang affiliation. Some gangs even require these tattoos. The tattoos will be in the gang's colors and often contain the gang's motto or logo.

★ *Hand signals/language.* Gangs commonly create their own methods of communication. They give gang-related meanings to everyday words or create codes. Hand signs provide quick identification among gang members, warn of approaching law enforcement, or show disrespect to other gangs. Gang members often perform signals so quickly that an uninformed outsider may not spot them, much less understand them.

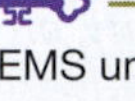

EMS uniforms should not resemble law enforcement uniforms.

EMS units venturing into gang territory must be extremely cautious. Danger is increased if your uniform looks similar to the uniform worn by police. Gangs with a history of arrest may in fact make every effort to prevent you from transporting one of their members to a hospital or any other place beyond the reach of the gang. Do not force the issue if your safety is at stake.

DRUG-RELATED CRIMES

The sale of drugs goes hand in hand with violence. Hundreds of people die each year in drug deals gone bad. In addition, drug dealers protect their drug stashes and "shooting galleries" with booby traps, weapons, and attack dogs. The combination of a high cash flow, addiction, and automatic weapons threatens anyone who unwittingly walks onto the scene of a drug deal or threatens to uncover an illicit drug operation.

Signs that can alert you to involvement of drugs at an EMS call include:

★ Prior history of drugs in the neighborhood of the call

★ Clinical evidence that the patient has used drugs of some kind

★ Drug-related comments by bystanders

★ Drug paraphernalia visible at the scene such as the following:

- Tiny zip-top bags or vials
- Sandwich bags with the corners torn off (indicating drug packaging) or untied corners of sandwich bags (indicating drug use)
- Syringes or needles

– Glass tubes, pipes, or homemade devices for smoking drugs
– Chemical odors or residues

Whenever you observe any of the preceding items, assume the use or presence of drugs at the scene. Even if the patient is not involved, others at the scene may still pose a danger. Keep in mind that not all patients who use drugs will be seeking to harm you. Some may, in fact, be looking for help. Evaluate each situation carefully. Above all else, remember to retreat and/or request police backup at the earliest sign of danger.

CLANDESTINE DRUG LABORATORIES

Drug dealers often set up "laboratories" to manufacture controlled substances or to otherwise refine or convert a substance to another more profitable or usable form such as tablets. One of the most common substances manufactured in drug laboratories is methamphetamine, also known by street names such as "crank," "speed," or "crystal." Other drugs include LSD and "crack."

Clandestine drug laboratories, or "clan labs," have three requirements: privacy, utilities, and equipment such as glassware, chemical containers, and heating mantles or burners. Most clan labs are uncovered by neighbors who report suspicious odors or activities. Raids on clan labs have a way of turning into hazmat operations. All too often, the labs contain toxic fumes and volatile chemicals. The people on scene complicate matters by fighting or shooting at the rescuers who come to extricate them from the toxic environment. As they retreat, drug dealers may also trigger booby traps or wait for police or EMS personnel to trigger them. If you ever come on a clan lab, take these actions:

★ Leave the area immediately.
★ Do not touch anything.
★ Never stop any chemical reactions already in progress.
★ Do not smoke or bring any source of flame near the lab.
★ Notify the police.
★ Initiate ICS and hazmat procedures.
★ Consider evacuation of the area.

Laboratories can be found anywhere—on farms, in trailers, in city apartments, and elsewhere. They may be mobile, roaming from place to place in a camper or truck. Or they may be disassembled and stored in a variety of locations. The job of raiding clan labs belongs to specialized personnel—not EMS crews.

DOMESTIC VIOLENCE

Domestic violence may be physical, emotional, sexual, verbal, or economic. It may be directed against a spouse or partner, or it may involve children and/or older relatives. When you go to the scene of domestic violence, the abuser may turn on you or other crew members. You have two main concerns: the safety of yourself and your crew and protection of the patient from further harm.

TACTICAL CONSIDERATIONS

As mentioned on several occasions, your best tactical response to violence is observation. Know the warning signs and stay out of danger in the first place. If the dispatcher alerts you to hazards, resort to staging until the appropriate authorities can resolve the situation. Nevertheless, you still may find yourself in situations with a potential for danger. In such instances, you must have a "game plan" in place. This section presents some of the actions you can take to protect your own safety while attempting to provide tactical patient care.

Content Review

Safety Tactics

- Retreat
- Cover and concealment
- Distraction and evasion
- Contact and cover
- Warning signals and communication

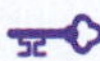

Nothing in the ambulance is worth your life. Retreat by foot or by whatever means possible to avoid violence that threatens your life.

SAFETY TACTICS

Dangerous situations mean extreme stress. As a result, your response to danger will be most effective if you practice tactical options frequently. Even on routine calls, think about safety, contact and cover, escape routes, and other strategies that can help you make a better decision when you are faced with actual danger. Borrowing a phrase from professional sports: "You will play the game the way you practice." If you have rehearsed the responses to danger before you actually need them, you will be more likely to use them successfully. The following sections describe some proven methods for EMS safety in dangerous situations.

Retreat

The prudent strategy is to retreat whenever you spot indicators of violence or potential physical confrontations, particularly with fleeing criminals or people with emotional disturbances. Retreat in a calm, but decisive manner. Be aware that the danger is now at your back and integrate cover into your retreat. Ideally you will retreat to the ambulance so you can summon help. However, if a dangerous obstacle such as a crowd blocks access to your rig, retreat by foot or by any means possible. Nothing in the ambulance is worth your life.

In deciding how far to retreat, your primary goal is to protect. You must be out of the immediate line of sight. You must also seek cover from gunfire. Finally, you must allow enough distance to react if a person or crowd attempts to move toward you again. You need time and space to respond to changing situations. As soon as possible, notify other responding units and agencies of the danger. Activate appropriate codes, SOPs, and/or interagency agreements, particularly with law enforcement. Be sure to document your observations of danger and your specific responses. Include information such as:

- ★ Actions taken while on scene
- ★ Reasons you retreated
- ★ Time at which you left and/or returned to the scene
- ★ Personnel or agencies contacted

Keep in mind that retreat does not mean the end of a call. As already mentioned, you should seek to stage at a safe area until police secure the scene and you can respond again. Staging, along with thorough documentation, will reduce liability and provide evidence to refute charges of abandonment.

concealment *hiding the body behind objects that shield a person from view but that offer little or no protection against bullets or other ballistics.*

Cover and Concealment

When faced with danger, two of your most immediate and practical strategies are cover and concealment (Figures 48-35a–b ■). **Concealment** hides your body, such as when you crouch behind bushes or vehicle doors. However, most common objects do not stop bullets. During armed en-

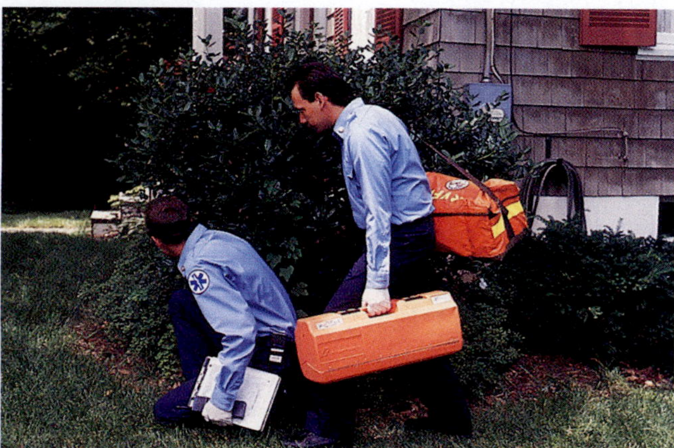

■ Figure 48-35a Concealing yourself means placing your body behind an object that can hide you from view.

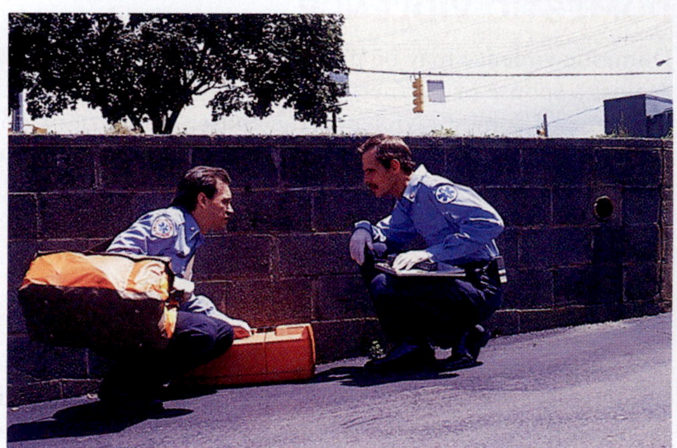

■ Figure 48-35b Taking cover is finding a position that both hides you and protects your body from projectiles.

counters, seek **cover** by hiding your body behind solid and impenetrable objects such as brick walls, rocks, large trees or telephone poles, or a vehicle engine block.

cover *hiding the body behind solid and impenetrable objects that protect a person from bullets.*

In applying these safety tactics, keep in mind these general rules:

- ★ As you approach any scene, remain aware of the surroundings and any potential sources of protection in case you must retreat or are "pinned down."
- ★ Choose your cover carefully. You may have only one chance to pick your protection. Select the item that hides your body adequately while shielding you against ballistics.
- ★ Once you have made your choice of cover, conceal as much of your body as possible. Be conscious of any reflective clothing that you may be wearing. Armed assailants can use it as a target, especially at night.
- ★ Constantly look to improve your protection and location.

Distraction and Evasion

Distraction and evasion can be integrated into any retreat. Some specific techniques to avoid physical violence include:

- ★ Throwing equipment to trip, slow, or distract an aggressor
- ★ Wedging a stretcher in a doorway to block an attacker
- ★ Using an unconventional path while retreating
- ★ Anticipating the moves of the aggressor and taking counter moves
- ★ Overturning objects in the path of the attacker
- ★ Using preplanned tactics with your partner to confuse or "throw off" an aggressor

Key to the success of these tactics is your own physical condition. Regular exercise and good health ensure that you will have the strength to outrun or, if necessary, defend yourself against an attacker. Some units provide basic training in self-defense or have protocols on its use. Make sure you take advantage of the training and know the protocols related to application of force.

Contact and Cover

The concept of contact and cover comes from a police procedure developed in San Diego, California, where several officers were injured or killed while interviewing suspects. Studies of the incidents revealed that the officers focused directly on the suspect, reducing their ability to observe the "big picture." This left them exposed to violence. To solve this problem, the San Diego Police Department adopted an interview approach in which one officer "contacts" the suspect while another stands 90 degrees to the side. By standing at a different angle, the second officer can provide "cover" to the officer dealing with the suspect.

When adapted to EMS practice, the procedure assigns the roles shown in Table 48–2. As with any tactic adopted from another discipline, contact and cover has obvious correlations and drawbacks for EMS. The tactic is ideal for street encounters with intoxicated persons or subjects acting in a suspicious manner. An obvious drawback is that two medics working on a cardiac arrest will not be able to designate one person to act solely as a "cover" medic.

Table 48–2 Contact and Cover

Contact Provider	Cover Provider
Initiates and provides direct patient care.	Observes the scene for danger while the "contact" provider cares for the patient.
Performs patient assessment.	Generally avoids patient care duties that would prevent observation of the scene.
Handles most interpersonal scene contact.	In small crews, may perform limited functions such as handling equipment.

Perhaps the best application of this police procedure to EMS is its emphasis on the importance of observation and teamwork. A crew that works well together will assign roles, formally or informally, to guarantee safety and patient care. In its most basic form, contact and cover means that you will watch your partner's back while your partner watches yours.

Warning Signals and Communication

In the case of "street survival," communication is an invaluable tool. Every team or crew should develop methods of alerting other providers to danger without alerting the aggressor. Devise prearranged verbal and nonverbal clues and then practice them. Be sure to involve dispatch in the process. Choose signals that will indicate a variety of circumstances while sounding harmless to an attacker. This can be a lifesaving technique in situations where you find yourself, the crew, and/or the patient held hostage. Your so-called "routine" radio reports can spell out the nature of the trouble and summon help from a **special weapons and tactics (SWAT) team**—a trained police unit equipped to handle hostage holders or other difficult law enforcement situations.

special weapons and tactics (SWAT) team *a trained police unit equipped to handle hostage holders and other difficult law enforcement situations.*

TACTICAL PATIENT CARE

The increased involvement of care providers in violent situations has raised discussion and debate over the tactical training and protection offered to the EMS community. Interagency planning is essential, especially for clarifying the duties and roles of EMS and law enforcement agencies at crime scenes, riots, or terrorist events. Other aspects of tactical patient care include the use of body armor by EMS providers and the training of special tactical EMS personnel.

Body Armor

Several years ago few EMS providers would have considered wearing **body armor,** or bulletproof vests, while on duty. Today more and more providers are taking "tactical patient care" seriously. An increasing number of EMS agencies have chosen to supply body armor or to provide a sum of cash toward its purchase. Body armor manufacturers have responded by designing and marketing vests specifically for the EMS community.

body armor *vest made of tightly woven, strong fibers that offer protection against handgun bullets, most knives, and blunt trauma; also known as "bulletproof vests."*

Unlike conventional armor, body armor is soft. Fibers such as Kevlar® are woven tightly together to form the vest. The tight weave and strength of the material offer protection from many handgun bullets, most knives, and blunt trauma. The number of layers of fiber determine the rating or "stopping power" of a vest. Most body armor is rated from level 1 (least protective) to level 3 (most protective). Specialty vests with steel inserts and other materials are available for use by the military or by SWAT teams.

Some critics of body armor claim that wearers may feel a false sense of security. They point out that body armor offers reduced protection when wet and that it provides little or no protection against high-velocity bullets, such as those fired by a rifle, or from thin or dual-edged weapons. An ice pick, for example, can penetrate between the fibers of most vests. Supporters of body armor feel it should be viewed just like any other PPE. They point to the new threats faced by emergency responders, such as paramilitary groups, terrorists, drug-related violence, and the widespread possession of handguns.

Whether you purchase or wear body armor is a personal decision. However, for it to be effective, you must follow several guidelines. They include:

- ★ Keep in mind the limitations of body armor. Never do anything you wouldn't do without it.
- ★ Remember that body armor doesn't cover the whole body. You can still get seriously injured or killed.
- ★ Even though body armor can prevent many types of penetration, you can still experience severe cavitation.
- ★ For body armor to work, it must be worn. The temptation not to wear it, especially in hot temperatures, can render even the best body armor useless.

Tactical EMS

As already mentioned, the provision of care in violent or tactically "hot" zones such as sniper situations necessitates risks far beyond those found on most EMS calls. Medical personnel assigned to such incidents require special training and authorization. Like hazmat teams, they must don special equipment, function with compact gear, and, in most cases, work as medical adjuncts to the police or military.

The patient care offered by a TEMS differs from routine EMS care in several ways. Differences include these:

- ★ A major priority is extraction of the patient from the hot zone.
- ★ Care may be modified to meet tactical considerations.
- ★ Trauma patients outnumber medical patients.
- ★ Treatment and transport interventions must almost always be coordinated with an Incident Commander.
- ★ Patients must be moved to tactically cold zones for complete assessment, care, and transport.
- ★ Metal clipboards, chemical agents, and other tools may be used as defensive weapons.

Local protocols, standing orders, and issues of medical direction must be resolved before employment of a TEMS unit, which may be composed of EMTs, paramedics, and/or physicians who operate as part of a tactical law enforcement team. Certification of SWAT-Medics and EMT-Tacticals (EMT-Ts) is offered by several organizations including the **CONTOMS** (Counter-Narcotics Tactical Operations) program and the National Tactical Officers Association (NTOA). The training required of EMT-Ts or SWAT-Medics involves strenuous physical activity under a variety of conditions. In a CONTOMS program, medics may be exposed to scenarios or skills such as:

- ★ Raids on clandestine drug laboratories
- ★ Emergency medical care in barricade situations
- ★ Wounding effects of weapons and booby traps
- ★ Special medical gear for tactical operations
- ★ Use of CS, CN (mace), capaicin (pepper spray), CR, or other riot-control agents
- ★ Blank-firing weapons
- ★ Helicopter operations
- ★ Pyrotechnics (smoke and distraction devices)
- ★ Operation under extreme conditions, darkness, and psychological stress
- ★ Firefighting and hazmat operations

In summoning or working with a TEMS unit, follow the same general approaches and procedures recommended in Parts 2, 3, and 4 of this chapter. If you have not had exposure to such a unit, find out more about EMT-Ts or SWAT-Medics from local law enforcement officials or from sites sponsored by CONTOMS or NTOA on the Internet.

EMT-Tacticals (EMT-Ts) *EMS personnel trained to serve with a Technical Emergency Medical Service or a law enforcement agency.*

CONTOMS *Counter-Narcotics Tactical Operations; program that manages the training and certification of EMT-Ts and SWAT-Medics.*

EMS AT CRIME SCENES

The goal of performing EMS at a crime scene is to provide high-quality patient care while preserving evidence. *NEVER* jeopardize patient care for the sake of evidence. However, do not perform patient care with disregard of the criminal investigation that will follow.

NEVER jeopardize patient care for the sake of evidence.

EMS AND POLICE OPERATIONS

Often police and EMS personnel respond to the same crisis but for different purposes. The EMS crew is there to treat patients and save lives. Law enforcement officers have come to protect the public and to solve a crime. These two goals sometimes create tension between the two teams. For example, police and paramedics often work under different time constraints. As a paramedic, you have a limited time at the scene. The police, in contrast, spend much more time at the location of a crime. In some major cases, police can remain at the scene for days or weeks as they methodically look for evidence.

The key to cooperation between EMS and law enforcement personnel is communication. You should become aware of the nature and significance of physical evidence at a crime scene and, if possible, keep that evidence intact. Police, however, should be aware that your responsibility is to save a life. However, police and paramedics can usually reach a common ground. By preserving evidence, you can help the police to lock up a criminal before the person hurts or kills someone else. Remember: EMS personnel and law enforcement are really on the same side. Talk to each other.

Remember: EMS personnel and law enforcement are really on the same side. Talk to each other.

PRESERVING EVIDENCE

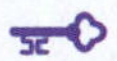

Whenever in doubt, save or treat an object as evidence.

Be aware that anything on and around the patient may be evidence. You never know when a seemingly unimportant item may in fact be evidence that could help solve a crime. Whenever in doubt, save or treat an object as evidence.

Anything you touch, walk on, pick up, cut, wipe off, or move could be evidence. Developing an awareness of evidence can affect the way you treat patients. For example, if clothing must be removed, never cut through a gunshot or knife hole. Instead, try to cut as far away from the wound as possible. Instead of placing the cut cloth or garment in a plastic bag, put it in a brown paper bag so condensation does not build up and destroy body fluid evidence.

Brown paper bags allow evaporation and prevent mold from forming. This makes them ideal for crime scene evidence collection.

Also, when examining a patient, remember that you may be at risk. The victim may have a concealed weapon, such as a knife or gun. Or the person who committed the crime may be intent on finishing it and reappear to attack the patient. As always, your first responsibility is to protect yourself. If you have any suspicions at all about the patient or the safety of the scene, wait for the police to frisk the patient and/or secure the scene.

Content Review

Types of Evidence

- Prints—fingerprints, footprints, tire prints
- Blood and blood splatter
- Body fluids
- Particulate evidence
- On-scene EMS observations

Types of Evidence

Although it is unrealistic to train EMS personnel in the details of police work, it is not unrealistic to ask them to develop an awareness of the general types of evidence that they may expect to encounter at a crime scene. Some of the main categories of evidence include: prints, blood and body fluids, particulate evidence, and your own observations at the scene.

Prints Prints include fingerprints, footprints, and tire prints. Of the three, fingerprints can be the most valuable source of evidence. As a paramedic, try not to disturb any fingerprint evidence that may be present. Second, do not leave behind your own fingerprints at a crime scene. The only way to preserve fingerprints is simply not to touch anything. Of course, this is impossible when treating a patient. However, you can and should minimize what you touch. If you must touch or move an item, remember to tell the police that you did so.

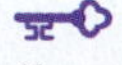

If you must touch or move an item, remember to tell the police.

You will be wearing disposable gloves as a part of infection control. These gloves prevent you from leaving your own fingerprints, but they will not prevent you from smudging existing prints. Again, touch as little as possible. Bring in only necessary equipment. The more equipment you have, the more evidence you can potentially disturb, including fingerprints. Also, scan the approach to the scene and the scene itself for footprints or tire prints and avoid disturbing them.

Blood and Body Fluids Blood and body fluids also give police a lot of information about a crime. Matching the DNA found in blood samples or other body fluids to the DNA of a suspect is nearly 100 percent accurate. Technologists need only a small sample to ascertain the genetic code. The way in which blood is splattered or dropped at the scene (called **blood spatter evidence**) provides additional clues for police.

blood spatter evidence *the pattern that blood forms when it is splattered or dropped at the scene of a crime.*

Preserving blood evidence can be performed in the following ways:

- ★ Avoid mixing samples of blood whenever possible. Cross-contamination of blood will render blood evidence useless.
- ★ Avoid tracking blood on your shoes. You will leave your own footprints, plus you risk contaminating other blood evidence.
- ★ If you must cut bloody clothing from a victim, place each piece in a separate brown paper bag. If the garment is wet, gently roll it in the paper bag to layer it. Place the entire contents in a second paper bag and then in a plastic bag for body fluid protection.
- ★ Do not throw clothes stained with blood or other body fluids in a single pile or in a puddle of blood.

★ Do not clean up or smudge blood spatter left at a scene.
★ If you leave behind blood from a venipuncture, notify police.
★ Because blood can be a biohazard, ask police whether the scene should be secured for evidence collection.

Particulate Evidence Particulate evidence, also known as microscopic or trace evidence, refers to evidence that cannot be readily seen by the human eye such as hairs or carpet and clothing fibers. Minimal handling of a victim's clothes by EMS personnel may help to preserve this evidence.

particulate evidence *evidence such as hairs or fibers that cannot be readily seen with the human eyes; also known as microscopic or trace evidence.*

On-Scene Observations Everything that you and other members of the EMS crew see and hear can serve as evidence. Your observations of the scene will become part of the police record—and ultimately part of the court record. Be sure to look for and record the following information:

Everything that you and other members of the EMS crew see and hear can serve as evidence.

★ Conditions at the scene (e.g., absence or presence of lights, locked or unlocked doors, open or closed curtains)
★ Position of the patient/victim
★ Injuries suffered by the patient/victim
★ Statements of persons at the scene
★ Statements by the patient/victim
★ Dying declarations
★ Suspicious persons at, or fleeing from, the scene
★ Presence and/or location of any weapons

If the victim is deceased by the time you arrive, any staff not immediately needed on the scene should leave to minimize the risk of disturbing evidence. If a gun is seen or found on the deceased victim, do not touch or move it unless it must be secured for the safety of others. Pick it up only as a last resort, and only touch it by the side grips or handles. The grips are coarse and will not generally leave good fingerprints. *NEVER* put anything into the barrel of the gun to lift or move it. The barrel of a gun can house the majority of the evidence used by the police: traces of gun powder, rifling patterns, and even flesh or blood.

NEVER put anything into the barrel of a gun to lift or move it.

Documenting Evidence

Record only the facts at the scene of a crime, and record them accurately. Use quotation marks to indicate the words of bystanders and any remarks made by the patient. Avoid opinions not relevant to patient care. If the patient has died, do not offer any judgments that might contradict later findings by the medical examiner. For example, a knife wound is not a knife wound until it is proven that a knife caused the laceration. Instead, describe the shape and anatomical location of the puncture or cut.

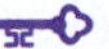
Record only the facts at the scene of a crime, and record them accurately.

Also keep in mind the protocols, local laws, and ethical considerations in reporting certain crimes such as child abuse, rape, geriatric abuse, and domestic violence. (For more on reporting abuse and assault see Chapter 44, "Abuse and Assault.") Finally, follow local policies and regulations regarding confidentiality surrounding any criminal case. Any offhand remarks that you make might later become testimony in a courtroom along with documents that you prepare at the scene.

Summary

As a paramedic, you should be familiar with standards that influence ambulance design, equipment requirements, and staffing. You should also regularly complete all checklists regarding onboard equipment and essential supplies. Be aware of items that require routine maintenance or calibration as well as the expiration dates on all drugs. Keep in mind OSHA safety requirements and know how to report equipment problems or failures. Be familiar with the profile of a typical ambulance

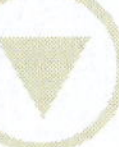

collision and to develop strategies for preventing it from occurring. Also be aware of the issues and policies surrounding the staging and staffing of ambulances. Appreciate the conditions or situations that merit air medical transport and the safety issues involved in packaging the patient, selecting a landing site, and approaching the aircraft.

Every paramedic should be thoroughly familiar with the procedures used in a typical Incident Management System. You should be able to follow these procedures at every multiple-patient, multiple-unit response—from the smallest incident to the largest. Expect to respond to several MCIs during your EMS career. A good preplan, regular use of the IMS, and MCI training will allow you to handle each event calmly and professionally.

Whenever you function in any phase of a rescue, you must be properly outfitted with protective equipment. You must also have training specific to the type of rescue. During the operational phases of a rescue, you must provide direct patient care and work with technical teams to assure optimal patient management. Any paramedic assigned to rescue duties should have training in the care of patients who may require prolonged management.

Every member of an EMS team should be prepared to face the challenges of the hazmat incident. As with any EMS operation, the primary consideration is your own safety. You become useless at a hazmat incident if you become contaminated yourself.

Similarly, your first priority at any crime scene is your own safety. To protect your life and the lives of others, you need to develop a "crime scene awareness." Do not needlessly expose yourself to dangers better left to professional emergency medical personnel such as SWAT-Medics or EMT-Ts. When you do treat the victim(s) at a crime scene, keep in mind that police and EMS personnel must work together to preserve the evidence. Touch only those items or objects that pertain directly to patient care.

Review Questions

1. Which of the following describes a Type II ambulance design?
   a. medium-duty ambulance rescue vehicle
   b. standard van, forward control integral cab-body ambulance
   c. specialty van, forward control integral cab-body ambulance
   d. conventional truck cab-chassis with a modular ambulance body
2. The strategy used by an EMS agency to maneuver its ambulances and crews in order to reduce response times is known as:
   a. assignment.
   b. calibration.
   c. deployment.
   d. maintenance.
3. Essentially ____________ exempts ambulance drivers from certain laws but at the same time holds them to a higher standard.
   a. due regard
   b. Good Samaritan laws
   c. negligence laws
   d. tiered response system
4. At the national level, ____________ provides a voluntary "gold standard" for the EMS community to follow.
   a. ACS
   b. NHTSA
   c. OSHA
   d. CAAS

5. Fixed-wing aircraft generally are employed when patients require transport over distances of more than ___________ miles.
   a. 50
   b. 100
   c. 300
   d. 500

6. In managing a multiple-casualty incident, which of the following is *not* one of the three main priorities?
   a. life safety
   b. incident stabilization
   c. property conservation
   d. cost/outlay evaluation

7. In a/an ___________ incident, the injuries have usually already occurred by the time you arrive on scene.
   a. open
   b. uncontained
   c. closed
   d. controlled

8. To ensure flexibility, an Incident Commander should radio a brief progress report approximately every ___________ minutes until the incident has been stabilized.
   a. 5
   b. 10
   c. 15
   d. 20

9. Because ___________ will drive subsequent operations, it is generally one of the first functions performed at a multiple-casualty incident.
   a. triage
   b. staging
   c. logistics
   d. transport

10. During triage, patients with respirations above 30 per minute should be tagged:
    a. red.
    b. green.
    c. black.
    d. yellow.

11. The best helmets have a ___________ suspension system.
    a. two-point, elastic
    b. two-point, nonelastic
    c. four-point, elastic
    d. four-point, nonelastic

12. ___________ triggers the technical beginning of the rescue.
    a. Access
    b. Arrival
    c. Size-up
    d. Hazard control

13. Examples of confined spaces include all of the following *except:*
    a. flat water.
    b. drainage culverts.
    c. wells and cisterns.
    d. grain bins and silos.

14. A/The ___________ is usually the easiest means of access to a motor vehicle.
   a. door
   b. window
   c. trunk
   d. windshield
15. As a rule, the primary role of EMS personnel in vehicle stabilization and removal is:
   a. extrication.
   b. scene control.
   c. patient care.
   d. communications.
16. Which of the following does *not* represent one of the three levels of training appropriate to EMS response at hazmat incidents?
   a. Awareness Level
   b. Paramedic Level 4
   c. EMS Level 1
   d. EMS Level 2
17. The basic IMS at a hazmat incident will require a:
   a. command post.
   b. Staging Area.
   c. decontamination corridor.
   d. all of the above
18. This source of information maintains a 24-hour, toll-free hotline, provides information on the chemical properties of a substance, and explains how the material should be handled.
   a. EPA
   b. NOAA
   c. CHEMTREC
   d. CAMEO
19. This control zone is the area where the incident operation takes place. It includes the command post, medical monitoring and rehabilitation, treatment areas, and apparatus staging.
   a. hot (red) zone
   b. warm (yellow) zone
   c. cold (green) zone
   d. exclusionary zone
20. ___________ is considered the universal decon solution, especially for reducing topical absorption.
   a. Water
   b. Potassium iodide
   c. Atropine
   d. Sodium nitrate
21. Which of the following is/are a warning of impending danger whenever a crowd is present?
   a. pushing or shoving
   b. rapid increase in crowd size
   c. inability of law enforcement officials to control bystanders
   d. all of the above
22. The contact-and-cover tactic is ideal to:
   a. escape from imminent danger.
   b. interview a victim on the street.
   c. signal incoming departments of potential danger.
   d. retreat and then return to the scene at a later time.
23. How should you hold your flashlight when approaching a dark house at a potential crime scene?
   a. behind you
   b. over your head
   c. to your side
   d. in front of you

24. At a crime scene, you should preserve evidence containing body fluids by placing it in a/an:
    a. sterile container.
    b. sealed plastic bag.
    c. brown paper bag.
    d. airtight container.
25. Which of the following is an appropriate way for the paramedic to avoid contaminating evidence at a crime scene?
    a. clean up blood spatter
    b. wear gloves while on scene
    c. place small articles of clothing in a plastic bag
    d. fold blood-stained clothes and place them in a single pile

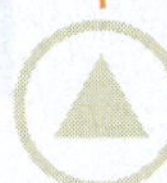

See Answers to Review Questions at the back of this book.

Chapter

49

Responding to Terrorist Acts

Objectives

After reading this chapter, you should be able to:

1. Identify the typical weapons of mass destruction likely to be used by terrorists. (pp. 1891–1902)
2. Explain the mechanisms of injury associated with conventional and nuclear weapons of mass destruction. (pp. 1892–1895)
3. Identify and describe the major subclassifications of chemical and biological weapons of mass destruction. (pp. 1895–1902)
4. List the scene evidence that might alert the EMS provider to a terrorist attack that involves a weapon of mass destruction. (pp. 1902–1903)
5. Describe the special safety precautions and safety equipment appropriate for an incident involving nuclear, biological, or chemical weapons. (pp. 1902–1903)
6. Identify the assessment and management concerns for victims of conventional, nuclear, biological, and chemical weapons. (pp. 1892–1902)
7. Given a narrative description of a conventional, nuclear, biological, or chemical terrorist attack, identify the elements of scene size-up that suggest terrorism and identify the likely injuries and any special patient management considerations necessary. (pp. 1891–1903)

**Note:* The objectives for this chapter are not included in the DOT Paramedic curriculum.

Key Terms

biological agents, p. 1900
biotoxin, p. 1897
dirty bomb, p. 1894
dosimeter, p. 1894
erythema, p. 1896
explosives, p. 1892
fallout, p. 1894
fasciculations, p. 1896
Geiger counter, p. 1894
incendiary agents, p. 1892
Mark I kit, p. 1896
miosis, p. 1896
nerve agents, p. 1895
nuclear detonation, p. 1893
pulmonary agents, p. 1897
rhinorrhea, p. 1896
specific gravity, p. 1895
terrorist act, p. 1891
vesicants, p. 1896
volatility, p. 1895
weapons of mass destruction (WMDs), p. 1891

INTRODUCTION

The events of September 11, 2001, have greatly impacted our society and our sensitivity to the threat of terrorist acts. The extensive planning and coordination needed to bring down the World Trade Center and achieve such a great loss of life show just how intent some people are on causing public harm. This new awareness forces the EMS community to prepare itself to respond to acts of terrorism. These acts can come in many forms.

The weapon of choice used by terrorist groups worldwide is the conventional explosive.

The weapon of choice used by terrorist groups worldwide is the conventional explosive. Conventional explosives have been used frequently in the Middle East and in the British Isles and were used by the Unabomber in the United States. We have also experienced major explosive events such as the destruction of the Physics Annex at the University of Wisconsin in the mid-1960s, the first attempt to destroy the World Trade Center in 1993, and the bombing of the Oklahoma City federal building in 1995. All of these incidents involved the use of vehicles filled with high nitrogen-content fertilizer soaked with diesel fuel and parked under or adjacent to the facility.

It is clear that the twenty-first century will bring new terrorism threats using more unconventional means, such as commercial aircraft to bring down structures (Figure 49-1 ■) and **weapons of mass destruction (WMDs)** including nuclear, biological, and chemical (NBC) weapons. Harbingers of such acts include the attack on the Tokyo subway system with sarin gas in 1996 and letters laced with anthrax spores sent through the mail in North America in 2001. Both events underscore the real potential for massive and widespread injury and death caused by those intending to incite terror using WMDs. With the increasing likelihood of a **terrorist act,** EMS personnel become responsible for maintaining a higher index of suspicion for such an event. As a paramedic, you also must prepare to protect yourself and your crew, your patients, and the public from the effects of such an attack.

weapons of mass destruction (WMDs) *variety of chemical, biological, nuclear, or other devices used by terrorists to strike at government or high-profile targets; designed to create a maximum number of casualties.*

terrorist act *the use of violence to provoke fear and influence behavior for political, social, religious, or ethnic goals.*

Terrorists may be of foreign or domestic origin. They are likely to target locations that are symbolic of the government (a federal building such as the Pentagon) or that represent a country's influence (such as an embassy). Domestic terrorists may further target corporations or their executives who represent a threat to their cause. They may also target their own employer or the public through their employer's products (as in tainted food or pharmaceuticals). The objective of both the domestic and the foreign terrorist is to incite terror in the public.

Weapons of mass destruction include explosive and incendiary agents, nuclear detonation or contamination, and the release of biological or chemical agents.

The likely mechanisms of mass destruction used by terrorists include explosive and incendiary agents, nuclear detonation or contamination, and the release of either chemical or biological agents.

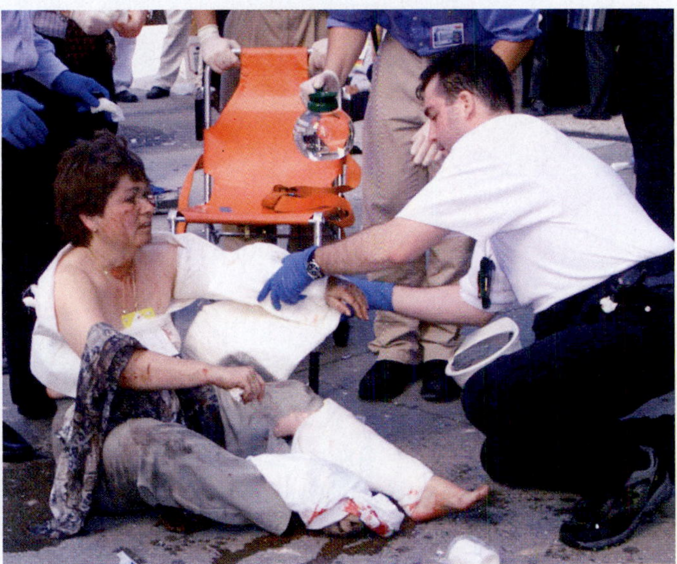

■ Figure 49-1 Providing treatment to a victim of the World Trade Center attack in New York City on September 11, 2001. *(Szenes Jason/Corbis Sygma)*

EXPLOSIVE AGENTS

explosives *chemical(s) that, when ignited, instantly generate a great amount of heat resulting in a destructive shock wave and blast wind.*

Be wary of secondary explosives set to disrupt rescue and injure emergency responders.

incendiary agents *a subset of explosives with less explosive power but greater heat and burn potential.*

Review

Content

Examples of Incendiary Agents

- Napalm
- Gasoline
- White phosphorus
- Magnesium

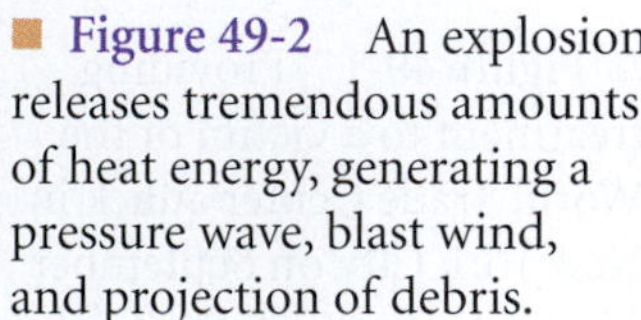

Explosives are the most likely method by which terrorists will strike. The method may range from a suicide bomber carrying a few sticks of dynamite to a large vehicle filled with highly explosive material. In an instant, the device detonates and causes damage to the human body through several mechanisms (Figure 49-2 ■). The blast pressure wave causes compression/decompression injury as it passes through the lungs, the ears, and other hollow, air-filled organs. This damage may be enhanced when the explosion occurs in a confined space, such as the interior of a building or other structure. Debris thrown by the blast produces penetrating or blunt injuries, and similar additional injury occurs as the victim is thrown by the blast wind. Secondary combustion induces burn injury, and structural collapse causes blunt and crushing injuries. After the initial explosion, associated dangers include structural collapse, fire, electrical hazard, and combustible or toxic gas hazards. *ALSO BE WARY OF SECONDARY EXPLOSIVES SET INTENTIONALLY TO DISRUPT RESCUE AND TO INJURE EMERGENCY RESPONDERS.* After the blast, emergency responders are left to locate, extricate, and provide medical care for the victims. (See Chapter 17, "Blunt Trauma," for a detailed explanation of the blast process, the associated mechanisms of injury, and assessment and care of the blast victim.)

Incendiary agents are a special subset of explosives with less explosive power and greater heat and burn potential. Napalm, used extensively during the Vietnam War, is a military example, whereas the Molotov cocktail or gasoline bomb is more of a terrorist weapon. Some incendiary agents are of special concern. White phosphorus may spontaneously combust when exposed to air and may be a part of military munitions or a terrorist weapon. It can be very difficult to extinguish when it contacts the skin. Often, fire-resistant oil is used to exclude the air and extinguish any flame. Another example is magnesium, a metal that burns vigorously and at a high temperature (3,000°C). It also is difficult to extinguish. Incendiary agents are likely to cause severe and extensive burn injuries. (For more information on burn injuries and their care, see Chapter 21, "Burns.")

Terrorists may choose to increase the effectiveness of their weapons by incorporating other agents with explosives. In some cases, they surround the explosive charge with old auto batteries, thereby contaminating the explosion scene with both lead and sulfuric acid. They may also surround the charge with scrap metal, nails, or screws that act as shrapnel. In some cases in the Middle East, terrorists have surrounded the explosive with nails coated with a form of rat poison, a derivative of coumadin, to increase the severity of wound hemorrhage associated with shrapnel wounds.

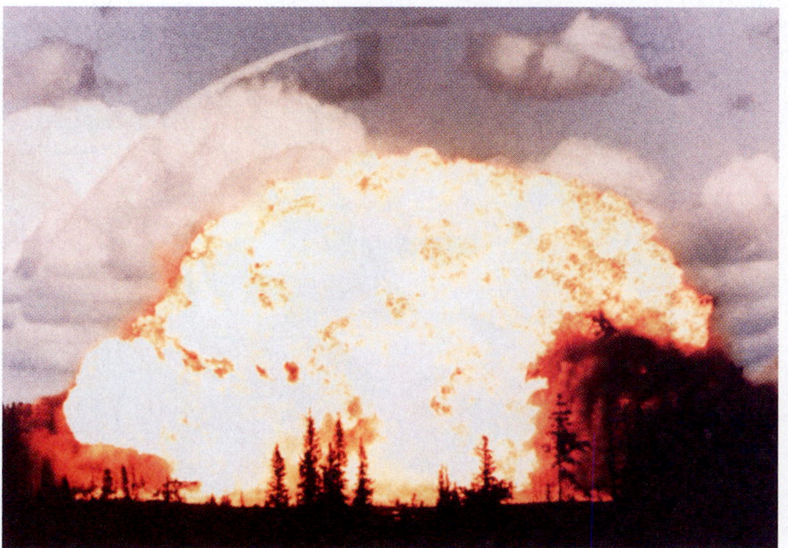

■ **Figure 49-2** An explosion releases tremendous amounts of heat energy, generating a pressure wave, blast wind, and projection of debris.

NUCLEAR DETONATION

Nuclear detonation is the release of energy that is generated when heavy nuclei split (fission) or light nuclei combine (fusion) to form new elements. The unleashed energy is tremendous and creates an explosion of immense proportion. In addition to the extremes of the injury-producing mechanisms associated with conventional explosions, radiant heat is likely to incinerate everything in the immediate vicinity of the blast and induce serious burn injury to exposed skin even at great distances from the blast epicenter. Burn injuries are likely to be the most lethal and debilitating injuries associated with a nuclear detonation.

nuclear detonation *the release of energy that is generated when heavy nuclei split (fission) or light nuclei combine (fusion) to form new elements. The unleashed energy is tremendous and creates an explosion of immense proportion.*

The damage associated with a typical nuclear detonation is extreme and results in concentric circles of total destruction and mortality, severe destruction and very high mortality, heavy destruction and moderate mortality, and light destruction and limited mortality (Figure 49-3 ■). The explosive energy disrupts communications, power, water and waste service, travel, and the medical, emergency medical, and public safety infrastructures. The destruction also disrupts access to the scene and limits the ability of the EMS system to identify, reach, and care for the seriously injured. It is an extreme disaster with great loss of life and injury and presents a great challenge to emergency responders.

The nuclear reaction also generates particles of debris and dust that give off nuclear radiation. Gases, heated by the explosion, draw these particles high into the atmosphere, where upper air currents carry the contamination until it falls to earth as fallout. This uplifting of irradiated debris leaves the scene almost radiation free from moments after the blast until about 1 hour post-ignition. Thereafter, there is a serious danger from fallout at the scene and downwind for many, many miles.

Nuclear radiation cannot be felt, seen, or otherwise detected by any of our senses.

Nuclear radiation cannot be felt, seen, or otherwise detected by any of our senses. However, it damages the cells of the human body as it passes through them. Radiation passage changes the structure of molecules and essential elements of the cells. Damaged cells then go on to repair themselves, to die, or to produce altered or damaged cells (cancer). As the intensity and duration of exposure increases, so do the degree and extent of cell damage and the risk to life. Nuclear radiation from the sun and other natural sources bombards us constantly. This exposure is very limited and the damage caused by it is minimal. However, the initial radiation produced by the nuclear chain

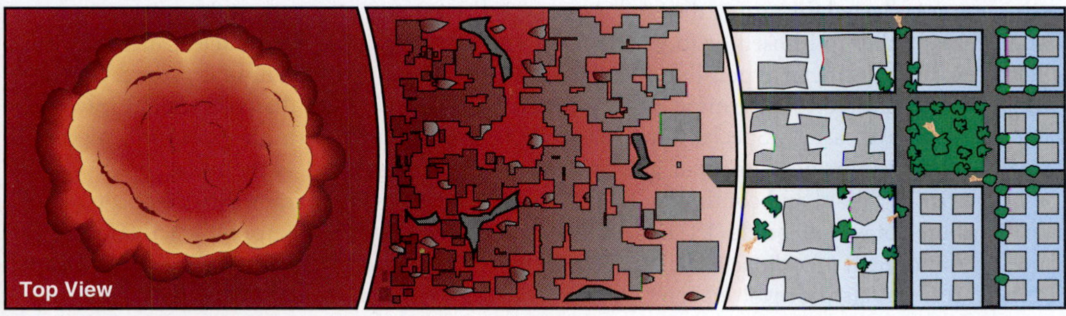

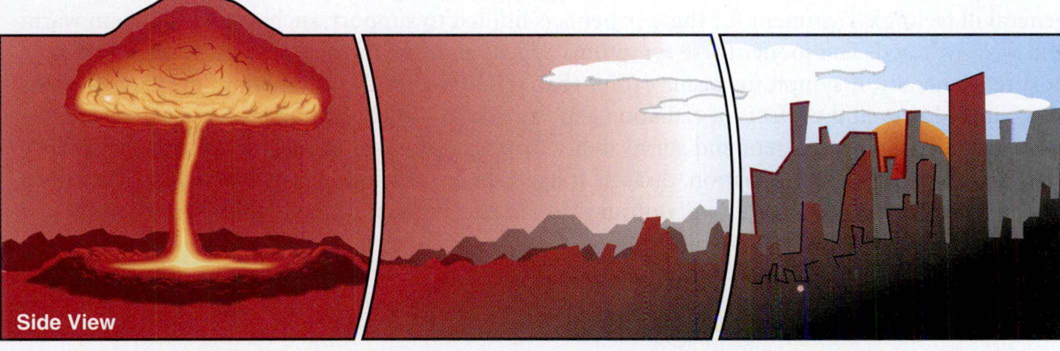

■ **Figure 49-3** The concentric circles of destruction following detonation of a nuclear weapon.

fallout *radioactive dust and particles that may be life threatening to people far from the epicenter of a nuclear detonation.*

reaction (the blast) and **fallout** can produce serious and life-threatening exposure. (See Chapter 21, "Burns," for the types of radiation, mechanisms of injury, and the assessment and care of the irradiated patient.)

A NUCLEAR INCIDENT RESPONSE

The first hour post-ignition is generally spent moving the injured into structures that will protect them from fallout. Ideally, they are moved into the central areas of large, structurally sound buildings or at least to some cover from the falling contaminated dust. Simultaneously, emergency responders organize, determine the direction of fallout movement, and begin to extricate the walking wounded and seriously injured from the outer perimeter of the explosion. During this time, evacuation of those in the anticipated path of fallout occurs. (They should remain outside the fallout pathway for at least 48 hours and until radiologic monitoring determines it is safe to return.) Entry into the scene is made from upwind and laterally to upper air movement in order to limit radioactive fallout exposure to rescuers.

As the response is organized, egress and evacuation routes are cleared, the injured are located and evacuated, and the response moves closer and closer to the blast epicenter. In general, some limited medical care is provided where the victims are found, but most emergency medical care is provided at treatment sectors that are remote from the seriously damaged areas and away from where fallout is expected. Patients are brought to a decontamination area, monitored for contamination, and decontaminated as needed before care begins.

Burns are the most common and most immediate life-threatening injuries associated with a nuclear detonation and will likely be the focus of most care.

Care for victims of a nuclear detonation involves decontamination (as necessary), treatment as for a conventional explosion (compression/decompression, blunt and penetrating injury care), and treatment for thermal burns. Burns are the most common and most immediately life-threatening injuries associated with a nuclear detonation and will likely be the focus of most care.

Geiger counter *an instrument used to detect and measure the radiation given off by an object or area.*

dosimeter *an instrument that measures the cumulative amount of radiation absorbed.*

Before victims of a nuclear detonation arrive at an emergency medical treatment sector, someone must monitor them for radioactive contamination. This monitoring is accomplished using a device called a **Geiger counter.** The Geiger counter measures the passage of radioactive particles or rays through a receiving chamber and requires some training to use properly. (Usually, someone specially trained—and other than EMS—provides radioactive monitoring and decontamination.) If any significant radioactivity is noted, the patient's clothing is removed and he is washed with soap, water, and gentle scrubbing and then rinsed. All contaminated clothing is bagged, and the wash water is collected for proper disposal. A properly decontaminated patient does not pose a radiation threat either to himself or to you. During a response to a suspected nuclear incident, you will likely wear a **dosimeter,** a pen-like device used to record your total radiation exposure. This device is then monitored to determine when your exposure level is such that you should leave the scene for your own safety. Specially trained scene responders or health physicists will monitor dosages and determine how long you, as a care provider, can safely work at the scene.

If the risk of fallout and continuing radiation exposure is serious, paramedics may be asked to help distribute potassium iodide (KI) tablets. These tablets reduce the uptake of radioactive iodine (a common component of radioactive fallout) by the thyroid, which reduces the risk of thyroid injury or cancer. You may also be involved in the effort to evacuate the public from the expected fallout path.

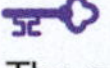

The sooner symptoms appear after radiation exposure, the more serious the incident. If they appear sooner than 6 hours afterward, the exposure was very high.

Generally, patients with serious radiation exposure present with nausea, fatigue, and malaise (a general ill feeling). Treatment for these patients is limited to support, such as keeping them warm and well hydrated. The sooner these symptoms appear after the incident, the more serious the exposure. Generally, if symptoms occur earlier than 6 hours after the detonation, the exposure was very high. However, the effects of radiation exposure differ widely among individuals, so early diagnosis of the exposure extent and survivability from symptoms is unreliable. Due to the severity and nature of a nuclear detonation, disaster triage is necessary and many serious-to-critical burn and radiation-exposure patients will not survive—in part because of the inability of a medical system to care for the sheer number of victims.

dirty bomb *a conventional explosive device that distributes radioactive material over a large area.*

RADIOACTIVE CONTAMINATION

Radioactive contamination may also be spread using conventional explosives (the "**dirty bomb**"). This type of blast is of conventional origin and does not cause the great magnitude of destruction that a nuclear detonation would. However, the explosion distributes radioactive material over a large area and into the surrounding air. The result is an explosion site with radioactive material contaminating the immediate vicinity. The greatest danger of this terrorist weapon is that the nature of the risk (the radiation) may not be recognized until well after the incident. Consequently, many more individuals and rescuers may be exposed or contaminated. Emergency care for victims of a recognized dirty bomb ignition includes radioactive decontamination and treatment (at a remote sector) for injuries that would be expected from a conventional bomb blast.

Emergency care for victims of a recognized "dirty bomb" includes decontamination and treatment for injuries that would be expected from a conventional bomb blast.

CHEMICAL AGENTS

Another terrorist weapon of mass destruction is the release of chemical agents. Potential chemical weapons range from simple hazardous materials common in our society, such as chlorine gas, to sophisticated chemicals, such as nerve agents specifically designed to harm humans. Because these chemical weapons are often gases or aerosols that will disperse in an open or windy area, the more common targets for their use are confined spaces such as subways or large buildings, which have central heating or air-conditioning, or areas where many people congregate such as arenas, shopping malls, and convention centers.

The concepts of volatility (vapor pressure) and specific gravity are important to understanding how chemical weapon agents are distributed. **Volatility** is the ease with which a chemical changes from a liquid to a gas. Most chemical weapons are liquids that are moderately volatile. They are often deployed by an explosion or sprayed into the atmosphere, creating an aerosol. A chemical that remains a liquid is said to be persistent and poses a contact or absorption threat, whereas vapors, gases, or aerosols present an inhalation danger. An example of a persistent chemical weapon is mustard agent. An example of a volatile, inhalable chemical weapon is lewisite.

volatility *the ease with which a chemical changes from a liquid to a gas; the tendency of a chemical agent to evaporate.*

Specific gravity refers to the density or weight of the vapor or gas as compared with air. A vapor or gas with a specific gravity less than air rises and quickly disperses into the atmosphere. This limits the effectiveness of the agent as a weapon. A gas with a specific gravity greater than air sinks beneath it, stays close to the ground, and accumulates in low places. Closed spaces, such as a basement, or low areas like a river valley resist dispersal of the vapor and maintain the danger. Common chemicals with high specific gravity include chlorine and phosgene.

specific gravity *refers to the density or weight of a vapor or gas as compared with air.*

Environmental conditions affect the dispersal of chemical weapons. In strong winds the gas or vapor mixes with large quantities of air and dilutes and disperses very quickly, limiting its concentration and effectiveness. Light wind moves the cloud downwind as a unit, increasing its effectiveness and the area involved. In windless conditions (which are infrequent) the cloud remains stationary, decreasing the area affected by it. Trees and buildings retard dispersion, whereas open spaces enhance dispersal. Precipitation, especially rain, may deactivate or absorb some agents, such as chlorine. Early morning and the time just before sunset are best for agent release because the winds are usually at their lowest velocity. The interior of a building with few open windows, especially when being heated or air-conditioned, is an especially controlled environment. Confined within a building, a chemical agent remains concentrated and deadly for a prolonged period.

Review

Content

Classifications for Chemical Weapons

- Nerve agents
- Vesicants
- Pulmonary agents
- Biotoxins
- Incapacitating agents
- Other hazardous chemicals

Chemical weapons are classified according to the way they cause damage to the human body. These chemicals include nerve agents, vesicants, pulmonary agents, biotoxins, incapacitating agents, and other hazardous chemicals.

NERVE AGENTS

Nerve agents and some insecticides damage nervous impulse conduction. These agents generally inhibit the degradation of a neurotransmitter (acetylcholine) and quickly cause a nervous system overload. This results in muscle twitching and spasms, convulsions, unconsciousness, and respiratory failure. Some common examples of nerve agents include GB (sarin), VX, GF, GD (soman), and GA (tabun). Although not designed as weapons, organophosphate (malathion, parathion) and carbamate (sevin) insecticides share a similar mechanism of action to nerve agents. They are much less potent, but they are still dangerous.

nerve agents *chemicals that inhibit the degradation of a neurotransmitter (acetylcholine) and quickly facilitate a nervous system overload.*

Nerve agents present as either vapor or liquid and are capable of being absorbed through the skin or inhaled and absorbed through the respiratory system. Exposure quickly leads to a series of signs and symptoms remembered as SLUDGE, or *S*alivation, *L*acrimation, *U*rination, *D*iarrhea, *G*astrointestinal distress, and *E*mesis. In addition to these signs, the patient may experience dyspnea, **fasciculations** (these are prominent), **rhinorrhea,** blurry vision, **miosis,** nausea, and sweating. Ultimately, the patient may become unconscious, seize, stop breathing, and die.

fasciculations *involuntary contractions or twitchings of muscle fibers.*

rhinorrhea *watery discharge from the nose.*

miosis *abnormal contraction of the pupils; pinpoint pupils.*

The actions of nerve agents can generally be reversed if the antidote is administered shortly after exposure. However, many nerve agents permanently bind to the agents, reabsorbing the neurotransmitters, and their effects become more difficult to reverse. The prognosis for a patient exposed to a nerve agent is good with aggressive artificial ventilation and quick administration of the antidote.

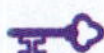

The actions of nerve agents can generally be reversed if the antidote is administered shortly after exposure.

Treatment for nerve agent exposure includes the administration of atropine and then pralidoxime chloride. The military currently has these medications available in a two-part auto-injector set called a **Mark I kit.** As the threat of nerve agent release to the civilian population becomes greater, these kits may become increasingly available to the EMS provider. The auto-injectors are designed for self-administration or buddy-administration (mainly for military personnel) or may be administered by rescue personnel. They are quick to use and may be necessary when confronted with numerous patients exposed to a nerve agent. The antidote combination is often followed by the administration of diazepam to reduce seizure activity. The auto-injector is a convenient way to administer this regimen of medications; however, the intravenous route is more rapid and preferred when available and as time permits.

Mark I kit *a two-part auto-injector set the military uses as treatment for nerve agent exposure; involves the administration of atropine and then pralidoxime chloride.*

The Mark I kit contains 2 mg of atropine and 600 mg of pralidoxime chloride (2-PAM). It is administered for the first and mild symptoms of exposure (blurry vision, mild dyspnea, and rhinorrhea) and repeated in 10 minutes if symptoms do not improve. If serious signs and symptoms are present, three doses of both atropine and pralidoxime chloride may be administered. Intravenous administration should provide 2 mg of atropine every 5 minutes (until drying of secretions or 20 mg is administered) and 1 g of pralidoxime chloride every hour (until spontaneous respirations return). A pediatric version of the Mark I kit is available overseas and may soon be available in the United States.

VESICANTS (BLISTERING AGENTS)

Vesicants are agents that damage exposed tissue, frequently causing vesicles (blisters). They are capable of causing damage to the skin, eyes, respiratory tract, and lungs, and are able to induce generalized illness as well. The mustard gas of World War I is an example of a vesicant. Other examples include sulfur mustard (HD), nitrogen mustard (HN), lewisite (L), and phosgene oxime (CX). With the exception of phosgene oxime, the vesicants are thick oily liquids that create a toxic vapor threat in warm temperatures. The liquid form, however, is highly toxic to the touch. Lewisite and phosgene oxime induce immediate irritation on contact or inhalation, whereas the mustards produce only slight discomfort that becomes more severe with time. The slow progression of signs and symptoms may prolong contact and increase the severity of exposure.

vesicants *agents that damage exposed skin, frequently causing vesicles (blisters).*

Patients exposed to vesicants present with the signs and symptoms of injury to the skin, mucous membranes, and lungs. Exposed skin exhibits the signs of a chemical burn including pain, **erythema,** and eventually blistering. The eyes and upper airway display a burning or stinging sensation with tearing and rhinorrhea. Respiratory tract exposure results in dyspnea, cough, wheezing, and pulmonary edema. Systemic signs and symptoms include nausea, vomiting, and fatigue. Signs and symptoms occur slowly with the mustard agents, which may prolong exposure.

erythema *general reddening of the skin due to dilation of the superficial capillaries.*

Emergency care for the patient exposed to a vesicant is immediate decontamination. Exposure of even a few minutes can result in permanent injury. The exposed areas should be irrigated immediately with water from a hose (using limited pressure if possible). Also irrigate the eyes, with a preference for saline over water, but do not delay irrigation to await the proper fluid. If blistering has occurred, treat the lesions as you would any chemical burn. Apply loose sterile dressings, gently bandage affected eyes, and medicate the patient for any serious pain.

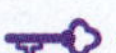

Emergency care for the patient exposed to a vesicant is immediate decontamination.

PULMONARY AGENTS

Pulmonary agents are those that cause chemical injury primarily to the lungs. They include phosgene, chlorine, hydrogen sulfide, and similar agents, and some of the by-products that are created when synthetics such as plastic combust. These agents attack the mucous membranes of the respiratory system from the oral pharynx and nasal pharynx to the smaller respiratory bronchioles and alveoli. They produce inflammation and pulmonary edema resulting in dyspnea and hypoxia. Early signs and symptoms of pulmonary agent exposure are related to irritation of the upper airway. They include rhinorrhea, nasal, oral, and throat irritation, wheezing, and cough. The victim may also experience tearing and eye irritation. Pulmonary edema is generally a late sign of exposure.

pulmonary agents *chemicals that primarily cause injury to the lungs; commonly referred to as choking agents.*

Emergency care for the individual exposed to a pulmonary agent is removal from the environment; exposure to fresh air; high-flow, high-concentration oxygen; and rest. Endotracheal intubation and ventilation may be required. In cases of moderate-to-severe respiratory distress, consider 0.5 mL of albuterol by nebulized inhalation.

Emergency care for pulmonary agent exposure is removal from the environment, administration of high-flow, high-concentration oxygen, and rest.

BIOTOXINS

Another type of agent that is classified as a biological agent but behaves more like a chemical agent is the **biotoxin.** These toxins are produced by living organisms but are themselves not alive. Such agents include ricin, staphylococcal enterotoxin B (SEB), botulinum toxin, and trichothecene mycotoxins (T2). Ricin, a by-product of castor oil production, inhibits the body's ability to synthesize proteins. It may be either aerosolized and inhaled or ingested. Ricin causes pulmonary edema when inhaled and gastric symptoms when ingested. Poisoning by both routes may cause shock and multiple organ failure.

biotoxin *poisons that are produced by a living organism but are themselves not alive.*

Staphylococcal enterotoxin is produced by a bacterium, *Staphylococcus aureus,* and is the agent most commonly responsible for food poisoning. Contamination may occur either orally, causing nausea and vomiting, or by inhalation, causing dyspnea and fever. Though only a small amount of toxin may cause symptoms and 50 percent of those contaminated may be incapacitated, SEB is rarely fatal.

Botulinum, the most toxic agent known, is an infrequent result of improper canning technique. It is 15,000 times more potent that VX, the most lethal nerve agent. Fortunately, the botulism toxin is very unstable, which limits its usefulness as a weapon of mass destruction. Like the nerve agents, botulinum attacks the nervous system. It interferes with impulse transmission and interrupts the central nervous system's control of the organs. The result is weakness, paralysis, and death by respiratory failure. Botulinum can be ingested or inhaled.

Trichothecene mycotoxins are a group of biotoxins produced by fungus molds. They prohibit protein and nucleic acid formulation and affect body cells that divide rapidly first. T2 acts very quickly, causing skin irritation (pain, burning, redness, and blistering), respiratory irritation (nasal and oral pain, rhinorrhea, epistaxis, wheezing, dyspnea, and hemoptysis), eye irritation (pain, redness, tearing, and blurry vision), and gastrointestinal symptoms (nausea, vomiting, abdominal cramping, and bloody diarrhea). T2 is most effective when absorbed through the skin. Generalized signs and symptoms include central nervous system signs, hypotension, and death.

Management of a victim of a biotoxin is supportive; antitoxins are generally not available. A special concern is directed to careful decontamination because even a very small amount of biotoxin can endanger rescuers and others.

Biotoxin exposure management is supportive. However, careful decontamination is necessary to prevent exposure of others.

INCAPACITATING AGENTS

Incapacitating agents include the riot control agents used by police and for personal protection as well as newer agents being investigated by the military. These agents are intentionally selected or designed to incapacitate, not injure or harm, the recipient.

Riot control agents include CS, CN (mace), capaicin (pepper spray), and CR. You may come into contact with these agents when they are released by police to suppress a large public disturbance or to subdue an assaultive or violent individual or are released by an individual for personal protection or possibly in the commission of a crime. These agents may, in the future, be used by those who wish to disrupt the public and incite terror.

The exposed patient often complains of eye irritation and tearing as well as rhinorrhea. If the agent is inhaled, these symptoms are often accompanied by airway irritation and dyspnea. These signs and symptoms are relieved by removal from the source, exposure to fresh air, and the administration of oxygen, when needed. The signs and symptoms further diminish with time.

The anticholinergic agents (atropine-like drugs) BZ and QNB are the prototype incapacitating agents for the military. The primary method of distribution of these agents is through the detonation of a mixture of explosive and agent. This explosion produces an aerosolized cloud. Exposure to BZ and QNB produces inappropriate affect, dry mucous beds, dilated pupils, slurred speech, disorientation, blurred vision, inhibition of the sweating reflex, elevated body temperature, and facial flushing. These effects become apparent after about 30 minutes of inhalation and last for up to 8 hours. The most dangerous effects of exposure include dysrhythmias and hyperthermia from the loss of the sweating reflex. The actions of BZ and QNB may be reversed by the administration of physostigmine.

OTHER HAZARDOUS CHEMICALS

Any toxic chemical has a potential for use as a weapon of mass destruction. Industry produces countless hazardous materials with the potential to cause great harm if released into the air or water supply or ignited to release toxic gases. The only difference between an accidental release and one that is intended to incite terror is that the intentional release will likely be optimized to affect the greatest number of people. It may also be more difficult to identify the agent used by a terrorist because the container will likely not identify the agent. The Department of Transportation's *Emergency Response Guidebook,* which should be carried on every ambulance and fire apparatus, is a good guide to most common hazardous materials that might be used as a weapon as well as information on other WMD agents. It can also be helpful in denoting isolation and evacuation distances and suggesting specific care management steps.

RECOGNITION OF A CHEMICAL AGENT RELEASE

A chemical weapon release may be visible as a cloud of mist, vapor, dust, or as puddles, or it may be completely unrecognizable. There may be an associated smell such as that of newly mown grass (phosgene), the smell of rotten eggs (hydrogen sulfide), or other strange or unusual odors. Suspect a chemical release if there are chemical odors when and where chemicals are not used or expected. However, never search out such an odor or touch any suspect liquid or material. You may also notice clusters of patients with chemical exposure symptoms or injured, incapacitated, or dead insects, birds, or animals. (You might remember that parakeets have been used in mines to detect toxic gas levels.) Given that the terrorist may be intent on optimizing the effect of the release, be especially wary of large public gatherings or large but confined spaces, such as public buildings, and low spaces that limit dissipation, such as subway terminals. Terrorists may also target food or water supplies with either chemical or biological agents. This may result in very widespread effects.

A cardinal sign of a chemical release is the manifestation of similar signs and symptoms occurring rapidly among a group of individuals.

A cardinal sign of a chemical release is the manifestation of similar signs and symptoms occurring rapidly among a group of individuals. Common signs of a chemical release include inflamed mucosa (eye, nasal, oral, or throat irritation), exposed skin irritation, chest tightness, burning and/or dyspnea, gastrointestinal signs (nausea, abdominal cramping, vomiting, and diarrhea), and central nervous system disturbances (confusion, lethargy, nausea/vomiting, intoxication, headache, and unconsciousness).

MANAGEMENT OF A CHEMICAL AGENT RELEASE

Approach the scene from upwind and higher ground and remain a good distance away from the site. Generally, evacuate the immediate area if the release is small and contained. However, if the release involves a great quantity of material, such as that in a railway tank car or large commercial storage container, evacuate the general population for a radius of 700 to 2,000 feet and 1.5 miles downwind during the day. If the release occurs at night, then evacuate a 2,000-foot radius and as much as 6 to 7 miles downwind (Figure 49-4 ■).

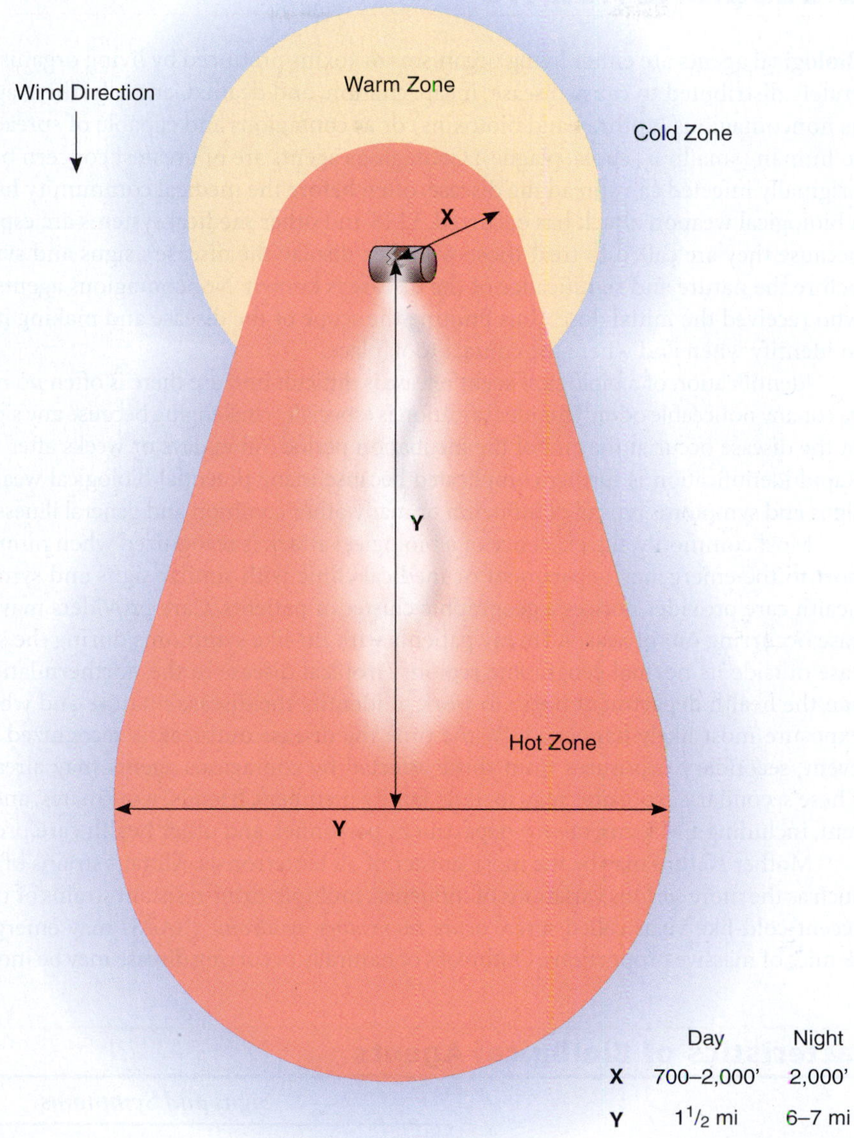

■ **Figure 49-4** Hot, warm, and cold zones associated with a hazardous materials release.

Once the public danger is reduced by scene isolation, make sure the injured are properly decontaminated before you begin care. Rescuers coming out of the danger zones must also be decontaminated. The agency that provides spill containment and decontamination at the hazardous materials incident generally provides decontamination for both nuclear and chemical weapons of mass destruction. This service is most commonly the fire department. (See the section on Hazardous Materials Incidents in Chapter 48, "Operations.")

In addition to the specific emergency care steps noted earlier, most patients require decontamination, exposure to fresh air, oxygen administration, and possibly respiratory support. As a precautionary measure, use personal protective equipment (PPE), including a well-fitting HEPA filter mask, nitrile gloves (latex gloves do not offer much protection against chemical agents), and a Tyvek® disposable suit. Be careful of leather clothing items. Belts, watch bands, and shoes made of leather absorb many chemical agents and will present a continuing exposure danger once contaminated. These precautions provide very minimal protection against chemical agents and do not constitute the PPE necessary to work in a warm or hot zone.

BIOLOGICAL AGENTS

biological agents *either living organisms or toxins produced by living organisms that are deliberately distributed to cause disease and death.*

Biological agents are either living organisms or toxins produced by living organisms that are deliberately distributed to cause disease, incapacitation, and death. Generally, these agents are grouped as noncontagious (anthrax and biotoxins) or as contagious and capable of spreading from human to human (smallpox, ebola, plague). Contagious agents are of greatest concern because the people originally infected can spread the disease, often before the medical community has recognized that a biological weapon attack has occurred. EMS and other medical systems are especially vulnerable because they are called to treat those who first display the disease's signs and symptoms, possibly before the nature and significance of the disease is known. Noncontagious agents affect only those who received the initial dose, thus limiting the scope of the disease and making it somewhat easier to identify when and where the contact took place.

Identification of a biological agent release is difficult because there is often no noticeable cloud of gas or any noticeable odor. This identification is especially challenging because any signs and symptoms of the disease occur at the end of the incubation period, often days or weeks after the initial contact. Rapid identification is further complicated because many potential biological weapons present with signs and symptoms typical of influenza or many other common and general illnesses (Table 49–1).

Most commonly, the existence of a biological attack is recognized when numerous patients report to emergency departments or clinics with similar signs and symptoms.

Most commonly, the existence of a biological attack is recognized when numerous patients report to the emergency department or medical clinic with similar signs and symptoms or when a health care provider notices a geographic cluster of patients. Care providers may also notice a disease occurring out of season (many patients with flu-like symptoms during the summer) or a disease outside its normal geographic regions (tropical disease in the northern latitudes). Only then can the health department begin to work to identify the disease's nature and when and where the exposure most likely happened. By the time the disease outbreak is recognized as a bioterrorism event, secondary exposures from those affected by contagious agents may already be occurring. These secondary exposures may include family members, friends, workmates, and the medical system, including EMS, emergency department personnel, and other health care providers.

Mother Nature may be the most sinister of all bioterrorists. Mutant strains of common diseases such as the more serious variations of influenza, multiple-drug-resistant strains of tuberculosis, or the recent cold-like virus called *severe acute respiratory syndrome (SARS)* may emerge and create epidemics of massive proportions. Outbreaks of naturally occurring disease may be more likely and more

Table 49–1 Characteristics of Biological Agents

Disease	Incubation Period	Mortality	*Signs and Symptoms*				
			Fever	Chills	Cough	Malaise	Nausea/ Vomiting
Anthrax	1 to 6 days	90%	✓		✓	✓	
Pneumonic plague*	1 to 6 days	57% to 100%	✓	✓	✓	✓	
Tularemia	3 to 5 days	35%	✓		✓	✓	
Q fever	2 to 14 days	1%	✓		✓	✓	
Smallpox*	12 days	30%	✓			✓	✓
Venezuelan equine encephalitis	1 to 5 days	1%	✓	✓	✓	✓	✓
Cholera	1 to 3 days	50%					✓
Viral hemorrhagic fever	3 to 7 days	5% to 20%	✓			✓	
Ebola*	3 to 7 days	80% to 90%	✓			✓	

*Human-to-human contagious disease.

severe than a terrorist's use of a biological weapon. Tracking the origin and combating these naturally occurring diseases is exactly like tracking and combating a biological weapon used by terrorists.

Currently the list of potential WMD diseases is extensive and contains pneumonia-like agents, encephalitis-like agents, and others.

PNEUMONIA-LIKE AGENTS

Pneumonia-like bioterror agents include anthrax, plague, tularemia, and Q fever and are the most likely agents for a terrorist attack. They generally cause cough, dyspnea, fever, and malaise. Anthrax and plague are the most deadly, with 90 to 100 percent mortality. Anthrax is a very effective biological agent, though it is not contagious, which limits any human-to-human transmission. The strain of plague most likely used for bioterrorism is pneumonic, which carries not only a very high mortality (100 percent untreated and about 57 percent when treated), but also has minimum victim survival when left untreated for the first 18 hours after signs and symptoms appear. Pneumonic plague incubates over 1 to 4 days and can be spread through droplets and inhalation. Tularemia (also known as rabbit fever or deerfly fever) may be aerosolized and presents with signs and symptoms in 2 to 10 days. It carries a mortality rate of up to 35 percent. Q fever may appear in 10 to 20 days after contact and lasts from 2 days to 2 weeks; however, it is more of an incapacitating disease with a very low death rate.

ENCEPHALITIS-LIKE AGENTS

Smallpox and Venezuelan equine encephalitis (VEE) are influenza-like diseases with headache, fever, and malaise and a higher mortality, probably because these diseases attack the central nervous system. They are very effective as biological weapons because small amounts of aerosolized agent can cause the disease. Smallpox is very contagious through airborne droplets via the respiratory route. Signs and symptoms usually appear after about 12 days in about 30 percent of those exposed, with about a third of that number dying within 5 to 7 days. Smallpox is considered eradicated as a naturally occurring disease, but it is thought that it may exist in the WMD programs of some countries. With VEE, human-to-human transmission does not occur, and mortality is generally less than 20 percent.

OTHER AGENTS

Cholera is a common disease in underdeveloped countries and is frequently linked to poor sanitation. It is most commonly transmitted by the fecal–oral route and primarily causes severe dehydration and shock because of profuse diarrhea. It is one of the few agents that is not transmitted by the inhalation route and may be delivered as a weapon by way of contamination of food or untreated water.

Viral hemorrhagic fever (VHF) is a class of disease that includes the deadly ebola virus. As the name suggests, hemorrhagic fever attacks the bloodstream and damages blood vessels, causing them to leak and the patient to bleed easily. The patient may bruise easily and display petechia (tiny red patches of dermal hemorrhage). Most diseases of this class can be spread through the inhalation route or through direct contact with infectious material. VHFs may carry a high mortality rate (90 percent) and are aerosolized easily, though they are difficult to cultivate.

Protection against biological agents used as weapons includes the prudent care steps used to prevent ordinary communicable disease transmission.

PROTECTION AGAINST BIOLOGICAL AGENT TRANSMISSION

Protection against the most common biological weapons includes the prudent care steps used to prevent ordinary communicable disease transmission. If there is a heightened alert status for a WMD release or terrorist event, employ a more aggressive use of Standard Precautions. Gloves are very effective in protecting against biological agent transmission from body fluids, as is rigorous and frequent hand washing. Almost all biological agents are transmitted by the respiratory route, so be sure to take droplet inhalation precautions. A properly fitted HEPA respirator is very effective in preventing agent transmission (Figure 49-5 ■). Consider applying a mask to your patient if he displays any signs or symptoms of respiratory disease. A sodium hypochlorite solution (0.5 percent) or other disinfectants are very effective in killing many biological agents. The ambulance interior and any equipment used or possibly contaminated should be vigorously cleaned with the solution.

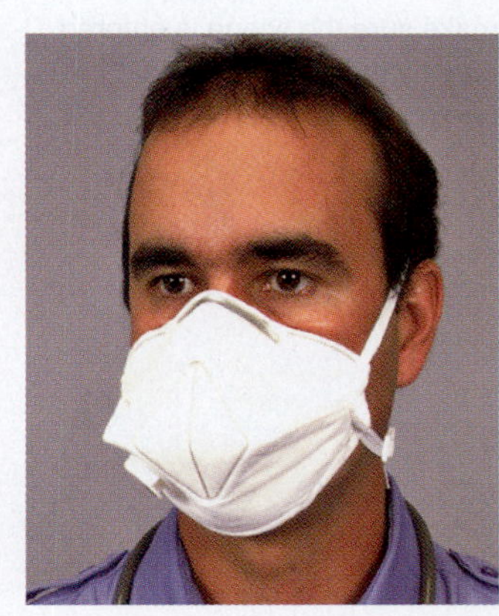

■ **Figure 49-5** A HEPA respirator.

Immunizations against many biological agents are not available. Those immunizations that are available usually carry a small risk of associated reaction. Hence, the prophylactic administration to a very large number of health care workers may not be warranted unless or until a significant risk becomes apparent. Consult with your medical director for your system's recommendations and the method used to provide you with immunizations if the need arises.

Emergency care for most patients affected by biological weapons is limited to supportive care.

Emergency care for most patients affected by biological weapons is limited to supportive care (maintain body temperature, administer oxygen, provide oral fluids, and, in some cases, administer IV fluids). Because some of the biological agents may produce respiratory compromise, protocols may call for an albuterol or other nebulized treatment. If practical, consider the use of metered-dose inhalers (MDIs) rather than nebulization, because MDIs limit aerosolized-droplet formation and subsequent risk of contaminating inhalation. Once the exact organism is isolated (after prehospital care), then a regimen of antibiotic therapy may be prescribed.

If a biological attack is suspected, health officials will interview the victims carefully. They will try to determine when the patients first noticed symptoms and identify any close personal contacts since that time. These people may be infected if the agent is indeed contagious. The public health approach to biological terrorism may also involve isolation and quarantine. The patient or caregiver exposed to a highly contagious disease may be quarantined through a restriction to home or may be confined within a commandeered facility such as a motel. A person with the signs and symptoms of the disease may be isolated through a similar arrangement. There is a danger associated with placing affected patients or caregivers in a hospital or other medical facility because they can then endanger other patients or care providers who are receiving or providing care there.

GENERAL CONSIDERATIONS REGARDING TERRORIST ATTACKS

SCENE SAFETY

One in every five victims of the World Trade Center collapse on September 11, 2001, was a member of an emergency response team. This great number of emergency personnel deaths underscores the need to recognize the dangers to EMS providers and ensure that safety is an active concern during the response to any potential act of terrorism.

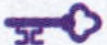

Carefully analyze an emergency scene to determine the risk to you and other rescuers. Then make sure the scene is entered only by those trained and equipped to do so.

Terrorists in other countries often set secondary explosive devices with the intent to disrupt any rescue attempt. A chemical release or radioactivity can linger and affect those who attempt unprotected rescue of patients. Biological agents are likely to affect the EMS provider as well. It is imperative that you carefully analyze a scene to determine the risk to you and other rescuers. Then ensure the scene is entered only by those properly equipped and trained to enter a hazardous or deadly environment.

RECOGNIZING A TERRORIST ATTACK

It is relatively easy to recognize a nuclear or conventional explosion. However, remember that radioactive fallout travels with the upper wind current (not just those at ground level), so watch cloud movement. Stay upwind. Remember, too, that terrorists may use the conventional explosion to distribute radioactive or other hazardous material (the "dirty bomb"), and they may set secondary detonations through booby traps or timers that are designed to target rescuers. Also be aware of structural collapse, because the explosion may weaken a building's structure. Do not enter the scene until you are sure it is safe from all hazards.

A chemical release may not be as obvious. There may or may not be a cloud of gas or aerosolized material. There also may or may not be any unusual odors. However, groups of victims will be complaining of similar symptoms, though symptom development may take some time. Suspect a chemical incident when you notice incapacitated small animals, birds, and insects. You may also be alerted to a possible chemical incident when confronted with chemical-exposure-like symptoms where chemicals are not usually used. Stay upwind and uphill of the site and request that victims and potential victims evacuate (or be evacuated) to you. Only personnel who are specially trained and equipped to deal with hazardous materials should enter the scene. However, to protect yourself, don nitrile gloves, a well-fitting HEPA filter mask, and a Tyvek® coverall when caring for a patient who has been decontaminated. These precautions provide only limited protection while working on decontaminated patients. They are not considered adequate for entry into the scene (warm or hot zone).

Identifying a biological agent at the time of release is probably impossible. There might be a cloud of dust or aerosolized material but there are no immediate signs and symptoms from those exposed. Such contamination also may be distributed by the mail (anthrax-laced letters, for instance) or other mechanisms. The incident is likely to be recognized after the incubation period and only after several patients report to the emergency departments or clinics with the disease. Then the local health department will investigate what all victims have in common to identify where the biological agent release took place. If you happen to notice many patients presenting with signs and symptoms of illness at or around the same time, consider a possible biological attack. As with any potential disease, don gloves and a well-fitted HEPA filter mask. (See Chapter 37, "Infectious Disease.") It is important to remember that you may be inadvertently exposed to a contagious agent, contract the disease, and then become a carrier. If you become aware of possible exposure or notice the signs and symptoms of a contagious disease, contact the proper health resource (your medical director, service infection control agent, or other person, according to protocols or your service policies) and ensure that you do not transmit the disease to others.

RESPONDING TO A TERRORIST ATTACK

Your first role in responding to a possible act of terrorism is to ensure your own safety and that of your patient, other rescuers, and the public. Once safety is ensured, make certain all patients are properly decontaminated (if need be) and then begin to provide the appropriate emergency medical care.

Your role as an emergency care provider for a terrorist attack is very similar to the other emergency responses you are more likely to encounter during your career. A nuclear incident is handled like a conventional explosion with a hazardous material (radiation) involved. The release of a chemical agent is a hazardous material incident. A biological weapon release is handled like an infectious disease outbreak. Although the location of the attack may maximize the number of people it affects, it is still a hazardous material incident (chemical or radiation agent), an infectious disease incident (biological event), a conventional explosion, or a combination. Use the training you already have for these situations and follow your system's protocols and disaster plans for each.

Once a WMD incident is identified, begin preparing for the casualties. Often this will entail instituting the incident command system and establishing extrication, decontamination, triage, treatment, and transport sectors. Carefully match the available resources against the nature, number, and severity of injuries. Review the section on Medical Incident Management in Chapter 48, "Operations."

Summary

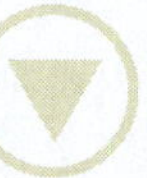

Many of the mechanisms of injury used by terrorists subtly induce their damage (toxic gases, radiation contamination, or biological agents) so that there is little scene evidence. Your responsibility is to maintain an enhanced lookout for any signs of NBC release or exposure and limit the contact you, the general population, and your patients have to such an agent. In general, it is not the role of EMS to deal with NBC agents. Your role as a paramedic is likely to be providing supportive care after patient decontamination.

Review Questions

1. __________ are the most common method by which terrorists strike.
   a. Explosives
   b. Chemical weapons
   c. Anthrax exposures
   d. Poisonings of public water supplies
2. After an initial explosion, associated dangers include:
   a. fire.
   b. electrical hazard.
   c. structural collapse.
   d. all of the above
3. __________ are likely to be the most lethal and debilitating injuries associated with a nuclear detonation.
   a. Burn injuries
   b. Inhalation injuries
   c. Blunt trauma injuries
   d. Penetrating trauma injuries
4. If there is serious risk of fallout and continuing radiation exposure, paramedics may be asked to help distribute __________ tablets.
   a. iron
   b. magnesium
   c. potassium iodide
   d. sodium chloride
5. Which of the following is not a common example of a nerve agent?
   a. GB (sarin)
   b. GD (soman)
   c. GA (tabun)
   d. carbamate (sevin)
6. Emergency care for the patient exposed to a vesicant is immediate:
   a. triage.
   b. fluid therapy.
   c. oxygenation.
   d. decontamination.
7. Which of the following agents is not considered contagious?
   a. ebola
   b. anthrax
   c. plague
   d. smallpox
8. __________ is a common disease in underdeveloped countries and is frequently linked to poor sanitation.
   a. Cholera
   b. SARS
   c. Tularemia
   d. VEE

See Answers to Review Questions at the back of this book.

Precautions on Bloodborne Pathogens and Infectious Diseases

Prehospital emergency personnel, like all health care workers, are at risk for exposure to bloodborne pathogens and infectious diseases. In emergency situations it is often difficult to take or enforce proper infection control measures. However, as a paramedic, you must recognize your high-risk status. Study the following information on infection control carefully.

Infection control is designed to protect emergency personnel, their families, and their patients from unnecessary exposure to communicable diseases. Laws, regulations, and standards regarding infection control include:

- ★ *Centers for Disease Control and Prevention (CDC) Guidelines.* The CDC has published extensive guidelines on infection control. Proper equipment and techniques that should be used by emergency response personnel to prevent or minimize risk of exposure are defined.
- ★ *The Ryan White Comprehensive AIDS Resources Emergency (CARE) Act.* The Ryan White CARE Act of 1990 allows emergency personnel to find out if they were exposed to an infectious disease while rendering patient care. Employers are required to name a "designated officer" to coordinate communications with the treating hospital.
- ★ *Americans with Disabilities Act.* This act prohibits discrimination against individuals with disabilities including those with contagious diseases. It guarantees equal employment opportunities and job protection if the infected individual can perform essential job functions and does not pose a threat to the safety and health of patients and coworkers.
- ★ *Occupational Safety and Health Administration (OSHA) Regulations.* OSHA has enacted a regulation titled Occupational Exposure to Bloodborne Pathogens, which classifies emergency response personnel as being at the greatest risk of occupational exposure to communicable diseases. This regulation requires employers to provide hepatitis B (HBV) vaccinations free of charge, maintain a written exposure control plan, and provide personal protective equipment. These requirements primarily apply to private employers. Applicability to local and state governmental employees varies by locality. Many states have developed their own OSHA plans.
- ★ *National Fire Protection Association (NFPA) Guidelines.* This is a national organization that has established specific guidelines and requirements regarding infection control for emergency response agencies, particularly fire departments and EMS services.

STANDARD PRECAUTIONS AND PERSONAL PROTECTIVE EQUIPMENT

Emergency response personnel should practice Standard Precautions, a strategy that considers ALL body substances potentially infectious. To achieve this, all emergency personnel should utilize personal protective equipment (PPE). Appropriate PPE should be available on every emergency vehicle. The minimum recommended PPE includes the following:

- ★ *Gloves.* Disposable gloves should be donned by all emergency response personnel BEFORE initiating any emergency care. When an emergency incident involves more than one patient, you should attempt to change gloves between patients. When gloves have been contaminated, they should be removed as soon as possible. To properly remove contaminated gloves, grasp one glove approximately 1 inch from the wrist. Without touching the inside of the glove, pull the glove halfway off and stop. With that half-gloved hand, pull the glove on the opposite hand completely off. Place the removed glove in the palm of the other glove, with the inside of the removed glove exposed. Pull the second glove completely off with the ungloved hand, only touching the inside of the glove. Always wash hands after gloves are removed, even when the gloves appear intact.
- ★ *Masks and Protective Eyewear.* Masks and protective equipment should be present on all emergency vehicles and used in accordance with the level of exposure encountered. Masks and protective eyewear should be worn together whenever blood spatter is likely to occur, such as during arterial bleeding, childbirth, endotracheal intubation, invasive procedures, oral suctioning, and cleanup of equipment that requires heavy scrubbing or brushing. Both you and the patient should wear masks whenever the potential for airborne transmission of disease exists.
- ★ *HEPA and N-95 Respirators.* Due to the resurgence of tuberculosis (TB), prehospital personnel should protect themselves from TB infection through use of an N-95 or a high-efficiency particulate air (HEPA) respirator, as approved by the National Institute of Occupational Safety and Health (NIOSH). It should fit snugly and be capable of filtering out the tuberculosis bacillus. An N-95 or HEPA respirator should be worn when caring for patients with confirmed or suspected TB. This is especially true when performing "high-hazard" procedures such as administration of nebulized medications, endotracheal intubation, or suctioning on such a patient.
- ★ *Gowns.* Gowns protect clothing from blood splashes. If large splashes of blood are expected, such as with childbirth, wear impervious gowns.
- ★ *Resuscitation Equipment.* Disposable resuscitation equipment should be the primary means of artificial ventilation in emergency care. Such items should be used once, then disposed of.

Remember, the proper use of personal protective equipment ensures effective infection control and minimizes risk. Use ALL protective equipment recommended for any particular situation to ensure maximum protection.

Consider ALL body substances potentially infectious and ALWAYS practice Standard Precautions.

Answers to Review Questions

The following are the correct answers to the Review Questions presented in each chapter of Essentials of Paramedic Care.

Chapter 1
1. *c*
2. *a*
3. *d*
4. *d*
5. *b*
6. *a*
7. *c*
8. *d*
9. *d*
10. *c*
11. *c*
12. *d*

Chapter 2
1. *a*
2. *d*
3. *b*
4. *a*
5. *c*
6. *c*
7. *d*
8. *c*
9. *d*
10. *d*

Chapter 3
1. *b*
2. *d*
3. *a*
4. *a*
5. *d*
6. *d*
7. *c*
8. *d*
9. *b*
10. *b*
11. *c*
12. *a*
13. *d*
14. *d*
15. *c*
16. *c*
17. *a*
18. *a*
19. *b*
20. *c*
21. *d*
22. *d*
23. *b*
24. *b*
25. *c*

Chapter 4
1. *d*
2. *d*
3. *a*
4. *d*
5. *b*
6. *b*
7. *d*
8. *d*
9. *b*
10. *d*
11. *a*
12. *c*
13. *c*
14. *b*
15. *c*

Chapter 5
1. *c*
2. *d*
3. *c*
4. *a*
5. *c*
6. *b*
7. *c*
8. *c*

Chapter 6
1. *c*
2. *b*
3. *b*
4. *c*
5. *b*
6. *a*
7. *a*
8. *b*
9. *d*
10. *c*
11. *c*
12. *d*
13. *a*
14. *c*
15. *b*
16. *d*
17. *d*
18. *b*
19. *b*
20. *b*

Chapter 7
1. *a*
2. *c*
3. *c*
4. *b*
5. *b*
6. *b*
7. *d*
8. *d*
9. *c*
10. *c*
11. *b*
12. *d*
13. *c*
14. *a*
15. *c*
16. *d*
17. *c*
18. *c*
19. *d*
20. *c*
21. *a*
22. *b*
23. *b*
24. *d*
25. *c*
26. *b*
27. *c*
28. *c*
29. *d*
30. *b*
31. *c*
32. *b*

Chapter 8
1. *b*
2. *d*
3. *c*
4. *c*

5. *d*
6. *d*
7. *b*
8. *b*
9. *d*
10. *c*
11. *c*
12. *b*
13. *c*
14. *a*
15. *a*
16. *d*
17. *c*
18. *d*
19. *b*
20. *a*

Chapter 9

1. *c*
2. *c*
3. *b*
4. *a*
5. *b*
6. *b*
7. *a*
8. *c*

Chapter 10

1. *d*
2. *d*
3. *d*
4. *d*
5. *a*
6. *c*
7. *d*
8. *c*
9. *c*
10. *c*

Chapter 11

1. *c*
2. *b*
3. *c*
4. *c*
5. *d*
6. *a*
7. *d*
8. *b*
9. *d*
10. *c*
11. *a*
12. *b*
13. *d*
14. *a*
15. *c*
16. *b*
17. *d*
18. *c*
19. *b*
20. *d*

Chapter 12

1. *c*
2. *d*
3. *d*
4. *d*
5. *b*
6. *a*
7. *b*
8. *c*
9. *a*
10. *a*
11. *d*
12. *c*
13. *b*
14. *d*
15. *a*

Chapter 13

1. *b*
2. *a*
3. *c*
4. *d*
5. *c*
6. *b*
7. *b*
8. *c*

Chapter 14

1. *c*
2. *b*
3. *b*
4. *d*
5. *a*
6. *d*
7. *c*
8. *b*

Chapter 15

1. *d*
2. *c*
3. *b*
4. *d*
5. *a*
6. *a*
7. *d*
8. *c*

Chapter 16

1. *c*
2. *d*
3. *d*
4. *b*
5. *a*
6. *a*
7. *b*
8. *c*
9. *c*
10. *c*

Chapter 17

1. *b*
2. *b*
3. *a*
4. *d*
5. *d*
6. *b*
7. *b*
8. *c*
9. *a*
10. *b*
11. *b*
12. *c*
13. *c*
14. *b*
15. *c*
16. *a*
17. *c*
18. *b*

Chapter 18

1. *b*
2. *c*
3. *d*
4. *b*
5. *b*
6. *a*
7. *a*
8. *d*
9. *d*
10. *b*

Chapter 19

1. *a*
2. *b*
3. *d*
4. *b*
5. *d*
6. *c*
7. *b*
8. *d*
9. *c*
10. *d*

Chapter 20

1. *d*
2. *b*
3. *c*

4. *c*
5. *d*
6. *a*
7. *a*
8. *d*
9. *a*
10. *b*

Chapter 21
1. *b*
2. *b*
3. *c*
4. *b*
5. *d*
6. *a*
7. *c*
8. *d*
9. *a*
10. *b*
11. *a*
12. *b*
13. *c*

Chapter 22
1. *d*
2. *b*
3. *c*
4. *d*
5. *c*
6. *d*
7. *d*
8. *b*
9. *b*
10. *a*
11. *d*
12. *b*

Chapter 23
1. *b*
2. *d*
3. *a*
4. *c*
5. *b*
6. *b*
7. *a*
8. *a*
9. *d*
10. *d*

Chapter 24
1. *a*
2. *c*
3. *a*
4. *b*
5. *d*
6. *a*
7. *a*
8. *b*
9. *d*
10. *a*

Chapter 25
1. *d*
2. *c*
3. *b*
4. *c*
5. *d*
6. *a*
7. *d*
8. *a*
9. *b*
10. *d*

Chapter 26
1. *b*
2. *b*
3. *a*
4. *a*
5. *b*
6. *d*
7. *c*
8. *a*
9. *d*
10. *c*

Chapter 27
1. *a*
2. *d*
3. *c*
4. *b*
5. *a*
6. *d*
7. *b*
8. *c*
9. *c*
10. *c*

Chapter 28
1. *b*
2. *c*
3. *b*
4. *a*
5. *a*
6. *b*
7. *c*
8. *c*
9. *a*
10. *d*
11. *a*
12. *c*
13. *c*
14. *c*
15. *d*
16. *b*
17. *d*
18. *c*
19. *a*
20. *a*

Chapter 29
1. *b*
2. *d*
3. *a*
4. *b*
5. *b*
6. *c*
7. *a*
8. *b*
9. *c*
10. *d*

Chapter 30
1. *b*
2. *c*
3. *b*
4. *d*
5. *a*
6. *d*
7. *c*
8. *c*
9. *a*
10. *c*

Chapter 31
1. *a*
2. *b*
3. *b*
4. *a*
5. *c*
6. *d*
7. *d*
8. *d*

Chapter 32
1. *a*
2. *b*
3. *d*
4. *c*
5. *a*
6. *c*
7. *b*
8. *c*
9. *a*
10. *d*

Chapter 33
1. *a*
2. *d*

3. *b*
4. *c*
5. *d*
6. *d*
7. *c*
8. *d*

Chapter 34

1. *b*
2. *c*
3. *d*
4. *b*
5. *c*
6. *a*
7. *b*
8. *b*
9. *b*
10. *d*

Chapter 35

1. *c*
2. *d*
3. *a*
4. *d*
5. *a*
6. *c*
7. *a*
8. *b*

Chapter 36

1. *c*
2. *c*
3. *c*
4. *d*
5. *a*
6. *a*
7. *c*
8. *c*
9. *a*
10. *d*
11. *b*
12. *c*
13. *c*
14. *b*
15. *b*

Chapter 37

1. *d*
2. *b*
3. *b*
4. *c*
5. *d*
6. *b*
7. *c*
8. *b*
9. *a*
10. *d*

Chapter 38

1. *c*
2. *d*
3. *c*
4. *b*
5. *c*
6. *b*
7. *d*
8. *b*
9. *a*
10. *c*

Chapter 39

1. *a*
2. *b*
3. *d*
4. *c*
5. *b*
6. *c*
7. *d*
8. *d*

Chapter 40

1. *b*
2. *d*
3. *b*
4. *c*
5. *c*
6. *c*
7. *a*
8. *a*
9. *c*
10. *d*

Chapter 41

1. *a*
2. *b*
3. *c*
4. *d*
5. *d*
6. *d*
7. *b*
8. *b*
9. *c*
10. *d*

Chapter 42

1. *b*
2. *c*
3. *b*
4. *b*
5. *b*
6. *b*
7. *a*
8. *b*
9. *a*
10. *d*
11. *a*
12. *d*
13. *b*
14. *a*
15. *c*
16. *c*
17. *c*
18. *d*
19. *b*
20. *c*

Chapter 43

1. *a*
2. *c*
3. *b*
4. *b*
5. *d*
6. *d*
7. *b*
8. *c*
9. *b*
10. *b*

Chapter 44

1. *c*
2. *b*
3. *b*
4. *c*
5. *a*
6. *b*
7. *d*
8. *d*

Chapter 45

1. *c*
2. *b*
3. *d*
4. *b*
5. *d*
6. *a*
7. *d*
8. *d*

Chapter 46

1. *d*
2. *c*
3. *b*
4. *d*
5. *b*
6. *c*

7. *a*
8. *b*
9. *b*

Chapter 47

1. *b*
2. *b*
3. *d*
4. *c*
5. *a*
6. *d*
7. *c*

Chapter 48

1. *b*
2. *c*
3. *a*
4. *d*
5. *b*
6. *d*
7. *c*
8. *b*
9. *a*
10. *a*
11. *d*
12. *a*
13. *a*
14. *a*
15. *c*
16. *b*
17. *d*
18. *c*
19. *c*
20. *a*
21. *d*
22. *b*
23. *c*
24. *c*
25. *b*

Chapter 49

1. *a*
2. *d*
3. *a*
4. *c*
5. *d*
6. *d*
7. *b*
8. *a*

Further Reading

General

Bledsoe, B. E., and R. W. Benner. *Critical Care Paramedic.* Upper Saddle River, N.J.: Pearson/Prentice Hall Health, 2006.

Bledsoe, B. E., R. S. Porter, and R. A. Cherry. *Paramedic Care: Principles and Practice.* 2nd ed. 5-volume set (Vol. 1, *Introduction to Advanced Prehospital Care;* Vol. 2, *Patient Assessment;* Vol. 3, *Medical Emergencies;* Vol. 4, *Trauma Emergencies;* Vol. 5, *Special Considerations/Operations*). Upper Saddle River, N.J.: Pearson/Prentice Hall Health, 2006.

EMT-Paramedic National Standard Curriculum. Washington, D.C.: U.S. Department of Transportation, National Highway Traffic Safety Administration, 1998.

Martini, F. H., E. F. Bartholomew, and B. E. Bledsoe. *Anatomy and Physiology for Emergency Care.* Upper Saddle River, N.J.: Pearson/Prentice Hall Health, 2002.

Division One: Introduction to Advanced Prehospital Care

Alonzo-Sierra, H., D. Blanton, and R. E. O'Connor. "Physician Medical Direction in EMS." *Prehospital Emergency Care* 2(2)(1998): 153–157.

The Ambulance Service Guide to HIPAA Compliance. Mechanicsburg, Pa.: Page, Wolfberg, & Wirth, 2003.

American College of Surgeons, Committee on Trauma. *Advanced Trauma Life Support Course: Student Manual.* 5th ed. Chicago, Ill.: American College of Surgeons, 2002.

Bailey, E. D., and T. Sweeney. "Considerations in Establishing Emergency Medical Services Response Time Goals." *Prehospital Emergency Care* 7(3) (2003): 397–399.

Beauchamp, T., and J. F. Childress, Eds. *Principles of Biomedical Ethics.* 5th ed. New York: Oxford University Press, 2001.

Bhende, M. S., and D. C. LaLovey. "End-Tidal Carbon Dioxide Monitoring in the Prehospital Setting." *Prehosital Emergency Care* 5 (2001): 208–213.

Bledsoe, B. E. "Critical Incident Stress Management (CISM): Benefit or Rise for Emergency Services." *Prehospital Emergency Care* 7(2) (2003): 272–329.

Bledsoe, B. E. "EMS Needs a Few More Cowboys." *Journal of Emergency Medical Services (JEMS)* 28(12)(2003): 112–113.

Bledsoe, B. E. "Searching for the Evidence behind EMS." *Emergency Medical Services (EMS)* 31(1)(2003): 63–67.

Bledsoe, B. E. "The Golden Hour: Fact or Fiction?" *Emergency Medical Services (EMS)* 31(6)(2002): 105.

Bledsoe, B. E. "Where Are the Wise Men?" *Emergency Medical Services (EMS)* 31(10) (2002): 172.

Bledsoe, Bryan E., and Dwayne Clayden. *Prehospital Emergency Pharmacology.* 6th ed. Upper Saddle River, N.J.: Pearson/Prentice Hall, 2005.

Campbell, John Emory, and the Alabama Chapter of the American College of Emergency Physicians. *Basic Trauma Life Support for Paramedics and Other Advanced Care Providers.* 5th ed. Upper Saddle River, N.J.: Pearson/Prentice Hall, 2004.

Chung, Michele B. *Math Principles and Practice: Preparing for Health Career Success.* Upper Saddle River, N.J.: Prentice Hall, 1999.

Cotran, Ramzi, Vinay Kumar, Tucker Collins, and Stanley Robbins. *Robbins Pathological Basis of Disease.* 7th ed. Philadelphia: W. B. Saunders, 2005.

Dacey, J., J. Travers, and D. Neuki. *Human Development Across the Lifespan.* 5th ed. Dubuque, Iowa: McGraw-Hill, 2004.

Dalton, Alice L., D. Limmer, J. J. Mistovich, and H. A. Werman. *Advanced Medical Life Support.* 3rd ed. Upper Saddle River, N.J.: Pearson/Prentice Hall, 2006.

DeVito, J. *Essentials of Human Communication.* 4th ed. New York City: Longman, 2002.

EMT-Paramedic: National Standard Curriculum. Washington, D.C.: U.S. Department of Transportation, National Highway Traffic Safety Administration, 1998.

Greenwood, M. D. "Community Cooperatives Combat Sexual Assault and Domestic Violence." *Emergency Medical Services (EMS)* 32(2)(2003): 60–61.

Guyton, Arthur, and John Hall. *Textbook of Medical Physiology.* 11th ed. Philadelphia: W. B. Saunders, 2006.

Heightman, A. J. "EMS Workforce. A Comprehensive Listing of Certified EMS Providers by State and How the Workforce Has Changed Since 1993." *Journal of Emergency Medical Services (JEMS)* 25(2)(2000): 108–112.

Jaslow, D., J. Ufberg, and R. Marsh. "Primary Injury Prevention in an Urban EMS System." *Journal of Emergency Medicine* 25(2)(2003): 167–170.

Katzung, Bertram G. *Basic and Clinical Pharmacology.* 9th ed. Stamford, Conn.: Appleton & Lange, 2004.

Kübler-Ross, E. *On Death and Dying.* (Originally published 1969.) Scribner Classics reprint edition. New York: Simon & Schuster, 1997.

Kuehl, A. E. *Prehospital Systems and Medical Oversight.* 3rd ed. Dubuque, Iowa: Kendall-Hunt Publishing, 2002.

Lee, N. G. *Legal Concepts and Issues in Emergency Care.* Philadelphia: W. B. Saunders, 2001.

Lehne, Richard A. *Pharmacology for Nursing Care.* 5th ed. Philadelphia: W. B. Saunders, 2004.

Limmer, D., M. F. O'Keefe, E. T. Dickinson, et al. *Emergency Care.* 9th ed. Fire Service Edition. Upper Saddle River, N.J.: Pearson/Prentice Hall, 2003.

Mappes, T., and D. Degrazia. *Biomedical Ethics.* 5th ed. Columbus: McGraw-Hill, 2000.

Martini, Frederick. *Fundamentals of Anatomy and Physiology.* 6th ed. San Francisco: Benjamin Cummings, 2004.

McCance, Kathryn, and Sue Huether. *Pathophysiology: The Biological Basis for Disease in Adults and Children.* 4th ed. St. Louis: Mosby, 2002.

McKenny, Leda M., and Evelyn Salerno. *Pharmacology in Nursing.* 21st ed. St. Louis: Mosby, 2003.

McNally, R. J., R. A. Bryant, and A. Ehlers. "Does Early Psychological Intervention Promote Recovery from Posttraumatic Stress?" *Psychological Science in the Public Interest* 4(2)(2003): 45–79 [available at http://www.psychologicalscience.org/journals/pspi/index.html].

McSwain, Norman E., and Scott Frame. *Prehospital Trauma Life Support.* 5th ed. St. Louis: Mosby, 2003.

Mikolaj, Alan A. *Drug Dosage Calculations for the Emergency Care Provider.* 2nd ed. Upper Saddle River, N.J.: Pearson/Prentice Hall, 2003.

Mistovich, Joseph J., Randall W. Benner, and Gregg Margolis. *Prehospital Advanced Cardiac Life Support.* 2nd ed. Upper Saddle River, N.J.: Pearson/Prentice Hall, 2004.

Mosesso, V. N., Jr., C. R. Packer, J. McMahon, T. E. Auble, and P. M. Paris. "Influenza Immunizations Provided by EMS Agencies: The MEDICVAX Project." *Prehospital Emergency Care* 7(1)(2003): 74–78.

National Academies of Emergency Dispatch. *Emergency Telecommunicator Course Manual.* Sudbury, Ma.: Jones and Bartlett Publishers, 2001.

National Academy of Sciences, National Research Council. *Accidental Death and Disability: The Neglected Disease of Modern Society.* Washington, D.C.: U.S. Department of Health, Education, and Welfare, 1966.

National Highway Traffic Safety Administration. *Emergency Medical Dispatch National Standard Curriculum, Instructor's Guide.* Washington, D.C.: National Highway Traffic Safety Administration, 1996.

National Highway Traffic Safety Administration. *The EMS Agenda for the Future.* Washington, D.C.: National Highway Traffic Safety Administration, 1996 [available at http://www.nhtsa.dot.gov/people/injury/ems/agenda/emsman.html].

Page, J. O. "Anatomy of a Lawsuit." *JEMS* 14 (1989).
Page, J. O. *Simple Advice.* San Diego, CA: JEMS Publishing, 2002.
Page, J. O. *The Magic of 3 AM.* San Diego, CA: JEMS Publishing, 2002.
Page, J. O. *The Paramedics.* Morristown, N.J.: Backdraft Publications, 1979. [No longer available for purchase except as a used book. Entire book can be viewed online at http://www.JEMS.com/Paramedics.]
Persse, D. E., C. B. Key, R. N. Bradley, C. C. Miller, and A. Dhingra. "Cardiac Arrest Survival as a Function of Ambulance Deployment Strategy in a Large Urban Emergency Medical Services System." *Resuscitation* 59(1)(2003): 97–104.
Roberts, James R., and Jerris R. Hedges. *Clinical Procedures in Emergency Medicine.* 4th ed. Philadelphia: W. B. Saunders Company, 2004.
Rogan, Dennis. *For Love of Life.* Sydney, NSW, Australia: NSW Ambulance Publishing Services, 1986.
Rosen, Peter, and Roger M. Barkin. *Emergency Medicine Concepts and Clinical Practice.* 5th ed. Philadelphia: W. B. Saunders Company, 2002.
Shannon, Margaret T., Billie Ann Wilson, and Carolyn L. Stang. *Prentice Hall's Health Professionals Drug Guide 2005–2006.* Upper Saddle River, N.J.: Pearson/Prentice Hall, 2005.
Sherwood, Lauralee. *Human Physiology: From Cells to Systems.* 5th ed. Belmont, Calif.: Wadsworth, 2004.
Stewart, Charles E. *Advanced Airway Management.* Upper Saddle River, N.J.: Pearson/Prentice Hall, 2002.
Streger, M. "Keeping Kids Safe: Injury Prevention Programs in EMS." *Emergency Medical Services (EMS)* 31(6)(2002): 24.
Streger, M. "Professionalism." *Emergency Medical Services (EMS)* 23(1)(2003): 35.
Walz, B. J. *Introduction to EMS Systems.* Albany, N.Y.: Delmar Thomson Learning, 2002.
Weiss, S. J., R. Chong, M. Ong, A. A. Ernst, and M. Balash. "Emergency Medical Services Screening of Elderly Falls in the Home." *Prehospital Emergency Care* 7(1) (2003): 79–84.
Williams, M. E. *The American Geriatrics Society's Complete Guide to Aging and Health.* New York: Harmony Books, 1995.
Yancey, A. H. 2nd, R. Martinez, and A. L. Kellermann. "Injury Prevention and Emergency Medical Services: The 'Accendents Aren't' Program." *Prehospital Emergency Care* 6(2)(2002): 204–209.

Division Two: Patient Assessment

Bates, Barbara, Lynn S. Bickley, and Robert A. Hoekelman. *A Guide to Physical Examination and History Taking.* 8th ed. Philadelphia: J. B. Lippincott, 2003.
Bradford, C. A. *Basic Ophthalmology for Medical Students and Primary Care Residents.* 7th ed. San Francisco: American Academy of Ophthalmology, 1999.
Campbell, John E. *Basic Trauma Life Support for Paramedics and Advanced EMS Providers.* 5th ed. Upper Saddle River, N.J.: Pearson/Prentice Hall, 2004.
Coulehan, John L., and Marian R. Block. *The Medical Interview: Mastering Skills for Clinical Practice.* 4th ed. Philadelphia: F. A. Davis, 2001.
Dalton, Alice L., D. Limmer, J. J. Mistovich, and H. A. Werman. *Advanced Medical Life Support.* 3rd ed. Upper Saddle River, N.J.: Pearson/Prentice Hall, 2006.
Eichelberger, Martin R., et al. *Pediatric Emergencies: A Manual for Prehospital Care Providers.* 2nd ed. Upper Saddle River, N.J.: Pearson/Prentice Hall, 1998.
Epstein, Owen, et al. *Clinical Examination.* 3rd ed. St. Louis: Mosby, 2003.
Foltin, George, et al. *Teaching Resource for Instructors in Prehospital Pediatrics for Paramedics.* New York: Center for Pediatric Medicine, 2002.
Hazinski, Mary Fran, Ed. *Textbook of Pediatric Advanced Life Support.* Dallas: American Heart Association, 2002.
Lipkin, Mack Jr., Samuel M. Putnam, and Aaron Lazare. *The Medical Interview: Clinical Care, Education, and Research.* New York: Springer, 1996.

Martini, Frederick. *Fundamentals of Anatomy and Physiology.* 6th ed. Upper Saddle River, N.J.: Pearson/Prentice Hall, 2004.

Netter, F. H. *Netter's Atlas of Human Anatomy.* 3rd ed. Icon Learning Systems, 2002.

Seidel, Henry M., et al. *Mosby's Guide to Physical Examination.* 5th ed. St. Louis: Mosby, 2003.

Yanoff, M., et al. *Ophthalmology.* 2nd ed. St. Louis: Elsevier Science, 2004.

Division Three: Trauma Emergencies

American College of Surgeons, Committee on Trauma. *Advanced Trauma Life Support Course: Student Manual.* Chicago: American College of Surgeons, 2003.

American College of Surgeons, Committee on Trauma. *Resources for Optimal Care of the Injured Patient.* Chicago: American College of Surgeons, 1998.

Bates, Barbara, Lynn S. Bickley, and Robert A. Hoekelman. *A Guide to Physical Examination and History Taking.* 8th ed. Philadelphia: J. B. Lippincott, 2003.

Baxt, William G. *Trauma, The First Hour.* Upper Saddle River, N.J.: Pearson/Prentice Hall, 1985.

Bledsoe, Bryan E., and Dwayne E. Clayden. *Pocket-Reference for ALS Providers.* 3rd ed. Upper Saddle River, N.J.: Pearson/Prentice Hall, 2006.

Bledsoe Bryan E., and Dwayne Clayden. *Prehospital Emergency Pharmacology.* 6th ed. Upper Saddle River, N.J.: Pearson/Prentice Hall, 2005.

Campbell, John E. *Basic Trauma Life Support for Paramedics and Other Advanced Providers.* 5th ed. Upper Saddle River, N.J.: Pearson/Prentice Hall, 2004.

Clemente, C. D. *Anatomy: A Regional Atlas of the Human Body.* 4th ed. Baltimore: Lippincott, Williams, & Wilkins, 1997.

Cooper, M. A. "Electrical and Lightning Injuries," in Rosen, P., and R. Barkin, Eds. *Emergency Medicine: Concepts and Clinical Practice.* 5th ed. St. Louis: Mosby, 2002.

De Lorenzo, Robert A., and Robert S. Porter. *Tactical Emergency Care: Military and Operational Out-of-Hospital Medicine.* Upper Saddle River, N.J.: Pearson/Prentice Hall, 1999.

Di Maio, Vincent J. *Gunshot Wounds: Practical Aspects of Firearms, Ballistics, and Forensic Techniques.* 2nd ed. New York: CRC Press, 1999.

Edlich, R. F, and J. C. Moghtader. "Chemical Injuries," in Rosen, P., and R. Barkin, Eds. *Emergency Medicine: Concepts and Clinical Practice.* 5th ed. St. Louis: Mosby, 2002.

Feliciano, D. V., et al. *Trauma.* 5th ed. New York: McGraw-Hill, 2004.

Hall-Craggs, E. C. B. *Anatomy as a Basis for Clinical Medicine.* 3rd ed. Baltimore: Lippincott, Williams, & Wilkins, 1995.

Ivatury R. R., and G. C. Cayten, eds. *Textbook of Penetrating Trauma.* Media, Pa.: Williams & Wilkins, 1996.

Markovchick, V. "Radiation Injuries," in Rosen, P., and R. Barkin, Eds. *Emergency Medicine: Concepts and Clinical Practice.* 5th ed. St. Louis: Mosby, 2002.

Martini, Frederic. *Fundamentals of Anatomy and Physiology.* 6th ed. San Francisco: Benjamin Cummings, 2004.

Maull, Kimball Kirby, and Jackie and Dennis Rowe. *Trauma Update for the EMT.* Upper Saddle River, N.J.: Pearson/Prentice Hall, 1992.

McManus, W. F., and B. A. Pruitt, Jr. "Thermal Injuries," in Feliciano, D. V., E. E. Moore, and K. L. Mattox, eds. *Trauma.* 5th ed. New York: McGraw-Hill, 2004.

McSwain, N. E., and S. B. Frame, Eds. *Prehospital Trauma Life Support.* 5th ed. St. Louis: Mosby, 2003.

Monafo, W. W. "Initial Management of Burns." *New England Journal of Medicine* 335 (1996): 1581–1586.

Rosen, P., and R. Barkin, Eds. *Emergency Medicine: Concepts and Clinical Practice.* 5th ed. St. Louis: Mosby, 2002.

Uman, Martin A. *All About Lightning.* Mineola, N.Y.: Dover Publications, 1987.

Division Four: Medical Emergencies

American Psychiatric Association. *Diagnostic and Statistical Manual of Mental Disorders-TR.* 4th ed. (*DSM-IV*-Text Revision). Washington, D.C.: American Psychiatric Press, 2000.

Atkinson, T. P., and M. A. Kaliner. "Anaphylaxis." *The Medical Clinics of North America* 6 (July 1992): 4.

Beasley, B. M. *Understanding 12-Lead EKGs: A Practical Approach.* 2nd ed. Upper Saddle River, N.J.: Pearson/Prentice Hall, 2001.

Beasley, B. M. *Understanding EKGs: A Practical Approach.* 2nd ed. Upper Saddle River, N.J.: Pearson/Prentice Hall, 2003.

Bledsoe, B. E. "Dealing with Diabetic Emergencies." *JEMS* 16(12)(1991): 40–50.

Bledsoe, B. E. "No More Coma Cocktails: Using Science to Dispel and Improve Patient Care." *JEMS* 27(11)(2002): 54–60.

Bledsoe, B. E., and D. Clayden. *Prehospital Emergency Pharmacology.* 6th ed. Upper Saddle River, N.J.: Pearson/Prentice Hall, 2005.

Braunwald, E., et al. *Harrison's Principles of Internal Medicine.* 15th ed. New York: McGraw-Hill, 2001.

Brooks, G. F., J. S. Butel, and S. A. Morse. *Jawetz, Melnick, and Adelberg's Medical Microbiology.* 22nd ed. Stamford, Conn.: Appleton & Lange, 2001.

Brunner, Lillian, et al. *Brunner and Suddarth's Textbook of Medical-Surgical Nursing.* 10th ed. Philadelphia: Lippincott, Williams, and Wilkins, 2003.

Canan, S., C. D. Miller, and M. Taigman. *Taigman's Advanced Cardiology (in Plain English).* Upper Saddle River, N.J.: Pearson/Prentice Hall, 1995.

Cecil, R. L., et al. *Cecil Essentials of Medicine.* 6th ed. Philadelphia: W. B. Saunders, 2004.

Chin, J. E., Ed. *Control of Communicable Diseases Manual.* 17th ed. Washington, D.C.: American Public Health Association, 2001.

Cunningham, F., et al. *Williams Obstetrics.* 21st ed. New York: McGraw-Hill, 2002.

Dalton, Alice L., D. Limmer, J. J. Mistovich, and H. A. Werman. *Advanced Medical Life Support.* 3rd ed. Upper Saddle River, N.J.: Pearson/Prentice Hall, 2006.

Garcia, T. B., and N. E. Holtz. *12-Lead ECG: The Art of Interpretation.* Sudburry, Mass.: Jones & Bartlett, 2001.

Gates, R. H. *Infectious Disease Secrets.* 2nd ed. Philadelphia: Hanley and Belfus, 2004.

Goldfrank, L. R., Ed., and Neal E. Flamenbau (contributor). *Goldfink's Toxicologic Emergencies.* 7th ed. New York: McGraw-Hill, 2002.

Gorbach, S., J. Bartlett, and N. Blacklow. *Infectious Diseases.* 2nd ed. Philadelphia: Saunders, 1998.

Greenspan, Francis S., and Gordon J. Strewler. *Basic & Clinical Endocrinology.* 7th ed. Stamford, Conn.: Appleton & Lange, 2004.

Guyton, A. C., and J. E. Hall. *Textbook of Medical Physiology.* 11th ed. Philadelphia: W. B. Saunders, 2006.

Isada, C. M., et al. *Infectious Diseases Handbook.* 5th ed. Hudson, Oh.: Lexi-Comp Inc., 2003.

Isselbacher, K. J., et al. *Harrison's Principles of Internal Medicine.* 15th ed. New York: McGraw-Hill, 2001.

Kidwell, C. S., S. Starkman, M. Eckstein, K. Weems, and J. L. Saver. "Identifying Stroke in the Field. Prospective Validation of the Los Angeles Prehospital Stroke Screen (LAPSS)." *Stroke* 31(1) (January 2000): 71–76.

Kothari, R. U., A. Pancioli, T. Liu, T. Brott, and J. Broderick. "Cincinnati Prehospital Stroke Scale: Reproducibility and Validity." *Annals of Emergency Medicine* 33(4) (April 1999): 373–378.

Ladewig, P. W., M. L. London, and S. B. Olds. *Contemporary Maternal-Newborn Maternal Care.* 5th ed. Menlo Park, Calif.: Addison Wesley Longman, Inc., 2001.

Marieb, E. N., Ed. "The Respiratory System," in *Human Anatomy and Physiology.* 6th ed. San Francisco: Benjamin Cummings, 2004.

McCance, K. L., and S. E. Huether. *Pathophysiology: The Biologic Basis for Disease in Adults and Children.* 4th ed. St. Louis: C. V. Mosby Company, 2001.

Mueller, P. D., and W. S. Korey. "Death by Ecstasy." *Annals of Emergency Medicine* 32(3) (1998).

National Association of EMS Physicians. "Patient Restraint in Emergency Medical Services Systems." *Prehospital Emergency Care* 6(3) (2002): 340–345.

National Institute of Neurological Disorders and Stroke. *Rapid Identification and Treatment of Acute Stroke.* Bethesda, Md.: National Institutes of Health, 1997.

Portier, P., and C. Richet. "De L'action Anphylactique de Certains Venins." *CR Soc Biol (Paris)* 6:170 (1902).

Rosen, P., et al. *Emergency Medicine Concepts and Clinical Practice.* 5th ed. St. Louis: Mosby, 2002.

Ross, C. "A Trauma Patient with Sickle Cell Disease." *Journal of Emergency Nursing* (June 1997): 211–213.

Runge, J. W., et al. "Histamine Antagonists in the Treatment of Acute Allergic Reactions." *Annals of Emergency Medicine* (March 1992): 21.

Salomone, J. A. "Anaphylaxis and Acute Allergic Reactions," in J. E. Tintinalli, et al., Eds., *Emergency Medicine: A Comprehensive Study Guide.* 6th ed. New York: McGraw-Hill, 2004.

Saunders, C. E., and R. Humphries. *Current Emergency Diagnosis and Treatment.* 5th ed. New York: McGraw-Hill, 2004.

Shah, K. H., R. K. Simons, T. Holbrook, D. Fortlage, R. J. Winchell, and D. B. Hoyt. "Trauma in Pregnancy: Maternal and Fetal Outcomes." *The Journal of Trauma* 45(1): 83–86.

Soreff, S. M., and R. T. Cadigan. *EMS Street Strategies.* Albany, N.Y.: Delmar Learning, 2004.

Spitzer, R. L., et al. *DSM-IV-TR Casebook.* Washington, D.C.: American Psychiatric Press, 2002.

Stewart, C. E. "Sexually Related Trauma: Female Injuries." *Emergency Medical Services* 24(4) (April 1995): 48–53.

Taylor, M. *Gastrointestinal Emergencies.* 2nd ed. Baltimore: Williams and Wilkins, 1997.

Thibodeau, G. A., and K. T. Patton, Eds. "Anatomy of the Respiratory System and Physiology of the Respiratory System," in *Anatomy and Physiology.* 5th ed. St. Louis: Mosby, 2003.

Tintanelli, J. E., et al. *Emergency Medicine: A Comprehensive Study Guide.* 6th ed. New York: McGraw-Hill, 2004.

Tortora, Gerard J., and Sandra Reynolds Grabowski. *Principles of Anatomy and Physiology.* 10th ed. New York: John Wiley & Sons, 2001.

Division Five: Special Considerations/Operations

Abrams, W. B., et al., Eds. *The Merck Manual of Geriatrics.* 3rd ed. Whitehouse Station, N.J.: Merck Research Laboratories, 2000.

American Academy of Pediatrics. *Pediatric Education for Prehospital Professionals.* Sudbury, Ma.: Jones and Bartlett Publishers, 2000.

American Geriatrics Society, National Council of State EMS Coordinators. *Geriatric Education for Emergency Medical Services.* Sudbury, Ma.: Jones and Bartlett Publishers, 2003.

American Heart Association. *Guidelines 2000 for Cardiopulmonary Resuscitation and Emergency Cardiovascular Care.* Dallas, Tex.: American Heart Association, 2000.

American Heart Association and American Academy of Pediatrics. *PALS Provider Manual.* 4th ed. Dallas, Tex.: American Heart Association, 2000.

ASTM F 1288–90. *Standard Guide for Planning and Responding to a Multiple Casualty Incident.* West Conshohocken, Pa.: ASTM International, 1998.

Auerbach, P. S. *Wilderness Medicine.* 4th ed. St. Louis, Mo.: Mosby-Year Book, 2001.

Barry, P. *Mental Health & Mental Illness.* 7th ed. Philadelphia: Lippincott, 2002.

Becker, L. R. "Ambulance Crashes: Protecting Yourself and Your Patient." *Journal of Emergency Medical Services* 28(5) (2003): 24–26.

Beers, M. H., et al. *The Merck Manual of Diagnosis and Therapy.* 17th ed. Whitehouse Station, N.J.: Merck Research Laboratories, 1999.

Behrman, R. E., et al. *Nelson Textbook of Pediatrics.* 17th ed. Philadelphia, Pa.: W. B. Saunders Company, 2004.

Bevelacqua, A., and R. Stilp. *Terrorism Handbook for Operational Responders.* Clifton Park, N.Y.: Delmar Learning, 2004.

Bledsoe, B., and D. Clayden. *Prehospital Emergency Pharmacology.* 6th ed. Upper Saddle River, N.J.: Pearson/Prentice Hall, 2005.

Braner, D., J. Kattwinkel, S. Denson, and S. Niermeyer, Eds. *Neonatal Resuscitation.* 4th ed. Elk Grove Village, Ill.: American Academy of Pediatrics, 2000.

Brennan, K. *Rope Rescue for Firefighting.* Saddlebrook, N.J.: Fire Engineering, 1998.

Buck, G. *Preparing for Biological Terrorism: An Emergency Services Guide.* Albany, N.Y.: Delmar Publishing, 2001.

Byrnes, M. E., D. A. King, and P. M. Tierno. *Nuclear, Chemical, and Biological Terrorism: Emergency Response and Public Protection.* Chelsea, Mi.: Lewis Publishers, 2003.

Christen, H., and P. Maniscalco. *The EMS Incident Management System: EMS Operations for Mass Casualty and High-Impact Incidents.* Upper Saddle River, N.J.: Pearson/Prentice Hall, 1998.

Cohn, B. M., A. J. Azzara, and R. Petrie. "EMS and Law Enforcement," in *Legal Aspects of Emergency Medical Services.* Philadelphia, Pa.: W. B. Saunders, Co., 1998.

Custalow, C. B., and C. S. Gravitz. "Emergency Medical Vehicle Collisions and Potential for Preventive Intervention." *Prehospital Emergency Care* 8(2) (2004): 175–184.

Dalton, Alice L., D. Limmer, J. J. Mistovich, and H. A. Werman. *Advanced Medical Life Support.* 3rd ed. Upper Saddle River, N.J.: Pearson/Prentice Hall, 2006.

DeBoer, J. L. *Emergency Newborn Care: The First Minutes of Life.* Chicago, Ill.: ACM Publications, 2004.

DeGraeve, K., K. F. Deroo, P. A. Calle, O. A. Vanhaute, and W. A. Buylaert. "How to Modify the Risk-Taking Behaviour of Emergency Medical Services Drivers?" *European Journal of Emergency Medicine* 10(2) (2003): 111–116.

DeLorenzo, Robert A., and Robert S. Porter. *Tactical Emergency Care: Military and Operational Out-of-Hospital Medicine.* Upper Saddle River, N.J.: Pearson/Prentice Hall, 1999.

DeLorenzo, Robert A., and Robert S. Porter. *Weapons of Mass Destruction: Emergency Care.* Upper Saddle River, N.J.: Pearson/Prentice Hall, 2000.

Dick, T. "Addressing the Need for Speed." *Emergency Medical Services* 33(6) (2004): 68.

Dickinson, E. T., D. Limmer, M. O'Keefe, et al. *Emergency Care.* 9th ed. Fire Service Edition. Upper Saddle River, N.J.: Pearson/Prentice Hall, 2003.

Dresser, R. *When Science Offers Salvation: Patient Advocacy and Research Ethics.* Oxford, UK: Oxford University Press, 2001.

Early Identification of Hearing Impairment in Infants and Young Children, Program and Abstracts. Bethesda, Md.: National Institutes of Health, 1993.

Eichelberger, M. R., et al. *Pediatric Emergencies.* 2nd ed. Upper Saddle River, N.J.: Pearson/Prentice Hall, 1998.

Eliopilos, L. N. *Death Investigator's Handbook: A Field Guide to Crime Scene Processing, Forensic Evaluation, and Investigation Techniques.* Expanded and Updated Edition. Boulder, Colo.: Paladin Press, 2003.

Emergency Program Manager. Washington, D.C.: Federal Emergency Management Agency, Emergency Management Institute IS-1.

Emergency Response Guidebook (ERG2004). Washington, D.C.: U.S. Department of Transportation, 2004.

Emergency Response to Terrorism: Basic Concepts Student Manual. Emmitsburg, Md.: U.S. Fire Administration, National Fire Academy, 1997.

Federal Bureau of Investigation. *Uniform Crime Statistics.* Washington, D.C.: FBI, 2003.

Final Report: Alfred P. Murrah Federal Building Bombing, April 19, 1995. The City of Oklahoma. Stillwater, Okla.: Fire Protection Publications, 1996.

Fitch, J., et al. *EMS Management: Beyond the Street.* 2nd ed. Carlsbad, Calif.: JEMS Publishing, 2004.

Friedman, H. H. *Problem Oriented Medical Diagnosis.* 7th ed. Philadelphia, Pa.: Lippincott, Williams, and Wilkins, 2000.

Gausche-Hill, M., et al. *Pediatric Airway Management for the Prehospital Professional.* Sudbury, Ma.: Jones and Bartlett Publishers, 2004.

"Geriatric Considerations," in Harwood-Nuss, A. L., et al., Eds. *Clinical Practice of Emergency Medicine.* 3rd ed. Philadelphia: Lippincott-Raven, 2000.

"Geriatric Trauma" and "Abuse in the Elderly and Impaired," in Tintinalli, J. E., et al., Eds. *Emergency Medicine: A Comprehensive Study Guide.* 6th ed. New York: McGraw-Hill, 2004.

Giardino, A. P., and E. R. Giardino. *Recognition of Child Abuse for the Mandated Reporter.* 3rd ed. St. Louis, Mo.: G. W. Medical Publishers, 2003.

Goldfarb, Z., and S. Kuhr. "EMS Response to the Explosion," in Manning, W., Ed. *The World Trade Center Bombing: Report and Analysis.* Washington, D.C.: Federal Emergency Management Agency, United States Fire Administration, National Fire Data Center.

Hankins, D. G. "Hazardous Materials," in Kuehl, A. E., Ed. *Prehospital Systems & Medical Oversight.* 3rd ed. Dubuque, Iowa: Kendall/Hunt, 2002.

Hawley, C. *Hazardous Materials Response and Operations.* Albany, N.Y.: Delmar Publishers, 2000.

Hendrick, W., and A. Zafares. *Surface Ice Rescue.* Saddlebrook, N.J.: Fire Engineering, 1999.

Hobbs, C. J., and J. M. Wynne. *Physical Signs of Child Abuse: A Colour Atlas.* 2nd ed. London: W. B. Saunders, 2002.

Holleran, R. S., et al. *Air and Surface Patient Transport: Principles and Practice.* 3rd ed. St. Louis: Mosby, 2003.

Illustrated Guide to Home Health Care. Springhouse, Pa.: Springhouse Corporation, 1995.

Incident Command System for Emergency Medical Services, Student Manual. Washington, D.C.: Federal Emergency Management Agency, United States Fire Administration, National Fire Academy.

Kehner, G. *Date Rape Drugs.* Broomall, Pa.: Chelsea House Publishers, 2004.

Kuehl, A. E. *Prehospital Systems and Medical Oversight.* 3rd ed. Dubuque, Iowa: Kendall/Hunt Publishing, 2002.

Leonard, J. E., and G. D. Robinson. *Managing Hazardous Materials.* Rockville, Md.: Institute of Hazardous Materials Management, 2002.

Lesak, D. M. *Hazardous Materials: Strategies and Tactics.* Upper Saddle River, N.J.: Pearson/Prentice Hall, 1999.

Lilja, G. P., M. A. Madsen, and J. Overton. "Multiple Casualty Incidents," in Kuehl, A. E., Ed., *Prehospital Systems & Medical Oversight.* 3rd ed. Dubuque, Iowa: Kendall/Hunt, 2002.

MacDonald, M., Ed. *Guidelines for Air and Ground Transport of Neonatal and Pediatric Patients.* Washington, D.C.: American Academy of Pediatrics, 1999.

Markenson, D. S. *Pediatric Prehospital Care.* Upper Saddle River, N.J.: Pearson/Prentice Hall, 2002.

Marks, M. E. *Emergency Responder's Guide to Terrorism.* Chester, Md.: Red Hat Publishers, 2003.

Martinette Jr., C. V. *Trench Rescue.* Sudbury, Ma.: Jones and Bartlett Publishers, 2002.

Merrick, C., Ed. *Rescue Technician: Operational Readiness for Rescue Providers.* St. Louis: Mosby-Year Book, 1998.

Meyer, E. *Chemistry of Hazardous Materials.* 4th ed. Upper Saddle River, N.J.: Brady Pearson, 1998.

Moore, R. E. *Vehicle Rescue and Extrication.* 2nd ed. St. Louis: Mosby Lifeline, 2003.

National Association of EMS Physicians Position Paper. "Guidelines for Air Medical Dispatch." *Prehospital Emergency Care* 7(2) (2003): 265–271.

National Incident Management System (NIMS). Washington, D.C.: U.S. Department of Homeland Security, 2004. NIMS information also available from the Department of Homeland Security website: http://www.dhs.gov (keyword: NIMS).

Neal, L. J., and S. E. Guillet. *Care of the Adult with a Chronic Illness or Disability: A Team Approach.* St. Louis, MO: Mosby-Year Book, 2004.

Noll, G. G., M. S. Hildebrand, and J. G. Yvorra. *Hazardous Materials: Managing the Incident.* 2nd ed. Stillwater, Okla.: Fire Protection Publications, 1995.

Page, J. "Silly Vests and Dunce Caps: Which Would You Rather Wear as an Incident Commander?" *Rescue* (January–February 1996): 6.

Patrick, R. W. "Emergency Vehicle Driving and Traffic Preemption." *Emergency Medical Services* 33(6) (2004): 78–79.

Peto, G. J., and W. J. Medve. *EMS Driving: The Safe Way.* Upper Saddle River, N.J.: Pearson/Prentice Hall, 1996.

Phipps, W., et al. *Medical-Surgical Nursing: Health and Illness Perspective.* St. Louis: Mosby-Year Book, 2003.

Ray, S. *Swiftwater Rescue: A Manual for the Rescue Professionals.* Ashville, N.C.: CPS Press, 1997.

Redman, B. K. *Patient Self-Management of Chronic Disease: The Health Care Provider's Challenge.* Sudbury, Ma.: Jones and Bartlett Publishers, 2003.

Reece, R. M. *Child Abuse: Medical Diagnosis and Management.* 2nd ed. Philadelphia: Lippincott, Williams, & Wilkins, 2002.

Rosen, P., et al. *Emergency Medicine: Concepts and Clinical Practice.* 5th ed. St. Louis: Mosby, 2002.

Sachs, G. *Terrorism Emergency Response: A Workbook for Responders.* Upper Saddle River, N.J.: Pearson/Prentice Hall, 2003.

Schmidt, C. A. "EMS on the Acute Interventions for Chronic-Care Patients." *JEMS* (December 1999): 68–76.

Smith, D. S., and S. J. Smith. *Water Rescue: Basic Skills for Emergency Responders.* St. Louis: Mosby Lifeline, 1994.

Spratt, S. J., et al., Eds. *Home Health Care: Principles and Practices.* Delray Beach, Fl.: GR/St. Lucie Press, 1997.

Strange, G., et al. *Pediatric Emergency Medicine: A Comprehensive Study Guide.* 2nd ed. New York: McGraw-Hill, 2002.

Stutz, D. R., and S. Ulin. *Haztox: EMS Response to Hazardous Materials Incidents.* Miramar, Fla.: GDS Communications, 1994.

Tilton, B., and F. Hubbell. *Medicine for the Backcountry.* 3rd ed. Guilford, Conn.: Globe Pequot, 2000.

Tintinalli, J. E., R. L. Krome, and E. Ruiz. *Emergency Medicine: A Comprehensive Study Guide.* 6th ed. New York: McGraw-Hill, Inc., 2004.

Tunik, M. G., et al. *Teaching Resource for Instructors in Prehospital Pediatrics.* New York: Center for Pediatric Medicine, 1998.

U.S. Department of Justice. *National Crime Victimization Survey.* Washington, D.C.: Bureau of Justice Statistics, 1996.

U.S. Department of Justice. *Violence against Women.* Washington, D.C.: Bureau of Justice Statistics, 1994.

Vines, T. *High-Angle Rescue Techniques.* 3rd ed. St. Louis: Mosby, 2004.

Wilkerson, J. A. *Medicine for Mountaineering & Other Wilderness Activities.* 5th ed. Seattle, Wash.: The Mountaineers, 2002.

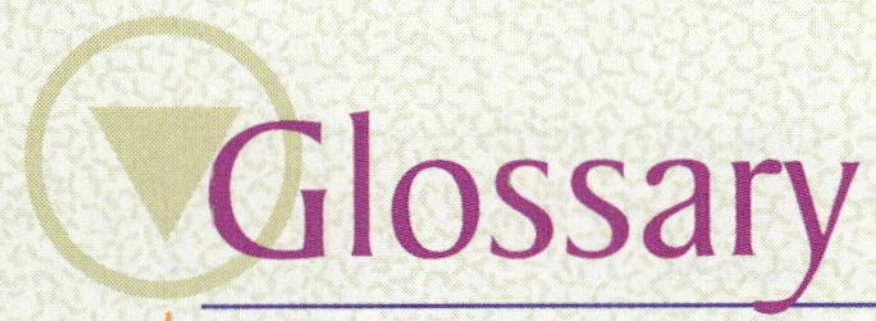

Glossary

10-code radio communications system using codes that begin with the word *ten.*

2,3-diphosphoglycerate (2,3-DPG) chemical in the red blood cells that affects hemoglobin's affinity for oxygen.

abandonment termination of the paramedic-patient relationship without assurance that an equal or greater level of care will continue.

ABCs airway, breathing, and circulation.

abduction movement of a body part away from the midline.

aberrant conduction conduction of the electrical impulse through the heart's conductive system in an abnormal fashion.

ABO blood groups four blood groups formed by the presence or absence of two antigens known as A and B. A person may have either (type A or type B), both (type AB), or neither (type O). An immune response will be activated whenever a person receives blood containing A or B antigen if this antigen is not already present in his own blood.

abortion termination of pregnancy before the 20th week of gestation. The term refers to both miscarriage and induced abortion. Commonly, *abortion* is used for elective termination of pregnancy and *miscarriage* for the loss of a fetus by natural means. A miscarriage is sometimes called a "spontaneous abortion."

abrasion scraping or abrading away of the superficial layers of the skin; an open soft-tissue injury.

abruptio placentae a condition in which the placenta separates from the uterine wall.

absence seizure type of generalized seizure with sudden onset, characterized by a brief loss of awareness and rapid recovery.

absolute refractory period the period of the cardiac cycle when stimulation will not produce any depolarization whatsoever.

acceleration the rate at which speed or velocity increases.

acclimatization the reversible changes in body structure and function by which the body becomes adjusted to a change in environment.

acetylcholinesterase (AChE) enzyme that stops the action of acetylcholine, a neurotransmitter.

acid a substance that liberates hydrogen ions (H^+) when in solution.

acidosis a high concentration of hydrogen ions; a pH below 7.35.

acquired immunity immunity that develops over time and results from exposure to an antigen or that is transferred to the person from an outside source.

acquired immunodeficiency syndrome *see* AIDS.

acrocyanosis cyanosis of the extremities.

action potential the stimulation of myocardial cells, as evidenced by a change in the membrane electrical charge, that subsequently spreads across the myocardium.

activated charcoal a powder, usually premixed with water, that will adsorb (bind) some poisons and help prevent them from being absorbed by the body.

active immunity acquired immunity that occurs following exposure to an antigen and results in the production of antibodies specific for the antigen.

active listening the process of responding to a person's statements with words or gestures that demonstrate your understanding.

active rescue zone area where special rescue teams operate; also known as the *hot zone* or *inner circle.*

active transport movement of a substance through a cell membrane against the osmotic gradient; that is, from an area of lesser concentration to an area of greater concentration, opposite to the normal direction of diffusion; requires the use of energy to move a substance.

actual damages refers to compensable physical, psychological, or financial harm.

acuity the severity or acuteness of a patient's condition.

acute arterial occlusion the sudden occlusion of arterial blood flow.

acute coronary syndrome (ACS) a spectrum of disease processes, from myocardial ischemia and injury to myocardial infarction.

acute effects signs and/or symptoms rapidly displayed on exposure to a toxic substance.

acute gastroenteritis sudden onset of inflammation of the stomach and intestines.

acute myocardial infarction (AMI) *see* myocardial infarction.

acute pulmonary embolism blockage that occurs when a blood clot or other particle lodges in a pulmonary artery.

acute renal failure (ARF) the sudden onset of severely decreased urine production.

acute respiratory distress syndrome (ARDS) respiratory insufficiency marked by progressive hypoxemia, due to severe inflammatory damage; also known as *adult respiratory distress syndrome.*

acute retinal artery occlusion a nontraumatic occlusion of the retinal artery resulting in a sudden, painless loss of vision in one eye.

acute tubular necrosis a syndrome characterized by the sudden death of renal tubular cells.

addendum addition or supplement to an original report.

addiction compulsive and overwhelming dependence on a drug; an addiction may be a physiological dependence, a psychological dependence, or both.

Addison's disease endocrine disorder characterized by adrenocortical insufficiency. Symptoms may include weakness, fatigue, weight loss, and hyperpigmentation of skin and mucous membranes.

Addisonian crisis form of shock associated with adrenocortical insufficiency and characterized by profound hypotension and electrolyte imbalances.

adduction movement of a body part toward the midline.

adenosine triphosphate (ATP) a high-energy compound present in all cells, especially muscle cells; when split by enzyme action it yields energy. Energy is stored in ATP.

adhesion union of normally separate tissue surfaces by a fibrous band of new tissue.

adjunct medication agent that enhances the effects of other drugs.

administration tubing flexible, clear plastic tubing that connects the solution bag to the IV cannula.

administrative law law that is enacted by governmental agencies at either the federal or state level. Also called *regulatory law.*

adrenergic pertaining to the neurotransmitter norepinephrine. *See also* sympathomimetic.

adult respiratory distress syndrome (ARDS) form of pulmonary edema that is caused by fluid accumulation in the interstitial space within the lungs; also known as *acute respiratory distress syndrome.*

advance directive a document created to ensure that certain treatment choices are honored when a patient is unconscious or otherwise unable to express his choice of treatment.

advanced life support (ALS) life-support activities that go beyond basic procedures to include adjunctive equipment and invasive procedures such as intravenous therapy, drug therapy, intubation, and defibrillation.

aerobic metabolism the second stage of metabolism, requiring the presence of oxygen, in which the breakdown of glucose (in a process called the Krebs or citric acid cycle) yields a high amount of energy. *Aerobic* means "with oxygen."

aeromedical evacuations transport by helicopter or fixed-wing aircraft.

affect visible indicators of mood.

affinity force of attraction between a drug and a receptor.

afterbirth the placenta and accompanying membranes that are expelled from the uterus after the birth of a child.

afterload the resistance against which the heart must pump.

against medical advice (AMA) when a patient refuses care even though he is told he needs it.

ageism discrimination against aged or elderly people.

aggregate to cluster or come together.

agonist drug that binds to a receptor and causes it to initiate the expected response.

agonist-antagonist (partial agonist) drug that binds to a receptor and stimulates some of its effects but blocks others.

AIDS acronym for *acquired immunodeficiency syndrome,* a group of signs, symptoms, and disorders that often develop as a consequence of HIV infection.

air embolism air in the vein.

airborne transmitted through the air by droplets or particles.

air-purifying respirator (APR) system of filtering a normal environment for a specific chemical substance, using filter cartridges.

albumin a protein commonly present in plant and animal tissues. In the blood, albumin works to maintain blood volume and blood pressure and provides colloid osmotic pressure, which prevents plasma loss from the capillaries.

algorithm schematic flow chart that outlines appropriate care for specific signs and symptoms.

alimentary canal *see* digestive tract.

alkali a substance that liberates hydroxyl ions (OH^-) when in solution; a strong base.

alkalosis a low concentration of hydrogen ions; a pH above 7.45.

allergen a substance capable of inducing allergy of specific hypersensitivity. Allergens may be protein or non-protein, although most are proteins.

allergic reaction an exaggerated response by the immune system to a foreign substance.

allergy exaggerated immune response to an environmental antigen.

allied health professions ancillary health care professions, apart from physicians and nurses.

alloimmunity *see* isoimmunity.

alveoli microscopic air sacs in the lungs where most oxygen and carbon dioxide gas exchanges take place.

Alzheimer's disease a degenerative brain disorder; the most common cause of dementia in the elderly.

amnesia *see* anterograde amnesia; retrograde amnesia.

amniotic fluid clear, watery fluid that surrounds and protects the developing fetus.

amniotic sac the membranes that surround and protect the developing fetus during intrauterine development.

ampere basic unit for measuring the strength of an electric current.

amphiarthrosis joint that permits a limited amount of independent motion.

ampule breakable glass vessel containing liquid medication.

amputation severance, removal, or detachment, either partial or complete, of a body part.

amyotrophic lateral sclerosis (ALS) progressive degeneration of specific nerve cells that control voluntary movement characterized by weakness, loss of motor control, difficulty speaking, and cramping. Also called *Lou Gehrig's disease.*

anabolism the constructive or "building up" phase of metabolism in which cells convert nonliving substances into living cytoplasm.

anaerobic able to live without oxygen.

anaerobic metabolism the first stage of metabolism, which does not require oxygen, in which the breakdown of glucose (in a process called glycolysis) produces pyruvic acid and yields very little energy. *Anaerobic* means "without oxygen."

analgesia the absence of the sensation of pain.

analgesic medication that relieves the sensation of pain.

anaphylactic shock *see* anaphylaxis.

anaphylaxis an unusual or exaggerated allergic reaction to a foreign protein or other substance; also called *anaphylactic shock. Anaphylaxis* means the opposite of *phylaxis,* which means "protection."

anastomosis communication between two or more vessels.

anatomy the structure of an organism; body structure.

anchor time set of hours when a night-shift worker can reliably expect to rest without interruption.

anemia a reduction in red blood cells or in the hemoglobin content within the red blood cells to a point below that required to meet the oxygen requirements of the body.

anesthesia the absence of all sensations.

anesthetic medication that induces a loss of sensation to touch or pain.

aneurysm the ballooning of an arterial wall, resulting from a defect or weakness in the wall.

anger hostility or rage to compensate for an underlying feeling of anxiety.

angina pectoris chest pain that results when the myocardial demand for oxygen exceeds the heart's ability to deliver an adequate supply of oxygenated blood to the myocardium.

angiocatheter *see* over-the-needle catheter.

angioneurotic edema marked edema of the skin that usually involves the head, neck, face, and upper airway; a common manifestation of severe allergic reactions and anaphylaxis.

anion ion with a negative charge—so called because it will be attracted to an anode, or positive pole.

anorexia lack of appetite.

anorexia nervosa psychological disorder characterized by voluntary refusal to eat.

anoxia the absence or near absence of oxygen.

anoxic hypoxemia an oxygen deficiency due to disordered pulmonary mechanisms of oxygenation.

antacid alkalotic compound used to increase the gastric environment's pH.

antagonist drug that binds to a receptor but does not cause it to initiate the expected response.

antepartum before the onset of labor.

anterior cord syndrome condition that is caused by bony fragments or pressure compressing the arteries of the anterior spinal cord and resulting in loss of motor function and sensation to pain, light touch, and temperature below the injury site.

anterior medial fissure deep crease along the ventral surface of the spinal cord that divides the cord into right and left halves.

anterograde amnesia inability to remember events that occurred after the trauma that caused the condition. *See also* retrograde amnesia.

antiadrenergic *see* sympatholytic.

antibiotic agent that kills or decreases the growth of bacteria.

antibody a substance produced by B lymphocytes in response to the presence of a foreign antigen that will combine with and control or destroy the antigen, thus preventing infection. *See also* immunoglobulin (IG).

anticholinergic *see* parasympatholytic.

anticoagulant drug that inhibits blood clotting.

antidiuresis formation and passage of a concentrated urine, preserving blood volume.

antidote a substance that will neutralize a specific toxin or counteract its effect on the body.

antidysrhythmic drug used to treat and prevent abnormal cardiac rhythms.

antiemetic medication used to prevent vomiting.

antigen a marker on the surface of a cell that identifies it as "self" or "non-self" and that is capable, under appropriate conditions, of inducing a specific immune response.

antihistamine medication that arrests the effects of histamine by blocking its receptors.

antihyperlipidemic drug used to treat high blood cholesterol.

antihypertensive drug used to treat hypertension, or high blood pressure.

antineoplastic agent drug used to treat neoplasms, or cancer.

antiplatelet drug that decreases the formation of platelet plugs.

antiseptic cleansing agent that destroys or inhibits pathogenic microorganisms but is not toxic to living tissue.

antitussive medication that suppresses the stimulus to cough in the central nervous system.

anuria no elimination of urine.

anxiety state of uneasiness, discomfort, apprehension, and restlessness.

anxiety disorder condition characterized by dominating apprehension and fear.

anxious avoidant attachment a type of bonding that occurs when an infant learns that his caregivers will not be responsive or helpful when needed.

anxious resistant attachment a type of bonding that occurs when an infant learns to be uncertain about whether or not his caregivers will be responsive or helpful when needed.

aortic dissection a degeneration of the wall of the aorta.

APGAR scoring a numerical system of rating the condition of a newborn. It evaluates the newborn's heart rate, respiratory rate, muscle tone, reflex irritability, and color.

aphasia absence or impairment of the ability to communicate through speaking, writing, or signing as a result of brain dysfunction. *Sensory aphasia* is when the person cannot understand the spoken word. *Motor aphasia* is when the person can understand what is said but cannot speak. *Global aphasia* is when the person has both sensory and motor aphasia.

apnea absence of breathing.

apneustic respiration breathing characterized by a prolonged inspiration unrelieved by expiration attempts, seen in patients with damage to the upper part of the pons.

apoptosis response in which an injured cell releases enzymes that engulf and destroy itself; one way the body rids itself of damaged and dead cells.

appendicitis inflammation of the vermiform appendix at the juncture of the large and small intestines.

appendicular skeleton bones of the extremities, shoulder girdle, and pelvis (excepting the sacrum).

aqueous humor clear fluid filling the anterior chamber of the eye.

arachnoid membrane middle layer of the meninges.

ARDS *see* acute respiratory distress syndrome; adult respiratory syndrome.

arrhythmia the absence of cardiac electrical activity; often used interchangeably with *dysrhythmia.*

arterial gas embolism (AGE) an air bubble, or air embolism, that enters the circulatory system from a damaged lung.

arteriosclerosis a thickening, loss of elasticity, and hardening of the walls of the arteries from calcium deposits.

arthritis inflammation of a joint.

articular surface surface of a bone that moves against another bone.

artifact deflection on the ECG produced by factors other than the heart's electrical activity.

artificially acquired immunity *see* induced active immunity.

ascending loop of Henle the part of the renal tubule beyond the descending loop of Henle.

ascending tracts bundles of axons along the spinal cord that transmit signals from the body to the brain.

ascites an accumulation of fluid in the peritoneal space and in the abdomen; often a result of congestive heart failure or liver failure.

asepsis a condition free of pathogens.

asphyxia a decrease in the amount of oxygen and an increase in the amount of carbon dioxide as a result of some interference with respiration.

aspiration inhaling foreign material, such as vomitus, into the lungs.

assault an act that unlawfully places a person in apprehension of immediate bodily harm without his consent.

assay test that determines the amount and purity of a given chemical in a preparation in the laboratory.

asthma a condition marked by recurrent attacks of dyspnea with wheezing due to spasmodic constriction of the bronchi, often as a response to allergens, or by mucous plugs in the arterial walls.

ataxic respiration poor respirations due to central nervous system damage, causing ineffective thoracic muscular coordination.

atelectasis alveolar collapse.

atherosclerosis a progressive, degenerative disease of the medium-sized and large arteries.

atrophy a decrease in cell size resulting from a decreased workload.

atypical angina *see* Prinzmetal's angina.

augmented limb leads another term for unipolar limb leads reflecting the fact that the ground lead is disconnected, which increases the amplitude of deflection on the ECG tracing. *See also* unipolar limb leads.

aural medication drug administered through the mucous membranes of the ear and ear canal.

auscultation listening with a stethoscope for sounds produced by the body.

authoritarian a parenting style that demands absolute obedience without regard to a child's individual freedom.

authoritative a parenting style that emphasizes a balance between a respect for authority and individual freedom.

autoimmune disease condition in which the body makes antibodies against its own tissues.

autoimmunity an immune response to self-antigens, which the body normally tolerates.

automatic collision notification (ACN) system data collection and transmission system that can automatically contact a national call center or local public safety answering point and transmit specific crash data.

automaticity capability of self-depolarization by pacemaker cells of the heart.

autonomic dysfunction an abnormality of the involuntary aspect of the nervous system.

autonomic ganglia groups of autonomic nerve cells located outside the central nervous system.

autonomic hyperreflexia syndrome condition associated with the body's adjustment to the effects of neurogenic shock; presentations include sudden hypertension, bradycardia, pounding headache, blurred vision, and sweating and flushing of the skin above the point of injury.

autonomic nervous system the part of the nervous system controlling involuntary bodily functions. It is divided into the sympathetic and the parasympathetic systems.

autonomic neuropathy condition that damages the autonomic nervous system, which usually senses changes in core temperature and controls vasodilation and perspiration to dissipate heat.

autonomy a competent adult patient's right to determine what happens to his own body.

autoregulation process that controls blood flow to the brain tissue by causing alterations in the blood pressure.

avulsion forceful tearing away or separation of body tissue; an avulsion may be partial or complete.

axial loading application of the forces of trauma along the axis of the spine; this often results in compression fractures of the spine.

axial skeleton bones of the head, thorax, and spine.

B lymphocytes white blood cells that, in response to the presence of an antigen, produce antibodies that attack the antigen, develop a memory for the antigen, and confer long-term immunity to the antigen.

Babinski's response a response in which the big toe dorsiflexes and the other toes fan out when sole is stimulated.

bacterial tracheitis bacterial infection of the airway, subglottic region; in children, most likely to appear after episodes of croup.

bactericidal capable of killing bacteria.

bacteriostatic capable of inhibiting bacterial growth or reproduction.

bacterium single-cell organism with a cell membrane and cytoplasm but no organized nucleus that binds to the cells of a host organism to obtain food and support; *plural:* bacteria.

bag-valve mask ventilation device consisting of a self-inflating bag with two one-way valves and a transparent plastic face mask.

ballistics the study of projectile motion and its interactions with the gun, the air, and the object it contacts.

barotrauma injury caused by pressure within an enclosed space.

basal metabolic rate (BMR) rate at which the body consumes energy just to maintain stability; the basic metabolic rate (measured by the rate of oxygen consumption) of an awake, relaxed person 12 to 14 hours after eating and at a comfortable temperature.

basic life support (BLS) basic lifesaving procedures such as artificial ventilation and cardiopulmonary resuscitation (CPR).

basophil type of white blood cell that participates in allergic responses.

battery the unlawful touching of another individual without his consent.

Battle's sign *see* retroauricular ecchymosis.

behavior a person's observable conduct and activity.

behavioral emergency situation in which a patient's behavior becomes so unusual that it alarms the patient or another person and requires intervention.

Bell's palsy one-sided facial paralysis with an unknown cause characterized by the inability to close the eye, pain, tearing of the eyes, drooling, hypersensitivity to sound, and impairment of taste.

bend fracture fracture characterized by angulation and deformity in the bone without an obvious break.

bends *see* decompression illness.

beneficence the principle of doing good for the patient.

benign prostatic hypertrophy a noncancerous enlargement of the prostate associated with aging.

bereavement death of a loved one.

bilateral periorbital ecchymosis black-and-blue discoloration of the area surrounding the eyes. It is usually associated with basilar skull fracture. Also called *raccoon eyes.*

bills of lading *see* shipping papers.

bioassay test to ascertain a drug's availability in a biological model.

bioavailability amount of a drug that is still active after it reaches its target tissue.

bioequivalence relative therapeutic effectiveness of chemically equivalent drugs.

bioethics ethics as applied to the human body.
biologic half-life time the body takes to clear one half of a drug.
biological agents either living organisms or toxins produced by living organisms that are deliberately distributed to cause disease and death.
biological/organic related to disease processes or structural changes in the body.
biotoxin poisons that are produced by a living organism but are themselves not alive.
biotransformation chemical alteration of a substance within the body; in the case of hazardous materials, the body works to create less toxic materials.
BiPAP bilevel positive airway pressure.
bipolar disorder condition characterized by one or more manic episodes, with or without periods of depression.
bipolar limb leads electrocardiogram leads applied to the arms and legs that contain two electrodes of opposite (positive and negative) polarity; leads I, II, and III.
birth injury avoidable and unavoidable mechanical and anoxic trauma incurred by the newborn during labor and delivery.
blast wind the air movement caused as the heated and pressurized products of an explosion move outward.
blepharospasm twitching of the eyelids.
blood pressure force of blood against artery walls as the heart contracts and relaxes.
blood spatter evidence the pattern blood forms when it is spattered or dropped at the scene of a crime.
blood tube glass container with color-coded, self-sealing rubber top.
blood tubing administration tubing that contains a filter to prevent clots or other debris from entering the patient.
bloodborne transmitted by contact with blood or body fluids.
blood–brain barrier tight junctions of the capillary endothelial cells in the central nervous system vasculature through which only non-protein-bound, highly lipid-soluble drugs can pass.
blunt trauma injury caused by the collision of an object with the body in which the object does not enter the body.
body armor vest made of tightly woven, strong fibers that offer protection against handgun bullets, most knives, and blunt trauma.
body language *see* nonverbal communication.
body surface area (BSA) amount of a patient's body affected by a burn.
Bohr effect phenomenon in which a decrease in PCO_2/acidity causes an increase in the quantity of oxygen that binds with the hemoglobin; conversely, an increase in PCO_2/acidity causes the hemoglobin to give up a greater quantity of oxygen.
bolus concentrated mass of medication.
bonding the formation of a close personal relationship (as between mother and child), especially through frequent or constant association.
borborygmi loud, prolonged, gurgling bowel sounds indicating hyperperistalsis.
bowel obstruction blockage of the hollow space within the intestines.
Bowman's capsule the hollow, cup-shaped first part of the renal nephron tubule.
bradycardia a heart rate less than 60 beats per minute.
bradypnea slow respiration.
brain abscess a collection of pus localized in an area of the brain.
brain attack *see* stroke.
brain ischemia injury to brain tissues caused by an inadequate supply of oxygen and nutrients.
brainstem the part of the brain connecting the cerebral hemispheres with the spinal cord. It is comprised of the medulla oblongata, the pons, and the midbrain.
branches functional levels within the Incident Management System based on primary roles and geographic locations.
breach of duty an action or inaction that violates the standard of care expected from a paramedic.
bronchi tubes from the trachea into the lungs.
bronchiectasis chronic dilation of a bronchus or bronchi, with a secondary infection typically involving the lower portion of the lung.
bronchiolitis viral infection of the medium-sized airways, occurring most frequently during the first year of life.
bronchophony abnormal clarity of patient's transmitted voice sounds.
Broselow tape a measuring tape for infants that provides important information regarding airway equipment and medication doses based on the patient's length.
Brown-Séquard syndrome condition caused by partial cutting of one side of the spinal cord resulting in sensory and motor loss to that side of the body.
Brudzinski's sign physical exam finding in which flexion of the neck causes flexion of the hips and knees.
bruit sound of turbulent blood flow around a partial obstruction; usually associated with atherosclerotic disease.
bubble sheet scannable run sheet on which boxes or "bubbles" are filled in to record assessment and care information.

buccal between the cheek and gums.
buckle fracture fracture characterized by a raised or bulging projection at the fracture site.
buffer a substance that tends to preserve or restore a normal acid–base balance by increasing or decreasing the concentration of hydrogen ions.
bulimia nervosa recurrent episodes of binge eating.
bundle branch block a kind of interventricular heart block in which conduction through either the right or left bundle branches is blocked or delayed.
bundle of Kent an accessory AV conduction pathway that is thought to be responsible for the ECG findings of preexcitation syndrome.
burette chamber calibrated chamber of Berutrol IV administration tubing that enables precise measurement and delivery of fluids and medicated solutions.
burnout a condition that occurs when coping mechanisms no longer buffer stressors, which may compromise personal health and well-being.
bursae sacs containing synovial fluid that cushion adjacent structures; *singular:* bursa.
bursitis acute or chronic inflammation of the small synovial sacs.
caliber the diameter of a bullet expressed in hundredths of an inch (.22 caliber = 0.22 inches); the inside diameter of the barrel of a handgun, shotgun, or rifle.
callus thickened area that forms at the site of a fracture as part of the repair process.
CAMEO® Computer-Aided Management of Emergency Operations; website developed by the EPA and NOAA as a source of information, skills, and links related to hazardous substances.
cancellous having a latticework structure, as in the spongy tissue of a bone.
cannula hollow needle used to puncture a vein.
cannulation *see* intravenous access.
capnography a recording or display of the measurement of exhaled carbon dioxide concentrations.
carboxyhemoglobin hemoglobin with carbon monoxide bound.
cardiac arrest the absence of ventricular contraction.
cardiac contractile force force of the strength of a contraction of the heart.
cardiac cycle the period of time from the end of one cardiac contraction to the end of the next.
cardiac depolarization a reversal of charges at a cell membrane so that the inside of the cell becomes positive in relation to the outside; the opposite of the cell's resting state in which the inside of the cell is negative in relation to the outside.
cardiac monitor machine that displays and records the electrical activity of the heart.
cardiac muscle *see* muscle tissue.
cardiac output the amount of blood pumped by the heart in 1 minute.
cardiac tamponade accumulation of excess fluid inside the pericardium.
cardiogenic shock shock caused by insufficient cardiac output; the inability of the heart to pump enough blood to perfuse all parts of the body.
cardiovascular disease (CVD) disease affecting the heart, the peripheral blood vessels, or both.
carrier-mediated diffusion process in which carrier proteins transport large molecules across the cell membrane; also called *facilitated diffusion.*
cartilage connective tissue providing the articular surfaces of the skeletal system.
case law *see* common law.
catabolism the destructive or "breaking down" phase of metabolism in which cells break down complex substances into simpler substances with release of energy.
cataracts medical condition in which the lens of the eye loses its clearness.
catatonia condition characterized by immobility and stupor, often a sign of schizophrenia.
catecholamine a hormone such as epinephrine or norepinephrine that strongly affects the nervous and cardiovascular systems, metabolic rate, temperature, and smooth muscle.
catheter inserted through the needle Teflon catheter inserted through a large metal stylet; also called *intracatheter.*
cation ion with a positive charge—so called because it will be attracted to a cathode, or negative pole.
cauda equina syndrome condition occurring when nerve roots at the lower end of the spinal cord are compressed, interrupting sensation and movement.
cavitation the outward motion of tissue due to a projectile's passage, resulting in a temporary cavity and vacuum.
cell the basic structural unit of all plants and animals; a membrane enclosing a thick fluid and a nucleus. Cells are specialized to carry out all of the body's basic functions.
cell-mediated immunity the short-term immunity to an antigen provided by T lymphocytes, which directly attack the antigen but do not produce antibodies or memory for the antigen.
cell membrane the outer covering of a cell; also called *plasma membrane.*
cellular immunity immunity resulting from a direct attack of a foreign substance by specialized cells of the immune system.
cellular swelling swelling of a cell caused by injury to or change in permeability of the cell membrane with resulting inability to maintain stable intra- and extracellular fluid and electrolyte levels.

cellular telephone system telephone system divided into regions, or cells, that are served by radio base stations.

cellulitis inflammation of cellular or connective tissue.

central cord syndrome condition usually related to hyperflexion of the cervical spine that results in motor weakness, usually in the upper extremities, and possible bladder dysfunction.

central IV line intravenous line placed into the superior vena cava for the administration of long-term fluid therapy.

central nervous system the brain and the spinal cord.

central neurogenic hyperventilation hyperventilation caused by a lesion in the central nervous system, often characterized by rapid, deep, noisy respirations.

central pain syndrome condition resulting from damage or injury to the brain, brainstem, or spinal cord characterized by intense, steady pain described as burning, aching, tingling, or a "pins and needles" sensation.

central venous access surgical puncture of the internal jugular, subclavian, or femoral vein.

cerebellum portion of the brain located dorsally to the pons and medulla oblongata. It plays an important role in the fine control of voluntary muscular movements.

cerebral perfusion pressure (CPP) the pressure moving blood through the brain.

cerebrospinal fluid fluid surrounding and bathing the brain and spinal cord.

cerebrovascular accident (CVA) *see* stroke.

cerebrum largest part of the brain. It consists of two hemispheres separated by a deep longitudinal fissure. It is the seat of consciousness and the center of the higher mental functions such as memory, learning, reasoning, judgment, intelligence, and emotions.

certification the process by which an agency or association grants recognition to an individual who has met its qualifications.

cerumen earwax.

C-FLOP mnemonic for the main functional areas with the Incident Management System—command, finance/administration, logistics, operations, and planning.

chain of evidence legally retaining items of evidence and accounting for their whereabouts at all times to prevent loss or tampering.

chancroid highly contagious sexually transmitted ulcer.

chemotactic factors chemicals released by white blood cells that attract more white blood cells to an area of inflammation.

chemotaxis the movement of white blood cells in response to chemical signals.

CHEMTEL, Inc. Chemical Telephone, Incorporated; maintains a 24-hour, toll-free hotline at 800-255-3024; for collect calls and calls from other points of origin, dial 813-979-0626.

CHEMTREC Chemical Transportation Emergency Center; maintains a 24-hour toll-free hotline at 800-424-9300; for collect calls and calls from other points of origin, dial 703-527-3887.

chest leads *see* precordial leads.

Cheyne-Stokes respirations respiratory pattern of alternating periods of apnea and tachypnea.

chickenpox *see* varicella.

chief complaint the pain, discomfort, or dysfunction that caused the patient to request help.

child abuse physical or emotional violence or neglect toward a person from infancy to 18 years of age.

chlamydia group of intracellular parasites that cause sexually transmitted diseases.

choanal atresia congenital closure of the passage between the nose and pharynx by a bony or membranous structure.

cholinergic pertaining to the neurotransmitter acetylcholine. *See also* parasympathomimetic.

chronic gastroenteritis non-acute inflammation of the gastrointestinal mucosa.

chronic obstructive pulmonary disease (COPD) a disease such as emphysema, chronic bronchitis, or asthma characterized by a decreased ability of the lungs to perform the function of ventilation.

chronic renal failure permanently inadequate renal function due to nephron loss.

chronotropy pertaining to heart rate.

chyme semifluid mixture of ingested food and digestive secretions found in the stomach and small intestine.

circadian rhythms physiological phenomena that occur at approximately 24-hour intervals.

circulation assessment evaluating the pulse and skin and controlling hemorrhage.

circulatory overload an excess in intravascular fluid volume.

circumduction movement at a synovial joint where the distal end of a bone describes a circle but the shaft does not rotate; movement through an arc of a circle.

cirrhosis degenerative disease of the liver.

civil law the division of the legal system that deals with noncriminal issues and conflicts between two or more parties.

claudication *see* intermittent claudication.

cleaning washing an object with cleaners such as soap and water.

cleft lip congenital vertical fissure in the upper lip.

cleft palate congenital fissure in the roof of the mouth, forming a passageway between oral and nasal cavities.

clinical judgment the use of knowledge and experience to diagnose patients and plan their treatment.

clitoris highly innervated and vascular erectile tissue anterior to the labia minora.

clonic phase phase of a seizure characterized by alternating contraction and relaxation of muscles.

closed fracture a broken bone in which the bone ends or the forces that caused it do not penetrate the skin.

closed incident an incident that is not likely to generate any further patients; also known as a *contained incident.*

closed questions questions that ask for specific information and require only very short or yes-or-no answers. Also called *direct questions.*

closed stance a posture or body position that is tense and suggests negativity, discomfort, fear, disgust, or anger.

clotting the body's response to stop the loss of blood.

coagulation the third step in the clotting process, which involves the formation of a protein called fibrin that forms a network around a wound to stop bleeding, ward off infection, and lay a foundation for healing and repair of the wound.

coagulation necrosis the process in which an acid, while destroying tissue, forms an insoluble layer that limits further damage.

cold zone location at a hazardous materials incident outside the warm zone; area where incident operations take place; also called the *green zone* or the *safe zone.*

colic acute pain associated with cramping or spasms in the abdominal organs.

collagen tough, strong protein that comprises most of the body's connective tissue.

collecting duct the larger structure beyond the distal tubule into which urine drips.

colloid intravenous solution containing large proteins that cannot pass through capillary membranes.

colloid osmotic pressure *see* oncotic force.

colostomy opening of a portion of the colon through the abdominal wall, allowing feces to be collected outside the body.

coma a state of unconsciousness from which the patient cannot be aroused.

Command the individual or group responsible for coordinating all activities and who makes final decisions at the scene of a multiple-casualty incident; often referred to as the *Incident Commander (IC)* or *Officer in Charge (OIC).*

Command Post (CP) place where command officers from various agencies can meet with each other and select a management staff.

Command Staff officers who report directly to the Incident Commander at a multiple-casualty incident; officers who handle public information, safety, outside liaisons, and critical stress debriefing; also known as the *Management Staff.*

comminuted fracture fracture in which a bone is broken into several pieces.

common law law that is derived from society's acceptance of customs and norms over time. Also called *case law* or *judge-made law.*

communicable capable of being transmitted to another host.

communicable period time when a host can transmit an infectious agent to someone else.

communication the exchange of common symbols—written, spoken, or other kinds such as signing and body language.

community-acquired infection an infection occurring in a nonhospitalized patient who is not undergoing regular medical procedures, including the use of instruments such as catheters. *See also* nosocomial infection.

comorbidity associated disease process; having more than one disease at a time.

compartment syndrome muscle ischemia that is caused by rising pressures within an anatomical fascial space.

compensated shock early stage of shock during which the body's compensatory mechanisms are able to maintain normal perfusion.

compensatory pause the pause following an ectopic beat where the SA node is unaffected and the cadence of the heart is uninterrupted.

competent able to make an informed decision about medical care.

competitive antagonism when one drug binds to a receptor and causes the expected effect while also blocking another drug from triggering the same receptor.

complex partial seizure type of partial seizure usually originating in the temporal lobe characterized by an aura and focal findings such as alterations in mental status or mood. *See also* partial seizures.

compliance the stiffness or flexibility of the lung tissue.

concealment hiding behind objects that shield a person from view but that offer little or no protection against bullets or other ballistics. *See also* cover.

concentration weight per volume.

concussion a transient period of unconsciousness. In most cases, the unconsciousness will be followed by a complete return of function.

conduction moving electrons, ions, heat, or sound waves through a conductor or conducting medium.

conductive deafness deafness caused when there is a blocking of the transmission of the sound waves through the external ear canal to the middle or inner ear.

conductivity ability of the cells to propagate the electrical impulse from one cell to another.

confidentiality the principle of law that prohibits the release of medical or other personal information about a patient without the patient's consent.

confusion state of being mentally unclear or unable to make a decision easily.

congenital present at birth.

congestive heart failure (CHF) condition in which the heart's reduced stroke volume causes an overload of fluid in the body's other tissues.

conjunctiva mucous membrane that lines the eyelids.

connective tissue the most abundant body tissue; it provides support, connection, and insulation. Examples: bone, cartilage, fat, blood.

consensual reactivity the response of both eyes to changes in light intensity that affect only one eye.

consensus standards widely agreed-on guidelines, such as those developed by the National Fire Protection Association and others.

consent a patient's granting of permission for treatment.

constitutional law law based on the U.S. Constitution.

contamination presence of an agent on the surface of the host without penetrating it.

contamination reduction zone *see* warm zone.

continuous quality improvement (CQI) a program designed to refine and improve an EMS system, emphasizing customer satisfaction.

CONTOMS Counter-Narcotics Tactical Operations; program that manages the training and certification of EMT-Tacticals and SWAT-Medics.

contractility ability of muscle cells to contract, or shorten.

contrecoup injury occurring on the opposite side; an injury to the brain opposite the site of impact. *See also* coup injury.

contusion closed wound in which the skin is unbroken, although damage has occurred to the tissue immediately beneath.

convection transfer of heat via currents in liquids or gases.

conventional reasoning the stage of moral development during which children desire approval from individuals and society.

convergent focusing on only the most important aspect of a critical situation.

COPD *see* chronic obstructive pulmonary disease (COPD).

cor pulmonale overload of the right ventricle of the heart resulting from pulmonary hypertension.

core temperature the body temperature of the deep tissues, which usually does not vary more than a degree or so from its normal 37°C (98.6°F).

cornea thin, delicate layer of tissue covering the pupil and the iris.

coronary heart disease (CHD) a type of cardiovascular disease; the single largest killer of Americans.

corrected QT (QTc) QT interval divided by the square root of the RR interval.

cortex the outer tissue of an organ such as the kidney.

cortisol a steroid hormone released by the adrenal cortex that regulates the metabolism of fats, carbohydrates, sodium, potassium, and proteins and also has an anti-inflammatory effect.

coup injury an injury to the brain occurring on the same side as the site of impact. *See also* contrecoup injury.

coupling interval distance between the preceding beat and the PVC.

cover hiding behind solid and impenetrable objects that protect a person from bullets. *See also* concealment.

CPAP continuous positive airway pressure.

crackles light crackling, popping, nonmusical sounds that may be heard, usually during inspiration.

cramping muscle pain resulting from overactivity, lack of oxygen, and accumulation of waste products.

cranial nerves twelve pairs of nerves that extend from the lower surface of the brain.

cranium vaultlike portion of the skull encasing the brain.

creatinine a waste product caused by metabolism within muscle cells.

crepitus crunching or crackling sounds of fracture bone ends or unlubricated joints rubbing against each other.

cricothyroid membrane membrane between the cricoid and thyroid cartilages of the larynx.

cricothyrotomy a surgical incision into the cricothyroid membrane, usually to provide an emergency airway; also called *cricothyrostomy.*

criminal law division of the legal system that deals with wrongs committed against society or its members.

critical thinking thought process involving analysis and evaluation.

Crohn's disease idiopathic inflammatory bowel disorder commonly affecting the distal portion of the small intestine.

croup laryngotracheobronchitis; a common viral infection of young children, resulting in edema of the sub-glottic tissues; characterized by barking cough and inspiratory stridor.

crowning the bulging of the fetal head past the opening of the vagina during a contraction. Crowning is an indication of impending delivery.

crumple zone the region of a vehicle designed to absorb the energy of impact.

crush injury mechanism of injury in which tissue is locally compressed by high pressure forces.

crush syndrome systemic disorder of severe metabolic disturbances resulting from the crush of a limb or other body part.

crystalloid intravenous solution that contains electrolytes but lacks the larger proteins associated with colloids. In solution, unlike a colloid, a crystalloid can diffuse through a membrane such as a capillary wall.

Cullen's sign discoloration around the umbilicus (occasionally the flanks) suggestive of intra-abdominal hemorrhage.

cultural imposition the imposition of one's beliefs, values, and patterns of behavior on people of another culture.

current the rate of flow of an electric charge.

Cushing's reflex response to cerebral ischemia characterized by an increase in systemic blood pressure, which maintains cerebral perfusion during increased intracranial pressure.

Cushing's syndrome pathological condition resulting from excess adrenocortical hormones. Symptoms may include changed body habits, hypertension, and vulnerability to infection.

Cushing's triad the combination of increasing blood pressure, slowing pulse, and erratic respirations in response to increased intracranial pressure.

cyanosis bluish discoloration of the skin due to a reduction of hemoglobin in the blood resulting from poor ventilation.

cystic fibrosis *see* mucoviscidosis.

cystic medial necrosis a death or degeneration of a part of the wall of an artery.

cystitis an infection and inflammation of the urinary bladder.

cytochrome oxidase enzyme complex, found in cellular mitochondria, that enables oxygen to create the adenosine triphosphate (ATP) required for all muscle energy.

cytoplasm the thick fluid that fills a cell; also called *protoplasm.*

deafness the inability to hear.

deceleration the rate at which speed or velocity decreases.

decerebrate posture sustained contraction of extensor muscles of the extremities resulting from a lesion in the brainstem. The patient presents with stiff and extended extremities and retracted head. *See also* decorticate posture.

decode to interpret a message.

decompensated shock advanced stages of shock when the body's compensatory mechanisms are no longer able to maintain normal perfusion; also called *progressive shock.*

decompression illness development of nitrogen bubbles within the body's tissues due to a rapid reduction of air pressure when a diver returns to the surface; also called *the bends.*

decontaminate to destroy or remove pathogens.

decontamination the process of minimizing toxicity by reducing the amount of toxin absorbed into the body.

decorticate posture characteristic posture associated with a lesion at or above the upper brainstem. The patient presents with the arms flexed, fists clenched, and legs extended. *See also* decerebrate posture.

deep frostbite freezing involving epidermal and subcutaneous tissues resulting in a white appearance, hard (frozen) feeling on palpation, and loss of sensation.

deep venous thrombosis a blood clot in a vein.

defamation an intentional false communication that injures another person's reputation or good name.

defibrillation the process of passing an electrical current through a fibrillating heart to depolarize a critical mass of myocardial cells. This allows them to depolarize uniformly, resulting in an organized rhythm.

degenerative neurological disorders a collection of diseases that selectively affect one or more functional systems of the central nervous system.

degloving injury avulsion in which the mechanism of injury tears the skin off the underlying muscle, tissue, blood vessels, and bone.

degranulation the emptying of granules from the interior of a mast cell into the extracellular environment.

dehydration excessive loss of body fluid.

delayed effects signs, symptoms, and/or conditions developed hours, days, weeks, months, or even years after the exposure.

delayed hypersensitivity reaction a hypersensitivity reaction that takes place after the elapse of some time following reexposure to an antigen. Delayed hypersensitivity reactions are usually less severe than immediate reactions. *See also* immediate hypersensitivity reaction.

DeLee suction trap a suction device that contains a suction trap connected to a suction catheter. The negative pressure that powers it can come either from the mouth of the operator or, preferably, from an external vacuum source.

delirium condition characterized by relatively rapid onset of widespread disorganized thought; an acute alteration in mental functioning that is often reversible.

delirium tremens (DTs) disorder found in habitual and excessive users of alcoholic beverages after cessation of drinking for 48–72 hours. Patients experience visual, tactile, and auditory disturbances. Death may result in severe cases.

delusions fixed, false beliefs not widely held within the individual's cultural or religious group.

demand valve device a ventilation device that is manually operated by a push button or lever.

dementia condition involving gradual development of memory impairment and cognitive disturbance; a deterioration of mental status usually associated with structural neurologic disease. It is often progressive and irreversible.

demobilized released for use outside the incident, as occurs when resources including personnel, vehicles, and equipment are no longer needed at the scene.

demographic pertaining to population makeup or changes.

demyelination destruction or removal of the myelin sheath of nerve tissue; found in Guillain-Barré syndrome.

denature alter the usual substance of something.

depersonalization feeling detached from oneself.

deployment strategy used by an EMS agency to maneuver its ambulances and crews in an effort to reduce response times.

depression profound sadness or feeling of melancholy; a mood disorder characterized by hopelessness and malaise.

dermatome topographical region of the body surface innervated by one nerve root.

dermis true skin, also called the *corium;* it is the layer of tissue producing the epidermis and housing the structures, blood vessels, and nerves normally associated with the skin.

descending loop of Henle the part of the renal tubule beyond the proximal tubule.

descending tracts bundles of axons along the spinal cord that transmit signals from the brain to the body.

desired dose specific quantity of medication needed.

detailed physical exam careful, thorough process of eliciting the history and conducting a physical exam.

devascularization loss of blood vessels from a body part.

diabetes mellitus disorder of inadequate insulin activity, due either to inadequate production of insulin or to decreased responsiveness of body cells to insulin.

diabetic coma *see* diabetic ketoacidosis.

diabetic ketoacidosis complication of diabetes caused by decreased insulin secretion or intake and characterized by high levels of blood glucose, metabolic acidosis, and, in advanced stages, coma; often referred to as *diabetic coma.*

diabetic retinopathy slow loss of vision as a result of damage done by diabetes.

dialysate the solution used in dialysis (blood cleansing process) that is hypoosmolar to many of the wastes and key electrolytes in blood.

diaphoresis sweatiness.

diaphragmatic hernia protrusion of abdominal contents into the thoracic cavity through an opening in the diaphragm.

diaphysis hollow shaft found in long bones.

diarthrosis a synovial joint.

diastole the period of time when the myocardium is relaxed and cardiac filling and coronary perfusion occur.

diastolic blood pressure force of blood against arteries when ventricles relax.

differential field diagnosis list of possible causes of a patient's symptoms.

difficult child an infant, who can be characterized by irregularity of bodily functions, intense reactions, and withdrawal from new situations. *See also* easy child.

diffuse axonal injury type of brain injury characterized by shearing, stretching, or tearing of nerve fibers with subsequent axonal damage.

diffusion movement of solute in a solution from an area of higher concentration to an area of lower concentration.

digestive tract internal passageway that begins at the mouth and ends at the anus; also called the *alimentary canal.*

digital communications data or sounds that are translated into a digital code for transmission.

dilation enlargement. In reference to the heart, an abnormal enlargement resulting from pathology.

diplopia double vision.

direct pressure method of hemorrhage control that relies on the application of pressure to the site of the bleeding.

direct questions *see* closed questions.

dirty bomb a conventional explosive device that distributes radioactive material over a large area.

disaster management management of incidents that generate large numbers of patients, often overwhelming resources and damaging parts of the infrastructure.

disease period the duration from the onset of signs and symptoms of disease until the resolution of symptoms or death.

disentanglement process of freeing a patient from wreckage to allow for proper care, removal, and transfer.

disinfect to destroy certain forms of microorganisms, but not all.

disinfectant cleansing agent that destroys or inhibits pathogenic microorganisms and is also toxic to living tissue.

disinfecting cleaning with an agent that can kill some microorganisms on the surface of an object.

dislocation complete displacement of a bone end from its position in a joint capsule.

dissecting aortic aneurysm aneurysm caused when blood gets between and separates the layers of the aortic wall.

disseminated intravascular coagulation (DIC) a disorder of coagulation caused by systemic activation of the coagulation cascade.

dissociate separate; break down. For example, sodium bicarbonate, when placed in water, dissociates into a sodium cation and a bicarbonate anion.

dissociative disorder condition in which the individual avoids stress by separating from his core personality.

distal tubule the part of the renal tubule beyond the ascending loop of Henle.

distributive shock marked decrease in peripheral vascular resistance with resultant hypotension; examples include septic shock, neurogenic shock, and anaphylactic shock.

diuresis formation and passage of a dilute urine, decreasing blood volume.

diuretic an agent that increases urine secretion and elimination of body water; drug used to reduce circulating blood volume by increasing the amount of urine.

divergent taking into account all aspects of a complex situation.

diverticula small outpouchings in the mucosal lining of the intestinal tract.

diverticulitis inflammation of diverticula.

diverticulosis presence of diverticula, with or without associated bleeding.

Do Not Resuscitate (DNR) order legal document, usually signed by the patient and his physician, that indicates to medical personnel which, if any, life-sustaining measures should be taken when the patient's heart and respiratory functions have ceased.

domestic elder abuse physical or emotional violence or neglect when an elder is being cared for in a home-based setting.

dosage on hand the amount of drug available in a solution.

dose packaging medication packages that contain a single dose for a single patient.

dosimeter an instrument that measures the cumulative amount of radiation absorbed.

DOT KKK 1822E specs the manufacturing and design specifications produced by the Federal General Services Administrative Automotive Commodity Center.

down-regulation binding of a drug or hormone to a target cell receptor that causes the number of receptors to decrease.

downtime duration from the beginning of the cardiac arrest until effective CPR is established. *See also* total downtime.

drag the forces acting on a projectile in motion to slow its progress.

drip chamber clear plastic chamber that allows visualization of the drip rate during intravenous adminsitration.

drip rate pace at which the fluid moves from the bag into the patient during intravenous administration.

dromotropy pertaining to the speed of impulse transmission.

drop former device that regulates the size of drops.

drowning asphyxiation resulting from submersion in liquid, with death occurring within 24 hours of submersion.

drug agent used to diagnose, treat, or prevent disease; medication.

drug overdose poisoning from a pharmacological substance in excess of that usually prescribed or that the body can tolerate.

drug-response relationship correlation of different amounts of a drug to clinical response.

ducted gland *see* exocrine gland.

ductless gland *see* endocrine gland.

ductus arteriosus channel between the main pulmonary artery and the aorta of the fetus.

due regard legal terminology found in the motor vehicle laws of most states that sets higher standards for the operators of emergency vehicles.

duplex system communication system that allows simultaneous two-way communications by using two frequencies for each channel.

dura mater tough layer of the meninges firmly attached to the interior of the skull and interior of the spinal column.

duration of action length of time the amount of drug remains above its minimum effective concentration.

duty to act a formal contractual or informal legal obligation to provide care.

dynamic steady state homeostasis; the tendency of the body to maintain a net constant composition although the components of the body's internal environment are always changing.

dysmenorrhea painful menstruation.

dyspareunia painful sexual intercourse.

dysphagia inability to swallow or difficulty swallowing.

dysphoria an exaggerated feeling of depression or unrest, characterized by a mood of general dissatisfaction, restlessness, discomfort, and unhappiness.

dysplasia a change in cell size, shape, or appearance caused by an external stressor.

dyspnea difficult or labored breathing; a sensation of "shortness of breath"; an abnormality of breathing rate, pattern, or effort.

dysrhythmia any deviation from the normal electrical rhythm of the heart.

dystonias a group of disorders characterized by muscle contractions that cause twisting and repetitive movements, abnormal postures, or freezing in the middle of an action.

dysuria painful urination often associated with cystitis.

easy child an infant, who can be characterized by regularity of bodily functions, low or moderate intensity of reactions, and acceptance of new situations. *See also* difficult child.

ecchymosis blue-black discoloration of the skin due to leakage of blood into the tissues.

echo procedure immediately repeating each transmission received during radio communications.

ectopic beat cardiac depolarization resulting from depolarization of ectopic focus.

ectopic focus nonpacemaker heart cell that automatically depolarizes; *plural:* ectopic foci.

ectopic pregnancy the implantation of a developing fetus outside of the uterus, often in a fallopian tube.

eddy water that flows around especially large objects and, for a time, flows upstream around the downside of an obstruction.

edema excess fluid in the interstitial space.

effacement the thinning and shortening of the cervix during labor.

efficacy a drug's ability to cause the expected response.

egophony abnormal change in tone of patient's transmitted voice sounds.

Einthoven's triangle the triangle around the heart formed by the bipolar limb leads.

ejection fraction ratio of blood pumped from the ventricle to the amount remaining at the end of diastole.

elderly a person age 65 or older.

electrical alternans alternating amplitude of the P, QRS, and T waves on the ECG rhythm strip as the heart swings in a pendulum-like fashion within the pericardial sac during tamponade.

electrocardiogram (ECG) the graphic recording of the heart's electrical activity. It may be displayed either on paper or on an oscilloscope.

electrolyte a substance that, in water, separates into electrically charged particles.

emancipated minor a person under 18 years of age who is married, pregnant, a parent, a member of the armed forces, or financially independent and living away from home.

embolus undissolved solid, liquid, or gaseous matter in the bloodstream that may cause blockage of blood vessels; *plural:* emboli.

emergency doctrine *see* implied consent.

emergency medical dispatcher (EMD) EMS person medically and technically trained to assign emergency medical resources to a medical emergency; usually the person who is contacted by anyone who calls the EMS system.

Emergency Medical Services for Children (EMSC) federally funded program aimed at improving the health of pediatric patients who suffer from life-threatening illnesses and injuries.

emergency medical services (EMS) system a comprehensive network of personnel, equipment, and resources established for the purpose of delivering aid and emergency medical care to the community.

Emergency Operations Center (EOC) a site from which civil government officials (municipal, county, state, and/or federal) exercise direction and control in an emergency or disaster.

emergent phase first stage of the burn process that is characterized by a catecholamine release and pain-mediated reaction.

emesis vomitus.

empathy identification with and understanding of another's situation, feelings, and motives.

EMS Communications Officer person who notifies hospitals of incoming patients from a multiple-casualty incident; reports to the Transportation Officer and may also be called the EMS COM or MED COM.

EMT-Tacticals (EMT-Ts) EMS personnel trained to serve with a Technical Emergency Medical Service or a law enforcement agency.

encephalitis acute infection of the brain, usually caused by a virus.

encode to create a message.

end-diastolic volume *see* preload.

endocrine gland gland that secretes chemical substances directly into the blood; also called a *ductless gland.*

endometriosis condition in which endometrial tissue grows outside of the uterus.

endometritis infection of the endometrium.

endometrium the inner layer of the uterine wall where the fertilized egg implants.

endotoxins molecules in the walls of certain gram-negative bacteria that are released when the bacterium dies or is destroyed, causing toxic (poisonous) effects on the host body.

endotracheal intubation passing a tube into the trachea to protect and maintain the airway and to permit medication administration and deep suctioning.

end-stage renal failure an extreme failure of kidney function due to nephron loss.

end-tidal carbon dioxide ($ETCO_2$) detector a device used in capnography to measure exhaled carbon dioxide concentrations.

enema a liquid bolus of medication that is injected into the rectum.

energy the capacity to do work in the strict physical sense.

enteral route delivery of a medication through the gastrointestinal tract.

enterotoxin an exotoxin that produces gastrointestinal symptoms and diseases such as food poisoning.

enucleation removal of the eyeball after trauma or illness.

environmental emergency a medical condition caused or exacerbated by the weather, terrain, atmospheric pressure, or other local factors.

epidemiology the study of factors that influence the frequency, distribution, and causes of injury, disease, and other health-related events in a population.

epidermis outermost layer of the skin comprised of dead or dying cells.

epididymis small sac in which sperm cells are stored.

epidural hematoma accumulation of blood between the dura mater and the cranium.

epiglottitis bacterial infection of the epiglottis, usually occurring in children older than age 4; a serious medical emergency.

epiphyseal fracture disruption in the epiphyseal plate of a child's bone.

epiphyseal plate area of the metaphysis where cartilage is generated during bone growth in childhood; the growth plate.

epiphysis end of a long bone, including the epiphyseal, or growth plate, and supporting structures underlying the joint.

epistaxis nosebleed.

epithelial tissue the protective tissue that lines internal and external body tissues. Examples: skin, mucous membranes, the lining of the intestinal tract.

epithelialization early stage of wound healing in which epithelial cells migrate over the surface of the wound.

erythema general reddening of the skin due to dilation of the superficial capillaries.

erythrocyte red blood cell.

erythropoiesis the process of producing red blood cells.

erythropoietin a hormone produced by kidney cells that stimulates maturation of red blood cells.

eschar hard, leathery product of a deep full-thickness burn; it consists of dead and denatured skin.

Esophageal Tracheal CombiTube (ETC) dual-lumen airway with a ventilation port for each lumen.

esophageal varices enlarged and tortuous esophageal veins; *singular:* esophageal varix.

essential equipment equipment/supplies required on every ambulance.

estimated date of confinement (EDC) the approximate day the infant will be born. This date is usually set at 40 weeks after the date of the mother's last menstrual period (LMP).

ethics the rules or standards that govern the conduct of members of a particular group or profession.

ethnocentrism viewing one's own life as the most desirable, acceptable, or best, and acting in a superior manner to another culture's way of life.

ETT endotracheal tube.

eustachian tube a tube that connects the ear with the nasal cavity.

evaporation change from liquid to a gaseous state.

evisceration a protrusion of organs from a wound.

excitability ability of the cells to respond to an electrical stimulus.

exclusionary zone *see* hot zone.

exertional metabolic rate rate at which the body consumes energy during activity. It is faster than the basic metabolic rate.

exocrine condition involving external secretions.

exocrine gland gland that secretes chemical substances to nearby tissues through a duct; also called a *ducted gland.*

exotoxins toxic (poisonous) substances secreted by bacterial cells during their growth.

expectorant medication intended to increase the productivity of cough.

explosives chemical(s) that, when ignited, instantly generate a great amount of heat resulting in a destructive shock wave and blast wind.

exposure any occurrence of blood or body fluids coming in contact with nonintact skin, mucous membranes, or parenteral contact (needle stick).

expressed consent verbal, nonverbal, or written communication by a patient that he wishes to receive medical care.

exsanguination the draining of blood to the point at which life cannot be sustained.

extension bending motion that increases the angle between articulating elements.

extension tubing IV tubing used to extend a macrodrip or microdrip setup.

extracellular fluid (ECF) the fluid outside the body cells. Extracellular fluid is comprised of intravascular fluid and interstitial fluid.

extrapyramidal symptoms (EPS) common side effects of antipsychotic medications, including muscle tremors and parkinsonism-like effects.

extrauterine outside the uterus.

extravasation leakage of fluid or medication from the blood vessel that is commonly found with infiltration.

extravascular outside the vein.

extravascular space the volume contained by all the cells (intracellular space) and the spaces between the cells (interstitial space); the volume not contained within the vascular system.

Extrication group or branch responsible for removing patients from entanglements at a multiple-casualty incident and transferring them to the treatment area; also known as *Rescue*.

extrication use of force to free a patient from entrapment.

extubation removing a tube from a body opening.

facilitated diffusion diffusion of a substance such as glucose through a cell membrane that requires the assistance of a "helper," or carrier protein; also called *carrier-mediated diffusion*.

Facilities Unit selects and maintains areas used for rehabilitation and command at a multiple-casualty incident.

facsimile machine (fax) device for electronically transmitting and receiving printed information.

factitious disorder condition in which the patient feigns illness in order to assume the sick role.

fallopian tubes thin tubes that extend laterally from the uterus and conduct eggs from the ovaries into the uterine cavity.

fallout radioactive dust and particles that may be life threatening to people far from the epicenter of a nuclear detonation.

false imprisonment intentional and unjustifiable detention of a person without his consent or other legal authority.

fascia a fibrous membrane that covers, supports, and separates muscles and may also unite the skin with underlying tissue.

fasciculations involuntary contractions or twitchings of muscle fibers.

fasciculus small bundle of muscle fibers.

fatigue condition in which a muscle's ability to respond to stimulation is lost or reduced through overactivity.

fatigue fracture break in a bone associated with prolonged or repeated stress.

fatty change a result of cellular injury and swelling in which lipids (fat vesicles) invade the area of injury; occurs most commonly in the liver.

fear feeling of alarm and discontentment in the expectation of danger.

febrile seizures seizures that occur as a result of a sudden increase in body temperature; occur most commonly between ages 6 months and 6 years.

fecal–oral route transmission of organisms picked up from the gastrointestinal tract (e.g., feces) into the mouth.

Federal Communications Commission (FCC) agency that controls all nongovernmental communications in the United States.

feedback a response to a message.

fibrin protein fibers that trap red blood cells as part of the clotting process.

fibrinolysis the process through which plasmin dismantles a blood clot.

fibrinolytic drug that acts directly on thrombi to break them down; also called *thrombolytic*.

fibroblasts cells that secrete collagen, a critical factor in wound healing.

fibrosis the formation of fiber-like connective tissue, also called scar tissue, in an organ.

field diagnosis prehospital evaluation of the patient's condition and its causes.

filtrate the fluid produced in Bowman's capsule within the kidney by filtration of blood.

filtration movement of molecules across a membrane from an area of higher pressure to an area of lower pressure; movement of water out of the plasma across the capillary membrane into the interstitial space.

Finance/Administration Section responsible for maintaining records for personnel, time, and costs of resources/procurement; reports directly to the Incident Commander at a multiple-casualty incident.

FiO_2 concentration of oxygen in inspired air.

first-pass effect the liver's partial or complete inactivation of a drug before it reaches the systemic circulation.

flail chest one or more ribs fractured in two or more places, creating an unattached rib segment; defect in the chest wall that allows a segment to move freely, causing paradoxical chest wall motion (motion in a direction opposite to that of the rest of the chest wall).

flanks the part of the back below the ribs and above the hip bones.

flat affect appearance of being disinterested, often lacking facial expression.

flechettes arrow-shaped projectiles found in some military ordnance.

flexion bending motion that reduces the angle between articulating elements.

fluid shift phase stage of the burn process in which there is a massive shift of fluid from the intravascular to the extravascular space.

food poisoning nonspecific term often applied to gastroenteritis that occurs suddenly and that is caused by the ingestion of food containing preformed toxins.

foreign body airway obstruction (FBAO) blockage or obstruction of the airway by an object that impairs respiration; in the case of pediatric patients, tongues, abundant secretions, and deciduous (baby) teeth are more likely to block airways.

free drug availability proportion of a drug available in the body to cause either desired or undesired effects.

French unit of measurement approximately equal to one-third millimeter.

frostbite environmentally induced freezing of body tissues, causing destruction of cells. *See also* deep frostbite; superficial frostbite.

frostnip *see* superficial frostbite.

fugue state condition in which an amnesic patient physically flees.

full-thickness burn burn that damages all layers of the skin; characterized by areas that are white and dry; also called *third-degree burn.*

functional impairment decreased ability to meet daily needs on an independent basis.

fungi plant-like microorganisms; *singular:* fungus.

gag reflex mechanism that stimulates retching, or striving to vomit, when the soft palate is touched.

galea aponeurotica connective tissue sheet covering the superior aspect of the cranium.

gangrene death of tissue or bone, usually from an insufficient blood supply; deep-space infection usually caused by the anaerobic bacterium *Clostridium perfringens.*

gangrenous necrosis *see* necrosis.

gastric lavage removing an ingested poison by repeatedly filling and emptying the stomach with water or saline via a gastric tube; also known as "pumping the stomach."

gastroenteritis generalized disorder involving nausea, vomiting, gastrointestinal cramping or discomfort, and diarrhea.

gauge the size of a needle's diameter.

Geiger counter an instrument used to detect and measure the radiation given off by an object or area.

general adaptation syndrome (GAS) a sequence of stress response stages: stage I, alarm; stage II, resistance or adaptation; stage III, exhaustion.

general impression the initial, intuitive evaluation of a patient.

generalized seizures seizures that begin as an electrical discharge in a small area of the brain but spread to involve the entire cerebral cortex, causing widespread malfunction. *See also* seizure.

genitourinary system the male organ system that includes reproductive and urinary structures.

geriatric abuse a syndrome in which an elderly person is physically or psychologically injured by another person.

geriatrics the study and treatment of diseases of the aged.

gerontology scientific study of the effects of aging and of age-related diseases on humans.

Glasgow Coma Scale (GCS) tool used in evaluating and quantifying neurological status or the degree of coma by determining the best motor, verbal, and eye-opening response to standardized stimuli.

glaucoma group of eye diseases that results in increased intraocular pressure on the optic nerve; if left untreated, it can lead to blindness.

glomerular filtration the removal from blood of water and other elements, which enter the nephron tubule.

glomerular filtration rate (GFR) the volume per day at which blood is filtered through capillaries of the glomerulus.

glomerulonephritis a form of nephritis, or inflammation of the kidneys; primarily involves the glomeruli, one of the capillary networks that are part of the renal corpuscles in the nephrons.

glomerulus a tuft of capillaries from which blood is filtered into a nephron.

glottic function opening and closing of the glottic space.

glottis liplike opening between the vocal cords.

glucagon substance that increases blood glucose level.

glucometer tool used to measure blood glucose level.

gluconeogenesis conversion of protein and fat to form glucose.

glucose intolerance the body cells' inability to take up glucose from the bloodstream.

glycogenolysis the breakdown of glycogen to glucose, primarily by liver cells.

glycosuria glucose in urine, which occurs when blood glucose levels exceed the kidney's ability to reabsorb glucose.

gold standard ultimate standard of excellence.

Golden Hour the 60-minute period after a severe injury; it is the maximum acceptable time between the injury and initiation of surgery for the seriously injured trauma patient.

gonorrhea sexually transmitted disease caused by a gram-negative bacterium.

Good Samaritan laws laws that provide immunity to certain people who assist at the scene of a medical emergency.

gout inflammation of joints and connective tissue due to buildup of uric acid crystals.

Gram stain method of differentiating types of bacteria according to their reaction to a chemical stain process.

granulocytes white blood cells charged with the primary purpose of neutralizing foreign bacteria.

granuloma a tumor or growth that forms when foreign bodies that cannot be destroyed by macrophages are surrounded and walled off.

Graves' disease endocrine disorder characterized by excess thyroid hormones resulting in body changes associated with increased metabolism; primary cause of *thyrotoxicosis.*

Gray (Gy) a unit of absorbed radiation dose equal to 100 rads.

gray matter areas in the central nervous system dominated by nerve cell bodies; the central portion of the spinal cord.

great vessels the large arteries and veins located in the mediastinum that enter and exit the heart; the aorta, superior and inferior vena cava, pulmonary arteries, and pulmonary veins.

greenstick fracture fracture characterized by an incomplete break in the bone.

green zone *see* cold zone.

Grey Turner's sign discoloration over the flanks suggesting intra-abdominal bleeding.

growth plate the area just below the head of a long bone in which growth in bone length occurs; the epiphyseal plate.

gtts drops (Latin *guttae,* drops [*gutta,* drop]).

guarding protective tensing of the abdominal muscles by a patient suffering abdominal pain; may be a voluntary or involuntary response.

Guillain-Barré syndrome acute viral infection that triggers the production of autoantibodies, which damage the myelin sheath covering the peripheral nerves; causes rapid, progressive loss of motor function, ranging from muscle weakness to full-body paralysis.

gynecology the branch of medicine that deals with the health maintenance and the diseases of women, primarily of the reproductive organs.

hairline fracture small crack in a bone that does not disrupt its total structure.

half-life time required for half of the nuclei of a radioactive substance to lose activity by undergoing radioactive decay. In biology and pharmacology, the time required by the body to metabolize and inactivate half the amount of a substance taken in.

hallucinations sensory perceptions with no basis in reality.

hantavirus family of viruses that are carried by the deer mouse and transmitted by ticks and other arthropods.

hate crime crime committed against a person wholly on the basis of the individual's actual or perceived race, color, national origin, ethnicity, gender, disability, or sexual orientation.

haversian canals small perforations of the long bones through which the blood vessels and nerves travel into the bone itself.

hazardous material (hazmat) any substance that causes adverse health effects on human exposure.

health care professionals properly trained and licensed or certified providers of health care.

heart failure clinical syndrome in which the heart's mechanical performance is compromised so that cardiac output cannot meet the body's needs.

heat cramps acute painful spasms of the voluntary muscles following strenuous activity in a hot environment without adequate fluid or salt intake.

Heat Escape Lessening Position (HELP) an in-water, head-up tuck or fetal position designed to reduce heat loss by as much as 60 percent.

heat exhaustion a mild heat illness; an acute reaction to heat exposure.

heat illness increased core body temperature due to inadequate thermolysis.

heatstroke acute, dangerous reaction to heat exposure, characterized by a body temperature usually above 105°F (40.6°C) and central nervous system disturbances. The body usually ceases to perspire.

HEENT acronym standing for *head, eyes, ears, nose, throat.*

hematemesis bloody vomitus.

hematochezia blood in the stool.

hematocrit the percentage of the blood occupied by erythrocytes.

hematology the study of blood and the blood-forming organs.

hematoma collection of blood beneath the skin or trapped within a body compartment.

hematopoiesis the process through which pluripotent stem cells differentiate into various types of blood cells.

hematopoietic system body system having to do with the production and development of blood cells, consisting of the bone marrow, liver, spleen, kidneys, and the blood itself.

hematuria blood in the urine.

hemoconcentration elevated numbers of red and white blood cells.

hemodialysis a dialysis (blood cleansing) procedure relying on vascular access to the blood and on an artificial membrane.

hemoglobin oxygen-bearing molecule in the red blood cells. It is made up of iron-rich red pigment called *heme* and a protein called *globin.*

hemoglobin-based oxygen-carrying solutions (HBOCs) intravenous fluids with the ability to transport oxygen.

hemolysis the destruction of red blood cells.

hemophilia a blood disorder in which one of the proteins necessary for blood clotting is missing or defective.

hemopneumothorax condition where air and blood are in the pleural space.
hemoptysis coughing up of blood.
hemorrhage an abnormal internal or external discharge of blood.
hemorrhoid small mass of swollen veins in the anus or rectum.
hemostasis the body's natural ability to stop bleeding, the ability to clot blood.
hemothorax accumulation in the pleural cavity of blood or fluid containing blood.
heparin lock peripheral IV port that does not use a bag of fluid.
hepatic alteration change in a medication's chemical composition that occurs in the liver.
hepatitis inflammation of the liver characterized by diffuse or patchy tissue necrosis.
hepatomegaly enlarged liver.
hernia protrusion of an organ through its protective sheath.
herniation protrusion or projection of an organ or part of an organ through the wall of the cavity that normally contains it.
herpes simplex virus organism that causes infections characterized by fluid-filled vesicles, usually in the oral cavity or on the genitals.
herpes zoster an acute eruption caused by a reactivation of latent varicella virus (chickenpox) in the dorsal root ganglia; also known as *shingles.*
hiatal hernia protrusion of the stomach upward into the mediastinal cavity through the esophageal hiatus of the diaphragm.
high-pressure regulator regulator used to transfer oxygen at high pressures from tank to tank.
hilum the notched part of the kidney where the ureter and other structures join kidney tissue.
histamine a product of mast cells and basophils that causes vasodilation, capillary permeability, bronchoconstriction, and contraction of the gut.
HIV *human immunodeficiency virus,* a virus that breaks down the immune defenses, making the body vulnerable to a variety of infections and disorders; organism responsible for acquired immunodeficiency syndrome (AIDS).
hives *see* urticaria.
hollow-needle catheter stylet that does not have a Teflon tube but is itself inserted into the vein and secured there.
homeostasis the natural tendency of the body to maintain a steady and normal internal environment.
hookworms parasites that attach to the host's intestinal lining.
hormone chemical substance released by a gland that controls or affects processes in other glands or body systems.
hospice program of palliative care and support services that addresses the physical, social, economic, and spiritual needs of terminally ill patients and their families.
hot zone location at a hazardous materials incident where the actual hazardous material and highest levels of contamination exist; also called the *red zone* or the *exclusionary zone.*
Huber needle needle that has an opening on the side of the shaft instead of the tip.
human immunodeficiency virus *see* HIV.
humoral immunity the long-term immunity to an antigen provided by antibodies produced by B lymphocytes.
hydrolysis the breakage of a chemical bond by adding water, or by incorporating a hydroxyl (OH^-) group into one fragment and a hydrogen ion (H^+) into the other.
hydrostatic pressure blood pressure or force against vessel walls created by the heartbeat. Hydrostatic pressure tends to force water out of the capillaries into the interstitial space.
Hymenoptera any of an order of highly specialized insects such as bees and wasps.
hyperbaric oxygen chamber recompression chamber used to treat patients suffering from barotrauma.
hyperbilirubinemia an excessive amount of bilirubin—the orange-colored pigment associated with bile—in the blood. In newborns, the condition appears as jaundice. Precipitating factors include maternal Rh or ABO incompatibility, neonatal sepsis, anoxia, hypoglycemia, and congenital liver or gastrointestinal defects.
hypercarbia excessive pressure of carbon dioxide in the blood.
hyperglycemia abnormally high concentration of glucose in the blood.
hyperglycemic hyperosmolar nonketotic (HHNK) coma complication of Type II diabetes due to inadequate insulin activity. Marked by high blood glucose, marked dehydration, and decreased mental function. Often mistaken for ketoacidosis.
hypermetabolic phase stage of the burn process in which there is increased body metabolism in an attempt by the body to heal the burn.
hyperosmolar a solution that has a concentration of the substance greater than that of a second solution.
hyperplasia an increase in the number of cells resulting from cell division caused by an increased workload.
hypersensitivity an exaggerated and harmful immune response; an umbrella term for allergy, autoimmunity, and isoimmunity.
hypertension blood pressure higher than normal.

hypertensive emergency an acute elevation of blood pressure that requires the blood pressure to be lowered within 1 hour; characterized by end-organ changes such as hypertensive encephalopathy, renal failure, or blindness.

hypertensive encephalopathy a cerebral disorder of hypertension indicated by severe headache, nausea, vomiting, and altered mental status. Neurological symptoms may include blindness, muscle twitches, inability to speak, weakness, and paralysis.

hyperthermia increase in the body's core temperature.

hyperthyroidism excessive secretion of thyroid hormones resulting in an increased metabolic rate.

hypertonic having a greater concentration of solute molecules; one solution may be hypertonic to another.

hypertrophy an increase in cell size or in the size or bulk of an organ or structure resulting from an increased workload.

hyphema blood in the anterior chamber of the eye, in front of the iris.

hypnosis instigation of sleep.

hypochondriasis an abnormal concern with one's health, with the false belief of suffering from some disease, despite medical assurances to the contrary; commonly known as *hypochondria.*

hypodermic needle hollow metal tube used with the syringe to administer medications.

hypoglycemia abnormally low concentration of glucose in the blood. Sometimes called *insulin shock.*

hypoglycemic seizure seizure that occurs when brain cells are not functioning normally due to low blood glucose.

hypoosmolar a solution that has a concentration of the substance lower than that of a second solution.

hypoperfusion inadequate perfusion of the body tissues, resulting in an inadequate supply of oxygen and nutrients to the body tissues. Also called *shock.*

hypotension blood pressure lower than normal.

hypothalamus portion of the diencephalon producing neurosecretions important in the control of certain metabolic activities, including body temperature regulation.

hypothermia decrease in the body's core temperature.

hypothyroidism inadequate secretion of thyroid hormones resulting in a decreased metabolic rate.

hypotonic having a lesser concentration of solute molecules; one solution may be hypotonic to another.

hypoventilation reduction in breathing rate and depth.

hypovolemic shock decreased amount of intravascular fluid in the body; often due to trauma that causes blood loss into a body cavity or frank external hemorrhage; in children, can be the result of vomiting and diarrhea.

hypoxemia decreased blood oxygen level.

hypoxia state in which insufficient oxygen is available to meet the oxygen requirements of the cells.

hypoxic drive mechanism that increases respiratory stimulation when blood oxygen falls and inhibits respiratory stimulation when blood oxygen climbs.

immediate hypersensitivity reaction a hypersensitivity reaction that occurs swiftly following reexposure to an antigen. Immediate hypersensitivity reactions are usually more severe than delayed reactions. The swiftest and most severe of such reactions is anaphylaxis. *See also* delayed hypersensitivity reaction.

immersion foot *see* trench foot.

immune response the body's reactions that inactivate or eliminate foreign antigens, pathogens, abnormal cells, or foreign molecules.

immune senescence diminished vigor of the immune response to the challenge and rechallenge by pathogens.

immune system the body system responsible for combating infection.

immunity [biological] the body's ability to respond to the presence of a pathogen; a long-term condition of protection from infection or disease. [legal] exemption from legal liability.

immunogens antigens that are able to trigger an immune response.

immunoglobulin (Ig) alternative term for antibody.

impacted fracture break in a bone in which the bone is compressed on itself.

impaled object foreign body embedded in a wound.

impetigo infection of the skin caused by staphylococci or streptococci.

implied consent consent for treatment that is presumed for a patient who is mentally, physically, or emotionally unable to grant consent. Also called *emergency doctrine.*

impulse control disorder condition characterized by the patient's failure to control recurrent impulses.

impulsive acting instinctively without stopping to think.

incendiary an agent that combusts easily or creates combustion.

incendiary agents a subset of explosives with less explosive power but greater heat and burn potential.

Incident Command System (ICS) *see* Incident Management System (IMS).

Incident Commander (IC) the person responsible for coordinating all activities at a multiple-casualty scene.

Incident Management System (IMS) a management program designed for controlling, directing, and coordinating emergency response resources; sometimes used as a synonym for *Incident Command System (ICS).*

incision very smooth or surgical laceration, frequently caused by a knife, scalpel, razor blade, or piece of glass.

incontinence inability to retain urine or feces because of loss of sphincter control or cerebral or spinal lesions.

incubation period the time between contact with a disease organism and the appearance of the first symptoms.

incubator *see* isolette.

index case the individual who first introduced an infectious agent to a population.

index of suspicion the anticipation of injury to a body region, organ, or structure based on analysis of the mechanism of injury.

induced active immunity immunity achieved through vaccination given to generate an immune response that results in the development of antibodies specific for the injected antigen; also called *artificially acquired immunity.*

inertia tendency of an object to remain at rest or remain in motion unless acted on by an external force.

infarction area of dead tissue caused by lack of blood.

infection presence of an agent within the host, without necessarily causing disease.

infectious disease any disease caused by the growth of pathogenic microorganisms, which may be spread from person to person.

infestation presence of parasites that do not break the host's skin.

inflammation complex process of local cellular and biochemical changes as a consequence of injury or infection; an early stage of healing. Also called *inflammatory response.*

inflammatory process a nonspecific defense mechanism that wards off damage from microorganisms or trauma.

inflammatory response *see* inflammation.

influenza disease caused by a group of viruses.

Information Officer (IO) the person who collects data about the incident and releases it to the press during a multiple-casualty incident.

informed consent consent for treatment that is given based on full disclosure of information.

infusion liquid medication delivered through a vein.

infusion controller gravity-flow device that regulates fluid's passage through an electromechanical pump.

infusion pump device that delivers fluids and medications under positive pressure.

infusion rate speed at which a medication is delivered intravenously.

ingestion entry of a substance into the body through the gastrointestinal tract.

inhalation entry of a substance into the body through the respiratory tract.

injection entry of a substance into the body through a break in the skin.

injury intentional or unintentional damage to a person resulting from exposure to mechanical or any other form of energy or from absence of essentials such as heat or oxygen.

injury risk a situation that puts people in danger of injury.

injury-surveillance program ongoing systematic collection, analysis, and interpretation of injury data important to public health practice.

innate immunity *see* natural immunity.

inotropy pertaining to cardiac contractile force.

insertion attachment of a muscle to a bone that moves when the muscle contracts.

inspection the process of informed observation.

institutional elder abuse physical or emotional violence or neglect when an elder is being cared for by a person paid to provide care.

insufflate to blow into.

insulin substance that decreases blood glucose level.

insulin shock *see* hypoglycemia.

integumentary system skin, consisting of the epidermis, dermis, and subcutaneous layers.

intercalated discs specialized bands of tissue inserted between myocardial cells that increase the rate in which the action potential is spread from cell to cell.

intermittent claudication severe pain in the calf muscle, resulting from an inadequate blood supply, that usually subsides with rest.

intermittent mandatory ventilation (IMV) respirator setting where a patient-triggered breath does not result in assistance by the machine.

interpolated beat a PVC that falls between two sinus beats without effectively interrupting this rhythm.

interstitial fluid the fluid in body tissues that is outside the cells and outside the vascular system.

interstitial nephritis an inflammation within the tissue surrounding the nephrons.

intervener physician a licensed physician, professionally unrelated to patients on scene, who attempts to assist EMS providers with patient care.

intervertebral disk cartilaginous pad between vertebrae that serves as a shock absorber.

intracatheter *see* catheter inserted through the needle.

intracellular fluid (ICF) the fluid inside the body cells.

intracerebral hemorrhage bleeding directly into the tissue of the brain.

intracranial pressure (ICP) pressure exerted on the brain by the blood and cerebrospinal fluid.

intractable resistant to cure, relief, or control.

intradermal within the dermal layer of the skin.

intramuscular within the muscle.

intraosseous within the bone.

intrapartum occurring during childbirth.

intrarenal abscess a pocket of infection within kidney tissue.

intravascular fluid the fluid within the circulatory system; blood plasma.

intravascular space the volume contained by all the arteries, veins, and capillaries and other components of the circulatory system.

intravenous access surgical puncture of a vein to deliver medication or withdraw blood. Also called *cannulation.*

intravenous fluid chemically prepared solution tailored to the body's specific needs.

intussusception condition that occurs when part of an intestine slips into the part just distal to itself.

involuntary consent consent to treatment granted by the authority of a court order.

ion a charged particle; an atom or group of atoms whose electrical charge has changed from neutral to positive or negative by losing or gaining one or more electrons. (In an atom's normal, nonionized state, its positively charged protons and negatively charged electrons balance each other so that the atom's charge is neutral.)

ionization the process of changing a substance into separate charged particles (ions).

ionize to become electrically charged or polar.

ionizing radiation electromagnetic radiation (e.g., X-ray) or particulate radiation (e.g., alpha particles, beta particles, and neutrons) that, by direct or secondary processes, ionizes materials that absorb the radiation. Ionizing radiation can penetrate the cells of living organisms, depositing an electrical charge within them. When sufficiently intense, this form of energy kills cells.

iris pigmented portion of the eye; the muscular area that constricts or dilates to change the size of the pupil.

irreversible antagonism when a competitive antagonist permanently binds with a receptor site.

irreversible shock final stage of shock in which organs and cells are so damaged that recovery is impossible and death is inevitable.

ischemia a blockage in the delivery of oxygenated blood to the cells.

isoimmunity an immune response to antigens from another member of the same species, for example Rh reactions between a mother and infant or transplant rejections; also called *alloimmunity.*

isolette a clear plastic enclosed bassinet used to keep prematurely born infants warm; also known as an *incubator.*

isometric exercise active exercise performed against stable resistance, where muscles are exercised in a motionless manner.

isosthenuria inability to concentrate or dilute urine relative to the osmolarity of blood.

isotonic equal in concentration of solute molecules; solutions may be isotonic to each other.

isotonic exercise active exercise during which muscles are worked through their range of motion.

J wave ECG deflection found at the junction of the QRS complex and the ST segment. It is associated with hypothermia and seen at core temperatures below 32°C, most commonly in leads II and V6; also called an *Osborn wave.*

Jackson's theory of thermal wounds explanation of the physical effects of thermal burns.

jargon language used by a particular group or profession.

joint area where adjacent bones articulate.

joint capsule the ligaments that surround a joint; also called a *synovial capsule.*

Joule's law the physical law stating that the rate of heat production is directly proportional to the resistance of the circuit and to the square of the current.

judge-made law *see* common law.

justice the obligation to treat all persons fairly.

keloid a formation resulting from overproduction of scar tissue.

Kernig's sign inability to fully extend the knees with hips flexed.

ketone bodies compounds produced during the catabolism of fatty acids, including acetoacetic acid, b-hydroxybutyric acid, and acetone.

ketosis the presence of significant quantities of ketone bodies in the blood.

kidney an organ that produces urine and performs other functions related to the urinary system.

kinetic energy the energy an object has while it is in motion. It is related to the object's mass and velocity.

kinetics the branch of physics that deals with motion, taking into consideration mass, velocity, and force.

Korotkoff's sounds sounds of blood hitting arterial walls.

Korsakoff's psychosis psychosis characterized by disorientation, muttering delirium, insomnia, delusions, and hallucinations. Symptoms include painful extremities, bilateral wrist drop (rarely), bilateral foot drop (frequently), and pain on pressure over the long nerves.

Kussmaul's respiration rapid deep respirations caused by severe metabolic and central nervous system problems.

kyphosis exaggeration of the normal posterior curvature of the spine.

labia structures that protect the vagina and urethra, including the labia majora and the labia minora.

labor the time and processes that occur during childbirth; the physiologic and mechanical process in which the baby, placenta, and amniotic sac are expelled through the birth canal.

labrynthitis inner ear infection that causes vertigo, nausea, and an unsteady gait.

laceration an open wound, normally a tear with jagged borders.

lacrimal fluid liquid that lubricates the eye.

lactic acid compound produced from pyruvic acid during anaerobic glycolyis.

laminae posterior bones of a vertebra that help make up the foramen, or opening, of the spinal canal.

laryngeal mask airway (LMA) airway with an inflatable distal end that masks the laryngeal opening.

laryngoscope instrument for lifting the tongue and epiglottis in order to see the vocal cords.

larynx the complex structure that joins the pharynx with the trachea.

latent period time when a host cannot transmit an infectious agent to someone else.

laxative medication used to decrease stool's firmness and increase its water content.

Le Fort criteria classification system for fractures involving the maxilla.

leading questions questions framed to guide the direction of a person's answers.

legislative law law created by law-making bodies such as the United States Congress and state assemblies. Also called *statutory law*.

lesion any disruption in normal tissue.

leukemia a cancer of the hematopoietic cells.

leukocyte white blood cell.

leukocytosis too many white blood cells.

leukopenia a low white blood cell count.

leukopoiesis the process through which stem cells differentiate into the white blood cells' immature forms.

leukotrienes substances synthesized by mast cells during inflammatory response that cause vasodilation, vascular permeability, and chemotaxis. Also called *slow-reacting substances of anaphylaxis (SRS-A)*.

liability legal responsibility.

Liaison Officer (LO) coordinates all incident operations that involve outside agencies.

libel the act of injuring a person's character, name, or reputation by false statements made in writing or through the mass media with malicious intent or reckless disregard for the falsity of those statements.

lice parasitic infestation of the skin of the scalp, trunk, or pubic area.

licensure the process by which a governmental agency grants permission to engage in a given occupation to an applicant who has attained the degree of competency required to ensure the public's protection.

life expectancy based on the year of birth, the average number of additional years of life expected for a member of a population.

ligament of Treitz ligament that supports the duodenojejunal junction.

ligaments connective tissue that connects bone to bone and holds joints together.

ligamentum arteriosum cordlike remnant of a fetal vessel connecting the pulmonary artery to the aorta at the aortic isthmus.

limb leads *see* augmented limb leads; bipolar limb leads; unipolar limb leads.

liquefaction necrosis the process in which an alkali dissolves and liquefies tissue.

living will a legal document that allows a person to specify the kinds of medical treatment he wishes to receive should the need arise.

local limited to one area of the body.

local effects effects involving areas around the immediate injury or burn site.

Logistics Section supports incident operations, coordinating procurement and distribution of all medical resources at a multiple-casualty incident.

Lou Gehrig's disease *see* amyotrophic lateral sclerosis (ALS).

lower gastrointestinal bleeding bleeding in the gastrointestinal tract distal to the ligament of Treitz.

Luer-sampling needle long, exposed needle that screws into the vacutainer and is inserted directly into the vein.

lumen the tunnel through a tube.

Lyme disease recurrent inflammatory disorder caused by a tick-borne spirochete.

lymphangitis inflammation of the lymph channels, usually as a result of a distal infection.

lymphatic system a network of vessels that drains fluid, called lymph, from the body tissues. Lymph nodes help filter impurities en route to the subclavian vein and thence to the heart.

lymphocyte a type of leukocyte, or white blood cell, that attacks foreign substances as part of the body's immune response.

lymphoma a cancer of the lymphatic system.

maceration process of softening a solid by soaking it in a liquid.

macrodrip tubing administration tubing that delivers a relatively large amount of fluid.

macrophage immune system cell that has the ability to recognize and ingest foreign pathogens.

Magill forceps scissor-style clamps with circular tips.

major basic protein (MBP) a larvacidal peptide.

major trauma patient person who has suffered significant mechanism of injury.

malfeasance a breach of duty by performance of a wrongful or unlawful act.

Mallory-Weiss tear esophageal laceration, usually secondary to vomiting.

mammalian diving reflex a complex cardiovascular reflex, resulting from submersion of the face and nose in water, that constricts blood flow everywhere except to the brain.

Management Staff *see* Command Staff.

mandible the jawbone.

manic characterized by excessive excitement or activity (mania).

manometer pressure gauge with a scale calibrated in millimeters of mercury (mmHg).

Marfan syndrome hereditary condition of connective tissue, bones, muscles, ligaments, and skeletal structures characterized by irregular and unsteady gait, tall lean body type with long extremities, flat feet, and stooped shoulders. The aorta is usually dilated and may become weakened enough to allow an aneurysm to develop.

Mark I kit a two-part auto-injector set the military uses as treatment for nerve agent exposure; involves the administration of atropine and then pralidoxime chloride.

mask a device for protecting the face.

mass a measure of the matter that an object contains; the property of a physical body that gives the body inertia.

mass-casualty incident *see* multiple-casualty incident.

mast cells large cells, resembling bags of granules, that reside near blood vessels. When stimulated by injury, chemicals, or allergic responses, they activate the inflammatory response by degranulation (emptying their granules into the extracellular environment) and synthesis (construction of leukotrienes and prostaglandins).

material safety data sheets (MSDS) sheets of detailed information about chemicals found at fixed facilities, intended to be easily accessible.

maxilla bone of the upper jaw.

maximum life span the theoretical, species-specific, longest duration of life, excluding premature or "unnatural" death.

McBurney's point common site of pain from appendicitis, 1 to 2 inches above the anterior iliac crest in a direct line with the umbilicus.

measles highly contagious, acute viral disease characterized by a reddish rash that appears on the fourth or fifth day of illness.

measured volume administration set IV setup that delivers specific volumes of fluid.

mechanism of injury the processes and forces that cause trauma.

meconium dark green material found in the intestine of the full-term newborn. It can be expelled from the intestine into the amniotic fluid during periods of fetal distress.

medical direction medical policies, procedures, and practices that are available to providers either on-line or off-line. *See also* medical director.

medical director a physician who is legally responsible for all of the clinical and patient-care aspects of an EMS system. Also referred to as *medical direction.*

Medical Supply Unit coordinates procurement and distribution of equipment and supplies at a multiple-casualty incident.

medically clean careful handling to prevent contamination.

medicated solution parenteral medication packaged in an IV bag and administered as an IV infusion.

medication *see* drug.

medication injection port self-sealing membrane into which a hypodermic needle is inserted for drug administration.

medulla the inner tissue of an organ such as the kidney.

medulla oblongata lower portion of the brainstem containing the respiratory, cardiac, and vasomotor centers.

medullary canal cavity within a bone that contains the marrow.

melena a dark, tarry stool caused by the presence of partially digested free blood.

menarche the onset of menses, usually occurring between ages 10 and 14.

Meniere's disease a disease of the inner ear characterized by vertigo, nerve deafness, and a roar or buzzing in the ear.

meninges three membranes that surround and protect the brain and spinal cord: dura mater, pia mater, and arachnoid membrane.

meningitis inflammation of the meninges, usually caused by an infection.

meningomyelocele herniation of the spinal cord and membranes through a defect in the spinal column.

menopause the cessation of menses and ovarian function resulting from decreased secretion of estrogen.

menorrhagia excessive menstrual flow.
menstruation sloughing of the uterine lining (endometrium) if a fertilized egg is not implanted. It is controlled by the cyclical release of hormones; commonly called a *period*.
mental status the state of the patient's cerebral functioning.
mental status examination (MSE) a structured exam designed to quickly evaluate a patient's level of mental functioning.
mesenteric infarct death of tissue in the peritoneal fold (mesentery) that encircles the small intestine; a life-threatening condition.
mesentery double fold of peritoneum that supports the major portion of the small bowel, suspending it from the posterior abdominal wall.
metabolic acidosis acidity caused by increased production of acids during metabolism or from causes such as vomiting, diarrhea, diabetes, or medication.
metabolic alkalosis alkalinity caused by an increase in plasma bicarbonate resulting from causes including diuresis, vomiting, or ingestion of too much sodium bicarbonate.
metabolism the sum of cellular processes that produce the energy and molecules needed for growth and repair; the total changes that take place during physiological processes.
metaphysis growth zone of a bone, active during the development stages of youth, located between the epiphysis and the diaphysis.
metaplasia replacement of one type of cell by another type of cell that is not normal for that tissue.
metered-dose inhaler handheld device that produces a medicated spray for inhalation.
microangiopathy a disease affecting the smallest blood vessels.
microdrip tubing administration tubing that delivers a relatively small amount of fluid.
midbrain portion of the brain connecting the pons and cerebellum with the cerebral hemispheres.
minimum effective concentration minimum level of drug needed to cause a given effect.
minimum standards lowest or least allowable standards.
minor depending on state law, usually a person under the age of 18.
minute volume amount of gas inhaled and exhaled in 1 minute.
miosis abnormal contraction of the pupils; pinpoint pupils.
miscarriage term commonly used to describe a pregnancy that ends before 20 weeks' gestation; also called *spontaneous abortion*.
misfeasance a breach of duty by performance of a legal act in a manner that is harmful or injurious.
mitosis cell division with division of the nucleus; each daughter cell contains the same number of chromosomes as the mother cell; the process by which the body grows.
mittelschmerz abdominal pain associated with ovulation.
Mix-o-Vial *see* nonconstituted drug vial/Mix-o-Vial.
mobile data terminal vehicle-mounted computer keyboard and display.
modeling a procedure whereby a person observes someone perform a model behavior and then attempts to imitate that behavior.
mononucleosis acute disease caused by the Epstein-Barr virus.
mons pubis fatty layer of tissue over the pubic symphysis.
mood disorder pervasive and sustained emotion that colors a person's perception of the world.
morals social, religious, or personal standards of right and wrong.
morgue area where deceased victims of an incident are collected.
Morgue Officer person who supervises the morgue; may report to the Triage Officer or the Treatment Officer at a multiple-casualty incident.
Moro reflex occurs when a newborn is startled, arms are thrown wide, fingers are spread, and a grabbing motion follows. Also called *startle reflex*.
motion the process of changing place; movement.
mucolytic medication intended to make mucus more watery.
mucous membranes tissues lining body cavities that communicate with the air; usually contain mucus-secreting cells.
mucoviscidosis disease so called because of the abnormally viscous mucoid secretions associated with it; also called *cystic fibrosis*.
mucus slippery secretion that lubricates and protects airway surfaces.
multi-infarct dementia *see* senile dementia.
multiple-casualty incident (MCI) incident that generates large numbers of patients and that often makes traditional EMS response ineffective because of special circumstances surrounding the event; also known as a *mass-casualty incident*.
multiple myeloma a cancerous disorder of plasma cells.
multiple organ dysfunction syndrome (MODS) progressive impairment of two or more organ systems resulting from an uncontrolled inflammatory response to a severe illness or injury.
multiple personality disorder manifestation of two or more complete systems of personality.
multiple sclerosis disease that involves inflammation of certain nerve cells followed by demyelination, or

the destruction of the myelin sheath, which is the fatty insulation surrounding nerve fibers.

multiplex system duplex communications system that can transmit voice and data simultaneously.

mumps acute viral disease characterized by painful enlargement of the salivary glands.

Murphy's sign pain caused when an inflamed gallbladder is palpated by pressing under the right costal margin.

muscle tissue tissue that is capable of contraction when stimulated. There are three types of muscle tissue: *cardiac* (myocardium, or heart muscle), *smooth* (within intestines, surrounding blood vessels), and *skeletal,* or *striated* (allows skeletal movement). Skeletal muscle is mostly under voluntary, or conscious, control; smooth muscle is under involuntary, or unconscious, control; cardiac muscle is capable of spontaneous, or self-excited, contraction.

muscular dystrophy a group of genetic diseases characterized by progressive muscle weakness and degeneration of the skeletal or voluntary muscle fibers.

mutual aid agreements agreements or plans for sharing departmental resources.

myasthenia gravis disease characterized by episodic muscle weakness triggered by an autoimmune attack of the acetylcholine receptors.

myocardial infarction (MI) death and subsequent necrosis of the heart muscle caused by inadequate blood supply; also called *acute myocardial infarction (AMI).*

myocardium *see* muscle tissue.

myoclonus temporary, involuntary twitching or spasm of a muscle or group of muscles.

myometrium the thick middle layer of the uterine wall made up of smooth muscle fibers.

myotome muscle and tissue of the body innervated by a spinal nerve root.

myxedema condition that reflects long-term exposure to inadequate levels of thyroid hormones with resultant changes in body structure and function.

myxedema coma life-threatening condition associated with advanced myxedema, with profound hypothermia, bradycardia, and electrolyte imbalance.

nares the openings of the nostrils.

nasal cannula catheter placed at the nares.

nasal flaring excessive widening of the nares with respiration.

nasal medication drug administered through the mucous membranes of the nose.

nasal septum cartilage that separates the right and left nasal cavities.

nasogastric tube/orogastric tube a tube that runs through the nose or mouth and esophagus into the stomach, used for administering liquid nutrients or medications or for removing air or liquids from the stomach. (*Nasogastric:* from the nose into the stomach; *orogastric:* from the mouth into the stomach.)

nasolacrimal duct narrow tube that carries into the nasal cavity tears and debris that have drained from the eye.

nasopharyngeal airway uncuffed tube that follows the natural curvature of the nasopharynx, passing through the nose and extending from the nostril to the posterior pharynx.

nasotracheal route through the nose and into the trachea.

National Incident Management System (NIMS) national system used for the management of multiple-casualty incidents, involving assumption of responsibility for command as well as designation and coordination of such elements as triage, treatment, transport, and staging.

natural immunity genetically predetermined immunity that is present at birth; also called *innate immunity.*

naturally acquired immunity immunity that begins to develop after birth and is continually enhanced by exposure to new pathogens and antigens throughout life.

near-drowning an incident of potentially fatal submersion in liquid which did not result in death or in which death occurred more than 24 hours after submersion.

nebulizer inhalation aid that disperses liquid into aerosol spray or mist.

necrosis cell death; a pathological cell change. Four types of necrotic cell change are coagulative, liquefactive, caseous, and fatty. *Gangrenous necrosis* refers to tissue death over a wide area.

needle adapter rigid plastic device specifically constructed to fit into the hub of an intravenous cannula.

needle cricothyrotomy surgical airway technique that inserts a 14-gauge needle into the trachea at the cricothyroid membrane.

negative feedback loop body mechanisms that work to reverse, or compensate for, a pathophysiological process (or to reverse any physiological process, whether pathological or nonpathological).

negligence deviation from accepted standards of care recognized by law for the protection of others against the unreasonable risk of harm.

neonatal abstinence syndrome (NAS) a generalized disorder presenting a clinical picture of central nervous system hyperirritability, gastrointestinal dysfunction, respiratory distress, and vague autonomic symptoms. It may be due to intrauterine exposure to heroin, methadone, or other less potent opiates. Nonopiate central nervous system depressants may also cause NAS.

neonate an infant from the time of birth to 1 month of age.

neoplasm literally meaning "new form"; a new or abnormal formation; a tumor.

neovascularization new growth of capillaries in response to healing.

nephrology the medical specialty dealing with the kidneys.

nephron a microscopic structure within the kidney that produces urine.

nerve agents chemicals that inhibit the degradation of a neurotransmitter (acetylcholine) and quickly facilitate a nervous system overload.

nerve tissue tissue that transmits electrical impulses throughout the body.

net filtration the total loss of water from blood plasma across the capillary membrane into the interstitial space. Normally, hydrostatic pressure forcing water out of the capillary is balanced by an oncotic force pulling water into the capillary for a net filtration of zero.

neuroeffector junction specialized synapse between a nerve cell and the organ or tissue it innervates.

neurogenic shock shock resulting from brain or spinal cord injury that causes an interruption of nerve impulses to the arteries with loss of arterial tone, dilation, and relative hypovolemia.

neuroleptanesthesia anesthesia that combines decreased sensation of pain with amnesia while the patient remains conscious.

neuroleptic antipsychotic (literally, "affecting the nerves").

neuron nerve cell.

neurotransmitter chemical messenger that conducts a nervous impulse across a synapse; a substance that is released from the axon terminal of a presynaptic neuron on excitation and that travels across the synaptic cleft to either excite or inhibit the target cell. Examples include acetylcholine, norepinephrine, and dopamine.

neutropenia a low neutrophil count.

neutropenic having an abnormally low neutrophil count in the blood (less than 2,000/mm^3).

newborn a baby in the first few hours of its life; also called a *newly born infant.*

nitrogen narcosis a state of stupor that develops during deep dives due to nitrogen's effect on cerebral function; also called *raptures of the deep.*

nocturia excessive urination during the night.

noncardiogenic shock types of shock that result from causes other than inadequate cardiac output.

noncompensatory pause pause following an ectopic beat when the SA node is depolarized and the underlying cadence of the heart is interrupted.

noncompetitive antagonism the binding of an antagonist causing a deformity of the binding site that prevents an agonist from fitting and binding.

nonconstituted drug vial/Mix-o-Vial vial with two containers, one holding a powdered medication and the other holding a liquid mixing solution.

nonfeasance a breach of duty by failure to perform a required act or duty.

nonmaleficence the obligation not to harm the patient.

non-ST-elevation myocardial infarction (NSTEMI) myocardial infarction without the presence of an elevated ST segment on the ECG.

nonverbal communication gestures, mannerisms, and postures by which a person communicates with others; also called *body language.*

normal flora organisms that live inside our bodies without ordinarily causing disease.

normal sinus rhythm the normal heart rhythm.

nosocomial infection an infection acquired in a hospital or other medical setting. *See also* community-acquired infection.

nuclear detonation the release of energy generated when heavy nuclei split (fission) or light nuclei combine (fusion) to form new elements. The unleashed energy is tremendous and creates an explosion of immense proportion.

nucleus the organelle within a cell that contains the DNA, or genetic material; in the cells of higher organisms, the nucleus is surrounded by a membrane.

obligate intracellular parasite organism that can grow and reproduce only within a host cell.

oblique having a slanted position or direction.

oblique fracture break in a bone running across it at an angle other than 90 degrees.

obstetrics the branch of medicine that deals with the care of women throughout pregnancy.

ocular medication drug administered through the mucous membranes of the eye.

Officer in Charge (OIC) *see* Command.

off-line medical direction refers to medical policies, procedures, and practices that medical direction has set up in advance of a call.

ohm basic unit for measuring the strength of electrical resistance.

Ohm's law the physical law stating that the current in an electrical circuit is directly proportional to the voltage and inversely proportional to the resistance.

old-old an elderly person age 80 or older.

oliguria decreased urine elimination.

omphalocele congenital hernia of the umbilicus.

oncotic force a form of osmotic pressure exerted by the large protein particles, or colloids, present in blood plasma. In the capillaries, the plasma colloids tend to pull water from the interstitial space across the capillary membrane into the capillary. Oncotic force is also called *colloid osmotic pressure.*

on-line medical direction occurs when a qualified physician gives direct orders to a prehospital care provider by either radio or telephone.

onset of action the time from administration until a medication reaches its minimum effective concentration.

open cricothyrotomy surgical airway technique that places an endotracheal or tracheostomy tube directly into the trachea through a surgical incision at the cricothyroid membrane.

open fracture a broken bone in which the bone ends or the forces that caused it penetrate the surrounding skin.

open incident an incident that has the potential to generate additional patients; also known as an uncontained incident.

open stance a posture or body position that is relaxed and suggests confidence, ease, warmth, and attentiveness.

open-ended questions questions that permit unguided, spontaneous answers.

Operations Section any unit or group that carries out directions from Command and does the actual work at a multiple-casualty incident.

ophthalmoscope handheld device used to examine the interior of the eye.

opportunistic pathogen ordinarily nonharmful bacterium that causes disease only under unusual circumstances.

opposition pairing of muscles that permits extension and flexion of limbs.

oral drug administration the delivery of any medication taken by mouth and swallowed into the lower gastrointestinal tract.

orbit the eye socket.

ordnance military weapons and munitions.

organ a group of tissues that function together. Examples: heart, liver, brain, ovary, eye.

organ system a group of organs that function together. Examples: the cardiovascular system, formed of the heart, blood vessels, and blood; the gastrointestinal system, comprising the mouth, salivary glands, esophagus, stomach, intestines, liver, pancreas, gallbladder, rectum, and anus.

organelles structures that perform specific functions within a cell.

organic brain syndrome *see* senile dementia.

organism the sum of all the cells, tissues, organs, and organ systems of a living being. Examples: the human organism, a bacterial organism.

organophosphates phosphorus-containing organic chemicals.

origin attachment of a muscle to a bone that does not move (or experiences the least movement) when the muscle contracts.

orogastric tube *see* nasogastric tube/orogastric tube.

oropharyngeal airway semicircular device that follows the palate's curvature.

orthopnea difficulty breathing while lying supine.

orthostatic hypotension a decrease in blood pressure that occurs when a person moves from a supine or sitting to an upright position.

Osborn wave *see* J wave.

osmolality the concentration of solute per kilogram of water. *See also* osmolarity.

osmolarity the concentration of solute per liter of water (often used synonymously with *osmolality*).

osmosis movement of solvent in a solution from an area of lower solute concentration to an area of higher solute concentration.

osmotic diuresis greatly increased urination and dehydration that results when high levels of glucose cannot be reabsorbed into the blood from the kidney tubules and the osmotic pressure of the glucose in the tubules also prevents water reabsorption.

osmotic gradient the difference in concentration between solutions on opposite sides of a semipermeable membrane.

osmotic pressure the pressure exerted by the concentration of solutes on one side of a membrane that, if hypertonic, tends to "pull" water (cause osmosis) from the other side of the membrane.

osteoarthritis a degenerative joint disease, characterized by a loss of articular cartilage and hypertrophy of bone.

osteoblast cell that helps in the creation of new bone during growth and bone repair.

osteoclast bone cell that absorbs and removes excess bone.

osteocyte bone-forming cell found in the bone matrix that helps maintain the bone.

osteoporosis weakening of bone tissue due to loss of essential minerals, especially calcium.

otitis media middle ear infection.

otoscope handheld device used to examine interior of ears and nose.

ovaries the primary female sex glands that secrete estrogen and progesterone and produce eggs for reproduction.

overdrive respiration positive-pressure ventilation supplied to a breathing patient.

overhydration the presence of retention of an abnormally high amount of body fluid.

overpressure a rapid increase, then decrease, in atmospheric pressure created by an explosion.

over-the-needle catheter semiflexible catheter enclosing a sharp metal stylet; also called an *angiocatheter.*

ovulation the release of an egg from the ovary.

oxidation the loss of hydrogen atoms or the acceptance of an oxygen atom. This increases the positive charge (or lessens the negative charge) on the molecule.

oxidizer an agent that enhances combustion of a fuel.

oxygen saturation percentage (SpO_2) the saturation of arterial blood with oxygen as measured by pulse oximetry expressed as a percentage.

PA alveolar partial pressure.

Pa arterial partial pressure.

pallor paleness.

palmar grasp a reflex in the newborn, which is elicited by placing a finger firmly in the infant's palm.

palpation using your sense of touch to gather information.

pancolitis ulcerative colitis spread throughout the entire colon.

panic attack extreme period of anxiety resulting in great emotional distress.

papilla the tip of a pyramid; it juts into the hollow space of the kidney.

paradoxical breathing assymetrical chest wall movement that lessens respiratory efficiency. *See also* flail chest.

parasites organisms that live in or on another organism.

parasympathetic nervous system division of the autonomic nervous system that is responsible for controlling vegetative functions. Parasympathetic nervous system actions include decreased heart rate and constriction of the bronchioles and pupils. Its actions are mediated by the neurotransmitter acetylcholine.

parasympatholytic drug or other substance that blocks or inhibits the actions of the parasympathetic nervous system; also called *anticholinergic.*

parasympathomimetic drug or other substance that causes effects like those of the parasympathetic nervous system; also called *cholinergic.*

parenchyma principle or essential parts of an organ.

parent drug *see* prodrug.

parenteral route delivery of a medication outside of the gastrointestinal tract, typically using needles to inject medications into the circulatory system or tissues.

Parkinson's disease chronic, degenerative nervous disease characterized by tremors, muscular weakness and rigidity, and a loss of postural reflexes.

paroxysmal nocturnal dyspnea (PND) sudden short episodes of difficult breathing that occur after lying down; usually at night, most commonly caused by left heart failure.

partial pressure the pressure exerted by each component of a gas mixture.

partial seizures seizures that remain confined to a limited portion of the brain, causing localized malfunction. Partial seizures may spread and become generalized. *See also* seizure.

partial-thickness burn burn in which the epidermis is burned through and the dermis is damaged; characterized by redness and blistering; also called a *second-degree burn.*

particulate evidence evidence such as hairs or fibers that cannot be readily seen with the human eyes; microscopic or trace evidence.

partner abuse physical or emotional violence from a man or woman toward a domestic partner.

passive immunity acquired immunity that results from administration of antibodies either from mother to the infant across the placental barrier (natural passive immunity) or through vaccination (induced passive immunity).

passive transport movement of a substance without the use of energy.

pathogen a microorganism capable of producing infection or disease.

pathology the study of disease and its causes.

pathophysiology the physiology of disordered function; the study of how disease affects normal body processes.

patient assessment problem-oriented evaluation of patient and establishment of priorities based on existing and potential threats to human life.

patient interview interaction with a patient for the purpose of obtaining in-depth information about the emergency and the patient's pertinent medical history.

PCO_2 partial pressure of carbon dioxide; (*partial pressure* defined—*see* PO_2).

peak load the highest volume of calls at a given time.

pedicles thick, bony struts that connect the vertebral bodies with the spinous and transverse processes and help make up the opening for the spinal canal.

PEEP *see* positive end-expiratory pressure (PEEP).

peer review an evaluation of the quality of emergency care administered by an individual, which is conducted by that individual's peers (others of equal rank). Also, an evaluation of articles submitted for publication.

pelvic inflammatory disease (PID) an acute infection of the reproductive organs that can be caused by a bacteria, virus, or fungus.

pelvic space division of the abdominal cavity containing those organs located within the pelvis.

penetrating trauma injury caused by an object breaking the skin and entering the body.

penis male organ of copulation.

peptic ulcer erosion caused by gastric acid.

percussion the production of sound waves by striking one object against another.

perforating canals structures through which blood vessels enter and exit the bone shaft.

perfusion the supplying of oxygen and nutrients to the body tissues as a result of the constant passage of blood through the capillaries.

pericardial tamponade filling of the pericardial sac with fluid, which in turn limits the filling and function of the heart.

perimetrium the serosal peritoneal membrane which forms the outermost layer of the uterine wall.

perinephric abscess a pocket of infection in the layer of fat surrounding the kidney.

perineum muscular tissue that separates the vagina and the anus.

period *see* menstruation.

periorbital ecchymosis black and blue discoloration surrounding the eye sockets.

periosteum the tough exterior covering of a bone.

peripheral arterial atherosclerotic disease a progressive degenerative disease of the medium-sized and large arteries.

peripheral nervous system part of the nervous system that extends throughout the body and is composed of the cranial nerves arising from the brain and the peripheral nerves arising from the spinal cord. Its subdivisions are the somatic and the autonomic nervous systems.

peripheral neuropathy any malfunction or damage of the peripheral nerves. Results may include muscle weakness, loss of sensation, impaired reflexes, and internal organ malfunctions.

peripheral vascular resistance the resistance of the vessels to the flow of blood; increased when the vessels constrict, decreased when the vessels relax.

peripheral venous access surgical puncture of a vein in the arm, leg, or neck.

peripherally inserted central catheter (PICC) line threaded into the central circulation via a peripheral site.

peristalsis wavelike muscular motion of the esophagus and bowel that moves food through the digestive system.

peritoneal dialysis a dialysis procedure relying on the peritoneal membrane as the semipermeable membrane.

peritoneal space division of the abdominal cavity containing those organs or portions of organs covered by the peritoneum.

peritoneum fine fibrous tissue surrounding the interior of most of the abdominal cavity and covering most of the small bowel and some of the abdominal organs.

peritonitis inflammation of the peritoneum, which lines the abdominal cavity, caused by chemical or bacterial irritation.

permissive a parenting style that takes a tolerant, accepting view of a child's behavior.

persistent fetal circulation condition in which blood continues to bypass the fetal respiratory system, resulting in ongoing hypoxia.

personal protective equipment (PPE) equipment used by EMS personnel to protect against injury and the spread of infectious disease.

personality disorder condition that results in persistently maladaptive behavior.

pertussis disease characterized by severe, violent coughing; whooping cough.

pH abbreviation for *potential of hydrogen.* A measure of relative acidity or alkalinity. Since the pH scale is inverse to the concentration of acidic hydrogen ions, the lower the pH the greater the acidity and the higher the pH the greater the alkalinity. A normal pH range is 7.35 to 7.45.

phagocytosis process in which a cell surrounds and absorbs a bacterium or other particle.

pharmacodynamics how a drug interacts with the body to cause its effects.

pharmacokinetics how a drug is absorbed, distributed, metabolized (biotransformed), and excreted; how drugs are transported into and out of the body.

pharmacology the study of drugs and their interactions with the body.

pharyngitis infection of the pharynx and tonsils.

pharyngo-tracheal lumen airway (PtL) a dual-lumen airway system.

pharynx a muscular tube that extends vertically from the back of the soft palate to the superior aspect of the esophagus.

phobia excessive fear that interferes with functioning.

phototherapy exposure to sunlight or artificial light for therapeutic purposes. In newborns, light is used to treat hyperbilirubinemia or jaundice.

physiological stress a chemical or physical disturbance in the cells or tissue fluid produced by a change in the external environment or within the body.

physiology the functions of an organism; the physical and chemical processes of a living thing.

pia mater inner and most delicate layer of the meninges. It covers the convolutions of the brain and spinal cord.

Pierre Robin syndrome unusually small jaw, combined with a cleft palate, downward displacement of the tongue, and an absent gag reflex.

pill-rolling motion an involuntary tremor, usually in one hand or sometimes in both, in which fingers move as if they were rolling a pill back and forth.

pinna outer, visible portion of the ear.
pinworms parasites that are 3–10 mm long and live in the distal colon.
pitting depression that results from pressure against skin when pitting edema is present.
placenta the organ that serves as a lifeline for the developing fetus. The placenta is attached to the wall of the uterus and the umbilical cord.
placental barrier biochemical barrier at the maternal/fetal interface that restricts certain molecules.
planning provides past, present, and future information about a potential incident.
plasma the liquid part of the blood.
plasma-level profile describes the lengths of onset, duration, and termination of action, as well as the drug's minimum effective concentration and toxic levels.
plasma membrane *see* cell membrane.
platelet phase second step in the clotting process in which platelets adhere to blood vessel walls and to each other.
pleura membranous connective tissue covering the lungs.
pleural friction rub the squeaking or grating sound of the pleural linings rubbing together.
pleuritic sharp or tearing, as a description of pain.
pluripotent stem cell a cell from which the various types of blood cells can form.
pneumatic anti-shock garment (PASG) garment designed to produce uniform pressure on the lower extremities and abdomen; used with shock and hemorrhage patients in some EMS systems.
pneumomediastinum the presence of air in the mediastinum.
pneumonia acute infection of the lung, including alveolar spaces and interstitial tissue.
pneumothorax a collection of air in the pleural space, causing a loss of the negative pressure that binds the lung to the chest wall. In an *open pneumothorax,* air enters the pleural space through an injury to the chest wall. In a *closed pneumothorax,* air enters the pleural space through an opening in the pleura that covers the lung. A *tension pneumothorax* develops when air in the pleural space cannot escape, causing a buildup of pressure and collapse of the lung.
PO_2 partial pressure of oxygen (*partial pressure* is the pressure exerted by a given component of a gas containing several components).
Poiseuille's law a law of physiology stating that blood flow through a vessel is directly proportional to the radius of the vessel to the fourth power.
poliomyelitis (polio) infectious, inflammatory viral disease of the central nervous system that sometimes results in permanent paralysis.
polycythemia an excess of red blood cells.
polypharmacy multiple drug therapy in which there is a concurrent use of a number of drugs.
polyuria excessive urination.
pons process of tissue responsible for the communication interchange between the cerebellum, the cerebrum, the midbrain, and the spinal cord.
portal pertaining to the flow of blood into the liver.
positional asphyxia death from positioning that prevents sufficient intake of oxygen.
positive end-expiratory pressure (PEEP) a method of holding the alveoli open by increasing expiratory pressure. Some bag-valve units used in EMS have PEEP attachments. Also EMS personnel sometimes transport patients who are on ventilators with PEEP attachments.
postconventional reasoning the stage of moral development during which individuals make moral decisions according to an enlightened conscience.
posterior medial sulcus shallow longitudinal groove along the dorsal surface of the spinal cord.
postganglionic nerves nerve fibers that extend from the autonomic ganglia to the target tissues. *See also* preganglionic nerves.
postpartum depression the "let down" feeling experienced during the period following birth occurring in 70–80 percent of mothers.
postrenal acute renal failure ARF due to obstruction distal to the kidney.
post-traumatic stress syndrome reaction to an extreme stressor.
posture position, attitude, or bearing of the body.
PPD purified protein derivative, the substance used in a test for tuberculosis.
prearrival instructions dispatcher's instructions to caller for appropriate emergency measures.
preconventional reasoning the stage of moral development during which children respond mainly to cultural control to avoid punishment and attain satisfaction.
precordial leads electrocardiogram leads applied to the chest in a pattern that permits a view of the horizontal plane of the heart; leads V1, V2, V3, V4, V5, and V6. Also called *chest leads.*
precordium area of the chest wall overlying the heart.
prefilled/preloaded syringe syringe packaged in a tamper-proof container with the medication already in the barrel.
preganglionic nerves nerve fibers that extend from the central nervous system to the autonomic ganglia. *See also* postganglionic nerves.
prehospital care report (PCR) the written record of an EMS response.

preload the pressure within the ventricles at the end of diastole, also called *end-diastolic volume.*

premenstrual syndrome (PMS) a variety of signs and symptoms, such as weight gain, irritability, or specific food cravings, associated with the changing hormonal levels that precede menstruation.

prerenal acute renal failure acute renal failure caused by decreased blood perfusion of the kidneys.

presbycusis progressive hearing loss that occurs with aging.

pressure ulcer ischemic damage and subsequent necrosis affecting the skin, subcutaneous tissue, and often the muscle; result of intense pressure over a short time or low pressure over a long time; a pressure sore or bedsore.

pressure wave area of overpressure that radiates outward from an explosion.

priapism a painful, prolonged erection of the penis.

primary area of responsibility (PAR) stationing of ambulances at specific high-volume locations.

primary assessment prehospital process designed to identify and correct life-threatening airway, breathing, and circulation problems.

primary care basic health care provided at the patient's first contact with the health care system.

primary contamination direct exposure of a person or item to a hazardous substance.

primary prevention keeping an injury or illness from ever occurring.

primary problem the underlying cause for a patient's symptoms.

primary response initial, generalized response to an antigen.

primary triage triage that takes place early in the incident, usually on first arrival.

Prinzmetal's angina variant of angina pectoris caused by vasospasm of the coronary arteries, not blockage per se; also called *vasospastic angina* or *atypical angina.*

prions particles of protein, folded in such a way that protease enzymes cannot act on them.

priority dispatching system that uses medically approved questions and predetermined guidelines to determine the appropriate level of response.

proctitis ulcerative colitis limited to the rectum.

prodrug medication that is not active when administered, but whose biotransformation converts it into active metabolites; also called *parent drug.*

profession a specialized body of knowledge or skills.

professionalism the conduct or qualities that characterize a practitioner in a particular field or occupation.

profile the size and shape of a projectile as it contacts a target; it is the energy exchange surface of the contact.

prognosis the anticipated outcome of a disease or injury.

progressive shock *see* decompensated shock.

prolonged QT interval QT interval greater than 0.44 second in an ECG.

prostaglandins substances synthesized by mast cells during an inflammatory response that cause vasodilation, vascular permeability, and chemotaxis and also cause pain.

prostate gland gland that surrounds the male urinary bladder neck and is a major source of the fluid that combines with sperm to form semen.

prostatitis infection and inflammation of the prostate gland.

protocol predetermined, written guidelines for patient care; the policies and procedures for all components of an EMS system.

protoplasm *see* cytoplasm.

prototype drug that best demonstrates the class's common properties and illustrates its particular characteristics.

protozoa single-celled parasitic organisms with flexible membranes and the ability to move.

proximal tubule the part of the renal tubule beyond Bowman's capsule.

proximate cause action or inaction of the paramedic that immediately caused or worsened the damage suffered by the patient.

pruritus itching; often occurs as a symptom of some systemic change or illness.

pseudo-instinctive learned actions that are practiced until they can be done without thinking.

psychogenic amnesia failure to recall, as opposed to inability to recall.

psychoneuroimmunological regulation the interactions of psychological, neurological/endocrine, and immunological factors that contribute to alteration of the immune system as an outcome of a stress response that is not quickly resolved.

psychosis extreme response to stress characterized by impaired ability to deal with reality.

psychosocial related to a patient's personality style, dynamics of unresolved conflict, or crisis management methods.

psychotherapeutic medication drug used to treat mental dysfunction.

public safety answering point (PSAP) an agency that takes emergency calls from citizens in a given region and dispatches the necessary emergency resources.

puerperium the time period surrounding the birth of the fetus.

pulmonary agents chemicals that primarily cause injury to the lungs; commonly referred to as choking agents.

pulmonary embolism (PE) blood clot in one of the pulmonary arteries.

pulmonary hilum central medial region of the lung where the bronchi and pulmonary vasculature enter the lung.

pulmonary overpressure expansion of air held in the lungs during ascent. If not exhaled, the expanded air may cause injury to the lungs and surrounding structures.

pulse oximeter noninvasive device that measures the hemoglobin oxygen saturation of hemoglobin.

pulse pressure the difference between the systolic and diastolic blood pressures.

pulse quality strength, which can be weak, thready, strong, or bounding.

pulse rate number of pulses felt in 1 minute.

pulse rhythm pattern and equality of intervals between beats.

pulsus paradoxus drop of greater than 10 mmHg in the systolic blood pressure during the inspiratory phase of respiration that occurs in patients with pericardial tamponade.

puncture specific soft-tissue injury involving a deep, narrow wound to the skin and underlying organs that carries an increased danger of infection.

pupil dark opening in the center of the iris through which light enters the eye.

pus a liquid mixture of dead cells, bits of dead tissue, and tissue fluid that may accumulate in inflamed tissues.

pyelonephritis an infection and inflammation of the kidney.

pyramids the visible tissue structures within the medulla of the kidney.

pyrexia fever, or above-normal body temperature.

pyrogen any substance causing a fever, such as viruses and bacteria or substances produced within the body in response to infection or inflammation.

QT interval period from the beginning of the QRS to the end of the T wave in an ECG.

quality assurance (QA) a program designed to maintain continuous monitoring and measurement of the quality of clinical care delivered to patients.

quality improvement (QI) an evaluation program that emphasizes service and uses customer satisfaction as the ultimate indicator of system performance.

quality of respiration depth and pattern of breathing.

rabies viral disorder that affects the nervous system.

raccoon eyes *see* bilateral periorbital ecchymosis.

radiation transfer of energy through space or matter.

radiation absorbed dose (rad) basic unit of absorbed radiation dose.

radio band a range of radio frequencies.

radio frequency the number of times per second a radio wave oscillates.

radioactive substance a substance that emits ionizing radiation; also called a *radionuclide* or *radioisotope.*

radioisotope *see* radioactive substance.

radionuclide *see* radioactive substance.

rape penile penetration of the genitalia or rectum without the consent of the victim.

Rapid Intervention Team ambulance and crew dedicated to stand by in case a rescuer becomes ill or injured.

rapid secondary assessment quick check for signs of serious injury.

rapid-sequence intubation giving medications to sedate (induce) and temporarily paralyze a patient and then performing orotracheal intubation.

raptures of the deep *see* nitrogen narcosis.

reabsorption the movement of a substance from a nephron tubule back into the blood.

reasonable force the minimal amount of force necessary to ensure that an unruly or violent person does not cause injury to himself or others.

rebound tenderness pain on release of the examiner's hands, allowing the patient's abdominal wall to return to its normal position; associated with peritoneal irritation.

receptor specialized protein that combines with a drug resulting in a biochemical effect.

reciprocity the process by which an agency grants automatic certification or licensure to an individual who has comparable certification or licensure from another agency.

recirculating currents movement of currents over a uniform obstruction; also known as a "drowning machine."

recompression resubmission of a person to a greater pressure so that gradual decompression can be achieved; often used in the treatment of diving emergencies.

red bone marrow tissue within the internal cavity of a bone responsible for manufacture of erythrocytes and other blood cells.

red zone *see* hot zone.

reduced nephron mass the decrease in number of functional nephrons that causes chronic renal failure.

reduced renal mass the decrease in kidney size associated with chronic renal failure.

reduction returning of displaced bone ends to their proper anatomical orientation.

referred pain pain that is felt at a location away from its source.

reflective acting thoughtfully, deliberately, and analytically.

refractory period the period of time when myocardial cells have not yet completely repolarized and cannot be stimulated again. *See also* relative refractory period.

registration the process of entering one's name and essential information within a particular record. In EMS this allows the state to verify the provider's initial certification and to monitor recertification.

regulatory law *see* administrative law.

relative refractory period the period of the cardiac cycle when a sufficiently strong stimulus may produce depolarization. *See also* refractory period.

remodeling stage in the wound healing process in which collagen is broken down and relaid in an orderly fashion.

renal pertaining to the kidneys.

renal ARF (renal acute renal failure) acute renal failure resulting from pathology within the kidney tissue itself.

renal calculi kidney stones.

renal dialysis artificial replacement of some critical kidney functions.

renal pelvis the hollow space of the kidney that junctions with a ureter.

renin an enzyme produced by kidney cells that plays a key role in controlling arterial blood pressure.

repair healing of a wound with scar formation.

repolarization return of a cell to its preexcitation resting state.

reportable collisions collisions that involve over $1,000 in damage or a personal injury.

res ipsa loquitur a legal doctrine invoked by plaintiffs to support a claim of negligence, a Latin term that means "the thing speaks for itself."

Rescue *see* Extrication.

reserve capacity the ability of an EMS agency to respond to calls beyond those handled by the on-duty crews.

reservoir any living creature or environment (e.g., water, soil) that can harbor an infectious agent.

resiliency the connective strength and elasticity of an object or fabric.

resistance [biological] a host's ability to fight off infection. [physical] property of a conductor that opposes the passage of an electric current.

resolution the complete healing of a wound and return of tissues to their normal structure and function; the ending of inflammation with no scar formation.

resolution phase final stage of the burn process in which scar tissue is laid down and the healing process is completed.

respiration exchange of gases between a living organism and its environment; exchange of oxygen and carbon dioxide in the lungs and at the cellular level.

respirator an apparatus worn that cleanses or qualifies the air that is breathed in.

respiratory acidosis acidity caused by abnormal retention of carbon dioxide resulting from impaired ventilation.

respiratory alkalosis alkalinity caused by excessive elimination of carbon dioxide resulting from increased respirations.

respiratory effort how hard a person works to breathe.

respiratory rate the number of times a person breathes in 1 minute.

respiratory syncytial virus (RSV) common cause of pneumonia and bronchiolitis in children.

response time time elapsed from when a unit is alerted until it arrives on the scene.

resting potential the normal electrical state of cardiac cells.

resuscitation provision of efforts to return a spontaneous pulse and breathing.

reticular activating system (RAS) a series of nervous tissues keeping the human system in a state of consciousness.

retina light- and color-sensing tissue lining the posterior chamber of the eye.

retinal detachment a condition that may be of traumatic origin and that presents with patient complaint of a dark curtain obstructing a portion of the field of view.

retinopathy any disorder of the retina.

retroauricular ecchymosis black-and-blue discoloration over the mastoid process (just behind the ear) that is characteristic of a basilar skull fracture; also called *Battle's sign.*

retrograde amnesia inability to remember events that occurred before the trauma that caused the condition. *See also* anterograde amnesia.

retroperitoneal space division of the abdominal cavity containing those organs that lie posterior to the peritoneal lining.

return of spontaneous circulation resuscitation resulting in the patient's having a spontaneous pulse.

review of systems a list of questions categorized by body system.

Rh blood group a group of antigens discovered on the red blood cells of rhesus monkeys that is also present to some extent in humans.

Rh factor an antigen in the Rh blood group that is also known as antigen D. About 85 percent of North Americans have the Rh factor (are Rh positive) while about 15 percent do not have the Rh factor (are Rh negative). Rh positive and Rh negative blood are incompatible; that is, a person who is Rh negative can experience a severe immune response if Rh positive blood is introduced, as through a transfusion or during childbirth.

rhabdomyolysis acute pathologic process that involves the destruction of skeletal muscle.

rheumatoid arthritis chronic disease that causes deterioration of peripheral joint connective tissue.

rhinorrhea watery discharge from the nose.

rhonchi continuous sounds with a lower pitch and a snoring quality.

rhythm strip electrocardiogram printout.

roentgen equivalent in man (rem) a gauge of the likely injury to the irradiated part of an organism.

rooting reflex occurs when a hungry infant's cheek is touched by a hand or cloth and the infant turns his head to the right or left.

rotation a turning along the axis of a bone or joint.

rouleaux group of red blood cells that are stuck together.

rubella (German measles) systemic viral disease characterized by a fine pink rash that appears on the face, trunk, and extremities and fades quickly.

rule of nines method of estimating amount of body surface area burned by a division of the body into regions, each of which represents approximately 9 percent of the total body surface area, plus 1 percent for the genital region.

rule of palms method of estimating amount of body surface area burned that sizes the area burned in comparison to the patient's palmar surface.

rules of evidence guidelines for permitting a new medication, process, or procedure to be used in EMS on the basis of proven efficacy.

Ryan White Act federal law that outlines the rights and responsibilities of agencies and health care workers when an infectious disease exposure occurs.

Safety Officer (SO) person who monitors all on-scene actions at a multiple-casualty incident and ensures that they do not create any potentially harmful conditions.

safe zone *see* cold zone.

saline lock peripheral IV cannula with a distal medication port used for intermittent fluid or medication infusions. Saline is injected into the device to maintain its patency.

scabies skin disease caused by mite infestation and characterized by intense itching.

scaffolding a teaching/learning technique in which one builds on what has already been learned.

scene safety doing everything possible to ensure a safe environment.

scene-authority law state or local statute specifying who has ultimate authority at a multiple-casualty incident.

schizophrenia common psychiatric disorder involving significant change in behavior often including hallucinations, delusions, and depression.

sclera the white of the eye.

scope of practice range of duties and skills paramedics are allowed and expected to perform.

scrambling climbing over rocks and/or downed trees on a steep trail without the aid of ropes. This can be especially dangerous when the surface is icy.

scree loose pebbles or rock debris that can form on the slopes or bases of mountains; sometimes used to describe debris in sloping dry stream beds.

scuba acronym for *self-contained underwater breathing apparatus.* Portable apparatus that contains compressed air, which allows the diver to breathe underwater.

sebaceous glands glands within the dermis that secrete sebum.

sebum fatty secretion of the sebaceous gland that helps keep the skin pliable and waterproof.

second messenger chemical that participates in complex cascading reactions that eventually cause a drug's desired effect.

secondary assessment problem-oriented assessment process based on initial assessment and chief complaint.

secondary contamination transfer of a hazardous substance to a noncontaminated person or item via contact with someone or something already contaminated by the substance.

secondary prevention medical care after an injury or illness that helps to prevent further problems from occurring.

secondary response response by the immune system that takes place if the body is exposed to the same antigen again; in secondary response, antibodies specific for the offending antigen are released.

secondary triage triage that takes place after patients have been moved to a treatment area to determine any change in status.

secretion the movement of a substance from the blood into a nephron tubule.

Section Chief officer who supervises major functional areas or sections at a multiple-casualty incident; reports to the Incident Commander.

sector interchangeable name for a branch, group, or division within the Incident Management System; does not, however, designate a functional or geographic area.

secure attachment a type of bonding that occurs when an infant learns that his caregivers will be responsive and helpful when needed.

sedation state of decreased anxiety and inhibitions.

seizure a temporary alteration in behavior due to the massive electrical discharge of one or more groups of neurons in the brain. Seizures can be clinically classified as generalized or partial.

Sellick maneuver pressure applied in a posterior direction to the anterior cricoid cartilage to occlude the esophagus.

semantic related to the meaning of words.

semicircular canals the three rings of the inner ear that sense the motion of the head and provide positional sense for the body.

semi-decontaminated patient another term for field-decontaminated patient.

semi-Fowler's position sitting up at a 45-degree angle.

semipermeable able to allow some, but not all, substances to pass through. Cell membranes are semipermeable.

Sengstaken-Blakemore tube three-lumen tube used in treating esophageal bleeding.

senile dementia general term for an abnormal decline in mental functioning in the elderly; also called *organic brain syndrome* or *multi-infarct dementia.*

sensitization initial exposure of a person to an antigen that results in an immune response.

sensorineural deafness deafness caused by the inability of nerve impulses to reach the auditory center of the brain because of nerve damage either to the inner ear or to the brain.

sensorium sensory apparatus of the body as a whole; also that portion of the brain that functions as a center of sensations.

sepsis *see* septicemia.

septic shock shock that develops as the result of infection carried by the bloodstream, eventually causing dysfunction of multiple organ systems.

septicemia the systemic spread of toxins through the bloodstream. Also called *sepsis.*

sequestration the trapping of red blood cells by an organ such as the spleen.

seroconversion creation of antibodies after exposure to a disease.

serotonin a substance released by platelets that, through constriction and dilation of blood vessels, affects blood flow to an injured or affected site.

serous fluid a cellular component of blood, similar to plasma.

serum solution containing whole antibodies for a specific pathogen.

sesamoid bone bone that forms in a tendon.

severe acute respiratory syndrome (SARS) highly infectious viral respiratory illness that first appeared in southern China in 2002.

sexual assault unwanted oral, genital, rectal, or manual sexual contact.

sexually transmitted disease (STD) illness most commonly transmitted through sexual contact.

sharps container rigid, puncture-resistant container clearly marked as a biohazard.

shipping papers documents routinely carried aboard vehicles transporting hazardous materials; ideally should identify specific substances and quantities carried; also known as *bills of lading.*

shock a state of inadequate tissue perfusion. *See also* hypoperfusion.

short haul an extrication technique where a person is attached to a rope that is, in turn, attached to a helicopter. The aircraft lifts off with the person attached to it.

shunt surgical connection that runs from the brain to the abdomen for the purpose of draining excess cerebrospinal fluid, thus preventing increased intracranial pressure.

Shy-Drager syndrome chronic orthostatic hypotension caused by a primary autonomic nervous system deficiency.

sick sinus syndrome a group of disorders characterized by dysfunction of the sinoatrial node in the heart.

sickle cell anemia an inherited disorder of red blood cell production, so named because the red blood cells become sickle-shaped when oxygen levels are low.

side effect unintended or unwanted response to a drug.

silent myocardial infarction a myocardial infarction that occurs without exhibiting obvious signs and symptoms.

simple diffusion the random motion of molecules from an area of high concentration to an area of lower concentration.

simple partial seizure type of partial seizure that involves local motor, sensory, or autonomic dysfunction of one area of the body. There is no loss of consciousness. *See also* partial seizures.

simplex system communication system that transmits and receives on the same frequency.

Singular Command process in which a single individual is responsible for coordinating a multiple-casualty incident; most useful in single-jurisdictional incidents.

sinus air cavity that conducts fluids from the eustachian tubes and tear ducts to and from the nasopharynx.

sinusitis inflammation of the paranasal sinuses.

skeletal muscle *see* muscle tissue.

slander act of injuring a person's character, name, or reputation by false or malicious statements spoken with malicious intent or reckless disregard for the falsity of those statements.

slow-reacting substance of anaphylaxis (SRS-A) substance released from basophils and mast cells that causes spasm of the bronchiole smooth muscle, resulting in an asthma-like attack and occasionally asphyxia. *See also* leukotrienes.

slow-to-warm-up child an infant who can be characterized by a low intensity of reactions and a somewhat negative mood.

smooth muscle *see* muscle tissue.

sociocultural related to the patient's actions and interactions within society.

solvent a substance that dissolves other substances, forming a solution.
somatic nervous system part of the nervous system controlling voluntary bodily functions.
somatic pain sharp, localized pain that originates in walls of the body such as skeletal muscles.
somatoform disorder condition characterized by physical symptoms that have no apparent physiological cause and are attributable to psychological factors.
span of control number of people or tasks that a single individual can effectively monitor.
spasm intermittent or continuous contraction of a muscle.
special weapons and tactics (SWAT) team a trained police unit equipped to handle hostage holders and other difficult law enforcement situations.
specific gravity the density or weight of a vapor or gas as compared with air.
sphygmomanometer blood pressure measuring device comprising a bulb, a cuff, and a manometer.
spike sharp-pointed device inserted into the IV solution bag's administration set port.
spina bifida (SB) a neural defect that results from the failure of one or more of the fetal vertebrae to close properly during the first month of pregnancy.
spinal canal opening in the vertebrae that accommodates the spinal cord.
spinal cord central nervous system pathway responsible for transmitting sensory input from the body to the brain and for conducting motor impulses from the brain to the body muscles and organs.
spinal nerves 31 pairs of nerves that originate along the spinal cord from anterior and posterior nerve roots.
spinous process prominence at the posterior part of a vertebra.
spiral fracture a curving break in a bone as may be caused by rotational forces.
spondylosis a degeneration of the vertebral body.
spontaneous abortion *see* miscarriage.
spontaneous pneumothorax a pneumothorax (collection of air in the pleural space) that occurs spontaneously, in the absence of blunt or penetrating trauma. *See also* pneumothorax.
spotter the person positioned behind the left rear side of the ambulance who assists the operator in backing up the vehicle.
sprain tearing of a joint capsule's connective tissues.
staff functions officers who perform supervisory roles in the Incident Management System rather than actually performing a specific task.
Staging Area location where ambulances, personnel, and equipment are kept in reserve for use at a multiple-casualty incident.
Staging Officer person who supervises the Staging Area and guards against premature commitment of resources and freelancing by personnel at a multiple-casualty incident; reports to the branch director.
standard of care the degree of care, skill, and judgment that would be expected under like or similar circumstances by a similarly trained, reasonable paramedic in the same community.
Standard Precautions a strict form of infection control that is based on the assumption that all blood and other body fluids are infectious.
standing orders preauthorized treatment procedures; a type of treatment protocol.
Starling's law of the heart law of physiology stating that the more the myocardium is stretched, up to a certain limit, the more forceful the subsequent contraction will be.
START acronym for the most widely used disaster triage system; stands for *Simple Triage and Rapid Treatment.*
startle reflex *see* Moro reflex.
status asthmaticus a severe, prolonged asthma attack that cannot be broken by aggressive pharmacological management.
status epilepticus prolonged seizure or multiple seizures with no intervening periods of consciousness.
statutory law *see* legislative law.
ST-elevation myocardial infarction (STEMI) myocardial infarction with the presence of an elevated ST segment on the ECG.
stenosis narrowing or constriction.
sterilization use of a chemical or physical method such as pressurized steam to kill all microorganisms on an object.
sterile free of all forms of life.
sterilize to destroy all microorganisms.
stethoscope tool used to auscultate sounds within the body.
stock solution standard concentration of a routinely used medication.
Stokes-Adams syndrome a series of symptoms resulting from heart block, most commonly syncope. The symptoms result from decreased blood flow to the brain caused by the sudden decrease in cardiac output.
stoma opening in the anterior neck and trachea through which the patient breathes.
strain injury resulting from overstretching of muscle fibers.
strainers partial obstructions that filter, or strain, the water, such as downed trees or wire mesh, causing an unequal force on the two sides of the obstruction.
stress a state of physical or psychological arousal to stimulus.
stress response changes within the body initiated by a stressor.

stressor the stimulus or cause of stress.

striated muscle *see* muscle tissue.

stridor predominantly inspiratory wheeze associated with laryngeal obstruction.

stroke injury to or death of brain tissue caused by either ischemic or hemorrhagic lesions to a portion of the brain. Commonly also called a *cerebrovascular accident (CVA)* or *brain attack.*

stroke volume the amount of blood ejected by the heart in one cardiac contraction.

stylet plastic-covered metal wire used to bend an endotracheal tube into a J or hockey-stick shape.

subarachnoid hemorrhage bleeding that occurs between the arachnoid and dura mater of the brain.

subcutaneous emphysema crackling sensation caused by air just underneath the skin.

subcutaneous tissue skin layer beneath the dermis; the layer of loose connective tissue between skin and muscle.

subdural hematoma collection of blood directly beneath the dura mater.

subendocardial infarction myocardial infarction that affects only the deeper levels of the myocardium; also called *non-Q wave infarction* because it typically does not result in a significant Q wave in the affected ECG lead.

subglottic referring to the lower airway.

sublingual beneath the tongue.

subluxation partial displacement of a bone end from its position in a joint capsule.

substance abuse misuse of chemically active agents such as alcohol, psychoactive chemicals, and therapeutic agents; typically results in clinically significant impairment or distress; use of a pharmacological substance for purposes other than medically defined reasons.

sucking reflex sucking response that occurs when an infant's lips are stroked.

suction to remove solids or fluids with a vacuum-type device.

sudden death death within 1 hour after the onset of symptoms.

sudden infant death syndrome (SIDS) fatal illness of unknown etiology that occurs during the first year of life, with the peak at ages 2–4 months.

sudoriferous glands glands within the dermis that secrete sweat.

superficial burn a burn that involves only the epidermis; characterized by reddening of the skin; also called a *first-degree burn.*

superficial frostbite freezing involving only epidermal tissues, resulting in redness followed by blanching and diminished sensation; also called *frostnip.*

suppository medication packaged in a soft, pliable form, for insertion into the rectum.

supraglottic referring to the upper airway.

surface absorption entry of a substance into the body directly through the skin or mucous membrane.

surfactant a compound secreted by cells in the lungs that regulates the surface tension of the fluid that lines the alveoli, which is important in keeping the alveoli open for gas exchange.

survival when a patient is resuscitated and survives to be discharged from the hospital.

sutures pseudojoints that join the various bones of the skull to form the cranium.

sympathetic nervous system division of the autonomic nervous system that prepares the body for stressful situations. Sympathetic nervous system actions include increased heart rate and dilation of the bronchioles and pupils. Its actions are mediated by the neurotransmitters epinephrine and norepinephrine.

sympatholytic drug or other substance that blocks the actions of the sympathetic nervous system; also called *antiadrenergic.*

sympathomimetic drug or other substance that causes effects like those of the sympathetic nervous system; also called *adrenergic.*

synapse space between nerves.

synarthrosis joint that does not permit movement.

synchronized cardioversion the passage of an electric current through the heart during a specific part of the cardiac cycle to terminate certain kinds of dysrhythmias.

syncope transient loss of consciousness due to inadequate flow of blood to the brain with rapid recovery of consciousness on becoming supine; fainting.

syncytium group of cardiac muscle cells that physiologically function as a unit.

synergism pharmacological principle in which two drugs or other substances work together to produce an effect that neither of them can produce on its own.

synovial capsule *see* joint capsule.

synovial fluid substance that lubricates synovial joints.

synovial joint joint that permits the greatest degree of independent motion.

syphilis bloodborne sexually transmitted disease caused by the spirochete *Treponema pallidum.*

syringe plastic tube with which liquid medications can be drawn up, stored, and injected.

system status management (SSM) a computerized personnel and ambulance deployment system.

systemic throughout the body.

systemic effects effects that occur throughout the body after exposure to a toxic substance.

systole the period of the cardiac cycle when the myocardium is contracting.

systolic blood pressure force of blood against arteries when ventricles contract.

T lymphocytes white blood cells that do not produce antibodies but, instead, attack antigens directly.

tachycardia a heart rate greater than 100 beats per minute.

tachypnea rapid respiration.

tactical emergency medical services (TEMS) a specially trained unit that provides on-site medical support to law enforcement.

tactile fremitus vibratory tremors felt through the chest by palpation.

teachable moment the time shortly after an injury when patients and observers may be more receptive to teaching about how similar injuries may be prevented in the future.

tenderness pain that is elicited through palpation.

tendonitis inflammation of a tendon and/or its protective sheath.

tension lines natural patterns in the surface of the skin revealing tensions within.

tension pneumothorax buildup of air under pressure within the thorax. The resulting compression of the lung severely reduces the effectiveness of respirations. *See also* pneumothorax.

teratogenic drug medication that may deform or kill the fetus.

terminal-drop hypothesis a theory that death in an elderly person is preceded by a 5-year period of decreasing cognitive functioning.

termination of action time from when the drug's level drops below its minimum effective concentration until it is eliminated from the body.

terrorist act the use of violence to provoke fear and influence behavior for political, social, religious, or ethnic goals.

tertiary prevention rehabilitation after an injury or illness that helps to prevent further problems from occurring.

testes primary male reproductive organs that produce hormones responsible for sexual maturation and sperm; *singular:* testis.

tetanus acute bacterial infection of the central nervous system.

thalamus switching station between the pons and the cerebrum in the brain.

therapeutic index ratio of a drug's lethal dose for 50 percent of the population to its effective dose for 50 percent of the population; the range between curative and toxic dosages; also called *therapeutic window.*

therapeutic window *see* therapeutic index.

therapy regulator pressure regulator used for delivering oxygen to patients.

thermal gradient the difference in temperature between the environment and the body.

thermogenesis the production of heat, especially within the body.

thermoregulation the maintenance or regulation of a particular temperature of the body.

thrill vibration or humming felt when palpating the pulse.

thrombocyte blood platelet.

thrombocytopenia an abnormal decrease in the number of platelets.

thrombocytosis an abnormal increase in the number of platelets.

thrombolytic *see* fibrinolytic.

thrombophlebitis inflammation of the vein.

thrombosis clot formation, which is extremely dangerous when it occurs in coronary arteries or cerebral vasculature.

thrombus blood clot.

thyroid storm *see* thyrotoxic crisis.

thyrotoxic crisis toxic condition characterized by hyperthermia, tachycardia, nervous symptoms, and rapid metabolism; also known as *thyroid storm.*

thyrotoxicosis condition that reflects prolonged exposure to excess thyroid hormones with resultant changes in body structure and function; toxic condition characterized by tachycardia, nervous symptoms, and rapid metabolism due to hyperactivity of the thyroid gland. *See also* Graves' disease.

tidal volume average volume of gas inhaled or exhaled in one respiratory cycle.

tiered response system system that allows multiple vehicles to arrive at an EMS call at different times, often providing different levels of care or transport.

tilt test drop in the systolic blood pressure of 20 mmHg or an increase in the pulse rate of 20 beats per minute when a patient is moved from a supine to a sitting position, a finding suggestive of a relative hypovolemia.

tinnitus the sensation of ringing in the ears.

tissue a group of cells that perform a similar function.

tocolysis the process of stopping labor.

tolerance the need to progressively increase the dose of a drug to reproduce the effect originally achieved by smaller doses.

tone state of slight contraction of muscles that gives them firmness and keeps them ready to contract.

tonic phase phase of a seizure characterized by tension or contraction of muscles.

tonic-clonic seizure type of generalized seizure characterized by rapid loss of consciousness and motor coordination, muscle spasms, and jerking motions.

tonicity solute concentration or osmotic pressure relative to the blood plasma or body cells.

topical medications material applied to and absorbed through the skin or mucous membranes.

tort a civil wrong committed by one individual against another.

total body water (TBW) the total amount of water in the body at a given time.

total downtime duration from the beginning of the arrest until the patient's delivery to the emergency department. *See also* downtime.

total lung capacity maximum capacity for air in the lungs.

touch pad computer on which data is entered by touching areas of the display screen.

tourniquet a constrictor used on an extremity to apply circumferential pressure on all arteries to control bleeding.

toxicology study of the detection, chemistry, pharmacological actions, and antidotes of toxic substances.

toxidrome a toxic syndrome; a group of typical signs and symptoms consistently associated with exposure to a particular type of toxin.

toxin any chemical (drug, poison, or other) that causes adverse effects in an organism that is exposed to it; any poisonous chemical secreted by bacteria or released following destruction of the bacteria.

trachea tube that connects the larynx to the mainstem bronchi.

tracheal deviation any position of the trachea other than midline.

tracheal tugging retraction of the tissues of the neck due to airway obstruction or dyspnea.

tracheobronchial tree the structures of the trachea and the bronchi.

tracheostomy a surgical incision from the anterior neck into the trachea held open by a metal or plastic tube.

trajectory the path a projectile follows.

transdermal absorbed through the skin.

transection cutting across a long axis; a cross-sectional cut.

transient ischemic attack (TIA) temporary, reversible interruption of blood flow to the brain; often seen as a precursor to a stroke.

transmural infarction myocardial infarction that affects the full thickness of the myocardium and almost always results in a pathological Q wave in the affected leads.

Transportation Unit Supervisor coordinates operations with the Staging Officer and the Transportation Supervisor at a multiple-casualty incident; gets patients into the ambulances and routed to the hospitals.

transverse fracture a break that runs across a bone perpendicular to the bone's orientation.

transverse process bony outgrowth of the vertebral pedicle that serves as a site for muscle attachment and articulation with the ribs.

trauma a physical injury or wound caused by external force or violence.

trauma center medical facility that has the capability of caring for the acutely injured patient. Trauma centers must meet strict criteria to use this designation.

trauma registry a data retrieval system for trauma patient information, used to evaluate and improve the trauma system.

trauma triage criteria guidelines to aid prehospital personnel in determining which trauma patients require urgent transportation to a trauma center.

Treatment Group Supervisor controls all actions in the Treatment Group/Sector at a multiple-casualty incident.

Treatment Unit Leaders EMS personnel who manage the various treatment units and who report to the Treatment Group Supervisor at a multiple-casualty incident.

trench foot a painful foot disorder resembling frostbite and resulting from exposure to cold and wet, which can eventually result in tissue sloughing or gangrene; also called *immersion foot.*

triage sorting patients based on the severity of their injuries.

Triage Group Supervisor person who supervises a Triage Group or Triage Sector at a multiple-casualty incident.

Triage Officer the person responsible for triage, or sorting patients into categories based on the severity of their injuries at a multiple-casualty incident.

triage tags tags containing vital information that are affixed to the patient during a multiple-casualty incident.

trichinosis disease resulting from an infestation of *Trichinella spiralis.*

trichomoniasis sexually transmitted disease caused by the protozoan *Trichomonas vaginalis.*

trocar a sharp, pointed instrument.

trunking communication system that pools all frequencies and routes transmissions to the next available frequency.

trust vs. mistrust refers to a stage of psychosocial development that lasts from birth to about 1H years of age.

tuberculosis (TB) disease that primarily affects the respiratory system, caused by the bacterium *Mycobacterium tuberculosis.*

turgor normal tension in a cell; the resistance of the skin to deformation.

turnover the continual synthesis and breakdown of body substances that results in the dynamic steady state.

two-pillow orthopnea the number of pillows—in this case, two—needed to ease the difficulty of breathing while lying down; a significant factor in assessing the level of respiratory distress.

ultrahigh frequency radio frequency band from 300 to 3,000 megahertz.

umbilical cord structure containing two arteries and one vein that connects the placenta and the fetus.

UN number a four-digit number specific to a given chemical; some UN numbers are assigned to a group of related chemicals, but with different characteristics, such as the UN 1203 designation for diesel fuel, gasohol, gasoline, motor fuels, motor spirits, and petrol. (The letters *UN* stand for "United Nations." Sometimes the letters *NA* for "North American" appear with or instead of the UN designation.)

Unified Command process in which managers from different jurisdictions—law enforcement, fire, EMS—coordinate their activities and share responsibility for command.

unipolar limb leads electrocardiogram leads applied to the arms and legs, consisting of one polarized (positive) electrode and a nonpolarized reference point that is created by the ECG machine combining two additional electrodes; also called augmented limb leads; leads aVR, aVL, and aVF. *See also* augmented limb leads.

unit predetermined amount of medication or fluid.

upper airway obstruction an interference with air movement through the upper airway.

upper gastrointestinal bleeding bleeding within the gastrointestinal tract proximal to the ligament of Treitz.

up-regulation a drug that causes the formation of more receptors than normal.

urea waste derived from ammonia produced through protein metabolism.

uremia the syndrome of signs and symptoms associated with chronic renal failure.

ureter a duct that carries urine from the kidney to the urinary bladder.

urethra the duct that carries urine from the urinary bladder out of the body; in men, it also carries reproductive fluid (semen) to the outside of the body.

urethritis an infection and inflammation of the urethra.

urinary bladder the muscular organ that stores urine before its elimination from the body.

urinary stasis a condition in which the bladder empties incompletely during urination.

urinary system the group of organs that produces urine, maintaining fluid and electrolyte balance for the body.

urinary tract infection (UTI) an infection, usually bacterial, at any site in the urinary tract.

urine the fluid made by the kidney and then eliminated from the body.

urology the surgical specialty dealing with the urinary/genitourinary system.

urosepsis septicemia originating from the urinary tract.

urostomy surgical diversion of the urinary tract to a stoma, or hole, in the abdominal wall.

urticaria the raised areas, or wheals, that occur on the skin, associated with vasodilation due to histamine release; commonly called *hives.*

uterus hollow organ in the center of the female abdomen that provides the site for fetal development.

vaccine solution containing a modified pathogen that does not actually cause disease but still stimulates the development of antibodies specific to it.

vacutainer device that holds blood tubes.

vagal response stimulation of the vagus nerve causing a parasympathetic response.

vagina canal that connects the external female genitalia to the uterus.

vallecula depression between the epiglottis and the base of the tongue.

valsalva maneuver forced exhalation against a closed glottis, such as with coughing. This maneuver stimulates the parasympathetic nervous system via the vagus nerve, which in turn slows the heart rate.

varicella viral disease characterized by a rash of fluid-filled vesicles that rupture, forming small ulcers that eventually scab; commonly called *chickenpox.*

varicose veins dilated superficial veins, usually in the lower extremity.

varicosities an abnormal dilation of a vein or group of veins.

vas deferens duct that carries sperm cells to the urethra for ejaculation.

vascular phase step in the clotting process in which smooth blood vessel muscle contracts, reducing the vessel lumen and the flow of blood through it.

vasculitis inflammation of blood vessels.

vasospastic angina *see* Prinzmetal's angina.

velocity the rate of motion in a particular direction in relation to time.

venous access device surgically implanted port that permits repeated access to central venous circulation.

ventilation the mechanical process that moves air into and out of the lungs.

Venturi mask high-flow, high-concentration face mask that uses a Venturi system to deliver relatively precise oxygen concentrations.
vertebrae the 33 bones making up the vertebral column; *singular:* vertebra.
vertebral body short column of bone that forms the weight-bearing portion of a vertebra.
vertigo the sensation of faintness or dizziness; may cause a loss of balance.
very high frequency (VHF) radio frequency band from 30 to 300 megahertz.
vesicants agents that damage exposed skin, frequently causing vesicles (blisters).
vial plastic or glass container with a self-sealing rubber top.
virulence an organism's strength or ability to infect or overcome the body's defenses.
virus an organism much smaller than a bacterium, visible only under an electron microscope. Viruses invade and live inside the cells of the organisms they infect.
visceral pain dull, poorly localized pain that originates in the walls of hollow organs.
visual acuity wall chart/card wall chart or handheld card with lines of letters used to test vision.
vital statistics height and weight.
vitreous humor clear watery fluid filling the posterior chamber of the eye. It is responsible for giving the eye its spherical shape.
volatility the ease with which a chemical changes from a liquid to a gas; the tendency of a chemical agent to evaporate.
voltage the difference of electric potential between two points with different concentrations of electrons.
volume on hand the available amount of solution containing a medication.
volvulus twisting of the intestine on itself.
von Willebrand's disease condition in which the vWF component of factor VIII is deficient.
warm zone location at a hazardous materials incident adjacent to the hot zone; area where a decontamination corridor is established; also called the *yellow zone* or *contamination reduction* zone.
warning placard diamond-shaped graphic placed on vehicles to indicate hazard classification.
washout release of accumulated lactic acid, carbon dioxide (carbonic acid), potassium, and rouleaux into the venous circulation.
weapons of mass destruction (WMDs) chemical, biological, nuclear, or other devices used by terrorists to strike at government or high-profile targets, designed to create a maximum number of casualties.
Wernicke's syndrome condition characterized by loss of memory and disorientation, associated with chronic alcohol intake and a diet deficient in thiamine.
wheezes continuous, high-pitched musical sounds similar to a whistle.
whispered pectoriloquy abnormal clarity of patient's transmitted whispers.
white matter material that surrounds gray matter in the spinal cord; made up largely of axons.
whole bowel irrigation administration of polyethylene glycol continuously at 1–2 L/hr through a nasogastric tube until the effluent is clear or objects are recovered.
window phase time between exposure to a disease and seroconversion.
windshield survey a survey of the emergency scene conducted through the windshield of an emergency vehicle as it arrives at the scene.
withdrawal referring to alcohol or drug withdrawal in which the patient's body reacts severely when deprived of the abused substance.
xiphisternal joint union between xiphoid process and body of the sternum.
yaw swing or wobble around the axis of a projectile's travel.
years of productive life age at death subtracted from 65.
yellow bone marrow tissue that stores fat in semiliquid form within the internal cavities of a bone.
yellow zone *see* warm zone.
Zollinger-Ellison syndrome condition that causes the stomach to secrete excessive amounts of hydrochloric acid and pepsin.
zone of coagulation area in a burn nearest the heat source that suffers the most damage and is characterized by clotted blood and thrombosed blood vessels.
zone of hyperemia area peripheral to a burn that is characterized by increased blood flow.
zone of stasis area in a burn surrounding the zone of coagulation and that is characterized by decreased blood flow.
zygoma the cheekbone.

Index